I0056136

Beumer's Maxillofacial Rehabilitation

BEUMER'S

MAXILLOFACIAL REHABILITATION

Prosthodontic and Surgical Considerations

Arun Sharma, BDS, MSc, FACP

Diplomate and Examiner American Board of Prosthodontics
Health Sciences Clinical Professor
Division Chair Prosthodontics
Director Advanced Education in Prosthodontics
School of Dentistry
University of California, San Francisco
San Francisco, California

Jay Jayanetti, DDS

Clinical Associate Professor
Program Director, Maxillofacial Prosthetics
Section of Special Patient Care & Maxillofacial Prosthetics
School of Dentistry
University of California, Los Angeles
Los Angeles, California

John Beumer III, DDS, MS

Distinguished Professor Emeritus
Section of Prosthodontics
School of Dentistry
University of California, Los Angeles
Los Angeles, California

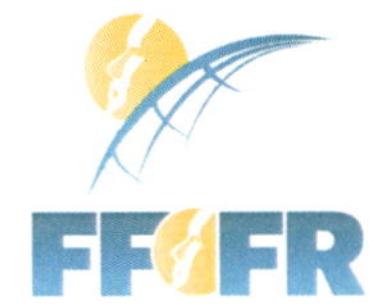

ISBN: 978-1-4956-1975-5 (print)
ISBN: 978-1-4956-1999-1 (ebook)

Printed in the United States of America

10 9 8 7 6 5 4 3 2 1

Contributors

Nadim AbouJaoude, DDS, CES, DU, FICD
Lecturer, Lebanese University
Clinical Associate, American University
Private Practice,
Beirut, Lebanon
nadimabj@yahoo.com
Chapter 7: Secondary author

Nabil J. Barakat, DDS, MS
Professor Emeritus and Chair
Department of Oral and Maxillofacial Surgery
School of Dentistry
Lebanese University
Private Practice
Beirut, Lebanon
nabilbarkat@gmail.com
Chapter 7: Secondary author

John Beumer III, DDS, MS
Distinguished Professor Emeritus
Section of Prosthodontics
School of Dentistry
University of California, Los Angeles
Los Angeles, California
jbeumeriii@gmail.com
Chapter 1: Secondary author
Chapter 3: Primary author
Chapter 4: Primary author
Chapter 5: Primary author
Chapter 7: Primary author
Chapter 10: Secondary author

Chris Butterworth, BDS (Hons), MPhil, FDSRCS, FDS (Rest Dent) RCS (Eng)
Professor
Consultant in Maxillofacial Prosthodontics
Liverpool Head & Neck Centre
University of Liverpool
United Kingdom
buttercj@liverpool.ac.uk
Chapter 3: Primary Section author "Zygomatic Implant Perforated technique."

Keith E. Blackwell, MD
Professor of Head and Neck Surgery
Chief of Facial Plastic and Reconstructive Surgery
David Geffen School of Medicine
University of California Los Angeles
KBlackwell@mednet.ucla.edu
Chapter 2: Secondary section author "Surgical treatment of mandibular tumors," "Microvascular free flaps" and "Reconstruction of tongue and lip."

Timothy C. Blood Jr., MD
Assistant Professor of Surgery
Uniformed Services University of the Health Sciences
Department of Otolaryngology-Head and Neck Surgery
Madigan Army Medical Center
Tacoma, WA USA
Chapter 2: Primary section author. "Oral swallowing function."

Lawrence Brecht, DDS
Director of Maxillofacial Prosthetics
Department of Dental Medicine & Oral and Maxillofacial Surgery
Department of Otolaryngology-Head & Neck Surgery
Northwell Health
Director of Maxillofacial Prosthetics
Adjunct Clinical Associate Professor
Advanced Education Program in Prosthodontics
NYU College of Dentistry
Private Practice Limited to Prosthodontics & Maxillofacial Prosthetics
New York, NY
lebrecht@nycpros.com
Chapter 6: Primary section author "Naso-Alveolar Molding"

Doke Buurman, DDS, PhD
Maxillofacial Prosthodontist
Department of Cranio-Maxillofacial Surgery
Maastricht University Medical Center
Maastricht, The Netherlands
doke.buurman@mumc.nl
Chapter 3: Secondary author.

Wanxing Chai-Ho, MD
Assistant Professor
Department of Medicine
Division of Hematology/Oncology
UCLA David Geffen School of Medicine
WChaiHo@mednet.ucla.edu
Chapter 10: Secondary author

Satinder Chander, BDS, MFDS RCS Edin, MSc, FDS RCS Edin
Consultant in Restorative Dentistry—Guy's and St Thomas' NHS Foundation Trust
Honorary Clinical Lecturer—Faculty of Dentistry, Oral & Craniofacial Sciences
King's College London
United Kingdom
Satinder.chander@kcl.ac.uk
Chapter 6: Primary section author "Resin Bonded bridges."

Ting Ling Chang, BDS, FACP
Diplomate American Board of Prosthodontics
Clinical Professor
Section Chair. Prosthodontics
Division of Regenerative and Reconstructive Sciences
UCLA School of Dentistry
Los Angeles, California
tichang@dent.ucla.edu
Chapter 6: Secondary Author

Denny S. Chao, DMD
Assistant Clinical Professor
Section of Prosthodontics
School of Dentistry
University of California, Los Angeles
Los Angeles, California
denchao@ucla.edu
Chapter 1: Secondary author
Chapter 2: Secondary author
Chapter 3: Secondary author
Chapter 5: Secondary author

Henry M. Cherrick, DDS, MSD
Professor and Dean Emeritus
UCLA School of Dentistry
Los Angeles, California
Chapter 5: Secondary section author "Neoplasms of the facial area."

Dinesh K. Chhetri, MD, FACS
Professor and Vice Chair
Department of Head and Neck Surgery
University of California, Los Angeles
DChhetri@mednet.ucla.edu
Chapter 2: Secondary section author "Oral Swallowing function."

Evelyn Chung, DDS
Clinical Professor
Section of Special Patient Care & Maxillofacial Prosthetics
Director, Postgraduate Programs
UCLA School of Dentistry
Los Angeles, CA
echung@dentistry.ucla.edu
Chapter 10: Primary author

Donald A. Curtis, DMD
Professor Emeritus
Graduate Prosthodontics
UCSF
don.curtis@ucsf.edu
Chapter 2: Primary section author "Morbidities and Physiology of oral function."

Kristen A. Echanique, MD
Resident Physician
Department of Head and Neck Surgery
UCLA
Chapter 2: Secondary section author "Oral swallowing function."

Michael Eggerstedt, MD
Assistant Professor
Facial Plastic & Reconstructive Surgery
Otorhinolaryngology—Head & Neck Surgery
Rush University Medical Center
MEggerstedt@mednet.ucla.edu
Chapter 2: Primary section author "Micro-vascular free flaps."

Andrew Erman, MA-SLP
Speech Pathology Clinic
University of California, Los Angeles
aerman@mednet.ucla.edu
Chapter 2: Secondary section author "Swallowing function."

Earl Freymiller, DMD
Clinical Professor emeritus
Section of Oral and Maxillofacial Surgery
UCLA School of Dentistry
Los Angeles, CA
efreymiller@dentistry.ucla.edu
Chapter 2: Primary section author "Avascular bone grafts"

Patrick K. Ha, MD
Irwin Mark Jacobs and Joan Klein Jacobs Distinguished Professor
Chief, Division of Head and Neck Surgical Oncology
Department of Otolaryngology Head and Neck Surgery
University of California San Francisco.
Patrick.Ha@ucsf.edu
Chapter 3: Secondary section author "Diagnosis and Management of Maxillary Tumors."

Peter S. Han, MD
Clinical Instructor
Facial Plastic and Reconstructive Surgery
David Geffen School of Medicine
University of California Los Angeles
Pshan@mednet.ucla.edu
Chapter 2: Primary section author "Reconstruction of tongue and lip."

Alan G. Hannam, BDS, PhD, FDSRCS
Professor Emeritus
Faculty of Dentistry
The University of British Columbia
Chapter 2: Secondary section author "Mastication"

Jay Jayanetti, DDS
Clinical Associate Professor
Program Director, Maxillofacial Prosthetics
Section of Special Patient Care & Maxillofacial Prosthetics
UCLA School of Dentistry
Los Angeles, California
jayanetti@ucla.edu
Chapter 2: Primary author
Chapter 3: Secondary author
Chapter 5: Secondary author

Minjee Kang, PhD
Postdoctoral Scholar
Division of Oral and Systemic Health Sciences
School of Dentistry
University of California, Los Angeles
mkang514@ucla.edu
Chapter 8: Secondary author

Rhorie P. R. Kerr, MD, FACS
Assistant Professor
Facial Plastic and Reconstructive Surgery
Department of Head and Neck Surgery
University of California, Los Angeles
rkerr@mednet.ucla.edu
Chapter 2: Secondary section author "Swallowing function."

Sudarat Kiat-amnuay, DDS, MS, FACP, FAAMP, FAADOCR, BCCA
Professor
Section Head, Houston Center for Biomaterials and Biomimetics
School of Dentistry
The University of Texas Health Science Center at Houston |
Houston, Texas
Kiat-Amnuay@uth.tmc.edu
Chapter 5: Primary section author "Prosthetic materials."

Lindsay Lanciault, MA-SLP
Speech Pathology Clinic
University of California, Los Angeles
llanciault@mednet.ucla.edu
Chapter 2: Secondary section author "Oral Swallowing function."

Min Lee, PhD
Professor
Division of Oral and Systemic Health Sciences
School of Dentistry
University of California, Los Angeles
mlee@dentistry.ucla.edu
Chapter 8: Primary author

Karl M. Lyons, BDS, MDS, PhD, FRACDS
Professor and Chair in Restorative Dentistry
Discipline of Prosthodontics
Department of Oral Rehabilitation
Faculty of Dentistry
University of Otago
karl.lyons@otago.ac.nz
Chapter 1: Secondary author

Reeva Mincer, DDS
Lecturer
Interim Program Director, General Practice Residency
Section of Special Patient Care & Maxillofacial Prosthetics
UCLA School of Dentistry
rmincer@g.ucla.edu
Chapter 1: Secondary author

Peter K. Moy, DDS
Nobel Biocare Chair, Surgical Implant Dentistry
Clinical Professor
Section Oral and Maxillofacial Surgery
UCLA School of Dentistry
Private practice
Los Angeles, CA
PMoy@mednet.ucla.edu
Chapter 7: Secondary author

Suresh Nayar, BDS, MDS, MFDSRCS, MRDRCSE, MRDRCPS, FDS (Rest Dent) RCS, MPhil
Associate Professor
Division of Otolaryngology Head and Neck Surgery
Maxillofacial Prosthodontist,
Institute for Reconstructive Sciences in Medicine, 16940,
Department of Surgery, Faculty of Medicine and Dentistry
University of Alberta, Edmonton, Canada.
Edmonton, Canada
svnayar@gmail.com
Chapter 2: Secondary section author "Virtual Surgical Planning."
Chapter 3: Secondary section author "Osteomyocutaneous flaps and conventional implants."

Sarah Panjwani, MA-SLP
Speech Pathology Clinic
University of California, Los Angeles
Chapter 2: Secondary section author "Oral Swallowing function."

Daniel Ramos, DDS, MS, PhD
Professor of Oral Medicine emeritus
Diplomate of the American Board of Oral Medicine
daniel.ramos@ucsf.edu
Chapter 2: Primary section author "Epidemiology of oral cancer."

David Rapkin, PhD
Voluntary Assistant Clinical Professor
Founding Director, Mind-Body-Medicine Group
Department of Head and Neck Surgery
David Geffen School of Medicine at UCLA
Los Angeles, California
Drapkin@mednet.ucla.edu
Chapter 9: Primary author

Jana Rieger, PhD, MSc, BSc
Professor, Faculty of Rehabilitation Medicine
Director of Research, Institute for Reconstructive Sciences in Medicine
University of Alberta
Edmonton, Alberta
jana.rieger@ualberta.ca
Chapter 2: Primary section author "Speech."
Chapter 4: Secondary author.

Arun Sharma, BDS, MSc, FACP
Diplomate and Examiner American Board of Prosthodontics
Health Sciences Clinical Professor
Division Chair Prosthodontics
Director, Residency in Advanced Prosthodontics
Director, Maxillofacial Prosthetics

Division of Preventive and Restorative Sciences
School of Dentistry
University of California, San Francisco
San Francisco, California
Arun.sharma@ucsf.edu
Chapter 4: Secondary author.
Chapter 6: Primary author.

Eric C. Sung, DDS
Professor of Clinical Dentistry
Chair
Section of Special Patient Care & Maxillofacial Prosthetics
UCLA School of Dentistry
Los Angeles, California
esung@dentistry.ucla.edu
Chapter 1: Primary author.
Chapter 10: Secondary author.

Robert M. Taft, DDS
Professor Emeritus
Uniformed Services University
robtaft1@me.com
Chapter 7: Secondary author.

Zhi Hui Tan Janice, BDS, MDS (Prosthodontics), MPros RCS (Edinburgh)
Associate Consultant
Department of Restorative Dentistry
National Dental Centre Singapore
janice.tan.z.h@ndcs.com.sg
Chapter 5: Secondary section author "Ocular defects."

Khim Hean Teoh, BDS, MDS (Prosthodontics), FAMS
Clinical Associate Professor
Academic Vice Chairman (Clinical Service)
Oral Health Academic Clinical Program
Duke-NUS Medical School
Deputy CEO (Clinical and Regional Health)
National Dental Centre Singapore
teoh.khim.hean@singhealth.com
Chapter 5: Primary section author "Ocular defects."

Ritchell R. Van Dams, MD
Instructor, Radiation Oncology, Harvard Medical School
Dana-Farber Brigham Cancer Center
Boston, Massachusetts
rvandams@bwh.harvard.edu
Chapter 1: Secondary author.

Karin Vargervik, DDS
Professor Emeritus and Former Director Center for Craniofacial Anomalies
School of Dentistry
University of California, San Francisco
San Francisco, California
Chapter 6: Primary section author "Growth and development and orthodontic treatment."

Andrew Weeks, DDS
Assistant Clinical Professor
Oral and Maxillofacial Surgery
University of California, San Francisco
San Francisco, California
Andrew.weeks@ucsf.edu
Chapter 6: Primary section author "Bone grafting."

Benjamin M. Wu DDS, PhD
Chief Science Officer and Senior Investigator,
The Forsyth Institute, Cambridge, Massachusetts
Director Emeritus, Weintraub Center for Reconstructive Biotechnology
Professor Emeritus and Former Chair, Division of Advanced Prosthodontics, School of Dentistry
Professor Emeritus and Former Chair, Department of Bioengineering, School of Engineering
Professor Emeritus, Department of Orthopedic Surgery, School of Medicine
Professor Emeritus, Department of Materials Science and Engineering, School of Engineering
University of California, Los Angeles, California
benwu@dentistry.ucla.edu
Chapter 8: Secondary author

Mary Jue Xu, MD
Clinical Instructor, Department of Otolaryngology-Head and Neck Surgery
Research Fellow, National Clinician Scholars Program
University of California San Francisco
MaryJue.Xu@ucsf.edu
Chapter 3: Primary section author "Diagnosis and Management of Maxillary Tumors."

Kenneth Yan, MD, PhD
Assistant Professor—Laryngology
Rutgers New Jersey Medical School
Chapter 2: Secondary section author "Oral swallowing function."

Contents

Preface

John Beumer III has devoted his professional life to Maxillofacial Rehabilitation. In 1976 he established and developed the Maxillofacial Prosthodontic center at the UCLA School of Dentistry which, over 4 decades, has trained more than 125 maxillofacial prosthodontists. His international distinction as a forerunner in the field is assured. Among his major contributions to this field, John co-authored the first edition of this textbook with Drs. Curtis and Firtell which earned prestigious distinction as the keystone for maxillofacial rehabilitation. He then edited subsequent editions together with Drs. Curtis, Marunick, and Esposito before mentoring Drs. Sharma and Jayanetti to become co-editors for the 4th edition in his position as Distinguished Professor Emeritus.

Rehabilitation of patients with disabilities of the head and neck secondary to acquired and congenital defects continues to be a challenging endeavor, requiring close interaction between many health care disciplines. Interdisciplinary care allows rehabilitation of most patients to near normal form and function, enabling them to lead useful and productive lives. The terms interdisciplinary and multidisciplinary are used interchangeably in the literature. The editors prefer the term interdisciplinary. "Multidisciplinarity draws on knowledge from multiple disciplines but stays within their boundaries. Interdisciplinarity synthesizes and harmonizes links between disciplines into a coordinated and coherent whole" (Choi et al., 2006).

We appeal to our readers to collaborate in an interdisciplinary manner for patient care and to promote and be involved in research endeavors. Surgeons, radiation, and medical oncologists must be made to appreciate the advantages of making their dental colleagues' equal members of the patient care and research teams. Despite progress, many challenges remain; for instance, we have yet to find effective means of minimizing the very significant long-term side effects of radiation and chemoradiation therapy.

Treatment strategies developed for Head and Neck cancer patients must always consider the need to maintain and restore oral function and health. No longer should we hear the cliché so often echoed in the past and even today, in reference to one of our patients: "the cure was worse than the disease."

The prosthodontist is highly knowledgeable in oral function and adept at restoring it, but to be an effective member of this interdisciplinary effort, they must not only comprehend their own role, but also those of the other team members. It is essential that they become conversant with the issues that are important to the cancer and reconstructive surgeons, and radiation and medical oncologists if they want to make sensible and pragmatic contributions to a patient's recovery. Everyone involved in the treatment and rehabilitation process must be familiar with the expertise of other personnel, making sure that all aspects of care are smoothly integrated. In an effort to encompass this interdisciplinary field we present insights into etiology and treatments and procedures for rehabilitation of the tongue, mandible, maxilla, and facial structures.

All chapters have undergone significant revision, reflecting the knowledge and sophistication we have gained over the last decade. Readers familiar with the 3rd edition will note that the chapter on "Digital technology in Maxillofacial Rehabilitation" has been deleted. Digital technology has become so integral to the diagnosis, treatment planning, treatment, design and manufacturing of maxillofacial prostheses that its discussion is appropriately distributed throughout this edition.

Chapter 2 on "Rehabilitation of tongue and mandible defects" has undergone major revision. Patients with non-reconstructed discontinuity defects are increasingly rare. For prosthodontic rehabilitation of these patients, the reader is directed to the 3rd edition of this book. The disabilities associated with resection of a portion of the tongue and the adjacent mandible are primarily dependent on the amount of the tongue resected and the method of surgical closure. In the first edition of this text, the authors frequently referred to patients with tongue and mandible resections as the "forgotten patients." The most reliable functional and occlusion-based reconstructions are obtained with collaborative virtual surgical planning and computer-aided manufacturing of models, guides, splints, and custom reconstruction plates.

Chapter 3 on "Rehabilitation of Acquired Maxillary Defects" has undergone a major revision. Occlusion-based virtual surgical planning allows for predictable immediate reconstruction of maxillary defects with vascularized osteomyocutaneous free flaps and osseointegrated implants. The use of zygomatic implants and subperiosteal implants with/without free flap closure of the defect as an alternative option are also discussed.

Chapter 7 "Restoration of traumatic defects" has been added. Reconstruction and rehabilitation of these patients can be complex and demanding most often requiring an interdisciplinary effort involving reconstructive surgeons, orthodontists, and prosthodontists. Complex deficits secondary to gunshot wounds frequently require surgical osteotomies and bone grafting to restore continuity defects and the placement of implants to retain and/or support dental prostheses.

Chapter 9 on "Psychosocial Perspectives in Maxillofacial Prosthodontic Treatment of Head and Neck Cancer Patients" has been rewritten to include the implication of the survivorship paradigm and the morbidities of head and neck cancer and its treatment effect on patients, caregivers, families and health care providers.

We would like to thank our many contributors. At their institutions they have embraced and through their contributions helped us expand our vision of interdisciplinary care. Finally, we would like to thank Brian Lozano, senior artist, UCLA School of Dentistry.

References

Choi BCK, Pak AWP. Multidisciplinarity, interdisciplinarity and transdisciplinarity in health research, services, education and policy: Definitions, objectives, and evidence of effectiveness. Clin Invest Med 2006 Dec;29(6):351–364.

Acknowledgments

Arun Sharma

I have been extremely fortunate to have had amazing mentors who have had an invaluable impact on my career and personal growth. Dr. Sabita Ram incited my desire to become a prosthodontist during dental school in India. Dr. Frank Kratochvil spent a sabbatical year at Guys Hospital in London, where I was enrolled in a Master's program. His guidance and encouragement is solely responsible for my coming to UCSF to train under Drs. Thomas Curtis and Galen Wagnild. Dr. John Beumer accepted me for the maxillofacial prosthetic fellowship at UCLA in 1989 and I have benefited from his mentorship ever since. Without these "giants" as my mentors and well-wishers I would not have been in the position that I am today. Their selfless commitment to education and patient care has been an inspiration. I am humbled that Dr. Beumer invited me to join him and Jay to serve as co-editors of the 4th edition of this textbook. I have also had the good fortune, to have had fantastic co-residents and over 75 residents at UCSF who have all challenged and driven me to continue learning. My sincere thanks to all my mentors who have made an indelible impact on my life.

Jay Jayanetti

I am immensely grateful to my mentors, Drs. Fritz Finzen, Arun Sharma, John Beumer, Brian Schmidt, Don Curtis, Mark Dellinges, Ruth Aponte and Arturo Mendez, for their formative influence in my professional development. Furthermore, it has been a great privilege and career honor to learn from and work alongside John and Arun as my co-editors. Additionally, I would like to acknowledge the extraordinary efforts and dedication of my 26 fellows, from 2015 to present, whose incredible photographic work provides visual examples that enrich this book. As my co-editors and fellows will attest, Tomomi Baba is an essential force behind the scenes in providing excellent care and training in our Maxillofacial Prosthodontic Center.

John Beumer III

I would like to pay tribute to my mentors, Dr. Sol Silverman Jr., Distinguished Professor of Oral Medicine, University of California, San Francisco (UCSF); Dr. Thomas A. Curtis, Professor of Prosthodontics, UCSF and one of the fathers of modern Maxillofacial Prosthetics; and Dr. F. J. Kratochvil, Professor of Prosthodontics, UCLA and the developer of the RPI system of removable partial design. They were selfless individuals and wonderful role models who are considered giants in their respective disciplines. Their personal integrity, commitment to excellence, and enthusiasm for education and research, has been inspiring for me, and countless others. They gave me the basic tools that have permitted me to forge the close professional relationships necessary for true progress. This being my last professional contribution to this fascinating and challenging field, I would also like to thank my patients, for their patience and forbearance, for they have been the true source of my inspiration.

Dedication

Arun Sharma

To my parents Dr. Badrinarayan Sharma and Rama Sharma for fostering an environment of independence and learning, to my wife Dr. Renu Sharma and our daughters Malini and Nithya for their love and unwavering never-ending support in my career development.

Jay Jayanetti

I owe a tremendous debt of gratitude to my parents Dr. Rogerio Jayanetti, and Bela Lemos de Moraes, my grandmother and aunt, Isalia Magalhães Leite and Dr. Rosana Jayanetti, for their unwavering support, lifelong nurture, and boundless love. While my father underwent stage III cancer treatment last autumn, I was able to make considerable progress in writing this book at his bedside. Through this experience, I gained an even greater appreciation of the plight of those afflicted with this illness. Lastly, I humbly dedicate this book to my spouse, my rock Dr. Daniela Orellana. Her tireless devotion, selflessness and unfaltering love for our two toddlers, Isabela and Luca, have been immeasurable.

John Beumer III

To Jan for her everlasting love and support.

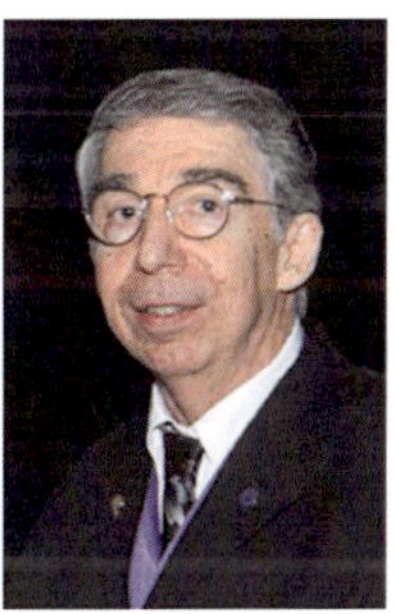

Mark T. Marunick, DDS MS

The fourth edition of this text is dedicated to Dr. Mark T. Marunick. Mark was a very special person who made significant contributions to our specialty. When the 2nd edition of this book was being prepared, Mark was an obvious choice to be a co-editor. Mark exemplified the ideal professional colleague and co-editor and we treasured the numerous interactions and collaborations that occurred during the preparation of the second edition and later the third edition and we fully expected Mark to play an active part in the preparation of the 4th edition. Mark's professionalism, high level of knowledge, attention to detail and his dedication to the work at hand, resulted in a significant improvement in the outcome. The stature that this publication has achieved world-wide during the last 25 years was in large measure due to Mark's efforts. However, it was not to be. As we prepared this edition, we missed his presence very much. We missed his dedication and willingness to spend the endless hours it takes to review chapters, his attention to detail, his expertise and willingness to engage in debate of contentious issues and his clarity of thought. But most of all, we missed our friend.

Arun Sharma
Jay Jayanetti
John Beumer

Oral Management of Patients Treated with Radiation Therapy and/or Chemoradiation

Eric C. Sung, John Beumer III, Reeva Mincer, Ritchell R. Van Dams, Denny S. Chao, Karl M. Lyons

Most patients with head and neck tumors will receive radiotherapy at some time during the course of their disease. For some tumors, radiation is employed alone whereas for others it is used in combination with surgery and, particularly in the treatment of oropharynx and nasopharynx tumors, with chemotherapy.

In recent years, biologic equivalent dose escalation has been employed in hopes of achieving higher rates of local regional control and overall survival; postoperative doses have risen from 50 Gy to 60 Gy and often are combined with chemotherapy. It has been estimated that chemoradiation therapy escalates the biologically equivalent dose to the tumor by 7 to 10 Gy (Fowler, 2008; Kasibhatla et al., 2007). Particularly in those patients treated with concomitant chemoradiation, the incidence and severity of preradiation and postradiation morbidity are increased. Fortunately, as the molecular basis of radiation injury becomes more understood, strategies to reduce the severity of post–chemoradiation therapy morbidities are evolving.

The task of the dental practitioner entering this field has become increasingly complex because he or she not only must keep abreast of the new methods of treatment (intensity-modulated radiation therapy [IMRT], volumetric-modulated arc therapy [VMAT], concomitant chemoradiation therapy, etc.) but also must be familiar with older technologies and approaches because a number of patients who were treated with conventional radiation therapy (CRT) may still require dental care. The role of the dental clinician is to minimize the postradiation morbidities associated with oral function that affect the patient's quality of life. With the new technologies and approaches to radiation delivery and the widespread use of chemoradiation therapy, many new questions have arisen while some of the old ones are still left unanswered. Quality clinical outcome studies are lacking and, given the size of the institutions and their limited patient populations, such studies probably will not be undertaken in the current funding environment. Clinicians responsible for preradiation assessments and postradiation dental maintenance and oral function must rely on clinical case series data and an in-depth knowledge and understanding of the literature and the biologic effects of radiation as the best levels of evidence to assist them in management decisions for patients who are about to be irradiated or who present postradiation.

Unfortunately, most of the current literature describing the means of minimizing morbidity, extraction of teeth prior to and following radiation, treatment of osteoradionecrosis (ORN), and restorative maintenance of the dentition is primarily retrospective and can be indeterminate and confusing. This chapter will summarize and collate the available data and clinical experience of those active in this field. The intent is to present a rational approach to minimizing the morbidity and a logical approach, based as much as possible on evidence available, to dental evaluation, dental care, and maintenance of oral health and function in patients undergoing tumoricidal doses of radiation therapy to the head and neck.

Principles of Radiation Therapy

Physical principles

It has become increasingly important for dentists who screen and treat patients undergoing radiation therapy, to have a basic understanding of radiation biology. Techniques of delivering high-energy photons to the gross tumor volume have undergone dramatic changes in recent years, but the response of tissues to these new modalities of radiation therapy has not changed. In addition, chemoradiation therapy has become the standard of care for the treatment of many pharyngeal and oropharyngeal tumors, resulting in more severe tissue reactions during therapy and increased severity of long-term side effects.

Radiation therapy is defined as the therapeutic use of ionizing radiation. Two broad categories of radiation are available. Electromagnetic waves of wavelengths less than 1 Å are called *photons*. They have neither mass nor charge. Their energy is measured in electron volts and varies from several thousand electron volts, *kiloelectron volts (keV)*, to several million electron volts, or *megaelectron volts (MeV)*. Photons that have energy equal or superior to 1 MeV are called *high-energy photons*.

Both X-rays and gamma rays are types of photons and are identical in nature. The difference between them lies in how they are produced. X-rays are generated by electric devices (X-ray machines, linear accelerators, betatrons, and so forth) when an electron beam of high energy bombards a target, usually of tungsten or gold. Gamma rays are produced by radioactive disintegration of unstable radioisotopes (cobalt 60, cesium 137, iridium 192, and so forth).

Particulate radiations, which have mass, are charged negatively (electrons, π mesons) or positively (protons, alpha particles) or are neutral (neutrons). The most commonly used particulate radiations are electrons and neutrons. Electrons are small negatively charged particles. These can be accelerated to high energy levels by means of the same electrical devices used to produce X-rays. Neutrons are particles with a mass similar to that of protons (hydrogen nuclei) but with no charge. Neutrons can be produced by fission or by means of a cyclotron.

All of these radiations produce similar biologic effects insofar as they produce ionization within tissues. Most ionization occurs when these rays give up energy by colliding with and ejecting electrons from atomic orbits.

Interactions of radiation in tissues

Radiation absorption by tissues is either directly or indirectly ionizing. When charged particles have sufficient energy, they are directly ionizing. In other words, as they pass through the target matter, they disrupt the atomic structure by producing chemical and biologic changes. On the other hand, photons and uncharged particles (neutrons) are indirectly ionizing as they give up their energy to produce fast-moving charged particles.

Photons entering tissues interact with orbital electrons and can be absorbed in three different ways: by *(1)* the photoelectric effect, *(2)* the Compton effect, and *(3)* pair production. In the photoelectric effect, the photon's entire energy is employed to eject an electron from its orbit. This type of absorption prevails for low-energy photons (orthovoltage) and increases with the atomic number of the absorber. The Compton effect prevails for high-energy photons at 1 to several MeV (cobalt 60, linear accelerator). In the Compton effect, one electron is ejected and the rest of the energy of the incident photon will generate a low-energy photon. Pair production occurs when very high–energy photons entering matter materialize into two charged particles of opposite signs, one negative electron and one positive electron (positron). The positron is short lived and reacts with another electron to produce a photon.

Unlike photons, which primarily produce secondary electrons, neutrons are essentially absorbed by colliding with hydrogen nuclei, which are most numerous in tissue. The neutron interactions set in motion fast recoil protons, alpha particles, and heavier fragments. Ionization is then produced by the secondary protons that are set in motion by the incident neutrons.

Biologic effects

The primary effect of radiation occurs within the nucleus. After irradiation, only a small amount of immediate cell death results from direct effects (e.g., damage to a key segment of the cell metabolism). Most of the damage is confined to intranuclear structures, such as the DNA and the mitotic apparatus. Damage to these structures may be lethal (irreparable) or sublethal and may not be apparent until at least one cell division is attempted (Fig 1-1). If enough time passes between the sublethal event and cell division, the damage may be corrected. Although the repair time varies with different tissues, a minimum safe clinical interval of six hours is necessary. This process is known as *repair of sublethal damage* (Elkind and Sutton, 1959). Lethal and unrepaired sublethal damage manifests as chromosomal abnormalities at the time of mitosis, when genetic material in daughter cells may be altered or lost. Occasionally, bridges occur between daughter cells, preventing the completion of cell division.

The biologic effects of radiation can occur through direct or indirect action. Direct action results when secondary particles (i.e., recoil electrons and protons) interact with the target molecule, while indirect action results from interaction with water to produce free radicals (hydroxyl and hydrogen), which in turn interact with the target molecule by oxidation-reduction reactions. In radiation biology, the target molecule is the DNA, which has a key role in cell life. However, DNA molecules are relatively scarce compared to the numbers of surrounding molecules of water. Therefore, photons have a higher probability of causing damage to DNA through indirect action. On the other hand, densely ionizing radiations, such as neutrons, interact primarily through direct action.

These biologic actions on target tissues are dependent on the level of oxygenation. When tissues are anoxic, they may be up to three times more resistant to radiation effects than they would be under full oxygenation. The role of oxygen can be explained, at least in part, by its combination with organic free radicals (R) to produce nonrestorable organic peroxides (RO_2) of the target molecule. This reaction leaves more hydroxyl free radicals, which can then interact with target molecules that would otherwise react with hydrogen to form inactive molecules of water. Thus, indirect action of radiation treatment, primarily in photon beam therapy, is dependent on oxygen in its fixing of organic free radicals. Therefore, it appears that the biologic effects in hypoxic tumors treated with photon beam

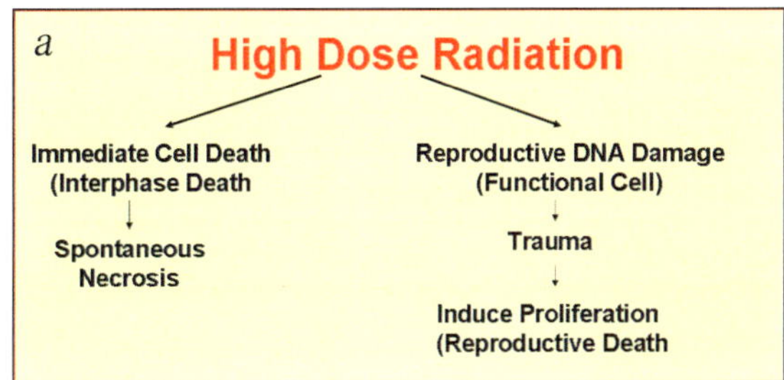

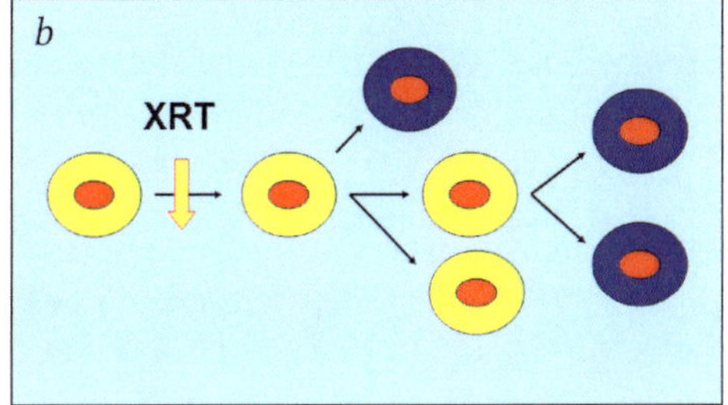

Figure 1-1 *(a and b)* Biologic effects of radiation (XRT) include induced proliferation and cell death. After irradiation, some cells undergo apoptosis or exhibit evidence of cell death. Residual cells remain viable and appear normal morphologically, but many lose the ability to divide. Inability to divide is known as *reproductive death* (Fajardo et al., 2001).

therapy are dependent on treatment strategies that increase the transport of oxygen to the tumor, a radiobiologic concept known as *reoxygenation* (Kaliman, 1972).

On the other hand, heavy particles such as neutrons have high kinetic energy, and the energy transferred per linear unit of track, or linear energy transferred, is sufficient to cause irreversible damage to the cells by direct action that happens to be on the track and perhaps "overkills" them. Consequently, the oxygen effect with these radiations is not as pronounced as it is for photons or light particles. Thus, these forms of radiation may be more effective in treating large, hypoxic tumors.

The effect on individual cells may vary according to the position the cell occupies in the cell cycle at the time of irradiation. It has been well demonstrated that cells are not uniformly radiosensitive during the different phases of their cycle. They are most vulnerable during gap 1 (G_1) phase and in mitosis and are relatively radioresistant at the beginning and end of DNA synthesis (Fajardo et al., 2001). Most cell populations, whether malignant or normal, are asynchronous; that is, the individual cells are in different phases of the cell cycle. If synchrony could be produced in neoplastic cells and radiation given during the most sensitive phase, cell killing would increase. This approach is known as *redistribution* of cells within the cell cycle. Theoretically, this can be accomplished with some chemotherapeutic agents, known as *cell cycle-dependent agents* (e.g., vinca alkaloids and hydroxyurea), or with timed fractionation of radiation therapy. However, to date there is no practical clinical way to produce synchrony and thereby take advantage of the phasic variation of cellular sensitivity.

Another radiobiologic principle is known as *repopulation*: Given enough overall treatment time, cells in irradiated tissue can proliferate and repopulate. In recent years, this seemingly simple concept has been modified by the observation that any cytotoxic agent, including radiation, can trigger clonogenic surviving cells in a tumor to divide faster than before. This *accelerated repopulation* is estimated to occur about four weeks after the initiation of treatment, when the tumor mass is coincidentally shrinking. Thus, to keep pace with the more rapid growth rate of tumor cells, a more rapid delivery of treatment may be needed.

The tolerance of normal tissues limits dose. In general tissues with rapid turnover rates such as oral mucosa exhibit acute reactions (e.g., oral mucositis), while tissues with extended turnover rates may not show evidence of tissue changes for months or years. New techniques such as IMRT and VMAT limit the volume of tissue exposed to the highest doses and theoretically should result in less severe late effects than CRT, in which large volumes of normal tissue were irradiated with doses equivalent to tumor doses.

Fractionation

Conventional fractionation

Radiation therapy is delivered in a series of treatments or fractions. Curative treatment regimens for squamous cell carcinomas of the head and neck region can vary. Conventional fractionation, prescribed by most radiation oncologists, consists of a total dose of 65.0 to 72.0 Gy given in daily fractions of 1.8 to 2.2 Gy fractions, Monday through Friday, over a 7-week period. The final total dose is limited by the radiation tolerance of critical normal tissues within the gross tumor volume and clinical target volume. This tolerance is determined by total dose, dose per fraction, overall treatment time, and frequency of dose fractions. Clinical experience has enabled the radiation therapist to establish the relationships among these treatment parameters and the severity of acute and late side effects.

Fractionation remains the most significant breakthrough in radiation therapy and its usefulness is apparent from the following lines of evidence. First, fractionated radiation allows the regular reoxygenation of the tumor during the course of treatment. Significant portions of the cell population in tumors are severely anoxic. Presumably, in fractionated radiation therapy, death of oxygenated cells allows oxygen to reach hypoxic cells, which therefore become more radiosensitive. Failure of reoxygenation may account for the resistance of some tumors to radiation. Second, fractionation offers more opportunities for the radiation to affect more tumor cells during the radiosensitive phase of their cell cycle. Third, between fractions, normal cells seem to recover more completely from sublethal damage than do tumor cells. This differential effect is most significant for late-responding tissues and least significant for early responding tissues, which react more like tumor tissue (Hall, 2006; Saberian et al., 2016).

Altered fractionation

IMRT, VMAT cyberknife, tomotherapy, and stereotactic radiosurgery are technological advances in radiation oncology. These types of high-technology equipment are designed to better sculpt the dose to the tumor and decrease the dose to the surrounding normal tissues compared to conventional and conformal radiation therapy. These newer technologies use multiple beams that "see" the tumor from multiple directions. The multileaf collimator moves during operation to modulate the dose so that large doses are given to the tumor volume while a smaller dose is given to the normal tissues.

In the absence of these technologies, attempts to increase the locoregional control and survival by altered fractionation regimens have been mostly replaced by chemoradiation schedules. However, patients who have received altered fractionation regimens may still present for follow-up and for treatment of dental disease. The incidence of morbidity, specifically ORN, in patients treated with these altered fractionation regimens is not sufficiently documented to allow a comparison with the incidence after conventional fractionation. Improved survival rates and local control have been well documented. Meta-analysis shows an increased survival rate of 6% (Bourhis et al., 2007; Pignon et al., 2009). There are four basic radiation plans:

1. *Conventional fractionation* is 1.7 to 2.0 Gy, five fractions per week, to 70.0 Gy.
2. *Hypofractionation* is reduction of the number of fractions with an increase of the daily fraction. An example is 2.5 Gy, five fractions per week, to 50.0 Gy.
3. *Hyperfractionation* involves increasing both the number of fractions and the total dose. An example is 1.1 Gy twice a day, six hours apart, five days a week, to 74.0 Gy.
4. *Accelerated fractionation* is a hybrid of hypofractionation and hyperfractionation and many of the altered fractionation schedules were hybrid (Bourhis et al., 2006).

A novel regimen still practiced in the United Kingdom is continuous hyperfractionation accelerated radiation therapy (CHART). In an examination of the CHART protocol, 3 fractions of 1.5 Gy each were delivered 7 days per week at 6-hour intervals without interruption for 12 days. The tumor and at-risk lymph nodes (the larger volume) received 42.0 Gy in 28 fractions. A boost was delivered to the tumor and palpable nodes (the smaller volume) with a dose of 12.0 Gy in 8 fractions, for a maximum total dose of 54.0 Gy in 36 fractions. The incidence of long-term severe morbidity 11 years after radiation therapy in about one-half of surviving patients was dysphagia, 12%; subcutaneous fibrosis, 3%; xerostomia, 15%; and mucosal ulcers, 18% (Saunders et al., 2010). Mandibular complications were not reported.

However, fewer complications affecting the oral cavity and oropharynx seem to be reported in randomized trials of conventional versus altered fractionation than are reported in studies of chemoradiation (Machetay et al., 2008). Despite claims that altered fractionation results in less late normal tissue damage than conventional fractionation, it is recommended that the identical oral precautions for preradiation extraction and preventive dental care be followed for both treatment regimens.

Radiation complications depend on the combination of total dose, daily dose, and volume of the tissue irradiated. Higher total dose, higher daily doses to large volumes, chemotherapy, and surgery will hurt the delicate balance between treatment needs and complications that was achieved with conventional fractionation schedules in 6.5 to 70 weeks. This balance has not been changed favorably by the altered fractionation schedules as was anticipated; therefore, no changes in dental care can be recommended.

It is hoped that the new technologies mentioned earlier will reduce the fragility of normal tissues to radiation. However, the total dose and daily doses have not changed, only the volumes. Furthermore, chemotherapy has been added to many treatment plans, which may alter the effects of modifications in radiation dose, fractionation, and volume.

Dosimetry

The purpose of dosimetry is to evaluate the amount of energy absorbed by the tissues subjected to radiation. The standard unit of the absorbed dose is the *gray*, which is the energy absorption of 1 J/kg of tissue. This unit has replaced the rad, which corresponds to an energy absorption of 100 ergs/g. Therefore, 1 rad = 1 cGy.

Accurate treatment planning must consider the beam characteristics for the different types of radiations, such as photons and electrons, used in clinical practice. These characteristics will vary with the type and energy of the radiation applied and can differ significantly among machines used to generate these beams. These distinctions include the penetration depth of the maximum dose (Dmax), the buildup region, the falloff region, and the isodose curves. When a radiation beam penetrates tissue, the dose decreases with depth of penetration after the maximum dose level is reached. The region from the surface to the depth of maximum dose is called the *buildup region*, while the region beyond is called the *falloff region*. The depth dose curves are visualized on a plane running along the axis of the beam where the points of equal dose are connected, yielding curves known as *isodose curves* (Fig 1-2).

Isodose curves for photon radiation

Single beam. For photons, as the energy of the beam is increased, the buildup region and Dmax extend to a greater depth. When low-energy X-rays such as orthovoltage are used, Dmax is located on the surface, making this an excellent treatment modality to treat superficial skin lesions. As photon energy increases, the surface dose decreases, the buildup region increases, and Dmax is located farther from the surface (Fig 1-2). For example, with a cobalt beam, Dmax is located at 4 to 5 mm, and as the photon beam becomes more energetic, it is located at greater depths (e.g., Dmax is 10 mm for 4 MeV photons and 25 mm for 10 MeV photons). Thus, with higher energy photons, there is a surface-sparing effect, which is more popularly described as the *skin-sparing effect*. The major advantage of high-energy photons, however, remains the increased percentage of depth dose. The falloff for photons is gradual, especially compared to that of electron beams.

Multiple beams. When a tumor is deeply located, it becomes necessary to use two or more beams (radiation ports) so that the dose delivered to the tumor is equal to or higher than the dose delivered to normal tissues. The goal of these field configurations is to maximize the tumor dose and to minimize the dose to normal tissues, especially sensitive tissues such as the spinal cord. Varying amounts of normal tissue are frequently treated to doses near or higher than the prescribed tumor dose, but, with modern equipment, this variation should seldom exceed 5%. Large dose inhomogeneities not only increase the total dose but also increase dose per fraction and, therefore, increase the biologic dose, especially with regard to late effects. Thus, treatment planning is essential.

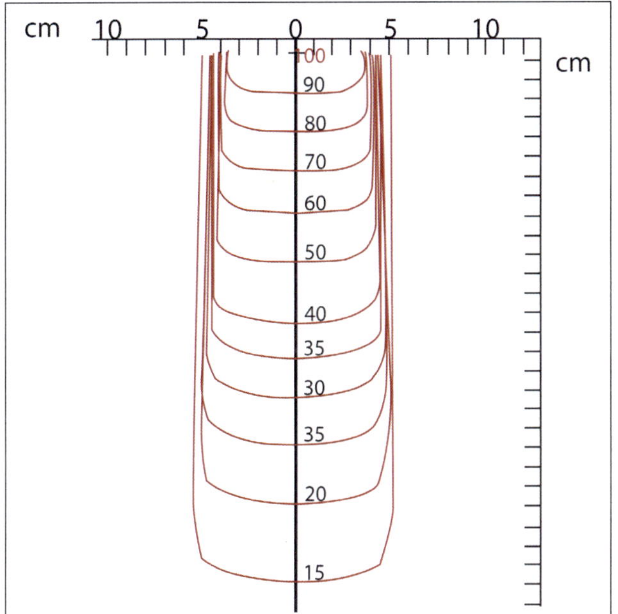

Figure 1-2 Isodose curves of a photon beam (cobalt 60). There is progressive falloff of tissue dose. Maximum dosage level (100%) is attained below the skin surface.

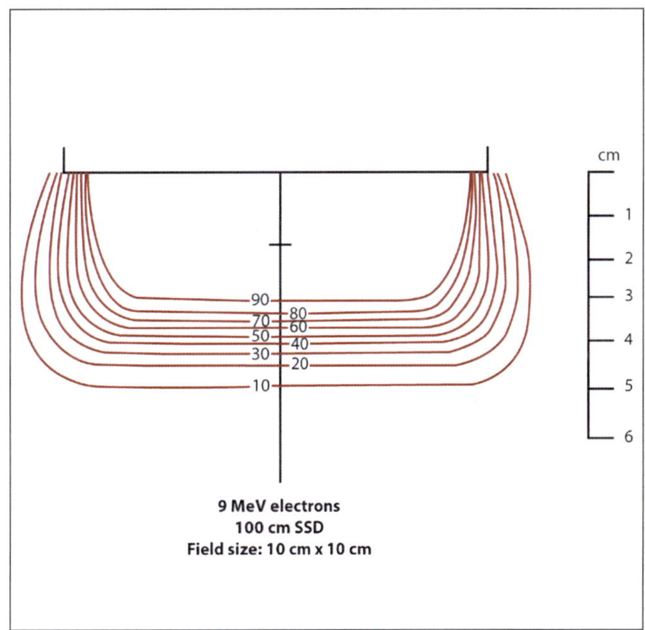

Figure 1-3 Isodose curves of an electron beam. There is a rapid falloff of tissue dose. SSD: source-skin distance.

To spare normal tissues, multiple beams with varying configurations can be applied. Beam configurations can vary from two simple opposed fields to two fields that are angled with respect to one another (wedge fashion), to three or more fields with different beam angles.

In addition, different beam energies can be used to manipulate the coverage of regions of interest. For example, if superficial areas such as lymph nodes need treatment, lower energy photon beams are applied. However, if the primary concern is for dose levels to reach deeply situated structures, higher energy photons should be used.

Isodose curves for particulate radiations

The dose distribution for an electron beam is similar to that of photons in that the higher the energy used, the greater the depth of penetration; however, electron beam dose distribution differs from that of photons in two significant ways. First, the electron beam exhibits a rapid falloff of the dose beyond the 80% to 90% isodose line (Fig 1-3). This permits treatment of superficial structures such as lymph node–bearing areas, yet spares deep structures such as the spinal cord. Hence, electron beam therapy is widely used in treatment of the posterior region of the neck during the "off-cord" portion of therapy.

The second difference applies to the buildup region. As the energy of the electron beam increases, the depth to Dmax decreases and a greater dose is applied to the skin, so the skin-sparing effect is reduced. As an alternative to orthovoltage therapy, these two qualities of electron beam therapy can be exploited to treat cutaneous lesions. However, superficial structures must not be underdosed when lower electron energies are used. A surface bolus, described later in this chapter, can be used to increase the dose level of the skin.

Modalities

Radiation therapy may be delivered via an external source or with the help of a radioactive material that may be surgically implanted locally within the area encompassed by the tumor. Implantation techniques usually result in less posttherapy morbidity because the radiation is more localized and, therefore, spares important structures such as major salivary glands and the mandible. External beam with CRT, IMRT, or VMAT therapy necessitates that the radiation traverse these structures, compromising their biologic integrity.

Conventional radiation therapy

Prior to the year 2000, most patients were treated with CRT, and in most patients, opposed parallel fields were employed. The patient was first positioned with the appropriate oral stent or shield, and then a face mask was placed. Structures of interest, such as palpable lymph nodes, were then outlined with wire and viewed under fluoroscopy. Afterward the fields were determined and planning (simulation) radiographs were taken (Fig 1-4a). Once the setup was deemed adequate for treatment by the radiation oncologist, ink markings of setup points were placed on the patient's skin or on the mask to facilitate reproducibility.

The standard beams produced by treatment machines were rectangular. These fields were converted into irregular shapes to conform to the shape of the individual tumor through the use of beam-shaping devices, most commonly customized blocks. These blocks were fabricated from an alloy with a low melting point. Before actual treatment commenced, setup and field blocking were verified with a radiograph (port film) of the patient that was taken with the block in place on the treatment machine (Fig 1-4b).

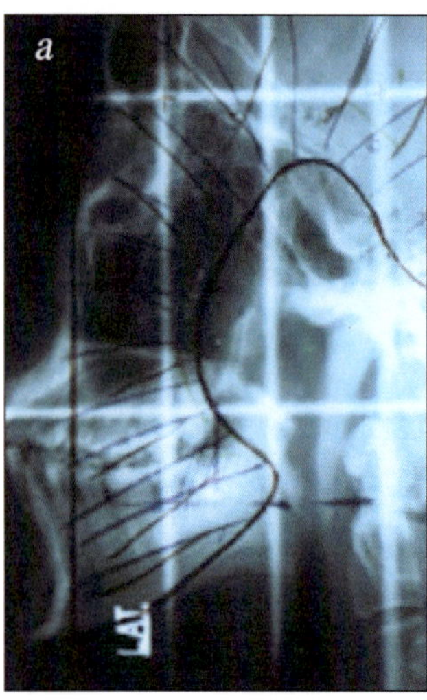

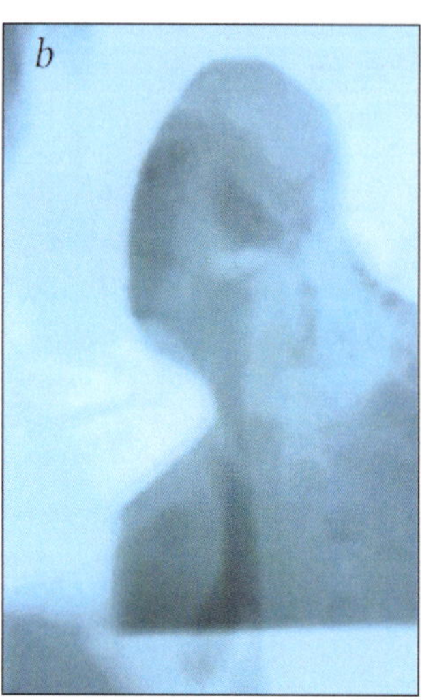

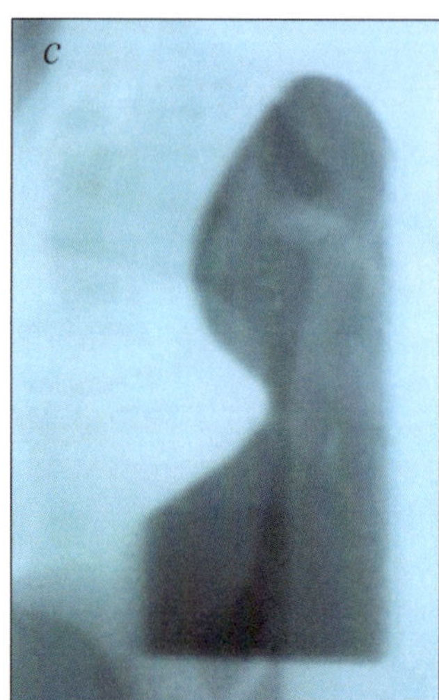

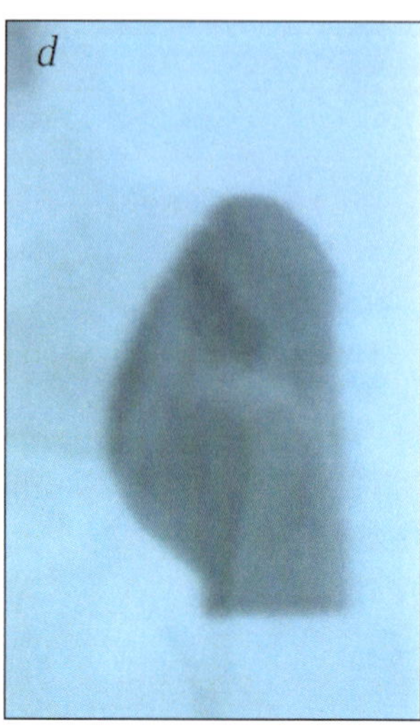

Figure 1-4 *(a)* Simulation radiograph of a patient to be treated for nasopharyngeal carcinoma. *(b)* Port film of the same patient. This field is treated to a level of 50 Gy. *(c)* Port film of the off-cord field. The dose is 55 to 60 Gy with this field. *(d)* Port film of the boost field. This field encompasses only the primary lesion, and the dose is brought to approximately 70 Gy.

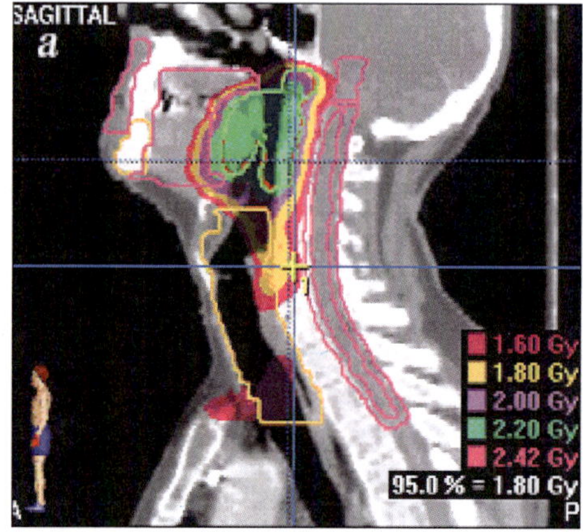

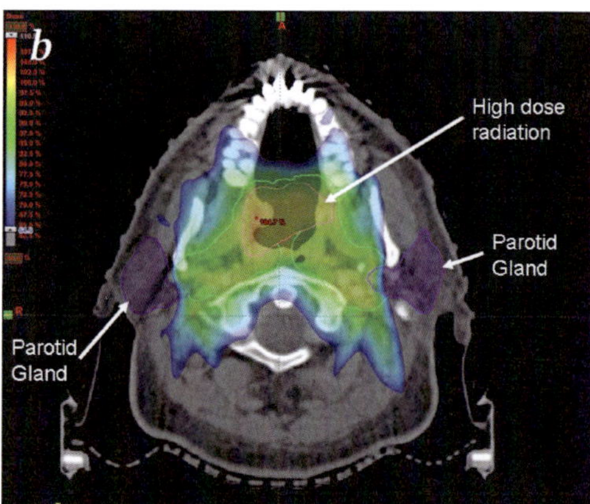

Figure 1-5 *(a)* IMRT dose distribution diagrams. Higher doses per fraction are centered on the clinical target volume. *(b)* Parotid tissues receive a lower dose. If the parotid dose can be kept less than 30 Gy, postradiation salivary flow will be close to normal one year after therapy.

The blocking could be modified during treatment as tissue tolerance was reached. For example, spinal cord tolerance is approximately 45 Gy; when this limit was reached, shielding could be placed to protect this structure from opposed lateral photon beam treatment directed at the off-cord field (Fig 1-4c and d). The cord block coincidentally shielded the posterior region of the neck. Treatment of the off-cord field could be continued with photon therapy; if a dose to the posterior region of the neck was needed, electron fields could be added to that area until an adequate dose was delivered.

Intensity-modulated radiation therapy (IMRT)

With IMRT, the delivered doses of radiation are defined for volumes as opposed to points (Fig 1-5). The volumes are drawn on the cross-sectional computed tomographic (CT) images. These circumscribed volumes are designated as *planning target volumes (PTVs)*: PTV1 is the cancer and the carcinomatous lymph nodes; PTV2 is the volume of nodes at high risk; and PTV3 is the subclinical nodes. A common prescription would be *PTV1: 7,029 cGy/33 fractions of 213 Gy, 5 days per week; PTV2: 6,303 cGy; PTV3: 5,709 cGy*. Unlike CRT, IMRT allows delivery of different doses to each volume at the same time, so that different daily doses are given to PTV1, PTV2, and PTV3 in 33 fractions, 5 days per week. A 5% to 10% variation of dose within a volume is common.

Although the calculation of normal tissue volume (e.g., spinal cord, parotid glands, and esophageal inlet) is an integral part of planning, the mandible may not be targeted for calculation. Tolerances for normal tissue can only be calculated if that tissue is drawn on the CT planning image, and drawing of the mandibular volume is not standard. In addition, the mandibular dose tolerance is often assumed to be 70 Gy, but the tolerance limit is much less if postradiation extraction or osseointegrated implants are planned and even lower if chemotherapy has been added during radiation.

The dose for the site of surgical intervention must be correlated with mandibular dose at that site. Because different regions of the mandible may receive different doses and the dose may vary across mandibular volume, a correlation of dose and volume to the surgical site is best made by the radiation oncologist, not a dosimetrist, physicist, or technician.

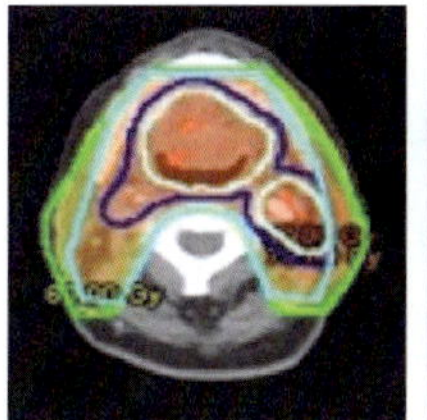
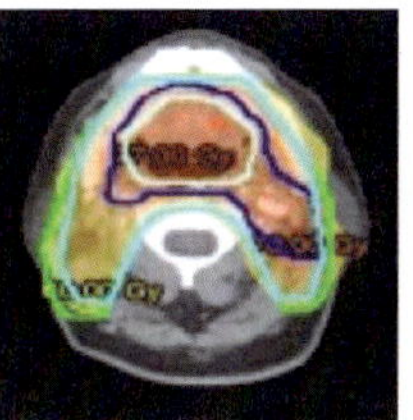
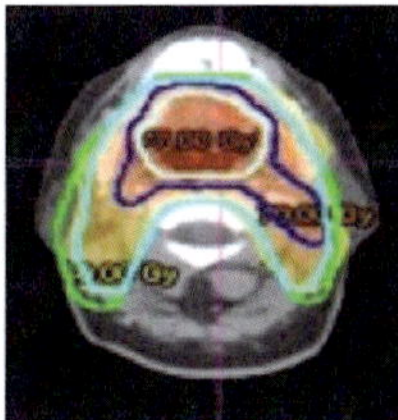

Figure 1-6 SBRT Dosimetry diagrams.

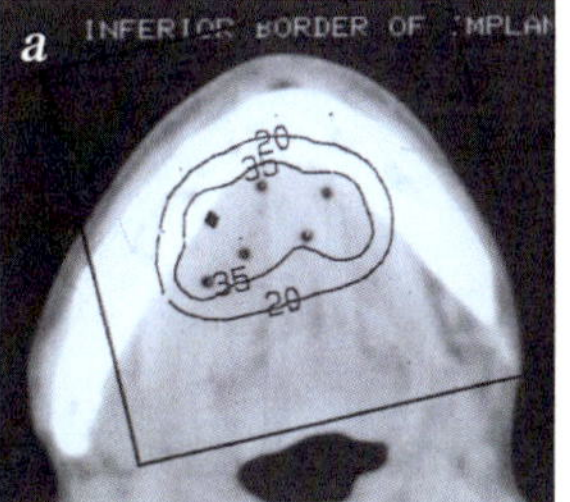

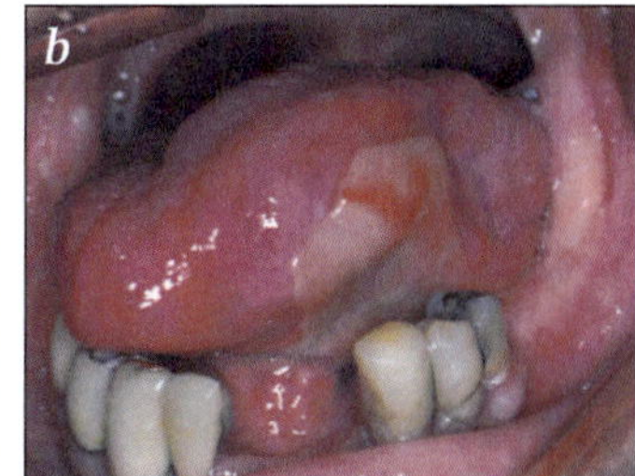

Figure 1-7 *(a)* Isodose curves of iridium implants positioned in the floor of the mouth. There is a rapid falloff of tissue dose as the distance from the sources increases. *(b)* Radiation mucositis is localized.

For IMRT, the PTV is the largest of the three building blocks that make up the volume that is finally irradiated. The first and smallest is known as the *gross tumor volume*. The gross tumor volume is defined by an image or a fusion of images such as a CT and magnetic resonance image (MRI) or a CT and a positron emission tomographic (PET) scan. The clinician adds a safety margin dependent on the potential subclinical extension. This margin is arbitrary but dependent on the size, grade, and site of origin of the tumor and the type of surgical procedure.

The gross tumor volume plus the margins for subclinical extension is termed the *clinical target volume*. The addition of a margin to the clinical target volume to allow for uncertainties associated with factors such as patient setup, motion, organ movement, and beam design finally defines the PTV. The established PTV varies among radiation oncologists, as does the dose delivered.

Volumetric-modulated arc therapy (VMAT)

An advanced form of IMRT is VMAT. VMAT utilizes a multileaf collimator (MLC), either delivering the radiation dose sequentially at various positions or continuously moving the MLC leaves while delivering the radiation. VMAT is becoming the mainstay treatment for head and neck tumors. Given the complexity of the structures in the head and neck, VMAT usually consists of a few partial arcs depending on the treatment targets. With the radiation given in a continuous form, there is improved conformal dose distribution to the target volume and improved homogeneity.

Stereotactic body radiation therapy (SBRT)

Similar to IMRT, this technique relies on sophisticated methods of radiation delivery that focus the highest doses to the local tissues in and around the tumor (Fig 1-6). Treatment plans are developed on the basis of CT and MRI data. SBRT is advantageous because the volume of tissue irradiated to high dose is minimized. SBRT delivers high doses per fraction (typically >5–8 Gy per fraction) with steep dose gradients and shorter treatment durations. With steep dose gradients, there are reduced radiation-related side effects in surrounding tissues and organs at risk (OARs).

SBRT has been utilized with both curative and palliative intent in patients with head and neck tumors. SBRT has shown to be particularly useful in patients with recurrent or unresectable head and neck malignancies, leading to more durable control while sparing normal adjacent tissues and previously irradiated tissues. Similar to IMRT, the highest doses are directed to tissues within the gross tumor volume, and intermediate doses are directed to areas where there is a high risk of microscopic disease (usually a clinical target volume).

Brachytherapy

Brachytherapy is a method of radiation treatment in which sealed radioactive sources are used to deliver the dose a short distance by interstitial (direct insertion into tissue), intracavitary (placement within a cavity), or surface application (molds). This method takes advantage of the rapid decrease in dose with distance from a radiation source (inverse square law). The intensity of radiation at a distance from the point source is inversely proportional to the square of the distance from the source. For example, if the dose received 1 cm from the source is 36 Gy, then at 3 cm, it would be approximately 4 Gy (one-ninth). Thus, a high-radiation dose can be given to the tumor while surrounding normal tissues are spared (Fig 1-7).

This technique does have potential disadvantages. The major concern is the potential for inhomogeneity of dose throughout the implanted volume. This can occur if the radioactive sources are spaced too closely together, resulting in a "hot spot," or too far apart, resulting in a "cold spot." Therefore, brachytherapy, particularly interstitial implantation, requires that the operator have adequate technical and conceptual skills to achieve good dose distribution. Other disadvantages are the need for general anesthesia and hospitalization of the patient as well as the potential exposure of operating room personnel and therapists to the radiation source.

Currently, the most commonly used radioisotope in the head and neck region is iridium 192. Other isotopes used include cesium 137 and radium 226. Generally, multiple sources are used, and their geometric arrangement is dictated preoperatively by the clinical circumstances of the particular lesion. The sources are ordered and received prior to the procedure and then placed surgically. After a prescribed period of time, the radiation sources are usually removed. Afterloading techniques, which are described later in the chapter, have been developed to avoid exposing the patient to radiation unnecessarily during the preloading period.

Localized tumors of the tongue are ideal candidates for a combination of external beam therapy followed by placement of removable radioactive implants. This approach results in a high rate of local control while maintaining structure and function. In Europe removable radioactive implants are often used alone for localized tumors of less than 3 cm. Because 20% of 3 cm lesions have or will have positive nodes, we use external beam radiation initially rather than wait for the neck disease to appear.

In the United States, a common recipe for combined treatment is the equivalent of 50 to 60 Gy in 25 to 30 fractions given to the oral cavity and level I, II, III, IV, and V lymph nodes. This is followed by a dose of 20 to 25 Gy delivered from the implant to the gross tumor volume and a margin of surrounding normal tissue at a dose rate of 0.2 to 0.4 Gy/h. Higher dose rates may be used in some centers, but no universal standards have been established. ORN occurs more often if the entire treatment is given with the implant (Murray et al., 1980a; Pierquin et al., 1970). The same radiation generalities apply to floor-of-the-mouth tumors, but to prevent ORN the implant should be positioned 5 mm or greater from the lingual surface of the mandible. Tumors classified as T3 and T4 are not well suited for this approach because of the large volumes that must receive a high dose.

Treatment planning

The intent of the radiation oncologist is to deliver a curative dose to the tumor while limiting the dose to the normal structures to a level that is within their tolerance. When a decision has been made to initiate therapeutic irradiation, the physician must first determine the extent of disease and the tumor volumes to be treated. A complete physical examination and appropriate laboratory studies, such as radiography, CT, MRI, PET, and triple endoscopy, must be completed for this assessment. In addition, the possible subclinical involvement of the tumor, based on the typical pattern of recurrences and the risk and site of regional lymph node involvement, is assessed to determine treatment volumes.

In general, a portion of the treatment must be given prophylactically to the areas at high risk for direct spread and lymph node involvement from subclinical disease. The remainder of the treatment delivers a dose to the gross tumor volume and, in certain instances, this is delivered using interstitial implantation. If the tumor is small and the risk of spread is minimal, then treatment of the primary site alone may be adequate.

Prescribed doses (in conventional fractionation) for the prophylactic volume range from 45 to 55 Gy, The total cumulative dose given to the gross tumor volume ranges from 65 to 72 Gy. However, the prescribed doses vary with the clinical situation and treatment techniques used. In the postoperative setting where tissue is hypoxic or if interstitial implantation is used, the prescribed dose to the tumor bed may be lower.

While these tumoricidal doses are delivered, normal tissues must be taken into consideration. These areas (e.g., spinal cord, salivary glands, and mandible) must be spared or at least the maximum permissible dose to these volumes must be considered. This can be determined from physical examination, radiographic studies, and CT scans and accomplished with careful planning procedures and simulation. The goal of the simulation is to simulate the patient setup during actual treatment. It is crucial that the patient position be exact and reproducible during the simulation. This consistency is achieved through the use of face masks and laser and field lights, which are available in the simulation and treatment rooms.

Indications

The majority of patients with head and neck cancer present with a tumor in an advanced stage. Loosening of teeth can be an early symptom of gingival carcinoma but a late symptom of sinus cancer. Trismus is a late symptom of tonsillar and maxillary cancer. Extensive lesions are associated with pain, otalgia, dysphagia, odynophagia, and/or problems with speech articulation and mastication.

The majority of malignant neoplasms of the mucosa of the head and neck are squamous cell carcinomas of various degrees of differentiation and radiosensitivity. Primary lymphomas arising in the nasopharynx or tonsil and adenocarcinomas of salivary and mucous glands are relatively rare. Lymphomas are radiosensitive, but the response of adenocarcinomas is less predictable. Sarcomas and melanomas are also rare and are primarily surgical diseases that require wide margins. These margins may not be possible to achieve in the head and neck region without undue morbidity, so treatment usually combines surgery and postoperative radiotherapy.

Radiation therapy, often supplemented by concomitant chemotherapy, is generally the treatment of choice for carcinomas arising in the nasopharynx, base of tongue, and soft palate. Carcinomas of the alveolar ridge and salivary glands (adenocarcinomas) should be treated surgically, because of the potential for bony infiltration, and then possibly by radiation therapy. Early carcinomas of the tongue and glottic larynx are equally well controlled by radiation or surgery, but radiation usually offers the better functional result. Hard, deeply infiltrating carcinomas of the tongue are less likely to be controlled by radiation, as are lesions causing fixation of the vocal cords. Superficial or exophytic lesions usually have a higher cure rate with radiation than do deeply infiltrating lesions.

Tumors exhibiting deep invasion of soft tissue or extension into bone or cartilage are far less likely to be controlled with radiation alone, and a combined approach with surgery followed by radiotherapy is advised. Other indications for postoperative radiotherapy include cancer cell–positive surgical margins, residual gross disease, tumor spillage, perineural invasion, and lymphovascular invasion. Indications for this treatment approach in the neck include multiple positive lymph nodes, extracapsular extension, and a known recurrence pattern. The 5-year disease-free control rates for radiation therapy vary according to the primary site, the size and extent of the tumor, and the distribution and size of involved lymph nodes.

Smaller carcinomas of the border of the tongue, the free portion of the epiglottis, and the floor of the mouth without infiltration into the tongue or mandible as well as early localized lesions of the soft palate, tonsil, and nasopharynx should be controlled by radiation in 60% to 80% of patients. Carcinomas of the pyriform sinus, subglottic area, and alveolar ridge are rarely controlled by radiation alone. Early lesions of the maxillary antrum, base of the tongue, hypopharynx, false vocal cords, and laryngeal ventricle have cure rates falling between these extremes. More advanced lesions and those with lymph node metastases have lower cure rates.

There is a risk that radiation-induced cancers will develop following definitive radiation therapy. Second primaries or other types of cancers such as sarcomas have been well documented. However, the incidence of radiation-induced second primaries appears to be less than 5% (Hall, 2006).

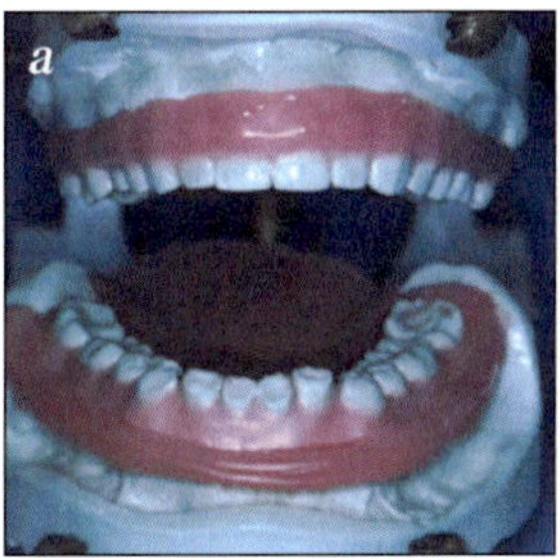

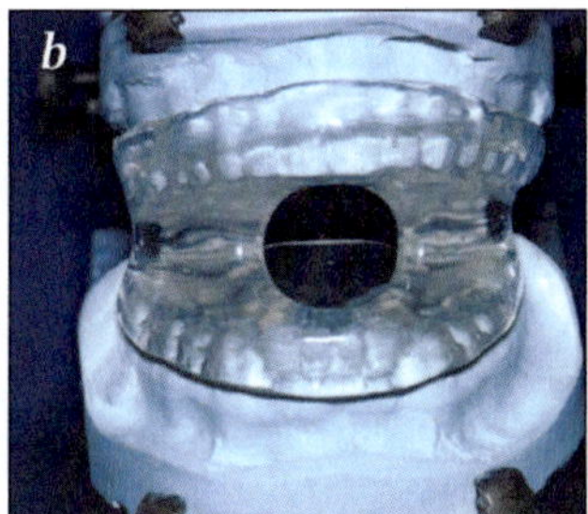

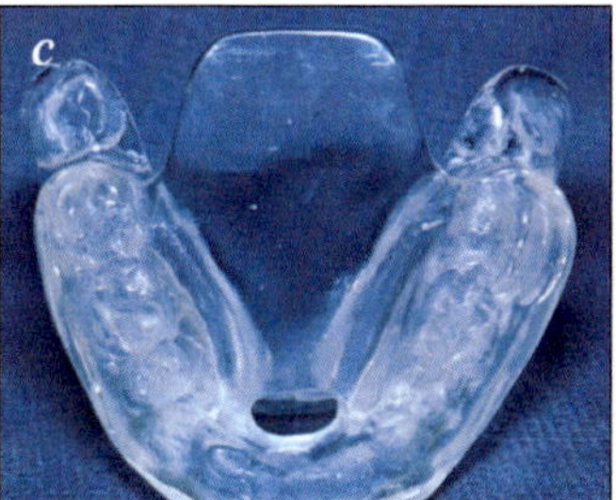

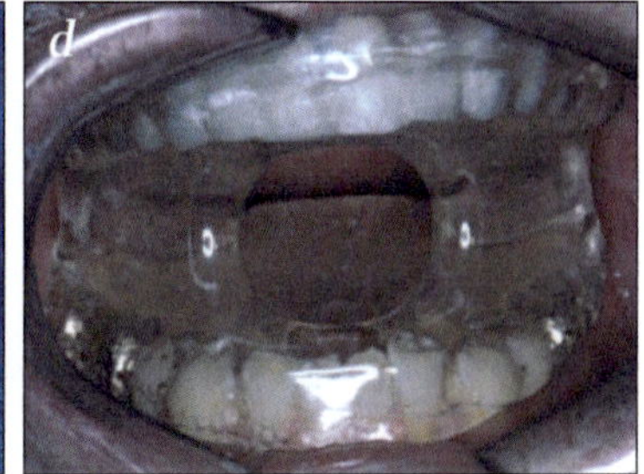

Figure 1-8 Stent for positioning the tongue in a repeatable and constant position. *(a)* Mounted casts with block-out wax. *(b and c)* Completed stent. The flat plane must extend to the second molar area to prevent the tongue from extending above the occlusal plane. *(d)* Stent positioned intraorally. The hole ensures a reproducible tongue position.

Use of Prosthodontic Stents and Splints during Therapy

As part of the preradiation dental evaluation process, the maxillofacial prosthodontist is often requested to fabricate prosthetic radiotherapy devices (splints, stents, shields, spacers, or positioners). These devices are used to shield, displace, and position tissues in an attempt to reduce radiation-induced tissue morbidity. For optimal treatment, these devices must allow repeatable positioning on a daily basis throughout the six to eight weeks of radiation therapy. The prosthetic devices are usually made from acrylic resin and are fabricated prior to the radiation simulation appointment to ensure that the radiation mask and calculated dosimetry take into account the position of the tissues when the patient is wearing the device. The request for a particular device is usually determined by the type of tumor, its location, and the method of radiation delivery.

Stents to displace the tongue and other tissues during treatment

This type of stent may be used to rearrange tissue topography within the radiation treatment volume and displace normal tissues away from the high-dose radiation treatment volume and has been shown to reduce postradiation morbidities (Kil et al., 2017; Stieb et al., 2020; Verrone et al., 2014). Patients treated with unilateral neck radiation therapy for localized tonsillar neoplasms with a tongue-deviating stent report less taste impairment and better appetite after treatment (Stieb et al., 2020).

Tongue-depressing stents are particularly useful for tongue and floor-of-the-mouth lesions. Separating the mandible from the maxilla and an inferior position of the tongue and mandible enables the radiation therapist to lower the clinical target volume, thus sparing the posterior palatine glands and significant portions of the parotid gland from radiation and thereby leading to higher levels of salivary output after therapy, and reduces radiation-induced xerostomia. This type of stent also results in less moderate/severe dysphagia (Kil et al., 2017; Stieb et al., 2020) and results in improved maintenance of mouth opening after radiation treatments (Nayar et al., 2016). Positioning stents also prevent the deviation of the mandible from its spatial relationship to the maxilla, thereby ensuring a repeatable positioning of the jaws from the time of simulation until the completion of radiation therapy. They can be fabricated with either analog techniques or CAD-CAM (Wilke et al., 2017; Zaid et al., 2019).

The traditional technique involves making reversible hydrocolloid impressions of the maxillary and mandibular teeth. Modeling wax is used to make an interocclusal record at an open vertical dimension of occlusion. The vertical extent of the interocclusal record is usually dependent on the patient's ability to open. It is usually one-half to two-thirds (18–20 mm) of the patient's maximal opening. Trismus is common in this patient population if the radiation clinical target volume encompasses the muscles of mastication and the temporomandibular joint, particularly if the patient is receiving concomitant chemotherapy. This may prevent seating the stent during therapy if the vertical opening is excessive.

Once the casts are mounted on an appropriate articulator, an interocclusal stent that engages the maxillary and mandibular teeth is fabricated from either heat-activated or autopolymerizing acrylic resin. A flat plate of acrylic resin extends lingually from both occlusal tables. This plate depresses the tongue within the lingual borders of the body of the mandible. A hole is made in the anterior horizontal segment, and the patient is instructed to maintain the tongue tip in this orientation hole during treatment. This will ensure that a consistent, reproducible tongue position is maintained during the treatment sequence (Fig 1-8).

Another method employs prefabricated stents made by pouring autopolymerizing acrylic resin into a master putty mold. The master putty molds can be made in different sizes such as small, medium, and large so stents can be fabricated to accommodate various arch widths. They are fitted and adjusted chairside to allow for one-half to two-thirds of the patient's maximal opening and then indexed to the dentition with temporary denture reline material (Fig 1-9).

Prefabricated stents can also be created with computer-aided design and computer-aided manufacturing (CAD/CAM) programs (Hong et al., 2019; Held et al., 2021; Herpel et al., 2021). With this method, design modifications can be easily made to the master Standard Tessellation Language (STL) file and produced via additive manufacturing (3D printing) without having to make new master putty molds. Our current design includes curved bite blocks based on Monson's spherical theory to accommodate for decreased interocclusal space posteriorly and increased interocclusal space anteriorly upon jaw opening. This design feature reduces chairside adjustments and increases stent stability when indexing the appliance to the natural dentition. This design permits the posterior teeth to consistently engage the bite blocks provided no excessive occlusal plane discrepancies exist. Digital prefabricated stents are

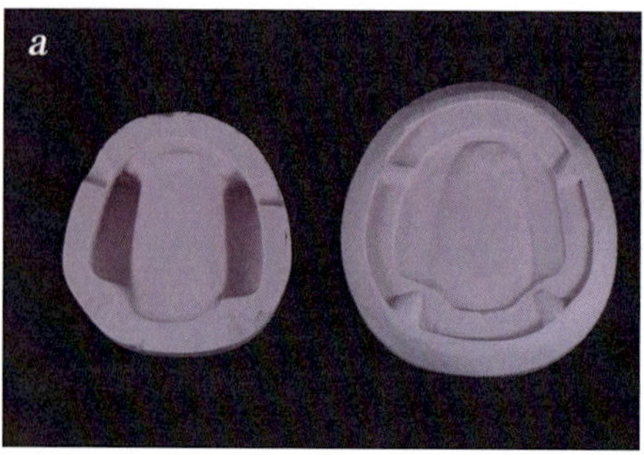
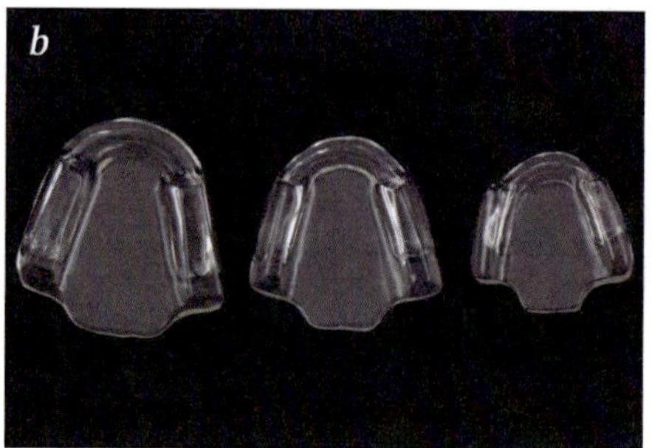
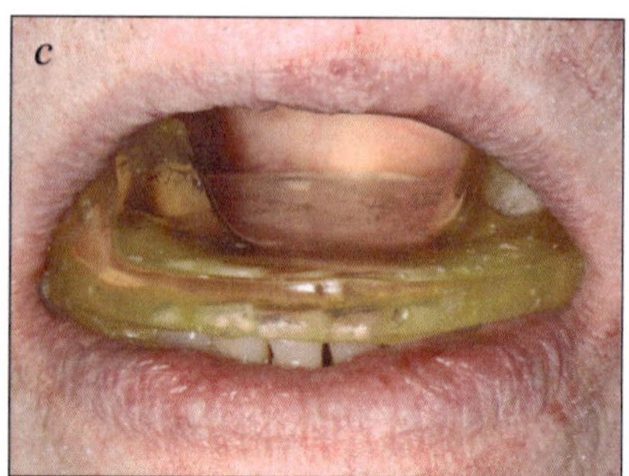

Figure 1-9 The Prefabricated stent technique. *(a)* Master putty mold. *(b)* Prefabricated stents of various sizes. *(c)* Stent positioned intraorally and indexed to the dentition with a temporary chairside reline material.

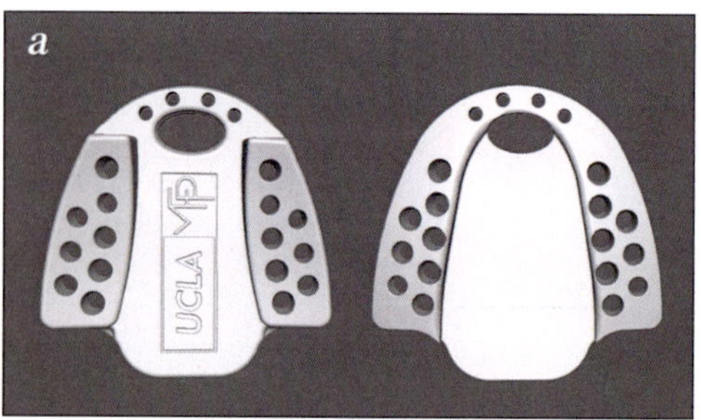

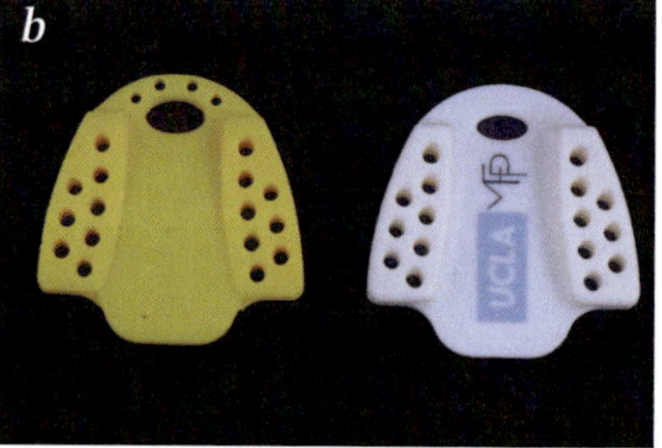

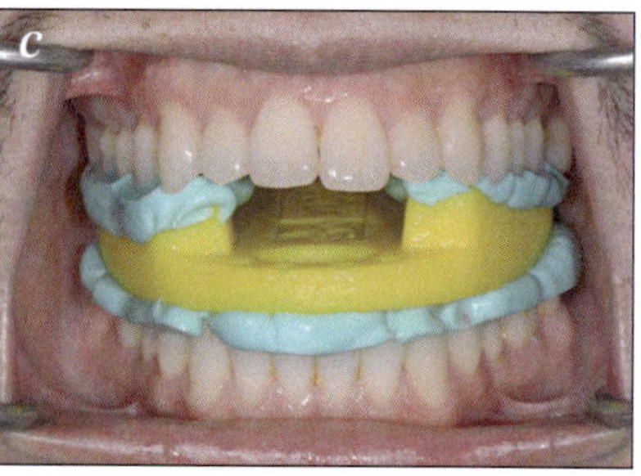

Figure 1-10 The digital prefabricated stent. *(a)* Master STL file. *(b)* 3D-printed prefabricated stent. *(c)* Stent positioned intraorally and indexed to the dentition with a quick-setting silicone material.

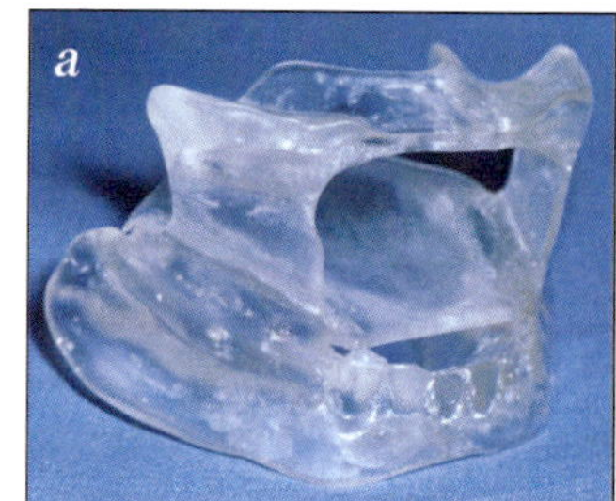
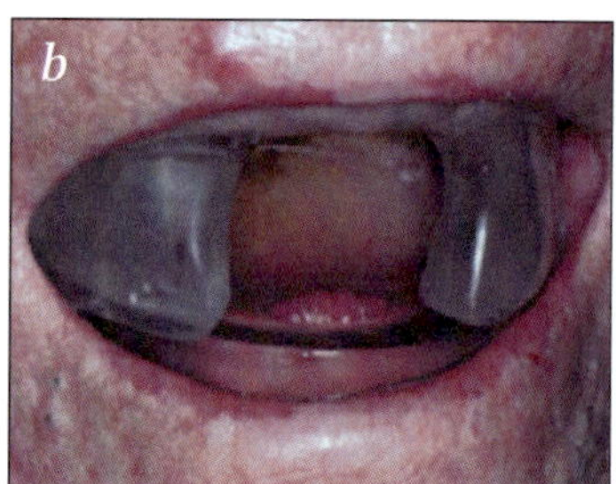

Figure 1-11 Tongue-positioning device. *(a)* Device for an edentulous patient with squamous cell carcinoma of the floor of the mouth. *(b)* Stent in position.

designed with retentive holes to engage the registration material. We suggest that a quick-setting dental silicone impression material be employed (Herpel et al., 2021) (Fig 1-10). It is possible to design and fabricate individualized positioning stents digitally that precisely engage the dentition, but an extra appointment is necessary for data acquisition.

Principles for fabrication of a positioning stent for the edentulous patient are similar to those used for the dentulous patient. Maxillary and mandibular impressions are made. Casts are fabricated, record bases are constructed, and an interocclusal record is prepared as described previously. The casts are mounted on a suitable articulator. Two thicknesses of baseplate wax are attached to the mandibular record base to form the portion of the stent that will depress the tongue. An occlusal index should be incorporated in the record bases to ensure patient comfort, stability of the stent, and consistent positioning of the mandible. If the existing dentures are adequate, duplication of the dentures can be a quick and easy way to begin fabrication. The duplicate dentures are returned to the mouth, lined with a temporary denture reline material when necessary, and the tongue-confining portion is fashioned as described previously (Fig 1-11).

A common problem observed during radiation is backscatter from large gold alloy dental restorations. Backscatter from these restorations enhances the dose locally by as much as 50% in tissues in direct contact with the restoration and approximately 22% 1 mm from its surface. The backscatter from dental restorations of zirconia (30% and 10.8%) and lithium disilicate (7.5% and 1.8%) is considerably less (Tso et al., 2019). As the data indicates, the intensity of the backscatter radiation decreases proportionally to the inverse square of the distance. This phenomenon can lead to severe mucosal ulcerations in adjacent tissues (Scrimger, 1977) (Fig 1-12). The effects of backscatter can be mitigated to some degree by having the patient wear empty custom-made fluoride trays during therapy. This simple stent creates sufficient space between the mucosa and metallic restorations to minimize the effects of backscatter (see Fig 1-51).

For some localized tongue tumors, many radiotherapists prefer to administer a moderate dose of external beam radiation therapy that includes the primary site and the regional lymph nodes, followed by use of low-dose-rate interstitial brachytherapy to boost the dose to the local primary site. In some instances, brachytherapy is used alone. If these radioactive implants are allowed to come in close

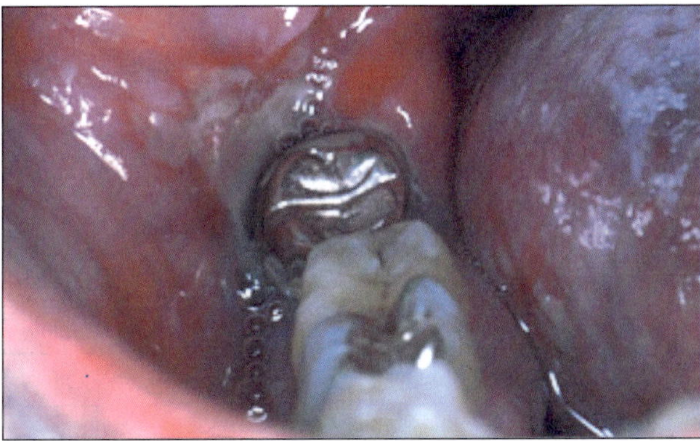

Figure 1-12 Backscatter from metallic restorations raises radiation exposure locally, resulting in more aggressive mucosal reactions. Prevention is easily accomplished by displacing the buccal mucosa or tongue away from the crown with a stent.

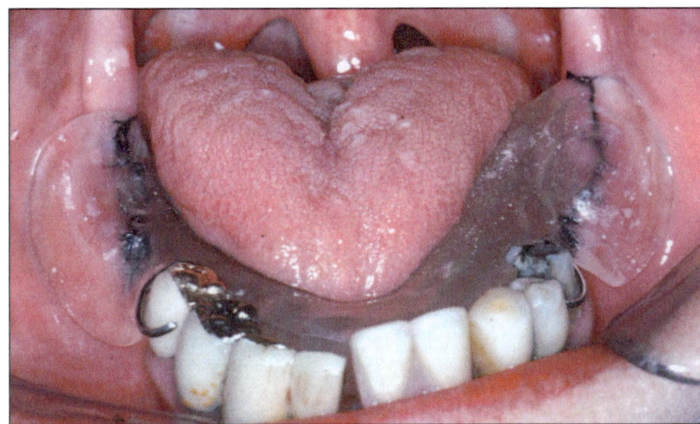

Figure 1-13 Displacing the tongue away from the lingual surface of the mandible with a lingual splint can reduce the radiation dose to the lingual of the mandible when brachytherapy is employed in treatment of localized lesions on the lateral surface of the tongue.

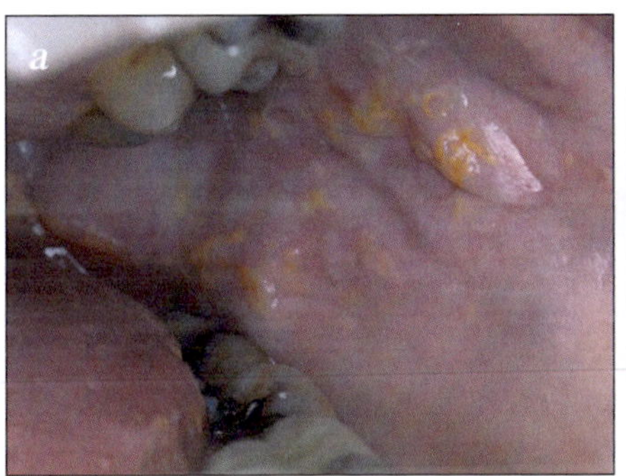

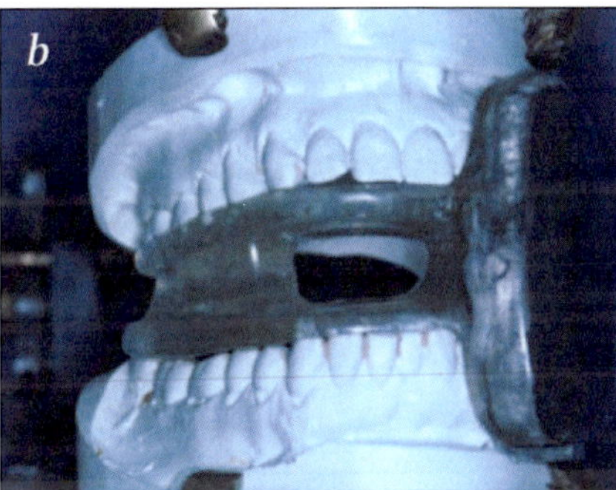

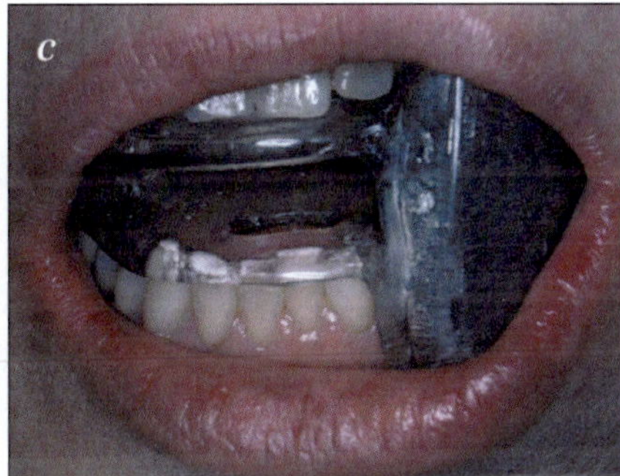

Figure 1-14 Shielding device to reduce exposure of normal tissues to high-energy electrons. *(a)* Squamous cell carcinoma of the buccal mucosa. *(b)* Completed shield. *(c)* Shield positioned intraorally.

proximity to the lingual surfaces of the mandible, the periosteum and lingual plate can receive a significant dose (up to 8,500 cGy) of radiation, which can lead to a high risk of osteoradionecrosis (Miura et al., 1998). A simple but effective stent (spacer) can be fabricated from autopolymerizing acrylic resin or light-curing resin. These resin stents are designed to rest between the lingual surface of the mandible and the tongue and should be at least 5 mm in thickness (Obinata et al., 2003). They can be fabricated for either dentulous (Fig 1-13) or edentulous patients. Because the radiation dose decreases rapidly with distance from the radioactive source, this simple device or variations thereof greatly reduces the dose absorbed by the lingual surface of the mandible and with it the risk of osteoradionecrosis (Obinata et al., 2003). Miura and colleagues (1998) showed that the incidence of osteoradionecrosis in patients with T1 or T2 carcinomas of the tongue treated with interstitial brachytherapy was 2.1% (1/48) with and 40.0% (22/55) without a spacer.

Shielding stents

Judicious placement of Cerrobend alloy can help reduce the radiation exposure to normal structures. Cerrobend alloy is a low-fusing alloy (158°F) composed of 50% bismuth, 26.7% lead, 13.3% tin, and 10% cadmium and is quite effective in shielding *high-energy electrons.* A 1 cm thickness of the alloy will prevent transmission of 95% of a unilateral 18 MeV electron beam. Shielding is most often possible in patients treated for tumors arising in the buccal mucosa (Yangchen et al., 2016a, 2016b) (Fig 1-14). The shield extends into the vestibule of both the mandible and the maxilla and is enclosed within a stent of acrylic resin that also serves to separate the mandible from the maxilla by about 20 mm.

Recontouring stents

A tissue-recontouring stent simplifies dosimetry when skin lesions associated with the upper and lower lips are treated. When the therapist adjusts the beam for the midline, the dosage delivered will be less at the corners of the mouth because of the convex curvature of the lips and face in this region. A stent can be employed to flatten the lip and corner of the mouth, thereby placing the entire lip in the same plane. Such stents often are combined with a shield. They are easily fabricated by forming dental modeling plastic to the desired dimensions. This pattern is invested and processed in acrylic resin.

Radiation-positioning stents

Brachytherapy delivers radiation over a short distance utilizing radioisotopes positioned in or close to the tumor. A radiation carrier can be

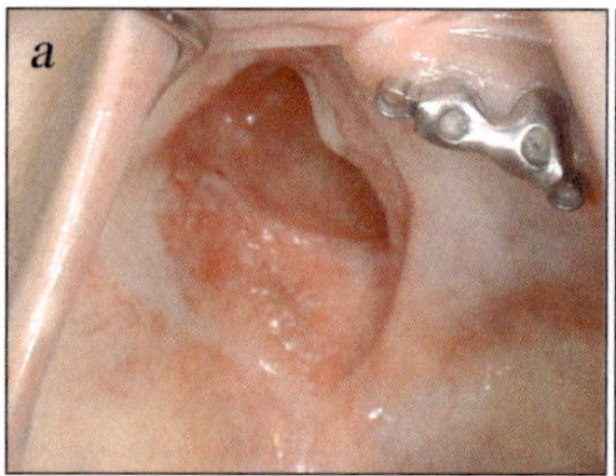

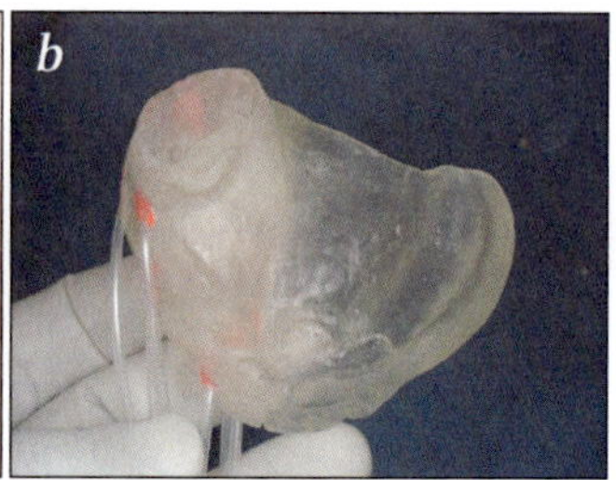

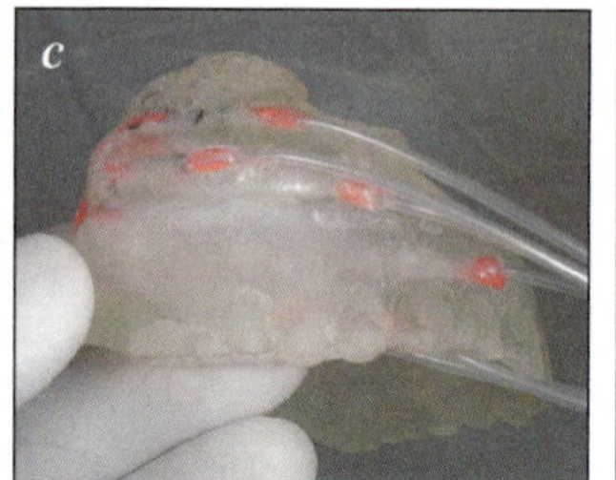

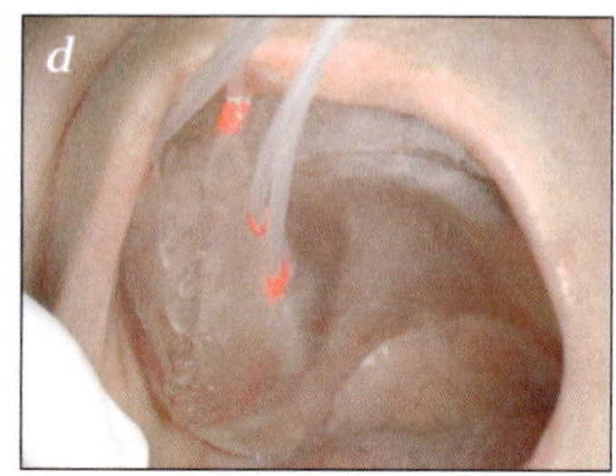

Figure 1-15 Radiation carrier. *(a)* Recurrent superficial squamous cell carcinoma on the posterolateral surface of a maxillectomy defect. The patient had previously received postoperative radiation following radical maxillectomy. *(b and c)* Tubing embedded within the device at prescribed intervals. The tubing will later receive the iridium seeds. *(d)* Device positioned intraorally. The device is retained with implant-retained tissue bar, and occlusal stops incorporated within the device help maintain consistent positioning.

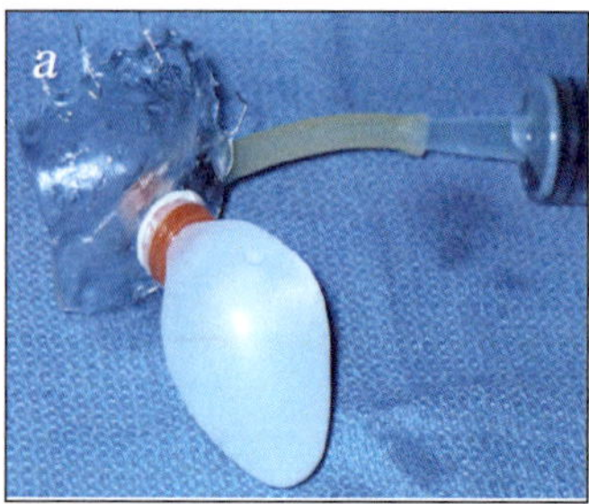

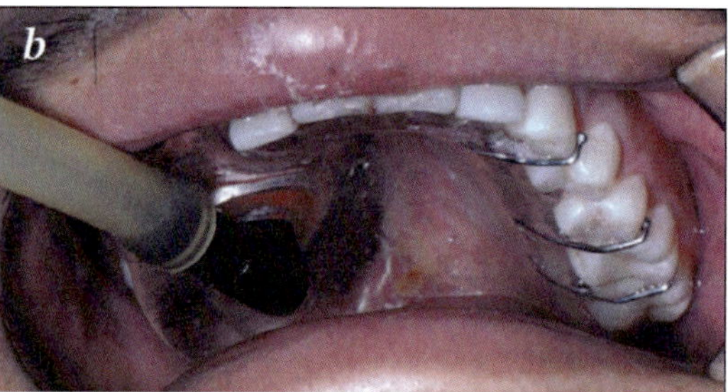

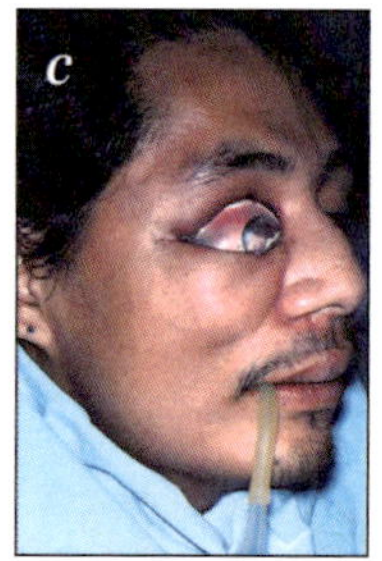

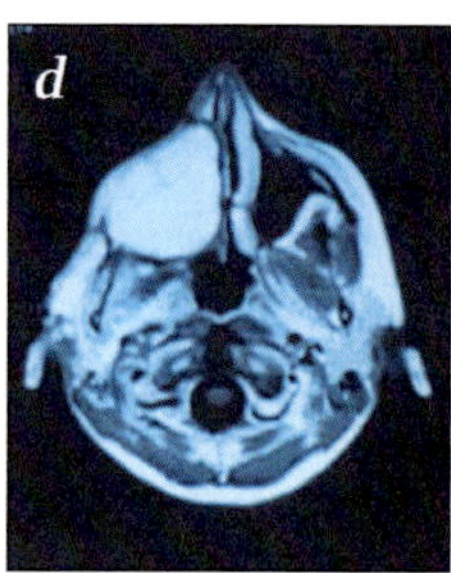

Figure 1-16 Tissue bolus device. *(a)* Bladder secured to a two-part connector. The assembly is embedded within a palatal stent. *(b)* Assembly positioned within the defect. *(c)* Resulting tissue distension when the bladder is filled with saline. *(d)* CT scan of a bladder filled with radiopaque material.

used to position the radioactive sources (cesium 132 or iridium 192) near the tumor site. Radiopaque shields and/or tissue positioners (stabilizers) can also be incorporated into the radiation carrier to spare surrounding tissues from unnecessary radiation exposure.

The radioactive sources may be either preloaded or afterloaded in the radiation carrier. When a carrier is preloaded, the radioactive source (typically cesium) is positioned within the prosthesis just prior to insertion of the carrier. The medical staff receives some radiation exposure when this technique is used. For afterloading techniques, the radiation carrier is designed with hollow catheters in predesigned locations. Once the radiation carrier is in position, radioactive isotopes (typically cesium 137 or iridium 192) are threaded in the hollow tubing. This technique reduces the exposure of the medical staff to radiation.

Techniques for fabricating radiation carriers vary, depending on the anatomical site being treated. Generally, an impression of the tumor site is made, and a master cast is generated from this impression. Once the master cast is retrieved, the radiation oncologist and/or radiation physicist determine the location of the radioactive sources. They also determine the dosimetry based on source location and isotope strength. Armed with this information, the prosthodontist fashions the carrier from acrylic resin. The completed carrier is positioned in the patient with dummy sources for simulation, and the final dosimetry is calculated by the radiation oncologist (Fig 1-15).

Tissue bolus devices

Irregular tissue contours create uneven radiation dose distributions and cause difficulty for the radiation oncologist. As a result, some areas within the clinical target volume may be undertreated, while other areas may develop isolated hot spots. A bolus is a tissue-equivalent material placed directly on or in irregular tissue contours to produce a more homogeneous dose distribution. The most commonly used materials for a bolus in the head and neck region are saline, wax, and acrylic resin.

Following orbital exenteration and maxillectomy, irregular contours and air spaces make it difficult to determine dose distribution, particularly when the size of the air spaces resulting from these surgical procedures is greater than the entry points through the orbit or palate. Tissues in greatest jeopardy of radiation injury are skin grafts within the defects, broad areas of thin mucosa over bone, and brain tissue that is in close approximation to the posterior borders of the defect.

A variety of methods have been employed to restore tissue density to facilitate radiation therapy. The placement of thermoplastic materials such as wax in the defect is one option. The physical properties of these thermoplastic materials allow the clinician to develop the desired shape. However, irritation of border tissues during insertion and removal of the materials and the unavoidable air spaces between the segments make their use time consuming as well as problematic.

Gauze boluses soaked in water can also be used to restore lost tissue density. However, water seeps through nasal passages and into the pharynx, leading to discomfort, coughing, and aspiration.

An innovative technique (Miyamoto et al., 1992; Singh et al., 2013) restores tissue density in maxillary defect air spaces with saline. The device consists of a palatal stent, a rubber bladder, and a hose connector (Fig 1-16). Normal saline is used to fill a flexible bladder placed in the tissue space. This method optimizes the dosimetry by restoring tissue density throughout the defect, particularly at the margins, and ensures uniform delivery of radiation to complex, irregularly shaped contours. The device is easy to insert and comfortable for the patient to wear.

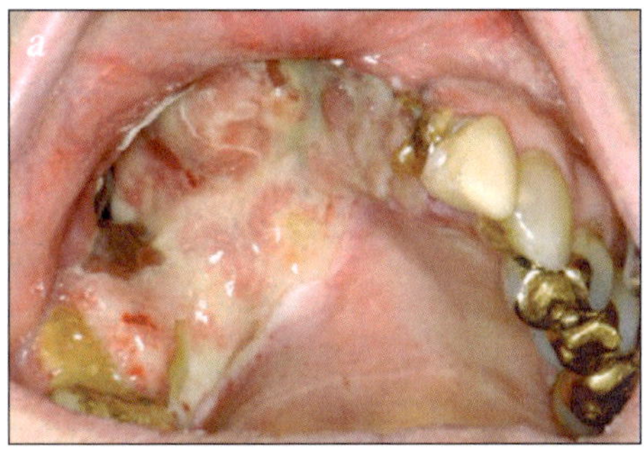
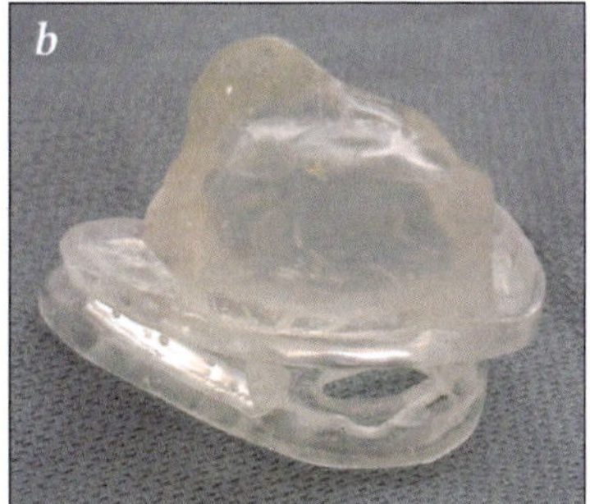
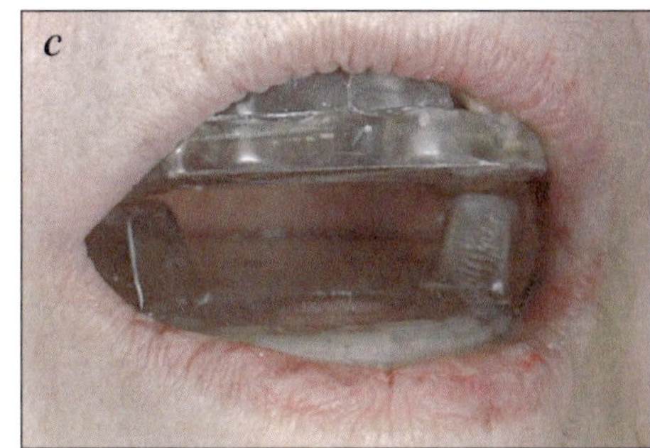

Figure 1-17 Combined positioner and tissue bolus device. *(a)* Status three weeks after partial palatectomy. The patient is to receive postoperative radiation therapy. *(b)* Stent made in two pieces to allow for easier insertion. *(c)* Device in position.

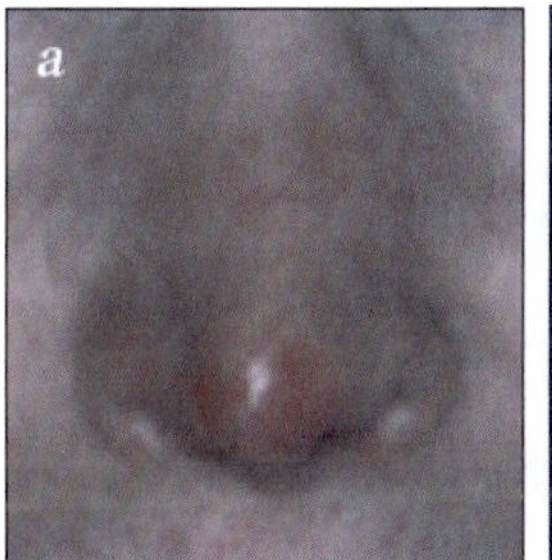
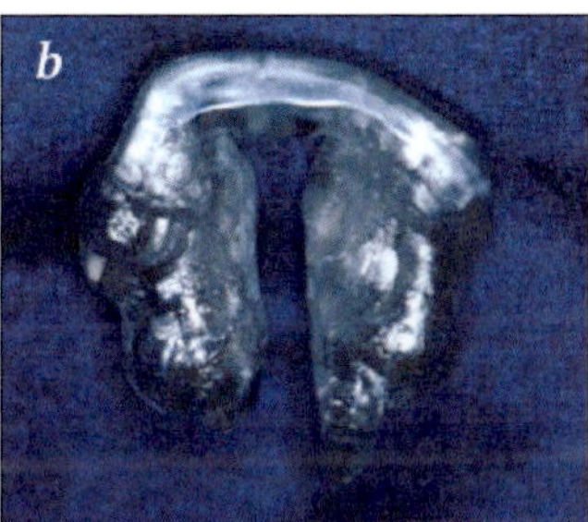
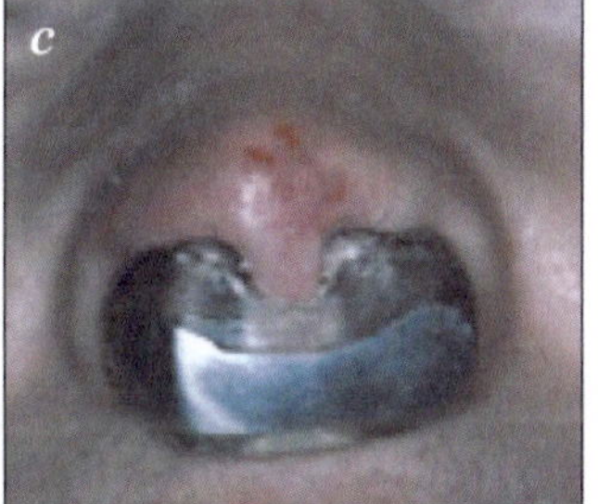
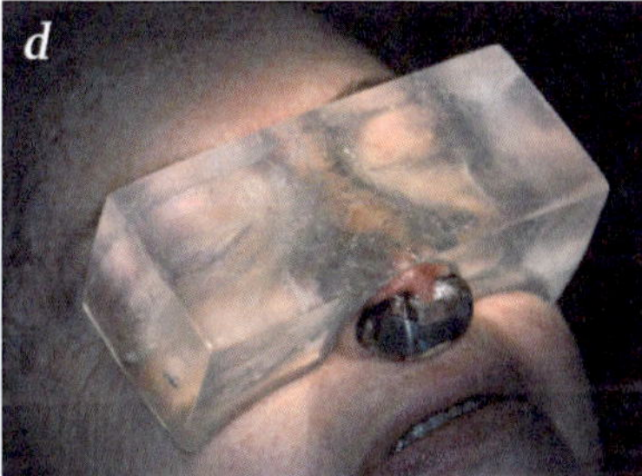

Figure 1-18 Radiation delivery to an extraoral structure. *(a)* Squamous cell carcinoma of the tip of the nose. *(b)* Cerrobend nasal stent. *(c)* Nasal stent in position. *(d)* Surface bolus of acrylic resin and Cerrobend nasal stent in position.

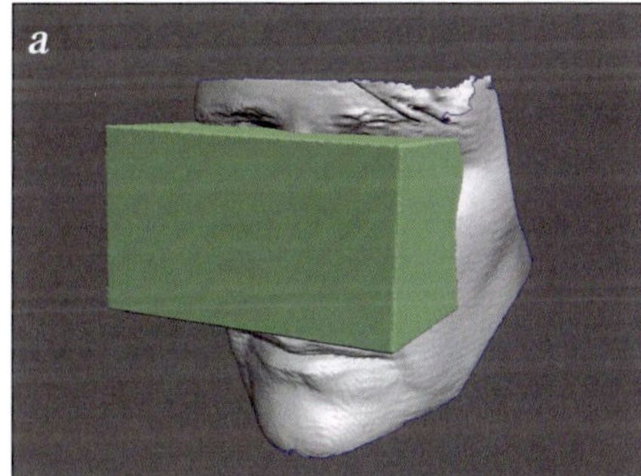
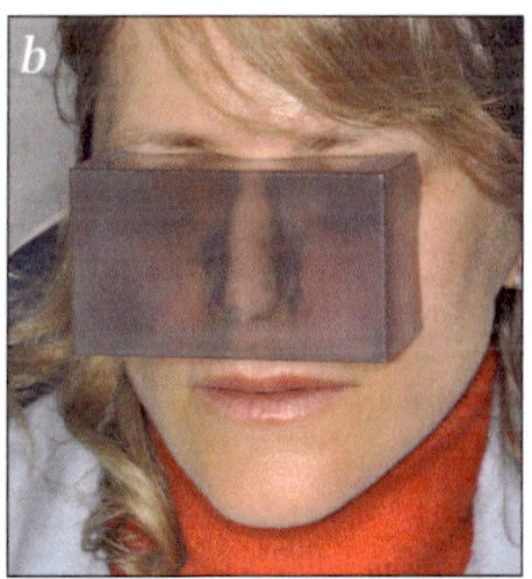

Figure 1-19 *(a)* Digitally designed tissue bolus device. *(b)* Printed device in position.

Pure gum latex rubber bladders, 3.5 inches in diameter, are used. Dimensionally compatible bladder and hose connectors are fabricated in polyurethane. A tissue surface–positioning stent is fabricated in autopolymerizing acrylic resin, to which the connector assembly is attached. A plastic or rubber hose is attached to the connector assembly and the bladder. The bladder is attached to the plug-shaped component of the two-part connector assembly. The central portion of the connector, with the bladder attached, is then pressed into the second portion of the connector, which is attached to the acrylic resin positioner. Adhesive felt is placed at the border of the stent to minimize the possibility of tissue irritation.

The bladder is inserted and positioned in the defect and stabilized by the opposing occlusion with an occlusal index. Once the palatal stent is positioned, a 50 mL syringe is used to fill the bladder. A finger-operated threaded clamp or a hemostat constricts the tubing beyond the radiation field and prevents fluid escape until completion of the treatment session. After the session is completed, the hose is placed below the level of the defect, the clamp is opened, and fluid is drained from the bladder.

Fig 1-17 shows a combination of positioning and bolus device. The stent separates the mandible from the maxilla by about 20 mm. The tissue bolus portion is fabricated of acrylic resin.

Radiation delivery to extraoral structures that display irregular tissue contours is also challenging. This process can be simplified by filling voids and/or overlaying the irregular contours with a bolus. Examples of such anatomical locations might be the nose, ear, or orbit. A facial moulage is made and poured into dental stone. The radiation oncologist is consulted as to the clinical target volume and the energy of the radiation to be delivered. This information is used to develop a bolus that extends beyond the edges of the clinical target volume, is of known thickness, fills voids, and smooths the tissue contours. These devices greatly simplify the dosimetry calculations for the radiation oncologist (Fig 1-18).

Extraoral tissue bolus devices can also be designed and manufactured digitally (Fig 1-19). A facial scan can be obtained with

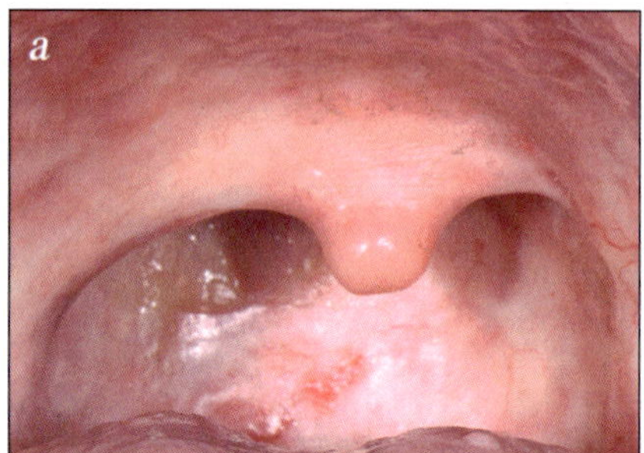

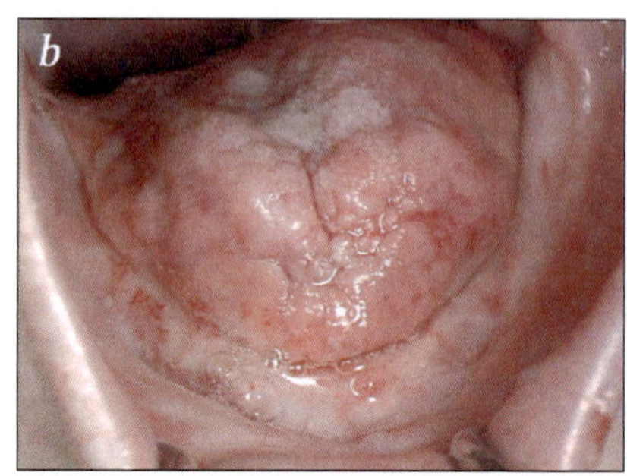

Figure 1-20 Examples of muscle wasting and fibrosis of heavily irradiated tissues. *(a)* A patient who was treated with chemoradiation of the left tonsillar fossa presents with velopharyngeal insufficiency, hypernasal speech, and nasal leakage during swallowing. *(b)* A patient who was treated with radiotherapy presents with compromised speech articulation secondary to a reduction in the bulk and mobility of the tongue.

structured-light 3D scanning or photogrammetry. Alternatively, the likeness of the face and involved structures can be extrapolated from computed tomography or magnetic resonance images. The tissue bolus with proper parameters is then designed with a CAD software program and manufactured with 3D printing. Such bolus devices are quick and easy to design and fabricate and fit precisely. Moreover, the printed material is more uniform, lacking the air inclusions often seen with devices made of autopolymerizing acrylic resin fabricated with conventional techniques (Pugh et al., 2017; Zhao et al., 2017; McCallum et al., 2021; Jreije et al., 2021).

Oral Effects of Radiation Therapy

General tissue effects

Any tumor can be destroyed by radiation if the dose delivered is sufficient. The limiting factor is the amount of radiation the adjacent normal tissue will tolerate. Tissues that exhibit rapid turnover rates are more readily affected. Reactions in the epithelium of the gastrointestinal tract, skin, and mucosa, because of their rapid turnover rates, appear very early but, if the dose is not excessive, healing is equally rapid. In tissues with slower turnover rates, damage may not become evident for months or years after therapy.

Immediately following initial exposure to tumoricidal doses of radiation, free radicals are formed within the cells and disruption of molecular bonds and breaks in DNA strands are noticed. Inflammatory cytokines and mediators are released, and intracellular signal pathways are altered, activating myofibroblasts and increasing the production of collagen. Early tissue changes noted include swelling, degeneration, and necrosis of the inner endothelial lining of small arteries and arterioles. Compromise of the endothelial lining leads to formation of thrombi that occlude the smaller vessels. These changes increase the permeability of vessel walls, which in turn leads to increased vascular congestion. Increased amounts of perivascular fluid exert pressure on the walls of small vessels, further impeding blood flow. Over time, medium-sized arteries such as the inferior alveolar artery may become occluded. These changes impair metabolic support for surrounding tissues and further increase fibroblastic activity and fibrosis. The process of fibrosis continues for years with resultant further narrowing and obliteration of vessel lumens. These responses are more severe and more permanent as the dose increases, particularly if combined with concomitant chemotherapy. Younger patients appear to be less affected with more potential for recovery following high-dose radiation therapy.

Radiation-induced fibrosis and the loss and impaired function of muscle stem cells (satellite cells) can lead to significant functional impairments in the head and neck (Jurdana et al., 2013; Zhou et al., 2017). High-dose radiation prevents mitosis of and reduces the population of the satellite stem cells, and muscle precursor myoblasts derived from these cells are responsible for muscle growth and regeneration. Muscle regeneration is responsible for maintaining the integrity of the muscle mass and function throughout life and particularly after muscle injury. It is assumed that a significant contributor to postradiation myopathy and muscle atrophy and fibrosis after high-dose radiation therapy may be the inability of muscle to regenerate (Jurdana et al., 2013). These effects appear to be dose dependent. Doses in excess of 60 Gy compromise muscle strength and decrease range of motion (Powers et al., 1991). Trismus, velopharyngeal insufficiency, chronic worsening dysphagia, and atrophy of the tongue musculature (Fig 1-20) are examples of the long-term effects associated with myopathy and muscle atrophy. Concomitant chemoradiation therapy appears to significantly increase the risk of these particular complications, and an increasing number of patients present with these symptoms (Eisbruch et al., 2002; Nguyen et al., 2008, 2009; Azzam et al., 2020). Numerous studies are currently being undertaken to minimize fibrosis and muscle-wasting prophylactically and promote muscle regeneration via a variety of drugs, free radical scavengers, injection of stem cells, and growth factors, but as yet none have proven to be even marginally effective.

Radiation-induced neuropathies probably potentiate some of the most notable postradiation functional morbidities occurring in the head and neck regions (dysphagia, trismus, etc.; Azzam et al., 2020). In the past, peripheral nerves were considered fairly resistant to the effects of radiation. Schwann cells were also thought to be radioresistant because of their low turnover rates. However, peripheral nerve radiosensitivity has been demonstrated in both experimental animal models and humans. Experimental evidence indicates that, following single doses of 20 to 25 Gy, both fibrosis of the endoneurium and impairment of the associated vasculature occur. Injury to Schwann cells, demyelination, and peripheral interstitial fibrosis have also been noted at these dose levels (Kinsella et al., 1991; Vujaskovic, 1997). The pathophysiological mechanisms are not well understood. No single target cell or tissue has been identified, but radiation injury to axons, myelin sheaths, and associated vasculature, plus the radiation-induced fibrosis, result in sufficient damage to explain the clinical manifestations (Fajardo et al., 2001). Nerve compression by radiation-induced fibrosis probably plays

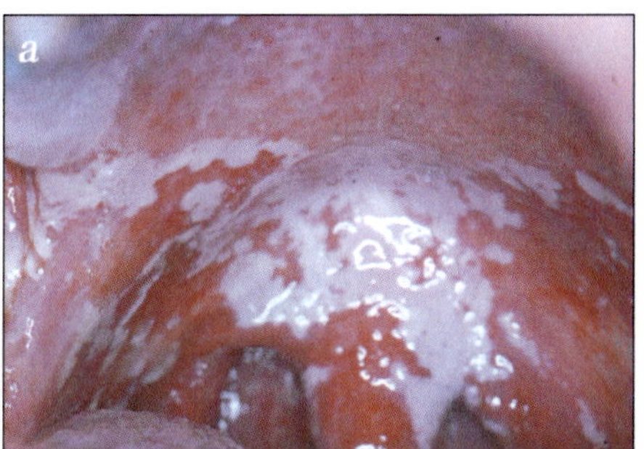

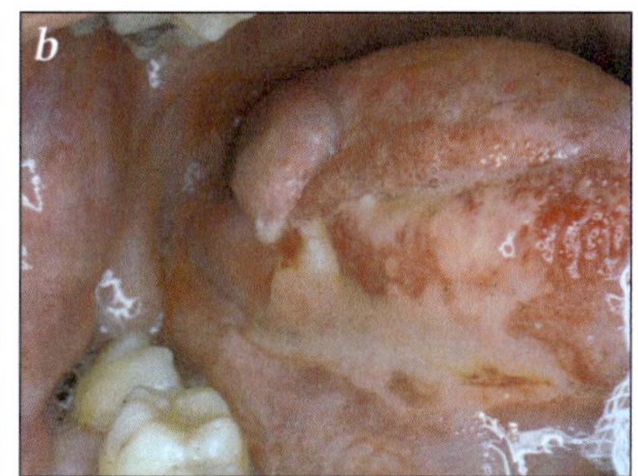

Figure 1-21 Acute radiation changes. Oral mucositis associated with *(a)* soft palate and *(b)* lateral border of the tongue.

an important role (Delanian et al., 2012), and so some researchers (Pradat et al., 2012) have suggested the use of drug combinations aimed at reducing radiation-induced fibrosis, ischemia, and inflammation (PENTO[CLO] protocol); however, the results of this study have not yet been reported.

Oral tissues effects

Early changes in oral mucous membranes

In oral mucosa, radiation effects appear early in the course of therapy. The severity of the local tissue reactions depends on the radiation dose, the size of each fraction, the volume of irradiated tissue, the fractionation scheme, and the type of ionizing radiation employed. An erythema appears that eventually leads to extensive ulceration and desquamation (Fig 1-21). These acute changes are secondary to radiation-induced mitotic death of the cells composing the basal layer of the epithelium and are rarely seen when the dose per fraction is less than 1.8 Gy (Scully and Epstein, 1996; Dumbrigue et al., 2000; Silverman, 2003). Most patients, however, are exposed to higher doses per fraction, generally 2.0 Gy or more. When the cumulative radiation dose is above 65 Gy, up to 90% develop mucositis (Vissink et al., 2003; Vera-Llonch et al., 2006; Elting et al., 2007).

Backscatter from gold alloy restorations can increase dose (up to 50%; Tso et al., 2019) to tissues in direct contact with the restoration and increase the severity of mucositis locally (see Fig 1-12). These secondary radiations travel short distances, and therefore the tissue reactions are prevented by use of a stent to deflect the adjacent mucosa away from the restoration. Backscatter is less of a concern in patients with titanium dental implants (see section below entitled "Dental Implants in Irradiated Tissues").

Oral mucositis is the result of damage to tissue mechanisms associated with both the epithelium and the underlying submucosa. Sonis (1998, 2004a, 2004b, 2009) proposed a model regarding the pathobiology of mucositis. He defined five stages: *(1)* initiation, *(2)* primary damage response, *(3)* signal amplification, *(4)* ulceration, and *(5)* healing. He proposed that delivery of the initial radiation fractions generates reactive oxygen species that result in breaks in DNA strands in the cells of the submucosa and epithelium; these breaks in turn initiate a chain of events that leads to stress-induced cell death of epithelial cells, fibroblasts, and epithelial stem cells in the region. Breaks in DNA strands activate nuclear factor kappa B (NF-*κ*B), which in turn upregulates multiple genes that lead to the production of proinflammatory cytokines, cytokine modulators, stress responders (i.e., COX-2, inducible NO-synthase, superoxide dismutase), and cell adhesion molecules, many of which have been linked to radiation-induced oral mucositis.

Pain, dysphagia, and resultant weight loss are common. Pseudomembranous mucositis begins to appear two to three weeks after the start of therapy but may appear earlier with altered fractionation schemes (Denham et al., 1999). It reaches a peak toward the end of treatment. Concurrent chemotherapy increases the incidence and severity (Elting et al., 2007; Chen et al., 2015), and these individuals occasionally require treatment interruption, hospitalization, and placement of gastric feeding tubes.

The severity of mucositis varies from patient to patient, and recent studies indicate that those with the most severe forms may be genetically predisposed (Brzozowska et al., 2018). The severity of mucositis depends on which tissues are included within the gross tumor volume and the clinical target volume, the dose per fraction, the fractionation pattern, and the total dose. Poorly keratinized mucosal surfaces of the nasopharynx and oropharynx are affected more severely than are keratinized surfaces such as the hard palate and attached gingiva. Elderly patients, those presenting with comorbidities, and patients treated with altered fractionation experience the most severe reactions. Patients with oral mucous membranes that are compromised secondary to alcoholism or insulin-dependent diabetes exhibit more severe mucosal changes. Chronically immunosuppressed patients—for example, those irradiated for oral tumors following organ transplantation—also develop more severe mucositis.

The role of oral microbiome changes associated with radiation therapy continues to be investigated. Changes in oral flora during radiotherapy are thought to exacerbate radiation mucositis (Almstahl et al., 2008; Schuurhuis et al., 2016). The radiation-induced death of the cells of the basal layer of the epithelium and subsequent ulceration of the mucosa plus the radiation-related reduction in microbial diversity predispose to colonization and invasion by preexisting oral bacteria and fungi. Cell wall products from bacteria lead to increased production of the proinflammatory cytokines, intensifying tissue damage. These changes appear to contribute to the severity of mucositis by altering the immune response leading to the production of additional inflammatory cytokines and toxins that cause further tissue damage (Reyes-Gibby, 2020; Zagury-Orly, 2021). Colonization by gram-negative bacilli, in particular, appears to induce more severe mucosal reactions during the later stages of radiation therapy (Spijkervet et al., 1989; Martin, 1993; Stokman et al., 2003).

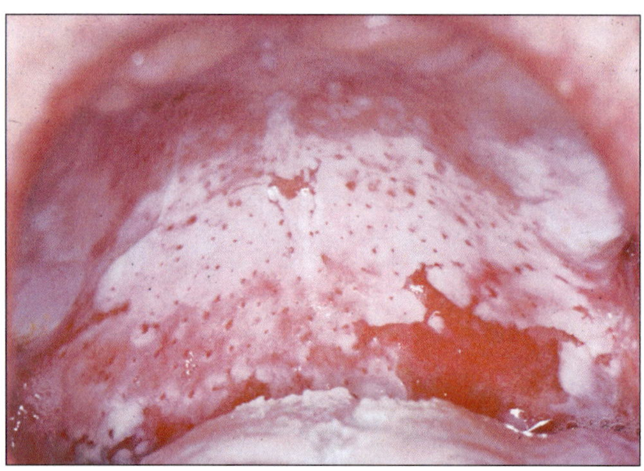

Figure 1-22 *Candida albicans* infection in a patient in the fifth week of external radiation therapy for treatment of squamous cell carcinoma of the tonsillar area.

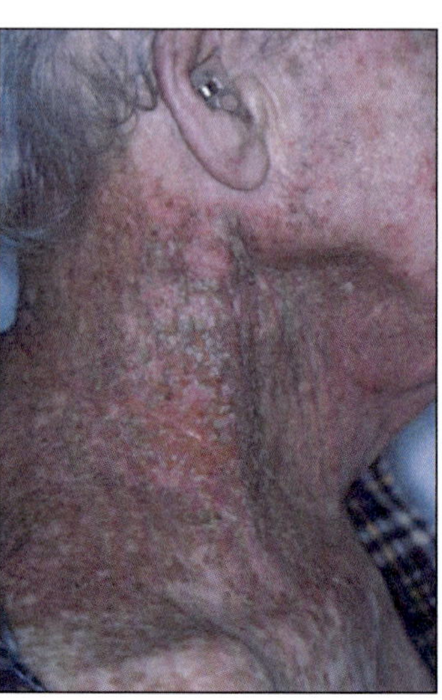

Figure 1-23 Acute skin reaction, including skin scaling and increased pigmentation.

Acute candidiasis may occur (Fig 1-22), triggered by the xerostomia and changes in salivary pH, reduction in salivary mucins, antimicrobial peptides, salivary proteins, and secretory IgA. About one-third of patients with oropharyngeal cancers treated with radiation therapy develop fungal infections during treatment. These opportunistic fungal infections intensify the discomfort and increase morbidity during and after radiation therapy (Ramirez-Amador et al., 1997; Suryawanshi et al., 2012). Candida albicans accounts for 80% of fungal infections (Bensadoun et al., 2011; Da Silva et al., 2017). The rate of those affected increases in patients treated with chemoradiation (Lalla et al., 2010). Topical antifungal medications (creams, lozenges, and mouthwashes of nystatins and azoles) administered during radiation treatments have been shown to reduce the incidence of these opportunistic fungal infections (Finlay et al., 1996; Epstein et al., 2002; Bensadoun et al., 2011; Silva et al., 2017). Sugar-sweetened nystatin preparations should be avoided because of the increased risk of caries. Systemic therapy with ketoconazole (200 mg daily) or fluconazole (100 mg daily) is favored by many clinicians and is preferred for the potentially noncompliant patient (Silverman, 2003). Prolonged use of antifungal medications is discouraged because of the risk of developing fungal resistance to these drugs.

Nutritional intake is adversely affected by the altered taste, partial xerostomia, and pain secondary to mucositis. Textured foods may exacerbate odynophagia, and patients will often shift to smooth-textured pureed foods and eventually to liquid intake. Liquid dietary supplements are useful but may be insufficient in patients with severe oral mucositis. In such patients, gastrostomy tubes or total parenteral nutrition may be required.

In patients receiving radiation alone, healing is rapid and is usually complete two to four weeks after the end of therapy. Resolution and restoration of mucosal integrity occur via signaling originating from the extracellular matrix of the submucosa and the surviving mucosal stem cells. In patients receiving concomitant chemoradiation, resolution of oral mucositis is prolonged and may take 6 to 12 months after the completion of radiation in some patients.

Similar changes are seen in skin, generally occurring about two weeks following the initiation of therapy. Erythema develops initially, and in some patients, leads to moist desquamation. Dry desquamation results if the therapy is temporarily halted. Dry desquamation is characterized by scaling and increased pigmentation (Fig 1-23). However, since the introduction of IMRT, the severity of radiation-induced skin toxicity has been reduced.

Palliation, prevention, and treatment. Treatment of radiation-induced mucositis in past years has been primarily palliative and symptomatic. Pain control with systemic analgesics has often been required. Appropriate oral hygiene practices lessen the severity of oral mucositis and include rinsing with saline, daily ultrasoft tooth brushing with fluoride toothpaste, maintaining a low-sugar and nonacidic food and drink diet, avoiding smoking and alcohol, and a dental prophylaxis prior to commencing radiotherapy. Mouth rinses with viscous lidocaine, doxepin, diphenhydramine-lidocaine-antacid (DLA), and gabapentin have been used for short-term relief of pain and in order to facilitate dietary intake. Unfortunately, the relief is short term, and there is no strong evidence for the routine use of these agents (Judge, 2021). Agents that bind to oral mucosa (mucosal protective agents) such as sulcrafate have been largely ineffective (Lalla et al., 2019).

As mentioned above, chemoradiation results in significantly more severe oral mucositis, and since it is being employed with increasing frequency, amelioration and prevention of mucositis have become urgent priorities. Mucositis secondary to chemoradiation significantly increases the cost of care because of the occasional need for additional procedures (hospitalization, use of gastric tubes, etc.) (Peterman et al., 2001).

Recent research has focused on strategies, based on the model proposed by Sonis (2004a, 2004b), that inhibit the development of tissue injury at the molecular level. Radioprotective agents such as amifostine, which act as reactive oxygen species inhibitors, have been tested (Antonadou et al., 2002; Law et al., 2007; Anderson et al., 2018). These agents act as free radical and reactive oxygen species scavengers, prevent the up-regulation of inflammatory pathways, and theoretically should minimize many of the deleterious effects of irradiation. Intravenous administration of amifostine has been tested the most, but the evidence is conflicting regarding the efficacy of this drug in reducing the incidence or severity of radiation-induced oral mucositis (Nicolatou-Galitis et al., 2013).

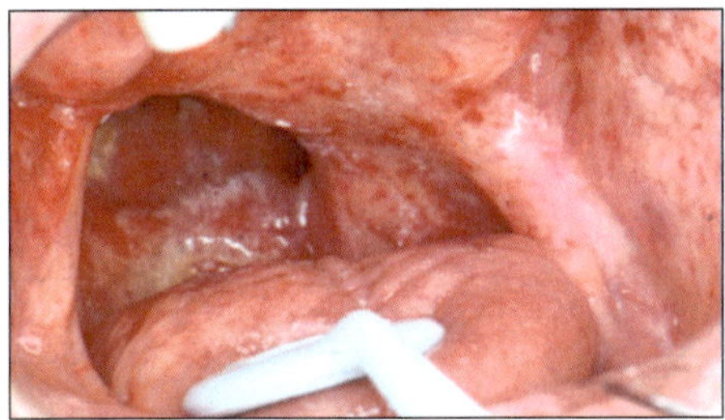

Figure 1-24 Severe mucosal changes. When telangiectasia extends beyond the gross tumor volume, it indicates that the patient tolerated radiation poorly and the dose was brought to the highest level of tissue tolerance. These widespread changes are less common with IMRT.

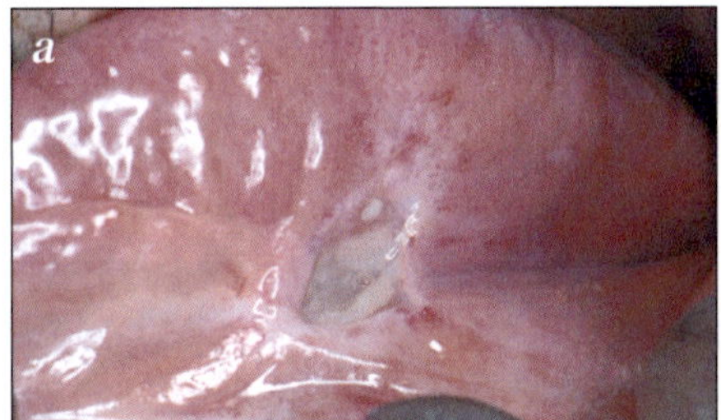

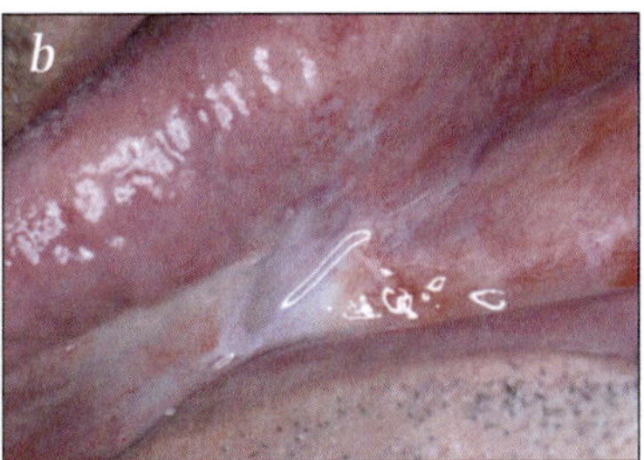

Figure 1-25 Soft tissue necrosis. *(a)* Squamous cell carcinoma of lateral border of tongue was treated with 55 Gy of external radiation followed by 25 Gy delivered by a radium implant. Nine months following therapy, a 2 × 3 mm ulceration developed at the tumor site. The results of the cytologic examination were negative for squamous carcinoma. *(b)* The lesion epithelialized nine months later.

As discussed earlier, the inflammatory response plays an important role in the initiation and progression of oral mucositis; drugs that suppress the inflammatory response theoretically should be beneficial. Benzydamine has received the most attention in recent years. It is a nonsteroidal anti-inflammatory drug with analgesic properties and has been shown to inhibit inflammatory cytokine production (Sironi et al., 2000) as well as to be a reactive oxygen species scavenger. It is administered as a mouthwash during radiotherapy, has been tested at a number of centers, and has been shown to reduce the severity of oral mucositis as well as the associated pain and dysphagia (Epstein et al., 2001; Cheng et al., 2006; Kazemian et al., 2009; Roopasshri et al., 2011; Rastogi et al., 2017).

Growth factors such as human keratinocyte growth factor (Palifermin) exercise cytoprotective effects on epithelial cells by reducing the levels of reactive oxygen species and have been shown to reduce the incidence and severity of oral mucositis in patients undergoing chemoradiation (Henke et al., 2011). However, data regarding safety are not yet available, and it is not approved for use in patients to be treated with radiation for tumors of the head and neck.

As mentioned earlier, secondary infection and the alteration in the oral microbiome are thought to worsen the severity of mucositis. Chlorhexidine mouth rinses have been tested extensively but have not been shown to be effective (Spijkervet et al., 1989; Epstein et al., 1992b; Foote et al., 1994; Dodd et al., 1996; Adamietz et al., 1998). However, therapies aimed at suppressing gram-negative bacilli with an oral lozenge consisting of polymyxin, tobramycin, and amphotericin B have been effective in minimizing the severity of oral mucositis (Spijkervet et al., 1990; Symonds et al., 1996; Wijers et al., 2001; McIlroy, 1996).

Photobiomodulation (low-level laser therapy) has been shown to reduce the severity of radiation-induced oral mucositis (Zadic et al., 2019). The biologic mechanisms for this treatment have yet to be clearly worked out, but it appears that they involve inhibition of the inflammatory response and promotion of cellular repair and wound healing. The optimum dose and energy deposition levels have been determined. Most researchers active in this field suggest that the most effective use of this technology is for prevention rather than for mitigation or correction (Zadic et al., 2019).

In summary, radiation-induced oral mucositis is a complex multifactorial phenomenon, and the palliative measures that have been employed have proven to be suboptimal. We are beginning to understand the pathogenesis of oral mucositis, but unfortunately, many of the cellular pathways involved are analogous to those in play in the destruction of tumor cells. We therefore face a dilemma. Will some of the strategies of mitigation that evolve from our increased level of understanding of these processes increase the risk of protecting tumor cells? Because of this risk, it follows that progress in this field will by necessity be slow and deliberate and will be based on specifically targeting the cellular pathways unique to oral mucositis.

Late changes in oral mucous membranes

After therapy there are significant changes in the field of radiation that predispose tissue to breakdown and delayed healing (Beumer et al., 1979; Cooper et al., 1995; Vissink et al., 2003). The overlying epithelium becomes thinned and exhibits less keratinization, and the submucosa becomes less vascular and more fibrotic. These changes appear to be irreversible. These late effects may be exacerbated by altered fractionation schemes and concomitant chemoradiation, predispose the oral mucosa to perforation, and as a result, make fabrication and tolerance of prosthetic restorations more challenging (see section below entitled "Complete Dentures for the Irradiated Patient").

The clinical appearance of irradiated mucous membranes is often a good indicator of the individual patient's tolerance and response. Transparent, pale mucosa with prominent telangiectasia are indicators of severe mucosal changes (Fig 1-24). In such patients, minimal trauma to tissues within the gross tumor volume can result in ulcerations that require months of healing and occasionally in exposure of bone. These soft tissue ulcerations generally occur at the tumor site and are most often associated with brachytherapy. In such patients, it is not unusual for the dose delivered to the local site to be in excess of 8,000 cGy. These so-called soft tissue necrosis may be difficult to differentiate from recurrent disease (Fig 1-25). They are nonindurated, lack the inflammatory halo observed in oral ulcerations at nonirradiated sites, and are quite painful. These clinical symptoms may be valuable aids in differentiating the lesions from tumor recurrence. Exfoliative oral cytology can be a useful supplement to clinical judgment in the evaluation of these lesions, but biopsy may be necessary to establish the diagnosis. PENTO(CLO) protocols have been used with some success to treat radiation-induced soft tissue necrosis (see section below entitled "Soft Tissue Necrosis").

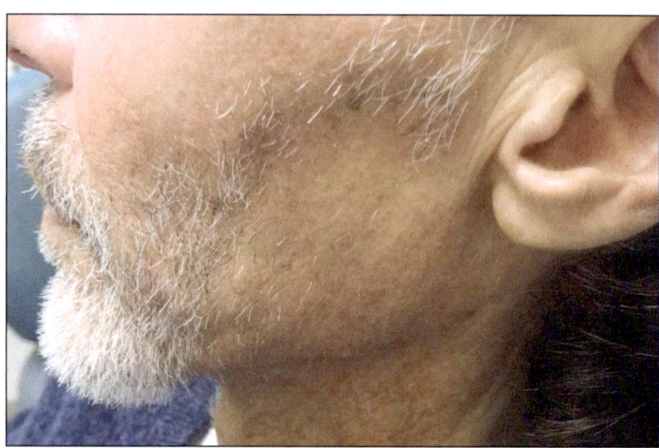

Figure 1-26 Late skin changes. Note the loss of hair within the clinical target volume (alopecia).

Chronic skin changes are characterized by atrophy, telangiectasia, and hair loss and may aid in determining the fields of radiation in a patient treated with CRT when records are not available (Fig 1-26).

Altered taste and olfaction

Taste buds are very sensitive to high-dose radiation, and since they are primarily found in the tongue, they are within the radiation treatment volume of most oral cavity cancers. Impairment of taste can have a profound effect on the quality of life of irradiated patients (Ruo et al., 2006; Epstein and Barasch, 2010; Asif et al., 2020), and its impairment may affect the nutritional status of the patient (Sandow et al., 2006). Significant alteration in taste has been found with sweet, salt, and bitter, but apparently less change has been found with sour (Asif et al., 2020). Patterns of food selection and intake change, and the patient may experience significant weight loss secondary to reduced appetite. Histologically, taste buds show signs of degeneration and atrophy at 10 Gy, and at tumoricidal levels of radiation, the architecture of the buds is almost obliterated (Conger and Wells, 1969; Conger, 1973; Silverman et al., 1983).

Most patients experience partial or complete loss of taste acuity during therapy. Alterations are discovered during the second week and continue until the end of treatment. Within six months, taste thresholds gradually return to near-normal levels, but taste impairment may linger years after radiation therapy (Sandow et al., 2006; Mirza et al., 2008). In experimental animals, when nerve fibers innervating the taste buds were severed, the buds rapidly disappeared; presumably, the changes observed in taste cells and buds are therefore due to both direct and indirect radiation effects on these epithelial structures (Yamashita et al., 2006).

Taste acuity may not return to normal levels in patients with severe xerostomia. Saliva is the solvent for gustatory stimuli and the presence of saliva plays an important role in regaining normal taste acuity (Matsuo, 2000). A significant reduction in saliva also appears to decrease the number of taste buds and may alter the form and function of the remaining buds (Henkin et al., 1972). Clinical trials with zinc supplements for such patients have shown some promise (Silverman et al., 1983; Matsuo, 2000; Ripamonti et al., 1998).

Olfactory loss can also occur in patients irradiated for head and neck cancer (Alvarez-Camacho et al., 2017; Gunn et al., 2021). Olfactory receptors receive odorant stimuli and transmit these stimuli via a series of interconnected neurons and brain structures, which then compute various associated stimuli into the notion of a specific smell. When patients with oral cavity cancers are treated with radiation therapy, the sense of smell is usually not affected because the olfactory receptors are located high in the nasal cavity above the superior turbinate and hence are not included within the radiation clinical target volume. However, when tumors arise in the nasopharynx, paranasal sinuses, pituitary glands, or sarcomas of the base of skull, the olfactory epithelium will be exposed to significant doses of radiation. Impairment in both odor sensitivity and identification of specific odors has been reported (Bramerson et al., 2013). Bramerson and colleagues (2013) have proposed that radiation may affect the olfactory epithelium both in the nasal cavity and on more central pathways. They noted that their data may also reflect an entirely peripheral effect, such as preventing the odor from reaching the olfactory region. The effects of radiation on olfaction appear to be dose dependent (Bramerson et al., 2013). When the olfactory epithelium is within the clinical target volume, Jalali and colleagues (2014) noted significant impairment of olfaction after the second week, and the decline continued until the end of treatment. In this study, no recovery of olfaction was recorded up to six months following completion of radiation. In the Bramerson report (2013), return of function after the completion of radiation treatments was sporadic. Of those patients in the high-dose category, one patient reported improvement and six reported a decline, while in the low-dose radiation group, four reported improvement and four reported a decline in olfactory capacity.

Lymphedema

Lymphedema of the tongue, buccal mucosa, and submental or submandibular areas occasionally can be clinically significant after completion of radiation therapy. Although direct effects of radiation are frequently implicated in lymphedema, it is also likely that radiation-induced fibrosis impairs the patency of both lymphatic and venous channels, resulting in lymphatic and venous obstruction (Ridner, 2013; Anand et al., 2018). A radical neck dissection may potentiate the effects and increase the edema. Lymphedema is most prominent in the submental areas following irradiation of tongue or floor of the mouth tumors and may make detection of recurrent local or regional disease difficult clinically. Lymphedema becomes apparent during the early postradiation period when scarring and fibrosis begin to appear. Occasionally it reaches proportions that compromise tongue mobility and impair salivary control, denture utilization, and speech articulation. It may also impact swallowing, vocal cord function, and neck mobility.

Recurrent tongue and cheek biting is a common complaint and may require occlusal alterations or alteration of the occlusal relationships of complete or removable partial dentures. A stent can also be fashioned to displace the tongue and/or buccal mucosa to alleviate this problem. This stent overlays the teeth and can be fashioned of mouthguard material on a dental stone cast. In some situations, the patient's fluoride carrier can serve the same purpose. In edentulous patients, when severe lymphedema occurs in the floor of the mouth, the floor of mouth is elevated, and the lingual denture extensions will be limited, impairing the stability of the prosthesis.

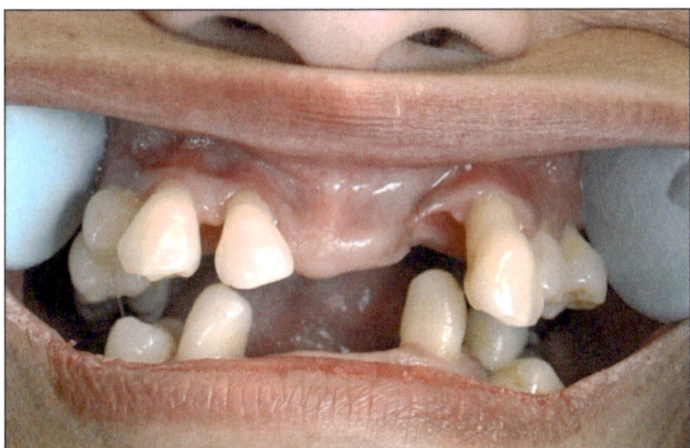

Figure 1-27 Maximum opening in a patient 13 years post radiotherapy for a nasopharyngeal carcinoma.

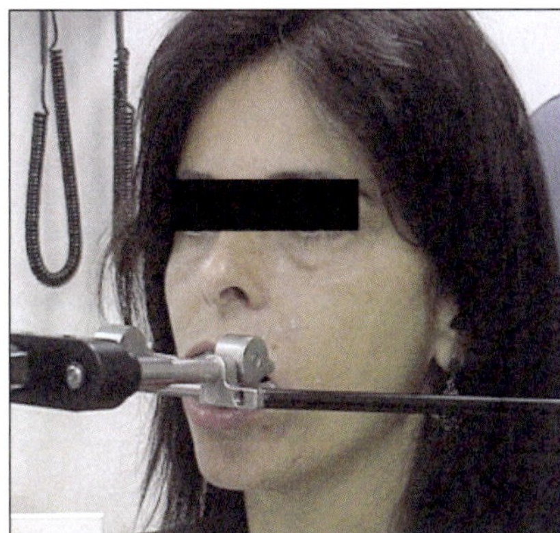

Figure 1-28 A dynamic bite opener (courtesy of Dyna Splint Severna Park, MD).

The severity of edema varies from day to day and with the time of day; it is most severe in the early morning hours and diminishes as the day progresses. This reduction in edema is probably a result of motor activities and the patient's assumption of an upright position. Occasionally massage and exercise of the affected area are useful.

Trismus, velopharyngeal incompetence, and dysphagia

A maximum mouth opening of 35 mm or less as measured from incisal edge to incisal edge has become the agreed-upon standard for moderate trismus (van der Geer et al., 2019). The incidence of clinical trismus in patients treated with radiation alone has been reported to be as low as 10% and as high as 45% (Louis et al., 2008; Watters et al., 2019). This risk increases in proportion to radiation dose and clinical target volume. The incidence in patients treated with concomitant chemoradiation therapy appears to be higher, but because of the lack of a standardized definition of trismus, comparisons between the two groups of patients are difficult to make at this time. Trismus is secondary to myopathy, muscle atrophy, and fibrosis of the muscles of mastication and often becomes noticeable at completion of radiation therapy. It is most noticeable following treatment of nasopharyngeal, tonsil, soft palate, and base of the tongue tumors, when the muscles of mastication receive high levels of radiation. Van der Geer et al. (2019) reported that mouth opening in such patients continues to worsen during the first year after therapy, and by the end of the year, trismus was noted in almost 40% of patients. Trismus can be exacerbated by the spread of odontogenic infection into myofascial spaces, which is an important consideration in this patient population, as they are at increased risk for developing caries and apical periodontitis (Abboud et al., 2020; Hommez et al., 2012).

The higher the radiation dose, the more severe the trismus (Goldstein et al., 1999; Kraaijenga et al., 2015; Rao et al., 2016). There is some evidence that IMRT, by reducing the dose to the muscles of mastication, may reduce the incidence and severity of trismus (Hsiung et al., 2008; Kraaijenga et al., 2015; Rao et al., 2016).

In some patients, the reduction of mouth opening becomes clinically significant (Fig 1-27). Maximum mandibular opening may be reduced to 5 to 15 mm, impairing mastication and preventing convenient oral access for the food bolus. Oral hygiene measures and dental treatment become problematic in such patients because of limited oral access, leading to an increased incidence of radiation caries and periodontal disease. Moreover, some clinical procedures have to be modified if an edentulous patient presents with clinically significant trismus. For example, when complete dentures are fabricated, the occlusal plane is lowered and the occlusal vertical dimension is reduced from the preradiation level to facilitate the insertion of the food bolus.

Trismus can be accentuated by some surgical resections. Following a total maxillectomy in combination with radiotherapy, trismus may be so severe that it impairs construction of an obturator of proper dimension and form (see Chapter 3, Fig 3-77). Border molding may be difficult, leading to an underextended prosthesis with compromised stability, support, and retention and an incomplete seal of the defect, resulting in hypernasal speech and escape of fluids into the nasal passages during swallowing.

The most predictable treatment outcomes result from structured exercise and use of jaw-mobilizing devices (Dijkstra et al., 2004; Pauli et al., 2014, 2016; Karlsson et al., 2021) (Fig 1-28) under the supervision of a physical therapist or a speech therapist. These devices are most effective in dentulous patients. They can be used in edentulous patients but require individual alteration. Best results are obtained when the patient is able to stretch for 30-minute sessions three times per day. Opening may be increased by as much as 10 to 15 mm, but such success requires a high level of patient cooperation because the discomfort associated with the required manipulation may prevent the patient from making meaningful progress (Dijkstra et al., 2004). Pain medications may be necessary as well as the use of Botox to counter muscle spasm.

In patients with a high risk of postradiation trismus (maxillectomy patients receiving postoperative radiation and those treated with concomitant chemoradiation), early manipulation and exercise of the mandible may lessen the severity of impairment. Tongue blades held together with tape and used as a lever can be effective at maintaining oral opening at preexisting levels but, in our experience, have not proven to be effective in significantly increasing oral opening following the onset of trismus after radiation. Delayed diagnosis impedes successful stretching therapy.

In patients where the soft palate and nasopharynx are within the clinical target volume, fibrosis and atrophy of the muscles of the soft palate and pharyngeal wall responsible for velopharyngeal closure and the pharyngeal phase of swallowing, can lead to velopharyngeal

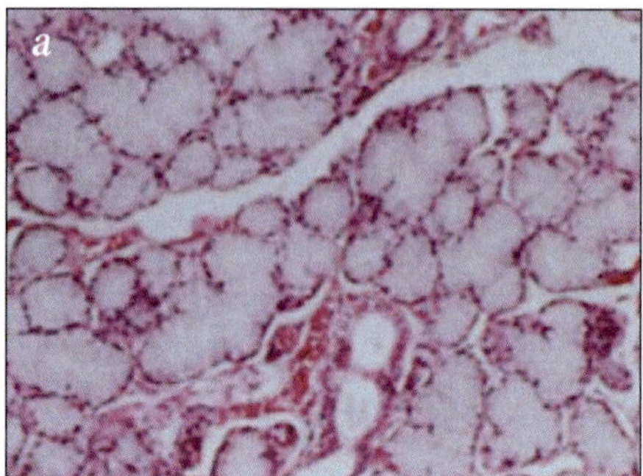
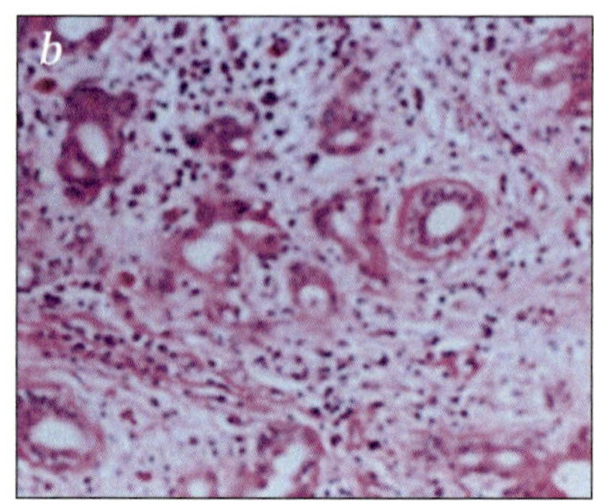

Figure 1-29 Radiation-induced changes in the salivary gland. *(a)* Normal salivary gland. *(b)* Irradiated salivary gland. Fibrosis and the lack of acini are apparent, but portions of the ductal system remain. Few stem cells remain (hematoxylin-eosin stain; original magnifications of ×40, and ×175, respectively; courtesy of Dr. Troy C. Daniels).

incompetence, velopharyngeal insufficiency, and dysphagia (see Fig 1-20a). These effects appear to be exacerbated in patients treated with concomitant chemoradiation therapy (Eisbruch et al., 2002; Nguyen et al., 2006, 2008, 2009). In such patients, swallowing dysfunction in particular appears to increase in incidence and severity, resulting in increased risk for aspiration pneumonia, which is associated with significant morbidity and mortality (Xu et al., 2015). As a result, an occasional patient must be fitted with a permanent feeding tube. Similar tissue changes can also lessen tongue bulk and impair its mobility when the radiation dose is excessive—for example, when brachytherapy is used with a large clinical target volume. In such patients, speech articulation and mastication are compromised as well as combined with xerostomia, the efficiency of bolus collection, and cohesion during oral transit and the overall efficiency of the oral preparatory and oral transit phases of swallowing (see Fig 1-20b).

As mentioned previously, concomitant chemotherapy escalates the biologically equivalent dose by 7 to 10 Gy (Kasibhatla et al., 2007; Fowler, 2008). When concomitant chemoradiation was first introduced, it was used in combination with CRT. Tumor response, local regional control, and overall survival appeared to be improved but the incidence of clinically significant late-occurring side effects and sequelae such as trismus, dysphagia, velopharyngeal incompetence, and ORN increased. Today, concomitant chemoradiation is most often employed with IMRT, and the incidence of these side effects appears to be less than that associated with combined chemotherapy and CRT.

New methods that offer the promise of improving the vitality of irradiated tissues are now evolving. The protocol proposed by Delanian et al. (2005) and Lyons and Ghazali (2008), which employs pentoxifylline and tocopherol (vitamin E), has yet to be employed in irradiated patients suffering from trismus and dysphagia, but recently this drug combination has been shown to reduce the risk of osteoradionecrosis in patients undergoing postradiation dental extractions (Aggarwal et al., 2017). Pentoxifylline is a vasodilator that facilitates blood flow by decreasing platelet aggregation and thrombus formation and inhibits fibrosis. Tocopherol is a free radical scavenger. Since the initial study, multiple iterations of this protocol have been tried using pentoxifylline and tocopherol (PENTO) in combination with other medications.

Salivary gland dysfunction

Given the slow turnover rates exhibited by the cells of the salivary gland parenchyma, these cells might be expected to be relatively resistant to the effects of radiation. However, within the first week of radiation therapy, dramatic reductions in salivary flow rates indicate that salivary glands are an acutely responding tissue. Changes in volume, viscosity, pH, and inorganic and organic constituents of saliva are manifest following irradiation of major salivary glands (Dreizen et al., 1977; Brown et al., 1975; Marks et al., 1981).

These changes predispose patients to fungal infections, caries, and periodontal disease that may lead to more serious bony infections and substantially diminish the quality of life. Increased viscosity and reduced flow of saliva also impair taste acuity and diminish tolerance for removable prostheses. Swallowing becomes difficult and the appetite is affected.

Early damage to the salivary glands is not apparent, and even at 40 Gy no apparent damage is detected histologically with light microscopy. However, at this level of irradiation, significant damage is visible with electron microscopy (Sodicoff et al., 1974). Early on, apoptosis is limited to 2% to 3% of all cell types following irradiation of salivary gland tissue (Paardekooper et al., 1998). However, irradiation dramatically compromises the function of the secretory cells, probably by impairing signal transduction of the plasma membrane (Paardekooper et al., 1998; Coppes et al., 2001). Although the architecture of the parenchyma remains relatively unchanged, the acinar cells cease to function normally and secretory responses are reduced by 50% immediately following the first few radiation fractions (Coppes et al., 2000).

During therapy and for a few months thereafter, there is evidence of varying degrees of recovery among acinar cells, as demonstrated by attempts at secretion or mitotic activity. However, these attempts are followed by a dramatic reduction in the number of acinar cells, accompanied by progressive fibrosis and continued degeneration of the fine vasculature. Loss of salivary gland function is due to loss of these parenchymal cells through apoptosis and varying degrees of inflammation and fibrosis. Cellular depletion is secondary to the lack of replenishment by glandular stem cells (Konings et al., 2005; Lombaert et al., 2017).

Ultimately, salivary glands exposed to high doses shrink and become adherent to adjacent tissues. Interstitial and interlobular fibrosis becomes advanced, with marked degeneration of acinar elements and loss of salivary stem cells. Reduced salivary output is ultimately secondary to the inability of stem cells to replace aging and dying parenchymal cells with functioning cells. Generally, all that remain are remnants of the ductal system (Fig 1-29).

Saliva originates from three sets of paired glands: the *(1)* parotid, *(2)* submandibular, and *(3)* sublingual, which are serous, mixed

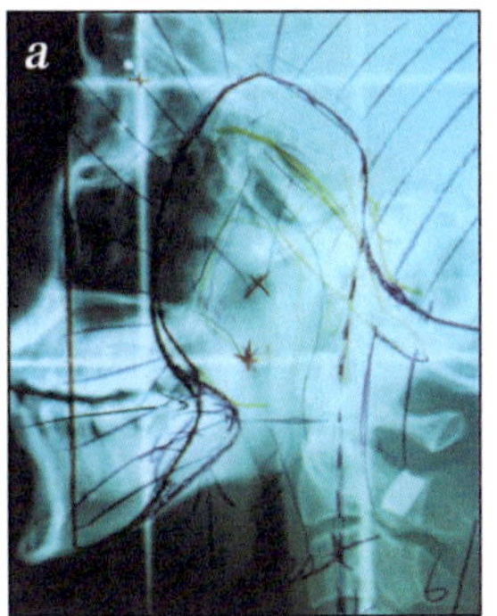

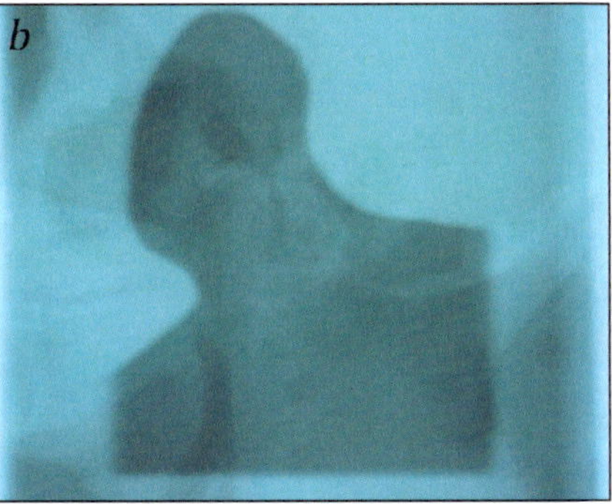

Figure 1-30 Typical fields used in CRT. *(a and b)* Initial bilateral posterior superior radiation fields used for nasopharyngeal carcinoma. High posterior radiation fields severely compromise salivary output, predisposing the patient to radiation caries. However, the risk of ORN is very low with these fields.

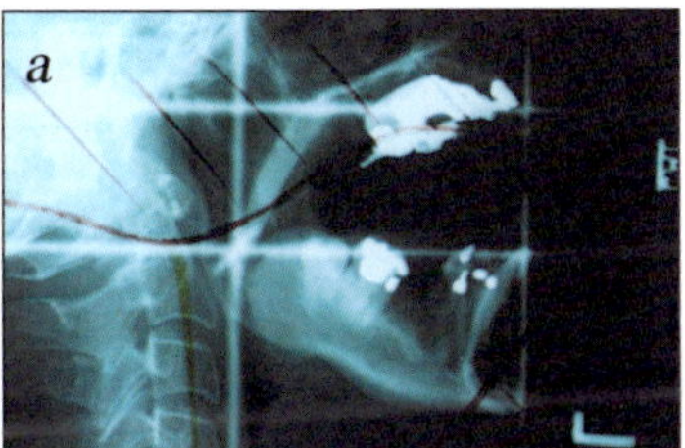

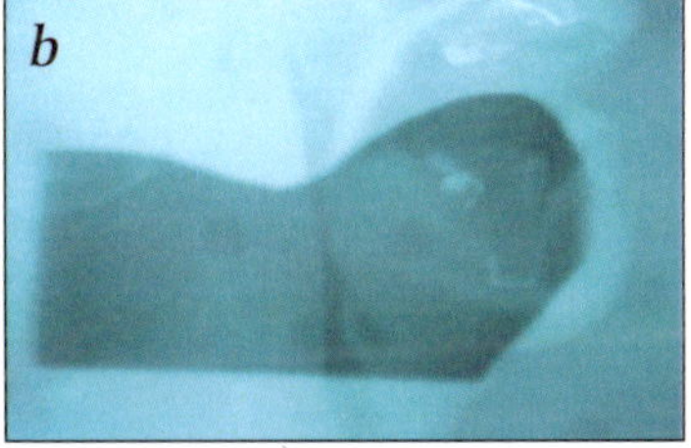

Figure 1-31 Typical fields used in CRT. *(a and b)* Initial radiation fields used for tongue carcinoma. These fields encompass most or all of the body of the mandible and predispose the patient to ORN.

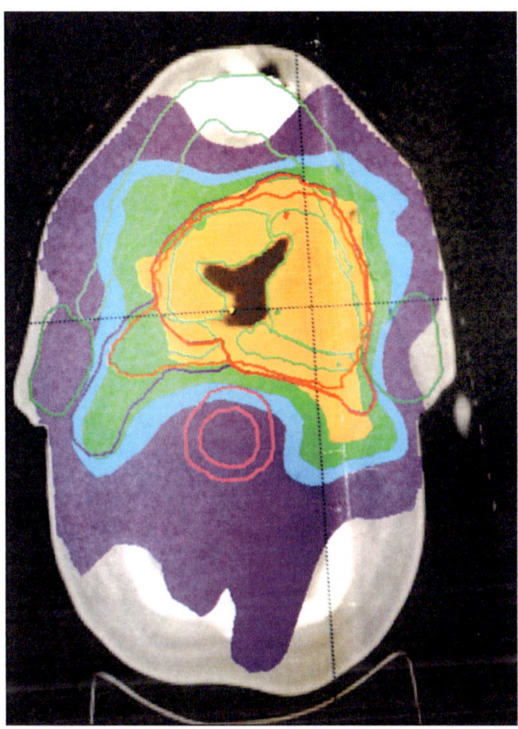

Figure 1-32 IMRT dosimetry diagram detailing the doses delivered to the tumor volume (right tonsil) and surrounding tissues. In this patient, contralateral and ipsilateral parotid glands are still exposed to doses in excess of 50 Gy.

serous and mucous, and mucous, respectively. Under stimulated conditions, the major glands produce more than 90% of salivary flow while the minor salivary glands account for the remainder. The minor salivary glands are responsible for most salivary production during nonstimulated periods. The parotid is the biggest producer under stimulated conditions. At moderate flow rates, it accounts for half the salivary output and at high flow rates can account for two-thirds of secretory production (Shannon et al., 1976). When CRT is given and all the major salivary glands are within the radiation clinical target volume (Fig 1-30), mean salivary output can be reduced by 86% to 93% (Dreizen et al., 1977; Curtis et al., 1976; Marunick et al., 1991).

Changes in salivary secretions are quickly apparent to the patient. Often within the first four or five treatments, patients notice the reduction in output and an increase in viscosity. In the past, when CRT was employed for lesions arising from the oropharynx or nasopharynx (retromolar trigone, tonsillar area, soft palate, base of tongue, and nasopharynx), most of the parenchyma of the major salivary glands were in the radiation field (Fig 1-30), and secretory output was almost immeasurable at the end of therapy. Return of salivary function was not significant in these patients, and consequently, the risk of caries was very high. Conversely, when CRT was employed for lesions of the floor of the mouth and oral tongue, the fields were quite low (if a tongue positioning stent was employed; see Figs 1-8–1-11), sparing the palatine glands at the junction of the hard and soft palate and significant amounts of parotid tissue and resulting in higher posttherapy salivary output (Fig 1-31). In addition, this group of patients often noted improved flow rates one to two years after radiation.

Today IMRT or VMAT is used in almost all circumstances. When these methods are employed for treatment of tumors arising from the oropharynx and nasopharynx, the dose to portions of the major salivary glands may be reduced (Fig 1-32), and there appears to be improvement of salivary flow (Murdoch-Kinch et al., 2008; Wang et al., 2011; Murphy et al., 2018). However, this is dependent on dose and the size and extent of the clinical target volume.

The dosage level of radiation required to effect irreversible damage to major salivary glands is complicated by many variables. Previous clinical reports are compromised by the difficulty in accurately assessing the dose distribution within the salivary gland parenchyma. Best estimates are that irreversible damage occurs in the range of 26 to 39 Gy and probably varies depending on the age of the patient and comorbidities present.

Posttherapy recovery and regeneration appear to be related to the size and extent of the radiation clinical target volume, the dosage, the age of the patient, and most importantly, the number of surviving salivary gland stem cells available for repair and repopulation (van Luijk et al., 2015). Eisbruch et al. (1999) reported that when the mean doses to the parotids were moderate (less than 26 Gy), flow rates were 50% of pretreatment levels in the initial weeks and months after radiation therapy but returned to pretreatment levels one year after radiation therapy. In addition, salivary glands that have received low to moderate doses (less than 26 Gy) show continued improvement in flow rates during the second year after radiation therapy, which in some patients actually exceed the preradiation therapy levels (Eisbruch et al., 2003). However, as the dose increases, tissue changes become irreversible. Dijkema and colleagues (2010) reported that at a mean dose of 39.9 Gy, there was a

50% probability that parotid gland flow would be reduced to <25% of the preradiotherapy outflow one year after therapy. At doses greater than 55 Gy there is little recovery of function (Eisbruch et al., 1999; Franzen et al., 1992; Roesink et al., 2001).

Age of the patient appears to be a key factor with regard to recovery of function. It is interesting to note that young patients treated with CRT who received doses of 35 to 45 Gy for lymphomas associated with the Waldeyer's ring, where both parotids were in the field, most of these patients experienced a return of salivary flow close to pretreatment levels within one year after CRT. The return of salivary output occurred even though these patients suffered moderate to severe xerostomia in the immediate post-CRT period.

In recent years the so-called mean dose concept has been the primary method used to predict postradiation salivary gland damage and output (Eisbruch et al., 1999; Roesink et al., 2001; Eisbruch et al., 2001). However, a complicating factor may be the so-called volume effect, and this concept raises questions about whether the mean dose concept is indeed the most reliable method of predicting radiation damage to major salivary glands and a predictor of postradiation salivary flow (Konings et al., 2005, 2006). Konings and associates (Konings et al., 2005, 2006), using a rat model, demonstrated that after partial irradiation of rat parotid glands, late damage to the shielded portion was caused by secondary events. Damage to the irradiated portions of the gland impacted the anatomical integrity and function of nonirradiated portions. In this animal model, radiation damage to blood vessels in the unshielded lobe that supplied the shielded portion of the gland and damage to the unshielded lobe's excretory ducts caused secondary damage to the shielded lobe. Moreover, van Luijk and colleagues (2015) have shown that salivary stem cells reside in the region of the parotid gland containing the major ducts. They demonstrated that the radiation dose to this region of the salivary gland was predictive of the function of the salivary glands one year postradiotherapy. Based on a preliminary study of select patients, they suggested that if this region of the salivary gland could be spared or the dose decreased, the severity of postradiotherapy xerostomia could be reduced. Presumably, limiting the dosage to this region resulted in the survival of a critical mass of stem cells that could be employed to repopulate the salivary gland acini.

All these data imply that best results in retaining reasonable salivary flow after radiation are achieved when salivary glands or key portions are spared from high-dose radiation. IMRT, which is now being used to treat a vast majority of patients, may reduce the dose to key portions of the major glands, particularly on the contralateral side of the tumor (Fig 1-32). However, substantial portions of the parotid and submandibular glands are still exposed to doses in excess of 50 Gy when tumors arising from the base of tongue tonsil and nasopharynx are treated with IMRT, and so moderate to severe xerostomia should be anticipated in such patients. However, it should be pointed out that attempts to reduce the dose to major salivary gland parenchyma may result in increasing the dose delivered to the mandible, elevating the risk of ORN. Theoretically, further dose reduction to strategic areas of the major salivary glands may be achieved with the use of proton beam therapy because of the superior dose distribution patterns that can be achieved (Kierkels et al., 2019). However, proton beam therapy is not yet widely available, and its efficacy for patients with head and neck cancer needs to be demonstrated in prospective randomized studies.

The viscous nature of secretions after radiation is quite bothersome to most patients. Swallowing and speech are both negatively impacted by these newly viscous secretions. When the radiosensitivity of the major and minor salivary glands is considered, the viscous nature of postradiation saliva is understandable. The minor salivary glands and the sublingual glands both have a greater percentage of mucous acini and appear to be more radiation resistant than the predominately serous parotid and submandibular glands. Moreover, when IMRT is employed, the sublingual gland, given its anterior position, is frequently exposed to doses below the 26–39 Gy threshold in patients treated for lesions arising from the base of tongue, tonsil, or nasopharynx. The result is that the ratio between the biologically viable mucous acini to serous acini is altered.

The changing nature of salivary secretions following tumoricidal doses of radiation therapy and the effect on the caries process is well established. There is no doubt that the reduced output alone results in an exceedingly high predisposition for dental caries, but recorded changes in organic and inorganic constituents and reduced pH also have important effects on the caries process. Until the work by Brown et al. (1975) salivary quantitative changes were assumed to be more important than the qualitative changes. Several investigators (Takei et al., 1994; Hashida et al., 1999; Kielbassa et al., 2006; Makkonen et al., 1986; Valdez et al., 1993; Almstahl et al., 2003; Laheij et al., 2015) have since confirmed that concentrations of peptides and proteins such as IgA, IgG, and lysozyme per unit volume were higher after radiation therapy. Nonetheless, the total daily salivary output was reduced sufficiently to create substantial deficits of these peptides and proteins, leading to changes in the oral flora balance favoring cariogenic organisms and a higher risk of dental caries. Immunologic mechanisms are also compromised, which increases the risk of caries and periodontal disease, the severity of oral mucositis, and perhaps the incidence and course of bone and soft tissue necroses. New methods are evolving that permit researchers to quantify a variety of peptides and proteins in saliva. As more insight is gained, it is reasonable to expect that it may be possible to identify specific biochemical markers in saliva that predispose to more severe forms of oral mucositis, candidiasis, and so on.

Deficits in bicarbonate load worsen as flow rates decline and the radiation dose increases, and this deficit is secondary to the radiation effects on the secretory duct system of the salivary glands. Reduced bicarbonate levels lead to a significant decrease in buffering capacity (Dreizen et al., 1976; Anderson et al., 1981) and, combined with a diminution of calcium and phosphate ions, preclude the regular and continuing process of remineralization of enamel that occurs in nonirradiated individuals with normal salivation. The result is that even in a compliant patient whose oral hygiene is meticulous, decalcification and erosion of the dentition is expected. This phenomenon can be partially counteracted by the use of remineralizing pastes and solutions (see section below entitled "Calcium phosphate remineralizing preparations").

Decreased output and increased viscosity have an important impact on the use of removable prostheses, especially complete dentures. Saliva is an effective lubricant at the denture-mucosa interface and is particularly important with regard to tolerance of mandibular complete dentures; when lesser amounts of saliva are present, more friction is produced as the mandibular denture slides over the mucosa-bearing surfaces during function. Changes in saliva, combined with irregular denture-bearing surfaces, are likely to increase the risk of mucosal irritation and perforation in patients using mandibular dentures. Furthermore, a peripheral seal may be difficult to obtain for maxillary complete dentures, compromising their retention (see section below entitled "Complete Dentures for the Irradiated Patient").

Agents to minimize radiation damage to salivary glands during radiation. Amifostine, a free radical scavenger known to accumulate in high concentrations in salivary glands, has been hypothesized by some investigators to limit the damage to acinar cells within the salivary glands during treatment. In some studies, it has been shown to moderately improve subjective symptoms (Antonadou et al., 2002; Law et al., 2007). However, in recent studies, there was no indication that pretreatment with amifostine made any difference in the incidence of radiation-induced xerostomia compared to a placebo (Lee et al., 2019; Riley et al., 2017; Ferraiolo and Veitz-Keenan, 2018). Side effects include hypotension, nausea, and vomiting. There has also been concern that this drug may have a protective effect on the tumor cells (Vissink et al., 2003; Jensen et al., 2019). However, in a recent Cochrane review, there was insufficient evidence to show that amifostine compromised the effects of cancer treatment when looking at patient survival (Riley et al., 2017).

Pilocarpine, administered during and after radiation, has been proposed as a means to limit radiation-induced damage (Roesink et al., 1999; Warde et al., 2002; Burlage et al., 2008). Animal experiments have shown some promise, but the human data are mixed and indeterminate. Some investigators feel there is little or no impact on salivary gland flow rates (Warde et al., 2002; Gornitsky et al., 2004), whereas others feel there is some benefit, particularly when the glands are exposed to doses in excess of 40 Gy (Burlage et al., 2008). In recent Cochrane literature reviews, there was insufficient evidence to demonstrate a difference in xerostomia or salivary flow rates as compared to placebo (Riley et al., 2017; Ferraiolo and Veitz-Keenan, 2018). Burlage and coworkers (2008) speculated that concomitant administration of pilocarpine may be of some benefit when patients are treated in institutions where advanced techniques are not available or when IMRT fails to spare sufficient portions of the salivary gland parenchyma. Others have suggested that the protective effect may be due to stimulation of the salivary gland parenchyma outside the radiation fields (Valdez et al., 1993). If this is the case, it follows that the use of pilocarpine concomitantly is probably only effective when significant portions of the salivary gland parenchyma are out of the clinical target volume or those areas that receive doses less than 26–39 Gy.

Several other preventive agents have shown potential in animal studies, but presently there is insufficient evidence to suggest their use in humans (Riley et al., 2017; Jensen et al., 2019).

Agents and strategies used to improve salivary flow after radiation therapy. Attempts to stimulate salivary activity have been disappointing in improving salivary flow and relieving subjective symptoms after therapy (Davies et al., 2015). However, in some studies, pilocarpine appeared to be partially successful in stimulating additional secretion in patients with residual salivary gland parenchyma (Fox et al., 1986; Greenspan and Daniels, 1989; Rieke et al., 1995; Johnson et al., 1993). In these reports, measured salivary flow may have been improved, but significant relief of subjective symptoms was rarely noted. Most of the benefit from postradiation pilocarpine usage is probably secondary to stimulation of residual minor salivary glands. They are more resistant to and recover more effectively from radiation damage than do the serous portions of the parotid or submaxillary glands (Niedermeier et al., 1998). Also, because of their wide distribution, some may have escaped exposure to levels above the threshold for permanent damage. Pilocarpine may be dispensed in liquid form and used as a mouth rinse (1 mg/mL, 5 mL per dose, four times per day) or in tablet form (5 mg, three times per day). Dosage levels greater than 20 mg daily may precipitate toxic side effects such as excessive sweating, lacrimation, nausea, urinary frequency, and gastric upset.

Cevimeline has a mechanism of action similar to that of pilocarpine and, like pilocarpine, may be useful in patients who have been treated in a manner that spares significant amounts of salivary gland parenchyma. It has been used with some success in patients with Sjögren's syndrome. Clinical trials involving postradiotherapy patients have been unremarkable (Davies et al., 2015; Riley et al., 2017).

Several other strategies have emerged aimed at increasing salivary production in patients with radiation-induced xerostomia. They include acupuncture, gustatory stimulus, extraoral and intraoral electrostimulation, and hyperbaric oxygen. The use of systemic sialogogues and the methods referred to above increase saliva secretion, but their efficacy depends on the amount of remaining functional salivary gland parenchyma, and as a result, none have shown to have a significant impact on this postradiation affliction.

Surgical relocation of the submandibular gland to the submental region prior to radiotherapy has been suggested for select patients, wherein one of the glands is transferred distant to the clinical target volume. The submandibular glands are mixed serous and mucous and, along with the numerous minor salivary glands present in the oral mucosa, are major contributors to saliva during resting conditions. This technique has been shown to be effective in partially mitigating the impact of postradiation xerostomia (Seikaly et al., 2004; Jha et al., 2012; Sood et al., 2014; Burgharz et al., 2016). Radiotherapy is begun within four to six weeks after surgery. The relocated gland is shielded after surgery, and radiotherapy is planned so as not to affect the radiation dose delivered to the primary disease areas or the neck nodes. The exclusionary criteria, which include carcinomas presenting in the oral cavity or nasopharynx, N3 neck disease, bilateral neck node involvement, preepiglottic space involvement, involvement of level I nodes on either side of the neck, and recurrent disease, render this option available to only a small group of patients.

Saliva substitutes. Attempts have been made to formulate saliva substitutes. Mouth rinses and sprays based on carboxymethylcellulose, glycerin, and mucin have received the most attention and have been tested by a number of investigators (Shannon et al., 1977, 1978; Vissink et al., 1983; Visch et al., 1986; Duxbury et al., 1989; Epstein et al., 1992a; Jellema et al., 2001; Momm et al., 2005). Those who have difficulty sleeping and/or speaking because of their xerostomia have reported the most benefit (Visch et al., 1986). Ideally, saliva substitutes should provide a protective coating for oral mucosa, maintain normal oral flora population patterns, be capable of remineralizing decalcified enamel, and be long lasting. All current formulations fall far short of achieving these objectives. These preparations provide only short-term relief and patient responses have been mixed. Most patients prefer frequently rinsing with water.

Stem cell transplantation and enhancement. Salivary gland parenchyma consists of acinar cells, myoepithelial cells, and a ductal system consisting of striated ducts and intercalated ducts. Primitive glandular stem/progenitor cells reside in the intercalated duct region and are responsible for regeneration of these cell populations (Takahashi et al., 2004; Katsumata et al., 2009; Cotroneo et al., 2010). Reduced production of saliva is ultimately secondary to sterilization of these glandular stem cells, which precludes replacement of aged and damaged ductal cells and saliva-producing acinar cells (Konings et al., 2005; Lombaert et al., 2008a, 2008b). The means of maintaining or refurbishing these glandular stem/progenitor cell populations are currently being studied by many institutions across the world. Mesenchymal stem cells from adipose tissue, labial mucosa, bone marrow, and the dental pulp and stem cells from human salivary glands, have shown promise.

Promising work has come from the Netherlands. Pringle and colleagues (2016) secured human salivary stem/progenitor cells via biopsy of submandibular glands resected during elective neck dissections and have shown them to be capable of self-renewal and differentiation. In vitro these cells were able to form salispheres (spherical clusters of cells) and to differentiate so as to form organoids (a miniaturized and simplified version of an organ produced in vitro in three dimensions that shows realistic microanatomy) containing both ductal and acinar cell lineages (Pringle et al., 2016). One month postradiation these salispheres were transplanted into both of the submandibular glands of irradiated mice. Each mouse received equal cell numbers so that a total of 1,000, 10,000, or 100,000 cells were transplanted per recipient mouse. At one, two, and three months postirradiation, whole stimulated saliva was collected from transplanted and control animals. In irradiated nontransplanted animals, production of stimulated saliva dropped to approximately 50% of preirradiation values. Stimulated saliva flow in mice transplanted with 100,000 human salisphere cells increased significantly to between 70–80% of preirradiation values. The authors also showed that significant numbers of salivary stem/progenitor cell populations reside within human salisphere cultures and replenished the salivary gland stem/progenitor cell populations of the mice that had received 100,000 human salisphere cells (Pringle et al., 2016). They also suggested that surviving endogenous salivary gland cells might additionally benefit from stimulation via transplanted salisphere cells to further increase salivary output.

Investigators have also demonstrated that bone marrow cells mobilized with different cytokines induce radiation-surviving stem cells to enhance repair of salivary parenchyma after irradiation (Lombaert et al., 2006, 2008c). Of great interest was the finding that this strategy induced significant angiogenesis and repair of the vasculature in the local tissues. Large vessels and capillaries showed improved morphology that was thought to be due to active replacement of the endothelium (Lombaert et al., 2008c). This finding is particularly significant since restoring the vascular network to a reasonable level is probably an important factor in the survival and function of transplanted stem/progenitor cells.

Research to date appears to indicate that when there is some retained salivary gland parenchyma and a reasonably viable vascular network, it is possible to recover salivary output to some degree in animal models with stem/progenitor cell transplants. If similar outcomes are to be obtained in humans, and such trials are underway, retaining some salivary gland parenchyma via IMRT or a similar approach—for example, with neutrons—and careful treatment planning would appear to be an important cofactor. Tissue engineering of functional salivary gland organoids and transplanting them successfully into patients whose vascular network has been all but obliterated by severe radiation damage would appear to be a challenge beyond reach at this time.

In summary, reducing the amount of salivary gland parenchyma exposed to high doses remains the most effective means of ensuring reasonable salivary flow after radiation. However, treatment of advanced tumors of the nasopharynx, oropharynx, and soft palate often requires large clinical target volumes, and even with the use of IMRT substantial portions of the major salivary gland parenchyma are exposed to doses in excess of 26–39 Gy, which theoretically is sufficient to cause irreversible damage in older patients. Many issues are yet to be resolved but in the future in such patients, the use of salivary stem/progenitor cell transplantation to increase the regenerative potential of irradiated salivary glands, combined with retaining some salivary gland parenchyma by means of careful radiation targeting, would seem to the offer the best hope for restoration of reasonable levels of salivary output for such patients.

Bone changes

Following tumoricidal doses of radiation, significant changes are observed in bone. It becomes a hypoxic, hypocellular, hypovascular tissue. Gross changes in bone after irradiation are primarily secondary to radiation-induced fibrosis. Several authors have proposed that radiation damage is the result of dysregulation of fibroblastic activity (Delanian and Lefaix, 2004; Lyons and Ghazali, 2008). Initially, endothelial cells are damaged by both the direct and the indirect effects of radiation. The injured endothelial cells produce cytokines that enhance the acute inflammatory response and, in turn, promote the release of inflammatory cytokines. Subsequently, the destruction of the endothelium combined with vascular thrombosis leads to substantial loss of the small vessel network in the irradiated tissues. During this process fibroblasts are transformed into myofibroblasts, and unregulated chronic activation of these myofibroblasts by a variety of growth factors leads to progressive fibrosis.

Progressive fibrosis and loss of vasculature within bone result in a dramatic reduction of the number of cells and destruction of the remodeling apparatus. The severity of these progressive changes depends on the dose. The late effects observed after radiation are similar to the natural changes that occur more slowly with aging but are much more profound. The marrow exhibits marked hypocellularity and hypovascularity, significant fibrosis, and fatty degeneration (Fig 1-33). Occlusion of the inferior alveolar artery has been demonstrated in animals and in humans (Rohrer et al., 1979). Lacunae become devoid of their osteocytes and the endosteum atrophies with significant loss of functioning osteoblasts and osteoclasts. The periosteum demonstrates significant fibrosis and a similar loss of remodeling elements (Rohrer et al., 1979; Silverman and Chierci, 1965). Such bone renders a poor response to trauma and infection, so the high incidence of ORN in irradiated patients is not surprising.

In addition, the biologic processes leading to osseointegration of titanium implants (the initiation of contact and distance osteogenesis that lead to implant anchorage) are severely compromised or may be entirely absent in heavily irradiated bone (see the section entitled "Dental Implants in Irradiated Tissues"). If the dose to the bone site exceeds 65 Gy, the implant anchorage that develops is most likely achieved by mechanical means as opposed to a biologically mediated phenomenon.

These tissue changes profoundly affect the repair and remodeling capability of bone. Adult bone changes continuously with the destruction of certain areas and the reconstruction of new areas and the jawbones exhibit a particularly high rate of remodeling and turnover. The basic multicellular unit, composed of osteoclasts and osteoblasts, is responsible for this phenomenon. This well-balanced process of destruction and reconstruction is disturbed

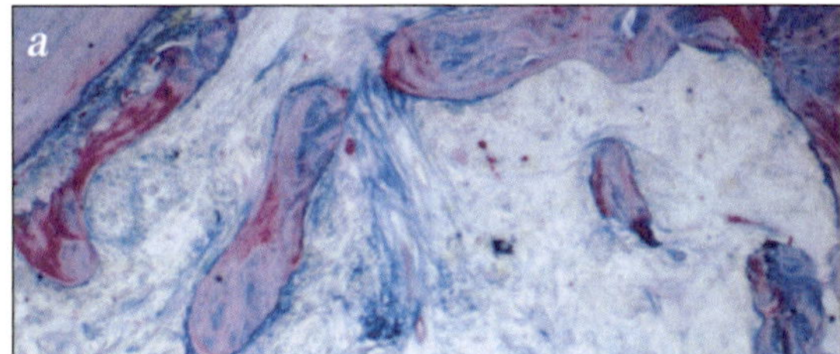

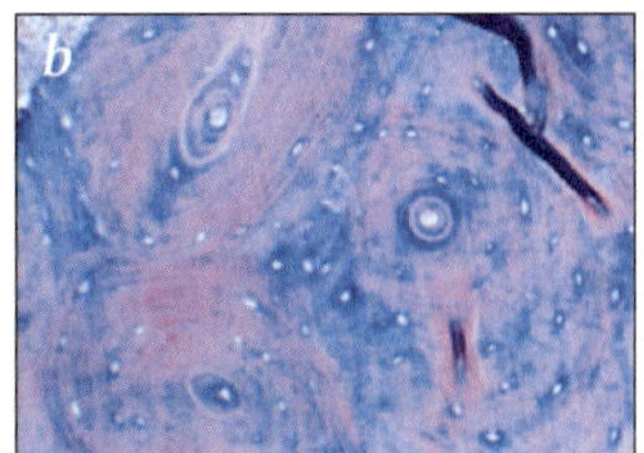

Figure 1-33 Radiation effects on bone in a patient who received a total 70 Gy dose for squamous cell carcinoma of the tonsillar pillar. *(a)* Changes include fibrosis, the hypocellular-hypovascular nature of the marrow, and the lack of endosteum. *(b)* Haversian systems. The central artery is often missing. Note the empty lacunae (Masson's trichrome stain; original magnification ×100).

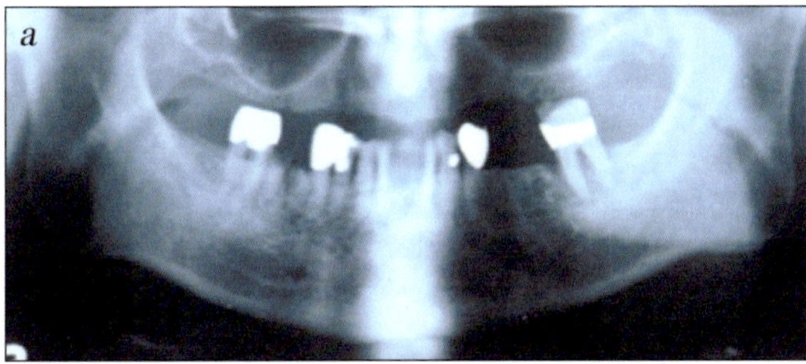

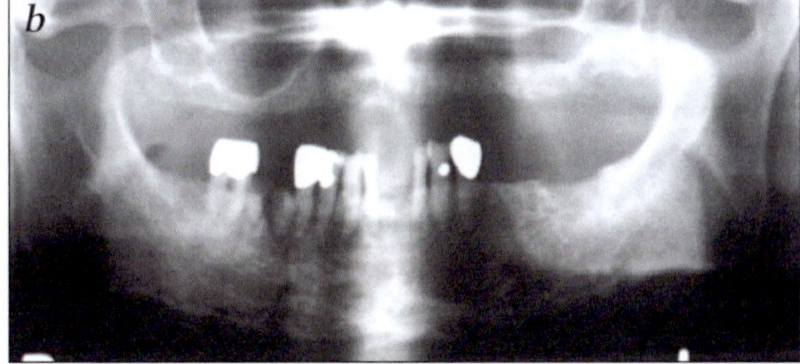

Figure 1-34 Radiation effects on bone in a patient who received external CRT (70.5 Gy) for a lateral floor of the mouth lesion. There was a dramatic change in trabecular patterns between preoperative *(a)* and postoperative *(b)* radiographs. The patient was asymptomatic.

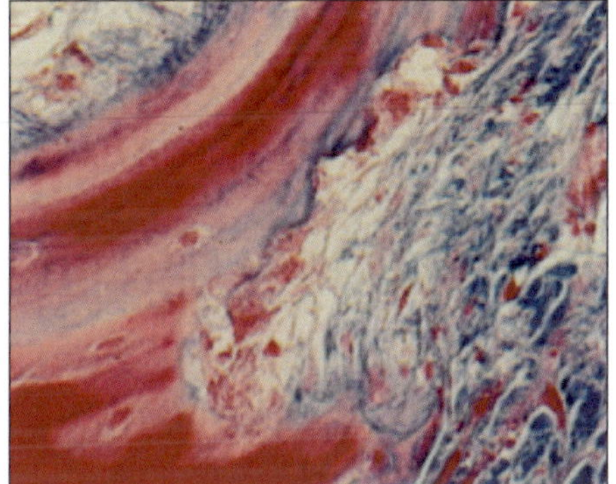

Figure 1-35 Isolated osteoclast in bone exposed to 70 Gy of radiation (Masson trichrome stain; original magnification ×200).

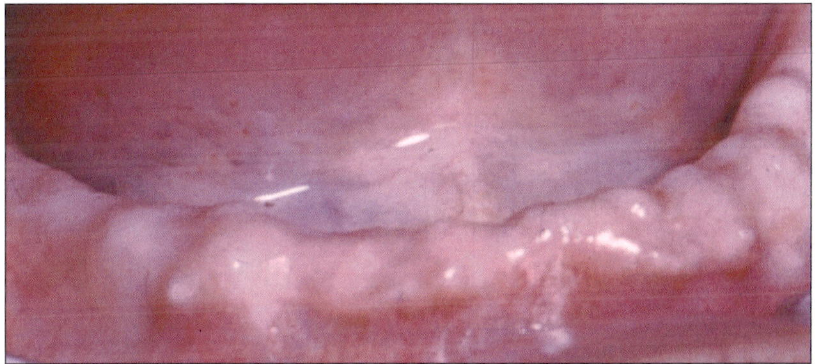

Figure 1-36 Results of an inadequate alveolectomy. Although the alveolar ridge is covered with healthy mucosa, its irregular morphology precludes the use of a mandibular denture at this time.

or totally eliminated by tumoricidal doses of radiation, and in many patients, there appears to be a dramatic increase in osteolytic activity (Fig 1-34). These osteolytic changes are caused by isolated osteoclasts (Fig 1-35). Whether these isolated osteoclasts represent the surviving remnants of the basic multicellular unit of the remodeling apparatus or find their way into irradiated bone via the circulation, mediated by macrophages, is not yet known. The osteolytic effect appears to be particularly prominent in patients treated with chemoradiation therapy.

Because of compromise of the remodeling apparatus, the dental surgeon must smoothly contour the alveolar ridge at the time of preradiation dental extractions when these sites are within the clinical target volume. If radical alveolectomies are not performed on such patients, the resulting alveolar ridge will not readily remodel and will be quite irregular (Fig 1-36). Construction and wearing of mandibular dentures on heavily irradiated irregular denture foundation areas within the clinical target volume is risky because mucosal perforations are likely and they may lead to exposed bone and subsequently to ORN.

Periodontal changes

The periodontium likewise exhibits change that predispose patients to infection. Radiographically, widening of the periodontal ligament space is often noted and there may also be loss of the lamina dura (Fugita et al., 1986). The rather specific network of fibers of the periodontal ligament becomes disoriented and the periodontal ligament thickens (Rohrer et al., 1979; Silverman and Chierci, 1965). It exhibits decreased cellularity and vascularity. The higher the dose, the more profound the tissue changes. Fig 1-37 shows the differences in periodontal ligaments exposed to 50 Gy and 70 Gy. The periodontal ligament exposed to 50 Gy retains much of its normal morphology and its regularly spaced vascular channels. These vascular channels are essentially absent in the 70 Gy specimens.

As a result, following radiation, attachment loss is accelerated in teeth exposed to high doses (Epstein et al., 1998; Marques and Dib, 2004; Ammajan et al., 2013; Schuurhuis et al., 2018). Chemoradiation appears to accelerate attachment loss as well as the progression of

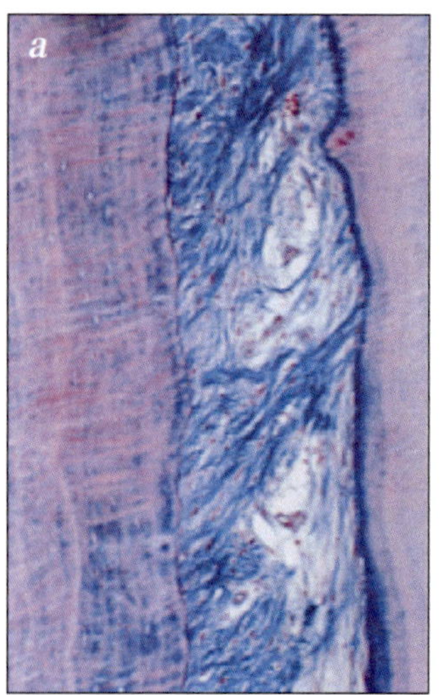

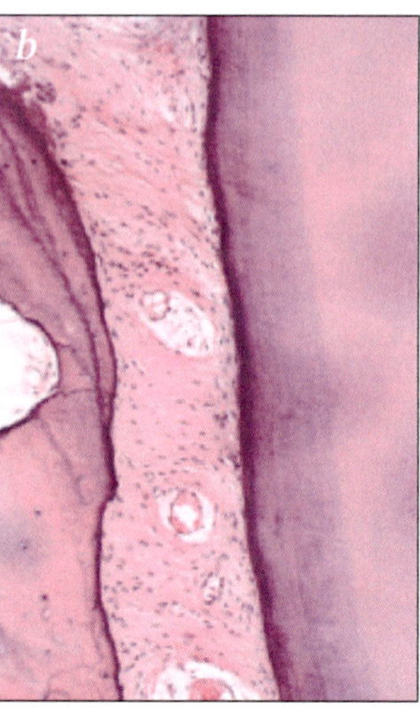

Figure 1-37 Effects of radiation therapy on the periodontal ligament. *(a)* Irradiated periodontal ligament that received 70 Gy of radiation. Note the changes in the arrangement of periodontal ligament fibers (Masson trichrome stain; original magnification ×150). *(b)* Irradiated periodontal ligament that received 50 Gy of radiation. The cellularity, the organization of fibril groups, and vascularity are better than those exhibited by the specimen that received 70 Gy (hematoxylin-eosin stain; original magnification ×150).

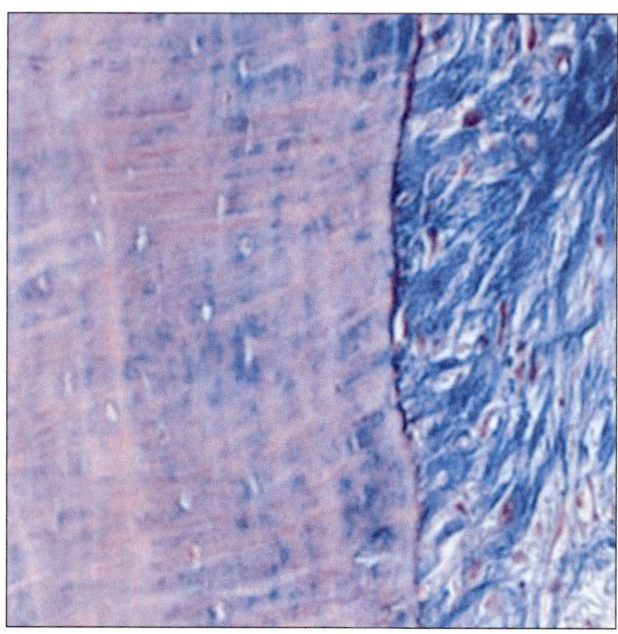

Figure 1-38 Cementum irradiated to 70 Gy. Note the empty lacunae (Masson trichrome stain; original magnification ×175).

pocket depths (Schuurhuis et al., 2011, 2016, 2018). Clinical reports indicate that many ORNs are preceded by periodontal infection associated with teeth within the clinical target volume exposed to tumoricidal doses of radiation (Beumer et al., 1984; Yusof and Bakri, 1993; Schuurhuis et al., 2018). Therefore, when teeth are evaluated for extraction prior to treatment, the periodontal status of the dentition is a most important dental consideration aside from preexisting acute infectious processes (Beumer et al., 1984; Ammajan et al., 2013; Schuurhuis et al., 2011, 2018; Spijkervet et al., 2021).

Cementum demonstrates changes similar to those observed in cortical bone. It becomes almost completely acellular and its capacity for repair and regeneration is severely compromised (Fig 1-38). Therefore, periodontal procedures such as flap surgery in the radiation field should be considered with caution, especially when the mandible is exposed to doses greater than 55 Gy. At these doses and higher, reattachment of the zonal epithelium will be compromised after most aggressive surgical procedures.

Changes to enamel, dentin, and pulp

Studies have shown that the microhardness and crystallinity (characterized by an increasingly disorganized prismatic structure) of both enamel and dentin are affected by cancerocidal doses of radiation therapy (Goncalves et al., 2014; de Siqueira et al., 2014; Lu et al., 2019). Irradiation damage at levels of 60 Gy appears to occur in the organic matrix portion of the enamel in the interprismatic spaces, via the oxidation of water molecules into hydrogen peroxide and hydrogen free radicals that denature the organic components, affecting the mechanical properties and integrity of the enamel. When dentin is exposed to 60 Gy, changes have been noted in the intertubular and peritubular dentin with a degradation of its collagen network. At this dosage level, the surface of dentin becomes amorphous, the dentinal tubules are difficult to visualize, and the collagen fiber networks become fragmented (de Siqueira et al., 2014; Goncalves et al., 2014). As the microhardness of dentin is decreased, the resulting softer dentin becomes less efficient in supporting enamel, predisposing to fractures and cracks in the enamel, especially at the dentino-enamel junction. These phenomena partially explain, in addition to radiation-induced xerostomia, the high rate of cervical caries observed in teeth within the clinical target volume of irradiated patients. The degradation of the organic portion of dentin also appears to degrade the adhesion of composite resins to dentin (Naves et al., 2012; Bernard et al., 2015; Soares et al., 2016).

There appear to be significant changes in the behavior of pulp tissue. Although odontoblasts may not be altered morphologically at the level of light microscopy by high-dose radiation therapy (Faria et al., 2014), their secretory metabolism may be affected (Gowgiel, 1960; Collett and Thonard, 1965; Koppang, 1967). Excessive formation of osteodentin has been observed in the pulp chambers in animal models and in humans (Gowgiel, 1960; Collett and Thonard, 1965; Koppang, 1967) (Fig 1-39). This phenomenon is thought to be secondary to radiation-induced premature differentiation of dental pulp stem cells into odontoblast-like cells, which then synthesize reparative tubular dentin (osteodentin; Havelek et al., 2013). These calcifications can make endodontic therapy problematic.

Human pulp tissue exposed to high-dose fractionated radiation therapy also shows a decrease in vascular elements, accompanied by fibrosis, and atrophy of the dental pulp (Gowgiel, 1960) (Fig 1-40). It follows that there is a progressive decrease in pulp sensitivity after completion of radiation treatments (Kataoka et al., 2012; Garg et al., 2015; Gupta et al., 2018). Clinical experience indicates that pulpal responses to infection, trauma, and various dental procedures appear compromised (Fawzi et al., 1985). Pulpal pain mechanisms appear to be altered, presumably because of the effect of high-dose radiation on the pulp's microvasculature and postradiation neuropathy. Pain is uncommon even in the presence of advanced caries with obvious

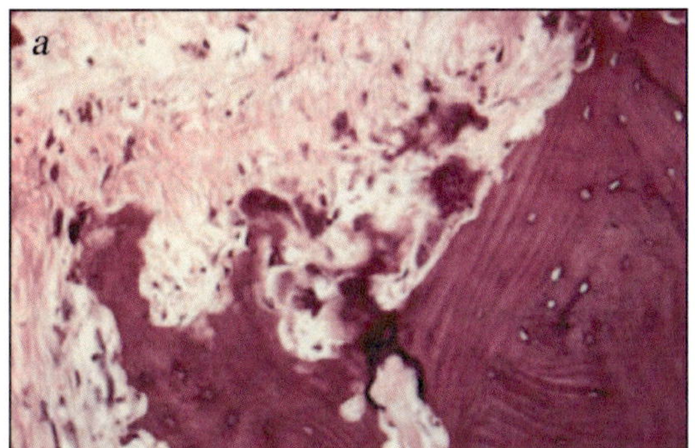
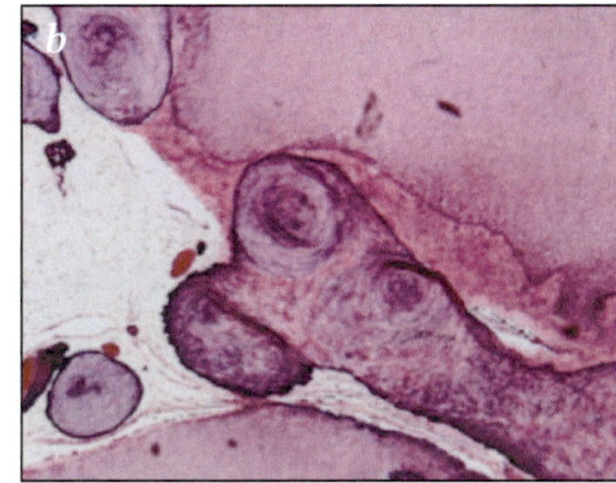

Figure 1-39 Specimens of human dental pulp that were exposed to 60 Gy. *(a)* Osteodentin has formed. *(b)* Pulp stones have formed (hematoxylin-eosin stain; original magnification ×40).

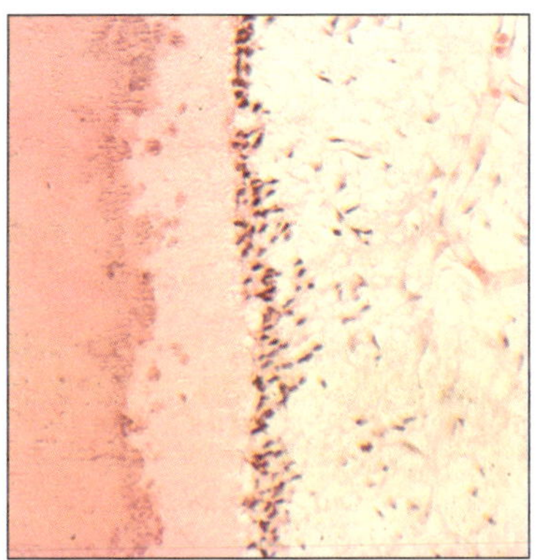

Figure 1-40 Pulp exposed to a radiation dose in excess of 60 Gy. (hematoxylin-eosin stain; original magnification ×150).

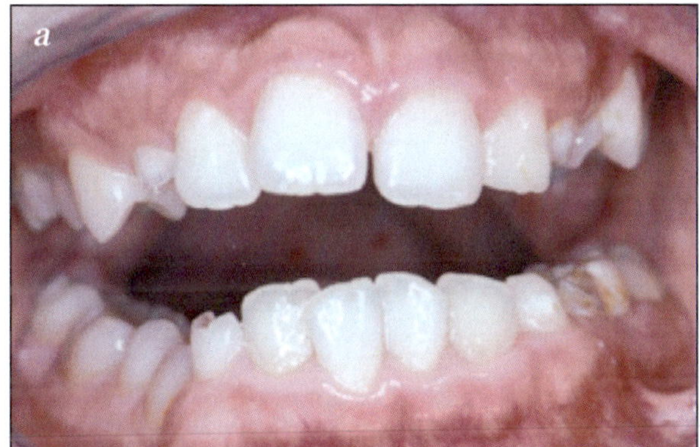

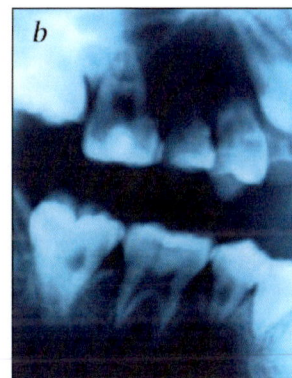

Figure 1-41 Effects of radiation therapy during growth and development. *(a and b)* At the age of three years, the patient received 30 Gy of radiation to the maxilla and mandible. The changes reflect a variety of defects that indicate the stages of development that existed during the course of radiotherapy.

pulpal exposure. In deep carious lesions where the pulp is encroached upon, MTA (mineral trioxide aggregate, a hydrophilic and biocompatible endodontic cement, capable of stimulating healing and osteogenesis) may be ineffective due to the compromised pulpal response and healing capacity.

Root sensitivity following full-course radiotherapy may be severe in the occasional patient. An explanation for this phenomenon has not been defined. The use of remineralizing pastes containing amorphous calcium phosphate or casein phosphopeptide–amorphous calcium phosphate (CPP-ACP) nanocomplexes has been effective. Remineralization of the tooth surface with topical fluoride gel has also been effective in reducing sensitivity.

During growth and development, any levels of radiation therapy significantly increase the risk of developing dental anomalies and the risk increases with dose. Levels of radiation exposure as low as 25 Gy can markedly effect tooth development (Gorlin and Meskin et al., 1963; Pietrokovski and Menczel, 1966; Dahllof et al., 1994; McGinnis et al., 1985). If radiation exposure occurs before significant calcification is complete, the tooth bud may be damaged or destroyed. Exposure at a later stage of development may arrest growth and may result in irregularities in enamel and dentin and shortened roots. The dentitions of those patients receiving moderate levels of radiation with a large clinical target volume will reflect a variety of defects that indicate the stages of development existing during the course of radiotherapy (Fig 1-41). Retarded root development impairs alveolar development and, combined with periodontal disease, often leads to premature tooth loss.

Irradiation of growth centers of the mandible and the maxilla predispose to agenesis of the maxilla and mandible that may require surgical correction at a later date (Denys et al., 1998; Gevorgyan et al., 2007). If the radiation dose is relatively low (less than 55 Gy) prospective bone implant sites remain viable and these patients are candidates for osseointegrated implants if a sufficient volume of bone is available.

Altered oral flora (microbiome) and posttreatment radiation caries and chronic candidiasis

Radiation-induced xerostomia, plus compromised buffering capacity and changes in the inorganic and organic components of the saliva that is produced, leads to significant changes in oral flora that predispose to dental caries. Pronounced population shifts in microbial oral flora have been reported in which cariogenic microorganisms gain at the expense of the noncariogenic microorganisms (Llory et al., 1971; Brown et al., 1975; Keene et al., 1981, 1987; Epstein et al., 1991; Almstahl et al., 2008; Shao et al., 2011; Schuurhuis et al., 2016; Zagury-Orly et al., 2021). Among aerobic organisms, significant increases have been noted in the relative numbers of *mutans streptococcus* and *lactobacillus* species at the expense of more benign species. Among anaerobic organisms, increases have been noted in *actinomyces* populations.

Changes in oral flora (microbiome) are long lasting. The amount of plaque per unit area increases as xerostomia becomes more profound. Total microorganisms per gram of plaque, however, remain constant; changes are noted only in the bacterial composition (Llory

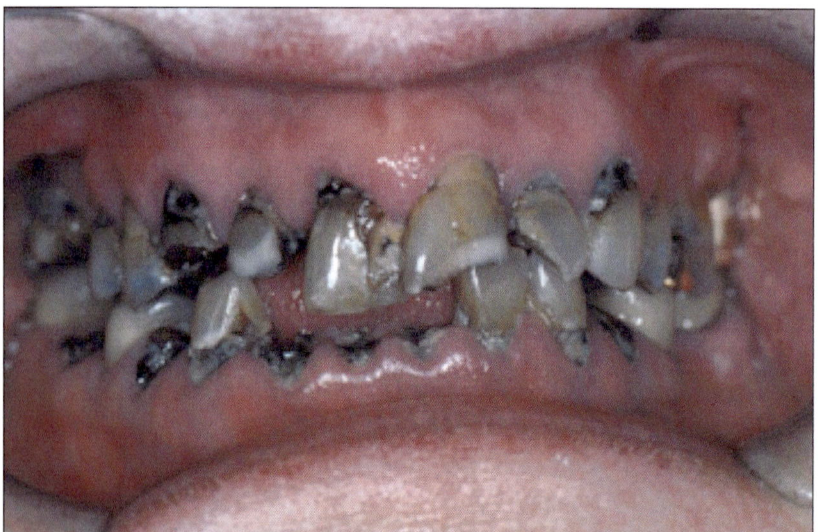

Figure 1-42 Radiation caries in a patient treated for nasopharyngeal carcinoma. The teeth were out of the field of radiation.

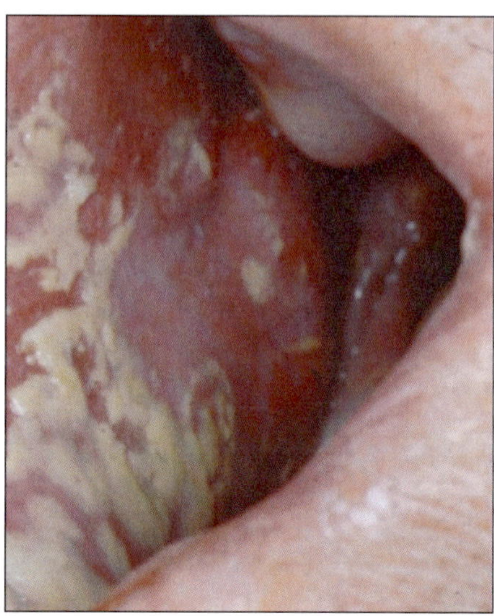

Figure 1-43 Acute candidiasis several years after external beam radiation.

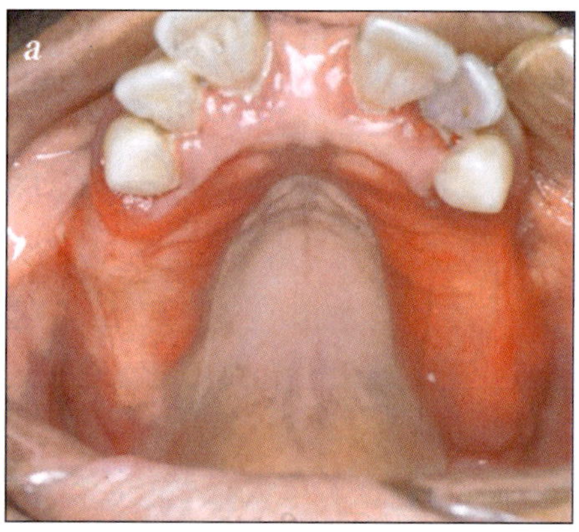

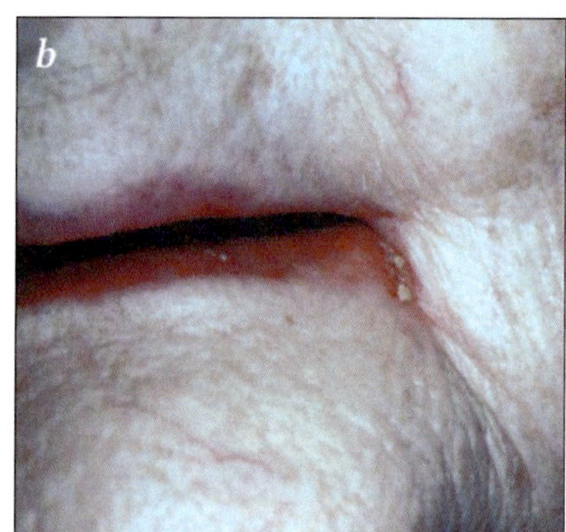

Figure 1-44 Chronic candidiasis in irradiated patients. *(a)* Lesion beneath a removable partial denture. *(b)* Lesion in the corner of the mouth.

et al., 1971; Brown et al., 1975; Keene et al., 1981, 1987; Epstein et al., 1991). In patients in whom a major portion of the oral cavity was in the field but substantial areas of salivary gland tissue were spared, little or no floral changes are noted (Llory et al., 1971; Brown et al., 1975; Keene et al., 1981, 1987; Epstein et al., 1991).

Strong evidence indicates that *mutans streptococci* is the predominant microorganism of dental caries. The striking increase in the *mutans streptococci* component of the streptococcal population in the plaque of patients with radiation-induced xerostomia, 1.6% of the total prior to radiation and 43.8% after radiation, provides additional evidence (Brown et al., 1975). Although *Actinomyces* probably plays a minimal role in caries, its increase in relative numbers cannot be ignored. It may be an important factor in lowering salivary pH. Changes observed in the oral microbiome in patients treated with chemoradiation mimic those treated with radiation alone (Schuurhuis et al., 2016).

These changes combined with the altered crystallinity of enamel and dentin (Goncalves et al., 2014; de Siqueira et al., 2014; Lu et al., 2019) predispose to a dramatic increase in the rate of caries. Cervical areas are most susceptible and patients often present with circumferential lesions (Fig 1-42). Caries progresses rapidly and, in many patients, becomes so extensive that the teeth so involved become nonrestorable. Eventually, such teeth fracture at the gingival margin and at this stage clinical care is directed toward preventing these teeth from triggering ORN (see section below entitled "Postradiation dental care"). It has been suggested that radiation dose is a significant predictor of caries rate and prevalence of apical periodontitis (Hommez et al., 2012).

The increase in fungal populations following completion of radiation therapy predisposes to acute and chronic candidiasis. The acute form presents as erythema and a burning sensation of the oral mucous membranes and is usually accompanied by the presence of discrete colonies of the organism on the oral mucosa (Fig 1-43). The chronic forms present as angular cheilitis and beneath removable prostheses, commonly referred to as denture stomatitis, and are frequently overlooked (Fig 1-44). Topical antifungal medications (creams, lozenges, and mouthwashes of nystatins and azoles) are quite effective at resolving these infections.

Polymicrobial biofilms containing Candida albicans are presumed to be the cause of the deterioration of silicone denture liners intraorally (Lyons et al., 2020). This material has been employed by some clinicians in the fabrication of large obturator prostheses to engage undercuts in patients with large maxillary defects in order to improve the retention of the prosthesis. In irradiated patients, the fungal-infested biofilms adherent to the silicone limit the life expectancy of the material to only a few months. The incorporation of antifungal agents or antiseptics in the soft liners does not significantly reduce *candida* adhesion or colonization (Nikawa et al., 2001).

Regional late sequelae

Other regions within the field of radiation can be affected. Given that the neck is often in the clinical target volume, the carotid arteries often are heavily irradiated. A report by Freymiller et al. (2000), using sequential panoramic radiographs, revealed a significant increase in carotid atheroma formation when radiation patients were compared to matched controls. These lesions narrow the lumen of the carotid, predispose the patient to ischemia in the carotid artery wall, and can form emboli (Zidar et al., 1997). Progressive fibrosis and radiation-induced peripheral neuropathy may also lead to difficulty in swallowing, dysphonia, aspiration pneumonia, and other associated morbidities (Nguyen et al., 2006, 2008, 2009; Eisele et al., 1991; Kang et al., 2000; Sharabi et al., 1994; Delanian et al., 2012; Azzam et al., 2020).

Dental Management of the Irradiated Patient

Criteria for preradiation extractions

Given their demographic profiles, most patients with oral cancer present with significant dental disease prior to therapy. Prophylactic extraction of diseased teeth in the radiation field has long been considered by most knowledgeable clinicians to be a means of reducing the long-term incidence of bone necrosis (Del Regato, 1939; Daland, 1941; Silverman and Chierici, 1965; Hayward et al., 1969; Beumer et al., 1983; Galler et al., 1992; Epstein et al., 1997; Bruins et al., 1999; Vissink et al., 2003; Oh et al., 2004). Recent studies continue to support this approach (Schuurhuis et al., 2011, 2018; Muraki et al., 2019; Spijkervet et al., 2021). However, evidence-based data supporting this position are few, and data may never be available to indicate the risks of ORN in relation to radiation alone or chemoradiation, timing of extractions and the start of radiotherapy or chemoradiation therapy, dosage levels, fractionation schemes, and clinical target volume. Clinicians responsible for preradiation assessments and postradiation dental maintenance must rely on clinical case series data and an in-depth knowledge of the biologic effects of radiation to assist in their management decisions. The authors continue to believe that a moderately aggressive policy of preradiation extraction, particularly for mandibular molars with Class II or III furcation involvement, will minimize the risk of ORN.

The downside of preradiation extractions is that, when the dentist becomes more aggressive about removing mandibular teeth with little or no periodontal bone loss within the gross tumor volume or clinical target volume, the surgical trauma resulting from these extractions probably increases the rate of bone necrosis (Daly and Drane, 1972; Beumer et al., 1983). On the other hand, if the clinician is too conservative regarding the removal of mandibular teeth within the field prior to therapy, the rate of posttherapy bone necrosis increases because of periodontal infections associated with the remaining teeth (Beumer et al., 1984, 1983; Thorn et al., 2000; Schuurhuis et al., 2018). The authors believe that the overall rate of bone necrosis is minimized when the clinician employs a philosophy of preradiation tooth removal somewhere between these extremes.

During recent times, significant changes in radiation delivery methods have evolved and concomitant chemotherapy has been used with increasing frequency, but the key issue determining the risk of ORN continues to be the dose, or the biologic equivalent dose, delivered to the mandibular dentition and investing bone and the volume of the mandibular body exposed to these tumoricidal doses (Tso et al., 2021; DeLuke et al., 2022). In recent years tumor doses have increased, but IMRT, SBRT, and proton therapy have limited the dose to normal tissues adjacent to the gross tumor volume; theoretically, the risk of ORN following irradiation of localized tumors should be reduced. Nevertheless, the risk of ORN in patients treated with IMRT or similar modalities ranges from 4% to 8% (Aarup-Kristensen et al., 2019; Kubota et al., 2021).

A complicating factor is the increased use of concomitant chemoradiation, which further compromises the vitality of the normal tissues within the clinical target volume (Kang et al., 2022). This combination appears to promote increased fibrosis and probably further compromises the vasculature of irradiated tissues. As mentioned previously, a course of concomitant chemotherapy theoretically adds the equivalent of 7 to 10 Gy to tumor effects, which would put most patients at an increased risk of developing ORN. When concomitant chemotherapy was combined with CRT and large volumes of the mandible were within the radiation field, this appeared to be the case. The incidence of ORN dramatically increased, and these ORNs did not respond to conservative forms of therapy as often as did those developing in patients treated solely with CRT. Almost all these patients required radical resection of the affected mandible and reconstruction with free vascularized flaps. Fortunately, the protocol of concomitant chemotherapy combined with CRT was employed for a relatively short period. IMRT has replaced CRT, and theoretically the rate of ORN should be reduced in this patient population. However, assessing the risk remains problematic because well-designed clinical outcome studies are still lacking in this patient group. The limits have been and will continue to be the tolerance of normal adjacent tissues, although radiation oncologists are also likely to continue to test these limits.

Accordingly, all patients scheduled for radiation therapy or chemoradiation therapy for tumors of the head and neck require a dental consultation. The purposes of the consultation are to *(1)* inform the patients of the anticipated tissue changes and reduction in salivary flow rate and that consequently he/she will be more susceptible to dental caries and dental and bony infection after radiation therapy, and that ultimately the response to infection will be compromised; *(2)* examine the dentition and determine which teeth are salvageable and which teeth have to be removed; and *(3)* explain to the patient the importance of dental compliance.

As mentioned above, even with the continued evolution of radiation therapy techniques that localize the highest dose levels to the gross tumor volume, most clinicians continue to believe that selected removal of teeth with a questionable prognosis will reduce the rate of ORN (Schuurhuis et al., 2011, 2018; Spijkervet et al., 2019, 2021). Hence, many questions arise concerning dental evaluations before the initiation of radiation treatment:

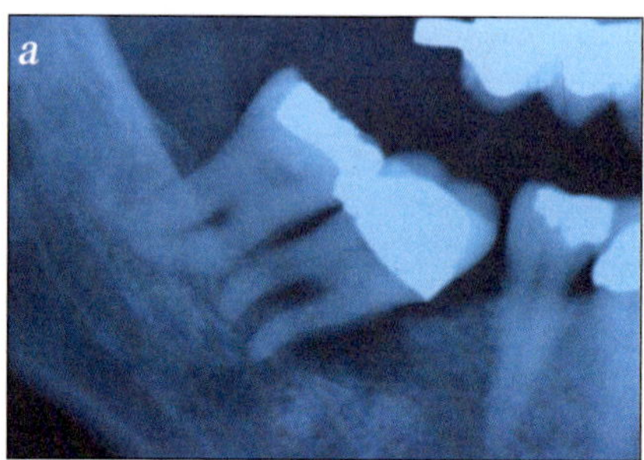

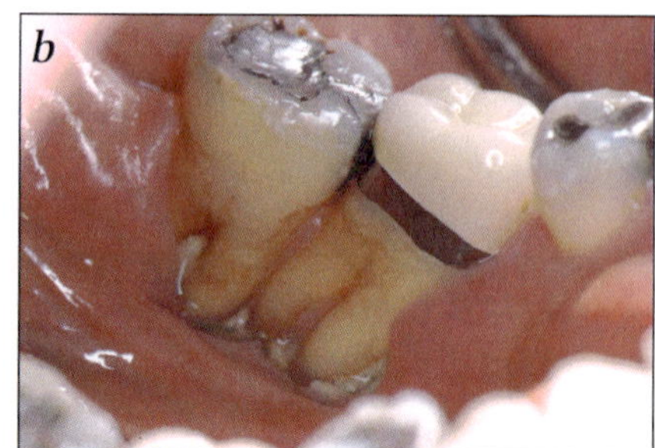

Figure 1-45 ORN precipitated by a periodontal infection. *(a)* Radiograph of the lesion. *(b)* Lingual view.

- Which teeth should be extracted?
- How does patient compliance impact these decisions?
- How should the teeth be extracted?
- How long should the patient wait to begin radiation therapy after tooth extraction?
- How can the remaining dentition be maintained during and after radiation therapy?

A number of factors should be considered before dental extractions are recommended for any particular patient. Before a final decision is made, consultation with the radiation oncologist is mandatory to gain insight into the dose to be delivered to key areas and the volume of tissues within the clinical target volume, particularly when IMRT or brachytherapy is used.

Several issues should be considered when the clinician is making decisions regarding extraction or retention of teeth. For purposes of discussion, they are divided into three categories: *(1)* patient-related factors, *(2)* radiation delivery factors, and *(3)* the impact of concomitant chemotherapy. Unless otherwise indicated, when dose is discussed, it should be assumed the radiation was delivered with conventional fractionation (approximately 2 Gy per fraction).

Patient-related factors

Condition of the residual dentition. The clinician's primary goal should be to place the dentition in optimal condition so that high-risk dental procedures need not be performed in the post-treatment period. All teeth with a questionable prognosis should be extracted before radiation. Teeth with advanced carious lesions in which excavation would lead to pulpal exposure, teeth exhibiting periapical infection, those teeth partially erupted and teeth with significant periodontal disease are most at risk. Mandibular teeth within the clinical target volume should receive the closest scrutiny.

Given the acceleration of attachment loss of teeth exposed to high-dose radiation and the risk that a periodontal infection will precipitate ORN (Fig 1-45), the patient's periodontal status is most important in this assessment. Studies have shown that patients presenting with periodontally affected teeth are predisposed to the development of ORN (Schuurhuis et al., 2011). Dentitions with significant periodontal disease are difficult to maintain, and an aggressive extraction philosophy is recommended in the management of dentitions with periodontal disease. To be specific, we believe that Class II or III furcation involvement of mandibular molar teeth in the radiation field is grounds for preradiation extraction in most patients, particularly if the dose with conventional fractionation to the immediate area is greater than 55 Gy. A recent prospective study reported that failure to remove such teeth prior to radiation therapy appears to increase the risk of ORN (Schuurhuis et al., 2018).

The presence of moderate caries is less important because in most instances it is restorable and in compliant patients can be controlled with appropriate oral hygiene measures and topical fluoride accompanied by the use of calcium phosphate preparations. When there are carious lesions in a region lower than 55 Gy and limited time prior to the start of radiation therapy, one may consider utilizing silver diamine fluoride (SDF) to stabilize caries until time permits to appropriately restore the affected teeth.

Mandible versus maxilla. Almost all ORN occurs in the mandible (Beumer et al., 1972, 1984; Murray et al., 1980a; Epstein et al., 1997; Oh et al., 2004). ORN in the maxilla is rare, and when it does occur it almost always resolves with conservative treatment. Because the maxilla has more favorable vasculature, a conservative approach to preradiation extraction of maxillary teeth is justified. Extraction of maxillary teeth within the gross tumor volume or clinical target volume can be performed after radiation therapy with little risk of a bony infection.

A far different situation exists in the mandible, where exposure of bone and infection after therapy may precipitate ORN and lead to the loss of large mandibular segments. Consequently, a more aggressive management approach is advocated when mandibular teeth are evaluated for extraction prior to therapy. Particular attention should be directed to the mandibular molars when they are exposed to doses in excess of 55 Gy radiation or its equivalent because this area is a common site of ORN (Beumer et al., 1984; Kubota et al., 2021).

Dental compliance of the patient. Dental compliance is a most important consideration when a patient is evaluated for dental extractions prior to therapy. High-dose radiation therapy predisposes the patient to caries and ORN, but with the proper use of the preventive measures developed in the last 40 years, the compliant patient can maintain his or her dentition in excellent health.

However, routine oral hygiene becomes increasingly difficult after treatment as trismus, impaired motor functions, and surgical morbidities compromise oral hygiene procedures. If oral and dental health are to be maintained, the patient must understand the implications of his or her radiation therapy and be disposed to carry out the prescribed procedures (Bichsel et al., 2016). These instructions must be reiterated constantly because patients often forget or fail to grasp the issues after a single presentation. Given the nature of the oral cancer population (e.g., increased smoking habits, socioeconomics), it is not surprising that substantial numbers of patients will be noncompliant; therefore, the less motivated the patient, the more aggressive the dentist should be in the preradiation extraction

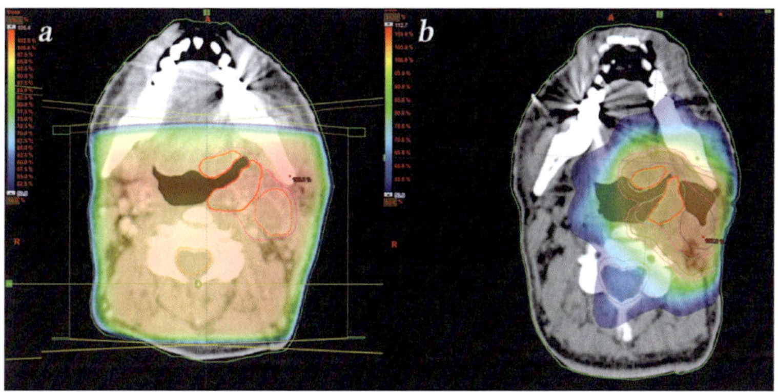

Figure 1-46 Dosimetry diagrams for CRT and IMRT. *(a)* CRT is less focused on the tumor compared to IMRT. *(b)* IMRT focuses radiation to the gross tumor volume so that adjacent tissues receive a lower dose.

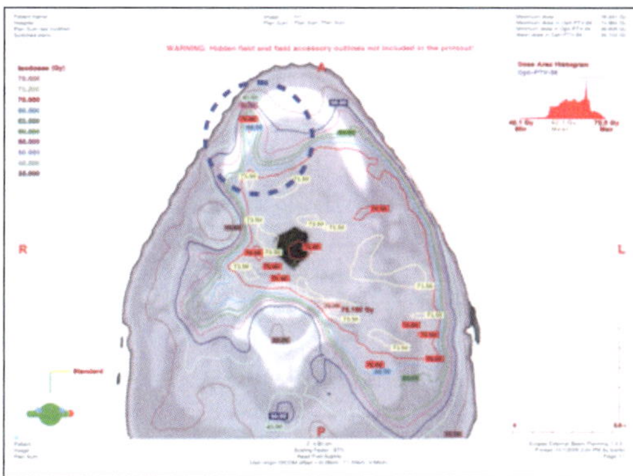

Figure 1-47 Hot spot of radiation on the anterior mandible *(circle)* from IMRT.

of mandibular teeth that will be exposed to a high dose of radiation (greater than 55 Gy). The patient's oral hygiene at the initial examination is probably the most reliable indicator of future performance.

Radiation delivery factors

Urgency of treatment. On rare occasions the status and behavior of the tumor may preclude preradiation dental extractions because delays in radiotherapy secondary to healing could significantly compromise control of the disease. The dentist, radiation therapist, and patient must accept the attendant risk of complications and must attempt to maintain oral health at an optimum level. Control of the tumor obviously is the most important consideration.

Mode of therapy

Intensity-modulated radiation therapy. Sophisticated methods of radiation delivery that focus the highest doses to the local tissues in and around the tumor have evolved (Fig 1-46). Treatment plans are developed on the basis of CT and MRI data. IMRT is advantageous because the volume of tissue irradiated to high dose is reduced considerably compared to that irradiated in CRT. In IMRT, the highest doses are directed to tissues within the gross tumor volume (usually about 70 Gy), and intermediate doses are directed to areas where there is a high risk of microscopic disease (usually a clinical target volume of 50 to 60 Gy). Because smaller volumes of the mandibular body receive a high dose, the incidence of ORN theoretically should be reduced (Bourhis et al., 2006; Ben-David et al., 2007). However, as mentioned above ORN still occurs in significant numbers following IMRT (Aarup-Kristensen et al., 2019; Kubota et al., 2021).

The risk of bone necrosis is highly dependent on the dose and volume of the body of the mandible exposed (Beumer et al., 1984; Glanzmann and Gratz, 1995; Kubota et al., 2021); therefore, the majority of ORNs will most likely occur in patients treated with tongue or floor of the mouth tumors. With IMRT, the gross tumor volume is important to consider when the dentition is evaluated prior to therapy. For instance, in lesions situated in the nasopharynx and soft palate or in the case of T1 lesions of the tonsil, the body of the mandible is rarely within the gross tumor volume. Small areas of the mandibular body may receive a tumoricidal dose, but this volume usually is very small (Fig 1-47). The risk of postradiation caries will be high in these patients because large portions of the salivary gland parenchyma will be exposed to doses in excess of 40 Gy; however, because little of the body of the mandible is within the gross tumor volume the incidence of bone necrosis is expected to be low. We advocate a conservative philosophy regarding extraction of teeth in such patients. In this group of patients, postradiation extractions in both the mandible and the maxilla may be performed with little risk of ORN.

Stereotactic body radiation therapy (SBRT). Similar to IMRT the highest doses are directed to tissues within the gross tumor volume and intermediate doses are directed to areas where there is a high risk of microscopic disease (usually a clinical target volume). Because smaller volumes of the mandibular body receive a high dose, the incidence of ORN theoretically should be reduced. However, one may expect tissue breakdown secondary to the boosted site, which may exceed the maximum level of tissue tolerance locally.

As mentioned previously, SBRT is often used in patients who have previously been irradiated and have developed recurrences. The retreatment will likely bring the entire site to the maximum tolerable dose. Extraction of teeth needs to be considered carefully, since prior irradiation may bring the local regional site to a level where a risk of ORN and delayed healing may already be a factor. In this patient population, extraction of teeth after radiation therapy will likely involve high risk of ORN because the dosage delivered by the multiple therapies will likely exceed 55 Gy and will also involve high volume of the mandible.

Brachytherapy. Brachytherapy has been used in combination with external beam radiation for accessible localized tumors of the tongue, tonsil, or floor of the mouth. Following a course of external beam radiation, which is generally limited to 50 to 55 Gy, radioactive sources are implanted in the gross tumor volume, delivering another 25 to 30 Gy. The tissues associated with and adjacent to the gross tumor volume receive doses up to 85 Gy. Tissue breakdown and ORN are thought to be secondary to the combined dosage from the implant and the external beam exceeding the maximum level of tissue tolerance locally, as opposed to dental disease.

In these patients, extraction of teeth after radiation therapy distant from the clinical target volume of the brachytherapy does not involve high risk unless the teeth and bone are adjacent to the site of the implant, because the dosage delivered by the external beam portion of therapy rarely exceeds 55 Gy. ORN, however, is common when the implant is located in close proximity to the lingual surface

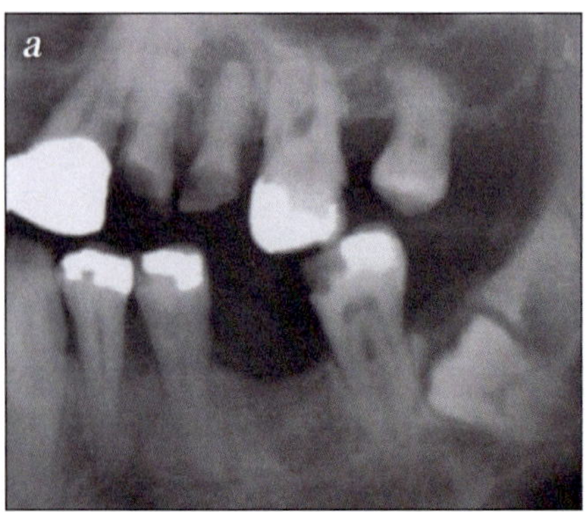
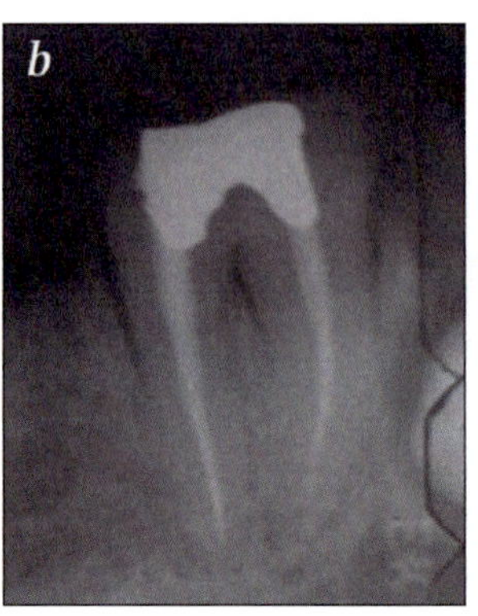
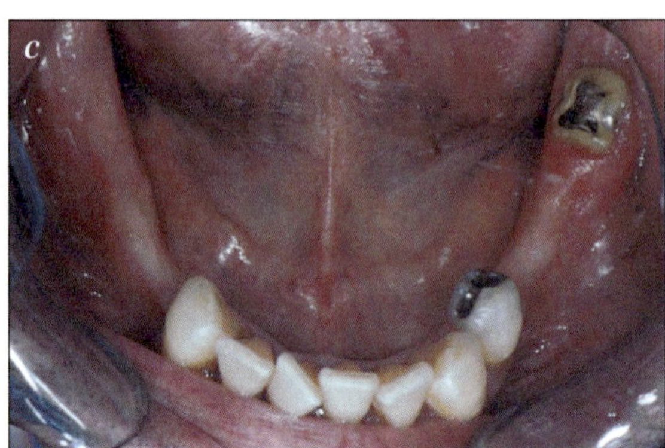

Figure 1-48 Endodontic therapy to avoid tooth extraction. *(a)* A diseased second molar is next to an impacted third molar, prior to radiation therapy. *(b)* Root canal therapy has been performed on the second molar, thereby avoiding extraction of the third molar. *(c)* The crown has been amputated and recontoured to facilitate oral hygiene.

of the mandible. For example, if a patient is to receive combined therapy (external beam [50 Gy] plus an interstitial implant [25 to 30 Gy]) for a carcinoma in the right side of the floor of the mouth, the lingual surface of the right side of the mandible is likely to receive more than 75 to 80 Gy. The presence of teeth in this region predisposes the patient to a high rate of bone necrosis following radiation therapy, and these teeth should probably be extracted. The opposite side of the mandible will generally receive less than 55 Gy from the external beam therapy plus a small amount from the interstitial implant. Because the dose to the mandible is less than 60 Gy on the left side, the risk of bone necrosis is low and teeth in this area need not be extracted unless they demonstrate advanced periodontal bone loss or periapical pathology. Postradiation extractions of mandibular teeth exposed to this dosage level can be carried out with a minimal degree of risk (Beumer et al., 1983).

Dose, volume of mandibular body within the clinical target volume, and fractionation schedules. The higher the dose, the higher the incidence of postradiation sequelae (Beumer et al., 1984; Morrish et al., 1981; Thorn et al., 2000). Almost all ORN occurs at doses equivalent to 65 Gy (with conventional fractionation) and greater. When ORN does occur in sites subjected to doses below this level, most heal with conservative measures without loss of mandibular continuity.

The type of tumor will dictate the radiation levels used in treatment. Patients treated for Hodgkin's disease receive dosage levels that reach 40 to 45 Gy, whereas patients with squamous cell carcinoma of the oral cavity receive 65 to 85 Gy. Although ORN has been reported at these lower radiation levels, occurrence is rare and heals without surgical assistance. In addition, lymphomas and Hodgkin disease occur in a younger population of patients whose capacity for repair of radiation damage is greater. Clinical experience indicates that postradiation extractions involve less risk in this particular patient population.

The volume of bone and soft tissue included in the gross tumor volume is also an important indicator of risk. For tumors treated to levels greater than 65 Gy, when large volumes of mandible are exposed to doses of this level or greater, a more aggressive approach to extracting teeth prior to therapy is indicated. Conversely, for tissues treated more conservatively, a less aggressive approach is indicated.

SBR, accelerated, and hyperfractionation treatment methods employ different total dose, time, and dose per fraction. For these patients, it is wise to consult the radiation oncologist to determine the cumulative radiation effect equivalent to that delivered with conventional time-dose and fractionation schedules. The cumulative radiation effect is calculated with formulas that consider the dose per fraction, time frame over which the radiation is delivered, and total dose (Fowler and Stern, 1963; Ellis, 1968). These indices represent an attempt to account for the variables of radiation delivery to indicate more accurately the true biologic response.

Prognosis for tumor control. Tumor prognosis can be of predominant importance in patients in whom palliation and relief of symptoms are the primary goals of the radiation therapist. Teeth that ordinarily would have been extracted in a patient with a more favorable prognosis are not extracted in terminally ill patients. If the clinician thinks that the remaining teeth will cause the patient unnecessary pain and discomfort during his or her remaining days, they probably should be extracted. However, if extractions could compromise the functional or emotional well-being of the patient, they probably should be deferred. Utilization of SDF in patients presenting with caries should also be considered in this patient population.

Concomitant chemotherapy

Concomitant chemoradiation induces an unknown factor of risk with regard to the dentulous patient. As stated previously, it has been suggested that concomitant chemoradiation therapy escalates the biologically equivalent dose to the tumor by 7 to 10 Gy (Kasibhatla, 2007; Fowler, 2008). Presently, in these patients, the authors treat teeth in the clinical target volume in the same manner as those within the gross tumor volume, even though the dose is generally about 10 Gy lower; namely, we consider extraction of mandibular molars with Class II or III furcation involvement as well as those with advanced periodontal disease or periapical infection.

Extraction of third molars

Extraction of bony and tissue-impacted mandibular third molars prior to radiation is not recommended unless a direct communication with the oral cavity can be demonstrated (Rothwell, 1987; Mealey et al., 1994; Spijkervet et al., 2021). Such extractions often

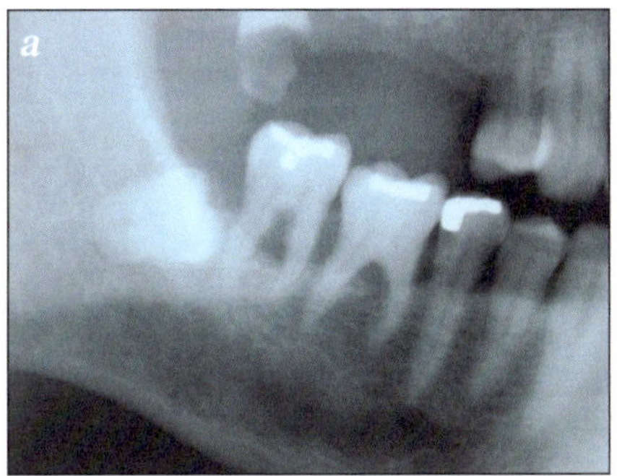

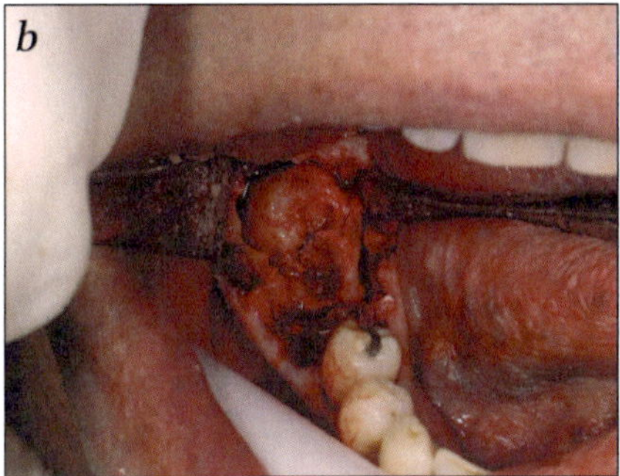

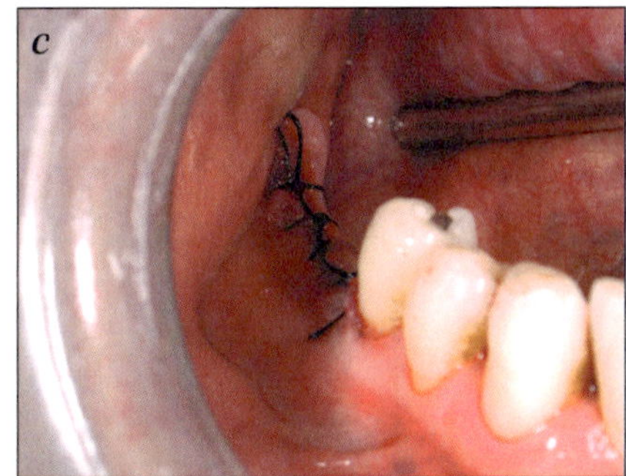

Figure 1-49 Tooth extraction prior to radiation therapy. *(a)* The third molar is partially impacted and the first and second molars present with advanced periodontal bone loss. *(b)* All three teeth have been extracted. *(c)* Primary closure has been obtained. Extra healing time will be allowed prior to radiation therapy.

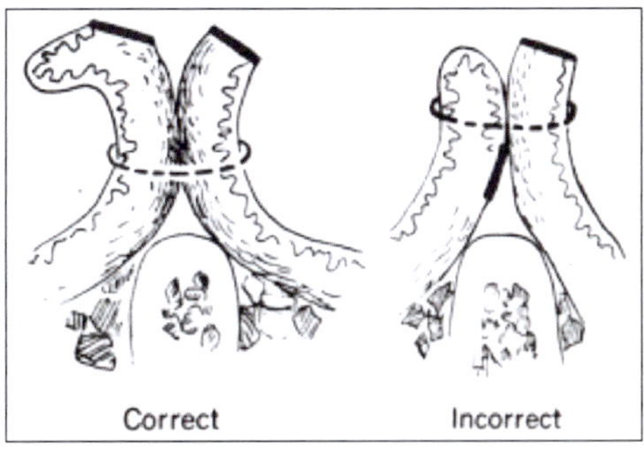

Figure 1-50 Everting the edges will promote more rapid epithelization following extraction and radical alveolectomy (reprinted from Moy et al., 2016, with permission).

necessitate removal of considerable bone, creating large bony defects that require prolonged periods for healing and delaying the onset of radiation therapy. A clinical report by Oh et al. (2004) indicated that 37 of 55 patients undergoing extraction of impacted third molars required 3 weeks or more for healing and 14 required 30 days or more of healing prior to initiation of radiation treatments. Most radiation oncologists are unwilling to wait for such long periods prior to therapy. When possible, the authors prefer to avoid extraction of such teeth. In the patient presented in Fig 1-48, the second molar presented with caries and furcation involvement. Exposure of the third molar was avoided by performing endodontic therapy on the second molar. The doming of the second molar also improved access to the furcation area improving hygiene access.

Patients with partially erupted mandibular third molars, however, represent a particularly difficult and perplexing problem. Trauma resulting from extraction may require prolonged healing periods. However, if these teeth are retained, there is significant risk of an episode of pericoronitis, which could lead to ORN. Most clinicians therefore recommend removal of partially erupted teeth or third molars that directly communicate with the oral cavity (Hayward et al., 1969; Oh et al., 2004; Spijkervet et al., 2021) (Fig 1-49).

Historically the majority of these patients are younger than 40 years of age and present with Hodgkin's disease or other types of lymphoma. The dosage and limited volume of the mandibular body within the gross tumor volume results in less compromise of the vasculature of the mandible. Clinical experience indicates that the incidence of ORN in patients receiving less than 50 Gy has been negligible, even in patients requiring extraction of teeth after radiation. Operculectomy is useful in selected cases presenting with pericoronitis. More recently, with human papillomavirus (HPV) positive oropharyngeal cancers being the fastest-growing subset of HNC in the United States, many of these younger patients are receiving high doses of radiotherapy to the posterior mandible. In these cases, preradiation removal of these partially impacted third molars is indicated in order to minimize the risk of ORN.

Surgical procedures

When extractions are performed in the preradiation period, clinical experience and the literature indicate that the following factors should be observed for best results.

When mandibular teeth are extracted, radical alveolectomies should be performed, the edges of the tissue flaps everted (Fig 1-50), and primary closure obtained. Closing the wound in this fashion will promote more rapid epithelialization. Radical alveolectomies are preferred for two reasons: *(1)* to enable primary closure and *(2)* to smooth the sharp edges of bone resulting from extraction. Because the remodeling apparatus is rendered nonfunctional by tumoricidal doses of radiation, alveolectomies are necessary so as to prepare the edentulous areas for complete or partial denture coverage. When maxillary teeth are extracted, primary closure is not required, and the need for recontouring the alveolus ridge is dependent on prosthodontic considerations.

Meticulous care should be exercised in the handling of the tissue flaps. Good surgical technique will pay dividends in reducing the incidence of complications. The periosteum will be the predominant source of vascularity in the surgical field, and all efforts should be made to avoid mishandling it during the surgical procedure. Perforation of the lingual flap in the mandible will almost always result in a bone exposure that may delay radiotherapy and increase the risk of postradiation ORN.

Mandibular teeth should be removed in segments in the field of radiation. It is far easier to perform an appropriate alveolectomy and attain adequate closure when teeth are extracted in segments. When individual teeth are extracted, closure is difficult to obtain without excessive tension on tissue flaps. Some clinicians advocate administration of antibiotics during the healing period. It is difficult to assess the benefits that prophylactic antibiotics provide in these situations. They probably are effective when extractions result in excessive trauma. Most clinicians continue to believe that 10 to 14 days are adequate for healing time before radiation therapy is begun (Beech et al., 2014; Spijkervet et al., 2021). This period may be extended or shortened depending on the progress made by the patient, accompanying medical comorbidities, the ease or difficulty of the surgery, the proposed dosage, the amount of mandible included within the clinical target volume, and the aggressiveness of the tumor.

When preradiation extractions are indicated, it is important to consider the restorative options available to the patient once medically stable postradiation. If complete dentures or removable dental prostheses are being considered, the clinician must also contemplate removing tori, bony exostoses, or enlarged maxillary tuberosities, as preprosthetic surgical intervention may be indicated at the time of preradiation extractions. If this is overlooked, preprosthetic surgery may no longer be possible after radiotherapy due to the risk of ORN, and as a result, the patient may not be a candidate for removable prostheses.

Postradiation dental care

Extraction of teeth

The risk of bone necrosis secondary to dental extractions in the postradiation period has been a topic of debate for many years. In recent years, with the use of topical fluoride, remineralizing preparations, regular dental care, and close follow-up, more patients have been allowed to retain teeth within the gross tumor volume and/or clinical target volume. However, it is difficult to predict the future dental compliance of a patient based on the initial dental examination and consultation prior to radiation therapy. Consequently, some patients may develop serious dental disease within the gross tumor volume or the clinical target volume after the completion of therapy. Some clinicians have proposed that diseased teeth within the gross tumor volume or the clinical target volume can be removed with little or no risk of bone necrosis (Solomon et al., 1968; Carl et al., 1973; Maxymiw et al., 1991), while others suggest that postradiation extraction of such teeth creates a significant risk (Daly and Drane, 1972; Murray et al., 1980a, 1980b; Beumer et al., 1983; Morrish et al., 1981; Marx et al., 1985; Thorn et al., 2000; Reuther et al., 2003). As is often the case, the truth lies somewhere between these two positions. The most important factors to consider are dose and the volume of the mandible within the gross tumor volume and the clinical target volume because the doses delivered are highest in this region. Continued tobacco use should also be considered when determining whether the patient is a candidate for postradiation extractions. As was the case with preradiation extractions, clinicians responsible for determining whether postradiation extractions are appropriate must rely on clinical case series data and an understanding of the biologic effects of radiation to assist in their treatment decisions. Interpretation of these case studies is difficult because of imprecise definitions of bone necrosis and poor documentation of radiation treatment methods and doses to extraction sites.

Based on the literature and clinical experience, we believe the best indicator of potential risk is the radiation dose administered to the bone supporting the dentition that is being considered for removal. Individual patient responses and comorbidities must also be taken into consideration. For the purpose of this discussion, dose levels refer to those achieved when 2 Gy fractions are administered five days per week. At UCLA, most patients who have completed radiation therapy fall into one of these treatment categories: *(1) high dose* (dose to the potential extraction sites greater than 65 Gy); *(2) intermediate dose* (dose to the potential extraction sites between 55 and 65 Gy); and *(3) low dose* (dose to the potential extraction sites of 55 Gy or less).

In the mandible, a dose in excess of 65 Gy to the potential extraction sites implies a significant risk of bone necrosis, probably in the range of 30–40%, especially when multiple teeth in a mandibular quadrant are considered for removal. For most such patients, root canal therapy for the affected teeth is the treatment of choice because it minimizes the risk of bone exposure. Root canal therapy allows the clinician to safely amputate the crowns of the teeth just above the epithelial attachment, reducing periodontal probing depths and exposing furcation areas for oral hygiene procedures. Most importantly, mucosal integrity is maintained. Any perforation of the mucosa, whether from trauma or a surgical procedure, predisposes the high-dose sites to great risk of bone necrosis. When endodontics is not an option and extractions of mandibular teeth are absolutely necessary, a planned combined course of HBO therapy (20 dives preextraction followed by 10 dives postextraction; Marx et al., 1985) is recommended. Another option is the PENTO(CLO) protocol developed by Delanian et al. (2005) and Lyons and Ghazali (2008; Patel et al., 2016a; Samani et al., 2021; see section entitled "PENTO(CLO) protocol").

In patients who receive low-dose therapy (less than 55 Gy), there appears to be little risk of bone necrosis secondary to postradiation extractions, even in the mandible. However, teeth should be removed atraumatically and with minimal reflection of the periosteum, from which most of the blood supply to the underlying bone is derived. Based on data from UCLA (Beumer et al., 1983) and Canada (Maxymiw et al., 1991), significantly less morbidity appears to be associated with extraction of a single mandibular tooth in the radiation field than with extraction of multiple teeth. The periosteum and overlying attached mucosa may suffer less damage and thus the limited available vasculature is better maintained during single-tooth extraction than during multiple-tooth extraction.

In the intermediate-dose category (55 to 65 Gy), individual patient factors become important. These factors include chemoradiation therapy; the amount of the body of the mandible in the clinical target volume; time elapsed since radiotherapy; a history of a radical neck dissection on the side of the proposed extraction; clinical signs of radiation-induced mucosal atrophy, such as scarring and telangiectasia; an altered radiographic appearance of the mandible; signs of acute infection; patient age; medical comorbidities; continued use of tobacco; and so forth. In these instances, endodontic therapy should be the first option considered. However, if root canal therapy is not applicable and extractions are unavoidable, the question becomes whether to use HBO or the PENTO(CLO) protocol as an adjunct. Any one of the aforementioned factors may increase the risk of bone necrosis in association with postradiation extractions and so when in doubt, it is wise to employ one or another of the adjunctive therapies suggested above.

There seems to be little risk of prolonged bone exposure following extraction of maxillary teeth in the field after radiation therapy because the maxilla has a more diverse blood supply. Even when prolonged exposure of bone occurs, rarely does significant morbidity ensue. Similar to preradiation extraction of maxillary teeth, postradiation extractions and bony recontouring of extraction sites in the maxilla should be directed toward prosthodontic considerations rather than the need for primary closure and rapid epithelialization of the wound.

Dental maintenance

The objective of dental maintenance is to bring the patient's remaining dentition to optimal levels prior to radiation therapy to minimize the need for invasive dental treatment during and following therapy. The risk of radiation caries and ORN is lifelong and increases with time. Regular recalls should extend indefinitely. In recent years, strict oral hygiene procedures in combination with regular application of topical fluoride and remineralization pastes have been quite effective in maintaining the health of the dentitions of irradiated patients if they are compliant. Remineralizing chewing gums containing CPP-ACP nanocomplexes may also be of benefit (Manton et al., 2008).

Prior to therapy, the patient is given oral hygiene instruction, and a thorough and aggressive oral prophylaxis is performed. The patient is reexamined at weekly intervals during radiation therapy and oral hygiene instruction is reinforced during these appointments. The use of disclosing tablets or solutions is helpful for both the dentist and the patient to monitor the effectiveness of oral hygiene.

After therapy is completed, the patient is placed on a regular recall schedule that usually requires visits every three months. The dentist must insist that the patient adhere strictly to oral hygiene procedures and follow the recommended preventive measures.

Topical fluorides

Since topical fluorides have been used in patients with radiation-induced xerostomia, a dramatic decrease in the incidence of radiation caries has been noted (Dreizen et al., 1976; Horiot et al., 1983; Jansma et al., 1989). Upon demineralization of tooth structure by the organic acids produced by oral bacteria, fluoride ions in the presence of calcium and phosphate ions unite to form fluorapatite (ten Cate, 1999). Most investigators now believe this is the primary mechanism of action by which fluoride ions prevent demineralization.

In existing caries lesions, the presence of fluoride is highly effective in accelerating surface remineralization, and this phenomenon is clinically well demonstrated in the effectiveness of caries arrest in patients with extensive radiation caries. Although caries arrest in vitro appears most effective in early enamel caries, clinical reports imply that remineralization does occur even in patients with advanced radiation caries (Matsuo, 2000). Recent reports indicate that remineralization of subsurface lesions may be enhanced with the addition of CPP-ACP (Reynolds et al., 2008). The role of topical applications of SDF in this population appears beneficial and continues to evolve (Manuschai et al., 2021; de Souza et al., 2021).

Fluoride uptake following topical application is primarily a surface phenomenon and is confined to the outer 30 to 50 μm of enamel. Recent studies suggest that with topical applications of SDF, the uptake of fluoride may be much deeper than the outer 30 to 50 μm (Manuschai et al., 2021).

Uptake and effectiveness are affected by a number of factors of which the patient and clinician must be cognizant. First, penetration into enamel is compromised in the presence of plaque or salivary residue on the tooth surface; consequently, application is most effective following thorough and effective oral hygiene procedures. Poor oral hygiene and the presence of debris prior to application dramatically impair penetration and therefore caries prevention (Jansma et al., 1989).

The acidulated phosphate fluoride solutions have gained some popularity because increased acidity facilitates fluoride uptake. However, in some patients, the low pH of these solutions results in significant mucosal discomfort that presents as burning pain with occasional erythema and ulceration. In addition, acidulated fluoride solutions will etch glazed porcelain, and therefore their use should be avoided in patients with this type of restoration (Copps et al., 1984). The form of topical fluoride used may impact patient tolerance and acceptance. As a result, most clinicians recommend the use of neutral preparations to improve compliance (Vissink et al., 2003).

Although fluoride diffuses into enamel when applied topically, it fails to rapidly form compounds that are stable in the oral environment, and much of it is lost within 24 hours (Gron, 1977). Therefore, to ensure maximum benefits, topical applications should be instituted on a daily basis. Increased application times and avoidance of rinsing the oral cavity for an extended period after application (30 to 60 minutes) likewise enhance fluoride uptake.

The application of SDF in this population is relatively new, and few studies have been reported. In extrapolating the studies, it can be surmised that should radiation caries be present, it may be beneficial to arrest the decay with SDF. It will stain the carious lesions black, but complaints in this population have been rare (Oliveira et al., 2018; McReynolds et al., 2018). Repeated applications appear to be needed. Studies using SDF at various intervals have been reported and range from three months to yearly applications (Manuschai et al., 2021; de Souza et al., 2021).

Numerous methods of fluoride application have been proposed, including highly concentrated fluoride toothpaste, gels carried to position by custom applicators, and mouth rinses (Dreizen et al., 1976; Horiot et al., 1983; Meyerowitz et al., 1991; Epstein et al., 1995). Compliance and the frequency of application are probably more important than the manner in which the fluoride is applied, but use of a gel in combination with custom-made carriers is popular among clinicians (Fig 1-51). The gel is confined to the dentition by these custom-made carriers and is held in position for five minutes once a day. As mentioned above, these devices are also an effective means of preventing the effects of backscatter during radiation therapy (see section entitled "Stents to displace the tongue and other tissues during treatment").

Fluoride treatments are continued for the lifetime of the patient but may be reduced if there is evidence of improved salivary function and continued good oral hygiene. This is especially true for those with low-dose radiation to the major salivary glands and otherwise healthy younger individuals where the salivary glands have increased capacity to recuperate from radiation therapy.

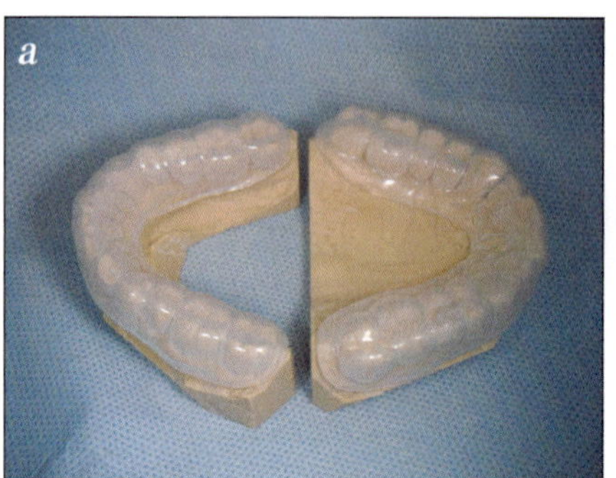

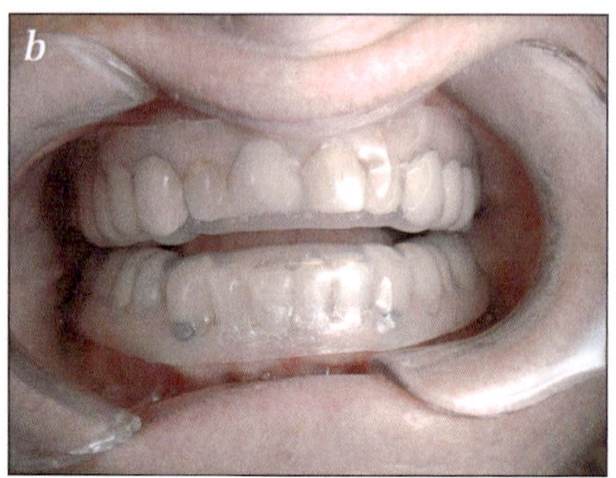

Figure 1-51 *(a and b)* Fluoride carriers. This method of topical fluoride application is favored by many clinicians and has been found to be clinically effective.

Calcium phosphate remineralizing preparations

Remineralizing preparations of calcium phosphate appear to be effective in irradiated patients if enamel demineralization is detected sufficiently early (Johansen et al., 1978; Papas et al., 2008; Deng et al., 2015; Sim et al., 2019). In irradiated patients with moderate to severe xerostomia, effective remineralization of early caries with topical fluoride applications may be limited by the lack of calcium and phosphate ions. Moreover, remineralization with topical fluorides is primarily a surface phenomenon, whereas calcium phosphate preparations can remineralize subsurface lesions (Reynolds et al., 1995). To form fluorapatite, 2 fluoride ions, 10 calcium ions, and 6 phosphate ions are required, but in patients with severe xerostomia levels of calcium and phosphate ions are insufficient. Several systems are available: one is based on unstabilized ACP (Arm and Hammer Enamel Care, Church & Dwight Co., Inc.), one on a casein phosphopeptide–stabilized ACP (Recaldent, GC America Inc.), and a third, a calcium phosphate powder designed to be dissolved in water and used as a mouthwash (SalivaMAX, Forward Science).

The CPPs (casein phosphopeptide) stabilize high concentrations of calcium and phosphate ions and fluoride ions at the surface of the tooth by adhering to plaque and the pellicle. The calcium, phosphate, and fluoride ions are stabilized by the CPP, preventing the formation of calculus. However, these ions diffuse down concentration gradients into subsurface caries lesions, promoting remineralization (Reynolds et al., 2008).

These CPP-ACP nanocomplexes have shown to be effective when incorporated within mouth rinses, chewing gum, and toothpaste and appear to work synergistically with fluoride (Reynolds et al., 1995, 2003; Cai et al., 2007; Sim et al., 2019). A dentifrice containing 2% CPP-ACP plus 1,100 ppm of fluoride was particularly effective at remineralizing subsurface caries (Reynolds et al., 2008; Sim et al., 2019). The study also showed that fluoride alone appears to promote remineralization of the surface, whereas CPP-ACP with fluoride promotes remineralization throughout the body of the lesion. Sugarless chewing gum containing CPP-ACP complexes has also been shown to be effective at remineralizing subsurface enamel lesions (Manton et al., 2008).

Patients afflicted with head and neck cancer tend to be noncompliant. A report by Epstein et al. (1995) showed that only 43% of patients with radiation-induced xerostomia used their fluoride daily as directed. However, of the patients examined regularly (every 3 to six months), 68% used their fluoride daily as directed. There was no correlation between toothbrushing and flossing and daily fluoride use. The fluoride gel was delivered with custom-made carriers, and the authors suggested that the inconvenience associated with the use of carriers may have a negative effect on compliance. A similar finding in an unpublished report at UCLA revealed only 33% of the patients continue to use the fluoride as directed. These reports clearly indicate the need for close follow-up and constant reinforcement if dental health is to be maintained in the irradiated patient.

Summary of preventive measures

Based on the literature and our own experience, we recommend that patients begin the use of daily topical fluoride applications immediately. This should be accompanied by the use of a remineralization paste and, if available, a remineralizing chewing gum. We suggest that the daily fluoride applications be performed one hour or so before bedtime. A remineralizing cream should be applied three times daily (Sim et al., 2019). Fluoride toothpastes should be employed for normal toothbrushing. Remineralizing chewing gum should be used during daytime hours. For optimal effect, the chewing gum is used four times a day and chewing is sustained for 20 minutes each time (Manton et al., 2008). Patients should be reexamined every three months, and hygiene instruction must be reinforced at each follow-up visit. Almost all patients who are reasonably compliant should be able to maintain a healthy dentition.

Follow-up and restorative care

The importance of close follow-up cannot be overemphasized. If preventive measures and stringent oral hygiene measures are not maintained, caries can destroy the entire dentition within six months. The changes in microflora persist and the risk of an aggressive caries attack remains indefinitely. Patients tend to forget the implications of their radiation treatments and constantly need to be reminded of the necessity for proper oral hygiene procedures and preventive measures.

Restorative dental care is provided as necessary. In the early posttreatment period, amalgam and composite resin restorations are favored. Complete-coverage gold restorations are inappropriate unless the patient has demonstrated that he or she can maintain oral hygiene at an acceptable level and properly use fluoride and remineralizing creams on a consistent basis.

When follow-up and oral hygiene are compromised, the patient inevitably will develop rampant dental caries. Most lesions occur in the gingival third of the teeth and in areas with extensive abrasion in which dentin is exposed, such as the incisal or occlusal surfaces. Cervical lesions may involve the entire circumference of the teeth, eventually leading to amputation of the crown. Incisal lesions can progress rapidly and soon involve the entire crown and result in a brownish-black discoloration. The histopathology of these lesions appears to be identical to that of caries in non-irradiated patients (Frank et al., 1965). Caries lesions in radiated patients, as in normal patients, exhibit high concentrations of *mutans streptococcus*. A past history of caries immunity is of little significance. All patients with radiation-induced xerostomia are susceptible to caries.

When caries is detected, the dentist should attempt to remove all caries and restore the affected teeth with provisional restorations using a remineralizing restorative material (such as IRM, Dentsply Caulk). If caries is extensive, one can apply SDF to stabilize the disease. Reapplication of SDF is required every three to four months. The patient should continue their topical fluoride applications in combination with the use of remineralizing creams and chewing gum. If the lesion is limited, it may not require placement of a provisional restoration.

Once caries has been arrested, the provisional restorative material is replaced with amalgam, composite resin, or glass ionomer. Amalgam is preferred because these restorations can be extended if recurrent caries develops. Amalgam restorations are also less sensitive to moisture contamination, and polished amalgam restorations promote better tissue responses.

When aesthetics is of concern, glass ionomer and composite resin are the materials of choice. However, all composite restorations are fraught with problems in the patient with radiation-induced xerostomia. First, during cavity preparation, margins frequently terminate in dentin or cementum; as a result, the risk of subsequent microleakage and recurrent caries is high. Second, moisture control is frequently less than optimal because of difficulty in controlling gingival hemorrhage. Given the amount of staining associated with SDF, it is not indicated under these circumstances. There are newer formulations of SDF with potassium iodide (KI) that seem to diminish the amount of staining when compared to SDF alone; however, studies suggest that regardless of application of KI staining will occur overtime (Roberts et al., 2020).

For small lesions, glass-ionomer cements may be preferred. Although microleakage is a significant problem with this material, glass-ionomer cements are ion releasing; when fluoride is incorporated within the material it is slowly released, resulting is an anticaries effect. CPP-ACP nanocomplexes have also been incorporated within glass-ionomer cements (Mazzaoui et al., 2003). As mentioned above, CPP-ACP nanocomplexes have decided anticariogenic and remineralizing capabilities. In addition to increasing the release of calcium, phosphate, and fluoride ions from the material after placement, the incorporation of CPP-ACP nanocomplexes also increased the microtensile bond strength and compressive strength of the material (Mazzaoui et al., 2003).

Surprisingly, most patients are relatively asymptomatic and voice few complaints, even when there is evidence of carious pulpal exposure. Often these initial restorative procedures can be performed without local anesthesia.

When the caries process proceeds to amputation of the crown, the clinician, in most instances, need only smooth the jagged edges resulting from the fracture. These teeth continue to be asymptomatic and the appearance on a periapical radiograph of the area will usually be within normal limits. If there is evidence of active infection, however, endodontic therapy may be employed for control (see section below entitled "Endodontic therapy as an alternative to postradiation extraction").

Extensive cervical caries is best restored with silver amalgam restorations. These lesions commonly involve the entire gingival area, although the buccal and labial surfaces are most often affected. If caries extends interproximally as well as buccally and lingually in posterior teeth, a conventional mesio-occlusodistal restoration is placed first; the restoration should be extended subgingivally. At a subsequent appointment, the buccal and/or lingual amalgam restorations are placed. Sequential restoration of circumferential lesions is advisable in anterior teeth. With large Class V restorations, a method that works well is to restore approximately one-half of the gingival area at the first appointment and restore the remaining gingival portion subsequently. If the caries extends to interproximal areas, placement of a small section of matrix band with a suitable interproximal wedge will simplify and improve the condensation of the amalgam.

Alternative techniques such as the silver-modified atraumatic restorative technique (SMART) have also been recently introduced in this population. This technique involves removing gross decay with a spoon excavator followed by placement of SDF and glass ionomer or composite restorative material. It is important to note that SDF does not interfere with bonding of restorative materials; however, studies have suggested that the dual application of SDF and KI leaves a precipitate that reduces bond strength (Knight et al., 2006). This is considered a temporary technique and may need to be repeated every few months to years.

Complete-coverage restorations may be considered for patients with good oral hygiene and caries control, for key teeth that serve as partial denture abutments, and for anterior restorations where aesthetics is of concern. Prosthetically, there are many advantages to restoring abutment teeth with complete-coverage restorations. Such teeth can be contoured for optimal placement of retainers, guiding planes, and rests. However, the judgment to provide extensive restorative procedures must be tempered by the prognosis for tumor control, general health, oral hygiene and compliance, the extent of radiation caries, and the patient's motivation. As a general rule for the patient with radiation-induced xerostomia, if crown restorations are necessary, complete coverage and subgingival margins are indicated. Three-quarter crowns or onlays should be used with caution unless the patient is compliant and exhibits excellent hygiene.

Margins should be exposed with retraction cord; care must be taken to avoid perforating the epithelial attachment. Although no sound evidence is available at this time, we believe the use of electrosurgery or laser therapy for gingival retraction should be avoided. Provisional restorations should be properly contoured to minimize gingival irritation. Although no substantiating evidence is available, some clinicians suggest that the patient should be given prophylactic antibiotics if multiple crowns are being prepared.

Pulpal procedures aimed at eliciting formation of secondary dentin are generally not successful. The compromised vascularity of the pulp and the impaired capabilities of odontoblasts predispose direct or indirect pulp capping techniques to failure. If carious or mechanical exposures are encountered during tooth preparation, endodontic therapy is suggested.

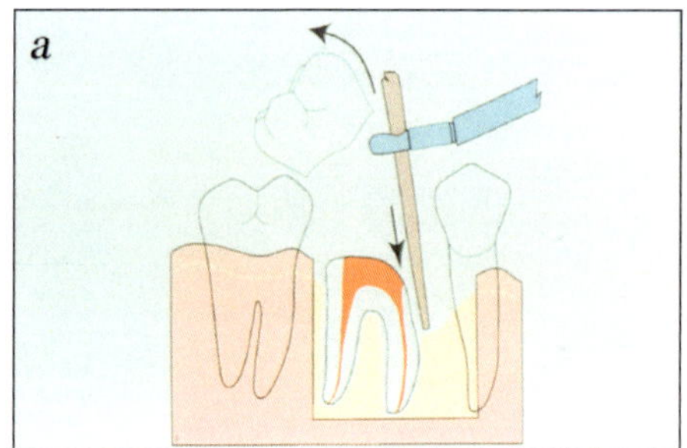
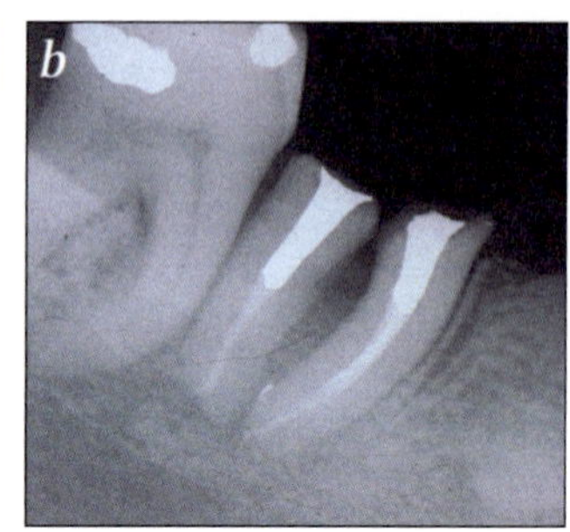

Figure 1-52 *(a and b)* Root canal therapy is used most often for treatment of periapical disease. However, when combined with crown amputation, it also is a means of eliminating deep periodontal pockets. This protocol is used instead of extraction when the risk of ORN secondary to postradiation extraction is high (i.e., the dose to bone was greater than 65 Gy).

Endodontic therapy as an alternative to postradiation extraction

As discussed previously, postradiation dental extraction of diseased teeth within the radiation field in high-risk patients leads to a high rate of ORN. Endodontic therapy, successfully employed, maintains mucosal integrity and should be considered in such circumstances.

The report by Seto et al. (1985) remains the most comprehensive. Sixteen postradiation patients who underwent endodontic therapy were followed. All patients were treated with CRT, and each of the teeth studied was in the radiation field. Ten patients (63%) received a tumor dose greater than 65 Gy and six (37%) received between 45 and 65 Gy. The researchers evaluated 11 teeth (13 canals) that were endodontically treated preradiation and 35 teeth (54 canals) that were endodontically treated postradiation. Follow-up, defined as the time between completion of endodontic therapy and the most recent recall visit, ranged from 6 months to 54 months (median of 21.6 months) for the postradiation group. The indications for postradiation root canal treatment were caries (80%), periodontal disease (17%), and periapical abscess (3%). Pretreatment periapical changes were evident in 31% of teeth and pain in 29%.

On follow-up (range of 6 to 54 months), 12 teeth and 2 roots of 35 teeth that were endodontically treated postradiation (40%) and 3 of 11 teeth that were endodontically treated preradiation (27%) did not have periapical changes, purulence, or pain. Periapical changes were demonstrated by 59% of the teeth (27 of 46), including 5 of 11 of the preradiation and 22 of 35 of the postradiation teeth. Three teeth (7%) had pain to percussion or palpation (1 of 11 preradiation and 2 of 35 postradiation teeth).

Examination of the relationships between endodontic length and postendodontic changes in teeth treated after radiation therapy showed no relationship between the length of the endodontic fill and subsequent periodontal disease, pain, or extractions. However, a significant relationship existed between periapical changes and the length of the endodontic fill. The short endodontic fills resulted in significantly fewer periapical changes than did either the long or normal fills. The overall retention of roots that received postradiation endodontic treatment was 85% (46 of 54 roots).

The criteria for endodontic success must be reconsidered for the irradiated patient. We define success as the prevention of ORN. If the criteria for success were defined as nonprogressive periapical changes and a lack of pain, a low success rate (40%) was obtained in the study reported by Seto et al. (1985). However, a high percentage of roots (85%) were retained with minor periapical changes and minimal pain. ORN was not associated with endodontic therapy. The success rate of treatment of severely diseased teeth in irradiated patients, in terms of the avoidance of extraction and prevention of ORN, was 100%. This is in contrast to the high incidence of ORN encountered when severely diseased teeth were extracted after radiation therapy (Beumer et al., 1983). Therefore, we believe that endodontic therapy is a reasonably predictable alternative to extraction for patients who have been irradiated for oral tumors.

Shorter endodontic fill lengths have the fewest postendodontic periapical changes (Seto et al., 1985). It is probable that fills close to the radiographic apex are overextended, thus precipitating the same pathologic responses as seen in long fills. Therefore, in the radiation patient, shorter fill lengths would appear to be more desirable than overextended fills; however, further study with a larger sample is needed for confirmation.

Endodontic treatment for postradiation patients may be difficult technically. Rubber dam isolation is complicated by a lack of coronal tooth structure and the risk of tissue trauma and resultant bone exposure. Oropharyngeal reflexes may be compromised by surgery and/or radiation therapy, predisposing the patient to a greater risk for aspiration of files. A throat screen, consisting of an open 2 × 2-inch piece of gauze, should be used whenever a rubber dam cannot be employed. Floss or thread should be attached to all files for easy retrieval if they are inadvertently dropped beyond normal reach.

Trismus and small pulp canals make access for instrumentation and filling difficult. When access is limited by trismus, the files can be bent along the noncutting portion of the shank to increase working space between the maxillary and mandibular dentitions. Hemostats can be used above the noncutting portion of the file to instrument the canals. Coronal amputation or creation of facial access can be helpful in the location and instrumentation of root canals in the presence of canal sclerosis and trismus.

Canals are obturated with gutta-percha condensed with finger spreaders and directed toward lateral condensation. Techniques that aid in the access, preparation, and completion of endodontic therapy can be used as long as the patient is protected from aspiration and soft tissue trauma.

Endodontic therapy of periodontally compromised teeth allows for coronal amputation and greater access to periodontal pockets (Fig 1-52). However, when multirooted teeth are amputated, care must be exercised to avoid exposure of the interradicular bone. The furcation should be opened short of the gingival attachment and incrementally fluted as the soft tissues recede. In this way, extraction of teeth that demonstrate moderate to severe periodontal disease can be avoided, and these teeth can be retained with hope of exfoliation, maintaining mucosal coverage.

Overall treatment approach

Our current approach to the management of dental disease in the mandible in the radiation field is dependent on three factors: *(1)* the dose to bone at the affected area, *(2)* the radiation modality used, and *(3)* the nature and severity of the dental infection. If the dose to bone locally is less than 55 Gy and the tooth or teeth in question are restorable, a number of conventional therapies, including root planing and curettage and root canal therapy, can be employed. Periodontal flap surgery and crown lengthening, however, are not recommended. If the tooth is nonrestorable, a simple extraction with appropriate antibiotic coverage is justified.

If a patient is treated with a combination of external beam and radiation implant, the therapeutic options are dependent on the site of the dental infection in relation to the site of the implant. The mandibular dose at any particular location is dependent on the dosimetry of the implant plus the external beam dose. If the patient presents with a serious dental infection associated with a molar on the side opposite the implant, the dose to bone in this region most likely was less than 55 Gy, and the options previously discussed could be employed. However, if the dental infection involves teeth adjacent to the implant, in the absence of exposed bone dental extractions are employed only as a last resort. Endodontic therapy is recommended to maintain mucosal integrity. If the infection is periodontal and/or extends to the bifurcation region following root canal therapy, the crown can be amputated, thereby providing access for oral hygiene in this area.

If the infection persists and dental extraction is deemed unavoidable, the decision to use adjunctive therapy is dependent on the dose distribution patterns of the implant. If the buccal plate, inferior border, and buccal slopes of the alveolus were not affected by the implant, dental extractions and removal of nonvital bone are appropriate. If the implant increases the dose in these regions to greater than 55 Gy, PENTO(CLO) or HBO may be considered.

If the patient is treated with external beam alone and the dose to the local bone sites in question was greater than 65 Gy, root canal therapy is again the first choice of therapy. If IMRT, SBRT, or VMAT was employed, the dosimetry diagrams must be carefully reviewed to determine the volume of the mandibular body receiving doses greater than 65 Gy. If root canal treatment is not successful in eliminating the infection and dental extractions are unavoidable, the use of PENTO(CLO) or HBO will improve the prognosis for healing.

If the dose to the local bone falls between 55 and 65 Gy, decisions for therapy should be based on individual patient factors, such as a history of a radical neck dissection, mucosal or radiographic changes, continued tobacco use, and so on. Comorbidities such as these would tend to recommend that adjuvant PENTO(CLO) or HBO be employed.

Additional factors such as the elapsed time since completion of radiation therapy should be considered. The greater the elapsed time, the greater the fibrosis and reduction of the vasculature with the clinical target volume. This can impair the effectiveness of both PENTO and HBO. The decrease in vasculature and the capacity of angiogenesis likely play a factor in the ability to heal from surgical interventions. Along with elapsed time, the age of the patient may also play a factor. The HPV head and neck cancer demographic tends to be younger, and these patients will likely experience less initial fibrosis vascular compromise. However, as time elapses, and these changes become more profound, these patients will increasingly be predisposed to a risk of caries and ORN.

Diet

During radiation therapy, loss of taste acuity, reduced salivary flow, and pain on swallowing predispose the patient to loss of appetite, nausea, and malaise. A 20 to 30 lb weight loss is common, particularly among patients treated with chemoradiation therapy. Enriched dietary supplements are useful during this period. Citrus juices and other acidic foods can result in oral discomfort and should be replaced with blander food items. As oral mucositis becomes more severe, coarse foods should be eliminated and the diet changed to a soft or semisoft consistency. While dietary supplements are useful, they should not be relied on exclusively. Should oral intake become inadequate, percutaneous gastrostomy tubes (G-tubes) can be used to support these patients. Some institutions choose to prophylactically place G-tubes to maintain weight and nutrition during treatment (Lee et al., 1998). After therapy, foods that favor an increase in the activity of cariogenic microflora should be avoided. Consultation with a dietitian prior to therapy is recommended.

Osteoradionecrosis (ORN)

ORN is defined by most clinicians as exposure of bone within the radiation treatment volume that persists for three months or longer. It is a dreaded complication of radiotherapy because it may progress to intractable pain and pathologic fracture of the mandible, often accompanied by orocutaneous fistulae and requiring resection of major portions of the mandible (Beumer et al., 1984; Peterson et al., 2010; Spijkervet et al., 2019).

As mentioned previously, following tumoricidal doses of radiation, bone becomes a hypoxic, hypocellular, hypovascular tissue, and these changes are primarily due to radiation-induced fibrosis. Radiation damage appears to be the result of dysregulation of fibroblastic activity (Delanian and Lefaix, 2004; Lyons and Ghazali, 2008). Initially, endothelial cells are damaged by both the direct and the indirect effects of radiation. The injured endothelial cells produce cytokines that enhance the acute inflammatory response and, in turn, promote the release of inflammatory cytokines. Subsequently, the destruction of the endothelium combined with vascular thrombosis leads to substantial loss of the small vessel network in the irradiated tissues. During this process fibroblasts are transformed into myofibroblasts, and unregulated chronic activation of these myofibroblasts by a variety of growth factors leads to progressive fibrosis. Tissue breakdown that occurs is not related to the normal infectious processes but rather to radiation-induced tissue damage that results in chronic nonhealing wounds in which metabolic demands exceed supply.

Bone necrosis may be spontaneous or induced by trauma or infection. Spontaneous bone necrosis is secondary to the inability of hard and soft tissues to sustain cell turnover and collagen synthesis following irradiation. This type of bone necrosis is associated with treatment of large volumes of the mandible with a high dose of radiation (70 Gy and greater with conventional fractionation), positioning of implant sources adjacent to bone (Fig 1-53), and neutron beam therapy (Beumer et al., 1984; Murray et al., 1980a; Thorn et al., 2000; Marx et al., 1983a, 1983b; Kluth et al., 1988; Costantino et al., 1995; Marunick et al., 2000). Spontaneous bone necrosis makes up to 35% of all necroses and may represent

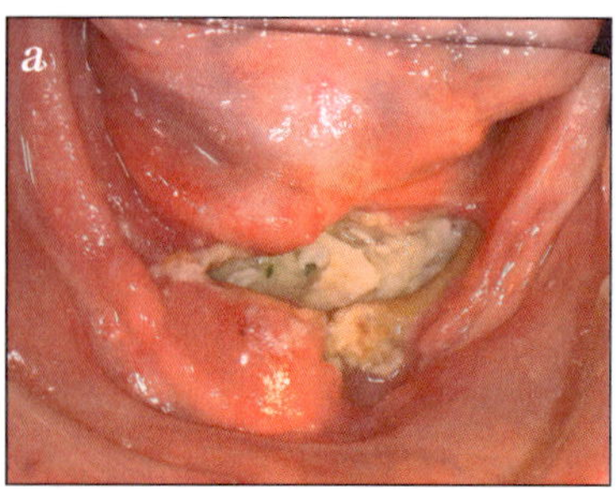
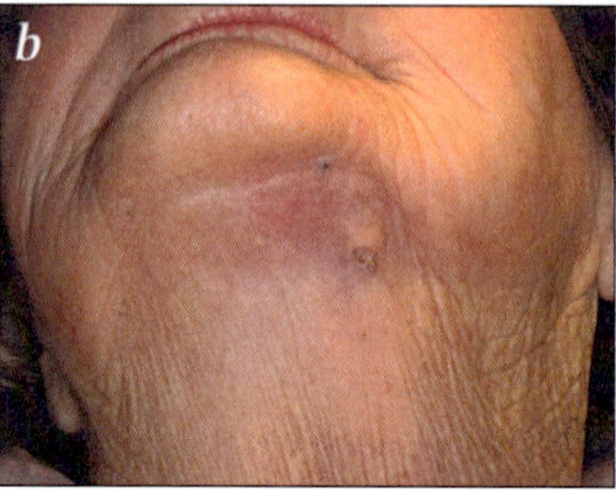

Figure 1-53 Sequela to the use of a high-dose rate iridium implant preceded by 50 Gy of external beam radiation. *(a)* Spontaneous ORN. *(b)* Fistula in the same patient.

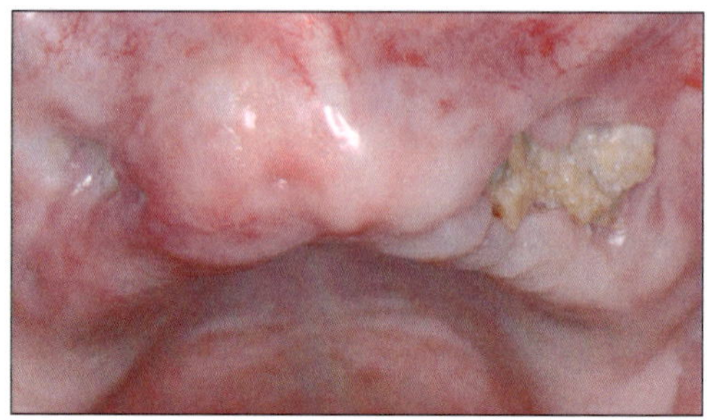

Figure 1-54 Spontaneous ORN in a patient treated with concomitant chemoradiation. The BED (biologic equivalent dose) to the maxilla approached 8,000 cGy. Eventually the entire maxilla was lost.

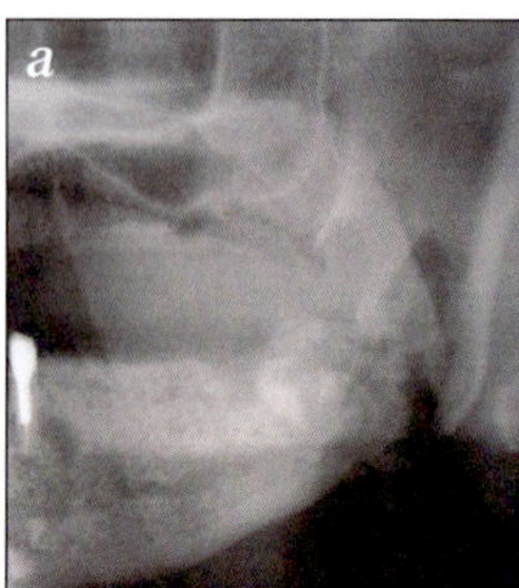
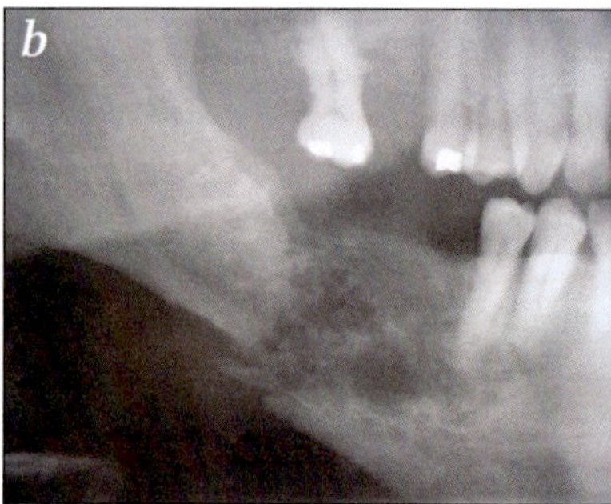
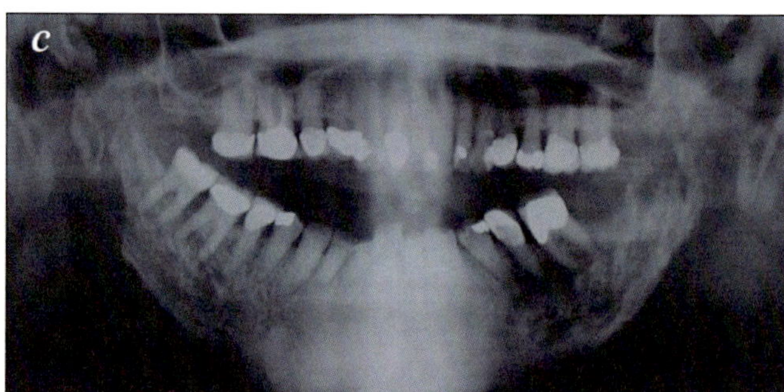

Figure 1-55 Spontaneous ORNs associated with concomitant chemotherapy and CRT. All patients received a total dose of 70 Gy. *(a and b)* Neither lesion was associated with the dentition. *(c)* Bilateral fractures through the ramus and angle secondary to chemoradiation therapy. The fractures were not related to or precipitated by the dentition.

an even higher percentage now that concomitant chemoradiation is used more frequently (Vissink et al., 2003) (Figs 1-54 and 1-55).

Trauma-induced ORN occurs as a result of compromised wound healing when the tissues become fibrotic and hypovascular. For example, if the patient develops a periodontal or periapical infection or requires postradiation extractions, the compromised healing capacity may lead to bone necrosis (see section below entitled "Contributing factors").

Most bone necroses occur in the mandible, which is particularly at risk when large volumes of the mandibular body are exposed to tumoricidal doses. Most patients that develop ORN are dentulous at the time of tumor diagnosis. Fewer than 5% of all ORNs occur in edentulous patients. The risk of ORN is higher in patients who have been treated with a combination of external therapy and brachytherapy and external beam and SBRT than in those treated with external therapy alone, but ORN associated with the brachytherapy and SBRT respond more predictably to conservative treatment than does ORN associated with external beam alone.

When patients were treated with CRT, the incidence varied, depending on total dosage, fractionation, volume of the mandibular body within the fields, and dental disease factors. It has been reported as low as 3% and as high as 37% but generally averaged 10% to 15% when high-energy photons were used (Grant and Fletcher, 1966; Beumer et al., 1972; Bedwinek et al., 1976; Murray et al., 1980a; Morrish et al., 1981; Thorn et al., 2000; Reuther et al., 2003; Studer et al., 2004). The great disparity in these numbers was probably due to the variety of fractionation schedules and total doses employed at the various centers. For example, several centers in the 1950s through the 1960s employed fractions of 175 cGy with total doses often limited to less the 6,500 cGy. The incidence was higher when brachytherapy was used and extremely high when neutron radiation therapy is used (Marunick et al., 2000). Increased risk has also been associated with concomitant chemotherapy and CRT (Kuhnt et al., 2006; Hehr et al., 2006).

Preliminary reports appear to indicate that the incidence of ORN is lower with IMRT, probably in the range of 4–8% (Aarup-Kristensen et al., 2019; Kubota et al., 2021). This reduced risk is probably secondary to the fact that smaller volumes of the mandible are exposed to tumoricidal doses or within the clinical target volume. However, the rate of bone necrosis appears to be increased to levels approaching 10% when IMRT is used in combination with a boost delivered via SBRT (Baker et al., 2019). The ORN risk associated with the use of VMAT is unknown, but the hopes of accurate dose prediction may be achieved using autocontours from pretherapy 18 FDG PET scans. The dose and volume of the mandible can be better controlled and possibly reduced. In addition, the planned three-dimensional visual displays of high mandibular dose may be useful for oral health practitioners to decide whether to prophylactically extract teeth.

Contributing factors

Diseased teeth present within the radiation treatment volume prior to radiation are the prime initiators of trauma-induced ORN (Beumer et al., 1984; Murray et al., 1980a, 1980b; Marx et al., 1985; Thorn et al., 2000). Preradiation extraction sites may dehisce if healing time is inadequate (Fig 1-56). A significant number of ORNs are precipitated by periodontal infections associated with mandibular

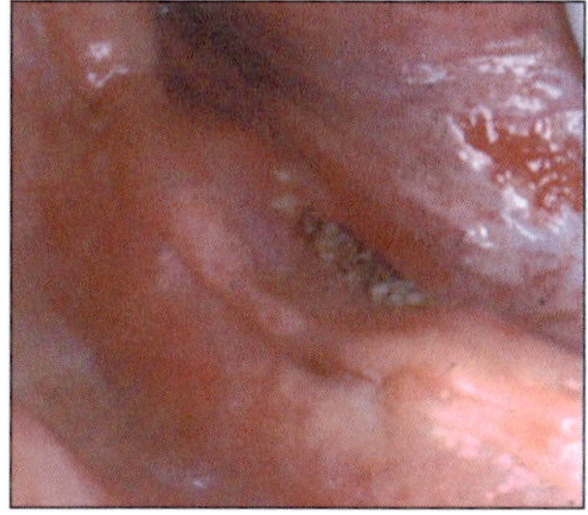

Figure 1-56 ORN at a preradiation extraction site.

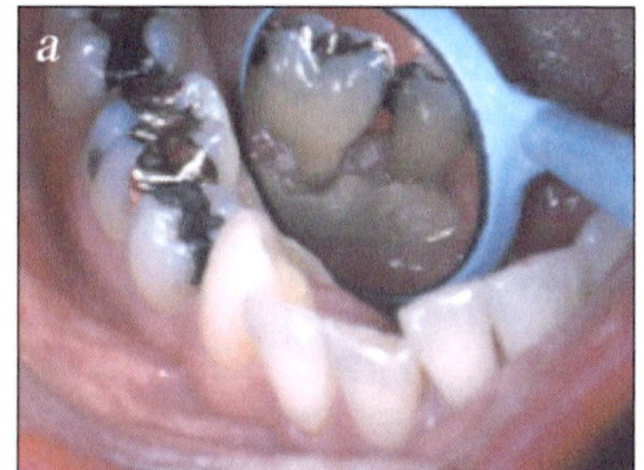
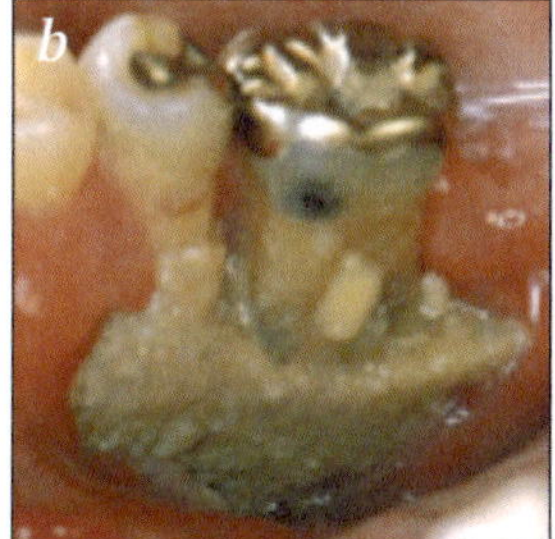
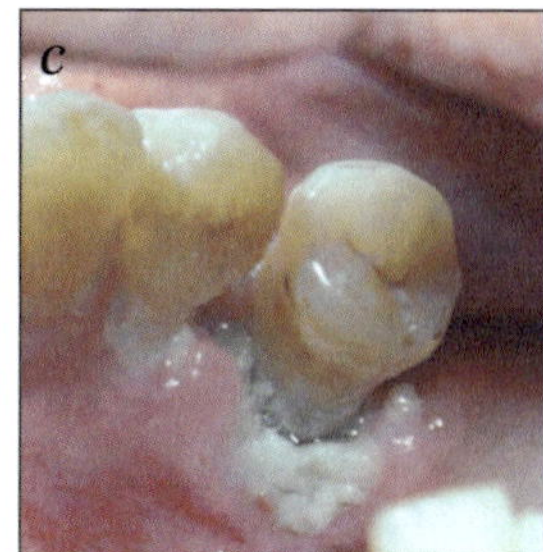

Figure 1-57 *(a, b, and c)* ORN precipitated by periodontal infections.

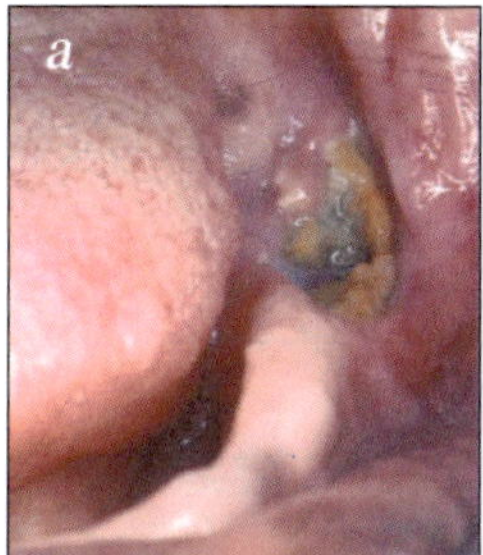
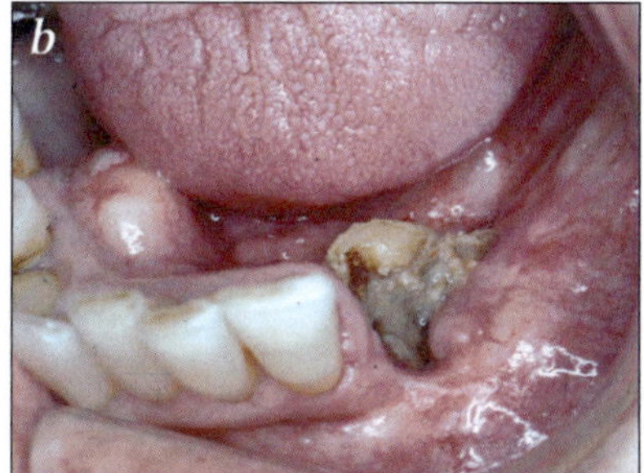
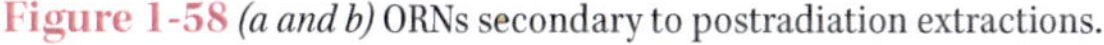

Figure 1-58 *(a and b)* ORNs secondary to postradiation extractions.

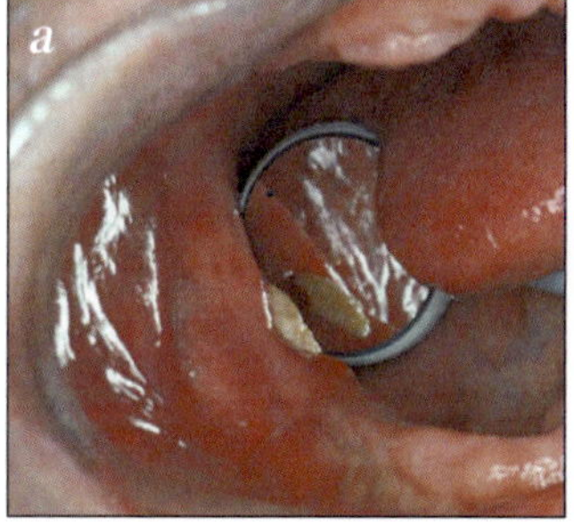
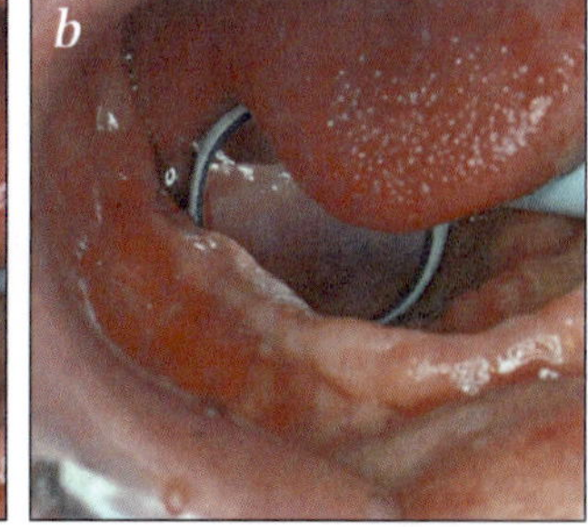

Figure 1-59 Bone necrosis at a preradiation extraction site. *(a)* ORN occurred beneath a complete denture, six months following completion of external radiation therapy for squamous cell carcinoma of the right tonsil and soft palate. *(b)* The bone exposure healed with conservative measures eight months later.

teeth left within the gross tumor volume (Fig 1-57). Postradiation extraction of teeth within the gross tumor volume leads to a significant number of bone necroses as well (Murray et al., 1980a, 1980b; Morrish et al., 1981; Beumer et al., 1983; Marx et al., 1985; Thorn et al., 2000; Reuther et al., 2003) (Fig 1-58). Bone necroses are rare in association with the use of removable partial dentures or complete dentures, but when they do occur, most are confined within the zone of attached keratinized mucosa and resolve with conservative treatment measures (Beumer et al., 1976, 1984) (Fig 1-58).

Therefore, we continue to believe that an aggressive policy of removal of diseased mandibular teeth within the radiation gross tumor volume, as described earlier, will minimize the incidence of bone necrosis (Schuurhuis et al., 2018; Spijkervet et al., 2021). Extraction of all remaining teeth in the radiation treatment volume, however, is not indicated and probably increases the risk of bone necrosis, particularly in those patients with healthy dentitions and a history of good dental compliance.

When the dose in the area exceeds 65 Gy, postradiation extraction of diseased teeth within the clinical target volume predisposes to a high risk of ORN (Morrish et al., 1981; Beumer et al., 1983; Marx et al., 1985; Thorn et al., 2000; Reuther et al., 2003). In addition, in the UCLA study, bone exposures caused by postradiation extractions appear to lead to a high rate of mandibular resection (45.4%; Beumer et al., 1983). If postradiation extractions of teeth within the clinical target volume cannot be avoided, the use of either HBO or the PENTO(CLO) protocol is suggested in association with the extractions. A more viable option for treatment of dental disease in the field after radiation treatment is root canal therapy. After endodontic therapy, teeth can be amputated at the gingival margins and the remaining tooth structure can be recontoured to improve access for oral hygiene.

ORN precipitated by the use of removable partial or complete dentures does not appear to be as significant, particularly if a patient has been edentulous for more than six months prior to radiotherapy (Beumer et al., 1976). Beumer et al. (1984) reported that only one of eight bone exposures that resulted from a removable prosthesis led to resection of the mandible; all others healed with conservative measures (Fig 1-59). However, seven of eight bone exposures occurred at either preradiation or postradiation extraction sites. Caution should be exercised before dentures are placed in these circumstances because the remodeling apparatus of bone is severely disrupted by tumoricidal doses of radiation therapy. In addition, as radiation-induced xerostomia becomes more severe, the risk of bone exposure from complete dentures also increases. Saliva is an important lubricant for mandibular complete dentures, and in its absence friction at the denture-mucosa interface may be increased as the denture slides over the mucosa during function (see section below entitled "Complete Dentures for the Irradiated Patient").

When the primary tumor is adjacent to or overlying bone, the risk of bone necrosis is increased. Rapid shrinkage of a tumor, particularly in large lesions, can result in a bone exposure. If the mucosa does resurface, the affected area is often thin and atrophic and thus more susceptible to perforation. More importantly, a large volume of the body of the mandible is irradiated in these lesions. As the dose increases tissue changes become more profound and irreversible, increasing the risk of bone necrosis. The greater the body of the mandible that is included within the clinical target volume, the greater the risk of ORN.

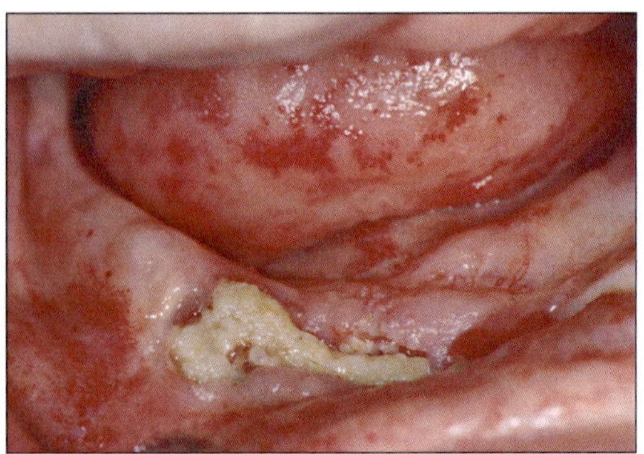

Figure 1-60 Localized ORN. Epithelium is beginning to undermine bone margins. Widespread telangiectasia indicates that the patient has been treated to the highest level of tolerance.

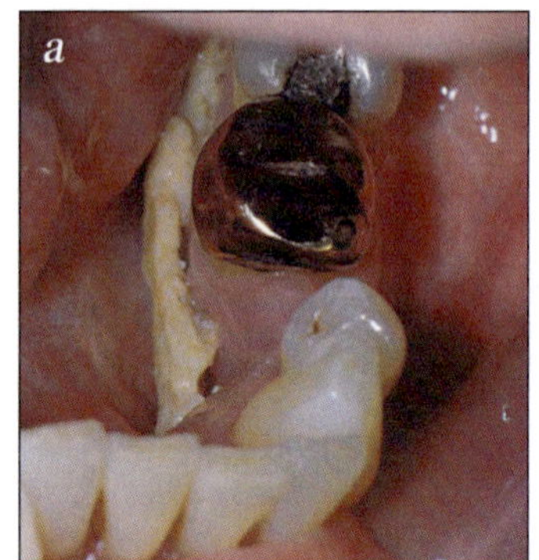

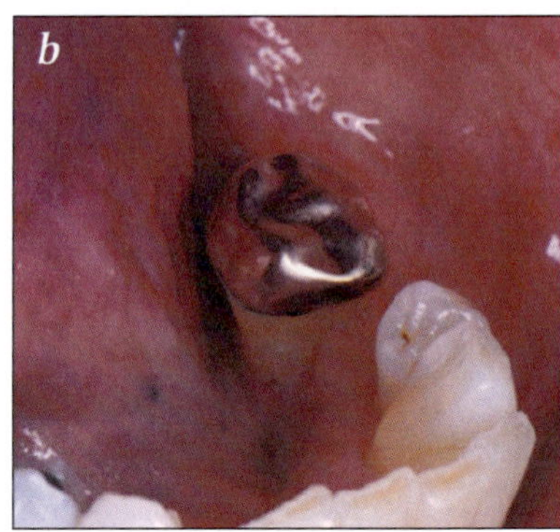

Figure 1-61 Bone exposure associated with iridium implants in a patient who received 55 Gy external beam therapy and 25–30 Gy therapy via an iridium implant. *(a)* He presented with ORN 24 months after radiation therapy. Nonvital exposed bone was removed with an air rotor under copious irrigation. *(b)* After several treatments, epithelial coverage has been attained.

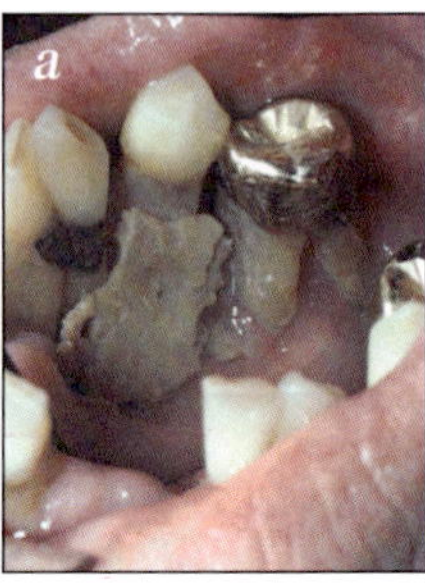

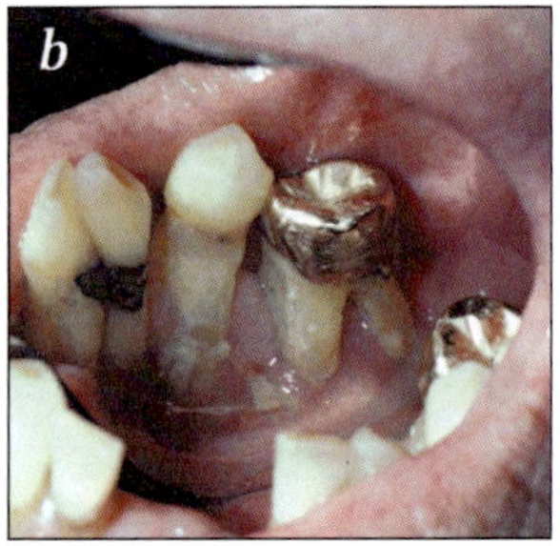

Figure 1-62 Bone exposure associated with iridium implants in a patient who received 55 Gy external beam therapy and 25–30 Gy therapy via an iridium implant. Patient refused extraction of teeth adjacent to the implant. *(a)* Several months later the patient presented with the lingual plate of the mandible exposed. *(b)* This area of nonvital bone was carefully removed. Eventually all these teeth exfoliated leaving this area mucosalized.

Treatment options

The treatment of mandibular ORN consists of *(1)* conservative measures (local irrigation, topical antibiotic packings, etc.; Beumer et al., 1984; Schwartz, 1995; Wong et al., 1997), *(2)* the pentoxifylline-tocopherol-clodronate protocol (PENTO[CLO]; Lyons and Ghazali, 2008; Delanian et al., 2005, 2011; Robard et al., 2014; Hayashi et al., 2015), *(3)* HBO, and *(4)* the combination of HBO with surgical debridement (Marx et al., 1983b; Hart and Mainous, 1976; Shaha et al., 1997) or (5) when necessary, resection and reconstruction with either a free graft (Marx et al., 1983a, 1983b; Hart and Mainous, 1976; Shaha et al., 1997) or a vascularized osteomyocutaneous flap (Notani et al., 2003; Pirak et al., 2008; Zaghi et al., 2014).

Conservative treatment

If the dose to the affected area is less than 70 Gy, most localized bone exposures presenting within the zone of attached gingiva, can be controlled with local irrigation of saline and chlorhexidine (Beumer et al., 1984; Wong et al., 1997). In some instances, it may also be possible to employ iodoform gauze packing impregnated with tincture of benzoin (Schwartz, 1995). When such conservative measures are successful, evidence of the epithelium undermining the bone exposure will be readily apparent (Fig 1-60). Stringent oral hygiene measures must be employed by the patient and close follow-up by the clinician is mandatory. These patients are monitored at intervals ranging from twice per week to once per month, depending on patient compliance and the extent and severity of the exposure. Sharp bony projections can traumatize adjacent soft tissues or contribute to plaque accumulation and should be smoothed. As the edges of the necrotic bone are undermined by oral mucosa, these bony edges should be removed carefully to avoid injury to underlying epithelium or granulation tissue.

If the necrosis remains limited to the local area and if pain and swelling of the adjacent soft tissues are not evident, conservative methods can be continued. Periodic radiographs are recommended to monitor the extent of the bone necrosis. Resolution of the lesion and restoration of mucosal coverage may take several months or years.

Healing is accomplished by natural sequestration and resorption of the nonvital bone. Antibiotics are necessary only to control local, acute infectious episodes involving the adjacent soft tissues. Routine administration of antibiotics for extended periods is not advised for such patients. Antibiotics provide little benefit because of the compromised vasculature of the local area and may lead to the development of drug-resistant organisms.

The previously described conservative measures are also recommended for ORN associated with brachytherapy. As mentioned previously, brachytherapy is frequently used in the treatment of localized tumors of the mobile tongue and floor of the mouth. The outcome of these ORNs is primarily dependent on the magnitude of the external beam dosage. In most patients, external beam dosage to the mandible is limited to 50 to 55 Gy. The interstitial implant boosts the dose to the gross tumor volume by approximately 30 Gy. The risk of bone necrosis is dependent on the number and distribution of the interstitial radiation sources. When the sources are in close proximity to the mandible, the risk of necrosis is high. However, because the dose delivered by the implant is confined to the lingual surface of the mandible, almost all exposures will heal with conservative measures and will not require aggressive surgery or HBO (Figs 1-61 and 1-62).

The outcomes of patients treated with external beam followed by a boost of SBRT behave in a similar manner. The risk of bone necrosis is dependent on the dose distribution patterns. The risk of bone necrosis and whether it is likely to respond to conservative forms of treatment depend on the dosimetry of the SBRT boost.

Wong et al. (1997) reported the results of conservative therapy in 32 patients, including 21 treated with CRT and 11 treated with CRT plus brachytherapy. Most external beam doses were less than 65 Gy. Of 28 patients available for follow-up, in 19 (65%) the lesion stabilized, improved, or completely resolved with conservative therapy. A similar response to conservative measures has been reported in several other studies (Beumer et al., 1984; Epstein et al., 1997; Harris, 1992).

PENTO(CLO) protocol. In recent years, pharmacological management has been used to enhance conservative therapy. The combination of pentoxifylline and tocopherol, with clodronate sometimes added, has been shown to be effective in promoting healing and mucosalization of localized ORNs (Delanian et al., 2003, 2005, 2011; Robard et al., 2014; Hayashi et al., 2015; Patel et al., 2016a; Dissard et al., 2019). Pentoxifylline is a vasodilator and increases erythrocyte flexibility, which improves blood flow. This drug also lessens postradiation-induced fibrosis by reducing the proliferation of dermal fibroblasts. Tocopherol is an antioxidant that acts as a free radical scavenger and also possesses antifibrotic activity. Clodronate is a bisphosphonate that reduces the numbers of osteoclasts and impairs their activity. This drug is also an anti-inflammatory agent. Pentoxifylline is administered orally (400 mg twice per day) as is tocopherol (1,000 IU once per day) and clodronate when included in the protocol (1,600 mg daily). Not all clinicians include clodronate in the treatment regimen (Hayashi et al., 2015; Patel et al., 2016a), and it is still not clear whether clodronate shortens the recovery time. In most studies, antibiotics, corticosteroids, and antifungal medications were administered prior to starting the PENTO(CLO) medical treatment.

In a retrospective report, Hayashi et al. (2015) enrolled 13 patients in a PENTO protocol (without clodronate) with ORN with 60 Gy or more of radiation, 9 of which also had chemotherapy. Eleven patients displayed resolution with an average treatment time of 13.5 months. One patient displayed no resolution after 22 months and eventually opted for mandibular resection. In another report that included the use of clodronate (Robard et al., 2014), healing was obtained in 16 of 21 patients. In a more recent report (Dissard et al., 2019), which included the use of clodronate, complete mucosal coverage was achieved in 76.5% of patients (27 patients) at a mean of 9.6 months. In this series one patient reported an undisplaced fracture of the mandibular body that healed following treatment. Several randomized prospective clinical trials are currently underway in the United States and Australia to test the efficacy of the PENTO(CLO) protocols. In our clinical experience, we find this approach most effective within the first five years since completion of radiotherapy.

When conservative measures are employed, compliance is an important predictor of clinical outcome. After the onset of necrosis, a pattern of poor oral hygiene compliance and continued tobacco use decreases the probability of a successful result (Hayashi et al., 2015; Robard et al., 2014). If conservative measures are to be successful, the local area of bone exposure must be meticulously cleansed by the patient several times per day.

Hyperbaric oxygen therapy

HBO has been the mainstay of treatment for advanced ORN since the 1970s. HBO promotes neovascular proliferation in marginally necrotic tissues, enhances fibroblastic proliferation, enhances the bactericidal activity of white blood cells, accelerates differentiation of osteoblasts, and promotes the formation of bone (Marx et al., 1983a, 1983b; Hunt and Pai, 1972; Knighton et al., 1984; Nilsson et al., 1988; Al Hadi et al., 2015). It has also been shown that HBO elevates the expression of vascular endothelial growth factor, one of the growth factors responsible for angiogenesis during wound healing (Fok et al., 2008).

The early work with HBO for irradiated patients was performed by Hart and Mainous (1976) and continued by Marx et al. (1983a, 1983b, 1985). Hart and Mainous (1976) reported on the first large series of patients with ORN of the mandible treated in a hyperbaric chamber. Patients with bone necrosis were exposed to 2 atm of oxygen in a hyperbaric chamber for two hours per session. Each course of therapy extended for 120 hours. All patients were housed on-site and available for daily wound care and monitoring. The local area was irrigated daily with 9-aminoacridine, an antibacterial rinse. The patients were prescribed systemic tetracycline once oral suppuration had been controlled. In addition, tocopherol (100 mg daily) was administered during the treatment. Neomycin packings were used in purulent oral wounds. Surgical procedures, such as extraction and surgical sequestrectomy, were performed between the 20th and 40th treatments.

All patients presented with advanced bone necrosis and would normally have been considered for mandibular resection according to a formula previously developed by Rankow and Weissman (1971). After the first series of hyperbaric treatments, 37 of 46 patients were free of symptoms, including elimination of all bony exposure intraorally. In 9 patients, teeth were extracted with a radical alveolectomy, and all sites healed without complication. Of these 9 patients, 5 received immediate dentures, and these dentures were employed without complication. In 4 patients, free bone grafts successfully restored mandibular discontinuity defects. It should be noted that this series of ORNs involved advanced and extensive bone exposures. For instance, 19 patients had pathologic fractures of the mandible and 15 had orocutaneous fistulae prior to hyperbaric therapy.

The results achieved by Hart and Mainous (1976) have never been duplicated, probably because daily wound care was provided and diet, tobacco use, and alcohol consumption were carefully controlled. As discussed earlier, the use of tocopherol (a free radical scavenger) has reemerged, and this drug may work synergistically with HBO to inhibit fibrosis.

Since then, several authors (Epstein et al., 1997; Oh et al., 2004; van Merkesteyn et al., 1993) have reported less than satisfactory results when HBO was used alone or in combination with surgical sequestrectomy; significant numbers of those patients required mandibulectomy even with adjunctive HBO therapy. The report by Oh et al. (2004) is representative. In their study, 79 of 114 patients received HBO. The exposures in 4 patients were resolved with HBO alone and those in 25 patients were resolved with a combination of HBO and surgical debridement. HBO was ineffective in the remaining 50 patients. In a prospective, randomized, double-blind clinical trial (Annane et al., 2004), HBO combined with conservative treatment was found to be of no additional benefit in the treatment of ORN compared to conservative treatment alone.

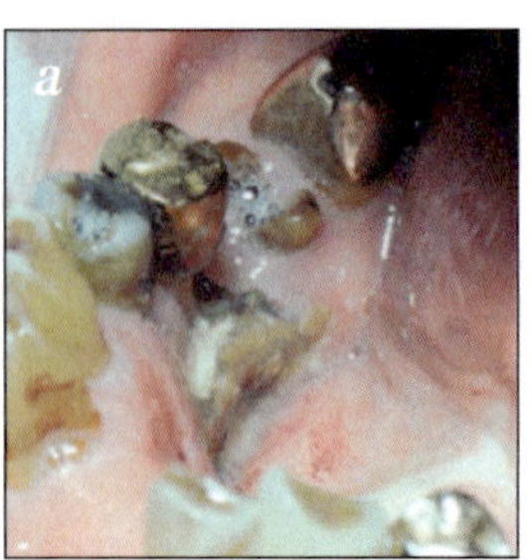
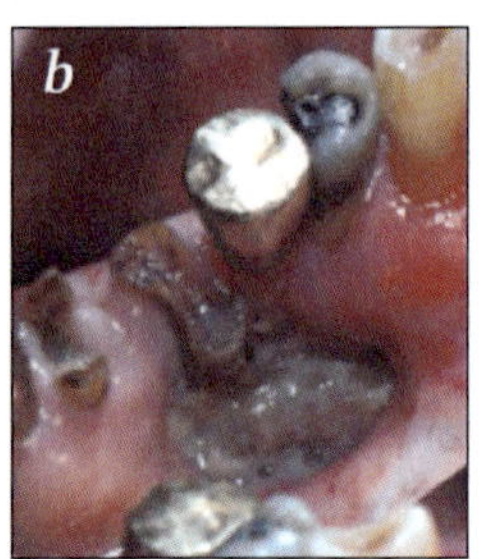
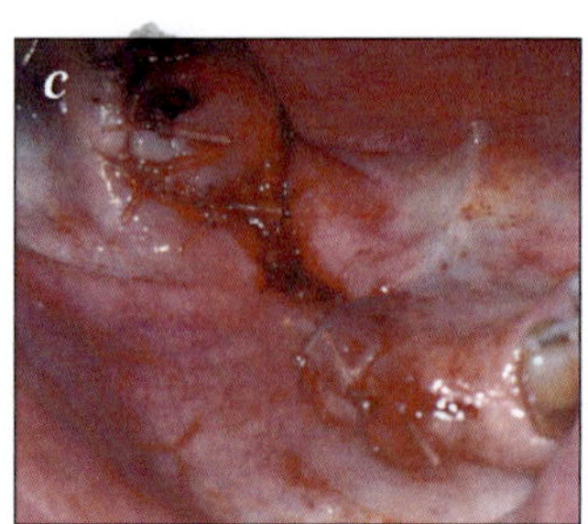
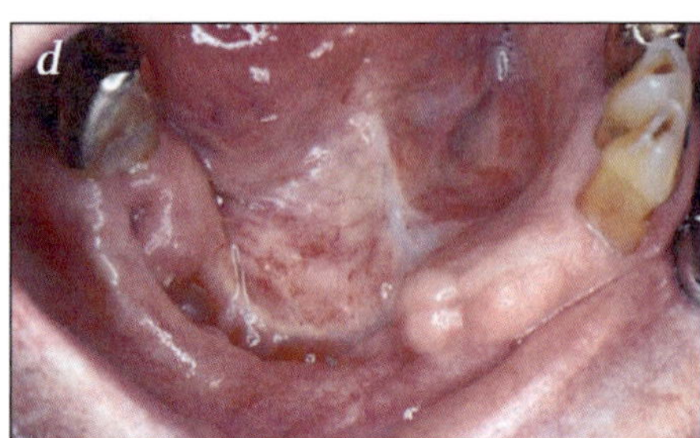

Figure 1-63 Combined HBO-surgical treatment of ORN. *(a)* Bone necrosis discovered 18 months following external radiation therapy for squamous cell carcinoma of the lateral floor of the mouth. The dose to bone in the region exceeded 71 Gy. *(b)* Status after HBO therapy according to the protocol described by Marx et al. (1983b). *(c)* Surgical resection of nonvital bone and primary closure. *(d)* Wound healing two months after resection.

Nevertheless, when patients present with extensive areas of necrotic bone or bone necrosis involving teeth, most clinicians continue to employ the Marx protocol (Marx et al., 1983b) in the hope of avoiding resection of a significant portion of the mandible, thus retaining its continuity (Fig 1-63).

Vascularized free flaps

Resection and immediate reconstruction with an osteomyocutaneous vascularized flap is recommended when patients present with advanced, diffuse ORN in which the full thickness of bone is necrotic, pathologic fracture of the mandible, or ORN associated with concomitant chemoradiation therapy (Shaha et al., 1997; Notani et al., 2003; Pirak-Arnnop et al., 2008; Zaghi et al., 2014). As mentioned previously, concomitant chemoradiation escalates the biologically equivalent dose to the tumor by 7 to 10 Gy (Kasibhatla et al., 2007; Fowler, 2008). When used in conjunction with external beam radiation, long-term side effects such as trismus, dysphagia, and velopharyngeal function increased dramatically. When concomitant chemotherapy was used with CRT, the increase in ORN was dramatic, and these ORNs did not respond to conservative treatment methods or HBO and required radical resection of the mandible and reconstruction with an osteomyocutaneous vascularized flap. However, a recent report that approximately 25% of patients with ORN of the mandible develop ongoing disease despite extensive mandible resection and reconstruction with vascularized flaps (Zaghi et al., 2021). The extent of resection in these surgeries was determined by excising necrotic bone until a bleeding edge was encountered. This report illustrates the difficulty in ascertaining viable bone in the surgical setting. Currently, methods are being developed that seek to ascertain the vascularity of the affected bone by means of dynamic contrast-enhanced (DCE) MRI scans using quantifiable biomarkers (Mohamed et al., 2020). These scans could be used to stage the severity of the disease as well as to determine appropriate surgical margins during resection.

Soft Tissue Necrosis

Soft tissue necrosis in the postradiation field is defined as a nonneoplastic mucosal ulceration that does not expose bone (Fig 1-64). These lesions occur most often following treatment with interstitial implants (Beumer et al., 1972) and, most recently, SBRT boosts (Lee et al., 2012; Baker et al., 2019). The incidence of soft tissue necrosis in these later two reports was 16% and 27%, respectively, and the risk of developing a soft tissue necrosis was dramatically increased by smoking. These techniques are used following a prescribed course of external beam therapy, allowing the radiation therapist to increase the local dose without compromising surrounding structures. Most of these necroses occur within one year after completion of radiation therapy.

Intense local discomfort is a clinical symptom that is sometimes useful in differentiating this lesion from persistent disease. A tumor recurrence usually presents with irregular indurated margins, whereas soft tissue necroses present with regular, nonindurated margins. Exfoliative cytology and incisional biopsy may be necessary to rule out persistent tumor.

Clinical experience indicates that an appreciable number of soft tissue necroses are precipitated by cheek and tongue biting. A misshaped oral cavity, compromised sensory and motor innervation of the tongue, lips, and buccal mucosa, and aberrant mandibular movements combine to predispose many patients to tongue and cheek trauma. Often occlusal adjustments in the dentulous patient or removal of the mandibular denture from the edentulous patient will alleviate the difficulty and reduce the chances of recurrent trauma.

Treatment consists of establishing the diagnosis and close follow-up. Most heal without intervention (Beumer et al., 1972). For severe cases, some clinicians believe that a course of HBO will accelerate healing. As mentioned previously, PENTO enhances blood flow in ischemic tissues and has also been proposed as a means to facilitate mucosalization (Dion et al., 1990; Futran et al., 1997; Oxford et al., 2021).

Complete Dentures for the Irradiated Patient

Risk of osteoradionecrosis

In view of the long-term changes associated with oral mucous membranes and bone and the reduction of output and compromise of the physical properties and biologic effectiveness of saliva, some radiotherapists have been reluctant to permit their patients to wear dentures after radiotherapy because of the risk of osteoradionecrosis. However, most studies (Beumer et al., 1976; Buurman et al., 2013; Abed et al., 2020) have shown that the risk of developing ORN is minimal, particularly if the patient was edentulous and an

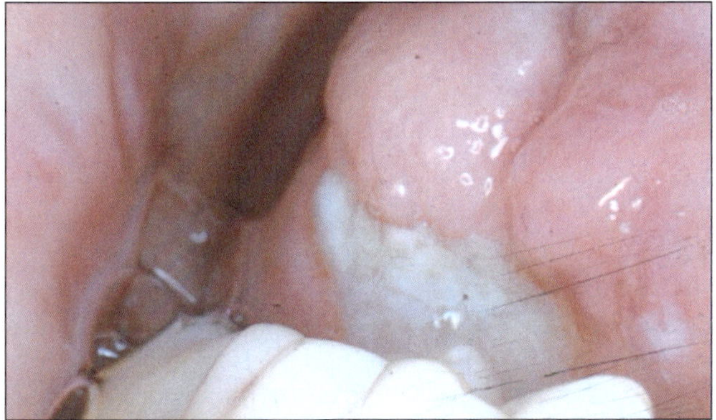

Figure 1-64 Soft tissue necrosis of the tongue.

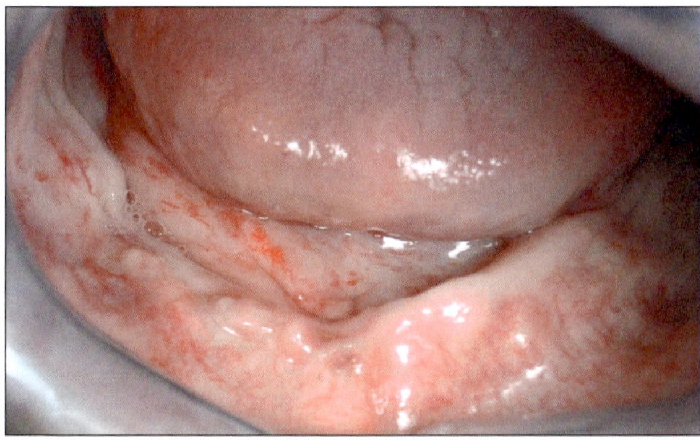

Figure 1-65 A combination of irregular bony bearing surfaces and telangiectasia of the oral mucosa predisposes the bearing surface mucosa to ulceration secondary to denture usage.

experienced denture user prior to radiotherapy. In one report from UCLA and UCSF (Beumer et al., 1976) of 92 edentulous irradiated patients who were fitted with new complete maxillary and mandibular dentures, none developed bone exposures, even though a portion of the denture-bearing surface was in the radiation field. In 87 of these patients, the mandibular denture-bearing surface was within the radiation field. It is important to note that this was a retrospective analysis of a carefully screened population of edentulous patients. If clinical examination indicated that the risk of ORN secondary to denture use was unacceptably high because of excessive and widespread radiation-induced telangiectasia combined with irregular denture-bearing surfaces and high dosage delivered to the mandibular body or a potential lack of compliance by the patient, the mandibular denture was not fabricated.

The risk of ORN is always greater in patients who require removal of teeth prior to or after completion of radiation therapy. In a joint report by UCLA and UCSF, 3 cases of bone necrosis were attributed to dentures in a group of 36 patients rendered edentulous by preradiation or postradiation extractions (Beumer et al., 1976) (see Fig 1-53). Two occurred in a group of 23 patients with preradiation extractions and 1 occurred in a group of 16 patients requiring postradiation extractions. All 3 bone necroses developed at an extraction site that had previously healed from the extraction. From a prosthodontic perspective, this finding appears to underscore the importance of adequate alveolectomies when teeth in the radiation target volume are extracted prior to or after radiation. The well-balanced process of bone remodeling is seriously disturbed by tumoricidal doses of radiation therapy. If a radical alveolectomy is not performed, the resulting alveolar ridge will be irregular and increases the risk of bony exposure in a patient wearing complete dentures, especially the mandibular denture (Fig 1-65). The mandibular denture slips and slides over the bearing surface during function and its stability is in large part dependent upon tongue control. If the denture is not properly centered on the bearing surface during a forceful closure, if the alveolar ridge is irregular, and if the bearing surface mucosa exhibits telangiectasia, the patient is at high risk of perforating denture-bearing mucosa during function.

The literature reveals few cases of bone necrosis associated with dentures that led to resection of the mandible. Almost all have been resolved with conservative treatment measures. Daly and Drane (1972) reported five cases of ORN in a group of 82 patients receiving intraoral prostheses after therapeutic radiotherapy to the head and neck region. Sixty-four patients received complete dentures and 18 received removable partial dentures. Four healed under conservative treatment and one still was present at the time of publication. Beumer et al. (1984) reported eight ORNs attributed to complete dentures or removable partial dentures. All but one occurred at either a preradiation or a postradiation extraction site. Seven healed with conservative measures and after sequestration of small amounts of nonvital bone (see Fig 1-59). The mandibular body of the eighth patient received in excess of 8,000 cGy, progressively expanded, and eventually required a partial mandibular resection. None of the patients received HBO.

Dentures and soft tissue necrosis

The risk of developing a soft tissue necrosis when complete dentures are worn following therapeutic doses of radiation appears to be relatively small and the resultant morbidity is insignificant. Rahn et al. (1968) reported observations of 50 patients for whom complete dentures had been constructed following irradiation. Two developed soft tissue necrosis. On removal of the dentures, both lesions healed without further complications. In another study, 6 of 128 edentulous patients wearing complete dentures patients developed soft tissue necroses (Beumer et al., 1976). Five of the six were attributable to the dentures. Three of the six had been treated with a combination of high-energy external radiation therapy followed by a radioactive implant. After removal of the dentures, five healed within six months without incident. The sixth patient died of a cardiovascular accident before resolution of the lesion. Consequently, when fabricating complete dentures precautions should be taken to avoid local trauma especially when border molding the peripheral extension areas. This is especially important at the tumor site because scarring and fibrosis are most severe in this region. The epithelium in this area will be quite thin and less keratinized as consequence of radiation treatments and easily perforated.

Use of silicone liners

Silicone liners have been suggested as a means of minimizing mucosal trauma in mandibular dentures (Griem et al., 1964; Rahn et al.,

1968). Clinical experience, however, has confirmed silicone to be less beneficial than polymethyl methacrylate. The silicones exhibit reduced wettability, and their hydrophobicity and inherent surface roughness contribute to increased drag that does not allow the mandibular denture to slide freely over the dry mucosal surface during function and predispose to mucosal abrasion. In patients with radiation-induced xerostomia, this phenomenon assumes added clinical significance. In a clinical report in which dentures with soft silicone liners were used in 25 patients, 8 developed soft tissue necrosis, and 1 developed ORN (Daly and Drane, 1972). The high risk of tissue abrasion plus the poor adjustability of silicone have influenced clinicians to abandon its use in irradiated patients. Moreover, as mentioned previously, the fungal-infested biofilms adherent to the silicone lead to material degradation and limit its life expectancy to only a few months (Nikawa et al., 1995, 2000a, 2000b). The incorporation of antifungal agents or antiseptics in the soft liners does not significantly reduce *Candida* adhesion or colonization (Nikawa et al., 2001; Lyons et al., 2020).

Timing of denture placement after radiation therapy

Complete dentures can be fabricated or reinserted soon after completion of radiation therapy in most patients (Beumer et al., 1976). For example, when CRT is used, if the radiation fields cover little of the mandibular denture-bearing surfaces, such as in treatment of a nasopharyngeal carcinoma, dentures can be inserted as soon as the mucositis resolves. For other patients with greater amounts of denture-bearing area in the fields, a slightly longer period of recovery is recommended. When IMRT is used for tumors in these areas, the dose to the bearing surfaces of the mandible, with some exceptions (see Fig 1-47), is generally not clinically significant, and dentures can be used on resolution of mucositis.

There are several reasons that this protocol can be recommended. Most patients who have been edentulous for extended periods (more than one year) prior to radiation therapy present with nicely remodeled denture-bearing surfaces. The bony irregularities associated with past dental extractions have long since resolved. In addition, when CRT or IMRT is employed with conventional fractionation and dosage, the kind of mucosal compromise (extensive telangiectasia, thinning, and atrophy of epithelium) that would predispose the mandibular denture-bearing surfaces to mucosal perforation from complete dentures is rare. Severe mucosal reactions to radiation are rare and found only in patients with long-standing mucosal atrophy prior to radiation, for example, secondary to diabetes mellitus or to chronic alcoholism combined with severe dietary deficiencies, or, most recently, in patients treated with chemoradiation that included CRT. In these patients, if telangiectasia is noted in the zone of the keratinized attached tissue of the mandible, use of mandibular dentures is not recommended.

Experienced complete denture wearers usually have developed the necessary neuromuscular coordination necessary for successful function with dentures and are less likely to exhibit tongue or cheek biting. Edentulous patients with a history of multiple complaints and difficulties associated with their dentures prior to radiation treatment may be at greater risk of complications with postradiation dentures. This possibility must be discussed frankly with the patient and a family member prior to prosthetic treatment and the patient must be well informed of the risks associated with dentures. Because most complaints are associated with mandibular complete dentures, rarely will these patients be pleased with their new mandibular denture.

For patients who submitted to extraction of teeth in conjunction with radical alveolectomies immediately prior to therapy or postradiation extractions, a more conservative approach is in order. In the UCLA-UCSF study of 23 patients edentulated with preradiation extractions, dentures were placed on the average of 22.2 months following completion of therapy (Beumer et al., 1976). Two cases of bone necroses developed in this group. For 13 patients (57%), dentures were delivered within one year of completion of radiation therapy. In this report (Beumer et al., 1976), 16 patients had complete dentures placed after postradiotherapy extractions were performed in the radiation field after being treated with CRT. Extractions were performed on an average of 26.1 months after therapy, and the dentures were inserted on the average of 11.8 months later. One patient developed ORN associated with his denture at a recent extraction site.

Based on this report and other studies (Rahn et al., 1968; Beumer et al., 1976), the status of the residual ridge is probably the most important clinical factor to be considered when calculating the risk of complete denture usage. Since the mandibular denture slips and slides over the bearing surfaces during function, patient presenting with an irregular mandibular ridge in which the entire body of the mandible is heavily irradiated may prompt the clinician to defer placement of dentures indefinitely. On the other hand, a smooth, well-contoured mandibular denture-bearing surface may enable the clinician to insert dentures quite soon after therapy.

In summary, clinicians should differentiate between those patients who are edentulous and have used dentures prior to therapy and those who underwent extraction of teeth in the field of radiation prior to therapy and have not subsequently used complete dentures. Long-term edentulous patients have little risk of developing significant complications from wearing dentures so, in most instances, it seems justified to provide dentures to these patients soon after radiation therapy, particularly if they were irradiated with IMRT. Deferring denture use in this group for the 12 to 18 months, as was often advocated in the past, is unnecessary (Rahn et al., 1968; Krajicek, 1969; Daly and Drane, 1972). The dentate patients rendered edentulous either before or after radiation therapy have a greater risk of developing complications from dentures, and deferment of dentures for extended periods may be in order for selected patients with irregular denture-bearing surfaces and widespread telangiectasia of the bearing surface mucosa.

When IMRT is used to irradiate tumors of the oropharynx or nasopharynx, the bearing surfaces of the mandible receive relatively low doses and therefore the risk of ORN is negligible. However, when tumors of the oral tongue and floor of the mouth are irradiated with IMRT, portions of the bearing surface may be within the gross tumor volume and exposed to high doses; this factor should be taken into consideration. If the high-dose volume is relatively small, the risk of ORN is probably very low in patients treated with IMRT. Likewise, for the same reasons, the risk of ORN secondary to placement of osseointegrated implants theoretically should be low when IMRT is used; if the patient presents with a compromised mandibular denture-bearing surface, a retruded tongue position, and unfavorable floor of the mouth contours and experiences difficulty tolerating dentures, implants should be considered because of the anticipated dramatic improvements in mastication.

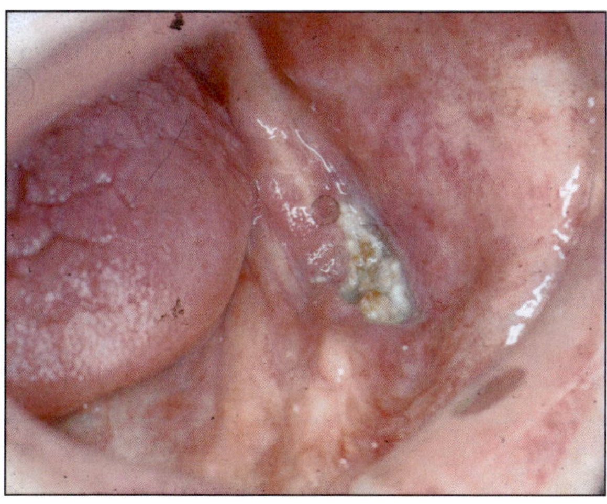

Figure 1-66 This ORN extends beyond the zone of attached mucosa. Denture use is contraindicated.

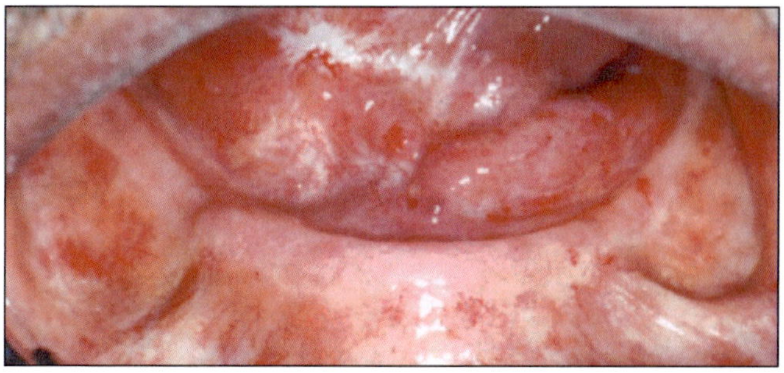

Figure 1-67 Severe radiation-induced mucosal atrophy. Note the prominent telangiectasia. The patient is a poor candidate for mandibular dentures.

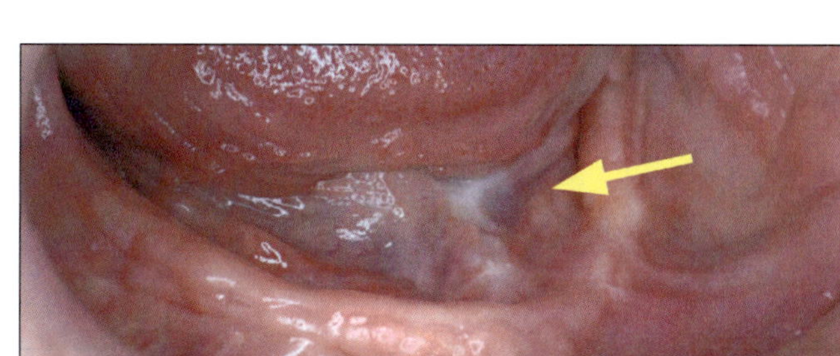

Figure 1-68 Patient who received 68 Gy of CRT via opposed mandibular fields. Note scarring at the tumor site *(arrow)*. Denture use is permitted, but overextension of the denture flange at this site may lead to ORN.

Dentures and preexisting bone necrosis

The possibility exists for selected patients to use mandibular or maxillary dentures over areas of exposed bone within the radiation field in compliant patients (Beumer, 1976). Ideally the bone exposures should be well localized with significant amounts of circumscribing attached mucosa (see Fig 1-59). If the bone exposure extends beyond the attached keratinized mucosa dentures should not be worn (Fig 1-66). Utmost caution, however, should be exercised when a patient is allowed to wear dentures over bone necroses. Proper relief must be provided in the denture, and the patient should understand the risks of denture use and be available for close follow-up.

Prosthodontic procedures

When dentures are considered for a patient, it must be remembered that ORN is a phenomenon confined almost exclusively to the mandible. Extreme care should be taken in construction of the mandibular denture base to ensure distribution of pressure as widely and as equally as possible over the mandibular denture bearing surface during function. Likewise, any occlusal scheme should attempt to minimize lateral movement of the mandibular denture base.

Exam findings of importance

Prior to the construction of complete dentures, the clinician must contact the radiation therapist who treated the patient and inform the therapist of the intention. Information collected from the therapist should include the type and site of the tumor, mode of therapy employed (external, interstitial, or combination), dose to the clinical target volume, dates of treatment, radiation fields if CRT was used, dose distribution if IMRT was employed, tumor response, and the prognosis for disease control.

When the patient is interviewed, a history of successful use of complete dentures prior to therapy is an accurate indicator of future success. The patient's attitude toward himself or herself and the disease is of prime importance. Many patients are emotionally distraught over the uncertainty regarding cure and the morbidity inflicted by their radiation treatment. These attitudes should be anticipated, and psychosocial counseling should be provided when appropriate (see Chapter 9). An uncooperative, poorly motivated patient is a poor candidate for postradiation denture service. The clinician must remember the objective of rehabilitation—in other words, the return of the patient to society. Without a prosthesis, this objective may not be realized (Curtis et al., 1976).

Initial oral examination will reveal important clinical manifestations of radiation treatment, including the appearance of oral mucous membranes, scarring and fibrosis at the tumor site, the degree of trismus, the presence and nature of lymphedema, and the status of salivary function. The appearance of oral mucous membranes is an important and valuable indicator of radiation response. A translucent, boggy mucosa with prominent telangiectasia implies poor tolerance to prosthodontic restorations and an increased risk of compromising mucosal integrity (Fig 1-67). If severe mucosal changes are present, use of dentures may be deferred indefinitely.

Scarring at the tumor site may be quite prominent, especially if brachytherapy was employed. Particular note should be taken when the tumor included floor-of-the-mouth lesions, because some limitation in extension of the mandibular lingual flange at the site of the tumor may be prudent. Scar tissue is unyielding, and the slightest overextension may result in a mucosal perforation (Fig 1-68).

Excessive trismus is often observed in patients with oropharyngeal and/or pharyngeal lesions treated with chemoradiation and

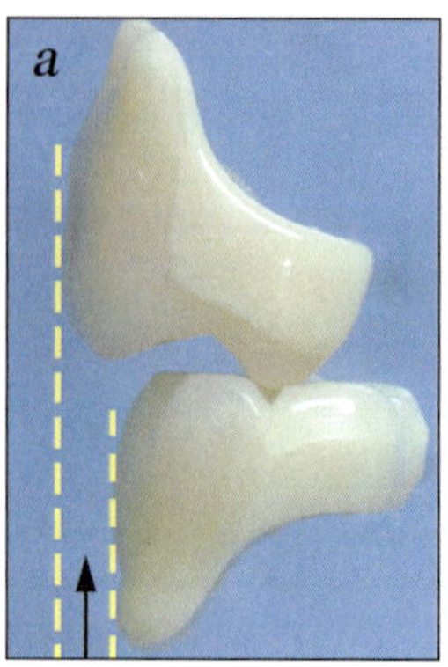

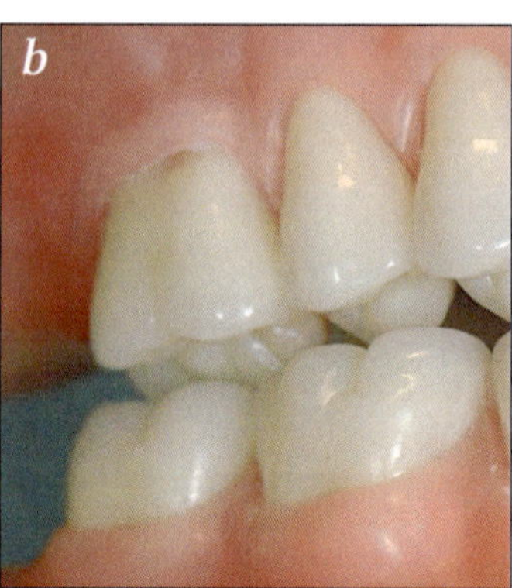

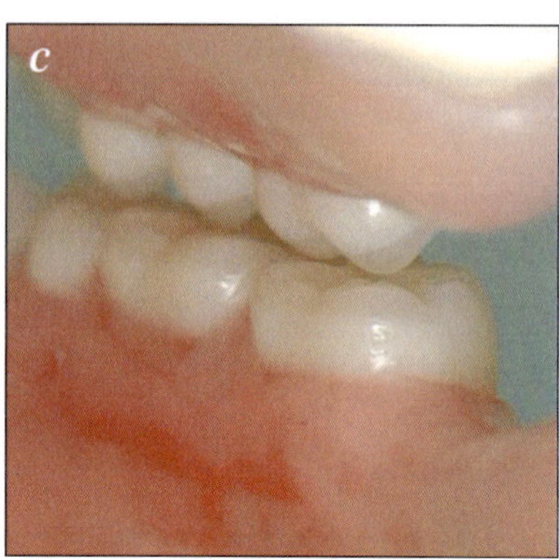

Figure 1-69 *(a, b, and c)* Use of a lingualized tooth form in the maxilla and a nonanatomic tooth form in the mandible will reduce the risk of cheek biting.

where the temporomandibular joint and the muscles of mastication were exposed to moderate to high doses. In these patients, an exercise program should be initiated as soon as possible after therapy. Dynamic bite openers are not as effective in edentulous patients as they are in dentulous patients but occasionally may be useful with modification.

As has been noted previously, the amount and viscosity of saliva are important determinants of prosthodontic success. Compromised salivary function leads to more friction at the denture mucosa interface and therefore more mucosal irritation. The less saliva, the more difficulty the patient will have tolerating dentures. In addition, the retention of the maxillary complete denture may be compromised because of the film thickness of the scanty and more mucinous saliva. The posterior palatal seal area should be carefully inspected. If the palatine salivary glands have been exposed to doses in excess of 40 Gy, these glands become replaced with fibrous connective tissue. Displacement of this area with the usual and customary postpalatal seal may be difficult, compromising peripheral seal of the maxillary denture.

No specific technique is advantageous over any other in the construction of dentures for these patients. The clinician should employ those methods with which he or she is most familiar and follow prosthodontic principles.

The clinician should also examine the denture foundation area thoroughly for undercuts, tori, high tissue attachments, enlarged maxillary tuberosities, flabby and redundant tissue, lack of attached gingiva, retruded tongue position, unfavorable floor of the mouth contours, and abnormal maxillomandibular relationships. Any condition that compromises the prosthetic prognosis in nonirradiated patients assumes added significance in irradiated patients. For example, patients who have mandibular ridges with severe bilateral undercuts or excessive ridge resorption with little attached mucosa are poor candidates for complete denture service following radiation therapy.

Impressions

Conventional border molding using a custom tray and impression compound is advocated for making impressions. Border molding should be performed with care to avoid overextension. If the patient's xerostomia is particularly profound, a thin coating of petrolatum may be applied over the soft modeling plastic to prevent its sticking to the dry mucosa. Particular attention should be paid to the lingual extension of the mandibular denture because overextension could result in a mucosal perforation.

Displacement of the tissues of the floor of the mouth in an attempt to obtain peripheral seal is not advocated. Peripheral seal is virtually impossible to obtain in these patients because of the curtailment of the patient's salivary flow. Efforts to develop the lingual flange should be directed toward gaining stability rather than retention.

Edema of the tongue and floor of the mouth, which is particularly prominent if the patient has undergone a radical neck dissection, will occasionally be sufficiently extensive to compromise tongue space, compromise floor-of-the-mouth posture, and limit the extent of the lingual flange.

Any of the traditional impression materials may be used with success. The clinician should use the material with which he or she feels most comfortable. The prime objective is to obtain an impression that displaces as little tissue as possible. The mylohyoid ridge is a critical area in which to avoid excessive pressure. How the clinician accomplishes this depends on what works best in his or her hands. Removal of residual viscous secretions with gauze or a mouth rinse immediately before the final impression is obtained will improve surface detail.

Determination of the occlusal vertical dimension

The completed impressions are boxed and poured into dental stone. Record bases and wax rims are prepared in the usual way and used to determine the vertical dimension of occlusion. The traditional methods of determining vertical dimension are applicable, such as phonetics, closest speaking distance, swallowing, neuromuscular perception, and vertical dimension of rest.

For some patients the clinician should consider reducing the vertical dimension of occlusion. In patients with clinically significant trismus, entrance of the bolus is more easily accomplished by increasing the interocclusal space. Occasionally patients present with severe scarring of the tongue and experience difficulty elevating the tongue, and in these patients, it may be useful to lower the occlusal plane.

Centric relation records are obtained in the usual manner. Wax, plaster, zinc oxide paste, and silicone are suitable media for obtaining the final registrations. Graphic recording devices can similarly be successfully employed. There is no evidence that a therapeutic course of radiation therapy results in changes of mandibular lateral border or intraborder movements during mastication.

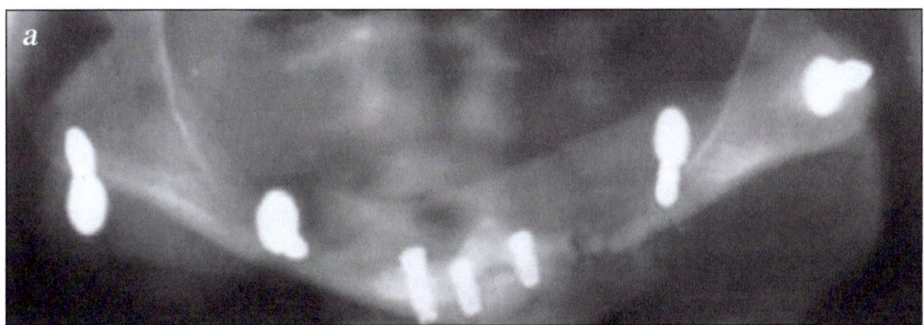

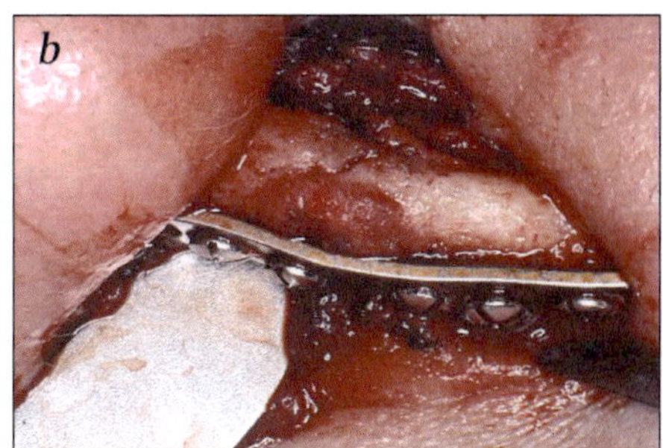

Figure 1-70 *(a)* This patient received a dose of 6,000 cGy to the body of the mandible prior to implant placement. The mandible fractured through the left posterior implant site two weeks after implant surgery. *(b)* The fracture was reduced with miniplates, and external fixation was used to stabilize the fragments. Ultimately the fracture site healed, probably because of the relatively low radiation dose delivered.

Occlusal forms

It is not possible with the information available to determine the relative efficacy of any particular occlusal scheme for the construction of complete dentures for irradiated patients. In our review of 128 patients, both anatomical teeth and nonanatomical forms with full balance were employed (Beumer et al., 1976). On a theoretical basis, however, we have come to favor lingualized or monoplane occlusal schemes in which the balance is facilitated with posteriorly situated balancing ramps. Studies in the past appear to indicate that less horizontal force is generated by a nonanatomical occlusal scheme and this, if true, would be of obvious advantage to irradiated patients (Frechette, 1955; Kydd, 1956; Sharry et al., 1960).

When posterior teeth are arranged, careful attention should be directed toward attaining proper buccal horizontal overlap. We favor a lingualized maxillary tooth form opposing a mandibular nonanatomic tooth form (Fig 1-69). Some clinicians use only three posterior teeth, one premolar and two molars. These two strategies will minimize the risk of cheek biting particularly posteriorly. In some patients, edema of the tongue and buccal mucosa is prominent, and tongue and cheek biting are not uncommon. Occlusal trauma may lead to soft tissue necrosis, particularly in patients whose tongue lesions were treated with brachytherapy. Whether anatomical or nonanatomical posterior teeth are used, balanced articulation is mandatory.

Delivery and postinsertion care

Occlusal discrepancies caused by processing errors should be eliminated before the dentures are removed from the cast. After removal, any rough projections on the tissue surface should be smoothed. Pressure indicator paste is used to identify areas of excessive pressure, and disclosing wax is useful in delineating overextension of denture flanges. Remounting the dentures on a suitable articulator with new maxillomandibular records made at the time of delivery is mandatory. Light polishing of the bearing surface of the mandibular denture is advisable.

The patient is given an instruction sheet detailing possible problems and precautions. Instructions concerning removal of the dentures if soreness develops, the necessity for periodic return visits, and the initial limited use of the prosthesis for mastication are provided. Complete dentures should never be worn while the patient is sleeping.

The care provided after delivery of dentures is critical and requires an understanding patient to avoid untoward complications. During the first week, 24 and 48-hour recall appointments are recommended, regardless of how well the patient is tolerating the dentures. At the end of the adjustment period, the patient is required to return four times during the first year. If the patient continues to present without complications, the interval between visits may be lengthened during succeeding years.

The risk of serious postradiation sequelae in denture wearers is small. However, individual reactions to therapeutic doses of radiation may vary greatly, and good judgment and sound technique are factors that can never be ignored in placement of prostheses in postradiation patients. Cooperation of the patient is a necessity. Without such cooperation, the best intentions of the dentist may result in bone or soft tissue necrosis. The patient must understand the tissue changes resulting from radiation treatments and must be available for close follow-up.

Dental Implants in Irradiated Tissues

Radiation effects on osseointegration

Irradiation of head and neck tumors predisposes to changes in mucosa and bone (Silverman and Chierici, 1965; Rohrer et al., 1979) that affect the predictability of osseointegrated implants (see Fig 1-33). Osseointegration requires initial implant anchorage and immobilization, the formation of a clot between the surface of the implant and the osteotomy site, release of growth factors, angiogenesis, migration of mesenchymal stem cells to the surface of the implant, and deposition of bone on the surface of the implant and the osteotomy site. However, these biologic processes may be compromised or absent in patients exposed to high-dose radiation. As a result, anchorage of implants in bone may be primarily mechanical as opposed to biologic, especially when the dose to the implant sites exceeds 5,500 cGy (Nishimura, 1996). Moreover, osteoclastic activity continues in some patients (see Fig 1-35), diminishing the mineral content of the jawbones within the clinical target volume and reducing the thickness of the cortical layers and the volume of individual trabeculae (see Fig 1-34). These changes make the mandible more susceptible to fracture secondary to implant placement (Fig 1-70). Moreover, it is more difficult to achieve initial primary stability of the implants (Karayazgan-Saracoglu et al., 2015) in sites that have been exposed to tumoricidal doses of radiation, particularly maxillary sites.

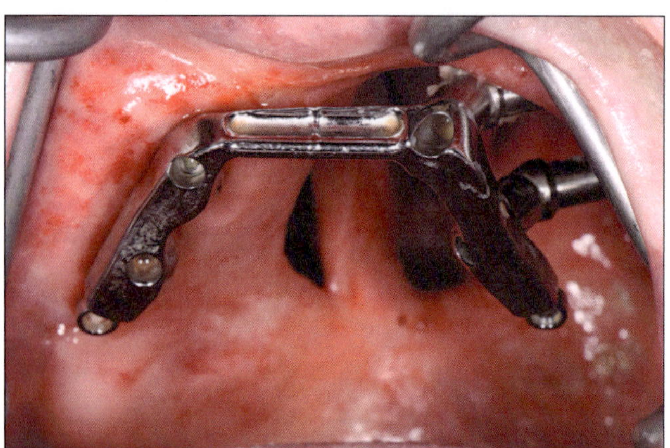

Figure 1-71 The addition of implants enables patients with major palatal resections to dramatically improve oral function. This implant connecting bar serves to retain a large complete denture-obturator prosthesis, effectively sealing the defect, but also provides sufficient support for reasonable levels of masticatory efficiency.

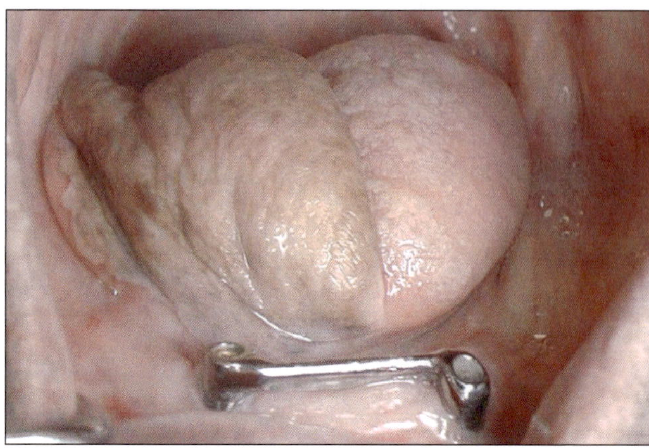

Figure 1-72 Patient who underwent a hemi-glossectomy and reconstruction of the tongue with a free vascularized flap. The patient received 5,500 cGy of radiation postoperatively. Without implants, given the compromise of the denture-bearing surfaces, the use of a mandibular complete denture would not be possible.

Furthermore, long-term function of osseointegrated implants is dependent on the presence of viable bone that is capable of remodeling and turnover as the implant is subjected to stresses associated with supporting, retaining, and stabilizing prosthetic restorations. These processes are compromised, or perhaps entirely lacking, in heavily irradiated bone (Nishimura et al., 1996; Bolind et al., 2006). Given the adverse effect of high doses of radiation, remodeling and turnover of bone are significantly compromised to the point that an implant subjected to functional stresses may not be sustained indefinitely.

Risks and potential benefits

Maxilla

The potential benefit provided by implants in patients with large palatal defects customarily outweighs the potential morbidity associated with implant placement or the higher rates of implant failure observed in heavily irradiated patients. Implants are highly beneficial for edentulous patients or those whose residual dentition is insufficient to properly retain, stabilize, and support obturator prostheses used to restore large palatal defects. In particular, complete denture-obturator prostheses in edentulous patients, designed to restore such defects, lack the retention, stability, and support to restore even a minimal level of mastication. Such prostheses primarily restore speech and swallowing but the masticatory performance score for these patients is essentially zero (Garrett, 2008). The addition of implants provides retention, stability, and support for the prosthesis so that masticatory performance is restored to presurgical levels in some patients (Garrett, 2008; Buurman et al., 2020a, 2020b) (Fig 1-71). The long-term survival rate of implants placed in edentulous maxillectomy patients whose implant sites have been irradiated is relatively low compared with that in nonirradiated patients (55% to 65% for irradiated sites versus 90% or greater for nonirradiated patients). Nonetheless, the placement of implants in these patients is justified on the basis that the risk of osteoradionecrosis (ORN) is extremely low in the maxilla and there is substantial functional benefit derived from implant-retained maxillary obturator prostheses.

Mandible

The primary concern with implant placement in the irradiated mandible is the risk of ORN, which is almost entirely dependent on the dose administered to the implant sites. If the patient is treated with radiation alone, and the implant sites are subjected to doses in excess of 6,500 cGy, the placement of implants for the purpose of improving masticatory performance is not easily justified because of the significant risk of osteoradionecrosis. If the dose is below 6,000 cGy, the risk of ORN secondary to implant placement is almost negligible and justified if the patient is having difficulty masticating with a conventional complete denture. In such patients an implant-assisted overdenture can dramatically improve masticatory efficiency and make a significant difference in their quality of life (Buurman et al., 2013), especially those presenting with unfavorable floor-of-mouth posture and a retruded tongue position. When the mandibular prosthesis is implant-retained, the patient can focus primarily on manipulating the food bolus as opposed to stabilizing and retaining a conventional denture.

The functional benefit obtained from implant placement in the irradiated reconstructed tongue and edentulous mandible is less clear and mostly dependent on the functional status of the reconstructed tongue. Frequently the mandibular bearing surfaces are compromised to the point where the use of a conventional denture is not possible. However, if the tongue bulk is restored and mobility of the unresected portion is maintained, an implant retained overdenture may significantly improve masticatory performance and the quality of life (Buurman et al., 2013). Such protheses can also serve to support and recontour the lower lip, permitting lip seal with the upper lip, leading to improved speech and control of saliva (see Chapter 2). Although the flaps used to reconstruct the tongue are essentially nonsensate, if the bolus is confined to the unresected side it can be manipulated effectively, and mastication can be maintained at reasonable levels with an implant retained overdenture (Fig 1-72). Moreover, the risk of osteoradionecrosis when the dose delivered is less than 6,000 cGy is almost negligible, and those that do develop are generally self-limiting and heal with conservative measures (Beumer et al., 1984). Implant-assisted overdenture

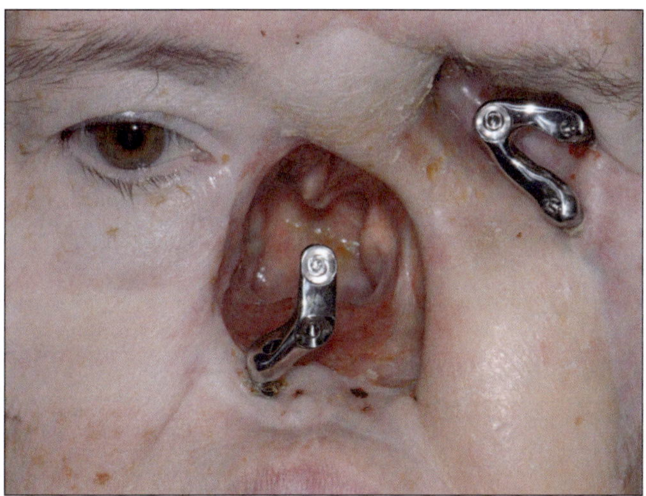

Figure 1-73 Implants dramatically improve the retention and stability provided for large facial prostheses.

designs are preferred because of compromised implant anchorage and the need to provide support for the lower lip, with a denture flange in such patients (see section below entitled "Recommendations for patient selection and treatment").

In dentate patients, when the resected mandible, tongue, and floor-of-mouth region have been reconstructed with a free osteomyocutaneous vascularized flap, the value of implants is less clear. Given the fact that these flaps are nonsensate, almost all effective mastication will be conducted on the unresected side. If the unresected residual mandible is dentate and these teeth are in reasonable condition, these teeth can be used to retain and stabilize a removable dental prosthesis. If needed, the prosthesis can be extended onto the resected side to provide support for the cheek and lower lip and replace the missing dentition, and these objectives can be easily accomplished with an RPD. Implants are placed only if the residual dentition is not up to the task. Implants in irradiated vascularized osteomyocutaneous flaps used to reconstruct the mandible appear to fare equally as well as in the irradiated native mandible, given equivalent doses.

Craniofacial sites

Irradiated patients with facial defects secondary to tumor ablation also will gain significant advantage from the placement of implants (Fig 1-73) (see Chapter 5, section entitled "Craniofacial Implants"). Implant-retained facial prostheses have changed patients' perceptions of rehabilitation, and patients favor implant-retained prostheses over adhesive-retained prostheses by a wide margin (Chang et al., 2005). In irradiated sites, with the exception of the irradiated orbit, success rates are good, and little morbidity is associated with implant failure (Granström et al., 1994; Roumanas et al., 1994, 2002; Beumer et al., 1995; Subramaniam et al., 2018).

Predictability of implants in irradiated bone

Clinical reports and animal studies indicate that the success-failure rate of osseointegrated implants in irradiated bone appears to be dependent on various factors, including the anatomical site, the dose to the site, the lengths of the implants used, and the use of hyperbaric oxygen (HBO). Dosage to the potential implant sites is dependent on the mode of radiation (CRT, IMRT, brachytherapy, etc.), the gross tumor volume, and the clinical target volume. The use of concomitant chemotherapy during radiation (chemoradiation) may also have a significant impact on the viability of tissues within the clinical target volume because of escalation of the biologically equivalent radiation dose.

Animal studies

As mentioned previously, the wound-healing potential of irradiated bone is severely compromised. In addition, the density of potential bone sites is diminished because the multicellular unit responsible for remodeling and repair of bone is compromised, and bone resorption continues, probably secondary to the presence of isolated osteoclasts (see Fig 1-35). Animal experiments have shown that when bone is irradiated, not only is the bone-implant contact area reduced, but also the quality of the bone that eventually anchors the implant is compromised (Jacobsson et al., 1988; Nishimura, 1996; Asikainen et al., 1998; Weinlander et al., 2006).

Weinlander et al. (2006) tested the feasibility of placing implants at the time of tumor resection followed by postoperative radiation. They tested three different types of implants using a dog model. Three implants (machined-surface implants, plasma spray–surface implants, and hydroxyapatite-coated implants) were placed on one side of the mandible in seven dogs. After three months of healing, 21 implants in the seven dogs were recovered with block section and served as controls. After a suitable period of healing, these three selected implants were positioned in the contralateral mandible of each of the seven dogs. Radiation commenced three weeks later. A dose equivalent to 5,000 cGy was delivered to these sites.

The specimens were recovered three months later, and studies conducted included histomorphometric analysis of the bone-implant contact area. For the machined-surface implants, the bone-implant contact area was 34% for the nonirradiated control specimens and 24% for the irradiated specimens; for the titanium plasma spray–surface implants, the contact area was 50% for nonirradiated controls and 45% for irradiated specimens.

Nishimura et al. (1996) tested the feasibility of placing implants in bone sites that had already been irradiated. The researchers assigned 44 adult New Zealand rabbits at random to six test groups (Fig 1-74). The animals received radiation to either the proximal or diaphyseal segment of both tibias. Equivalent doses ranged from 4,000 to 7,000 cGy. Three months after completion of radiation treatment, 5 mm screw-type, machined-surfaced implants were placed in each half of the left tibia of the surviving 38 rabbits. Polyfluorochrome labeling was performed three months after implant placement and two days prior to sacrifice. Ground nondecalcified sections were prepared and evaluated. Results revealed a steady decrease in the label, especially with the equivalent dosage of 5,800 cGy and greater, indicating reduced cellular activity. At these dose levels, there was virtually no contact osteogenesis on the implant surface. In addition, when viewed under polarized light, the specimens receiving doses equivalent to 5,200 cGy and greater showed a preponderance of woven bone, in contrast to the dense lamellar bone observed in the control specimens (Nishimura et al., 1996) (Fig 1-75). The quality of bone in the implant appositional zone was compromised at radiation dose

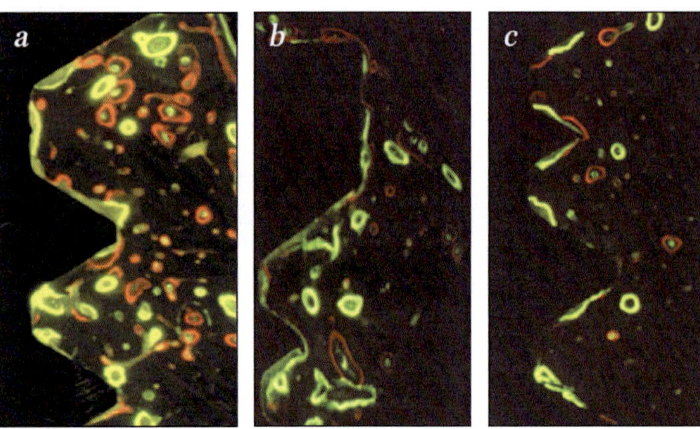

Figure 1-74 *(a)* Normal control specimen. Note both contact and distance osteogenesis (×40). *(b)* Specimen exposed to equivalent to 52 Gy. Note dramatic reduction in osteogenesis (×40). *(c)* Specimen exposed to 58 Gy. Note further reduction of osteogenesis (×40) (courtesy of Dr. R. Nishimura).

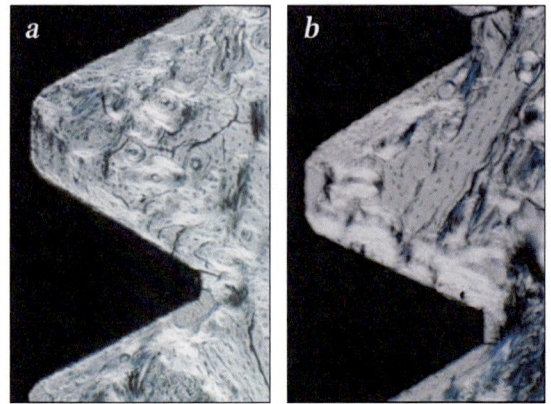

Figure 1-75 *(a)* Specimen received the equivalent of 49 Gy. Normal lamellar bone is seen in the appositional zone (×40). *(b)* Specimen received equivalent to 66 Gy (×40). Note the woven bone in the appositional zone (courtesy of Dr. R. Nishimura).

levels as low as the equivalent of 5,200 cGy. At the highest levels of radiation, very little (if any) bone was deposited on the surface of the implants and little distance osteogenesis was observed.

To summarize the most significant animal studies, at radiation levels equivalent to tumoricidal doses (greater than 6,500 cGy), little or no bone is deposited on the implant surface, and the remodeling apparatus is severely compromised. Implant anchorage is essentially mechanical as opposed to biologic. At doses equivalent to those used for postoperative radiation therapy (5,000 to 6,000 cGy), a greater component of woven bone is observed at the interface, and the compromise or absence of remodeling elements makes it less likely that this immature bone will be replaced by mature lamellar bone in the usual time frame, if ever.

At these doses, even if the implant becomes osseointegrated, the bone-implant contact area is decreased compared with that observed in nonirradiated controls, compromising the load-bearing capacity of the implant. In the event an implant does achieve osseointegration (e.g., if it is placed prior to radiation), late postradiation changes in bone (i.e., occlusion of medium-sized arteries, compromise of the microcirculation, death of osteocytes, and loss of the multicellular unit composed of osteoclasts and osteoblasts responsible for remodeling of bone) mean that bone remodeling is severely compromised; eventually the bone anchorage will be degraded, and the response of the implant to occlusal forces will be compromised. Diminished blood supply and fibrosis in the marrow and mucoperiosteum predispose sites to peri-implantitis and implant loss and, in the mandible exposed to doses equivalent to 6,500 cGy and greater, may lead to ORN (see Fig 1-77).

However, no animal model truly reflects human biology. The tissues and vascular systems of lower-form vertebrates are more tolerant of radiation damage than humans. Also, use of the mathematical biologic equivalent of human doses in a single administration, or use of fewer fractions with large doses, serves a mathematical purpose but does not guarantee biologically equivalent outcomes. In addition, animal studies are yet to report the impact of adjuvant chemotherapy on osseointegration. Nevertheless, based on animal studies it is reasonable to make the following assumptions regarding the use of osseointegrated implants in humans:

The success rates of implants in

- irradiated bone will be lower than rates in nonirradiated bone. The higher the dose, the more likely it is that the long-term success rates will be lower.
- As the dose to the implant sites increases and anchorage becomes more mechanical as opposed to biologic, the load-carrying capacity of implants in irradiated bone will be lower than the load-carrying capacity of implants in nonirradiated bone.
- Because of compromise in the remodeling apparatus of bone, a significant number of late failures should be anticipated, even in bone sites with good quality, such as the anterior mandible (Brasseur et al., 2006).
- Because of persistent osteoclastic activity secondary to residual, isolated functioning osteoclasts, the quality of the irradiated bone is compromised (less dense) and initial anchorage of the implants may be more difficult to achieve, especially in the maxilla.
- In the mandible, the risk of ORN becomes significant at higher doses (greater than 6,500 cGy with conventional fractionation or its biologic equivalent).
- Because of the above (compromised remodeling apparatus and impaired anchorage, etc.), long-term clinical observations (more than five years of follow-up) will be needed to properly assess the success-failure rates of implants in response to various radiation doses.

Human studies

The trends observed in human studies appear to substantiate the concerns raised in the animal studies (Jacobsson et al., 1988; Parel and Tjellström, 1991; Granström et al., 1992, 1994, 2005a, 2005b; Roumanas et al., 1994, 1997, 2002; Esser et al., 1997; Nimi et al., 1993; Visch et al., 2002; Yerit et al., 2006; Visser, 2008; Chambrone et al., 2013; Dholam et al., 2013; Chrcanovic et al., 2016; Shugaa-Addin et al., 2016; Pellegrino et al., 2018; Subramaniam et al., 2018). The report by Granström (2005a) remains the largest series in the literature and is especially revealing. He analyzed the failures of 631 implants placed in 107 irradiated patients over a 25-year period. He compared the patterns of failure in this group of patients with those in a group of 100 nonirradiated patients with similar profiles in whom 614 implants were placed.

In the irradiated group, tumors were most commonly associated with the orbit (24), followed by the maxillary sinus (23), ear (17), skin (8), floor of the mouth (5), tonsil (4), tongue (4), maxilla (3), nasal cavity (2), palate (1), oropharynx (1), and buccal mucosa (1). Ten additional patients presented with tumors in other sites. These patients were treated with high-energy CRT. Ninety-three patients received their CRT prior to surgical ablation, and 14 were irradiated postoperatively.

In the study population, 528 implants were placed within the clinical target volume after radiation, 58 implants were irradiated after implant installation, and 14 others were placed in irradiated tissues and then were exposed to a second course of radiation. Doses were calculated for each implant site. Adjuvant chemotherapy was used in 29 patients, and 141 implants were placed in these patients. Granström (2005a) placed 53.8% (340) of the implants in conjunction with HBO treatments. Screw-type machined-surface implants were used in all patients.

In the irradiated group, 146 implants (23.1%) failed: 117 of 291 in the non-HBO group (40.2%) and 29 of 340 in the HBO group (8.5%). The shortest implants demonstrated the lowest survival rates, and the author suggested that this was probably due to the inability of these implants to withstand the loading forces. The use of longer "oral-type" implants in craniofacial sites reduced the implant failure rate.

Granström (2005a) noted that the higher the radiation dose, the poorer the results. Particularly high losses were observed in patients who received two courses of radiotherapy, one before implant placement and one after. He added that the longer the time after radiation therapy, the poorer the results. The highest failure rates were observed in the frontal bone, followed by the zygoma, mandible, and nasal maxilla. Failure rates for osseointegrated implants were substantially reduced with the use of HBO for all sites except the temporal-parietal region.

The craniofacial implant data reported by the UCLA team (Roumanas et al., 1994, 2002) are consistent with the pattern and distribution of failures reported by Granström (2005a). Roumanas et al. (2002) reported the outcomes of 207 implants placed in craniofacial defects in 72 patients (follow-up of 5 to 14 years). Of the implants followed for at least five years, only 52% placed in irradiated bone were still present, as opposed to 85% in nonirradiated sites. Only 27% of the implants placed in an irradiated supraorbital rim survived five years, while implants placed in a nonirradiated supraorbital rim had a 70% survival rate. Doses delivered to all irradiated sites exceeded 5,000 cGy.

Data reported by Parel and Tjellström et al. (1991), Visser et al. (2008), and Subramaniam et al. (2018) suggest similar trends. In an attempt to reverse these trends, in recent years clinicians have used longer dental implants without flanges to retain facial prostheses (Flood and Downie, 2009; Proops et al., 2009). The initial data appear favorable, but the long-term results of this practice have yet to be determined. Others have attempted to improve implant success rates in craniofacial sites with adjuvant HBO (Granström, 2005b).

In the maxilla, the implant failure rate has been substantially higher in irradiated patients than in nonirradiated patients (Roumanas et al., 1997; Nimi et al., 1993; Visch et al., 2002; Sammartino et al., 2011; Carr, 2010). A significantly higher failure rate at stage-two surgery has been reported for the irradiated maxilla compared with the nonirradiated maxilla, but many of the failures occurred after the implants were placed in function (Carr, 2010). Roumanas et al. (1997) reported on the results of 33 implants placed in the irradiated maxillae of 13 patients. All patients received at least 5,000 cGy to the implant sites. The researchers reported that 11 of 33 failed to osseointegrate or were lost after loading and 2 others were buried beneath the mucosa for a success rate of 63.6%. Many of the surviving implants demonstrated moderate to severe bone loss (bone loss extending to at least the level of the fourth thread), particularly those placed in the premaxillary segment.

In the mandible, initial reports indicated higher short-term success rates, but subsequent studies with long-term follow-up, indicate that the numbers of failures increase as a function of time, a pattern seen previously in the craniofacial and maxilla sites. For example, Yerit et al. (2006) reported long-term results of 316 implants placed in 71 patients. All patients were treated with chemotherapy (mitomycin C and 5-fluorouracil) presurgically followed by CRT. The patients received 200 cGy per fraction and 25 fractions for a total of 5,000 cGy. Following radiation, the local tumor site was surgically removed in combination with a neck dissection. The site was immediately reconstructed, as needed, with local flaps or free vascularized flaps. Free vascularized flaps from the iliac crest, radial forearm, and jejunum were used, depending on whether the defect consisted of soft tissue or combined bone and soft tissue. Most patients presented initially with T2 to T4 squamous cell carcinomas. The implants were placed at various intervals (0.34 to 6.35 years) following surgery. Based on a careful review of the radiation treatment records of these patients, implants were identified as positioned in the irradiated residual mandible, the nonirradiated residual mandible, or in grafted sites. Implant success was defined by the absence of implant mobility and bone loss less than one-third the length of the implant. The success rate of 154 implants placed in the irradiated residual mandibular sites was 93% at one year, 90% at two years, 84% at five years, and 72% at eight years. The success rate of 84 implants placed in the non-irradiated residual mandibular sites was 99% at one year, 99% at two years, 99% at five years, and 95% at eight years. The success rate of 78 implants placed in grafted mandibular sites was 96% at one year, 96% at two years, 96% at five years, and 54% at eight years.

What phenomenon is responsible for the differences in success rates among the different sites? Given sufficient follow-up time, will the success rates be relatively equal? For example, why is the success rate of implants placed in the irradiated mandible higher than that in the irradiated maxilla, given the fact that the post-radiation blood supply is less impaired in the maxilla (which has an initially better blood supply) than in the mandible? The most likely explanation is that the high short-term success rates in the mandible can be attributed to the better initial implant anchorage and stabilization achieved in the anterior mandible, while the large number of long-term mandibular failures is suggestive of mechanical anchorage as opposed to biologic. Osseointegration in the usual sense probably does not occur because the mesenchymal stem cells are either absent or substantially reduced in number, and the activity of those still present is impaired.

Of note was the fact that in many of the early studies, machined-surface, straight-wall implants were used in the irradiated maxilla. The use of tapered implants with variable thread patterns available today permits better initial implant stabilization in poor-quality bone sites and may improve patient outcomes in radiated sites, especially in the maxilla.

Some clinicians have attempted to improve the viability of periosteum and bone with adjuvant HBO (Marx, 1993; Granström, 2005b, 2006; Salinas et al., 2010; Shah et al., 2017). HBO promotes

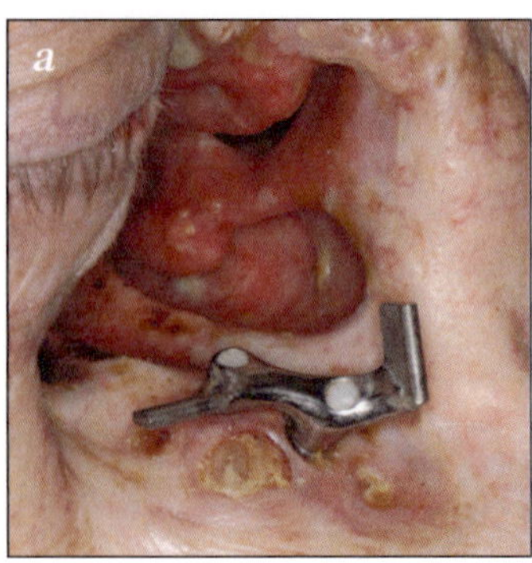
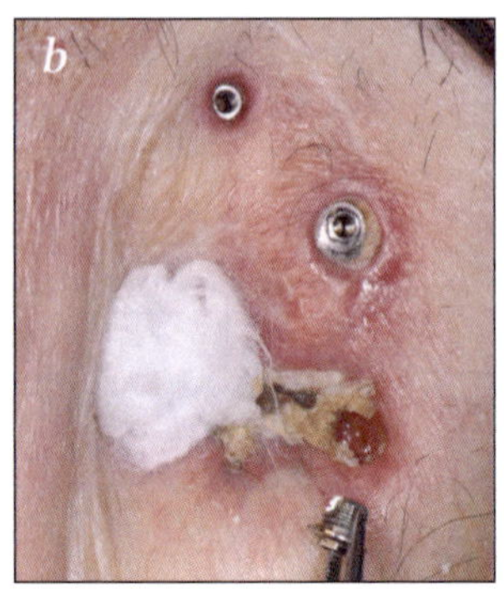
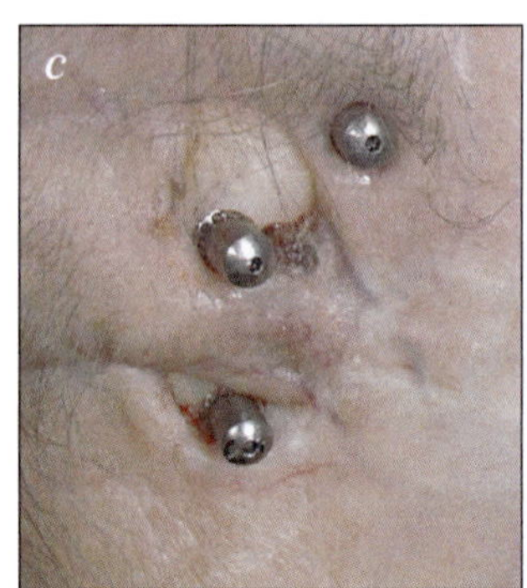
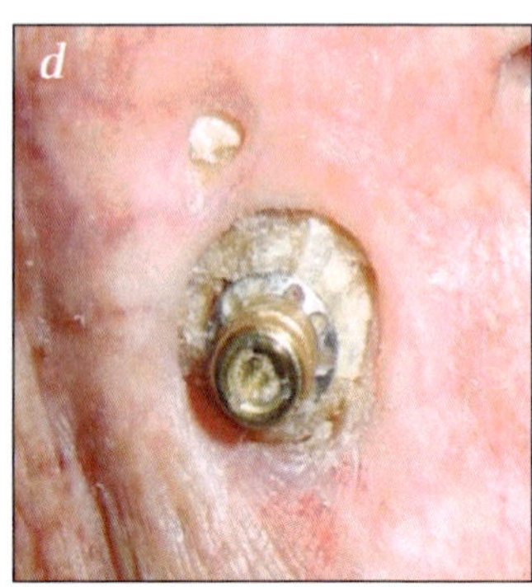

Figure 1-76 ORN associated with implants in the *(a)* floor of the nose and *(b, c, and d)* the mastoid area. All patients had received radiation doses of at least 6,000 cGy. All lesions healed with conservative measures following sequestration of necrotic bone.

angiogenesis in irradiated tissues. Expression of vascular endothelial growth factor is suppressed in irradiated tissues, but this suppression can be reversed by HBO (Dudziak et al., 2000; Fok et al., 2008). In addition, HBO has been shown to interact with other growth factors to stimulate bone growth and bone turnover (Granström, 2005b). Granström (2005b) noted that 117 (40.2%) of 291 implants placed in irradiated sites without HBO failed, whereas 29 (8.5%) of 340 implants placed in the HBO group failed. Similar outcomes have been reported by Salinas (2010) and Shah (2017) in the native mandible and fibula-free flaps used to reconstruct the mandible in irradiated patients receiving HBO.

The use of adjuvant HBO remains controversial, so in 2006, the *Journal of Oral Maxillofacial Surgery* invited Professor Gosta Granström, of Gothenburg University (pro), and Professor Bruce Donoff, of the Harvard School of Dental Medicine (con), to debate the issue. Dr. Donoff expressed concern regarding the lack of randomized clinical trials but did admit that "Evidence supports enhanced long-term survival in all sites." He added: "But the clinician must weigh the availability, complications and added cost in the decision-making process." He also questioned the necessity of HBO therapy when the dose to the implant sites is less than 5,000 cGy (Donoff, 2006).

The critical question is not whether adjuvant HBO is useful but rather whether HBO is necessary for any individual patient. Unfortunately, currently, it is not possible to answer this question for individual patients. Currently, methods are being developed that seek to ascertain the vascularity of the affected bone by means of dynamic contrast-enhanced (DCE) MRI scans using quantifiable biomarkers (Mohamed et al., 2020). These scans could be used to determine the viability of potential implant sites.

New methods that show promise of improving the vitality of irradiated tissues are now evolving. The protocol proposed by Delanian et al. (2005) and Lyons and Ghazali (2008), which employs pentoxifylline, tocopherol (vitamin E), and clodronate, has been investigated the most. Pentoxifylline is a vasodilator that facilitates blood flow by decreasing platelet aggregation and thrombus formation and inhibits fibrosis. Tocopherol is a free radical scavenger. Clodronate inhibits osteoclastic activity. This drug combination has yet to be employed in irradiated patients scheduled for implant placement, but given its success in treating ORN and preventing ORN secondary to postradiation extraction (Aggarwal et al., 2017), its use would appear to be potentially beneficial.

In summary:

- The success rates in irradiated sites are lower than those achieved in nonirradiated sites.
- Success rates are lower in the maxilla than in the mandible.
- Implant failures are infrequent when doses to the implant sites are less than 5,000 cGy, but the success rates diminish as the dose to the implant sites increases.
- A high percentage of implants in irradiated tissues demonstrate advanced bone loss at an early stage.
- Implant failure rates increase with time, even in sites with high-quality bone where good initial implant anchorage can be achieved, such as the anterior mandible.
- The higher rate of stage-one failures indicates the difficulty in achieving initial implant anchorage, particularly in sites such as the maxilla.
- The use of longer implants is encouraged in irradiated sites.
- In heavily irradiated sites (doses in excess of 6,000 cGy), HBO will improve success rates and reduce the risk of ORN.

Risk of osteoradionecrosis

There are few reported cases of ORN secondary to osseointegrated implants (Figs 1-76 and 1-77). Esser and Wagner (1997) reported that 2 (3.4%) of a group of 60 patients developed ORN in the mandible. All patients received postoperative radiation after surgical resection of oral tumors. They were all treated with CRT and opposed mandibular fields to 6,000 cGy.

The risk of ORN in the mandible secondary to implant surgery is probably best determined by an analysis of the bone necrosis rate observed following postradiation extractions (Morrish et al., 1981; Beumer et al., 1983; Marx et al., 1985). Based on these data, it should be relatively safe to place implants in irradiated mandibular sites if the dose is less than 5,500 cGy. The risk would be significantly greater for sites exposed to doses greater than 6,500 cGy (Fig 1-76). In the mandible, when the potential bone sites are exposed to doses between 5,500 and 6,500 cGy, individual patient factors (e.g., the dose per fraction, a previous radical neck dissection, concomitant chemoradiation) may be important cofactors for the clinician to consider when assessing the risk.

If implants are desirable in patients who have received doses greater than 6,500 cGy to the desired implant sites, the authors recommend a course of HBO as described by Granström et al. (2005b,

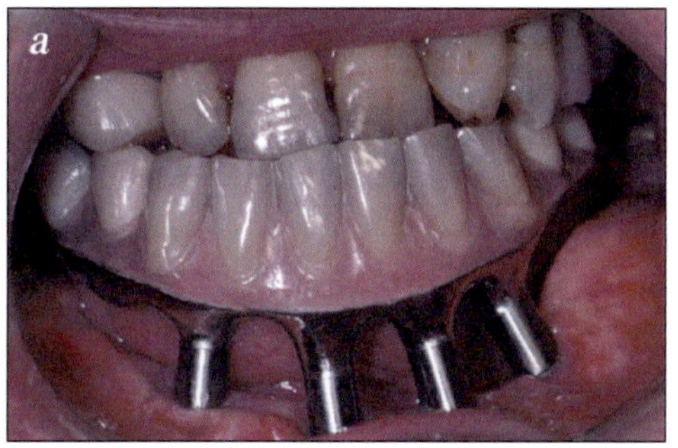
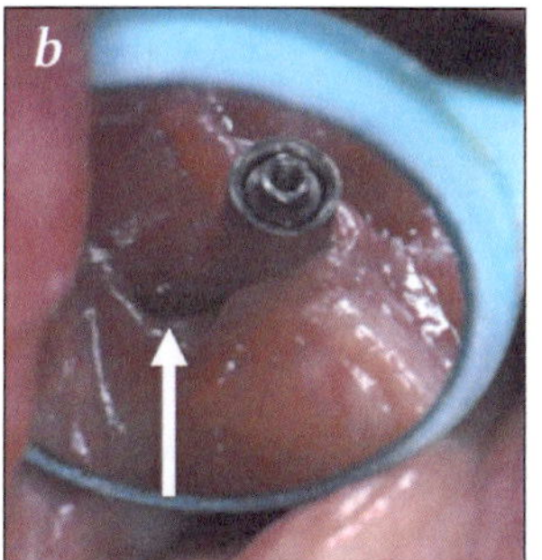
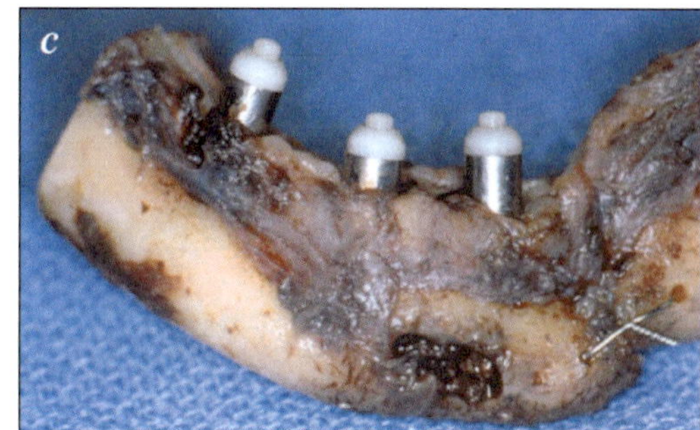

Figure 1-77 *(a)* Patient received 6,600 cGy prior and three years later implants were placed. *(b)* Three years later the patient developed infection on lingual side of implant as shown. *(c)* Infection led to osteoradionecrosis and loss of mandible.

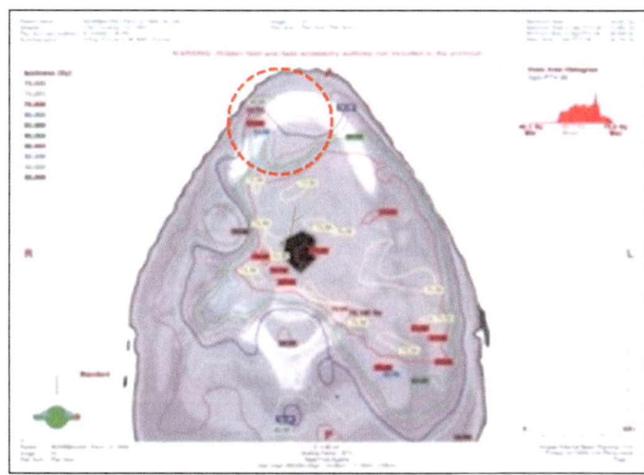

Figure 1-78 Hot spot of radiation on the anterior mandible from IMRT *(circle)*. This area received in excess of 7,000 cGy of radiation.

2006). Most patients who were treated with CRT do not receive radiation to the symphyseal region, and patients treated with IMRT may receive relatively low doses to the symphysis of the mandible and the premaxilla. Therefore, implants can be placed with a high degree of predictability in these regions in many irradiated patients. In the maxilla, the risk of bone necrosis is not significant even at high dose levels until the dose exceeds 7,500 cGy. The use of HBO can be justified on the basis of improving success rates (Granström et al., 2005b, 2006).

Recommendations for patient selection and treatment

Edentulous mandible

When the clinician is assessing the feasibility of mandibular implant placement in a patient who has undergone radiation therapy, there are several issues to consider, including the risk of ORN, the short- and long-term implant success rates, the potential life span of the patient, the potential benefit for the patient, and so on. The risk of ORN is primarily dependent on dose to the implant sites, although individual patient factors such as a history of a radical neck dissection or continuation of a heavy tobacco habit may be important to consider. In addition, concomitant chemotherapy accentuates the tissue effects and must be taken into account (Kasibhatla et al., 2007; Fowler, 2008). For the purposes of this discussion, when doses are discussed, the levels cited refer to doses delivered with conventional fractionation (200 cGy fractions, 5 fractions per week). When considering implant treatment for a patient treated with hyperfractionation or accelerated fractionation, the clinician should employ formulas that take into consideration dose per fraction, number of fractions, total dose, and time frame over which the therapy is delivered (Kirk et al., 1971).

Doses of less than 5,500 cGy or its equivalent imply an almost negligible risk of ORN at the implant sites, unless concomitant chemotherapy is employed; in contrast, doses greater than 6,500 cGy or its equivalent to the implant site imply a high risk of ORN unless the patient is treated with HBO or perhaps with one of the emerging therapies being tested in the treatment of ORN (pentoxifylline plus tocopherol). Under these guidelines, most patients with an edentulous mandible will be good candidates and have much to gain from implant therapy, particularly if the patient has had a surgical procedure that compromises the denture-bearing surfaces or negatively affects the patient's ability to control the denture with the tongue and cheeks.

If the patient was treated with CRT, in most cases the symphysis would have been out of the field, or the dose delivered to this region would have been less than 5,000 cGy. The exception is for tumors of the anterior floor of the mouth. In these patients, the dose to the symphysis usually matches the tumor dose and will almost always exceed 6,500 cGy or its equivalent. If the patient is treated with IMRT, the symphyseal region will almost always be irradiated, regardless of the site of the tumor, but the doses to the potential implant sites usually are less than 5,500 cGy. There usually will be hot spots where the dose exceeds 6,500 cGy, but the volume of these local areas exposed to high-dose radiation is usually quite small (Fig 1-78).

Tumor prognosis is an important factor in the potential success of implant therapy. Most recurrences take place within the first year, so the authors generally wait for this period to elapse before

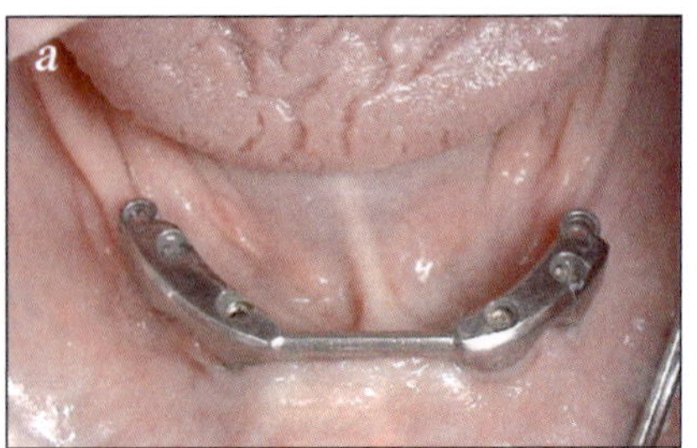

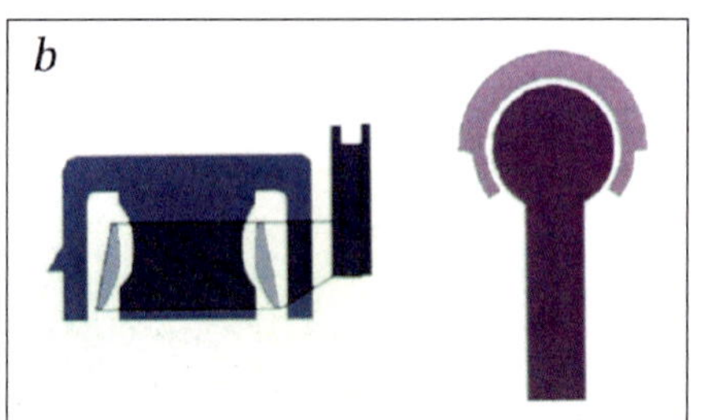

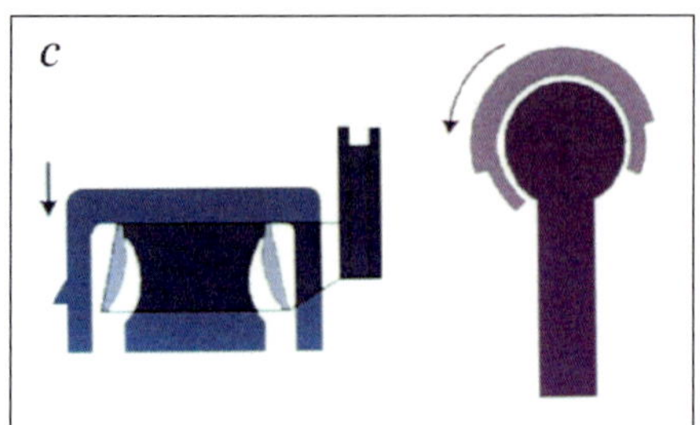

Figure 1-79 *(a)* Implant-assisted tissue bar. *(b and c)* ERA attachments are positioned adjacent to the distal implants and a "Hader" bar used to connect the two anterior implants. The "Hader" bar segment provides retention and serves as the axis of rotation. When posterior occlusal forces are applied to the overdenture, the ERA attachments permit the prosthesis to rotate around the bar and engage the primary denture support areas thereby minimizing the bending moments applied to the distal implants.

considering implants. Most patients who are tumor-free after this period are expected to survive approximately 10 years; if implants are expected to have a positive impact on function and the patient's quality of life, they should be considered.

Short-term success rates are quite favorable, but long-term rates are less than expected because as the dose to the implant sites increases implant anchorage becomes increasingly mechanical predisposing to late failures (Granström, 2005a; Yerit et al., 2006). However, HBO therapy appears to improve long-term success rates (Granström et al., 2005b; Granström, 2006). Therefore, when a plan of implant treatment is developed, implant loss rates and factors associated with implant failures in the irradiated mandible must be taken into account. The prosthodontic treatment should be tailored to anticipate these failures and to reduce the impact of factors leading to implant failure (avoidance of fixed prostheses, splinting multiple implants together, use of implants of maximum length, use of implant-assisted overdenture designs versus implant-supported designs).

The authors prefer the placement of 2–4 implants in the symphysis and the fabrication of an overdenture retained with an implant-assisted connecting bar (Fig 1-79). Individual overdenture attachments are discouraged as is the use of implant-supported designs because of the compromise of implant anchorage. The placement of additional implants is suggested when the anatomic configuration of the mandible permits. When four implants are placed, they should be positioned so that there is sufficient room between the two anterior implants for a Hader bar segment that will receive two clips. An ERA attachment (Sterngold) is secured to the distal portion of the implant connection bar. With this design, when posterior occlusal forces are applied to the posterior teeth of the overlay denture during mastication, the Hader segment acts as the axis of rotation, and the ERA attachments, being resilient, permit the posterior forces to be absorbed by the primary mandibular support areas (retromolar pad and the buccal shelf). Splinting of implants helps distribute stresses among the implants more equitably during function and parafunction, and if the experience in nonirradiated patients is taken into account, splinting implants together should increase success rates (Yilmaz et al., 2011; Mendonca et al., 2014; de Souza Batista et al., 2019).

Edentulous maxilla

All edentulous patients with maxillectomy or palatectomy defects derive significant benefit from implant-retained obturator prostheses, and the authors recommend their use even though the success rates are suboptimal in irradiated sites (Roumanas et al., 1997; Schmidt et al., 2004; Garrett, 2008; Chambrone et al., 2013). The risk of ORN is negligible and, if it does occur, is generally self-limiting. Success rates depend on radiation dose and the quantity and quality of bone associated with the implant site. As mentioned previously, when implant sites are exposed to doses greater than 5,500 cGy, initial implant anchorage is especially critical because it is highly unlikely that significant amounts of bone will be deposited on the surface of the implant following implant placement and because long-term anchorage is probably mechanical as opposed to biologic. A careful review of the dosimetry diagrams is useful prior to implant placement, for some implant sites may have been exposed to relatively low doses, whereas other sites may have been exposed to doses equivalent to the tumor dose (see Fig 1-83). This information is especially useful to the implant surgeon because dose can impact the density of the implant site and the difficulty that might be encountered in achieving initial implant stability at the site.

Some implant failures in the irradiated maxilla are the result of the difficulty in achieving initial implant anchorage at stage-one surgery, but a substantial number also occur after loading. As a result, when designing the implant connecting bar and selecting and positioning the attachments, the clinician should anticipate probable implant failures and the overdenture should be designed so that the prosthesis can be easily modified upon loss of a key implant. In most implant configurations, the implant connecting bar designs should be implant-assisted as opposed to implant-supported, especially if edentulous extension areas are subjected to significant occlusal forces. The primary purpose of the retentive apparatus, in such situations, should be to provide retention and stability for the prosthesis as opposed to support (Fig 1-80).

Success rates will be improved by careful preparation of the osteotomy site, by use of the longest implants possible given the vertical dimension of the bone site, and by the achievement of bicortical stabilization during implant surgery. Individual attachments should be avoided. When possible, implants should be splinted together with rigid implant connecting bars, and designs should be tailored to minimize the bending moments delivered to the implants. In all probability, success rates probably will be improved with the use of adjuvant HBO treatments (Granström, 1999, 2005b, 2006). Augmentation of heavily irradiated maxillary sites with autogenous bone grafts is not feasible because of the compromised blood supply.

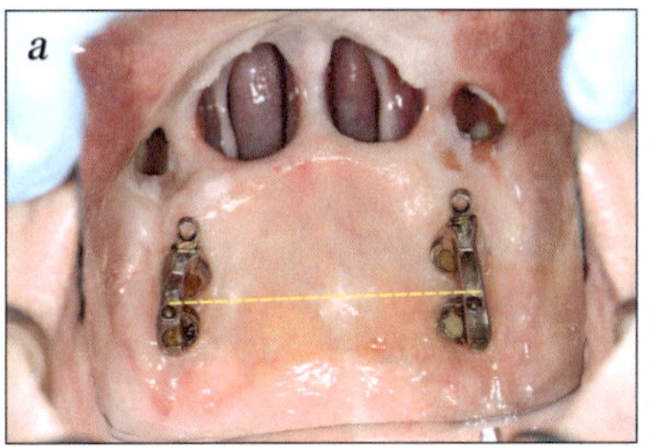

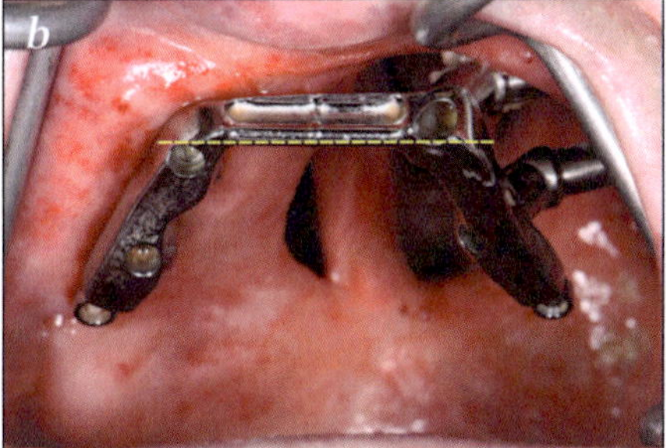

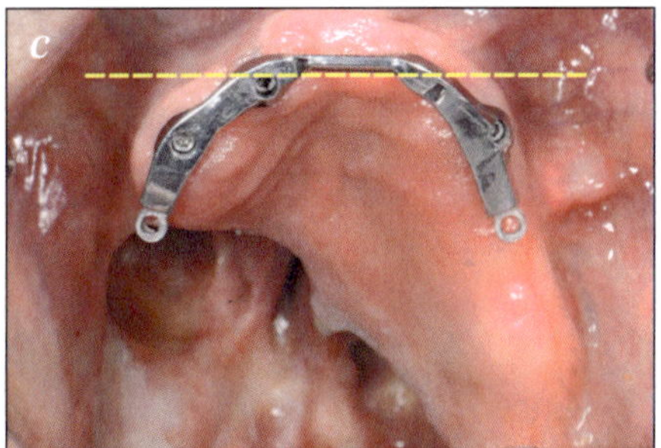

Figure 1-80 Implant-assisted connecting bar designs are suggested when the maxillary implant sites are irradiated and edentulous extension areas are used to support the forces of occlusion. The axis of rotation (dotted lines) is established by either strategic placement of rests *(a)* or the position of the *(b and c)* "Hader" bar segment.

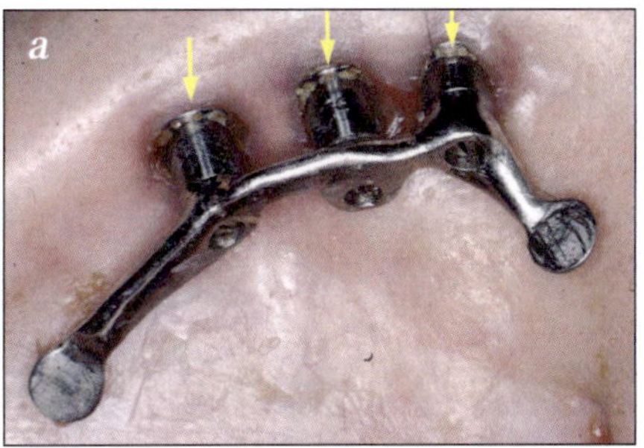

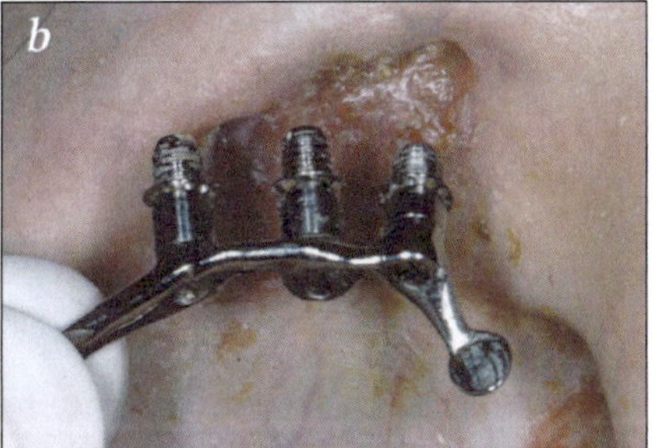

Figure 1-81 *(a and b)* This patient received a dose of more than 6,000 cGy to implant sites. Flange exposure *(arrows)* eventually led to loss of the implants.

Craniofacial sites

Retention of facial prostheses is dramatically improved with implants, and patients prefer implant retention to adhesive retention by a wide margin (Chang et al., 2005). Long-term success rates in irradiated sites, however, vary widely and range from 25% to 30% in the orbit to 75% to 80% in the floor of the nose (Parel and Tjellström, 1991; Roumanas et al., 1994, 2002; Karakoca et al., 2008; Subramaniam et al., 2018). Anchorage becomes increasingly mechanical as the dose increases, so it is not surprising that short implants have a higher failure rate. In addition, when the flange of the short craniofacial implant becomes exposed, it is impossible to keep this area clean, leading to persistent irritation of the peri-implant skin or mucosa (Fig 1-81). As a result, most clinicians have resorted to the use of longer dental-type implants, particularly in the floor of the nose and orbital sites. Success rates at these sites appear to be improved by the use of adjuvant HBO treatments (Granström et al., 2005b, 2006). ORN is a concern but usually is self-limiting and resolved with conservative measures.

Implants placed immediately after tumor ablation in patients planned to receive postoperative radiotherapy

Most of the oncologic resection patients in the series reported in the literature to date received straight-wall machined-surface implants after their radiotherapy. However, because of the relatively high failure rates in the irradiated maxilla, many clinicians are now placing tapered, self-tapping implants with microrough surfaces at the time of tumor ablation, with the expectation of improving survival rates (Wetzels et al., 2017; Butterworth, 2019; Alberga et al., 2021; Butterworth et al., 2022). Tapered, self-tapping implants with variable thread patterns enable improved initial mechanical implant stability. Microrough surface implants accelerate the biologic processes associated with osseointegration, and since postoperative radiation usually begins four to six weeks following tumor resection, there is sufficient time to allow microrough surface implants to become reasonably well osseointegrated. Moreover, the dosimetry may be manipulated to limit the dose to the implant sites without compromising the dosage delivered to the proposed tumor volume. Moreover, after surgical ablation and postoperative radiation therapy, many patients present with trismus limiting access to the desired implant sites and making implant placement more challenging. For these and other reasons (fewer surgical interventions, reduced cost, accelerated rehabilitation), the authors prefer, when possible, to place implants at the time of tumor ablation and prior to radiation therapy. However, it should be noted that long-term follow-up data documenting the efficacy of this approach is not yet available.

Timing of implant surgery in relation to completion of radiation therapy

It has become increasingly clear that bone irradiated to high doses does not recover with time; indeed, the opposite is likely: with time, irradiated bone becomes more fibrotic and less vascular with few, if any, surviving mesenchymal stem cells. There is no evidence to support the practice of delaying implant placement in order to enable the vascularity and vitality of the proposed implant sites to recover. Granström (2005a) has reported that failure rates increase as a function of the time elapsed after radiotherapy.

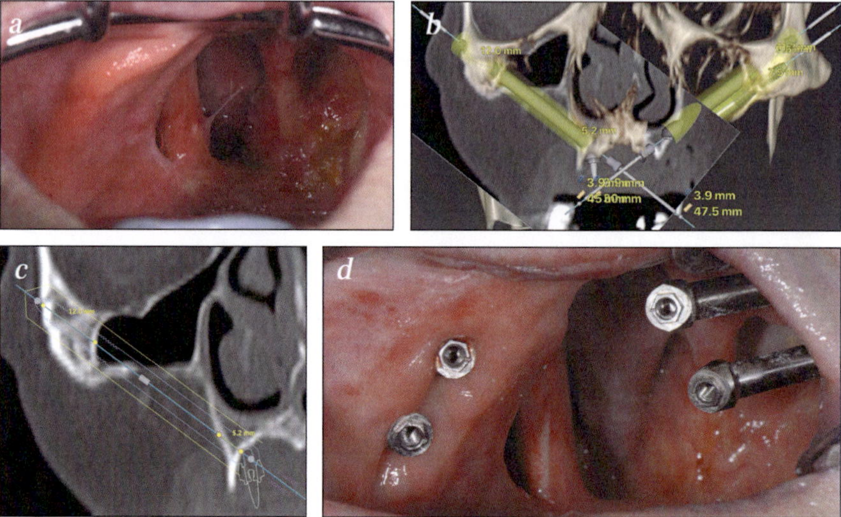

Figure 1-82 *(a)* Edentulous patient with a total maxillectomy defect. *(b and c)* CBCT scans allow visualization of potential implant sites in 3D. Four zygomatic implants are planned. *(d)* The implants in position.

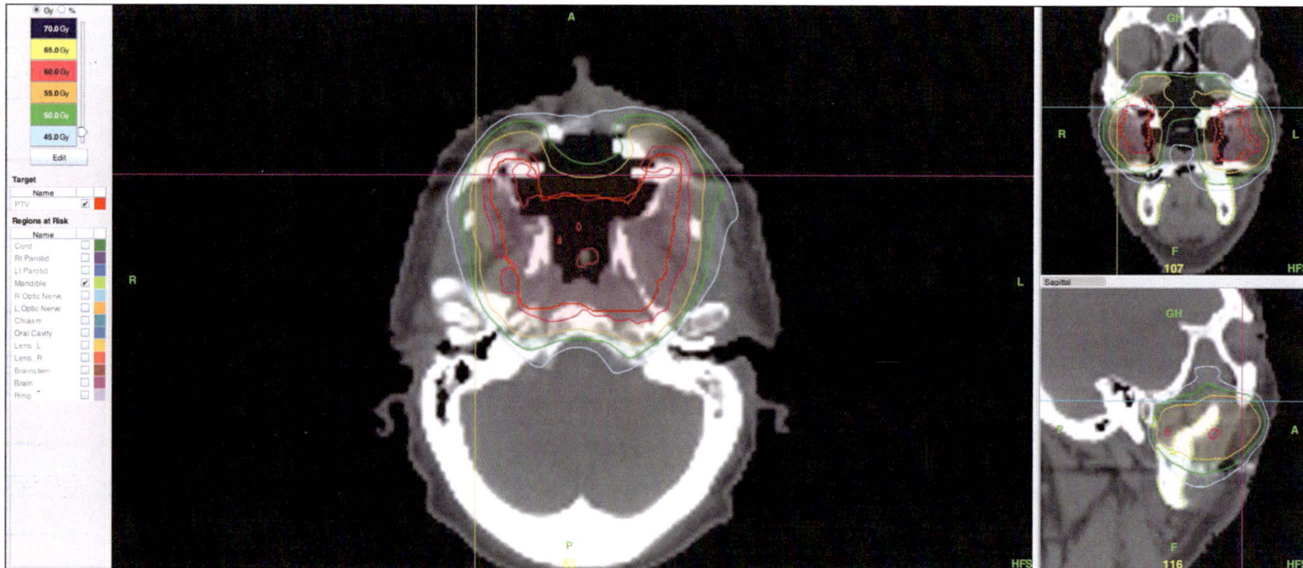

Figure 1-83 Dosimetry diagrams of a patient with a large palatal defect who is being considered for implants. The doses to the potential implant sites can be evaluated.

Pretreatment workup for irradiated sites, use of dosimetry diagrams, and selection of implant designs

CBCT scans with the associated software are recommended in order to assess the possible implant sites in three dimensions. Implant placement is more challenging in irradiated patients and alignment must be precise, and therefore implant placement with semiguided or fully guided drill guides is suggested. Computer-guided planning tools are rapidly becoming the standard of care, and the precision that can be achieved with these methods represents a sophisticated treatment planning tool that ensures that implant placement is directed by the demands of the prosthesis while making maximum advantage of the bone sites available. Moreover, these methods are rapidly becoming cost-effective. CBCT scans allow visualization of the bone contours of the potential bony implant sites and adjacent structures in three dimensions. The lengths, diameter, position, and probable angulation of the implants can be determined prior to implant placement (Fig 1-82). See Chapters 2, 3, and 5 for detailed descriptions for designing radiographic guides and surgical templates.

Dosimetry diagrams based on the radiotherapy plan of treatment are obtained in order to assess the dosage delivered to the potential implant sites (Fig 1-83). Sites are favored where the doses delivered are less than 5,500 cGy. Sites exposed to doses in excess of 6,500 cGy imply that these sites will present with decreased bone density, that implant anchorage will be primarily mechanical as opposed to biologic, and as a result, that increased long-term failure rates will result. In the case of the mandible, implant placement in such highly irradiated sites predisposes to a significant risk of ORN unless accompanied by HBO treatments.

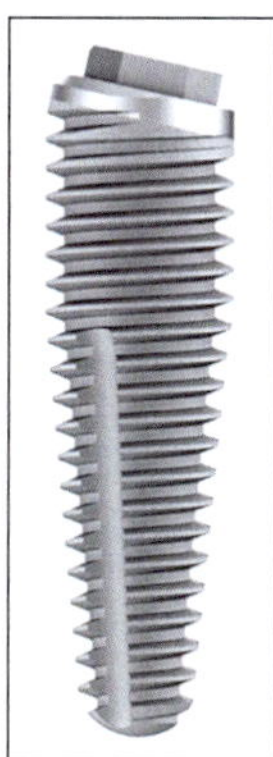

Figure 1-84 Tapered self-tapping implants with variable thread patterns are suggested for most irradiated sites.

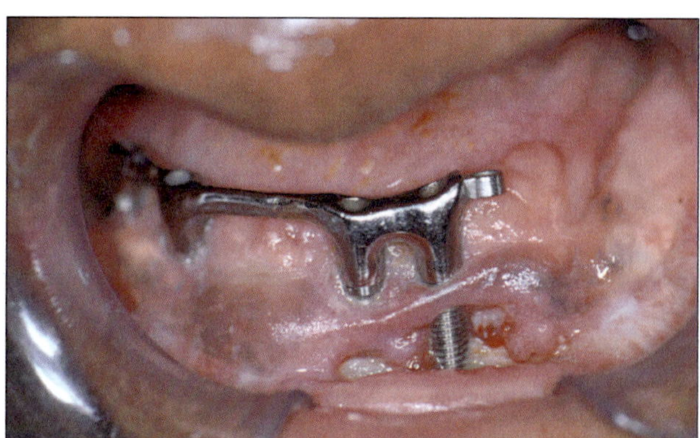

Figure 1-85 Following implant placement, the patient received 6,000 cGy of radiation. Backscatter increased the dose administered to the bone anchoring the implants by 15% to 20%. Subsequently, the patient developed ORN accompanied by loss of the two anterior implants. Eventually the necrosis healed with conservative measures, and an implant-assisted overdenture was fabricated for the patient.

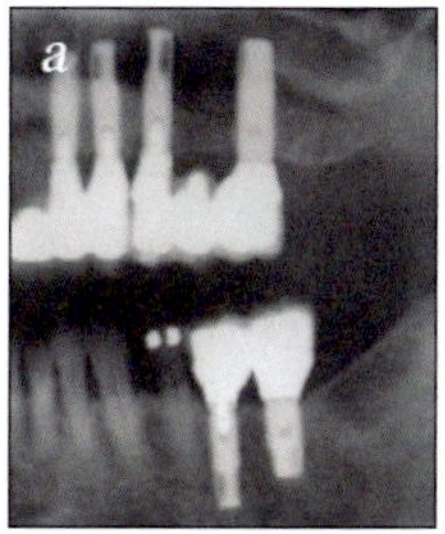

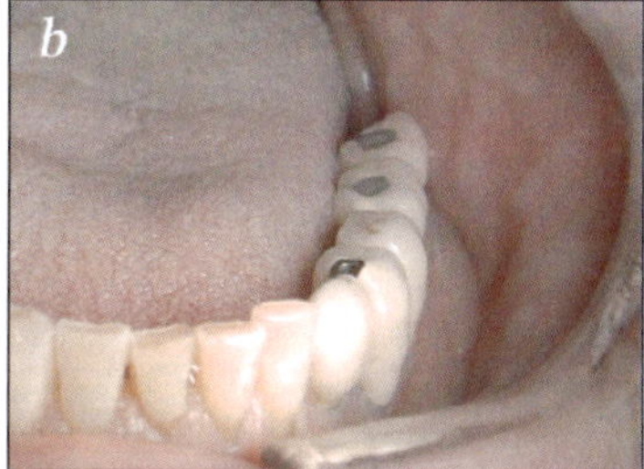

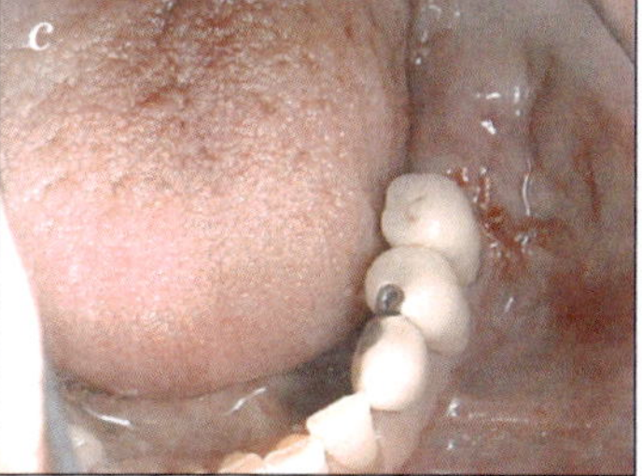

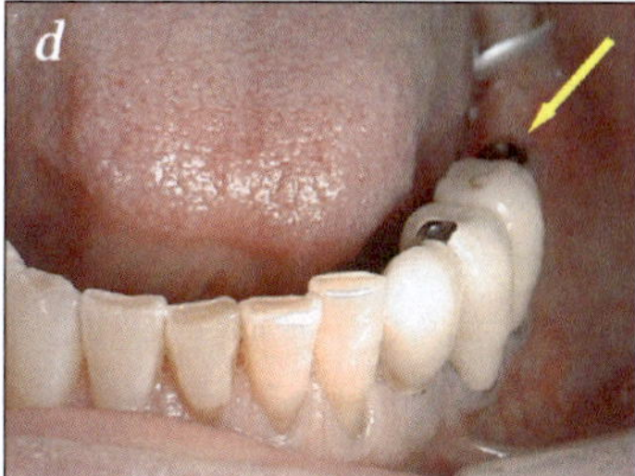

Figure 1-86 *(a and b)* A patient presenting with squamous carcinoma of the left base of the tongue is scheduled to receive a 7,000 cGy dose via IMRT. An implant-supported fixed partial denture restores the left posterior quadrant. *(c)* The prosthesis has been removed, and the implants have been buried beneath mucosa. *(d)* After radiation therapy, the cover screws have become exposed *(arrow)*.

Tapered, self-tapping implants with variable thread patterns, prepared with microrough surfaces (Fig 1-84), should improve implant success rates in patients with the poor-quality bone sites frequently encountered in irradiated patients. In irradiated sites exposed to moderate doses (less than 5,500 cGy), there may be sufficient vasculature and bone vitality available to permit a limited version of osseointegration, and the microrough implant surfaces will accelerate the process by upregulating and accelerating the expression of genes of the differentiating osteoblasts associated with the osseointegration process (Ogawa and Nishimura, 2006). These surfaces also upregulate and accelerate the genes that improve the quality (density) of bone that eventually anchors implants (Butz et al., 2006; Takeuchi et al., 2005). Self-tapping, tapered implants with variable thread patterns result in improved initial mechanical stability of the implant. With these designs, during insertion of the implant, the trabecular bone of the implant site is condensed around the implant improving the initial mechanical anchorage of the implant and this phenomenon should reduce the risk of early implant failure. These designs have proven their worth in poor-quality bone sites in normal patients, such as the posterior maxilla, and should be used in most heavily irradiated sites, with the exception of heavily corticated bone sites in the symphysis of the edentulous mandible. Such sites may still require tapping and the use of straight-wall implants.

Irradiation of existing implants

Irradiation of titanium implants that are already in place results in backscatter; as a result, the tissues on the radiation-source side of the implants receive a higher dose than the other tissues in the field (Friedrich et al., 2012). The dose is increased by about 15% to 18% in the zone 1 mm from the implant surface (Schwartz et al., 1979). The increase in dose locally may subject these tissues to ulceration, exposure of the underlying bone, and loss of the implants (Teramoto et al., 2016) (Fig 1-85).

Of additional concern is the backscatter created by noble metals, because frequently alloys of these metals are used to fabricate implant-connecting bars and implant restorations. These restorations may extend subgingivally and attach directly to the implant. Under these circumstances, the dose enhancement secondary to backscatter and to bone and mucosa immediately adjacent to the implants may approach 80% (Tso et al., 2019).

Because of backscatter and the increased numbers of patients presenting with implants at the time of tumor diagnosis, clinicians question whether osseointegrated implants should be removed in patients about to be irradiated for head and neck tumors. Surgical removal prior to radiation has been discouraged by most knowledgeable clinicians because of the significant trauma resulting from the trephination procedure required to remove an osseointegrated implant bonded to bone. Granström et al. (1995) addressed these issues in a report of 11 patients with 33 existing titanium implants who were scheduled to be irradiated. Dosages ranged from 5,000 to 6,600 cGy. Based on their findings, they recommended that all abutments and superstructures be removed prior to radiation and that skin and/or mucosa be closed over the implants. They suggested that radiation therapy can begin when healing is complete. However, primary closure may be difficult to accomplish, and frequently there is significant tension at the suture line. Often, the wound dehisces, and the implants and their cover screws become exposed (Fig 1-86).

As a result, the following protocol has evolved. Namely, that the restoration be removed and that titanium healing abutments be attached to the implants prior to initiation of radiation therapy. Following completion of radiation, the restoration may be reattached in many instances. However, in the mandible, this decision is based on a number of factors, including the dose to the implant sites, the type of prosthesis, its hygiene access, and the patient's level of compliance. For example, the implant retained fixed dental prostheses that were removed prior to radiation therapy in the patient shown in Fig 1-86 were not reinserted. The dose to the implant sites exceeded 6,500 cGy and given the dose enhancement secondary to backscatter and the oral hygiene challenges, the risk of developing an ORN from peri-implantitis was felt to be substantial. Therefore, the prosthesis was not reinserted. There are no data to guide the clinician in this matter when implant restorations in the mandible are considered for reinsertion. Individual patient factors drive the decision such as probable oral hygiene compliance, the functional benefit provided, whether the implant restoration exits through poorly keratinized mobile mucosa (a negative factor) or a healthy zone of attached keratinized mucosa (a positive factor), the dose to the sites in question (accumulated doses in excess of 6,500 are a negative factor) and whether chemoradiation was employed (a negative factor). Such decisions are difficult and must be made following a thorough discussion with the patient outlining the risks and benefits of retaining the implant-retained prosthesis.

Patients scheduled to receive radiation therapy with a history of bisphosphonate use

A significant number of patients with osteoporosis are being treated with oral bisphosphonates, and in the future, some will develop oral tumors requiring radiation therapy. These drugs have a strong affinity for calcium phosphate and rapidly accumulate in bone. During remodeling the bisphosphonates are internalized by osteoclasts, which induce apoptosis. Moreover, in animal models, bisphosphonate or similar therapies have been shown histologically to increase osteocyte necrosis, especially in the presence of periapical (Rao et al., 2017, 2019) and/or periodontal lesions (Li et al., 2016). Long-duration bisphosphonate administration also appears to substantially increase the death of osteocytes. Osteocytes are the most plentiful cells in mature bone and their death and replacement are normally the result of natural metabolic processes and remodeling. Many of the bisphosphonates are also potent inhibitors of angiogenesis. The result is that the jawbones of patients exposed to these drugs may be less vascular and less cellular.

A critical question as yet unanswered, given the known effects of high-dose radiation on bone and mucosa, is the impact of these drugs on patients with quiescent peri-apical infection and chronic periodontal disease that are scheduled to be irradiated for cancers of the head and neck and are such patients at increased the risk of developing ORN. These issues remain unresolved, including how aggressive the clinician should be in extracting diseased teeth within the gross tumor volume and clinical target volume and the appropriate treatment of those patients developing ORN in patients with such a drug profile. Resolution of these issues awaits completion of long-term clinical outcome studies.

Summary

This chapter presents the available data and clinical experience of those active in this highly complex and rapidly evolving field in order to present a logical approach, based on the evidence available, to dental evaluation, dental care, and maintenance of oral health and function of those receiving tumoricidal doses of radiation therapy to the head and neck region. Much has changed since the last edition of this book was published, including the introduction and widespread use of chemoradiation and IMRT, VMAT, SBRT, and so on. In addition, we better understand the basic biologic mechanisms of radiation-induced short-term and long-term tissue injury. Improved methods of caries control have evolved, and there is hope that, based on additional insights gained regarding radiation-induced tissue injury, some of the well-known and intractable vascular and fibrotic changes seen within radiated tissues that can lead to ORN can be minimized or reversed with medical therapy.

However, much research is still necessary. Because of the lack of well-designed clinical outcome studies, clinicians responsible for preradiation assessments and postradiation dental maintenance and restoration of oral function must still rely on clinical case series data and an in-depth understanding of the biologic effects of radiation as the best levels of evidence to assist them in management decision for patients about to be irradiated or those that present post-radiation for oral rehabilitation and dental care.

Most clinical decisions, whether it be the removal of teeth prior to or after radiation treatments, the wisdom of implant placement, the methods used to treat ORN, the risks and predictability of surgical interventions and reconstruction, and so on, are still best based on the level of dosage delivered to the tissues in question. In this chapter, we have attempted to guide the clinician by basing most of our clinical recommendations on the tumor dose and the volume of adjacent tissues receiving doses above 65 Gy or its equivalent.

References

Aarup-Kristenson S, Hansen CR, Forner L, et al. Osteoradionecrosis of the mandible after radiotherapy for head and neck cancer: Risk factors and dose-volume correlations. Acta Oncol 2019;58:1373–1377.

Abboud WA, Hassin-Baer S, Alon EE, et al. Restricted mouth opening in head and neck cancer: Etiology, prevention, and treatment. JCO Oncol Pract 2020 Oct;16(10):643–653.

Abed H, Burke M, Scambler S, et al. Denture use and osteoradionecrosis following radiotherapy for head and neck cancer: A systematic review. Gerodontology 2020;37:102–109.

Adamietz IA, Rahn R, Böttcher HD, et al. Prophylaxe der radiochemotherapeutisch bedingten mukositis. Strahlenther Onkol 1998;174:149–155.

Aggarwal K, Goutam M, Singh M, et al. Prophylactic use of pentoxifylline and tocopherol in patients undergoing dental extractions following radiotherapy for head and neck cancer. Niger J Surg 2017 Jul–Dec;23(2):130–133. http://doi.org/10.4103/njs.NJS_40_16.

Al Hadi H, Smerdon GR, Fox SW. Hyperbaric oxygen therapy accelerates osteoblast differentiation and promotes bone formation. J Dent 2015;433:382–388.

Almståhl A, Wikstrom M. Electrolytes in stimulated whole saliva in individuals with hyposalivation of different origins. Arch Oral Biol 2003;48:337–344.

Almståhl A, Wikström M, Fagerberg-Mohlin B. Microflora in oral ecosystems in subjects with radiation-induced hyposalivation. Oral Dis 2008;14:541–549.

Alvarez-Camacho M, Gonella S, Campbell S, et al. A systematic review of smell alterations after radiotherapy for head and neck cancer. Cancer Treat Rev 2017 Mar;54:110–121. http://doi.org/10.1016/j.ctrv.2017.02.003. Epub 2017 Feb 16.

Ammajan RR, Joseph R, Rajeev R, et al. Assessment of periodontal changes in patients undergoing radiotherapy for head and neck malignancy: A hospital-based study. J Cancer Res Ther 2013;9:630–637.

Anand A, Balasubramanian D, Subramanian N, et al. Secondary lymphedema after head and neck cancer therapy: A review. Lymphology 2018;51:109–118.

Anderson CM, Sonis ST, Lee CM, et al. Phase 1b/2a trial of the superoxide dismutase mimetic GC4419 to reduce chemoradiotherapy-induced oral mucositis in patients with oral cavity or oropharyngeal carcinoma. Int J Radiat Oncol Biol Phys 2018;100:427–435.

Anderson MW, Izutsu KT, Rice JC. Parotid gland pathophysiology after mixed gamma and neutron irradiation of cancer patients. Oral Surg Oral Med Oral Pathol 1981;52:495–500.

Annane D, Depondt T, Aubert P, et al. Hyperbaric oxygen therapy for radionecrosis of the jaw: A randomized, placebo-controlled, double-blind trial from the ORN96 group. J Clin Oncol 2004;22:4893–4900.

Antonadou D, Pepelassi M, Synodinou M, et al. Prophylactic use of amifostine to prevent radiochemotherapy-induced mucositis and xerostomia in head-and-neck cancer. Int J Radiat Oncol Biol Phys 2002;52:739–747.

Asif M, Moore A, Yarom N, et al. The effect of radiotherapy on taste sensation in head and neck cancer patients—a prospective study. Radiation Oncology 2020 Jun 5;15:144. http://doi.org/10.1186/s13014-020-01578-4.

Asikainen P, Klemetti E, Kotilainen R, et al. Osseointegration of dental implants in bone irradiated with 40, 50, or 60 Gy doses: An experimental study with beagle dogs. Clin Oral Implants Res 1998;9:20–25.

Azzam P, Mroueh M, Francis M, et al. Radiation-induced neuropathies in head and neck cancer: Prevention and treatment modalities. ecancer 2020;14:113. http://doi.org/10.3332/ecancer.2020.1133.

Baker S, Verduijn GM, Petit S, et al. Long-term outcomes following stereotactic body radiotherapy boost for oropharyngeal squamous cell carcinoma. Acta Oncol 2019;58:926–933.

Bedwinek JM, Shukovsky LJ, Fletcher GH, et al. Osteoradionecrosis in patients treated with definite radiotherapy for squamous cell carcinoma of the oral cavity and naso- and oropharynx. Radiology 1976;119:665–667.

Beech N, Robinson S, Porceddu S, et al. Dental management of patients irradiated for head and neck cancer. Australian Dent J 2014;59:20–28.

Ben-David MA, Diamante M, Radawski JD, et al. Lack of osteoradionecrosis of the mandible after intensity-modulated radiotherapy for head and neck cancer: Likely contributions of both dental care and improved dose distribution. Int J Radiat Oncol Biol Phys 2007;68:396–402.

Bensadoun RJ, Patton LL, Lalla RV, et al. Oropharyngeal candidiasis in head and neck cancer patients treated with radiation: Update 2011. Support Care Cancer 2011;19:737–744.

Bernard C, Villat C, Abouelleil H, et al. Tensile bond strengths of two adhesives on irradiated and nonirradiated human dentin. Biomed Res Int 2015. Article ID 798972. http://doi.org/10.1155/2015/798972.

Beumer J III, Curtis TA, Harrison RE. Radiation therapy of the oral cavity: Sequelae and management. Head Neck Surg 1979;1:301–312.

Beumer J III, Curtis TA, Morrish RB Jr. Radiation complications in edentulous patients. J Prosthet Dent 1976;36:193–203.

Beumer J III, Harrison R, Sanders B, et al. Osteoradionecrosis: Predisposing factors and outcomes of therapy. Head Neck Surg 1984;6:819–827.

Beumer J III, Harrison R, Sanders B, et al. Postradiation dental extractions: A review of the literature and a report of 72 episodes. Head Neck Surg 1983;6:581–586.

Beumer J III, Roumanas E, Nishimura R. Advances in osseointegrated implants for dental and facial rehabilitation following major head and neck surgery. Semin Surg Oncol 1995;11:200–207.

Beumer J III, Silverman S Jr, Benak SB Jr. Hard and soft tissue necroses following radiation therapy for oral cancer. J Prosthet Dent 1972;27:640–644.

Bichsel D, Lanfranchi M, Attin T, et al. Evaluation of oral prophylaxis during and after intensity-modulated radiotherapy due to head and neck cancer: A retrospective study. Clinical Oral Invest 2016;20:721–726.

Bolind P, Johansson CB, Johansson P, et al. Retrieved implants from irradiated sites in humans: A histologic/histomorphometric investigation of oral and craniofacial implants. Clin Implant Dent Relat Res 2006;8:142–150.

Bourhis J, Le Maître A, Baujat B, et al. Individual patients' data meta-analysis in head and neck cancer. Curr Opin Oncol 2007;19:188–194.

Bourhis J, Overgaard J, Audry H, et al. Hyperfractionated or accelerated radiotherapy in head and neck cancer: A meta-analysis. Lancet 2006;368:843–854.

Bramerson A, Nyman J, Nordin S, et al. Olfactory loss after head and neck cancer radiation therapy. Rhinology 2013;51:206–209. http://doi.org/10.4193/Rhino12.120.

Brasseur M, Brogniez V, Gregoire V, et al. Effects of irradiation on bone remodeling around mandibular implants: An experimental study in dogs. Int J Oral Maxillofac Surg 2006;35:850–855.

Brown LR, Dreizen S, Handler S, et al. The effect of radiation-induced xerostomia on human oral microflora. J Dent Res 1975;54:740–750.

Bruins HH, Jolly DE, Koole R. Preradiation dental extraction decisions in patients with head and neck cancer. Oral Surg Oral Med Oral Pathol Oral Radiol Endod 1999;88:406–412.

Brzozowska A, Miak R, Homa-Miak R, et al. Polymorphism of regulatory region of APEH gene (c.-521G>C, rs4855883) as a relevant predictive factor for radiotherapy induced oral mucositis and overall survival in head neck cancer patients. Oncotarget 2018 Jul 3;9(51):29644–29653.

Burgharz M, Ginzkey C, Hackenberg S, et al. Two-stage autotransplantation of the human submandibular gland: First long-term results. Laryngoscope 2016;126:1551–1555.

Burlage FR, Roesink JM, Kampinga HH, et al. Protection of salivary function by concomitant pilocarpine during radiotherapy: A double-blind, randomized, placebo-controlled study. Int J Radiat Oncol Biol Phys 2008;70:14–22.

Butterworth CJ. Primary vs secondary zygomatic implant placement in patients with head and neck cancer—a 10-year prospective study. Head Neck 2019 Jun;41(6):1687–1695.

Butterworth CJ, Lowe D, Rogers SN. The Zygomatic Implant Perforated (ZIP) flap reconstructive technique for the management of low-level maxillary malignancy—clinical & patient related outcomes on 35 consecutively treated patients. Head Neck 2022;44(2):345–358.

Butz F, Aita H, Wang CC, et al. Harder and stiffer osseointegrated bone to roughened titanium. J Dent Res 2006;85:560–565.

Buurman DJM, Speksnijder CM, de Groot RJ, et al. Masticatory performance and oral health-related quality of life in edentulous maxillectomy patients: A cross-sectional study to compare implant-supported obturators and conventional obturators. Clin Oral Implants Res 16 January 2020a. http://doi.org/10.1111/clr.13577.

Buurman DJM, Vaassen LA, Bockman R, et al. Prosthetic rehabilitation of head and neck cancer patients focusing on mandibular dentures in irradiated patients. Int J Prosthodont 2013;26:557–562.

Buurman DJM, Speksnijder CM, de Groot RJ, et al. Mastication in maxillectomy patients: A comparison between reconstructed maxillae and implant supported obturators: A cross-sectional study. J Oral Rehabil 2020b Jul 2. http://doi.org/10.1111/joor.13043.

Cai F, Manton D, Shen P, et al. Effect of addition of citric acid and casein phosphopeptide-amorphous calcium phosphate to a sugar free chewing gum on enamel remineralization in situ. Caries Res 2007;41:377–383.

Carl W, Schaaf NG, Sako K. Oral surgery and the patient who has had radiation therapy for head and neck cancer. Oral Surg Oral Med Oral Pathol 1973;36:651–659.

Carr AB. Implant location and radiotherapy are the only factors linked to 2-year implant failure. J Evid Based Dent Pract. 2010 Mar;10(1):49-51. doi: 10.1016/j.jebdp.2009.11.025. PMID: 20230970.

Chambrone L, Mandia J Jr, Shibli JA, et al. Dental implants installed in irradiated jaws: A systematic review. J Dent Res 2013;92(12 suppl):119S–130S.

Chang TL, Garrett N, Roumanas E, et al. Treatment satisfaction with facial prostheses. J Prosthet Dent 2005;94:275–280.

Chen SC, Lai YH, Huang BS, et al. Changes and predictors of radiation-induced oral mucositis in patients with oral cavity cancer during active treatment. Eur J Oncol Nurs 2015;19:214–219.

Cheng KKF, Ka Tsui Yuen J. A pilot study of chlorhexidine and benzydamine oral rinses for the prevention and treatment of irradiation mucositis in patients with head and neck cancer. Cancer Nurs 2006;29:423–430.

Chrcanovic BR, Albrektsson T, Wennerberg A. Dental implants in irradiated versus nonirradiated patients: A meta-analysis. Head Neck 2016;38:448–481.

Collett WK, Thonard JC. The effect of fractional radiation on dentinogenesis in the rat. J Dent Res 1965;44:84–90.

Conger AD, Wells MA. Radiation and aging effect on taste structure and function. Radiat Res 1969;37:31–49.

Conger AD. Loss and recovery of taste acuity in patients irradiated to the oral cavity. Radiat Res 1973;53:338–347.

Cooper JS, Fu K, Marks J, et al. Late effects of radiation in therapy in the head and neck region. Int J Radiat Oncol Biol Phys 1995;31:1141–1164.

Coppes RP, Roffel AF, Zeilstra LJ, et al. Early radiation effects on muscarinic receptor-induced secretory responsiveness of the parotid gland in the freely moving rat. Radiat Res 2000;153:339–346.

Coppes RP, Zeilstra LJ, Kampinga HH, et al. Early to late sparing of radiation damage to parotid gland by adrenergic and muscarinic receptor agonists. Br J Cancer 2001;85:1055–1063.

Copps DP, Lacy AM, Curtis TA, et al. Effects of topic fluoride on five low-fusing porcelains. J Prosthet Dent 1984;52:340–343.

Costantino PD, Friedman CD, Steinberg MJ. Irradiated bone and its management. Otolaryngol Clin North Am 1995;28:1021–1038.

Cotroneo E, Proctor GB, Carpenter GH. Regeneration of acinar cells following ligation of rat submandibular gland retraces the embryonic-perinatal pathway of cytodifferentiation. Differentiation 2010;79:120–130.

Curtis TA, Griffith MR, Firtell DN. Complete denture prosthodontics for the radiation patient. J Prosthet Dent 1976;36:66–76.

Dahllöf G, Rozell B, Forsberg CM, et al. Histologic changes in dental morphology induced by high dose chemotherapy and total body irradiation. Oral Surg Oral Med Oral Pathol 1994;77:56–60.

Daland EM. Surgical treatment of postirradiation necrosis. Am J Roentgenol 1941;46:287–301.

Daly TE, Drane JB. Management of Dental Problems in Irradiated Patients [thesis]. Houston: University of Texas; 1972.

Davies AN, Thompson J. Parasympathomimetic drugs for the treatment of salivary gland dysfunction due to radiotherapy. Cochrane Database Syst Rev 2015 Oct;2015(10):CD003782.

Da Silva EM, Mansano ESB, Miazima ES, et al. Radiation used for head and neck cancer increases virulence in Candida tropicalis isolated from a cancer patient. BMC Infect Dis 2017;17:783.

Delanian S, Chatel C, Porcher R, et al. Complete resolution of refractory mandibular osteoradionecrosis by prolonged treatment with a pentoxifylline-tocopherol-clodronate combination (PENTOCLO): A phase II trial. Int J Radiat Oncol Biol Phys 2011;803:832–839.

Delanian S, Depondt J, Lefaix JL. Major healing of refractory mandible osteoradionecrosis after treatment combining pentoxifylline and tocopherol: A phase II trial. Head Neck 2005;27:114–123.

Delanian S, Lefaix JL. The radiation-induced fibroatrophic process: Therapeutic perspective via the antioxidant pathway. Radiother Oncol 2004;73:119–131.

Delanian S, Lefaix JL, Pradar PF. Radiation-induced neuropathy in cancer survivors. Radiother Oncol 2012;105:273–282.

Delanian S, Porcher R, Balla-Mekias S, et al. Randomized placebo-controlled trial of combined pentoxifylline and tocopherol for regression of superficial radiation-induced fibrosis. J Clin Oncol 2003;21:2545–2550.

Del Regato JA. Dental lesions observed after roentgen therapy in cancer of the buccal cavity, pharynx, and larynx. Am J Roentgenol 1939;42:404–410.

DeLuke D, Carrico C, Ray C, et al. Is dose volume a better predictor of osteoradionecrosis risk than total dose for patients who have received head and neck radiation? J Oral Maxillofac Surg 2022 Sep 25;80(9):1557–1563. http://doi.org/10.1016/j.joms.2022.04.009. Epub 2022 Apr 25.

Deng J, Jackson L, Epstein J, et al. Dental demineralization and caries in patients with head and neck cancer. Oral Oncology 2015;51:824–831.

Denham J, Peters L, Johansen J, et al. Do acute mucosal reactions lead to consequential late reactions in patients with head and neck cancer? Radiother Oncol 1999;52:157–164.

Denys D, Kaste SC, Kun LE, et al. The effects of radiation on craniofacial skeletal growth: A quantitative study. Int J Pediatr Otorhinolaryngol 1998;45:7–13.

de Siqueira-Mellara MT, Palma-Dibb RG, de Oliveira HF, et al. The effect of radiation therapy on the mechanical and morphological properties of enamel and dentin of deciduous teeth—an in vitro study. Radiat Oncol 2014 Jan 22;9(30). http://doi.org/10.1186/1748-717X-9-30.

de Souza BM, Silva MS, Braga AS, et al. Protective effect of titanium tetrafluoride and silver diamine fluoride on radiation-induced dentin caries in vitro. Sci Rep 2021 Mar 16;11(1):6083. http://doi.org/10.1038/s41598-021-85748-8. PMID: 33727650; PMCID: PMC7966395.

de Souza Batista VE, Verri FR, Lemos CA, et al. Should the restoration adjacent implants be splinted or nonsplinted? A systematic review and meta-analysis. J Prosthet Dent 2019;121:41–51.

Dholam KP, Pusalkar HA, Yadav PS, et al. Implant-retained dental rehabilitation in head and neck cancer patients: An assessment of success and failure. Implant Dent 2013;22:604–660.

Dijkema T, Raaijmakers CPJ, Ten Haken R, et al. Parotid gland function after radiotherapy: The combined Michigan and Utrecht experience. Int J Radiat Oncol Biol Phys 2010;78:449–453.

Dijkstra PU, Kalk WW, Roodenburg JL. Trismus in head and neck oncology: A systematic review. Oral Oncol 2004;40:879–889.

Dion MW, Hussey DH, Doornbos JF, et al. Preliminary results of a pilot study of pentoxifylline in the treatment of late radiation soft tissue necrosis. Int J Radiat Oncol Biol Phys 1990;19:401–407.

Dissard A, Dang NP, Barthelemy I, et al. Efficacy of pentoxifylline–tocopherol–clodronate in mandibular osteoradionecrosis. Laryngoscope 2020 Nov;130(11): E559–E566. http://doi.org/10.1002/lary.28399. Epub 2019 Nov 20.

Dodd MJ, Larson PJ, Dibble SL, et al. Randomized clinical trial of chlorhexidine versus placebo for prevention of oral mucositis in patients receiving chemotherapy. Oncol Nurs Forum 1996;23:921–927.

Donoff RB. Treatment of the irradiated patient with dental implants: The case against hyperbaric oxygen treatment. J Oral Maxillofac Surg 2006;64:819–822.

Dreizen S, Brown LR, Daly TE, et al. Prevention of xerostomia-related dental caries in irradiated cancer patients. J Dent Res 1977;56:99–104.

Dreizen S, Brown LR, Handler S, et al. Radiation-induced xerostomia in cancer patients: Effect on salivary and serum electrolytes. Cancer 1976;38:273–278.

Dudziak ME, Saadeh PB, Mehrara BJ, et al. The effect of ionizing radiation on osteoblast-like cells in vitro. Plast Reconstr Surg 2000;106:1049–1061.

Dumbrigue HB, Sandow PL, Nguyen KH, et al. Salivary epidermal growth factor levels decrease in patients receiving radiation therapy to the head and neck. Oral Surg Oral Med Oral Pathol Oral Radiol Endod 2000;89:710–716.

Duxbury AJ, Thakker NS, Wastell DG. A double-blind cross-over trial of a mucin-containing artificial saliva. Br Dent J 1989;166:115–120.

Eisbruch A, Kim HM, Terrell JE, et al. Xerostomia and its predictors following parotid-sparing irradiation of head-and-neck cancer. Int J Radiat Oncol Biol Phys 2001;50:695–704.

Eisbruch A, Lyden T, Bradford CR, et al. Objective assessment of swallowing dysfunction and aspiration after radiation concurrent with chemotherapy for head and neck cancer. Int J Radiat Oncol Biol Phys 2002;53:23–28.

Eisbruch A, Rhodus N, Rosenthal D, et al. How should we measure and report radiotherapy-induced xerostomia? Semin Radiat Oncol 2003;13:226–234.

Eisbruch A, Ten Haken RK, Kim HM, et al. Dose, volume, and function relationships in parotid salivary glands following conformal and intensity-modulated irradiation of head and neck cancer. Int J Radiat Oncol Biol Phys 1999;45:577–587.

Eisele DW, Kock DG, Tarazi AE, et al. Case report: Aspiration from delayed radiation fibrosis of the neck. Dysphagia 1991;6:120–122.

Elkind M, Sutton H. X-ray damage and recovery in mammalian cells in culture. Nature 1959;184:1293–1295.

Ellis R. Relationship of biologic effect to dose-time: Fractionation factors in radiotherapy. In Current topics in radiation research. Vol 4. Ed. M Ebert, A Howard. Amsterdam: North-Holland; 1968. pp. 357–397.

Elting LS, Cooksley CD, Chambers MS, et al. Risk, outcomes, and costs of radiation-induced oral mucositis among patients with head and neck malignancies. Int J Radiat Oncol Biol Phys 2007;68:1110–1120.

Epstein J, van der Meij E, McKenzie M, et al. Postradiation osteonecrosis of the mandible: A long-term follow-up study. Oral Surg Oral Med Oral Pathol Oral Radiol Endod 1997;83:657–662.

Epstein JB, Barasch A. Taste disorders in cancer patients: Pathogenesis, and approach to assessment and management. Oral Oncol 2010;46:7781. http://doi.org/10.1016/j.oraloncology.2009.11.008.

Epstein JB, Gorsky M, Caldwell J. Fluconazole mouth rinses for oral candidiasis in postirradiation, transplant and other patients. Oral Surg Oral Med Oral Path Endod 2002;93:671–675.

Epstein JB, Lunn R, Le N, et al. Periodontal attachment loss in patients after head and neck radiation therapy. Oral Surg Oral Med Oral Pathol Oral Radiol Endod 1998;86:673–677.

Epstein JB, McBride BC, Stevenson-Moore P, et al. The efficacy of chlorhexidine gel in reduction of *Streptococcus mutans* and *Lactobacillus* species in patients treated with radiation therapy. Oral Surg Oral Med Oral Pathol 1991;71:172–178.

Epstein JB, Silverman S Jr, Paggiarino DA, et al. Benzydamine HCl for prophylaxis of radiation-induced oral mucositis: Results from a multicenter, randomized, double-blind, placebo-controlled clinical trial. Cancer 2001;92:875–885.

Epstein JB, Stevenson-Moore P. A clinical comparative trial of saliva substitutes in radiation-induced salivary gland hypofunction. Spec Care Dentist 1992a;12:21–23.

Epstein JB, van der Meij EH, Emerton SM, et al. Compliance with fluoride gel use in irradiated patients. Spec Care Dentist 1995;15:218–222.

Epstein JB, Vickars L, Spinelli J, et al. Efficacy of chlorhexidine and nystatin rinses in prevention of oral complications in leukemia and bone marrow transplantation. Oral Surg Oral Med Oral Pathol 1992b;73:682–689.

Esser E, Wagner W. Dental implants following radical oral cancer surgery and adjuvant radiotherapy. Int J Oral Maxillofac Implants 1997;12:552–557.

Fajardo LG, Bertrong M, Anderson R. Nervous system. In Radiation pathology. Ed. LG Fajardo, M Bertrong, R Anderson. Oxford: Oxford University; 2001. pp. 362–363.

Faria KM, Brandao TB, Ribeiro AC, et al. Micromorphology of the dental pulp is highly preserved in cancer patients who underwent head and neck radiotherapy. J Endod 2014;40:1553–1559.

Fawzi MI, Shklar G, Krakow AA. The effect of radiation on the response of the dental pulp to operative and endodontics procedures. Oral Surg Oral Med Oral Pathol 1985;59:405–413.

Ferraiolo DM, Veitz-Keenan A. Insufficient evidence for interventions to prevent dry mouth and salivary gland dysfunction post head and neck radiotherapy. Evid Based Dent 2018;19:30–31.

Finlay PM, Richardson MD, Robertson AG. A comparative study of the efficacy of fluconazole and amphotericin B in the treatment of oropharyngeal candidosis in patient undergoing radiotherapy for head and neck tumors. Br J Oral Maxillofac Surg 1996;34:23–25.

Flood T, Downie I. Prosthetic reconstruction following rhinectomy: Evolution of bone-anchored epistheses and adjunctive surgical techniques in nasal reconstruction from one unit. Presented at the Second International Symposium on Bone Conduction—Craniofacial Osseointegration, Gothenburg, Sweden, 11–13 Jun 2009.

Fok TC, Jan A, Peel SA, et al. Hyperbaric oxygen results in increased vascular endothelial growth factor (VEGF) protein expression in rabbit calvarial critical-sized defects. Oral Surg Oral Med Oral Pathol Oral Radiol Endod 2008;105:417–422.

Foote RL, Loprinzi CL, Frank AR, et al. Randomized trial of a chlorhexidine mouthwash for alleviation of radiation-induced mucositis. J Clin Oncol 1994;12:2630–2633.

Fowler JF, Stern B. Fractionation and dose-rate: II. Dose-time relationships in radiotherapy and the validity of cell survival curve models. Br J Radiol 1963;36:163–173.

Fowler JF. Correction to Kasibhatla et al. How much radiation is the chemotherapy worth in advanced head and neck cancer? (Int J Radiat Oncol Biol Phys 2007;68:1491–1495). Int J Radiat Oncol Biol Phys 2008;71:326–329.

Fox PC, van der Ven PF, Baum BJ, et al. Pilocarpine for the treatment of xerostomia associated with salivary gland dysfunction. Oral Surg Oral Med Oral Pathol 1986;61:243–248.

Frank RM, Herdly J, Philippe E. Acquired dental defects and salivary gland lesions after irradiation for carcinoma. J Am Dent Assoc 1965;70:868–883.

Franzén L, Funegård U, Ericson T, et al. Parotid gland function during and following radiotherapy of malignancies in the head and neck. A consecutive study of salivary flow and patient discomfort. Eur J Cancer 1992;28:457–462.

Frechette AR. Masticatory forces associated with the use of various types of artificial teeth. J Prosthet Dent 1955;5:252–267.

Freymiller EG, Sung EC, Friedlander AH. Detection of radiation-induced cervical antheromas by panoramic radiograph. Oral Oncol 2000;36:175–179.

Friedrich RE, Todorovic M, Heiland M, et al. Scattering effects of irradiation on surroundings calculated for a small dental implant. Anticancer Res 2012;32:2043–2046.

Fugita M, Tanimoto K, Wada T. Early radiographic changes in radiation bone injury. Oral Surg Oral Med Oral Pathol 1986;61:641–644.

Futran ND, Trotti A, Gwede C. Pentoxifylline in the treatment of radiation-related soft tissue injury: Preliminary observations. Laryngoscope 1997;107:391–395.

Galler C, Epstein JB, Guze KA, et al. The development of osteoradionecrosis from sites of periodontal disease activity: Report of 3 cases. J Periodontol 1992;63:310–316.

Garg H, Grewal MS, Rawat S, et al. Dental pulp status of posterior teeth in patients with oral and oropharyngeal cancer treated with concurrent chemoradiotherapy. J Endod 2015;41:1830–1833.

Garrett N. Outcomes of maxillectomies with conventional and implant restorations. Presented at the International Congress on Maxillofacial Rehabilitation, Bangkok, Thailand, 24–27 Sep 2008.

Gevorgyan A, La Scalia G, Neligan PC, et al. Radiation-induced craniofacial bone growth disturbances. J Craniofac Surg 2007 Sep;18:1001–1007.

Glanzmann C, Grätz KW. Radionecrosis of the mandible: A retrospective analysis of the incidence and risk factors. Radiother Oncol 1995;36:94–100.

Goldstein M, Maxymiw WG, Cummings BJ, et al. The effects of antitumor irradiation on mandibular opening and mobility: A prospective study of 58 patients. Oral Surg Oral Med Oral Pathol Oral Radiol Endod 1999;88:365–373.

Goncalves LM, Palma-Dibb RG, Paula-Silva FW, et al. Radiation therapy alters microhardness and microstructure of enamel and dentin of permanent human teeth. J Dent 2014;42:986–992.

Gorlin R, Meskin L. Severe irradiation during odontogenesis: Report of a case. Oral Surg Oral Med Oral Pathol 1963;16:35–38.

Gornitsky M, Shenouda G, Sultanem K, et al. Double-blind randomized, placebo-controlled study of pilocarpine to salvage salivary gland function during radiotherapy of patients with head and neck cancer. Oral Surg Oral Med Oral Path Oral Radiol Endod 2004;98:45–52.

Gowgiel JM. Experimental radio-steonecrosis of the jaws. J Dent Res 1960;39:176–197.

Granström G. Osseointegration in irradiated cancer patients: An analysis with respect to implant failures. J Oral Maxillofac Surg 2005a;63:579–585.

Granström G. Pathophysiologic basis for HBO in the treatment of healing disorders in radio-injured tissues. In The ECHM collection. Vol 2. Ed. A Marroni, D Mathieu, F Wattel. Flagstaff, AZ: Best; 2005b. pp. 3101–3110.

Granström G. Placement of dental implants in irradiated bone: The case for using hyperbaric oxygen. J Oral Maxillofac Surg 2006;64:812–818.

Granström G, Bergström K, Tjellström A, et al. A detailed analysis of titanium implants lost in irradiated tissues. Int J Oral Maxillofac Implants 1994;9:653–662.

Granström G, Jacobsson M, Tjellström A. Titanium implants in irradiated tissue: Benefits from hyperbaric oxygen. Int J Oral Maxillofac Implants 1992;7:15–25.

Granström G, Tellstrom A, Albrektsson T. Post implant irradiation of osseointegrated implants. In Proceeds of first international congress on maxillofacial prosthetics. Eds. I Zlotolow, S Esposito, J Beumer. New York: Memorial Sloane-Kettering Cancer Center; 1995. pp. 292–295.

Granström G, Tellstrom A, Branemark PI Osseointegrated implants in irradiated bone: A case controlled study using adjunctive hyperbaric oxygen therapy. J Oral Maxillofac Surg 1999;57:493–497.

Grant BP, Fletcher GH. Analysis of complications following megavoltage therapy for squamous cell carcinomas of the tonsillar area. Am J Roentgenol Radium Ther Nucl Med 1966;96:28–36.

Greenspan D, Daniels TE. Effectiveness of pilocarpine in postradiation xerostomia. Cancer 1989;59:1123–1125.

Griem ML, Robinson JE Jr, Barnhart GW. The uses of a soft denture-base material in management of the post-radiation denture problem. Radiology 1964;82:320–321.

Grøn P. Chemistry of topical fluorides. Caries Res 1977;11(suppl 1):172–204.

Gunn L, Gilbert J, Nenclares P, et al. Taste dysfunction following radiotherapy to the head and neck: A systematic review. Radiother Oncol 2021;157:130–140. http://doi.org/10.1016/j.radonc.2021.01.021. Epub 2021 Feb 3.

Gupta N, Grewal M, Gairola M, et al. Dental pulp status of posterior teeth in patients with oral and oropharyngeal cancer treated with radiotherapy: 1-year follow-up. J Endod 2018;44:549–554.

Hall EJ, Giaccia AJ. Radiobiology for the radiologist. 6th ed. Philadelphia: Lippincott, Williams, and Wilkins; 2006.

Harris M. The conservative management of osteoradionecrosis of the mandible with ultrasound therapy. Br J Oral Maxillofac Surg 1992;30:313–318.

Hart GB, Mainous EG. The treatment of radiation necrosis with hyperbaric oxygen (OHP). Cancer 1976;37:2580–2585.

Hashida T, Kamemoto H, Fuchihata H, et al. The effect of X-ray irradiation on the function and saliva composition of rat parotid and submandibular/sublingual glands. Oral Radiol 1999;15.

Havelek R, Soukup T, Cmielova J, et al. Ionizing radiation induces senescence and differentiation of human dental pulp stem cells. Folia Biologica (Praha) 2013;59:188–197.

Hayashi M, Pellecer M, Chung E, et al. The efficacy of pentoxifylline/tocopherol combination in the treatment of osteoradionecrosis. Spec Care Dentist 2015 Nov–Dec;35(6):268–271.

Hayward JR, Kerr DA, Jesse RH, et al. The management of teeth related to treatment of oral cancer. CA Cancer J Clin 1969;19:98–106.

Hehr T, Classen J, Welz S, et al. Hyperfractionated, accelerated chemoradiation with concurrent mitomycin-C and cisplatin in locally advanced head and neck cancer, a phase I/II study. Radiother Oncol 2006;80:33–38.

Held T, Herpel C, Schwindling FS, et al. 3D-printed individualized tooth-borne tissue retraction devices compared to conventional dental splints for head and neck cancer radiotherapy: A randomized controlled trial. Radiation Oncology 2021;16(1):75.

Henke M, Alfonsi M, Foa P, et al. Palifermin decreases severe oral mucositis of patients undergoing postoperative radiochemotherapy for head and neck cancer: A randomized, placebo-controlled trial. J Clin Oncol 2011;29:2815–2829.

Henkin RI, Talal N, Larson AL, et al. Abnormalities of taste and smell in Sjögren's syndrome. Ann Intern Med 1972;76:375–383.

Herpel C, Schwindling FS, Held T, et al. Individualized 3D-printed tissue retraction devices for head and neck radiotherapy. Front Oncol 2021 Mar 23;11:628743. http://doi.org/10.3389/fonc.2021.628743. eCollection 2021.

Hommez GM, De Meerleer GO, De Neve WJ, et al. Effect of radiation dose on the prevalence of apical periodontitis—a dosimetric analysis. Clin Oral Investig 2012 Dec;16(6):1543–1547.

Hong CS, Oh D, Ju SG, et al. Development of a semi-customized tongue displacement device using a 3D printer for head and neck IMRT. Radiation Oncology 2019;14(1):79.

Horiot JC, Schraub S, Bone MC, et al. Dental preservation in patients irradiated for head and neck tumors: A 10-year experience with topical fluoride and a randomized clinical trial between two fluoridation methods. Radiother Oncol 1983;1:77–82.

Hsiung CY, Huang EY, Ting HM, et al. Intensity-modulated radiotherapy for nasopharyngeal carcinoma: The reduction of radiation-induced trismus. Br J Radiol 2008;81:809–814.

Hunt TK, Pai MP. The effect of varying ambient oxygen tensions on wound metabolism and collagen synthesis. Surg Gynecol Obstet 1972;135:561–567.

Jacobsson M, Tjellström A, Thomsen P, et al. Integration of titanium implants in irradiated bone. Histologic and clinical study. Ann Otol Rhinol Laryngol 1988;97:337–340.

Jalali MM, Gerami H, Rahimi A, et al. Assessment of olfactory threshold in patients undergoing radiotherapy for head and neck malignancies. Iran J Otorhinolaryngol 2014 Oct;26(77):211–217.

Jansma J, Vissink A, Gravenmade EJ, et al. In vivo study on the prevention of post-radiation caries. Caries Res 1989;23:172–178.

Jellema AP, Langendijk H, Bergernhenegouwen L, et al. The efficacy of Xialine in patients with xerostomia resulting from radiotherapy for head and neck cancer: A pilot-study. Radiother Oncol 2001;59:157–160.

Jensen SB, Vissink A, Limesand KH, et al. Salivary gland hypofunction and xerostomia in head and neck radiation patients. Natl Cancer Inst Monogr 2019 Aug 1;2019(53):lgz016.

Jha N, Seikaly H, Harris J, et al. A phase II study of submandibular gland transfer prior to radiation for prevention of radiation-induced xerostomia in head and neck cancer (Rtog 0244)s. Int J Radiat Oncol Phys 2012;84:437–442.

Johansen E, Sobel S. Dental management of patients with head and neck cancer. Presented at the Sixtieth Annual Meeting of the American Radium Society, New Orleans, 26–30 Apr 1978.

Johnson JT, Ferretti GA, Nethery WJ, et al. Oral pilocarpine for post-irradiation xerostomia in patients with head and neck cancer. N Engl J Med 1993;329:390–395.

Jreije A, Keshelava L, Ilickas M, et al. Development of patient specific conformal 3D-printed devices for dose verification in radiotherapy. Applied Sciences 2021;11(18):8657.

Judge LF, Farrugia MK, Singh AK. Narrative review of the management of oral mucositis during chemoradiation for head and neck cancer. Ann Transl Med 2021 May;9(10):916. http://doi.org/10.21037/atm-20-3931. PMID: 34164550; PMCID: PMC8184418.

Jurdana M, Cermazar M, Pegan K, et al. Effect of ionizing radiation on human skeletal muscle precursor cells. Radiol Oncol 2013 Dec;47(4):376–381.

Kaliman R. The phenomenon of reoxygenation and its implication for fractionated radiotherapy. Radiology 1972;105:135–142.

Kang MY, Holland JM, Stevens KR Jr. Cranial neuropathy following curative chemotherapy and radiotherapy for carcinoma of the nasopharynx. J Laryngol Otol 2000;114:308–310.

Kang Z, Jin T, Li X, et al. Progression and postoperative complications of osteoradionecrosis of the jaw: A 20-year retrospective study of 124 non-nasopharyngeal cancer cases and meta-analysis. BMC Oral Health 2022 May 28;22(1):213. http://doi.org/10.1186/s12903-022-02244-9. PMID: 35643546; PMCID: PMC9148447.

Karakoca S, Aydin C, Yilmaz H, et al. Survival rates and peri-implant soft tissue evaluation of extraoral implants over a mean follow-up period of three years. J Prosthet Dent 2008;100:458–464.

Karayazgan-Saracoglu B, Atay A, Zulfikar H, et al. Assessment of implant stability on patients with and without radiotherapy using resonance frequency analysis. J Oral Implantol 2015 Feb;41(1):30–35. http://doi.org/10.1563/AAID-JOI-D-12-00107.

Karlsson O, Karlsson T, Pauli N, et al. Jaw exercise therapy for the treatment of trismus in head and neck cancer: A prospective three-year follow-up study. Support Care Cancer 2021;29:3793–3800.

Kasibhatla M, Kirkpatrick JP, Brizel DM. How much radiation is chemotherapy worth in advanced head and neck cancer? Int J Radiat Oncol Biol Phys 2007;68:1491–1495.

Kataoka SH, Setzer FC, Fregnani ER, et al. Effects of 3-dimensional conformal or intensity-modulated radiotherapy on dental pulp sensitivity during and after the treatment of oral or oropharyngeal malignancies. J Endod 2012;38:148–152.

Katsumata O, Yu-Ichi Sato Y, Sakai Y, et al. Intercalated duct cells in the rat parotid gland may behave as tissue stem cells. Anat Sci Int 2009;84:148–154.

Kazemian A, Kamian S, Aghili M, et al. Benzydamine for prophylaxis of radiation-induced oral mucositis in head and neck cancers: A double-blind placebo-controlled randomized clinical trial. Eur J Cancer Care (Engl) 2009;18:174–178.

Keene HJ, Daly T, Brown LR, et al. Dental caries and *Streptococcus mutans* prevalence in cancer patients with irradiation-induced xerostomia: 1–13 years after radiotherapy. Caries Res 1981;15:416–427.

Keene HJ, Fleming TJ. Prevalence of caries-associated microflora after radiotherapy in patients with cancer of the head and neck. Oral Surg Oral Med Oral Pathol 1987;64:421–426.

Kielbassa AM, Hinkelbein W, Hellwig E, et al. Radiation-related damage to dentition. Lancet Oncol 2006;7:326–335.

Kierkels RG, Fredriksson A, Both S, et al. Automated robust proton planning using dose-volume histogram-based mimicking of the photon reference dose and reducing organ at risk dose optimization. Int J Radiat Biol Phys 2019;103:251–258. http://doi.org/10.1016/j.ijrobp.2018.08.023.

Kil WJ, Kulasekere C, Hatch C, et al. Tongue-out versus tongue-in position during intensity-modulated radiotherapy for base of tongue cancer: Clinical implications for minimizing post-radiotherapy swallowing dysfunction. Head and Neck 2017;39(8):E85–E91. http://doi.org/10.1002/hed.24809.

Kinsella TJ, DeLuca AM, Barnes M, et al. Threshold dose for peripheral nerve following intraoperative radiotherapy (IORT) in a large animal model. Int J Radiat Oncol Biol Phys 1991;20:697–701.

Kirk J, Worthley BW. Cumulative radiation effect: I. Fractionated treatment regimes. Clin Radiol 1971;22:145–155.

Kluth EV, Jain PR, Stuchell RN, et al. A study of factors contributing to the development of osteoradionecrosis of the jaws. J Prosthet Dent 1988;59:194–201.

Knight GM, McIntyre JM, Mulyani M, et al. The effect of silver fluoride and potassium iodide on the bond strength of auto cure glass ionomer cement to dentine. Aust Dent J 2006;51(1):42–45. http://doi.org/10.1111/j.1834-7819.2006.tb00399.

Knighton DR, Halliday B, Hunt TK. Oxygen as an antibiotic: The effect of inspired oxygen on infection. Arch Surg 1984;119:199–204.

Konings AW, Coppes RP, Vissink A. On the mechanism of salivary gland radiosensitivity. Int J Radiat Oncol Biol Phys 2005;62:1187–1194.

Konings AW, Faber H, Cotteleer F, et al. Secondary radiation damage as the main cause for unexpected volume effects: A histopathologic study of the parotid gland. Int J Radiat Oncol Biol Phys 2006;64:98–105.

Koppang HS. Studies on the radiosensitivity of the rat incisor. Odontol Tidskr 1967;75:413–450.

Kraaijenga SAC, Oskam IM, van der Molen, et al. Evaluation of long term (10-years+) dysphagia and trismus in patients treated with concurrent chemo-radiotherapy for advanced head and neck cancer. Oral Oncol 2015 Aug;51(8):787–794. http://doi.org/10.1016/j.oraloncology.2015.05.003. Epub 2015 May 28.

Krajicek DD. Oral radiation in prosthodontics. J Am Dent Assoc 1969;78:320–322.

Kubota H, Miyawaki D, Mukumoto N, et al. Risk factors for osteoradionecrosis of the jaw in patients with head and neck squamous cell carcinoma. Radiat Oncol 2021;16:1. http://doi.org/10.1186/s13014-020-01701-5.

Kuhnt T, Becker A, Bloching M, et al. Phase II trial of a simultaneous radiochemotherapy with cisplatinum and paclitaxel in combination with hyperfractionated-accelerated radiotherapy in locally advanced head and neck tumors. Med Oncol 2006;23:325–333.

Kydd WL. Complete denture base deformation with varied occlusal tooth form. J Prosthet Dent 1956;6:714–718.

Laheij AM, Rasch CN, Brandt BW, et al. Proteins and peptides in parotid saliva of irradiated patients compared to that of healthy controls using SELDI-TOF-MS. BMC Res Notes 2015;8:639. http://doi.org/10.1186/s13104-015-1641-7.

Lalla RV, Brennan MT, Gordon SM, et al. Oral mucositis due to high-dose chemotherapy and/or head and neck radiation therapy. JNCI Monographs 2019;53:lgz011. http://doi.org/10.1093/jncimonographs/lgz011.

Lalla RV, Latortue MC, Hong CH, et al. A systematic review of oral fungal infections in patients receiving cancer therapy. Support Care Cancer 2010;18:985–992.

Law A, Kennedy T, Pellittieri P, et al. Efficacy and safety of subcutaneous amifostine in minimizing radiation-induced toxicities in patients receiving combined modality treatment for squamous cell carcinoma of the head and neck. Int J Radiat Oncol Biol Phys 2007;69:1361–1368.

Lee DS, Kim YS, Cheon JS, et al. Long-term outcome and toxicity of hypofractionated stereotactic body radiotherapy as a boost treatment for head and neck cancer: The importance of boost volume assessment. Radiat Oncol 2012;7:85.

Lee JH, Machtay M, Unger LD, et al. Prophylactic gastrostomy tubes in patients undergoing intensive irradiation for cancer of the head and neck. Arch Otolaryngol Head Neck Surg 1998;124(8):871–875. http://doi.org/10.1001/archotol.124.8.871.

Lee M, Freeman AR, Roos DE, et al. Randomized double-blind trial of amifostine versus placebo for radiation-induced xerostomia in patients with head and neck cancer. J Med Imaging Oncol 2019;63:142–150.

Li CL, Lu WW, Jayampath LC, et al. Role of periodontal disease in bisphosphonate-related osteonecrosis of the jaws in ovariectomized rats. Clin Oral Implants Res 2016;27:1–6. http://doi.org/10.1111/clr.12502.

Llory H, Dammron A, Frank RM. Changes in the aerobic oral flora following buccal pharyngeal radiotherapy [in French]. Arch Oral Biol 1971;16:617–630.

Lombaert I, Movahednia M, Adine C, et al. Concise review: Salivary gland regeneration: Therapeutic approaches from stem cells to tissue organoids. Stem Cells 2017;35:97–105 http://doi.org/10.1002/stem/2455.

Lombaert IM, Brunsting JF, Wierenga PK, et al. Cytokine treatment improves parenchymal and vascular damage of salivary glands after irradiation. Clin Cancer Res 2008a;14:7741–7750.

Lombaert IM, Brunsting JF, Wierenga PK, et al. Keratinocyte growth factor prevents radiation damage to salivary glands by expansion of the stem/progenitor pool. Stem Cells 2008b;26:2595–2601.

Lombaert IM, Brunsting JF, Wierenga PK, et al. Rescue of salivary gland function after stem cell transplantation in irradiated glands. PLoS One 2008c;3(4):e2063.

Lombaert IM, Wierenga PK, Kok T, et al. Mobilization of bone marrow stem cells by granulocyte colony-stimulating factor ameliorates radiation-induced damage to salivary glands. Clin Cancer Res 2006;12:1804–1812.

Louis M, Brennan MT, Noll JL, et al. Radiation-induced trismus in head and neck cancer patients. Support Care Cancer 2008;16:305–309.

Lu H, Zhao Q, Guo J, et al. Direct radiation-induced effects on dental hard tissue. Radiat Oncol 2019 Jan 11;14(1):5. http://doi.org/10.1186/s13014-019-1208-1.

Lyons A, Ghazali N. Osteoradionecrosis of the jaws: Current understanding of its pathophysiology and treatment. Br J Oral Maxillofac Surg 2008;46:653–660.

Lyons KM, Cannon RD, Beumer J, et al. The role of biofilms and material surface characteristics in microbial adhesion to maxillary obturator materials: A literature review. Cleft Palate Craniofac J 2020;57:487–498.

Machetay M, Moughan J, Trottie A, et al. Factors associated with severe late toxicity after concurrent chemoradiation for locally advanced head and neck cancer: An RTOG analysis. J Clin Oncol 2008;26:3582–3589.

Makkonen TA, Tenovuo J, Vilja P, et al. Changes in the protein composition of whole saliva during radiotherapy in patients with oral or pharyngeal cancer. Oral Surg Oral Med Oral Pathol 1986;62:270–275.

Manton DJ, Walker GD, Cai F, et al. Remineralization of enamel subsurface lesions in situ by the use of three commercially available sugar-free gums. Int J Paediatr Dent 2008;18:284–290.

Manuschai J, Talungchit S, Naorungroj S. Penetration of silver diamine fluoride in deep carious lesions of human permanent teeth: An in vitro study. Int J Dent 2021 Dec 22;2021:3059129. http://doi.org/10.1155/2021/3059129. PMID: 34976061; PMCID: PMC8716243.

Marks JE, Davis CC, Gottsman VL, et al. The effects of radiation on parotid salivary function. Int J Radiat Oncol Biol Phys 1981;7:1013–1019.

Marques M, Dib L. Periodontal Changes in Patients Undergoing Radiotherapy. J Periodontol 2004;75:1178–1187.

Martin MV. Irradiation mucositis: A reappraisal. Eur J Cancer B Oral Oncol 1993;29B:1–2.

Marunick MT, Bahu SJ, Aref A. Osteoradionecrosis of the maxillary-orbital complex after neutron beam radiotherapy. Otolaryngol Head Neck Surg 2000;123:224–228.

Marunick MT, Seyedsadr M, Ahmad K, et al. The effect of head and neck cancer treatment on whole salivary flow. J Surg Oncol 1991;48:81–86.

Marx R. Preprosthetic surgery in a radiated cancer patient [abstract 61]. In Proceedings of the Fifth International Congress on Preprosthetic Surgery, 15–18 Apr 1993. Ed. W Lill, H Spiekermann, G Watzek. Chicago: Quintessence; 1993. p. 75.

Marx RE. A new concept in the treatment of osteoradionecrosis. J Oral Maxillofac Surg 1983a;41:351–357.

Marx RE. Osteoradionecrosis: A new concept of its pathophysiology. J Oral Maxillofac Surg 1983b;41:283–288.

Marx RE, Johnson RP, Kline SN. Prevention of osteoradionecrosis: A randomized prospective clinical trial of hyperbaric oxygen versus penicillin. J Am Dent Assoc 1985;111:49–54.

Matsuo R. Role of saliva in the maintenance of taste sensitivity. Crit Rev Oral Biol Med 2000;11:216–229.

Maxymiw WG, Wood RE, Liu FF. Postradiation dental extractions without hyperbaric oxygen. Oral Surg Oral Med Oral Pathol 1991;72:270–274.

Mazzaoui SA, Burrow MF, Tyas MJ, et al. Incorporation of casein phosphopeptide-amorphous calcium phosphate into a glass-ionomer cement. J Dent Res 2003;82:914–918.

McCallum S, Maresse S, Fearns P. Evaluating 3D-printed bolus compared to conventional bolus types used in external beam radiation therapy. Curr Med Imaging 2021;17(7):820–831.

McGinnis JP, Hopkins KP, Thompson EJ, et al. Tooth root growth after mantle radiation in long-term survivors of Hodhkin's disease. JADA 1985;111:584–588.

McIlroy P. Radiation mucositis: A new approach to prevention and treatment. Eur J Cancer Care 1996;5:153–158.

McReynolds D, Duane B. Systematic review finds that silver diamine fluoride is effective for both root caries prevention and arrest in older adults. Evid Based Dent 2018 Jun;19(2):46–47. http://doi.org/10.1038/sj.ebd.6401304. PMID: 29930359.

Mealey BL, Semba SE, Hallmon WW. The head and neck radiotherapy patient: 2. Management of oral complications. Compendium 1994;15:442, 444, 446–452 passim; quiz 458.

Mendonca JA, Franischone CE, Senna PM, et al. A retrospective evaluation of the survival rates of splinted and non-splinted short dental implants posterior partially edentulous jaws. J Periodontol 2014;85:787–794.

Meyerowitz C, Featherstone JD, Billings RJ, et al. Use of intra-oral model to evaluate 0.05% sodium fluoride mouthrinse in radiation-induced hyposalivation. J Dent Res 1991;70:894–898.

Mirza N, Machtay M, Devine PA, et al. Gustatory impairment in patients undergoing head and neck irradiation. Laryngoscope 2008;118:24–31.

Miura M, Takeda M, Sasaki T, et al. Factors affecting mandibular complications in low dose rate brachytherapy for oral tongue carcinoma with special reference to spacer. Int J Radiat Oncol Biol Phys 1998;41:763–770.

Miyamoto RH, Fleming TJ, Davis MG. Radiotherapeutic management of an orocutaneous defect with a balloon-retaining stent. J Prosthet Dent 1992;68:115–117.

Mohamed ASR, He R, Ding Y, et al. Quantitative dynamic contrast-enhanced MRI identifies radiation-induced vascular damage in patients with advanced osteoradionecrosis: Results of a prospective study. Int J Radiat Oncol Biol Phys 2020;108:1319–1328.

Momm F, Volegova-Neher N, Schulte-Monting J, et al. Different saliva substitutes for treatment of xerostomia following radiotherapy: A prospective crossover study. Strahlenther Onkol 2005;181:231–236.

Morrish RB Jr, Chan E, Silverman S Jr, et al. Osteoradionecrosis in patients irradiated for head and neck carcinoma. Cancer 1981;47:1980–1983.

Muraki Y, Akashi M, Ejima Y. Dental intervention against osteoradionecrosis of the jaws in irradiated patients with head and neck malignancy: A single-arm prospective study. Oral Maxillofac Surg 2019;23:297–305.

Murdoch-Kinch CA, Kim HM, Vineberg KA, et al. Dose-effect relationships for the submandibular salivary glands and implications for their sparing by intensity modulated radiotherapy. Int J Radiat Oncol Biol Phys 2008;72:373–382.

Murphy V, Lewis S, Kannan S, et al. Submandibular function recovery after IMRT in head and neck cancer: A prospective dose modelling study. Radiother Oncol 2018;129:38–43.

Murray CG, Herson J, Daly TE, et al. Radiation necrosis of the mandible: A 10-year study: Part 1. Factors influencing the onset of necrosis. Int J Radiat Oncol Biol Phys 1980a;6:543–548.

Murray CG, Herson J, Daly TE, et al. Radiation necrosis of the mandible: A 10-year study: Part II. Dental factors; onset, duration and management of necrosis. J Radiat Oncol Biol Phys 1980b;6:549–553.

Naves LZ, Novals VR, Armstrong SR, et al. Effect of gamma radiation on bonding to human enamel and dentin. Support Care Cancer 2012;20:2873–2878.

Nayar S, Brett R, Clayton N, et al. The effect of a radiation positioning stent (RPS) in the reduction of radiation dosage to the opposing jaw and maintenance of mouth opening after radiation therapy. Eur J Prosthodont Restor Dent 2016;24:71–77.

Nguyen NP, Frank C, Moltz CC, et al. Analysis of factors influencing aspiration risk following chemoradiation for oropharyngeal cancer. Br J Radiol 2009;82:675–680.

Nguyen NP, Frank C, Moltz CC, et al. Aspiration rate following chemoradiation for head and neck cancer: An underreported occurrence. Radiother Oncol 2006;80:302–306.

Nguyen NP, Frank C, Moltz CC, et al. Dysphagia severity and aspiration following postoperative radiation for locally advanced oropharyngeal cancer. Anticancer Res 2008;28:431–434.

Nicolatou-Galitis O, Sarri T, Bowen J, et al. Systematic review of amifostine for the management of oral mucositis in cancer patients. Support Care Cancer 2013;21:357–364.

Niedermeier W, Matthaeus C, Meyer C, et al. Radiation-induced hyposalivation and its treatment with oral pilocarpine. Oral Surg Oral Med Oral Pathol Oral Radiol Endod 1998;86:541–549.

Nikawa H, Chen J, Hamada T, et al. Candida albicans colonization on thermal cycled maxillofacial polymeric materials in vitro. J Oral Rehabil 2001;28:526–533.

Nikawa H, Jin C, Hamada T, et al. Interactions between thermal cycled resilient denture lining materials, salivary and serum pellicles and Candida albicans in vitro: Part II. Effects on fungal colonization. J Oral Rehabil 2000a;27(2):124–130.

Nikawa H, Jin C, Hamada T, et al. Interactions between thermal cycled resilient denture lining materials, salivary and serum pellicles and Candida albicans in vitro: Part I. Effects on fungal growth. J Oral Rehabil 2000b;27(1):41–51.

Nikawa H, Yamamoto T, Hamada T. Effect of components of resilient denture-lining materials on the growth, acid production and colonization of Candida albicans. J Oral Rehabil 1995;22(11):817–824.

Nilsson P, Albrektsson T, Granström G, et al. The effect of hyperbaric oxygen treatment on bone regeneration. An experimental study in the rabbit using the bone harvest chamber (BHC). Int J Oral Maxillofac Implants 1988;3:43–48.

Nimi A, Ueda M, Kaneda T. Maxillary obturator supported by osseointegrated implants placed in irradiated bone: Report of cases. J Oral Maxillofac Surg 1993;51:804–809.

Nishimura R. Implants in irradiated tissues. In Maxillofacial rehabilitation: Prosthodontic and surgical considerations. Ed. J Beumer, T Curtis, M Marunick. St Louis, MO: Ishiyaku EuroAmerica; 1996. pp. 103–106.

Notani K, Yamazaki Y, Kitada H, et al. Management of mandibular osteoradionecrosis corresponding to the severity of osteoradionecrosis and the method of radiotherapy. Head Neck 2003;253:181–186.

Obinata K, Ohmori K, Tuchiya K, et al. Clinical study of a spacer to help prevent osteoradionecrosis resulting from brachytherapy for tongue cancer. Oral Surg Oral Med Oral Path Oral Radiol Endod 2003;95:246–250.

Ogawa T, Nishimura I. Genes differentially expressed in titanium healing. J Dent Res 2006;85:566–570.

Oh HK, Chambers MS, Garden AS, et al. Risk of osteoradionecrosis after extraction of impacted third molars in irradiated head and neck cancer patients. J Oral Maxillofac Surg 2004;62:139–144.

Oliveira BH, Cunha-Cruz J, Rajendra A, et al. Controlling caries in exposed root surfaces with silver diamine fluoride: A systematic review with meta-analysis. J Am Dent Assoc 2018 Aug;149(8):671–679.e1. http://doi.org/10.1016/j.adaj.2018.03.028. Epub 2018 May 24. PMID: 29805039; PMCID: PMC6064675.

Oxford K, Feschuk A, Tibbo J. Treatment of soft-tissue necrosis of the pyriform sinus using pentoxyllifylline and tocopherol. Cureus 2021 Nov;13(11):e19234. Published online 2021 Nov 3. http://doi.org/10.7759/cureus.19234.

Paardekooper GM, Cammelli S, Zeilstra LJ, et al. Radiation apoptosis in relation to acute impairment of rat salivary gland function. Int J Radiat Biol 1998;73:641–648.

Papas A, Russel D, Singh M, et al. Caries clinical trial of a remineralising toothpaste in radiation patients. Gerodontology 2008;25:76–88.

Parel SM, Tjellström A. The United States and Swedish experience with osseointegration and facial prostheses. Int J Oral Maxilllofac Implants 1991;6:75–79.

Patel V, Gadiwalla Y, Sassoon I, et al. Prophylactic use of pentoxifylline and tocopherol in patients who require dental extractions after radiotherapy for cancer of the head and neck. Br J Oral Maxillofac Surg 2016a;54:547–550.

Pauli N, Fagerberg-Mohlin B, Andrél P, et al. Exercise intervention for the treatment of trismus in head and neck cancer. Acta Oncol 2014;53:502–509.

Pauli N, Svennson U, Karlsson T, et al. Exercise intervention for the treatment of trismus in head and neck cancer—a prospective two-year follow-up study. Acta Oncol 2016;55:686–692.

Pellegrino G, Tarsitano A, Ferri M, et al. Effectiveness of hyperbaric oxygen therapy in irradiated maxillofacial dental implant patients: A systematic review with meta-analysis. Clin Implant Dent Relat Res 2018;20:852–859.

Peterman A, Cella D, Glandon G, et al. Mucositis in head and neck cancer: Economic and quality-of-life outcomes. J Natl Cancer Inst Monogr 2001;29:45–51.

Peterson DE, Doerr W, Hovan A, et al. Osteoradionecrosis in cancer patients: The evidence base for treatment dependent frequency, current management strategies, and future studies. Support Care Cancer 2010;188:1089–1098.

Pierquin B, Chassagne D, Cachin Y, et al. Carcinomes épidermoides de la langue mobile et du plancher buccal: Étude de 245 cas traités á l'institut gustave-roussy. Acta Radiol Ther Phys Biol 1970;9:465–480.

Pietrokovski J, Menczel J. Tooth dwarfism and root underdevelopment following irradiation. Oral Surg Oral Med Oral Pathol 1966;22:95–99.

Pignon JP, Le Maître A, Maillard E, et al. Meta-analysis of chemotherapy in head and neck cancer (MACH-NC): An update on 93 randomised trials and 17,346 patients. Radiother Oncol 2009;92:4–14.

Pirak-Arnnop P, Sader R, Dhanuthai K, et al. Management of osteoradionecrosis of the jaws: An analysis of evidence. Eur J Surg Oncol 2008;34:1123–1134.

Powers BE, Gillette EL, Gillette SL, et al. Muscle injury following experimental intraoperative irradiation. Int J Radiat Oncol Biol Phys 1991;20:463–471.

Pradat PF, Maisonobe T, Psimaras D, et al. Radiation-induced neuropathies: Collateral damage of improved cancer prognosis. Rev Neurol 2012;168:939–950.

Pringle S, Maimets M, van der Zwaag M, et al. Human salivary gland stem cells functionally restore radiation damaged salivary glands. Stem Cells 2016;34:640–652.

Proops D, Worrollo S, Jeynes P, et al. Head and neck reconstruction in adults—the Birmingham experience. Presented at the Second International Symposium on Bone Conduction Hearing-Craniofacial Osseointegration, Gothenburg, Sweden, 11–13 June 2009.

Pugh R, Lloyd K, Collins M, et al. The use of 3D printing within radiation therapy to improve bolus conformity: A literature review. Journal of Radiotherapy in Practice 2017;16(3):319–325.

Rahn AO, Matalon V, Drane JB. Prosthetic evaluation of patients who have received irradiation to the head and neck regions. J Prosthet Dent 1968;19:174–179.

Ramirez-Amador V, Silverman S, Mayer P, et al. Candidal colonization and oral candidiasis in patient undergoing pharyngeal radiation therapy. Oral Surg Oral Med Oral Pathol Oral Radiol Endod 1997;84:149–153.

Rankow RM, Weissman B. Osteoradionecrosis of the mandible. Ann Otol Rhinol Laryngol 1971;80:603–611.

Rao JR, Wang JY, Leung YY, et al. Role of periapical diseases in medication-related osteonecrosis of the jaws. Biomed Res Int 2017. http://doi.org/10.1155/2017/1560175. PMID: 29109954; PMCID: PMC5646299.

Rao NJ, Yu RQ, Wang JY, et al. Effect of periapical diseases in development of MRONJ in immunocompromised mouse model. Biomed Res Int 2019 Sep 22:1271492. http://doi.org/10.1155/20191271492. eCollection 2019.

Rao SD, Saleh ZH, Setton J, et al. Dose-volume factors correlating with trismus following chemoradiation for head and neck cancer. Acta Oncol 2016;55(1):99–104.

Rastogi M, Khurana R, Revannasiddaiah S, et al. Role of benzydamine hydrochloride in the prevention of oral mucositis in head and neck cancer patients treated with radiotherapy (>50 Gy) with or without chemotherapy. Support Care Cancer 2017;25:1439–1443.

Reuther T, Schuster T, Mende U, et al. Osteoradionecrosis of the jaws as a side effect of radiotherapy of head and neck tumour patients—a report of a thirty year retrospective review. Int J Oral Maxillofac Surg 2003;32:289–295.

Reyes-Gibby CC, Wang J, Zhang L, et al. Oral microbiome and onset of oral mucositis in patients with squamous cell carcinoma of the head and neck. Cancer 2020 Dec 1;126(23):5124–5136. http://doi.org/10.1002/cncr.33161. Epub 2020 Sep 5. PMID: 32888342; PMCID: PMC8191575.

Reynolds EC, Cai F, Cochrane NJ, et al. Fluoride and casein phosphopeptide-amorphous calcium phosphate. J Dent Res 2008;87:344–348.

Reynolds EC, Cai F, Shen P, et al. Retention in plaque and remineralization of enamel lesions by various forms of calcium in a mouthrinse or sugar-free chewing gum. J Dent Res 2003;82:206–211.

Reynolds EC, Cain CJ, Webber FL, et al. Anticariogenicity of calcium phosphate complexes of tryptic casein phosphopeptides in the rat. J Dent Res 1995;74:1272–1279.

Ridner SH. Pathophysiology of lymphedema. Semin Oncol Nurs 2013;29:4–11.

Rieke JW, Hafermann MD, Johnson JT, et al. Oral pilocarpine for radiation-induced xerostomia: Integrated efficacy and safety results from two prospective randomized clinical trials. Int J Radiat Oncol Biol Phys 1995;31:661–669.

Riley P, Glenny AM, Hua F, et al. Pharmacological interventions for preventing dry mouth and salivary gland dysfunction following radiotherapy. Cochrane Database Syst Rev 2017 Jul 31;7(7):CD012744. http://doi.org/10.1002/14651858.CD012744.

Ripamonti C, Zecca E, Brunelli C, et al. A randomized, controlled clinical trial to evaluate the effects of zinc sulfate on cancer patients with taste alterations caused by head and neck irradiation. Cancer 1998;82:1938–1945.

Robard L, Louis MY, Blanchard D, et al. Medical treatment of osteoradionecrosis of the mandible by PENTOCLO: Preliminary results. Eur Ann Otorhinolaryngol Head Neck Dis 2014;131:333–338.

Roberts A, Bradley J, Merkley S, et al. Does potassium iodide application following silver diamine fluoride reduce staining of tooth? A systematic review. Australian Dent J 2020;65:109–117. http://doi.org/10.1111/adj.12743.

Roesink JM, Konings AW, Terhaard CH, et al. Preservation of the rat parotid function after radiation by prophylactic pilocarpine treatment: Radiation dose dependency and compensatory mechanisms. Int J Radiat Oncol Biol Phys 1999;45:483–489.

Roesink JM, Moerland MA, Battermann JJ, et al. Quantitative dose-volume response analysis of changes to parotid gland function after radiotherapy in the head-and-neck region. Int J Radiat Oncol Biol Phys 2001;51:938–946.

Rohrer MD, Kim Y, Fayos JV. The effect of cobalt-60 irradiation on monkey mandibles. Oral Surg Oral Med Oral Pathol 1979;48:424–440.

Roopashri G, Jayanthi K, Guruprasad R. Efficacy of benzydamine hydrochloride, chlorhexidine, and povidone iodine in the treatment of oral mucositis among patients undergoing radiotherapy in head and neck malignancies: A drug trial. Contemp Clin Dent 2011;2:8–12.

Rothwell BR. Prevention and treatment of the orofacial complications of radiotherapy. J Am Dent Assoc 1987;114:316–322.

Roumanas ED, Freymiller EG, Chang TL, et al. Implant-retained prostheses for facial defects: An up to 14-year follow-up report on the survival rates of implants at UCLA. Int J Prosthodont 2002;15:325–332.

Roumanas ED, Nishimura R, Beumer J III, et al. Craniofacial defects and osseointegrated implants: Six-year follow-up report on the success rates of craniofacial implants at UCLA. Int J Oral Maxillofac Implants 1994;9:579–585.

Roumanas ED, Nishimura RD, Davis BK, et al. Clinical evaluation of implants retaining edentulous maxillary obturator prostheses. J Prosthet Dent 1997;77:184–190.

Ruo Redda MG, Allis S. Radiotherapy-induced taste impediment. Cancer Treat Rev 2006;32:541–547.

Saberian F, Ghate A, Kim M. Optimal fractionation in radiotherapy with multiple normal tissues. Math Med Biol 2016;332:211–252.

Salinas TJ, Desa VP, Katsnelson A, et al. Clinical evaluation of implants in radiated fibula flaps. J Oral Maxillofac Surg 2010;68:524–529.

Samani M, Beheshti S, Cheng H, et al. Prophylactic pentoxifylline and vitamin E use for dental extractions in irradiated patients with head and neck cancer. Oral Surg Oral Med Oral Pathol Oral Radiol 2022 Mar;133(3):e63–e71. http://doi.org/10.1016/j.oooo.2021.08.007. Epub 2021 Aug 21. PMID: 34753695.

Sammartino G, Marenzi G, Cioffi I, et al. Implant therapy in irradiated patients. J Craniofac Surg 2011;22:443–445.

Sandow PL, Hejrat-Yazdi M, Heft MW. Taste loss and recovery following radiation therapy. J Dent Res 2006;85:608–611.

Saunders MI, Rojas AM, Parmar MK, et al. Mature results of a randomized trial of accelerated hyperfractionated versus conventional radiotherapy in head-and-neck cancer. Int J Radiat Oncol Biol Phys 2010;77:3–8.

Schmidt BL, Pogrel MA, Young CW, Sharma A. Reconstruction of extensive maxillary defects using zygomaticus implants. J Oral Maxillofac Surg 2004 Sep;62(9 Suppl 2):82–9. doi: 10.1016/j.joms.2004.06.027. PMID: 15332185.

Schuurhuis JM, Stokman MA, Roodenburg JLN, et al. Efficacy of routine pre-radiation dental screening and dental follow-up in head and neck oncology patients on intermediate and late radiation effects: A retrospective evaluation. Radiother Oncol 2011;101:403–409.

Schuurhuis JM, Stokman MA, Witjes MJ, et al. Head and neck intensity modulated radiation therapy leads to an increase of opportunistic oral pathogens. Oral Oncol 2016;58:32–40.

Schuurhuis JM, Stokman MA, Witjes MJ, et al. Patients with advanced periodontal disease before intensity-modulated radiation therapy are prone to develop bone healing problems: A 2-year prospective follow-up study. Supp Care Cancer 2018;26:1133–1142.

Schwartz H. Treatment of osteoradionecrosis with measures other than hyperbaric oxygen. In Proceedings of the First International Congress on Maxillofacial Prosthetics. Ed. IM Zlotolow, S Esposito, J Beumer III. New York: Memorial Sloan-Kettering Cancer Center; 1995. pp. 192–198.

Schwartz HC, Wollin M, Leake DL, et al. Interface radiation dosimetry in mandibular reconstruction. Arch Otolaryngol 1979;105:293–295.

Scrimger JW. Backscatter from high atomic number materials in high energy photon beams. Radiology 1977;124:815–817.

Scully C, Epstein J. Oral health care for the cancer patient. Eur J Cancer B Oral Oncol 1996;32B:281–292.

Seikaly H, Jha N, Harris JR, et al. Long-term outcomes of submandibular gland transfer for prevention of postradiation xerostomia. Arch Otolaryngol Head Neck Surg 2004;130:956–961.

Seto BG, Beumer J III, Kagawa T, et al. Analysis of endodontic therapy in patients irradiated for head and neck cancer. Oral Surg Oral Med Oral Pathol 1985;60:540–545.

Shah DN, Chauhan CJ, Solanki JS. Effectiveness of hyperbaric oxygen therapy in irradiated maxillofacial dental implant patients: A systematic review with meta-analysis. J Indian Prosthodot Soc 2017;17:109–119.

Shaha AR, Cordeiro PG, Hidalgo DA, et al. Resection and immediate microvascular reconstruction in the management of osteoradionecrosis of the mandible. Head Neck 1997;19:406–411.

Shannon I, Suddick R. Saliva. In Dental biochemistry. Ed. E Lazzari. Philadelphia: Lea & Febiger; 1976. pp. 201–242.

Shannon IL, McCrary BR, Starcke EN. A saliva substitute for use by xerostomic patients undergoing radiotherapy to the head and neck. Oral Surg Oral Med Oral Pathol 1977;44:656–661.

Shannon IL, Wescott WB, Starcke EN, et al. Laboratory study of cobalt-60-irradiated human dental enamel. J Oral Med 1978;33:23–27.

Shao ZY, Tang ZS, Yan C, et al. Effects of intensity-modulated radiotherapy on human oral microflora. J Radiat Res 2011;52(6):834–839.

Sharabi Y, Dendi R, Holmes C, et al. Baroreflex failure as a late sequela of neck irradiation. Hypertension 1994;42:110–116.

Sharry JJ, Askew HC, Hoyer H. Influence of artificial tooth forms on bone deformation beneath complete dentures. J Dent Res 1960;39:253–266.

Shugaa-Addin B, Al-Shamiri HM, Al-Maweri S, et al. The effect of radiotherapy on survival of dental implants in head and neck cancer patients. J Clin Exp Dent 2016;8:194–200.

Silva FC, Marto JM, Salgado AM, et al. Nystatin and lidocaine pastilles for the local treatment of oral mucositis. Pharm Dev Technol 2017;22:266–274.

Silverman JE, Weber CS, Silverman S Jr. Zinc supplementation and taste in head and neck cancer patients undergoing radiation therapy. J Oral Med 1983;38:14–16.

Silverman S. Complications of treatment. In Oral cancer. 5th ed. Ed. S Silverman. Hamilton, ON: BC Decker; 2003. pp. 113–128.

Silverman S Jr, Chierici G. Radiation therapy of oral carcinoma: 1. Effects on oral tissues and management of the periodontium. J Periodontol 1965;36:478–484.

Sim CP, Walker GD, Manton DJ, et al. Anticariogenic efficacy of a saliva biomimetic in head-and-neck cancer patients undergoing radiotherapy. Aust Dent J 2019;47:47–54.

Singh BP, Vero N, Singh PK, et al. A simplified technique to fabricate tissue bolus device to manage dose distribution in maxillectomy patient with orbital exenteration. J Oral Biol Craniofac Res 2013;3:102–104.

Sironi M, Massimiliano L, Transidico P, et al. Differential effect of benzydamine on pro- versus anti-inflammatory cytokine production: Lack of inhibition of interleukin-10 and interleukin-1 receptor antagonist. Int J Clin Lab Res 2000;30:17–19.

Soares EF, Naves LZ, Correr AM, et al. Effect of radiotherapy, adhesive systems and doxycycline on the bond strength of the dentin-composite interface. Am J Dent 2016;29:352–356.

Sodicoff M, Pratt NE, Sholley MM. Ultrastructural radiation injury of rat parotid gland. Radiat Res 1974;58:196–208.

Solomon H, Marchetta FC, Wilson RO, et al. Extraction of teeth after cancercidal doses of radiation therapy to the head and neck. Am J Surg 1968;115:349–351.

Sonis ST. Mucositis as a biological process: A new hypothesis for the development of chemotherapy-induced stomatotoxicity. Oral Oncol 1998;34:39–43.

Sonis ST. Mucositis: The impact, biology and therapeutic opportunities of oral mucositis. Oral Oncol 2009;45:1015–1020.

Sonis ST. The pathobiology of mucositis. Nat Rev Cancer 2004a;44:277–284.

Sonis ST, Elting LS, Keefe D, et al. Perspectives on cancer therapy-induced mucosal injury: Pathogenesis, measurement, epidemiology, and consequences for patients. Cancer 2004b;100:1995–2025.

Sonis ST, Haddad R, Posner M, et al. Gene expression changes in peripheral blood cells provide insight into the biological mechanisms associated with regimen-related toxicities in patients being treated for head and neck cancers. Oral Oncol 2007;43:289–300.

Sood AJ, Fox NF, O'Connell BP. Salivary gland transfer to prevent radiation-induced xerostomia: A systematic review and meta-analysis. Oral Oncol 2014;50:77–83.

Spijkervet FK, Brennan MT, Peterson DE, et al. Research frontiers in oral toxicities of cancer therapies: Osteoradionecrosis of the jaws. JNCI Monographs 2019 Aug 1;2019(53):lgz006. http://doi.org/10.1093/jncimonographs/lgz006.

Spijkervet FK, Schuurhuis JM, Stokman MR. Should oral foci of infection be removed before onset of radiotherapy or chemotherapy. Oral Diseases 2021;27:7–13.

Spijkervet FK, van Saene HK, Panders AK, et al. Effect of chlorhexidine rinsing on the oropharyngeal ecology in patients with head and neck cancer. Oral Surg Oral Med Oral Pathol 1989:67:154–161.

Spijkervet FK, van Saene HK, van Saene JJ, et al. Mucositis prevention by selective elimination of oral flora in irradiated head and neck cancer patients. J Oral Pathol Med 1990;19:486–489.

Stieb S, Perez-Martinez I, Mohamed A, et al. The impact of tongue-deviating and tongue-depressing oral stents on long-term radiation-associated symptoms in oropharyngeal cancer survivors. Clin Translational Radiat Oncol 2020;24:71–78.

Stokman MA, Spijkervet FK, Burlage FR, et al. Oral mucositis and selective elimination of oral flora in head and neck cancer patients receiving radiotherapy: A double-blind randomized clinical trial. Br J Cancer 2003;88:1012–1016. http://doi.org/10.1038/sj.bjc.6600824.

Studer G, Gratz KW, Glanzmann C. Osteoradionecrosis of the mandibula in patients treated with different fractionations. Strahlenther Onkol 2004;180:233–240.

Subramaniam SS, Breik O, Cadd B, et al. Long-term outcomes of craniofacial implants for the restoration of facial defects. Int J Oral Maxillofac Surg 2018;47:773–782.

Suryawanshi H, Ganvir SM, Hazarey VK, et al. Oropharyngeal candidosis relative frequency in radiotherapy patient for head and neck cancer. J Oral Maxillofac Pathol 2012;16:31–37.

Symonds RP, McIlroy P, Khorrami J, et al. The reduction of radiation mucositis by selective decontamination antibiotic pastilles: A placebo-controlled double-blind trial. Br J Cancer 1996;74:312–317.

Takahashi S, Shinzato K, Domon T, et al. Mitotic proliferation of myoepithelial cells during regeneration of atrophied rat submandibular glands after duct ligation. J Oral Pathol Med 2004;33:430–434.

Takei T, Aono W, Nagashima S. Change of salivary IgA secretion and caries development in irradiated rats. J Dent Res 1994;73:1503–1508.

Takeuchi K, Saruwatari L, Nakamura H, et al. Enhancement of biomechanical properties of mineralized tissue by osteoblasts cultured on titanium with different surface topographies. J Biomed Mater Res 2005;72A:296–305.

ten Cate J. Current concepts on the theories of the mechanism of action of fluoride. Acta Odontol Scand 1999;57:325–329.

Teramoto Y, Kurita H, Kamata T, et al. A case of peri-implantitis and osteoradionecrosis arising around dental implants placed before radiation therapy. Int J Implant Dent 2016 Dec;2(1):11. Epub 2016 Apr 5.

Thorn JJ, Hansen HS, Specht L, et al. Osteoradionecrosis of the jaws: Clinical characteristics and relation to the field of radiation. J Oral Maxillofac Surg 2000;58:1088–1093.

Tso TV, Blackwell KE, Sung EC. Predictive factors of osteoradionecrosis necessitating segmental mandibulectomy: A descriptive study. Oral Surg Oral Med Oral Pathol Oral Radiol 2022 Jul;134(1):e8–e13. http://doi.org/10.1016/j.oooo.2021.08.024. Epub 2021 Sep 3. PMID: 34758937.

Tso TV, Hurwitz M, Margalit DN, et al. Radiation dose enhancement associated with contemporary dental materials. J Prosthet Dent 2019;121:703–707.

Valdez IH, Atkinson JC, Ship JA, et al. Major salivary gland function in patients with radiation-induced xerostomia: Flow rates and sialochemistry. Int J Radiat Oncol Biol Phys 1993;25:41–47.

van der Geer SJ, van Rijn PV, Kamstra J, et al. Criterion for trismus in head and neck cancer patients: A verification study. Support Care Cancer 2019;27:1129–1137.

Van Luijk P, Pringle S, Deasy JO, et al. Sparing the region of the salivary gland containing stem cells preserves saliva production after radiotherapy for head and neck cancer. Sci Trans Med 2015;7(305):305ra147. http://doi.org/10.1126/scitranslmed.aac4441.

van Merkesteyn JP, Bakker DJ, Borgmeijer-Hoelen AM. Pathogenesis and treatment of osteoradionecrosis of the jaws. Presented at the Annual Meeting of the International Association of Oral Oncology, Amsterdam, May 1993.

Vera-Llonch M, Oster G, Hagiwara M, et al. Oral mucositis in patients undergoing radiation treatment for head and neck carcinoma. Cancer 2006;106:329–336. http://doi.org/10.1002/cncr.21622.

Verrone JR, Alves FA, Prado JD, et al. Benefits of an intraoral stent in decreasing the irradiation dose to oral healthy tissue: Dosimetric and clinical features. Oral Surg Oral Med Oral Path Oral Radiol 2014;118:573–578.

Visch LL, Gravenmade EJ, Schaub RM, et al. A double-blind crossover trial of CMC- and mucin-containing saliva substitutes. Int J Oral Maxillofac Surg 1986;15:395–400.

Visch LL, van Waas MA, Schmitz PI, et al. A clinical evaluation of implants in irradiated oral cancer patients. J Dent Res 2002;81:856–859.

Visser A, Raghoebar GM, van Oort RP, et al. Fate of implant-retained craniofacial prostheses: Life span and aftercare. Int J Oral Maxillofac Implants 2008;23:89–98.

Vissink A, Burlage FR, Spijkervet FK, et al. Prevention and treatment of the consequences of head and neck radiotherapy. Crit Rev Oral Biol Med 2003;14:213–225.

Vissink A, Gravenmade EJ, Panders AK, et al. A clinical comparison between commercially available mucin- and CMC-containing saliva substitutes. Int J Oral Surg 1983;12:232–238.

Vujaskovic Z. Structural and physiological properties of peripheral nerves after intraoperative irradiation. J Peripher Nerv Syst 1997;2:343–349.

Wang ZH, Yan C, Zhang ZU, et al. Impact of salivary gland dosimetry on post-IMRT recovery of saliva output and xerostomia grade for head-and-neck cancer patients treated with or without contralateral submandibular gland sparing: A longitudinal study. Int J Radiat Oncol Biol Phys 2011;81:1479–1487.

Warde P, O'Sullivan B, Aslanidis J, et al. A phase III placebo-controlled trial of oral pilocarpine in patients undergoing radiotherapy for head and neck cancer. Int J Radiat Oncol Biol Phys 2002;54:9–13.

Watters AL, Cope S, Keller MN, et al. Prevalence of trismus in patients with head and neck cancer: A systematic review with meta-analysis. Head Neck 2019;41:3408–3421.

Weinlander M, Beumer J III, Kenney EB, et al. Histomorphometric and fluorescence microscopic evaluation of interfacial bone healing around 3 different dental implants before and after radiation therapy. Int J Oral Maxillofac Implants 2006;21:212–224.

Wetzels JW, Meijer GJ, Koole R, et al. Costs and clinical outcomes of implant placement during ablative surgery and postponed implant placement in curative oral oncology: A five-year retrospective cohort study. Clin Oral Implants Res 2017;28:1433–1444.

Wijers OB, Levendag PC, Harms ER, et al. Mucositis reduction by selective elimination of oral flora in irradiated cancers of the head and neck: A placebo-controlled double-blind randomized study. Int J Radiat Oncol Biol Phys 2001;50:343–352.

Wilke C, Zaid M, Chung C, et al. Design and fabrication of a 3D-printed oral stent for head and neck radiotherapy from routine diagnostic imaging. Printing in Medicine 2017;3:12. http://doi.org/10.1186/s41205-017-0021-4.

Wong JK, Wood RE, Mclean M. Conservative management of osteoradionecrosis. Oral Surg Oral Med Oral Pathol Oral Radiol Endod 1997;84:16–21.

Xu B, Boero IJ, Hwang L, et al. Aspiration pneumonia after concurrent chemoradiotherapy for head and neck cancer. Cancer 2015 Apr 15;121(8):1303–1311.

Yamashita H, Nakagawa K, Tago M, et al. Taste dysfunction in patients receiving chemotherapy. Head Neck 2006;28:508–516.

Yangchen K, Siddharth R, Singh SV, et al. A pilot study to evaluate the efficacy of cerrobend shielding stents in preventing adverse radiotherapeutic effects in buccal carcinoma patients. J Cancer Res Ther 2016a;12:314–317.

Yangchen K, Singh SV, Aggarwal H, et al. Cerrobend shielding stents for buccal carcinoma patients. J Cancer Res Ther 2016b;12:1102–1103.

Yerit KC, Posch M, Seemann M, et al. Implant survival in mandibles of irradiated oral cancer patients. Clin Oral Implants Res 2006;17:337–344.

Yilmaz B, Seidt JD, McGlumphy EA, et al. Comparison of strains for splinted and nonsplinted screw-retained prostheses on short implants. Int J Oral Maxillofac Implants 2011;26:1176–1182.

Yusof ZW, Bakri MM. Severe progressive periodontal destruction due to radiation tissue injury. J Periodontol 1993;64:1253–1258.

Zadic Y, Arany PR, Fregnani ER, et al. Systematic review of photobiomodulation for the management of oral mucositis in cancer patients and clinical practice guidelines. Support Care Cancer 2019;27:3969–3983.

Zaghi S, Danesh J, Hendizadeh L, et al. Changing indications for maxillomandibular reconstruction with osseous free flaps: A 17-year experience with 620 consecutive cases at UCLA and the impact of osteoradionecrosis. Laryngoscope 2014;1246:1329–1335.

Zaghi S, Miller M, Blackwell K, et al. Analysis of surgical margins in cases of mandibular osteoradionecrosis that progress despite extensive mandible resection and free tissue transfer. Am J Otolaryngol 2021;225:576–580.

Zagury-Orly I, Khaouam N, Noujaim J, et al. The effect of radiation and chemoradiation therapy on the head and neck mucosal microbiome: A review. Front Oncol 2021 Dec 2;11:784457. http://doi.org/10.3389/fonc.2021.784457. PMID: 34926301; PMCID: PMC8674486.

Zaid M, Bajaj N, Burrows H, et al. Creating customized oral stents for head and neck radiotherapy using 3D scanning and printing. Radiat Oncol 2019;14:148. http://doi.org/10.1186/s13014-019-1357-2.

Zhao Y, Moran K, Yewondwossen M, et al. Clinical applications of 3-dimensional printing in radiation therapy. Med Dosim 2017;42(2):150–155.

Zhou Y, Sheng X, Deng F, et al. Radiation-induced muscle fibrosis rat model: Establishment and valuation. Radiation Oncology 2018;13:160. http://doi.org/10.1186/s13014-018-11.

Zidar N, Ferluga D, Hvala A, et al. Contribution to the pathogenesis of radiation-induced injury to large arteries. J Laryngol Otol 1997;111:988–990.

Chapter 2

Rehabilitation of Tongue and Mandibular Defects

Jay Jayanetti, Denny S. Chao, Daniel Ramos, Keith Blackwell, Michael Eggersted, Suresh Nayar, Earl Freymiller, Peter Han, Donald Curtis, Alan Hannam, Timothy C. Blood Jr., Kenneth Yan, Kristen Echanique, Arman Danielian, Rhorie Kerr, Lindsay Lanciault, Sarah Panjwani, Andrew Erman, Dinesh K. Chhetri, Jana Rieger

The management of malignant tumors associated with the tongue, floor of mouth (FOM), mandible, and adjacent structures represents a difficult challenge for the surgeon, radiation oncologist, and prosthodontist in terms of both control of the primary disease and rehabilitation. The most common intraoral sites for squamous cell carcinoma (SCC) are the lateral margin of the tongue and the floor of mouth (FOM). Both locations predispose the mandible to tumor invasion, often necessitating a composite resection of the tongue, mandible, and the FOM.

Disabilities resulting from such resections may include impaired speech, difficulty in swallowing, problems with mastication, altered mandibular movements, compromised control of salivary secretions, and cosmetic disfigurement.

Vascularized free tissue transfers (free flaps) and dental implants have resulted in considerable improvement in the form and function of these patients. With these surgical and prosthodontic methods, more patients with defects of the tongue and mandible can have their appearance and function restored to levels that approach their presurgical condition. These rehabilitative techniques are complex and require the efforts of an interdisciplinary team of surgical oncologists and microvascular surgeons, radiation and medical oncologists, prosthodontists, speech and swallow therapists, social workers, and biomedical engineers. Virtual surgical planning (VSP) provides a predictable, accelerated, and occlusion-based rehabilitation.

In rare situations, free flaps and the placement of dental implants may not be indicated or possible. In such instances, rehabilitation efforts will be challenging, and functional outcomes are frequently diminished.

Treatment of malignant neoplasms that include the mandible or contiguous soft tissues impacts many vital and life-sustaining functions. A partially resected tongue compounds the problem because it will not function like a normal tongue. A mandible reconstructed with an osteomyocutaneous free flap can demonstrate relatively normal mandibular movements and appearance, but altered sensory status may still result in less-than-optimal function. Adjuvant radiation therapy may further impact the hard and soft tissues of the native and/or reconstructed mandible.

It is preferable to reconstruct the mandible and soft tissue defect immediately following tumor ablation. From the perspective of oral function and prosthodontic rehabilitation, reconstruction of the tongue should receive the highest priority, and we believe that flaps should be selected and tailored with this priority in mind. The tongue is the most important oral structure with regard to mastication, saliva control, speech, and swallowing. Its bulk should be restored and the reconstruction designed to maximize the mobility of the tongue remnant. If the tongue is not reconstructed adequately, the patient will be severely disabled even if the continuity of the mandible has been retained or restored.

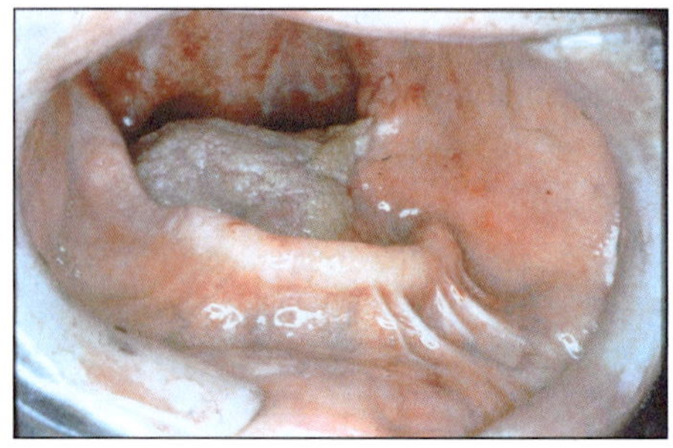

Figure 2-1 Tongue mandible defect. Residual tongue sutured to the buccal mucosa. Tongue mobility is limited, compromising oral competence.

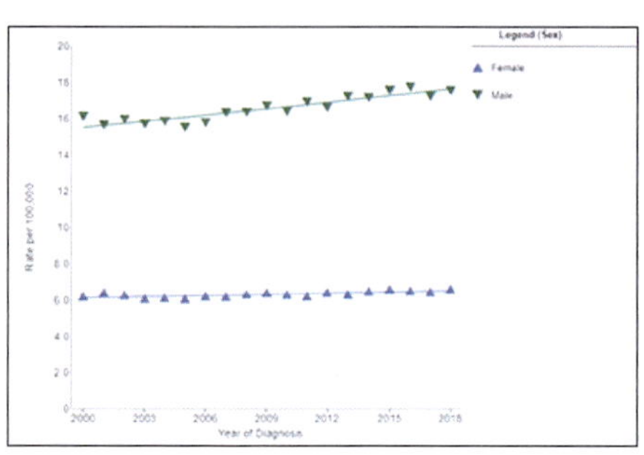

Figure 2-2 Recent trends in Surveillance Epidemiology End Results (SEER) age-adjusted incidence rates 2000–2018 oral cavity and oropharynx of all races (including Hispanic).

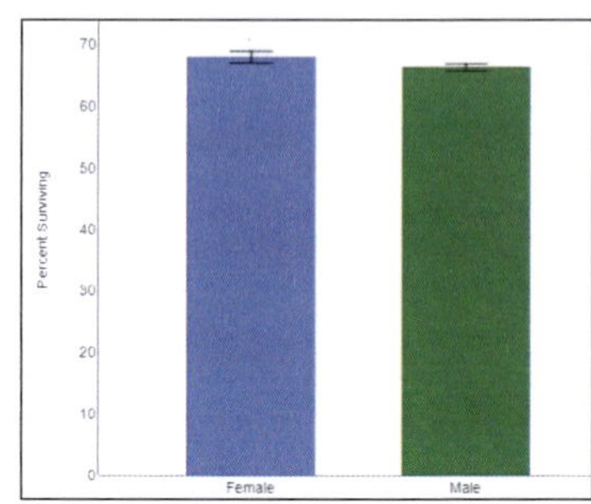

Figure 2-3 SEER five-year survival rates 2011–2017 by sex; inclusive of all races (including Hispanic), all ages, and all stages.

The functional disabilities associated with the tongue and mandible resections are dependent on the amount of tongue resected and the method of closure. If the surgical wound is closed primarily (e.g., connecting the midline of the residual tongue to the buccal mucosa), the functional disabilities are compounded (Fig 2-1). Patients may be unable to control their saliva, speak, swallow, or appear presentable.

It is unrealistic to discuss functional impairment without reference to the psychosocial factors that affect patients with mandibular resections. Those involved in the rehabilitation of these patients must be sensitive to the emotional trauma precipitated by cancer and its treatment (see Chapter 9). Distortions in self-image, inability to communicate, and altered family and vocational roles require support from or referral to appropriate professionals to handle these new demands.

Epidemiology of Oral Cancer

Prevention is the best approach to successfully manage oral cancer. This requires that oral health care providers take a more proactive role in the early identification of this disease. General dentists must be better educated in how to recognize and refer/treat/manage precancerous/cancerous lesions. Leukoplakia/erythroplakia are common precancerous lesions that can be managed. In addition to identifying and managing suspicious lesions, the dentist needs to promote/support healthy lifestyle choices by our patients, such as decreasing alcohol use and total abstinence from any tobacco products. Patients need to understand the risk factors associated with certain lifestyle choices. The human papillomavirus (HPV) is the most common sexually transmitted disease (STD). HPV is the leading cause of oropharyngeal cancers, primarily in the tonsils, tonsillar crypt, and the base of the tongue. There are multiple forms of HPV with HPV16/18 serving as the high-risk forms and most responsible for oropharyngeal carcinogenesis and affects both males and females.

Although the exact pathway of HPV carcinogenesis is not clear, it is thought that individuals with a weakened immune system may be more susceptible to oropharyngeal carcinoma. Transformation is more likely to occur if HPV is not cleared but allowed to sit in the tonsillar tissue (Fakhry et al., 2008).

High-risk HPV, particularly HPV-16/18, has been established as a causative agent for a significant proportion of oropharyngeal squamous cell carcinomas (Gillison et al., 2000), and the incidence of these HPV head and neck squamous cell carcinomas (HPV-HNSCC) is on the rise (Ramqvist and Dalianis, 2010). The incidence of HPV oropharyngeal cancer is so widespread that it has been called an epidemic (Ramqvist and Dalianis, 2010).

HPV-HNSCC represents a distinct biological and clinical subtype of *Oropharyngeal carcinoma.* HPV-HNSCC has a much better prognosis than non-HPV-HNSCC. HPV-positivity correlates with a lower risk of tumor progression and death, reflecting in part an enhanced sensitivity to ionizing radiation with or without chemotherapy (Ang et al., 2010). Individual genetics also influences susceptibility. A greater understanding of the occurrence, demographics, and risk factors—as well as education, research, and patient care—will improve patient prognosis.

Incidence

Oral and oropharyngeal cancer is the sixth most common cancer in the world and the fourth most common cancer in men (behind prostate, skin, and lung). Worldwide, there are more than 600,000 cases of head and neck cancer diagnosed annually. This includes 260,000 cases of oral cavity, 213,000 thyroid gland, 150,000 larynx, 130,000 pharynx, and 85,000 nasopharynx per year (Joseph and D'Souza, 2012). Nasopharynx is considered separately because of a distinct etiology: infection by HH4 (Epstein-Barr virus).

In 2018, there were an estimated 396,937 people living with oral cavity and oropharyngeal cancer in the United States. According to the National Cancer Institute (NIH, 2019), 54,000 individuals will be diagnosed with oral and oropharyngeal cancer in 2021 in the United States. This represents 2.8% of all cancers diagnosed in the United States (NIH, 2019) (Table 2-1) (Fig 2-2).

In the United States, oral cavity cancer has a five-year survival rate of 66.9% for the period of 2011–2017. In 2021, 10,860 people are expected to die from this disease, representing 1.8% of all cancer deaths.

Head and neck cancers are the most common cancers in some developing countries, especially in Southeast Asia (Joshi et al., 2014). Head and neck cancers are more common in males compared to females (Fig 2-3). This is mainly attributed to tobacco, areca nut, and alcohol use, which are predominantly used by males.

Late-stage diagnosis of most oral cancers (stage III or IV) results in decreased survival and leads to a deterioration in patient quality of life (Wangsa et al., 2008; Jung et al., 2010).

Oral cancers are most common among all head and neck squamous cell cancers (HNSCC). HNSCC in the developing world differs from those in the Western world in terms of age, site of disease, etiology, and molecular biology. Poverty, illiteracy, advanced stage at presentation, lack of access to health care, and poor treatment infrastructure pose a major challenge in the management of these cancers in developing countries (Joshi et al., 2014).

Etiology and Predisposing Factors

Cellular events leading to carcinogenesis take time. Another contributing factor is the age of the patient. Several oncogenes have been implicated in oral carcinogenesis. The aberrant expression of the protooncogene epidermal growth factor receptor (EGFR/c-erb 1)—members of the ras gene family, c-myc, int-2, hst-1, PRAD-1, and bcl-1—is believed to contribute toward cancer development (Todd et al., 1997).

Based on a significant amount of evidence in the literature, TGF-β signaling is currently considered to have paradoxical impacts on cancer, acting both as a tumor suppressor or as a tumor promoter in the epithelium depending on the stage of exposure (Pickup et al., 2013).

The use of tobacco or alcohol significantly increases the risk of oral cancer. To complicate matters, everyone reacts differently to these stimuli as a result of heredity, age, sex, and many other factors. Death rates from around the world suggest marked differences within populations.

The immune system and cancer

Immune surveillance is one of the most important factors in fighting cancer. The competence of the immune system, which includes immune surveillance, diminishes with age. This likely contributes to increased cancer occurrence with aging. Other studies have shown that there is an increased risk of cancer developing in individuals whose immune system is either congenitally defective or suppressed by chemotherapy or by specific diseases. The association between immunosuppression and increased cancer risk has been shown in those with HIV. It is not clear whether differences found in some immunologic variables are a *cause or a result* of the malignancy.

Viruses

The main factors associated with head and neck cancer are smoking and alcohol, which account for about 75% of all cases. Viruses have also been shown to be an important factor. The most common viruses related to head and neck cancers are those capable of cell transformation. These include the human papillomavirus (HPV) (Doorbar et al., 2012), herpesviruses, adenoviruses (Johnson, 1991), and hepatitis C viruses (Alibek et al., 2014).

Although many factors can promote cell transformation, viruses are now the focus of a great deal of research, since HPV was shown to be causative for oropharyngeal carcinoma.

Herpes viruses

Herpes is an enveloped double-stranded DNA virus with an icosahedral capsid. Six of these cause human disease: Human Herpes Virus type-1 (HHV-1 [*previously HSV-1*]), Human Herpes Virus type-2 (HHV-2 [*previously HSV-2*]), Human Herpes Virus type-3 (HHV-3 [*previously Herpes Zoster*]), Human Herpes Virus type-4 (HHV-4 [*previously Epstein-Barr*]), Human Herpes Virus type-5 (HHV-5 [*previously CMV*]), and Human Herpes Virus type-6 (HHV-6). Each of these viruses causes an acute human infection, and HHV-1, -2, -4, and -5 have been associated with certain malignant diseases as well (Wołącewicz et al., 2020).

HHV-4 causes Burkitt's lymphoma and nasopharyngeal carcinoma. HHV-4 is epidemiologically associated with those diseases and can transform the target cell type. HHV-4 is not associated with oral squamous cell carcinomas.

Carcinogenicity of HHV

Laboratory manipulation allows HHV to transform hamster cells in culture. When these transformed cells were placed back into hamsters, the cells grew as carcinomas.

However, no evidence of HHV was detected in the harvested tumors. Therefore, it is possible that HHV may act in a transient role promoting carcinogenesis.

Tobacco

Tobacco use may be viewed as a worldwide pandemic, causing serious disease and immense health problems. In addition to mortality, smoking carries considerable morbidity, resulting in loss of working days, decreased productivity, increased demand for medical services, and expenses (Wołącewicz et al., 2008).

Smoking tobacco is regarded as the main cause of oral cancer. The American Cancer Society (2021) indicates that 20% of *all* cancers can be traced to smoking tobacco. *Eighty percent of all lung cancers are a direct response to tobacco use.* All forms of tobacco smoking are linked to oral cancer. Pipes and cigars are more closely associated with lip and palatal cancer, likely due to the constant heat generated in the oral cavity. "Reverse Smoking" is quite popular in India and Southeast Asia. Since society in many parts of Asia frowns on women smoking, they have taken to the habit of "Reverse Smoking." Keeping the lit end of the cigarette in the mouth generates constant heat to the palatal and lingual tissue.

The longtime use of smokeless tobacco (snuff or chewing tobacco) is also thought to increase the risk of oral cancer, although lower than smoking.

Smokeless tobacco also has its own associated risks, such as periodontal disease, soft tissue hyperkeratosis (leukoplakia), and root caries. Many smokeless tobacco products contain cancer-causing chemicals. The most harmful chemicals are tobacco-specific nitrosamines, which form during the growing, curing, fermenting, and aging of tobacco. The amount of these chemicals varies by product. The higher the levels of these chemicals, the greater the risk for cancer.

Other chemicals found in tobacco can also cause cancer. These include the radioactive element (polonium-210) found in tobacco fertilizer. The curing of tobacco with heat generates polynuclear aromatic hydrocarbons—also known as polycyclic aromatic hydrocarbons, which are highly carcinogenic. Smokeless tobacco also contains harmful metals (arsenic, beryllium, cadmium, chromium, cobalt, lead, nickel, mercury).

Many of those using smokeless tobacco also continue to smoke and use alcohol, which synergistically raises the risk of oral cancer. Smokeless tobacco is not a safe alternative to smoking.

Tobacco components

There are approximately 600 ingredients in cigarettes, and when burned, cigarettes create more than 4,000 chemicals. At least 70 of these chemicals are known to cause cancer, and many are toxic (American Lung Association, 2020). There is evidence that mainly two, specifically nicotine and carbon monoxide, exert toxic effects on the heart and blood vessels (Leone, 2015).

Interestingly, many of these chemicals are also found in different products, such as rat poison, and carry a warning label. No such warning label is given for tobacco smoke. Some of the chemicals found in tobacco smoke include nicotine, hydrogen cyanide, formaldehyde, lead, arsenic, ammonia, carbon monoxide, tobacco-specific nitrosamines, and polycyclic aromatic hydrocarbons.

A lit cigarette releases 92% gas and 8% particulate matter. Eighty-five percent of the gas is carbon dioxide, oxygen, and nitrogen. Although the percentage of carbon monoxide is very low, it is still high enough to exert a negative effect on the hemoglobin exchange mechanism. Nicotine affects platelet adhesion and contributes to cardiovascular disease and hypertension (Ambrose and Barua, 2004; Leone, 2015).

The aromatic hydrocarbons (tars) are the most carcinogenic component of tobacco combustion. In a typical cigarette, the nicotine concentration ranges from less than 1 mg to more than 3 mg and is an addiction mechanism.

E-Cigarettes

E-cigarettes, or "vaping," refer to the use of a wide variety of electronic, battery-operated devices that aerosolize liquids to release nicotine and other substances. E-cigarettes are regulated as "tobacco products" by the FDA because the nicotine is derived from the tobacco plant. The use of vaping products has rapidly increased among young people; with an effort targeting high school students. The new generation of e-cigarettes more effectively delivers larger amounts of nicotine to the brain. Many e-cigarettes sold in the United States contain far more nicotine than e-cigarettes sold elsewhere, which is a conscious attempt to quickly addict a new generation of smokers. The long-term risks of the exclusive use of e-cigarettes are not fully known, but evidence is accumulating that e-cigarette use has negative effects on the cardiovascular system and lungs.

The e-cigarette aerosol, which users breathe from the device and exhale, can contain harmful and potentially harmful substances, including nicotine. In addition to nicotine, ultrafine particles such as diacetyl, a chemical linked to a serious lung disease; propylene glycol and/or vegetable glycerin, cancer-causing chemicals; and heavy metals such as nickel, tin, and lead can be inhaled into the lung tissue. Like smokeless tobacco, e-cigarettes are not a safe option as a nicotine delivery system.

Tobacco use and health

Cigarette smoking is responsible for more than 480,000 deaths per year in the United States, including more than 41,000 deaths resulting from secondhand smoke exposure. This is about 1 in 5 deaths annually, or 1,300 deaths every day. On average, smokers die 10 years earlier than nonsmokers (World Health Organization, 2017).

The total economic cost of smoking is more than $300 billion a year, including

- More than $225 billion in direct medical care for adults
- More than $156 billion in lost productivity due to premature death and exposure to secondhand smoke

The Center for Disease Control (CDC) reports that **4.6%** of all high school students are current smokers (5.4% of males and 3.9% of females) (Wang et al., 2019).

Also, among smokers, the numbers increase in those with lower levels of education. There are also ethnic differences, with Caucasians and African Americans being the heaviest users.

Other carcinogenic habit forms

Social customs that can lead to cancer are complex and far-reaching. Some customs, such as betel- and tobacco-dipping, are widespread. In the areas of the world where these habits are practiced, the incidence of oral carcinoma is comparatively high. There are considerable variations in prevalence in different countries, depending on the way the ingredients are prepared for chewing.

Oral cancer ranks among the three most common cancers in India and, in some areas, accounts for almost 40% of total cancer deaths. In most regions of India, oral cancer is the second most common malignancy diagnosed in men, accounting for up to 20% of cancers, and the fourth most common in women (Elango et al., 2009).

A relationship appears to exist between this extremely high occurrence of oral malignancy and the use of various forms and combinations of tobacco, slaked lime, betel nuts, and spices.

Summary

In conclusion, the use of tobacco in all forms—cigarettes, e-cigarettes, cigars, pipes, chewing preparations, and snuff—increases the risk of eventually developing oral carcinoma, which appears to be causally related. This is based on the following facts:

- Carcinogenic agents have been isolated from tobacco condensates.
- Tobacco can induce cellular change and tissue atypia.
- There is a greater use of tobacco in patients with oral carcinoma than among persons in control groups.
- Tobacco used in various forms has been associated with an unusually high prevalence of carcinoma at specific oral sites.
- Continued smoking is a factor in the development of multiple oral carcinomas.
- There is an increased mortality ratio from oral carcinoma for smokers as compared with nonsmokers.

While tobacco-use cessation is difficult to achieve, approaches to assessing a patient's willingness to stop is the first step. Consultation and assisting in this process is critical and presents a role for dental professionals in health care. Nicotine replacement forms and pharmacotherapeutics, along with consultation, are extremely useful. Effectiveness is dependent upon good follow-up and motivation.

Second primary tumors

Compared to the general population, patients with HNSCC have an increased risk of second primary malignancies (SPM). The most common site for an SPM is the head and neck, lung, and esophagus. The incidence of an SPM in HNSCC patients is about 3% to 7% every year, with an estimated 20-year cumulative risk of 36% (Adjei Boakye et al., 2018). However, patients whose initial tumor was HPV-positive have a lower risk of an SPM than those whose initial diagnosis was HPV-negative (Adjei Boakye et al., 2018).

Approximately one-third of HNSCC deaths are attributable to second primary malignant neoplasms. Second primary malignant neoplasms cause the death of three times as many patients with HNSCC than those who die of metastatic disease. SPM represents the second leading cause of mortality in patients with HNSCC (Baxi et al., 2014). This cause of mortality is greater in HPV-negative HNSCC. SPM are associated with a poor prognosis, are the leading cause of long-term morbidity and mortality, and represent an impediment to survival in patients with HNSCC (Garavello et al., 2006).

HNSCC remains the leading cause of death over time (Baxi et al., 2014). One-quarter to one-third of deaths in these patients are attributable to SPM (Siegel, 2020; Noone et al., 1975–2015), highlighting the importance of SPM in the successful management of HNSCC.

Persistent tobacco smoking and alcohol drinking after treatment of an HNSCC contributed to the risk of the appearance of a second neoplasm (Siegel et al., 2020). According to the attributable risk estimation, persistent tobacco and alcohol consumption would be responsible for one-third of the second neoplasms in the patients with an HNSCC tumor index.

Field cancerization

The concept of field cancerization was first described in 1953 when pathologic changes in the epithelium surrounding the oropharyngeal SCC were identified (Slaughter et al., 1953). In that report, the authors observed that all cases of oropharyngeal SCC had pathologic dysplasia and foci of SCC *in situ* in the adjacent normally appearing mucosa. Many of these changes were not contiguous with the primary tumor and represented separate islands of dysplastic epithelium. In addition, 11% of oropharyngeal SCCs presented with two separate primary lesions, a rate 10-fold greater than expected based on disease prevalence.

Cancer begins with multiple cumulative epigenetic (i.e., *methylation or histone modification*) and genetic changes that can transform a cell or a group of cells in a tissue/organ. These early genetic "changes" may promote the clonal expansion of precancerous cells. Genomic changes in some of these cells drive them toward the malignant phenotype. These transformed cells are diagnosed histologically as cancers due to their morphology. Daughter cells with these same genetic changes, not examined histologically, can remain in the tissue/organ indefinitely or become cancer (Jaiswal et al., 2013).

These findings support the independent or co-incident development of multiple lesions rather than the linear progression of a single mutant clone. This suggests that the "normal" epithelium in the vicinity of a primary SCC is not normal. The cells are primed to become malignant and are simply awaiting the appropriate signals to complete the transformation process.

Recent studies show that the risk of HNSCC attributed to tobacco and alcohol exposure differs. Alcohol is most strongly associated with risk for oral cavity and oropharyngeal cancers, and tobacco is most strongly associated with laryngeal tumors (Hashibe et al., 2009; Purdue et al., 2009).

Human papillomaviruses (HPV)

HPV is the most common sexually transmitted infection in the United States. There are more than 100 types of HPV. Of these, about 40 types can spread through direct sexual contact to genital areas, as well as the oropharynx. Most HPV is cleared by the immune system within one to two years but can persist in some individuals. HPV is so common that almost every person who is sexually active will get HPV at some time in their life if they don't get the HPV vaccine. There were about 43 million HPV infections in 2018, many among people in their late teens and early 20s. Human papillomaviruses (HPVs) are strictly epitheliotropic and infect either cutaneous or mucosal squamous epithelium (Conway and Meyers, 2009; Feller et al., 2009). HPV promotes carcinogenesis through protein E6, inhibiting the tumor suppressor p53 (Odar et al., 2014).

HPV has been recovered in over 85% of anal cancer cases. HPV 16/18 has been recovered in greater than 70% of cervical dysplasia and cancer. While HPV 16/18 does not apparently contribute to oral cavity carcinogenesis, it's a well-known contributing factor in oral pharyngeal carcinoma (Ang et al., 2010).

Since the late 1990s, tobacco-related cancers, including oral cavity and laryngeal cancers, have decreased due to public awareness of the health risks. During this same period, rates of oropharyngeal cancers increased (Frisch et al., 2000). HPV associated with oropharyngeal cancer increased from 20% in the 1980s to 70% by 2005.

High-risk HPV 16 and 18 are clearly risk factors / causative for oropharyngeal cancer (Da Silva et al., 2007; Sturgis and Cinciripini, 2007; McNeil, 2000; Chen et al., 2008). Not all individuals infected with HPV will go on to develop cancer. Likely, there are unidentified cofactors, such as smoking or using smokeless tobacco, that may contribute to HPV carcinogenesis. The association between oropharyngeal cancer and HPV is strongest in the tonsils. More than 70% of all tonsil cancers are positive for HPV 16/18.

This preferential targeting likely reflects complex biological interactions between HPV and the highly specialized lympho-epithelium lining the tonsillar crypts known as the reticulated epithelium.

The microscopic features of the reticulated epithelium lining the tonsillar crypts are unique and may provide an immune-privileged site.

HPV-SCC presents a different molecular profile when compared with HPV-negative SCC (Ang et al., 2010). The most clinically relevant difference is that the presence of HPV in the tumor provides a positive impact on patient survival (Ang et al., 2010).

HPV that infects the mucosal epithelium is characterized as high-risk (e.g., HPV-16, 18, 31, 33, and 35) or low-risk types (HPV-6, 11, 13, and 32) based on their epidemiological association with cervical carcinoma. The most highly carcinogenic is HPV 16, which inhibits the tumor suppressor protein p53 through the protein E6.

HPV-positive oropharyngeal carcinomas present with a better prognosis when compared to HPV-negative SCC and appear to

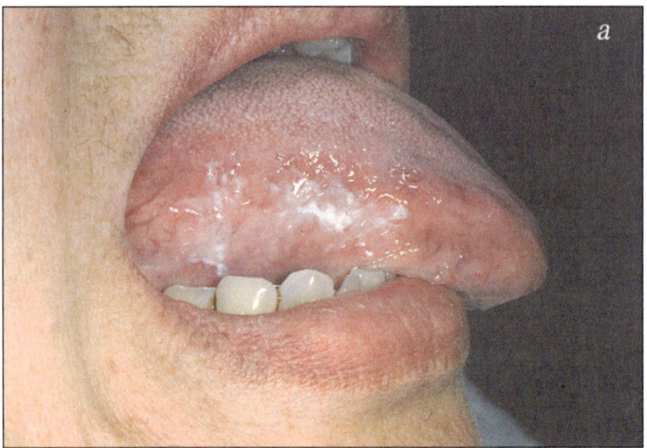

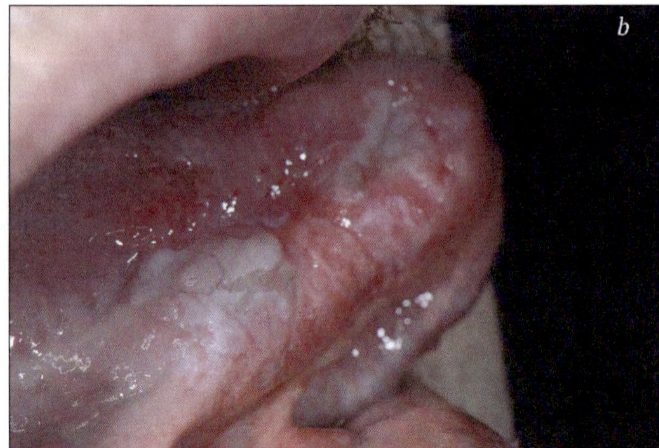

Figure 2-4 *(a)* Leukoplakia cluster on the lateral tongue. *(b)* Erythroplakia; mixed red/white lesion.

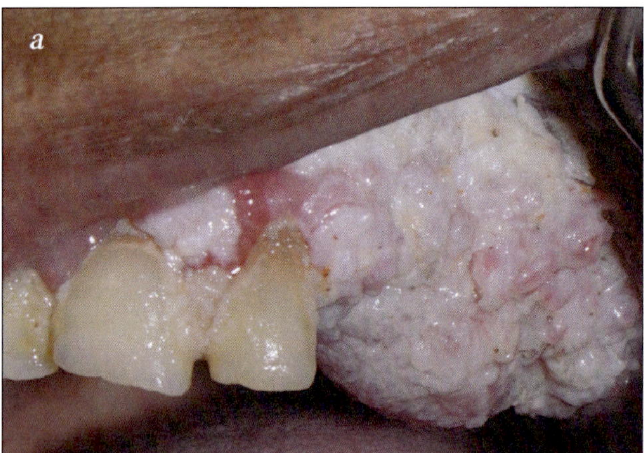

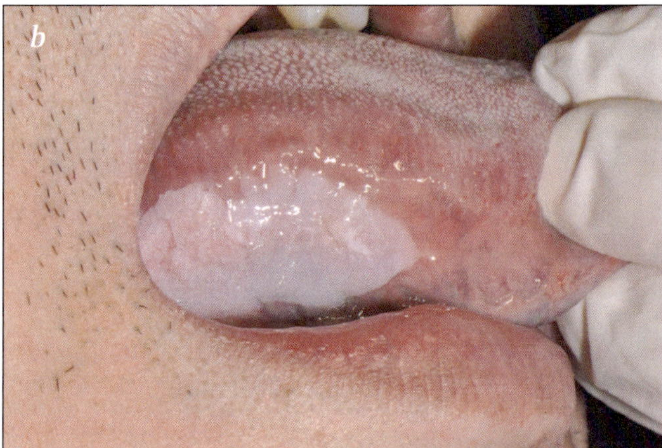

Figure 2-5 Example of different appearances of PVL. *(a)* PVL can present as a thick nodular-appearing mass as seen here on the anterior gingiva. *(b)* PVL can also appear as a flat corrugated-type lesion as seen on the lateral border of the tongue.

respond better to treatment (Ang et al., 2010). HPV may play a role in some oral leukoplakia for which there are no obvious etiologic factors, such as habits and age.

Leukoplakia is the most common potentially malignant lesion of the mouth. It may unpredictably regress, remain stable, or undergo carcinomatous transformation.

The nature of the link between HPV infection and oral leukoplakia is yet unknown.

Leukoplakia

Oral leukoplakia is categorized into two main types based on the clinical appearance as homogenous or heterogeneous. Either type may occur as an isolated lesion or a cluster. Leukoplakia can vary in size from a few millimeters to several centimeters.

Typically, homogeneous leukoplakia is a smooth white plaque. Heterogeneous leukoplakia may be nodular or verrucous, having a wrinkled or corrugated surface (Fig 2-4a). Heterogenous lesions may be a mixture of white and red areas termed *erythroleukoplakia*/specked (Fig 2-4b) (Lodi et al., 2006; Reibel, 2003).

The clinical appearance of oral leukoplakia may change over time. Some homogeneous lesions may become larger, or nonhomogeneous, but most oral leukoplakia will remain stable or regress, while very few will undergo carcinomatous transformation (Napier and Speight, 2008).

Proliferative verrucous leukoplakia

Proliferative verrucous leukoplakia (PVL) is considered separately from other leukoplakia. PVL is a rare form of oral leukoplakia, which was first described in 1985 by Hansen et al. Since then, various published case series have presented PVL as a disease with high biological behavior and consequently a high recurrence rate. Malignant transformation to verrucous carcinoma or squamous cell carcinoma runs close to 70% (Munde and Karle, 2016). The buccal mucosa and tongue (Fig 2-5) are the most frequently involved sites. It develops initially as hyperkeratosis that eventually becomes a multifocal disease, which can become locally invasive. Tobacco use is not a factor and occurs in both smokers and nonsmokers (Munde and Karle, 2016). Although greater than 70% of PVL become malignant, regional lymph node metastasis is rare.

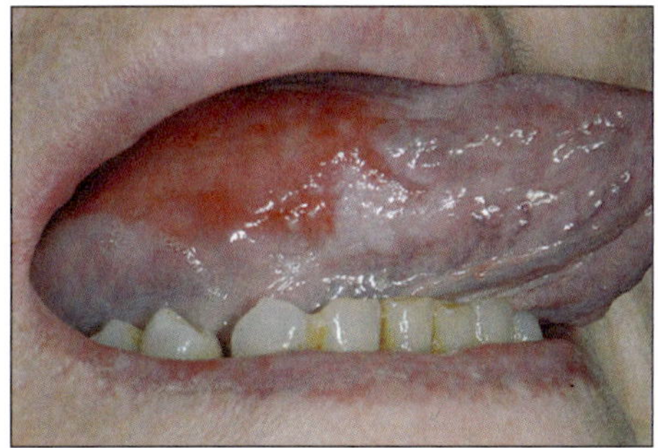

Figure 2-6 Example of erythroplakia on the lateral posterior border of the tongue. The red lesion on the lateral tongue represents a high-risk lesion and most of the time represents a high-grade dysplasia or SCC. This lesion transformed into an SCC.

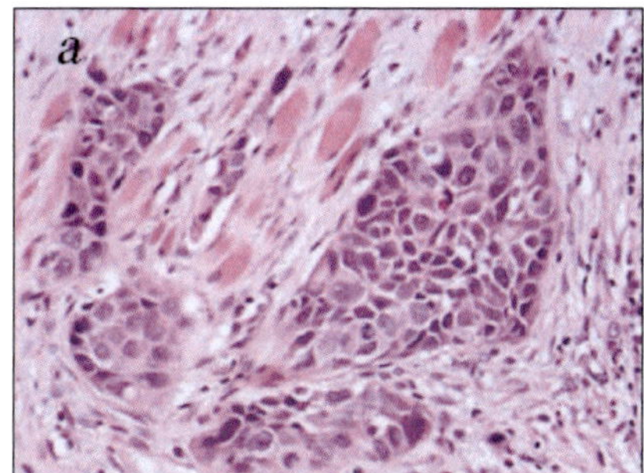

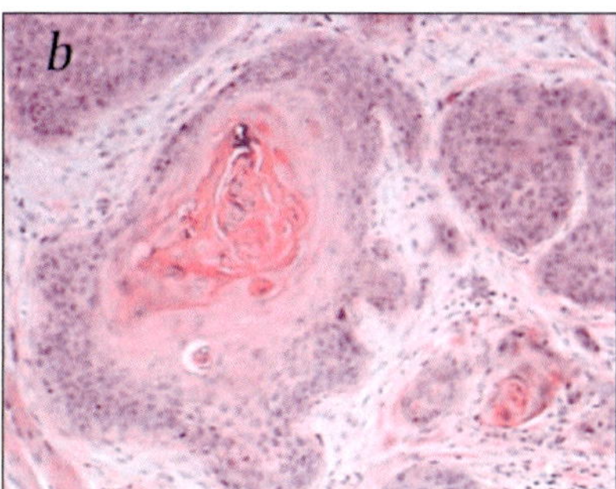

Figure 2-7 Distinct morphology of HPV-positive and HPV-negative SCC. *(a)* HPV-positive SCC form tight clusters without keratinization (magnification: ×400), whereas HPV-negative SCC *(b)* have extensive keratinization (magnification: ×200) (micrograph courtesy of Dr. Richard Jordan).

Red lesions

Oral erythroplakia (Fig 2-6) is the most worrisome of all precursor/precancerous oral lesions, as it has the greatest threat of malignant transformation. About 40% of all erythroplakia is already a squamous cell carcinoma at the time of diagnosis.

Oral erythroplakia is a purely clinical term and refers to a red patch in the oral cavity. Ninety percent of erythroplakia represents either severe dysplasia (50%) or squamous cell carcinoma (40%) at the time of diagnosis. Less than 10% represent mild or moderate dysplasia. It is thought that the same risk factors responsible for squamous cell carcinoma contribute to oral erythroplakia (tobacco and alcohol use).

Oral erythroplakia has the highest risk of malignant transformation compared to all other oral "precancerous" mucosal lesions. Initial histology is typically high-grade dysplasia/microinvasive carcinoma (Reichart and Phillipsen, 2008).

Separation of oropharyngeal and oral cavity tumors

The oral cavity is made up of the lips, gingiva, retromolar trigone, hard palate, buccal mucosa, oral (mobile) tongue, and the floor of mouth (Westra and Lewis, 2017). The oropharynx is made up of the palatine tonsils, soft palate, base of the tongue / lingual tonsils (posterior to circumvallate papillae), and posterior pharyngeal wall (Westra and Lewis, 2017). Historically, malignancies of the oral cavity and oropharynx were described as oral cancer. Although the oral cavity and oropharynx form one continuous "tube" of stratified squamous epithelium, they are dissimilar in many significant respects: The oropharynx is rich in *lymphoid tissue* (lingual and palatine tonsils). The lymphoepithelium lining the tonsillar crypts is highly specialized and provides a more permissive environment for HPV infection (Lyford-Pike et al., 2013).

Interestingly, even as overall rates of oral cancer have plateaued and even declined, there has been a significant increase in the diagnosis and treatment of HPV-positive cancer in the last 15 to 20 years (Chaturvedi, 2012). This is likely due to the overall decrease in cigarette smoking. HPV is a highly transmissible sexually transmitted disease. CDC reports that likely 74% of sexually active adults in the United States have been exposed to HPV. CDC also reports that 60% of female college students have had an HPV infection at some point. Most HPV infections are cleared by the immune system within two years, defined as an absence of HPV DNA detection on follow-up swabs (Giuliano et al., 2011). At 12 months, 66% of infections are cleared; this increases to 90% at 24 months. However, in men, HPV-16 has been identified as one of the slowest viral types to be cleared and takes nearly two times longer (12 months) to be cleared than other high-risk viral types (Guliani et al., 2011). This is an interesting finding, since HPV-16 is the viral type, which accounts for over 90% of HPV-related oropharyngeal cancer in the United States, and this disease is more prevalent in men as compared to women, suggesting possible gender differences in the ability to mount immunologic responses against this viral type (Best et al., 2012). These HPV-positive oropharyngeal cancers have unique demographic profiles and unique genetic features distinct from the typical squamous cell carcinoma of the head and neck (Hayes et al., 2015). These tumors have distinct clinical and morphological features (Gillison et al., 2015; Gondim et al., 2016), and they have a more favorable clinical outcome (Ang et al., 2010).

Morphology of HPV-positive oropharnygeal carcinoma

Although both oral and oropharyngeal SCC are squamous epithelium, their morphologies are different. HPV-positive SCC typically arise within a rich lymphoid background, the tonsillar crypts. HPV-positive SCC (Fig 2-7a), unlike their HPV-negative counterparts (Fig 2-7b), are not associated with keratinizing dysplastic surface lesions. Most HPV-positive SCC are nonkeratinizing (Fig 2-7a).

This suggests that HPV-positive SCC are less well differentiated than HPV-negative SCC. Nonkeratinizing-HPV-SCC typically present as a large, advancing bordered nest of tumor cells with little stroma. The HPV-SCC cells may be embedded in a dense lymphoid stroma (Fig 2-8b).

HPV-SCC cells (Fig 2-9) are predominantly nuclear (hyperchromatic) with minimal cytoplasm (Lewis, 2017). There is a lack of maturation/differentiation with less than 10% of the tumor keratinized (Gondim et al., 2016).

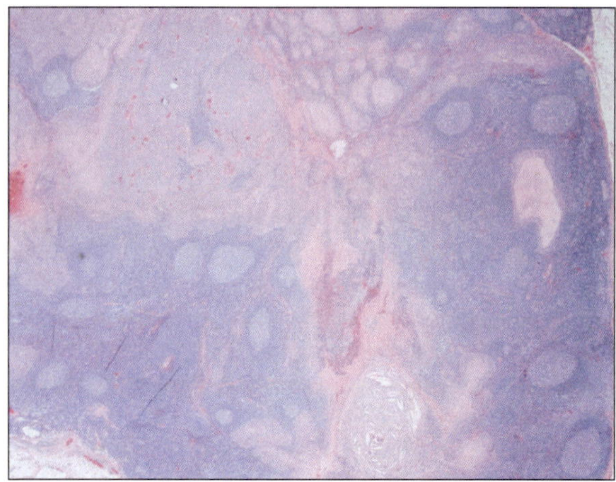

Figure 2-8 HPV oropharyngeal cancer in a lymph node. Note the cystic nature of the lymph node (magnification: ×200).

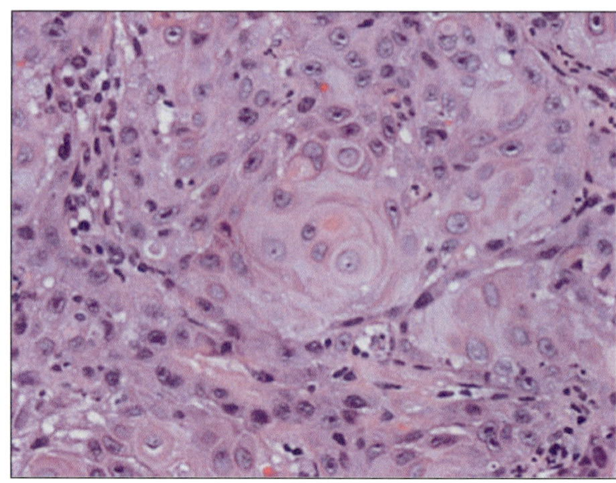

Figure 2-9 Hyperchromatic and multinucleated HPV-SCC cells. Note poorly differentiated, hyperchromatic, multinucleated SCC cells (magnification: ×400).

Table 2-1 Number of deaths per 100,000 people oral/oropharyngeal cancer

Males		Females
3.9	All Races	1.3
3.9	White	1.4
4.4	**African American**	1.2
3.2	Asian / Pacific Islander	1.1
3.5	American Indian / Alaska Native	1.1
2.4	Hispanic	0.8

Table 2-2 Estimated new cases and mortality for the year 2018 in the United States [1]

	Estimated new cases	Estimated deaths
Oral cavity and pharynx	51,540 (M: 37,160; F: 14,380)	10,030 (M: 7,280; F: 2,750)
Tongue	17,111 (M: 12,490; F: 4,620)	2,510 (M: 1,750; F: 760)
Floor of mouth	13,580 (M: 7,980; F: 5,600)	2,650 (M: 1,770; F: 880)
Other sites of the oral cavity	3,260 (M: 2,440; F: 820)	1,640 (M: 1,280; F: 360)

Age and gender

Oral cancer is more common in men than women, among those with a history of tobacco or heavy alcohol use, and individuals infected with HPV. In 1950, the male/female ratio was more than 6:1. Currently, the M/F ratio is now about 2:1.

One explanation for this may be the great increase in smoking among women. In addition, considering cancer as an age-related disease, it should be noted that in the over-65 age group in the general population, the number of women exceeds the number of men by 45%.

Oral cancer, like most cancers, is a disease of older individuals. About 95% of all oral cancer occurs in persons over 40 years of age, and the average age at the time of onset is about 60 (Sapp et al., 2004). This is important as the population of the United States continues to age. Over the past 10 years, the population age 65 and over increased from 37.2 million in 2006 to 54 million in 2019 (United States Census Bureau, Population). There is an increase in the incidence of oral cancer in patients under the age of 40, and this is likely a result of HPV-influenced SCC.

For oral cancer, death rates are higher among males, particularly those of African American descent. The death rate was 2.5 per 100,000 men and women per year based on 2014–2018 deaths, age-adjusted (American Cancer Society, 2021).

Sites

- The most common locations for cancer in the oral cavity are the tongue, tonsils, and oropharynx.

Data from the American Cancer Society (March 2021) indicate that the most common site for oral cancer is the tongue, followed by the tonsil and floor of mouth (Table 2-2). The tongue is the most common site for oral cancer for both men and women. Oral tongue malignancies (located in the anterior two-thirds) account for about 53% of tongue cancers. Since about half of tongue cancers occur in the base of the tongue, the problems regarding recognition of signs and symptoms and early diagnosis are apparent. Base-of-tongue cancers are often manifested by a chronic sore throat, dysphagia, and/or metastatic neck node. Many times, there are no symptoms until the patient notices a swelling in the neck.

Stage at diagnosis and survival

Greater than 90% of all oral cancers are squamous cell carcinomas. It becomes obvious at the present time that early diagnosis is a key factor in oral cancer control and a positive outcome. Oral cancer can mimic a variety of benign lesions (Fig 2-10), and therefore, careful evaluations as routine dental visits are essential.

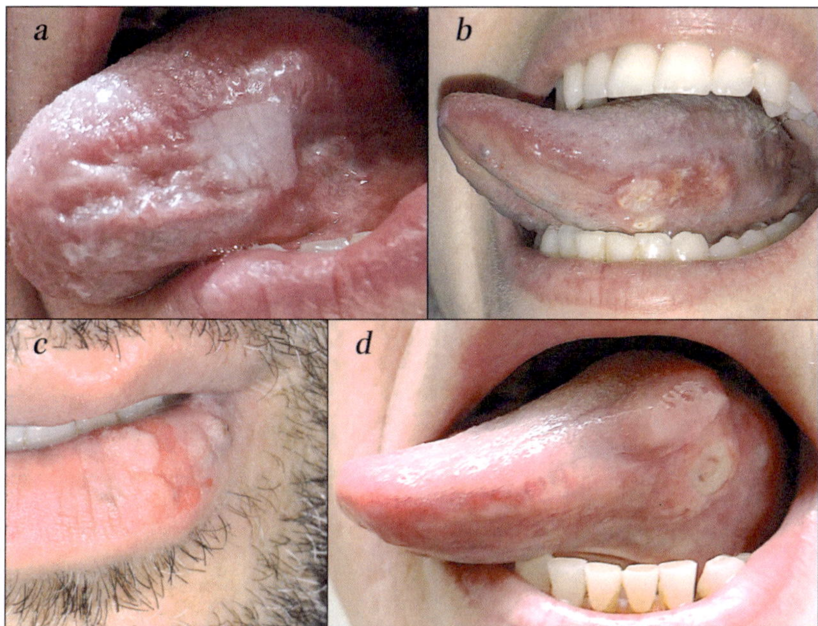

Figure 2-10 Multiple presentation of SCC leading to a delay in diagnosis. *(a)* White patch, which could represent hyperkeratosis. *(b)* Multiple aphthous-like ulcers in a 22-year-old individual without risk factors. *(c)* Lip lesion that could represent healing HSV or solar cheilitis. *(d)* Demonstrates ulceration adjacent to a sharp lingual cusp.

Clinical presentations are varied and confusing, which can lead to a delay in diagnosis. Frictional hyperkeratosis is a common oral lesion resulting from a parafunctional thrusting of the tongue or rubbing on a fractured tooth or dental filling. In Fig 2-10a, white changes on the ventral tongue could be the result of continued friction of the tongue on the adjacent tooth. However, an incisional biopsy revealed this to be squamous cell carcinoma. In Fig 2-10b, the patient is a 22-year-old individual with no risk factors and a history of aphthous-like ulcers related to Celiac disease. The biopsy revealed this to be squamous cell carcinoma. Fig 2-10c can be confused with either HSV infection or solar cheilitis. The biopsy in Fig 2-10c also revealed it to be squamous cell carcinoma. Fig 2-10d can be confused with trauma from sharp mandibular teeth. However, the biopsy of this area also proved to be squamous cell carcinoma. Improving the prognosis for oral cancer requires the recruitment of the dental community. A moment spent by the dentist can save an individual's life.

Race and genetics

Ethnic background is known to influence many types of cancer. For example, overall cancer rates in African Americans are increasing at a faster rate than in American whites. African Americans have proportionately higher rates of oropharyngeal cancer than do other racial groups. Like other familial cancers, a family history of oral cancer was associated mostly with an early age of onset of the disease. Family members without habits such as tobacco chewing, smoking, or alcohol consumption were also affected (Ragin et al., 2010). Cancer of the nasopharynx is 20 to 30 times as prevalent in Chinese as in whites and other ethnic groups. The rate of nasopharyngeal carcinoma is highest in Chinese who have remained in Asia. For example, in Southeast Asia, it is one of the most common cancers in both men and women.

The link between nasopharyngeal cancer and HHV-4 (Epstein-Barr virus) was first observed in 1966 (Old et al., 1966). Genetic susceptibility has also been proposed as a risk factor for the development of nasopharyngeal cancer. Haplotypes that have been associated with the malignancy include certain human leukocyte antigens (HLA), such as HLA-A2, HLA-B46, and HLA-B58 (Ren and Chan, 1996). Environmental factors such as salt-preserved fish and vegetables, which are known to release nitrosamine, have also been implicated in this disease.

Several of these cellular oncogenes are homologous of retroviral oncogenes (e.g., the ras gene); others are new oncogenes. Several oncogenes have been implicated in oral carcinogenesis. An aberrant expression of the protooncogene epidermal growth factor receptor (EGFRI c-erb 1), members of the ras family—as well as c-myc, int-2, hst-1, PRAD-l, and bel—is believed to contribute to oral cancer development (Usman et al., 2021).

Oral lichen planus

Lichen planus is a complex, chronic, inflammatory disease (Fig 2-11). Both the keratinized and nonkeratinized mucosa may be affected. The etiology of lichen planus is unknown. However, the mechanism of action appears to be the destruction of the basal keratinocytes by the band of adjacent T lymphocytes characteristically found beneath the basement membrane.

The degree of lymphocytic infiltration may vary. This has a direct effect on the presentation of the oral lesions. As much as 1% of the adult population may have some degree of lichen planus.

Lichen planus is typically a disease of adults (>40 years old) and is relatively common (0.2–1% of the population). Lichen planus runs a persistent course. The best management is to keep ahead of it by making simple lifestyle changes. For example, avoiding stress and a specific type of food, such as citrus, cinnamon, and tomatoes.

Bilateral, white reticulations on the buccal mucosa represent the classical appearance of lichen planus (Fig 2-11a). Striations can also appear on the FOM, dorsal and ventral tongue, and the gingiva. Lichen planus is divided into types—reticular, erosive/ulcerative (Fig 2-11b), plaque (Fig 2-11c), papular, and erythematous/atrophic (Fig 2-11d). There is considerable overlap between the "types."

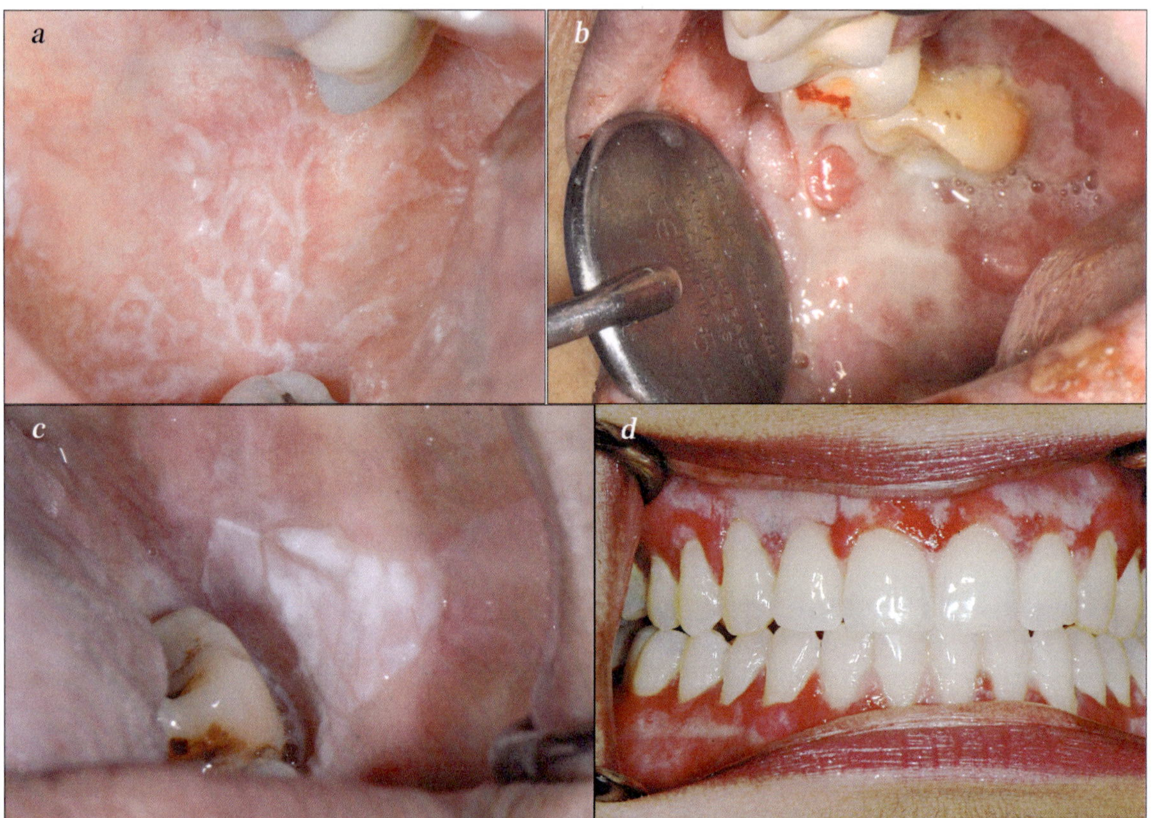

Figure 2-11 Distinct manifestations of lichen planus, of oral lichen planus. *(a)* Represents the reticular form of lichen planus. *(b)* Represents the erosive form of lichen planus. *(c)* Is the plaque form of lichen planus, and *(d)* represents the atrophic form.

Pain is usually only associated with the erosive and erythematous forms; although many individuals with long-standing oral lesions become tolerant of the pain.

The risk of carcinoma transformation is controversial and rare (0.4–2.5% of cases). It is not clear whether the erosive form of lichen planus can transform or if it is a lichen planus mimic, termed epithelial dysplasia with lichenoid features (Fig 2-12). This lesion needs to be entirely excised, as it is aggressive and transforms into oral SCC quickly. An intermittent biopsy is recommended for patients with lichen planus that may change in appearance or location.

Pathology of lichen planus. There is an obvious band of lymphocytes in the connective tissue directly beneath the basement membrane (Fig 2-13a).

Using immunofluorescence (Fig 2-13b), one can also see a thick band of fibrinogen beneath the basement membrane in greater than 70% of specimens. One Thai study has the shaggy BMZ presentation of fibrinogen at 82.9% (Buajeeb et al., 2015), but generally, it's considered to be 75% positive.

Treatment

Depending on the severity of the disease, topical corticosteroids (Fluocinonide mixed 1:1 with orabase paste) or systemic corticosteroids (prednisone) may be utilized. Several forms of lichen planus exist. The most common is the reticular form in which the typical Wickham's striae are usually found on the buccal mucosa (bilaterally). The oral lesions are frequently asymptomatic and chronic, persisting indefinitely in most patients. Lichen planus is primarily a disease of adults, with the average age of onset being about 40 years. It is rarely found in persons less than 30 years old. Women predominate, about 2 to 1. Lichen planus can be found in all ethnic groups, and there is little evidence of familial clustering.

Mimics of lichen planus

The discussion of lichen planus is controversial. One such mimic of lichen planus, which is precancerous, is epithelial dysplasia with lichenoid features. It clinically mimics lichen planus, but the resolution of inflammation first needs to be addressed and then reevaluated and biopsied if necessary. However, epithelial dysplasia with lichenoid features is a precancerous condition that can mimic lichen planus. This lesion requires excision and close observation.

Surgical Treatment of Tongue and Mandible Tumors

Optimal results are obtained when an interdisciplinary approach is applied, including VSP in the reconstruction of mandibular defects. Vascular and avascular osseous grafts should be tailored to support the desired prosthesis, whether it be fixed or removable.

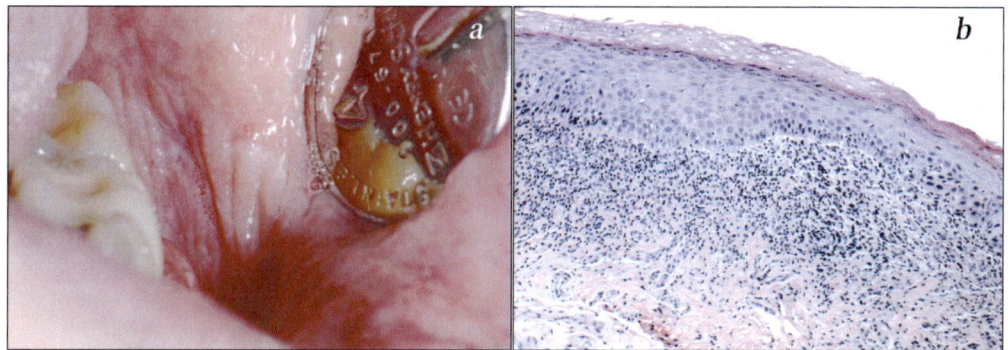

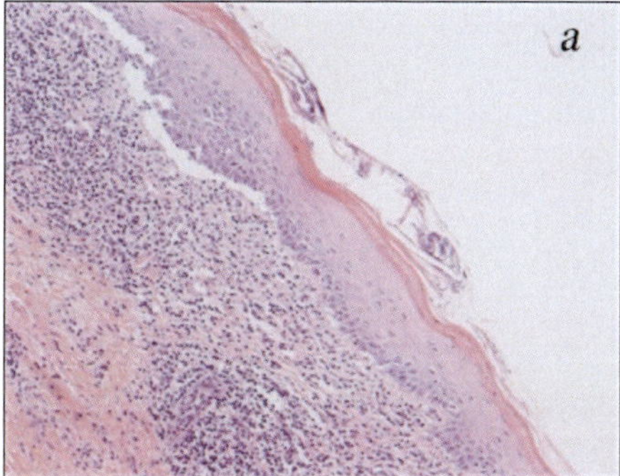
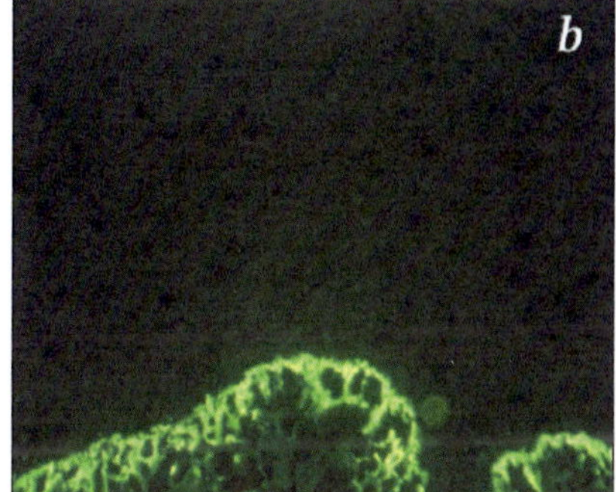

Figure 2-12 Epithelial Dysplasia with lichenoid features. *(a)* Example of a patient referred for lichen planus. *(b)* The biopsy indicated was a lichen planus mimic. Dysplasia with lichenoid features. Notice dysplastic epithelium with the lymphocytic infiltrate seen in lichenoid reactions/lichen planus (magnification: ×200).

Figure 2-13 Histopathology and direct immunofluorescence on lichen planus. *(a)* Note the dense lymphocytic infiltrate directly beneath the epithelium and the extensive keratinization (magnification: ×200). *(b)* When processed by direct immunofluorescence, note the high degree of fibrinogen deposition (courtesy of Dr. Troy Daniels and Richard Jordan).

Because osseointegrated implants play such an important role in retaining, supporting, and stabilizing the prosthesis, the graft that is selected should provide suitable bone volume and contours for proper implant position and angulation. The oral portions of the osseous grafts should be surfaced with keratinized attached epithelium, regardless of whether a conventional or implant restoration will be used. Computer-aided design and computer-aided manufacturing (CAD/CAM) techniques that enable the team to better accomplish these goals continue to evolve. Osteotomies can be planned virtually and duplicated at surgery with prefabricated surgical guides, and implant drill guides can be prepared with CAD-CAM technologies. Custom-designed reconstruction plates can be milled prior to surgery, as can provisional prostheses for early rehabilitation.

The prognosis for oral function is closely linked to the postoperative status of the tongue, more so than the continuity of the osseous mandible. Accordingly, reconstructive priority should be given to the tongue. The subsequent sections will be dedicated to the reconstruction of the tongue, mandible, and lips.

Presurgical Prosthodontic Consultation and Evaluation

Obtaining optimal results begins with the understanding that the treatment of tongue and mandible disease often requires an interdisciplinary team. At cancer centers, a patient is reviewed by a tumor board where all pertinent services meet to discuss the clinical, radiologic, and pathologic findings. If upfront radiotherapy or chemoradiation is prescribed, a referral to a dentist or prosthodontist would include a request for a radiation splint or stent. These custom-made appliances are discussed in the previous chapter (see Chapter 1) For surgical treatment, the surgical oncologist will make a referral to the prosthodontist, including a description and depiction of the extent of the resection (Fig 2-14). At UCLA, we ask our colleagues to delineate on a diagram the approximate margins of the resection or, in cases of a mandibulotomy, the location of the mandibular split. Because we lack a universal mandibulectomy classification (Brown et al., 2016), a simple drawing and a statement of tongue involvement are important for the prosthodontist to be able to elaborate to the patient on the dental and oral functional ramifications of the oncologic resection and rehabilitation. It also allows the dental examination to be focused on the teeth that will remain and also on the fabrication of any prescribed surgical templates, such as an interocclusal splint or split-thickness skin graft and vestibuloplasty stent (see the section below titled "Secondary Surgical Procedures"; see Fig 2-21 for healed split-thickness skin graft).

The dental examination includes dental radiographs to rule out any emergent dental needs, prophylactic dental cleaning, the making of either diagnostic casts or intraoral scans, and maxillomandibular relation records and photographs. A psychosocial evaluation is also done at the time (see Chapter 9).

Although the patient has met with the surgical team, patients commonly have additional questions regarding their treatment. The dental visit is another opportunity to reaffirm the collaborative effort to the patient's care. Learning that one has cancer is liable to constrain one's ability to absorb or retain information. The authors encourage at least one family member or close friend to be chairside during the initial consultation with the prosthodontist. Even though

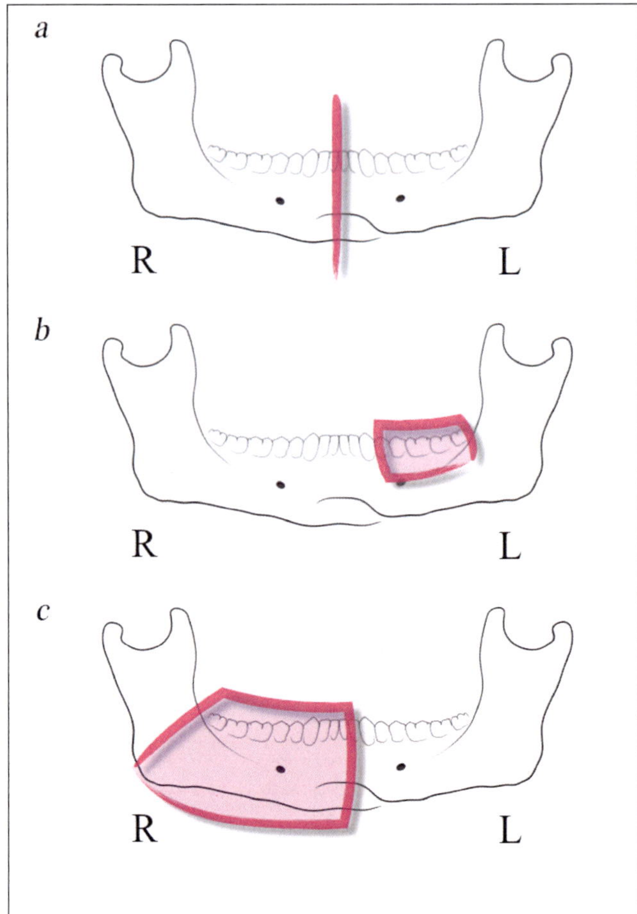

Figure 2-14 Delineations of proposed procedures involving the mandible. *(a)* Median mandibulotomy for access to the base of the tongue. *(b)* Marginal (monocortical) mandibulectomy. *(c)* Segmental mandibulectomy.

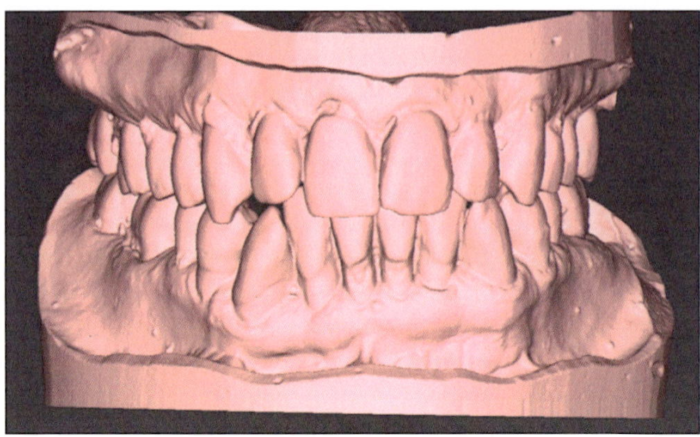

Figure 2-15 Opposing digitized diagnostic casts.

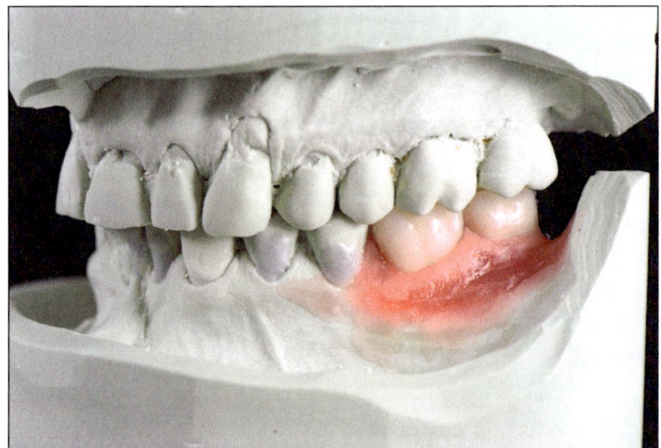

Figure 2-16 Opposing diagnostic casts. Because of the missing mandibular teeth, a diagnostic wax-up was performed prior to VSP.

the patient is informed that a significant portion of the mandible would be removed to eradicate the tumor, or secondary to treatment of osteoradionecrosis (ORN), the patient may need reminding that the associated teeth in the resection will be lost.

If optimal rehabilitation is to be achieved, it is essential that the dentist examine the patient and discuss with the surgeon the proposed surgical resection and the plan for and the timing of rehabilitation. Given the broad array of rehabilitative options, timing, costs, and impact on quality of life, every effort should be made to facilitate an informed decision by the patient.

If dental implants are to be considered for primary placement at the time of microvascular reconstruction, much presurgical planning is necessary. A fully dentate patient with acceptable occlusion requires either opposing dental casts that are digitized (Fig 2-15) or an intraoral scan exported into a Standard Tessellation Language (STL) file format. For the partially edentulous patient with missing teeth in the area to be reconstructed, an analog or digital tooth setup is needed (Fig 2-16). Completely edentulous patients who don't already have complete dentures, would need additional appointments for maxillomandibular records with record bases and a trial denture appointment so that ideal tooth positions and prosthetic space can be accounted for. The biomedical engineers who will conduct the virtual surgical planning (VSP) will need an STL file of the dentition, a medical-grade computer tomograph (CT) of the head, and a CT angiogram (CTA) of the proposed donor site, most often the leg for a fibula free flap (FFF). Once these are available, a VSP session can be scheduled (see the subsection titled "Virtual Surgical Planning" on page 116).

Cases of advanced disease or small posterior defects with few teeth lost are scenarios where it may be prudent to delay the placement of dental implants. Under these circumstances, dental implants can be placed secondarily, provided that the flap selection and position are conducive to implant therapy. The caveat is that the placement of implants in irradiated flaps is subject to greater failure rates and the risk of ORN and loss of the reconstructed mandible.

Interocclusal splints

Whether implants are placed or not, it is advisable that an interocclusal splint is made presurgically to help reestablish and preserve the dental occlusion (Markowitz and Calcaterra, 1994). Outcomes are less predictable when a splint is not used (Fig 2-17b). The fewer teeth remaining, the more challenging it is to reorient the residual mandibular segments and the interposed osseous graft.

To fabricate splints, casts are mounted in the maximum intercuspal position and surveyed, heights of the contour are delineated,

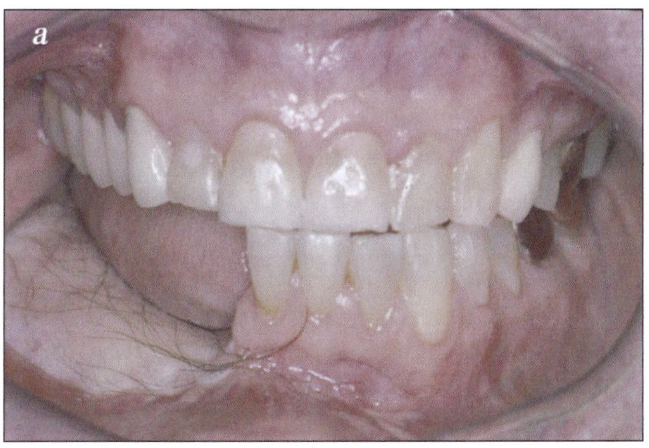

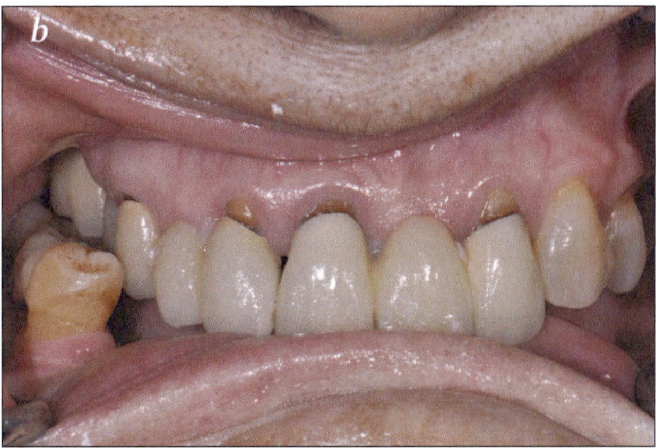

Figure 2-17 *(a)* Lateral mandibular defect with acceptable dental occlusion. *(b)* Severe malocclusion resulting from the insetting of a FFF without the use of an interocclusal splint.

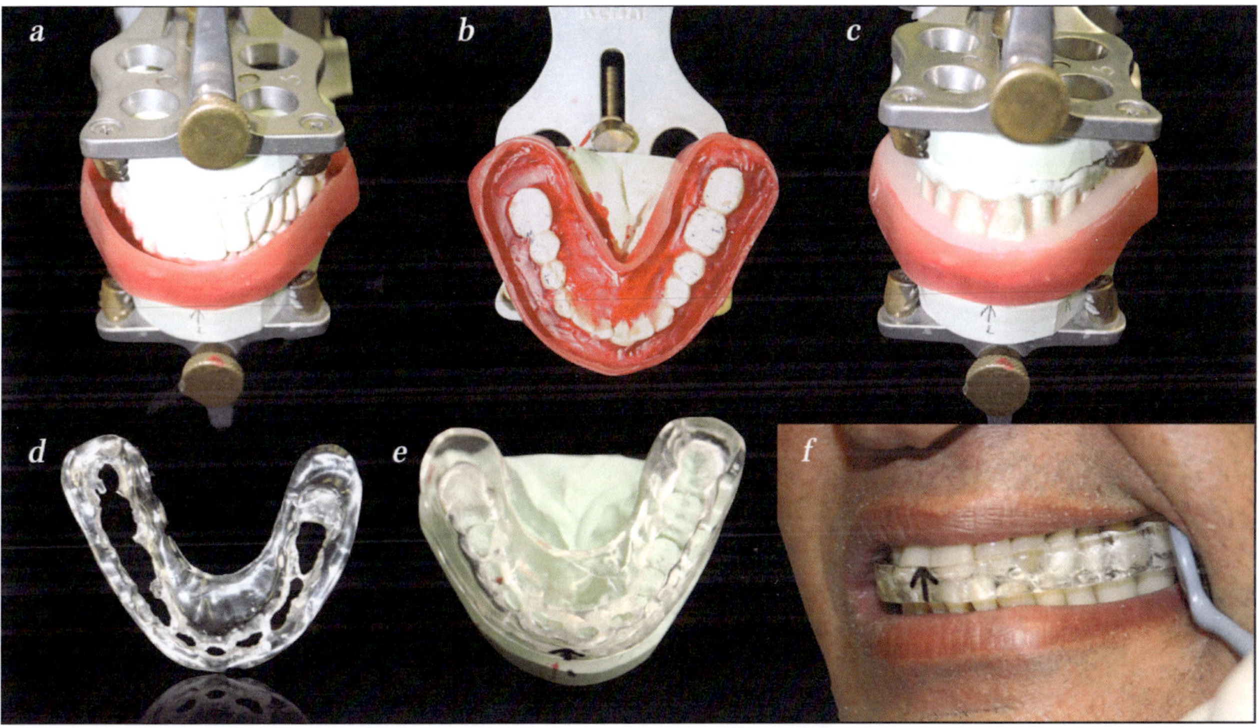

Figure 2-18 Analog fabrication of interocclusal splint. *(a)* Mounted casts on a plaster-less hinge articulator. *(a and b)* Wax blockout to the height of contour and boxing to contain fluid PMMA. *(c)* Poured clear PMMA and closed articulator to maximum intercuspation. *(d)* Cured under pressure, trimmed, and polished splint. Note that tight occlusion will result in perforations indicating tooth contacts. *(e and f)* Confirming full seating of the splint onto the stone cast and intraorally prior to surgery.

and parallel wax blockout is performed. The mandibular cast is boxed to contain poured vacuum-mixed autopolymerizing polymethylmethacrylate (PMMA) (Fig 2-18). Casts are lubricated with petroleum jelly, and the mounted maxillary casts are closed to maximum intercuspation. The PMMA is allowed to polymerize under 20 PSI before removing, trimming, and polishing. Alternatively (Fig 2-19), digital models are made by direct intraoral scanning or indirectly with a desktop scan of mounted casts. The models are digitally blocked out based on a user-defined path of insertion. Similar to virtually designing implant surgical guides, the maxillary surface of the interocclusal splint is automatically generated by the software. The mandibular surface is created by the computer command Boolean Difference. Once the design is completed, the interocclusal splint is printed in a biocompatible photopolymer. Prior to surgery, it is critical to verify the complete and accurate seating of the splint.

Care must be taken during the reconstruction to maintain the patient's dental occlusion or maxillomandibular relationship in its original state (Fig 2-20). The patient and clinician should be cognizant that even with the use of an interocclusal splint, muscle imbalances and scar contracture can lead to discrepancies that may require an occlusal adjustment.

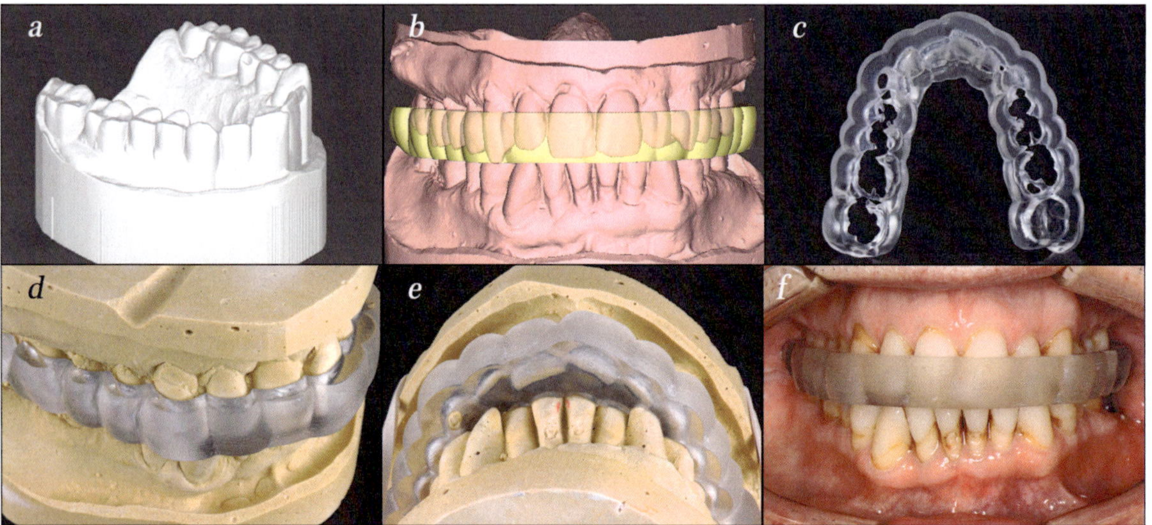

Figure 2-19 CAD/CAM fabrication of interocclusal splint. *(a)* Digital blockout. *(b)* Designing follows a similar protocol to implant surgical guides. *(c)* Once the design is completed, the interocclusal splint is 3D printed in a photopolymer. *(d–f)* The fit of the splint should be confirmed on the gypsum cast and intraorally prior to surgery.

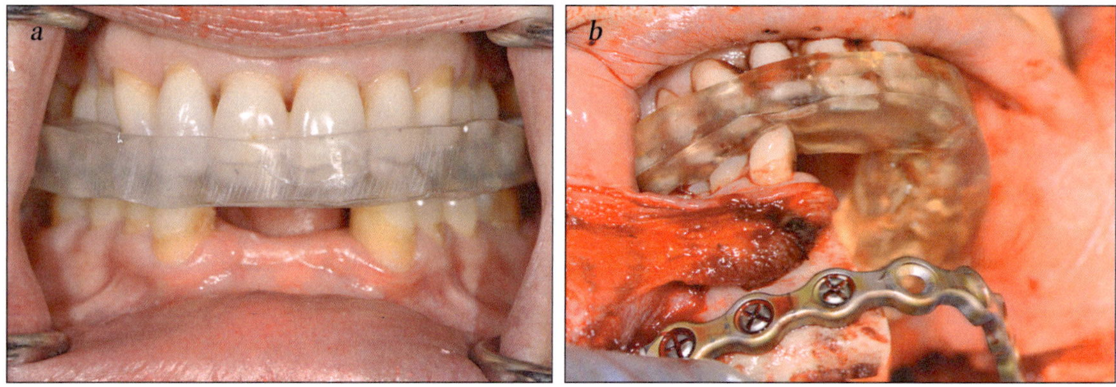

Figure 2-20 *(a)* Interocclusal splints should be made and fit-checked prior to mandibulectomy. *(b)* During the insetting of an osseous flap, care is taken to maintain dental occlusion.

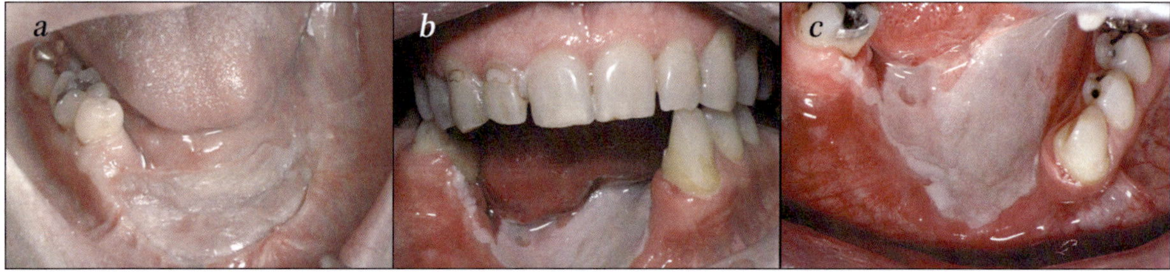

Figure 2-21 Use of a split-thickness skin grafts following marginal mandibulectomy. *(a)* Note the ideal denture-bearing surfaces and preserved buccal and lingual sulci. *(b and c)* When the resection extends lingually, the split-thickness skin graft also prevents the tethering of the tongue.

Marginal mandibulectomies

In patients undergoing a marginal mandibulectomy, primary soft tissue closure should be avoided. It is prudent to line the raw tissue surfaces with a split-thickness skin graft (Fig 2-21) and bolster them with a prefabricated splint. A skin graft preserves the buccal and lingual sulci, avoids primary closure, and optimizes the denture-bearing area.

Patients will invariably ask if their lost dentition can be replaced with dental implants. Lateral marginal mandibulectomies are generally not candidates for primary placement of dental implants due to inadequate bone height above the infra-alveolar (IA) nerve. In some situations, however, it may be possible to place implants secondarily by tilting the fixture buccally above IA nerve (Fig 2-22).

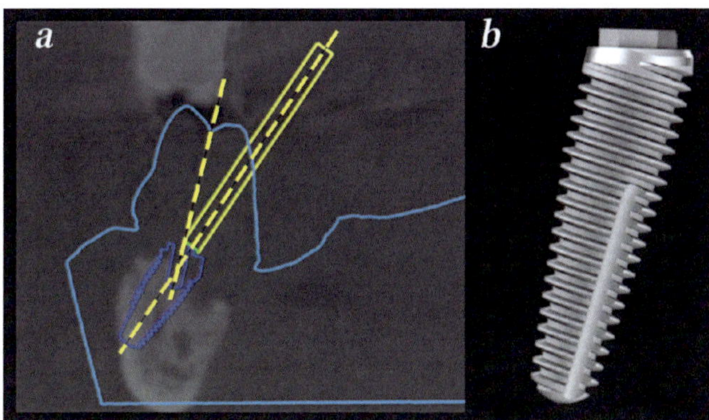

Figure 2-22 Planning for secondary placement of dental implant postmarginal mandibulectomy. *(a)* Screenshot of the buccolingual slice of an implant tilted over the IA nerve. Note the angle correction *(dotted line)*. *(b)* Subcrestal angle-correcting fixture.

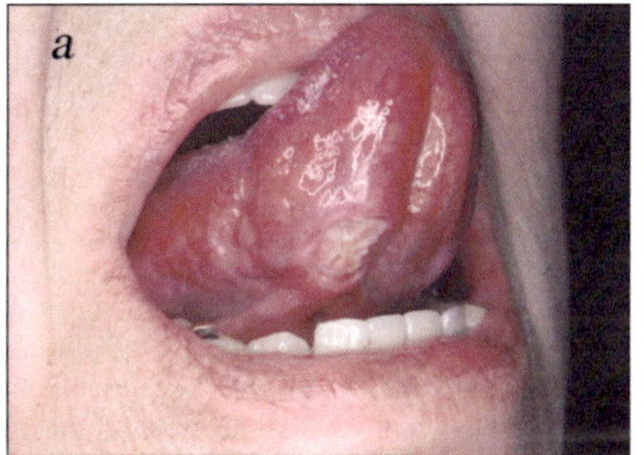

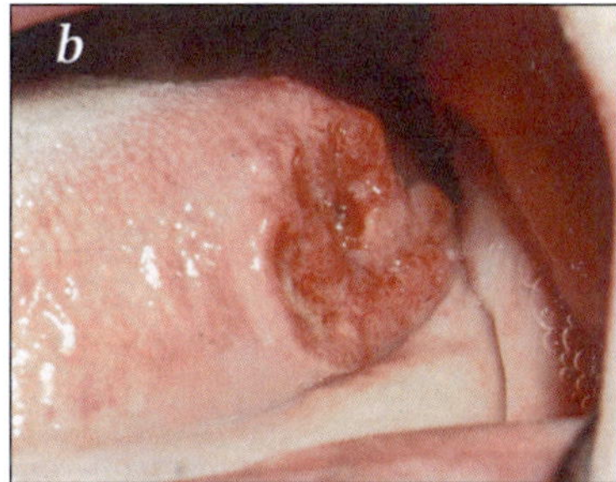

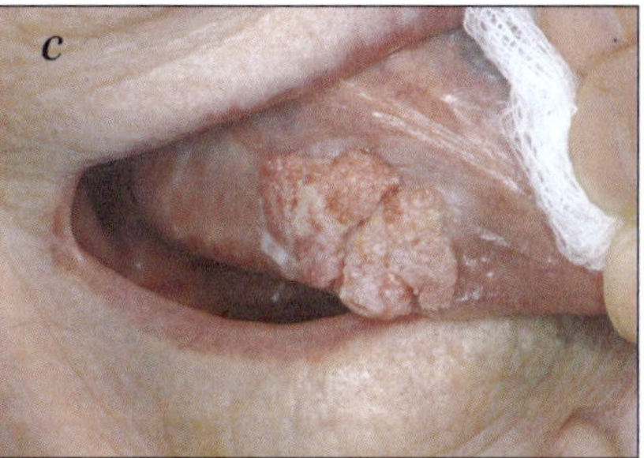

Figure 2-23 Epidermoid carcinomas of the oral tongue. Lesions may be *(a)* ulcerative, *(b)* infiltrative, or *(c)* exophytic.

Surgical Oncology

As previously mentioned, epidermoid carcinomas account for more than 90% of all oral tumors. Many of these carcinomas are located in areas that require resecting some combination of the tongue, FOM, and mandible. The degree of functional disability and cosmetic disfigurement is dependent on the location of the tumor and the extent of the surgical resection. Similarly, the prognosis varies by anatomic location, extent, and differentiation of the tumor. The categories discussed in this section will be (1) carcinomas confined to the oral tongue, (2) carcinomas confined to the anterior FOM, (3) carcinomas confined to the oropharynx, (4) carcinomas confined to the mandible and/or alveolar ridges, and (5) carcinomas confined to the gingiva.

Carcinoma of the oral tongue

Clinical and pathologic considerations

Squamous cell carcinoma (SCC) of the oral tongue has traditionally been associated with the elderly. However, an increasing number of cases are occurring in significantly younger individuals and, therefore, obtaining a biopsy specimen of all suspicious tongue lesions in young patients is of paramount importance (Shiboski et al., 2005).

The tongue is divided into the anterior and posterior segments. This division is not arbitrary, because tumors developing in different areas of the tongue exhibit distinct histologic patterns, require different modalities of treatment, and have different associated prognoses. The anterior segment constitutes the oral cavity or mobile tongue, representing the anterior two-thirds of the tongue. It includes the tip, the ventral surface, the lateral borders, and the dorsum of the tongue anterior to the circumvallate papillae. The posterior segment, or base of the tongue, represents the posterior third of the tongue and is the portion situated posterior to the circumvallate papillae. This section of the tongue is considered part of the oropharynx, as are the palatine tonsils.

Patients with oral tongue cancer are most likely to complain of a painful mass (Gorsky et al., 2004). Therefore all chronic, nonhealing lesions of the tongue and painful, palpable lesions warrant biopsy. Oral tongue SCC may exhibit an infiltrative, ulcerative, or exophytic behavior and have a variable growth rate (Fig 2-23). The average delay between the onset of symptoms and establishment of the diagnosis has been reported as four months (Wildt et al., 1995).

Oral tongue SCC may infiltrate the intrinsic musculature as well as nearby local subsites. Tumors arising on the ventral surface tend to involve the mucosa of the FOM. Lateral lesions of the oral tongue readily gain access to the lateral FOM, alveolar ridge, glossopalatine folds, and the retromolar trigone mucosa. Posterior extension may involve the base of the tongue, the tonsil and/or its fossa, and in some cases, the soft palate. All of these extensions carry increased morbidity with resection and present their own difficulties during rehabilitation.

Cervical metastases are of great concern in the treatment of oral tongue SCC because their presence has a negative impact on survival rates. Findings of pathologically positive lymph nodes obtained in elective neck dissections of patients with a clinically negative neck examination have been reported to be greater than 30% (Greenberg et al., 2003). Histopathologic tumor characteristics help predict the presence of occult cervical metastasis. A tumor depth of greater than 4 mm, a tumor diameter of greater than 2 cm, perineural invasion, angiolymphatic invasion, and poorly differentiated histology have all been indicated as independent factors in occult nodal metastasis (Sparano et al., 2004). As such, for patients with oral tongue SCC, an ipsilateral elective neck dissection is recommended for all clinically palpable nodes and when the neck examination is clinically negative but at least T_2 disease is present (tumor greater than 2 cm in diameter), tumor depth is greater than 4 mm, or other concerning histologic features are present.

In select patients with T1-T2 and clinically N_0 necks, consideration may be given to performing sentinel lymph node biopsy (SLNB). This can be especially useful in patients with small, superficial tumors near the midline, who may qualify for procedures ranging from no neck dissection to bilateral neck dissection. The negative predictive value of SLNB ranges from 88% to 97%, and it has been found to have the additional benefit of uncovering contralateral sentinel lymph nodes in a minority of cases (Bree et al., 2021).

There are instances where treatment of the contralateral neck must also be considered. Metastasis to contralateral lymph nodes has been shown to be significantly higher in all oral cavity cancers where advanced invasion has been demonstrated, there is ipsilateral lymph node involvement, or there is extension across the midline (Koo et al., 2006). Furthermore, delayed time to diagnosis, advanced TNM (tumor, nodes, and metastasis) staging, close surgical margins, and perineural infiltration have also been associated with contralateral lymph node metastasis (González-García et al., 2008). The use of positron emission tomography may assist with diagnosis and surveillance of primary, locoregional, and distant spread of disease, yet its role as a substitute for surgery in contralateral neck staging has not yet been defined.

In addition to imaging, genetic profiling may offer both prognostic information as well as information regarding metastatic potential in the clinically negative neck (Mendez et al., 2007). This may be the determining factor in the near future regarding whether to perform elective neck dissections in the clinically negative neck. For patients with a disease that has low metastatic risk (stages I and II), genetic profiling offers hope of avoiding the potential morbidity of overtreatment.

Conversely, the detection of occult metastasis has a direct impact on survival. The comparison of tumor cells from the lymph nodes of metastatic carcinoma with those from node-negative primary tumors revealed a differential expression of 160 genes. Analysis of this 160-gene set showed that the node-negative samples were distinguishable from both node-positive primary tumors and tumors in the lymph nodes. This suggests the presence of a global "metastatic signature" that will be found in primary tumors with the potential to metastasize but will be absent in stage I or II, or nonmetastatic, primary tumors (Mendez et al., 2007).

Table 2-3 Classification and staging

American joint committee on cancer staging of oral cavity squamous cell carcinoma

Primary tumor			
T_X	Unable to assess primary tumor		
T_0	No evidence of primary tumor		
T_{is}	Carcinoma in situ		
T_1	Tumor ≤2 cm and DOI ≤5 mm		
T_2	Tumor ≤2 cm, DOI >5 mm, and ≤10 mm ***OR*** tumor >2 cm and ≤4 cm and DOI ≤10 mm		
T_3	Tumor >4 cm ***OR*** any tumor with DOI >10 mm		
T_{4a} (oral)	Tumor invades adjacent structures only (e.g., through cortical bone of mandible or maxilla or involves the maxillary sinus or skin of the face)		
T_{4b} (oral)	Tumor invades masticator space, pterygoid plates, or skull base or encases the internal carotid artery		
Regional lymphadenopathy			
N_X	Unable to assess regional lymph nodes		
N_0	No evidence of regional metastasis		
N_1	Metastasis in a single ipsilateral lymph node ≤3 cm and ENE-		
N_{2a}	Metastasis in a single ipsilateral lymph node >3 cm and ≤6 cm and ENE-		
N_{2b}	Metastases in multiple ipsilateral lymph nodes ≤6 cm and ENE-		
N_{2c}	Metastases in bilateral or contralateral lymph nodes ≤6 cm and ENE-		
N_{3a}	Metastasis in a lymph node >6 cm and ENE		
N_{3b}	Metastasis in any lymph node(s) with ENE+ clinically		
Distant metastases			
M_X	Unable to assess for distant metastases		
M_0	No distant metastases		
M_1	Distant metastases		
TMN staging			
Stage 0	T_{is}	N_0	M_0
Stage I	T_1	N_0	M_0
Stage II	T_2	N_0	M_0
Stage III	T_3	N_0	M_0
	T_{1-3}	N_1	M_0
Stage IVa	T_{4a}	N_0	M_0
	T_{4a}	N_1	M_0
	T_{1-4a}	N_2	M_0
Stage IVb	Any T	N_3	M_0
	T_{4b}	Any N	M_0
Stage IVc	Any T	Any N	M_1

DOI: depth of invasion; ENE: extranodal extension
(Amin et al., 2017)

Classification and staging

The classification of tumors of the tongue is based on the TNM Staging System established by the American Joint Committee on Cancer (American Joint Committee, 2009) in accordance with the criteria listed in Table 2-3.

Prognosis

Several factors may influence the prognosis associated with oral tongue SCC. An increased disease-specific mortality has been associated with increasing age (Davidson et al., 2001). Early stage grouping, clear margins, and surgery as a primary treatment modality have been associated with improved disease-specific survival

(Sessions et al., 2002). Conversely, the use of radiotherapy, increasing tumor size, positive lymph node status, close or involved margins, advanced stage grouping, and ultimately tumor recurrence are associated with decreased survival (Davidson et al., 2001; Sessions et al., 2002). Therefore, obtaining clear surgical margins is crucial because it influences not only recurrence but survival. One of the most important factors in determining the outcome is the status of margins. An appropriate margin, given the patterns of histologic tumor spread, is 1.5 to 2.0 cm (Yuen et al., 1998). P16, a biomarker for human papillomavirus (HPV)–related carcinomas, is known to be associated with improved survival in oropharyngeal SCC patients; however, its relationship to oral cavity SCC has offered mixed reports (Li et al., 2018; Chakravarthy et al., 2016).

Schiff et al. (2005) reported a 10% local recurrence rate and a 5.9% recurrence rate in the ipsilateral neck. Sessions et al. (2002) reported a recurrence rate of 34% at the primary site and 31% in the neck; furthermore, no correlation was found linking treatment modality and recurrences. Patients whose disease recurred more than six months after completion of their primary treatment had better survival rates than those who recurred within six months of initial treatment. The overall salvage cure rate was 21% (Li et al., 2018; Schwartz et al., 2000).

Treatment

There are three basic approaches for the successful management of oral tongue SCC: (1) surgery, (2) radiation therapy, and (3) combined treatment, namely surgery followed by radiation therapy. Glossectomy, whether partial, hemi, or total, is the usual mode of surgical resection. Wedge excision plays a role in small, superficial, well-circumscribed lesions arising on the tip, dorsum, or lateral margin of the tongue.

In general terms, irradiation has the advantages of preserving tongue function while avoiding the cosmetic deformity associated with radical surgery. However, irradiation is not free of complications and appears to be less effective than surgery in the management of bulky lesions, tumors involving bone or cartilage, and tumors in which nodal metastases are clinically evident. Chemotherapy is only useful in combination with radiation therapy to provide radiosensitization and to assist in controlling regional and, more often, distant metastases. However, it is less often required for oral cavity cancers than for other cancers of the upper aerodigestive tract.

Because oral tongue SCC has a high propensity for regional metastasis, neck disease is best treated in conjunction with the primary tumor. The basic operation for these lesions is a partial glossectomy or hemiglossectomy in continuity with an ipsilateral selective neck dissection. Surgical treatment of the primary has improved survival whether neck dissection is performed or not (Davidson et al., 1999; Wushou et al., 2021a). However, neck dissection alongside primary surgical management has also been shown to have increased the survival rate (Wushou et al., 2021b; Haddadin et al., 1999; Myers et al., 2000). Older studies have shown that elective delayed neck dissection once cervical metastasis becomes apparent does not have a negative impact on the rate of survival (Schiff et al., 2005; Vandenbrouck et al., 1980).

Patients with a positive ipsilateral neck dissection are at high risk for contralateral nodal involvement as well. Thus, it is recommended that patients with ipsilateral nodal involvement undergo contralateral completion neck dissection or postoperative radiotherapy of the contralateral neck.

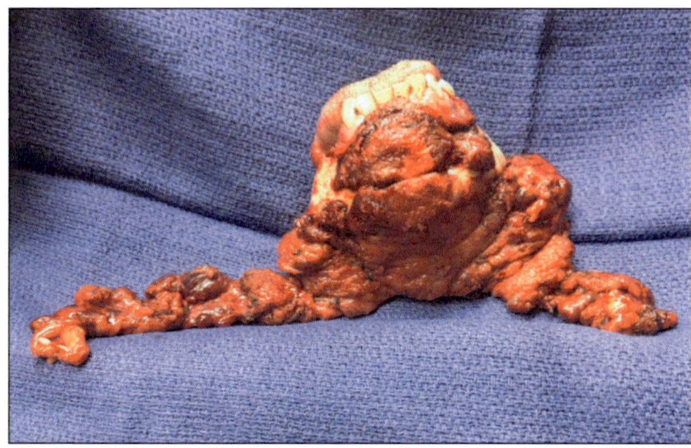

Figure 2-24 En bloc resection of a primary tongue cancer, portion of the mandible and associated lymphatics.

Radiation treatment to the primary site can be administered by brachytherapy implants or traditional irradiation methods. Brachytherapy employs interstitial or intracavitary implantation of radioactive sources to irradiate tumors. This method focuses most of the dose to the tumor volume, while delivering minimal radiation to the surrounding normal tissues, thereby allowing for further future irradiation if needed. Although infrequently utilized, brachytherapy may be a good option in a subset of patients in whom surgical margins are questionable (Harrison, 1997). Reports comparing standard radiation techniques and intensity-modulated radiation therapy (IMRT) have demonstrated similar survival benefits, while IMRT patients have been shown to have significantly reduced postradiation morbidity (Foster et al., 2018; Eisbruch et al., 2004).

Primary resection

Partial glossectomy and hemiglossectomy are used for excision of oral tongue SCCs. Mucosal cuts may be made with either a scalpel or cutting electrocautery techniques. Deeper muscular cuts must be made at depths with appropriate margins as done on the mucosa. This must often be approximated by palpation of the tumor. In situations of nonindurated oral tongue SCC, frozen margins offer tumor localization and assist in maintaining required margins.

Composite resection

The surgical treatment of oral SCC when it lies abutting the mandible is based on the principle of en bloc resection (Fig 2-24) of the primary tumor in continuity with a portion of the mandible to remove the tumor without tumor spillage but with appropriate margins. This technique is applicable to tumors involving the tongue, FOM, mandibular alveolar ridge, retromolar trigone, and tonsillar area and occasionally to tumors of the buccal mucosa and deeply infiltrative lesions of the skin overlying the mandible. When extensive disease is present or a wide excision is required to achieve clear margins, resection of the mandible may become necessary. Such extirpative procedures are termed *composite resections* because more than one tissue type is involved in the resection.

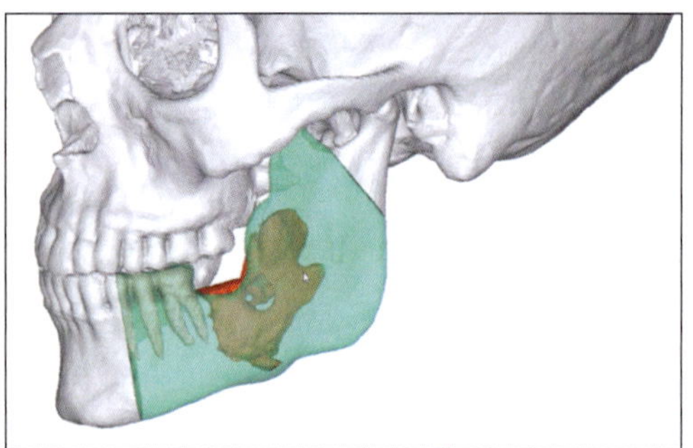

Figure 2-25 Digital planning segmental mandibular osteotomies. Note the intraseptal osteotomy though the first premolar to preserve periodontal support around the adjacent canine.

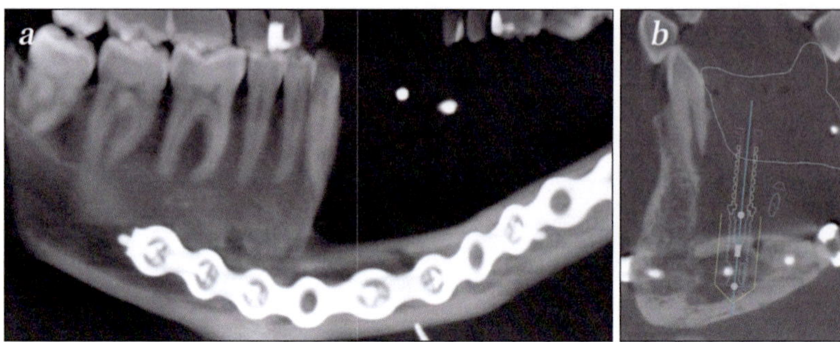

Figure 2-26 Mandibulectomy reconstructed with a FFF. *(a)* Postoperative computer tomograph shows that the osteotomy ran interproximally. *(b)* A buccolingual slice reveals that the resection clipped the apex of the canine.

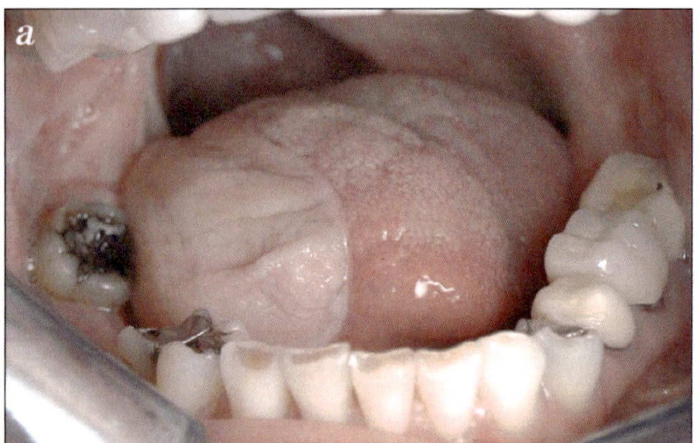

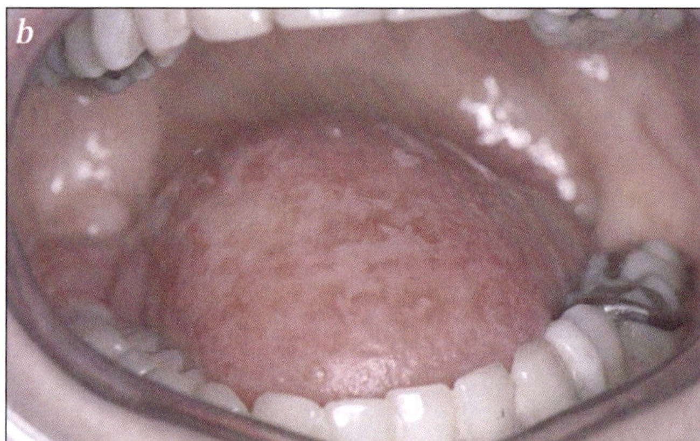

Figure 2-27 *(a)* Lateral third of tongue reconstructed with a RFFF. *(b)* Scapular free flap used to reconstruct a total glossectomy.

The indications for mandibular resection and the extent of surgery depend on the size and location of the primary tumor. As for other head and neck malignancies, the ideal tumor-free margin should be 2 cm. Natural barriers to cancer spread, such as fascial layers, periosteum, or bone, are also important when the resection is planned. As already noted, for all malignancies of the oral cavity, margin status is of utmost importance. For malignancies abutting the periosteum but without frank bony invasion, obtaining clear margins dictates a marginal mandibulectomy, in which monocortical cuts of bone are made and margin-appropriate bone is resected, leaving mandibular continuity, and hence dental occlusion, intact. When the tumor grossly invades the mandible, a segmental mandibulectomy is required. This requires bicortical cuts of the bone, removal of the involved segment, and reestablishment of both mandibular continuity and occlusion.

As in a maxillectomy, osteotomies through the dentulous portion of the mandible should be through a tooth socket (Fig 2-25) rather than interproximal (Fig 2-26). This will result in higher levels of bone for the tooth adjacent to the surgical defect, thus making the tooth more suitable as a partial denture abutment. In addition, bony resections through the body of the mandible should be made as far posteriorly as safe oncologic margins will allow. The more of the mandible remaining, the better the prosthetic prognosis, particularly in edentulous patients.

The presence and the condition of teeth profoundly influence the rehabilitation of patients, regardless of whether they present with a mandibular discontinuity defect. If mandibular continuity has been maintained or restored, teeth are used to retain, support, and stabilize mandibular resection prosthesis (MRP). Key teeth to be salvaged should be identified prior to surgery. Retention of the mandibular canines is especially beneficial.

It is difficult to assess mandibular margins intraoperatively because frozen sections cannot be taken from mineralized bone, although Forrest et al. (1995) have described one technique that may be useful. As such, clinical and radiographic assessment becomes critical in assessing tumor invasion. Invasion of the inferior alveolar canal is also an important consideration because the tumor may exhibit perineural spread, seemingly sparing the bone. In the instance of an expectant nerve transection for a segmental mandibulectomy, it is important to take a frozen margin of the inferior alveolar nerve to assess the neurotropic behavior of the malignancy and avoid late recurrence of the tumor intraosseously or at the skull base. Elsewhere in the resection, all mucosal and soft tissue margins must be evaluated with multiple frozen sections.

Once the decision has been made to resect the mandible for oncologic purposes, it is necessary to consider how mandibular continuity may be restored (see the next section). The development of microvascular free flaps has allowed restoration of mandibular continuity, reconstruction of the tongue, return of vital oral functions, and limitation of cosmetic deformity (see Fig 2-27).

Neck dissection

Historically, cervical disease was treated by performing a radical neck dissection. However, refinements in technique and a better understanding of how tumors spread via the cervical lymphatics have resulted in modifications of this operation that preserve function without oncologic compromise. A basic knowledge of the classic neck dissection is necessary before newer modifications are discussed.

The principles and technique of this operation were first described by George Washington Crile, in 1906 (Crile, 1906). He outlined an operation, still in use today, that effectively removes, en bloc, the cervical nodal basins at risk for or afflicted by tumor metastases. The operation aims to eradicate nodal metastases enveloped within the superficial and deep layers of the cervical fascia.

The lymphatics included within these fascial layers drain all the structures of the head and neck. Terminal lymphatic vessels collect the lymph in a capillary system and transfer it to larger afferent vessels. Following passage through a node, the lymph passes via efferent vessels toward the thoracic duct on the left side of the neck and a smaller lymphatic duct on the right side of the neck. Cells may escape from the node into the systemic circulation thus bypassing the efferent system.

There are approximately 150 nodes in the neck, divided into closely interrelated deep and superficial systems. The superficial lymphatics are located immediately deep in the fibers of the platysma muscle, and they drain the skin and its appendages. The deep system has a principal lymphatic chain and several accessory groups. The principal chain is composed of the nodes adjacent to the internal jugular vein.

Among the accessory systems, the most anterior is composed of a small group of submental nodes just lateral to the midraphe and attached to the fascia of the anterior belly of the digastric muscle. This submental group drains the upper lip and the superficial structures within the nasolabial fold. Immediately posterior to the submental nodes is the submandibular group. This group is adjacent to the facial artery. The submandibular nodes primarily drain the lower lip, the FOM, the alveolar ridge, and portions of the mobile tongue. Of greatest importance, especially in nasopharyngeal and scalp tumors, is the lymphatic chain associated with the accessory nerve. These nodes are located in the posterior triangle of the neck, anterior to the trapezius muscle.

In an effort to standardize nomenclature, Robbins et al. (2002) designated the nodal groups of the head and neck into six regions or levels to better classify neck dissections (Fig 2-28). Level I is the submental and submandibular group; levels II, III, and IV are the upper, middle, and lower jugular groups, respectively; level V is the posterior triangle group; and level VI is the anterior compartment group. The lymph nodes associated with oral cavity carcinomas tend to involve levels I, II, III, and occasionally IV. The incidence of isolated level IV metastases is low; however, inclusion of level IV confers a relatively small increased risk of morbidity, and thus level IV nodes are often included based on the surgeon's preference (Altuwaijri et al., 2021).

Radical neck dissection removes lymph nodes from levels I through V, including the submandibular gland, the sternocleidomastoid and omohyoid muscles, the internal jugular vein, and the spinal accessory nerve. These structures are removed en bloc, much like the resection of the primary lesion, to prevent a lymphatic spillage of possible metastatic carcinoma.

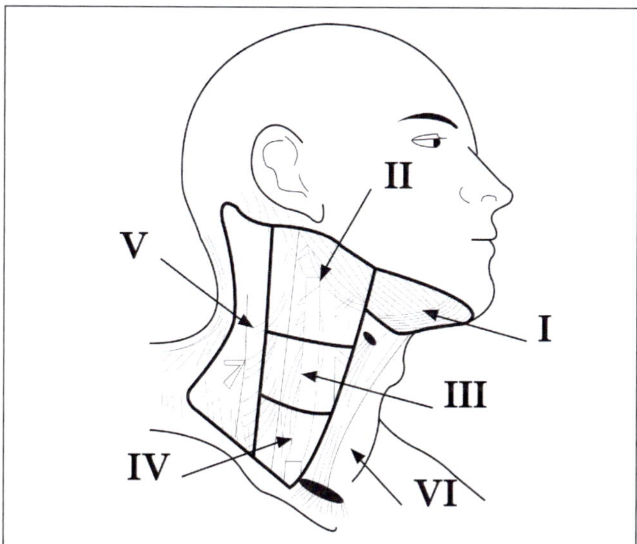

Figure 2-28 Level system for describing the position of neck nodes. Level I—submental and submandibular nodes; level II—upper jugular nodes; level III—middle jugular nodes; level IV—lower jugular nodes; level V—posterior triangle nodes; level VI—paratracheal nodes.

Surgical removal of three of the aforementioned structures can have profound postoperative morbidity. Transection of the accessory nerve results in a functional inability to raise the ipsilateral arm above the level of the shoulder. At rest, there is a noticeable drop in the affected shoulder because of muscle atrophy, and the accompanying "shoulder syndrome" consists of chronic pain in the shoulder (Larsen et al., 2020). Cross-clamping of the internal jugular vein may result in long-term edema of the face when combined with extensive lymphadenectomy and radiation fibrosis. Sternocleidomastoid muscle resection results in cosmetic deformity, as well as weakness with head turn. Thus, the radical neck dissection is not without significant morbidity.

Without sacrificing oncologic principles, modifications of the radical neck dissection are undertaken when possible. *Modified radical neck dissection* refers to one of three variations of the radical neck dissection, namely, sparing of any one of the following structures: the accessory nerve, the internal jugular vein, or the sternocleidomastoid muscle. *Selective neck dissection* refers to any type of cervical neck dissection in which one or more lymph node groups normally removed during a radical neck dissection is preserved. The four subtypes of selective dissections and the corresponding levels of nodes removed are *supraomohyoid dissection* (levels I through III), *posterolateral dissection* (levels II through V), *lateral dissection* (levels II through IV), and *anterior compartment dissection* (level VI). The determination of which selective neck dissection technique to employ is largely dependent on the subsite location of the primary tumor and its most probable nodal basin.

Surgical complications

Although extensive surgery may be effective in treating oral tongue SCC, these procedures are not without serious complications. One important postoperative complication related to composite resections is the potential development of an orocutaneous or pharyngocutaneous fistula because, intraoperatively, continuity exists between the oral cavity and neck. Prior radiotherapy has been shown to significantly increase the risk of perioperative complications and wound infection following clean-contaminated head and neck surgical procedures (Girod et al., 1995). Major complications are associated with an elevated comorbidity level, as outlined by the American Society of Anesthesiology, and with the T stage of the recurrent tumor (Agra et al., 2003; Kim et al., 2007). Late complications—such as ORN, nonhealing oral ulcers, xerostomia, and wound dehiscence—may be seen in irradiated patients.

In the immediate setting, the patient's airway must be considered in preoperative planning to avoid complications at the time of induction and, more often, at arousal. Airway obstruction is rarely a complication because composite resections are often planned with tracheostomy procedures and eventual decannulations. Published indications for consideration of tracheostomy include large tongue-base or pharyngeal defects, bilateral neck dissection, and central mandibular resection (Moubayed et al., 2015; Wu et al., 2022a).

Complications related to the radical neck dissection may also occur intraoperatively or during the early postoperative period. Davidson et al. (1999) reported complications in up to 38% of all neck dissections. Furthermore, they found that preoperative radiotherapy was associated with complications in 58% of patients when the dose was greater than 70 Gy but only in 29% of patients when the dose was less than 70 Gy. This trend was reflected primarily in wound complications. These complications include nerve injury, such as injury to the hypoglossal, vagus, phrenic, and laryngeal nerves; branches of the facial nerve, particularly the marginal mandibular nerve; and portions of the brachial plexus. Though more common in left-neck dissections, chylous fistulae can occur on either side. Excessive bleeding, pneumothorax, and damage to the subclavian vessels are uncommon. Among postoperative complications, hemorrhage or hematoma, skin flap necrosis, seroma, and infection are relatively frequent. Carotid artery rupture is a rare but often lethal complication associated with carotid sheath exposure and either radiation therapy or residual tumor.

Oral tongue and oral cavity SCCs may often be adequately exposed without mandibulotomy (mandibular split) unless a segmental mandibulectomy is required to achieve clear margin status. Similarly, the advent of transoral robotic surgery (TORS) has alleviated the need for mandibulotomy for select tongue-base and hypopharyngeal tumors. If mandibulotomy is performed for exposure purposes, the mandible is sectioned either through the symphysis or the mandibular body in a straight or stepladder fashion. Following resection of the tumor, the two ends are reapproximated and held in position with fixation plates (Fig 2-29). If further exposure is required, a lip-split incision may be utilized. Care is taken to conceal the incision around the chin. Meticulous reapproximation of the mucosa is extremely important.

Following surgery, the patient is maintained with nasogastric tube feedings for the first 7 to 10 days and then started on a mechanical soft diet to prevent fibrous union of the osteotomy site. Maxillomandibular fixation (MMF) is usually not necessary.

Preservation of the outer cortex of the mandible is used only in carefully selected cases where the tumor has limited extension in the FOM and is not contiguous with the mandible. However, mandibular height is an important consideration. In the edentulous patient, a marginal mandibulectomy may place the patient at risk for pathologic fracture, especially in the setting of postoperative irradiation. Therefore, in such circumstances, the placement of a free vascularized bone graft should be considered.

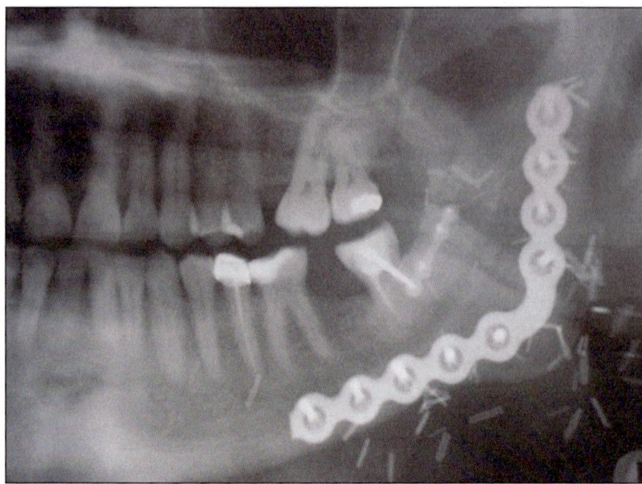

Figure 2-29 Mandibulotomy to achieve better exposure. The mandible is reapproximated and fixated with a reconstruction plate.

If a marginal mandibulectomy is to be undertaken, the closure must be planned preoperatively. Coverage of the raw bony surface may require STSG and bolstered with a prefabricated stent, mobilization of a local, regional, or free flap.

Postoperative care

The patient who has undergone composite resection is initially monitored in an intensive care unit setting. Vigilant tracheostomy care is initiated and is maintained until the patient has met the criteria for decannulation (Pandian et al., 2014). Serial evaluations of the free flap are undertaken to ensure viability of the transferred tissue. Initially this is done at frequent intervals because any delay in diagnosis of a nonviable flap prolongs ischemic time or delays the diagnosis of flap congestion. Multiple methods of free tissue monitoring are available, including a transcutaneous Doppler ultrasound, implantable Doppler ultrasound, and continuous tissue pulse-oximetry.

Local wound care such as dressings and topical antibiotic ointment must be applied in a timely fashion. Drain output is followed diligently to detect impending hematomas or bleeding in the postoperative course. Donor site evaluations must be carried out regularly. Prophylactic antibiotic usage is mandatory in clean-contaminated major oncologic head and neck surgery to reduce the risk of infection (Simó and French, 2006).

Routine postoperative prophylactic milestones should be met in a timely fashion whenever possible, including Foley catheter removal, early ambulation with or without weight bearing, and standard hygiene. Speech pathology specialists who are also versed in swallowing rehabilitation are involved in patient rehabilitation both in the inpatient setting and during outpatient care.

Carcinoma of the anterior floor of mouth (FOM)

Clinical and pathologic considerations

Clinically, FOM is described as a U-shaped space overlying the mylohyoid and hypoglossus muscles. It extends from the inner surface of the mandibular alveolar ridge to the root of the tongue and is

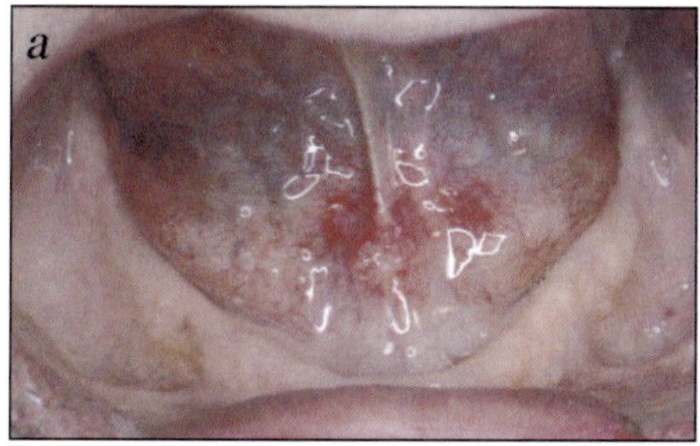
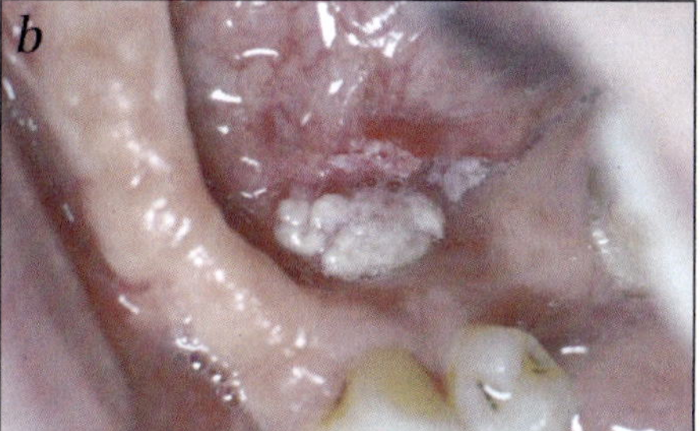
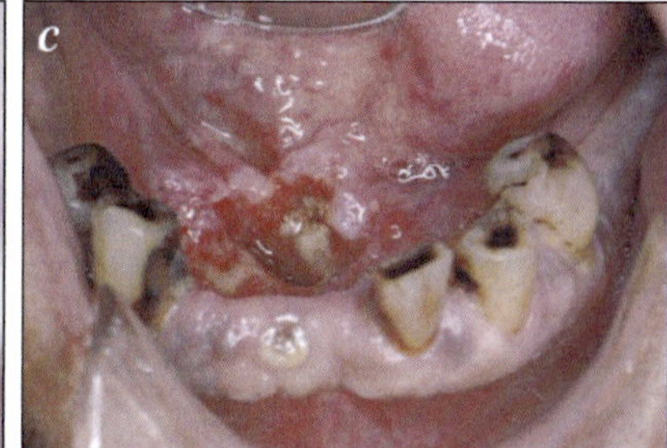

Figure 2-30 *(a)* Early SCC of anterior FOM. *(b)* Small exophytic SCC. *(c)* Large infiltrative SCC.

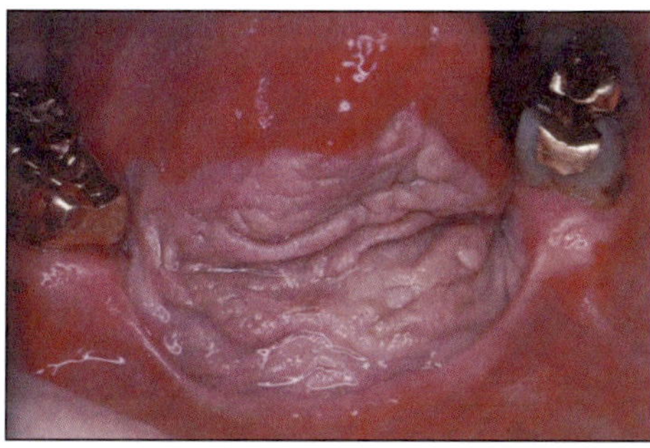

Figure 2-31 FOM and ventral tongue surface lined with a split-thickness skin graft. Primary closure would have tethered the tongue to the residual alveolar mucosa.

limited posteriorly by the anterior tonsillar pillar. Tumors arising from the posterior half of the FOM are managed in a manner similar to those arising from the middle third of the tongue, whereas those lesions involving the anterior half present unique treatment and rehabilitation problems.

The most common presenting symptom is a painful mass or ulcer (Nason et al., 1989). Anterior lesions can involve the frenulum and submandibular ducts. Frequently the tumor infiltrates the mucosa of the alveolar ridge and neighboring tongue. Advanced tumors are characterized by invasion of the root of the tongue, into the extrinsic lingual musculature, and along the mandibular periosteum. Eventually the tumor may extend directly into the submandibular triangle (Fig 2-30).

Regional metastases are commonly encountered. Even when examinations are clinically negative, there is a reported 25% to 30% incidence of occult nodal disease (Nason et al., 1989; McGuirt et al., 1995). The most commonly involved regional nodes are the perifacial nodes and nodal levels I, II, and III. The incidence of nodal metastases correlates with T stage at time of presentation (McGuirt et al., 1995). Furthermore, there is a 20% incidence of contralateral nodal disease (McGuirt et al., 1995). Distant metastases eventually develop in 12% to 30% of patients (McGuirt et al., 1995; Sessions et al., 2000).

Second primary tumors are not uncommon with FOM SCC. Rates of 17% to 35% for both synchronous and metachronous tumors have been reported (Nason et al., 1989; Session et al., 2000; Pernot et al., 1995; Shaha et al., 1984), mandating a thorough assessment, including positron emission tomography to evaluate for hypermetabolic tissue sites throughout the body.

Classification and staging

The TNM system is used to classify FOM tumors. The guidelines for classification and staging are similar to those previously described for oral tongue SCC (see Table 2-3).

Prognosis

Nason et al. (1989) found that, for 198 patients with FOM SCC with uninvolved margins, survival at 5 years was 69%, 64%, 46%, and 26% for stages I, II, III, and IV cancers, respectively, whereby survival was directly correlated with stage at presentation. Sessions et al. (2000) found significantly better 5-year disease-specific survival in patients with clear margins, early T stage, and negative nodes. Recurrence at the primary site (41%) was the most common reason for treatment failure, while 19% of patients had recurrence in the neck. The researchers also reported that 88% of initial recurrences occurred within 60 months after the onset of treatment (Sessions et al., 2000).

Treatment

Surgery, with or without adjuvant radiation, remains the primary treatment modality for FOM SCC. Chemotherapy is reserved for the palliative treatment of advanced lesions or distant metastasis. Although disease-specific survival does not significantly correlate to any particular treatment approach, the accessibility of small (T_1 or T_2) lesions mandates excision (Sessions et al., 2000).

There are conflicting findings regarding radiation therapy for treatment of the primary disease site. Magge et al. (2003) found that the incremental benefit in terms of control of tumor at the primary site for patients receiving postoperative radiation therapy was between 0% and 7%. Surgery alone controlled 80% to 85% of primary tumors. Furthermore, the dose of postoperative radiation therapy did not correlate with local control (Magge et al., 2003). Other investigators have found that postoperative irradiation appears to improve local control in advanced lesions, but evidence of improved survival remains unclear (Guillamondegui et al., 1980; Rodgers et al., 1993). In all cases of FOM SCC, an interdisciplinary team must carefully evaluate the potential benefits and detriments of each treatment approach for a given patient.

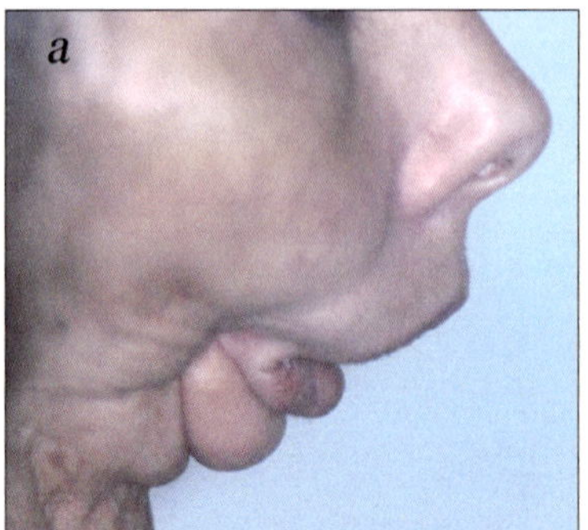

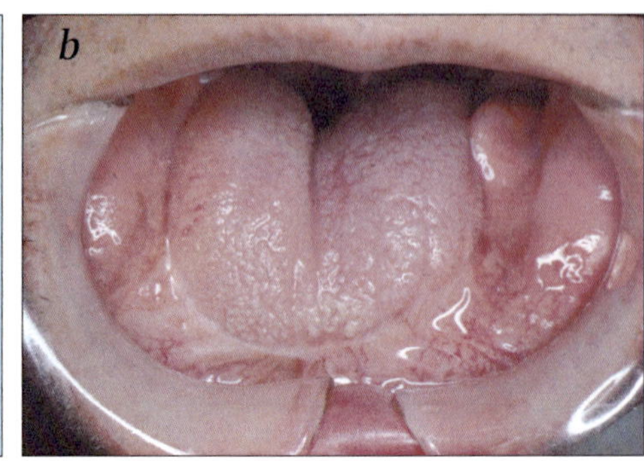

Figure 2-32 *(a)* Severe facial deformity resulting from symphyseal mandibular resection and multiple failed attempts at reconstruction. *(b)* Typical result of resection of the anterior FOM lesion when the wound is closed primarily.

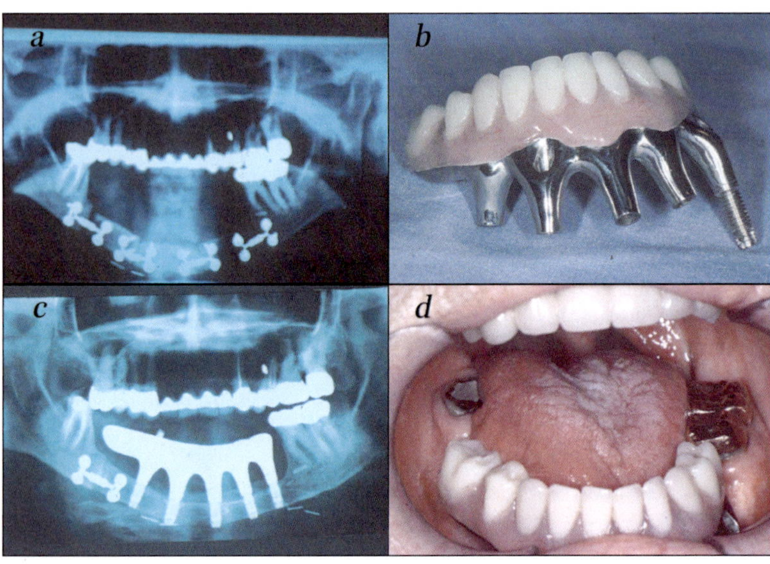

Figure 2-33 *(a)* FFF used to reconstruct a symphyseal defect. *(b–d)* Implants were placed secondarily one year later and used to support a fixed metal-acrylic mandibular resection prosthesis (MRP).

Primary resection

Much like oral tongue SCC, mucosal cuts may be performed with either a scalpel or cutting electrocautery techniques. Deeper muscular cuts must be made at depths with appropriate margins, as on the mucosa. Such deeper margins are best assessed by direct palpation. Frozen section margins offer tumor localization and assist in guaranteeing full tumor excision.

Secondary intention via granulation, primary closure, and local mucosal flaps have all been used successfully in defect closure when size and/or depth permits. However, a split-thickness skin graft is often favored because the other methods often impair tongue mobility (Fig 2-31).

As in oral tongue SCC resection defects, application of bolster may warrant placement of a tracheostomy. Alternatively, if extensive mucosal resection is needed, a microvascular free transfer may be undertaken. Whichever technique is used, the positioning of the margins must be considered in follow-up surveillance examinations.

Composite resection and surgical variations

The major disadvantage of surgery in the management of tumors involving the anterior FOM has been the tremendous disability created by extensive resection. The tendency of these tumors to invade periosteum and bone often necessitates sacrifice of the anterior mandibular arch, which results in the most debilitating defect encountered in the management of intraoral malignancies (Fig 2-32). Fortunately, the use of free flaps has dramatically altered this situation. Microvascular free tissue from the fibula, scapula, ilium, or rib can be used to immediately restore mandibular continuity and resected soft tissues, and many patients emerge with acceptable function and appearance (Fig 2-33).

In early lesions without evidence of bony invasion, resection of anteriorly situated cancers may be adequately accomplished with preservation of the mandibular arch. The primary concern in resection of FOM lesions by marginal mandibulectomy is the potential for local recurrence; therefore, patients must be carefully selected. The adjacent dentition must often be extracted. It is a serious mistake to simply dissect the mucosal lesion from the adjacent periosteum. Adequate resection always requires generous margins, and in these cases it is important to include neighboring bone.

Primary closure over exposed bone may be difficult when a marginal mandibulectomy is performed. The use of mucosal flaps and circumdental sutures may be of assistance, but this places patients at relatively high risk for orocutaneous fistula. In nonirradiated patients, placement of a split-thickness skin graft with a mandibular denture or surgical stent molded to the surgical defect, used as a bolster, may have favorable results even in the absence of periosteum (Figs 2-21 and 2-31).

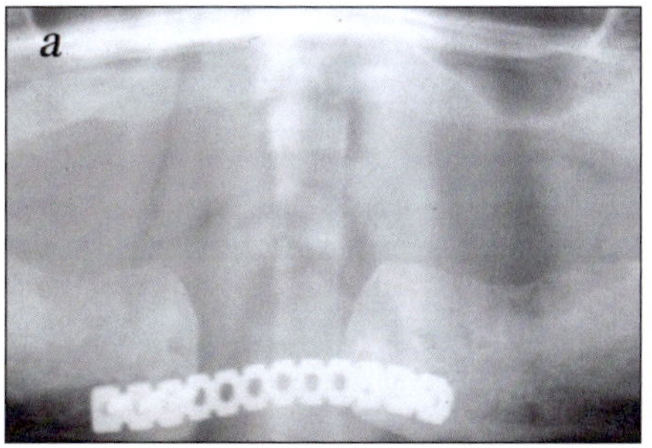
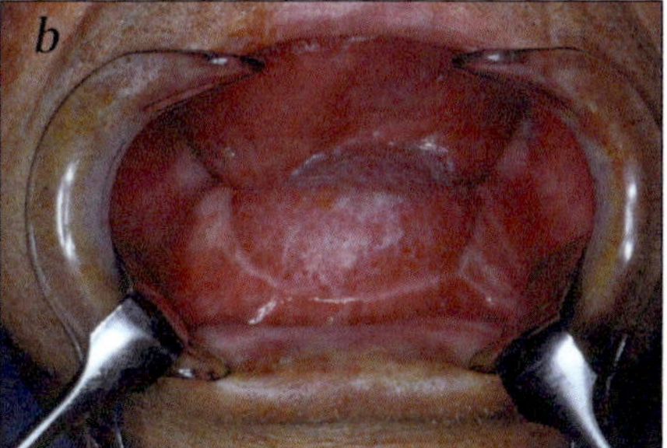
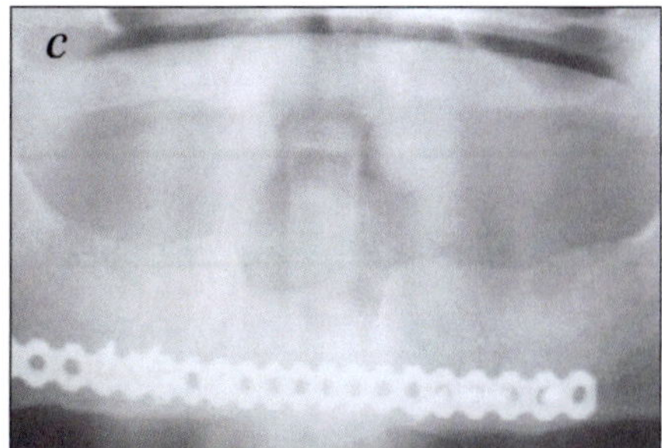

Figure 2-34 *(a)* Lateral mandibular segments maintained in position with a reconstruction plate. *(b)* The pectoralis major, myocutaneous flap provides adequate soft tissue coverage. *(c)* Secondary bone graft.

In most advanced cases, a conventional composite resection of the mandible and soft tissue is needed. In addition to the loss of the mandibular arch, which is usually sacrificed from one mental foramen to the other, resection of the submental structures, including the digastric muscle and extrinsic muscles of the tongue along with portions of its intrinsic musculature, compounds the functional problems and the difficulties of reconstruction. Such resections violate the insertion of the genioglossus muscle, which places patients at a higher risk for respiratory compromise during the recovery period. Composite resections are described more fully in the section titled "Composite resection" under "Carcinoma of the oral tongue."

Neck dissection

The incidence of occult metastasis appears to be less than 20% for a stage I or II tumor (Shaha et al., 1984; Mohit-Tabatabai et al., 1986; Patterson et al., 1984). Although no statistically significant difference in survival has been found when patients with N_0 whose initial treatment was observation and in whom neck treatment was reserved for subsequent neck disease were compared with patients whose necks were treated at the same time as the primary lesion (Pernot et al., 1995), many believe that elective neck dissection is indicated in cases of the clinically negative neck for staging purposes. For anterior lesions crossing or approximating the midline, bilateral neck dissections should be considered, and SLNB may be a viable option in such lesions.

The nodal basins involved in cervical metastasis for FOM SCC tend to be levels I to IV (Shaha et al., 1984). Strong consideration should also be given to excision of the facial perivascular lymphatics. Most T_1 and T_2 lesions have correlating N_0 necks, whereas more than 50% of T_3 and T_4 primary FOM SCCs will have N-positive disease (Magge et al., 2003).

Extensive neck disease isolated in cervical lymphatic specimens may warrant irradiation of the neck as well, but given that the risk of secondary carcinomas in this population is quite high, reserving such treatment for future usage must also be considered.

Initial reconstructive steps

Reconstruction of the mandibular defect should be undertaken at the time of initial resection. Given the predictability of free tissue transfers and the propensity for skin envelope contraction in this area, it is highly preferable to reconstruct discontinuity defects of the anterior mandible primarily. The fibula is the preferred donor site. The osteotomized fibula provides sufficient length and bulk of bone, and endosseous implants can be placed to retain and support a resection prosthesis at a later date (Fig 2-33).

If bony reconstruction is to be delayed, two objectives must be achieved to prepare the area for reconstruction: (1) stabilization of the mandibular fragments by placement of a fixation device or reconstruction plate (Fig 2-34) and (2) adequate soft tissue coverage. These objectives can be achieved with the use of a myocutaneous or a free flap.

Carcinoma of the tonsil and oropharynx

Clinical and pathologic considerations

The oropharynx includes four contiguous sites: (1) the base of the tongue; (2) the soft palate; (3) the palatine tonsillar region (fossa and pillars); and (4) the posterior pharyngeal wall. The oropharynx is limited superiorly by a horizontal line parallel to the superior surface of the soft palate and inferiorly by the superior surface of the hyoid bone (adjacent to the deepest aspect of the vallecula). The anterior borders of the oropharynx include the soft palate and uvula, the anterior tonsillar pillars, and the circumvallate papillae of the tongue base.

The tonsillar region is formed by the tonsil proper and bordered by the anterior tonsillar pillar or palatoglossus muscle and the posterior tonsillar pillar or palatopharyngeus muscle. Lesions arising from these structures have different clinical behaviors and likely different etiologies, despite their proximity. Tumors originating in the tonsil itself are the most common. In most clinical situations these lesions are advanced such that it is difficult to identify their exact site of origin (Fig 2-35).

The tonsil and base of the tongue comprise the majority of oropharyngeal tumors (Shiboski et al., 2005; Magge et al., 2003), with most being SCC (89% to 98%), followed by lymphoma and adenocarcinoma (Mak-Kregar et al., 1995; Zhen et al., 2004). Oropharyngeal SCC is most common among white males, and the majority of cases occur in individuals older than 55 years (Shiboski et al., 2005; Zhen et al., 2004).

Oropharyngeal SCC is one of the very few cancers that has increased in incidence since 1990 (Chaturvedi et al., 2011). This is related to the increasing proportion of these cancers related to the human papillomavirus (HPV) infection and not related to other associated risk factors, such as tobacco, alcohol, and betel nut use.

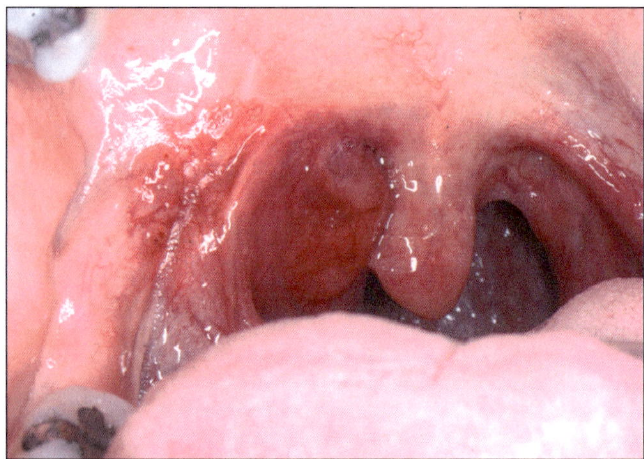

Figure 2-35 Carcinoma of the tonsil involving the palate.

Incidence is rising more quickly among younger cohorts of males (under 55 years); however, as stated above, the majority of cases are still diagnosed in older adults. Over 70% of HPV-associated oropharyngeal carcinomas will demonstrate the overexpression of the P16 biomarker (Fakhry et al., 2018). This is an important factor in prognostication and treatment planning for oropharyngeal SCC, in that P16-positive tumors portend significantly improved responsiveness and survival.

Oropharyngeal SCC may be exophytic or infiltrative. Extension from the tonsil to the tonsillar pillars, base of the tongue, and soft palate may develop rapidly. Involvement of the lateral pharyngeal wall, retromolar trigone, and buccal mucosa are common in advanced cases. SCC of the base of the tongue is often insidious and may only be diagnosed once local spread occurs into the tonsils, lateral pharyngeal walls, and/or supraglottic larynx.

Early symptoms of oropharyngeal carcinoma include throat irritation, neck lump, and odynophagia. Referred ipsilateral otalgia is common. Hemoptysis or oral bleeding can occur with tonsillar cancers. Late symptoms include dysphagia, dysarthria, trismus, obstructive airway symptoms, serous otitis media secondary to eustachian tube obstruction and middle ear effusion, and weight loss.

Because of delays in diagnosis and a propensity for early nodal metastasis, oropharyngeal carcinoma is often at an advanced stage at the time of presentation. Although much of the oropharynx can be inspected and palpated without special instrumentation, many individuals may harbor cancer of the oropharynx for some time before a diagnosis is made.

Oropharyngeal SCC tends to metastasize early to regional nodes (Shiboski et al., 2005; Zhen et al., 2004; Lim et al., 2006a; Ho et al., 2004). For base of the tongue SCC, there is a pattern of bilateral cervical lymphatic metastases due to its midline location and bilateral lymphatic drainage. Furthermore, any cervical metastatic lymphadenopathy may be clinically occult. Lim et al. (2006a) found that, in patients with oropharyngeal SCC and necks that were clinically N_0, 24% of ipsilateral elective neck dissections and 21% of contralateral elective neck dissections harbored occult metastasis.

The probability of distant metastasis for oropharyngeal SCC is relatively low (6% to 11%) (Lim et al., 2006a; Fein et al., 1996).

Table 2-4 Classification and staging
American Joint Committee on cancer staging of P16+ oropharynx SCC

Primary tumor			
T_X	Unable to assess primary tumor		
T_0	No evidence of primary tumor		
T_{is}	Carcinoma in situ		
T_1	Tumor ≤2 cm in large axis		
T_2	Tumor >2 cm and ≤4 cm in large axis		
T_3	Tumor >4 cm in large axis or infiltration of the lingual surface of the epiglottis		
T_4	Invasive tumor: larynx, extrinsic tongue muscles (genioglossus, mylohyoid, styloglossus, palatoglossus), medial pterygoid muscle, hard palate, mandible, lateral pterygoid muscle, pterygoid apophysis, lateral wall of the nasopharynx, base of skull, or internal carotid		
Regional lymphadenopathy			
N_X	Unable to assess regional lymph nodes		
N_0	No evidence of regional metastasis		
N_1	Metastasis in a single or several ipsilateral lymph nodes ≤6 cm		
N_2	Metastasis in a single or several bilateral or contralateral lymph nodes ≤6 cm		
N_3	Metastasis in a single lymph node >6 cm		
Distant metastases			
M_X	Unable to assess for distant metastases		
M_0	No distant metastases		
M_1	Distant metastases		
TMN staging			
Stage 0	T_{is}	N_0	M_0
Stage I	T_{1-2}	N_{0-1}	M_0
Stage II	T_{1-2}	N_2	M_0
	T_{3-4}	N_{0-1}	M_0
Stage III	T_{3-4}	N_2	M_0
Stage IV	Any T	Any N	M_1

DOI: depth of invasion; ENE: extranodal extension
(Amin et al., 2017)

However, when local or regional recurrence has occurred, the risk of distant metastasis is significantly increased (26% to 28%) (Lim et al., 2006a; Fein et al., 1996). Stage has been found to correlate with distant metastasis; furthermore, the presence of pathologic positive lymph nodes, especially bilateral neck metastases, is an independent risk factor for distant metastasis (Lim et al., 2006a).

Classification and staging

The staging system used is based on the TNM system established by the American Joint Committee on Cancer. P16 positive and negative oropharyngeal SCC are staged on different scales. Similarly, pathology-based staging exists for both entities; however, this is not currently discussed (see Tables 2-4 and 2-5).

Table 2-5 Classification and staging
American Joint Committee on cancer staging of P16– oropharynx SCC

Primary tumor			
T_X	Unable to assess primary tumor		
T_0	No evidence of primary tumor		
T_{is}	Carcinoma in situ		
T_1	Tumor ≤2 cm in large axis		
T_2	Tumor >2 cm and ≤4 cm in large axis		
T_3	Tumor >4 cm in large axis or infiltration of the lingual surface of the epiglottis		
T_{4a}	Invasive tumor: larynx, extrinsic tongue muscles (genioglossus, mylohyoid, styloglossus, palatoglossus), medial pterygoid, hard palate, or mandible		
T_{4b}	Invasive tumor: lateral pterygoid muscle, pterygoid apophysis, lateral wall of the nasopharynx, base of skull, internal carotid		
Regional lymphadenopathy			
N_X	Unable to assess regional lymph nodes		
N_0	No evidence of regional metastasis		
N_1	Metastasis in a single ipsilateral lymph node ≤3 cm and ENE-		
N_{2a}	Metastasis in a single ipsilateral lymph node >3 cm and ≤6 cm and ENE-		
N_{2b}	Metastases in multiple ipsilateral lymph nodes ≤6 cm and ENE-		
N_{2c}	Metastases in bilateral or contralateral lymph nodes ≤6 cm and ENE-		
N_{3a}	Metastasis in a lymph node >6 cm and ENE-		
N_{3b}	Metastasis in any lymph node(s) with ENE+ clinically		
Distant metastases			
M_X	Unable to assess for distant metastases		
M_0	No distant metastases		
M_1	Distant metastases		
TMN staging			
Stage 0	T_{is}	N_0	M_0
Stage I	T_1	N_0	M_0
Stage II	T_2	N_0	M_0
Stage III	T_3	N_0	M_0
	T_{1-3}	N_1	M_0
Stage IVa	T_{4a}	N_{0-1}	M_0
	T_{1-4a}	N_2	M_0
Stage IVb	Any T	N_3	M_0
	T_{4b}	Any N	M_0
Stage IVc	Any T	Any N	M_1

DOI: depth of invasion; ENE: extranodal extension
(Amin et al., 2017)

Prognosis

A wide body of literature exists regarding the outcome and prognosis of oropharyngeal SCC. Prognosis varies depending on stage, P16 status, site, treatment modality, and salvage outcomes. Furthermore, various centers have distinct advantages over others with respect to a given treatment modality based on the merits of the available resources, making interinstitutional comparisons difficult. Meta-analysis studies attempt to overcome this confounding variable. However, variations in techniques, whether regarding surgery, administration of radiation, or follow-up surveillance, will affect outcome data. Certain consistent findings regarding improved survival were found across multiple studies with regard to early stage (Sessions et al., 2000; Mak-Kregar et al., 1995; Zhen et al., 2004; Gourin and Johnson, 2001; Mendenhall et al., 2000; Sundaram et al., 2005), clinically negative neck disease or lesser N stage (Denittis et al., 2001; Newkirk et al., 2001), and P16 status (Fakhry et al., 2008; Ang et al., 2010). Of note, patients with P16+ disease have a 58% reduction in the risk of death, as well as a greater than 50% reduction in the risk of disease progression following treatment (Ang et al., 2010).

Treatment

The definitive treatment of base of the tongue SCC is controversial and evolving. Small, localized tumors have traditionally been treated with surgical intervention, followed by postoperative low-dose radiation therapy; however, some centers advocate chemoradiation therapy as a primary therapeutic modality. They maintain that chemoradiation therapy offers high locoregional control rates and possibly better function with regard to speech and swallowing (Harrison et al., 1997). IMRT, because it focuses the radiation, results in less injury to the adjacent tissues than does conventional external beam therapy (Chao et al., 2004). However, recent reports indicate that the long-term side effects of chemoradiation therapy can be quite debilitating. An increasing number of patients treated in this manner present with severe trismus, velopharyngeal incompetence, and difficulty in swallowing three to five years after completion of therapy (Laccourreye et al., 2005). De-escalation trials for upfront chemoradiation are ongoing.

Others advocate surgery as the primary treatment modality because it offers important histologic, biologic, and prognostic information that can guide the decision to use adjuvant therapies (Galati et al., 2000). Minimally invasive TORS has greatly reduced the morbidity associated with surgically approaching tumors of the oropharynx. This has led to multiple trials of TORS with de-escalated chemoradiotherapy aimed only at controlling regional disease (Swisher-McClure et al., 2020; Owadally et al., 2015; Ferris et al., 2022).

In addition, the surgical defect secondary to the resection of the base of the tongue can be effectively reconstructed with vascularized free flaps. The stage of the disease may also dictate the treatment.

The locoregional control rate with surgery for early (stage I or II) base of the tongue SCC exceeds 80% (Gourin and Johnson, 2001). Some centers have reported similar survival rates for advanced (stage III or IV) base of the tongue cancers (Azizzadeh et al., 2002). The locoregional control rates are more variable by institution when irradiation is the primary treatment (Mendenhall et al., 2000). In instances of radiation failure, subsequent salvage surgical therapy of the base of the tongue SCC is often difficult and demonstrates poor outcomes (Goodwin, 2000).

Several reports have demonstrated improved locoregional control rates with combined therapy: surgery plus postoperative radiation, radiation followed by chemoradiation, suggesting that integrated multimodality therapy is superior to any single modality treatment plan alone (Denittis et al., 2001; Gourin and Johnson, 2001).

For tonsillar SCC, definitive radiation therapy is thought to be as effective as surgery in controlling the primary site for early (stage I and II) lesions (Mendenhall et al., 2006). Some centers are performing transoral lateral oropharyngectomy procedures, often using induction chemotherapy and postoperative radiation therapy, depending on margin status and extracapsular spread (Laccourreye et al., 2005; Galati et al., 2000). For such procedures, patient selection is critical, because those best suited for the procedure are patients with anterior T_1 to T_2 tonsillar SCC without posterior anatomical spread. It is thought that this approach may avoid complications related to the use of radiation therapy or chemoradiation and reserves these therapeutic options for subsequent management if needed, based on histologic results or should recurrence or metachronous cancers develop.

Extensive tonsillar lesions invading the base of the tongue or those with extensive metastatic cervical lymphadenopathy have less satisfactory tumor control and survival rates. For disease that is an advanced stage (III or IV), combination therapy may have an advantage over either therapy alone (Perez et al., 1998; Poulsen et al., 2007); however, meta-analysis results may suggest otherwise (Parson et al., 2002). The addition of chemotherapy for locoregional disease is generally reserved for evidence of extranodal extension or a positive surgical margin (Bernier et al., 2005). Currently, advanced tumors of the tonsils continue to challenge radiation oncologists and surgeons. Combined modalities, including chemoradiation therapy, are generally preferred in such cases.

Neck dissection

Although it is evident that at least a comprehensive neck dissection must be performed for all N-positive disease, controversy exists regarding the N_0 neck. Unlike other primary sites, no consensus exists regarding which lymph node groups to remove in elective management of the N_0 neck in patients with oropharyngeal SCC. Shah and Andersen (Shah and Andersen, 1994) found that the majority of occult cervical lymphatic metastases were to levels II through IV and that occult metastases occurred 7% of the time in both levels I and V. On the other hand, Spiro et al. (1988) recommend elective supraomohyoid neck dissection (levels I through III) for the treatment of patients with a N_0 neck with oropharyngeal SCC.

We prefer to perform a neck dissection that encompasses levels I through IV in both the clinically N_0 neck as well as when node-positive disease is present. Level V lymphatics are removed only if they are involved clinically. The level I dissection permits access to the facial artery, which is frequently the recipient artery for microvascularized free tissue transfer.

Appraisal of QOL issues following treatment requires large population studies that use specific, validated head and neck QOL instruments. Only through such studies regarding treatment outcomes can patients be provided with the information necessary to give their fully informed consent.

Composite resection

A composite resection may be needed for the surgical treatment of oropharyngeal SCC. The posterior location of these tumors makes access an important consideration for surgical planning. Multiple surgical approaches may be considered, including direct transoral, TORS, transhyoid, lateral pharyngotomy, and mandibular swing approaches. The choice among these approaches may be based on tumor size, infiltration, location, vascular proximity, and prior irradiation therapy.

The direct transoral and TORS approach is the least invasive. Tumors may be resected with the carbon dioxide laser, electrocautery (as in TORS), or cold steel.

The remainder of surgical approaches are less commonly used in the current era, due to the propensity for upfront chemoradiation therapy in locally and locoregionally advanced diseases. Despite this, they remain useful for salvaging surgical approaches. A transhyoid or suprahyoid approach involves division of the suprahyoid musculature, which provides direct access to the vallecular mucosa. The pharyngotomy must take into account the need for an oncologic margin and must, therefore, be made opposite the tumor. For this reason, this approach is often combined with a lateral pharyngotomy approach to improve contralateral access. The lateral pharyngotomy is made through a lateral incision in pharyngeal mucosa. Retraction of the thyroid ala and transsection of the superior laryngeal muscle fibers allow access to tumors of the lateral pharyngeal wall or posterolateral tongue base. Inadvertent injury to the hypoglossal and superior laryngeal nerves may occur during this procedure, and their respective neurovascular bundles must be identified initially.

The greatest exposure to the oropharynx is provided by the mandibular swing approach. A mandibulotomy is made at the symphysis or parasymphysis and the proximal incisor is extracted. The FOM mucosa and musculature are divided, providing adequate mucosa on either side for future closure; the tissues are divided carefully to protect the lingual and hypoglossal nerves. The wide exposure allows for removal of high retropharyngeal nodes and for en bloc resection of the primary tumor with the ipsilateral neck dissection. Once the defect is closed or covered with a rotational or microvascular free flap, the mucosa in the FOM is closed and the mandible is reapproximated with a previously prepared reconstruction plate. Occlusion and speech are often unaffected by this approach.

Mandibular involvement of the primary lesion may be assessed preoperatively by radiographic techniques, but frozen sections of the bone cortex are generally not performed. As discussed for oral tongue and FOM tumors, for oropharyngeal lesions a composite resection may include bicortical portions of the mandible or be performed with marginal (monocortical) mandibulotomy alone if the tumor adheres to periosteum.

The defects resulting from these resections are best surfaced with vascularized free flaps. Reconstructive techniques and vascularized free flaps are described in detail later in this chapter. Velopharyngeal defects may be restored with an obturator prosthesis. Most patients are capable of near-normal speech, swallowing, and mastication (Fig 2-36).

Complications

The complications arising from surgical management of oropharyngeal SCC are similar to those described for the treatment of posteriorly located lingual tumors. As in all tumors in close proximity to the mandible, osteitis and ORN are serious and debilitating problems that frequently fail to respond to any form of treatment. At surgery, care should be taken to avoid unnecessary trauma to the mandible and to provide healthy soft tissue coverage to prevent postoperative bone exposure. Pharyngocutaneous fistulae

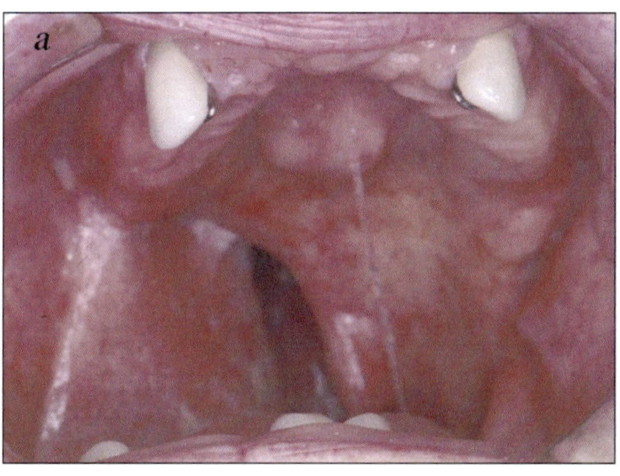

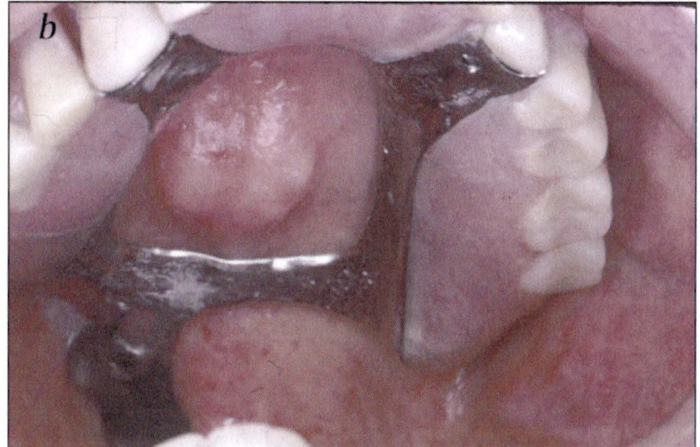

Figure 2-36 *(a)* Large defect of the tonsil, soft palate, and base of tongue resurfaced with a pectoralis major myocutaneous flap. *(b)* Velopharyngeal function was restored with a soft palate obturator and partial denture.

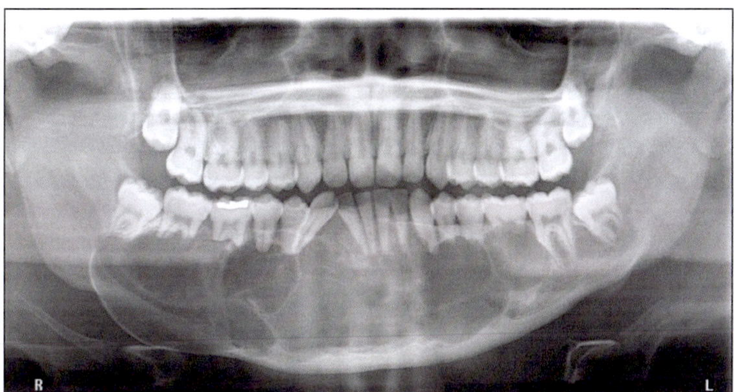

Figure 2-37 Panoramic radiograph demonstrating an ameloblastoma of the mandible.

and wound infection remain formidable threats during the postoperative period. Nasogastric or gastric tube feeding is necessary to ensure nutrition postoperatively without compromising the wound bed. Complications of neck dissection were delineated previously in the section addressing carcinoma of the oral tongue.

Carcinoma of the mandible and alveolar ridge

Intraosseous tumors requiring marginal or segmental resection of the mandible can arise from the periosteum, bone of the mandible, or dental elements. Ameloblastoma and osseous sarcomas figure most prominently among these lesions.

Ameloblastoma

Ameloblastoma is a rare odontogenic tumor arising from the enamel organ. Although ameloblastoma tends to be locally invasive, it is not commonly known to have metastatic potential. However, malignant forms have been described (Verneuil et al., 2002; Zarbo et al., 2003). Ameloblastoma of the mandible usually presents as an indolent mass in the parasymphyseal or body region of the mandible. All ages may be affected, but the disease is most prevalent during the second to fifth decades. There is nearly equal incidence among males and females, with a slight male preponderance (Lim et al., 2006b; Reichart et al., 1995).

Clinical and pathologic considerations

The typical radiographic finding is that of a rounded, multilocular radiolucent area (Fig 2-37). Unilocular ameloblastoma is biologically less aggressive. A panoramic radiograph is not considered diagnostic but may have a typical appearance. A biopsy is needed to confirm the diagnosis and to differentiate this from other benign mandibular lesions. These tumors are relatively slow growing, but they exhibit a marked tendency to destroy the involved bone. The most common presentation is a painless, gradually growing mass (McClary et al., 2016).

Treatment based on type. There are three types of ameloblastoma, based on radiography: (1) *solid* (or multicystic), (2) *unicystic*, and (3) *peripheral*. Conservative treatments have come under scrutiny in terms of controlling local recurrences. Reported recurrence rates with conservative curettage are often in excess of 70%, while those of radical resection are typically 10% to 20% (Sehdev et al., 1974; Shatkin and Hoffmeister, 1965; Mehlisch et al., 1972). More recent studies have demonstrated a narrower discrepancy between the two modalities (Eckardt et al., 2009; Nakamura et al., 2002).

The solid or multicystic ameloblastoma characteristically infiltrates the trabeculae of cancellous bone, causing the tumor to extend beyond its radiologically apparent margin. This characteristic increases the risk of recurrence if the tumor is excised based on such a guide. The risk of recurrence increases with increasing size and in lesions that extend beyond the bony confines of the

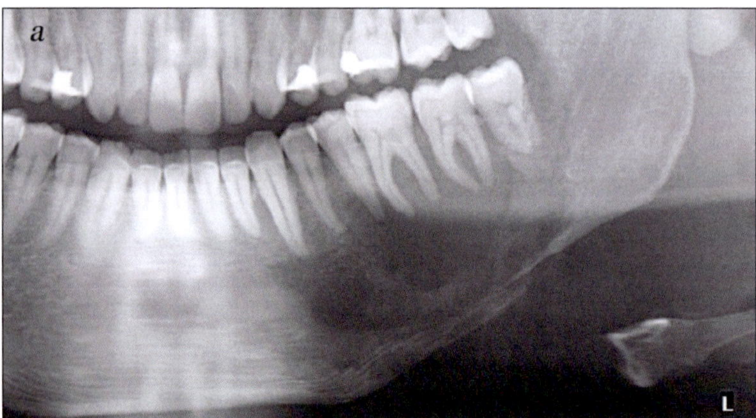

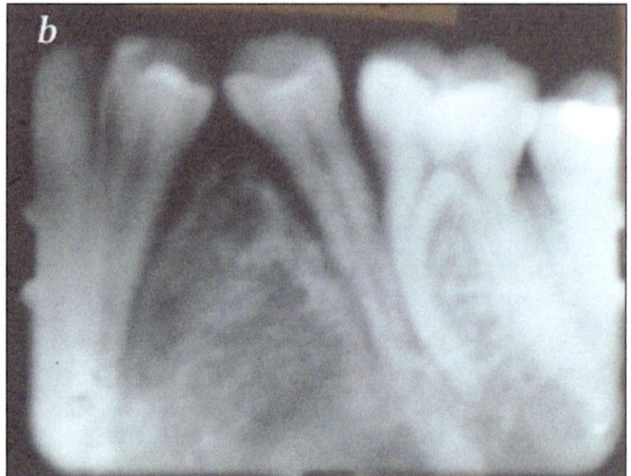

Figure 2-38 *(a)* Panoramic radiograph demonstrating an osteosarcoma of the mandible. *(b)* Periapical radiograph of a different patient showing displacement of teeth.

mandible (Yang et al., 2019). Complete excision, including removal of an extensive margin of apparently unaffected bone, is the definitive treatment for multicystic mandibular ameloblastomas.

Smaller, accessible tumors may undergo curettage, provided that both the surgeon and the patient realize that there is a chance of recurrence and that close follow-up is mandated. In a compliant and informed patient, recurrence may be treated with multiple curettage procedures to preserve function and esthetics. Other ameloblastoma subtypes fare better with conservative management.

Unicystic ameloblastomas occur more often in younger persons, mainly in the second and third decades, than do classic multicystic ameloblastomas (Kim and Jang, 2001). Unicystic ameloblastoma is both unilocular, clinically and radiologically, and cystic on histologic examination, which reveals that the epithelial lining consists of ameloblastomic cells (Gardner, 1996). Most small unicystic ameloblastomas are diagnosed clinically and radiologically as dentigerous cysts and, as such, are enucleated. Pathologic examination yields the diagnosis of unicystic ameloblastoma. Conservative therapies such as curettage appear to be quite effective at preventing recurrence of unicystic ameloblastomas (Nakamura et al., 2002).

Several reports indicate that a radical resection for all ameloblastomas offers better results in terms of recurrence than a conservative approach (marsupialization, enucleation, or curettage; Kim and Jang, 2001; Sehdev et al., 1974; Muller and Slootweg, 1985). However, many considerations must be taken into account when the appropriate management is decided, including the tumor subtype and the patient's compliance with follow-up and tolerance for aesthetic disruption.

Osteosarcoma

Osteogenic sarcoma or *osteosarcoma* is the most common primary osseous malignancy. Osteosarcoma involves the mandible or maxilla in only 5% of cases and represents approximately 15% of all head and neck sarcomas, although this may be underestimated (Patel et al., 1996). Although the cause of these tumors is unknown, it has been established that osteosarcoma is a malignancy of mesenchymal origin, particularly of the cells that produce osteoid, or immature bone. The peak age of onset in the head and neck is between 25 and 40 years, approximately 10 to 20 years later than the analogous tumor involving long bones (Sturgis and Potter, 2003).

Predisposing factors for osteosarcoma include a prior history of radiation exposure and Paget disease of the bone (Maghami et al., 2005). Other associated, but not necessarily causative, factors include fibrous dysplasia, multiple osteochondromatosis, chronic osteomyelitis, myositis ossificans, and trauma (Shao et al., 2010; Mendenhall et al., 2011; Ogunlewe et al., 2006; van Es et al., 1997). Several hereditary disorders are associated with an increased risk of these neoplasms, including Li-Fraumeni syndrome and the hereditary form of retinoblastoma (Sturgis and Potter, 2003).

Clinical and pathologic considerations. Many patients with osteosarcoma present with a painless mass, but dental pain, loose teeth, and ulceration may occur. Numbness within the distribution of the inferior alveolar nerve can occur in up to 35% of patients, indicating neural involvement of the tumor (Sturgis and Potter, 2003; Fernandes et al., 2007; Mardinger et al., 2001). The duration of symptoms averages between two and six months before initial evaluation (Sturgis and Potter, 2003).

On radiographic examination, osteosarcoma appears as a destructive, poorly defined, intraosseous lesion with or without an adjacent soft tissue mass. The bony lesion may be characterized as lytic, sclerotic, or mixed (Fig 2-38). A prominent sunburst appearance may be seen as well.

Treatment

Surgical resection is the treatment of choice for mandibular osteosarcoma. A segmental resection of the mandible with removal of adjacent involved soft tissues is required. Osteosarcoma of the mandible is characterized by frequent local recurrence and late metastases. A substantial cuff of normal tissue is recommended to obtain an adequate margin. Although the amount of normal tissue in the margin is not established, we recommend resection of at least 2 cm around the apparent diseased area, irrespective of original lesion size.

Elective operative treatment of cervical lymph nodes is unnecessary, because osteosarcoma spreads hematogenously and not to regional lymphatics. More recently, multimodal treatment has been implemented based on the success of neoadjuvant chemotherapy in the treatment of osteosarcoma of long bones (Jaffe et al., 1995). In examining the effect of chemotherapy on osteosarcoma of the head and neck, Smeele et al. (1997) found that patients who underwent complete surgical resections had a more favorable overall survival

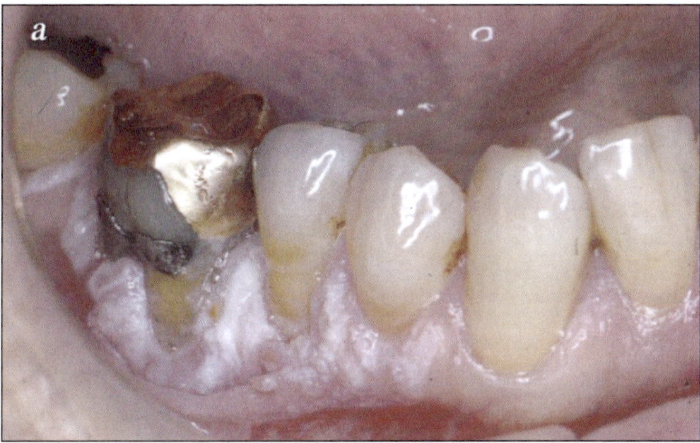

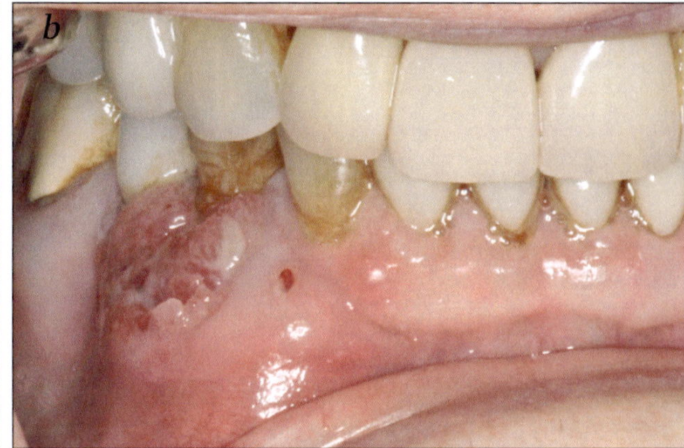

Figure 2-39 *(a)* Localized SCC of the alveolar ridge (courtesy of Dr. Sol Silverman Jr., San Francisco, CA). *(b)* Gingival SCC with mandibular involvement.

rate than did those who were left with residual disease. The addition of adjuvant chemotherapy may improve early survival; it does not appear to affect long-term survival (Guadagnolo et al., 2009; Smith et al., 2003). There remains some uncertainty as to the radiosensitivity of osteosarcoma (Sturgis and Potter, 2003); however, adjuvant irradiation may assist in local control (Patel et al., 1996; Laskar et al., 2008).

Distant metastases occur less frequently when the head and neck is the primary site than when osteosarcoma occurs in long bones. Distant disease is seen in up to 18% of patients and mainly occurs in the lungs (Mardinger et al., 2001). However, local recurrence is an utmost concern. Up to 40% of patients develop local disease recurrence after treatment (Patel et al., 1996; Ha et al., 1999; Oda et al., 1997). Younger patients, especially those with a previous retinoblastoma diagnosis, those with tumors greater than 4 cm, and patients with positive surgical margins have a significantly greater risk of local failure (Patel et al., 1996).

Various reports suggest different survival rates. In a meta-analysis conducted by Mardinger et al. (2001), five-year survival ranged from 20% in earlier reports to more than 70% more recently (Patel et al., 1996; Ha et al., 1999; Cady and Catlin, 1969). This range may be attributable to improved assessment of tumors with modern imaging techniques, to refinement of reconstruction that permits more aggressive margin resection, or to the recent multimodal approach to treatment. However, most studies underscore that positive surgical margins are a significant predictor of worse disease-specific survival rates (Sturgis and Potter, 2003; Jaffe et al., 1995; Ha et al., 1999).

Carcinoma confined to the gingiva

SCCs of the gingiva and the alveolar mucosa comprise about 10% of all oral malignancies. They occur more frequently in the mandible and affect primarily the molar gingiva (Fig 2-39a). These tumors are more common in men (about 4:1). Cady and Catlin (1969) reported that in 88% of male patients the tumor occurred between the ages of 50 and 80 years.

Clinical and pathologic considerations

The presence of an ulcer, bleeding gum, and pain are the most common symptoms. The lesions may be flat, ulcerative, or exophytic and tend to spread rapidly. Their pattern of spread is often radial before diving deeply. They are usually well differentiated histologically (Willen et al., 1975). The search for a second primary tumor is important in these patients because the incidence of additional intraoral epidermoid carcinomas has been reported to be 11% to 18% due to the concept of field cancerization (Cady and Catlin, 1969). Mandibular involvement occurs in about 50% of the cases, and it does not always correlate with radiographic findings (Fig 2-39b).

The tumors tend to expand to the FOM and buccal mucosa. Regional metastases are present initially in approximately 30% of the patients and first involve the submandibular nodes.

Classification and staging

These lesions are classified according to the TNM system in the same manner as other oral cancers (see Table 2-3).

Prognosis

The prognosis for SCC of the gingiva varies according to the stage of the disease. Overall survival rates have been reported to be as high as 65% (Cady and Catlin, 1969; Wald and Calcaterra, 1983) The expected two-year survival rate is 80% for stage I disease and 70% for stage II disease (Cady and Catlin, 1969; Wald and Calcaterra, 1983). For stage III and stage IV disease, the two-year survival rates are 60% and 50%, respectively (Wald and Calcaterra, 1983).

Treatment

The treatment of SCC of the mandibular alveolar ridge is predominantly surgical, usually involving a marginal mandibular resection for early lesions and a segmental resection for advanced lesions with extensive bony involvement (Wald and Calcaterra, 1983). The resection should be performed in conjunction with a supraomohyoid neck dissection if regional metastasis is suspected. In advanced cases, postoperative radiation therapy may be indicated.

For most patients, resections do not require the sacrifice of large amounts of soft tissue. Repair can be accomplished with primary closure or skin grafts (Fig 2-40). With large segmental bony defects, immediate reconstruction with a FFF is recommended by most clinicians.

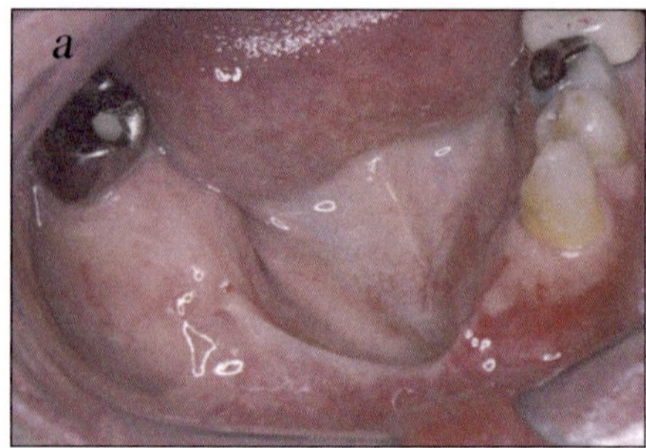

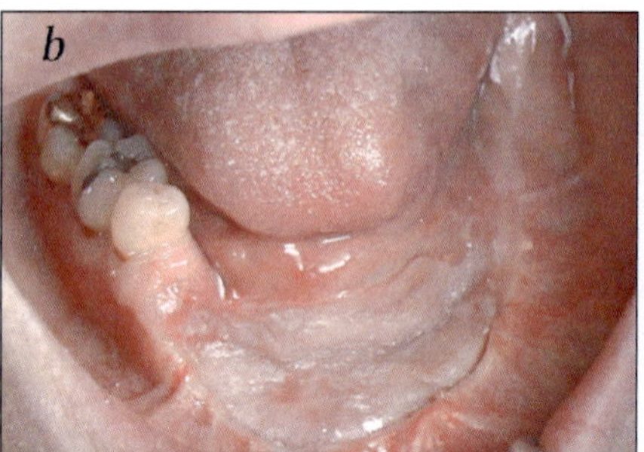

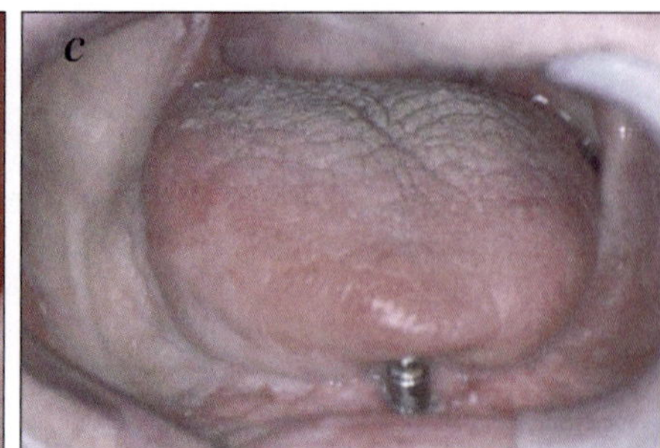

Figure 2-40 Soft tissue management following marginal mandibular resections. *(a)* Primary closure of the oral mucosa. *(b)* Closure with a split-thickness skin graft. *(c)* Closure with a radial forearm free flap (RFFF).

Avascular Bone Grafts

Mandibular reconstruction poses a significant challenge for both the surgeon and the patient. The primary goals are to restore facial form and mandibular continuity so that both aesthetic and functional goals are met. However, these play a secondary role to making certain that the disease process leading to the need for the reconstruction has been appropriately managed. Surgical advances have improved the surgeon's ability to achieve these goals, and the use of dental implants further enhances the functional potential of the patient. It has been shown that dental implants successfully osseointegrate with grafted bone (Dodson and Smith, 1987; Listrom and Symington, 1988; Keller, 1991; Habal and Rasmussen, 1993; Chana et al., 2004; Roumanas et al., 2006a). Consideration must be given not only to restoring mandibular continuity but also to providing appropriate volume and quality of bone for the placement of dental implants.

Vascularized free tissue transfer has revolutionized the reconstruction of composite tongue and mandible defects. For defects larger than 6 cm, or composite defects that require soft tissue coverage, or in poorly vascularized beds (e.g., prior to or after radiation therapy), vascularized free flaps are preferable (Foster et al., 1999; Paley et al., 2005; Lonie et al., 2016). However, an avascular bone graft is still a predictable reconstructive option, especially in patients who have a well-vascularized soft tissue recipient bed. Avascular bone grafts yield excellent results and, in some instances, offer several advantages over vascularized free flaps. Avascular bone grafts require less extensive surgery. The procedures are less technique sensitive and do not rely on specialized equipment, skill, training, or instrumentation. Finally, a bone graft can be more easily shaped to meet the final geometric goals.

Many patients can be reconstructed immediately. This can improve the final reconstructive result because scarring and tissue contraction will not impede the placement of the avascular bone graft, which would adversely affect the recipient graft site. In the past, reconstructive procedures were delayed to allow clinical monitoring of the tumor resection site. With the routine availability of computed tomography, magnetic resonance imaging, and positron emission tomography, recurrent disease can be detected within the grafted tissues and will have less chance of going undetected. However, immediate reconstruction with bone grafts increases the risk of infection due to the contamination of the nonvascularized graft by oral bacteria.

Goals of mandibular reconstruction

The two main goals of mandibular reconstruction are the restoration of (1) form and (2) function. The mandible maintains facial contours through support of the overlying soft tissues. The shape, size, and position of the final grafted mandible are crucial factors in maximizing esthetics. The grafted bone must be positioned as close to the original native mandible as possible.

The most important anatomical consideration is the position of the graft along the lower border of the mandibular body and symphysis, because the soft tissue drape over the lower border contributes significantly to facial form. In addition, if the bone graft is properly positioned and contoured, prosthetic rehabilitation of the alveolus and teeth will be easier, resulting in more accurate support of the cheeks and lips to further improve esthetics.

The challenge for the reconstructive surgeon rests with the height of the reconstructed mandible. Although form is improved when the bone is positioned along the lower border, implant potential may be compromised if the grafted bone is not of substantial size. Consideration must be given to the type of grafted bone used; this decision depends on the surgeon's preferences and the configuration of the potential donor sites.

If an avascular bone graft is considered, extraoral and intraoral soft tissue defects must be addressed first to provide a vascularized recipient tissue bed for the future bone graft. This can be accomplished with pedicled myocutaneous flaps. In the absence of significant soft tissue defects, the accurate repositioning of the overlying muscle, fascia, and connective tissue layers following a tumor resection will facilitate future reconstructive procedures.

Proper positioning of the mandibular bone graft is essential for a good functional result. Both the grafted bone and the remaining native mandibular segments must be in the proper three-dimensional location. This will ensure accurate intercuspation and occlusion of remaining teeth and establish the necessary relationships required for future prosthetic reconstruction. This will also result in correct positioning of the condyles within the glenoid fossae, thus minimizing temporomandibular joint dysfunction.

Consideration for future dental implants affects the way that mandibular bone graft reconstruction is planned and executed. The grafted bone must be accurately positioned if implants are to be placed in their proper locations. If not executed correctly, a functional prosthesis may be compromised or even impossible.

The reconstructive surgeon must also consider the final volume and quality of the grafted bone. This will affect the choice of donor sites for both vascularized free flaps and avascular bone grafts. For example, if a significant amount of bone is required for reconstruction, the posterior iliac crest should be considered instead of the anterior iliac crest, since the posterior iliac crest yields a greater quantity of bone.

Dental implants have also changed the way that the reconstructive surgeon approaches the intraoral soft tissues. The health of the peri-implant soft tissues is more easily maintained if these tissues are thin, keratinized, and attached to the periosteum. Delayed split-thickness skin grafting may be required to obtain this result. Therefore, the reconstructive surgeon and prosthodontist must be aware of the potential and limitations of mandibular reconstruction and work together to achieve the best possible results for patients requiring mandibular resection and reconstruction.

Biology of avascular bone grafting

The biology of bone regeneration after autogenous avascular grafting is complex, but the concept is relatively straightforward. If bone is harvested and placed in a distant recipient bony defect that is surrounded by a well-vascularized soft tissue bed, new living bone will form to bridge the defect. The bone cells come from the adjacent native bone (osteoconduction), are induced from pluripotential cells located in the surrounding blood or soft tissue (osteoinduction), or come from the few donor cells that survive the transplant (osteogenesis). Likely, all three processes play a role, but the predominant factors may depend on the type of bone transplanted (i.e., cortical versus packed cancellous bone).

The two-phase theory of osteogenesis proposes that some bone cells survive transplantation and form the initial osteoid in a random pattern during the first phase (Axhausen, 1956). This is followed by the second phase, during which the osteoid is resorbed and replaced by bone derived from cells in the recipient bed. Therefore, the initial cellular concentration of the bone graft is very important, because the higher the density of transplanted cells, the greater the numbers of cells that will survive to deposit bone during phase one. For this reason, a cancellous-marrow bone graft has a greater osteogenic potential.

When cortical bone is grafted, fewer cells are transplanted, so fewer cells survive. The final living bone is probably the result of resorption of the graft by osteoclasts from the adjacent native bone, followed by new bone deposition by osteoblasts from the adjacent viable bone.

The concept of osteoinduction implies that growth factors in the grafted bone induce pluripotential mesenchymal cells from the surrounding tissues to transform into osteoblasts. This process is well documented, and the proteins responsible for the induction, found in the organic demineralized bone, were termed *bone morphogenetic proteins* by Urist (1968). Bone morphogenetic proteins are members of the transforming growth factor βfamily, and recombinant human BMP-2 is commercially available (INFUSE). Although it is FDA approved for sinus grafting and for localized alveolar ridge augmentation for defects associated with extraction sockets, it has been used off-label for larger mandibular reconstruction (Fisher et al., 2019). Due to its lack of structural integrity when used alone on a collagen sponge, it is commonly used in combination with other grafting materials to maintain the graft volume (autologous bone, allogenic bone, demineralized bone, etc.). Other advances in bone grafting include the addition of autologous growth factors found in platelets for improved and faster bone healing. Platelet concentrates, such as platelet-rich plasma and platelet-rich fibrin, can be mixed with the bone graft to improve outcomes (Marx et al., 1998). For the reader interested in a more detailed review of mandibular reconstruction, an excellent overview has been published by Konopnicki and Troulis (2015).

Donor sites

Although bone substitutes or synthetic bone grafting materials have been used, the most common graft material used for mandibular reconstruction is autogenous bone harvested from the patient. Sources for bone include the outer table of the cranium, rib, tibia, and iliac crest. Of these, the iliac crest is used most commonly, although for smaller defects, cancellous tibial grafting can provide ample bone volume with minimal postoperative morbidity and offers the potential for successful harvest under local anesthesia (Kirmeier et al., 2007; Geressen et al., 2008; Walker et al., 2009). Advantages of the iliac crest include the overall amount of either cancellous or cortical bone that can be obtained (Burk et al., 2016) and the relative safety and minimal morbidity of the procedure (Marx and Morales, 1988).

Calvarial bone is used for onlay grafting and orbital reconstruction, especially when smaller amounts of purely cortical bone are needed. Rib bone undergoes a greater amount of resorption than the other two sources but is beneficial when a cartilaginous cap covering the cut end of the bone is desired, such as in reconstruction of the mandibular condyle. This is especially important in children when future growth is needed.

Bone can be harvested from either the anterior or posterior ilium, and each has its advantages and disadvantages. The primary advantage of the posterior iliac crest is the greater amount of bone that is available. Morbidity is minimal with respect to gait disturbances, pain, and blood loss (Marx and Morales, 1988). The primary disadvantage is the need to have the patient in the prone position to harvest the bone and in the supine position for the resection and reconstruction of the mandible. This necessitates turning the anesthetized patient in the middle of the operation. The advantage of the anterior ilium is its convenient location (which does not require intraoperative patient repositioning when the mandible is being reconstructed) and the ability to have two surgical teams working simultaneously with one at the head and the other at the ilium. However, the anterior ilium does not possess sufficient quantities of bone required to reconstruct large defects.

The surgical techniques involved in procurement of the various autogenous bone grafts are beyond the scope of this text, but this information can be found in a technical article by Marx (1993).

Techniques of bone graft reconstruction

The technique used for bone graft reconstruction of the resected mandible depends on the type of bone selected by the surgeon for the reconstruction. If the surgeon chooses an autogenous block graft (Fig 2-41), as opposed to a compressed cancellous-marrow graft, the graft is shaped and adapted to span the bony mandibular defect, approximating as closely as possible the position of the original resected mandible (Fig 2-41c). This may involve using multiple large blocks of bone for large body or ramus defects or several smaller blocks for curved defects, such as for the mandibular

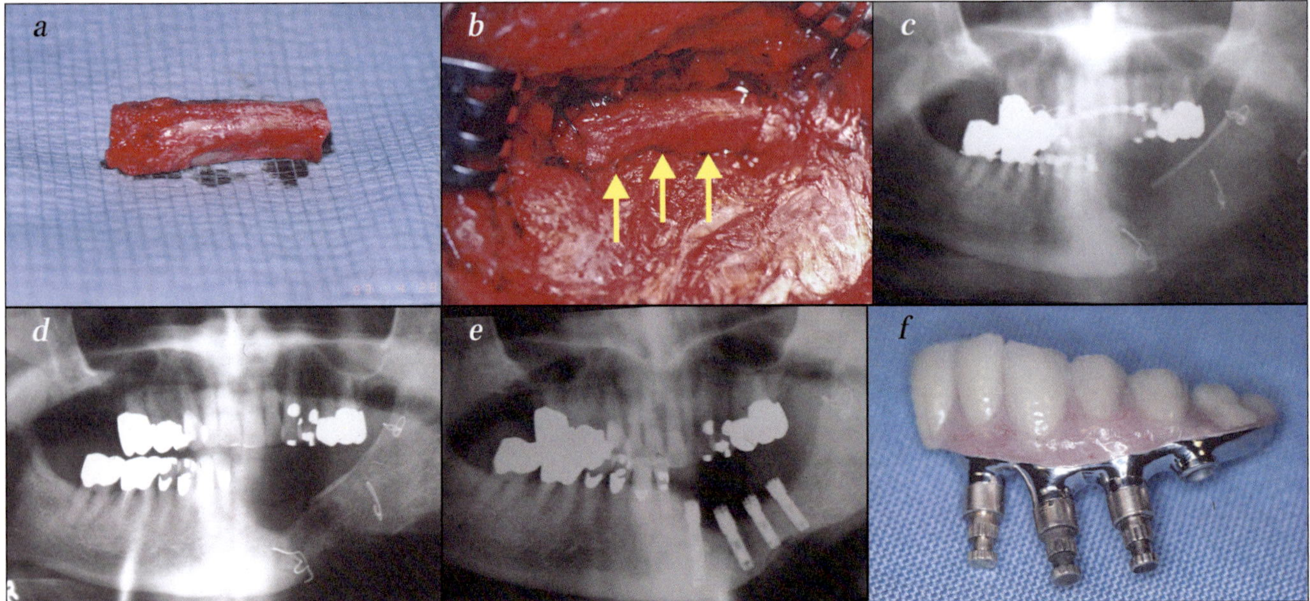

Figure 2-41 Left-body defect restored with block graft. *(a)* Harvested iliac crest block graft. *(b)* Inset graft *(arrows)* fixated with wires. Note the extraoral approach to avoid oral contamination. *(c)* The radiograph shows a close approximation of mandibular defect. Note the need for MMF. *(d)* Remodeling changes. *(e)* Implants were placed after 12 months of graft maturation. *(f)* Implant-supported, fixed MRP.

symphysis. Most frequently, the block grafts are fixed to a large reconstruction plate spanning the defect. The reconstruction plate can be bent intraoperatively, prebent on a three-dimensional model of the mandible, or custom fabricated using CAD/CAM technology. The block graft is fixated with screws to the medial aspect of the plate. If reconstruction is to be delayed in order to decrease the risk of infection, the reconstruction plate is still placed at the time of the initial tumor resection to maintain the correct positions of the two segments of the mandible. During the subsequent reconstructive procedure, the block bone graft is harvested and placed behind the reconstruction plate from a sterile extraoral approach, avoiding oral bacterial contamination.

It is crucial that there be no mobility between the grafted and native bone during healing of the bone graft. Reconstruction plates offer sufficient rigidity to prevent this mobility, especially custom plates that are reinforced at the osteosyntheses. Other forms of fixation, such as miniplates and wire (Fig 2-41), do not provide the necessary stability, so supplemental MMF with arch bars (Fig 2-42) or external pin fixation devices are needed.

When the reconstructive surgeon opts for bony reconstruction of a mandibular defect with a compressed cancellous-marrow graft, some type of conformer, such as a tray (Fig 2-42), may be beneficial to provide both contour and rigidity to the harvested amorphous cancellous bone and marrow. Prefabricated titanium reconstruction trays of various sizes or custom-made trays are available (Singare et al., 2004). These are fixed to the remaining mandibular segments with multiple small bone screws. Alternatively, the corticocancellous bone can be packed medial to a reconstruction plate.

Others advocate the use of cadaveric bone from a bone bank to hold the harvested autogenous bone. Trays can be fabricated from cadaveric mandibles, or cadaveric ribs can be bent, shaped, and adapted to hold the compressed, autogenous bone graft (Marx, 1991).

Regardless of the type of bone or fixation chosen by the surgeon, three important principles must be followed. First, the bone graft must be surrounded by a well-vascularized soft tissue bed to enhance graft survival and minimize resorption. Second, the graft must be protected from ongoing contamination by being isolated from the oral cavity. Third, the bone graft must be immobilized during the healing phase through either rigid fixation or MMF.

If insufficient soft tissue is available to cover the graft as a result of the surgical resection, then soft tissues must be augmented with either a pedicled or free myocutaneous flap before avascular bone grafting takes place. If there is sufficient soft tissue coverage for the graft but vascularity is limited, as is common after mandibular resection for ORN, hyperbaric oxygen (HBO) therapy may be considered prior to bone grafting, with success rates reported at over 90% (Marx and Ames, 1982). However, with the introduction of bony free flaps, most mandibular reconstructions in irradiated tissue beds are now performed with free flaps.

Timing of reconstruction and implant placement

Two decisions regarding timing must be made. First, should the bony reconstruction be performed at the time of the resection, or should it be delayed? Second, if dental implants are to be placed, how much time should be allowed for bone graft healing and maturation prior to the dental implant reconstructive procedure?

The answers to these and other questions must be addressed by the surgeon-prosthodontic team preoperatively. The answers will depend on individual patient factors, the nature of the tumor to be resected, and the skill and experience of the surgeon-prosthodontist team.

Any discussion of primary versus delayed mandibular reconstruction must weigh the risks and benefits for the patient. Advocates of delayed bony reconstruction with bone grafts argue that the increased risk of infection with possible loss of the graft due to oral contamination that occurs at the time of resection—coupled with the risk of tumor recurrence requiring further resection, radiation, or chemotherapy, which could adversely lead to graft failure—outweighs the benefits of immediate reconstruction. One study demonstrated a greater than 40% infection rate in grafts that communicate with the oral cavity (Manchester, 1977). Lawson et al. reported that immediate bone grafting is only about half as successful as delayed grafts, primarily because of infection (1982). If delayed reconstruction is planned, the residual native bone segments should be maintained in proper anatomical location by use of a reconstruction plate.

Proponents of immediate reconstruction believe that the risk of infection is greatly decreased if sufficient tissue remains after the resection to allow a tight, meticulous, multilayer oral closure that is not under tension. These surgeons claim that immediate reconstruction will provide a superior cosmetic result because scar contracture is limited or prevented. Furthermore, the more vascular, unscarred soft tissue bed will serve as a better recipient site for the avascular bone graft. The psychologic benefits with respect to the patient's appearance and self-esteem and the elimination of a second major operation are additional arguments used by those in favor of immediate reconstruction.

Most surgeons prefer to delay implant placement for 6 to 12 months to allow the graft to become vascularized and viable. During this period, a provisional dental prosthesis designed entirely for cosmetic purposes and lip support can be fabricated, so long as it does not put undue pressure on the underlying graft. This delay is preferred not only for increased implant success but also for the ability to plan and position the implants more ideally. If a provisional prosthesis is used, the soft tissues overlying the bone graft must be monitored closely to minimize the chance of soft tissue perforation and graft exposure. Reconstruction using vascularized free flaps does not require a delay in implant placement. With VSP, the precise location for future implants can be determined and implants placed into the viable bone of the free flap at the same time as the reconstruction.

Prior to implant placement, a surgical template is fabricated by a prosthodontist to ensure that the implants are positioned properly. If removal of a reconstruction plate or tray is desired, this can be performed during the implant surgery. Excessive soft tissue overlying the graft can be debulked at this time. Final debulking and thinning of the tissues overlying the implants can be accomplished using a staged implant procedure. At the time of implant uncovering and abutment placement, consideration can be given to repositioning the buccal mucosa and FOM to more ideal locations. A split-thickness skin graft vestibuloplasty will allow for more natural positioning of the buccal and lingual sulci and improve the amount of attached, keratinized tissue around the implants.

The need to remove the reconstruction plate or tray is somewhat controversial. Some surgeons believe that there is no need to remove hardware unless it presents a problem or if fixation screws interfere with proper implant placement. Others believe that the large reconstruction plates are so rigid that they shield the underlying bone graft from the normal physiologic forces that act to maintain it, resulting in disuse atrophy of the bone. This concept, known as *stress shielding*, is also of concern in orthopedics (Raffa et al., 2021). Others recommend plate removal only if it would become exposed during vestibuloplasty or limit the buccal flange of the prosthesis.

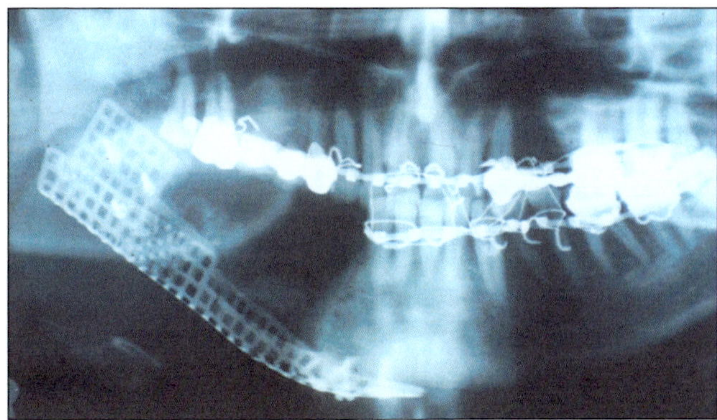

Figure 2-42 Postreconstruction radiograph shows a prefabricated titanium tray fixated with multiple bone screws. Note the need for MMF for added immobilization.

Some surgeons who use compressed cancellous bone grafts in titanium trays (Fig 2-42) also electively remove the tray after the graft has consolidated. However, these trays are not nearly as rigid as the reconstruction plates, and some flexion of the tray can occur. During chewing, especially in patients with dental implants, the mandible flexes slightly because of the increase in occlusal force. Although these natural forces are probably beneficial for the maturation and maintenance of the volume of the bone graft, the constant flexion and extension of the tray can weaken the metal and lead to eventual fatigue and subsequent fracture. Even large reconstruction plates will fracture over time in the absence of an underlying bone graft.

Complications

Wound infection is the most worrisome complication in the immediate postgrafting period, because it may lead to the loss of the entire bone graft. Even after the patient has apparently recovered from the surgical procedure, close attention should continue because late infection can occur. If the prosthodontist has any concern about infection, the surgeon should be contacted immediately because early intervention is crucial. If infection occurs, appropriate antibiotics, early drainage of any localized fluid, meticulous irrigation, and possible debridement should be employed in an attempt to salvage most of the graft.

Soft tissue dehiscence is another concern, especially for patients who wear mucosa-borne prostheses over the grafted area. Wound dehiscence can introduce oral bacteria to the grafted site and result in infection. The underlying soft tissues must be monitored closely if a prosthesis is to be worn early. Frequently, initial areas of soft tissue breakdown may go unnoticed by the patient if the area is insensate from prior treatment. The prosthodontist and surgeon must follow the patient closely and adjust the prosthesis or remove it if problems develop.

Fracture of the graft is always a concern but is a relatively rare complication. Graft fracture is usually the result of a graft of inadequate quantity and poor quality, although even the most robust graft will fracture under sufficient force. As with other mandibular fractures, reduction and fixation to immobilize the fracture segments are required.

Exposure of a titanium plate or tray used in combination with the avascular bone graft during the immediate postsurgical period can

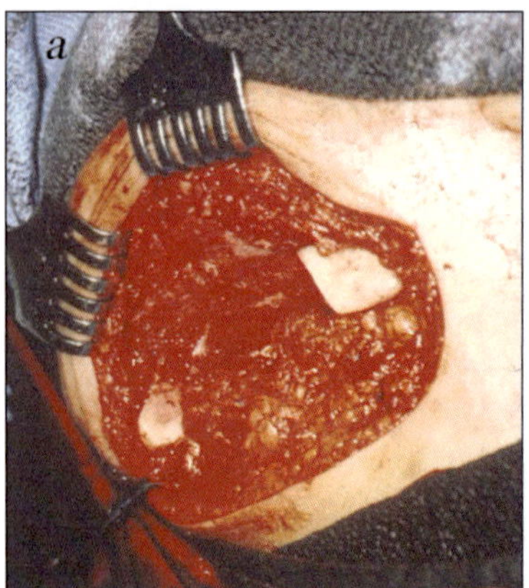
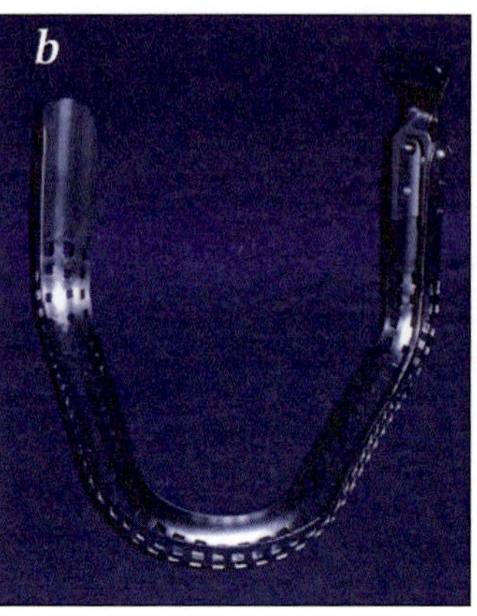
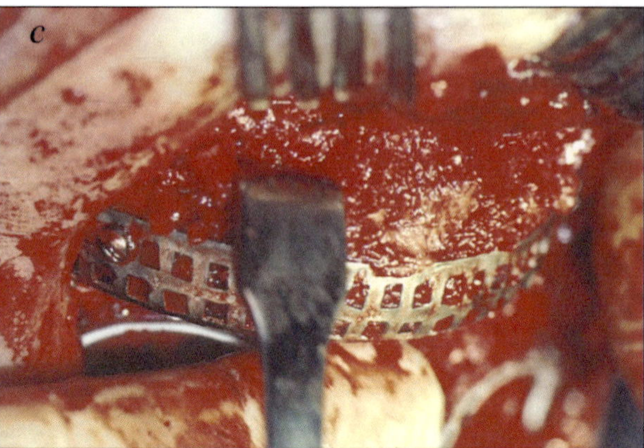

Figure 2-43 Symphyseal defect restored with a titanium tray and compacted cancellous bone marrow graft. *(a)* Exposed anterior edges of the mandibular segments. *(b)* A titanium tray is used to contain the graft and rigidly fixate the native mandible. *(c)* Compaction of cancellous marrow graft into the tray.

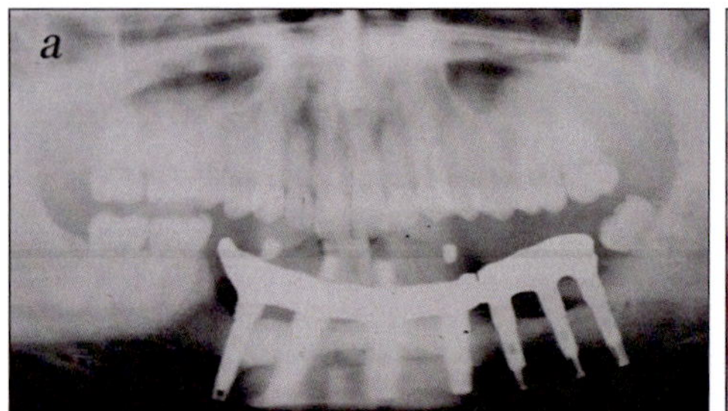
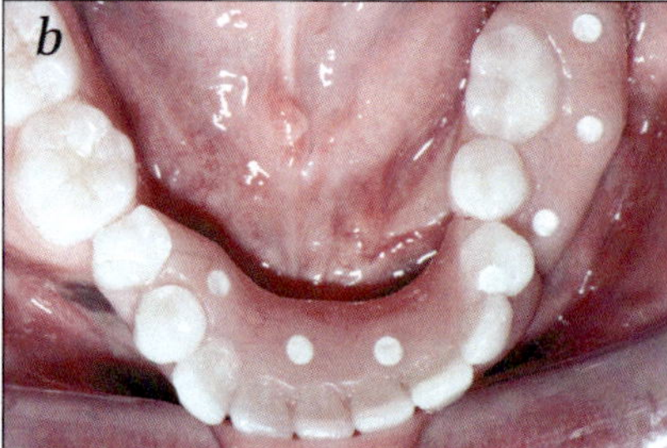
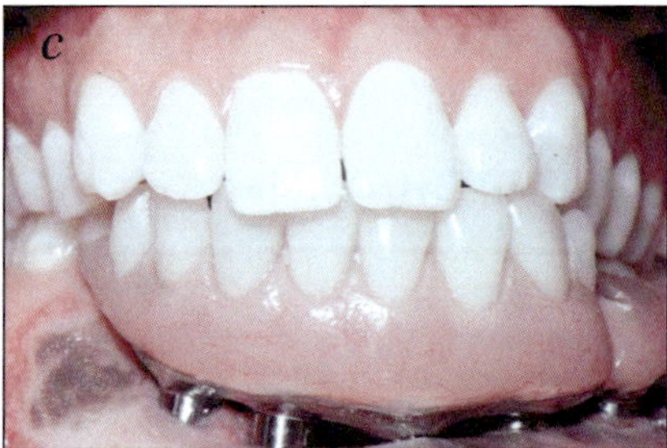

Figure 2-44 Ameloblastoma resection restored with an avascular bone graft. *(a)* Panoramic radiographs after rehabilitation. *(b)* The occlusal view shows the posterior implant positions buccal to the occlusal table. *(c)* Completed restoration in occlusion.

lead to loss of the graft. Conservative management (irrigation, antibiotics, etc.) should be attempted for up to eight weeks in the hope that osteogenesis will occur. The tray can then be removed, leaving the grafted bone. This therapy is indicated for both intraoral and extraoral exposures. External fixation devices such as MMF may be required for a period following removal of the tray to provide stability for the graft. The delay in the removal of the plate or tray allows the graft time to mature. Early removal may disrupt osteogenesis and nonunion or loss of graft may result.

Rates of successful bony union in nonvascularized bone grafts have been reported to be only 69%, compared with 96% in vascularized free flaps (Foster et al., 1999). Treatment of a nonunion requires additional bone grafting and immobilization to achieve a union. A functional malunion (e.g., leading to malocclusion) would also require reoperation and repositioning of the misaligned segments, with or without further grafting.

Complications can be associated with the bone graft donor site. A complete discussion of these complications is beyond the scope of this text, but the interested reader is referred to articles by Dodson and Kaban (1990) and Cricchio and Lundgren (2003).

Reconstruction of the mandibular body

Surgical resection of a carcinoma of the lateral tongue may require resection of a portion of the body of the mandible if the tumor is extensive. The relatively straight contour of the mandible between the angle and the canine makes it one of the easier areas to reconstruct with avascular bone grafts. A reconstruction plate or tray can be utilized to stabilize the bone graft. As with all mandibular resection and reconstruction, appropriate care must be taken to ensure that the remaining native mandibular segments maintain their original positions for the best cosmetic and functional results.

The grafted bone is placed at the position of the original inferior border of the mandible to enhance esthetics. Molars lie somewhat lingual to the lower border of the mandible; this concept is important to remember during mandibular reconstruction, especially when dental implants are being considered. If the graft is not extended to the lingual, the most posterior dental implants will exit buccal to the ideal tooth position (Fig 2-44). This will result in off-axis loading forces.

Reconstruction of the symphysis

The symphyseal region is more difficult to reconstruct than the mandibular body because of its abrupt curvature. If ample amounts of well-vascularized soft tissue are available, compacted cancellous bone graft can be effectively packed and molded around the curve of the symphysis with the aid of a tray (Fig 2-43).

The bilateral native mandibular segments should be fixated to and maintained in their original location. This can be accomplished in a variety of ways, including MMF, locking reconstruction plates, splinting, or external fixation devices (for edentulous patients). Care must be taken to ensure that the native mandibular segments do

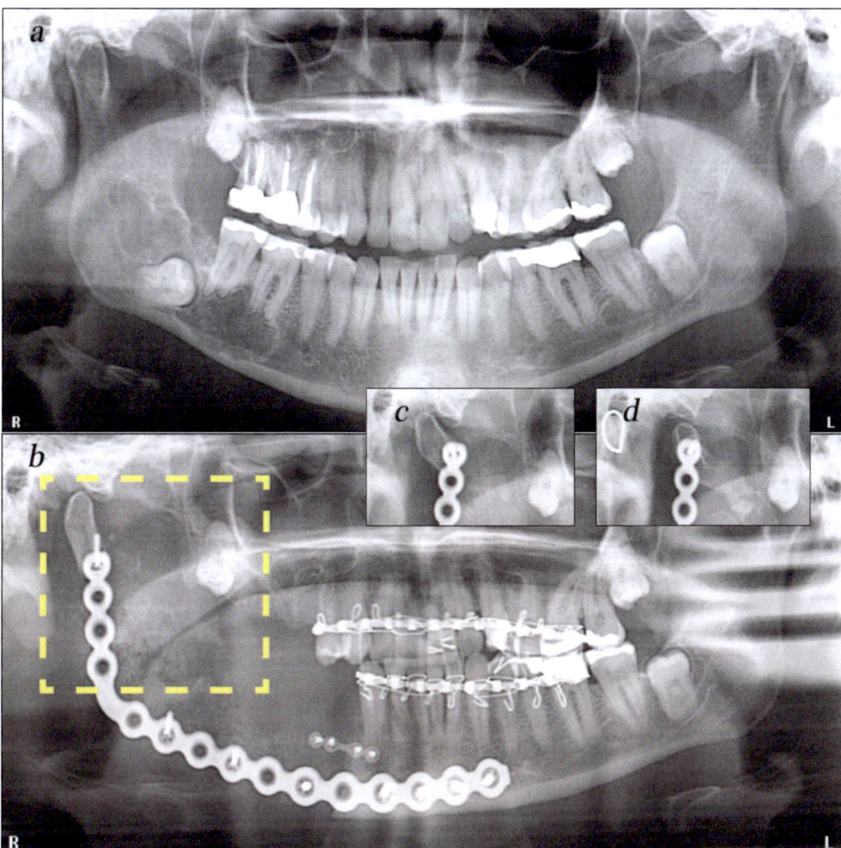

Figure 2-45 Odontogenic myxoma requiring segmental resection of the right mandibular body, angle, and ramus. Posterior iliac crest graft used for reconstruction. *(a)* Preoperative panoramic radiograph showing radiolucent lesion. *(b)* Immediate postoperative radiograph. Note the use of a stock reconstruction plate and MMF. *(c and d)* Progressive iatrogenic rotation of the remnant condyle about the single fixation screw.

not rotate buccally or lingually during insetting, fixation, or healing by the action of muscles inserting into the native mandible.

Buccal rotation is a particular risk with the use of MMF, because the wires used to keep the mandibular teeth in correct occlusion with the maxillary teeth are on the buccal aspect of the teeth. The direction and location of the resulting forces have a natural tendency to rotate the mandibular segments buccally. This problem has been avoided with the use of internal fixation. If nonrigid fixation is used, MMF usually remains for around three months to allow for initial bone stabilization and to prevent progressive shifting during healing.

The bone graft for the symphyseal reconstruction should be placed in the same position as the original mandible and chin for the best aesthetic result. Because the normal mentum always lies anterior to the mandibular incisors, implants in this region may have a significant lingual inclination unless this geometry is reproduced at the time of bone graft reconstruction. Increasing the anterior-posterior width of the grafted bone in the symphyseal region will prevent this problem.

Every effort should be made to attach the genioglossus and suprahyoid musculature to the reconstruction tray or plate to maintain adequate anterior tongue position and superoanterior hyoid suspension. Both are important factors in maintaining the airway. In addition, muscular resuspension aids in the swallow function, reducing the risk of aspiration by providing a more anterior location of the larynx during swallowing, and it gives a better aesthetic contour to the neck line.

Reconstruction of the angle and ramus

The angle and ramus of the mandible are often resected during treatment of a tonsillar carcinoma or benign osseous tumors, such as ameloblastoma, odontogenic myxoma (Fig 2-45), or odontogenic keratocyst (Fig 2-46). If the native condyle can be spared from an oncologic standpoint, mandibular movement will be enhanced following the grafting procedure. This benefit derives from the preservation of functional muscular attachments of the lateral pterygoid muscle and, in some cases, the temporalis muscles, in addition to maintaining the native meniscus. Enough of the condylar neck must remain to allow fixation with two screws for antirotation. If only a single screw is accommodated, the condyle must be removed lest the remnant rotate out of position (Fig 2-45 c and d), resulting in nonunion to the graft and affecting mandibular movement.

Although the natural mandibular ramus is flat and wide, excellent cosmetic and functional results can be obtained with the reconstruction of only the posterior border of the ramus and angle.

If the resection is so extensive that it includes the condyle, a costochondral rib graft or prosthetic total joint is indicated. If a rib graft is placed, the joint must be mobilized early. However, if a compressed cancellous bone graft is also needed to reconstruct the ramus and angle regions, this part of the graft should be relatively immobile during healing. This conflict can be resolved by staging the reconstruction.

During the first reconstructive procedure, a titanium tray packed with compressed cancellous bone or a reconstruction plate with graft packed to the medial side can be used to reconstruct the posterior border of the mandibular ramus and angle. Then either the

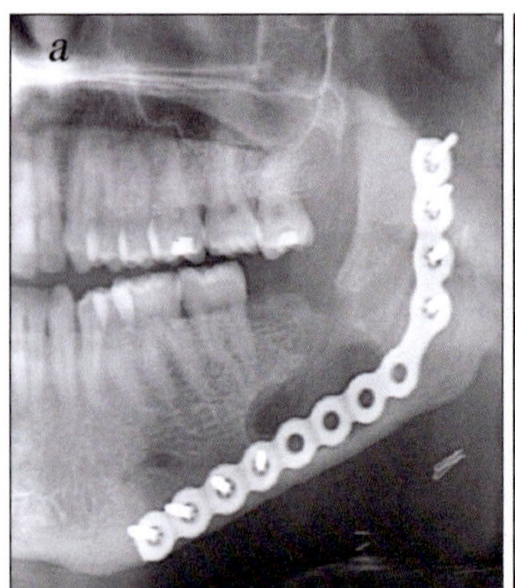

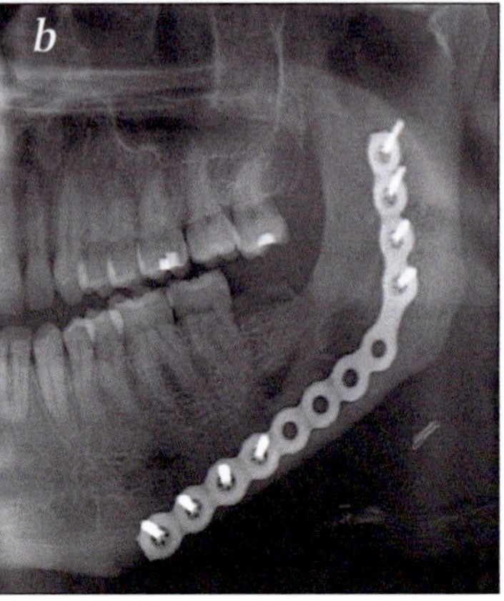

Figure 2-46 Left posterior mandibular odontogenic keratocyst treated with enucleation and 5-fluorouracil. *(a)* A reconstruction plate was placed to prevent fracture of a thin residual inferior border. *(b)* After partial consolidation of the bone graft.

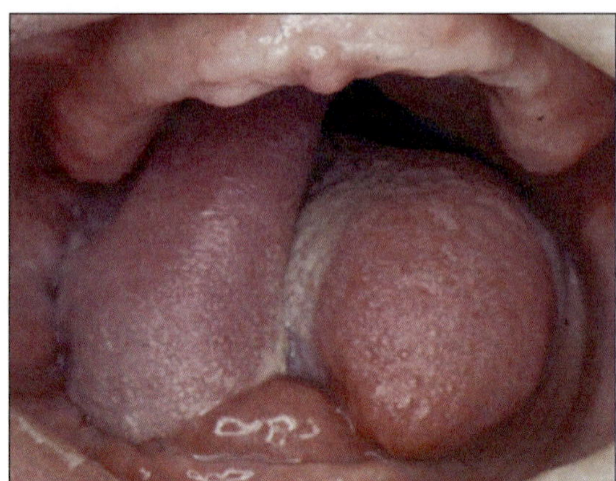

Figure 2-47 Tonsil defect resurfaced with a tongue flap.

reconstruction plate or tray can be fitted with a titanium condyle placed in the glenoid fossa. This artificial condyle will function within the fossa and maintain a space for a future costochondral rib graft or prosthetic joint.

A second procedure is performed 6 to 12 months later to remove the original metal plate or tray with the titanium condyle and to secure a costochondral rib graft to the posterior aspect of the now solid ramus bone graft or to place a custom-fitted total prosthetic joint. The cartilaginous cap of the rib is shaped and positioned to fit into the fossa. Physical therapy is then instituted.

Reconstruction following marginal mandibulectomy

For some pathologic lesions, a more limited resection may be indicated. A marginal resection that spares the inferior border of the mandible is an excellent situation in which to employ a nonvascularized bone graft. The native inferior border of the mandible will maintain the appropriate contours and positions of the segments of the mandible anterior and posterior to the resection. It will also provide increased rigidity to help prevent micromotion of the segments during healing, thus reducing the risk of a nonunion. In the event that the inferior border no longer has sufficient rigidity and is at risk for fracture during function prior to consolidation of the bone graft, a reconstruction plate can still be placed across the defect to help stabilize the thin inferior border (Fig 2-46).

Microvascular Free Flaps

It is preferable to reconstruct the mandible and soft tissue defect immediately upon tumor ablation. From the perspective of oral function and prosthodontic rehabilitation, reconstruction of the tongue should receive the highest priority, and we believe that flaps should be selected and tailored with this priority in mind. The tongue is the most important oral structure with regard to mastication, saliva control, speech, and swallowing. Its bulk should be restored and the reconstruction designed to maximize the mobility of the tongue remnant. If the tongue is not reconstructed in a proper manner, the patient will be severely disabled even if the continuity of the mandible has been retained or restored.

The introduction of the pedicled myocutaneous flap in the late 1970s ameliorated some of the disabilities and deformities, and this flap became a popular means of wound closure following tongue and mandible resections during the 1970s and 1980s. From a prosthodontic perspective, these flaps were preferred over the methods previously available. They replaced the resected tissues, such as the missing portion of the tongue, thus resulting in less mandibular deviation. The residual and reconstructed portion of the tongue is centered more normally beneath palatal structures (Fig 2-49). However, the reconstructed portion of the tongue was scarred and relatively immobile. The overall result is improved speech, swallowing, and saliva control. Skin paddles of appropriate size can be left attached to the muscle pedicle and used to reline extensive areas of the oral cavity. The muscle portion of the flap provides the bulk necessary to replace the resected tissues, which in some combined tongue and mandibular resections, can be quite extensive.

Tumors of the tonsil often extend to the soft palate and lateral tongue. In the past, defects secondary to resection of these tumors were closed either with tongue flaps (Fig 2-47) or occasionally with a pedicled forehead flap of forehead flap. These methods of closure predisposed the patient to such functional disabilities and/or significant cosmetic deformity that they have mostly been abandoned. The use of tongue flaps was particularly disabling. A large portion of the tongue was no longer available for function, and that which remained was relatively immobile and not properly centered beneath the palate. Speech, swallowing, and salivary control were inevitably compromised.

In the early 1980s, myocutaneous pedicle flaps were used to close and reconstruct tonsil defects. The most common pedicle flap was based on the pectoralis major muscle. These have mostly been replaced by vascularized free flaps. The radial forearm free flap (RFFF) is preferred for its thinness and suppleness, making it very applicable to reconstruct tonsillar defects that extend to the soft palate or tongue. When the resection includes a significant portion of the soft palate, the resulting velopharyngeal defects are best restored with obturator prostheses. The functional results

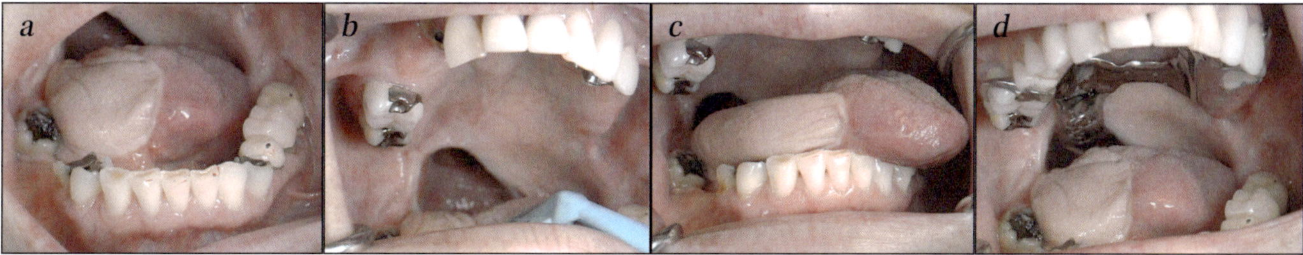

Figure 2-48 Successful reconstruction with a RFFF. *(a)* Tongue and tonsil defects restored. *(b)* The soft palate is free of the flap. *(c)* Excellent tongue mobility. *(d)* Velopharyngeal defect was restored with an obturator. Speech has been restored to nearly normal.

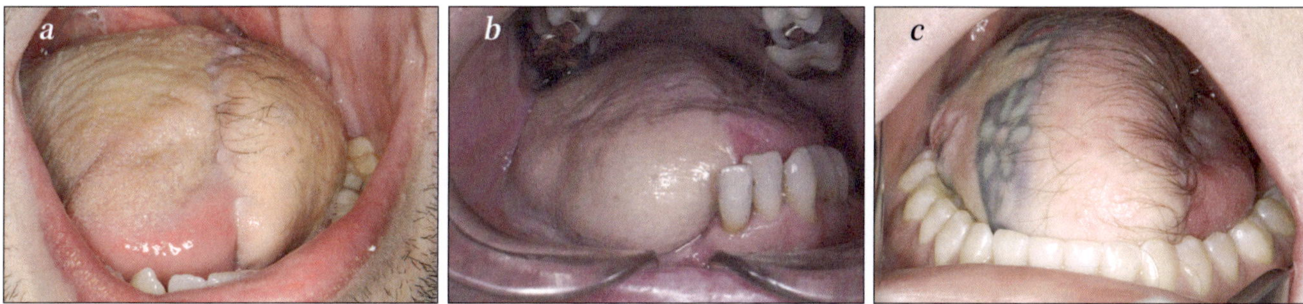

Figure 2-49 Tongue defects restored with free flaps. *(a)* Radial forearm flap. *(b)* Scapula flap. *(c)* Anterior lateral thigh flap. All these patients are excellent candidates for prosthodontic rehabilitation.

are quite acceptable, and most patients are capable of normal speech, swallowing, and nearly normal mastication (Fig 2-48). As mentioned previously, the residual soft palate should not be tied to the flap.

Microvascular free tissue transfer (free flaps) was introduced in the mid-1980s as a means of restoring the large soft and hard tissue defects associated with the resection of tongue and mandible tumors. Like the pedicle myocutaneous flaps, the technique provides replacement of the tissues lost to the resection of the tumor. The most significant advantage of this flap over the others is its improved blood supply, not only for the tissue being transferred but also to the recipient site, which in turn ensures that the reconstructed portion of the tongue is less scarred and more mobile. The result is that the residual tongue musculature is able to move and shape the flap portion. In many patients, speech approaches normal limits (Figs 2-55 and 2-56). The improved blood supply also improves wound healing and ensures the survival of the flap even in irradiated tissues.

Free flaps are suitable for restoring the tongue as well as a combination of tongue and mandible defects. A number of donor sites have been used to restore oral cavity defects, including the radial forearm, iliac crest, scapula, thigh, and fibula.

A major advance in mandibular reconstruction has been the development of improved techniques in microvascular surgery that allow composite grafting of larger volumes of tissue. In free flaps, various combinations of bone, muscle, fascia, and skin can be autogenously grafted and remain viable with a high degree of success (Urken et al., 1998). This has greatly improved reconstructive outcomes because the grafted tissues are no longer limited to the anatomical constraints of adjacent pedicled flaps yet have a robust blood supply to facilitate wound healing. Previously, bone grafting procedures were staged to follow soft tissue reconstruction by pedicled flaps. Simultaneous grafting of hard tissue, soft tissue, and skin can now be accomplished.

Reconstruction with traditional avascular bone grafts requires a well-vascularized soft tissue recipient bed. This was a limiting factor when significant soft tissue defects existed or when vascularity was compromised by prior surgery or radiation therapy. The application of microvascular surgical techniques and rigid internal osseous fixation have greatly facilitated the reconstruction of these complex head and neck defects. The advantages of immediate reconstruction using well-vascularized osseous and soft tissue are well documented. Predictable healing, particularly in the face of radiated tissue and oral contamination, allows the early return of form and function, greatly enhancing the QOL for patients.

Numerous variables, including the patient's age, tumor stage, physical condition, and psychologic status, must be carefully evaluated prior to embarking on major ablative and reconstructive surgery of the head and neck. Although many patients undergoing composite resections are elderly and have compromised health, the majority are candidates for free flap reconstruction (Urken et al., 1998; Urken et al., 1991a). Patients with a good prognosis and life expectancy are aggressively reconstructed; the goal is complete oral and facial rehabilitation, that is, restoration of articulate speech, the ability to chew and swallow solid foods, and control of saliva. Their reconstruction employs a composite osseous flap and, at a later stage, prosthetic rehabilitation.

Patients with a short-segment mandibular resection who are elderly, edentulous, or those with a poor prognosis can be selectively managed with locking mandibular reconstruction plates covered by free or pedicle soft tissue flaps (Fig 2-50).

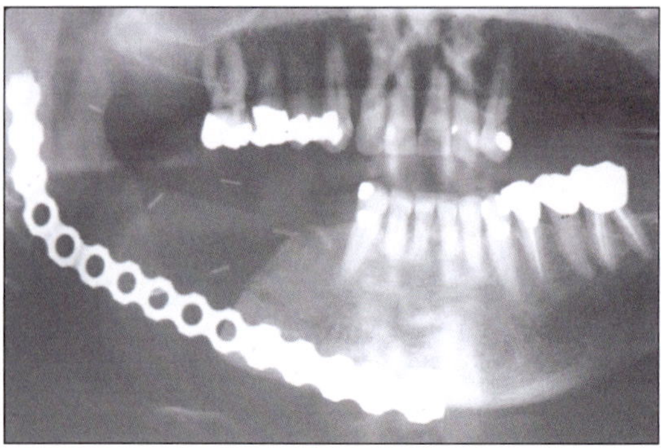

Figure 2-50 Lateral mandibular defect restored with a reconstruction plate.

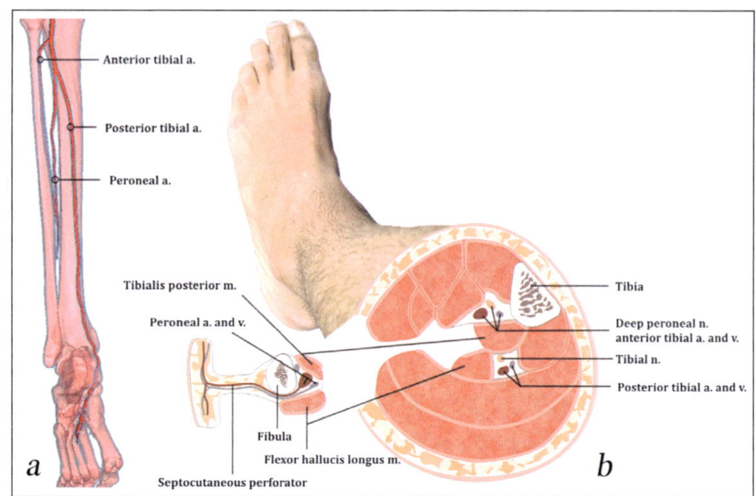

Figure 2-51 Blood supply for the composite FFF. *(a)* The principal blood supply to the fibula is the peroneal artery. Segmental periosteal vessels cycle the fibula along its length. *(b)* Schematic axial slice of the lower leg. Note the perforating septocutaneous vessels. A skin island is centered over these vessels.

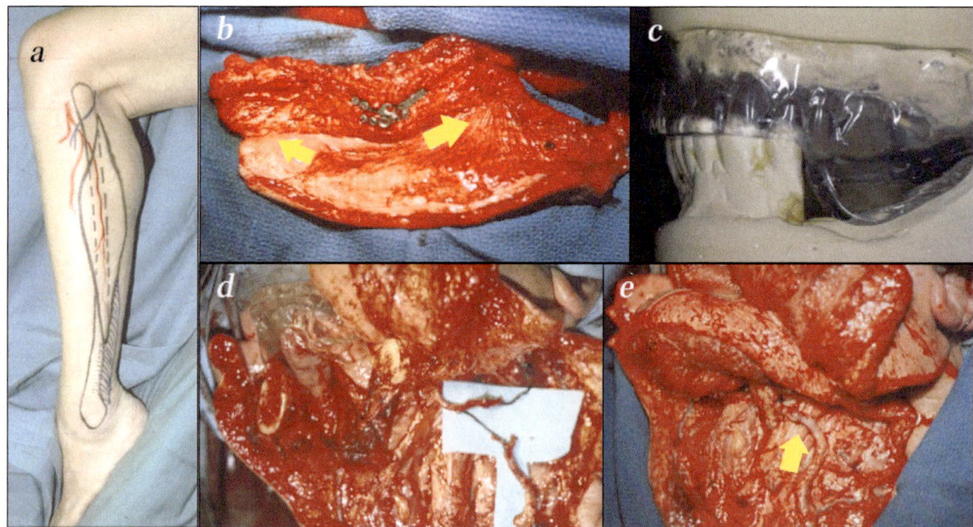

Figure 2-52 *(a)* Outline of an osteomyocutaneous FFF. Note the fusiform skin island and the course of the peroneal artery. *(b)* Flap perfused in situ. Osteotomies are performed inside with the flap vascularized. Osteotomies are stabilized with miniplates and screws. The arrow points to vessel anastomosis. *(c)* Template prepared for use. *(d)* Composite symphyseal and lateral mandibular defect. A posterior mandibular fragment has been positioned in the template. *(e)* FFF inset with the skin island rotated over the occlusal aspect of the osseous graft for intraoral soft tissue closure. The flexor hallucis muscle had been used to replace resected submental musculature and separate the oral cavity from the neck, where the microvascular anastomosis *(arrow)* has been performed.

Bony donor sites

Numerous free flaps have been described for the reconstruction of mandibular defects. Herein, we focus on the most commonly utilized free flaps for mandibular reconstruction.

Fibula

The fibula is the preferred donor site. The fibula provides a sufficient length and bulk of bone. Either primarily or secondarily at a later date, dental implants can be placed to retain and support a prosthesis designed to replace the missing dentition.

The composite fibula flap is nourished by the peroneal (fibular) vessels (Fig 2-51). The flap may be transferred with bone alone or with skin and muscle (Figs 2-51b and 2-52). The composite flap may include up to 25 cm of bone, more than 250 cm of lateral leg skin surface, a portion of the soleus muscle, and the entire flexor hallucis longus muscle if needed for complex defects.

The bone's length and extensive periosteal blood supply allows the reconstruction of the entire mandible, if necessary (Hidalgo, 1989). Multiple osteotomies may be performed to replicate the contour of the resected mandible, and most authors maintain 1.5–2 cm as the minimum segment length, as this corresponds to an 84% and 94% chance of containing a periosteal arterial branch, respectively (Fry et al., 2016). At least 6 cm of bone is left proximally and distally to prevent injury to the common peroneal nerve and ankle joint instability, respectively. The fibula's cortical nature and thickness make it an excellent recipient of endosseous implants, and success rates for implant stability are excellent (Roumanas et al., 1997; Kramer et al., 2005; Wu et al., 2008). Either leg may be utilized as a donor site, although the choice may be determined by the vascularity of the lower extremity, the side, location, and extent of the tumor

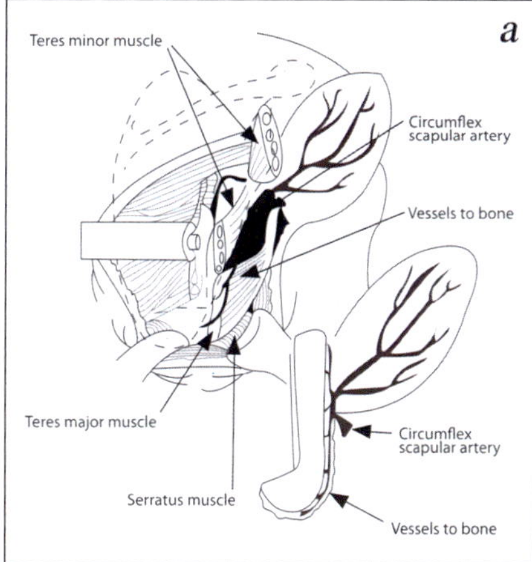

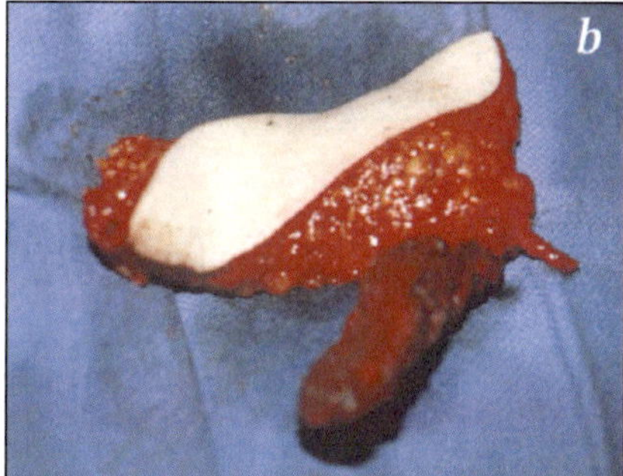

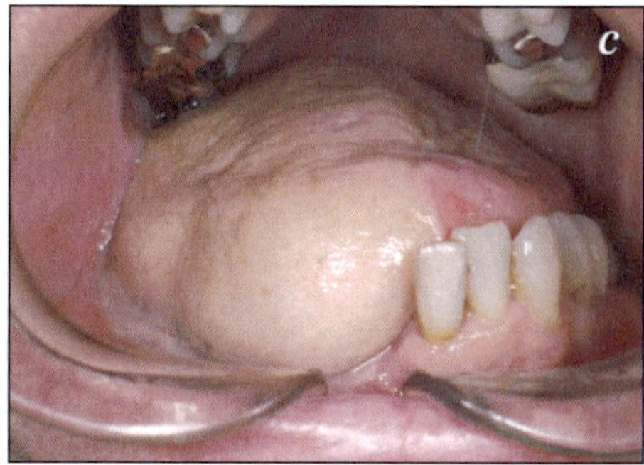

Figure 2-53 Composite scapula flap. *(a)* Dissection of the osteocutaneous scapula free flap (SFF). *(b)* The flap is retrieved and ready for insetting. *(c)* Hemimandibulectomy/hemiglossectomy defect reconstructed with the free flap. Speech and swallowing were restored to within normal limits.

resection, and the reconstructive surgeon's preference. When the ipsilateral neck is vessel depleted, the pedicle may be lengthened by using the distal bone (closest to the ankle) and maintaining the proximal periosteum (toward the knee) as an additional pedicle.

The skin island is based on septocutaneous perforators, emanating through the posterior crural septum from the peroneal vasculature. The cutaneous portion of the flap may be used for intraoral, cutaneous, or combined defects. Harvesting a 2 cm cuff of flexor hallucis longus can enhance the vascular supply to the skin paddle by preserving musculocutaneous perforators traversing this location. In the event of no septocutaneous perforators to the skin paddle, a cuff of soleus muscle may be maintained and used as a vascularized soft tissue graft.

The composite fibula flap is the preferred donor site for most complex orofacial-mandibular defects. For defects of the lateral mandible that do not involve a significant amount of oral mucosa, the osseous flap may suffice. The addition of a skin island allows for absolute tension-free intraoral closure that enhances tongue mobility. It also improves the monitoring of an otherwise buried flap. The donor site may be closed directly when less than 4 to 5 cm of skin are included with bone, but split-thickness skin grafting to the site must be considered in the majority of situations.

The fibula osteomyocutaneous flap is also recommended for lateral and symphyseal composite defects that include substantial amounts of intraoral mucosa, tongue, and facial skin. As the mucosal defect enlarges, so do the harvested skin paddle requirements. Skin islands 10 to 12 cm wide are available for more extensive defects. A skin graft is necessary to close the distal donor site.

Scapula

The composite scapula or parascapular flap is supplied by the circumflex scapular artery through its terminal deep branches, the transverse and descending cutaneous branches, and venae comitantes (Fig 2-53). Approximately 12 to 14 cm of lateral scapular bone, 400 cm of the back skin, and the latissimus dorsi and serratus anterior muscles may be included in the flap for large and complex defects. The thoracodorsal vessels must be included when the scapular tip bone, latissimus muscle, or serratus muscle is harvested. The pedicle may be traced to the parent subscapular artery and vein for additional pedicle length and increased vessel caliber.

The lateral border of the scapula is dependent on the terminal intramuscular (deep) branch of the circumflex scapular artery for its periosteal blood supply. The bone's robust blood supply allows multiple osteotomies but its thickness limits its use in extensive mandibular defects. Its contours, thin cortices, and calcification pattern make it a poor recipient of dental implants.

The cutaneous portion of the flap may be directed in any plane but is usually planned horizontally or obliquely. The axial transverse and descending cutaneous branches run in the subcutaneous tissues to supply their respective territories, and the independent mobility of the skin relative to the bone makes it a prime donor site for complex defects. The skin island is particularly well suited for composite defects involving large portions of the tongue and through-and-through resections (see Fig 2-53). Massive craniofacial defects may be reconstructed with the fasciocutaneous and muscle flap.

The major drawback of the scapular flap is that flap harvest must usually be performed after the resection is completed. This adds significant time to an already lengthy and arduous procedure. Complex regional anatomy also plays a factor in the surgeon's comfort with this donor site.

Serratus-rib

The serratus-rib free flap is another useful source of vascularized bone, which is not typically affected by peripheral vascular disease as the FFF may be. Additionally, this donor site allows for a simultaneous resection and free flap harvest, in contrast to the scapular free flap (Kim and Blackwell, 2007). This bony flap can be raised with a myocutaneous latissimus dorsi component on one thoracodorsal artery pedicle. Its ability to be successfully implanted for dental rehabilitation, however, has not yet been elucidated in the literature (Brown et al., 2017).

Virtual surgical planning (VSP)

Printed models are one method to facilitate preoperative plate adaptation when bulky tumors are present or to use operative time efficiently. Similarly, preoperative planning can be done in the virtual space to mirror unaffected sides; evaluate occlusion; plan (donor and recipient) osteotomy sites; develop custom, patient-specific plates; and plan dental implants (Fig 2-54). When these techniques

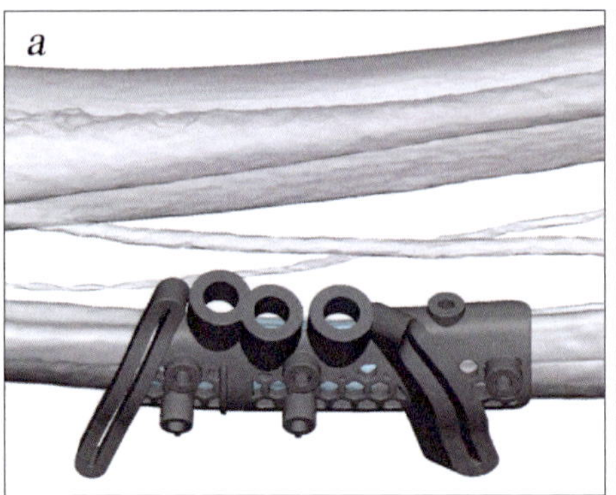

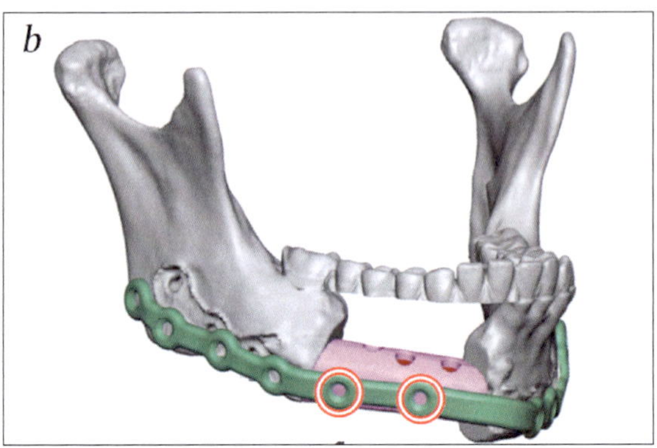

Figure 2-54 Verification images of a completed virtual surgical plan. *(a)* Completed CAD of a combination fibula-implant osteotomy guide *(b)* Planned reconstruction with a uni-segment fibula, three dental implants, and a custom plate.

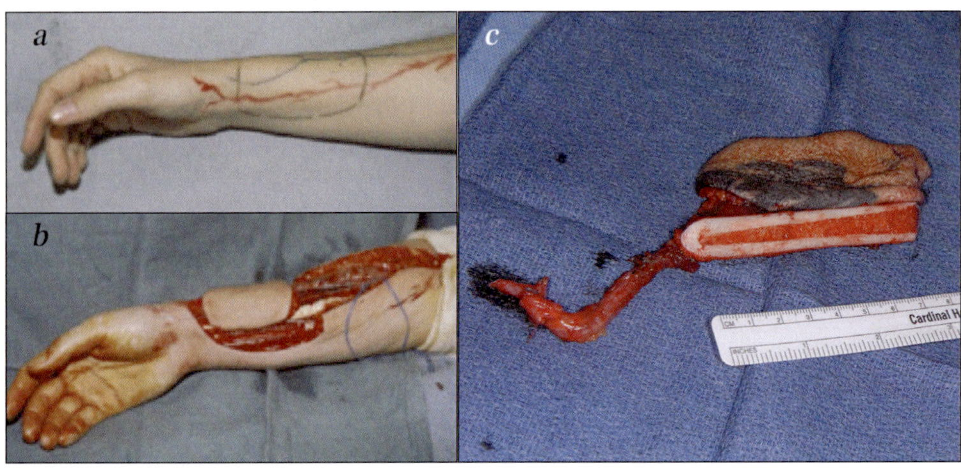

Figure 2-55 Radial forearm free flap (RFFF). *(a)* Fasciocutaneous RFFF planned for the reconstruction of a subtotal tongue defect; the flap is based on the radial artery, vena comitans, and cephalic vein. *(b)* Flap elevated in situ. *(c)* Example of a RFFF harvested as an osteofasciocutaneous free flap.

are combined, cutting guides can be applied to both the mandible and donor bone, implant osteotomies are predictively drilled, and dental implants can be placed prior to initiating ischemia time. For an in-depth discussion of VSP, see a later section titled "Virtual Surgical Planning."

Soft tissue donor sites

Radial forearm

The radial forearm fasciocutaneous flap is supplied by the radial artery, its venae comitantes, and superficial veins (Fig 2-55). The flap may be harvested with up to 12 cm of monocortical radial (osteocutaneous) or with brachioradialis muscle (myocutaneous). The composite flap may include 10 to 12 cm of bone, the entire skin of the volar and radial forearm, the palmaris longus tendon, and parts of the flexor radialis and flexor pollicis longus muscles. The medial and lateral cutaneous nerves may be included to make it a sensate flap.

Approximately one-third of the circumference (radial aspect) of the radius may be harvested as a monocortical graft (Fig 2-55c). Several radial artery perforators traverse the flexor pollicis longus muscle in this region to supply the bone's periosteum. This maintains the viability of the bone graft, but a single osteotomy is all that is advised because of the concerns about interrupting the blood supply. The bone can be folded on itself to increase its thickness, although its stock is not well suited for dental implants. Due to its relatively small bone stock, this bony site is useful only for lateral mandibular defects, whereas it offers robust fasciocutaneous soft tissue reconstruction and thus has been classified as a soft tissue flap in the current description.

The skin island is centered between the radial artery and cephalic vein (when present) and includes volar ulnar extension when necessary. If the cephalic vein is not available, the flap is moved toward the ulna, and a superficial volar vein as well as the venae comitantes may be used for venous outflow. The cutaneous paddle is nourished by perforators traversing the lateral intermuscular septum. The fasciocutaneous component of the flap is thinner distally where the perforators are also more numerous.

The radial forearm skin island is an ideal substitute for intraoral lining and can also be used for external and combined defects (see Figs 2-48, 2-49a, and the subsequent sections titled "Reconstruction of the Tongue" and "Reconstruction of the Lip"). The nondominant upper extremity is the preferred site for flap harvest, although either side may be used because there is a minimal long-term impact on function. A nondominant harvest site also allows better communication via writing for patients in the immediate postoperative period, when they are unable to speak because of the location of the surgery and the presence of a tracheotomy in many instances.

The fasciocutaneous soft tissue–only flap with a mandibular reconstruction plate is selectively used for the reconstruction of composite posterolateral defects in patients with advanced disease and finite life expectancies or those edentulous patients whose anticipated masticatory forces are less than would warrant bony reconstruction (see Fig 2-50). The composite (osteofasciocutaneous) flap is used

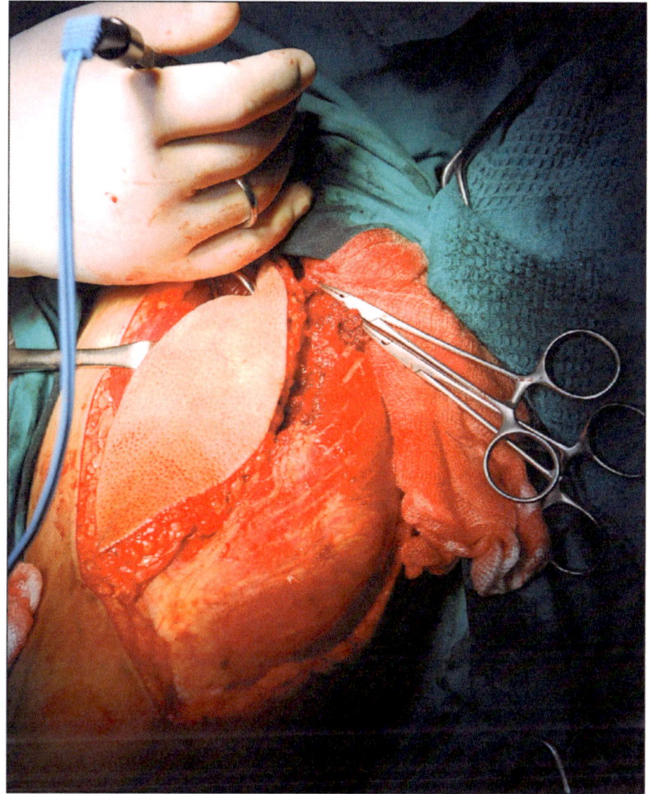

Figure 2-56 Anterolateral thigh free flap offers a large skin island. Drawbacks include a relatively short pedicle length and narrow pedicle diameter.

(more sparingly) for straight lateral segmental osseous defects that include buccal mucosa and/or FOM (Militsakh and Werle, 2005).

The thinness and suppleness of the tissue are this flap's major advantage and disadvantage. It is an excellent substitute for intraoral lining but does not have sufficient volume for more extensive composite resections and cannot reliably obliterate significant dead space in the neck. In addition, the bone is not of sufficient thickness for dental implants, long segment defects, anterior defects, or defects requiring multiple osteotomies.

Anterolateral thigh

The anterolateral thigh free flap is a fasciocutaneous and/or fasciomusculocutaneous soft tissue flap that offers a large skin paddle (Fig 2-56), the ability to harvest a separate muscle (vastus lateralis) component, and minimal donor-site morbidity. The descending branch of the lateral circumflex femoral artery and vein supplies this flap, and it may be innervated via the lateral femoral cutaneous nerve. Drawbacks include a relatively short pedicle length, narrow pedicle diameter, and challenges in raising a thin flap.

Free flap monitoring

Multiple methods of anastomotic monitoring have been successfully utilized during the immediate postoperative period following free flap reconstruction. These have included clinical evaluation (color, warmth, turgor, bleeding with scratching), handheld Doppler ultrasonography, implantable (arterial and/or venous) ultrasonography, and tissue pulse-oximetry. Regardless of the monitoring method utilized, rapid (<1 hour) identification of arterial compromise and urgent (<4 hours) identification of venous compromise are paramount in any attempt to salvage an ischemic free flap.

Complications

Complications of these major reconstructive procedures are divided into those related to the systemic manifestations of the surgery and those that occur at the recipient and donor sites. In this patient population, the cardiovascular, respiratory, and cerebrovascular systems are at greatest risk. Issues at the surgical sites are related to infection, bleeding, vessel thrombosis, and wound healing. It is rather remarkable that these long operative procedures, in radiated, orally contaminated environments, are so well tolerated.

Recipient site complications include partial or total flap loss, wound dehiscence, fistulae, cellulitis, airway obstruction, and hematoma. Donor site complications vary by site but are similar to those listed for the recipient site, in addition to physical and functional limitations in range of motion of the donor extremity.

Reconstruction of the Tongue

Tongue defect morbidities

The prognosis for oral function is closely linked to the postoperative status of the tongue, more so than the continuity of the osseous mandible. Accordingly, reconstructive priority should be given to the tongue. The degree to which speech, mastication, saliva control, and deglutition are adversely affected depends on the extent of ablative surgery and the method of surgical closure and reconstruction of the tongue.

In normal patients, the tongue rapidly changes shape to touch or nearly touch the dentition, the hard and soft palate, in order to articulate plosive and fricative phonemes. The tongue, in concert with the cheeks and lips, helps position the food bolus on the occlusal tables and sweeps residue from the lingual and buccal sulci. In concert with the soft palate, the tongue directs the bolus posteriorly to the oral pharynx with a synergistic squeezing action. The tongue and lips detect pooling saliva and direct it posteriorly for swallowing. All these actions are performed with far less efficiency in patients with tongue resections.

The loss of large portions of the tongue, without concomitant reconstruction (Fig 2-57), prevents appropriate valving and/or interaction with other oral structures. This structural loss, combined with the loss of motor and sensory innervation and impaired mobility, further compromises the articulation of speech phonemes. The deviated tongue mound with reduced mobility and bulk is unable to manipulate the food bolus; patients cannot elevate the tongue sufficiently to position the bolus onto the occlusal table for mastication or propel or transit the food bolus or saliva posteriorly for deglutition. Saliva control therefore is dramatically compromised and results in pooling, and ultimately, drooling. The same oral incompetence is seen with large defects that are closed laterally to buccal mucosa (Fig 2-58), effectively tethering the remnant to the cheek and further immobilizing the tongue.

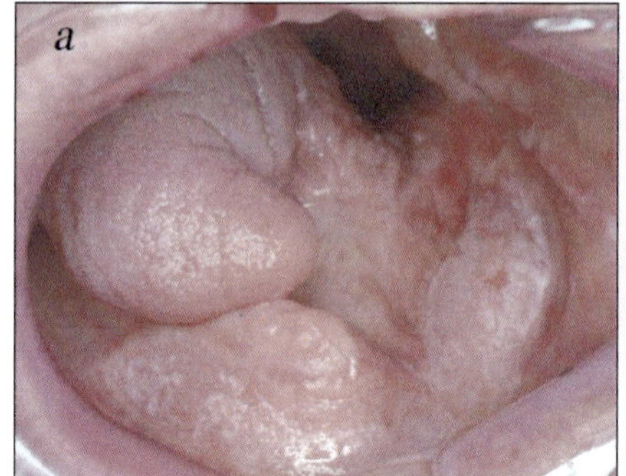

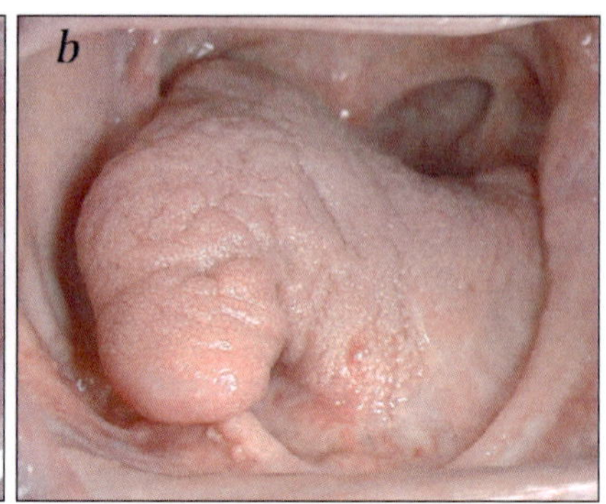

Figure 2-57 Failure to restore bulk following hemiglossectomy. *(a)* Hemiglossectomy defect. Initially the wound was closed but later the mandible was reconstructed with an avascular graft and a skin graft-vestibuloplasty. *(b)* Partial glossectomy defect with primary closure. Marginal mandibular resection without the need for osseous reconstruction. Oral function is severely compromised in both patients.

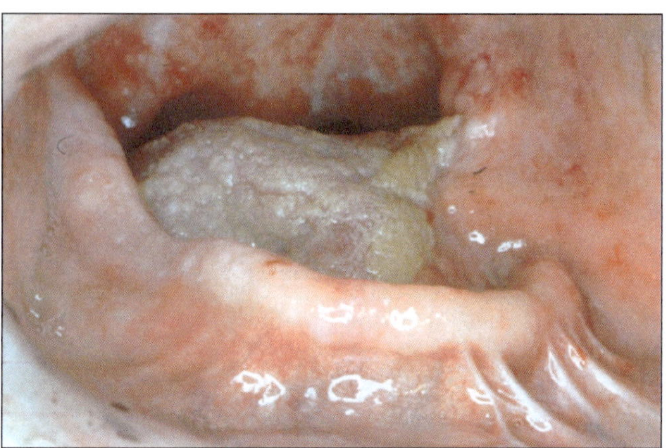

Figure 2-58 Tongue sutured to the buccal mucosa following hemiglossectomy. Tongue mobility is limited, compromising oral competence.

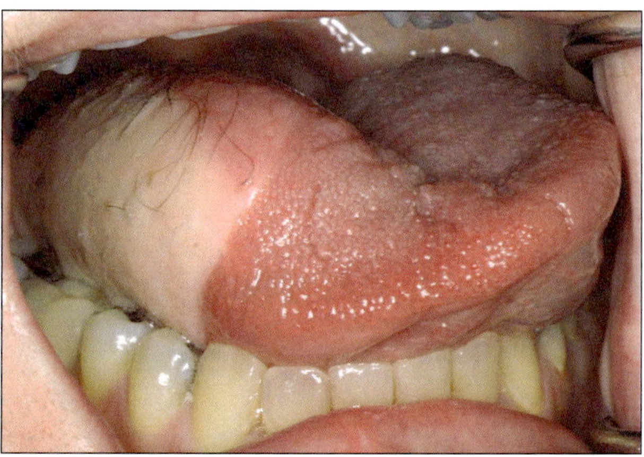

Figure 2-59 Partial glossectomy defect lined with a split-thickness skin graft.

Moderate to large glossectomies must include a reconstructive plan to restore tongue bulk, preserve tongue mobility, and center its position under the palatal vault. Failure to heed this recommendation has resulted in crippling resections (Figs 2-57 and 2-58).

Lastly, these deficits are also seen when using a free flap to purely close a defect as opposed to restoring lost shape and volume. If inadequately small skin paddles are harvested, the resulting tongue mound is flat and nonfunctional (Figs 2-65 and 2-66).

Minor tongue defects

Small tongue defects can be successfully managed with several conservative techniques. Because oral tongue defects have a great propensity for granulation formation, healing by secondary intention is a viable method for small superficial defects of the lateral tongue.

In cases where the resection includes a segment of the FOM, a split-thickness skin graft or acellular dermal matrix is necessary to avoid adherence of the raw surfaces (Fig 2-59) (Alsini et al., 2020) and to accelerate healing by assisting in mucosalization of the defect. Application of a bolster may be warranted as well as placement of a tracheostomy if not already necessary.

Primary closure techniques are equally appropriate with small defects less than one-quarter of the oral tongue, and they include tongue tip rotation, V-Y flap closure (Fig 2-60), and local mucosal flaps. Whichever technique is used, the positioning of the margins must be considered in follow-up examinations.

Pedicled flaps

Small regional pedicled flaps, such as the facial artery myomucosal (FAMM) flap or submental island flap, can be utilized when thin pliable tissues that preserve tongue mobility are desired. Because these flaps lack bulk, they are most appropriate for small defects less than one-third of the oral tongue. Some authors express concern regarding the oncologic soundness of the submental island flap, in that level I nodal basins can be transposed to the recipient site.

Large glossectomy defects necessitate either large pedicled flaps, such as a rotated latissimus myocutaneous flap or pectoralis major myocutaneous flap (Fig 2-61), or a free myocutaneous or fasciocutaneous free flap via microvascular surgical techniques (Figs 2-62, 2-63, and 2-64).

Large pedicle flaps allow restoration of moderate to large soft tissue defects. Historically, the pectoralis major myocutaneous pedicle flap was the "workhorse" of flaps because of its reliable blood supply, relative ease in raising, and large surface area available for closure of oropharyngeal and glossectomy defects (Fig 2-61). This flap, first described by Ariyan (1979), is based on the pectoral branch of the thoracoacromial artery. Because its blood supply is well away from the tumor, the pectoralis major myocutaneous flap is an ideal closure method in previously irradiated patients.

The thick, fan-shaped pectoralis muscle is elevated from the ribs and fascia of the pectoralis minor muscle. Multiple variations in the shape and size of the overlying skin paddle are possible, depending on the resected defect. Care is taken to preserve the fascia surrounding the

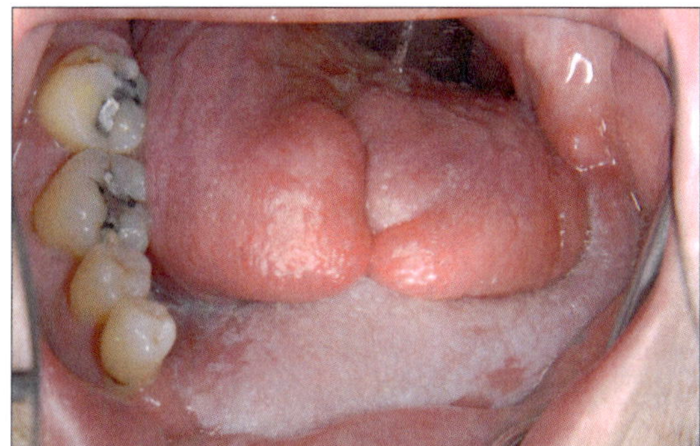

Figure 2-60 Composite resection of the anterior mandible, FOM, and anterior oral tongue. The mandible and FOM were reconstructed with a FFF, however the partial glossectomy was closed primarily with a V-Y advancement flap.

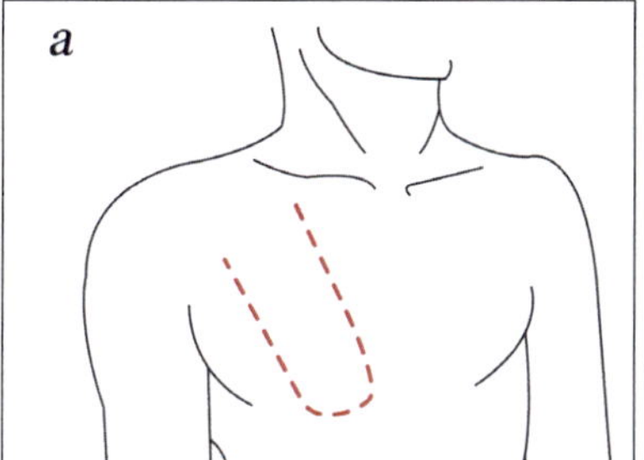

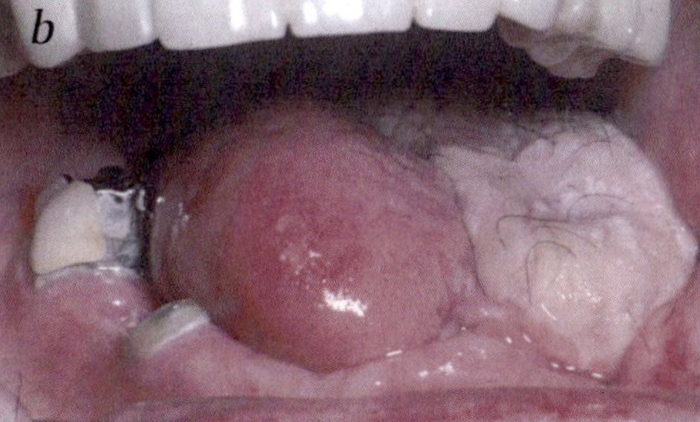

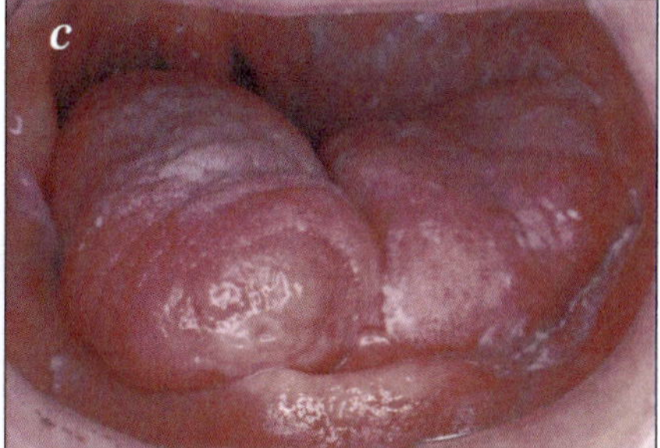

Figure 2-61 *(a)* Pectoralis major myocutaneous flap. All or part of the outlined area can be carried by a thin layer of muscle. Its vascular supply is provided by the thoracoacromial artery. This pedicled flap can be used to resurface and reconstruct many oral cavity defects. *(b and c)* Hemiglossectomy defects reconstructed with a pectoralis major pedicle flap.

neurovascular pedicle as the flap is tunneled underneath the chest wall skin and brought over the clavicle into the previously dissected neck.

The muscle portion of the flap provides coverage for the cervical portion of the carotid artery and restores the defect created by the neck dissection and partial mandibulectomy. The skin paddle is rotated into the oral cavity and meticulously sutured in place to prevent orocutaneous fistula formation. The donor site is almost always closed primarily. When bulk is a problem, the flap can be de-epithelialized, creating a myofascial flap that can be covered with a split-thickness skin graft or allowed to epithelialize by secondary intention.

Other large pedicled flaps that have been utilized include the deltopectoral, latissimus dorsi, sternocleidomastoid, platysma, and trapezius. The trapezius, and occasionally the latissimus dorsi flaps, requires intraoperative repositioning. The platysma and sternocleidomastoid flaps are used less frequently because of their tenuous variable blood supplies. In addition, the sternocleidomastoid muscle may be included in the neck dissection. The deltopectoral flap, although popular in the past, has the disadvantage of requiring a multistage procedure, and the blood supply is less reliable than that of the pectoralis flap.

Pedicle flaps, however, become scarred and immobile and thus limit the mobility of the residual tongue, and speech articulation may remain poor (see Fig 2-61). This adverse result improved with the introduction of free flaps.

Free flaps

Currently, when a significant bulk of the tongue is removed, it is suggested that bulk be restored with a vascularized free tissue transfer (free flaps), provided the patient is a candidate for microvascular surgery.

Like pedicle flaps, free flaps restore lost bulk. The residual tongue and flap are centered beneath the palatal structures, permitting the reconstructed tongue to articulate speech phonemes more effectively.

Most patients whose tongues are reconstructed with free flaps have the potential to achieve near-normal speech. The free flap restores lost bulk, as does the pedicle myocutaneous flap, but it does not become heavily scarred and immobile. Thus, the mobility of the residual tongue is improved dramatically. With speech therapy, the patient learns to manipulate the residual tongue musculature and flap quite effectively, to the point that the quality of speech articulation approaches normal limits in many patients (Fig 2-62).

For tongue-only defects, the options include a RFFF (Fig 2-63a), scapula myocutaneous free flap (Fig 2-63b), and anterior lateral thigh free flap (ALT; Fig 2-63c). Composite defects of the tongue and mandible are restored with an osteomyocutaneous FFF (Fig 2-64a) or osteomyocutaneous scapula free flap (SFF; Fig 2-64b).

Well-designed and configured vascularized free flaps can effectively restore mandibular continuity and the bulk of the tongue (Fig 2-64) and, in many patients, restore oral functions such as speech articulation, swallowing, and mastication to acceptable levels; consequently, many patients are able to resume their careers and reengage socially.

Too frequently, however, tongue bulk is not properly restored. This inadequacy can be the result of prioritizing the hard tissue reconstruction over the soft tissue bulk needed for the tongue. We believe that the priority should be the reverse, especially for posterior-lateral defects. In such scenarios, the first priority should be to restore the bulk and shape of the tongue. If necessary, the continuity of the

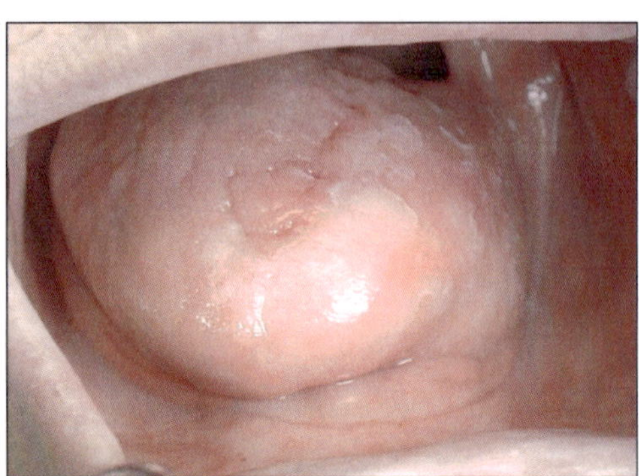

Figure 2-62 Hemiglossectomy defect restored with a RFFF. Mandibular continuity was maintained. The mandible and FOM were reconstructed with a FFF, however the partial glossectomy was closed primarily with a V-Y advancement flap.

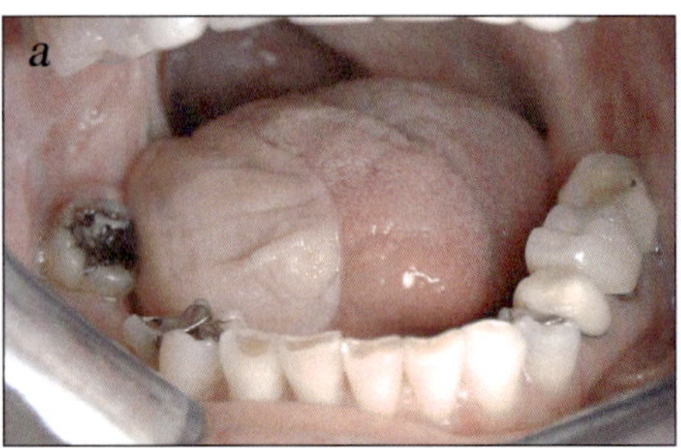

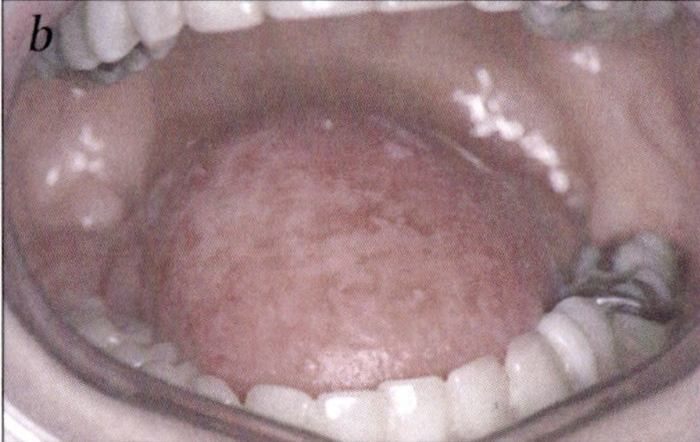

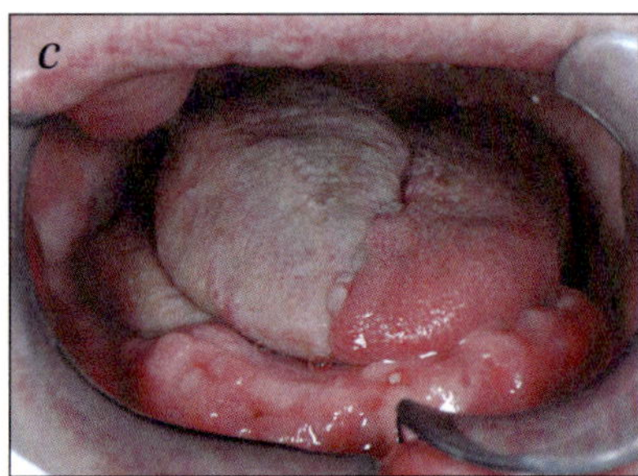

Figure 2-63 Examples of tongue-only reconstructions. *(a)* The lateral third of the tongue is reconstructed with a RFFF. *(b)* Scapular free flap used to reconstruct a total glossectomy defect. *(c)* ALT flap used for a hemiglossectomy.

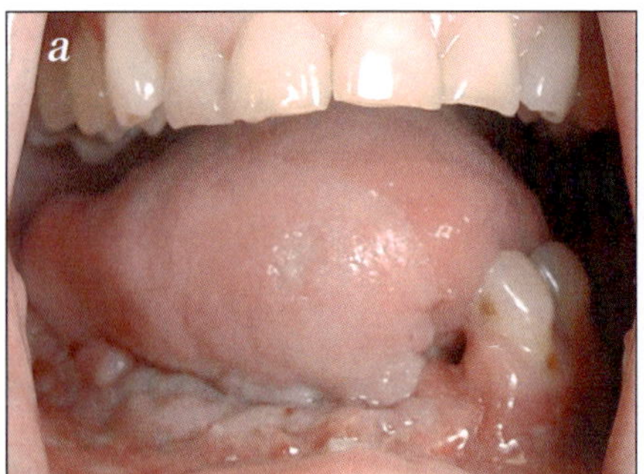

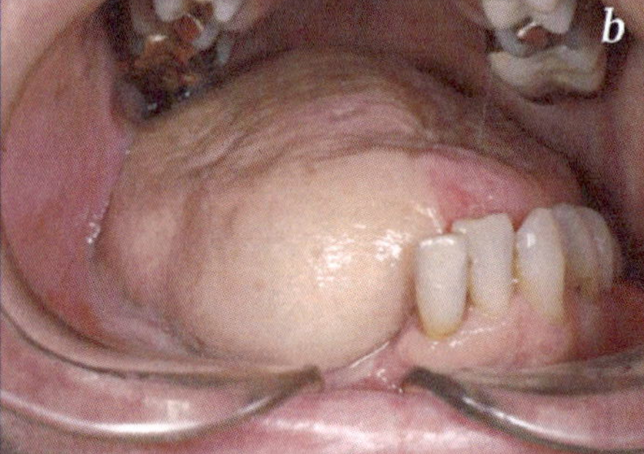

Figure 2-64 Tongue bulk and mandibular continuity restored with free flaps. *(a)* FFF. *(b)* Scapular free flap. With proper anchorage for the removable prosthesis, oral function can be restored to nearly normal.

mandible can be maintained with a reconstruction plate, and a bone graft can be used to reconstruct the mandible at a later date. Figs 2-65 and 2-66 show examples of such misdirected priorities, where mandibular continuity was achieved, while the tongue reconstruction was grossly inadequate. When delineating the skin island for a tongue defect, it is best to overestimate and aim to completely obliterate the oral cavity with the folded skin flap (Fig 2-67). Given the atrophy of flap reconstructions as well as the frequent need for postoperative radiation, which further decreases volume over time, various techniques are utilized to overcorrect the volume defect at the time of tumor extirpation. It is recommended that the neotongue reconstruction be oversized by about 30% (Hsiao et al., 2003).

Flap choices and alternatives

Flap choice in tongue reconstruction is dependent on a number of factors, including the type of glossectomy, presence, and length of neck recipient vessels for anastomosis, the existence of FOM involvement, and the existence of mandible involvement. Other considerations include the size and width of potential donor sites, such as the wrist and thigh.

For tongue (Thompson et al., 2022) defects up to 25% of the tongue volume without FOM involvement, primary closure may have similar outcomes to that of flap reconstruction in defects that do not involve the tip or base of the tongue (Sun et al., 2007). For those same defects that involve the FOM, biologic dressings and split-thickness skin grafts can provide coverage while limiting the amount of postsurgical tethering and contracture (Thompson et al., 2022; Sun et al., 2007).

Tongue defects from 25% to 50% of the tongue volume without mandible involvement require additional volume, and the RFFF is the primary reconstructive option for these defects if there are available recipient vessels. The RFFF has reliable and predictable anatomy during harvest and produces a thin and flexible skin paddle with a long vascular pedicle for anastomosis. Additional bulk can be garnered by harvesting a proximal area of subcutaneous tissue,

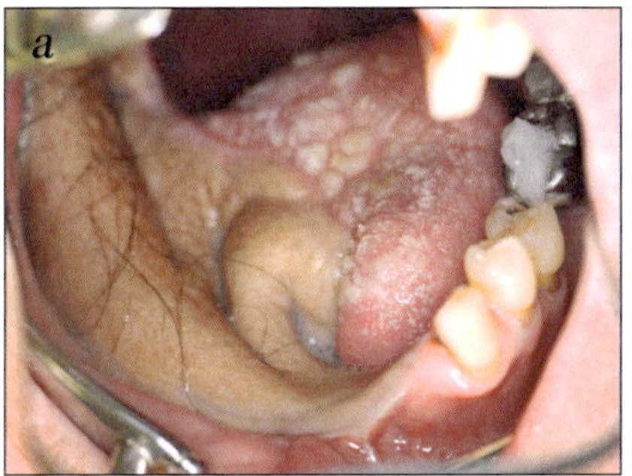
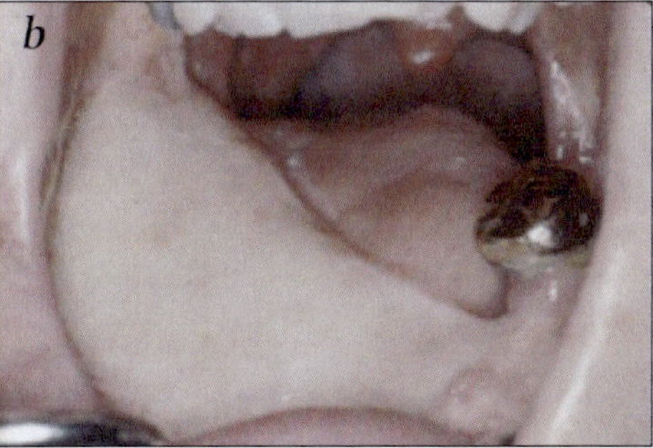
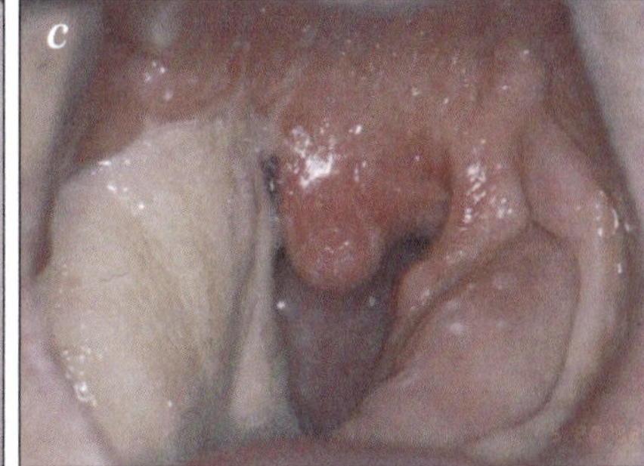

Figure 2-65 *(a–c)* Three examples of inadequate myocutaneous paddles harvested along with the respective FFFs. Mandibular continuity has been restored, but the tongue bulk has not been properly restored. The result is that oral function cannot be restored.

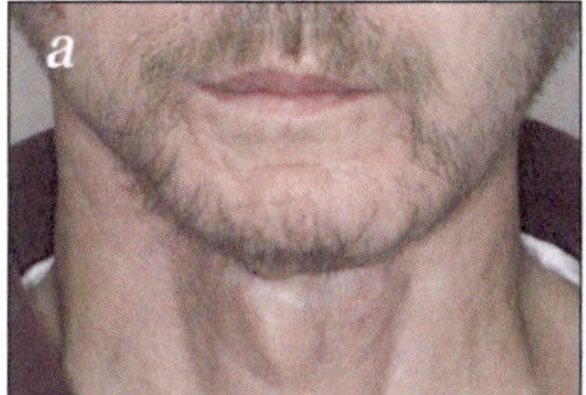
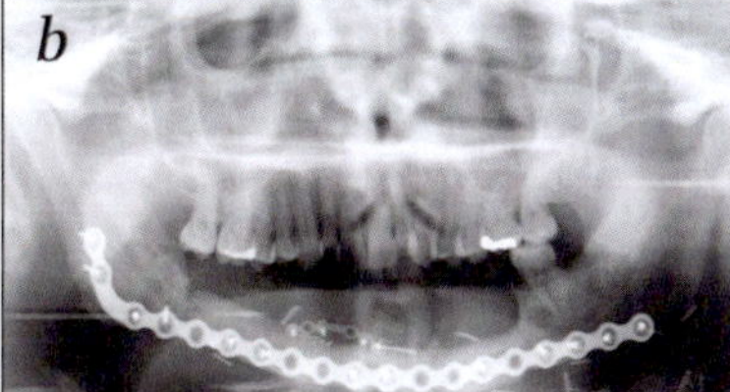
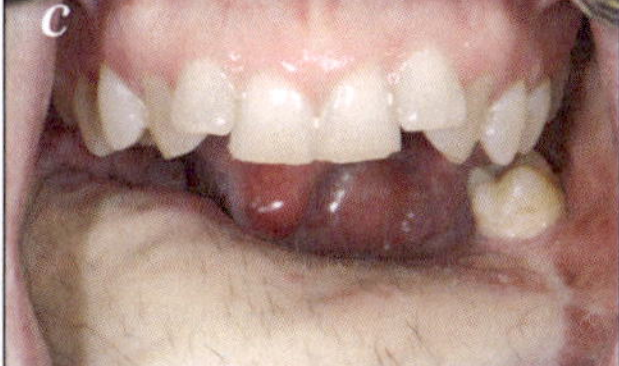
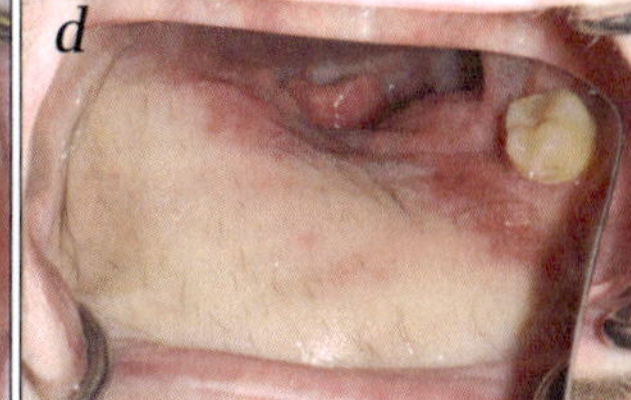

Figure 2-66 Segmental mandibulectomy and total glossectomy restored with a FFF. *(a)* Reconstruction resulted in reasonable facial contours. *(b)* Panoramic radiograph shows the extent of the reconstructed mandible. *(c)* Lack of reconstructed tongue bulk fails to provide volume to articulate speech. *(d)* The occlusal view shows no discernible neoridge for an MRP. Note that the epiglottis is directly visible.

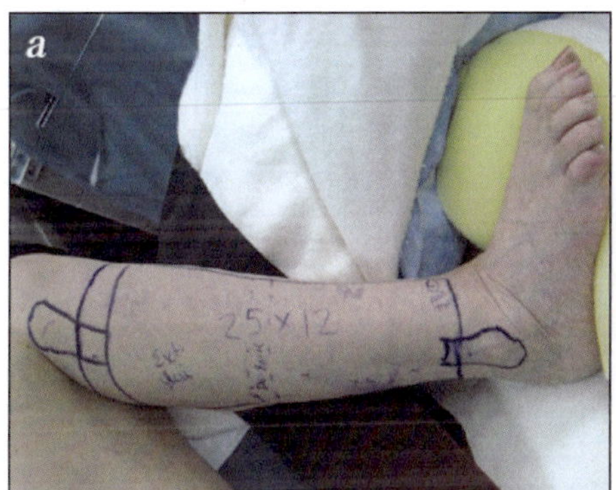

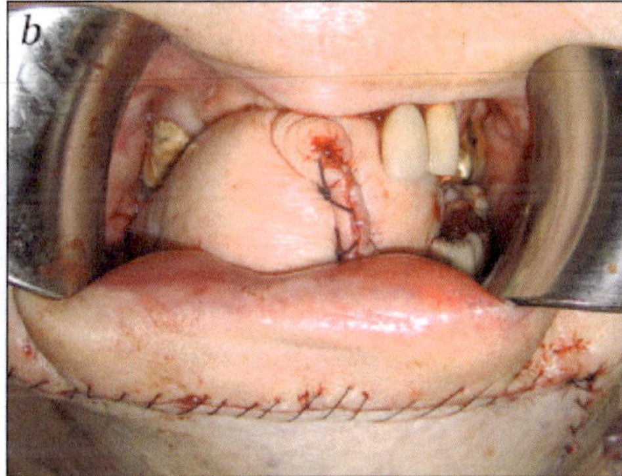

Figure 2-67 *(a)* Two delineated skin islands on the lower leg. *(b)* Tongue, mandible cutaneous defect reconstructed with a FFF.

or *beavertail*, which is especially advantageous in defects with a concurrent base-of-tongue defects (Seikaly et al., 2009). Bulk can also be generated by harvesting a large skin paddle with subsequent de-epithelialization and imbrication of the de-epithelialized portion underneath the neotongue. The RFFF is fed by the radial artery, and an Allen's test must be performed preoperatively to ensure that blood supply to the hand can be maintained with the remaining ulnar artery. Free flap alternatives to the RFFF include the ALTFF, in patients with thin wrists in which additional bulk is needed, or the medial sural artery perforator (MSAP) flap, which has a mean skin thickness between that of the RFFF and ALTFF with a pliable skin paddle suitable for oral tongue reconstruction.

Oral tongue defects from 50% to 100% of the tongue volume are commonly reconstructed with the ALTFF, provided there are recipient vessels. The ALTFF is fed by the descending branch of the lateral circumflex artery; however, the route of its perforators to the skin paddle is variable, making for a more difficult harvest. Its thickness depends on the patient's BMI but is significantly thicker than the RFFF, making it well suited to provide the bulk needed for total glossectomy defects. Other free flap options include the rectus abdominus free flap or flap based on the subscapular system.

Oral tongue defects with cortical bone involvement require osteocutaneous reconstruction. The FFF is preferred for this reconstruction due to the amount and quality of bone stock and its ability to support a skin paddle up to 550 cm^2 (Blackwell, 1999). Larger defects with large soft tissue reconstruction requirements in addition to bone can be addressed with chimeric flaps based on the subscapular artery system or a combination of free and pedicled flaps.

In cases where recipient vessels are sacrificed for oncologic control or where recipient vessels are distant from the tongue defect, pedicled artery flaps—such as the submental island flap, the supraclavicular island flap, and pectoralis major flap—are options as well and can also be reserved for use for salvage reconstruction as needed.

While a number of free flaps have an associated nerve that can be harvested, sensate free flap tongue reconstruction has not been shown to make a functional difference (Uwiera et al., 2004).

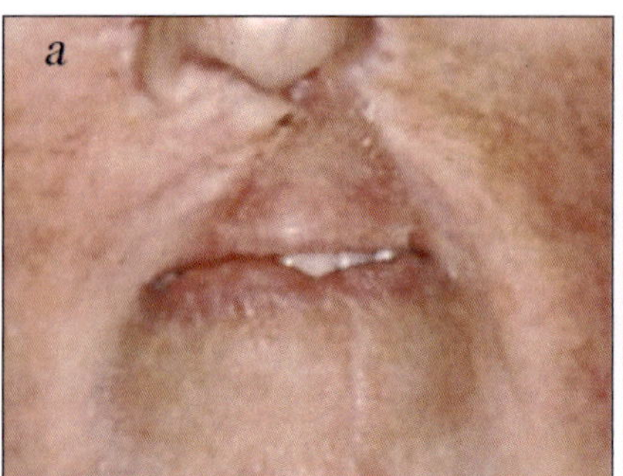

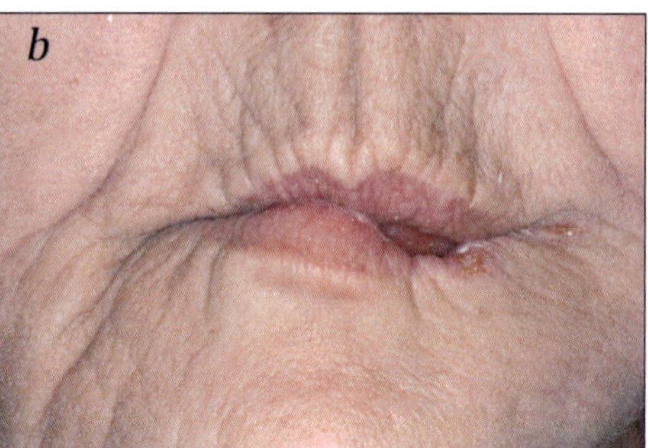

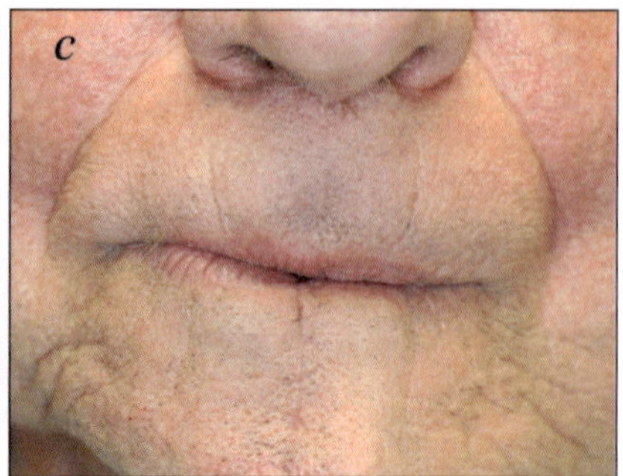

Figure 2-68 *(a)* Appearance following resection of 60% of the upper lip and reconstructed with advancement flaps and Abbe flap. *(b)* Appearance following composite resection of the mandible. The lip is retracted and the commissures lowered. *(c)* Postoperative scarring and resection of the marginal mandibular nerve may result in lip incompetence.

Functional outcomes after tongue reconstruction

A functional outcome after tongue reconstruction is dependent on the size of the oral tongue defect and, by extension, the involvement of the base of the tongue, FOM, and mandible. As such, larger defects have poorer outcomes in regard to speech and swallowing. There is a lack of consensus in the literature that suggests that one type of free flap is advantageous to another in regard to speech and swallowing outcomes, especially with larger defects. While the majority of studies looking at functional outcomes of defects isolated to the oral tongue or base of the tongue have used the RFFF, larger defects have more variability in reconstructive choices, making it difficult to draw a unified conclusion on functional outcomes (Lam and Samman, 2013).

The volume and protuberance of the tongue reconstruction have been proposed to be correlated with speech intelligibility (Manrique et al., 2016), while postoperative radiation and larger defects have been found to prognosticate worse speech outcomes (Lam and Samman, 2013). For patients with defects involving the oral tongue up to a subtotal glossectomy, single-word intelligibility preoperatively was found to be 90.0%, 69.2% at 1 month after surgery, and 79.6% at 6 months after surgery (Uwiera et al., 2004). When hemiglossectomy patients were graded on an intelligibility scale from one to seven, six months after surgery, the mean score was 4.8, corresponding between "intelligible but with noticeable errors" and "intelligible with careful listening" (Hsiao et al., 2003). Speech in subtotal to total glossectomy patients 10 months after surgery, on average, was found to be good in 29.4%, acceptable in 52.9%, and poor in 17.7% of patients (Yanai et al., 2008).

Not surprisingly, improved swallowing ability is associated with improved speech intelligibility as well as tongue volume and protuberance (Yun et al., 2010). Thirty-three percent of free-flap reconstructed hemiglossectomy patients were found to tolerate a regular diet after 6 months, while 66% tolerated a soft diet (Hsiao et al., 2003). In a systematic review, 14% of patients who underwent total glossectomy and free flap reconstruction were reliant on G-tube nutrition 6 to 12 months after surgery, which increased to 24% 12 months after surgery (Dziegielewski et al., 2012). Similarly, when total glossectomy patients were graded on a scale from 1 to 7 for their swallowing, the mean value was 3.4 points, corresponding between "those who could consume a liquid diet" and "those who felt discomfort with a soft diet" (Yun et al., 2010).

Functional outcomes have also been shown to improve with consistent follow-up with speech-language pathologists and physicians as well as good family support and positive motivation (Manrique et al., 2016).

Reconstruction of the Lip

The lips may be directly affected by resection of a primary disease (Fig 2-68a) or indirectly affected due to injury or resection of the marginal mandibular or inferior alveolar nerves (Fig 2-68b). Postoperative scarring may also impact lip function and cosmesis (Fig 2-68c).

Lesions that compromise the lips, preventing functional lip seal and salivary control, can be disabling. These patients often demonstrate deficits in speech articulation, drooling, and slurred speech secondary to pooling of saliva and inadequate lip seal. Incompetent lip seal, whether sensory, motor, or structurally related, can be a major disability affecting speech, mastication, and self-esteem and frequently challenges the prosthetic rehabilitation of the patient.

When considering lip reconstruction, the various tissues that compose this facial subunit must be considered, including skin, subcutaneous tissue, muscle, as well as oral mucosa and wet and dry lips. During reconstructive planning, the functional and aesthetic architecture of the lip must be considered while attempting to minimize the less desirable outcomes, such as gross asymmetry, microstomia, and a lack of lip competence.

When contemplating a reconstructive plan for a lip resection, one must prioritize form and function. Cutaneous and mucosal lip defects that are partial thickness can be left closed by secondary intention, closed primarily, or reapproximated with the aid of local flaps (Nabili and Knott, 2008). The decision of the closure technique is dictated by the size and depth of the defect relative to the size of the upper and lower lip subunits. Primary surgical closure can be performed for defects that are equal to or lesser than one-fourth of the upper lip and one-third of the lower lip. Defects ranging from one-third to two-thirds of the total lip length may be closed using the Abbe (Fig 2-69) or Estlander flaps. The choice of flap is based on the involvement of the oral commissure, with the former used to reconstruct medial defects that spare the oral commissure and the latter for defects involving the oral commissure (See et al., 2022). The Abbe flap, however, requires a second-stage surgery to take down the pedicle. Defects ranging from one-half

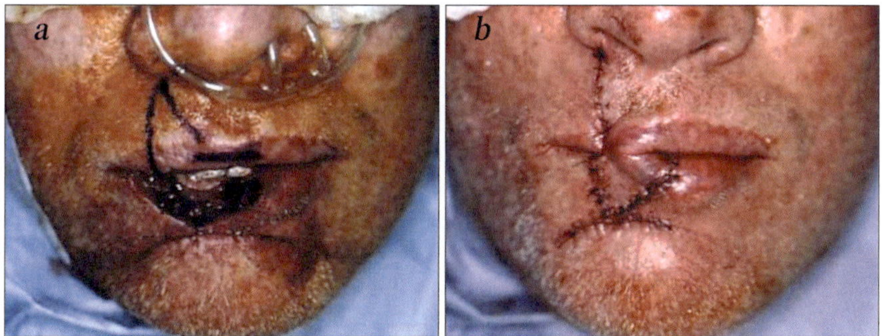

Figure 2-69 Abbe flap. *(a)* Patient with a 50%, full-thickness defect of the right lower lip that spares the lateral commissure. *(b)* Completed initial phase with a superiorly based Abbe flap. Note the releasing incisions along the mentolabial crease to provide bilateral advancement for closure. This technique requires a second stage revision.

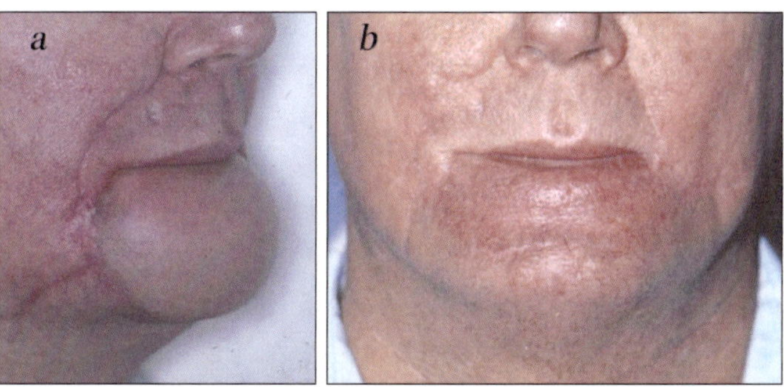

Figure 2-70 Radial forearm free flap (RFFF). *(a)* Total lower lip defect reconstructed with a RFFF. *(b)* Final result after flap revision (figures courtesy of Dr. John Lorant, Los Angeles, CA).

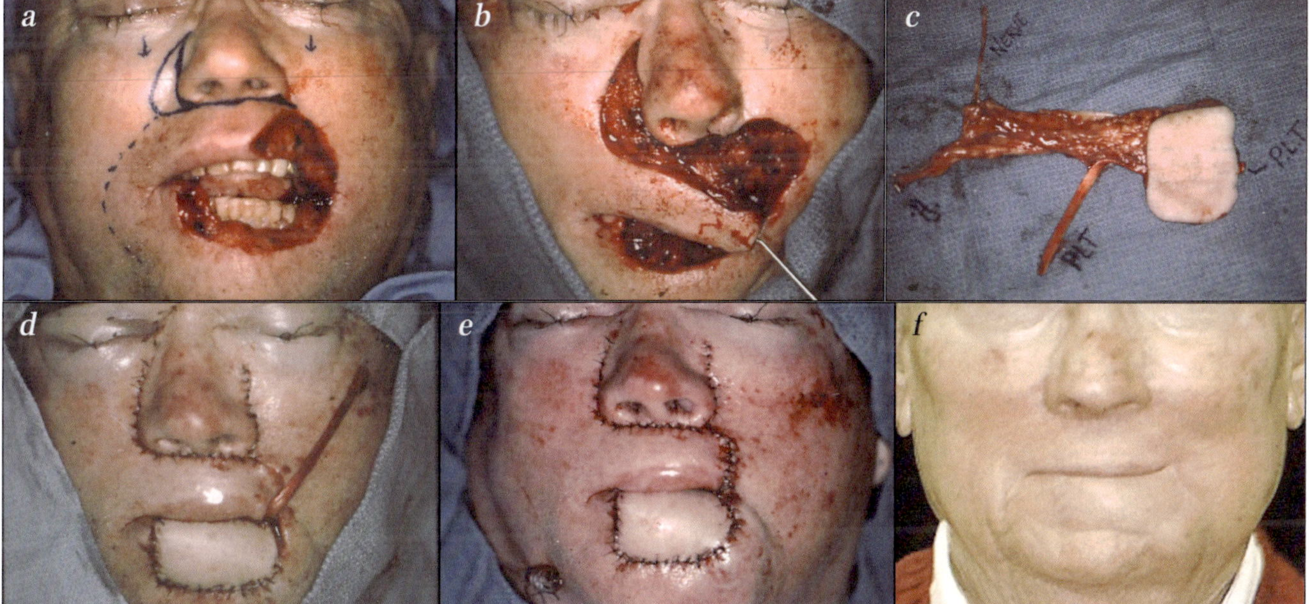

Figure 2-71 Radial forearm free flap (RFFF). *(a)* Patient with a defect of one-half the upper lip and nearly the entire lower lip after Mohs skin cancer excision. In cases that involve multiple subunits, a mixture of local and free flaps is often needed. Care is taken to hide incision lines and flaps within the boundaries of the lip and facial subunits. *(b)* A right-sided upper lip advancement (perialar crescent flap) is performed in addition to *(c)* a RFFF with palmaris longus. *(d)* The palmaris longus tendon was used to suspend the flap to the left zygomatic arch in a static sling fashion. *(e)* Completed reconstruction. *(f)* Final results.

to two-thirds in size can be managed using Gillies or Karapandzic flaps that borrow adjacent tissue and maximize incisions by placing them in relaxed skin tension lines. The repair of defects greater than 75% generally requires the Bernard-Burrow, the Webster modification of the Bernard-Burrow, or a free flap (Nabili and Knott, 2008). Reconstruction of a near-total lip defect with a free flap is not perfect, as it lacks dynamic functional motion with the absence of the motor and sensory innervation of the native lip (Fig 2-70).

The two commonly used free flaps for lip reconstruction are the RFFF for thinner defects and the anterior lateral thigh flap (ALTF) for larger and more complex defects requiring more bulk (Sanniec et al., 2018). The RFFF is the most commonly used given its pliable nature and ability to incorporate the palmaris longus tendon

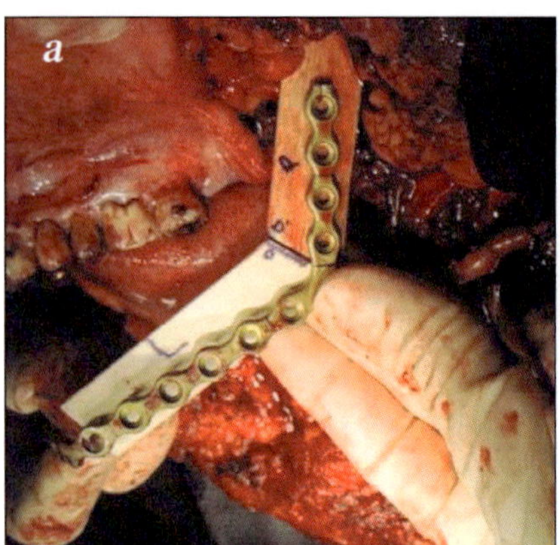

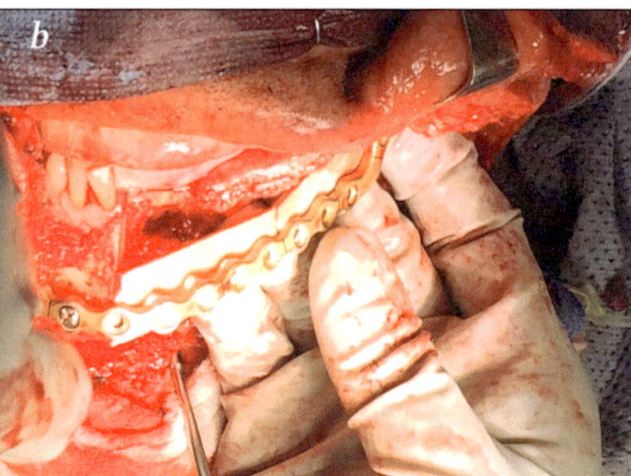

Figure 2-72 Tongue depressor blades trimmed to fit the medial border of the stock reconstruction plate and then used as templates for fibula osteotomies.

(Fig 2-71c) as a static sling to suspend the new lower lip and prevent future ptosis of the reconstruction (Nabili and Knott, 2008). These techniques are fundamental for obtaining oral competence and preserving an oral diet. The FFF with adequate skin paddle may also be used if there is a concurrent bony defect.

Ratios of defect size to lip size are not hard rules, and clinical judgment is required when determining the selection of reconstruction of borderline defects. Incorporating a functional orbicularis muscle into the reconstructive paradigm is more important than obtaining size parity. An adynamic lip is often more problematic from a functional standpoint than microstomia. However, microstomia can interfere with the placement of an oral prosthetic device. Avoiding microstomia is particularly important for edentulous patients who are dependent on removable dentures for esthetics and oral function.

Virtual Surgical Planning

With the increasing sophistication of CAD/CAM technologies and the pioneering work of Rohner and his colleagues (2003 and 2013), several centers (Sharaf et al., 2010; Antony et al., 2011; Berrone et al., 2014; Kim et al., 2016; Seikaly et al., 2019; Patel et al., 2019) have developed surgical approaches geared toward harvesting the osteomyocutaneous flap, reconstructing the mandible, and placing dental implants simultaneously. As was the case with the method developed by Rohner et al. (2003 and 2013), the configuration and positioning of the flap is based on dental occlusion. The orientation and position of the dental implants and the osseous portion of the flap are preplanned based on the anticipated position of the prosthesis in the three-dimensional (3D) virtual surgical environment.

Prior to digital planning capabilities, microvascular reconstruction was based on intraoperative intuitive decision-making. This creates a spatial design challenge when using dental implants for oral rehabilitation. Reconstructions were based on bone-driven approaches that generally used the lower and lateral border of the mandible as the templates for reconstruction, since these contours are deemed critical to the eventual cosmetic outcomes (Fig 2-72). Moreover, the position and angulation of the implants frequently are not "prosthetically driven." The patient is then referred to a prosthodontist for oral rehabilitation. As a result, in many patients, the functional occlusal reconstruction is suboptimal because the arrangement of the bony portions of the flap and the positioning of implants are not ideal. In addition, with this approach, up to a quarter of the implants could not be used because of malpositioning or improper angulation, even though they were osseointegrated (Hundepool et al., 2008; Fenlon et al., 2012).

Presurgical planning based on dental occlusion represents a significant advance. This type of occlusal and functional reconstruction utilizes virtual surgical planning (VSP) and starts with the development of proper occlusion for the proposed prosthesis. Based on the existing dentition, wax-ups, or a trial denture, the prosthodontists can determine the most ideal positions for the dental implants. Once the implant positions are determined, the 3D location of the osseous graft can be finalized. The VSP reconstruction is then converted into a physical plan and implemented in the operating room (OR) using various surgical templates and resection guides. As a result, the use of dental implants becomes prosthetically driven.

Timing of implant placement

If mandibular resection is secondary to the removal of a malignant tumor from the oral cavity, the benefits of the primary placement of implants must be carefully weighed against the risks. Sophisticated CAD/CAM protocols enable the accurate placement of implants simultaneously with the free flap reconstruction of the mandible. One must consider that the five-year survival of oral cancer patients with lymphatic spread is about 50%. Additionally, because 80% of tumor recurrences occur within the first year, an argument can be made to wait 12 months following tumor ablation before undertaking implant placement (Garrett et al., 2006).

Furthermore, most of these patients will receive postoperative radiation. The backscatter from the radiation increases the dosage delivered to the bone anchoring the implant by approximately 15% to 18% (Tso et al., 2019; Schwartz et al., 1979; Mian et al., 1987). This increases the risk of complications (Fig 2-73).

The case for an interdisciplinary approach

Treatment and rehabilitation of jaw resection and reconstruction are highly specialized, and an interdisciplinary team with specialists across various disciplines is essential in achieving a successful

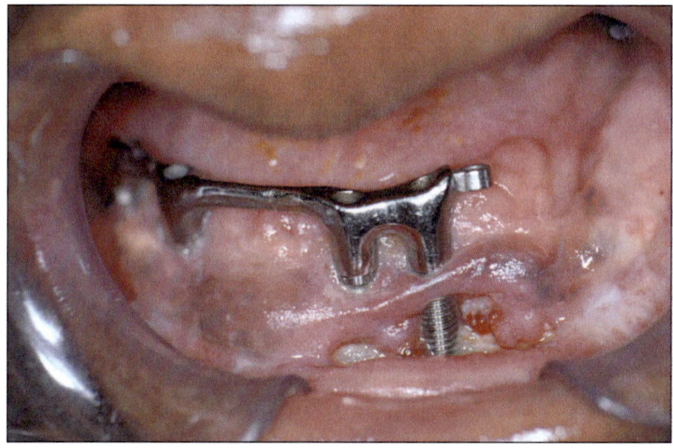

Figure 2-73 Primarily placed implants into a FFF reconstruction of a body-symphyseal defect. The patient received 60 Gy of adjuvant radiotherapy. Several months later and just after the delivery of the implant connecting bar, tissues on the labial surface of the implants dehisced.

outcome (Berrone et al., 2014; El Saghir et al., 2014; Patel et al., 2019; Pfister et al., 2020). This collaborative planning is crucial in the various aspects of the workflow. The surgeons are responsible for planning the soft and hard tissue resection margins, the type of defect reconstruction, the flap donor site, the length of the bone reconstruction segment(s), the positioning of the bony segment(s) within the soft tissue envelope, the access to vascular structures for the microvascular anastomoses, the effect of dental implant placement on the surgery and adjunctive treatment, and the type of plating systems. The prosthodontist needs to consider the edentulous defect and propose oral rehabilitation, identify the position of the dentition, and determine the position, angulation, and number of the implants, the prosthetic space needed for the future prosthesis, mouth opening and access issues, the 3D positioning of the reconstruction bone segments, and how that will affect the prosthodontic outcome.

The most reliable functional and occlusion-based reconstructions in patients with jaw defects are obtained with printed models, resection guides, flap osteotomy guides, implant guides, articulation splints, and custom reconstruction plates. This can be achieved using different approaches that require virtual surgical planning.

Surgical factors

The main requirement for achieving a consistent functional outcome is to place the bony reconstruction in the correct 3D spatial position based on the dental occlusion (Patel et al., 2019; Seikaly et al., 2019). The use of VSP has increased in prevalence over the past decade and provides superior outcomes. Compared to intraoperative surgical design or analog planning, VSP results in a decrease in surgical time (Weitz et al., 2016; Seruya et al., 2013; Hanasono et al., 2008; Toto et al., 2015) and improved 3D spatial relationships of the reconstruction (Okay et al., 2013; Toro et al., 2007; Antony et al., 2011; Ueda et al., 2001; Zheng et al., 2013) and has been shown to be more accurate (Weitz et al., 2016; Wu et al., 2016; Ochi et al., 2013; Zhang et al., 2016). Studies also suggest that there is no increase in rates of surgical complications (Weitz et al., 2016; Toto et al., 2015), morbidity, and flap survival (Seruya et al., 2013; Toto et al., 2015).

Limitations

A limitation of VSP is the uncertainty in planning the resection margins preoperatively, especially in oncologic cases. However, in instances where the resection margins must be extended beyond the virtual planning, the relevant parts of the plan can still be used and augmented with conventional reconstructive techniques. Unfortunately, one can never fully predict the nature of the disease and how rapidly it can spread, and in those scenarios, a return to conventional resection and reconstructive techniques is warranted.

Indications and contraindications

The indications and contraindications of VSP-centered resection and reconstruction are no different than those of conventional resection and reconstruction. Patients without significant medical comorbidities who can undergo a lengthy microvascular reconstructive surgery are good candidates for reconstruction. The mandibular defect must be a minimum of 2 cm in size (Fry et al., 2016). The procedure is contraindicated in patients who are unable to tolerate prolonged surgery, have poor or abnormal vascularity of the proposed donor sites, or are not motivated for treatment. In addition, hypercoagulability states—such as factor V Leiden thrombophilia, protein C or S deficiency, and antiphospholipid syndrome—can pose significant problems in microvascular reconstruction.

Virtual surgical planning (VSP) workflow

With the introduction and evolution of VSP, an optimal pathway has been created for a digital workflow in the surgical—prosthodontic continuum for head and neck cancer patients.

Presurgical medical consultation

The surgical team obtains a CT of the head and a donor-site contrast CT angiography (CTA). The purpose of a routine CTA of the leg is to rule out peripheral vascular disease, congenital absence of the anterior tibial artery, posterior tibial artery, or the presence of peroneal arteria magna. While the latter congenital conditions present a normal pedal pulse, they are contraindications for utilizing the fibula.

Presurgical prosthodontic consultation

During the presurgical prosthodontic consultation, impressions or direct intraoral scans of the dental arches must be obtained. If the area to be resected and reconstructed is dentate, the existing dentition can be utilized for planning. However, if the area of interest is partially edentulous, an analog or digital wax-up of the missing teeth is a prerequisite for occlusion-based VSP. If analog impressions were made, the gypsum casts and wax-up of the missing dentition can be digitized with a scanner and sent to the design team electronically. The digitized casts or scans are then aligned to the head CT based on common reference points (remaining dentition). Proper alignment is critical for the precision of the bony and oral rehabilitation and for the accuracy of any planned tooth-borne surgical guides. Tooth-borne surgical guides must be designed from digitized casts or digital scans and not from CT reconstructions of the dentition

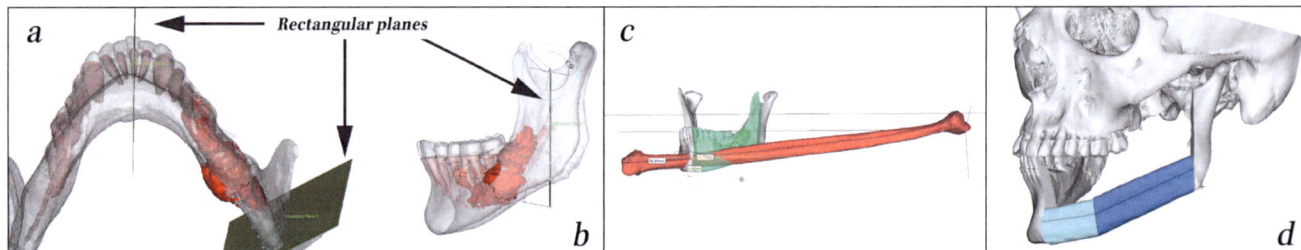

Figure 2-74 *(a and b)* Two rectangular osteotomy planes represent proposed resection margins for the patient presenting with a tumor of the mandible. Resection through a tooth-bearing portion of the mandible is planned through a tooth socket. *(c)* The left fibula overlayed as the proposed bony reconstruction. Note that the same symphyseal osteotomy plane defines the distal fibula osteotomy. *(d)* Completed bisegmental fibula reconstruction.

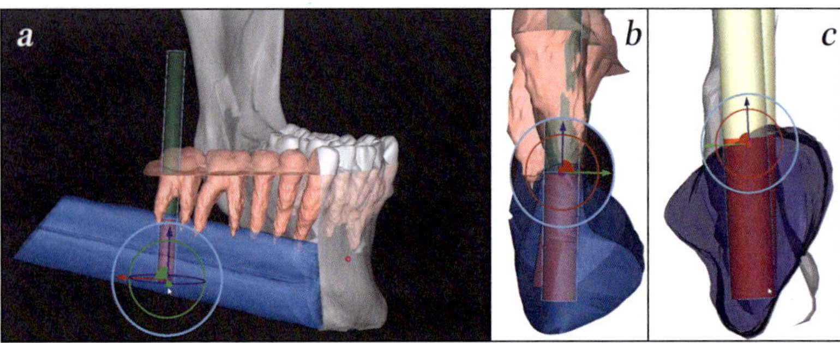

Figure 2-75 *(a and b)* Buccolingually, the fibula is positioned to encompass the tooth roots. *(b)* Notice how a 4 mm wide implant cannot be housed within the osseous spine found in the ventral border of the middle fibula. *(c)* The dorsal fibula border rotated occlusally to better house dental implants.

because CT data of the teeth are often riddled with radiographic artifacts, especially in patients with metallic restorations.

In edentulous patients, the dual scan protocol is employed with a trial complete denture laced with fiducial markers. The dual scan protocol consists of two scans, one of the patients wearing the trial complete denture and another of the trial prosthesis. The two scans are aligned later via common points (fiducial markers) prior to the planning process.

Virtual surgical planning process

Prior to the planning session, the biomedical engineer aligns the dental data with the CT data. The biomedical engineer, reconstructive surgeon(s), and prosthodontist collaborate and plan the mandibular resection and occlusion-based reconstruction via video conferencing. The biomedical engineer assists in the planning process and operates the advanced digital planning software. The ablative surgeon finalizes the resection margins. Subsequently, the microvascular surgeon determines the size and position of the osseous segments to be used in the reconstruction. Finally, the prosthodontist determines the planned oral rehabilitation and the position, depth, and angulation of the proposed dental implants.

Resection

The first step in the VSP process is to identify the surgical resection margins. The biomedical engineer will import rectangular planes, which represent surgical cuts, and position them along the mandible as directed by the ablative surgeon. As demonstrated in Fig 2-74, two rectangular planes representative of the proximal and distal osteotomies are brought in to simulate the en block resection. Once the positions of the planes are finalized, they are used to separate and remove the intermediate osseous specimen, effectively creating the surgical defect. Once the surgical defect is known, osseous reconstruction planning can begin.

Osseous reconstruction

Choice of reconstruction flap

Several potential vascularized bone flaps exist, including the FFF, the deep circumflex iliac artery (DCIA) flap, and the SFF. The FFF is the most common choice for mandibular reconstruction, preferred by most clinicians (Seikaly et al., 2003; Ide et al., 2015; Patel et al., 2019), and will be our main focus.

Orientation of the reconstruction flap

The biomedical engineer is asked to toggle on the native mandible, the native mandible after virtual resection, and the teeth, wax-ups, or trial complete dentures to aid in the orientation of the fibula reconstruction. The proximal fibula is oriented toward the side of the recipient neck vessels ipsilateral to the defect. As shown in the left mandibulectomy scenario in Fig 2-74, the proximal fibula is positioned toward the left ramus, while the distal fibula is positioned toward the mandibular symphysis. In bilateral mandibulectomy defects, however, either neck vessels can be an option.

Buccolingually, the fibula should be positioned within the defect to restore facial projection while also encompassing the root apices of the ipsilateral dentition (Fig 2-75). Occlusoapically, the fibula should be positioned within the defect, congruent to the inferior border of the native mandible. The primary complaint for the FFF is that its height is representative of an edentulous atrophic mandible (14 mm on average) and about half the height of a dentate mandible (Fig 2-76).

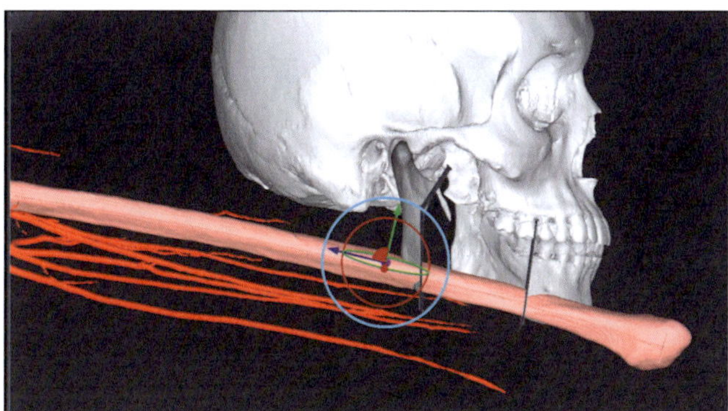

Figure 2-76 Fibula superimposed on a proposed mandibular defect. The peroneal vessels are passed into the neck, and the matched vessels of the neck are identified for the anastomoses. Note the height discrepancy between the fibula and the dentate mandible.

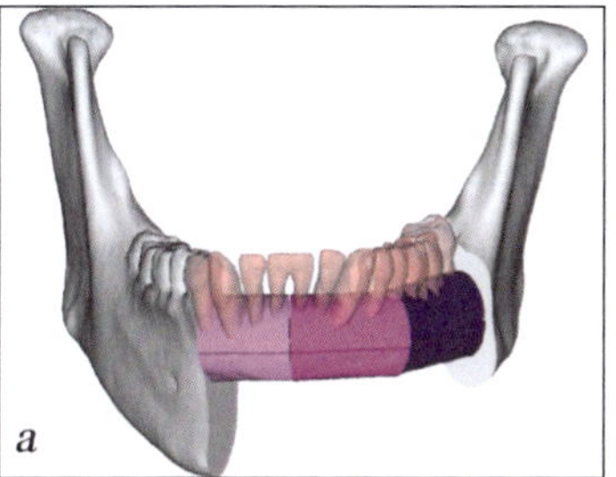

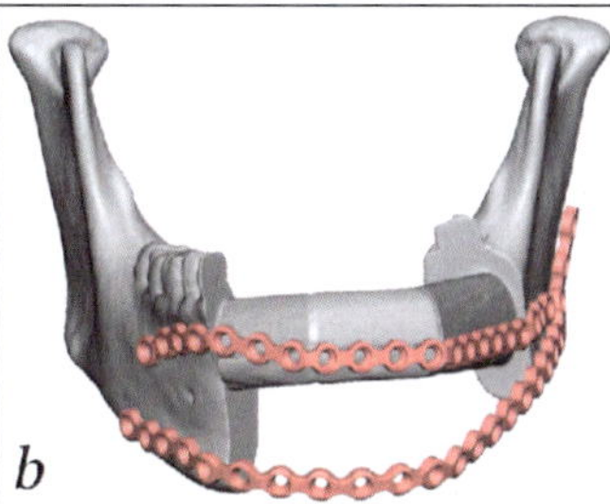

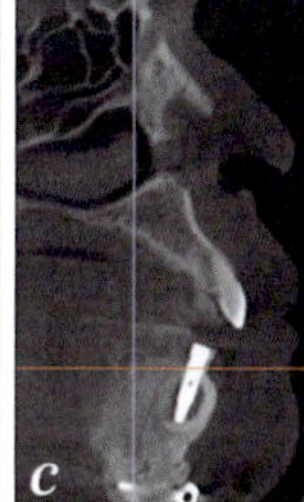

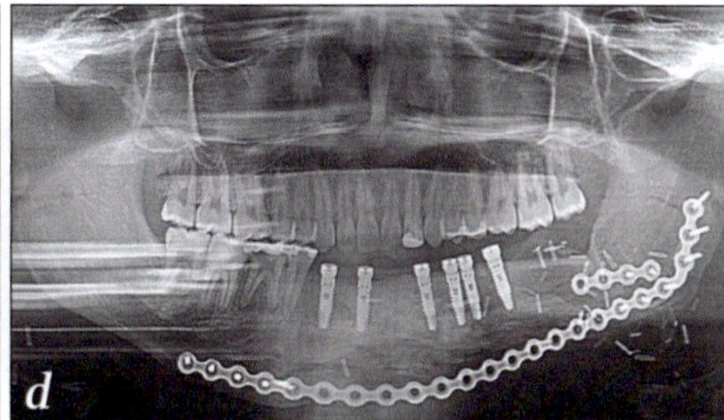

Figure 2-77 Combined microvascular and guided tissue regeneration for full mandibular height reconstruction in benign osseous lesions. *(a and b)* FFF virtually planned to reconstruct the alveolar arch. The inferior mandibular border was planned for corticocancellous bone grafting. Note the need for two reconstruction plates. *(c and d)* The superior plate was removed six months after healing for the secondary placement of dental implants.

While there are few consequences to this height discrepancy, multiple techniques have been developed to address this concern. For short uni-segmental and lateral defects, the fibula segment can be raised up from the inferior border of the native mandible by 5 mm with little to no cosmetic compromise (Seikaly et al., 2003). However, raising the fibula segment more than 5 mm could produce facial asymmetry, especially after adjuvant radiotherapy as the soft tissues atrophy. In situations where adjuvant radiation is not needed, the fibula segment(s) may be raised to the height of the alveolar ridge, and the inferior border can be reconstructed with an autologous corticocancellous bone graft (Fig 2-77) or remaining fibula graft.

Alternatively, the inferior border can also be reconstructed via the double-barrel technique. This has three major challenges and also increases ischemia time and therefore overall OR time. First, the orientation of the skin paddle becomes more challenging (Brown and Shaw, 2010). Second, the pedicle length becomes shorter, making it difficult to reach the recipient neck. Third, if not performed with great care, the switch back could introduce a kink in the pedicle, impairing its vasculature. Additionally, defects greater than 10 cm are not candidates for this procedure, thus reducing the applicability of this technique to uni- or bisegment defects. Moreover, from a prosthodontic perspective, a double-barrel approach can encroach on prosthetic space and limit restorative options.

In addition, the vertical positioning of the fibula segment can be altered based on prosthodontic needs. Sufficient prosthetic space is important for hygiene access and ensuring adequate strength of the definitive prosthesis. When a fixed or removable metal-acrylic prosthesis is planned for a patient with a benign osseous neoplasm where the native gingiva will be retained for primary closures, the occlusal surface of the osseous graft restoring the alveolar ridge should be placed at least 16 mm apical to the occlusal plane. However, when a skin paddle is needed for closing composite defects, additional prosthetic space (18 mm or more) is advised (Fig 2-78). When implants emerge through thick skin paddles, the soft tissues overlying the osseous graft must be thinned via a secondary debulking procedure to reduce the thickness of the peri-implant soft tissues. Patients who received postoperative radiation or chemoradiation and need debulking warrant special considerations in order to avoid devascularizing the osteomyocutaneous flap (see below, section entitled "Stage II implant surgery"). While fixed monolithic or layered zirconia prostheses and metal-ceramic prostheses require less prosthetic space, debulking and the reduction of deep peri-implant pockets are still critically important for the long-term maintenance of the fibula and dental implants.

The fibula graft is best situated with its ventral border facing the occlusally and its lateral border facing the buccally. Because these two borders (Fig 2-79) are overlaid by only the periosteum without muscles, arteries, or veins, they are the most ideal for the placement of dental implants and reconstruction plates. However, the osseous spine found in the ventral border of the middle portion of the fibula can be thin and complicate dental implant placement (Figs 2-75b and 2-80). Five options are available to the reconstructive surgeon and prosthodontist to address this situation. The first three options are best-case scenarios when the thinness of the osseous spine is moderate, while the latter two options carry an increased risk to the perforator vessels and periosteal blood supply.

1. Rotating the fibula on its long axis to direct the osseous spine in the direction of the implant axis or deliberately away may allow the implant to emerge toward the lateral border of the fibula.

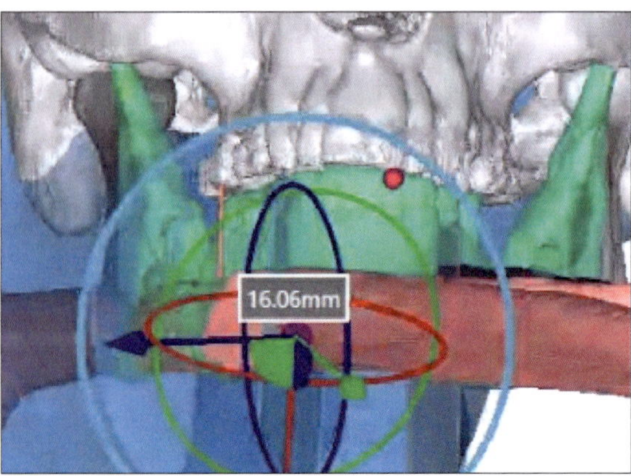

Figure 2-78 The prosthetic space can be determined during the virtual planning stage. Note that 16 mm is measured from the opposing occlusal table to the fibula.

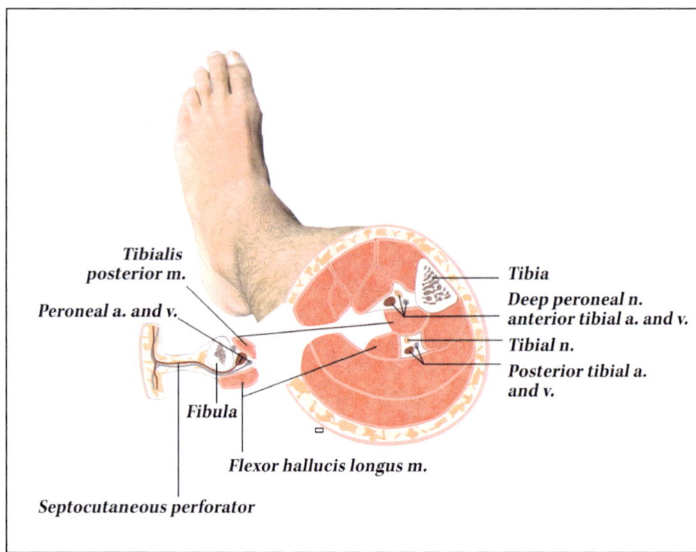

Figure 2-79 This axial cut through the lower left leg shows the harvested osteomyocutaneous FFF. Note that the superior-lateral borders are free of vessels and muscle tissues. The medial (deep) and dorsal borders a closely associated with the peroneal artery and vein, septocutaneous perforator vessels and tibialis posterior, and flexor hallucinate longus muscles.

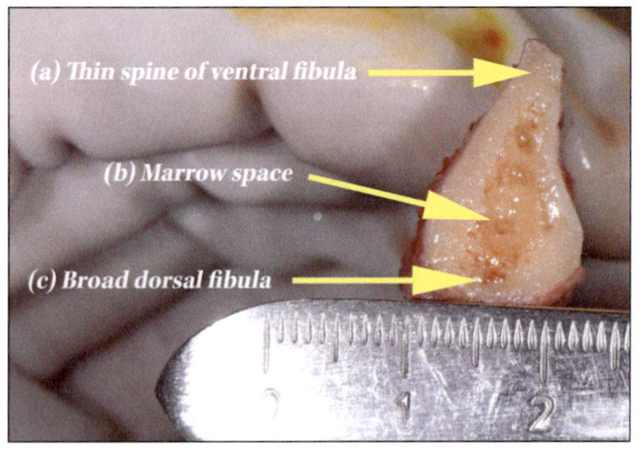

Figure 2-80 *(arrow a)* The osseous spine found in the ventral border of the middle fibula can be too thin for implant placement. Osteoplasty of the spine to create a platform may expose the marrow space *(arrow b)* and compromise primary implant stability. For this patient, the fibula was flipped to allow implant placement into the *(arrow c)* broader dorsal fibula border.

2. Using a narrower implant with a diameter less than the recommended standard of 4 mm. This is the simplest alternative when the spine is moderately thin (approximately 6 mm), so a narrow implant (3.5 mm) can be placed with a minimum of 1 mm of bone remaining on either side. The surgical guide used to place these implants, however, needs to fit very intimately to ensure accurate placement. Because narrow implants carry an additional risk of fracture, an implant-assisted design should be considered for the final prosthesis.
3. Using a subcrestal implant and countersinking the implant. It is critical to utilize a countersink drill to develop an appropriate emergence so implant abutments can be connected without bony impediments.
4. Switching to the contralateral leg and rotating the fibula on its axis so the dental implant enters the broader dorsal border of the fibula (see Fig 2-75). This technique requires a modification to the combination fibula-implant surgical guide in that the guide, which normally seats on the anterolateral borders of the fibula, must have implant surgical sleeves that extend around the fibula to the dorsal border (Fig 2-100).
5. Performing osteoplasty of the spine until a wide enough platform is achieved. Ide et al. (2015) investigated the anatomical characteristics and available bone volume in fibulas for installing dental implants. They concluded that the cross section of the middle part of the fibula is triangular and will need osteoplasty to flatten the surface for implant placement. Because this technique reduces the periosteal blood supply to the fibula segment, its benefit must be weighed against the increased risk of flap failure. Additionally, if the bone marrow is exposed following osteoplasty, bicortical engagement with dental implants will be compromised to some degree, and primary stability may be reduced. An osteoplasty guide is strongly advised for this technique, and the length of the selected implants should be based on the height and width of the fibula postosteoplasty.

Once the fibula axis rotation and the decision to flatten the osseous spine (or not) is finalized, the biomedical engineer uses the same rectangular planes for the mandibulectomy to make the fibula osteotomies (Fig 2-74). In order to maintain ankle stability, 6–8 cm of distal fibula is usually preserved. The subsequent fibula cuts are made as wedge osteotomies to produce the desired angle between the fibula segments. The final and most proximal fibula cut is made with the same rectangular plane used for the posterior mandibulectomy margin.

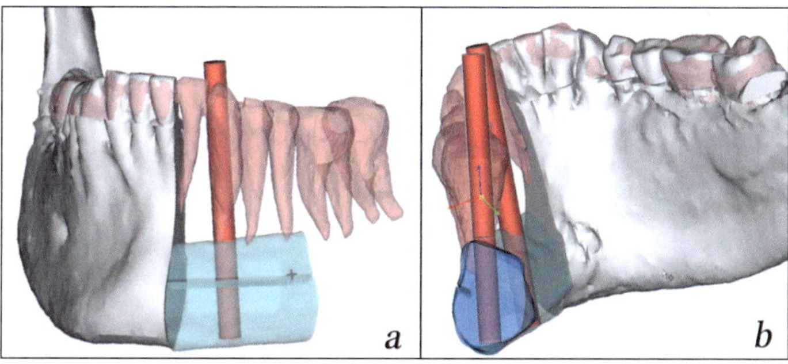

Figure 2-81 Midline mandibulectomy reconstructed with a bisegment fibula. Cylinders representing the implants are positioned along the long axis of the native dentition. *(a)* Right canine. *(b)* Molar.

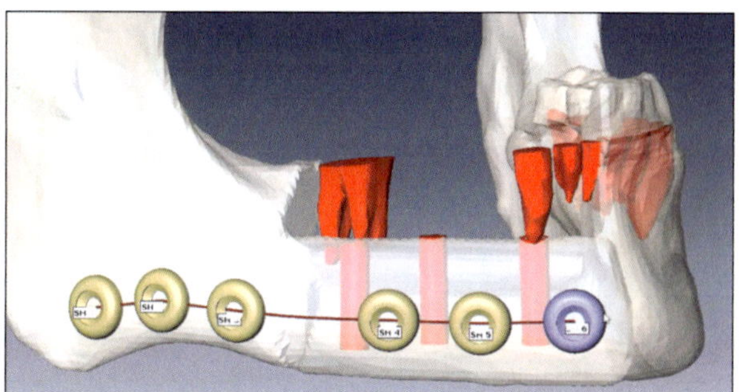

Figure 2-82 Providing 5 mm between implants allows adequate room for screw holes (SH) when planning for a custom reconstruction plate.

Dental implants

Following the virtual osseous reconstruction, the prosthodontist can proceed with planning the oral rehabilitation. The biomedical engineer is asked to toggle on the native dentition, wax-up, or scan of the trial prosthesis and import cylinders representing implants so they can be simulated at prosthetically driven positions. The occlusal edge of the cylinders is extended past the occlusal tables of the proposed prosthesis so that the angulation and position of the screw access holes can be visualized (Figs 2-81, 2-84, and 2-86). The prosthodontist then directs the biomedical engineer to position the cylinders along the long axis of the tooth and tooth roots while following the occlusal curves of Spee and Wilson (Figs 2-81 and 2-86). Similar to conventional implant prosthodontics, the choice of the implant macro design, length, diameter, spacing, number of implants, implant distribution, and angulation should not be an afterthought and must be planned at this point in time. However, due to several factors—including but not limited to implant spacing (to each other and to the end of a fibula segment), prosthetic space, and minimum fibula segment length—the team may find it necessary to backtrack and adjust the previously positioned osseous reconstruction for the best occlusion-based outcome.

Macro design

The use of tapered self-tapping implants should be avoided if the fibula is chosen to reconstruct the mandibular defect. When tapered, self-tapping implants are inserted, the stresses can be excessive and, in some cases, trigger cracks in the fibula adjacent to the implant osteotomy sites, leading to fractures of the fibula. Implants with parallel walls are preferred, and the osteotomy sites are prepared in the usual manner and tapped prior to inserting the implants.

Length

When the fibula is used, bicortical stabilization of the dental implants is recommended. Therefore, the length of the aforementioned cylinders is chosen based on the dorsoventral height of the fibula so that both cortices can be engaged. The length of the implants selected needs to be slightly longer than the height of the fibula. As a result, the implants will protrude slightly out of the inferior surface of the fibula following placement (see section on VSP surgery). This protrusion, however, is inconsequential, as it will be covered by soft tissue.

Diameter

The diameter of the cylinders is by default 4 mm unless narrower implants are being planned due to the limited width of the bone stock. Wide-diameter implants should not be used when the fibula is chosen. Creating a large osteotomy in the fibula and engaging both the facial and lingual cortices will weaken the fibula, predisposing the peri-implant bone to cracks and fractures, which can lead to resorption of bone around the implant.

Spacing

Implants placed in the native alveolar bone are generally positioned at least 3 mm apart. However, in order to avoid undue stresses on the fibula during osteotomy preparation and to mitigate the impact of microfractures adjacent to the osteotomy sites, a minimum of 5 mm of interimplant spacing is recommended. Additionally, because peri-implantitis is more prevalent when implants emerge through the skin, the additional spacing facilitates hygiene access and resolution of peri-implantitis (see below, section entitled "Stage II implant surgery"). Lastly, there is less concern about nicking the dental implants with fixation screws used to secure reconstruction plates when 5 mm of interimplant spacing is available (Fig 2-82).

The distance from the implant to the cut edge of a fibula segment should be no less than 3 mm. Additional spacing is advised if the height difference between the native mandible and the fibula creates a vertical bony wall (Fig 2-83). This geometry tends to tent the soft tissue so that implants placed within a right isosceles triangle are usually surrounded by excessively deep peri-implant soft tissues. Therefore, we recommend that no implants be planned within the base of this triangle as shown in Fig 2-83. To illustrate, if the vertical bony wall from the alveolar crest to the fibula crest is 6 mm, then the first implant should be planned 6 mm away from that vertical wall. This precaution means that the implant is aligned with the second or third prosthetic tooth, and a cantilever is needed to extend from the implant to the natural tooth adjacent to the vertical bony wall (Fig 2-84).

Number of implants and distribution patterns

When the implants are arranged in a linear configuration, at least three should be considered. The addition of a third implant dramatically improves the biomechanics of the restoration (Rangert et al., 1997; Wu et al., 2022b) and the clinical outcomes (Lekholm

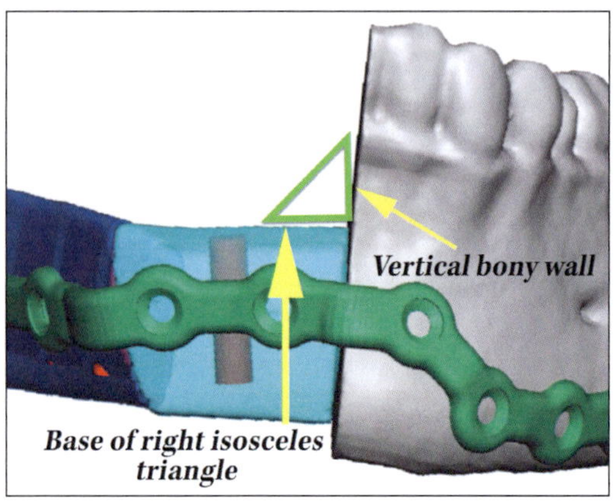

Figure 2-83 Implant adjacent to a vertical alveolar defect should be positioned outside the right isosceles triangle formed by the height of the vertical bony wall from the occlusal fibula crest.

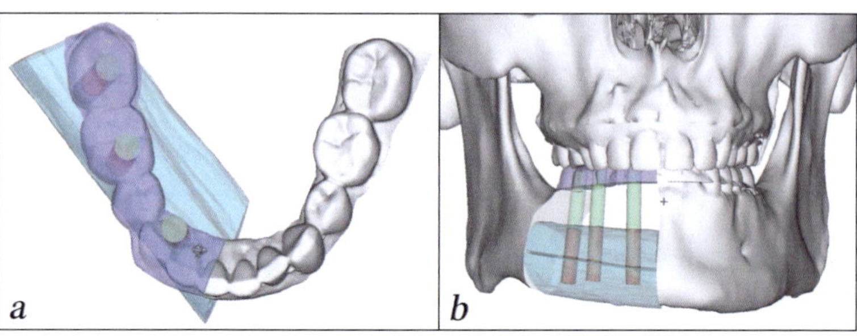

Figure 2-84 *(a)* Implant sites are "prosthetically driven." *(b)* When implants are arranged in a linear configuration, at least 3 implants should be considered.

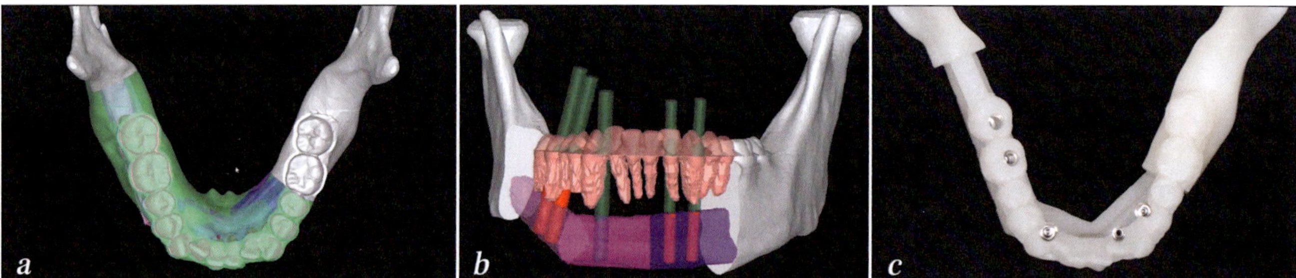

Figure 2-85 The defect will encompass the anterior curvature of the mandible. Implant distribution should idealize the A-P spread. *(a)* Planned resection and tri-segment fibula reconstruction. *(b)* Five planned implants. *(c)* Printed model of the reconstructed mandible. Note the implant analogs pressed into the implant osteotomies and connected titanium cylinders engaging the printed dentition.

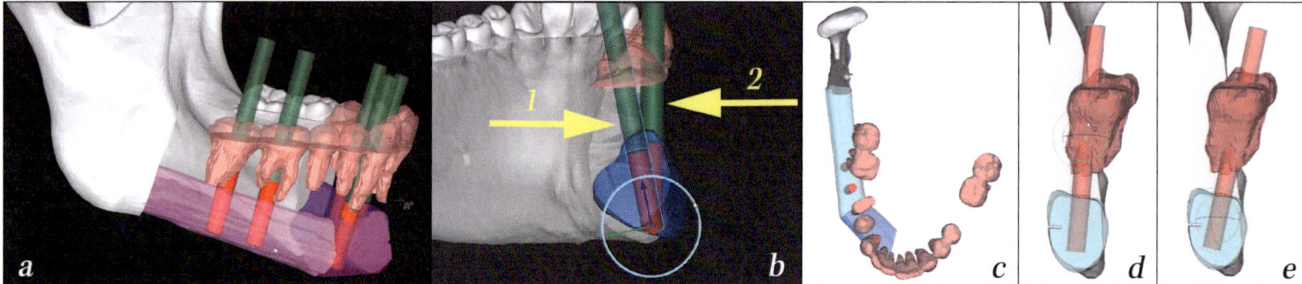

Figure 2-86 Implants restoring posterior teeth should be aligned compatible with the curve of Spee *(a)* and the curve of Wilson *(b)* so that posterior occlusal forces will be directed along their long axis. *(c)* Notice that because the fibula must project toward the ramus, molar implants must tilt lingually *(arrow 1)*. Otherwise, they emerge buccal to the tooth *(arrow 2)*. *(d and e)* Another example of angulating the implant in accordance with the curve of Wilson.

et al., 1999; Gunne et al., 1994) (Fig 2-84). When the defect extends anteriorly to encompass the curvature of the mandibular arch, additional implants are needed. In addition, every effort should be made to maximize the A-P spread so as to idealize biomechanics and enhance the effects of cross-arch stabilization (Wu et al., 2022b) (Fig 2-85).

Angulation

Implants restoring the posterior dentition should be angled such that occlusal forces are directed along their long axes and compatible with the curve of Wilson and the curve of Spee (Fig 2-86). This is particularly important when the implants are aligned in a linear configuration where cross-arch stabilization is not possible (Fig 2-84). Similarly, implants restoring anterior dentition should be oriented parallel to the long axes of the teeth in a coronal and sagittal view (Fig 2-87a and b). From an occlusal view, the implant should emerge through the cingulum of an anterior tooth (Fig 2-87c).

Custom plating

Once the prosthodontist approves the implant positions, the biomedical engineer is asked to assist with the digital design of a custom reconstruction plate. This process involves the placement

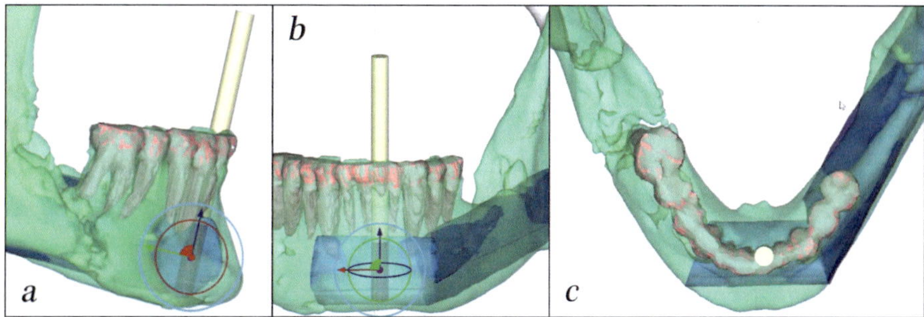

Figure 2-87 *(a and b)* Implants restoring anterior teeth should be aligned compatible with their long axes. *(c)* From an occlusal view, the implant should emerge through the cingulum of the anterior teeth.

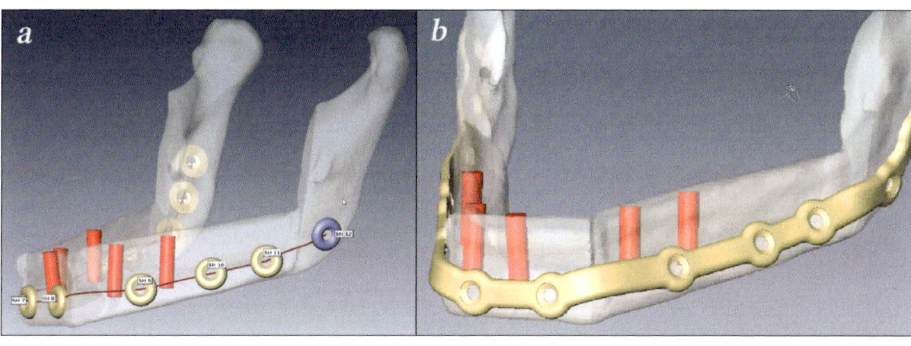

Figure 2-88 Custom reconstruction plate for an angle-to-angle mandibulectomy planned as a tri-segment fibula. *(a)* Screw holes (SH) are positioned at least two per fibula segment and three on either end onto the residual mandibular fragments. In this example, there are three SH in each ascending ramus. The SH are spaced to avoid the planned dental implants. *(b)* CAD of customized, 2.0 mm profile plate. Note the increased occlusal-apical height of the plate in the osteosyntheses for additional strength.

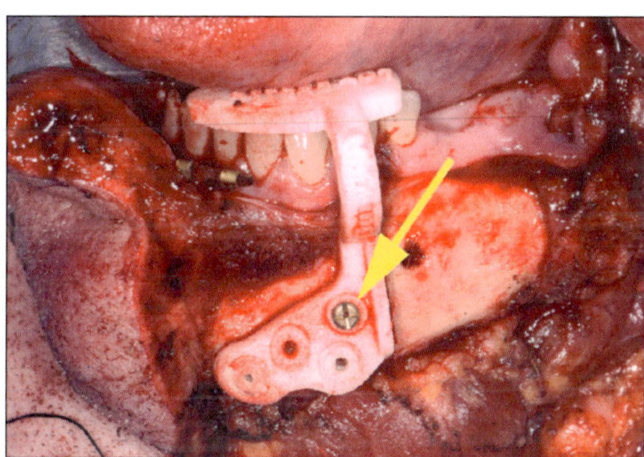

Figure 2-89 Seated tooth and bone-supported mandibulectomy guide, retained with one bone screw *(arrow)*.

of fixation screw holes along the fibula segment(s) to generate a bushing around each of the screw holes (Fig 2-88a). The screw holes are carefully placed to avoid collision with the planned dental implants, retained teeth, and intact inferior alveolar nerves, all of which are clearly visualized within the software. At the minimum, two screw holes are recommended per fibula segment to reduce rotation (pitch and roll), and three or more screw holes are recommended for the native mandibular fragments. If two screws per fibula segment are not possible, some backtracking and modifications to the spacing and number of dental implants may be required. After all screw holes have been defined, the software will connect the bushings automatically and design the custom reconstruction plate (Fig 2-88b). To reduce the likelihood of intraoral exposure, the plate should be placed at least 5 mm below the occlusal crest of the fibula segment. For added rigidity and strength, plates can be thickened in the occlusoapical dimension at the osteosyntheses (Fig 2-88b). The custom reconstruction plate is then manufactured.

CAD/CAM mandibulectomy, fibula, and implant surgical guides

After completing the virtual surgical plan, and before terminating the collaborative session, a list of the 3D-printed models and guides are prescribed.

Tooth-supported mandibulectomy guide

The tooth-supported mandibulectomy guide is intended to index available teeth adjacent to the resection margin for stabilization purposes so the surgical cuts can be executed as closely to the plan as possible (Fig 2-89). As mentioned before, because the dentition reconstructed via the head CT may be riddled with radiographic artifacts, a computer-aided design of the surgical guide requires a properly aligned direct intraoral scan of the dental arch or scan of a physical cast. A chimeric model is then created by merging the dentition from the surface scan and the mandible from the head CT prior to

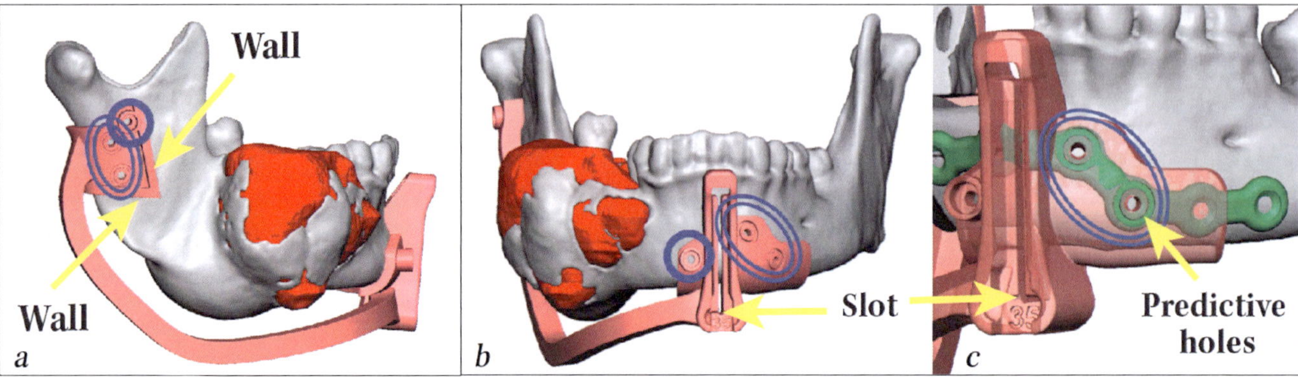

Figure 2-90 CAD of a connected bone-supported, mandibular osteotomy guide. *(a)* The posterior mandibular resection contains two walls to guide an angular osteotomy. This is done to retain the condylar neck. *(b)* The symphyseal margin has a slot that allows a press fit metal insert. *(c)* Two of the screw holes are called "predictive" (double blue circles) because they coincide with the reconstruction plate screw holes.

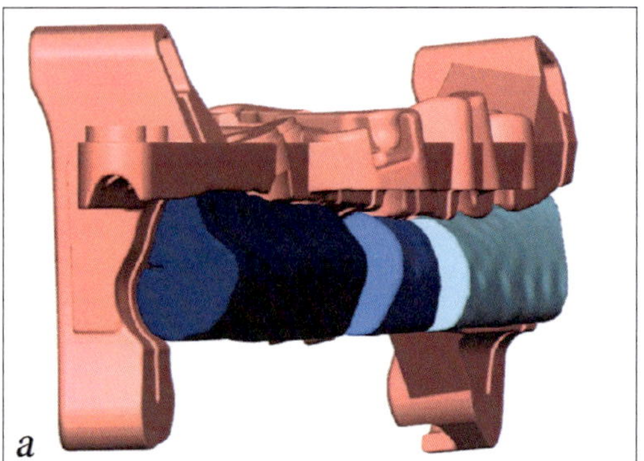

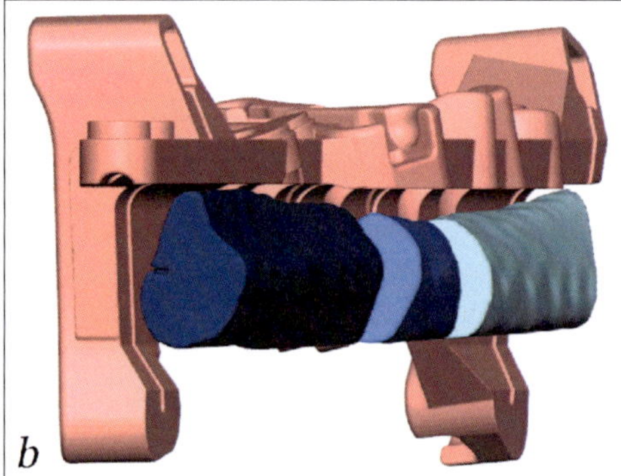

Figure 2-91 For the same case, compare the adaptation of the inner surface of the combination fibula-implant guide to the graft. *(a)* An "anatomic" fit is patient specific and offers the best indexing. *(b)* A "generic" and L-shaped inner surface to allow the microvascular surgeon maximum freedom to slide the guide along the length of the fibula.

designing the guide. Undercuts are eliminated via virtual parallel blockout, and a slight relief space is incorporated to ensure that the guide seats completely, without binding. The same rectangular osteotomy planes used during planning are brought back to generate saw guiding walls (Fig 2-89) or slots for metal surgical inserts (Fig 2-90b and c). The actual inserts are cemented or press-fitted following the 3D printing of the guide. Metal surgical inserts work well in guiding the reciprocating saw when access to the site is unhindered; however, when access is restricted, such as with osteotomies at or near the condylar neck, saw guiding walls are recommended. While periodontally stable teeth are extremely helpful in accurately indexing surgical guides, many patients are either completely edentulous or present with resection margins far away from the dentition. In such circumstances where guide support cannot be derived from natural dentition, bone-supported mandibulectomy guides are used (Fig 2-90).

Bone-supported mandibulectomy guide

The process of designing a bone-supported mandibulectomy guide is similar to that of a tooth-supported mandibulectomy guide. The biggest difference between the two is that a chimeric model is not needed, as guide support is solely derived from osseous structures. The bone-supported mandibulectomy guide is designed to index to the inferior or posterior borders of the mandible after raising a full-thickness flap. Retention of these guides is achieved with bone fixation screws. Ideally, the screw holes for the mandibulectomy guide should correspond with the screw holes for the custom titanium reconstruction plate. When the two screw holes coincide, they are called "predictive holes" (Fig 2-90c).

Combination fibula-implant surgical guide

The next guide to be designed digitally is the combination fibula-implant osteotomy guide. This guide is responsible for directing the surgeon in cutting the fibula and placing the dental implants. There are four components to this guide that must be considered during the design process, including features that allow for guide indexing, guide fixation, fibula osteotomy guidance, and implant osteotomy guidance.

1. **Guide Indexing:** The guide is designed to saddle the fibula barrel on its ventral and lateral borders where the soft tissue is thinnest (Fig 2-91a and b). The guide should not be designed to saddle the medial border because the peroneal vascular bundle and the dissected tibialis posterior muscle run adjacent to it. Likewise, the dorsal border should not be saddled due to the presence of the septocutaneous perforator vessels and the flexor hallucis longus muscle (see Fig 2-79).

   Once the design is finalized, it may be helpful to obtain a measurement in the software from the distalmost portion of the guide to the lateral malleolus of the fibula (Fig 2-93a) so the surgical guide can be indexed intraoperatively at the intended position

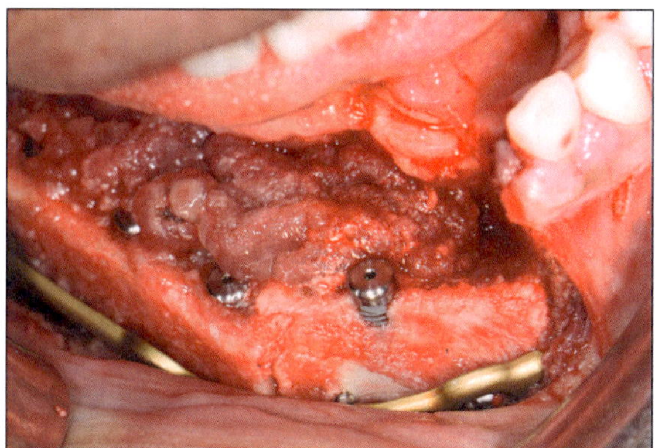

Figure 2-92 Implants entering the ventral fibular spine risk exposed threads.

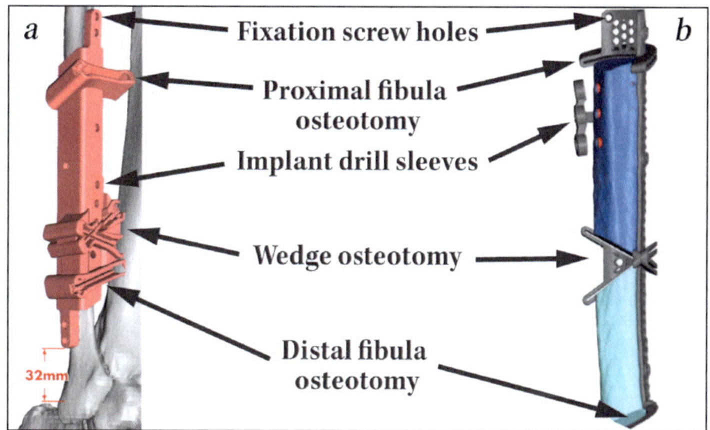

Figure 2-93 *(a)* CAD of a nylon fibula-implant guide seated. Notice the 32 mm measurement from the malleolus to the guide helps intraoperative orientation. *(b)* CAD of a metal guide. Notice that metal inserts are not needed. Multiple fixation screw holes retain the guide during instrumentation. Implant drill sleeves enable fully guided implant placement. Note that the implants for example (a) enter the ventral fibula border, and for example (b), they enter the dorsal fibula border.

along the fibula. However, because the exact position of the perforator vessels is identified intraoperatively with an arterial Doppler, the microvascular surgeon may need to slide the surgical guide proximally or distally from the planned location in order to best position the vessels and skin paddle over the fibula.

Because the cross-sectional geometry of the fibula changes considerably along its length and becomes more triangular toward the knee (Ide et al., 2015), moving the guide proximally from the intended location may result in dental implants being placed through the ventral spine and result in implant thread fenestrations (Fig 2-92). This is especially common in large, angle-to-angle mandibular defects that require more fibula length. Intimate indexing of the guide in such scenarios is even more important to prevent the rotation of the fibula axis.

Due to the reasons mentioned above, microvascular surgeons may prefer surgical guides of varying levels of adaptation to the fibula. The most intimate fit is achieved with a level of adaptation called "anatomic" and allows for the best precision. The generic option, with a cross section shaped like an L offers the guide the most freedom to slide along the length of the fibula (Fig 2-91). A third hybrid option is also available, which offers an intermediate level of both indexing and sliding.

2. **Guide Fixation:** The combination fibula-implant surgical guide needs to be secured to the fibula prior to surgical instrumentation. Fixation of the surgical guide is achieved via fixation screws (Fig 2-93). At least three well-distributed screw holes should be incorporated to prevent movement or unseating of the guide, regardless of how well the guide is indexed.
3. **Fibula Osteotomy Guidance:** The rectangular planes used to simulate the mandibulectomy and fibula osteotomies are toggled back on when designing the combination fibula-implant surgical guide. For polymer-based surgical guides, a slot is generated over each rectangular plane. Once the guide is 3D printed, metal surgical sleeves are cemented or press-fitted into each individual slot. For metal-based surgical guides, no separate metal inserts are required because the sleeves are designed and 3D printed as part of the guide in a monolithic fashion. The biggest advantage of metal surgical guides is rigidity, which allows for guides of lower profile and smaller size to be produced. Examples of combination fibula-implant surgical guides are shown in Fig 2-93. The fibulas in both cases will be cut into two segments for mandibular reconstruction and require four osteotomy planes: the distal fibula plane, the proximal fibula plane, and two planes for a wedge osteotomy between the two fibula segments.
4. **Implant Osteotomy Guidance:** Digital implant drill sleeves are imported over the positions of the proposed dental implants. If fully guided implant surgery is considered, the drill sleeve models of proper dimensions specific to the implant system of choice must be selected. For polymer-based surgical guides, a recess slightly larger in diameter than the drill sleeve is generated so the actual sleeve can be cemented or press-fitted into the recess after guide manufacturing. For metal-based surgical guides, this is not necessary, as the sleeve can be printed as part of the guide.

A combination fibula-implant surgical guide where the implant drill sleeves are suspended over the dorsal surface of the fibula, remote from the ventral and lateral surfaces where the actual guide is indexed, is shown in Fig 2-93b. As mentioned before, this is sometimes done to avoid placing dental implants through the thin osseous spine of some fibulas. Additionally, because the dorsal border of the fibula is where the septocutaneous perforators and flexor hallucis longus muscle are located, a larger relief space needs to be prescribed to avoid potential impediments to seating the guide. This is why the implant drill sleeves are suspended rather than contacting the fibula. Lastly, due to the increased distance from the top of the implant drill sleeves to the fibula cortex, longer twist drills may need to be made available in the OR.

The completed designs are forwarded to the prosthodontist and surgeons for final verification. After approval, the guides are 3D printed. Quality assurance is carried out by assessing the fit and accuracy of the biomedical engineer, surgeon, and prosthodontist followed by sterilization.

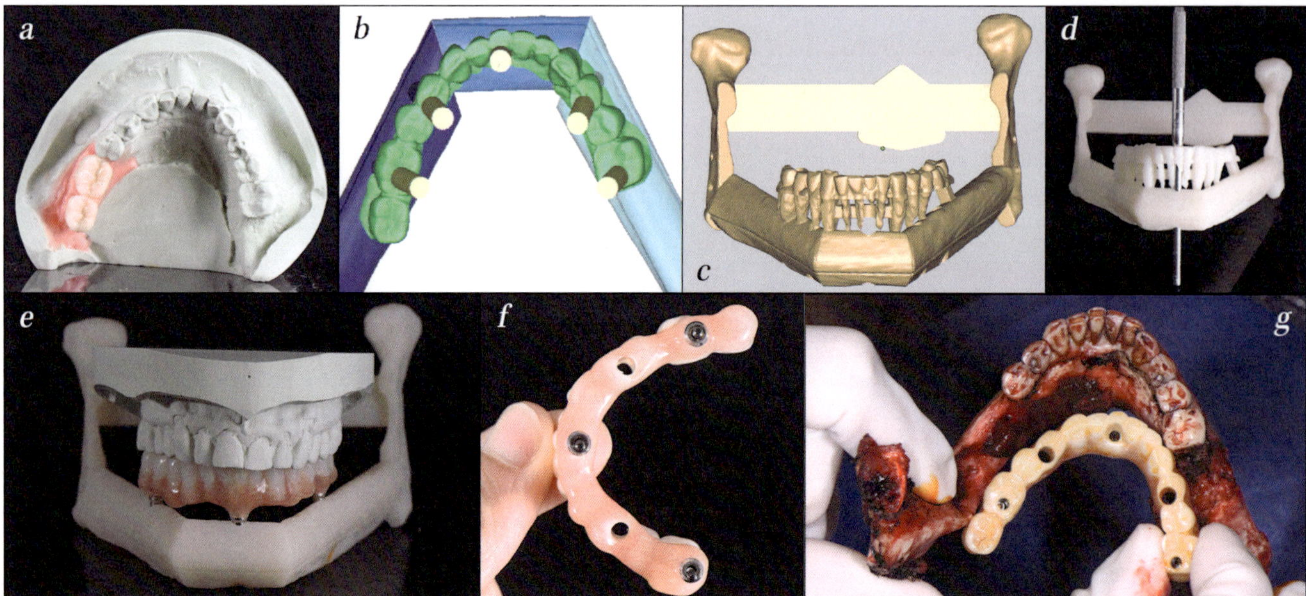

Figure 2-94 Sequence for making an implant-borne articulation splint (IBAS). *(a)* The diagnostic cast is digitized in a lab scanner and merged with the head CT prior to planning. Note the tooth arrangement in the edentulous area. *(b)* Completed plan with five cylinders as placeholders for the implants extending through the occlusal table. *(c)* CAD of the reconstructed mandible with floating native dentition. *(d)* Printed reconstructed mandible and dentition, with cylinders Boolean-subtracted from the fibula and teeth. Note the dental instrument fits through the lateral incisor and the neomandible. *(e)* Implant analogs seated into the planned osteotomies, followed by connection of titanium cylinders. Autopolymerizing acrylic resin is used to lute the titanium cylinders to the printed teeth and to fill in the interdental spaces. *(f)* Completed and polished IBAS. Note that the second implant site in the lateral fibula segments was left empty for intraoperative use. *(g)* IBAS adjacent to the resected specimen.

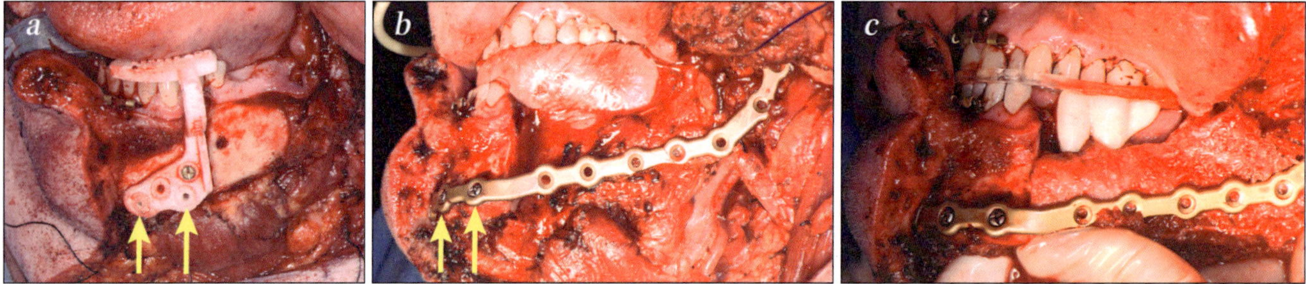

Figure 2-95 *(a)* Seated tooth and bone-supported mandibulectomy guide, retained with one bone screw. Note that two predictive screw holes *(arrows)* match the screw holes of the custom plate. *(b and c)* The IBAS-fibula complex is articulated to the opposing dentition via an interocclusal splint.

Implant-borne articulation splint (IBAS)

An implant-borne articulation splint (IBAS; Sukato et al., 2023) is crucial for orienting the osteotomized fibula segment(s) that houses the dental implants during insetting. The biomedical engineer is asked to "subtract" the cylinders (representative of the proposed dental implants) from the reconstructed neomandible and the native dentition, wax-ups, or trial denture setup with the computer operation Boolean Difference to generate implant osteotomies in the 3D-printed model. When using a 4 mm wide implant analog, the authors have requested a 4.15 mm wide osteotomy in the reconstruction model to allow a comfortable press fit of the implant analog. One implant analog per fibula segment is press-fitted into the printed model to the planned depth. Titanium cylinders are screwed into the analogs and luted to the printed teeth with autopolymerizing acrylic resin. Prosthetic gingiva can then be created using pink autopolymerizing acrylic resin followed by polishing. Figure 2-94 shows the full sequence of fabricating an IBAS.

Intraoperatively, the IBAS is screwed directly to the implants with abutment screws. The fibula-IBAS complex is articulated against the maxillary dentition while the reconstructive surgeon fixates the fibula segment(s) with a custom reconstruction plate. A more detailed description of its intraoperative utilization can be found in the section below entitled "Surgical phase."

Surgical phase

The sterilized models, guides, and articulation splint are then transferred to the OR. A full-thickness flap is raised to expose the mandible and allow the seating of the bone-supported or combination tooth- and bone-supported osteotomy guide (Fig 2-95a). Fixation is

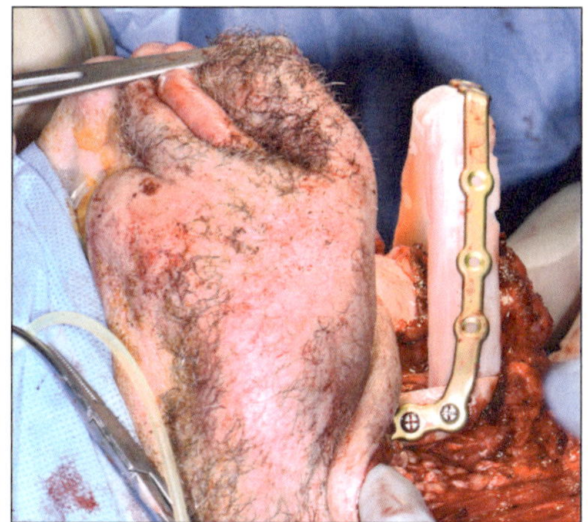

Figure 2-96 Custom-milled plate is fixated using predictive holes. Note that the reconstruction model is checked to fit.

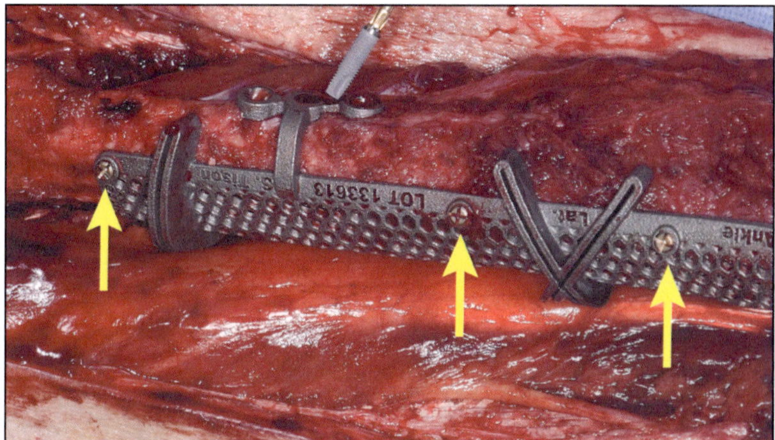

Figure 2-97 Fibula raised. Fibula-implant guide seated and secured with bone screws *(arrows)*. Fully guided implant surgery is performed while the vascular pedicle is still intact.

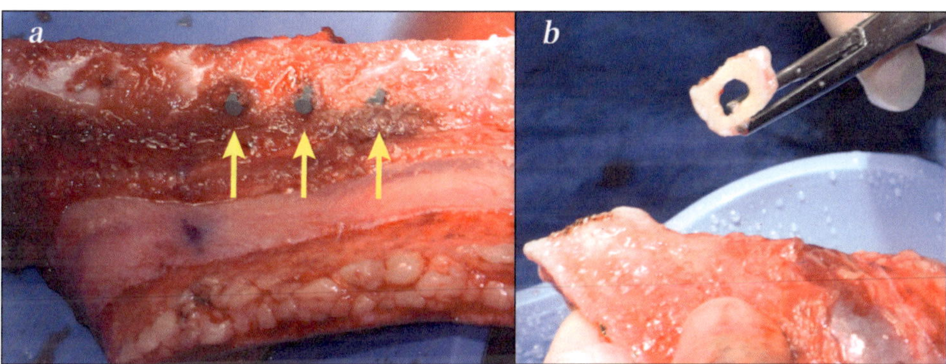

Figure 2-98 Effective bicortical engagement of the fibula requires perforating the inferior cortex. *(a)* Notice the implant apices *(arrows)* on this fibula prior to wedge osteotomies. *(b)* Notice the empty marrow space of the discarded wedge osteotomy.

achieved with monocortical bone screws. If "predictive holes" were planned, then these osteotomies are made to align and secure the custom-milled reconstruction plate (Fig 2-95a and b). The mandible osteotomies are completed with a reciprocating saw using either a wall or slot guide. Once the specimen is removed, the custom reconstruction plate is seated and fixated using the predictive holes on either end (Fig 2-95b). Prior to making the graft osteotomies, the fit of the neomandible reconstructed model can be verified (Fig 2-96).

While the ablative surgeon resects the lesion, the reconstruction team raises the osteomyocutaneous flap. When the fibula is employed, the ablative and reconstructive teams work simultaneously. Before seating the combination fibula-implant osteotomy guide, an arterial Doppler is used to auscultate and locate the perforator vessels at the dorsal border of the fibula. Because bicortical osteotomies are prepared for the implants, it is important that the twist drills do not damage this/these vessel(s), especially when a skin paddle will be used to close a soft tissue or glossectomy defect. In situations where the implant osteotomies are initiated at the dorsal border, auscultation of the perforators is even more critical. The combination fibula-implant osteotomy guide is secured to the fibula, using a predetermined measurement from the lateral malleolus for orientation.

Once the guide is oriented and seated to the ventrolateral border of the fibula, it is secured with bone screws (Fig 2-97). Using the implant drill sleeves, the implant osteotomies are performed, followed by implant installation in a fully guided fashion. The implant osteotomy begins with a 2 mm twist drill to place the first pilot osteotomy using the implant osteotomy guide secured on the fibula. The drill will perforate both fibula cortices for bicortical stabilization. Wider osteotomy drills are used sequentially until the implant osteotomy diameter is near the planned implant width. Then a screw tap of the same width as the planned implant is used to the full depth, engaging both cortices (Fig 2-98). This is followed by the use of a countersink to widen the crestal area of the fibula to allow passive seating of the implant head, and subsequently, the abutment. Of note, the tactile feedback of placing an implant into the prepared fibula osteotomy is different from alveolar bone, since the fibula has a hollow marrow space (Fig 2-98b). Because these guides are made for a fully guided approach, they maintain the implant trajectory across the hollow marrow space and ensure the apex enters the second fibular cortex.

With the guide still secured, the reconstructive surgeon sections off the fibula with an oscillating saw. Because a guide diminishes the tactile feedback perceived when the saw blade completes the cut—particularly when both sides of the cut are secured to a rigid guide—great care is needed to avoid damaging the peroneal vessels. Some surgeons may prefer to perform two-thirds of each osteotomy guided and then remove the guide and complete the osteotomies freehand. While free-handing can incur some inaccuracy, it is balanced against the full tactile feedback of completing the osteotomy and protecting the pedicle. Next, the intersegment wedges are dissected out to maintain soft tissue connection between segments (Fig 2-99a).

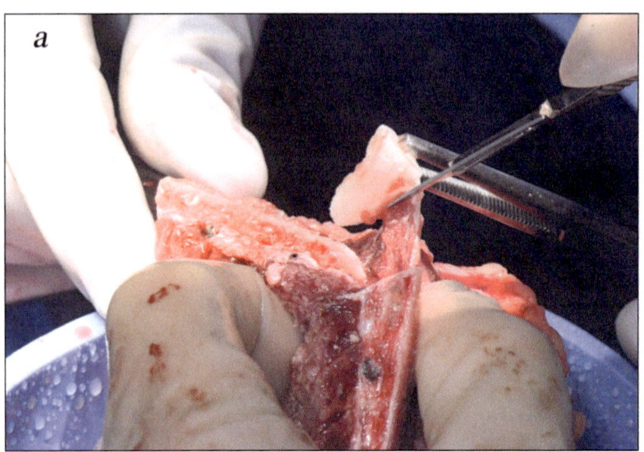
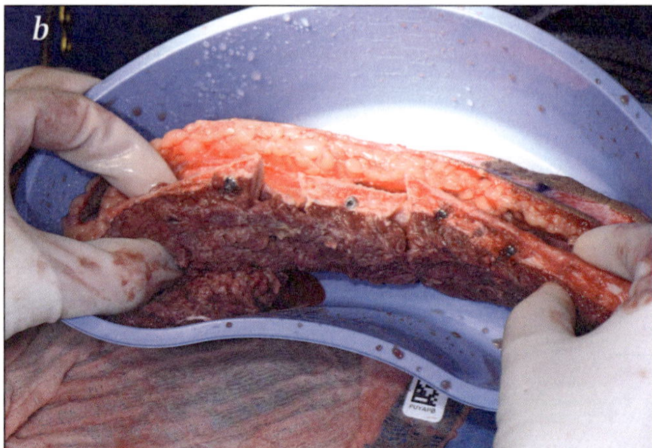

Figure 2-99 Preparing the fibula graft. *(a)* Wedge osteotomy is dissected out from between two fibula segments. *(b)* Tri-segment fibula ready to receive IBAS.

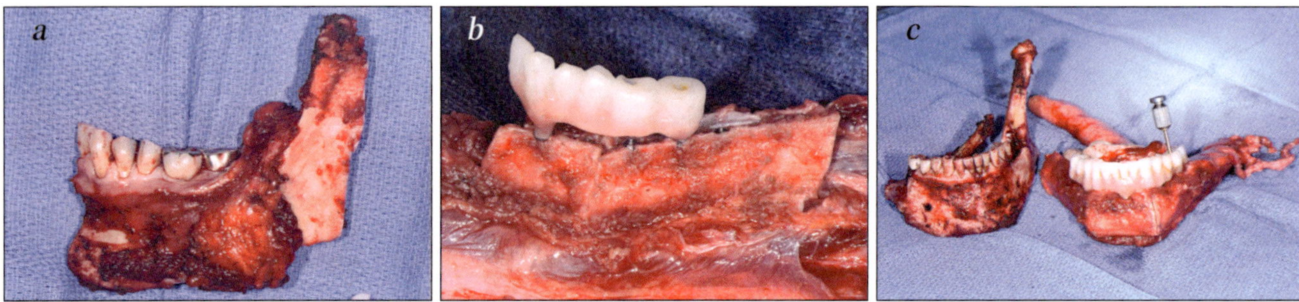

Figure 2-100 Example of *(a and b)* a midline-to-angle and *(c)* angle-to-angle mandibulectomy specimen adjacent the fibula-IBAS complex ready to articulate with the maxillary dentition for insetting of the osteomyocutaneous free flap. Abutment screws were used to secure the IBAS direct to implants in graft to articulate the bi- and tri-segment fibula reconstruction. Note that the prosthetic teeth for the IBAS are the patients' 3D-printed dentition.

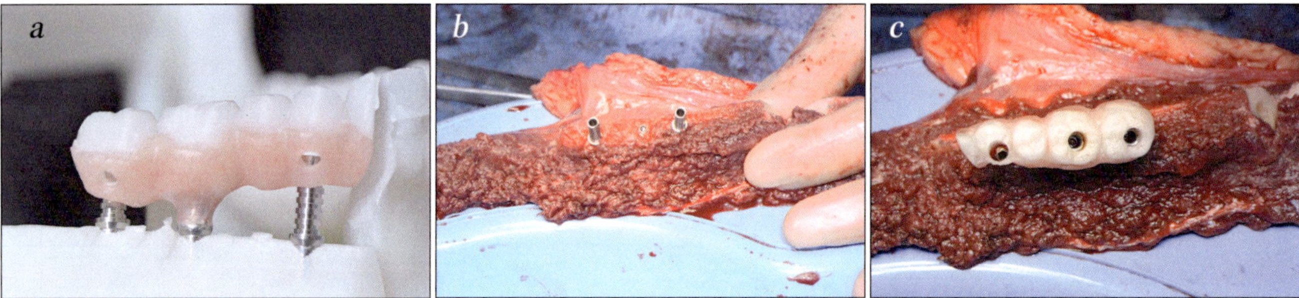

Figure 2-101 Example of lateral mandibulectomy requiring a uni-segment fibula. *(a)* Completed IBAS on the model. Notice that only one titanium cylinder was luted, and two were free. *(b)* The two free titanium cylinders were seated directly to the fixture. *(c)* The IBAS slips into position, and all three abutment screws were hand tightened. At this point, the fibula-IBAS complex was ready to articulate with the maxillary dentition for insetting of the osteomyocutaneous free flap.

The prosthodontist seats the IBAS directly to the implant fixtures and hand tightens the abutment screws (Figs 2-100b and c). This effectively splints the bi- and tri-segment fibulas; limits freedom in pitch, roll, and yaw; and allows the complex to articulate as one unit with the opposing maxillary dentition directly, or, in conjunction with an interocclusal splint, at the correct occlusal vertical dimension (OVD).

When a uni-segment fibula is planned, antirotation of the IBAS to the graft is achieved by employing one other titanium cylinder. Because preluting more than one cylinder would make it unlikely that they would seat passively, instead, additional cylinders in any one segment are left free (Fig 2-101a). At the time of surgery, the free titanium cylinders are seated first (Fig 2-101b), followed by slipping the IBAS over them (Fig 2-101c). Finally, all abutment screws are hand tightened. Because the titanium cylinders fit snugly into the printed channels, they provide antirotation of the IBAS.

The entire composite flap with the IBAS is then transferred to the oral cavity defect and articulated to the remaining maxillary dentition (Fig 2-102). Once the fidelity of the articulation is verified, the microvascular surgeon completes the insetting to the native mandible using fixation screws and either prebent, or custom, locking mechanism reconstruction plates. The IBAS is removed, and cover screws or healing abutment are seated (Fig 2-103a). Healing abutments are preferred over cover screws because they are more easily

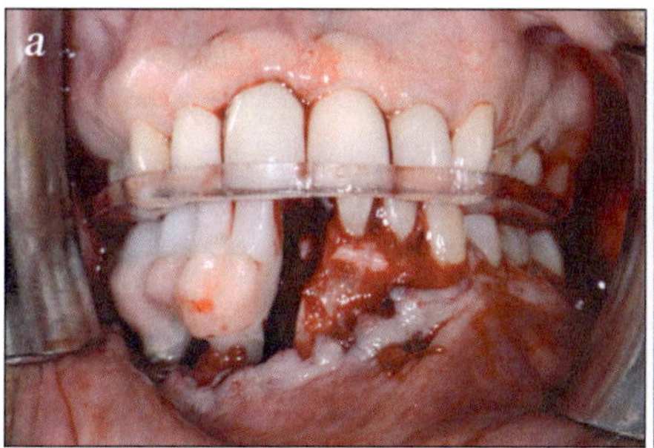
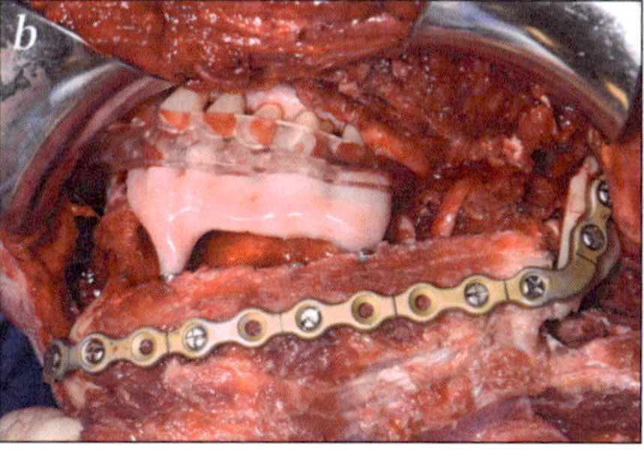
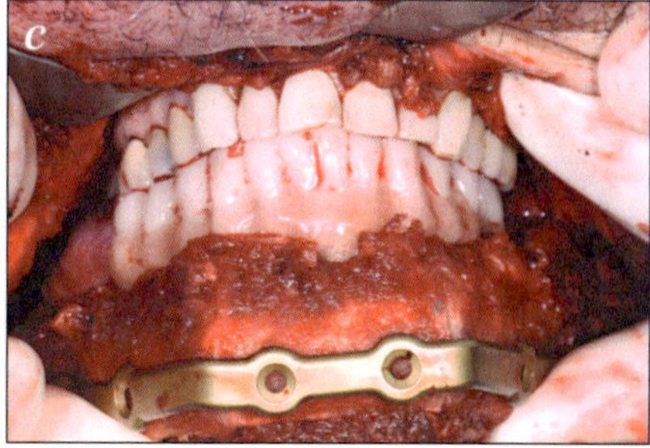

Figure 2-102 Three examples of using an IBAS to inset FFFs. *(a)* Uni-segment fibula for an ameloblastoma. *(b)* Bisegment fibula for a clear cell odontogenic carcinoma. *(c)* Tri-segment fibula for bilateral ORN. Notice that articulation with full-arch IBAS was adequately stabilized without the use of an interocclusal splint.

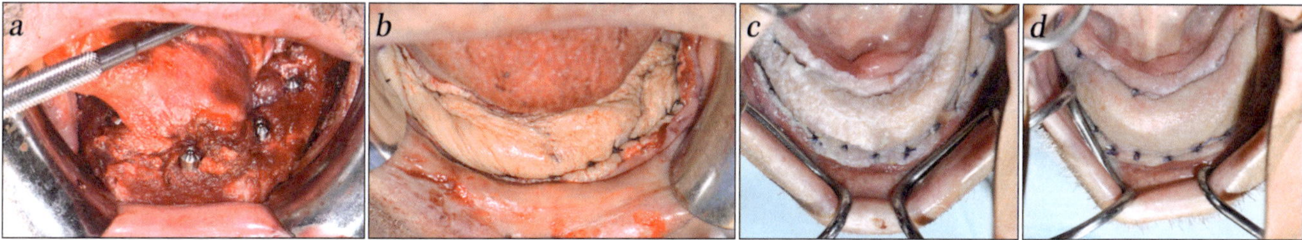

Figure 2-103 Reconstruction of an angle-to-angle mandibulectomy with a FFF. *(a)* Five mm tall healing abutments torqued into place. *(b)* Soft tissue closure with the skin paddle. *(c and d)* Fifteen and thirty days post surgery.

palpated through the skin paddle during stage II implant surgery. Notice that in Fig 2-103a, a 5 mm tall healing abutment is at an even height with the dissected muscle when implants enter the dorsal fibula border. Cover screws are preferred when a skin paddle is not needed, and the soft tissue defect is closed primarily. The microvascular surgeon then proceeds to complete the anastomosis of the donor vessels to the recipient counterparts before finally completing soft tissue closure (Fig 2-103b).

The patient remains under hospital care for an average of 10 days. The patient returns for a follow-up with the surgeon one month after surgery, and necessary adjunctive treatments are arranged. At this time, the patient should also be seen by the prosthodontist to evaluate the dental condition, reinforce oral hygiene practices, evaluate occlusion of any remaining teeth, and evaluate maximum incisal opening. If the patient is to undergo adjuvant radiotherapy (see Chapter 1), the patient undergoes a preradiation evaluation, which inevitably includes a radiation stent, such as a tongue depressor and the fabrication of custom fluoride carriers.

Postsurgical Phase and Interim Mandibular Resection Prostheses

The interim phase is defined as the period after tumor ablation until a definitive prosthesis is delivered. The first step is an assessment of tongue function, as it is the prime predictor of future oral function. If tongue function and mobility are compromised, aspiration or silent aspiration into the lungs must be assessed by a speech and swallow specialist (see later section "Oral Swallow Function in the Head and Neck Cancer Patients"). Some patients will require the fitting of an interim palatal augmentation prosthesis (PAP; see later section titled "Speech and deglutition aids").

Second, the extent of the defect, hard and soft tissue reconstruction, and healing associated with the surgical site are evaluated. Prosthetic space is assessed especially when soft tissue defects are closed with a skin paddle. Scapula, iliac crest, and FFF can result in the complete obliteration of prosthetic space (Fig 2-104a and b). The number, distribution, and status of remaining dentition, occlusion, and maximum interincisal opening (MIO) need to be evaluated. When patients present with trismus, the use of a dynamic jaw-mobilizing device is prescribed, and until one is available, instructions for assisted opening exercises should be given. Lastly, the need for adjuvant radiotherapy will affect how to move forward with secondary surgeries, such as the debulking of skin flaps or whether implants can be considered postradiation (see Chapter 1, the section on "Dental Implants in Irradiated Tissues," and the section on "Secondary Surgical Procedures" below)—if they were not placed primarily at the time of surgical reconstruction. Patients with few or no remaining teeth have the most to gain from dental implants. Patients who are rendered completely edentulous, especially when they lack prior experience with a denture, unless tongue function is nearly normal, are not candidates for an interim prosthesis until there is complete soft tissue healing, debulking, and vestibuloplasty. Dental implants should be considered after carefully scrutinizing isodose curves. Sites that receive over 65 Gy should be avoided.

The prosthodontist should plan for any necessary restorative procedures and occlusal adjustments. For patients with small lateral segmental or marginal resections with no involvement of the tongue, a shortened dental arch can be an acceptable outcome. If anterior teeth are not involved in the resection, some mandibulectomy patients will prefer not to wear a removable prosthesis, especially in the interim period of healing, or during postsurgical radiotherapy when acute

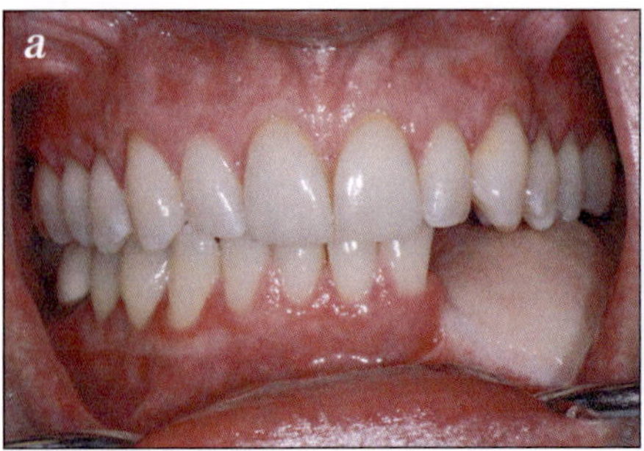
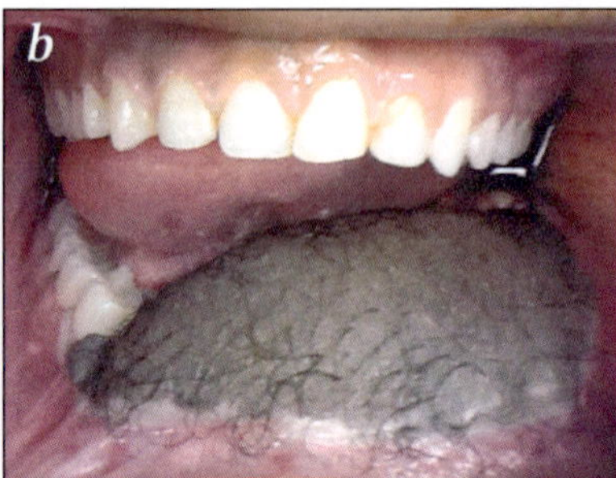
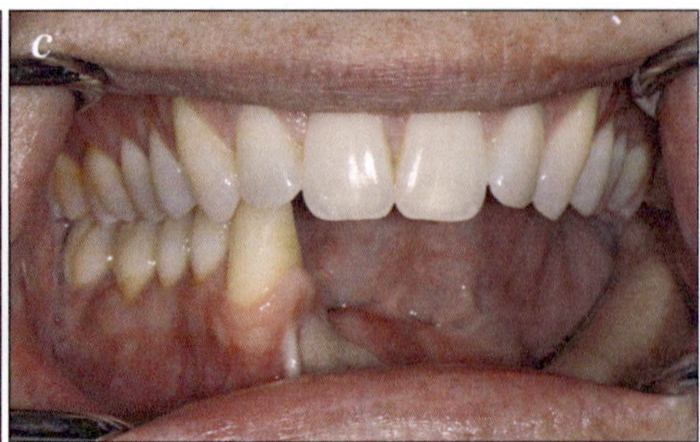

Figure 2-104 Varying presentations status postmandibulectomy and FFF reconstruction. *(a)* Lateral segmental resection of an SCC. Excellent postop occlusion, little compromise in esthetics; however, no prosthetic space until flap debulking is performed. *(b)* Latero-symphyseal resection of an ameloblastoma. The bulk of soft tissue interferes with occlusion and obliterates prosthetic space. Paradoxically, the excess bulk masks the lack of anterior teeth by providing lip support. *(c)* Latero-symphyseal segmental resection of an osteosarcoma. The lack of lip support affects resting and smiling cosmesis. This patient is a good candidate for an interim MRP (see Fig 2-105b).

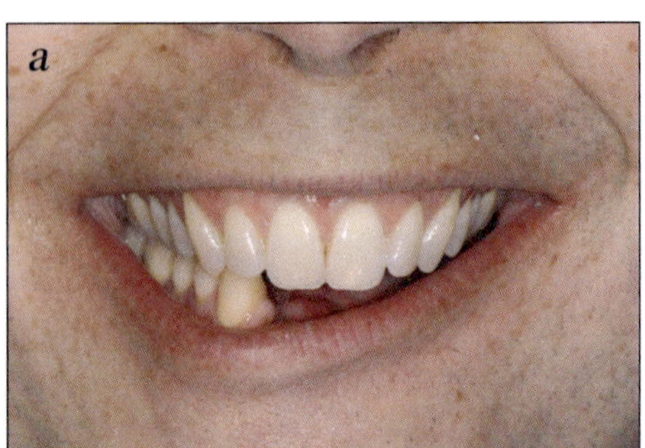
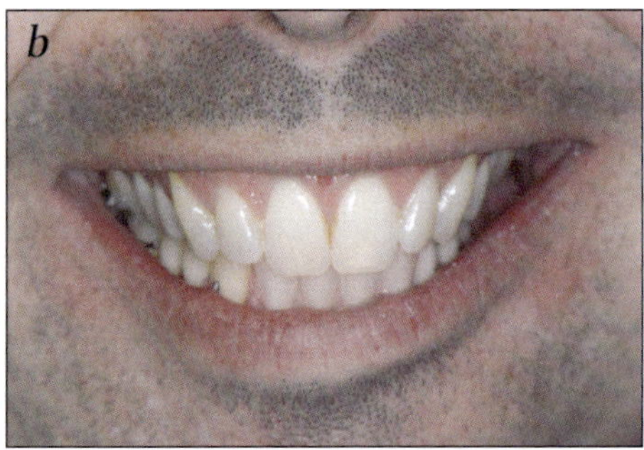

Figure 2-105 Lateral and symphyseal segmental mandibular resection of an osteosarcoma, restored with a FFF. *(a)* Postoperative presentation, lacking anterior and left posterior dentition. Note the lack of lip support. *(b)* Interim MRP restoring smile esthetics, providing lip support, and improving lip valving.

effects of radiation and caries may be a major consideration. Because interim prostheses can complicate oral hygiene, they may be contraindicated if esthetics are not a major concern. A lateral defect that does not extend to the ipsilateral canine will gain little from an interim mandibular resection prosthesis (MRP). They are also advised to delay prosthetic rehabilitation until the flap has fully healed.

In contrast, segmental mandibulectomies that cross the midline are better candidates for an interim MRP. These patients incur greater morbidities, including a bilateral loss of lower lip sensation, complete loss of lip support, and sequela, such as compromised salivary control and speech, altered lower facial third esthetics, and an aged appearance (Fig 2-105).

When too few teeth remain, especially when they are in poor periodontal health, the interim MRP may worsen their condition by exerting additional forces. The situation is exacerbated when the extension base rests on a redundant and bulky tissue flap. In these situations, it would be prudent to await full healing of the flap reconstruction—6 months—followed by flap debulking. The best candidates for an interim MRP are partially dentate patients with latero-symphyseal or symphyseal defects with reasonably good occlusion and periodontally sound dentition (Figs 2-105 through 2-108).

Purposes and benefits of an interim mandibular resection prosthesis

An interim MRP is an important diagnostic tool for determining the design of the definitive prosthesis. It may be an option during the extended healing phase in order to improve esthetics and lip support, which in turn helps with lip valving, seal, and saliva control. The interim prosthesis is also used to assess whether a patient will adapt to and be satisfied with a removable prosthesis (Fig 2-106). When a removable prosthesis is supported by displaceable tissue, a trampoline effect may cause an unseating of the prosthesis. While Some patients will develop the necessary neuromuscular control to retain the extension base, others will grow intolerant of the unstable prosthesis and direct the treatment to debulking the flap. Furthermore, the interim MRP may elucidate the need for additional prosthetic space, to allow proper extensions and thicknesses of restorative materials. Finally, the interim prosthesis can be used in the planning of secondary dental implants.

An interim prosthesis can be worn prior to, during, and after debulking or dental implant surgeries. In situations when debulking is warranted, the existing interim prosthesis can be relined intraoperatively and used as a stent for a vestibuloplasty (see subsequent section titled "Secondary Surgical Procedures").

Lastly, an interim prosthesis is beneficial when definitive treatment will be delayed for an extensive period. The interim MRP may prevent supraeruption of the opposing maxillary dentition.

Glossectomy patients will require coordinated therapy with speech and swallow specialists and the fabrication of palatal augmentation prostheses (see section titled "Speech and Deglutition Aids").

Fabrication of interim mandibular resection prostheses

Tooth modification is performed to create proximal and lingual guide planes (Fig 2-107). Because of the natural lingual tilt of mandibular molars (curve of Wilson), preparing a long lingual guide

Figure 2-106 *(a)* Symphyseal marginal mandibular resection of an ameloblastoma. Notice the lack of attached soft tissues secondary to the primary closure of the mucosa. *(b)* Interim MRP restoring smile esthetics, providing lip support.

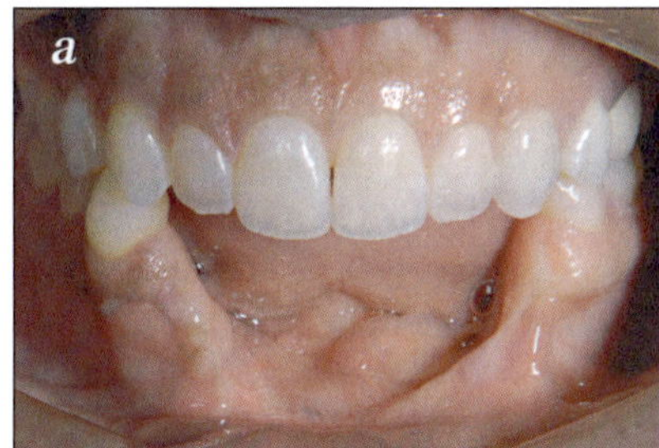

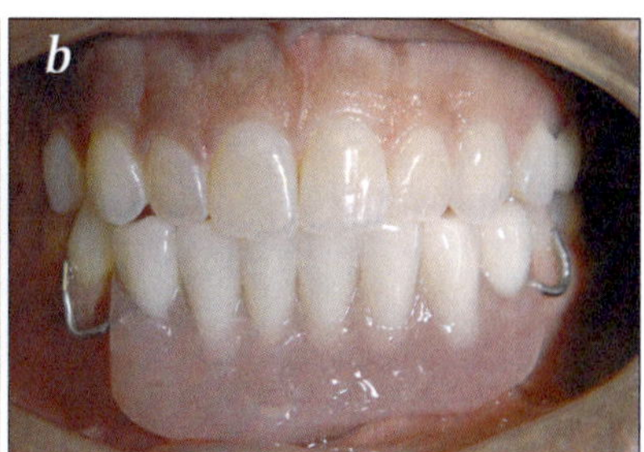

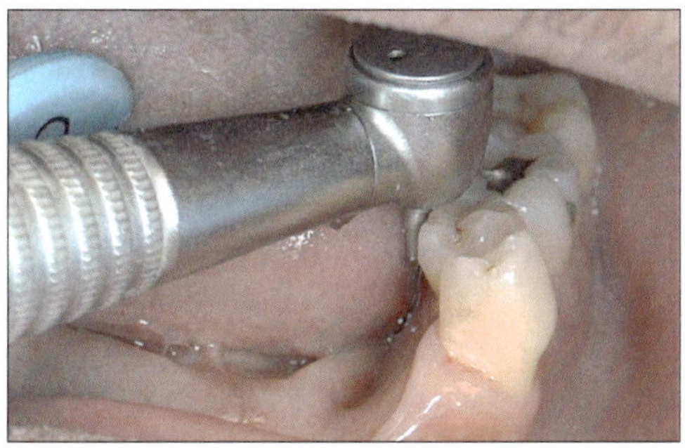

Figure 2-107 Proximal and lingual guide planes are critical to maximizing bracing and indirect retention of interim and definitive, removable MRPs.

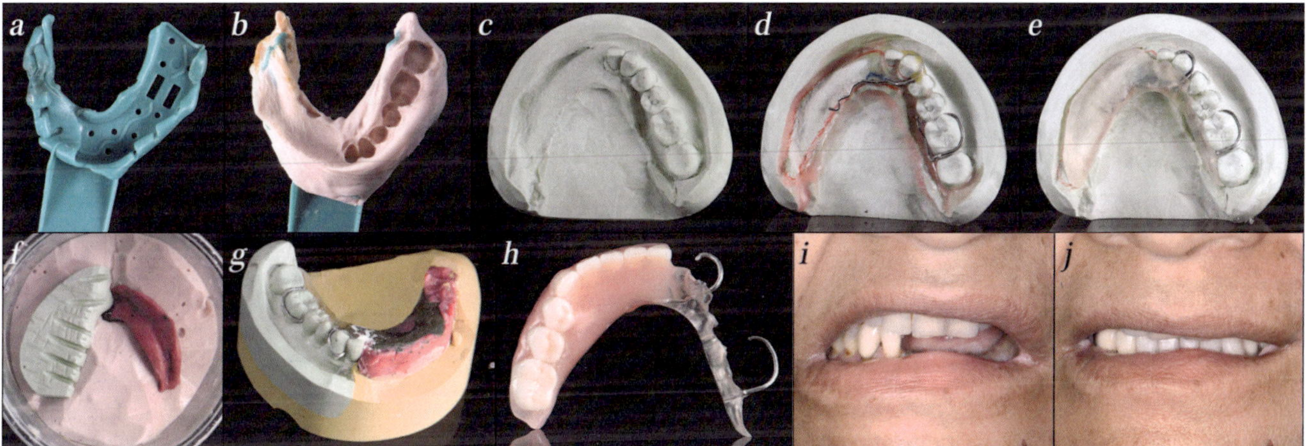

Figure 2-108 Latero-symphyseal segmental mandibular resection of an epidermoid carcinoma, restored with a FFF. *(a)* A plastic stock tray is thermoplastically customized. *(b)* Alginate impression. *(c, d, and e)* Initial type V stone cast is surveyed, heights of contour marked, undercuts measured, prosthesis design drawn, wire clasps adapted, parallel wax blockout applied, tinfoil substituted applied, and a base fabricated with autopolymerizing PMMA. *(e and f)* The base is tried, adjusted, and used to make a corrected impression and interocclusal record. *(g)* The altered cast is made and mounted. *(h)* Prosthetic teeth are waxed up and processed onto the previously made base with autocuring PMMA. *(i and j)* Before and after smiles. Notice the improved cosmesis.

plane will establish a more definite path of insertion, improve stability, and resist lifting of the contralateral side. Lastly, occlusal embrasure rests should be considered so that a minimum of two wrought wire retainers can be adapted without interfering with the occlusion. Avoid retainers on mandibular incisors.

Given the altered denture-bearing anatomy and/or presence of trismus, a plastic stock tray allows for thermoplastic customization to optimally impress the hard and soft tissues (Fig 2-108a). In the presence of trismus, avoid trimming tray flanges to shorten them. This makes an already flexible plastic tray even more so. Instead, consider flaming the flanges with an alcohol torch and folding them occlusally. This achieves the goal of shortening the flange while maintaining some rigidity (Fig 2-108a). A reinforced stone cast is surveyed, and the interim MRP is designed. Wire clasps are adapted to engage 0.02″ undercuts (Fig 2-108d). Parallel wax blockout is applied, and clear autopolymerizing PMMA is used to make a base (Fig 2-108e). The extension base is used to make an altered cast impression and an initial interocclusal record (Fig 2-108f and g). Attention is paid during the border molding to the idealized lip support on the defect side. After verifying the occlusion, esthetics, and phonetics, denture teeth are processed onto the base with autopolymerizing PMMA (Fig 2-108h).

The patient is followed, and the functional benefits are assessed. Procedures that can improve retention, stability and support, and ultimately comfort and performance include single or splinted surveyed abutment crowns, skin flap debulking and vestibuloplasty, and finally, osseointegrated implants.

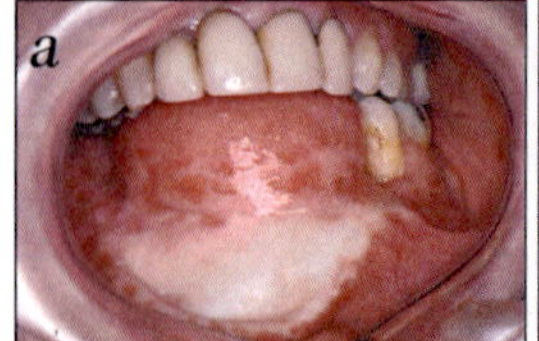
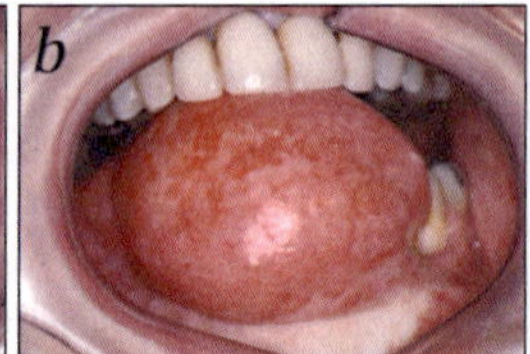
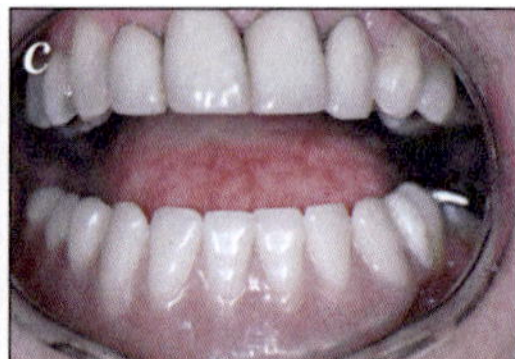
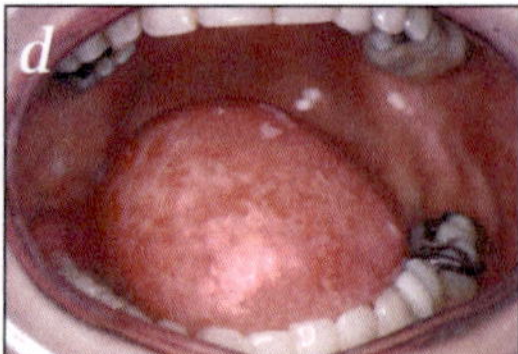
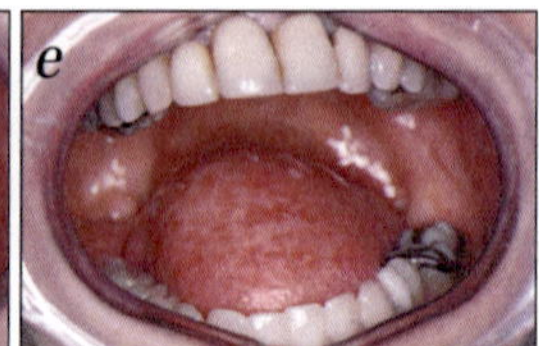

Figure 2-109 *(a)* Total glossectomy restored with free flap with tongue at rest. *(b)* Reconstructed tongue valving with maxillary anterior teeth during speech. *(c)* Prosthesis inserted. Note the position of the reconstructed tongue during the production of the /S/ sound. *(d)* Reconstructed tongue elevated with prosthesis in position. *(e)* Prosthesis in position, tongue at rest. Speech was intelligible.

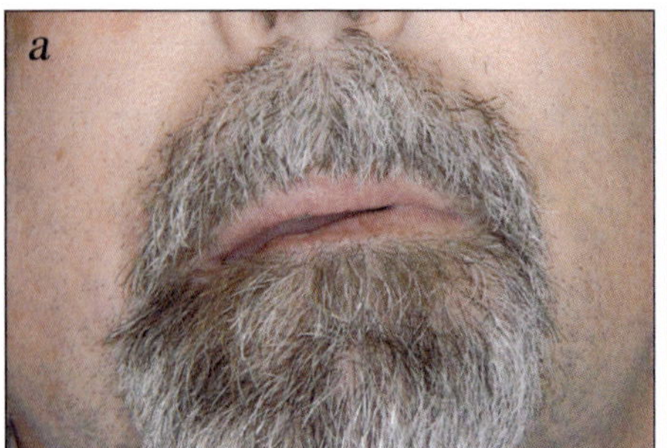
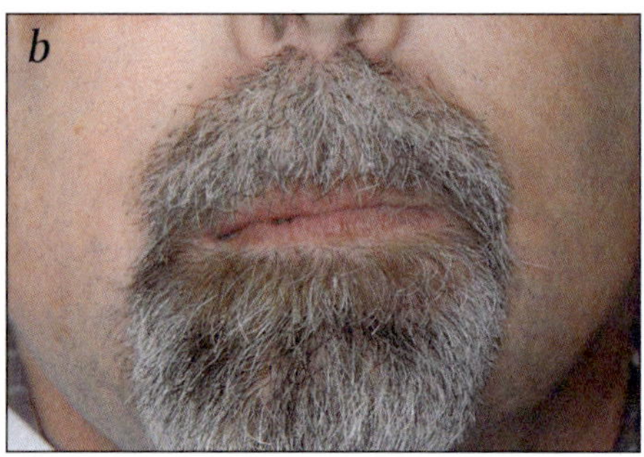

Figure 2-110 Right mandibulectomy with free flap reconstruction. Resection of, or injury to the marginal mandibular nerve resulted in lip incompetence. *(a)* Note the lip is retracted and the commissures lowered in repose. *(b)* Attempt to purse the lips results in incomplete lip closure.

Morbidities and Physiology of Oral Function Following Resections

The nature and extent of the disability is dependent upon the location and size of the tumor, the impact of radiation and/or chemotherapy, the structures and volume of tissue resected, the design of the surgical resection, and the method of reconstruction.

Prior to the development of modern microvascular surgical techniques, reconstructive efforts of the mandible were staged, and bone grafting was performed after soft tissue reconstruction via pedicled flaps.

However, due to improved outcomes and reliability, microvascular free flaps are currently considered the standard of care for the reconstruction of composite defects of the tongue and mandible (Patel et al., 2019). Because grafted tissues are no longer limited by anatomical constraints of regional pedicled flaps, the grafting of soft and hard tissues can be accomplished primarily following tumor ablation, avoiding many of the morbidities seen with the primary closure of soft tissue deficits, which would lead to tethering and immobile tongue, deviation of the remnant mandible, and so on. Therefore, delayed surgical reconstruction of the mandible and discontinuity defects are seldom observed.

Given the effectiveness of free flaps when they are properly configured, disabilities secondary to the resection of the tongue and lateral FOM tumors have been dramatically reduced.

In general, posterior lesions involving large portions of the base of the tongue, tonsillar fossa, and soft palate with extension onto the posterior pharyngeal wall, mandible, or combinations of these structures often result in the most significant disabilities. In these instances, the loss of large portions of the tongue, FOM, and mandible with subsequent loss of innervation from glossopharyngeal, hypoglossal, lingual, inferior alveolar, and marginal mandibular nerves complicate oral function.

On the other hand, large portions of the anterior tongue (50–60%) can be lost without significant functional deficits. The sensory and mobility status of the remaining tongue and the integrity of the mandible are key factors in functional rehabilitation. As larger volumes of tongue tissue are lost, compromise of oral functions is usually encountered with the accompanying risk of aspiration. The total glossectomy patient without flap reconstruction is infrequently encountered. Most of the flaps used to reconstruct the tongue are insensate and demonstrate varying degrees of mobility. However, if the bulk is carefully managed, they usually enhance functional rehabilitation when accompanied by a physiologically designed palatal augmentation prosthesis (PAP; Fig 2-109). With the use of this prosthesis, the improvement of speech is most frequently observed, followed by swallowing and, to a much lesser extent, mastication.

Anterior lesions involving the tongue, FOM, and mandible usually result in less severe functional impairment than posterior ones because of a lesser compromise to structural, sensory, or motor innervation. However, larger lesions that compromise the lips, preventing functional lip seal and salivary control, can be quite disabling (Fig 2-110). Control of saliva is profoundly affected by most resections of the tongue and mandible. These resections obliterate the lingual and buccal sulci and consequently are a means of collecting and channeling secretions posteriorly that no longer exist. In addition, the motor and sensory innervation of the lower lip on the resected side is often lost, adversely affecting oral competency and preventing the patient from detecting secretions escaping from the mouth. Impaired sensory innervation and poor tongue control and mobility also contribute to poor control of saliva. Individuals with unimpaired tongue function are capable of identifying escaping secretions and using the tongue to direct these secretions posteriorly to be swallowed. With compromised tongue function, this manipulation often is impossible. Drooling is compounded on the defect side by the drooping of the corner of the mouth. Cracking and large fissures develop, and these may become infected with Candida albicans (Fig 2-111).

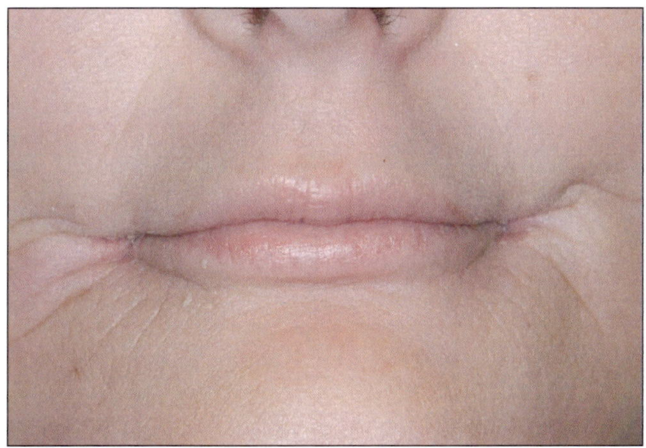

Figure 2-111 Candida albicans infections. Infection develops at the corner of the mouth, where cracks and fissures develop.

These patients often demonstrate deficits in speech articulation, drooling, and slurred speech secondary to the pooling of saliva and inadequate lip seal. Incompetent lip seal—whether sensory, motor, or structurally related—can be a major disability, affecting speech, mastication, and self-esteem and frequently challenging the prosthetic rehabilitation of the patient.

A number of structures resected during the course of a classic radical neck dissection may have prosthetic implications. The internal jugular vein is resected, predisposing to local venous congestion and edema that elevate the FOM, which may compromise the lingual extension of a mandibular complete denture into the retromylohyoid space. Resection of the marginal mandibular branch of the facial nerve results in a unilateral loss of the motor innervation of the muscles that control movements of the lower lip. Consequently, additional prosthetic support may be required for the lower lip.

For functional purposes, the mandible is considered to be the mobile stabilizing framework, which supports the tongue functions. The evolution of sound oncological surgical principles of preserving mandibular continuity whenever possible has done much to enhance postsurgical tongue status and oral functions. These procedures include median and lateral mandibulotomies to gain access to tumors and subsequent reapproximation of the mandibular segments along with plating them to maintain continuity. Inner table, superior, and inferior marginal mandibulectomies also maintain the integrity of the mandible. Surgeries so designed and executed result in a decreased volume of tissue loss, more normal mandibular movements, improved relationship with opposing structures in the maxillary arch, and an intact stabilizing framework for the tongue and adjacent tissues.

When the size of tumor and resection allows for primary closure, attention should be given to the tightness of wound closure and the potential limitation of mobility and volume of remaining tissue and their effects on function. When remaining volume of tissue is reasonable, split-thickness skin grafts can be used to enhance mobility and restrict scar contracture. When indicated, proponents of this approach (Conley, 1954; LaFerriere et al., 1980; Schramm et al., 1983) report good functional results. The size and extent of resection may preclude this approach. There are very few instances where tongue flaps should be used for surgical closure if functional rehabilitation is planned for the patient. This flap has been used in the past because it is convenient, reliable, and provides viable tissue for areas of exposed bone that are to be irradiated. These factors are outweighed by the disabilities that tongue flaps are capable of producing for speech, mastication, and swallowing.

Mastication

Normal masticatory function involves the synchronous interaction of the hard and soft tissues to manipulate, triturate, and consolidate a food bolus prior to deglutition. Following a partial mandibular resection, the trituration, or grinding phase of mastication is often adversely affected by the loss of mandibular structure, altered maxillomandibular relationships, and decreased tooth-to-tooth contacts. The sensory and soft tissue deficits following a partial mandibular resection compromise both the patient's ability to manipulate a bolus to the occlusal table for trituration and the ability to retrieve and consolidate the bolus prior to deglutition (Kapur et al., 1990). All three components of mastication (manipulation, trituration, and consolidation) are required to masticate efficiently and a deficiency in one area can result in diminished global measures of masticatory function. For example, when the ability to manipulate a bolus to the occlusal table is compromised due to a partial loss of tongue volume and/or sensation, masticatory inefficiency results, even if the patient can effectively triturate a food bolus.

The difficulty patients have in mastication following mandibular resection is influenced by numerous factors, some of which the surgeon and prosthodontist can control to improve mastication. Although tumor control and survival should be primary concerns regarding treatment decisions, rehabilitation strategies and timing of rehabilitation are important because these decisions impact masticatory function and quality of life (de Graeff et al., 2000; Schliephake et al., 1995; Bundgaard et al., 1993) Optimal individual rehabilitation requires an understanding of the variables that impact masticatory function, which should include an understanding of normal masticatory function and how anatomic loss impacts function.

Identifying and ranking by importance the variables contributing to masticatory impairment in patients with a mandibular resection is difficult for many reasons. First, techniques to measure masticatory performance have not been adequately standardized, and investigators often disagree on the interpretation of results (Olthoff et al., 1984) Second, variability has been reported between and within subjects using the same experimental protocol (Gunne, 1985), and test foods that are acceptable with denture patients are sometimes not suitable for oral cancer patients (Marunick and Mathog, 1990). Often there is no correlation or only a weak correlation when using two accepted measures of masticatory performance on the same individual (Olthoff et al., 1984; Krysiński et al., 1981). Additionally, it is generally recognized that different tests of masticatory function measure different aspects of mastication (Krysinski et al., 1981). Accurately assessing masticatory performance in head and neck cancer patients is also difficult because of the heterogeneous patient population. Variables of age, gender, skeletal form, modality of treatment and rehabilitation, and the willingness of the patient to work toward rehabilitation are variables difficult to control and make comparisons within and between groups challenging. Additionally, pretreatment measurements of masticatory performance are often impacted by the patient's psychological state (Schliephake et al., 1995), pain (Namaki et al., 2004), and the impact of disease, yet longitudinal randomized clinical trials remain the best opportunity for better understanding the variables that impact function in mandibular resection patients.

Variables contributing to masticatory impairment in mandibular resection patients

Integrity of the mandible

The mandible plays an important role in controlling oral competence in mastication, swallowing, and speech. An intact mandible provides symmetry for proper function and esthetics. When a segment of the mandible is removed, symmetry and balance are sacrificed. Joint loading, mandibular movement, occlusal contact time and the angle of occlusal contact are altered (Curtis et al., 1999). The residual mandible shifts toward the surgical defect with both retrusion and rotation (Fig 2-112). Protrusive movement and incising are especially difficult (Curtis et al., 1975). Although the patient's mandibular movements and functional disability are influenced by numerous factors including the patient's level of depressive symptoms prior to surgery (de Graeff et al., 2000) volume of hard and soft tissue removed (Bozec et al., 2008; Marunick et al., 1992a), whether radiation is used (Bozec et al., 2008; Epstein et al., 1999) and the type of reconstruction completed (Urken et al., 1991b), continuity of the mandible as an independent variable has an impact on masticatory function (Marunick et al., 1992a; Curtis et al., 1997). These clinical findings showing the importance of continuity of the mandible are consistent with modeling data of jaw biomechanics (Hannam et al., 2010).

A segmental mandibular resection should be reconstructed primarily to avoid deviation of the mandible secondary to scar contracture and muscle imbalances. With no tongue involvement, normal bulk and unimpaired motor control, salivary control, speech, or swallowing are unaffected. Saliva control, if affected, is usually secondary to compromised motor and sensory innervation of the lower lip on the resected side. The deviation of the mandible is secondary to muscle imbalance and compromised proprioception.

Benign tumors that require osseous resection likewise result in little soft-tissue loss and have a similar favorable prognosis for rehabilitation. Disability is almost entirely related to the amount of mandible resected. The prognosis for immediate bony reconstruction with either avascular bone grafts or vascularized free flaps is excellent.

Reconstruction that reestablishes the continuity of the mandible provides the obvious benefit in esthetics but also facilitates the potential for improved function (Hannam et al., 2010; Flynn et al., 2015). When continuity of the mandible is reestablished, it is much easier to create an occlusal platform and the patient has an easier time occluding to a repeatable position. The number of opposing tooth-to-tooth contacts has been shown to be highly correlated with masticatory efficiency (Helkimo et al., 1977; Helkimo et al., 1978). The increase in stable posterior occlusal contacts is one reason patients with reestablished continuity of the mandible report improved masticatory function (Urken et al., 1991a; Curtis et al., 1997; Bozec et al., 2008; Kumar et al., 2016; Hannam et al., 2010; Flynn et al., 2015). Bozec et al. (2008), in a prospective study

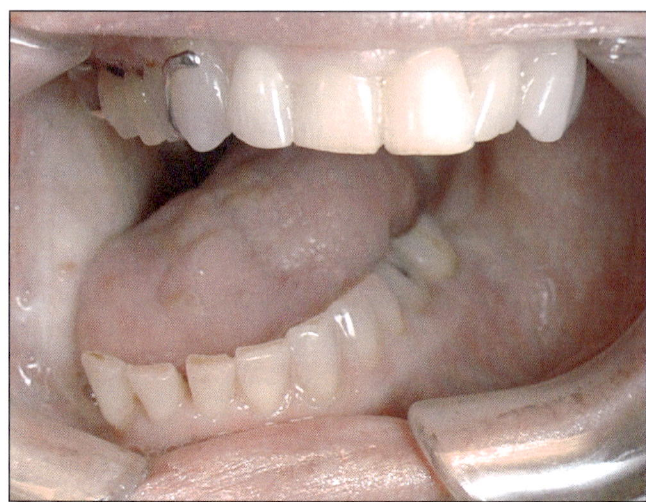

Figure 2-112 Defects of the tongue and mandible. Failed osseous reconstruction, leaving the patient with a discontinuity defect.

of 95 patients, showed that reconstructed patients, compared to nonreconstructed patients, had higher levels of physical and social functioning and more confidence in social eating, which becomes important because approximately 25% of oral cancer patients avoid social eating situations.

A number of studies have been completed comparing masticatory function in mandibular resection patients with mandibular reconstruction to mandibular resection patients without reconstruction (Marunick and Mathog, 1990; Urken et al., 1991b; Marunick et al., 1992a; Marunick et al., 1992b; Patel et al., 1996; Curtis et al., 1997; Namaki et al., 2004; Hannam et al., 2010) Although differences in study design, methods to evaluate function, surgical technique and rehabilitation strategies make comparisons between studies difficult, several general trends can be seen.

When the neoplasm is confined to the alveolar ridge, resection of the tumor results in minimal soft-tissue loss. Consequently, the resulting disabilities are less severe. In a simple marginal resection in which mandibular continuity is retained, if the inferior alveolar nerve is not resected, little morbidity results other than the obliteration of the buccal or lingual sulci (Fig 2-113). Such defects are easily restored with conventional mandibular resection prostheses (MRP).

The effect of unilateral occlusion was studied by Namaki et al. (2004) and included three treatment groups: glossectomy, marginal mandibular resection, and segmental mandibular resection without continuity. Namaki also included two noncancer control groups: intact dentition and a second control with patients missing a posterior quadrant (Namaki et al., 2004). The authors concluded that discontinuity of the mandible limited diet and adversely impacted the quality of life as compared to a marginal mandibular resection (Namaki et al., 2004). The authors also found no difference in chewing efficiency between the two control groups, which included an intact dentition group and a second group with one missing posterior quadrant. These findings suggest that reconstruction efforts allowing unilateral occlusion may be acceptable. Also of interest was the finding that patient reports of eating ability improved from the third month to the twelfth month testing period for the glossectomy and marginal resection patients but not for the segmental mandibular resection group. The clinical implication is that soft

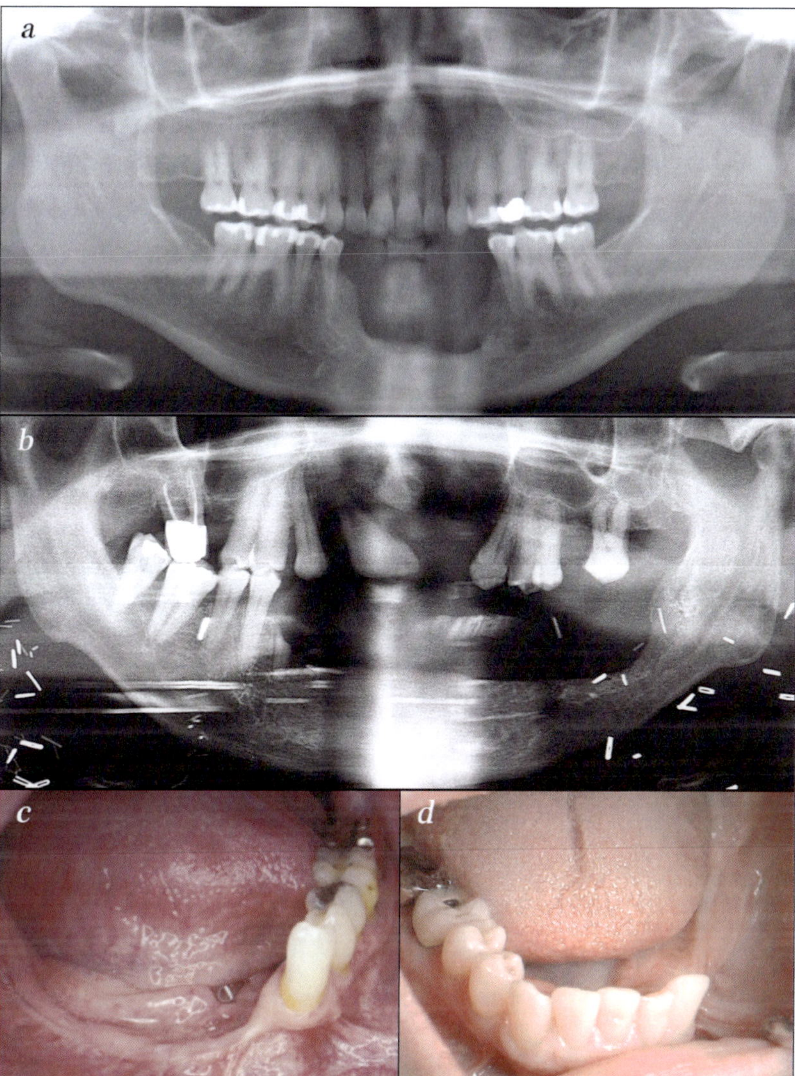

Figure 2-113 Marginal mandibular resections. *(a and b)* Postoperative panoramic radiographs of anterior and anterior lateral marginal resections. *(b and c)* Clinical examples of marginal mandibular defects secondary to the resection of localized SCC. These can be restored with a conventional MRP or an implant-assisted or -supported resection prosthesis.

tissue adaptation and masticatory improvement are less likely to occur in individuals who do not have continuity of the mandible (Namaki et al., 2004). Other studies evaluating oral symptoms in mandibular resection patients with reconstruction have shown that levels of reported pain tend to decrease from the time of surgery to 12 months postoperation, but the restricted diet and comfort in eating in public do not appreciably improve from 6 to 12 months postoperatively (Bozec et al., 2008; Kumar et al., 2016; Hannam et al., 2010).

Marunick et al. (1992a, 1992b) in a study of 5 mandibular resection patients and 10 controls, evaluated masticatory function pre- and postsurgery using sieve analysis. Using Frito corn chips as a test substrate and having each participant act as their own control, the authors found surgery results in a measurable impairment in mastication that cannot always be reversed by prosthetic rehabilitation. Marunick found a test-retest reliability of 0.59 for the measure of masticatory performance and 0.84 for the swallowing threshold. Marunick et al. determined the extent of mandibular resection and loss of continuity tended to decrease masticatory function levels. Urken et al. (1991a)—in a study of reconstructed, nonreconstructed, and control patients—evaluated patients who had microvascular surgery to reconstruct mandibular continuity. The objective measures of masticatory function included occlusal force, chewing cycle, a global measure of masticatory performance, as defined by Manly and Braley (1950), and a subjective questionnaire that asked patients to report performance. Results indicate that patients with reconstructed mandibles had significantly improved occlusal force levels, improved masticatory performance levels, and a more vertical masticatory cycle.

Occlusal force may be a predictor of successful masticatory performance as Urken found, but other investigators have not always shown occlusal force to be important in predicting masticatory performance (Hagberg, 1987a; Hagberg, 1987b; Curtis et al., 1997; Ikebe et al., 2006). In elderly noncancer edentulous patients, Ikebe et al. showed occlusal force and salivary flow were strong predictors of a patient's masticatory function. However, Curtis et al. (1997), in a study of 10 reconstructed and 10 nonreconstructed mandibular resection patients, found that occlusion force was poorly correlated to patient reports of food they could masticate. The typical Western diet requires less than 40 N of occlusal force, whereas harder to eat foods, such as nuts and carrots, require an average of 66 N (Haraldson et al., 1979). Curtis et al. (1997) found that the nonreconstructed patients in his study had an average first molar occlusal force of 76 N and would probably not be limited in their ability to masticate because of occlusal force alone. In the study by Urken et al. (1991b), nonreconstructed edentulous patients had an average of only 23 N, and in this group, the diet would likely be limited because of a low occlusal force. The value of measuring occlusal force in mandibular resection patients is in establishing a base threshold. Patients above this threshold, who have limitations in masticatory ability, are probably compromised for reasons other than a lack of occlusal force.

Tooth-to-tooth stops or implant equivalent. The number of opposing tooth-to-tooth contacts has been shown to be highly correlated with masticatory efficiency (Helkimo et al., 1977; Helkimo et al., 1978) in people with intact dentition without oral cancer. In patients with oral cancer, it has been shown that stable posterior tooth-to-tooth contacts result in better functional measures. Patel et al. (1996), in a subgroup of 47 nonreconstructed patients, found patients with dentition functioned at a much higher level than those without dentition; the clinical significance being that having tooth-to-tooth stops or equivalent with implants tends to help patients with function (Fig 2-114).

Support and retention of dental prosthesis / dental implants. Following surgery and radiation treatment many edentulous patients have difficulty wearing a mandibular prosthesis (Petrovic et al., 2018). Schoen et al. (2008) determined that over 50% of oral cancer patients who were edentulous were dissatisfied and wore their mandibular prostheses at most a few hours a day. Therefore, dental implants have been advocated as a way to improve retention, support and stability in hopes of improving function for patients (Roumanas et al., 1997). The use of dental implants in edentulous noncancer patients has been systematically reviewed by Fueki et al. (2007) who found that implant overdentures in edentulous patients provided significant improvement in masticatory performance compared to patients wearing conventional dentures, especially for patients with an atrophic mandible. The most comprehensive study evaluating masticatory function and the potential benefits of dental implants following mandibular reconstruction in cancer patients was completed by Garrett et al. (2006), Roumanas et al. (2006b), and Petrovic et al. (2018). In these longitudinal prospective studies, patients with a partial mandibulectomy had an immediate FFF reconstruction. The study included 23 patients (16 partially dentate and 7 edentulous) receiving conventional prostheses (CP) and 15 (12 partially edentulous and 3 edentulous) of the CP patients having implants added for an implant-supported prosthesis (IP). All patients completed sensory and functional tests before and after surgery, after CP treatment, and after IP treatment. Results indicate that IP prostheses offered several advantages over CP, especially when patients chewed on the defect side. Roumanas et al. did not find a statistically significant difference in masticatory function between the CP and IP on the nondefect side, but this could be because 12 of the 15 IP patients had some dentition, which could influence the independent variable of potential benefits from dental implants.

Tongue, cheek, and peri-oral function

The tongue plays an important role in mastication because of its mobility, tactile sensitivity, and ability to manipulate a bolus of food.

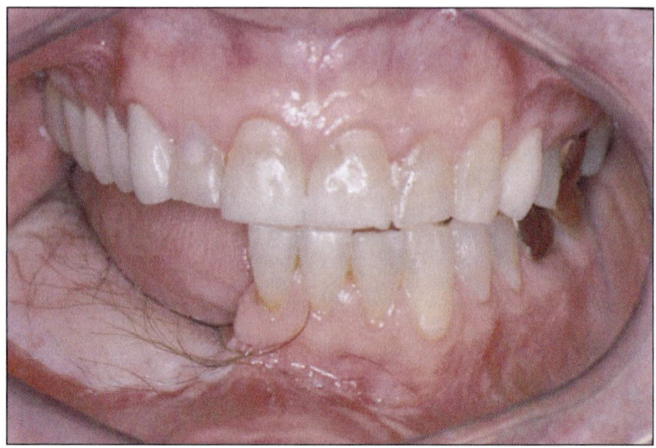

Figure 2-114 Lateral mandibular defect reconstructed with FFF and preserving tooth-to-tooth stops (image same as 2-17a).

The tongue can crush by pressing a food substrate against the rugae of the palate, manipulate a bolus to the occlusal surface, and help mix food with saliva. The tongue also functions with the buccinator to help manipulate and maintain a bolus of food on the occlusal table. In addition, the tongue can discriminate particle size so larger food particles requiring crushing are selectively placed on the occlusal platform (Kapur et al., 1990) Additionally, the tongue can help stabilize a mandibular prosthesis.

A high percentage of surgical procedures for oral cancers directly or indirectly affect the motor and/or sensory innervation, mobility, or volume of the tongue. With loss of motor innervation, the tongue cannot move to the ipsilateral side, so function becomes difficult on the affected side. With sensory loss, the patient cannot discriminate particle size of food and manipulation of food to the occlusal platform becomes less predictable (Kapur et al., 1990). With a compromise in mobility or volume of the tongue, clearing a bolus from the buccal vestibule or crushing food against the palate is difficult (Curtis et al., 1997).

In a study comparing three methods of reconstruction, McConnel et al. concluded that tongue mobility was a critically important factor in predicting good oral function (McConnel et al., 1987). McConnel's finding is consistent with others who have shown that normal tongue volume, sensation (Kapur et al., 1990; Urken et al., 1991b; Aviv et al., 1992), and mobility (Urken et al., 1991b) are important to masticatory function.

Radiation therapy

Independent of surgical management, radiation has been shown to significantly impact masticatory function (Beumer et al., 1979; Epstein et al., 1999; Bozec et al., 2008). Epstein et al. (1999) showed that 50% of edentulous patients who received radiation alone stated a decrease in masticatory ability. The direct effects of radiation and indirect effects of xerostomia often result in fragile mucous membranes that can often be painful to the effects of wearing a prosthesis. Epstein et al. also showed that the most common patient concerns following radiation alone were oral dryness (84%), pain (70%), lack of taste (97%), and diminished appetite (70%) while following surgery. Langius and Lind (1995) reported that patient complaints were primarily difficulty eating (82%), swallowing (81%), chewing (68%), and disfigurement (55%).

Garrett et al. (1996) stated that a patient's perception of chewing ability is often influenced by comfort rather than objective measures of chewing performance, so patient reports of discomfort are important feedback when evaluating a new prosthesis. Because most patients receive both radiation and surgery, the additive impact can be a daunting task to manage. Bozec et al. (2008) showed that patients with both surgery and radiation had significantly more concerns related to function than did patients receiving surgery alone.

Computer modeling of jaw biomechanics in oral cancer patients

The major problems studying mandibular resection patients and patients having reconstructive surgery are related to the lack of sample size and the heterogeneous nature of this patient population. Tumor sizes vary, surgical approaches differ by surgeon and region, and the resulting functional limitations are specific to each patient. Often, the presurgical recordings are influenced by the presence of the disease. Computer modeling offers the opportunity to simulate an anatomic deficit, make quantitative determinations about joint loading and vectors of occlusal force, and make predictions about the potential impact of prosthodontic intervention. Investigators have developed both mechanical and mathematical models to help answer questions of occlusal force, vectors of muscle force, and temporomandibular joint loading (Hatcher et al., 1986; Faulkner et al., 1987; Hannam et al., 2008; Stavness et al., 2010; Stavness et al., 2014). Models have ranged from simple, one-dimensional models with two muscles represented to more advanced dynamic models (van Eijden et al., 1995; Langenbach et al., 1999; Langenbach et al., 2002; Koolstra, 2002).

The computer modeling program initially used to study mandibular resection patients was developed by Nelson (1986) and was designed as a three-dimensional model with nine pairs of muscles represented (Curtis et al., 1999). Calculations were completed on an existing database representing a normal patient having an intact mandible to determine the maximum clenching force at the first molar and incisal edge as well as the joint force / tooth force ratio. The computer modeling program was then altered to simulate the anatomic deficit characteristically seen in a mandibular resection patient with the tests of clenching force and joint force / tooth force measures duplicated.

Computer simulations of normal and mandibular resection patients predicted that mandibular resection patients would have 35% less incisal clenching force (187 vs. 339) and 45% less first molar clenching force (251 vs. 454), have an unfavorable joint force / tooth force ratio, and have rotation of the mandible with occlusal instability. Clinical trials showed that the computer simulations provide slightly lower values for molar clenching and high values for incisal clenching. The unfavorable joint force / tooth force ratio prediction from computer modeling cannot be validated clinically but makes sense that without bilateral articulation, the joint is heavily loaded. The rotation of the mandible was predicted to occur because the masseter on the nondefect side serves to rotate the mandible and is not balanced unilaterally by the medial pterygoid (Curtis et al., 1999).

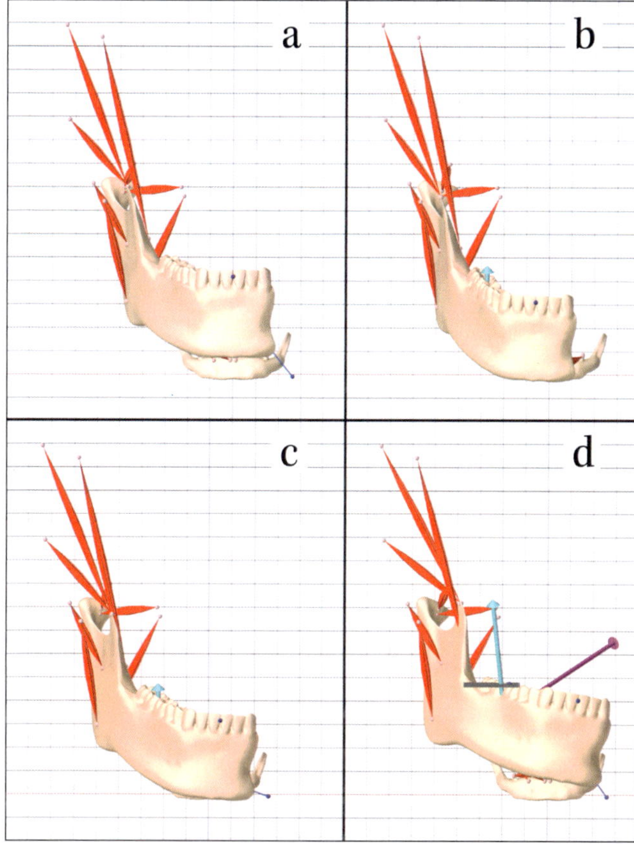

Figure 2-115 Dynamic simulation of a mandible without continuity. The model illustrates the jaw and scar vector (blue) in maximum intercuspation. *(a)* At rest without scarring. *(b)* At rest with a scar stiffness of 200N/cm. *(c)* And during the activation of the right masseter muscle on the right molar contact with the same scar stiffness. *(d)* In the latter case, both rotation and translation of native fragments are evident. Arrows indicate the direction of total muscle force (cyan) and torque (purple) expressed at the jaw's center of mass. The calibration grid represents 10 mm. The model is described in detail elsewhere (Hannam et al., 2008).

Dynamic modeling

The physical principles of normal jaw function are well defined and can be demonstrated by more advanced programs using dynamic modeling (van Eijden et al., 1995; Koolstra and van Eijden, 1995; Peck et al., 2000; Peck et al., 2002; Koolstra, 2002; Hannam et al., 2008; Stavness, 2010; Stavness et al., 2014). Sophisticated models include active and passive muscle properties with various articular and occlusal constraints. The movements and forces modeled generally correspond well to averaged experimental data (Curtis et al., 1999), suggesting that simulation can be a plausible predictor of structural and functional interactions. Importantly, modeling allows changes to structural and functional parameters and the estimation of parameters difficult to measure in living subjects.

Biomechanics of mandibles without continuity

Mandibles lacking continuity are severely compromised biomechanically (Fig 2-115). The depleted musculature on the defect side has a profound effect, since many jaw muscles cannot be activated bilaterally, thus changing the lines of action of the resultant muscle force vector and its torque on the mandible. Moreover, all jaw positioning and movement (e.g., resting posture, protrusion, opening, and closing into dental contact) must take place with the remaining muscles working around a single load-bearing joint, within an environment of passive closing-muscle tensions on the native side and soft tissue forces significantly influenced by wound-healing and radiation-scarring on the defect side.

A modeling study of a left-side mandibular resection patient in a rest position showed that passive forces in the remaining elevator muscles would tend to rotate the resting jaw clockwise (when viewed frontally) as expected but that the lower incisor region would be drawn toward the nondefect side, which would not be expected clinically (Hannam et al., 2010). Modeling suggested that soft tissue scarring and wound-closure tightness counteract the effects of the elevator muscles and result in the commonly observed deviation toward the defect side.

Modeling the effect of an operator-induced downward pressure on the lower incisors in mandibular resection patients can help explain the impact of scarring. Incisor-point movement as a result of operator-induced downward force on the mandibular incisors reflects the interaction of the applied force, passive muscle tensions, and scar forces. If the latter are insignificant, an incisal force less than 5 N in the fully relaxed jaw is enough to achieve incisal gapes of 30 mm without major lateral deviation.

Simulation studies confirm clinical observations of lateral deviation to the deficit side which results from asymmetric lateral pterygoid activity on jaw opening. The digastrics and geniohyoids, which initially help open the jaw, rapidly lose their biomechanical effectiveness unless the head is simultaneously rotated backward to improve their lines of action and can actually reduce the lateral jaw motion induced by the lateral pterygoid.

Mandibular resection patients often have difficulty with occlusion. The lines of action of the closing muscles distribute around the axis joining the single articulation and the occlusion point. Vectors from the temporalis and masseter pass laterally to this axis and are associated with complex rotations of the native fragment. These include a clockwise component when viewed frontally, for which the only reaction force available is provided by scarring on the defect side. In addition, the middle and posterior temporalis and deep masseter have a marked a lateral-displacing action on the ipsilateral condyle, for which the only natural restraint is the temporomandibular ligament (Koolstra and van Eijden, 1995; van Eijden et al., 1995; Hannam et al., 2008; Stavness, 2010; Stavness et al., 2014; Petrovic et al., 2018). In contrast, the medial pterygoid's line of action encourages counterclockwise jaw rotation viewed frontally, especially with attempted molar occlusion on the normal side. Its medial-displacing effect on the condyle is likely resisted by the upper and medial surfaces of the articular fossa.

The various forces and torques produced by individual jaw-closing muscles can sometimes seem counterintuitive (van Eijden et al., 1995; Koolstra, 2002). Nevertheless, they explain jaw instability during unilateral occluding, where patients with mandibles lacking continuity are challenged to find patterns of muscle use that permit the generation of occlusal force without rotation of the native fragment. Here, inverse dynamic modeling (where displacements and/or forces are inputs, and muscle recruitment patterns are outputs) is a promising simulation method, since it can include potential contributions from auxiliary inframandibular muscles and the tongue.

Biomechanics of mandibles with continuity

Patients with vascular and avascular bone grafts to restore mandibular continuity have improved functional stability with or without muscles on the defect side. During opening, some jaw guidance is offered by the defect-side condyle working against the posterior slope of the articular eminence. On jaw closure, the articulation can resist compressive forces bilaterally, thereby preventing any counterclockwise jaw rotation caused by medial pterygoid activity on the normal side. Also, any functioning elevator musculature retained on the deficit side will help bring the muscle resultant within the resistance triangle offered by the condyles and occlusion-point (thus loading the grafted condyle). Grafted condyles are not necessarily effective however in preventing the clockwise jaw rotation induced by temporalis and masseter muscle activity acting on the normal side; in this state, the deficit-side articulation is in traction rather than compression.

Dental occlusion

To date, dynamic modeling studies have not addressed the role of dental occlusion. Occlusion is especially relevant in mandibular-resection patients where occlusal restoration is often performed to improve oral function. Workable prosthetic approaches have been developed more by trial and error than from designs based on the biomechanics of specific deficits. During chewing, movements and interocclusal forces occur simultaneously, and the occlusal interface is constantly modified by a changing food bolus. In the normal subject, early closing starts close to the midline, and the jaw swings laterally toward the side of the food bolus, rotating around its ipsilateral condyle. In late closing, as the bolus is engaged, the jaw rotates medially as the contralateral condyle returns to its articular fossa, creating shearing forces through or near the dental intercuspal position. The stroke continues into a short lingual phase before jaw opening recommences.

This situation is likely very different in a mandible without continuity, where the closing stroke is most likely medially directed from an already deviated starting location on the deficit side, resembling a reversed chewing stroke. Muscle actions normally used to start the normal upward and lateral stroke will cause clockwise jaw rotation, since there are no effective participants (such as the medial pterygoid and superficial masseter) on the deficit side, and as soon as contact is made between the molars or on the bolus, the muscles usually employed to drive the mandible medially are either absent (the temporalis and deep masseter on the deficit side) or likely to cause clockwise jaw rotation (the superficial masseter on the normal side) or counterclockwise rotation (if indeed the medial pterygoid could be activated in isolation). The dynamics involved in successfully creating interocclusal shearing forces are clearly complex, not only requiring patients to experiment with any remaining muscles but possibly needing contributions from muscles in the submandibular region. Relearning may prove difficult for some patients and arguably impossible for others.

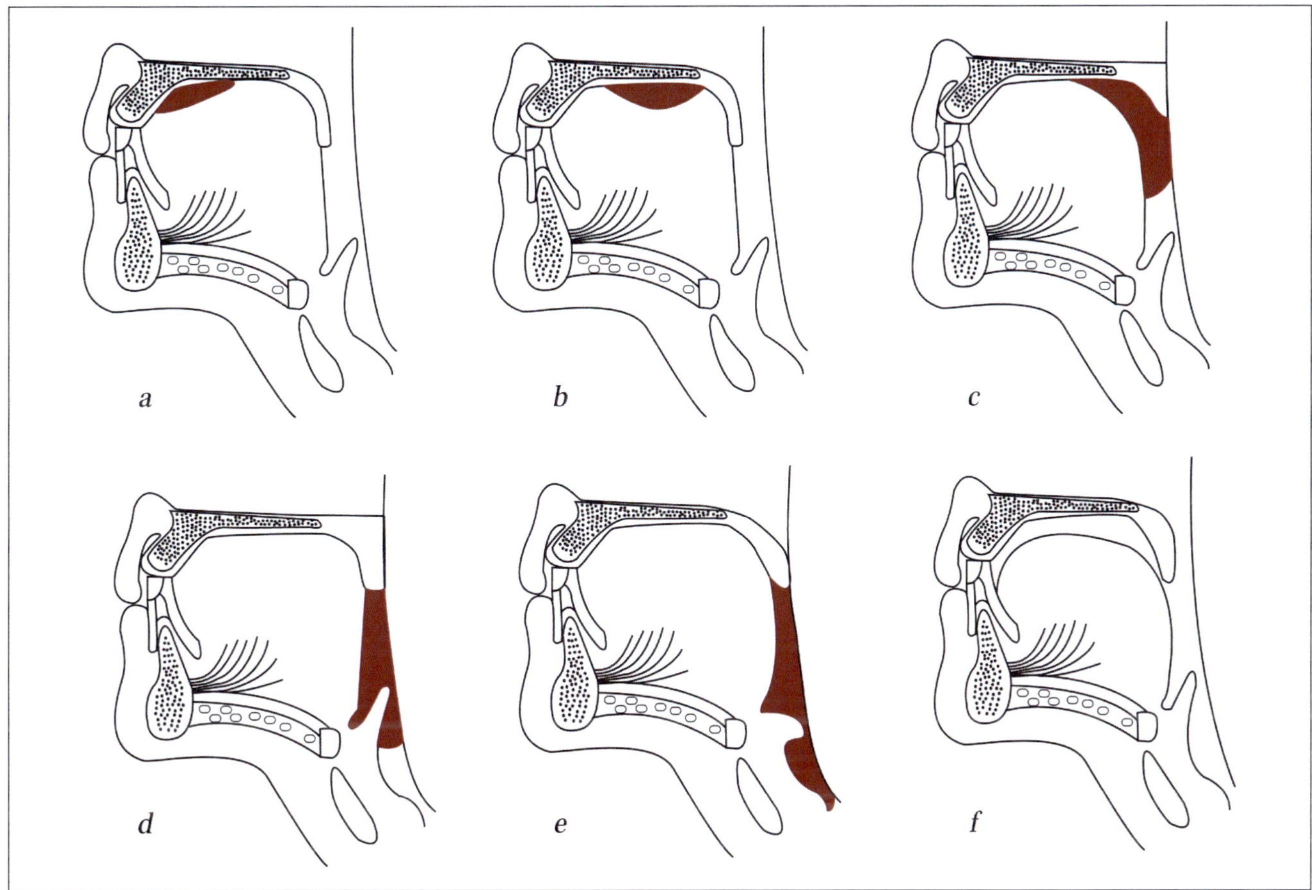

Figure 2-116 Normal swallowing sequence. *(a)* Oral preparatory phase. Bolus is prepared for oral transit. *(b)* Oral transit phase. Bolus is transported by the tongue to the pharyngeal introitus. *(c)* Pharyngeal phase. Initiation of swallow reflex and soft palate elevation. *(d)* Pharyngeal bolus transport. *(e)* Laryngeal protection with epiglottic rotation and glottic closure. *(f)* Esophageal phase. Bolus is transported to the stomach by esophageal musculature.

Oral Swallow Function in the Head and Neck Cancer Patient

Introduction

The oral portion of deglutition normally leads seamlessly to the pharyngeal and then esophageal swallowing phases (Fig 2-116). Oral cavity cancer and its treatments can impair an individual's ability to masticate, form a bolus, and transport that bolus to the pharynx. Dysfunctional oral bolus control can significantly impact oropharyngeal swallow safety and efficiency. Additionally, abnormal oral swallowing can reduce a person's eating and drinking enjoyment and thus affect quality of life. Therefore, it is critical that prosthodontists seeking to improve oral swallowing in head and neck cancer survivors understand normal and abnormal oral swallow function in this patient population.

Normal oral swallow physiology

The initial two phases of swallowing are the oral preparatory phase and the oral transit phase. The pharyngeal and esophageal phases of swallowing are beyond the scope of this textbook. The main goal of the oral preparatory phase, regardless of the consistency to be swallowed, is to form a bolus on the tongue. The oral transit stage involves propelling the bolus into the pharynx. The oral preparatory and oral phases of swallowing are considered volitional. However, these phases can occur without awareness, most notably with saliva swallows (Johnson, 2006). In the following, we will review the normal components of these two oral swallowing phases. Oral cavity anatomy separate from physiology is not discussed in this section, as it is assumed that the reader has sufficient background in the muscular, neural, and bony anatomy of the oral cavity.

Oral preparatory phase

A normal oral preparatory phase requires adequate sensory and motor function. The lips are sealed to prevent anterior oral leakage during swallowing, and therefore, respiration occurs via the nasal passages (Logemann, 1998). Oral cavity movement patterns vary depending on the bolus type (e.g., chewable food vs pureed food vs liquids), bolus size, taste, and temperature (Logemann, 1998; Sonies, 2003). Mastication of chewable food precedes bolus formation. Normal mastication requires rotary-lateral movement of the mandible. Food is pushed by the tongue laterally between the upper and lower teeth; the food falls out of the occlusal table as the mandible occludes and is pushed back in by the tongue for further crushing by the teeth until the food is sufficiently chewed (Logemann, 1998). Saliva is mixed with the masticated food and helps form a cohesive bolus. The buccinators remain taut during mastication to prevent food from entering the buccal sulci. Food, liquid, and/or saliva are formed into a bolus on the dorsal tongue in preparation for oral transit. There are two normal lingual positions for holding food and thick liquid boluses—midline on the tongue with the tongue tip elevated to the anterior alveolar ridge or on the anterior oral tongue with the tongue tip lowered (Logemann, 1998). A thin liquid bolus is held between the anterior hard palate and the body of the tongue. It is contained laterally by the sides of the tongue contacting the lateral alveolus and anteriorly by the tongue tip opposing the anterior alveolar ridge. The posterior oropharyngeal isthmus (bounded superiorly by the velum, laterally by the palatoglossal arches, and inferiorly by the tongue) contracts to prevent premature spillage of the bolus into the pharynx (Chhetri, 2019).

Oral transit phase

Oral transit refers to the propulsion of a bolus (saliva, liquid, or food) from the oral cavity to the pharynx. This occurs by an anterior-to-posterior lingual stripping wave that opposes the palate and generates pressure to move the bolus. The tongue blade forms a central groove, which acts as a chute to direct the bolus into the pharynx (Logemann, 1998). Lateral spillage during oral transit is avoided by the sides of the tongue contacting the lateral alveolus. Greater tongue-to-palate pressure is required as bolus viscosity increases. The required level of pressure for a successful oral transit is modulated by sensory feedback from the tongue (Youmans and Stierwalt, 2006). The velum, which was previously pulled down and forward for bolus containment, elevates during oral transit. The oral phase appears to terminate after the leading edge of the bolus passes the posterior edge of the mandible (mandibular ramus; Martin-Harris et al., 2007). There should be little to no residue after swallowing. The lingual movement pattern that occurs during oral transit is consistent among individuals (Chi-Fishman and Stone, 1996; Chi-Fishman et al., 1998).

Impact of radiation on oral bolus control

Radiation is frequently employed to treat HNSCC as a primary treatment, as an alternative to surgery in poor surgical candidates, or as adjuvant therapy for late-stage tumors (Caudell et al., 2022). Radiation can have significant effects on oral bolus control. These effects can be divided into early versus late treatment sequelae, with early effects occurring within weeks and late effects occurring months or even years after completion of radiation. Because of the possibility of late side effects of radiation, patients should be followed long-term for these potential sequelae of radiation.

Early effects of radiation

Early effects of radiation (during treatment and up to 2 months post-treatment) that can impact oral bolus control include mucositis, dysgeusia, pain, and xerostomia (Brook, 2021; Togni et al., 2021) These decrease pleasure derived from oral intake and can contribute to malnutrition and dehydration. Furthermore, decreased peroral intake can negatively impact an individual's ability to participate in posttreatment rehabilitation.

Many patients who undergo radiation therapy to the oral cavity will struggle with mucositis (Mercadante et al., 2015). The addition of certain chemotherapeutic agents such as cisplatin can increase the incidence and severity of mucositis (Dewan, 2020). Erythema and ulcerations related to mucositis can precipitate oral pain, which will consequently lead to food aversion and reduced oral intake. Oral mucositis may be graded using the World Health Organization Oral Mucositis Scale (scale 0–4: 0 = no mucositis, 1 = oral soreness, erythema, 2 = oral erythema, ulcers, solid diet tolerated, 3 = oral ulcers, liquid diet only, 4 = oral alimentation impossible; Villa et al., 2021).

Xerostomia is another well-described early sequela of radiation, with decreased salivary flow in irradiated patients (Rogus-Pulia et al., 2016; Nichols et al., 2022). Lack of saliva impairs mastication and cohesive food bolus formation and is also associated with dental caries. Xerostomia has been shown to correlate directly with patient-reported dysphagia (Vainshtein et al., 2016), which is understandable given saliva's role in moistening the oral cavity and food bolus for efficient oral transit.

Sensory changes are common following radiation treatment. The tongue contains a combination of normal sensory fibers as well as special sensory fibers that carry the sensation of taste. Radiation may cause neuroepithelial disruption, affecting both types of sensory fibers, leading to increased mucosal sensitivity and dysgeusia (Leitzen et al., 2012). This impairment can persist after the resolution of mucositis and can be found in two-thirds of patients at the one-year follow-up (Leitzen, 2012; Epstein et al., 1999; Hovan et al., 2010). As with other radiation side effects, dysgeusia will decrease the pleasure derived from deglutition, potentially decreasing oral intake.

Late effects of radiation

Late effects of radiation therapy (from months to decades) are secondary to fibrosis and the atrophy of irradiated structures (Brook, 2021). The pathophysiology of radiation fibrosis is described in detail in Chapter 1. The most well-described swallowing sequela of radiation fibrosis is trismus, which impairs a patient's ability to sufficiently lower the mandible to place food in the mouth or to masticate. Trismus is present in 17.3% of head and neck cancer patients prior to treatment and in 44.1% of patients 6 months after radiation. Up to 32.6% of patients have been diagnosed with trismus 10 years after treatment (Watters et al., 2019).

Tongue fibrosis and atrophy also occur as a late complication of radiation (Fig 2-117). This leads to tongue weakness, which will affect the patient's ability to propel the food bolus to the level of the faucal arches (Rogus-Pulia et al., 2016). Measures of oral tongue endurance are significantly impaired in irradiated patients (Rogus-Pulia et al., 2016).

Impact of surgery on oral bolus control

Per the most recent guidelines from the National Comprehensive Cancer Network (NCCN), the gold standard of treatment for oral squamous cell carcinoma continues to be surgical resection with intraoperative assessment of surgical margins. A selective neck dissection is often performed to improve survival and minimize the

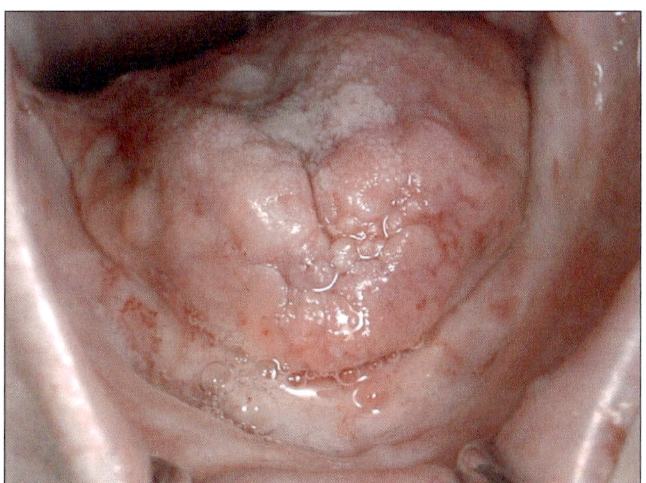

Figure 2-117 Example of muscle wasting and fibrosis of heavily irradiated tissues. A patient who was treated with radiotherapy presents with compromised speech articulation secondary to a reduction in the bulk and mobility of the tongue.

field for adjuvant radiation therapy (Bertlich et al., 2022; Wushou et al., 2021a). The degree and characteristics of swallowing dysfunction relate to the site and degree of resection.

Adequate labial competence is required to prevent spillage of the bolus from the oral commissure. Resection of lip cancers or damage to the marginal mandibular nerve during selective neck dissection can impair labial competence. In addition, lip resections can lead to microstomia as well as impaired speech, denture malposition, and impaired facial expression. See the prior section "Reconstruction of the Lip."

Tongue movement is essential for mastication, bolus collection, and oral transit. Consequently, anterior oral tongue and FOM resections may affect sensation and movement of the tongue, with larger resections leading to more morbidity and difficulties with oral bolus control (Ihara et al., 2021; Dzioba et al., 2017) Partial glossectomies may have minimal functional sequelae, while larger resections with reconstructive surgery may tether and decrease residual tongue mobility and impact the ability to manipulate the oral bolus. Finally, the sacrifice of the hypoglossal nerve in a neck dissection due to tumor involvement will lead to severe atrophy of the tongue following surgery with resulting disruption in oral bolus control (Chambers et al., 2016). See the prior section "Reconstruction of the Tongue."

Tumors involving the mandible may be treated with marginal or segmental mandibulectomies. While marginal resections often have little functional impact, segmental mandibulectomies present unique challenges in regard to preserving the functionality of the mandible in mastication and swallowing. Ohkoshi et al. (2018) found that the anterior and extensive mandibular bone resection was an independent predictor of poor chewing and swallowing outcomes. Furthermore, the masseter is not reattached to the mandible following resection and reconstruction, and this will lead to changes in occlusal forces. Mandible resection can impact pharyngeal swallowing due to the detachment of suprahyoid muscles from the mandible. However, this topic is beyond the scope of this textbook.

The mandible has important aesthetic and functional characteristics that must be accounted for during reconstruction. The mandible serves an important role in chewing, as all muscles of mastication are attached to it. In addition, tumors that necessitate a surgical resection of the lateral pterygoid muscles or a portion of the buccal mucosa can lead to trismus. A primary goal of reconstructing the buccal mucosa is the prevention of postoperative trismus. Reconstruction of this functional unit is a challenging balance between pliability, adequate tissue bulk, and postsurgical scarring. Common locoregional flaps include the nasolabial flap, submental flap, buccal mucosal flap, and buccal fat pad flap (Patel et al., 2017). If a flap is required to reconstruct the defect, a thin pliable flap like the RFFF can be considered (Gilbert, 2020). If buccal mucosa and extraoral facial skin are involved simultaneously, a chimeric flap model to line the inner and outer layers of the defect can be used (Huang et al., 2002).

While the primary outcome of head and neck cancer treatment is oncologic control, preserving postablation function remains paramount for patients' quality of life and daily activities. As with all reconstructions, the goal is to replace resected tissue(s) with those of similar quality and characteristics. The reconstruction of various oral cavity defects follows the principles of the reconstructive ladder and will be discussed herein.

Impact on recurrence and retreatment on swallow function

Initial treatment for oral cavity cancer with surgery (with or without reconstruction) or radiation affects oral cavity anatomy and function. However, resumption of an oral diet is achievable in the majority of patients. Chen et al. documented a 7.3% rate of dysphagia after oral cavity cancer treatment (2018). However, they note that dysphagia severity is related to the cancer subsite, with the oral tongue having worse swallowing outcomes than other oral cavity subsites (Chen et al., 2018; Schache et al., 2009).

Treatment of recurrent oral cavity cancer can severely impact residual swallow function due to further surgical resection or repeat radiation therapy. Obtaining tumor resection with clear margins is paramount in oncologic surgery. Structures that may have been spared in the primary surgery are at increased risk of sacrifice with each subsequent operation, resulting in potential sensorimotor dysfunction (Lubbers et al., 2014; Speksnijder et al., 2011; Bearelly et al., 2017). The addition of concurrent chemotherapy to radiation therapy can intensify mucositis and increase oral cavity dysphagia (Lubbers et al., 2014).

Surgical defects can be managed via healing by secondary intention, primary closure, or reconstruction with local, regional, or free flap techniques. Regardless of the chosen reconstruction, volume deficits significantly impact mastication and oral bolus manipulation. Retreatment can increase scar tissue and/or tethering of mobile oral structures with functional consequences. In addition, both surgical scarring and radiation effects may worsen trismus, which can be profoundly problematic for normal oral function and hygiene.

Assessment of the oral swallow

Oropharyngeal swallow evaluations assess both the oral swallow and the pharyngeal swallow. For the purpose of this chapter, only the oral swallow portion of exams will be discussed. Velar assessment will be included, given prosthodontists' interest in the structure, even though it is anatomically grouped in the pharyngeal swallow. Before beginning a discussion of oral swallow evaluations, we should consider the usual scope of oropharyngeal assessments, which is to address how efficiently and safely a person swallows. Efficiency relates to how quickly and thoroughly a bolus moves through the oral cavity and pharynx. Swallow safety relates to how well a person prevents swallowed material from entering the trachea and lungs during the act of swallowing. Oropharyngeal swallow evaluations largely focus on the pharynx and larynx, because swallow deficits in these areas are most closely related to aspiration. Less attention is usually given to the oral portion of the swallow, as it is less commonly the proximal cause of aspiration. Therefore, the oral swallow may be considered to be somewhat neglected in swallowing examinations (Sonies, 2003).

Following is a description of commonly used swallow assessments, including the clinical swallow exam, modified barium swallow study (MBSS), and fiber-optic endoscopic evaluation of swallowing (FEES). Prior to the administration of liquid and food, the patient should be interviewed to elicit a description of the swallowing problem, and an examination of oral structures should be performed; both of these areas will be discussed. Medical/surgical history that may be associated with the patient's dysphagia needs to be obtained. It is important to understand the dysphagia etiology to anticipate the expected swallowing problem as well as the course of progression or recovery. For example, if a patient was irradiated, it is important to understand when the radiation occurred, the dose given, and what parts of the swallowing anatomy were in the radiation field. Swallow deficits for which there is no corresponding medical history may prompt further assessment.

Patient's description of swallowing issues

For both instrumental and noninstrumental examinations, it is necessary to obtain the patient's description of the swallowing problem. It should be noted that many individuals treated for head and neck cancer have some degree of sensory impairment, and therefore, the ability to self-describe swallow dysfunction may be limited. The following questions are recommended:

- What is the nature of your swallowing problem?
- Do you cough when you eat/drink?
- When did your swallowing problem begin?
- What are typical foods you eat?
- Are there any foods/liquids you avoid because they are a challenge to swallow?
- Do you finish meals after others? If so, how long does it usually take to eat a meal?
- Do food and liquid taste as you would expect?
- Is your mouth dry?
- Is it painful to swallow? When did the pain begin? Where do you experience the pain? Rate your pain on a 10-point scale, with 10 being the most painful.
- Have you been losing weight for unexplained reasons? If so, how many pounds have you lost and over what period of time?

Oral peripheral exam

Regardless of swallow exam type, it is important to examine the patient's oral structures prior to giving food or liquid to answer the following questions:

- Are any possible lesions noted?
- Is the patient able to create a labial seal (to contain saliva, liquid, and/or food)?
- Is trismus present and to what degree? Is oral opening adequate for feeding and/or placement/removal of a dental prosthesis?
- Are there any anatomical abnormalities that could impact swallowing (e.g., changes related to head and neck cancer treatments, including flaps, missing structures, and/or edema)?
- Is the dental rehabilitation adequate for mastication?
- Is tongue volume normal in appearance?
- Are lingual fasciculations present, indicating possible denervation?
- Is tongue movement restricted, and if so, is it unilateral or bilateral?
- Does velar elevation appear restricted? If so, is it unilateral or bilateral? Does the velum appear shortened?
- Is there excess saliva or food debris in the oral cavity? If so, where?
- Are there signs of oral sensory loss as indicated by a lack of awareness with drooling, excess saliva, and/or liquid/food residue?
- Does the oral cavity appear to be dry, indicating xerostomia?
- If the patient's speech is abnormal, are there atypical oral exam findings that correlate with the perceived speech deficit (e.g., reduced tongue movement observed and dysarthria perceived; possible reduced velar elevation observed and hypernasality perceived)?

The answers to all of these questions should be considered in context with swallow exam results, since this may help explain the pathophysiology of the abnormal oral swallow.

Noninstrumental evaluation—clinical swallow examination

The clinical swallow exam is noninstrumental, meaning that no imaging technology or instruments are used to observe swallowing. The oral and pharyngeal portions of swallowing are not observed. Instead, signs and symptoms indicating dysphagia are assessed. This exam is most commonly used in the acute inpatient setting, to determine if a patient is safe for a diet or requires an instrumental assessment (i.e., to visualize the swallowing act). However, the clinical swallow exam has utility in the ambulatory environment, depending on the clinical question one wishes to answer (e.g., does modifying a PAP result in less oral cavity residue when puree is swallowed?).

Following is a brief description of how the test is conducted: Liquid and/or food are provided to the patient. Labial continence is assessed, as well as oral residue after the swallow. The oral cavity stasis pattern may indicate the nature of the oral dysphagia. For example, food residue on the palate may suggest inadequate tongue-to-palate stripping wave verses xerostomia. Sensory deficits may be evident, as indicated by drooling or oral residue for which the patient is unaware. The time from the introduction of food or liquid to the end of the swallowing effort is monitored. Mandibular movement during mastication is observed. Coughing or wet vocal quality are signs of aspiration suggesting that an instrumental swallow evaluation is indicated.

Instrumental evaluations—modified barium swallow study (MBSS)

An MBSS is a videofluoroscopic procedure. In this study, patients swallow liquid and food and sometimes pills while sitting upright.

Barium contrast is added to these materials so that swallowed items may be discerned radiographically. The oropharyngeal swallow may be observed in the lateral, anterior-posterior, and oblique planes. Anatomy observed includes the oral cavity, nasal cavity, pharynx, larynx, upper trachea, and upper portion of the cervical esophagus. If dysphagia is noted, techniques to improve swallowing may be tested. For example, a patient having difficulty containing an oral bolus, with premature spillage of the material into the pharynx, may be asked to lower the chin to shift the bolus forward to the anterior oral cavity. This study's strength in evaluating the oral swallow is the ability to visualize lingual, velar, and mandibular behavior and nasal penetration. Weaknesses include the following: (1) seeing images in a two-dimensional plane, which makes it difficult to perceive depth (to compensate for this, a view of the same structures from a different angle while swallowing must be obtained); (2) inability to visualize discrete anatomical structures; and (3) the need to keep exams short because of radiation exposure. The following are some of the important oral swallow behaviors as well as examples of dysphagia that may be observed during an MBSS:

- Mastication: mastication is best observed in the anterior-posterior view. Rotary-lateral mandibular movement is observed. Abnormal findings include limited mandibular movement with insufficient crushing of the chewable food or limited lateralization of food onto the occlusal table.
- Forming a bolus: this means taking liquid or food, which may be spread diffusely in the oral cavity, and collecting it into a bolus on the tongue. Possible abnormal findings include reduced ability to form a bolus due to restricted tongue-blade movement and/or sensory deficits and oral cavity residue after the swallow (Logemann, 1998).
- Holding a bolus: when performed correctly, an individual retains a liquid or food bolus on the tongue (as described in the normal anatomy and physiology section) until oral transit is initiated. Dysfunctions include premature loss of a portion of the bolus into the pharynx, which sometimes results in aspiration, and spillage of the bolus out of the mouth if there is poor oral and labial sensation and reduced labial seal.
- Propelling a bolus (oral transit): this refers to propelling a bolus from the oral cavity to the pharynx. Abnormal findings include excess lingual motion for bolus transit, reduced tongue-to-palate contact, oral cavity residue, and multiple swallows per bolus.
- Bolus clearance: normally, an oral transit results in a fairly complete bolus clearance from the oral cavity. An abnormal finding is an oral residue after the swallow. This may result from lingual weakness or ineffective tongue-to-palate contact. Xerostomia may contribute to oral cavity food residue.
- Nasal penetration via the velopharyngeal port: nasal penetration by way of the velopharyngeal port can be observed most easily in the lateral view and is typically associated with the pharyngeal phase of swallowing. Nasal penetration most commonly occurs because of a pharyngeal obstruction to bolus flow (e.g., a nondeflecting epiglottis or reduced upper esophageal sphincter opening) that together with pharyngeal contraction squeezes the bolus upward. The material enters the nasal cavity under pressure. This usually occurs with large boluses and most commonly with liquids. Velar closure with swallowing and phonation may be grossly viewed in the lateral plane.

Instrumental evaluations—fiber-optic endoscopic evaluation of swallowing (FEES)

FEES is performed by the transnasal passage of a flexible videoendoscope into the oropharynx. Swallows of food and liquid are observed on a video monitor. The weakness of FEES in regard to the oral swallowing phases is that the oral cavity cannot be observed. One may note the loss of bolus control from the oral cavity into the pharynx or extra lingual motion (inferred by excess tongue-base movement prior to the pharyngeal phase of swallowing). FEES is primarily a test for the pharynx and larynx. The FEES strength includes the ability to visualize the adequacy of velopharyngeal port closure during swallowing and speech (Vanderwegen, 2008). One may also see swallowed material penetrating the nasal cavity secondary to reduced upper esophageal sphincter opening, velopharyngeal incompetence or insufficiency (see Chapter 4), or a leaking obturator (see Chapter 3).

Treatment for oral dysphagia

Dysphagia treatment typically focuses on the pharyngeal swallow, as this phase is most closely associated with aspiration. The following content will focus specifically on swallow treatments designed to improve oral swallowing. Dysphagia treatment planning should stem from a comprehensive swallowing evaluation. Treatments may be medical, surgical, or behavioral.

Behavioral treatments

Behavioral treatment options may be categorized as compensations or exercise. Compensatory techniques alter swallowing function but do not change swallow physiology in a lasting manner. Exercise-based treatments aim to improve the patient's swallow physiology (Adult Dysphagia, 2022). It is important to note that compensatory behaviors can negatively impact swallow function and cause more residue and/or aspiration. Thus, compensations should only be recommended after they have been tested and found efficacious during an imaging study, such as MBSS or FEES.

Compensatory techniques include postural adaptations and bolus modification. The following are postural adaptations that may improve oral swallowing:

- Chin-to-chest posture: Patients may aspirate due to premature spillage of liquid from the oral cavity into the larynx. This may occur because of insufficient tightening of the oropharyngeal isthmus, reduced lingual range of motion, disorganized lingual movement, and/or poor oral cavity sensation. This premature liquid spillage into the pharynx may be prevented or reduced if the patient lowers the chin toward the chest so that the bolus is positioned in the anterior oral cavity prior to oral transit.
- Head extension (otherwise known as chin elevation): Some patients have severely limited tongue mobility and consequently are largely unable to create tongue-to-palate pressure to propel a bolus to the pharynx. These patients may benefit from elevating their chin to move the bolus from the oral cavity to the pharynx via gravity. This compensation works best with thin liquids and nectar-thick liquids.
- Head tilted to the right or left: Tilting the head to one side may be utilized for patients with unilateral lingual weakness. For

example, a patient with left lingual weakness may have difficulty clearing some of the bolus through the oral cavity because of reduced left-sided tongue-to-palate pressure generation. This could result in left-sided oral cavity residue. Tilting the head to the right will position more of the bolus in the region of the stronger right hemi-tongue, which has a better capacity to oppose the palate and generate pressure to drive the bolus into the pharynx.

- Bolus modification: Some patients have difficulty forming and maintaining a thin liquid bolus due to lingual dysfunction. These patients may improve oral control if liquid viscosity is increased, since thicker liquids may be more cohesive and move more slowly. Other patients have mastication challenges and may benefit from a diet with less chewing requirements. There is a range of solid food textures from thin puree textures to minced and moist textures and soft and bite-sized textures (International Dysphagia Diet Standardization Initiative, 2019). Unfortunately, patients may not enjoy the experience of modified liquids and foods and therefore may be reluctant to abandon their usual diet. An adept speech pathologist will assess the use of behavioral techniques and modified food/liquid textures during an instrumental swallow exam to develop recommendations that will balance swallow safety and efficiency with eating and drinking pleasure, as much as this is possible.

Patients may be asked to engage in exercise-based treatment to improve their oral swallow. This can include performing lip, tongue, and mandible range-of-motion exercises during radiation therapy to preserve the range of motion of these structures if they are in the treatment field. These exercises may be employed after radiation or surgery as well if oral structure mobility is limited. The relationship between these range-of-motion exercises and oral swallowing function is not well understood (McCauley et al., 2009).

Treatment-related trismus can impact a patient's ability to eat, drink, swallow, talk, and maintain oral hygiene (Loorents et al., 2014). Interestingly, a recent meta-analysis performed by Charters et al. found no evidence that trismus prevention exercises performed during radiation therapy decreased the incidence of trismus (2022). However, the authors did find that posttreatment trismus did respond to therapy with similar results between stacked tongue blades vs commercially available mandible mobilizing devices. Patients undergoing radiation treatment for head and neck cancer at our institution are typically seen weekly in the speech pathology clinic for therapy designed to preserve swallow function (Hutcheson et al., 2013). A maximum incisal opening is measured weekly and therapy is instituted to improve the mandible range of motion when a patient's oral opening reaches the trismus threshold levels described below. Additionally, after radiation therapy, we routinely assess the mouth opening during clinic encounters and aggressively refer to trismus treatment as needed.

Trismus may be treated by a speech pathologist or a physical therapist. The clinician should obtain an objective assessment of the patient's baseline jaw opening prior to initiating treatment. This can be done using a range-of-motion scale, which allows measurement of the space between the incisors during maximum mandibular opening. A patient with intact dentition is considered to have trismus if the MIO is <35 mm (Loorents et al., 2014; Dijkstra et al., 2006). If the patient is missing maxillary or mandibular central incisors, the clinician should measure from the edentulous ridge and add 10 mm if missing one set of incisors or 20 mm if missing both sets. Trismus can be treated with a combination of manual massage and passive and active range-of-motion therapies. Various devices can be used to passively range the mandible, including Therabite, Orastretch, Dynasplint, and stacked tongue depressor blades. Active range-of-motion exercises include functional tasks (such as eating foods that require greater interincisal opening) and strengthening exercises. Trismus treatment is most effective if started when the condition is mild (Karlsson et al., 2021). Because trismus resulting from radiation treatment is progressive, the patient must work to maintain the gains made in therapy with regular exercise in perpetuity (Karlsson et al., 2021).

Tongue strength may be reduced in some patients who have undergone surgery, radiation, or chemoradiation for head and neck cancer. Tongue weakness may also occur because of non-cancer-related insult to the brain or cranial nerves. Tongue-strengthening therapy employs resistance exercises, with the tongue pressing against an object, such as the palate. Biofeedback devices have been developed for this type of exercise. The Iowa Oral Pressure Instrument (IOPI) is one such device. An air-filled bulb is placed between the hard palate and the tongue. The bulb connects via a catheter to the IOPI device. The IOPI produces data based on how much tongue-to-bulb pressure the patient applies. These readings are utilized to determine if goal levels are reached. An exercise algorithm that aligns with exercise physiology principles is employed to systematically increase the effort used by the patient. The use of the IOPI has been validated in many studies (Adams et al., 2013). Exercise to strengthen the oral tongue may also have a benefit on pharyngeal pressure generation for bolus transit (Adams et al., 2013).

Surgical and prosthetic treatments

While oral dysphagia can have many different etiologies, the goal of the treating provider is to normalize the function as much as possible. Glossectomy defects can be managed via surgical reconstruction (see the section titled "Reconstruction of the Tongue") and further aided with a prosthesis (see section titled "Speech and deglutition aids"). Reduced tongue-to-palate contact may result from oral cancer treatment or neurologic damage unrelated to cancer. These patients may experience difficulty propelling the bolus to the pharynx because of insufficient intraoral pressure generation. Palatal augmentation prostheses improve oral transit by creating a surface the tongue can oppose for oral transit. The palatal augmentation prostheses have mainly been studied with patients who have had partial or total glossectomy surgeries and have been shown to restore some degree of tongue-to-palate contact with improved oral transit efficiency for some patients (Pauloski et al., 1996). The degree of oral transit improvement conferred by an oral prosthesis appears to relate to the size of the surgical defect with less benefit for larger resections (Vickers and Shapiro, 1967). Patients may require swallow therapy in addition to the use of an intraoral prosthesis to meet their dysphagia goals (Kuniyuki et al., 2021).

Speech

Production of intelligible speech relies on the controlled movement of air from the lungs through the larynx, hypopharynx, pharynx, and oral cavity. The production of phonemes, or unique sounds in a language, is highly dependent on the shape that those structures assume as the air passes through the various chambers. Articulation of phonemes is accomplished by discreet and precise positional changes of the tongue, lips, and cheeks in relation to the palate, teeth, and other oral structures. While all these structures are important to the intelligible production of speech, the tongue is the major articulator during the production of all phonemes with the exception of the bilabial and labiodental sounds. The tongue shapes the oral and pharyngeal cavities for vowel and consonant production. For example, it restricts airflow in the oral cavity to produce the linguovelar consonants /*k*/ and /*g*/; the linguoalveolar consonants /*s*/, /*z*/, /*t*/, and /*d*/; the interdental variants of /*th*/; and palatoalveolar consonants such as /*sh*/ and /*ch*/. The basic tongue movements necessary for articulation are controlled by both intrinsic and extrinsic musculature of the tongue. The intrinsic tongue musculature creates changes in form and shape of the tongue, such as elevation or depression of the blade or tip. The intrinsic musculature has the potential to make discreet rapid changes in the shape and position of the tongue independent of mandibular movements or contraction of the extrinsic musculature. The extrinsic musculature, on the other hand, is primarily responsible for gross movements related to the elevation, depression, and retraction of the tongue. The tongue is richly endowed with both motor and sensory innervation in order to accomplish the task of speech production.

Surgical resection that alters the volume and restricts the movement of the tongue can have an adverse effect on the quality of speech. Consequently, resection of mandibular lesions that encroach upon the tongue musculature may adversely affect articulation. As discussed earlier, this group of patients is not homogenous. Lesions vary in their size and location and therefore, the surgical and radiological treatment will vary, as will the impact on oral structure and function. In general, following mandibular resections, the oral cavity may be reduced in size and a portion of the tongue may be excised. The sensory and motor innervation of the tongue can be compromised, as can innervation of the lower lip and cheek. Teeth may be lost as a result of the mandibular resection, which may compromise articulation and result in sound distortions. Mandibular movements may be significantly altered, especially if the temporomandibular joint is affected or any of the muscles of the jaw are resected. If the patient receives radiation therapy, changes in the volume and consistency of saliva can make prolonged discourse difficult. All of these factors, either alone or in combination, predispose the patient to misarticulation of speech sounds.

In general, research shows us that the speech exhibited by most mandibulectomy patients will be highly understandable when only the osseous structures are involved in resection. The degree of impairment is related primarily to the status of tongue function. If only the osseous structures are affected, reported speech results have been promising. For example, a scoping review by Lam-Tang and colleagues in 2008 of functional outcomes revealed that the majority of patients who had undergone mandibular reconstruction and who had either received no prosthetic dental rehabilitation or had been rehabilitated with either a tissue-borne or implant-retained prosthesis experienced speech results that were rated as highly intelligible or "near normal." In the studies that were reviewed, restricted tongue mobility was indicated as a potential contributing factor to decreased intelligibility. The review also indicated that when there was no tongue involvement, satisfactory speech outcomes were achieved regardless of the method of prosthetic rehabilitation (Tang et al., 2008). Since the time of that review, research results have continued to confirm similar outcomes for speech related to osseous resection (Dholam et al., 2011) and that an influential factor in speech intelligibility is the number of opposing teeth (Tsuchiya et al., 2013). Finally, although there may not be differences in speech intelligibility scores from the pre- to postoperative state in patients undergoing mandibular resection, research has shown that patient satisfaction with speech outcomes may be decreased, especially in cases where tumors are malignant (Mochizuki et al., 2014).

While speech results are generally favorable when cancers of the mandible affect only the osseous structures, those that include the soft tissue of the tongue may be associated with varying degrees of speech dysfunction depending on the size of the resection, its proximity to the lower jaw (Stelzle et al., 2011), and the method of reconstruction. With extensive resections of the tongue and FOM, the remaining portion of the tongue may exhibit limited and imprecise movements. Sensory loss compromises proprioceptive mechanisms of the residual tongue, requiring that contiguous structures with unimpaired sensory innervation serve to monitor tongue position. When functional outcomes were first reported for resections of extensive portions of the FOM and tongue, few controlled studies were available and results were somewhat equivocal. For example, Duguay described two patients following total glossectomy who produced intelligible speech without a tongue (1964). He reported that substitutions for tongue motion were made by the buccinator muscles and the muscles of the FOM. Consonant substitutes were used to produce acceptable speech. Kalfuss reported on the speech of 22 patients following mandibulectomy and glossectomy surgery (1968). The patients were divided into 4 groups based on the degree of tongue resection. There was a direct correlation between the amount of lingual tissue that was resected and the impairment of articulation. Skelly et al. studied and provided speech therapy for 14 total glossectomy and 11 partial glossectomy patients (1971). They studied this patient population with cineradiography and reported different compensation patterns between patient groups. Partial glossectomy patients made use of the residual tongue to perform adaptive movements approximating the normal ones, whereas the total glossectomy patients developed truly compensatory patterns of speech. Both patient groups benefited from speech therapy if dysphagia was not a problem. Bloomer and Hawk described a patient with a total glossectomy and reported that speech was understandable, although it had a "Donald Duck" quality (1973). Rentschler and Mann studied 20 patients, 2 with total glossectomies and 18 with partial glossectomies (1980). The majority of these patients also had partial mandibulectomies. They found that the rate of speech for most of these patients was slower than normal. Speech and oral discrimination were more severely impaired in patients who had more extensive surgical excisions.

Since that time, advances in microvascular free flap reconstruction have advanced functional outcomes in patients with extensive tongue defects, and speech results have been reported. Yanai and colleagues reported on 17 patients who underwent either total or subtotal glossectomy followed by free flap reconstruction (2008). Speech ratings by speech-language pathologists revealed that speech was good, with only occasional misunderstandings, in 30% of patients. In the majority of patients (53%), speech was understood only when the content was known. In the remaining 18% of patients, speech was either unintelligible or only occasionally understood. Lin et al. reported on a multi-institutional study of 55 patients who underwent total glossectomy, where 76% of patients retained the ability to communicate verbally with varying degrees of speech intelligibility (2015). Similar results were found by Keski-Santti and colleagues, who reported that 59% of their total glossectomy patients were able to communicate verbally; however, the degree of speech intelligibility was not reported. Finally, in a prospective study of speech intelligibility in total glossectomy, Dziegielewski and colleagues reported that patients' sentence intelligibility was 66% one year after oncological intervention (Dziegielewski et al., 2012).

In addition to the size of the defect, the type of flap used for reconstruction has been considered an influential factor in speech outcomes. For example, Wong et al. reported that free flap reconstruction with the radial forearm, anterolateral thigh, or latissimus dorsi resulted in better speech outcomes than did reconstruction with a myocutaneous pectoralis flap or primary closure (2007). These authors also examined other factors that had the potential to affect speech outcomes. The time of assessment (i.e., less than 12 months versus more than 12 months) did not reveal a difference in speech outcomes. However, a history of radiation therapy and a higher T stage (i.e., III and IV) at diagnosis were related to poorer speech outcomes. Su and colleagues similarly reported that patients reconstructed with a RFFF had better speech outcomes than did those reconstructed with a pectoralis major free flap (2003). These authors also demonstrated that total glossectomies resulted in significantly poorer speech outcomes than hemiglossectomy; hemiglossectomy resulted in only occasional sound errors, while total glossectomy resulted in severely unintelligible speech. Matsui and colleagues also reported that the RFFF results in better speech outcomes than other flaps, but only for patients with lateral defects. In their study, speech results for patients who had anterior defects, or a combination of anterior and lateral defects, were similar whether a radial forearm flap, pectoralis major myocutaneous flap, rectus abdominus myocutaneous flap, or anterior lateral thigh flap was used (Matsui et al., 2009). In other comparisons of the RFFF to the anterolateral thigh flap, Farace and colleagues and de Vicente and colleagues found no differences in speech outcomes between these two types of flaps in hemiglossectomy reconstruction (Farace et al., 2007; de Vicente et al., 2008). In consideration of the results of all of the aforementioned studies, there is no one type of flap that appears to result unequivocally in better speech outcomes. This has led researchers to begin to study other factors that may be influential in outcomes related to tongue reconstruction.

Two factors that may affect functional outcomes related to tongue reconstruction are the size and shape of the flap. Sakakibara et al. (2019) studied the effect of the size of the reconstructive flap. Their research suggested that postoperative function, including speech, could be optimized if a flap with a surface area that is 1.3 to 1.8 times greater than the area of resection is used. With respect to the shape of the flap, Wang and colleagues studied outcomes in relation to flaps that were customized using a "tip, body, root" approach versus those that did not consider these aspects of normal tongue anatomy. The authors did not find an advantage in speech intelligibility when patients were treated with a customized flap. The majority of their patients (68%) achieved good speech intelligibility, with the remaining achieving acceptable results (Wang et al., 2016). The results of these studies suggest that the size of the flap that is used may be an important factor in functional outcomes and, as such, warrants future study.

Some attention has also been paid to speech results after free flap closure versus a local or primary closure. Sun and colleagues compared speech outcomes in patients with forearm free flaps to those in patients with adjacent flaps. Intelligibility scores for the patients in the adjacent flap group ranged between 92.0% and 99.5% postoperatively; the largest decline in any one patient was 7.5%. Conversely, patients who underwent forearm free flap reconstruction demonstrated intelligibility scores between 79.5% and 99.0%, and the largest decline in any one patient was 20.5%. Not surprisingly, T stage predicted speech outcome, and lower stages were associated with better outcomes (Sun et al., 2007). Similarly, Konstantinović and Dimić showed that patients with local flaps had better speech outcomes than did those with pectoralis major myocutaneous flaps (1998). Hsiao et al. and Chuanjun et al. reported that speech results were better with primary closure than with reconstruction with a RFFF. These authors attributed the decline in speech function in the reconstruction group to restriction of the movement of the remaining tongue tissue by the bulky flap (Hsiao et al., 2002; Chuanjun et al., 2002). Conversely, Bressmann and colleagues did not reveal any differences in consonant intelligibility or tongue motility between patients who underwent local closure of their defect and those who underwent reconstruction with a platysma flap. In fact, these authors reported fewer consonant errors in patients who had flap closure than in patients with local closure (Bressmann et al., 2003). Thus, whether speech outcomes are better with primary closure or flap closure is still up for debate. One variable that must be considered in these comparisons is the size of the defect, because it may dictate whether a patient will undergo reconstruction or primary closure. Several authors have reported on speech outcomes for patients with partial glossectomy (i.e., removal of <40% of the tongue) who either received a flap or were allowed to heal via secondary intention. The patients who received flaps had poorer speech outcomes than the patients who healed via secondary intention (Pai et al., 2021; Ji et al., 2017; Tsuchiya et al., 2013; Lam-Tang et al., 2008). When Ji and colleagues studied their patients with defects that were larger (i.e., hemiglossectomy), the authors found that speech intelligibility was substantially better in patients who received a flap versus those who received primary closure (Ji et al., 2017). Thus, it appears that flaps may interfere with speech outcomes when defects are small but are vital to good speech outcomes when a larger portion of the tongue is resected.

Most of the aforementioned studies relied on listener judgments to rate speech outcomes. These types of assessments are important because they lend face validity to the outcomes. In order to provide a more objective evaluation of speech outcomes, some authors have focused on the acoustic characteristics of speech output. For example, Salibian and colleagues reported on patients with total and subtotal glossectomy who underwent reconstruction. Their results revealed that spectrograms of several vowels produced in the postoperative period were quite normal, indicating that patients were able to move the flap tissue within the oral cavity to approximate correct positioning for such production. Consonants appeared to be affected to a greater degree, with the expected bursts and closures being absent for many such sounds (Salibian et al., 1990). Whitehill et al. reported on patients with partial glossectomies. Their results indicated that certain vowel formant frequencies were affected, whereas others were not, when compared to controls. The authors concluded that the deviations from normal may be related to a limited range of lingual motion in the anterior-posterior plane in patients (Whitehill et al., 2006). Laaksonen et al. reported acoustic outcomes across the course of a year in patients who underwent partial glossectomy of the anterior two-thirds of the tongue followed

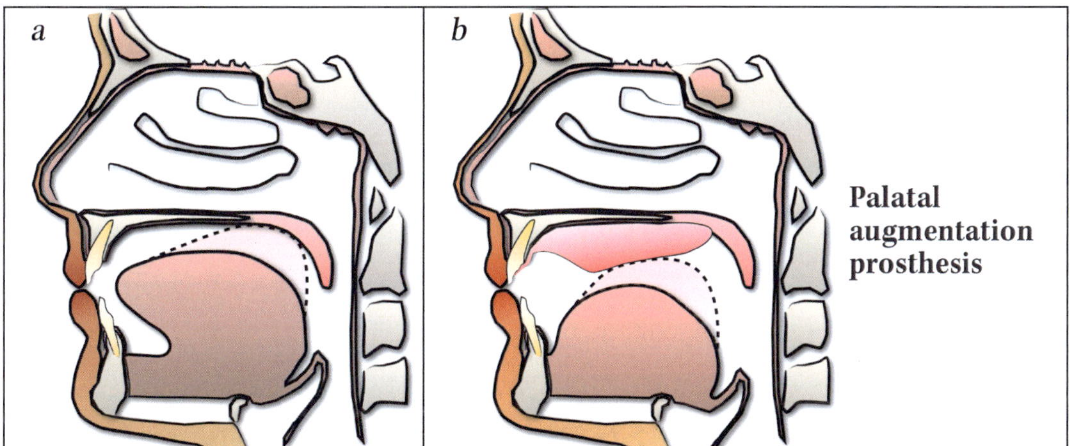

Figure 2-118 *(a)* Production of many speech phonemes requires the tongue to elevate and interact with the palate and/or maxillary dentition. *(b)* Insertion of a PAP (blue). The dorsum of the reconstructed tongue can valve against the prosthetic palate.

by reconstruction with a RFFF. Their study found that the acoustic characteristics in speech changed more dramatically from the preoperative state in males than in females. The authors reported many individual changes in the extent of the acoustic adaptations across the year and in the speech sounds that were affected. They suggested that their results reflect speaker-specific abilities for adaptation and/or compensation for altered conditions after tongue reconstruction (Laaksonen et al., 2010). Future acoustic studies of speech output likely will shed more light on the fine articulatory changes that take place after glossectomy.

Speech and deglutition aids

An approach to the improvement of the articulation for mandibulectomy patients was originally suggested by Cantor et al. They noted that consonant sounds such as /*k*/ and /*g*/ required valving by the posterior part of the tongue with the posterior part of the hard palate and the anterior portion of the soft palate and that these consonant sounds were particularly difficult for mandibulectomy patients to make properly (Cantor et al., 1969). Herberman also noted distortion of these phonemes (Herberman, 1958).

Cantor et al. reasoned that if the palatal vault were lowered prosthetically into the space of Donders to accommodate restricted tongue movements, speech might improve (Cantor et al., 1969; Fig 2-118). To test this hypothesis, 10 patients with restricted tongue movements were selected. Five patients had extreme restriction of movement of the tongue and 5 had moderate restriction. Extreme restriction was defined as the inability to contact either the palate or the maxillary teeth with the residual tongue. Moderate restriction was defined as partial or frequent tongue contact with the teeth or the palate during speech. The palate was lowered by means of a retainer for dentulous patients and a palatal acrylic resin extension to the maxillary denture for edentulous patients. A functional impression of the dorsal surface of the tongue was molded during attempts at speech production and a hollow palatal speech prosthesis was constructed. Speech samples were recorded before placement of the prosthesis and again after a 2-week period. The test sample contained 10 words with /*k*/ and /*g*/ sounds. No speech therapy was used during the test period. The speech samples were randomized and rated by five trained speech pathologists in a double-blind evaluation. The results showed a significant improvement for patients with severely restricted tongue movements, but the prosthesis slightly hampered speech for patients with moderate movement. Although Chierici and Lawson questioned the value of these prostheses for sustained speech (1973), Cantor et al. demonstrated that, in patients with severely restricted tongue movements, specific sounds can be improved by a palatal speech aid (1969).

Subsequent to the study of speech outcomes in 1969, the palatal prosthesis has been evaluated for its effects on both speech and swallowing. Wheeler et al., Davis et al., and Robbins et al. objectively evaluated the effects of a palatal prosthesis on speech and deglutition in 10, 1, and 10 patients, respectively, who had partial or total glossectomies with or without mandibular involvement. The prosthesis was designed to accommodate the required range of motion of the residual tongue. Voice recordings were used to evaluate speech and videofluoroscopy techniques were applied to study deglutition. All patients were evaluated and received speech and swallowing therapy prior to the insertion of the prosthesis. The authors of all three studies reported improvement in speech and deglutition following the placement of the prosthesis (Wheeler et al., 1980; Davis et al., 1987; Robbins et al., 1987).

Leonard and Gillis evaluated the differential effects of a speech prosthesis in five glossectomy patients. Three patients, all of whom had 50% or more remaining tongue with good mobility, were treated with a palatal prosthesis. One patient was treated with a mandibular prosthesis and one patient had both palatal and mandibular prostheses. The mandibular prosthesis was used if little or no residual tongue remained. Recordings with and without the prosthesis were evaluated by a practicing speech pathologist. All subjects demonstrated varying degrees of improvement in the speech measures evaluated (intelligibility, number of consonants in error, and the acoustic characteristics of vowels). The effects of these prostheses on swallowing was not studied, nor was it determined if the same results could have been achieved with a palatal prosthesis in the two patients who had a mandibular prosthesis (Leonard and Gillis, 1990).

In a case study, Shimodaira et al. reported speech outcomes for a patient with total glossectomy. The results from 10 listeners showed that intelligibility scores on a standard Japanese speech test increased from 19% correct without a PAP to 74% correct with the prosthesis.

In addition, listener judgments of a conversational speech sample revealed that speech improved from unintelligible without the prosthesis to adequate but not normal with the prosthesis. These authors also evaluated swallowing in this patient with the use of durational measures for swallowing a thin or thick paste. Oral transit duration time for a thin paste decreased from 72 seconds without the prosthesis to 27 seconds with the prosthesis. The patient was unable to swallow the thick paste without the prosthesis and subsequently able to swallow it in 116 seconds with the prosthesis. The swallowing durations with the prosthesis deviated from normal; nonetheless, the improvement was substantial (Shimodaira et al., 1998).

Marunick and Tselios conducted a review of studies published between 1966 and 2002 on palatal augmentation prostheses for individuals who had severe restrictions in tongue-palate contact after tongue resection for cancer. Nine of 130 studies met their inclusion criteria, leading to results for 50 subjects (42 had swallowing data and 37 had speech data). The results from the swallowing data suggested that a PAP promoted improved swallowing ability in 86% of patients (36 of 42 subjects). The speech data indicated that a prosthesis also was advantageous for 86% of patients (32 of 37 subjects; Marunick and Tselios, 2004).

Using spectrograms, de Carvalho-Teles et al. analyzed intelligibility and acoustic characteristics in Brazilian Portuguese vowel sounds in 36 patients who had undergone differing degrees of glossectomy and who were rehabilitated with a PAP. Their results revealed that spontaneous speech intelligibility and the number of correctly identified syllables improved with the use of a PAP. In addition, the formant values for several vowels were reported to be closer to normal with the use of a prosthesis than without it (de Carvalho-Teles et al., 2008).

Laaksonen et al. reported on acoustic speech outcomes in a patient who underwent resection of the anterior third of the tongue followed by reconstruction with a RFFF. The authors reported on outcomes one year after the resection without a prosthesis and two years after resection with the prosthesis. Acoustic changes of the vowels and the spectral moments of the sibilants indicated that the tongue resection and reconstruction distorted speech from the normal state. Treatment with a PAP improved the production of sibilants /s/ and /z/. The effect of the PAP on vowel production was less pronounced (Laaksonen et al., 2009).

Speech therapy

Speech therapy may be effective in improving articulation in these patients; however, there is little information published in the literature on the efficacy of speech rehabilitation in patients with glossectomy or mandibulectomy. Scott investigated the potential benefit of intensive speech therapy for mandibulectomy patients. Twenty patients were selected for study; 10 wore palatal augmentation prostheses and 10 did not. The patients were divided into 4 groups. Two groups of 5 patients (5 with and 5 without prostheses) received 6 weeks of intensive speech therapy and the control groups received no speech therapy. Although the groups were small, the study does offer two valid conclusions: (1) placement of a PAP, although improving the quality of specific sounds may not improve discourse, and (2) intensive speech therapy improves speech significantly for patients both with and without prostheses (Scott, 1970).

Furia and colleagues studied the effect of speech therapy in 27 patients who had differing degrees of glossectomy. Therapy goals over the course of 16 planned sessions included maximizing residual tongue movement and developing appropriate articulatory adaptations and compensations. The authors reported significant improvements in patients with total and subtotal resections; however, there were no significant improvements for patients with partial resections. In the absence of a patient control group, it is unclear whether their results were due to the therapeutic intervention or to spontaneous recovery over time (Furia et al., 2001).

Pauloski and colleagues did not formally assess a specific therapy program but did evaluate whether better speech outcomes were associated with a history of speech therapy in patients who had surgical intervention for both oral and oropharyngeal cancers. Their results revealed that 28 of 38 patients received speech therapy during their first postoperative year. Of these, 70% of the patients received therapy within one month following surgical intervention. The results did not show any significant improvements in speech outcomes across time in these patients. The authors suggested that this lack of improvement could be related to the small amount of therapy that the patients received (Pauloski et al., 1994).

The lack of standardization of speech therapy targeted at hemiglossectomy was reported in a 2015 systematic review (Blyth et al., 2015). The authors of that review reported that interventions for speech rehabilitation generally targeted new methods of articulation that would lead to clear sound production. The studies that were included in the review generally used multiple exercises and techniques at the same time, leading to uncertainty regarding which behavior actually was responsible for meaningful changes. As a start in addressing some of these limitations, Blyth and colleagues (2016) reported on two patients who underwent speech therapy using ultrasound for biofeedback in a multiple baseline design study. There was a significant improvement in the percentage of consonants correct after therapeutic intervention. It is clear that there is a need for more systematic, well-designed studies to assess the effect of speech therapy in patients with oral resection and reconstruction.

Fabrication of Speech and Deglutition Aids

The determination of whether a speech and deglutition aid should be placed in the maxilla as a PAP, or in the mandible as a tongue prosthesis, has been based primarily on (1) the volume and mobility of the residual or reconstructed tongue (2) and the patient's chief complaint (speech, swallowing, or both). These factors may influence the treatment options, as well as trismus and patient motivation. A thorough examination and appropriate tests and radiographic studies should be completed before treatment is initiated.

Mandibular-based tongue prostheses are best indicated on dentate arches where a total glossectomy resulted in a low, flat, and immobile FOM, which will serve as a seat for the prosthetic tongue. Residual mobility of the tongue mound could dislodge the tongue prosthesis that overlays it. A good mandibular range of motion is another requisite because it provides a means for the patient to control the approximation or contact of the prosthetic tongue to the palate as necessary for articulating speech or oral transit of the food bolus. Normal cheek and lip mobility allow the patient to control the shape of the oral cavity as a resonating chamber.

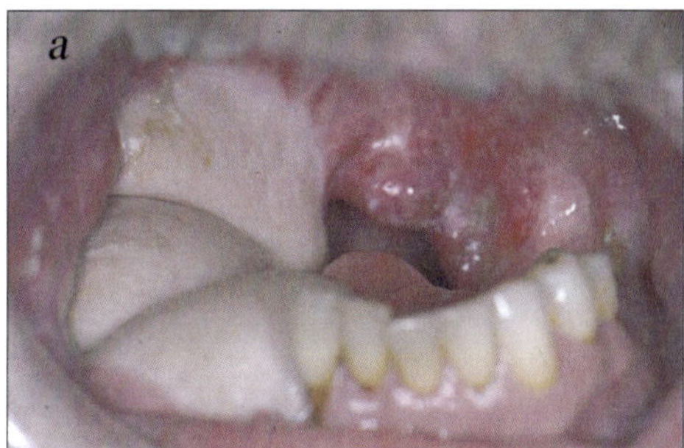

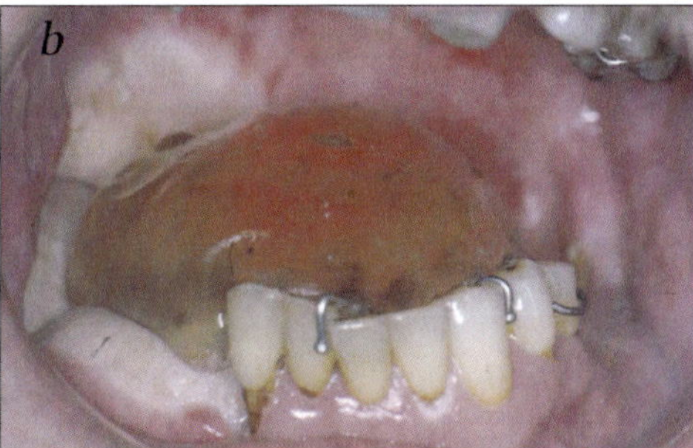

Figure 2-119 Mandibular-based tongue prosthesis made of acrylic resin. *(a)* Total glossectomy defect. *(b)* Speech is intelligible with the tongue prosthesis.

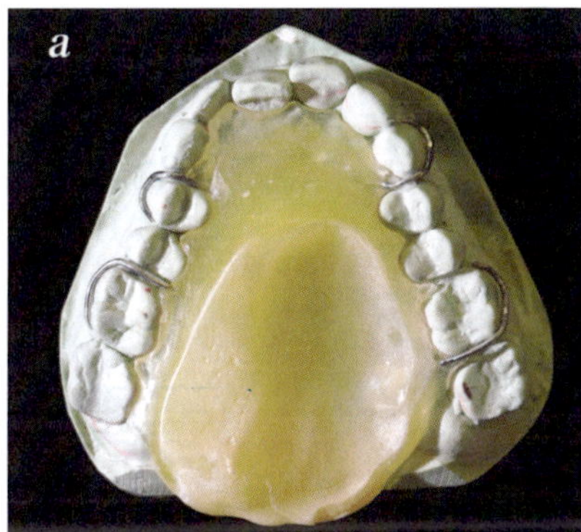

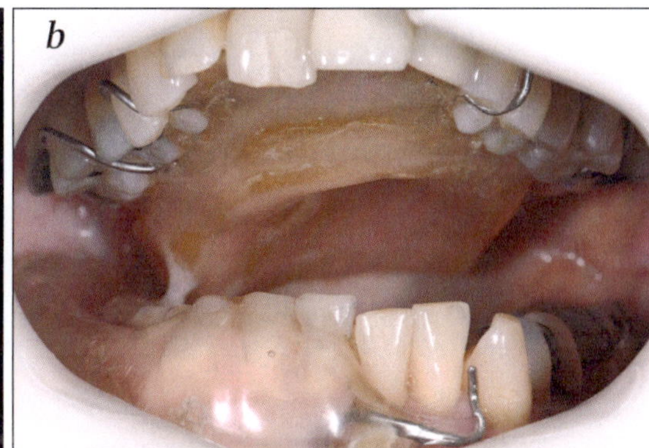

Figure 2-120 Interim PAP for a dentate patient. *(a)* The prosthesis returned to the cast after molding. Note the extension onto the soft palate beyond the vibrating line. *(b)* Prosthesis in position. When the mandible is in the closed position, the tongue interacts with the prosthetic palate.

A mandibular-based tongue prosthesis following surgery has improved the quality of speech and assisted in deglutition (Moore, 1972; Lauciello et al., 1980; Aramany et al., 1982) (Fig 2-119). The support for this intervention, however, has been based on case reports of a small number of patients who have been evaluated in a research setting. With the refinement of microvascular free flaps for tongue reconstruction, the use of the tongue prosthesis has generally fallen out of favor.

Maxillary-based speech and deglutition aids—namely, a PAP (previously referred to as a palatal-drop prosthesis)—are best indicated when a residual tongue mound or free flap reconstructed tongue retains some mobility yet fails to valve against the palate and/or dentition. As with any removable prosthesis, healthy abutment teeth improve prosthesis stability and retention; however, complete denture PAPs are possible (Fig 2-124). A good mandibular range of motion improves the patient's ability to approximate or contact the residual tongue to the prosthetically augmented palate.

Interim prostheses are used as therapy while the tongue recovers its function. This period allows patients and clinicians follow-up appointments for adjustments to accommodate specific adaptations, including increased mobility or hypertrophy of the articulating tissues. This approach does require multiple appointments with trial-and-error modifications that are based on input from the patient, family members, and the speech pathologist. Computerized analysis and simulation techniques may prove to be helpful in patient selection for prosthetic intervention and design of speech and deglutition prostheses. Follow-up with modifications are often necessary (Leonard, 1991).

Interim PAPs are more effective in dentate patients because the superior retention permits the prosthesis to be extended more posteriorly on the soft palate, thereby facilitating oral airflow during speech (Fig 2-120). Hand-adapted wire clasps and an acrylic resin denture base are made on an accurate cast. The denture base is fitted and adjusted chairside as needed before the augmentation is functionally generated with either low-fusing impression compound, impression waxes, slow-setting acrylic resins, or tissue conditioning materials. These modifications must be made to accommodate residual tongue and mandibular movements during speech, swallowing, or both, depending on the planned function of the prosthesis. Because of their ease of handling, adjustment, and long working time to allow functional impressions, the authors prefer either tissue conditioners or slow-setting acrylic resins (Fig 2-120). The latter has the added advantage that it can be polished and added to at subsequent follow-up appointments. Tissue conditioners need to be completely replaced after a month of use, as they quickly become rough and delaminate. Either material used is mixed to a thick, moldable consistency for an initial tracing. If small additions are necessary, subsequent mixtures are prepared with slightly more liquid to increase flow. Runny mixtures should be avoided to prevent the material from flowing posteriorly and being swallowed.

If tongue function returns to acceptable limits during a therapy/healing period and is only marginally compromised, a PAP may no longer make discernible improvements. In these circumstances, the use of the interim prosthesis can be discontinued.

Definitive prostheses. Some patients may require an indefinite use of a PAP. When long-term use is deemed necessary, it is recommended that a definitive prosthesis be made. The interim prosthesis is reviewed to help design the metal framework. Notice that in the interim prosthesis shown in Fig 2-120a, all teeth are plated on their palatal surfaces and that the molded acrylic extends to just shy of the occlusal table. This requires that the metal-acrylic junction on the metal framework be defined as a sharp external finish line with an undercut to retain the acrylic resin (Fig 2-121). A metal base is

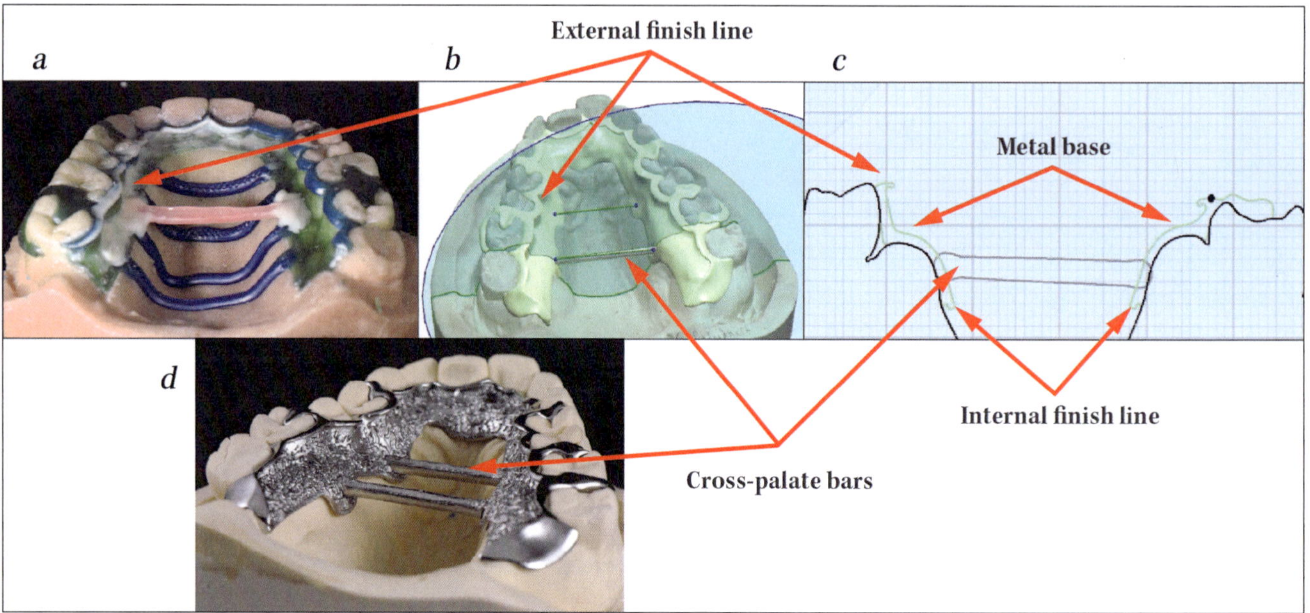

Figure 2-121 Two different PAP frameworks for dentate patients. Note the occlusal placement of the external finish lines for a clear demarcation of the metal-acrylic junction. Note the metal base along the teeth and cross-palatal bars. *(a)* Conventional wax-up onto the refractory cast. Note the idealization of the external finish line. *(b and c)* Digital designs. Note the 2D cross-sectional evaluation of the components. *(d)* Completed metal framework.

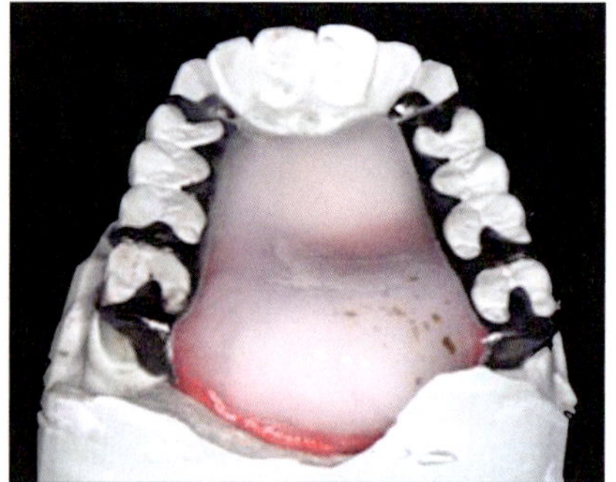

Figure 2-122 Molded PAP onto a metal framework. Note that the final tracing was made in tissue conditioner. The patient was allowed to functionally generate the final contours over a few days.

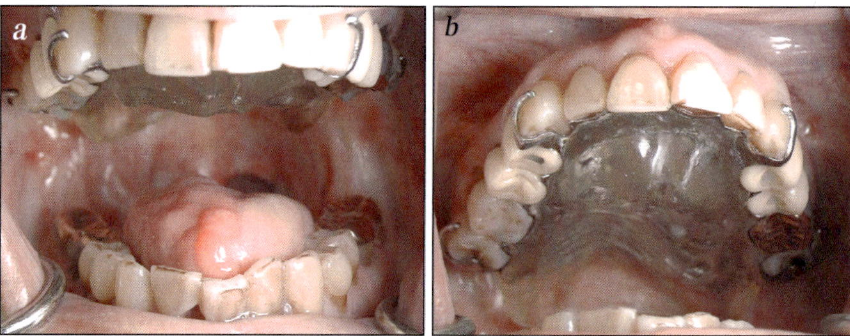

Figure 2-123 Definitive palatal augmentation prosthesis in a dentate patient. *(a)* Prosthesis in position with maximum tongue elevation. When the mandible is in the closed position, the tongue interacts with the prosthetic palate. *(b)* Improved retention with a metal framework allows extension to the soft palate, facilitating oral functions.

preferred to contact the palatal surface of the dentition and the first 6 mm of the gingiva, placing the internal finish line away from the free gingival margins. In the presence of palatally tipped or restoratively defective teeth, surveyed crowns should be considered to allow ideal modifications and the addition of palatal guide planes. Across the palate, an open lattice is designed to retain the acrylic resin. Cross-palate bars raised off the palatal vault are added when a significant volume of augmentation is needed. Once the metal framework is fabricated, it is fitted and adjusted as customary for any RPD framework prior to molding the augmentation. The interim prosthesis is reviewed to guide the volume and contours of the definitive counterpart. Because the molded PAP will be invested into stone for conversion to acrylic resin, it is advisable to functionally generate the palatal contours with materials that are either thermoplastic or flexible to allow either boiling out or teasing out from the stone investment (Fig 2-122). The advantage of using a tissue conditioner as the final tracing is that the patient can functionally generate the final contours over a few days. Once the contours are verified, the trial prosthesis is invested for processing in heat-activated acrylic resin (Fig 2-123).

For the edentulous patient, if a complete denture already exists, the palatal vault of the prosthesis is modified and functionally generated as described above (Fig 2-124). After a trial period, when the optimum contours have been achieved and patient expectations managed, the interim material is converted to laboratory-processed acrylic resin (Fig 2-124d).

In the presence of a trismus, new complete denture prostheses should be considered so that the OVD can be decreased and the occlusal plane lowered. These modifications have three advantages: (1) Improved reach of the tongue to the palate, which in turn decreases the volume of palatal augmentation. (2) Increased interocclusal rest space, which effectively improves the vertical range of motion of the mandible and tongue. (3) Lowered occlusal plane to improve the ability of the tongue remnant to manipulate the food bolus onto the occlusal table.

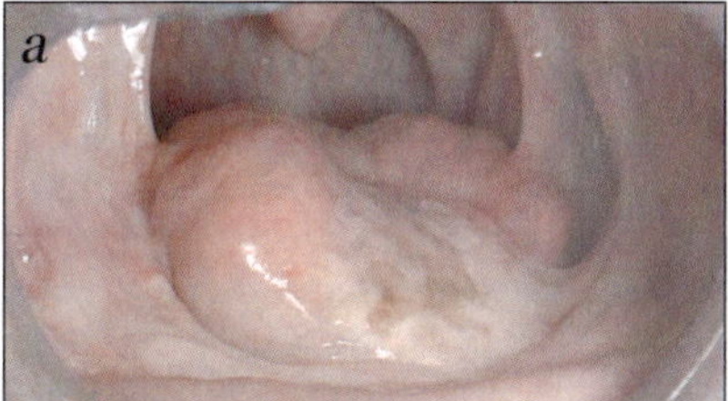

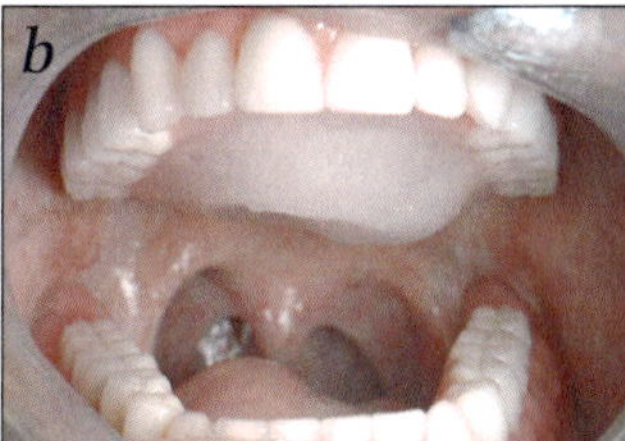

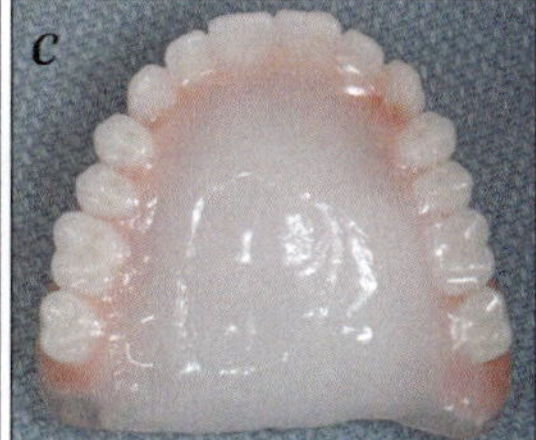

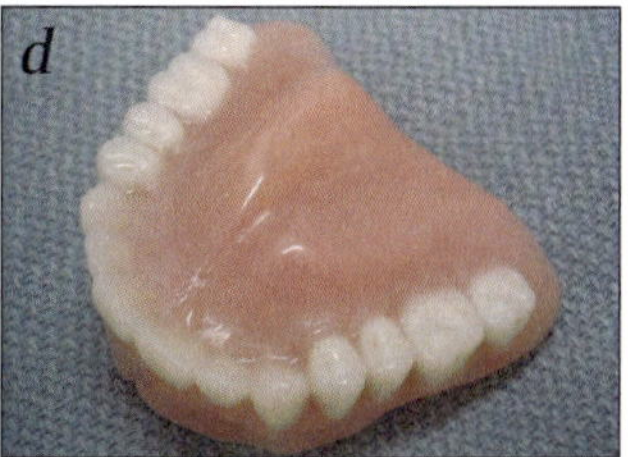

Figure 2-124 PAP. *(a)* Partial glossectomy defect. Tongue elevation was deficient secondary to tethering. *(b)* A thick mix of tissue conditioner material was added to the palatal vault area followed by asking the patient to speak and swallow. *(c)* Resulting palatal contour after functional molding. *(d)* Optimized contours invested and lab-processed with acrylic resin.

Secondary Surgical Procedures

This section covers several surgical procedures commonly needed secondary to the tumor ablation (Box 2-1) to improve oral function by optimizing the defect for prosthodontic rehabilitation.

If the patient has been irradiated, the treatment dose and clinical target volume need to be known, since the predictability of osseointegration is affected (see Chapter 1, section "Dental Implants in Irradiated Tissues"). Isodose curves (Fig 2-125) are reviewed, and a target volume that received greater than 60 Gy is considered a poor candidate for invasive surgery and risks devitalizing the free flap (Ch'ng et al., 2016). As described previously, the use of an interim MRP for an extended period will help assess functional deficits and help weigh the potential benefit of secondary surgery against the potential risks. Patients with a few missing teeth, reasonable tongue function, and high-dose radiation should not be considered for additional surgery, as there would be little functional gain. Edentulous resection patients with reasonable tongue function but who are unable to retain and manipulate a conventional soft tissue–borne MRP have the most to gain by the placement of dental implants and skin paddle debulking if indicated.

Radiation or chemoradiation therapy does not preclude the use of dental implants. If the patient was treated with external beam radiotherapy or brachytherapy, implant therapy can be considered in sites known to have received 55 Gy or less; at this dosage, reasonably good viability remains in the bone to permit osseointegration. By contrast, implant placement in areas that received a dose of 65 Gy or more is at significant risk of implant failure and ORN. We view areas of 60 Gy as a gray zone (see Chapter 1, section "Dental Implants in Irradiated Tissues").

A radiographic evaluation should be performed. Minimally, a panoramic radiograph is ordered (Fig 2-126) to assess the osteosyntheses, the soft tissue reconstruction, and plate and screw positions. In Figure 2-126a, the plate is occlusal to the osseous reconstruction, which would requre removal of the hardware should any debulking procedure be considered to avoid exposures intraorally (Patel et al., 2019). However, this same patient has a right para-symphyseal malunion, making hardware removal a contraindication.

Periapical radiographs could also be considered, especially of any terminal abutments adjacent to the alveolar resection margins. One should perform a clinical evaluation, measure probing depth and attachment loss, and assess periodontal support and widened periodontal ligament, mobility, and fremitus. With the loss of periodontal attachment comes exposed root surfaces and a high risk of root caries. Always keep in mind that preserving the remaining

Box 2-1 List of secondary surgical procedures

- Debulking and vestibuloplasty
- Split-thickness skin grafts
- Palatal grafts
- Tongue release
- Secondary dental implants
- Stage II implant surgery

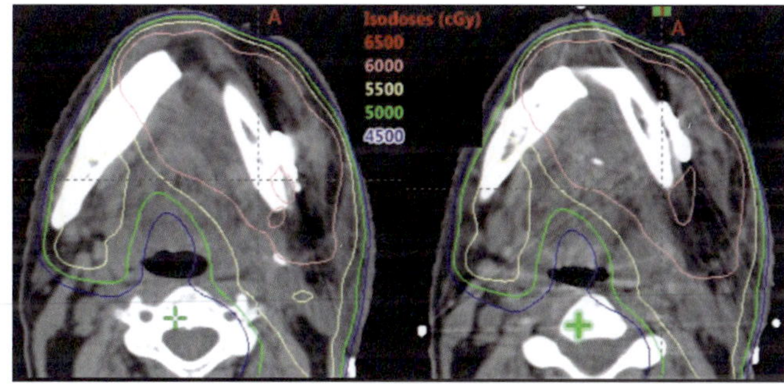

Figure 2-125 CT planning example of postmandibulectomy adjuvant IMRT. Notice that the entire fibula flap will receive 60 Gy. The site of the right second molar will receive 55 Gy.

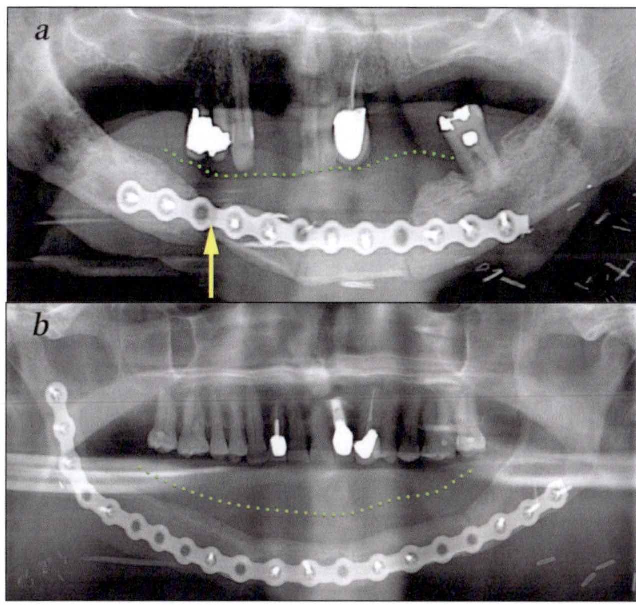

Figure 2-126 *(a)* Symphyseal ORN defect reconstructed with a two-piece SFF. Notice the malunion of the graft to the native mandible *(arrow)*, the plate position occlusal to the scapula graft, and the bulk of the soft tissue flap *(dotted line)*. *(b)* Angle-to-angle mandibulectomy of gingival SCC, reconstructed with a three-piece FFF. Notice the appropriate apical position of the plate and the four complete osseous unions.

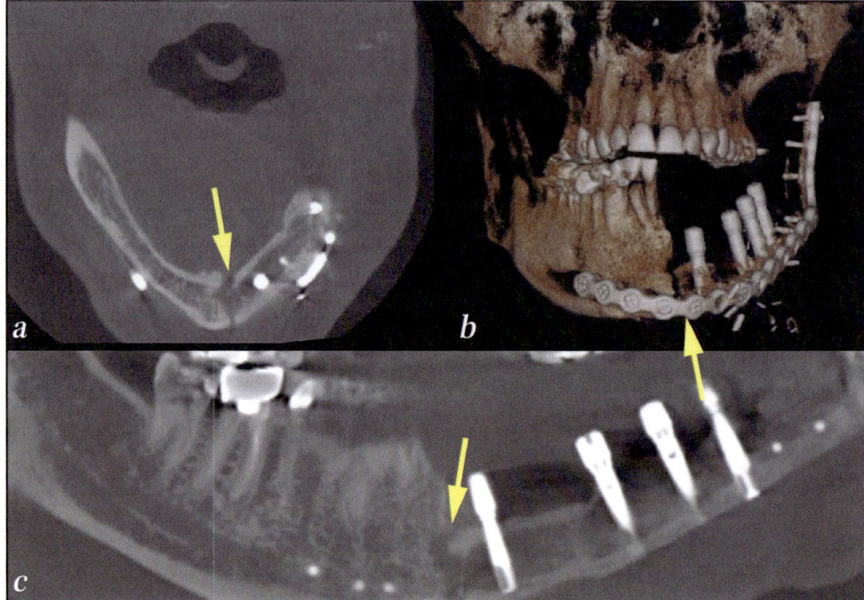

Figure 2-127 CBCT evaluation of the osteosyntheses and primarily placed dental implants in a FFF. *(a)* Axial slice showing bucco-lingual malunion. *(b)* 3D rendering showing malunion. *(c)* Panoramic rendering of the CT data showing malunion *(arrow)*.

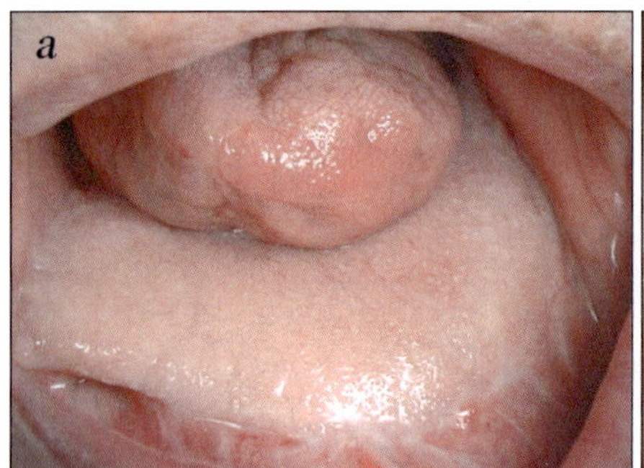

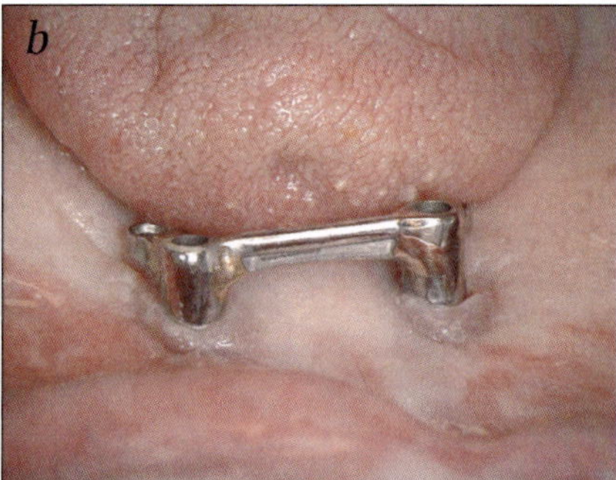

Figure 2-128 *(a)* Symphyseal defect reconstructed with an osteomyocutaneous free flap. *(b)* Soft tissues that were not sufficiently thinned resulting in peri-implantitis.

dentition is as important if not more so than replacing those lost secondary to the tumor ablation.

Computer tomography is critical for the planning of secondary dental implants and for assessing the osteosyntheses when a two-dimensional radiograph is inconclusive (Fig 2-127). If malunion is the result of high-dose radiation, then bone grafting is unlikely to ameliorate the problem. In these situations, close monitoring is suggested and surgical intervention is avoided unless the patient becomes symptomatic.

Debulking and vestibuloplasty

Defects restored with osteomyocutaneous free flaps generally present with an excess of soft tissue overlying the osseous graft (Figs 2-26, 2-28, and 2-130a). In most patients, a skin paddle has been used to replace the soft tissues removed during tumor extirpation. Skin flaps covering the graft—and implants if implants were placed primarily—can be 1.5 cm thick or more depending on the patient's body habitus and donor site. Figure 2-135 shows an extreme case of a scapula skin flap measuring 2 cm in height occlusal to the osseous graft, displacing the tongue posteriorly. These tissues must be thinned (even if dental implants will not be employed) in order to provide prosthetic space and to create a proper denture-bearing surface for mucosa-borne or tooth-mucosa-borne MRPs. When dental implants emerge through a cutaneous flap, two options are available to create appropriately thin and attached peri-implant soft tissues:

- Supraperiosteal dissection, careful debulking, and reattachment of the skin to the periosteum (Figs 2-128 and 2-130) or
- Supraperiosteal excision of the skin paddle with concurrent split-thickness skin grafting (Figs 2-131 and 2-134)

The goal for either technique is to create thin, attached tissues around the implants so as to minimize the risk of peri-implantitis. Ideally, the thickness of the soft tissues circumscribing the implants should not exceed 4 mm. If the tissues are not thinned sufficiently, deep peri-implant pockets that predispose the site to infection, granulation tissue formation, and hypertrophy will result. These soft tissue infections can spread to the bone, leading to loss of bone and ultimately implant failure (Fig 2-129).

Stent fabrication

The process of stent fabrication has evolved. Conventionally, a cast made from an overextended impression is modified using intuition

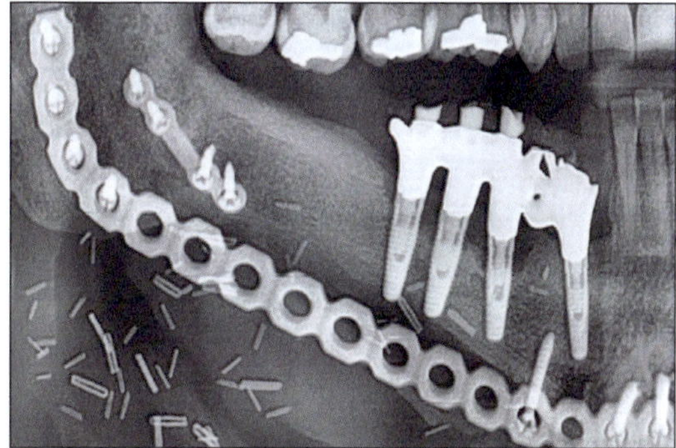

Figure 2-129 Panorex of a patient with persistent granulation and hypertrophic soft tissues under a fixed, metal-acrylic MRP. Note the cratered bone loss around the three posterior implants.

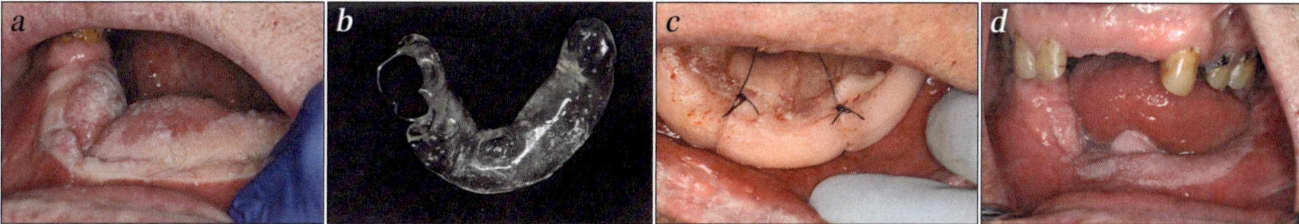

Figure 2-130 *(a)* FFF reconstruction of a defect secondary to removal of a sarcomatoid carcinoma. *(b)* Conventional surgical splint with wire clasps. *(c)* After a supraperiosteal dissection and thinning of the skin paddle, the splint is relined and secured with circum-mandibular nylon sutures *(d)* Several weeks following debulking surgery.

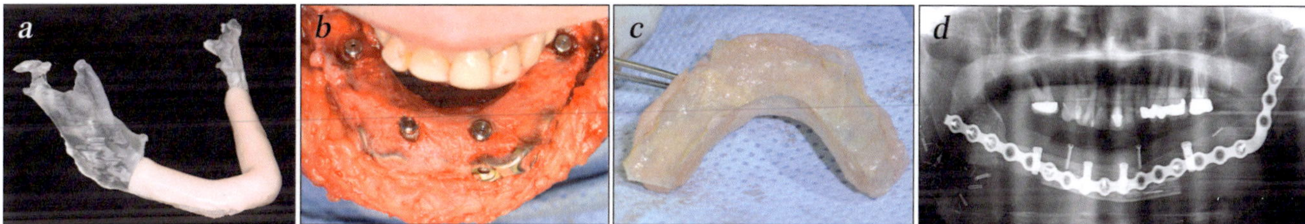

Figure 2-131 *(a)* 3D-printed model of the reconstructed mandible. Relief wax is adapted to account for the thickness of the soft tissue over the periosteum. Autocuring PMMA was used to fabricate a stent. *(b)* Vestibuloplasty dissection completed. Care was taken not to tear the periosteum. *(c)* PMMA stent was relined with a soft denture liner. Harvested STSG is laid into the relined stent. *(d)* Panorex shows two lag screws securing the stent in place.

about the position of the neomandible. Autopolymerizing PMMA is cured under 20 PSI with or without wire clasps adapted to available dentition. After raising a supraperiosteal flap and debulking, the stent is relined with a soft denture liner (Fig 2-130).

If VSP was used in the mandibular reconstruction, then the printed model of the reconstructed mandible, which mimics the osseous graft, is used—assuming the reconstruction went according to the VSP. Instead of subtractive changes to the model, the addition of two to three layers of baseplate wax, about 4 mm, approximates the thickness of the soft tissue (Fig 2-131a). As with the conventional method, acrylic resin is used to form the stent. The periphery should end 3 mm short of the reconstruction plate if one is present and have a rounded periphery. Intraoperatively, the stent is relined as described above. In comparison to the conventional methods, the amount of reline material should be considerably less (Fig 2-131).

The fully digital technique utilizes postreconstruction CT and 3D-modeling software to design the stent after the addition of a 4 mm digital spacer. Screw holes or channels can also be designed to allow fixation of the stent, which is printed in a biocompatible material (Fig 2-132). Stents should be left in situ for three to four weeks.

Figures 2-130, 2-131, and 2-132 illustrate three techniques for stent fabrication; notice, however, that two different surgical approaches were employed to achieve thinner attached soft tissues over the osteocutaneous graft: (1) thinning of the skin paddle by the removal of muscle and adipose tissue (Figs 2-128 and 2-130) and (2) excision of the myocutaneous flap and reepithelialization with a split-thickness skin graft (Figs 2-131 and 2-134). The latter is described in more detail below and is preferred because it will achieve thinner tissues more appropriate for dental implants, with one surgical intervention. In irradiated tissues, however, this may be contraindicated for fear of reducing vascularity to the fibula. By comparison, the former technique frequently results in modest thinning, inadequate for dental implants to emerge through, and requires a second or third round of debulking (see Fig 2-146).

Split-thickness skin grafts (STSG)

The successful use of split-thickness skin grafts (STSG) as a free epithelial graft over supraperiosteal dissections has been well documented in the literature. Schuchardt suggested that the periosteal

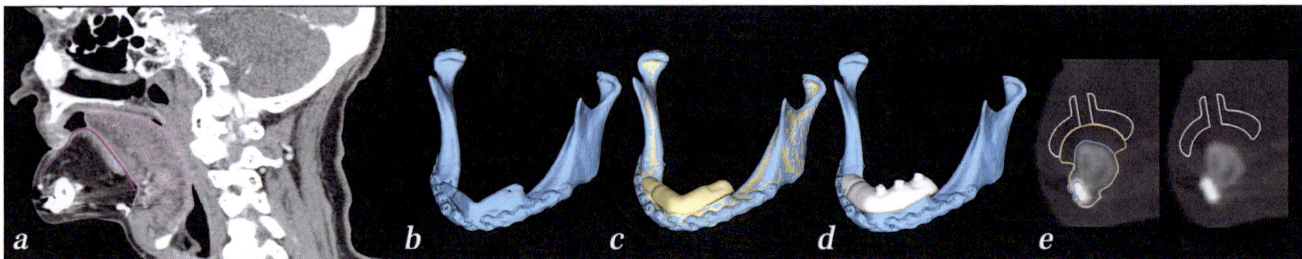

Figure 2-132 Reconstruction of a symphyseal mandibulectomy with an SFF *(a)* Sagittal CT shows soft tissue bulk over the osseous scapula *(purple outline)* measuring 2 cm in height. Notice the displaced position of the oral tongue *(pink outline)*. *(b)* CAD of the reconstructed mandible. *(c)* Digital spacer 4 mm thick. *(d)* CAD of debulking/vestibuloplasty stent. *(d and e)* Facio-lingual section shows the juxtaposition of the graft, the soft tissue spacer, and the stent. Notice that fixation screw holes are also designed.

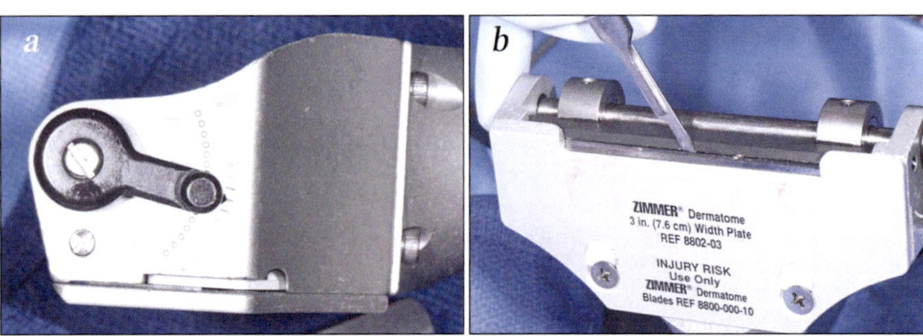

Figure 2-133 *(a)* Dermatome thickness setting to 0.012 inches or 0.30 mm. *(b)* This is equivalent to the thickness of a scalpel blade, which is used to double-check the spacing of the Dermatome blade.

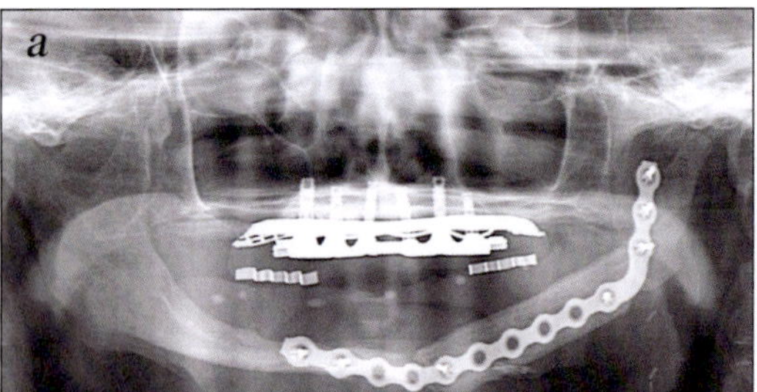

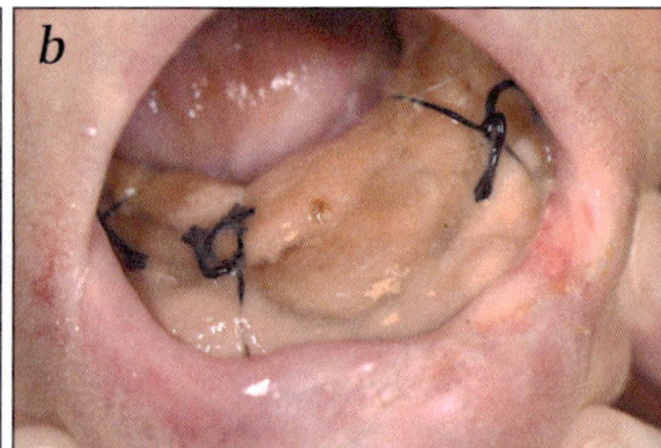

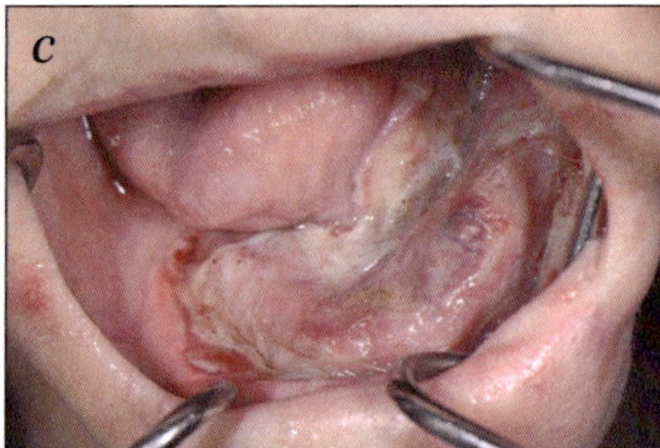

Figure 2-134 *(a)* Panoramic radiograph of a patient post right mandible reconstructed with a FFF, who will undergo debulking and vestibuloplasty. *(b)* Stent carrying the split-thickness skin graft secured with circum-mandibular sutures. *(c)* Clinical presentation after removing the splint three weeks after surgical procedures.

surface, but not the soft tissue bed, be covered with skin. To achieve this, he sutured the free mucosal edge to the periosteum in the depth of the newly created vestibule (Schuchardt, 1952).

The combination of vestibuloplasty with skin grafting and concomitant lowering of the FOM was described by Trauner, Rehrmann, and Obwegeser (Trauner, 1952; Rehrmann, 1953; Obwegeser, 1963). The major advantage of skin grafting is that the depth of the sulcus does not regress following surgery. Tissue contraction is the major reason for the regression of the sulcus, and the wound contracts when the margins are free to migrate or when granulation tissue forms (Donoff, 1976). The placement of an STSG minimizes the formation of the granulation tissue. As long as the surgery is technically correct, contraction is prevented if the margins of the incision are secured. Skin grafting also allows healing to progress more rapidly.

Split-thickness skin grafting for vestibuloplasty usually utilizes skin from the patient's thigh. The graft must be thin to avoid including hair follicles located in the dermis and to improve perfusion by the recipient bed. The patient's thigh is isolated, the skin is lubricated with mineral oil, and a dermatome is used to harvest a 0.3 mm thin graft (Fig 2-133).

Attention is next directed toward the vestibular extension procedure. A detailed description of the surgical procedure is beyond the scope of this text, but an excellent description has been provided by Davis et al. (1995).

Following the dissection, an impression of the extended alveolar ridge (or neoridge, in cases of mandibular reconstruction) and deepened vestibule is made with a previously fabricated stent and a soft denture reline material (Fig 2-131c). The relined and readapted stent is cleansed and painted with a tincture of benzoin that will act as an adhesive for the skin graft. After the adhesive has dried, the skin graft is placed on the stent so that the raw side will be in contact with the periosteum, and the skin graft is trimmed.

The stent carrying the graft is carefully seated and secured with circum-mandibular sutures (Fig 2-134b) or bone screws through the stent (Fig 2-135b). If circum-mandibular sutures are used, care must be paid to avoid compressing the pedicle vasculature of the fibula. Three to four weeks later, the stent is removed (Fig 2-134c), and the excess necrotic skin is trimmed with scissors. In order to prevent relapse of the gained vestibular depth, an existing denture or interim prosthesis is relined chairside and worn by the patient.

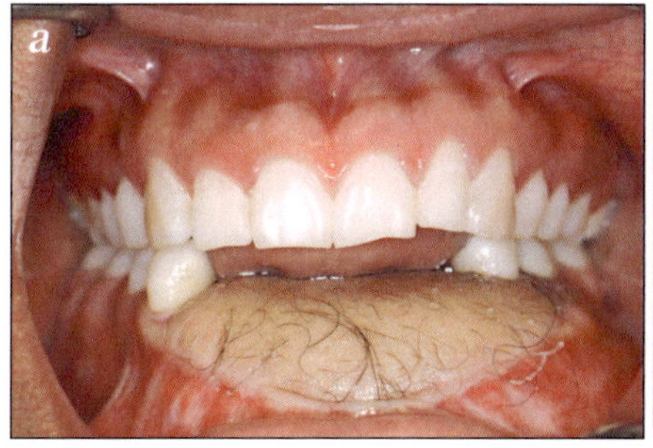
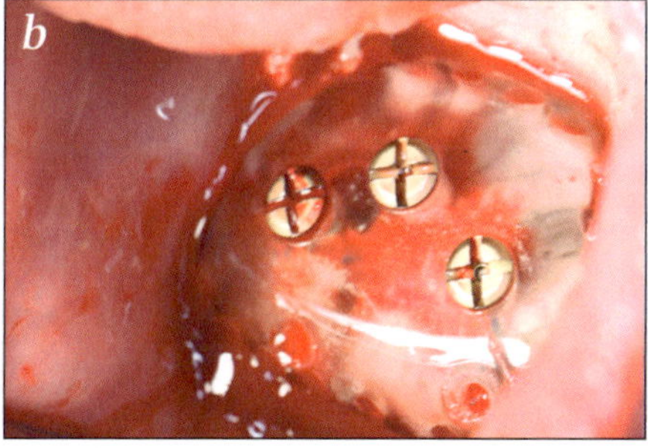
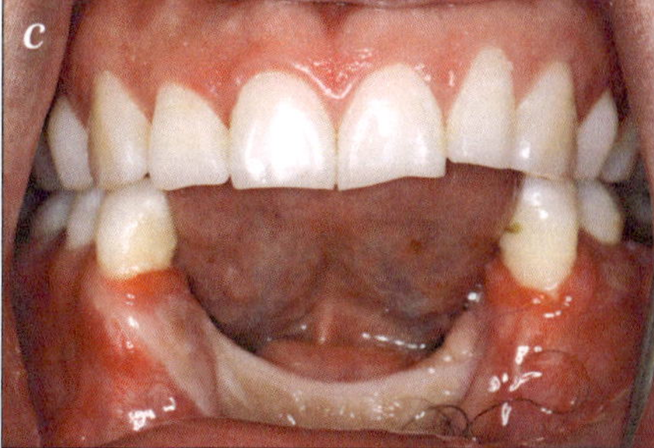

Figure 2-135 *(a)* Segmental symphyseal defect reconstructed with a FFF. *(b)* Six months after confirming good osseous union debulking is performed using a CAD/CAM vestibuloplasty stent, fixated with bone screws for three to four weeks. *(c)* Result after debulking and vestibuloplasty.

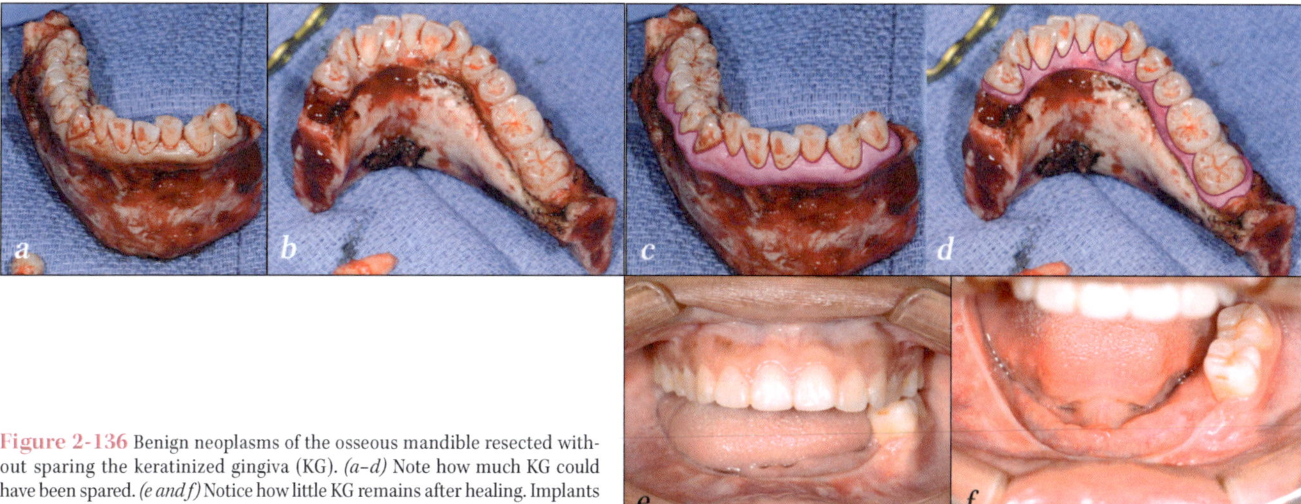

Figure 2-136 Benign neoplasms of the osseous mandible resected without sparing the keratinized gingiva (KG). *(a–d)* Note how much KG could have been spared. *(e and f)* Notice how little KG remains after healing. Implants emerging through little to no KG have a worse long-term prognosis.

Follow-up appointments are scheduled to adjust the peripheral extensions as needed.

Skin grafts will not take well on exposed cortical bone (Anderson et al., 1969). Acceptance of a graft depends on rapid revascularization, and bone denuded of periosteum presents a poorly vascularized bed (Converse, 1964). The periosteal surface of the vestibular extension must remain intact, or the success of the skin graft in this region will be jeopardized (Steinhauser, 1971). A drill may be used to bur the bare bone and stimulate bleeding of the outer cortex of the bone but attempts to directly graft to bare bone should be limited.

A technical mishap, such as a tearing of the periosteum during vestibuloplasty, is a very real possibility for even the experienced surgeon. If a large tear that cannot be mended is created in the periosteum during a vestibuloplasty, it may be advisable to decorticate the denuded site before the skin graft is placed (Sanders and McKelvy, 1976).

The donor site usually heals in about three weeks without complications. However, because a scar will remain, an inconspicuous area ought to be chosen as the donor site. In rare occasions, if the graft is too thick, skin appendages (hair follicles) will become apparent after the graft has healed. The chances for the presence of appendages increase with the thickness of the skin graft, which is why it is best to double-check that the dermatome setting matches the thinness of a scalpel blade (Fig 2-133b).

Palatal grafts

Palatal grafts are preferred to skin grafts, when the facial and lingual vestibules are adequate, otherwise a vestibuloplasty and STSG are required.

In situations of benign osseous neoplasm, such as ameloblastomas and odontogenic keratocysts, when the attached mucosa is not involved, care should be taken during tumor ablation to make intracrevicular incisions to preserve the gingiva. This will save the patient from needing a secondary grafting procedure and allow additional soft tissue to aid in a tension-free primary closure over a vascular or avascular bone graft. Fig 2-136 shows an example where the gingiva could have been better preserved—owing to the benign nature of the tumor—to avoid the need for secondary soft tissue management. Fig 2-137 illustrates a second example of a benign neoplasm reconstruction with a FFF. The resulting narrow strip of keratinized attached mucosa required a secondary palatal graft.

Following mandibular resection for a malignant neoplasm, there is often a significant soft tissue deficit. In some instances, the wound is closed primarily (Fig 2-138), which risks tethering the tongue or lip. Primary closure results in displaceable, poorly keratinized, and friable tissues inadequate for supporting a denture base. Those closed primarily almost always require secondary surgical intervention with vestibuloplasty in which the proximating soft tissues are supplemented with an STSG or palatal graft.

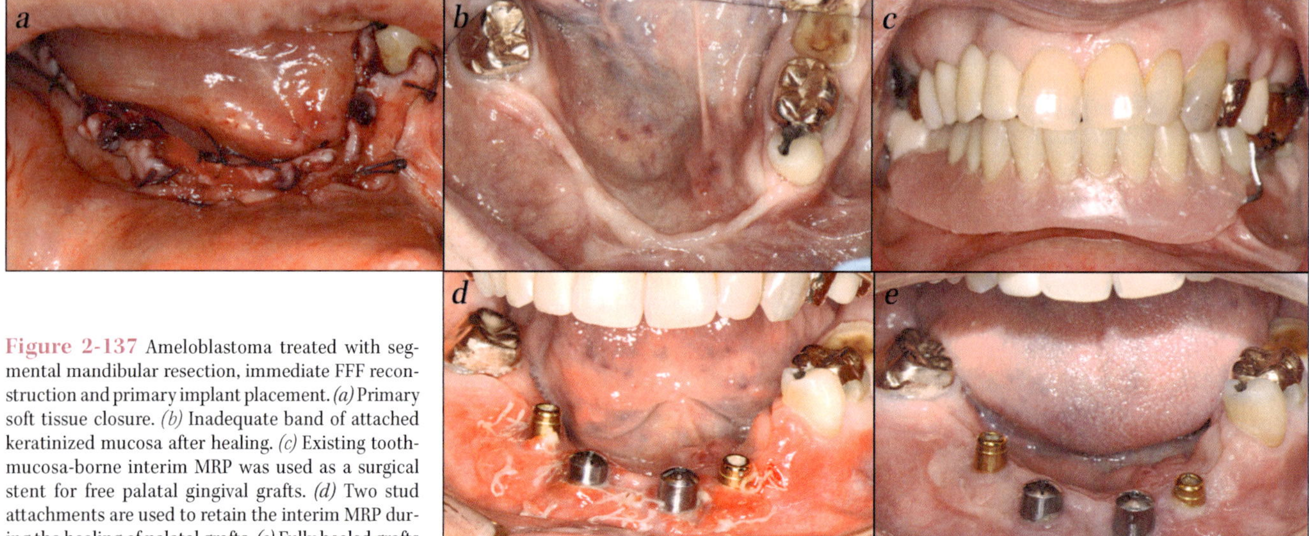

Figure 2-137 Ameloblastoma treated with segmental mandibular resection, immediate FFF reconstruction and primary implant placement. *(a)* Primary soft tissue closure. *(b)* Inadequate band of attached keratinized mucosa after healing. *(c)* Existing tooth-mucosa-borne interim MRP was used as a surgical stent for free palatal gingival grafts. *(d)* Two stud attachments are used to retain the interim MRP during the healing of palatal grafts. *(e)* Fully healed grafts and improved peri-implant tissues.

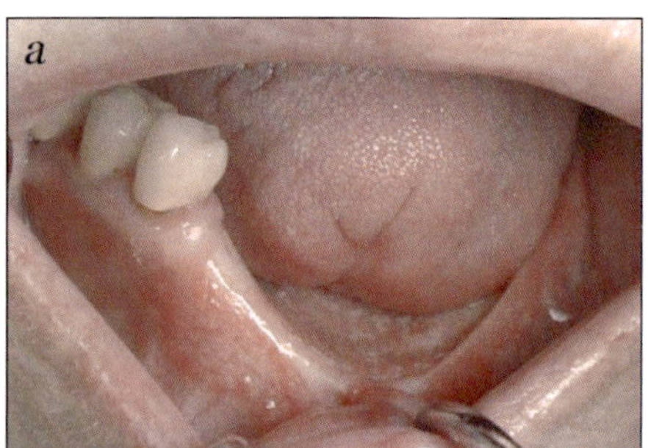

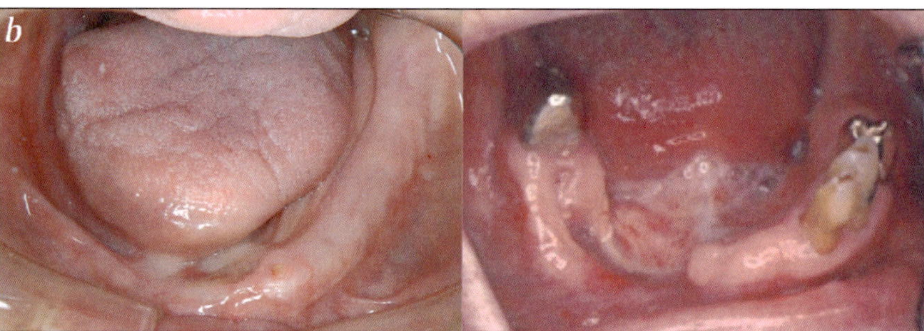

Figure 2-138 *(a and b)* Segmental mandibular defect restored with a FFF. Primary closure of the soft tissue resulted in displaceable, poorly keratinized mucosa covering most of the denture-bearing surface. *(b)* Marginal mandibular resection. Continuity was retained and the wound closed primarily.

The need for secondary split-thickness skin grafting can be eliminated if done primarily. With some forethought by the prosthodontist and ablative surgeon, a prefabricated surgical stent can be relined with a soft liner as described above and secured in place to bolster the STSG (Fig 2-139). The approach may not be advisable, however, for soft tissue closure over a free flap reconstruction due to questionable watertightness needed to prevent saliva contamination of the osseous free flap during initial healing. These situations therefore are necessary in addressing secondarily as described above.

The objective of an STSG or palatal graft whether performed primarily or secondarily is to create a broad band of keratinized soft tissues that are attached to the periosteum of the mandible—or neomandible. The creation of attached mucosa on the ridge surface with either a skin or palatal graft enhances the stability, support, and retention of a prosthesis. Esthetics may also be improved because a prosthesis now can be molded to provide contour and support for the lower lip and cheek. When dental implants are planned, a vestibule and attached mucosa are just as important. When implants emerge through a healed and attached STSG or palatal graft, oral hygiene measures are easier to perform by the patient, and the risk of peri-implantitis is reduced.

Tongue release

Tongue release is of value when mandibular continuity has been maintained or restored (Schramm et al., 1983). The creation of vestibules enables the patient to pool salivary secretions more efficiently and allows for the extension of denture flanges, thus providing a more stable dental prosthesis.

Improvement of speech is less noticeable except in the case of anterior soft tissue defects (Fig 2-140). In these patients, usually, the motor and sensory innervation of the tongue is intact, and any tongue dysfunction is generally related to limited mobility of the tongue.

Secondary dental implants

Minimally, complete denture MRPs should improve esthetics by providing lip support. Restoring mastication for patients with a complete denture MRP is difficult when there are compromised denture-bearing surfaces, impaired motor and sensory innervation of remaining tissues, and most importantly, compromised tongue function. These patients are required to stabilize and retain their complete denture MRPs with the tongue while at the same time

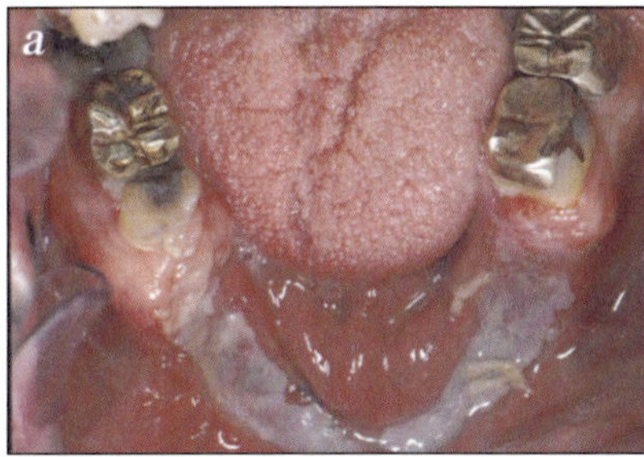
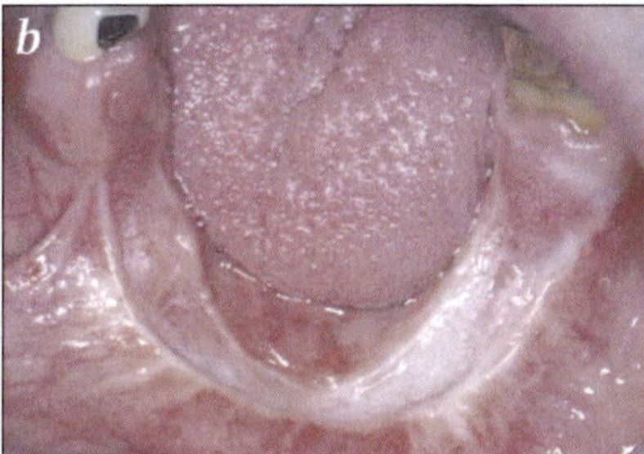

Figure 2-139 Marginal mandibular resection closed with a split-thickness skin graft. *(a)* Nascent skin graft after unpacking three weeks after mandibulectomy. *(b)* Matured skin graft.

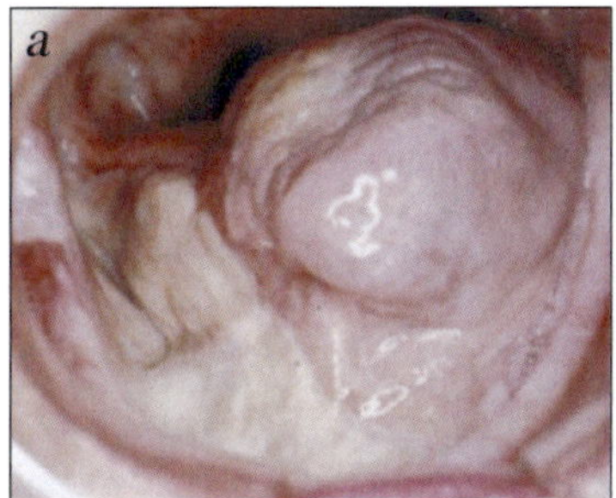
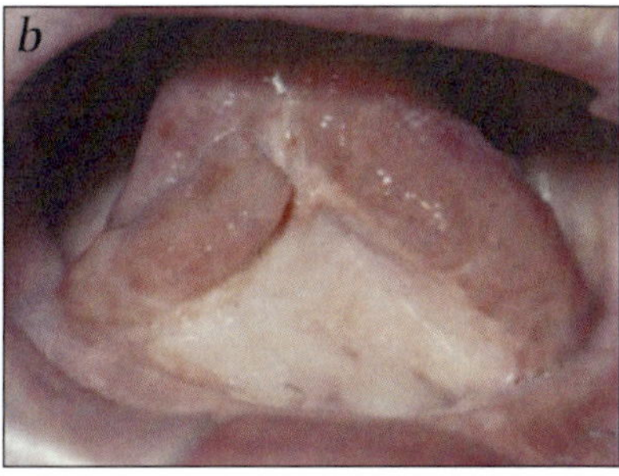

Figure 2-140 Comparison of vestibuloplasty for lateral and anterior tongue defects. *(a)* In this patient, half of the tongue was resected. Mandibular continuity was maintained. Tongue release and vestibuloplasty, using STSG, have enabled the patient to control salivary secretions more efficiently and permitted the construction of a complete denture MRP. Speech articulation has been improved only slightly. *(b)* Tongue release and vestibuloplasty with STSG have given this patient relatively normal tongue functions. Tongue mobility is almost completely restored.

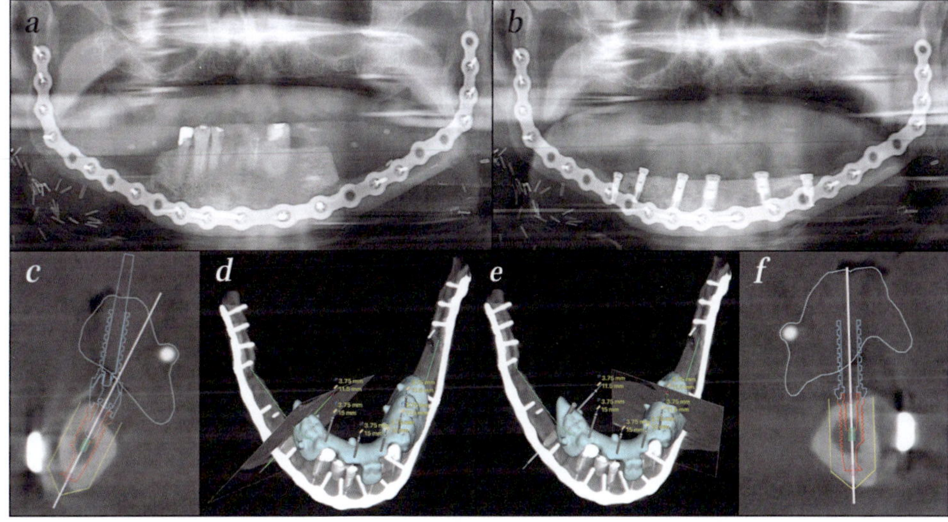

Figure 2-141 Bilateral ORN segmental resection restored with a FFF, sparing the native symphysis. *(a and b)* Pre- and post-secondary implant surgery. Notice the terminal dentition was extracted and alveolectomy performed. *(c–f)* Trial denture was used to plan implant positions. *(c)* Notice that the right fibula segment is triangular in cross-section and is buccally positioned relative to the trial tooth, requiring a lingual tilt of the implant and an angle-correction abutment. *(f)* Notice the left fibula is quadrilateral and positioned vertically beneath the proposed molar. *(c and f)* Implants placed into the fibula are planned for bicortical anchorage.

using the tongue to manipulate the bolus. This maneuver is beyond the capability of almost all patients. Knowing this, implants are more critical for the patient who will become edentulous after mandibular reconstruction.

Primary placement of dental implants shortens overall treatment time, and when postsurgical radiation is needed, implants are given five to six weeks to osseointegrate while recovering from the free flap reconstruction. By comparison, one should wait a minimum of six months before considering implants secondary to flap reconstruction regardless of whether adjuvant radiation is needed. It may be prudent to wait a full year because recurrence happens most often in the first 12 months (Carvalho et al., 2005; Kowalski et al., 2005; Fan et al., 2011).

If implants are to be placed secondarily in the resected mandible to retain and stabilize an MRP, then the placement of maxillary implants should also be considered for the edentulous patient for the following reasons. Resection margins may alter the peripheral tissues of the maxilla. In particular, a soft tissue flap may obliterate the maxillary buccal vestibule (Fig 2-142a–b). In addition, xerostomia secondary to radiotherapy or chemoradiation may compromise the peripheral seal. Two implants placed in the canine positions will provide the necessary retention and stability (Fig 2-142c).

The placement of endosteal implants enables the fabrication of well-retained and stable overlay prostheses. The support derived from the implants and the residual denture-bearing surfaces and the retention and stability provided by the implants are more than sufficient to allow effective mastication if the patient presents with reasonable tongue function. Patients with sufficient tongue bulk and mobility and with motor and sensory innervation intact on at least one side will benefit the most from implant-retained overlay prostheses. The tongue is no longer required to control the denture, so it can now be used solely for control and manipulation of the bolus during mastication and swallowing.

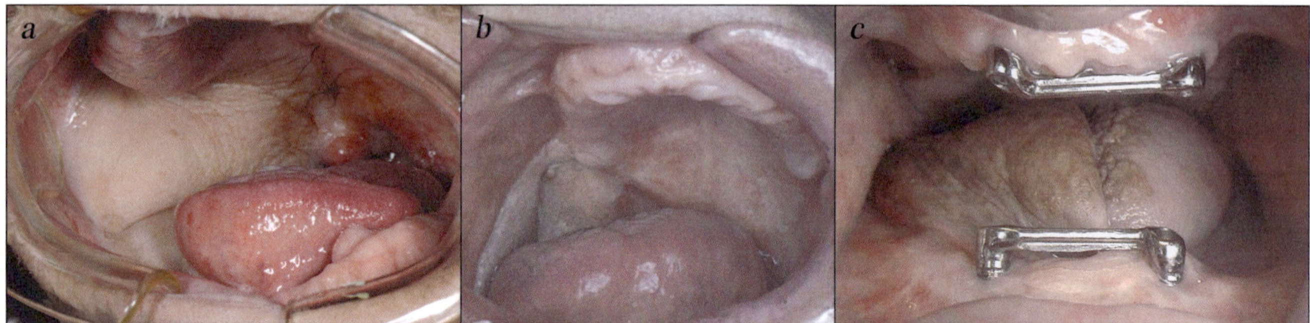

Figure 2-142 Edentulous patients with tongue and mandible tonsillar pillar defects reconstructed with soft tissue flaps. *(a and b)* Flaps extend to and alter peripheral tissues of the maxilla. *(c)* Implants are placed into canine positions to assist in the retention and stability of complete dentures.

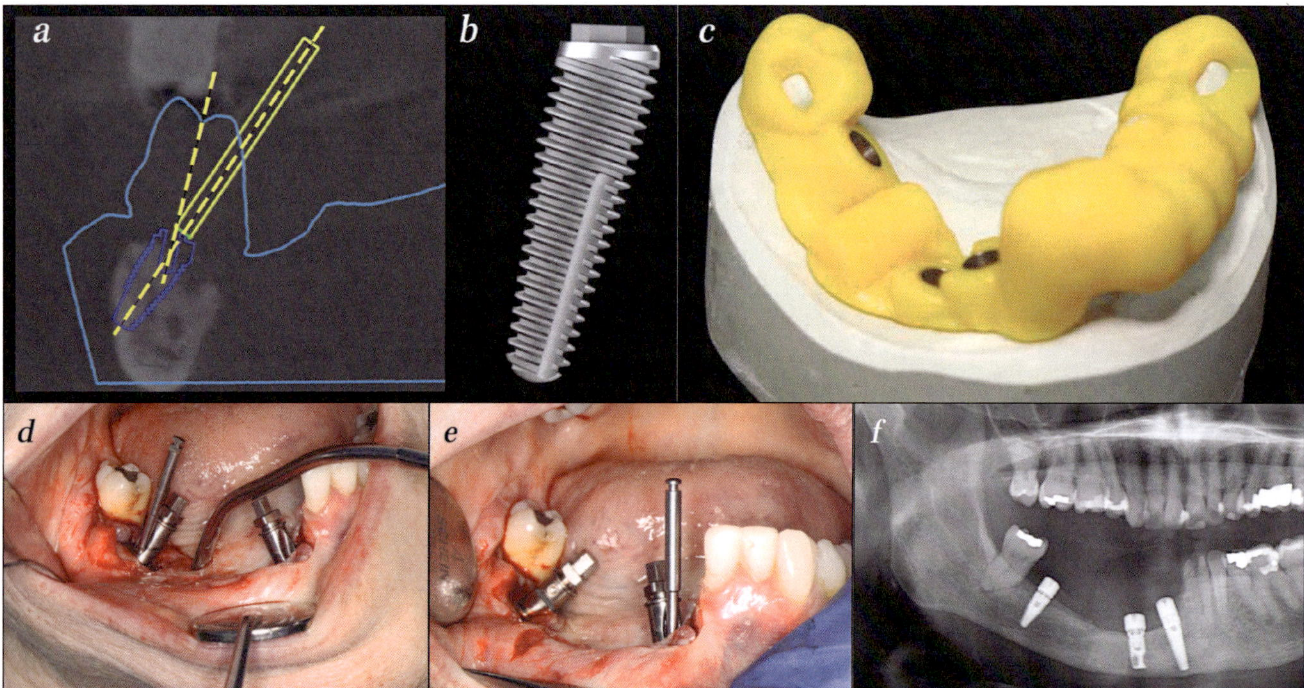

Figure 2-143 Marginal resection defect of the mandible secondary to removal of a verrucous carcinoma. *(a)* A trial denture was used to plan implant positions. Notice the lingual tilt with the implant apex extending into the oblique mandibular ridge to avoid the intact inferior alveolar nerve. *(b)* Dual axis implant. *(c)* Printed implant guide. *(d and e)* This dual-axis implant provided 24° of subgingival angulation correction. *(f)* Postplacement panoramic radiograph. Note the molar implant is superimposed on the IA nerve.

Preparations for secondary implant surgery follow established conventions for the prosthodontic patient. A trial denture is verified for occlusion, OVD, and esthetics. A dual scan protocol is performed, the CT and dental scan data are aligned, and the digital implant planning is completed (Figs 2-141 and 2-143).

Implants should be placed perpendicular to the occlusal plane when possible. Tilted implants splinted to additional fixtures are needed either when posterior grafts are buccal to the dental arch (Fig 2-141c) or when marginal resections require the tilting of the fixture to avoid the inferior alveolar nerve (Fig 2-143). Angle correction can be achieved conventionally with the use of angled abutments or by utilizing a subgingival angle-corrected implant. With either approach, care is needed to keep the emergence within the zone of the residual attached gingiva. The prognosis for implants that emerge through the mobile tissues of the FOM is poor and usually requires them to be buried beneath the mucosa.

Guides are printed and made available for either semi- or fully guided implant surgery. Implant surgery is performed in the usual way. During the two- to three-month healing period, care should be taken to avoid exposing the implants to occlusal forces through the mucosa. During this early stage of healing, the bone-implant interface is not prepared to accept significant loading.

Patients who have undergone marginal mandibulectomies, are candidate for dental implants (Karayazgan-Saracoglu et al., 2017; Petrovic et al., 2019). Implants placed in avascular bone grafts used to reconstructed this region are also successful (Keller et al., 1988). Once matured, bone grafts demonstrate a homogenous calcification pattern that results in an excellent bone-implant interface (Marx,

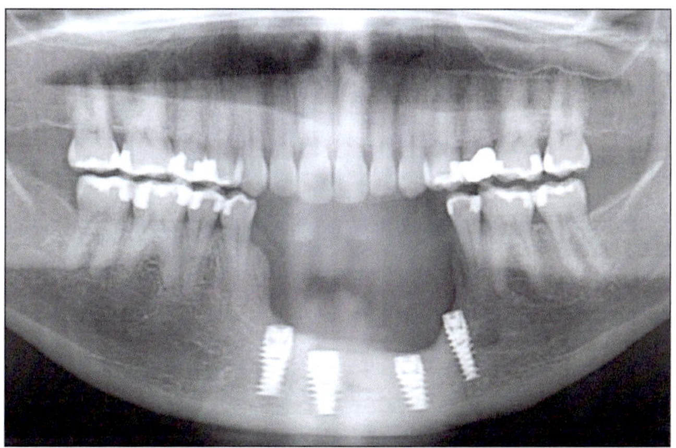

Figure 2-144 *(a)* Marginal anterior mandibulectomy for an ameloblastoma. More than 10 mm of residual mandible height allowed for the placement of dental implants.

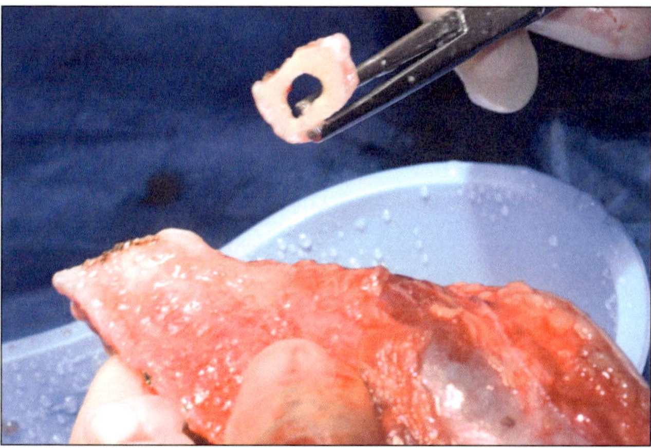

Figure 2-145 *(a)* Discarded osteotomized wedge of fibula. Notice the thick coteries but hollow marrow space. Anchorage of the implant is dependent on engaging both cortices.

1993). Osteocutaneous free flaps, particularly the fibula, present with prominent cortical plates that (Fig 2-145), when properly engaged, provide excellent stabilization for implants; reports of their outcomes are equally favorable (Roumanas et al., 1997; Garrett et al., 2006).

Stage II implant surgery

Stage II implant surgery can take different approaches depending on the nature of the overlaying soft tissues. On one hand, the most ideal situation is when all of the gingivae have been spared and no skin island is needed to reconstruct a composite defect. Stage II is not unlike a conventional nonresection patient. When primary closure is achieved and no attached mucosa is present, a free palatal graft should be considered to improve the peri-implant tissues as described above (Fig 2-137). This can be done simultaneously with stage II or in sequence. The advantage of having the implants exposed is the ability to utilize them as a means of retention for a surgical stent.

In the presence of a thick skin paddle, debulking procedures can happen prior to implant uncovering or concurrently. If, however, inadequate debulking is performed, deep pockets around healing abutments inevitably lead to soft tissue hypertrophy and granulation tissue formation.

Stage II with concurrent debulking of skin paddle

A supraperiosteal flap is raised. Care is taken with the subcutaneous dissection to thin the tissues over the neoridge and around the implants. An ideal result is the presence of a cuff of attached keratinized peri-implant tissue that does not exceed 4 mm in thickness. Healing abutments are placed, and a strict hygiene regimen is implemented. When an interim MRP is available, it is relined, modified, and used as a stent to hold the peri-implant tissues in position during healing (Fig 2-146). If an interim MRP is not available, then a dedicated surgical stent can be made as described above. With either method, the objective is to ensure that the lining epithelium remains adherent to the underlying periosteum during healing. After a suitable period of healing (three to four weeks), the stent is removed and the areas cleaned. It may be necessary to change the height of the healing abutments at this time.

If the submucosal resections are not properly executed and the tissues around the implants are not properly thinned and tacked down, the peri-implant pockets will be excessive and the peri-implant tissues will be susceptible to inflammation, resulting in granulation tissue formation and hypertrophy (Fig 2-146c; Roumanas et al., 1997).

Soft tissue complications in the immediate period following stage II surgery consist mainly of soft tissue hypertrophy and granulation tissue formation. Reinforcing oral hygiene and the use of an antiplaque mouth rinse is recommended. Occasionally, electrocautery or surgical excision of the hypertrophic tissue is required. Silver nitrate can also be used to chemically cauterize the wound following excision. When soft tissues are deeper than 4 mm, additional debulking of the flap may be required.

If the patient has undergone postoperative radiation or chemoradiation, the tissues overlying the implants should be minimally manipulated during the second stage of surgery and exposure of the implants. The clinician should realize that failure to thin the peri-implant soft tissues will predispose the patient to a higher risk of inflammation and hypertrophy of the peri-implant soft tissues. However, inadvertent exposure of the bony portion of the flap and postoperative soft tissue breakdown in this patient population is a significant concern, and if it occurs, it can lead to infection and necrosis of the bony portion of the flap. In such patients, soft tissue healing can be enhanced with HBO treatments (Dauwe et al., 2014; Hoggan and Cameron, 2014).

Choice of abutments

Highly polished abutment surfaces will reduce the incidence of soft tissue problems around the implants. Frequently implants in these patients exit through skin, and in the presence of plaque accumulation, the skin surrounding the implants becomes highly inflamed. Conventional healing abutments with their machined surfaces retain plaque and calculus quite readily and should be used with

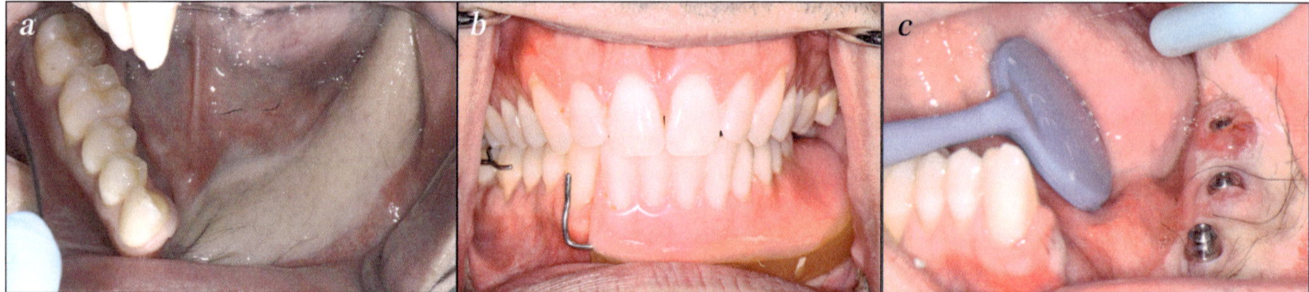

Figure 2-146 *(a)* Six months post-FFF reconstruction of a segmental mandibular resection secondary to removal of an osteosarcoma. *(b)* The implants were exposed with a supraperiosteal dissection, skin paddle thinned, healing abutments attached, and the existing interim MRP was relined to stent the peri-implant soft tissues in position during healing. *(c)* Several weeks following second stage surgery. Notice the peri-implant inflammatory response. The peri-implant tissues require additional thinning before a definitive MRP is fabricated.

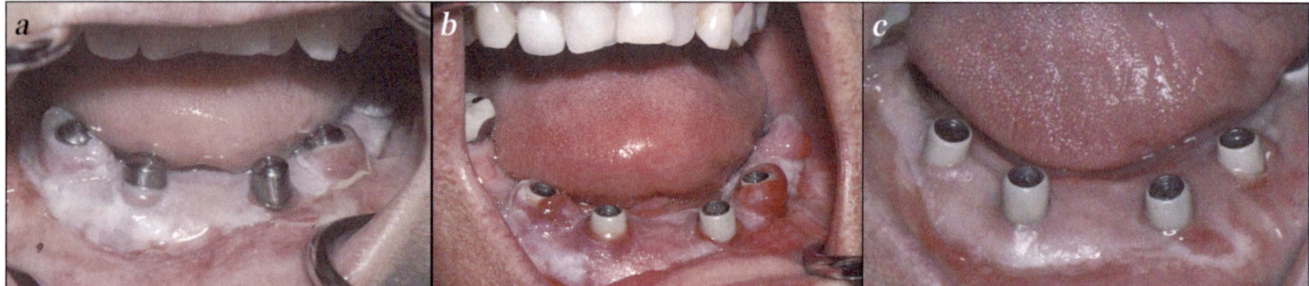

Figure 2-147 Inflammatory response to machined titanium implants. *(a)* Soft tissue hypertrophy around implants following stage II surgery and the placement of healing abutments. *(b)* Conventional healing abutments were replaced with ceramometal healing abutments made from UCLA abutments. *(c)* Complete resolution within three weeks.

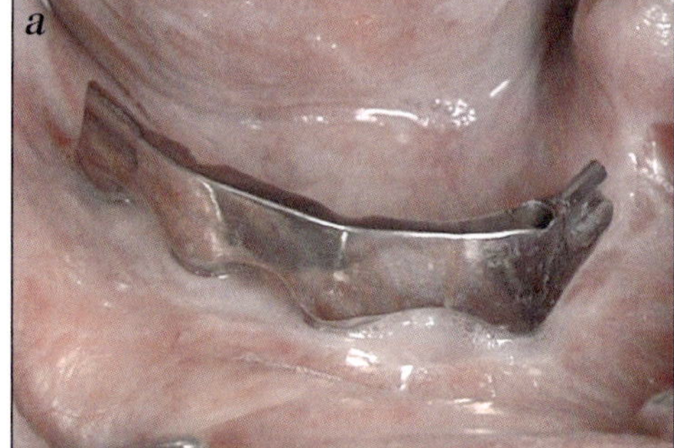

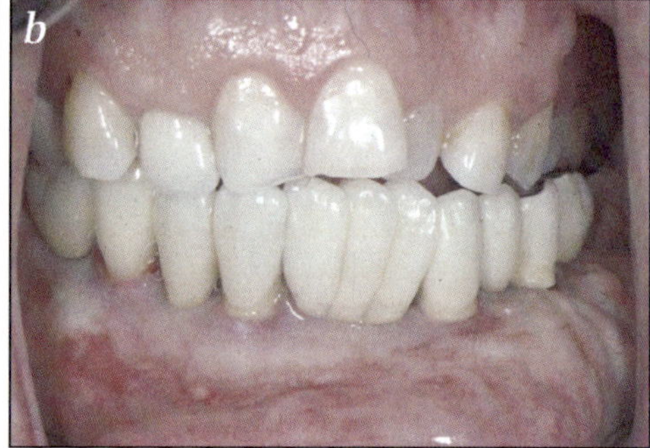

Figure 2-148 Prevention of soft tissue reactions. *(a)* Free palatal grafts were used to create a zone of attached keratinized peri-implant tissues. In addition, the implant connecting bar extending subgingivally directly to the fixture is highly polished. *(b)* A fixed ceramometal MRP allows for a polished and glazed feldspathic porcelain emerging through the fibula skin paddle.

caution during the healing period after stage II surgery (Figs 2-154a and 2-156a).

We also recommend against the use of machined abutments in the final prosthesis. When implants exit through the skin, we prefer to fabricate implant connecting bars or fixed prostheses directly to the implant fixture. In such situations, this ensures that either highly polished metal (Fig 2-148a) or glazed porcelain (Fig 2-148b) will abut the tissues in the peri-implant sulcus.

Machined titanium implant surfaces that perforate skin in the oral cavity have a tendency to precipitate inflammatory tissue reactions (Fig 2-147a and 2-149a). These tissue responses can usually be eliminated by the use of polished healing abutments. In the patient shown in Fig 2-147, customized ceramometal healing abutments made from the UCLA abutment resolved the tissue problems. Alternatively, custom-milled zirconia healing abutments that are highly polished can be used (Fig 2-149b). A sufficiently tall abutment and occlusal divergence is recommended to help resist the overgrowth of the soft tissues.

Definitive MRPs for Edentulous Patients

Patients in this category have either undergone a marginal mandibulectomy or had successful osseous reconstruction of a segmental resection of the mandible. A portion of their denture-bearing surfaces have been affected to some degree. Some patients may have had portions of the tongue resected. Most of these patients are best served if dental implants are utilized to assist with retention, stability, and support. Treatment of patients who are unable to undergo primary reconstruction of the mandible is addressed in a subsequent section.

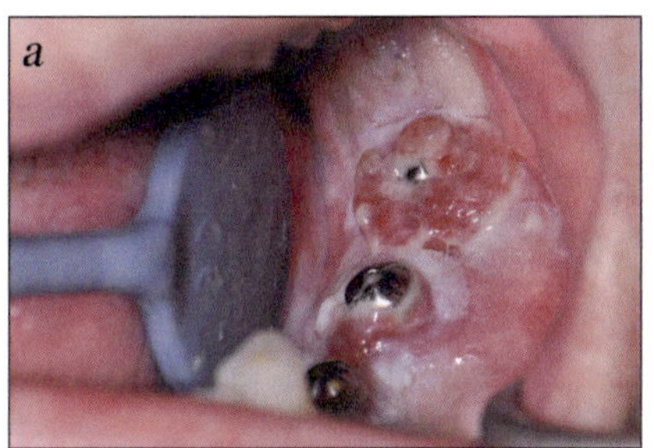
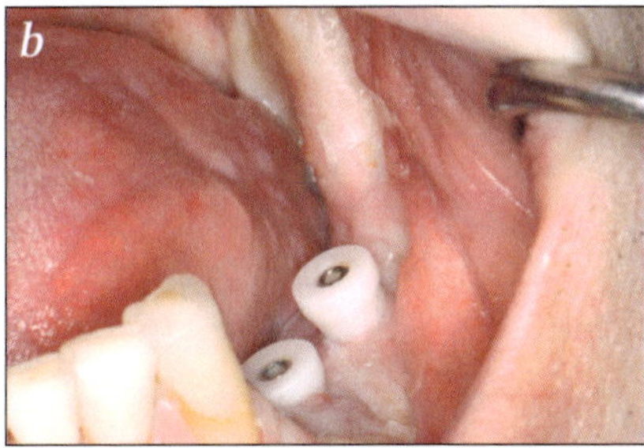

Figure 2-149 Inflammatory response to machined titanium Abutments. *(a)* Soft tissue hypertrophy around implants following stage II surgery and the placement of healing abutments. *(b)* Conventional healing abutments were replaced with custom highly polished zirconia healing abutments. Complete resolution around two of the three implants. The third implant had to be buried.

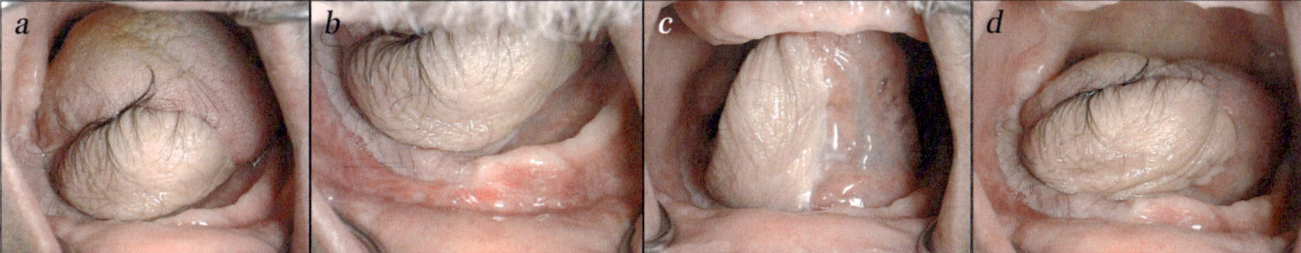

Figure 2-150 *(a)* Partial glossectomy defect restored with a radial forearm flap. A portion of the denture-bearing surface was also resurfaced with the flap. *(b–d)* Movement of the tongue is excellent. The prosthodontic prognosis is excellent, particularly if implants are employed to retain and stabilize the mandibular denture.

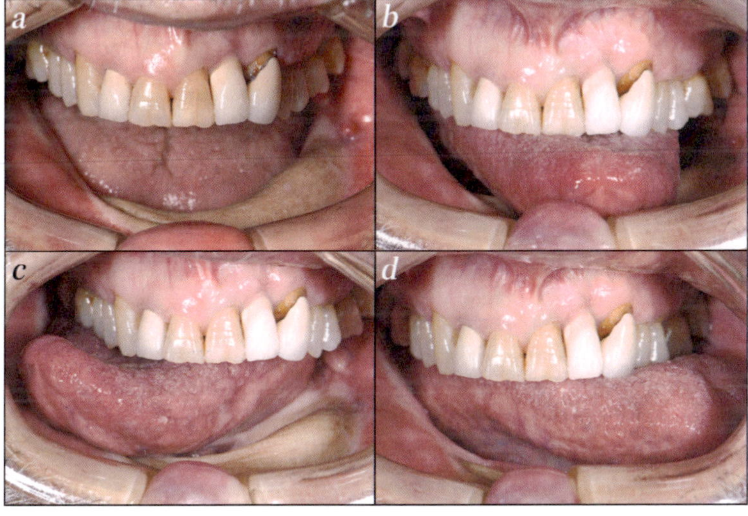

Figure 2-151 Patients with mandibular defects and no tongue involvement will have a favorable prognosis. *(a–d)* Tongue at rest, protruded, and lateral positions.

Prosthetic prognosis

The prosthetic prognosis for patients with resections of the tongue and mandible is quite variable. In some patients, only esthetics can be improved, with minor functional benefits, whereas in other patients, particularly those reconstructed with properly configured vascularized free flaps, improved mastication is a reasonable objective. The prosthetic prognosis in these patients is primarily dependent on the status of tongue function. When the tongue volume is favorable and motor and sensory innervation is intact on the unresected side, the prosthetic prognosis for mastication becomes quite favorable (Fig 2-150).

Secondary prognostic indicators include the extent of the bony and soft tissue resection, the status of the lip, and a history of radiation. Excellent functional and esthetic prosthetic prognosis is expected when there is no tongue involvement (Fig 2-151), when the composite resection is minimal, when the lip is unaffected, and when adjuvant radiation is not needed. Inadequate tongue bulk and immobility cannot be overcome surgically at this stage, but deficiencies in denture-bearing surfaces can be addressed with skin and palatal grafts, vestibuloplasty, and the placement of endosteal implants (see section "Secondary Surgical Procedures").

Tongue

The key to the restoration of oral functions—mastication, saliva control, swallowing, and speech—is the bulk, mobility, neuromuscular control, and sensory innervation of the tongue. For this reason, if possible, resected tongue tissue and mandibular continuity should always be restored at the time of tumor ablation, preferably with a free flap. Free flaps are preferred over myocutaneous flaps because the reconstructed tissues retain their volume and are

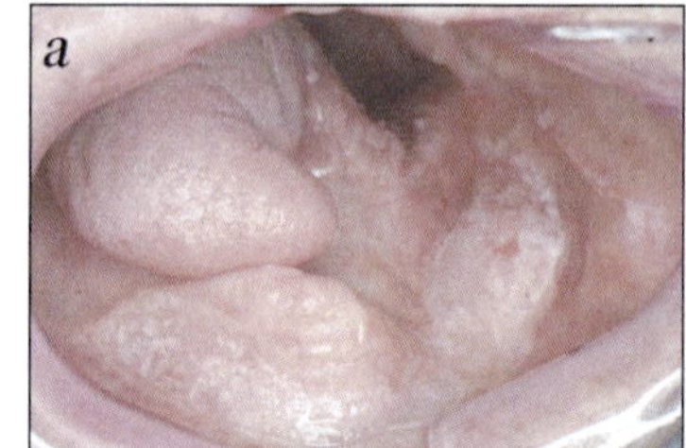

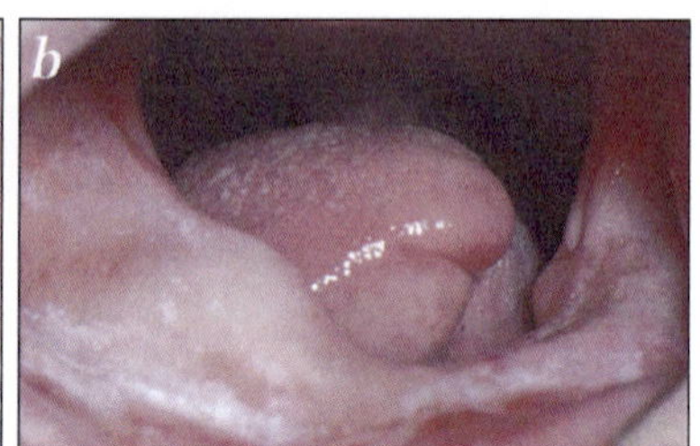

Figure 2-152 Patients in whom the mandible has been reconstructed but the tongue has not. *(a)* The tongue is immobilized. *(b)* The tongue is unable to elevate to the level of the occlusal plane. The prognosis for mastication with complete dentures is very poor for both patients, even if implants are employed.

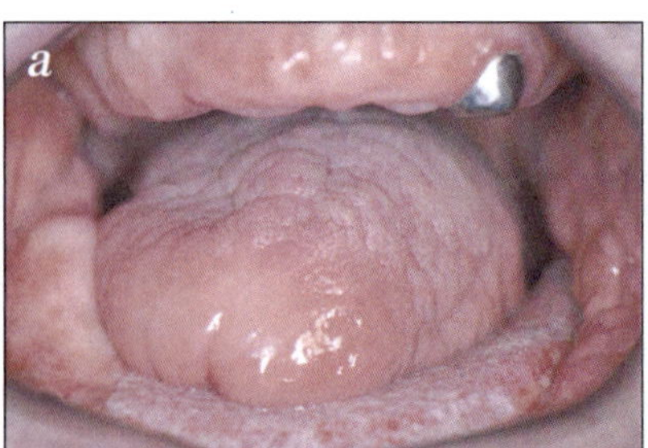

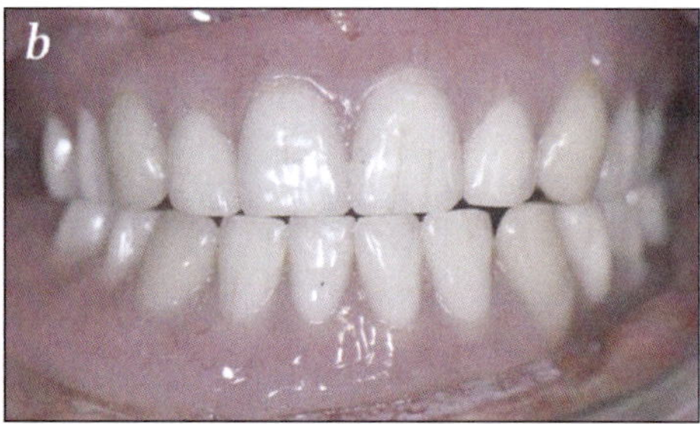

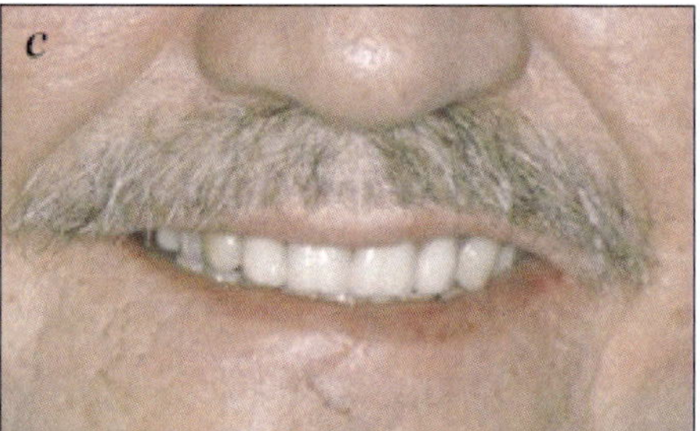

Figure 2-153 Effect of good denture-bearing surfaces on prosthetic outcome. *(a)* Symphyseal defect restored with a FFF. The tongue is intact and has retained motor and sensory innervation bilaterally. *(b and c)* Maxillary overlay complete denture opposing a conventional CD-MRP inserted.

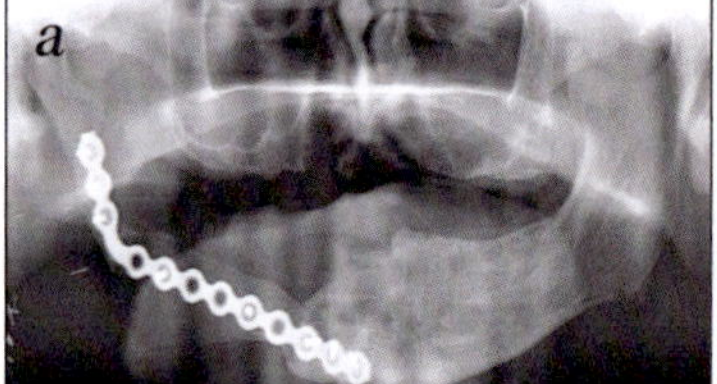

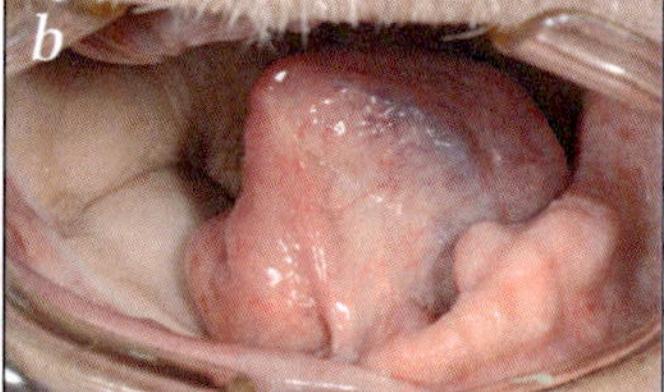

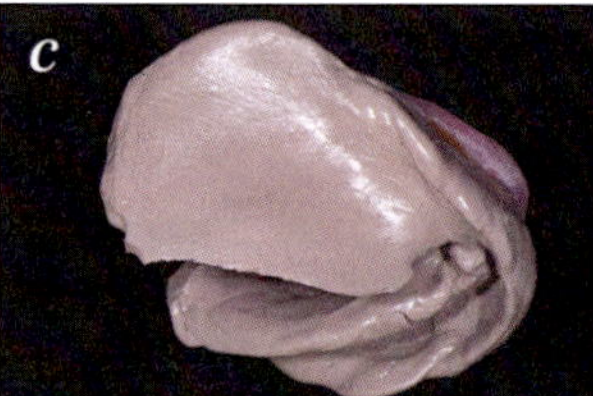

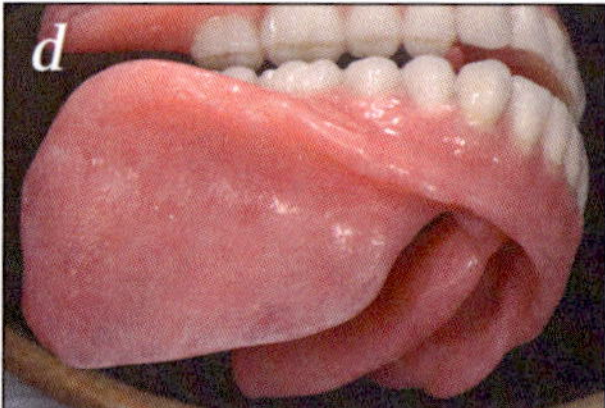

Figure 2-154 *(a and b)* Right segmental mandibulectomy defect reconstructed with an SFF. *(c and d)* Extension of the denture onto the reconstructed mandible will improve the stability and retention of the CD-MRP.

more flexible. If the patient is capable of elevating and moving the tongue in a number of directions (Fig 2-151), he or she probably will be successful in stabilizing the mandibular denture during function. For the patient to masticate with a reasonable degree of efficiency, the tongue must be able to manipulate the food bolus and place it on the occlusal surfaces of the mandibular teeth.

If the resection extends to the base of the tongue, the remaining portion of the oral tongue may be immobilized in a retruded position and lack the ability to elevate and interact with dental and palatal structures. The two patients shown in Figure 2-152 present with mandibular continuity. However, their ability to detect, control, and manipulate the food bolus has been compromised by the lack of tongue bulk and mobility, by the use of the tongue to obtain wound closure, or by reconstruction efforts that were compromised by scarring and lack of tissue volume. Paradoxically, immobility of the tongue, particularly an inability to elevate the tongue, creates a minor anatomical advantage: it often enables more aggressive extension of the lingual flange on the nonsurgical side, thus facilitating stability and retention.

Denture-bearing surfaces

If the bearing surface is favorable, either following the resection of benign tumors or an epidermoid carcinoma confined to the alveolar ridge or following free flap reconstruction and secondary revisions, we attempt to satisfy the needs of the patient with a conventional complete denture (Fig 2-153).

Free flap reconstruction can sometimes create a lingual sulcus lined in the skin that can be aggressively engaged by a denture flange, which will enhance stability and retention, and enables the patient to control the denture more effectively (Fig 2-154).

If a conventional MRP is not successful in such patients, because the denture-bearing surface is unfavorable, or the tongue is partially immobilized or reduced in bulk, the authors would consider the preprosthetic surgical procedures referred to earlier in the chapter followed by the placement of dental implants. See a subsequent section titled "Definitive Implant-Assisted and Implant-Supported MRP."

Lip

Postsurgical lip posture and control, although less important prognostically than tongue function, do have important prosthodontic implications (Fig 2-155). As previously mentioned, most composite resections compromise the motor control and sensory innervation of the corner of the mouth, cheek, and the lower lip on the resected side because of resection of the marginal mandibular and inferior alveolar nerves. This predisposes the patient to cheek biting and poor control of salivary

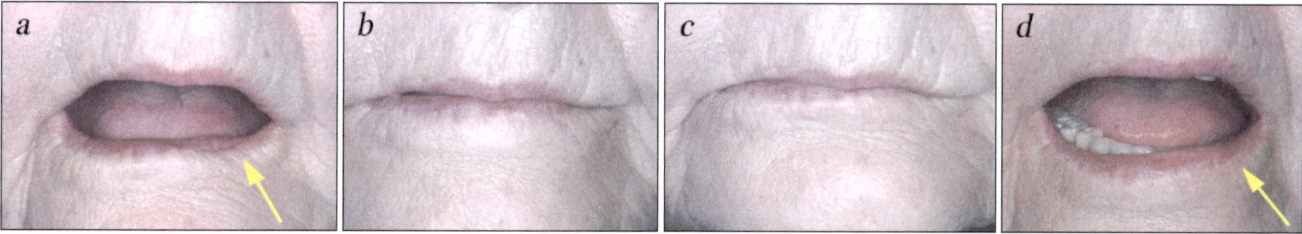

Figure 2-155 Effect of lip posture on prosthetic outcome. *(a)* Note the contour of the lower lip, particularly on the resected side *(arrow)*. *(b and c)* The patient has difficulty obtaining the lip seal on both the resected and unresected sides. *(d)* Prosthesis in place. On opening, the lip on the resected mandible *(arrow)* is displaced posteriorly, tending to dislodge the denture.

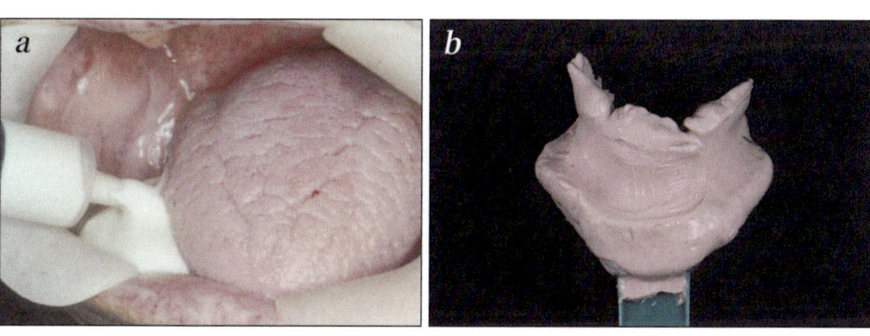

Figure 2-156 *(a)* Disposable syringe used to inject irreversible hyrocollooid into the lingual vestibule prior to the seating of the tray. *(b)* Impression of a mandibulectomy, FFF reconstructed defect.

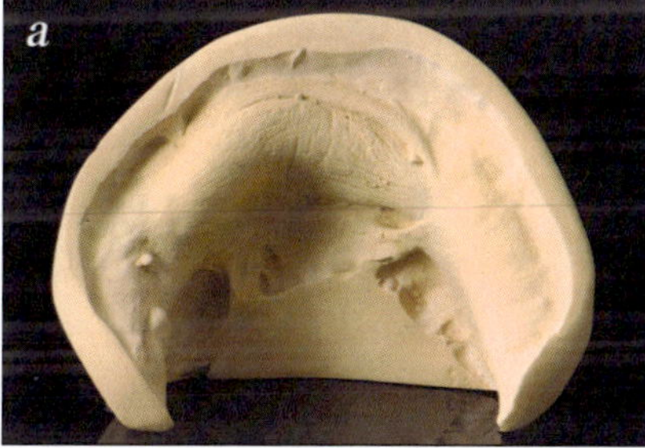

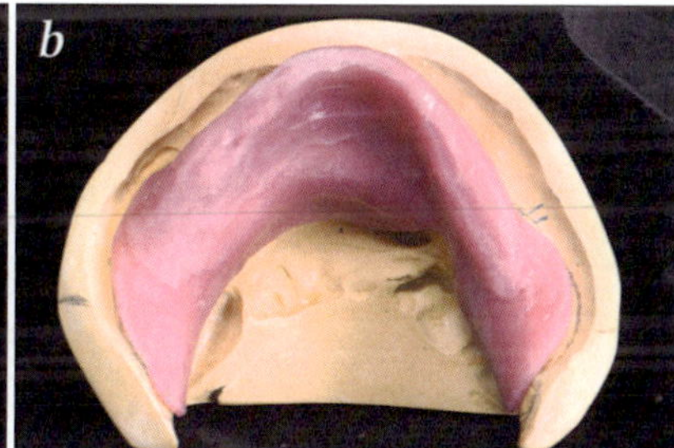

Figure 2-157 *(a)* Diagnostic cast of a FFF reconstructed mandibular defect. *(b)* Custom tray. Notice the asymmetry of the tray. A continuous handle and finger rests are made to occupy the neutral zone, which also provides rigidity where the ridge is thin. This handle design allows for a closed mouth impression technique (see Fig 2-158).

secretions. In some patients, the lip may be retracted posteriorly, significantly compromising the extent of the labial and buccal flanges and necessitating a more lingual placement of the denture teeth.

Radiation

If the patient has received a definitive course of radiation therapy, tolerance of complete dentures is further compromised (see Chapter 1).

Prior to therapy the prosthodontist must consider all these factors and inform the patient of the prognosis for the complete dentures. This is an important discussion that must be handled in a delicate and supportive manner. As with other types of prosthodontics, those problems affecting the prognosis that are discussed with the patient prior to fabrication are usually accepted by the patient.

Impressions

Maximum extension and tissue coverage should be recorded with the preliminary impression. Irreversible hydrocolloid is used in combination with a modified stock tray. Plastic trays can be thermoplastically altered when the situation calls for it. Periphery wax or an impression compound may be useful to extend the stock tray in areas of difficult access. This may be true for the lingual flange on the unresected side due to the tongue's close proximity to the alveolar ridge. A disposable syringe with a cut tip is often used to inject an impression material into areas of difficult access before the stock tray with the impression material is seated (Fig 2-156a). Special attention should also be paid to recording the soft tissue areas on the reconstructed side. When a free flap reconstructs the FOM, the lingual sulcus can be quite extensive (Fig 2-156b).

Custom impression trays are fabricated. Handles and finger rests should occupy the neutral zone and allow for border movements (Fig 2-157). The objectives of the master impressions are the same as in conventional prosthodontics: to establish retention, to provide support and stability, and to create the appropriate esthetics support for the lips and cheeks. Because experience and training vary, clinicians should employ the techniques they prefer for making the master impression. We advocate conventional border molding with an impression compound to establish peripheral extensions. This border-molded impression is then refined with an elastomeric impression material (Fig 2-158).

Retention in the mandible is achieved by obtaining close adaptation of the prosthesis with the denture-bearing surface and by

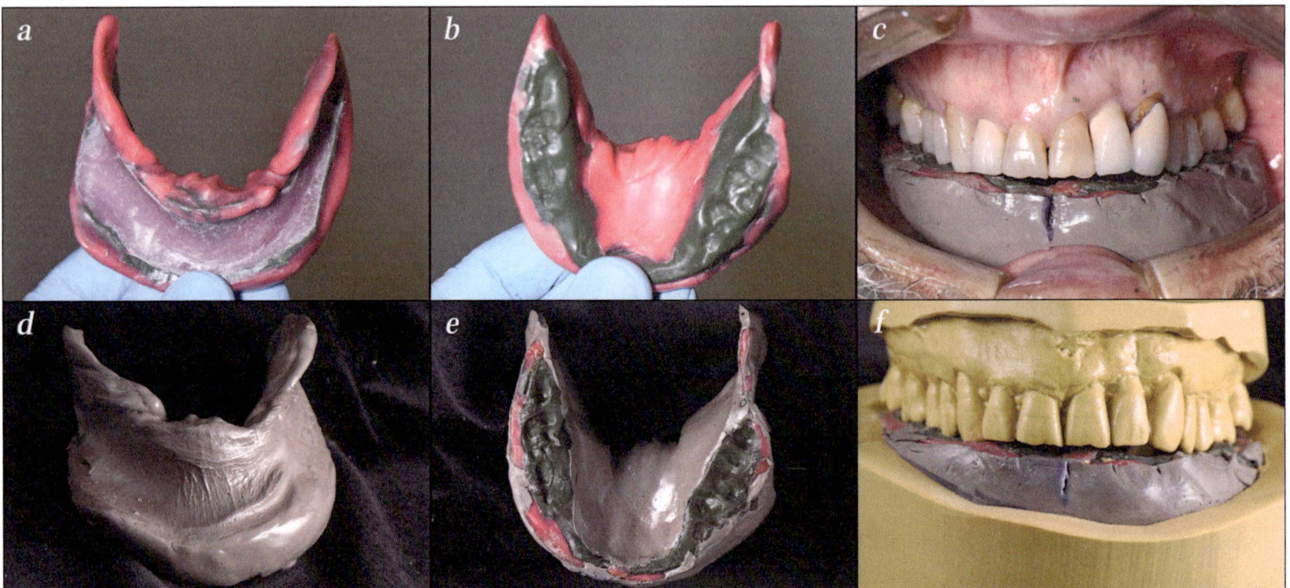

Figure 2-158 Completed mandibular impression. *(a and b)* Note the development of the lingual flange. Both cameo and intaglio surfaces have been recorded. *(c)* Occlusal registration was made to allow a closed-mouth impression technique. *(d and e)* Wash impression with an elastomeric material. *(f)* Mounted master cast prior to harvesting the final impression.

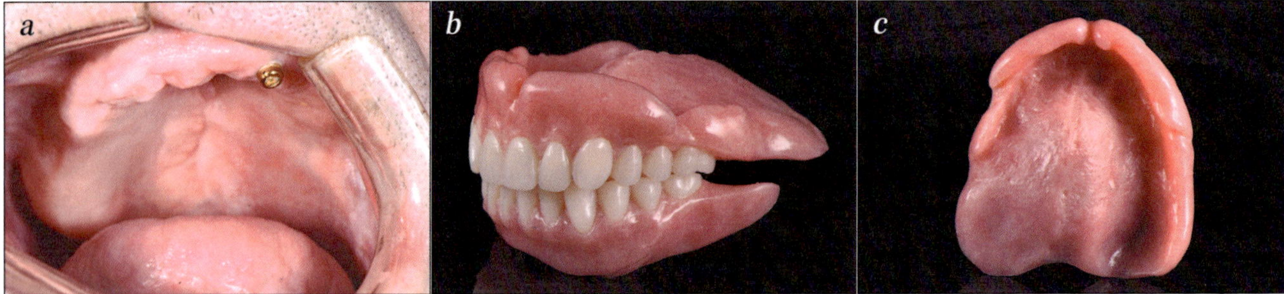

Figure 2-159 *(a–c)* A lateral marginal mandiblectomy with soft tissue resection extending to the buccal mucosa, the maxillary vestibule, alveolar ridge, and hard palate. The soft tissue defect was reconstructed with a faciocutaneous RFFF. The resulting soft tissue contours compromise the ideal buccal flange extension and peripheral seal of the maxillary denture. A single implant survived in the anterior maxilla, which will assist in the maintenance of peripheral seal.

extending the lingual periphery on the unresected side to the maximal extent compatible with functional and anatomical limitations. The degree of peripheral seal created may be greater than expected because many patients may have difficulty elevating the FOM and tongue.

An accurate recording of the contour of the cameo surfaces of the denture is an important consideration, especially the lingual flanges on the resected and unresected sides. If these cameo surfaces are recorded accurately, the tongue will be able to control and retain the mandibular denture in position more efficiently during function (Cantor and Curtis, 1971; Fig 2-158).

Support for the mandibular prosthesis can be obtained from the buccal shelf, the crest of the ridge, the retromolar pad, and when possible, the soft tissue bed over the reconstructed mandible. The stability of the definitive prosthesis is facilitated if the clinician appropriately develops the contours of the lingual flange on the unresected side. Careful contouring of the lingual flange on the reconstructed side will also help resist the lateral forces exerted on the prosthesis during mastication.

As previously mentioned, the lower lip on the resected side is often retracted posteriorly, predisposing the patient to cheek and lip biting. If the lower lip can be repositioned labially with the denture flange, this frustrating and disconcerting side effect may be negated. Proper support for the lower lip will also enhance control of salivary secretions. However, if the lip and cheek on the resected side are heavily scarred and unyielding, this extension can create a dislodging force on the prosthesis. Consequently, this flange must be carefully molded to obtain appropriate lip support without compromising retention. We prefer to develop this flange, sometimes referred to as a *lip plumper*, after delivery of the denture when its effect on the stability of the denture can be assessed more accurately.

In conventional prosthodontics, some clinicians advocate the fabrication of a functional impression of the cameo surfaces of the mandibular prosthesis (Fish, 1966; Lott and Levin, 1966; Beresin and Scheisser, 1978). This concept has special application for mandibulectomy patients and enhances the stability and retention of the prosthesis and enables the patient to control the denture more effectively (Fish, 1966). The clinician can record the cameo surfaces

Figure 2-160 *(a and b)* Both patients have undergone a right mandibular resection with osteomyocutaneous reconstruction. Both have lower right lip motor and sensory deficits. Decreasing the OVD can help improve lip competence.

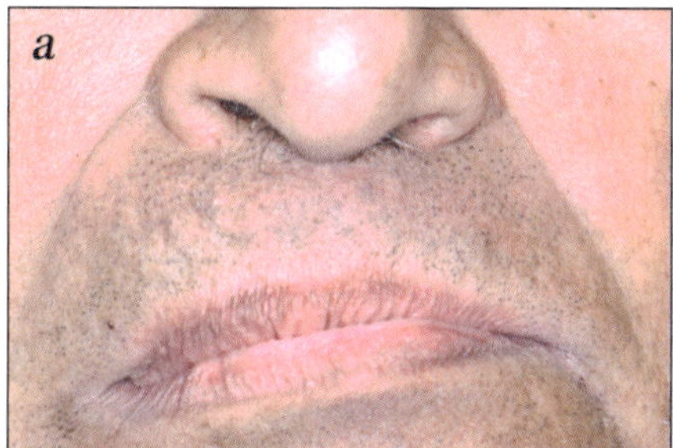

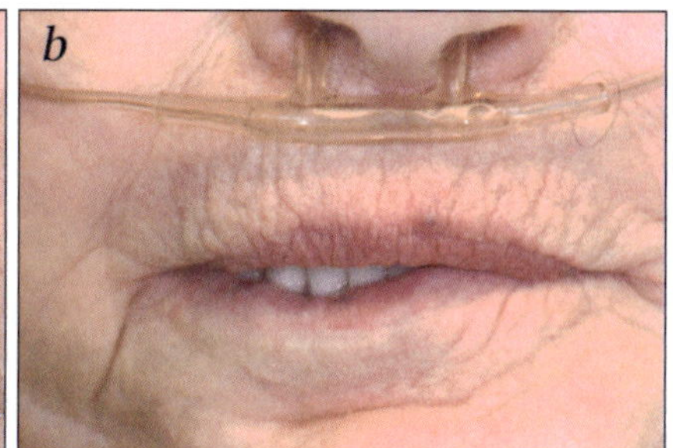

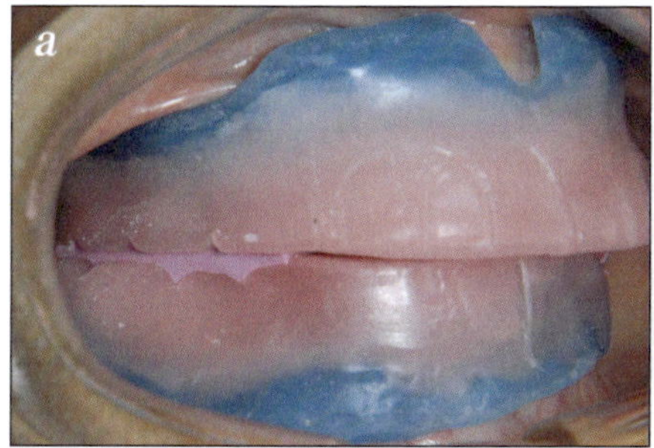

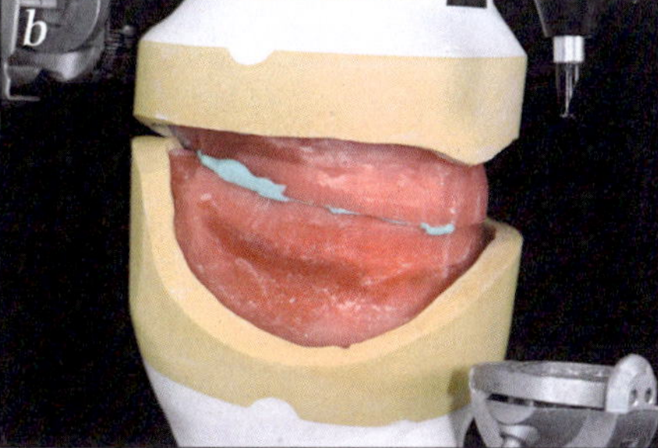

Figure 2-161 Centric relation registration. *(a)* CR registration was obtained with wax occlusion rims and polyvinyl siloxane. *(b)* Maxillomandibular records are used for mounting to an articulator (different patient).

when molding the master impression (Fig 2-158) during try-in or at delivery. If these surfaces are recorded at the impression stage, care should be taken to bead and box the impression in order to maintain the imprint of the cameo surfaces.

The peripheral seal of the maxillary denture may be difficult to achieve in some patients. Pedicle flaps or free flaps used to reconstruct soft tissue defects that extend superiorly may compromise the denture extension around the maxillary tuberosity (Fig 2-159). If denture extensions are compromised, consideration should be given to placement of implants in the anterior maxilla to retain and stabilize the maxillary complete denture (Fig 2-159a).

Maxillomandibular records

Record bases and wax occlusion rims are constructed in the usual way. Processed bases may be indicated to maximize the stability and retention and improve the accuracy of the records made (Brewer, 1963; Langer, 1981; Jacob and Yen, 1991).

The OVD may be difficult to determine. Altered proprioceptive mechanisms, trismus, impaired motor and sensory function, lip incompetence, and muscle imbalances make it difficult to obtain accurate and repeatable registrations. If the patient has nearly normal tongue bulk, mobility, and control, the resting vertical dimension (RVD) and OVD are best evaluated with phonetics, the closest speaking space, and the unstrained ability to approximate the lips (Fig 2-160). Some clinicians advocate for the evaluation of swallowing during the records and trial appointments for assessing OVD.

In patients who exhibit reduced tongue bulk and compromised tongue mobility, particularly with poor tongue elevation, OVD should be reduced as much as possible and the plane of occlusion lowered. The tongue needs to raise 5 mm above the mandibular occlusal plane if it's expected to position the bolus on the occlusal table. Reestablishing the original OVD in these patients will prevent the tongue from effectively interacting with the teeth and palatal structures during speech and swallowing.

After adjusting the maxillary wax occlusion rim for lip support, incisal edge display, and parallelism to the interpupillary and alatragus plane, the mandibular wax rim is softened in a hot water bath, seated intraorally, and the patient is asked to occlude naturally until the lips approximate without straining the mentalis muscle. The patient is also asked to swallow. The rim is softened as needed.

This technique is particularly useful in patients with moderately restricted tongues. If the tongue is very restricted, consideration should be given to the functional augmentation of the palatal surface of the maxillary complete denture with a PAP.

If the softened mandibular wax occlusion rim technique is used, then the opposing planes will parallel (Fig 2-161), and a centric relation (CR) can be made.

The more normal the maxillomandibular relationship, the more favorable the prosthodontic prognosis. Reconstructed edentulous mandibles, especially those performed without CAD/CAM technologies, can present with altered maxillomandibular relationships. Moderate arch discrepancies can be addressed by reversing the occlusion posteriorly (Fig 2-162). More severe discrepancies may require formulating a functionally generated palatal ramp (Cantor and Curtis, 1971; Swoope, 1969).

Facebow records: A facebow record is made in the usual fashion: it records the orientation of the maxilla to the terminal hinge axis, the chosen horizontal reference plane, and the interpupillary plane (Fig 2-163).

Processing, delivery, and follow-up

After the trial prostheses have been perfected, they are processed with the customary procedures (Fig 2-164). When a processed base is used, it is recommended that a longer and slightly lower temperature

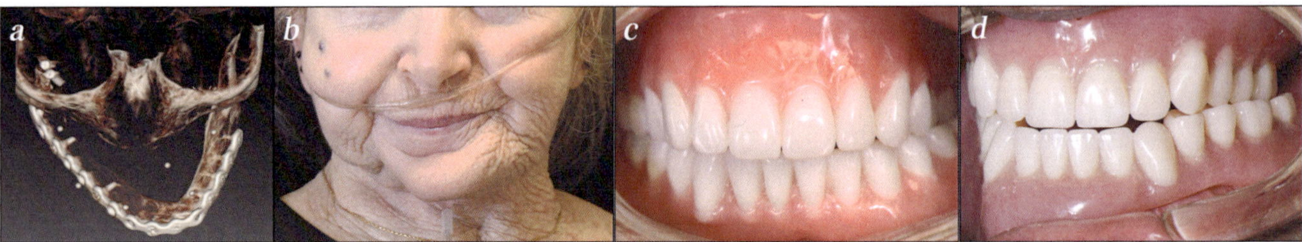

Figure 2-162 Resulting asymmetry may require reversed occlusion to account for moderate left lateral deviation of the reconstructed mandible. *(a)* Top-down view of a 3D rendering of CBCT, postreconstruction, *(b)* resulting in facial asymmetry with deviated chin point. *(c)* Transition from normal to reversed occlusion. *(d)* Example of a more severe deviation that required edge-to-edge anterior occlusion and reversed occlusion posteriorly.

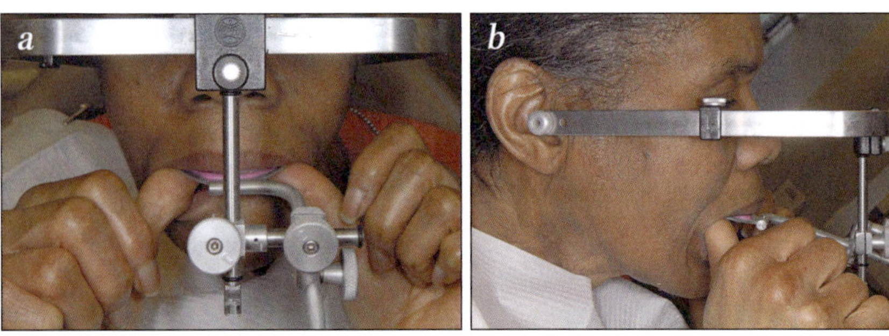

Figure 2-163 Facebow record. *(a)* Earbow parallel to the interpupillary plane. *(b)* When using orbitale as the anterior point of reference, the earbow is made parallel to the Frankfort horizontal plane.

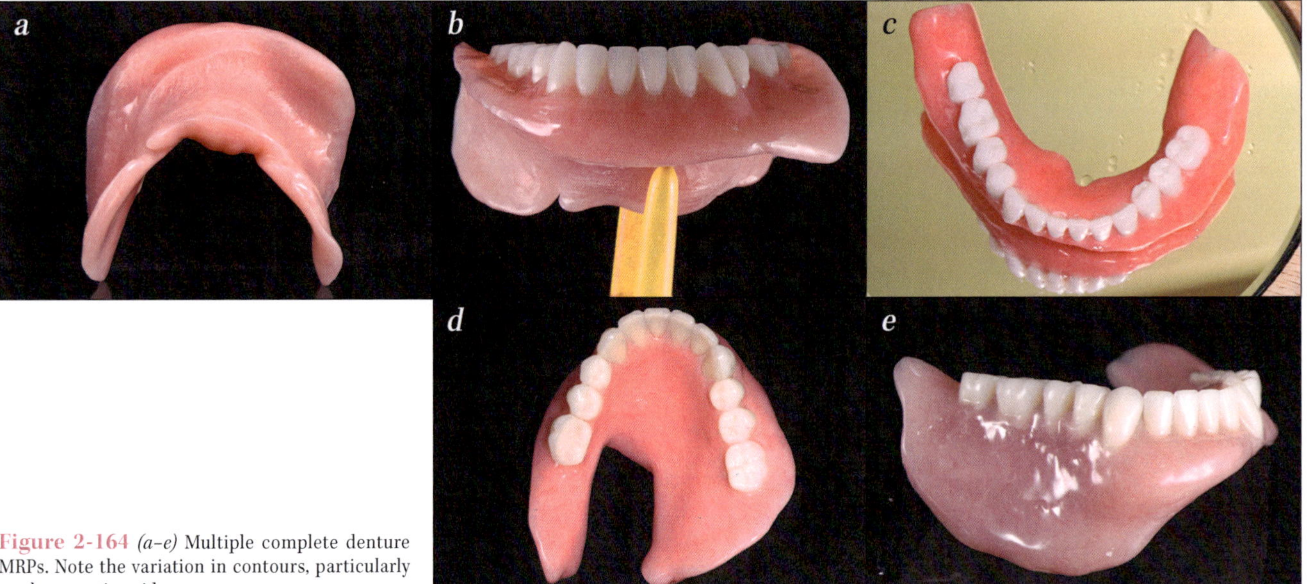

Figure 2-164 *(a–e)* Multiple complete denture MRPs. Note the variation in contours, particularly on the resection side.

be used to avoid distortion of the base during the second processing (Jacob and Yen, 1991). The prostheses are delivered, remounted, and adjusted in accordance with conventional prosthodontic guidelines. Disclosing wax is useful in identifying areas of excessive tissue pressure or displacement (Fig 2-165).

As a side note, both pressure indicating paste (PIP) and disclosing wax are increasingly difficult to find for purchase, and the authors have resorted to making both in-house. PIP is made by mixing approximately a 1:1 ratio of shortening and zinc dioxide. Disclosing wax is made by warming up impression wax in a metal crucible and mixing in PIP until the desired consistency is achieved (courtesy of Blanca Lozano, RDA, UCLA).

Patients should be monitored closely during the postinsertion period, particularly if the patient has received radiation therapy. In addition, many patients require continual support and encouragement. The use of the prosthesis for mastication should be deferred for at least 1 week.

Lip support

In most patients, the lower lip on the defect side will be flaccid, retracted posteriorly, and the vermilion inverted (Figs 2-166 and 2-167). Prosthetic lip support may be required to produce normal

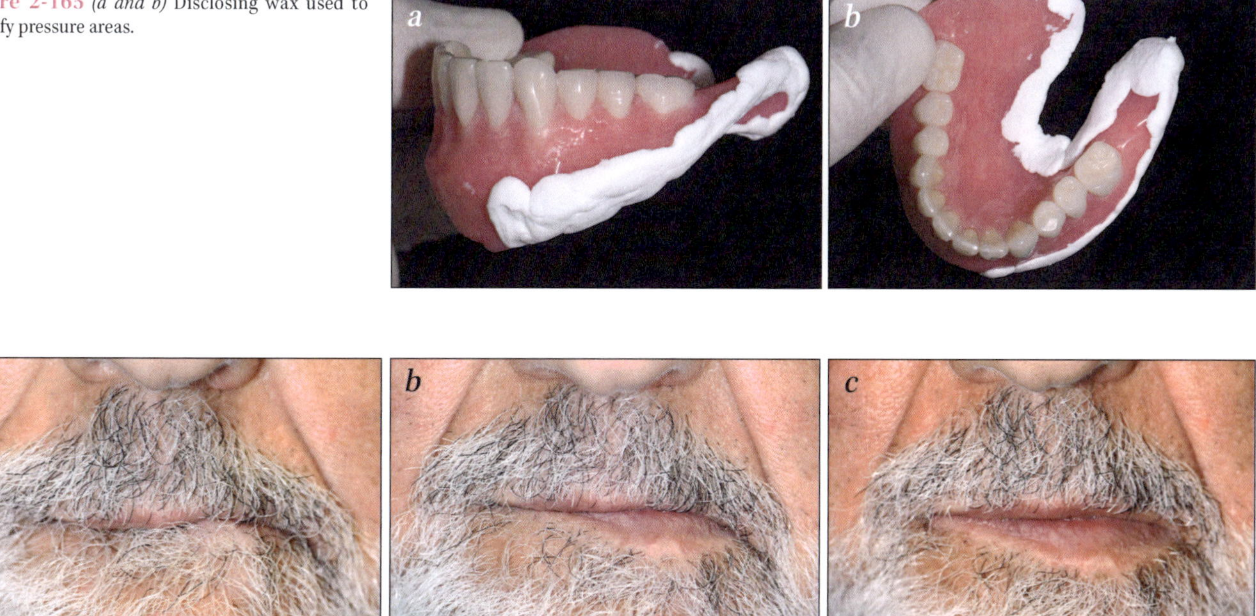

Figure 2-165 *(a and b)* Disclosing wax used to identify pressure areas.

Figure 2-166 Effect of a prosthetic lip plumper on lip contours. *(a)* Patient presentation status post gonion-to-gonion mandibular resection defect reconstructed with a FFF. Note the absence of lower lip support. *(b)* Improved appearance with the insertion of a CD-MRP. *(c)* Appearance after the addition of the plumper to the CD-MRP.

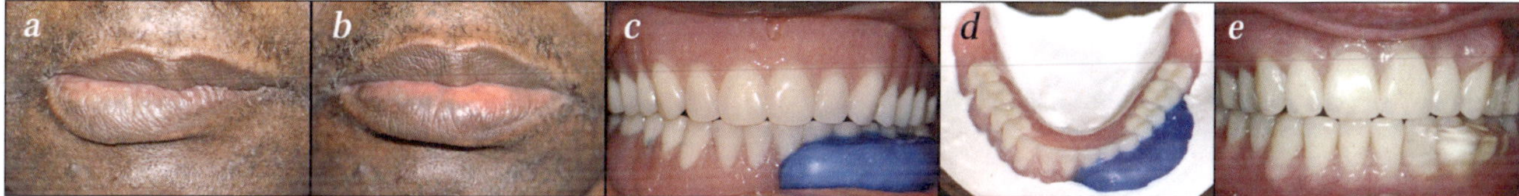

Figure 2-167 Prosthetic lip plumper added onto an MRP. *(a and b)* Appearance before and after the addition of the plumper. *(c)* Molding of the plumper with softened wax. Notice the wax is kept apical to the occlusal table. *(d)* Investment of the denture for boil out and heat processing using clear PMMA. *(e)* Completed lip plumper.

contours and eliminate lip biting. Proper contours are developed with a soft wax or tissue conditioner. Care is taken to avoid overextension, which could displace the denture. The lip plumper should be short of the plane of occlusion, or lip and cheek biting is likely to occur. By processing a lip plumper secondarily with clear heat-activated acrylic resin (Fig 2-167), the prosthetic teeth can be visualized.

Definitive RPD-MPRs

Partial denture design

Patients in this category range from those with small marginal defects to bilateral segmental defects with a single molar remaining. Manufacturing of the metal framework can be accomplished by conventional lost-wax and casting techniques. However, we have seen a shift toward CAD/CAM, either by selective laser melting (SLM) or by computer numerical control (CNC) milling. The usual principles of a metal framework design apply to all methods of manufacturing and to all defect sizes: the major connectors should be rigid (Fig 2-168), occlusal rests must direct occlusal forces along the long axis of the teeth, guiding planes should be employed to enhance stability and bracing, retention must be within the limits of physiologic tolerance of the periodontal ligament, and maximum support should be gained from the adjacent soft tissues. Clasp assemblies should consider the biomechanics of shared tooth and soft tissue support and be designed to minimize the effects of occlusal forces on the remaining teeth during function. Designs should also consider the need for cleanability, especially in light of the compromised oral hygiene and predisposition to plaque accumulation exhibited by patients treated for head and neck cancers.

Anterior defects

Included in this category are patients with marginal and segmental symphyseal resections. Both types of patients have posterior teeth bilaterally and an extensive edentulous area anteriorly, creating the need for a Kennedy Class IV, tooth-mucosa-borne partial denture. The length of the edentulous area depends on the extent of the surgery and the number and location of posterior teeth. Following these resections, the occlusion of the posterior teeth is rarely altered, and the pattern of mandibular movements is usually normal. Segmental defects restored surgically may display occlusal

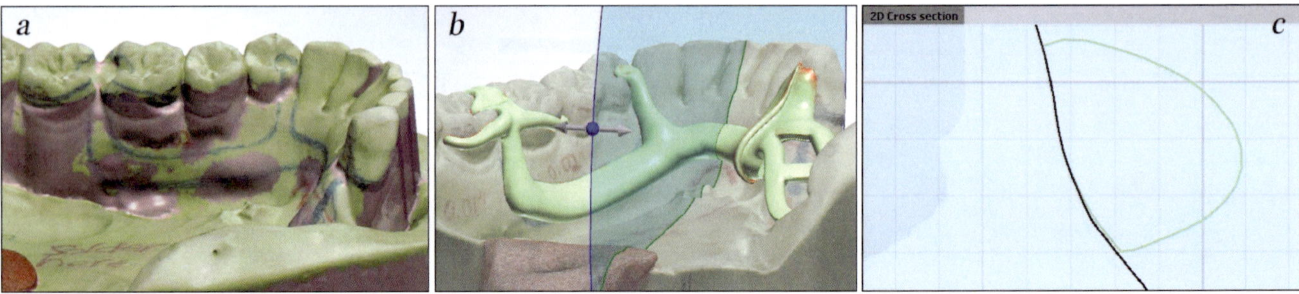

Figure 2-168 CAD evaluation of a sublingual bar major connector. *(a)* The lingual view shows the captured analog design. *(b)* Placing of a cross-section tool onto the completed CAD. *(c)* 2D cross-section evaluation of the major connector. Note that the grid scale is 1 mm, which means the 1/2 pear cross-section measures nearly 4 by 4 mm.

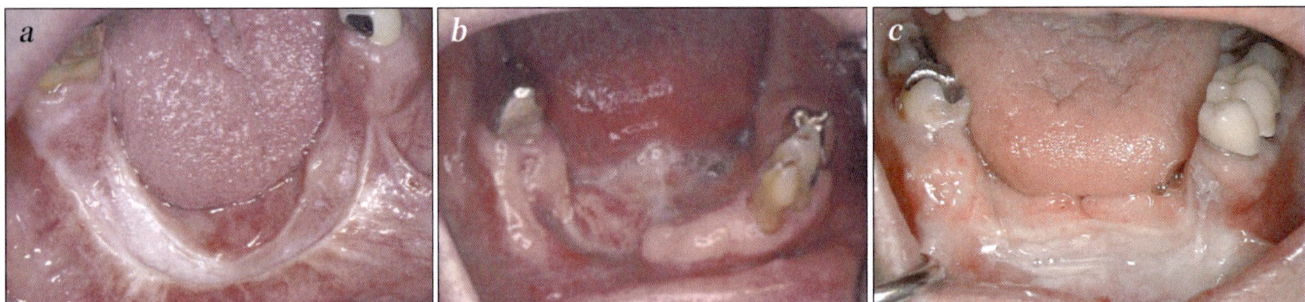

Figure 2-169 Anterior defects presenting with a number of different configurations. *(a)* Continuity of the mandible has been restored with an avascular bone graft. *(b)* Marginal mandibular resection. Continuity was retained and the wound closed primarily. *(c)* Marginal resection closed with a splint-thickness skin graft.

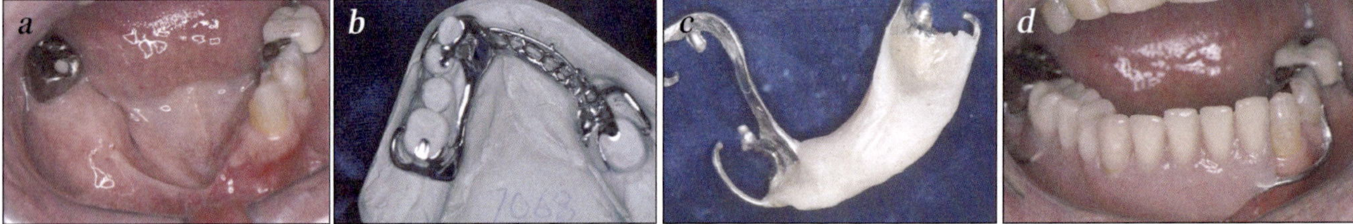

Figure 2-170 Adjusting for tissue mobility. *(a)* Symphyseal defect following marginal mandibular resection. *(b)* RPD framework. *(c)* Altered cast impression refined with mouth-temperature wax. *(d)* Completed RPD-MRP in situ. Mastication is effectively restored because of the support provided by the left canine.

abnormalities because of graft contracture or inaccurate positioning of the residual mandibular fragments at the time of insetting and fixating the graft. Once bony continuity is reestablished, the occlusion cannot be changed except with occlusal equilibration or placement of extracoronal restorations.

The anterior edentulous segment for both types of patients will usually display unusual soft tissue configurations and compromised bony support (Fig 2-169). There is considerable variation in the size and length of these defects. In large defects, the lack of attached mucosa and the obliteration of vestibules may necessitate a vestibuloplasty and split-thickness skin graft. If the radiation dose and field allow for them, dental implants should be considered. Frequently, bands of scar tissue cross the residual anterior alveolar ridge (Fig 2-170a) between the lip and tongue. Unless preprosthetic surgery is performed to optimize the denture-bearing surfaces, these tissue bands are frequently displaced on the movement of either the lip or tongue, preventing the efficient engagement of this bearing surface by the prosthesis. The clinician can account for tissue mobility by making an altered cast impression (Fig 2-170c).

Conventional RPD-MRPs for these patients enhance esthetics, provide support for the lower lip and cheek, frequently improve articulation of speech, and enhance the control of saliva. In small defects in which a canine has been retained, mastication is effectively restored (Fig 2-170).

In larger defects, the primary benefit of the prosthesis is to provide lip support for the patient (Fig 2-171). Masticatory efficiency is compromised because of the movement and length of the anterior edentulous section of the partial denture, exacerbated by poor soft tissue support. Implants positioned in the symphyseal region will provide the necessary support, and their placement should be considered for these defects (see section titled "Definitive Implant-Assisted and Implant-Supported MRP").

Partial denture designs must consider soft tissue displacement and tissue-ward movement of the anterior extension of the prosthesis (Fig 2-172). Designing distal rests effectively distalize the fulcrum line and position the infrabulge retainers and extension base on the same side of the axis of rotation. This allows the I bar to disengage the abutment undercuts during occlusal loads (Fig 2-172b). Particular care

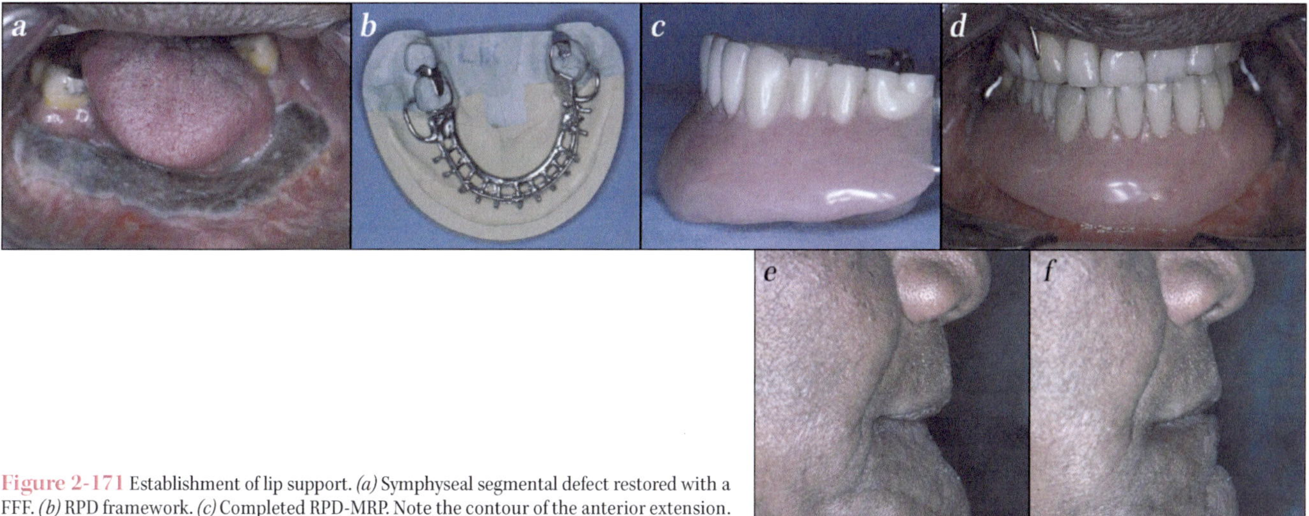

Figure 2-171 Establishment of lip support. *(a)* Symphyseal segmental defect restored with a FFF. *(b)* RPD framework. *(c)* Completed RPD-MRP. Note the contour of the anterior extension. *(d)* Prosthesis inserted. *(e and f)* Preinsertion and postinsertion facial contours.

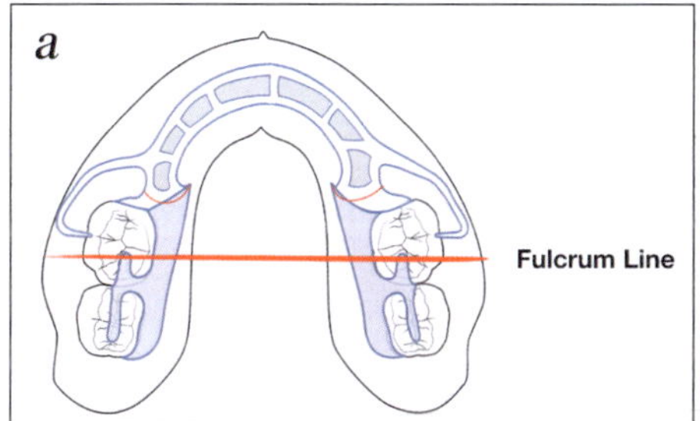

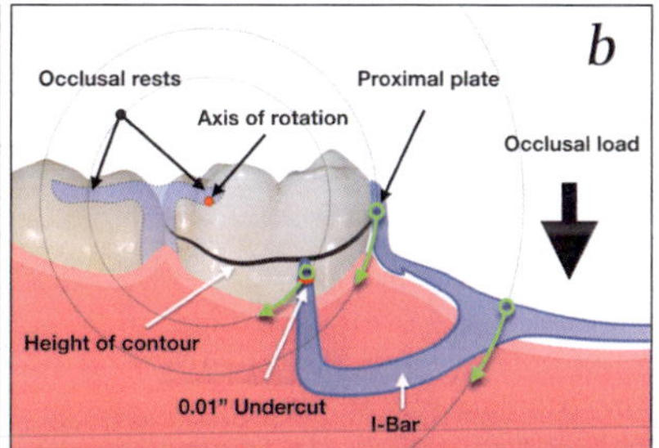

Figure 2-172 Suggested framework design for symphyseal defect: *(a)* occlusal view, *(b)* buccal view. Note the axis of rotation. The I bar and proximal plate will disengage *(green arrows)* when occlusal force is applied anteriorly. When the extension base lifts away from the tissues, the long rest on the second molar acts as an indirect retainer.

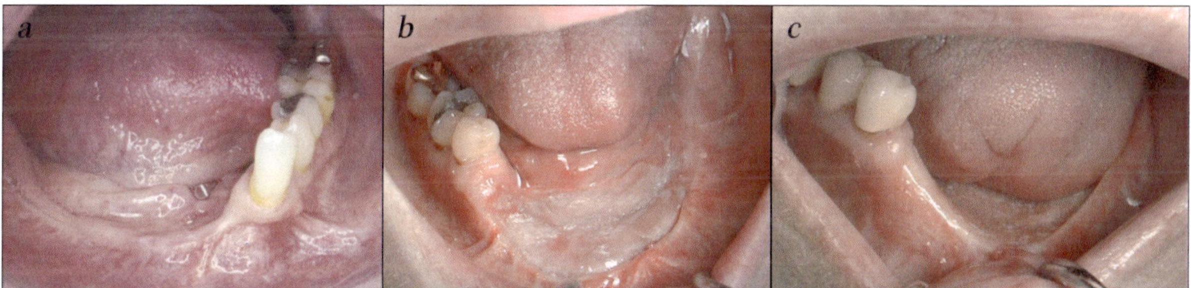

Figure 2-173 Lateral and symphyseal defects in which mandibular continuity was maintained or restored with a FFF. *(a)* Marginal mandibular defect with some attached keratinized mucous remaining. *(b)* Marginal mandibular defect closed with a split-thickness skin graft. *(c)* Segmental mandibular defect restored with a FFF. Primary closure of the soft tissue resulted in displaceable, poorly keratinous tissues covering most of the denture-bearing surface.

should be taken to relieve the proximal plates and the distal aspect of the minor connectors during physiologic adjustment to allow for the expected movement of the framework during function. Indirect retention is provided by extending a long mesial-occlusal rest on the second molars (Fig 2-172) and by preparing longer proximal guide planes on the first molars. Both these components will resist the unseating of the extension base in pure rotation around the fulcrum line.

The edentulous areas are recorded with an altered cast impression. Impression waxes are especially well suited for the anterior edentulous segment because they allow a functional impression of movable tissue beds. At the trial appointment, esthetics, occlusion, and speech should be assessed; particular attention should be paid to establishing the contour of the lower lip. These prostheses are processed, polished, delivered, and adjusted in accordance with conventional prosthodontic guidelines, and the patient is enrolled in a recall system for periodic monitoring and professional prophylactic hygiene.

Lateral defects

Lateral defects, in which the posterior dentition remains on only one side of the arch, are more challenging to restore than the defects described above for several reasons. Many of these patients have undergone large mandibular resections in which the body of the mandible and a portion of the symphysis were reconstructed with a vascularized free flap. The long lever arms and compromised denture-bearing surfaces contribute to the excessive movement of the prosthesis during function (Fig 2-173). The teeth retained in the residual

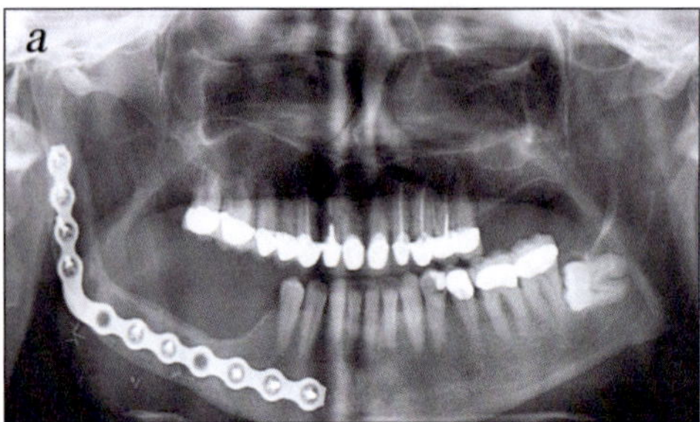

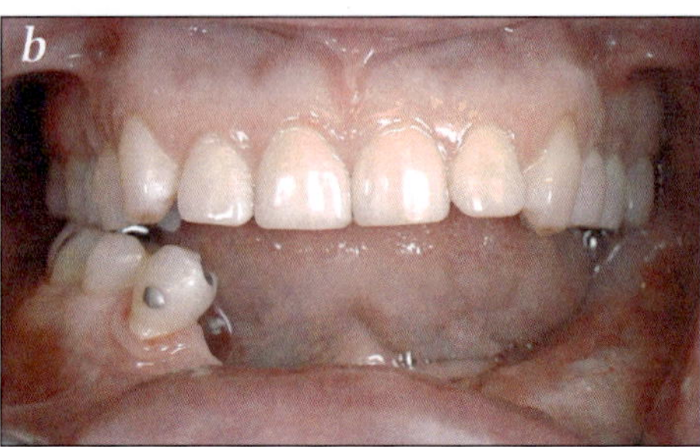

Figure 2-174 Small and large mandibular defect reconstructed with a FFF. Note that both show some degree of occlusal discrepancies. *(a)* The panoramic radiograph shows the lack of occlusion on the terminal abutment. *(b)* The clinical photograph shows a tilted occlusal plane of the mandible.

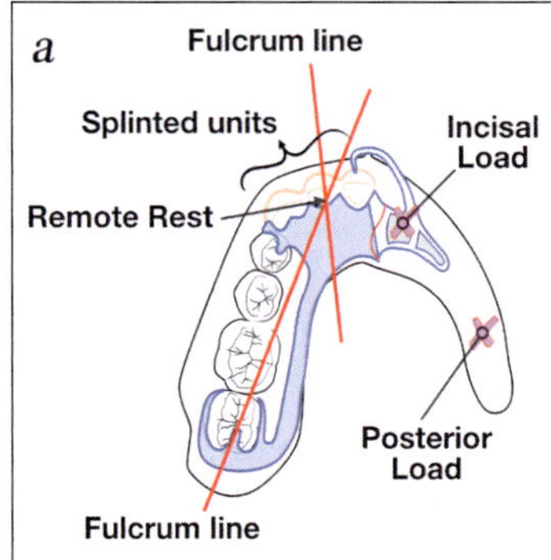

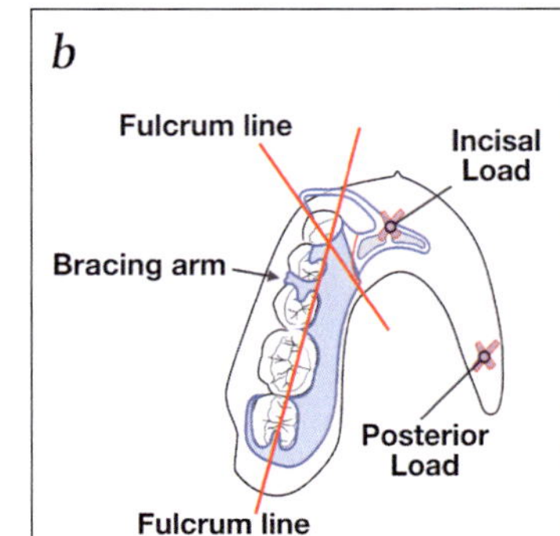

Figure 2-175 Suggested RPD framework design for a lateral mandibular defect. Notice the dynamic fulcrum lines dependent on the location of the occlusal load. *(a)* Incisors are splinted to the canine and designed with a remote rest concept for the RPI clasp assembly. *(b)* Larger defects with fewer teeth and less favorable edentulous denture-bearing surfaces are designed with more bracing of the abutment teeth by plating.

mandibular segment may not be in an ideal occlusion (Fig 2-174). Patients have lost the inferior alveolar nerve and possibly the lingual nerve and consequently cannot detect or manipulate the bolus on the resected side even if the continuity of the mandible is restored.

These patients present with unique partial denture design challenges. The fulcrum line is dynamic in that it changes depending on the point of force application on the extension base (Fig 2-175) Patients tend to confine the bolus to the dentate side during the chewing cycle because of the loss of sensory input on the defect side, but they may generate considerable load when incising a bolus of food. The abutment adjacent to the edentulous space is subjected to the greatest stresses, and therefore, the rests on these teeth should be positive and opposite the extension base. If this tooth is a canine, a cingulum rest is recommended. If a premolar or molar represents the most anterior abutment, the rest should be placed on the distal of the abutment or opposite the extension base.

Mandibular incisors make the worse terminal abutments given their short, narrow, and tapered roots. Frequently, the periodontal support on the defect side of the tooth is compromised, and if the area was irradiated, extraction could precipitate an ORN. If greater-than-class-II mobility is noted, and the site received tumoricidal doses of radiation, the tooth should undergo elective endodontic therapy with subsequent decoronation and conversion to an overlay abutment (Fig 2-176). These procedures serve many advantages. The mobility will decrease as the crown-to-root ratio will significantly improve. Support can be gained when the retained root is domed, proprioception within the PDL is retained, and the risk of ORN is abated. Root caries is avoided by the daily use of 5000 ppm fluoride gel or acidulated calcium phosphate in the wells of the metal overlay framework (Fig 2-176e) (Toolson and Smith, 1983).

When the mobility of an incisor is more moderate, splinted, full-coverage restorations are recommended to distribute occlusal forces and forces experienced by the removable prosthesis (Fig 2-177). If the abutment is a central incisor, splinting with the adjacent lateral and canine is advised. In addition to force distribution by rigid splinting, surveyed restorations allow control of the contours. Proximal and lingual guide planes can be milled parallel to the path of insertion. This not only improves bracing but effectively eliminates the black triangle often seen adjacent to a triangular-shaped abutment. Positive cingulum rests can be made, which can be nearly impossible on a mandibular incisor. Ideal undercuts can be designed. These surveyed features are assessed on either a full contour wax-up or a milled PMMA prototype (Fig 2-177c, d, and e). Lastly, a near-perfect color, texture, and contour match can be expected when a trial tooth arrangement is used to mirror the image using CAD/CAM.

Because splinted crowns function as a single unit, the components of a clasp assembly (proximal plate, rest, and retainer) can be distributed to different crowns. By distalizing the rest to the next splinted abutment and keeping the retainer on the abutment closer to the extension base, the biomechanics of the RPI clasp assembly are optimized, since the axis of rotation is farther from the retainer. This concept was described by Krol et al. and termed a *remote rest* (1999). Fig 2-177 shows that the rests are positioned on the lateral and canine but not the terminal, central incisor. Fig 2-178 is another example of a splinted central-lateral canine with remote rest on the cinguli of the lateral and canine and the retainer on the central.

A third option for addressing the mobility of an incisor as the terminal abutment is to simply not clasp it; instead, a retainer can be designed for the adjacent canine (Fig 2-179).

Fig 2-175 shows two RPD designs. Both employ minimal retention but multiple rests, guide planes, and proximal plates. When the edentulous-bearing surface is unfavorable on the defect side, a more generalized use of bracing with lingual plating is recommended to distribute lateral forces as widely as possible among the remaining dentition (Fig 2-175b). Because an anterior I bar is insufficient to keep the RPD from rotating toward the defect side,

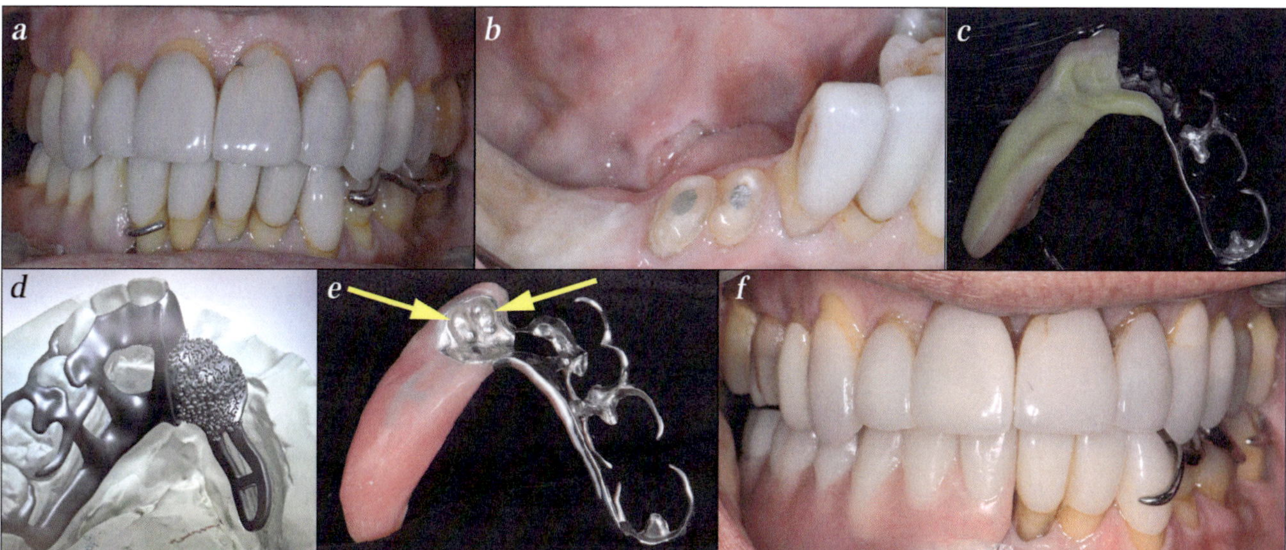

Figure 2-176 Right lateral mandibular defect reconstructed with a FFF. *(a)* RPD-MRP with a wrought wire engaged on the right lateral incisor. Greater than class II mobility is seen on the terminal abutment and adjacent central incisor. Note generalized attachment loss. *(b)* Elective endodontic therapy, decoronation, amalgam plugs, and doming of the retained roots. *(c)* MRP was made into a transitional prosthesis, while splinted crowns were made for the retained incisors and canine. *(d)* CAD of the metal framework. *(e)* New MRP. Note the overlay abutments are covered in a metal base. Fluoride is applied daily to the overlay wells of the MRP *(arrows)*.

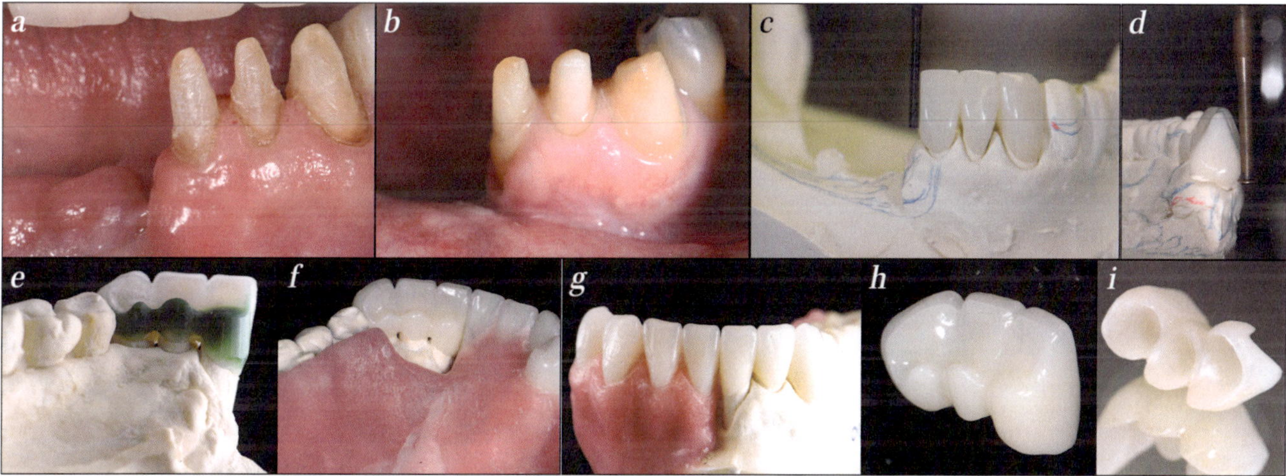

Figure 2-177 Splinted surveyed crowns for lateral mandibular defects. *(a and b)* Tooth preparations. *(c–e)* Milled PMMA prototypes are checked by a surveyor and modified as needed. *(e)* Notice the added wax to create positive rests and parallel lingual and proximal guide planes. *(f–i)* Completed layered zirconia restorations. *(g)* Notice the fidelity in replicating the shade, texture, and contours of the diagnostic tooth setup. *(h and i)* Two examples of finished splinted crowns.

a bracing arm in the embrasure between the premolars or first premolar and cuspid is employed to resist the described medial displacement (Fig 2-175b). Proximal plates should move freely during function without torquing the abutments. This is accomplished by a physiologic adjustment at the framework trial appointment. An RPI clasp assembly is designed for the teeth adjacent to the edentulous area, engaging a measured 0.01″ labial undercut. A distal or remote rest will allow the infrabulge clasp to disengage and rotate farther into the undercut when the patient incises the food bolus. Ribbon occlusal rests or overlay rests (Fig 2-195e, next section) are often employed to idealize the posterior occlusal plane or restore occlusal contacts. If possible, the occlusion should be refined to achieve contact in maximum intercuspation position; otherwise, balanced articulation is recommended. The patient should be instructed to masticate on the nondefect side with the residual mandibular dentition. We recommend the posterior retainer be a circumferential clasp because this design provides additional bracing. The retentive clasp measures 1.5 mm at the shoulder with the minor connector and is half round in cross section. This measurement tapers uniformly to half that proportion with only the terminal one-third dropping into a measured undercut located in either the buccal or lingual surface. Maximum coverage of the edentulous-bearing area is always an objective to minimize torsional moments. However, notice that the open lattice minor connector for the extension base need not extend more than two to three struts.

The patient in Fig 2-178 had a lateral mandibular defect reconstructed with a FFF. The skin paddle overlying the fibula was about 1.5 cm thick and displaceable. The tongue was intact, but the lingual

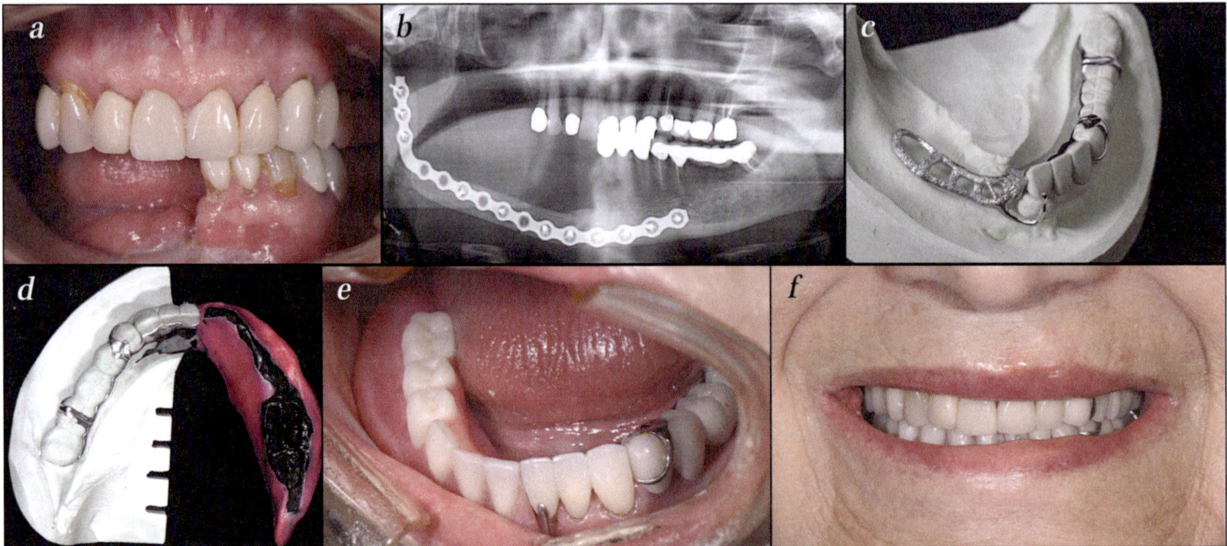

Figure 2-178 Hemimandibulectomy secondary to resection of a gingival SCC with osseous invasion, immediately reconstructed with a FFF. *(a and b)* Clinical and radiographic presentation. *(c)* Suggested RPD framework design. Note the bracing with the lingual plate major connector. Notice that the retainer on the central incisor is employed because it is splinted to the lateral and canine with fixed dental prosthesis. *(d)* Altered cast impression with interocclusal registration. *(e and f)* Completed RPD-MRP seated.

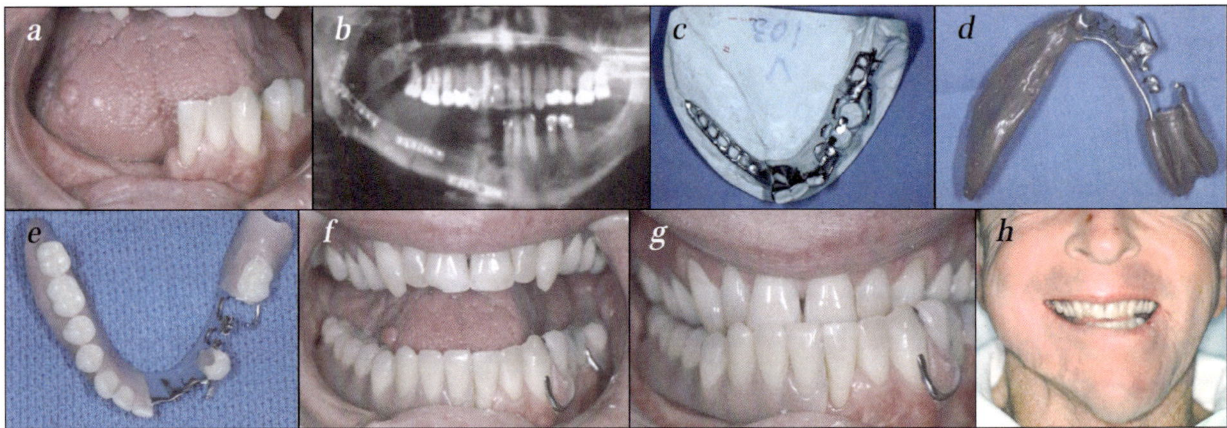

Figure 2-179 Hemimandibulectomy, reconstructed with a bisegmental FFF. *(a and b)* Clinical and radiographic presentation. *(c)* Cast metal framework. Note the position of rests, proximal plates, and retainers. *(d)* Altered cast impression. *(e)* Completed restoration. *(f to h)* Prosthesis in position. Note the reversed anterior and posterior occlusion. *(h)* Note the asymmetry of the lower facial third secondary to the suboptimal graft size and position.

and hypoglossal nerves had been resected. The residual mandibular segment was tipped, resulting in hyperocclusion of the anterior teeth. The existing single crown restorations could not be adjusted without destroying them. New splinted restorations were made for the central, lateral, and canine.

The RPD was designed with a remote cingulum rest on the lateral incisor controlling the axis of rotation when a force was applied anteriorly during the incision of the bolus. The axis changes depending on the point of load application. Because of the loss of sensory input on the defect side, the patient tended to masticate the bolus on the unresected side. The clasp on the premolar was purely for bracing and resisting medial displacement toward the defect. The circumferential clasp on the molar pontic engaged a 0.01″ undercut even though it is theoretically on the so-called wrong side of the fulcrum line. It is our opinion that the potential extraction force delivered to the posterior teeth when the patient incised the food bolus would not be clinically significant. Typically, the last molar is clasped from a distal minor connector; however, in this situation, the ascending ramus was too close to the distal-buccal line angle of the third molar to accommodate a clasp.

The casting was physiologically adjusted to account for the most common and clinically significant axes of rotation generated during mastication. An altered cast impression of the edentulous area was made to idealize support in the extension area (Fig 2-178d).

The patient in Fig 2-179 illustrates an issue encountered when the remaining mandibular segment is malaligned. The fibula segments were cut longer than the defect, and the left mandibular body was pushed laterally. While this creates skeletal and occlusal disharmony, patients are most concerned about the resulting compromise in facial appearance. The occlusal discrepancy is evaluated on properly mounted diagnostic casts followed by occlusal equilibration before the RPD design is developed.

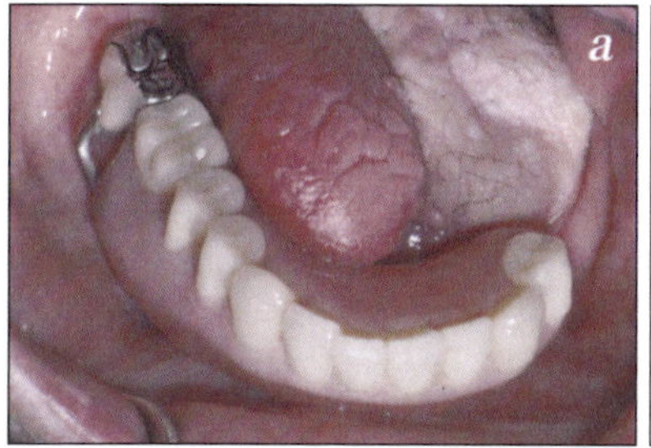

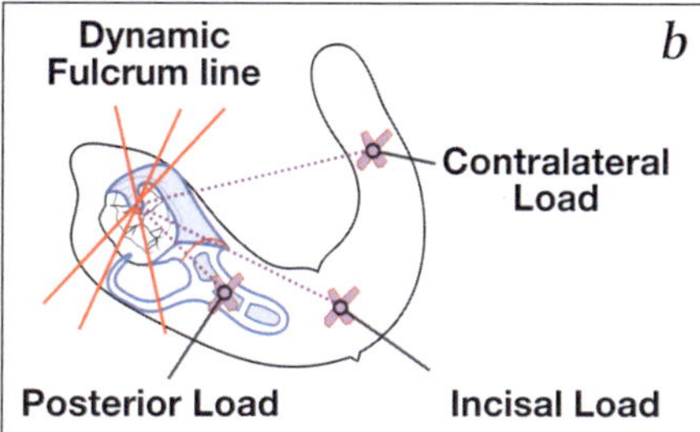

Figure 2-180 Tongue-mandible defect. *(a)* RPD-MRP in position. *(b)* Schematic of framework design. Note the dynamic fulcrum line dependent on load location and how the I bar becomes on the wrong side when the load is applied to the contralateral side.

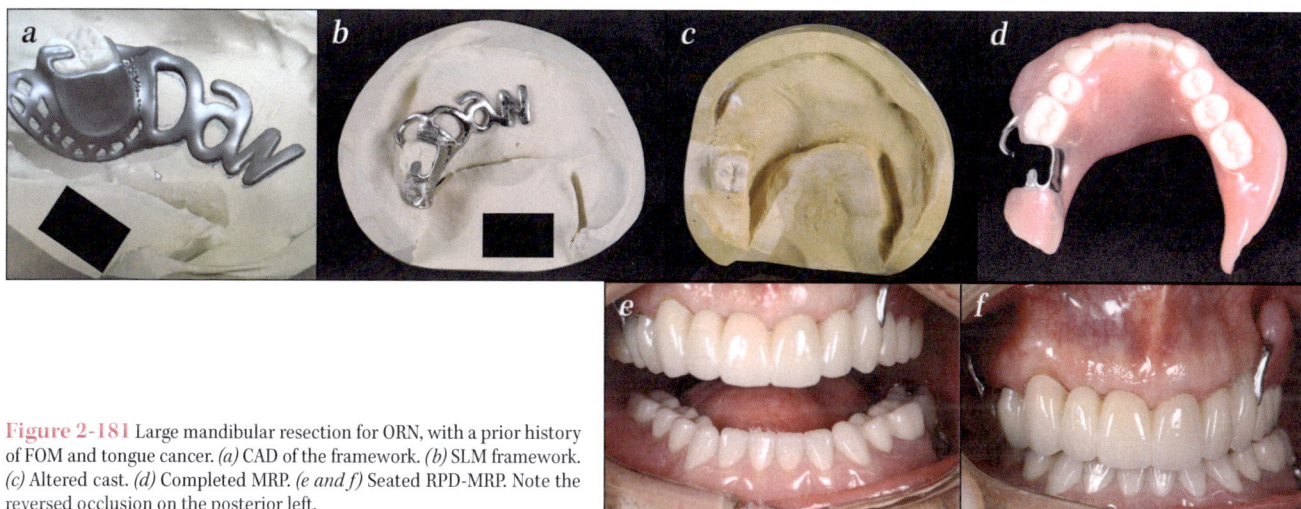

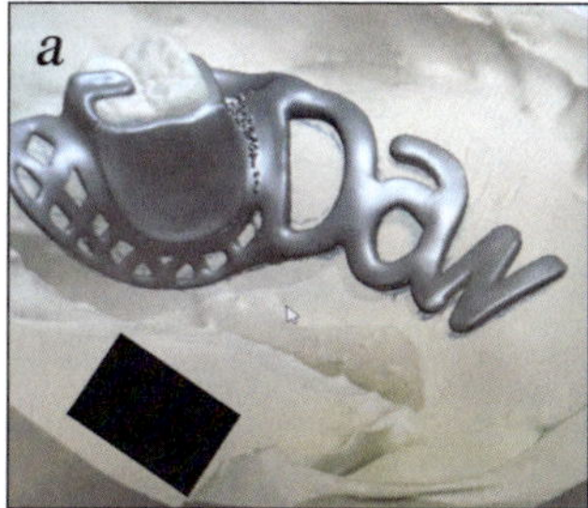

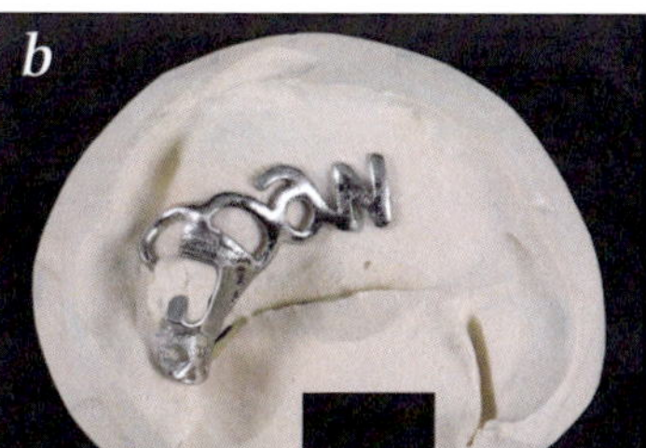

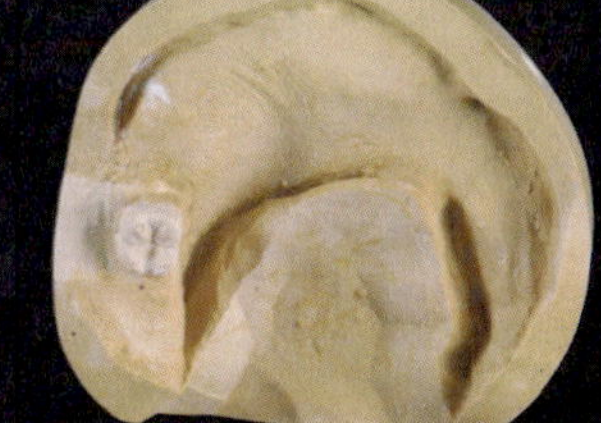

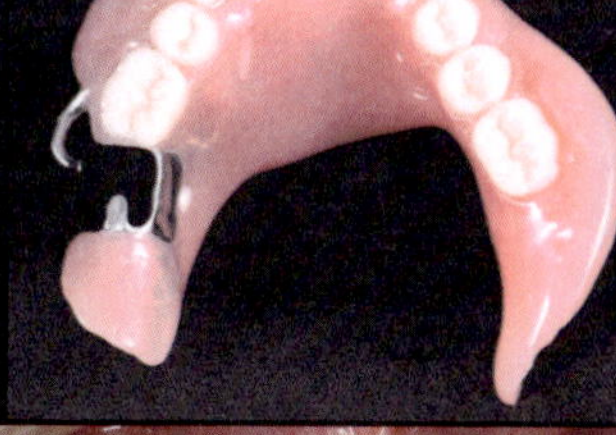

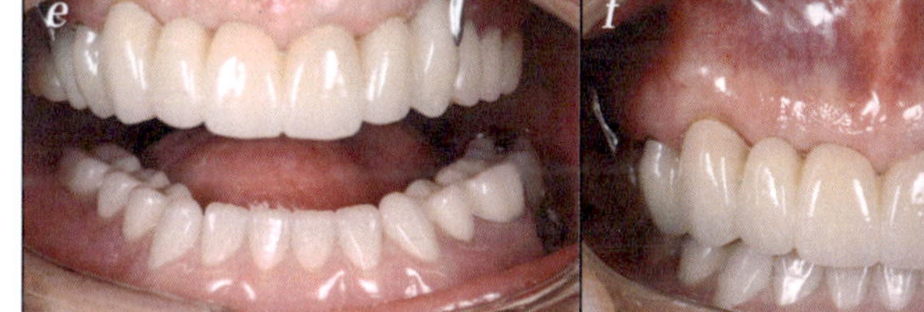

Figure 2-181 Large mandibular resection for ORN, with a prior history of FOM and tongue cancer. *(a)* CAD of the framework. *(b)* SLM framework. *(c)* Altered cast. *(d)* Completed MRP. *(e and f)* Seated RPD-MRP. Note the reversed occlusion on the posterior left.

Bracing was provided by minor connectors, guide planes, and proximal plates. The lingual plate engaging the remaining mandibular teeth further enhanced bracing. The mesial rest on the second premolar controlled the axis of rotation when an occlusal force was applied to the distal extension on the unresected side. The cingulum rest on the canine controlled the axis of rotation when the bolus was incised. Notice that no retainer was designed for the incisor.

The patient was insensate on the defect side and was encouraged to masticate on the unresected side. Therefore, the framework was physiologically adjusted to account for the axis that resulted when the bolus was incised as well as the axis that resulted when the bolus was masticated in the extension area on the unresected side.

Bilateral defects

Bilateral defects in which few teeth remain are particularly difficult to restore. These patients have undergone large mandibular resections in which portions of both bodies and symphysis of the mandible are reconstructed with a vascularized free flap. Ideally, at least two implants would be placed in the symphyseal area at the time of reconstruction to address the long lever arms and compromised edentulous denture-bearing surfaces that contribute to excessive movement of the prosthesis during function (Fig 2-180). Many patients will have lost the inferior alveolar nerves bilaterally and may have incurred injury to the lingual nerves. Total loss of sensation to the lower lip will surely compromise saliva control. Patients will have difficulty detecting and manipulating the bolus.

Patients tend to confine the bolus close to the remaining teeth, and the abutment adjacent to the defect is subjected to the greatest stresses. The loss of the remaining teeth that would result is an even greater deficit described in the Definitive MRPs for edentulous patients section above, so it is critical to utilize the abutment tooth in a manner that minimizes torsional forces.

Part of the challenge is that while we endeavor to replace the missing teeth, we must place as much effort into preserving the remaining dentition. This is complicated by the fact that these prostheses are borne on tissues of two different resiliencies—the displaceable skin flap verses a relatively rigid tooth, which creates a fulcrum located at the occlusal rest. The juxtaposition of the distal rest and I bar on a single molar allows the retainer to rotate farther into the undercut when the occlusal forces are applied to the adjacent portion of the extension base. Additionally, physiologic adjustment of the proximal plates should be performed to allow free movement during function without torquing the abutment.

Two examples (Figs 2-180 and 2-181) exemplify the design for patients who underwent bilateral mandibular resections. The skin paddle was used to close the soft tissue defect, and in the case of glossectomy, simultaneous reconstruction of the tongue was performed.

The RPD was designed so that the distal rest on the single molar controlled the axis of rotation when a force is applied anterior to the abutment. The axis changes depending on the point of load application (Fig 2-180). Because of the loss of sensory input, mastication is best performed adjacent to the remaining tooth. An altered cast impression of the edentulous area was made to idealize support in the extension area.

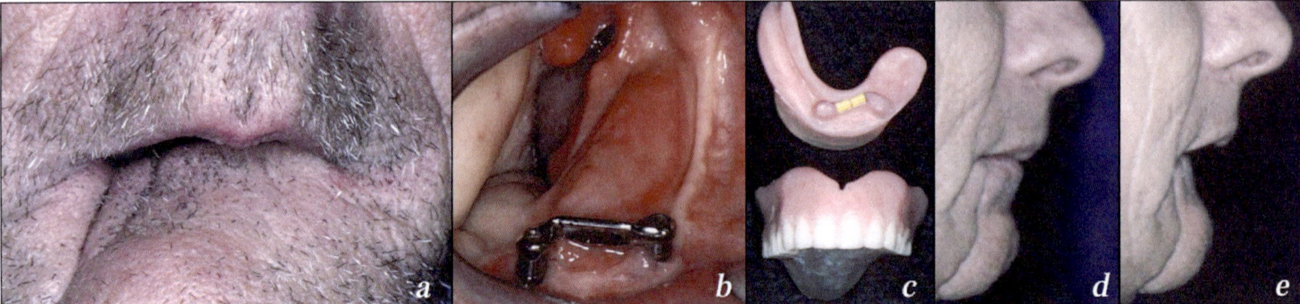

Figure 2-182 Patient who lacked the ability to achieve lip closure and presented with inarticulate speech and an inability to control saliva. *(a)* Lip posture without prosthetic rehabilitation. *(b)* Total glossectomy defect with an implant-assisted connecting bar in the anterior mandible. *(c)* Maxillary complete denture with palatal augmentation and MRP with a lip plumper. *(d)* A profile without prosthesis. *(e)* Improved profile with prosthesis in place. Oral competence is improved, and speech has become intelligible to family and friends.

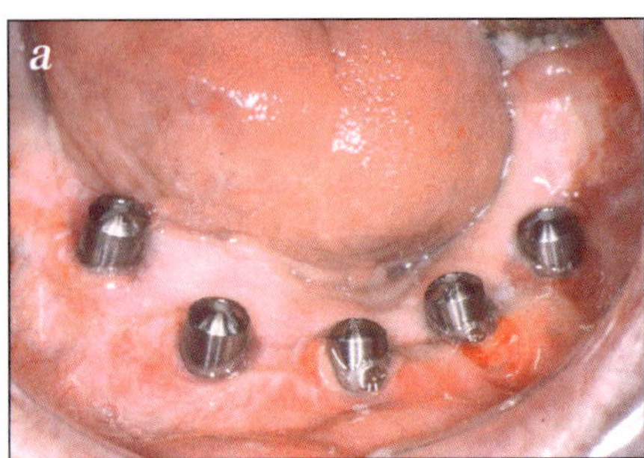

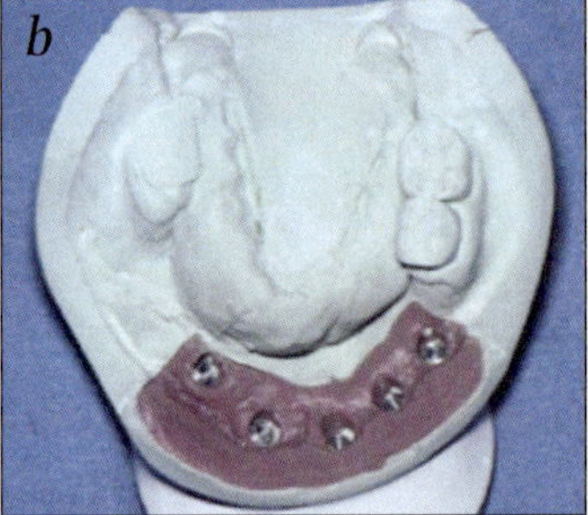

Figure 2-183 Curved arrangement of implants for an implant-supported fixed restoration. *(a)* Five implants have been placed. *(b)* Note the anterior-posterior spread of implants.

Definitive Implant-Assisted and Implant-Supported Mandibular Resection Prostheses (MRP)

Introduction

The prosthodontist should establish a prognosis for the treatment options as a good measure of managing patient expectations. To that end, the prosthodontist must reevaluate the history of the present illness and perform a thorough clinical and radiographic evaluation with close attention to the status of the tongue, lips, and function of nerves such as the marginal mandibular, inferior alveolar, lingual and hypoglossal nerves, the number and distribution of implants, dose and field of radiation, hard and soft tissue reconstruction, and peri-implant tissue health. How the patient has functioned with an interim prosthesis is the most tangible assessment of how the definitive prosthesis will perform. Only then can the prosthodontist and patient decide on the definitive prosthesis design: (a) implant assisted and removable, (b) implant supported and removable, (c) or implant supported and fixed. While patients may desire a fixed solution, it may not in reality offer the best long-term prognosis. A removable prosthesis in many scenarios is preferred for several reasons, discussed below. The best predictor of masticatory performance is tongue function. We must raise the patient's awareness that with compromised tongue function, implants alone may not improve masticatory performance.

Patients who have reasonable tongue function can expect significant improvement in masticatory function with implant-anchored prostheses. If the hypoglossal and lingual nerves are intact, the patient will be able to detect and manipulate the food bolus sufficiently well on the resected side to permit reasonable mastication. By contrast, patients who have lost these nerves and have poor tongue function have little to gain, no matter the number of implants. These findings would not necessarily preclude the use of implants in such patients because there are other benefits to be gained from a well-retained prosthesis, such as restoration of lip competence and improved appearance (Fig 2-182). In the face of poor tongue function, two implants are an adequate number to retain an implant-assisted prosthesis as shown in Fig 2-182.

A fixed MRP requires an adequate number and distribution of implants for ideal biomechanics. If the edentulous space extends to the molar region, a minimum of four well-distributed implants is critical. The arc of curvature of the arrangement must result in at least a 1 cm anterior-posterior spread (Fig 2-183). This arrangement will enable the implants and the prosthesis to effectively withstand the forces of mastication. Fixed restorations with a smaller anterior-posterior spread have a higher rate of implant failure and a greater number of complications associated with the prosthesis, such as screw and implant fracture (Fig 2-184) (Wu et al., 2022b). An implant-supported fixed prosthesis may not be indicated if the implant positions and angulations are not ideal. As discussed previously, malalignment of the reconstructed mandible may require that the denture teeth be positioned buccal to the ridge on the unresected side and lingual to the ridge on the reconstructed side. The osseous reconstruction and implant positions may be less than ideal (Fig 2-185), complicating the design of fixed restoration. Implants should be positioned so that the screw access channels exit through

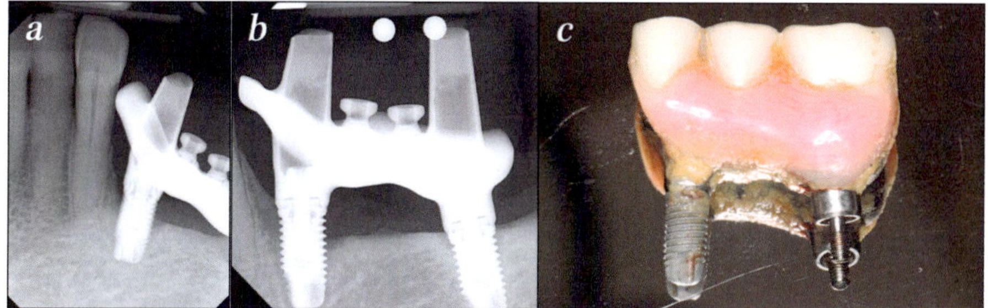

Figure 2-184 Two implant-fixed MRP. *(a and b)* Radiographs show peri-implant bone loss. *(c)* Failed implant, failed prosthesis, likely due to unfavorable implant biomechanics, and poor oral hygiene.

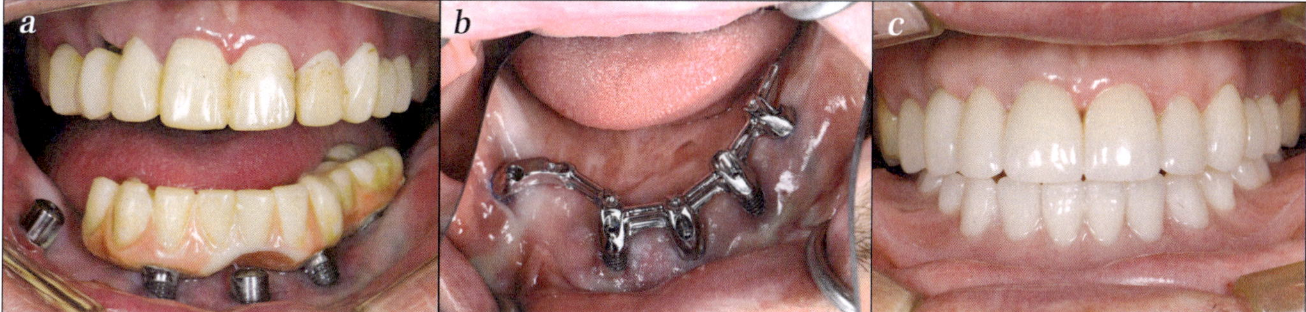

Figure 2-185 *(a)* Suboptimal osseous reconstruction, poor implant positions, and early crestal bone loss require a redesign from a fixed to a removable prosthesis. *(b)* Completed implant supported connecting bar. *(c)* Definitive implant supported MRP.

the cingulum area of the anterior teeth and the central fossa of the posterior teeth.

When a fixed restoration is contemplated, the authors recommend a trial period with a fixed, interim prosthesis (Fig 2-187a–b)—a prototype prosthesis—to evaluate and prognosticate the efficacy of a fixed design. Three major issues require evaluation. Peri-implant soft tissue health, esthetics, and function. The final decision is made in conjunction with the patient and based on how the interim prosthesis fares at the end of a four-month trial.

The patient must demonstrate the ability to maintain soft tissue health with a fixed, interim prosthesis. Impeccable hygiene practice alone may not be sufficient. Many of these patients have undergone soft tissue reconstruction with a myocutaneous flap. If the soft tissues are not adequately tailored, persistent inflammation or infection (Fig 2-187c–f) to the peri-implant soft and hard tissues could culminate in tissue breakdown and loss of implants. If radiotherapy is a part of the patient's oncologic treatment, soft tissue management is further compromised, and loss of the vascularized flap is a real risk. Owing to their narrower profile, implant connecting bars make it easier for patients to conduct proper hygiene measures. This is an important factor because most resection patients are elderly and may have impaired vision and poor manual dexterity.

Function and esthetics of the lower lip are affected when patients lose their marginal mandibular nerve. The lip on the resected side loses its muscle tonus and becomes retracted. Patients are quick to report this esthetic compromise. A weak lower lip also compromises the patient's ability to control saliva, which manifests as drooling from the ipsilateral lip commissure (Roumanas et al., 1997). Patients, however, are less inclined to associate this neuralgic deficit with their compromised ability to articulate plosive consonants, such as /b/ and /p/. The clinician can evaluate the status of the marginal mandibular nerve from an esthetic viewpoint and functionally by asking the patient to read a sentence laden with plosives such as "**p**ick u**p** the **p**u**pp**y." Lastly, a weak lower lip affects lip competence and lip seal, so one might ask a patient to demonstrate through the use of a straw. A patient won't be able to generate negative pressure to draw water from a straw if the opposing lips cannot purse around the implement. A denture flange, or perhaps a prosthetic lip plumper, features appropriate only for a removable prosthesis, are necessary to provide support for the lower lip and restore the lip seal (Fig 2-182).

It may be impossible to introduce a tall driver into a molar screw channel, especially when the osseous reconstruction follows a lower border of the mandible. The ability to negotiate a tall driver into a long screw channel in patients with limited mouth opening needs to be assessed. The stackable nature of an overlay and removable prosthesis effectively shortens the screw channel length to the height of the implant connecting bar instead of the occlusal table. The overlay prosthesis has the added benefit of eliminating screw access holes through the prosthetic teeth.

In situations when the number and distribution of implants are suboptimal, the prosthesis design should incorporate shared support with denture-bearing tissues and/or adjacent teeth. Additional resistance to vertical and lateral masticatory forces can be obtained by incorporating a removable partial denture framework within the overlay removable prosthesis that engages the residual dentition with positive rests, guide planes, and lingual plating (Fig 2-186d). Additional findings may influence the design for an implant-assisted prosthesis, including early crestal bone loss (Fig 2-185), early or late implant failure, implants in irradiated bone, emergence through a bulky skin flap, or questionable osseous union between the graft and native mandible. Under these circumstances, a removable MRP design with shared support from available dentition and/or denture-bearing tissues provides for possible contingencies.

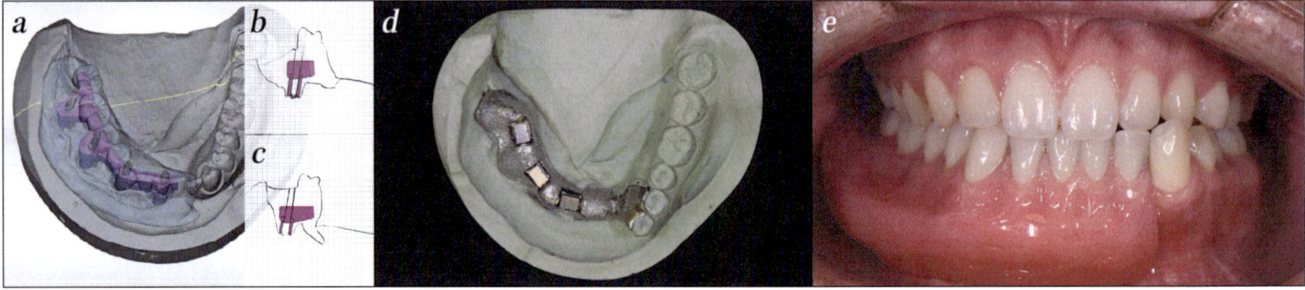

Figure 2-186 Suboptimal implant positions as a reason to employ a removable prosthesis. *(a)* Buccally positioned implants require an implant-supported, removable prosthesis. *(b and c)* Note the 2D cross-sectional evaluation of the implant position and the trial tooth position. *(d)* Overlay framework with positive rest on the adjacent canine. *(e)* Completed implant-supported MRP.

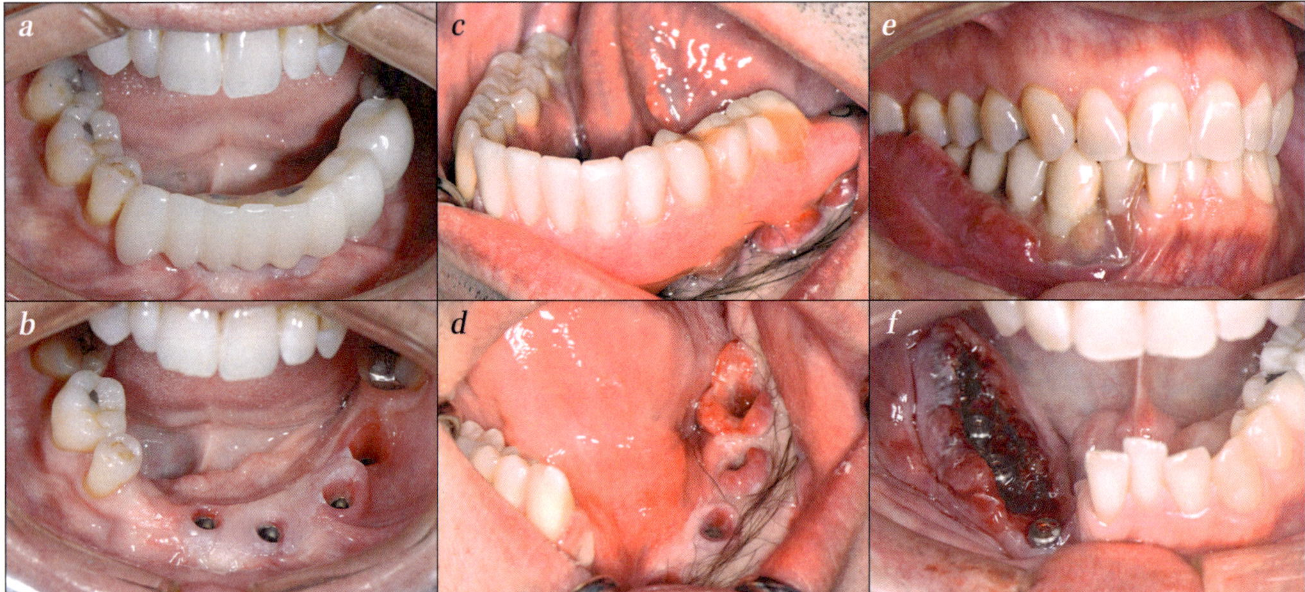

Figure 2-187 Three patients with FFF reconstructions, with varying presentations of the peri-implant soft tissues. *(a and b)* Interim fixed MRP after a trial period of over four months. Note the reasonable peri-implant soft tissue health. *(c–d)* Interim fixed MRP after a trial period of over four months. Note the poor soft tissue health. *(e and f)* Definitive fixed MRP four years postinsertion. Note the extensive soft tissue hypertrophy.

Designing implant connecting bars

When the peri-implant tissues are well healed, implant positions can be recorded with either conventional or digital methods (Davodi et al., 2022), but the authors still prefer conventional methods. Nonengaging pickup-type impression copings are secured to the implants and are connected to one another (Fig 2-188b–d). When the span of implants is large, it is prudent to add additional struts to supplement the rigidity of the impression apparatus (Fig 2-188c). An open-tray impression is made with heavy and light-body elastomeric impression material (Fig 2-188e and f). If soft tissue support or a flange is needed, then the extension base and periphery will be redefined with a corrected impression at a later date.

Implant analogs are secured to the impression copings embedded within the impression, and the impression is boxed and poured. It is prudent to verify the accuracy of the master cast. The authors fabricate a provisional implant connecting bar made by connecting titanium abutments with resin struts and pattern resin. This bar can also serve to make an interocclusal record (Fig 2-189) or retain a record base and trial denture. The trial denture is required to assess prosthetic space based on the tooth arrangement. With the record base/trial denture effectively retained, the proper OVD is determined and the CR record proven, or redone as necessary, before making the definitive implant connecting bar.

At the initial trial appointment, it may become apparent, especially if an interim MRP was not previously used as a prototype, that the occlusal relationship of remaining mandibular teeth requires modification. Fig 2-190 shows the gross supraeruption of the incisors adjacent to the defect. While in some cases, elective endodontic therapy may be required, in the elderly patient, the pulp may have receded sufficiently to prepare the teeth to correct the vertical and horizontal overlap with full-coverage restorations.

For a CAD/CAM workflow, the cast and trial dentures are both scanned. The two digital files are aligned with the CAD software and then used by the clinician/technologist to complete the initial design of the implant connecting bar (Fig 2-191). Alternatively,

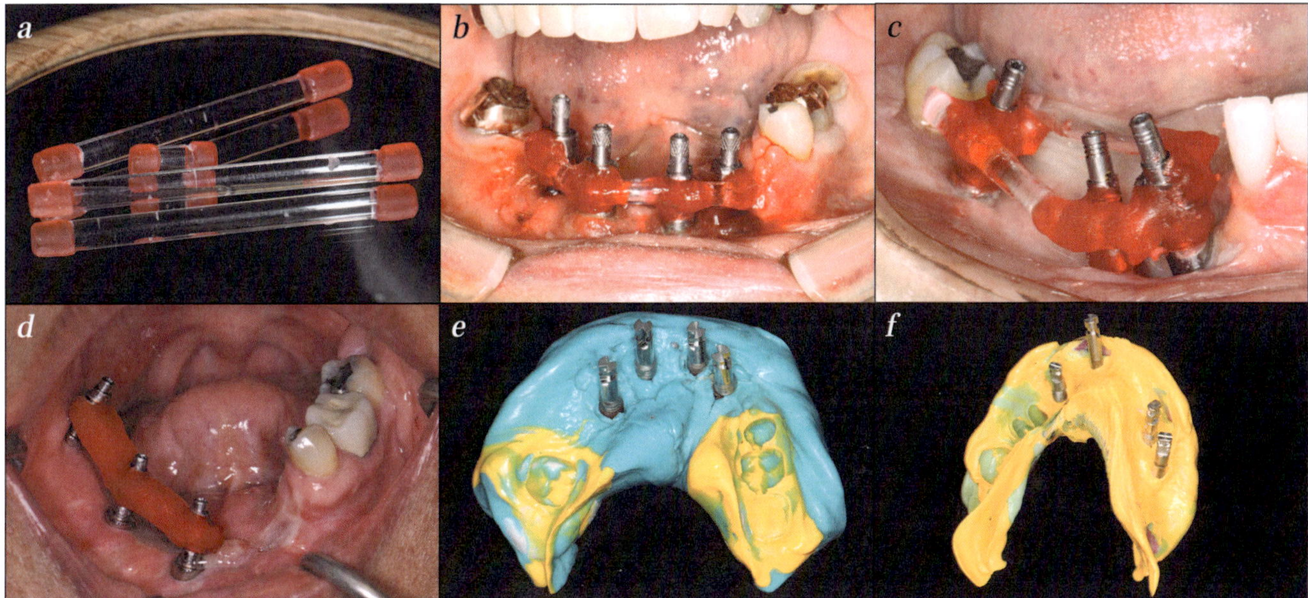

Figure 2-188 *(a)* Resin struts are connected to pickup-type implant impression copings and united together with pattern resin. *(e and f)* Open-tray impressions made with additional silicone.

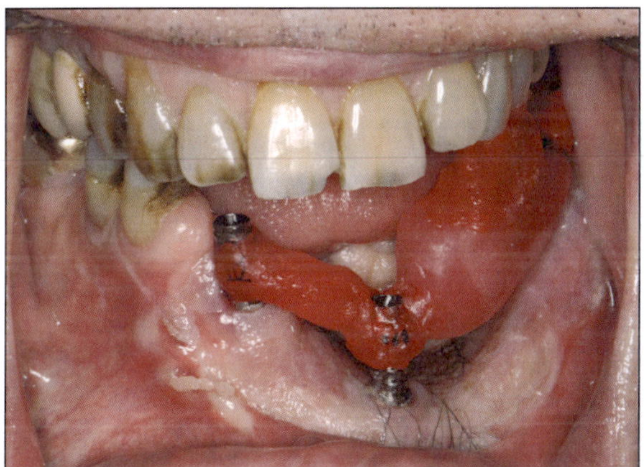

Figure 2-189 Provisional implant connecting bar used to verify implant impression and aid in maxillomandibular records.

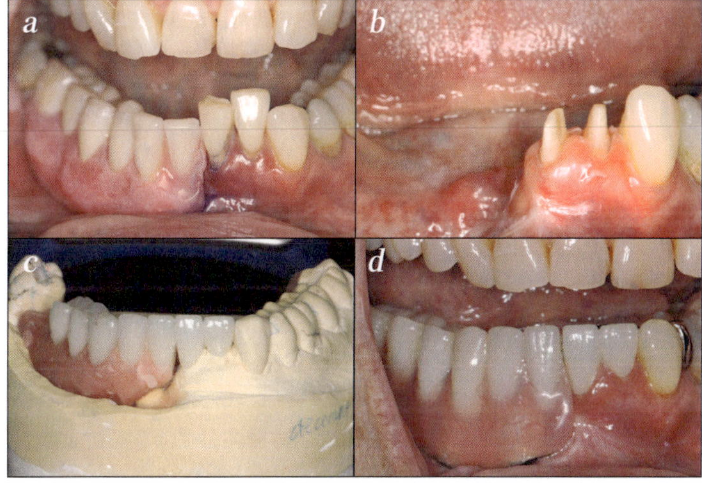

Figure 2-190 Correction of supraeruption. *(a)* Supraerupted incisors adjacent trial MRP. *(b)* Tooth preparations. *(c)* The final crown contours matched to the ideal tooth setup. *(d)* Completed rehabilitation.

a stone index is made of the tooth arrangement and keyed to the cast (Fig 2-192b). After boiling out the wax, silicone putty is used to impress the prosthetic space between the implant analog and the necks of the prosthetic teeth (Fig 2-192c). This silicone matrix and the cast are dual scanned and aligned to design the implant connecting bar (Fig 2-192d and e).

If conventional methods are used to fabricate the bar, a similar stone index is made (Fig 2-193a). The position of the denture teeth in relation to the master cast and UCLA abutments is physically evaluated while waxing the implant connecting bar Plastic patterns of the attachment are arranged with the help of a surveyor (Fig 2-193b). Prosthetics space is evaluated simply by replacing the stone index. Later, after the bar and overlay framework are made, the stone index is used to transfer the teeth onto the overlay metal framework (Fig 2-193c).

Whatever the method used to design and fabricate the implant connecting bar, when portions of the bar overlay the residual alveolar ridges, the design should conform to basic principles previously developed for normal patients (Beumer et al., 2022b). The bar must be rigid and allow for appropriate hygiene access between the implants and on the tissue side of the bar. The tissue surface of the bar should be rounded and smoothed, and the bar, and attachments connected to the terminal ends, should be located 1 to 2 mm above the tissues. The bar must be positioned and contoured so that there is ample room for the denture teeth, denture resin, and the metal overlay framework.

For an implant-supported connecting bar, titanium alloy is a suitable material. If an implant-assisted connecting bar is designed, it must be made of a wear-resistant alloy such as cobalt-chrome.

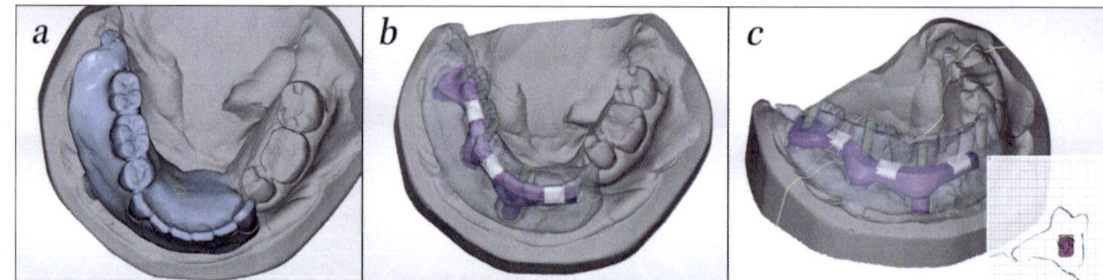

Figure 2-191 *(a, b, and c)*. The master cast and the trial denture setup are scanned, and the files are aligned. An implant-supported implant connecting bar is designed with CAD software. Before milling, the prosthodontist must inspect the design from all angles to ensure that it conforms to the design standards.

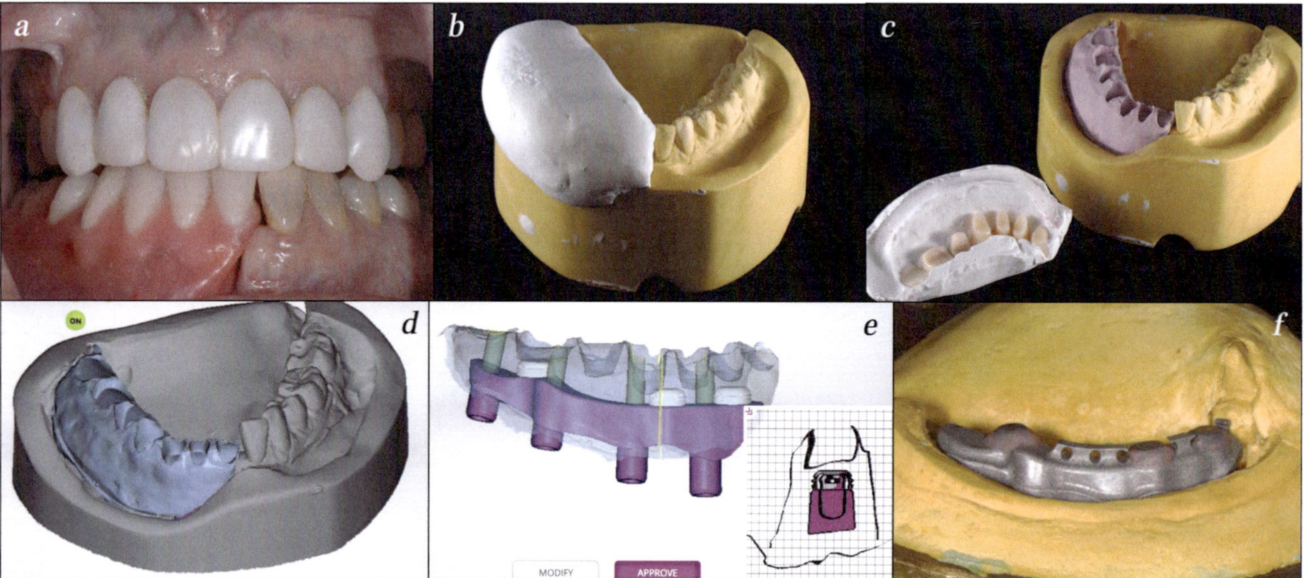

Figure 2-192 Right hemimandibulectomy reconstructed with a FFF. *(a)* Trial denture verification. *(b)* Plaster index of the prosthetic teeth. *(c)* Wax boil out. Silicone putty captures the space from the implant analogs to the necks of the denture teeth. *(d and e)* The bar is designed in the available prosthetic space. Note that the attachment is positioned apical to the neck of the denture tooth. *(f)* The overlay framework is milled to fit intimately with the milled titanium bar. Note that the plaster index is used to transfer the denture teeth onto the overlay framework.

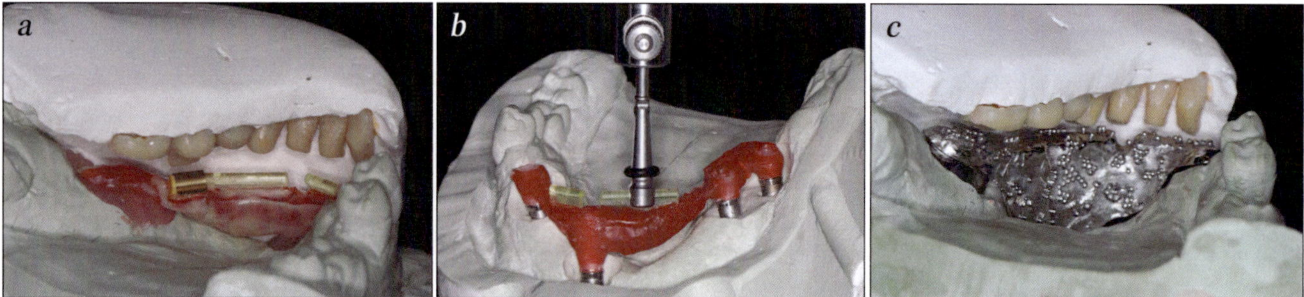

Figure 2-193 Conventional methods of relating tooth positions to the master cast while developing the contours and position of the implant connecting bar. *(a)* A plaster index with the denture teeth secured with wax, which is keyed to the master cast. *(b)* The attachment patterns are positioned parallel to the path of insertion using a surveyor. *(c)* The same stone index is later used to transfer the prosthetic teeth to the overlay framework.

Implant-supported bar designs

Partially or fully edentulous patients with mandibulectomy defects may be restored with implant-supported designs. By definition, an implant-supported design suggests a rigid connection between the overlay prosthesis and the bar. However, most bar attachment systems have some resilience. Therefore, additional design features must be employed to counteract any axes of rotation provided by resilient attachments.

The plunger attachment is an example of a rigid connection between the overlay prosthesis and the bar; however, it can only be used in full arch prostheses. Furthermore, plungers require excellent patient dexterity. Given the older patient population and often reduced mouth opening, this option may be contraindicated.

Large defects that cross the midline benefit from a favorable arched distribution of implants and attachments (Fig 2-194a). In these scenarios, the attachments will naturally resist any hinge and tipping resilience and provide a near-rigid connection. In a curvilinear implant arrangement (Fig 2-194b), when at least three attachments can be arranged as a right-angled triangle, hinging resilience

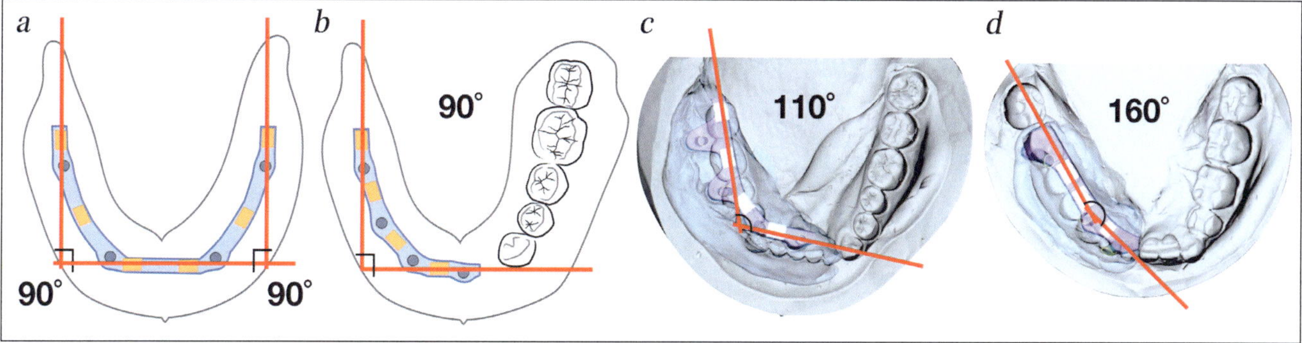

Figure 2-194 *(a–b)* Large defects that cross the midline benefit from a favorable distribution of implants and attachments. In theses scenarios the multiple attachments arranged in an arch will naturally resist hinge and tipping resilience. *(c and d)* As implant distribution becomes more linear and the angle between the attachments more obtuse, additional features to resist and counteract buccolingual tipping forces is considered. The overlay metal frameworks for both c and d incorporated rests on adjacent dentition.

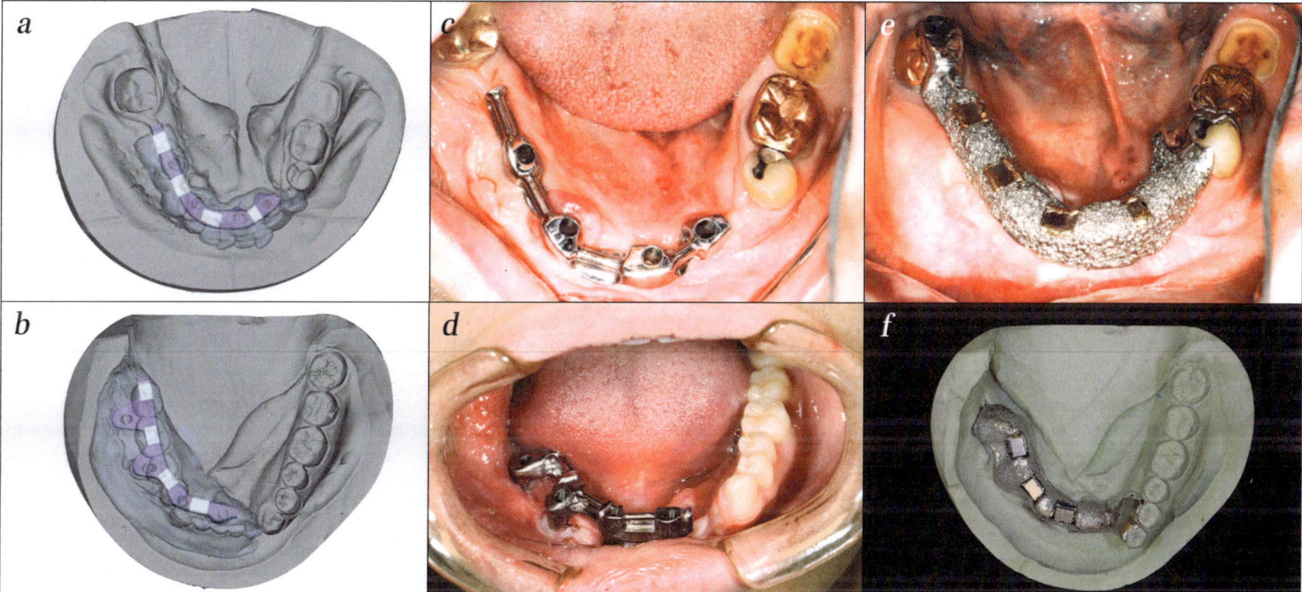

Figure 2-195 *(a and b)* Large mandibulectomy defects that cross the midline. Four implants arranged to provide support. *(c and d)* Milled implant connecting bars. *(e and f)* The overlay metal framework in both patients derives support from implants and dentition adjacent to the defect. The metal framework in the first example was printed with SLM (Zedan Dental Lab, Detroit, MI); the other was cast.

is also canceled just as is seen in a curved arch form. In situations when the bar becomes more linear, and the angle between the attachments is more obtuse (Fig 2-194c and d), one should consider incorporating additional features to resist and counteract buccolingual tipping forces.

When residual dentition is available on the contralateral side, the prosthesis can be designed to receive support from both the implant bar in the neomandible and abutment teeth. The two implant connecting bars shown in Fig 2-195 demonstrate the use of this concept. Both cases were restored with FFF and four implants. The overlay metal frameworks engage the residual dentition with positive rests and lingual plating, providing additional support and bracing (resistance to lateral displacement) for the overlay RPD. Note how an overlay rest was used to reestablish occlusal contact for a right molar in infraocclusion in Fig 2-195e.

A second design feature that will resist rotation is to prescribe a 3° taper to the buccal and lingual walls of the milled bar, for a total occlusal convergence (TOC) of 6° (Fig 2-196a). For bars that are taller than 4 mm, the TOC may be increased to 8° (Fig 2-196b). Just as important, the overlay framework must be made to engage the tapered walls of the bar (Fig 2-204).

If the bar is shorter than 4 mm, resistance and retention form can be enhanced by adding resistance grooves or boxes (Fig 2-197). The implant connecting bar shown in Fig 2-197 presents a linear arrangement of three implants. A combination of rest seats on the adjacent incisors and multiple resistance grooves were employed.

Implant-assisted bar designs for edentulous patients when implants are positioned in the lateral alveolar ridge

When implants are placed unilaterally, either on the unresected side or into the neomandible (Fig 2-198), implant-assisted designs are employed. The implants are used to enhance the retention and stability of the resection prosthesis but do not serve as the primary means of support. Provided that the soft tissues are optimized as

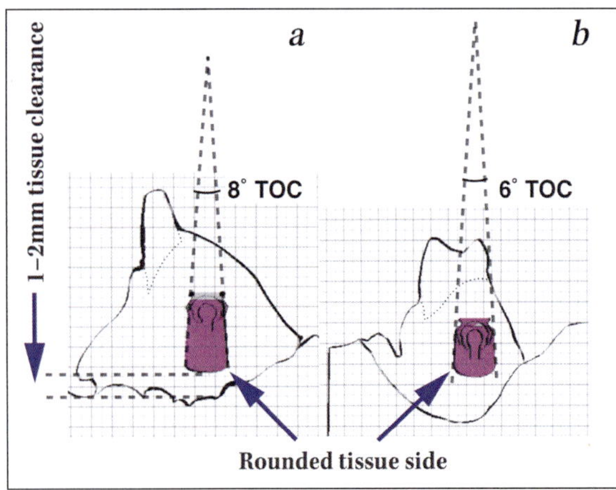

Figure 2-196 Cross-section evaluation of two bar designs. Taller bars *(a)* may require more total occlusal convergence (TOC) than shorter bars. *(b)* For cleanability, a rounded tissue side is designed as well as 1 to 2 mm of clearance.

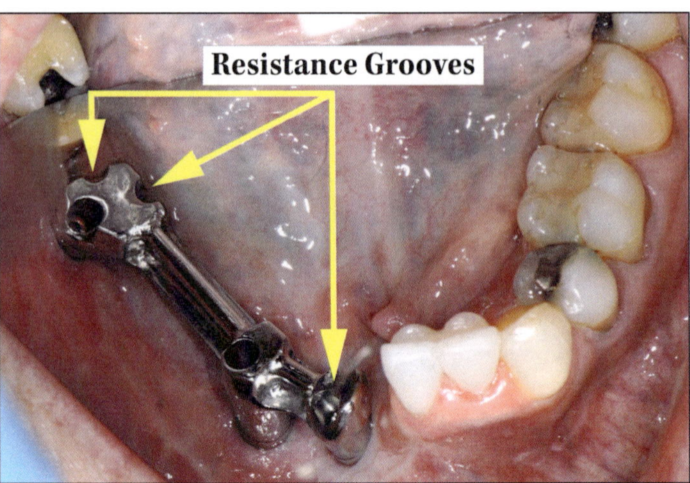

Figure 2-197 Resistance grooves added to resist buccolingual movement on a short and linear implant connecting bar.

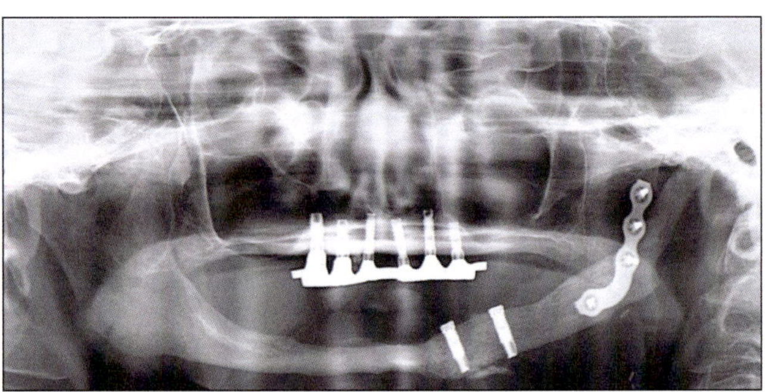

Figure 2-198 Left segmental mandibulectomy reconstructed with a FFF. Note that an inadequate bone in the native mandible meant that implants were only placed in the neomandible.

previously discussed, all denture-bearing tissues should be engaged to supplement retention, stability, and support. Based on the studies conducted by Davis and colleagues (Davis et al., 1995), and our own clinical experience, we recommend the implant-assisted bar design shown in Fig 2-199. With these designs, when occlusal forces are applied on the extension bases, support is shared between the implants and the residual denture-bearing surfaces.

The RPI clasp assembly permits rotation around an axis, allowing the edentulous ridges to provide support. Similarly, the design of the implant connecting bar–attachment apparatus should allow rotation of the prosthesis around a fulcrum. The implant connecting bars, along with their attachments, should be designed to minimize bending moments and direct these posterior occlusal forces along the long axis of the implants. When designing the bar, the axis of rotation (resulting from the generation of posterior occlusal forces on the unresected side) should be anticipated and the bar, rests, and attachments be positioned and designed to permit rotation of the prosthesis around this axis (Fig 2-199).

Forces generated during the incision of the bolus are one-quarter to one-fifth of those generated posteriorly during mastication and are less of a concern. For large defects extending across the midline, lateral bending moments applied to the implants secondary to lateral displacement of a large prosthesis, for example, during lateral movements of the mandible or contracture of the muscles of facial expression also need to be taken into account by extending the prosthesis into those areas, which resist these forces. The clinician should not forget that with these implant configurations, cross-arch stabilization is lacking, and so resistance to these lateral forces should be enhanced by an appropriate extension of the denture flanges and adaptation to the denture-bearing surfaces in the defect and the unresected side (see above, section entitled "Definitive MRPs for the edentulous patient").

Numerous factors complicate the design of the bar and affect the distribution of occlusal forces. Occlusal loads produce multiple axes of rotation of the resection prosthesis. These axes are dependent on the position of the implants and the point of load application (position of the bolus) on the prosthesis during mastication. When implants are only present unilaterally, the two key factors in the design that has evolved at UCLA are the placement of rest seats on the occlusal surface of the bar and the use of attachments on either end of the bar that provides both vertical and pivoting resilience (Fig 2-199) (Davis et al., 1995).

The most suitable choice is the extracoronal resilient attachment, or ERA (Davis et al., 1995). The ERA's 0.40 mm of vertical resiliency is indicated for distal extension RPDs to allow the extension base to depress and transmit the occlusal forces to the denture-bearing tissues. Unlike other bar attachments that are tapped onto the occlusal surface, the ERA is cast or milled on the same plane of the bar, which does not impinge on prosthetic space.

The Hader attachment is also positioned on the same plane of the bar and can be added between the occlusal rests as a means to provide stability as well as hinge resiliency when cross-arch loads

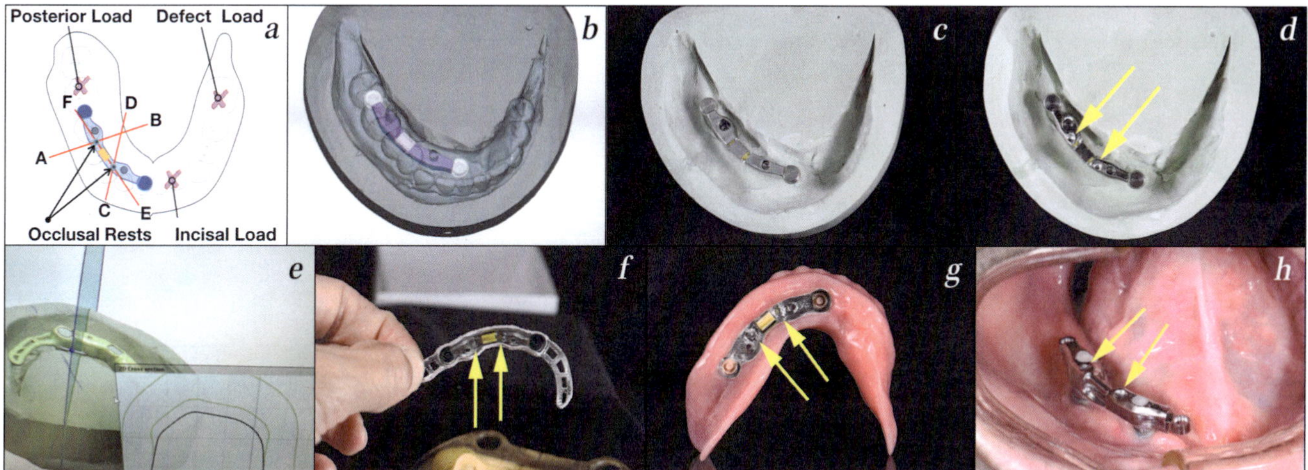

Figure 2-199 Function of resilient attachments. *(a)* Schematic of vertical compression of the prosthesis and the dynamic nature of a fulcrum. When a posterior load is applied, the prosthesis will rotate around fulcrum AB, which passes through the distal occlusal rest. When an incisal load is applied, the prosthesis will rotate around fulcrum CD, which passes through the anterior occlusal rest. When defect load is applied, the prosthesis will rotate around fulcrum FE, which passes through both occlusal rests. *(b and c)* CAD and milled implant connecting bar: extracoronal resilient attachments (ERA) are designed for each side of the bar. One Hader is designed between the abutments. *(d and h)* Postmilling modifications: rest seats *(arrows)* are created on the occlusal surface of the bar; additionally, occlusal line angles are rounded. *(e, f, and g)* CAD, SLM overlay framework, and completed prosthesis. Note the designed occlusal relief between the bar and framework. *(g)* Rests on the metal framework control the axis of rotation and allow the ERA attachments to function as designed. *(h)* Clinical photo of the seated implant connecting bar.

are applied (Fig 2-199a). It also provides a necessary third point of orientation when using the overlay framework as a tray for a corrected impression (see Fig 2-205).

Properly positioned and contoured rest seats serve to direct occlusal forces along the long axis of the implants, while the use of the ERA permits the extension bases to depress as they rotate around an axis determined by the position of the rests. The principle is similar to the biomechanics of the RPI concept of the removable partial denture design developed by Kratochvil (Kratochvil, 1963; Chang et al., 2019). However, it is important to note that when using this design concept for extension-based RPDs, the RPD framework must be "physiologically adjusted" to ensure that the RPD rotates around the rest as intended during function. Likewise, the overlay framework, like the RPD framework, must be similarly adjusted to allow the prosthesis to rotate around the rests when occlusal forces are applied. Furthermore, because the framework overlays the entire bar, digital or analog relieve blockout is needed over the occlusal aspect of the bar except for the rest seats (Fig 2-199e). As shown in Fig 2-199a, when posterior load is applied, the prosthesis will rotate around fulcrum AB, which passes through the distal occlusal rest. In this situation, most of the occlusal load is absorbed by the residual denture-bearing surfaces posteriorly when an occlusal force is applied in the posterior edentulous extension area, and these forces are directed more favorably along the long axis of the implants. The concave rest, contoured as a half sphere, is prepared onto the occlusal surface of the bar. Without the rests, the attachments on either side of the bar would serve as rotation points, leading to rapid wear of the attachments and exposing the implants to significant bending moments. This design allows the prosthesis to rotate around these rests, reduces wear on the attachments, and directs most of the occlusal forces along the long axes of the implants.

The patient should be advised against applying occlusal forces on the defect side (Fig 2-199a) if an excessively thick myocutaneous flap overlays the reconstructed mandible; the easily displaceable flap is unable to counteract these forces. Excessive occlusal loads in such situations will result in rapid wear of the attachments. Since the ERA only allows 0.40 mm of vertical movement before bottoming out, the resulting bending moments to the implants may trigger the resorption remodeling of the bone anchoring the implants. With these designs, the ERA attachments need to be replaced every six months.

Implant-assisted bar designs for edentulous patients when implants are positioned in the symphysis

If the mandibular symphysis remains, the number of implants, their distribution, and the design of the retention bar follow more conventional prosthodontic guidelines (Beumer et al., 2022b). Two to four implants are placed to retain and stabilize the resection prosthesis. When the AP spread is limited (Fig 2-200), an implant-assisted design is required with support provided posteriorly by the residual denture-bearing surfaces and reconstructed mandible—if the soft tissues have been optimized—and anteriorly by the dental implants.

Two Hader clips across the midline is ideal, which require 14 mm from center-to-center of two implants if the bar is cast, or 16 mm if the bar is milled; due milling tool path limitations.

The Hader bar hinge resilience serves as the axis of rotation. The ERA connected to the distal portion of the bar allows for the compression of the distal-extension area of the prosthesis into the denture-bearing surfaces without applying excess bending moments to the implants. For this design to function as planned, the paths of insertion of the Hader bar segment and the two ERA attachments should be identical and compatible with the path of insertion of the prosthesis. In addition, the Hader bar segment should be parallel to the

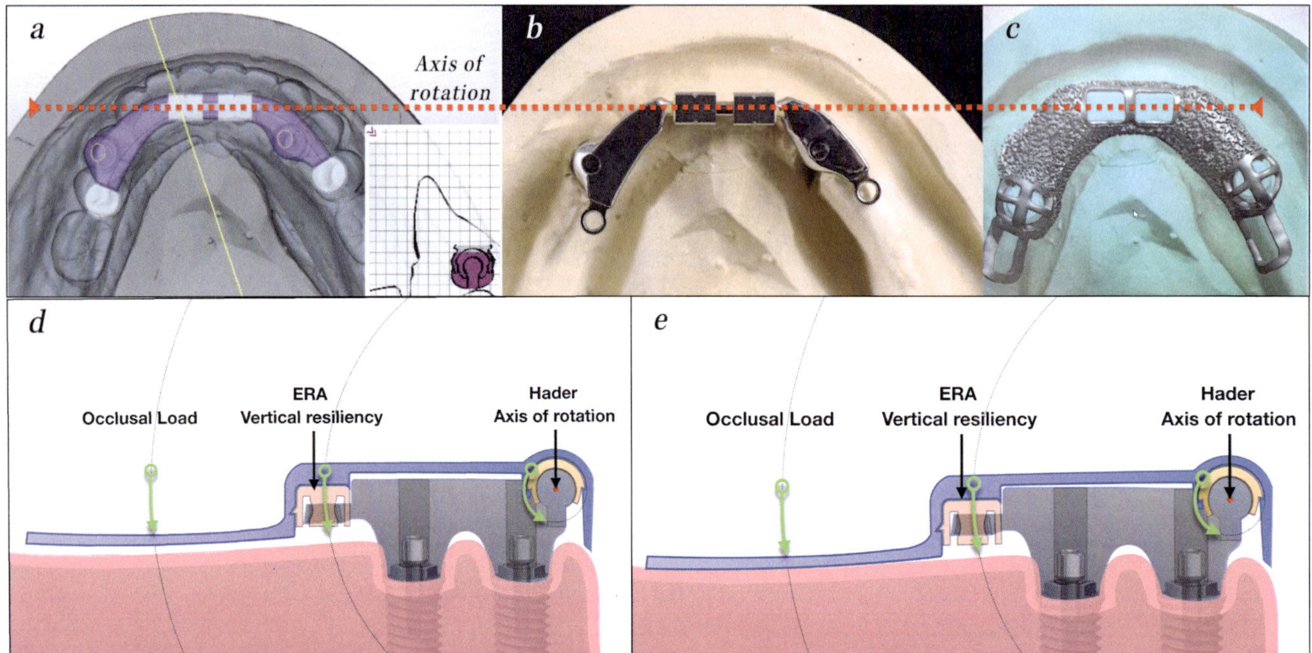

Figure 2-200 When the symphysis of the mandible remains, two to four implants are placed, and a conventional implant-assisted implant connecting bar design using a combination of a Hader bar and ERA attachments is suggested. *(a)* CAD of the bar. *(a, b, and c)* Note that ERA attachments are cantilevered posteriorly, and a Hader segment crosses the midline. *(b)* Milled CoCr bar. *(c)* CAD of the overlay framework. *(d and e)* Cross-sectional schematic of the biomechanics: the circular cross section of the Hader bar allows hinging resiliency (curved arrows) and acts as the axis of rotation. When a posterior occlusal load is applied to the prosthesis, the vertical resiliency of the ERA permits the extension bases to depress and engage the posterior denture support areas, thereby minimizing the bending moments applied to the implants.

plane of occlusion and perpendicular to the midline. This will ensure a relatively pure rotation around the Hader bar when occlusal forces are applied in the posterior region and will minimize the wear of the clips. When prosthetic space over the bar is limited, it is advisable to overlay the bar with a metal framework (Fig 2-200c) to prevent the acrylic resin overlying the bar from crazing and fracturing (Beumer et al., 2022a). With this design, attachments need to be replaced every 6 to 12 months depending on the resilience of the posterior denture-bearing surfaces.

When using an attachment that allows hinging or vertical resiliency, it is important to design relief between the overlay framework and the occlusal surface of the bar. This can be accomplished when fabricating this framework with CAD/CAM (Fig 2-199e) or by traditional blockout techniques when conventional means are employed. In the example shown (Fig 2-200), a fulcrum line is created by the two Hader clips. The incorporated gap over the occlusal surface of the bar allows the prosthesis to hinge on the Hader attachments and depress posteriorly into the ERAs. Because the ERAs provide 0.40 mm of vertical resiliency, the relief space over the implant bar can be digitally designed for the same height.

Suggested designs and materials for implant connecting bars and their overlay frameworks

Implant connecting bars can be designed and fabricated either with conventional techniques or by digital means, but the latter has become the preferred method. A trial denture is scanned and the data aligned with that of the scanned master cast. The design should conform to the principles described previously. Implant-supported implant connecting bars are best milled to a 3° taper. The attachment selected is determined by the nature of the prosthetic space. The authors favor Hader- or Locator-type attachments for implant-supported bars, since they have no or little vertical resiliency, respectively. There are four considerations when choosing between the two: method of fabrication, prosthetic space, wear, and cost. When cast conventionally, a Hader or Locator plastic pattern is waxed up and burnt out. If CAD/CAM technology is used, the Hader is milled of the same metal as the bar, either titanium alloy or cobalt-chrome, and so there is no additional cost to fabrication when a Hader is used. By contrast, the Locator is screwed into position after abutment threads are tapped onto the occlusal surface of the bar. As an added component to the bar, Locator attachments incur an additional cost per abutment. In an implant-supported design, wear is not a real concern, but if the Locator were to wear, it could be unscrewed from the bar and replaced without having to change the entire bar. Last, Figure 2-201 compares the difference in prosthetic space needed for each. The Hader insert and corresponding metal housing stands 0.67 mm proud of the occlusal surface of the bar (Fig 2-201c) compared to 2.22 mm when a Locator is used (Fig 2-201d). As discussed above, a combination of ERA and Hader attachments are used for implant-assisted implant connecting bars. Because the ERA is designed off the ends of the bar, the insert and housing lie flush with the occlusal surface of the bar (Fig 2-201e).

Bars must be rigid and allow for appropriate hygiene access between the implants and beneath the bar. As mentioned previously, the undersurface of the bar segment should be rounded and highly polished and the bar and ERA attachments positioned at least 1 to 2 mm above the tissues for hygiene access. The path of insertion of the resection prosthesis as it engages the implant connecting bar

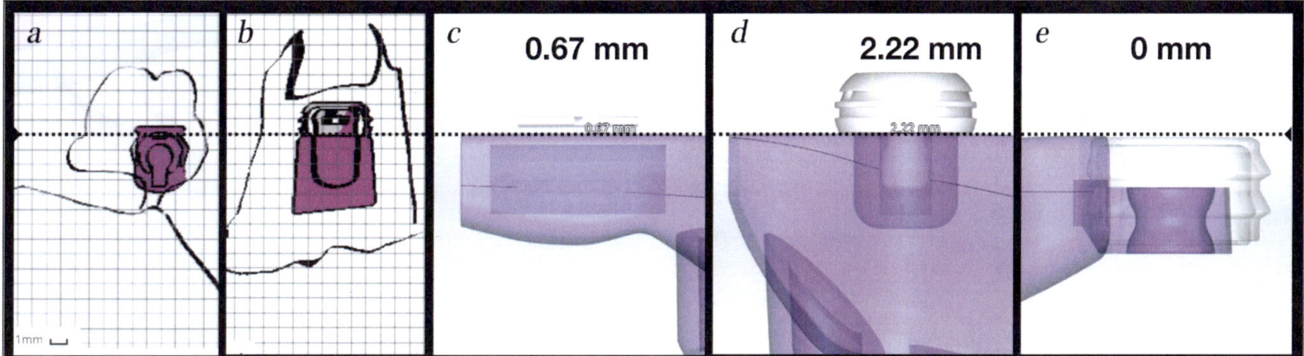

Figure 2-201 Side-by-side cross section and 3D renderings of three bar attachment options. *(a and b)* Cross section of Hader and Locator, respectively. *(c–e)* Side-by-side 3D rendering of Hader, Locator, and ERA, respectively. Note that when used as a bar attachment, the Hader insert and housing stand 0.67 mm proud of the occlusal surface of the bar, the Locator is 2.22 mm, and the ERA is designed flush. *(a and c)* For milling purposes, the Hader segment is positioned just below the occlusal surface of the bar.

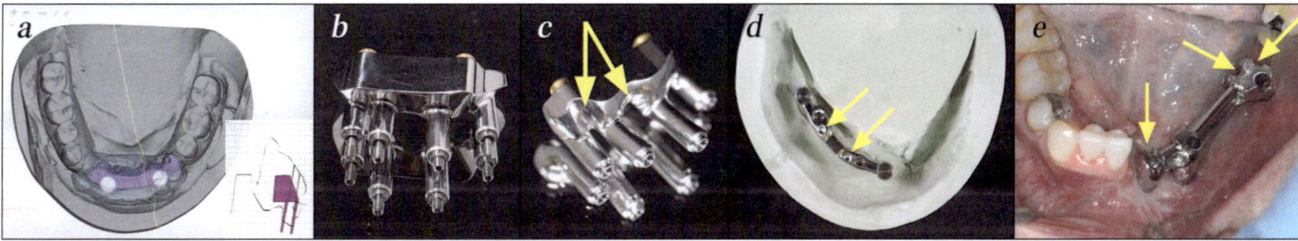

Figure 2-202 Because of the limitations of the CAD software, digitally designed implant connecting bars often require postmilling modifications. *(a)* Cross-section evaluation of CAD. Notice the square soft tissue side of the bar. *(b)* Milled bar. Note that the contours are not conducive to hygiene access. *(c)* Note that the bar has been altered to enhance hygiene access between the implants *(arrows)*. *(d)* Addition of rest seats *(arrows)* are added postmilling. *(e)* Resistance grooves *(arrows)* have been milled with a tapered bur into this milled implant-supported bar.

and the attachments should be along the same plane. The bar must be positioned and contoured so that there is ample room to house and retain denture teeth with a sufficient volume of acrylic resin to retain them.

When designed digitally, it may not be possible, because of the limitations of the software and/or the milling/printing apparatus, to incorporate all the necessary design features into the implant connecting bar (Fig 2-202). After milling/printing, the edges of the tissue surface of the bar may need to be rounded, or portions of the bar engaging the implants must be slightly recontoured to facilitate the removal of plaque and debris from the bar and between the implants (Fig 2-202c). Rests or resistance grooves may need to be milled into the bar after printing/milling (Fig 2-202d and e).

Implant-assisted bars should be milled or printed from a wear-resistant metal. Titanium alloy should not be used for such bars because the constant movement and rotation of the overdenture resection prosthesis during function will result in rapid wear of the bar, rendering the MRP nonretentive. Cobalt-chromium is the material of choice for implant-assisted implant connecting bars.

As mentioned previously, implant-supported connecting bars are usually milled with titanium alloy. There is little risk of wear of such bars because the prosthesis does not move or rotate during occlusal function. All bars must be confirmed intraorally. If the precision of fit is unsatisfactory, they can be sectioned and laser welded.

CAD software is used to design an overlay framework that engages the implant connecting bar in a specific manner. For an implant-supported design, where no movement or rotation is desired, an intimate fit between the vertical and occlusal surfaces of the bar is designed accordingly (Fig 2-204c).

If, however, the bar is implant assisted, the overlay framework should be designed to allow pivoting and rotational movement. As such, the bar should be rounded and the relief blockout specifically designed over the occlusal surface of the bar (Fig 2-203b), allowing only the occlusal rest to be in contact (Fig 2-203c). Once manufactured, the overlay framework must be "physiologically adjusted" clinically to enable the prosthesis to rotate around the implant connecting bar as intended. When designing the extension base latticework over redundant and displaceable tissues in the defect, extra relief blockout is prescribed (Fig 2-203d). The extra relief helps account for the anticipated soft tissue displacement during the initial impression.

If the metal attachment housings are to be laser welded, widows in the overlay framework are virtually opened to the occlusal edges of the metal housings (Fig 2-203a). Alternatively, a lattice or receptacle (Fig 2-204a) is designed, overlaying the metal housings to allow pickup with acrylic resin (Fig 2-204d).

Lastly, either ivory (Fig 2-203f) or pink opaque (Fig 2-204) coating is recommended to decrease the graying of the overlaying denture tooth or pink acrylic resin, respectively.

Remaining prosthodontic procedures

Implant-assisted designs that require precisely recorded denture-bearing tissues may require a new border-molded impression.

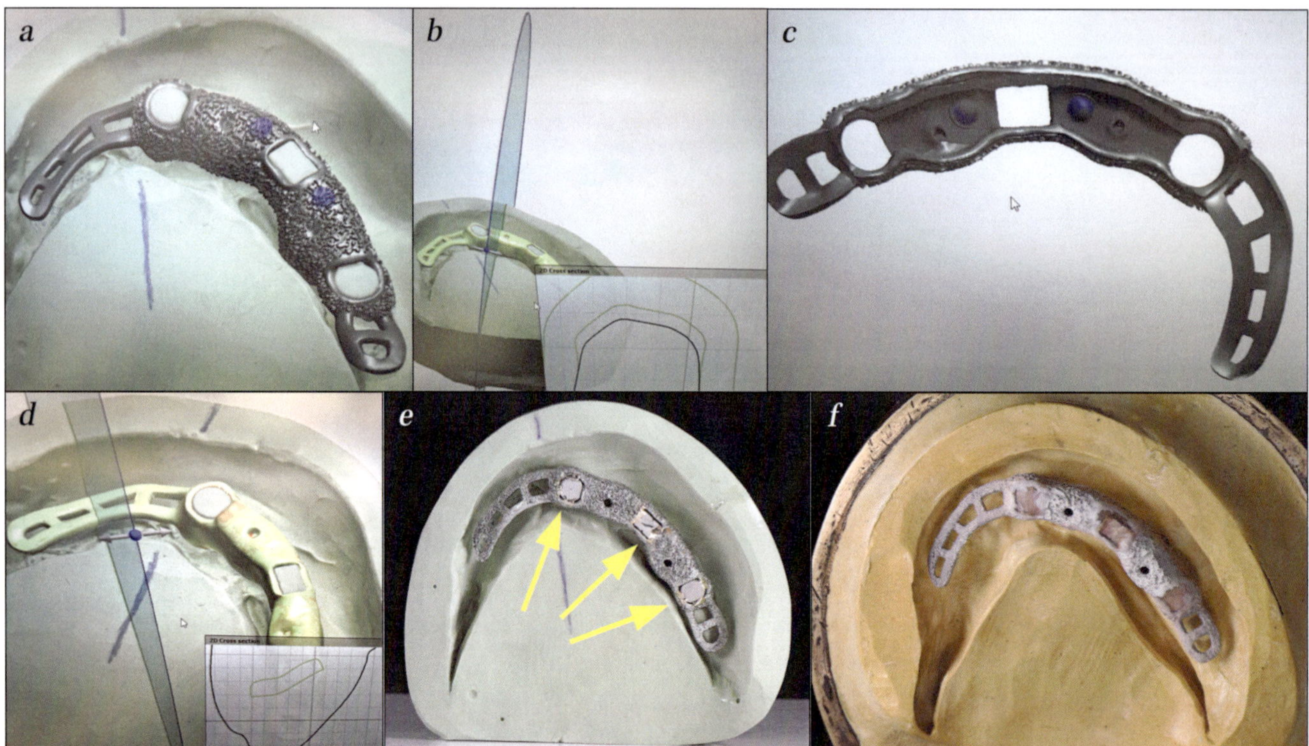

Figure 2-203 This implant-assisted overlay framework has been designed and fabricated with CAD/CAM. *(a)* The overlay framework is designed to engage the bar and the metal housing of the attachments. *(b)* Cross-section evaluation of an implant bar overlay framework. Note the relief space over the occlusal surface of the implant bar. *(c)* Intaglio surface of the overlay framework. Note the two occlusal rests. *(d)* Extension latticework is designed with extra relief to account for highly displaceable tissues. *(e)* SLM of CoCr was used for manufacturing this framework, after which the metal housings were laser welded to position *(arrows)*. *(f)* A tooth-colored opaque coating was added.

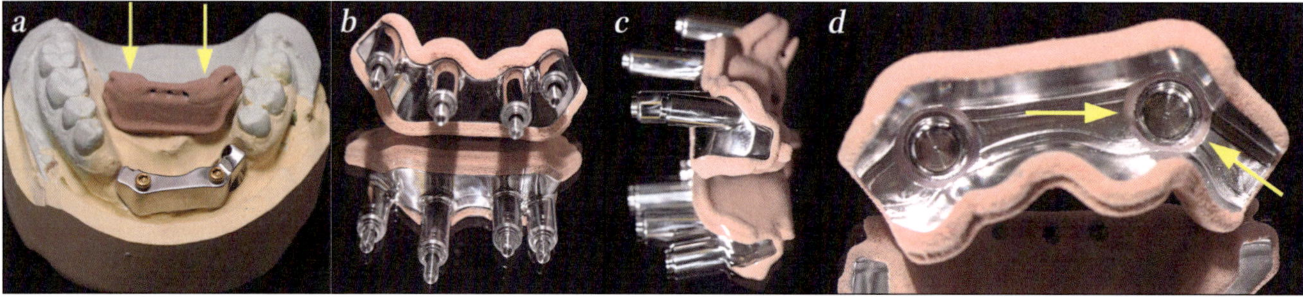

Figure 2-204 *(a–c)* This implant-supported overlay framework has been designed and fabricated with CAD/CAM. The manufacturing was accomplished with CNC milling of titanium. The attachment housings have been picked up with acrylic resin. A pink opaque coating was added. *(b and c)* Notice the intimate fit of the overlay to the milled bar.

Impression trays are added to the overlay framework to allow them to be retained by the implant connecting bar. At the onset, an interocclusal registration is made (Fig 2-205e) to keep the tray completely seated during the refinement of the impression with the thermoplastic material. Note that the tray handle, if present, must not prematurely contact the opposing dentition in centric at the established OVD. These design features will also allow the patient to be able to speak and swallow in a relatively normal manner while performing a closed-mouth impression technique.

Once the bar is verified, a border-molded impression is made to engage all residual edentulous extensions and denture-bearing surfaces as well as those of the defect (Fig 2-205). This is especially important when the implant connecting bar/attachment apparatus is designed to be implant assisted.

A new record base with the metal framework incorporated is fabricated in order to perform the final try-in. During this appointment, the esthetic, phonetics, OVD, and CR records should be verified.

It is also possible to defer capturing the peripheral extensions during the trial appointment. This option is best used for refining a denture flange of an implant-supported prosthesis and not capturing an extension base. Once the tooth arrangement is finalized, a low-fusing thermoplastic material is added to the periphery and functionally trimmed (Fig 2-206). The impression is boxed, and a

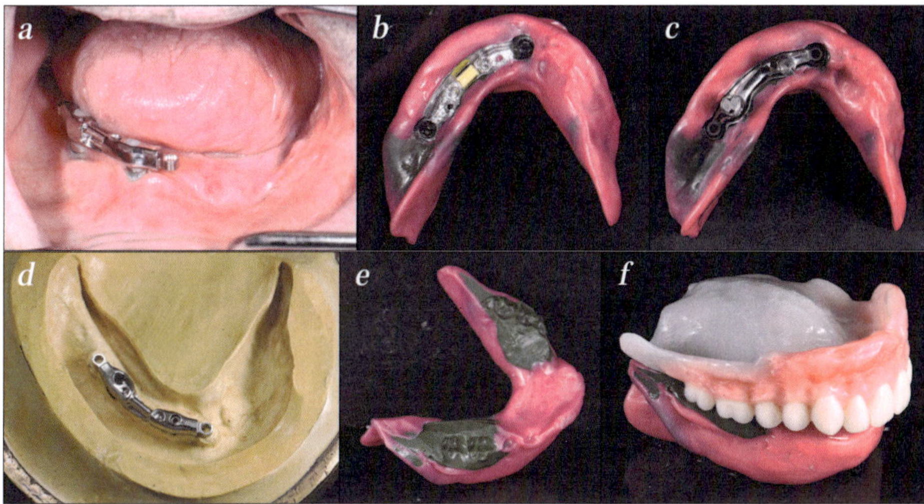

Figure 2-205 *(a)* Milled CoCr bar with ERA and Hader attachments. *(b)* Border-molded impressions using the overlay framework as a custom tray with attachment inserts to secure the tray in position. Note the extension on the defect side. *(c)* Bar and analogs transferred to the impression for making the *(d)* master cast. *(e)* Note that occlusal stops have been incorporated at the desired OVD to help stabilize the tray while correcting the impression with impression compound. *(f)* The corrected impression is ready for mounting with the maxillary trial denture.

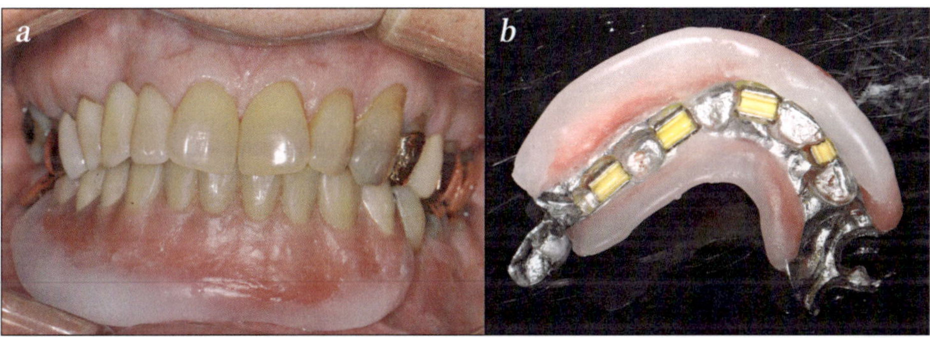

Figure 2-206 *(a and b)* Secondary impression of peripheral tissues captured at the trial appointment. Note that impression wax was used. *(b)* The border-molded trial denture is boxed, and a new master cast is made.

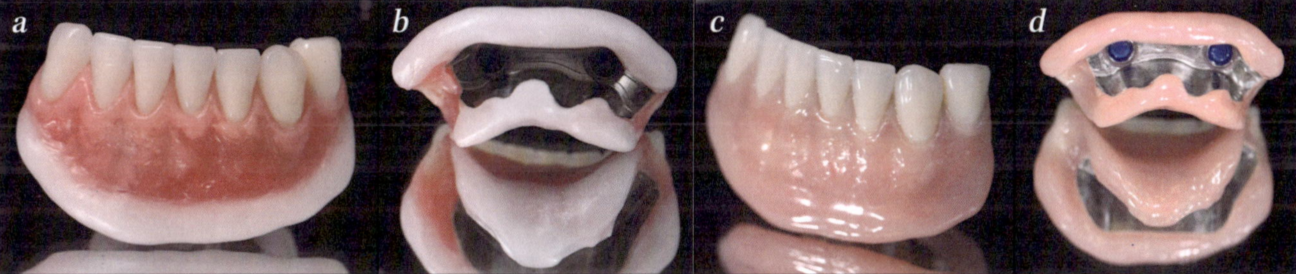

Figure 2-207 *(a and b)* Secondary impression of the peripheral tissues captured at the tooth trial appointment. Note that impression wax was used. *(c and d)* The border-molded trial denture is invested and processed.

new master cast is made. If occlusion and wax festooning have been perfected, then the border-molded trial prosthesis is invested and prepared for processing (Fig 2-207).

The occlusion should be designed either balanced articulation when an implant-assisted bar is employed or group function when an implant-supported bar is used to retain the prosthesis. A comprehensive discussion of occlusal design concepts used for implant-retained overdentures is found in Wu et al. (2022b).

The prosthesis is processed (Fig 2-208) and delivered in the usual fashion using PIP and disclosing wax to refine extensions and tissue adaptation (Fig 2-209). A clinical remount record is performed if indicated, the occlusion refined as needed, and the prosthesis delivered (Fig 2-217).

It is critically important that the patient keep the implant/abutment surfaces emerging through the peri-implant tissues free of plaque and debris as well as the undersurfaces of an implant connecting bar. Otherwise, inflammatory fibrous hyperplasia of the peri-implant tissues, peri-implantitis, and hyperplasia of the mucosal tissues underneath the bar will be the inevitable result. Implant patients should be followed up with every three months for the first year. This period may be extended depending on the hygiene compliance of the patient. Attachments are replaced as needed and primarily depend on the movement of the prosthesis during function. Attachments associated with an implant-supported implant connecting bar need to be replaced only every two to three years, but those associated with implant-assisted implant connecting bars require replacement every three to six months.

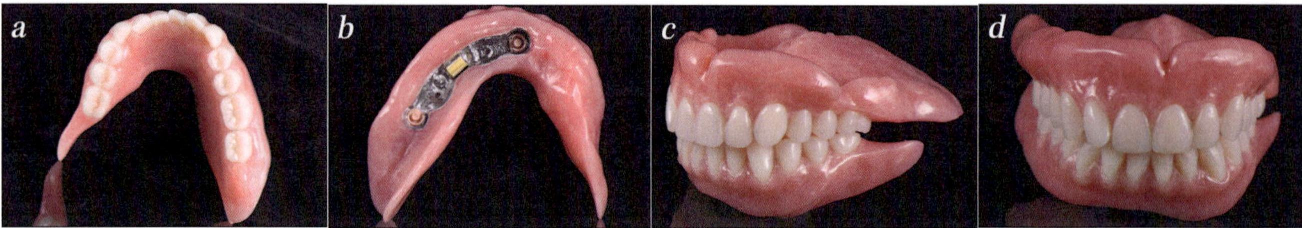

Figure 2-208 *(a)* An MRP restoring defect seen in Figure 2-205. Completed implant-assisted overlay prosthesis retained by two implants in the residual mandible. *(b)* Intaglio side of the prosthesis. *(c and d)* Lateral and anterior views of the MRP and opposing complete denture. Note the altered contours of the maxillary denture flange.

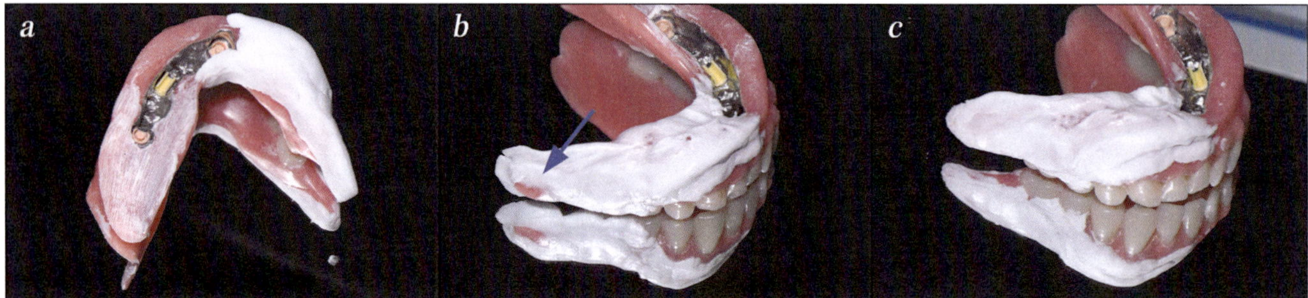

Figure 2-209 Disclosing pressure area. *(a)* PIP is applied to the intaglio corresponding to the residual denture-bearing area. Disclosing wax is preferred for the periphery and highly mobile tissues found within the defect. *(b)* Note the burn-through area *(arrow)* indicating excessive pressure. *(c)* After adjustment.

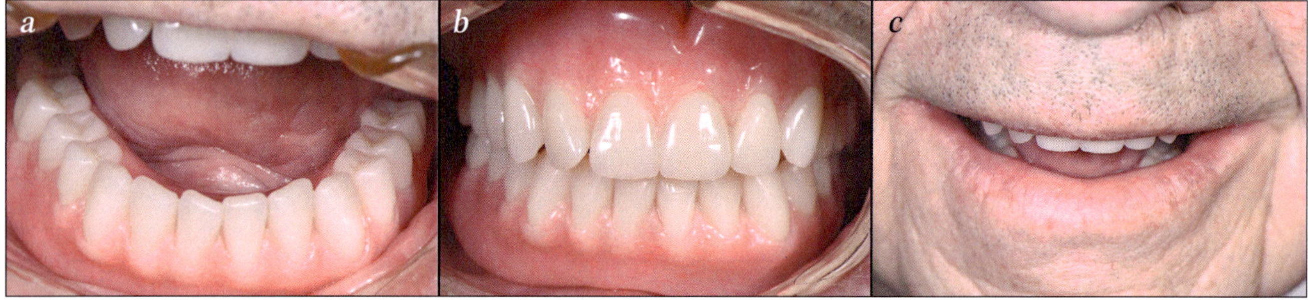

Figure 2-210 *(a and b)* The definitive MRP in position. *(c)* The contours of the lips are reasonably restored.

Definitive MPRs for glossectomy patients

Because the posture of the tongue and the lower lip may have been altered during the resection and reconstruction, careful placement of the mandibular anterior teeth and careful development of flange contour in this area are required. If the mobility of the tongue is compromised, particularly the ability to elevate above the level of the projected plane of occlusion, the OVD should be reduced and the occlusal plane lowered.

The placement of implants improves the prosthetic prognosis dramatically for most of these patients. With a well-retained and stable denture, the patient is able to direct attention toward manipulating the food bolus. If the opposing maxilla is edentulous and compromised by resorption, or if the clinician is unable to obtain peripheral seal because of postradiation xerostomia, placement of implants in the maxillary anterior teeth region should be considered, as referred to earlier. Usually, two maxillary implants are sufficient for retention. In the mandible, the number of implants required depends primarily on the status of the opposing maxilla. If the maxilla is edentulous, two mandibular implants are sufficient. If the opposing arch is dentate, four or more mandibular implants are recommended.

The patient shown in Fig 2-211 exemplifies the expected outcome in most patients presenting with a partial glossectomy defect restored with a free flap where mandibular continuity has been retained. Half of the oral tongue was removed in continuity with a selective neck dissection, and the tongue bulk was restored with a RFFF. Following mandibulotomy, the mandible was reopposed with a reconstruction plate.

Postsurgical examination revealed that the bulk of the tongue was restored, and its mobility was good. Sensory and motor innervation of the tongue however, had been lost on the resected side. The mandibular denture-bearing surface was largely unaffected by the surgery. The reconstructed tongue demonstrated good mobility, but its elevation was compromised.

Sufficient bone was available for the placement of two implants in the anterior portion of both the maxilla and mandible. After a

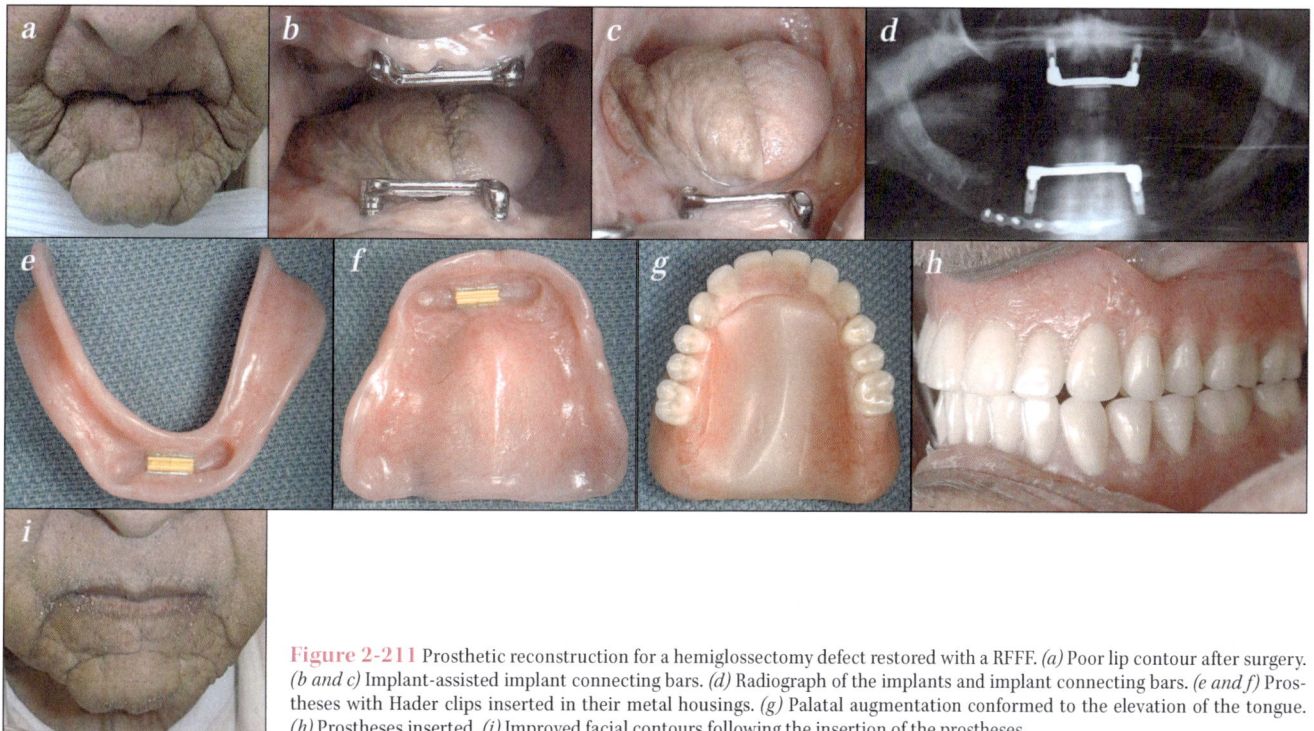

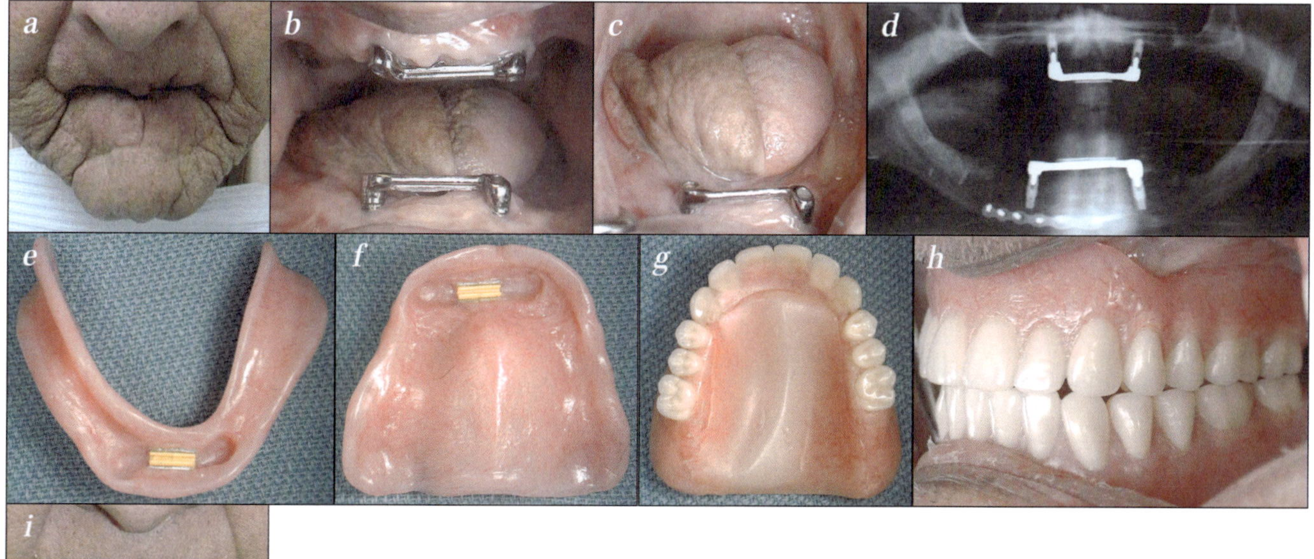

Figure 2-211 Prosthetic reconstruction for a hemiglossectomy defect restored with a RFFF. *(a)* Poor lip contour after surgery. *(b and c)* Implant-assisted implant connecting bars. *(d)* Radiograph of the implants and implant connecting bars. *(e and f)* Prostheses with Hader clips inserted in their metal housings. *(g)* Palatal augmentation conformed to the elevation of the tongue. *(h)* Prostheses inserted. *(i)* Improved facial contours following the insertion of the prostheses.

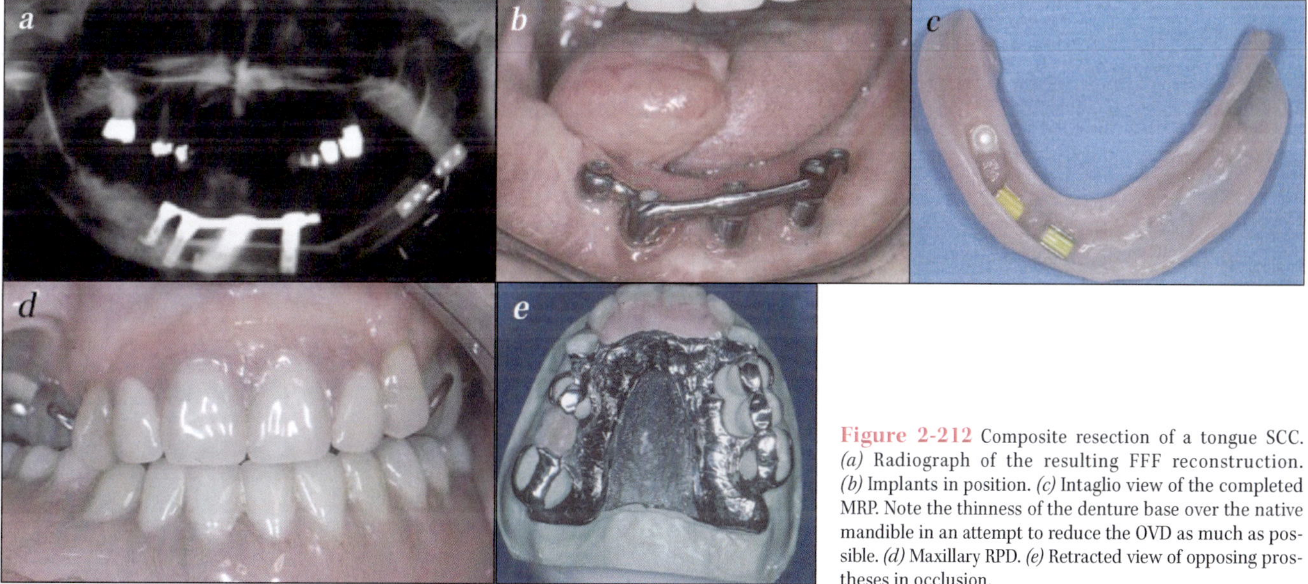

Figure 2-212 Composite resection of a tongue SCC. *(a)* Radiograph of the resulting FFF reconstruction. *(b)* Implants in position. *(c)* Intaglio view of the completed MRP. Note the thinness of the denture base over the native mandible in an attempt to reduce the OVD as much as possible. *(d)* Maxillary RPD. *(e)* Retracted view of opposing prostheses in occlusion.

suitable period was allowed for the implants to osseointegrate, the prosthodontic procedures were initiated. Implant-assisted connecting bars were fabricated using Hader attachments for retention. On fabrication of the overlay dentures, the OVD was reduced, and the plane of occlusion was lowered as much as feasible. The palatal contours were altered to create a PAP and idealize the interaction between the reconstructed tongue and the maxillary denture.

The patient shown in Fig 2-212 is typical of the outcome in most patients presenting with a partial glossectomy defect restored with a free flap where mandibular continuity has been reconstructed. Following a composite resection and selective neck dissection in which half of the oral tongue was resected for an SCC, the tongue and mandible defect were reconstructed with a FFF. The hypoglossal and lingual nerves were sacrificed on the resected side.

Examination revealed a reasonable bulk and contour of the reconstructed tongue and good tongue mobility. The OVD was reduced sufficiently that a PAP was not needed on the maxillary RPD. Four implants were placed in the native and reconstructed mandible. An implant-assisted connecting bar and overlay MRP were fabricated. The maxilla was restored with a tooth-supported RPD.

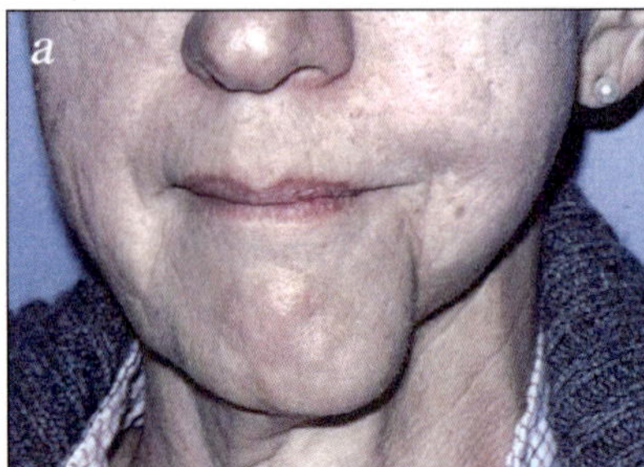

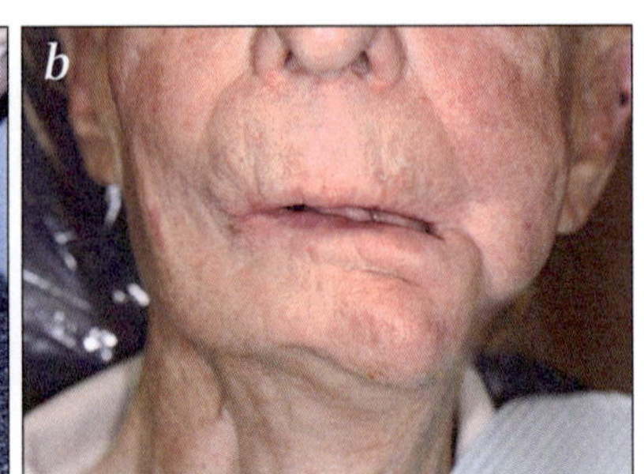

Figure 2-213 Discontinuity defects. *(a)* Composite resection defect. The intraoral wound was closed primarily. *(b)* Failed free flap reconstruction.

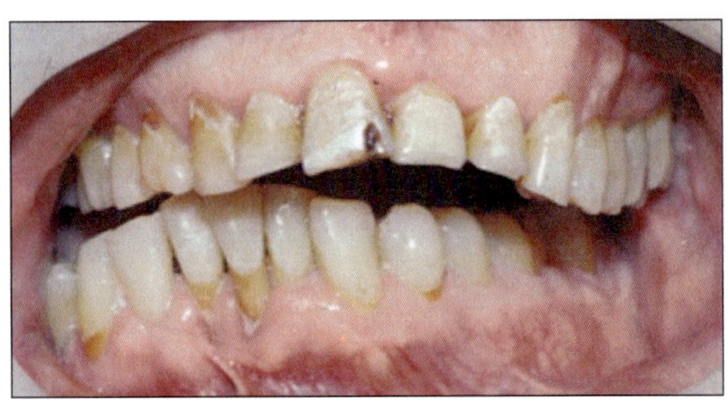

Figure 2-214 Severe deviation of the mandible secondary to the composite resection of the lateral FOM lesion, without primary reconstruction.

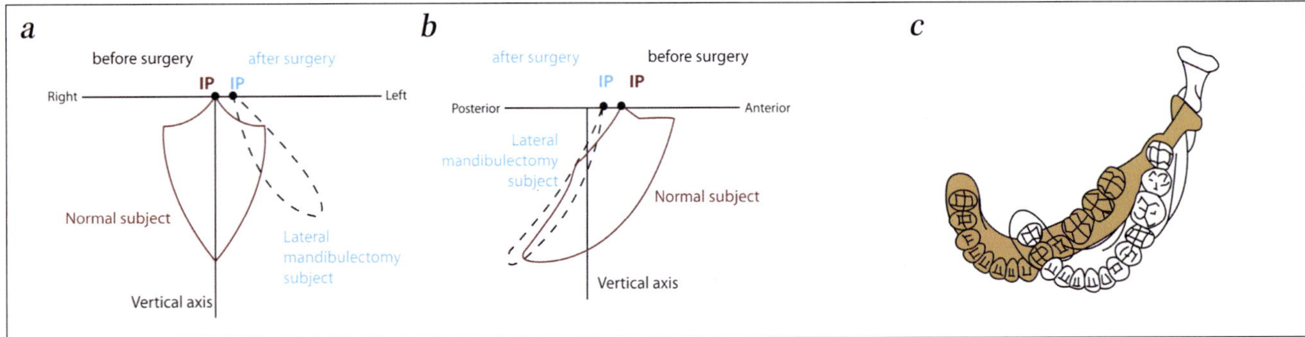

Figure 2-215 Envelope of motion as viewed in the *(a)* frontal and *(b)* sagittal planes in a normal patient (solid lines) and a patient who has undergone lateral mandibular resection (broken lines). IP interocclusal position. *(c)* Position of the remaining mandible in open (shaded) and closed (white) positions. Note the character of lateral movements toward the resected side. This lateral movement is somewhat reproducible.

Mandibular Discontinuity

With the widespread use of vascularized free flaps, few patients in the modern era will present with mandibular discontinuity defects. However, if mandibular continuity is not reconstructed, or if the osteomyocutaneous free flap fails, significant complications and disabilities will result. The extraoral presentation includes a concave facial defect created by the large hard and soft tissue deficiencies as a result of a composite mandible and tongue resection (Fig 2-213). The degree of facial disfigurement varies with the extent of surgery, the facial form exhibited by the patient, and the method of wound closure.

The intraoral presentation includes a retruded mandibular segment with a deviation toward the surgical side at the resting vertical dimension (Fig 2-214). The severity and permanence of mandibular deviation are highly variable and dependent on several factors, such as the amount of soft and hard tissue resected, the method of closure, scar contracture, muscle imbalances secondary to the primary resection, and so forth. Mandibular deviation is most severe following the primary closure, especially of the base of the tongue lesions. In these patients, an appropriate and stable maxillomandibular relationship cannot be achieved. Moreover, the deviation increases when these patients open, leading to an angular pathway of opening and closing. It is not uncommon to note a 1 to 2 cm deviation laterally and a 2 to 4 mm retrusion posterior to the chin point during maximum opening. When the incisal point of the mandible is traced, this oblique pathway of closure is obvious (Curtis et al., 1975). During mastication, the entire envelope of motion occurs on the surgical defect side (Curtis et al., 1975) (Fig 2-215), and some patients are unable to affect lateral movements toward the nondefect side and are incapable of making protrusive movements. Patients whose resections are closed with a myocutaneous flap demonstrate much less deviation and are more likely to attain an acceptable interocclusal relationship, regardless of whether mandibular continuity is restored.

In addition, the loss of a proprioceptive sense of occlusion leads to uncoordinated, imprecise movements of the mandible. The

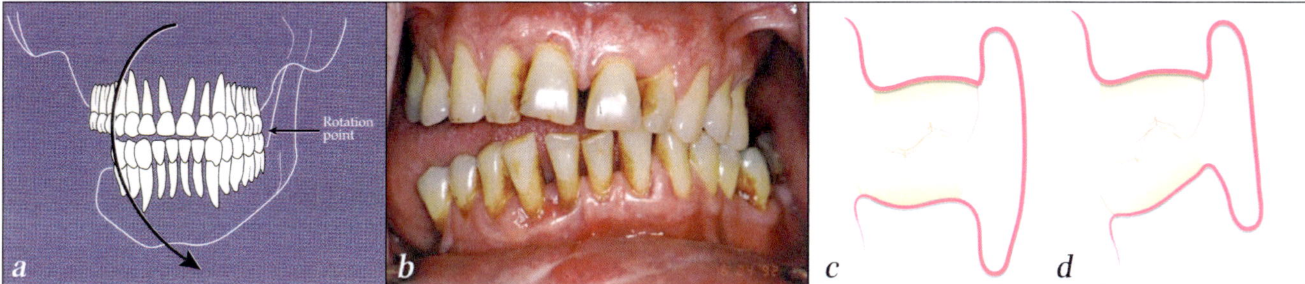

Figure 2-216 *(a and b)* Frontal plane rotation. As the force of the mandibular closure is increased, the mandible rotates around occlusal contacts on the unresected side, and the remaining teeth on the resected side drop farther out of occlusion. *(c)* Note the difference in occlusal relationship before (c) and after (d) mandibulectomy without reconstruction.

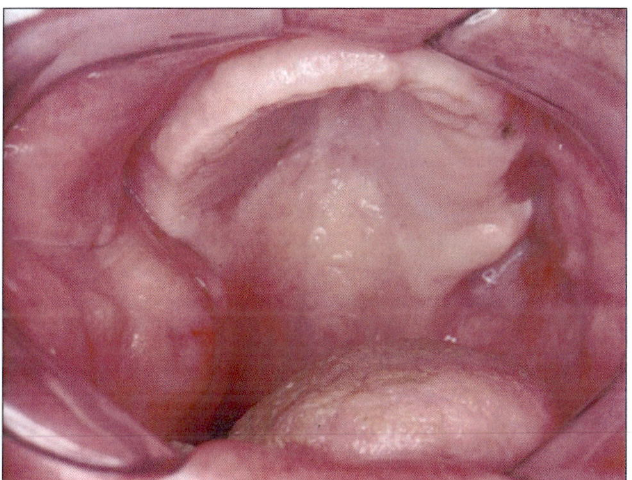

Figure 2-217 The condyle and ramus fragment have been retained but not maintained in position, with the result that the right buccal pouch area is obliterated.

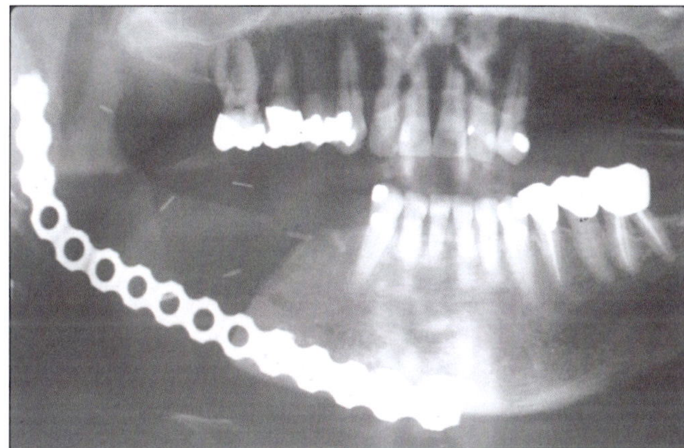

Figure 2-218 Lateral mandibular defect restored with a reconstruction plate.

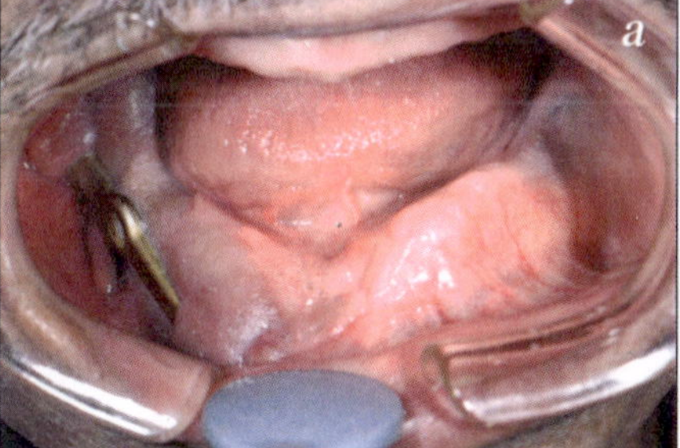

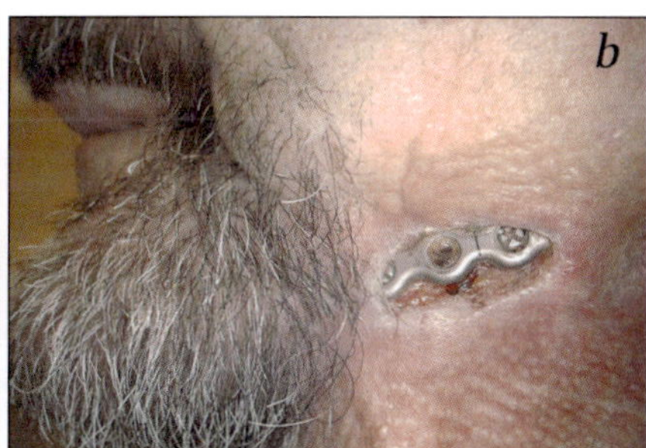

Figure 2-219 *(a)* Reconstruction plate exposed in the buccal vestibule. *(b)* Reconstruction plate exposed through the skin.

absence of the attachments of the muscles of mastication on the surgical side results in a significant rotation of the mandible on a forceful closure. When viewed from the frontal plane, the teeth on the surgical side of the mandible move away from the opposing maxillary teeth after initial contact on the nonsurgical side has been established. As the force of closure is increased, the remaining mandible rotates through the frontal plane, leading to the term *frontal plane rotation* (Fig 2-216). This factor, with the addition of impaired tongue function, may totally compromise mastication in some patients. Frontal plane rotation is observed in most patients with lateral mandibular discontinuity defects, regardless of whether the site has been closed primarily or with a myocutaneous pedicle flap or free flap. Nevertheless, patients whose resections are closed with a myocutaneous pedicle flap or free flap are more likely to achieve a usable occlusal relationship. However, the mandibular teeth will likely occlude distal to the presurgical pattern of cuspal interdigitation. On the nonsurgical side, the buccal slopes of the mandibular buccal cusps function with the central fossae of the maxillary teeth due to the mandibular frontal plane rotation (see Fig 2-216c).

If, for some reason, mandibular reconstruction is not anticipated or cannot be achieved at the time of tumor ablation, surgical alterations may improve the prospects of rehabilitating the patient prosthetically. In edentulous patients, the condyle and remaining portion of the ascending ramus should be removed. If a condylar-coronoid fragment remains, it is often retracted medially and anteriorly and approximates the maxillary tuberosity. This prevents the proper extension of the maxillary complete denture into the buccal vestibule and will compromise the retention and stability of the maxillary prosthesis (Fig 2-217).

If mandibular reconstruction is planned at a later date, it is vital to maintain the presurgical position of each mandibular fragment with a reconstruction plate (Fig 2-218), and the plate must be covered by a myocutaneous flap. These reconstruction plates serve only as provisional means of fixation, because if left over an extended period of time, they can fracture, loosen, or become exposed (Fig 2-219). The risk for failure is related to the position in the arch, the length of the missing segment (greater than 5 cm; Arden et al., 1999), and postoperative radiation (Mariani et al., 2006).

Several methods can reduce deviation, including maxillomandibular fixation (MMF) and mandibular or palatally based guidance prostheses in conjunction with occlusal equilibration. For best results, these methods and restorations should be combined with a well-organized mandibular exercise regimen initiated immediately following surgery and prior to, during, and following radiation therapy. The method of choice depends on numerous factors.

Guidance prostheses

Mandibular guidance therapy begins when the acute postsurgical sequelae have subsided, usually by week three. Initially, the patient should be introduced to an exercise program. Following the maximum opening, the patient manipulates the mandible by grasping the chin and moving the mandible away from the surgical side. These movements tend to loosen scar contracture, reduce trismus, and improve maxillomandibular relationships. Exercise should be carefully demonstrated to the patient, and notes should be made periodically to describe the progress made by the patient.

The earlier mandibular guidance therapy is initiated, the more successful the result. If the patient has undergone an extensive resection that included a classic radical neck dissection and received radiation therapy, and a considerable period has elapsed since surgery, guidance procedures are much more difficult, and a compromised occlusal relationship may result. Unfortunately, those patients suffering the most severe deviations of the mandible because of extensive soft tissue loss, tight wound closure, radiation therapy, and classic radical neck dissection are most susceptible to the complications of fistula formation, flap necrosis, and other postsurgical morbidities that delay the beginning of mandibular guidance therapy. Consequently, some of these patients may never achieve normal maxillomandibular relationships (Fig 2-220).

In the absence of primary wound complications, placement of a resection guidance prosthesis can be considered. There are several approaches that can be utilized to guide the mandible to an improved interocclusal relationship. Unfortunately, if no teeth are present, guidance will not be effective. The excessive lateral forces generated during the guidance of the mandible will only serve to dislodge complete dentures. If only mandibular teeth are present, then guidance is possible but less effective compared to when teeth are present in both arches.

The guidance prosthesis may be constructed for either the mandible or the maxilla. All guidance prostheses are utilized on an interim basis until acceptable occlusal relationships and proper proprioception are reestablished. Once an acceptable occlusal relationship is established, the guidance prosthesis may be discarded or used occasionally to reinforce the proprioceptive mechanism.

If the mandible can be manipulated into an acceptable maxillomandibular relationship but the patient lacks the motor control to bring the mandible into occlusion, a cast mandibular resection guidance prosthesis as described by Robinson and Rubright is appropriate (1964). This mandibular guidance prosthesis consists of an RPD framework with a flange extending 7 to 10 mm laterally and superiorly on the buccal aspect of the premolars and molars on the nondefect side. This flange engages the maxillary teeth during mandibular closure, thereby directing the mandible to an improved interocclusal position (Fig 2-221). The RPD framework must be suitably stable and retained to counteract the lateral forces generated on the prosthesis during closure.

The guidance ramp may be constructed in metal alone or in acrylic resin processed onto a meshed metal flange. The material choice will depend on the existing occlusal relationship and the need for adjustability. If the mandible can be manipulated comfortably into an acceptable occlusal position and minimal adjustments are anticipated, then a metal guidance ramp is appropriate. However, if resistance is encountered in the positioning of the mandible, or if changes in the mandibular range of motion or occlusal relationship are expected, then a guidance ramp ought to be formed in acrylic resin. The acrylic resin can be periodically adjusted as occlusal relationships change.

Fabrication begins with the retrieval of suitable maxillary and mandibular casts. The clinician needs to guide the mandible into the best possible interocclusal relationship and obtain a wax interocclusal record at this position in order to mount the diagnostic casts on an appropriate articulator. This mounting is used to examine the occlusal relationship carefully. If a considerable period has elapsed since surgery, the patient may exhibit some extrusion of teeth due to the lack of opposing occlusal contacts, and selective occlusal equilibration may permit closure in a more favorable occlusal relationship.

The mandibular diagnostic cast is surveyed, and the design of the RPD framework is outlined. To prevent movement of individual teeth, the framework should be designed to positively engage most of the remaining dentition (see Fig 2-221). The guidance ramp is usually designed to extend from a continuous clasp along the buccal surfaces of the molars. Because of the angular pathway of mandibular closure, this extension must extend superiorly and laterally in a diagonal manner and must allow normal horizontal and vertical overlap of the maxillary teeth.

The exact angulation of the guidance ramp is difficult to determine with a conventional articulator. A second interocclusal record obtained while the posterior teeth are separated approximately 3 to 4 mm (where the mandible is allowed to deviate) will give the prosthodontist an approximate angulation. To communicate the desired height and angulation of the ramp to the lab technician, wax is shaped and added by the prosthodontist to the land area of the master cast buccal to the premolar and molar teeth on the nondefect side. The technician will either digitally scan this wax-up and master cast complex as shown in Fig 2-221 for digital framework design or duplicate this complex into a single refractory cast for conventional framework fabrication.

Because most dental laboratories are not acquainted with the principles of resection guidance prostheses, the clinician must be particularly critical of aspects of the framework design—namely, the guidance ramp and the retentive features of the framework. The

Figure 2-220 *(a and b)* After the patient underwent severe months of guidance therapy, an RPD framework with palatal occlusal indices was fashioned. Note the frontal plane rotation.

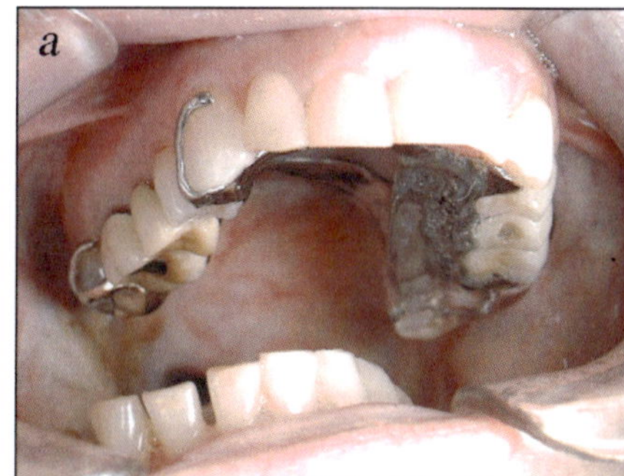

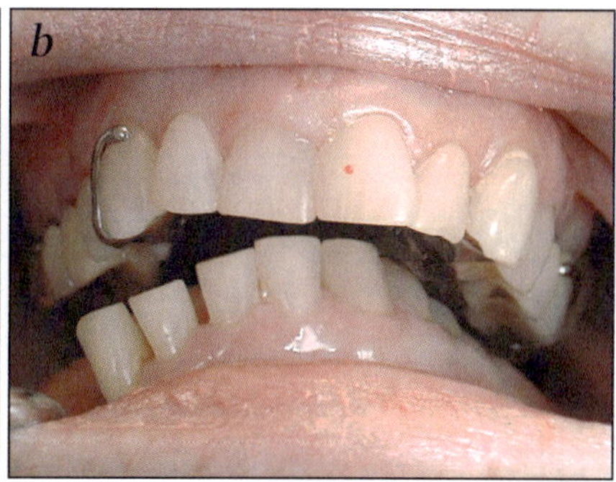

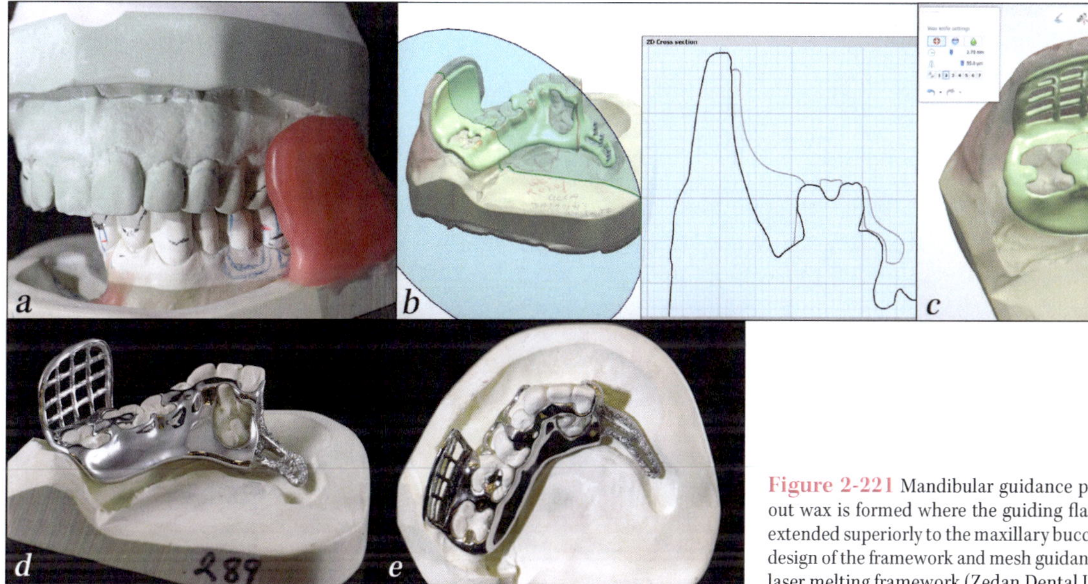

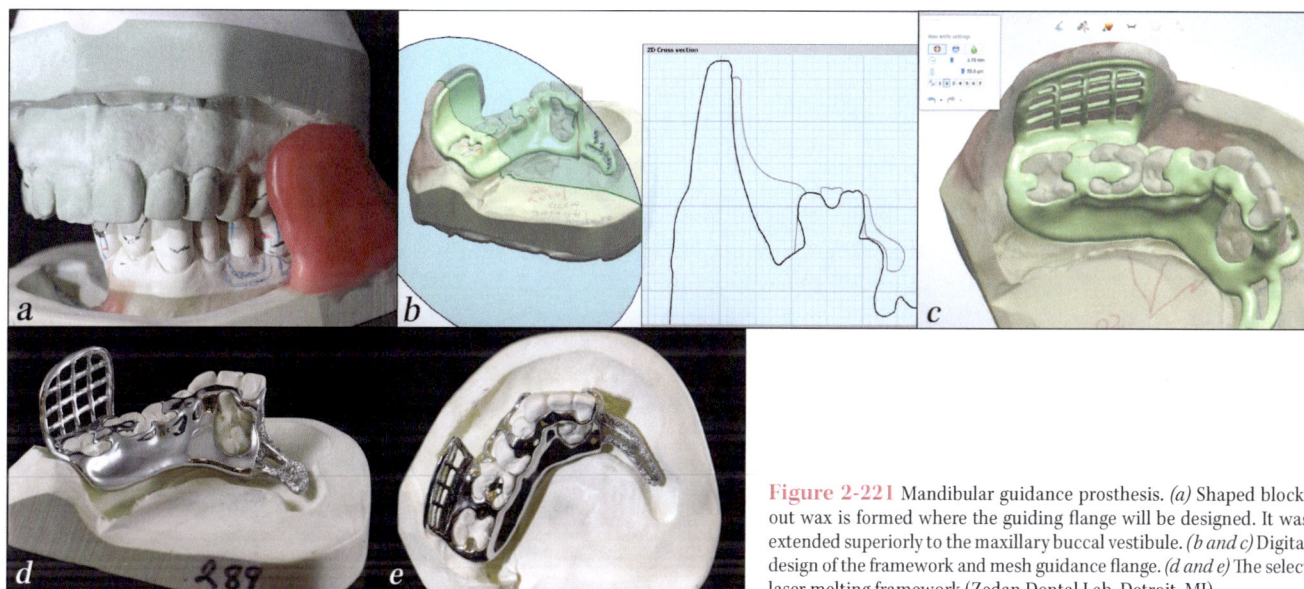

Figure 2-221 Mandibular guidance prosthesis. *(a)* Shaped blockout wax is formed where the guiding flange will be designed. It was extended superiorly to the maxillary buccal vestibule. *(b and c)* Digital design of the framework and mesh guidance flange. *(d and e)* The select laser melting framework (Zedan Dental Lab, Detroit, MI).

screenshots of the proposed design (Fig 2-221b and c) or the wax patterns on the refractory cast should be reviewed prior to manufacturing. The metal framework is produced by either conventional casting or additively manufactured via SLM. Following production, the technician will fit the framework onto the master cast and return it to the prosthodontist. The clinician will then verify the fit of the metal framework intraorally and adjust it accordingly, utilizing chloroform and rouge, an aerosol marking spray, disclosing wax, or similar materials.

If the guidance ramp is to be formed in acrylic resin, the acrylic resin retentive network should not touch or interfere with the maxillary teeth during guided closure. Impression compound and wax during the altered cast impression are used to form the guidance ramp (Fig 2-222). The thermoplastic material is applied to the retention network, and the prosthesis is seated intraorally. The mandible is manipulated into the desired interocclusal relationship several times. The resulting ramp should extend 7 to 10 mm superiorly. The prosthesis is removed from the mouth and chilled. The prosthesis is then placed back into the mouth to verify the guidance.

Some patients will experience initial difficulty in engaging the ramp with the buccal surfaces of the maxillary teeth, and manual manipulation of the mandible may be necessary for the patient to sense this position. If this position cannot be assumed by the patient with manual manipulation of the mandible, it may be necessary to warm the impression compound and reestablish the ramp, allowing for a more medial position of the mandible at closure. The molded ramp and altered cast are invested and heat processed.

The advantage of acrylic resin ramps over metal ones is that periodic revisions and adjustments are possible, and the final desired position does not have to be achieved with the initial application of acrylic resin. After the patient has adjusted to the initial position, the acrylic resin ramp can be reformed to guide the mandible farther laterally into an improved occlusal relationship.

A maxillary-based guidance prosthesis is indicated for patients with more severe mandibular deviation, who cannot be manipulated to an acceptable interocclusal relationship. In these patients, mandibular buccal guidance ramps become severely angulated and fall outside of the neutral zone, so maxillary guidance ramps, which emerge palatally, are utilized instead. Interim maxillary guidance prostheses are usually recommended and constructed with autopolymerizing acrylic resin and wrought wire clasps. They are used only on an interim basis until an acceptable occlusion can be established or until definitive use is deemed necessary, at which point a metal framework is indicated.

The interim maxillary guidance prosthesis is constructed following conventional prosthodontic guidelines and then fitted and adjusted in the mouth. The mandible is manipulated laterally toward the desired position until occlusal contact with the palatal prosthesis

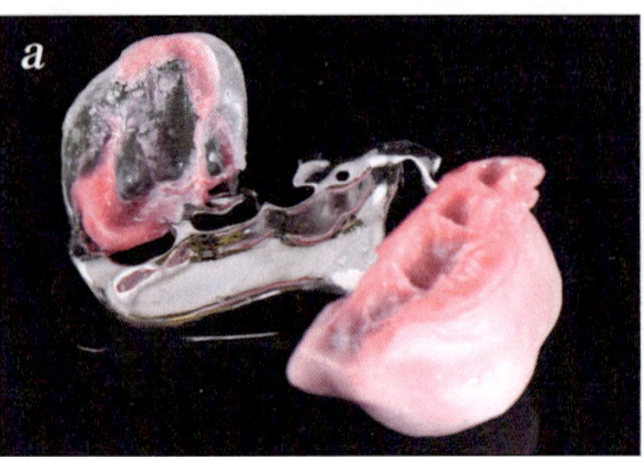
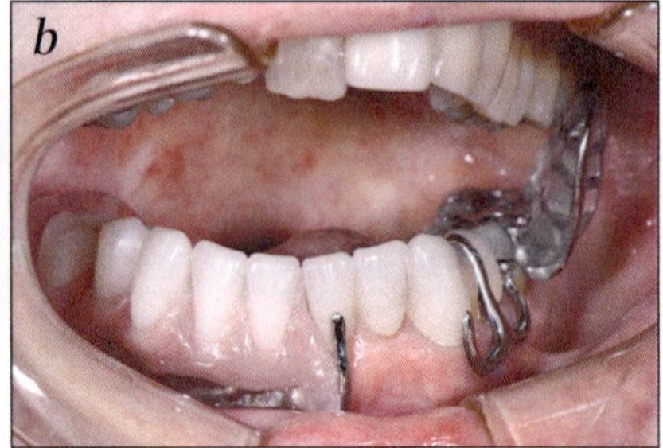
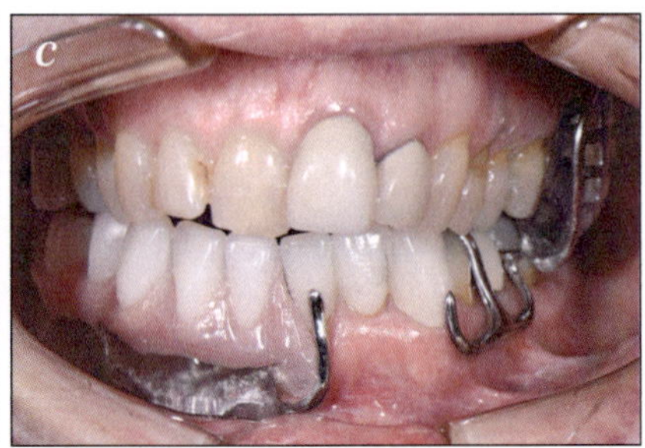

Figure 2-222 Mandibular guidance prosthesis. *(a)* Thermoplastic impression compound and wax were used to make an altered cast impression, occlusal recorder on the defect side, and functionally generated guidance flange. *(b)* On maximum opening, the occlusal reach of the flange catches the maxillary mandibular buccal cusps. *(c)* Note the angular path of closure as the flange guides the mandible into maximum intercuspation. Because mandibular incisors make poor RPD abutments, the mandibular lateral and central incisors and canine were splinted with a surveyed zirconia fixed dental prosthesis.

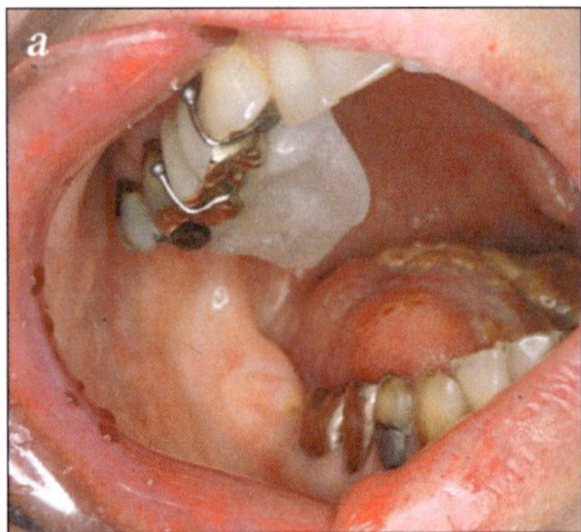
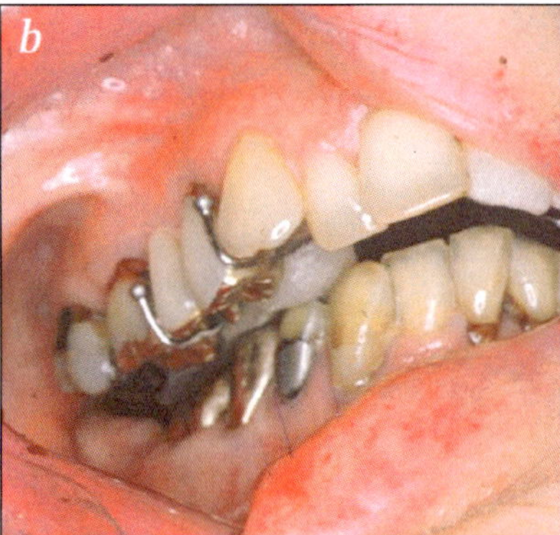
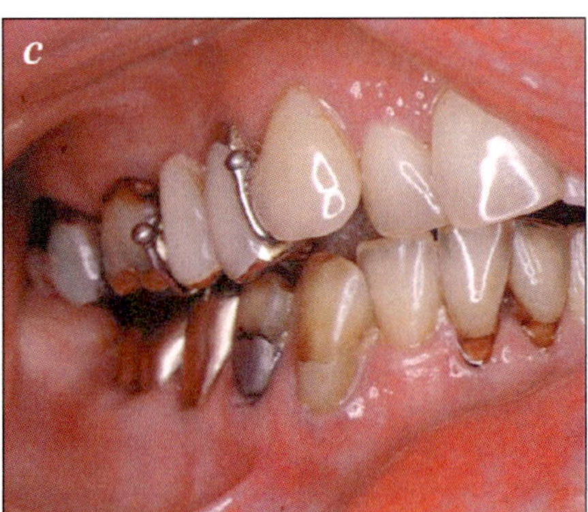

Figure 2-223 *(a)* Severity of mandibular deviation did not permit the establishment of an appropriate maxillomandibular relationship with a guidance ramp. *(b)* When palatal prosthesis was formulated and delivered, mandibular teeth still occluded lingual to the desired position. *(c)* As scar contracture loosened, the ramp and occlusal index were modified.

is noted. The prosthesis is removed, and a mix of autopolymerizing acrylic resin is prepared and added to the palatal prosthesis along its lateral and anterior borders on the nondefect side. The prosthesis is replaced in the mouth, and the mandible is manipulated to the desired position, thus establishing an index in the palate. At the first appointment, this index is usually lingual to the maxillary teeth (see Fig 2-223a and b).

The movement is repeated several times until the resin begins to polymerize. The prosthesis is then removed to allow for the complete polymerization of the acrylic resin. After adjustments and smoothing, the prosthesis is reinserted. The patient should be able to close into the index with an appropriate manual manipulation of the mandible. The prosthesis is then polished, and the patient is instructed to wear the prosthesis continuously. The objectives of the prosthesis are explained to the patient, and exercise instructions are outlined.

The index should not extend below the level of the maxillary teeth. If it does, speech, deglutition, and other oral functions requiring tongue manipulation may be affected. In select patients with limited tongue motion, this may not be of any concern.

When the patient returns, the mandible will usually exhibit more freedom of movement laterally toward the nonsurgical side, requiring an adjustment of the palatal guidance ramp so the mandible can assume a more desired maxillomandibular relationship (see Fig 2-223c). As the index approaches the maxillary teeth, it may be necessary to equilibrate select teeth to eliminate cuspal interferences. When an acceptable interocclusal position is achieved, occlusal equilibration is generally necessary to maintain the mandibular position.

The success of mandibular guidance therapy varies and depends on the nature of the surgical defect, the timing of the initiation of guidance therapy, patient cooperation, and other factors. Patients with an extensive posterior base-of-tongue lesions that have resulted in significant soft tissue resection in addition to radiation therapy are frequently unable to achieve useful interocclusal relationships. Guidance therapy is most successful in patients in whom the resection involves only bony structures with minimal sacrifice of the tongue, FOM, and adjacent soft tissues. The absence of a radical neck dissection also improves the prognosis for guidance therapy. Similarly, those patients who have not been irradiated have a better chance of obtaining a useful interocclusal position. However, even if guidance therapy is successful and an appropriate interocclusal position is reestablished, efficient mastication may still not be possible in those with compromised tongue mobility and control.

Occlusal equilibration

Occlusal equilibration is often necessary after mandibular guidance therapy has been completed. In most patients, the mandible assumes a different postural position at closure than it did prior to surgery. Occlusal equilibration is challenging because of the imprecise nature of mandibular movements and the nonreproducibility of CR records.

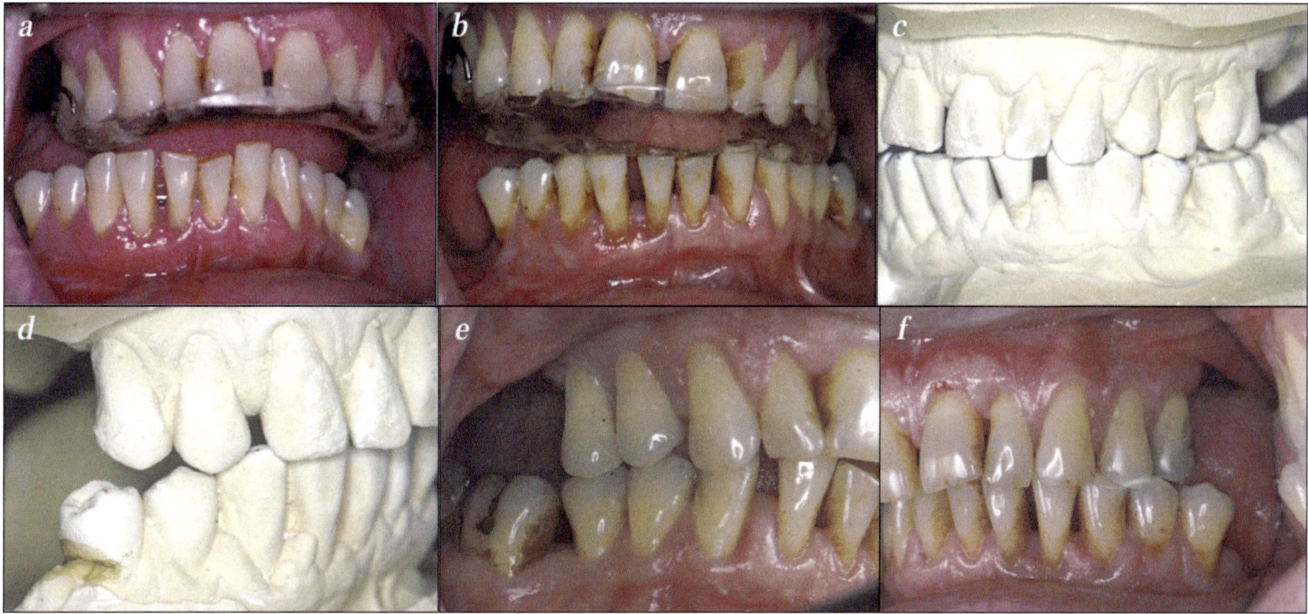

Figure 2-224 *(a)* Patient at the beginning of mandibular guidance therapy. Occlusal splint in position but index has not been formed. *(b)* The index formed and refined. Patients can achieve this position on a repeatable basis. *(c and d)* Casts are made and mounted on an articulator. Casts are equilibrated and sequence noted. *(e and f)* Equilibration completed. It may take two or three sessions to achieve a stable occlusion.

Centric occlusion records are made and transferred to a suitable articulator. The occlusal relationships are carefully examined, and prematurities are identified and noted. Reductions are made on the teeth of the mounted casts, and the sequence of the reductions is recorded. The sequence is repeated on the patient, and on completion, new impressions and interocclusal records are made. The casts are mounted and studied as before, and the entire sequence is repeated. Two or three sessions may be required before a stable occlusion is obtained (Fig 2-224). Often, selective crown placement may be required to achieve appropriate interocclusal relationships.

The patient should be informed that, as the mandibular deviation is reduced, the facial disfigurement on the defect side will be accentuated because the deviation of the mandible toward the surgical side will tend to camouflage the defect. The ultimate occlusal relationships established will depend on the reduction of mandibular deviation, the amount of frontal plane rotation, and the limitations imposed by the status of the remaining structures (tongue, lips, cheeks, FOM, soft palate, and flaps). The reestablished occlusal stops must not interfere with speech or deglutition and must provide freedom for the patient to masticate food and position the bolus in a manner that is consistent with the existing adaptive limitations.

The motivation of the patient should not be discounted when attempts are made to rehabilitate these patients. Many patients can overcome difficult obstacles, and if given a stable occlusion, many learn to masticate in a reasonable fashion.

Prosthetic Rehabilitation

Because the number of patients with nonreconstructed discontinuity defects is increasingly rare, the authors have decided that this section did not require updating. This group includes those with guarded prognoses for tumor control and patients with major health problems that prelude major reconstructive efforts. For prosthodontic rehabilitation of patients who have mandibular discontinuity defects, the reader is directed to the third edition of this book, where these procedures are well described and illustrated.

Summary

The functional disabilities associated with the resection of a portion of the tongue and the adjacent mandible are primarily dependent on the amount of the tongue resected and the method of surgical closure. In the first edition of this text, the authors frequently referred to patients with tongue and mandible resections as the "forgotten patients" because of the difficulty associated with restoring their form and function after tumor ablation. However, the refinement of vascularized free flaps to reconstruct the tongue and mandible and the use of dental implants to restore the dentition have enabled highly specialized, interdisciplinary teams to effectively restore the oral form and function for such patients. Well-integrated teams composed of surgical oncologist, microvascular surgeons, prosthodontists, and speech and swallowing therapists obtain the most predictable results. The most reliable functional and occlusion-based reconstructions are obtained with collaborative virtual surgical planning and computer-aided manufacturing of models, guides, splints, and custom reconstruction plates.

Missing portions of the tongue and mandible can be replaced at the time of tumor ablation, and dental implants are placed primarily for comprehensive rehabilitation. The soft tissues of vascularized flaps must be tailored so that the bulk and contour of the tongue can be restored to nearly normal conditions, while the osseous components of these flaps used to preserve the complex maxillomandibular relationships that are necessary to provide patients with functional occlusion. The first priority should be the selection and tailoring of the free flap to restore bulk and maximize tongue mobility. Restoration of mandibular continuity and placement of dental implants have minimal impact on oral function if the bulk of the tongue is not restored and its mobility is not maintained.

References

Adams V, Mathisen B, Baines S, et al. A systematic review and meta-analysis of measurements of tongue and hand strength and endurance using the Iowa Oral Performance Instrument (IOPI). Dysphagia 2013;28(3):350–369.

Adjei Boakye E, Buchanan P, Hinyard L, et al. Incidence and risk of second primary malignant neoplasm after a first head and neck squamous cell carcinoma. JAMA Otolaryngol Head Neck Surg 2018 Aug 1;144(8):727–737.

Adult Dysphagia. American Speech-Language-Hearing Association. Accessed 10 June 2022. http://www.asha.org/Practice-Portal/Clinical-Topics/Adult-Dysphagia/.

Agra IM, Carvalho AL, Pontes E, et al. Postoperative complications after en bloc salvage surgery for head and neck cancer. Arch Otolaryngol Head Neck Surg 2003;129:1317–1321.

Alibek K, Baiken Y, Kakpenova A, et al. Implication of human herpesviruses in oncogenesis through immune evasion and supression. Infect Agent Cancer 2014 Jan 20;9(1):3.

Alsini AY, Sayed S, Alkaf HH, et al. Tongue reconstruction post partial glossectomy during the COVID-19 pandemic. A case report. Ann Med Surg (Lond) 2020;59:53–56.

Altuwaijri AA, Aldrees TM, Alessa MA. Prevalence of metastasis and involvement of level IV and V in oral squamous cell carcinoma: A systematic review. Cureus 2021;13(12):e20255.

Ambrose JA, Barua RS. The pathophysiology of cigarette smoking and cardiovascular disease: An update. J Am Coll Cardiol 2004 May 19;43(10):1731–1737.

American Cancer Society. March 2021. https://amp.cancer.org/research/cancer-facts-statistics.

American Cancer Society. Head and Neck Cancers. 2021. https://www.cancer.org/cancer/types/head-neck-cancer.html.

American Joint Committee on Cancer Staging Manual. 7th ed. Chicago: American Joint Committee on Cancer; 2009.

American Lung Association. 2020. https://www.lung.org/.

Amin MB, Greene FL, Edge SB, et al., eds. AJCC Cancer Staging Manual. 8th ed. New York: Springer International Publishing; 2017.

Anderson JO, Benson D, Waite DE. Intraoral skin grafts: An aid to alveolar ridge extension. J Oral Surg 1969;27(6):427–430.

Ang KK, Harris J, Wheeler R, et al. Human papillomavirus and survival of patients with oropharyngeal cancer. N Engl J Med 2010 Jul 1;363(1):24–35.

Antony AK, Chen WF, Kolokythas A, et al. Use of virtual surgery and stereolithography-guided osteotomy for mandibular reconstruction with the free fibula. Plast Reconstr Surg 2011;128(5):1080–1084.

Aramany MA, Downs JA, Beery QC, et al. Prosthodontic rehabilitation for glossectomy patients. J Prosthet Dent 1982;48(1):78–81.

Aramany MA, Myers EN. Intermaxillary fixation following mandibular resection. J Prosthet Dent 1977;37(4):437–444.

Arden RL, Rachel JD, Marks SC, et al. Volume-length impact of lateral jaw resections on complication rates. Arch Otolaryngol Head Neck Surg 1999;125(1):68–72.

Ariyan S. The pectoralis major myocutaneous flap. A versatile flap for reconstruction in the head and neck. Plast Reconstr Surg 1979;63:73–81.

Aviv JE, Hecht C, Weinberg H, et al. Surface sensibility of the floor of the mouth and tongue in healthy controls and in radiated patients. Otolaryngol—Head Neck Surg 1992;107(3):418–423.

Axhausen W. The osteogenic phases of regeneration of bone: A historical and experimental study. J Bone Joint Am Surg 1956;38:593–600.

Azizzadeh B, Enayati P, Chhetri D, et al. Long-term survival outcome in transhyoid resection of base of tongue squamous cell carcinoma. Arch Otolaryngol Head Neck Surg 2002;128:1067–1070.

Baxi SS, Pinheiro LC, Patil SM, et al. Causes of death in long-term survivors of head and neck cancer. Cancer 2014 May 15;120(10):1507–1513.

Bearelly S, Wang SJ, Cheung SW. Oral sensory dysfunction following radiotherapy. Laryngoscope 2017;127(10):2282–2286.

Beresin V, Scheisser FJ. The neutral zone in complete dentures. St Louis, MO: Mosby; 1978.

Bernier J, Cooper JS, Pajak TF, et al. Defining risk levels in locally advanced head and neck cancers: A comparative analysis of concurrent postoperative radiation plus chemotherapy trials of the EORTC and RTOG. Head Neck 2005;27:843–850.

Berrone M, Crosetti E, Succo G. Repositioning template for mandibular reconstruction with fibular free flaps: An alternative technique to pre-plating and virtual surgical planning. Acta Otorhinolaryngol Ital 2014;34(4):278–282.

Bertlich M, Zeller N, Freytag S, et al. Factors influencing outcomes in selective neck dissection in 661 patients with head and neck squamous cell carcinoma. BMC Surg 2022;22(1):196.

Best SR, Niparko KJ, Pai SI. Biology of HPV infection and immune therapy for HPV-related head and neck cancers. Otolaryngol Clin North Am 2012 August;45(4):807–822.

Beumer J, Curtis T, Harrison RE. Radiation therapy of the oral cavity: Sequelae and management, part 2. Head Neck 1979;1(5):392–408.

Beumer J, Faulkner RF, Lyons KM, et al. Restoration of the edentulous maxilla with implant retained overdentures. In Fundamentals of implant dentistry—prosthodontic principles. 2nd ed. Eds. J Beumer, R Faulkner, K Shah, et al. Chicago: Quintessence; 2022a. pp. 202–243.

Beumer J, Lyons K, Kahensa N, et al. Implants in irradiated tissues, patients with osteoporosis and patients treated with bisphosphonates. In Fundamentals of implant dentistry—prosthodontic principles. 2nd ed. Eds. J Beumer, R Faulkner, K Shah, et al. Chicago: Quintessence; 2022b. pp. 498–515.

Blackwell KE. Unsurpassed reliability of free flaps for head and neck reconstruction. Archives of Otolaryngology–Head & Neck Surgery 1999;125(3):295.

Bloomer HH, Hawk AH. Speech considerations: Speech disorders associated with ablative surgery of the face, mouth, and pharynx—ablative approaches to learning. In Orofacial Anomalies: Clinical and Research Implications. ASHA Reports 8. Ed. Wertz RT. Washington, DC: American Speech and Hearing Association; 1973. pp. 42–61.

Blyth KM, McCabe P, Madill C, et al. Speech and swallow rehabilitation following partial glossectomy: A systematic review. Int J Speech Lang Pathol 2015;17(4):401–410. http://doi.org/10.3109/17549507.2014.979880. Epub 2014 Dec 17. PMID: 25515427.

Blyth KM, Mccabe P, Madill C, et al. Ultrasound visual feedback in articulation therapy following partial glossectomy. J Commun Disord 2016 May–Jun;61:1–15. http://doi.org/10.1016/j.jcomdis.2016.02.004. Epub 2016 Mar 2. PMID: 26994583.

Bozec A, Poissonnet G, Chamorey E, et al. Free-flap head and neck reconstruction and quality of life: A 2-year prospective study. Laryngoscope 2008;118(5):874–880.

Bree R, Keizer B, Civantos FJ, et al. What is the role of sentinel lymph node biopsy in the management of oral cancer in 2020? Eur Arch Otorhinolaryngol 2021 Sep;278(9):3181–3191.

Bressmann T, Sader R, Whitehill TL, et al. Consonant intelligibility and tongue motility in patients with partial glossectomy. J Oral Maxillofac Surg 2003;62:298–303.

Brewer AA. Prosthodontic research in progress at the School of Aerospace Medicine. J Prosthet Dent 1963;13:49–69.

Brook I. Early side effects of radiation treatment for head and neck cancer. Cancer Radiother 2021;25(5):507–513.

Brown JS, Barry C, Ho M, et al. A new classification for mandibular defects after oncological resection. Lancet Oncol 2016;17(1):e23–30.

Brown JS, Lowe D, Kanatas A, et al. Mandibular reconstruction with vascularised bone flaps: A systematic review over 25 years. Br J Oral Maxillofac Surg 2017;55(2):113–126.

Brown JS, Shaw RJ. Reconstruction of the maxilla and midface: Introducing a new classification. Lancet Oncol 2010 Oct;11(10):1001–1008. http://doi.org/10.1016/S1470-2045(10)70113-3.

Buajeeb W, Okuma N, Thanakun S, et al. Direct immunofluorescence in oral lichen planus. J Clin Diagn Res 2015 Aug;9(8):ZC34.

Bundgaard T, Tandrup O, Elbrønd O. A functional evaluation of patients treated for oral cancer. A prospective study. Int J Oral Maxillofac Surg 1993;22(1):28–34.

Burk T, Del Valle J, Finn R, et al. Maximum quantity of bone available for harvest from the anterior iliac crest, posterior iliac crest, and proximal tibia using a standardized surgical approach: A cadaveric study. J Oral Maxillofac Surg 2016;74:2532–2548.

Cady B, Catlin D. Epidermoid carcinoma of the gum: A 20-year survey. Cancer 1969;23:551–569.

Cantor R, Curtis TA. Prosthetic management of edentulous mandibulectomy patients. I. Anatomic, physiologic, and psychologic considerations. J Prosthet Dent 1971;25(4):446–457.

Cantor R, Curtis TA, Shipp L, et al. Maxillary speech prostheses for mandibular surgical defects. J Prosthet Dent 1969;22:253–260.

Carvalho AL, Kowalski LP, Agra IM, et al. Treatment results on advanced neck metastasis (N3) from head and neck squamous carcinoma. Otolaryngol Head Neck Surg 2005;132:862–868. http://doi.org/10.1016/j.otohns.2005.01.034.

Caudell JJ, Gillison ML, Maghami E, et al. NCCN Guidelines® insights: Head and neck cancers, version 1.2022. J Natl Compr Canc Netw 2022;20(3):224–234.

Ch'ng S, Skoracki RJ, Selber JC, et al. Osseointegrated implant-based dental rehabilitation in head and neck reconstruction patients. Head Neck 2016;38(Suppl 1):E321–E327.

Chakravarthy A, Henderson S, Thirdborough SM, et al. Human papillomavirus drives tumor development throughout the head and neck: Improved prognosis is associated with an immune response largely restricted to the oropharynx. J Clin Oncol 2016;34(34):4132–4141.

Chambers KJ, Anthony DC, Randolph GW, et al. Atrophy of the tongue following complete versus partial hypoglossal nerve transection in a canine model. Laryngoscope 2016;126(12):2689–2693.

Chana JS, Chang YM, Wei FC, et al. Segmental mandibulectomy and immediate free fibula osteoseptocutaneous flap reconstruction with endosteal implants: An ideal treatment method for mandibular ameloblastoma. Plast Reconstr Surg 2004;113:80–87.

Chang TL, Orellana D, Beumer J. Kratochvil's fundamentals of removal partial dentures. Chicago: Quintessence; 2019.

Chao KS, Ozyigit G, Blanco AI, et al. Intensity-modulated radiation therapy for oropharyngeal carcinoma: Impact of tumor volume. Int J Radiat Oncol Biol Phys 2004;59:43–50.

Charters E, Dunn M, Cheng K, et al. Trismus therapy devices: A systematic review. Oral Oncol 2022;126:105728.

Chaturvedi, AK. Epidemiology and clinical aspects of HPV in head and neck cancers. Head and Neck Pathology 2012;6(1):16–24.

Chaturvedi AK, Engels EA, Pfeiffer RM, et al. Human papilloma-virus and rising oropharyngeal cancer incidence in the UnitedStates. J Clin Oncol 2011;29(32):4294–4301.

Chen SC, Huang BS, Hung TM, et al. Swallowing ability and its impact on dysphagia-specific health-related QOL in oral cavity cancer patients post-treatment. Eur J Oncol Nurs 2018;36:89–94.

Chen X, Sturgis EM, Etzel CJ, et al. p73 G4C14-to-A4T14 polymorphism and risk of human papillomavirus-associated squamous cell carcinoma of the oropharynx in never smokers and never drinkers. Cancer 2008 Dec 15;113(12):3307–3314.

Chhetri D. Anatomy and physiology of swallowing. In Dysphagia evaluation and management in otolaryngology. 1st ed. Ed. Chhetri DK. Amsterdam: Elsevier; 2019. pp. 2.

Chierici G, Lawson L. Clinical speech considerations in prosthodontics: Perspectives of the prosthodontist and speech pathologist. J Prosthet Dent 1973;29:29–39.

Chi-Fishman G, Stone M. A new application for electropalatography: Swallowing. Dysphagia 1996;11(4):239–247.

Chi-Fishman G, Stone M, McCall GN. Lingual action in normal sequential swallowing. J Speech Lang Hear Res 1998;41(4):771–785.

Chuanjun C, Zhiyuan Z, Shaopu G, et al. Speech after partial glossectomy: A comparison between reconstruction and nonreconstruction patients. J Oral Maxillofac Surg 2002;60:404–407.

Conley JJ. Free skin grafting in the sinus, oral, and pharyngeal areas in radical surgery of the head and neck. Cancer 1954;7(3):444–454.

Converse JM. Reconstructive plastic surgery. Philadelphia: Saunders; 1964.

Conway MJ, Meyers C. Replication and assembly of human papillomaviruses. Journal of Dental Research 2009;88(4):307–317.

Cricchio G, Lundgren S. Donor site morbidity in two different approaches to anterior iliac crest bone harvesting. Clin Implant Dent Relat Res 2003;5:161–169.

Crile G. Excision of cancer of the head and neck with special reference to the plan of dissection based on one hundred thirty-two operations. J Am Med Assoc 1906;47:1780–1785.

Curtis DA, Plesh O, Hannam AG, et al. Modeling of jaw biomechanics in the reconstructed mandibulectomy patient. J Prosthet Dent 1999;81(2):167–173.

Curtis DA, Plesh O, Miller AJ, et al. A comparison of masticatory function in patients with or without reconstruction of the mandible. Head Neck 1997;19(4):287–296.

Curtis TA, Taylor RC, Rositano SA. Physical problems in obtaining records of the maxillofacial patient. J Prosthet Dent 1975;34(5):539–554.

Da Silva DM, Fausch SC, Verbeek JS, et al. Uptake of human papillomavirus virus-like particles by dendritic cells is mediated by Fcγ receptors and contributes to acquisition of T cell immunity. Journal of Immunology 2007;178(12):7587–7597.

Dauwe PB, Pulikkottil BJ, Lavery L, et al. Does hyperbaric oxygen therapy work in facilitating acute wound healing: A systematic review. Plast Reconstr Surg 2014;133(2):208e–215e.

Davidson BJ, Newkirk KA, Harter KW, et al. Complications from planned, post-treatment neck dissections. Arch Otolaryngol Head Neck Surg 1999;125:401–405.

Davidson J, Root WA, Trock BJ. Age and survival from squamous cell carcinoma of the oral tongue. Head Neck 2001;23:273–279.

Davis B, Roumanas E, Hong S, et al. Stress distributions of implants used for retention of maxillary obturators. In Proceedings of the First International Congress on Maxillofacial Prosthetics. Eds. I Zlotolow, S Esposito, J Beumer. New York: Memorial Sloan-Kettering Cancer Center; 1995. pp. 204–208.

Davis JW, Lazarus C, Logemann JA, et al. Effect of maxillary glossectomy prosthesis on articulation and swallowing. J Prosthet Dent 1987;57:715–719.

Davis WH, Davis CL, Delo R, et al. Surgical management of soft tissue problems. In Reconstructive preprosthetic oral and maxillofacial surgery. 2nd ed. Ed. R Fonseca, H Davis. Philadelphia: Saunders; 1995. pp. 767–820.

Davodi A, Beumer J, Faulkner RF, et al. Restoration of edentulous maxillae with fixed prostheses. In Fundamentals of implant dentistry—Prosthodontic principles. 2nd ed. Ed. J Beumer, R Faulkner, K Shah, et al. Chicago: Quintessence; 2022. pp. 244–295.

de Carvalho-Teles V, Sennes LU, Gielow I. Speech evaluation after palatal augmentation in patients undergoing glossectomy. Arch Otolaryngol Head Neck Surg 2008;134:1066–1070.

de Graeff A, de Leeuw JR, Ros WJ, et al. Pretreatment factors predicting quality of life after treatment for head and neck cancer. Head Neck 2000;22(4):398–407.

de Vicente JC, de Villalain L, Torre A, et al. Microvascular free tissue transfer for tongue reconstruction after hemiglossectomy: A functional assessment of radial forearm verses anterolateral thigh flap. J Oral Maxillofac Surg 2008;66:2270–2275.

Denittis AS, Machtay M, Rosenthal DI, et al. Advanced oropharyngeal carcinoma treated with surgery and radiotherapy: Oncologic outcome and functional assessment. Am J Otolaryngol 2001;22:329–335.

Dewan K. Chemotherapy and dysphagia: The good, the bad, the ugly. Curr Opin Otolaryngol Head Neck Surg 2020;28(6):385–391.

Dholam KP, Bachher GK, Yadav PS, et al. Assessment of quality of life after implant-retained prosthetically reconstructed maxillae and mandibles postcancer treatments. Implant Dent 2011 Feb;20(1):85–94. http://doi.org/10.1097/ID.0b013e31820031ab. PMID: 21278531.

Dijkstra PU, Huisman PM, Roodenburg JL. Criteria for trismus in head and neck oncology. Int J Oral Maxillofac Surg 2006;35(4):337–342.

Dodson TB, Kaban LB. Donor site morbidity: Diagnosis, treatment, and prevention. Oral Maxillofacial Surg Clin North Am 1990;2:489–498.

Dodson TB, Smith RA. Mandibular reconstruction with autogenous and alloplastic materials following resection of an odontogenic myxoma. Int J Oral Maxillofac Implants 1987;2:227–229.

Donoff RB. Biological basis for vestibuloplasty procedures. J Oral Surg 1976;34(10):890–896.

Doorbar J, Quint W, Banks L, et al. The biology and life-cycle of human papillomaviruses. Vaccine 2012 Nov 20;30(Suppl 5):F55–70.

Duguay MJ. Speech after glossectomy. NY State Med 1964;64:1836–1838.

Dziegielewski PT, Ho ML, Rieger J, et al. Total glossectomy with laryngeal preservation and free flap reconstruction: Objective functional outcomes and systematic review of the literature. Laryngoscope 2012;123(1):140–145.

Dzioba A, Aalto D, Papadopoulos-Nydam G, et al. Functional and quality of life outcomes after partial glossectomy: A multi-institutional longitudinal study of the head and neck research network. J Otolaryngol Head Neck Surg 2017;46(1):56.

Eckardt AM, Kokemuller H, Flemming P, et al. Recurrent ameloblastoma following osseous reconstruction—a review of twenty years. J Craniomaxillofac Surg 2009;37(1):36–41.

Eisbruch A, Schwartz M, Rasch C, et al. Dysphagia and aspiration after chemoradiotherapy for head-and-neck cancer: Which anatomic structures are affected and can they be spared by IMRT? Int J Radiat Oncol Biol Phys 2004;60(5):1425–1439.

El Saghir NS, Keating NL, Carlson RW, et al. Tumor boards: Optimizing the structure and improving efficiency of multidisciplinary management of patients with cancer worldwide. Am Soc Clin Oncol Educ Book 2014:e461–e466.

Elango J, Sundaram KR, Gangadharan P, et al. Factors affecting oral cancer awareness in a high-risk population in India. Asian Pac J Cancer Prev 2009 Oct–Dec;10(4):627–630.

Epstein JB, Emerton S, Kolbinson DA, et al. Quality of life and oral function following radiotherapy for head and neck cancer. Head Neck 1999;21(1):1–11.

Fakhry C, Lacchetti C, Perez-Ordonez B. Human papillomavirus testing in head and neck carcinomas: ASCO clinical practice guideline endorsement summary of the CAP guideline. J Oncol Pract 2018;14(10):613–617. Published correction appears in J Oncol Pract 2019 Jan;15(1):60.

Fakhry C, Westra WH, Li S, et al. Improved survival of patients with human papillomavirus-positive head and neck squamous cell carcinoma in a prospective clinical trial. J Natl Cancer Inst 2008 Feb 20;100(4):261–269.

Fan S, Tang QL, Lin YJ, et al. A review of clinical and histological parameters associated with contralateral neck metastases in oral squamous cell carcinoma. Int J Oral Sci 2011;3:180–191. http://doi.org/10.4248/IJOS11068.

Farace F, Fois VE, Maconi A, et al. Free anterolateral thigh flap versus free forearm flap: Functional results in oral reconstruction. J Plast Reconstr Aesthet Surg 2007;60:583–587.

Faulkner MG, Hatcher DC, Hay A. A three-dimensional investigation of temporomandibular joint loading. J Biomech 1987;20(10):997–1002.

Fein DA, Lee WR, Amos WR, et al. Oropharyngeal carcinoma treated with radiotherapy: A 30-year experience. Int J Radiat Oncol Biol Phys 1996;34:289–296.

Feller L, Khammissa RA, Wood NH, et al. Epithelial maturation and molecular biology of oral HPV. Infectious Agents and Cancer 2009 Dec;4(1):1–9.

Fenlon MR, Lyons A, Farrell S, et al. Factors affecting survival and usefulness of implants placed in vascularized free composite grafts used in post-head and neck cancer reconstruction. Clin Implant Dent Relat Res 2012;14(2):266–272.

Fernandes R, Nikitakis NG, Pazoki A, et al. Osteogenic sarcoma of the jaw: A 10-year experience. J Oral Maxillofac Surg 2007;65:1286–1291.

Ferris RL, Flamand Y, Weinstein GS, et al. Phase ii randomized trial of transoral surgery and low-dose intensity modulated radiation therapy in resectable p16+ locally advanced oropharynx cancer: An ecog-acrin cancer research group trial (E3311). J Clin Oncol 2022;40(2):138–149.

Fish EW. Principles of full denture prosthesis. Springfield (IL): Charles C. Thomas; 1966.

Fisher M, Yee K, Alba N, et al. Applications of bone morphogenetic protein-2: Alternative therapies in craniofacial reconstruction. J Craniofac Surg 2019;30: 1952–1959.

Flynn C, Stavness I, Lloyd J, et al. A finite element model of the face including an orthotropic skin model under in vivo tension. Comput Methods Biomech Biomed Engin 2015;18(6):571–582.

Forrest LA, Schuller DE, Lucas JG, et al. Rapid analysis of mandibular margins. Laryngoscope 1995;105:475–477.

Foster CC, Melotek JM, Brisson RJ, et al. Definitive chemoradiation for locally-advanced oral cavity cancer: A 20-year experience. Oral Oncol 2018;80:16–22.

Foster RD, Anthony JP, Sharma A, et al. Vascularized bone flaps versus nonvascularized bone grafts for mandibular reconstruction: An outcome analysis of primary bony union and endosseous implant success. Head Neck 1999;2:66–71.

Frisch M, Hjalgrim H, Jæger AB, et al. Changing patterns of tonsillar squamous cell carcinoma in the United States. Cancer Causes & Control 2000 Jul;11(6):489–495.

Fry AM, Laugharne D, Jones K. Osteotomising the fibular free flap: An anatomical perspective. Br J Oral Maxillofac Surg 2016;54(6):692–693.

Fueki K, Kimoto K, Ogawa T, et al. Effect of implant-supported or retained dentures on masticatory performance: A systematic review. J Prosthet Dent 2007;98(6):470–477.

Furia CL, Kowalski LP, Latorre MR, et al. Speech intelligibility after glossectomy and speech rehabilitation. Arch Otolaryngol Head Neck Surg 2001;127:877–883.

Galati LT, Myers EN, Johnson JT. Primary surgery as treatment for early squamous cell carcinoma of the tonsil. Head Neck 2000;22:294–296.

Garavello W, Ciardo A, Spreafico R, et al. Risk factors for distant metastases in head and neck squamous cell carcinoma. Arch Otolaryngol Head Neck Surg 2006 Jul;132(7):762–766.

Gardner DG. Some current concepts on the pathology of ameloblastomas. Oral Surg Oral Med Oral Pathol Oral Radiol Endod 1996;82:660–669.

Garrett NR, Kapur KK, Perez P. Effects of improvements of poorly fitting dentures and new dentures on patient satisfaction. J Prosthet Dent 1996;76(4):403–413.

Garrett N, Roumanas ED, Blackwell KE, et al. Efficacy of conventional and implant-supported mandibular resection prostheses: Study overview and treatment outcomes. J Prosthet Dent 2006;96(1):13–24.

Geressen M, Prescher A, Riediger D, et al. Tibial versus iliac bone grafts: A comparative examination if 15 freshly preserved adult cadavers. Clin Oral Implants Res 2008;19:1270–1275.

Gilbert RW. Reconstruction of the oral cavity; past, present and future. Oral Oncol 2020;108:104683.

Gillison ML, Chaturvedi AK, Anderson WF, et al. Epidemiology of human papillomavirus–positive head and neck squamous cell carcinoma. J Clin Oncol 2015;33(29):3235.

Gillison ML, Koch WM, Capone RB, et al. Evidence for a causal association between human papillomavirus and a subset of head and neck cancers. J Natl Cancer Inst 2000 May 3;92(9):709–720.

Girod DA, McCulloch TM, Tsue TT, et al. Risk factors for complications in clean-contaminated head and neck surgical procedures. Head Neck 1995;17:7–13.

Giuliano AR, Lee JH, Fulp W, et al. Incidence and clearance of genital human papillomavirus infection in men (HIM): A cohort study. Lancet 2011;377(9769):932–940.

Gondim DD, Wesley H, Xiaowei W, et al. Histologic typing in oropharyngeal squamous cell carcinoma. Am J Surg Pathol 2016;40(8):1117–1124.

González-García R, Naval-Gías L, Rodríguez-Campo FJ, et al. Contralateral lymph neck node metastasis of squamous cell carcinoma of the oral cavity: A retrospective analytic study in 315 patients. J Oral Maxillofac Surg 2008;66:1390–1398.

Goodwin WJ Jr. Salvage surgery for patients with recurrent squamous cell carcinoma of the upper digestive tract: When do the ends justify the means? Laryngoscope 2000;110:1–18.

Gorsky M, Epstein JB, Oakley C, et al. Carcinoma of the tongue: A case series analysis of clinical presentation, risk factors, staging, and outcome. Oral Surg Oral Med Oral Pathol Oral Radiol Endod 2004;98:546–552.

Gourin CG, Johnson JT. Surgical treatment of squamous cell carcinoma of the base of the tongue. Head Neck 2001;23:653–660.

Greenberg JS, El Naggar AK, Mo V, et al. Disparity in pathologic and clinical lymph node staging in oral tongue carcinoma. Implication for therapeutic decision making. Cancer 2003;98:508–515.

Guadagnolo BA, Zagars GK, Raymond AK, et al. Osteosarcoma of the jaw/craniofacial region: Outcomes after multimodality treatment. Cancer 2009;115:3262–3270.

Guillamondegui OM, Oliver B, Hayden R. Cancer of the anterior floor of the mouth. Selective choice of treatment and analysis of failures. Am J Surg 1980;140:560–562.

Gunne HS. Masticatory efficiency and dental state. A comparison between two methods. Acta Odontol Scand 1985;43(3):139–146.

Gunne J, Jemt T, Linden B. Implant treatment in partially edentulous patients. A report on prostheses after 3 years. Int J Prosthodont 1994;7:143–148.

Ha PK, Eisele DW, Frassica FJ, et al. Osteosarcoma of the head and neck: A review of the Johns Hopkins experience. Laryngoscope 1999;109:964–969.

Habal MB, Rasmussen RA. Osseointegrated implants in cranial bone grafts for mandibular reconstruction. J Craniofac Surg 1993;4:51–57.

Haddadin KJ, Soutar DS, Olvier RJ, et al. Improved survival for patients with clinically T1/T2, N0 tongue tumors undergoing a prophylactic neck dissection. Head Neck 1999;21:517–525.

Hagberg C. Assessment of bite force: A review. J Craniomandib Disord 1987a;1(3):162–169.

Hagberg C. EMG versus force relationship in painful masseter muscles before and after intramuscular anesthetics and saline injections. Scand J Dent Res 1987b;95(3):259–265.

Hanasono MM, Weinstock YE, Yu P. Reconstruction of extensive head and neck defects with multiple simultaneous free flaps. Plast Reconstr Surg 2008;122:1739–1746.

Hannam AG, Stavness I, Lloyd JE, et al. A dynamic model of jaw and hyoid biomechanics during chewing. J Biomech 2008;41(5):1069–1076.

Hannam AG, Stavness IK, Lloyd JE, et al. A comparison of simulated jaw dynamics in models of segmental mandibular resection versus resection with alloplastic reconstruction. J Prosthet Dent 2010;104;191–198.

Hansen LS, Olson JA, Silverman S Jr. Proliferative verrucous leukoplakia: A long-term study of thirty patients. Oral Surg Oral Med Oral Pathol 1985 Sep;60(3):285–298. http://doi.org/10.1016/0030-4220(85)90313-5.

Haraldson T, Carlsson GE, Ingervall B. Functional state, bite force and postural muscle activity in patients with osseointegrated oral implant bridges. Acta Odontol Scand 1979;37(4):195–206.

Harrison LB. Applications of brachytherapy in head and neck cancer. Semin Surg Oncol 1997;13:177–184.

Harrison LB, Zelefsky MJ, Pfister DG, et al. Detailed quality of life assessment in patients treated with primary radiotherapy for squamous cell cancer of the base of the tongue. Head Neck 1997;19:169–175.

Hashibe M, Brennan P, Chuang SC, et al. Interaction between tobacco and alcohol use and the risk of head and neck cancer: Pooled analysis in the International Head and Neck Cancer Epidemiology Consortium. Cancer Epidemiol Biomarkers Prev 2009 Feb;18(2):541–550.

Hatcher DC, Faulkner MG, Hay A. Development of mechanical and mathematic models to study temporomandibular joint loading. J Prosthet Dent 1986;55(3):377–384.

Hayes DN, Van Waes C, Seiwert TY. Genetic landscape of human papillomavirus–associated head and neck cancer and comparison to tobacco-related tumors. J Clin Oncol 2015;33(29):3227.

Helkimo E, Carlsson GE, Helkimo M. Bite force and state of dentition. Acta Odontol Scand 1977;35(6):297–303.

Helkimo E, Carlsson GE, Helkimo M. Chewing efficiency and state of dentition. A methodologic study. Acta Odontol Scand 1978;36(1):33–41.

Herberman MA. Rehabilitation of patients following glossectomy: Attempts to reestablish articulation and maintain normal nutrition. Arch Otolaryngol 1958;67:182–183.

Hidalgo DA. Fibula free flap: A new method of mandible reconstruction. Plast Reconstr 1989;84:71–79.

Ho T, Zahurak M, Koch WM. Prognostic significance of presentation-to-diagnosis interval in patients with oropharyngeal carcinoma. Arch Otolaryngol Head Neck Surg 2004;130:45–51.

Hoggan BL, Cameron AL. Systematic review of hyperbaric oxygen therapy for the treatment of non-neurological soft tissue radiation-related injuries. Support Care Cancer 2014;22(6):1715–1726.

Hovan AJ, Williams PM, Stevenson-Moore P, et al. A systematic review of dysgeusia induced by cancer therapies. Support Care Cancer 2010;18(8):1081–1087.

Hsiao HT, Leu YS, Lin CC. Primary closure versus radial forearm flap reconstruction after hemiglossectomy: Functional assessment of swallowing and speech. Ann Plast Surg 2002;49:612–616.

Hsiao HT, Leu YS, Lin CC. Tongue reconstruction with free radial forearm flap after hemiglossectomy: A functional assessment. J Reconstr Microsurg 2003 Apr;19(3):137–142.

Huang WC, Chen HC, Jain V, et al. Reconstruction of through-and-through cheek defects involving the oral commissure, using chimeric flaps from the thigh lateral femoral circumflex system. Plast Reconstr Surg 2002;109(2):433–441, discussion 442–433.

Hundepool AC, Dumans AG, Hofer SOP, et al. Rehabilitation after mandibular reconstruction with fibula free-flap: Clinical outcome and quality of life assessment. Int J Oral Maxillofac Surg 2008;37(11):1009–1013.

Hutcheson KA, Bhayani MK, Beadle BM, et al. Eat and exercise during radiotherapy or chemoradiotherapy for pharyngeal cancers: Use it or lose it. JAMA Otolaryngol Head Neck Surg 2013;139(11):1127–1134.

Ide Y, Matsunaga S, Harris J, et al. Anatomical examination of the fibula: Digital imaging study for osseointegrated implant installation. J Otolaryngol Head Neck Surg 2015 Feb 3;44(1):1. http://doi.org/10.1186/s40463-015-0055-9.

Ihara Y, Tashimo Y, Nozue S, et al. Changes in oral function and quality of life in tongue cancer patients based on resected area. Asian Pac J Cancer Prev 2021;22(8):2549–2557.

Ikebe K, Matsuda K, Morii K, et al. Association of masticatory performance with age, posterior occlusal contacts, occlusal force, and salivary flow in older adults. Int J Prosthodont 2006;19(5):475–481.

Vanderwegen J. Clinical benefits of FEES in the diagnosis and management of dysphagia patients. B-ENT 2008;4:7–16.

Jacob RF, Yen TW. Processed record bases for the edentulous maxillofacial patient. J Prosthet Dent 1991;65(5):680–685.

Jaffe N, Patel SR, Benjamin RS. Chemotherapy in osteosarcoma: Basis for application and antagonism to implementation; early controversies surrounding its implementation. Hematol Oncol Clin North Am 1995;9:825–840.

Jaiswal G, Jaiswal S, Kumar R, et al. Field cancerization: Concept and clinical implications in head and neck squamous cell carcinoma. J Exp Ther Oncol 2013;10(3):209–214.

Ji YB, Cho YH, Song CM, et al. Long-term functional outcomes after resection of tongue cancer: Determining the optimal reconstruction method. Eur Arch Otorhinolaryngol 2017 Oct;274(10):3751–3756. http://doi.org/10.1007/s00405-017-4683-8. Epub 2017 Jul 26. PMID: 28748261.

Johnson HSA. Saliva Management. In Dysphagia: Foundation, Theory and Practice. Eds. JAY Cichero, BE Murdoch. Chichester, UK: John Wiley & Sons; 2006. pp. 126–146.

Johnson NW. Risk markers for oral diseases. 1st ed. Cambridge: Cambridge University Press; 1991.

Joseph AW, D'Souza G. Epidemiology of human papillomavirus-related head and neck cancer. Clin North Am 2012 Aug;45(4):739–64.

Joshi P, Dutta S, Chaturvedi P, et al. Head and neck cancers in developing countries. Rambam Maimonides Med J 2014 April 28;5(2): e0009.

Jung DW, Che ZM, Kim J, et al. Tumor-stromal crosstalk in invasion of oral squamous cell carcinoma: A pivotal role of CCL7. Int J Cancer 2010 Jul 15;127(2):332–344.

Kalfuss AH. Analysis of the speech of the glossectomy patient [master's thesis]. Detroit: Wayne State University; 1968.

Kapur KK, Garrett NR, Fischer E. Effects of anaesthesia of human oral structures on masticatory performance and food particle size distribution. Arch Oral Biol 1990;35(5):397–403.

Karayazgan-Saracoglu B, Atay A, Korkmaz C, Gunay Y. Quality of life assessment of implant-retained overdentures and fixed metal-acrylic resin prostheses in patients with marginal mandibulectomy. J Prosthet Dent 2017 Oct;118(4):551–560.

Karlsson O, Karlsson T, Pauli N, et al. Jaw exercise therapy for the treatment of trismus in head and neck Cancer: A prospective three-year follow-up study. Support Care Cancer 2021;29(7):3793–3800.

Keller EE. Mandibular discontinuity reconstruction with composite grafts: Free autogenous iliac bone, titanium mesh trays, and titanium endosseous implants. Oral Maxillofac Surg Clin North Am 1991;3:877–878.

Keller EE, Desjardins RP, Eckert SE, et al. Composite bone grafts and titanium implants in mandibular discontinuity reconstruction. Int J Oral Maxillofac Implants 1988;3(4):261–267.

Kim AJ, Suh JD, Sercarz JA, et al. Salvage surgery with free flap reconstruction: Factors affecting outcome after treatment of recurrent head and neck squamous carcinoma. Laryngoscope 2007;117:1019–1023.

Kim BB, Zaid W, Spagnoli D, et al. Reconstruction of major maxillary and mandibular defects with implants. In Fundamentals of implant dentistry—Surgical principles. Ed. PK Moy, A Pozzi, J Beumer. Chicago: Quintessence; 2016. pp. 259–289.

Kim PD, Blackwell KE. Latissimus-serratus-rib free flap for oromandibular and maxillary reconstruction. Arch Otolaryngol Head Neck Surg 2007;133(8):791–795.

Kim SG, Jang HS. Ameloblastoma: A clinical, radiographic, and histopathologic analysis of 71 cases. Oral Surg Oral Med Oral Pathol Oral Radiol Endod 2001;91:649–653.

Kirmeier R, Payer M, Lorenzoni M, et al. Harvesting of cancellous bone from the proximal tibia under local anesthesia: Donor site morbidity and patient experience. J Oral Maxillofac Surg 2007;65:2235–2241.

Konopnicki S, Troulis M. Mandibular tissue engineering: Past, present, future. J Oral Maxillofac Surg 2015;73:S136–S146.

Konstantinović VS, Dimić ND. Articulatory function and tongue mobility after surgery following by radiotherapy for tongue and floor of the mouth cancer patients. Br J Plast Surg 1998;51:589–593.

Koo BS, Lim YC, Lee JS, et al. Management of contralateral N0 neck in oral cavity squamous cell carcinoma. Head Neck 2006;28:896–901.

Koolstra JH. Dynamics of the human masticatory system. Critical Reviews in Oral Biology & Medicine 2002;13(4):366–376.

Koolstra JH, van Eijden TM. Biomechanical analysis of jaw-closing movements. J Dent Res 1995;74(9):1564–1570.

Kowalski LP, Carvalho AL, Martins Priante AV, et al. Predictive factors for distant metastasis from oral and oropharyngeal squamous cell carcinoma. Oral Oncol 2005;41:534–541 http://doi.org/10.1016/j.oraloncology.2005.01.012.

Kramer FJ, Dempf R, Bremer B. Efficacy of dental implants placed into fibula free flaps for orofacial reconstruction. Clin Oral Implants Res 2005;16:80–88.

Kratochvil FJ. Influence of occlusal rest position and clasp design on movement of abutment teeth. J Prosthet Dent 1963;13:114–124.

Krol AJ, Jacobson TE, Finzen FC. Removable partial denture design: Outline syllabus. 5th ed. San Rafael, CA: Indent; 1999.

Krysiński Z, Ludwiczak T, Mucha J. Comparative investigations of selected methods of evaluating the masticatory ability. J Prosthet Dent 1981;46(5):568–574.

Kumar BP, Venkatesh V, Kumar KAJ, et al. Mandibular reconstruction: Overview. J Maxillofac Oral Surg 2016;15(4):425–441.

Kuniyuki I, Hisaoka T, Ikeda R, et al. Changes in tongue pressure and dysphagia at oral cancer patients by palatal augmentation prosthesis. Cancer Rep (Hoboken) 2021:e1516.

Laaksonen JP, Loewen I, Wolfaardt JF, et al. Speech after tongue reconstruction and use of a palatal augmentation prosthesis: An acoustic case study. Can J Speech Language Pathol Audiol 2009;33:196–203.

Laaksonen JP, Rieger JM, Happonen RP, et al. Speech after radial forearm free flap reconstruction of the tongue: An acoustic follow-up study. Clin Linguist Phon 2010;24:41–54.

Laccourreye O, Hans S, Ménard M, et al. Transoral lateral oropharyngectomy for squamous cell carcinoma of the tonsillar region: II. An analysis of the incidence, related variables, and consequences of local recurrence. Arch Otolaryngol Head Neck Surg 2005;131(7):592–599.

LaFerriere KA, Sessions DG, Thawley SE, et al. Composite resection and reconstruction for oral cavity and oropharynx cancer. A functional approach. Arch Otolaryngol 1980;106(2):103–110.

Lam L, Samman N. Speech and swallowing following tongue cancer surgery and free flap reconstruction—a systematic review. Oral Oncol 2013;49(6):507–524.

Lam-Tang JA, Rieger JM, Wolfaardt JF. A review of functional outcomes related to prosthetic treatment after maxillary and mandibular reconstruction in patients with head and neck cancer. Int J Prosthodont 2008 Jul–Aug;21(4):337–354.

Langenbach GEJ, Hannam AG. The role of passive muscle tensions in a three-dimensional dynamic model of the human jaw. Archives of Oral Biology 1999;44(7):557–573.

Langenbach GEJ, Zhang F, Herring SW, et al. Modelling the masticatory biomechanics of a pig. J Anatomy 2002;201(5):383–393.

Langer A. The validity of maxillomandibular records made with trial and processed acrylic resin bases. J Prosthet Dent 1981;45(3):253–258.

Langius A, Lind MG. Well-being and coping in oral and pharyngeal cancer patients. Eur J Cancer B Oral Oncol 1995;31B(4):242–249.

Larsen MH, Lorenzen MM, Bakholdt V, et al. The prevalence of nerve injuries following neck dissections—a systematic review and meta-analysis. Dan Med J 2020;67(8):A08190464.

Laskar S, Basu A, Muckaden MA, et al. Osteosarcoma of the head and neck region: Lessons learned from a single-institution experience of 50 patients. Head Neck 2008;30:1020–1026.

Lauciello FR, Vergo T, Schaaf NG, et al. Prosthodontic and speech rehabilitation after partial and complete glossectomy. J Prosthet Dent 1980;43(2):204–211.

Lawson W, Loscalzo LJ, Baek SM, et al. Experience with immediate and delayed mandibular reconstruction. Laryngoscope 1982;92:5–10.

Leitzen C, Bootz F, Herberhold S, et al. Changes in taste during IM/IMRT radiotherapy for head and neck cancer patients. Paper presented at Strahlentherapie Und Onkologie, 2012.

Lekholm U, Gunne J, Henry P, et al. Survival of the Brånemark implant in partially edentulous jaws: A 10-year prospective multicenter study. Int J Oral Maxillofac Implants 1999;14:639–645.

Leonard RJ. Computerized design of speech prostheses. J Prosthet Dent 1991;66(2):224–230.

Leonard RJ, Gillis R. Differential effects of speech prostheses in glossectomized patients. J Prosthet Dent 1990;64:701–708.

Leone A. Toxics of tobacco smoke and cardiovascular system: From functional to cellular damage. Curr Pharm Des 2015.

Lewis, James S. Morphologic diversity in human papillomavirus-related oropharyngeal squamous cell carcinoma: Catch me if you can! Modern Pathology 2017;30(1):S44–S53.

Li H, Torabi SJ, Yarbrough WG, et al. Association of human papillomavirus status at head and neck carcinoma subsites with overall survival. JAMA Otolaryngol Head Neck Surg 2018;144(6):519–525.

Lim YC, Koo BS, Lee JS, et al. Distributions of cervical lymph node metastases in oropharyngeal carcinoma: Therapeutic implications for the N0 neck. Laryngoscope 2006a;116:1148–1152.

Lim YC, Lee JS, Koo BS, et al. Treatment of contralateral N0 neck in early squamous cell carcinoma of the oral tongue: Elective neck dissection versus observation. Laryngoscope 2006b;116:461–465.

Lin DT, Yarlagadda BB, Sethi RK, et al. Long-term functional outcomes of total glossectomy with or without total laryngectomy. JAMA Otolaryngol Head Neck Surg 2015 Sep;141(9):797–803. http://doi.org/10.1001/jamaoto.2015.1463. PMID: 26291031.

Listrom RD, Symington JM. Osseointegrated dental implants in conjunction with bone grafts. Int J Oral Maxillofac Surg 1988;17:116–118.

Lodi G, Sardella A, Bez C, et al. Interventions for treating oral leukoplakia. Cochrane Database Syst Rev 2006 Oct 18;(4).

Logemann JA. Evaluation and treatment of swallowing disorders. 2nd ed. Austin: Pro-Ed; 1998. pp. 24–29.

Lonie S, Herle P, Paddle A, et al. Mandibular reconstruction: meta-analysis of iliac- versus fibula-free flaps. ANZ J Surg 2016;86:337–342.

Loorents V, Rosell J, Karlsson C, et al. Prophylactic training for the prevention of radiotherapy-induced trismus—a randomised study. Acta Oncol 2014;53(4): 530–538.

Lott F, Levin B. Flange technique: An anatomic and physiologic approach to increased retention, function, comfort, and appearance of dentures. J Prosthet Dent 1966;16(3):394–413.

Lubbers HT, Kruse AL, Ettlin DA. Postradiation xerostomia and oral pain. J Am Dent Assoc 2014;145(9):964–965.

Lyford-Pike S, Peng S, Young GD, et al. Evidence for a role of the PD-1:PD-L1 pathway in immune resistance of HPV-associated head and neck squamous cell carcinoma. Cancer Res 2013 Mar 15;73(6):1733–41.

Magge KT, Myers EN, Johnson JT. Radiation following surgery for oral cancer: Impact on local control. Laryngoscope 2003;113(6):933–935.

Maghami EG, St-John M, Bhuta S, et al. Postirradiation sarcoma: A case report and current review. Am J Otolaryngol 2005;26:71–74.

Mak-Kregar S, Hilgers FJ, Levendag PC, et al. A nationwide study of the epidemiology, treatment and survival of oropharyngeal carcinoma in the Netherlands. Eur Arch Otorhinolaryngol 1995;252:133–138.

Manchester WM. Immediate reconstruction of the mandible and temporomandibular joint. Br J Plast Surg 1977;18:291.

Manly RS, Braley LC. Masticatory performance and efficiency. J Dent Res 1950;29(4): 448–462.

Manrique O, Leland H, Langevin C-J, et al. Optimizing outcomes following total and subtotal tongue reconstruction: A systematic review of the contemporary literature. J Reconstr Microsurg 2016;33(02):103–111.

Mardinger O, Givol N, Talmi YP, et al. Osteosarcoma of the jaw. The Chaim Sheba Medical Center experience. Oral Surg Oral Med Oral Pathol Oral Radiol Endod 2001;91:445–451.

Mariani PB, Kowalski LP, Magrin J. Reconstruction of large defects postmandibulectomy for oral cancer using plates and myocutaneous flaps: A long-term follow-up. Int J Oral Maxillofac Surg 2006;35(5):427–432.

Markowitz BL, Calcaterra TC. Preoperative assessment and surgical planning for patients undergoing immediate composite reconstruction of oromandibular defects. Clin Plast Surg 1994;21:9–14.

Martin-Harris B, Brodsky MB, Michel Y, et al. Delayed initiation of the pharyngeal swallow: Normal variability in adult swallows. J Speech Lang Hear Res 2007;50(3):585–594.

Marunick MT, Tselios N. The efficacy of palatal augmentation prostheses for speech and swallowing in patients undergoing glossectomy: A review of the literature. J Prosthet Dent 2004;91:67–74.

Marunick MT, Mathes BE, Klein BB, et al. Occlusal force after partial mandibular resection. J Prosthet Dent 1992a;67(6):835–838.

Marunick MT, Mathes BE, Klein BB. Masticatory function in hemimandibulectomy patients. J Oral Rehabil 1992b;19(3):289–295.

Marunick MT, Mathog RH. Mastication in patients treated for head and neck cancer: A pilot study. J Prosthet Dent 1990;63(5):566–573.

Marx RE. Current advances in reconstruction of the mandible in head and neck cancer surgery. Semin Surg Oncol 1991;7:47–57.

Marx RE. Philosophy and particulars of autogenous bone grafting. Oral Maxillofac Surg Clin North Am 1993;5:599–611.

Marx RE, Ames JR. The use of hyperbaric oxygen therapy in bone reconstruction of the irradiated and tissue deficient patient. J Oral Maxillofac Surg 1982;40:412–420.

Marx RE, Morales MJ. Morbidity from bone harvest in major jaw reconstruction: A randomized trial comparing the lateral anterior and posterior approaches to the ilium. J Oral Maxillofac Surg 1988;48:196–203.

Marx RE, Carlson ER, Eichstaedt RM, et al. Platelet-rich plasma: Growth factor enhancement for bone grafts. Oral Surg Oral Med Oral Pathol Oral Radiol Endod 1998 Jun;85(6):638–646.

Matsui Y, Shirota T, Yamashita Y, et al. Analyses of speech intelligibility in patients after glossectomy and reconstruction with fasciocutaneous/myocutaneous flaps. Int J Oral Maxillofac Surg 2009;38:339–345.

Mazzone A, Cusa C, Mazzucchelli I, et al. Cigarette smoking and hypertension influence nitric oxide release and plasma levels of adhesion molecule. Clin Chem Lab Med 2001 Sep;39(9):822–826.

McCauley RJ, Strand E, Lof GL, et al. Evidence-based systematic review: Effects of nonspeech oral motor exercises on speech. Am J Speech Lang Pathol 2009;18(4):343–360.

McClary AC, West RB, McClary AC, et al. Ameloblastoma: A clinical review and trends in management. Eur Arch Otorhinolaryngol 2016;273(7):1649–1661.

McConnel FM, Teichgraeber JF, Adler RK. A comparison of three methods of oral reconstruction. Arch Otolaryngol Head Neck Surg 1987;113(5):496–500.

McGuirt WF Jr, Johnson JT, Myers EN, et al. Floor of mouth carcinoma. The management of the clinically negative neck. Arch Otolaryngol Head Neck Surg 1995;121:278–282.

McNeil C. HPV in oropharyngeal cancers: New data inspire hope for vaccines. J Natl Cancer Inst 2000 May 3;92(9):680–681.

Mehlisch DR, Dahlin DC, Masson JK. Ameloblastoma: A clinicopathologic report. J Oral Surg 1972;30(1):9–22.

Mendenhall WM, Fernandes R, Werning JW, et al. Head and neck osteosarcoma. Am J Otolaryngol 2011;32:597–600.

Mendenhall WM, Morris CG, Amdur RJ, et al. Definitive radiotherapy for tonsillar squamous cell carcinoma. Am J Clin Oncol 2006;29:290–297.

Mendenhall WM, Stringer SP, Amdur RJ, et al. Is radiation therapy a preferred alternative to surgery for squamous cell carcinoma of the base of tongue? J Clin Oncol 2000;18:35–42.

Mendez E, Fan W, Choi P, et al. Tumor-specific genetic expression profile of metastatic oral squamous cell carcinoma. Head Neck 2007;29:803–814.

Mercadante S, Aielli F, Adile C, et al. Prevalence of oral mucositis, dry mouth, and dysphagia in advanced cancer patients. Support Care Cancer 2015;23(11):3249–3255.

Mian TA, Van Putten MC, Kramer DC, et al. Backscatter radiation at bone-titanium interface from high-energy X and gamma rays. Int J Radiat Oncol Biol Phys 1987;13(12):1943–1947.

Militsakh ON, Werle A, Mohyuddin N, et al. Comparison of radial forearm with fibula and scapula osteocutaneous free flaps for oromandibular reconstruction. Arch Otolaryngol Head Neck Surg 2005;131:571–575.

Mochizuki Y, Omura K, Harada H, et al. Functional outcomes and patient satisfaction after vascularized osteocutaneous scapula flap reconstruction of the mandible in patients with benign or cancerous tumours. Int J Oral Maxillofac Surg 2014 Nov;43(11):1330–1338. http://doi.org/10.1016/j.ijom.2014.06.012. Epub 2014 Jul 22. PMID: 25062550.

Mohit-Tabatabai MA, Sobel HJ, Rush BF, et al. Relation of thickness of floor of mouth stage I and II cancers to regional metastases. Am J Surg 1986;152:351–353.

Moore DJ. Glossectomy rehabilitation by mandibular tongue prosthesis. J Prosthet Dent 1972;28(4):429–433.

Moubayed SP, Barker DA, Razfar A, et al. Microvascular reconstruction of segmental mandibular defects without tracheostomy. Otolaryngol Head Neck Surg 2015;152(2):250–254.

Muller H, Slootweg PJ. The growth characteristics of multilocular ameloblastomas: A histological investigation with some inferences with regard to operative procedures. J Oral Maxillofac Surg 1985;13:224–230.

Munde A, Karle R. Proliferative verrucous leukoplakia: An update. J Cancer Res Ther 2016 Apr–Jun;12(2):469–73.

Myers JN, Elkins T, Roberts D, et al. Squamous cell carcinoma of the tongue in young adults: Increasing incidence and factors that predict treatment outcomes. Otolaryngol Head Neck Surg 2000;122:44–51.

Nabili V, Knott PD. Advanced lip reconstruction: Functional and aesthetic considerations. Facial Plast Surg 2008;24(1):92–104.

Nakamura N, Higuchi Y, Mitsuyasu T, et al. Comparison of long-term results between different approaches to ameloblastoma. Oral Surg Oral Med Oral Pathol Oral Radiol Endod 2002 Jan;93(1):13–20.

Namaki S, Matsumoto M, Ohba H, et al. Masticatory efficiency before and after surgery in oral cancer patients: Comparative study of glossectomy, marginal mandibulectomy and segmental mandibulectomy. J Oral Sci 2004;46(2):113–117.

Napier SS, Speight PM. Natural history of potentially malignant oral lesions and conditions: An overview of the literature. J Oral Pathol Med 2008 Jan;37(1):1–10.

Nason RW, Sako K, Beecroft WA, et al. Surgical management of squamous cell carcinoma of the floor of the mouth. Am J Surg 1989;158:292–296.

Nelson GJ. Three dimensional computer modeling of human mandibular biomechanics. Vancouver: University of British Columbia; 1986.

Newkirk KA, Cullen K, Harter W, et al. Planned neck dissection for advanced primary head and neck malignancy treated with organ preservation therapy: Disease control and survival outcomes. Head Neck 2001;23:73–79.

Nichols AC, Theurer J, Prisman E, et al. Randomized trial of radiotherapy versus transoral robotic surgery for oropharyngeal squamous cell carcinoma: Long-term results of the ORATOR trial. J Clin Oncol 2022;40(8):866–875.

Noone AM, Howlader N, Krapcho M, et al., editors. SEER Cancer Statistics Review. Bethesda (MD): National Cancer Institute; 1975–2015.

Obwegeser HL. Chirurgie pre-prosthetique: Vestibuloplasties. Prat Odontol Stomatol 1963:1357.

Ochi M, Kanazawa M, Sato D, et al. Factors affecting accuracy of implant placement with mucosa-supported stereolithographic surgical guides in edentulous mandibles. Comput Biol Med 2013;43:1653–1660.

Oda D, Bavisotto LM, Schmidt RA, et al. Head and neck osteosarcoma at the University of Washington. Head Neck 1997;19:513–523.

Odar K, Kocjan BJ, Hošnjak L, et al. Verrucous carcinoma of the head and neck—not a human papillomavirus-related tumour? J Cell Mol Med 2014 Apr;18(4):635–645.

Ogunlewe MO, Ajayi OF, Adeyemo WL, et al. Osteogenic sarcoma of the jaw bones: A single institution experience over a 21-year period. Oral Surg Oral Med Oral Pathol Oral Radiol Endod 2006;101:76–81.

Ohkoshi A, Ogawa T, Nakanome A, et al. Predictors of chewing and swallowing disorders after surgery for locally advanced oral cancer with free flap reconstruction: A prospective, observational study. Surg Oncol 2018;27(3):490–494.

Okay DJ, Buchbinder D, Urken M, et al. Computer-assisted implant rehabilitation of maxillomandibular defects reconstructed with vascularized bone free flaps. JAMA Otolaryngol Head Neck Surg 2013;139:371–81.

Old LJ, Boyse EA, Oettgen HF, et al. Precipitating antibody in human serum to an antigen present in cultured Burkitt's lymphoma cells. Proc Natl Acad Sci USA 1966;56(6):1699.

Olthoff LW, van der Bilt A, Bosman F, et al. Distribution of particle sizes in food comminuted by human mastication. Arch Oral Biol 1984;29(11):899–903.

Owadally W, Hurt C, Timmins H, et al. PATHOS: A phase II/III trial of risk-stratified, reduced intensity adjuvant treatment in patients undergoing transoral surgery for human papillomavirus (HPV) positive oropharyngeal cancer. BMC Cancer 2015;15:602.

Pai P, Tuljapurkar V, Balaji A, et al. Comparative study of functional outcomes following surgical treatment of early tongue cancer. Head Neck 2021 Oct;43(10):3142–3152. http://doi.org/10.1002/hed.26811. Epub 2021 Jul 24. PMID: 34302408.

Paley MD, Lloyd CJ, Penfold CN. Total mandibular reconstruction for massive osteolysis of the mandible (Gorham-Stout syndrome). Br J Oral Maxillofac Surg 2005;43:166–168.

Pandian V, Miller CR, Schiavi AJ, et al. Utilization of a standardized tracheostomy capping and decannulation protocol to improve patient safety. Laryngoscope 2014;124(8):1794–1800.

Parsons JT, Mendenhall WM, Stringer SP, et al. Squamous cell carcinoma of the oropharynx: Surgery, radiation therapy, or both. Cancer 2002;94:2967–2980.

Patel A, Harrison P, Cheng A, et al. Fibular reconstruction of the maxilla and mandible with immediate implant-supported prosthetic rehabilitation: Jaw in a day. Oral Maxillofac Surg Clin North Am 2019;31(3):369–386.

Patel SG, Deshmukh SP, Savant DN, et al. Comparative evaluation of function after surgery for cancer of the alveolobuccal complex. J Oral Maxillofac Surg 1996;54(6):698–703, discussion 703–704.

Patel UA, Hartig GK, Hanasono MM, et al. Locoregional flaps for oral cavity reconstruction: A review of modern options. Otolaryngol Head Neck Surg 2017;157(2):201–209.

Patterson HC, Dobie RA, Cummings CW. Treatment of the clinically negative neck in floor of the mouth carcinoma. Laryngoscope 1984;94:820–824.

Pauloski BR, Logemann JA, Colangelo LA, et al. Effect of intraoral prostheses on swallowing function in postsurgical oral and oropharyngeal cancer patients. American Journal of Speech-Language Pathology 1996;5:31–46.

Pauloski BR, Logemann JA, Rademaker AW, et al. Speech and swallowing function after oral and oropharyngeal resections: One-year follow-up. Head Neck 1994;16:313–322.

Peck CC, Langenbach GE, Hannam AG. Dynamic simulation of muscle and articular properties during human wide jaw opening. Arch Oral Biol 2000;45(11):963–982.

Peck CC, Sooch AS, Hannam AG. Forces resisting jaw displacement in relaxed humans: A predominantly viscous phenomenon. J Oral Rehabil 2002;29(2):151–160.

Perez CA, Patel MM, Chao KS, et al. Carcinoma of the tonsillar fossa: Prognostic factors and long-term therapy outcome. Int J Radiat Oncol Biol Phys 1998;42:1077–1084.

Pernot M, Hoffstetter S, Peiffert D, et al. Epidermoid carcinomas of the floor of mouth treated by exclusive irradiation: Statistical study of a series of 207 cases. Radiother Oncol 1995;35:177–185.

Petrovic I, Ahmed ZU, Huryn, JM, et al. Oral rehabilitation for patients with marginal and segmental mandibulectomy: A retrospective review of 111 mandibular resection prostheses. J Prosthet Dent 2019 Jul;122(1):82–87.

Petrovic I, Rosen EB, Matros E, et al. Oral rehabilitation of the cancer patient: A formidable challenge. J Surg Oncol 2018;117:1729–1735.

Pfister DG, Spencer S, Adelstein D, et al. Head and neck cancers, version 2.2020, NCCN Clinical Practice Guidelines in oncology. J Natl Compr Canc Netw 2020;18(7):873.

Pickup M, Novitskiy S, Moses HL. The roles of TGFβ in the tumour microenvironment. Nat Rev Cancer 2013 Nov;13(11):788–799.

Poulsen M, Porceddu SV, Kingsley PA, et al. Locally advanced tonsillar squamous cell carcinoma: Treatment approach revisited. Laryngoscope 2007;117:45–50.

Purdue MP, Hashibe M, Berthiller J, et al. Type of alcoholic beverage and risk of head and neck cancer—a pooled analysis within the INHANCE Consortium. Am J Epidemiol 2009 Jan 15;169(2):132–142.

Raffa M, Nguyen V, Hernigou P, et al. Stress shielding at the bone-implant interface: Influence of surface roughness and of the bone-implant contact ratio. J Orthop Res 2021;39;1174–1183.

Ragin CC, Langevin S, Rubin S, et al. Review of studies on metabolic genes and cancer in populations of African descent. Genet Med 2010;12(1):12–18.

Ramqvist T, Dalianis T. Oropharyngeal cancer epidemic and human papillomavirus. Emerg Infect Dis 2010;16:1671–1677.

Rangert BR, Sullivan RM, Jemt TM. Load factor control for implants in the posterior partially edentulous segment. Int J Oral Maxillofac Implants 1997;12:360–370.

Rehrmann A. Beutragzur alveolarkammplastik am unterfiefer. Zahnartzl Rundsch 1953;62:505–512.

Reibel J. Prognosis of oral pre-malignant lesions: Significance of clinical, histopathological, and molecular biological characteristics. Crit Rev Oral Biol Med 2003;14(1):47–62.

Reichart PA, Philipsen HP. Oral erythroplakia—a review. Oral Oncol 2005;41(6):551–561.

Reichart PA, Philipsen HP, Sonner S. Ameloblastoma: Biological profile of 3677 cases. Eur J Cancer B Oral Oncol 1995;31B(2):86–99.

Ren EC, Chan SH. Human leucocyte antigens and nasopharyngeal carcinoma. Clinical Science 1996;91(3):256–258.

Rentschler GJ, Mann MB. The effects of glossectomy or intelligibility of speech and oral perceptual discrimination. J Oral Surg 1980;38:348–354.

Robbins KT, Bowman JB, Jacob RF. Postglossectomy deglutitory and articulatory rehabilitation with palatal augmentation prosthesis. Arch Otolaryngol Head Neck Surg 1987;113:1214–1218.

Robbins KT, Clayman G, Levine PA, et al. Neck dissection classification update: Revisions proposed by the American Head and Neck Society and the American Academy of Otolaryngology—Head and Neck Surgery. Arch Otolaryngol Head Neck Surg 2002;128:751–758.

Robinson JE, Rubright WC. Use of a guide plane for maintaining the residual fragment in partial or hemi-mandibulectomy. Journal of Prosthetic Dentistry 1964;14(5):992–999.

Rodgers LW Jr, Stringer SP, Mendenhall WM, et al. Management of squamous cell carcinoma of the floor of mouth. Head Neck 1993;15:16–19.

Rogus-Pulia NM, Larson C, Mittal BB, et al. Effects of change in tongue pressure and salivary flow rate on swallow efficiency following chemoradiation treatment for head and neck cancer. Dysphagia 2016;31(5):687–696.

Rohner D, Bucher P, Hammer B. Prefabricated fibular flaps for reconstruction of defects of the maxillofacial skeleton: Planning, technique, and long-term experience. Int J Oral Maxillofac Implants 2013;28(5):e221–229.

Rohner D, Jaquiéry C, Kunz C, et al. Maxillofacial reconstruction with prefabricated osseous free flaps: A 3-year experience with 24 patients. Plast Reconstr Surg 2003;112(3):748–757.

Roumanas ED, Chang TL, Beumer J III. Use of osseointegrated implants in the restoration of head and neck defects. J Calif Dent Assoc 2006a;34:711–718.

Roumanas ED, Garrett N, Blackwell KE, et al. Masticatory and swallowing threshold performances with conventional and implant-supported prostheses after mandibular fibula free-flap reconstruction. J Prosthet Dent 2006b;96(4):289–297.

Roumanas ED, Markowitz BL, Lorant JA, et al. Reconstructed mandibular defects: Fibula free flaps and osseointegrated implants. Plast Reconstr Surg 1997;99(2):356–365.

Sakakibara A, Kusumoto J, Sakakibara S, et al. Effect of size difference between hemiglossectomy and reconstruction flap on oral functions: A retrospective cohort study. J Plast Reconstr Aesthet Surg 2019 Jul;72(7):1135–1141. http://doi.org/10.1016/j.bjps.2019.03.015. Epub 2019 Mar 23. PMID: 30930123.

Salibian AH, Allison GR, Rappaport I, et al. Total and subtotal glossectomy: Function after microvascular reconstruction. Plast Reconstr Surg 1990;85:513–524.

Sanders B, McKelvy B. Split-thickness skin grafts transplanted over exposed maxillary bone in dogs. J Oral Surg 1976;34(6):510–513.

Sanniec KJ, Carboy JA, Thornton JF. Simplifying lip reconstruction: An algorithmic approach. Semin Plast Surg 2018;32(2):69–74.

Sapp JP, Eversole LR, Wysocki GP. Contemporary oral and maxillofacial pathology. Vol. 450. St. Louis (MO): Mosby; 2004.

Schache AG, Lieger O, Rogers P, et al. Predictors of swallowing outcome in patients treated with surgery and radiotherapy for advanced oral and oropharyngeal cancer. Oral Oncol 2009;45(9):803–808.

Schiff BA, Roberts DB, El-Naggar A, et al. Selective vs modified radical neck dissection and postoperative radiotherapy vs observation in the treatment of squamous cell carcinoma of the oral tongue. Arch Otolaryngol Head Neck Surg 2005;131:874–878.

Schliephake H, Neukam FW, Schmelzeisen R, et al. Long-term quality of life after ablative intraoral tumour surgery. J Craniomaxillofac Surg 1995;23(4):243–249.

Schoen PJ, Raghoebar GM, Bouma J, et al. Prosthodontic rehabilitation of oral function in head-neck cancer patients with dental implants placed simultaneously during ablative tumour surgery: An assessment of treatment outcomes and quality of life. Int J Oral Maxillofac Surg 2008;37(1):8–16.

Schramm VL Jr, Johnson JT, Myers EN. Skin grafts and flaps in oral cavity reconstruction. Archives of Otolaryngology 1983;109(3):175–177.

Schuchardt K. Epidermis transplantation in plastic surgery of the mouth atrium. Dtsch Zahnarztl Z 1952;7(7):364–369.

Schwartz GJ, Mehta RH, Wenig BL, et al. Salvage treatment for recurrent squamous cell carcinoma of the oral cavity. Head Neck 2000;22:34–41.

Schwartz HC, Wollin M, Leake DL, et al. Interface radiation dosimetry in mandibular reconstruction. Arch Otolaryngol 1979;105:293–229.

Scott L. Speech rehabilitation for oral cancer patients—a pilot investigation [master's thesis]. Santa Barbara (CA): University of California; 1970.

See M, Morritt A, Jallali N. Lip reconstruction. In Plastic surgery—principles and practice. Ed. RD Farhadieh, NW Bulstrode, BJ Mehrara, et al. Amsterdam: Elsevier; 2022. pp. 398–410.

National Cancer Institute (NIH). Surveillance, Epidemiology and End Results (SEER) Program. 2019. https://seer.cancer.gov/.

Sehdev MK, Huvos AG, Strong EW, et al. Proceedings: Ameloblastoma of maxilla and mandible. Cancer 1974;33(2):324–333.

Seikaly H, Chau J, Li F, et al. Bone that best matches the properties of the mandible. J Otolaryngol 2003;32:262–265.

Seikaly H, Idris S, Chuka R, et al. The alberta reconstructive technique: An occlusion-driven and digitally based jaw reconstruction. Laryngoscope 2019;129(Suppl 4):S1–S14.

Seikaly H, Rieger J, O'Connell D, et al. Beavertail modification of the radial forearm free flap in base of tongue reconstruction: Technique and functional outcomes. Head & Neck 2009;31(2):213–219.

Seruya M, Fisher M, Rodriguez ED. Computer-assisted versus conventional free fibula flap technique for craniofacial reconstruction: an outcomes comparison. Plast Reconstr Surg 2013;132:1219–1228.

Sessions DG, Spector GJ, Lenox J, et al. Analysis of treatment results for floor-of-mouth cancer. Laryngoscope 2000;110:1764–1772.

Sessions DG, Spector GJ, Lenox J, et al. Analysis of treatment results for oral tongue cancer. Laryngoscope 2002;112:616–625.

Shah JP, Andersen PE. The impact of patterns of nodal metastasis on modifications of neck dissection. Ann Surg Oncol 1994;1:521–532.

Shaha AR, Spiro RH, Shah JP, et al. Squamous carcinomas of the floor of the mouth. Am J Surg 1984;148:455–459.

Shao Z, He Y, Wang L, et al. Computed tomography findings in radiation—induced osteosarcoma of the jaws. Oral Surg Oral Med Oral Pathol Oral Radiol Endod 2010;109:e88–e94.

Sharaf B, Levine JP, Hirsch DL, et al. Importance of computer-aided design and manufacturing technology in the multidisciplinary approach to head and neck reconstruction. J Craniofac Surg 2010;21(4):1277–1280.

Shatkin S, Hoffmeister FS. Ameloblastoma: A rational approach to therapy. Oral Surg Oral Med Oral Pathol 1965;20(4):421–435.

Shiboski CH, Schmidt BL, Jordan RC. Tongue and tonsil carcinoma: Increasing trends in the U.S. population ages 20–44 years. Cancer 2005;103:1843–1849.

Shimodaira K, Yoshida H, Yusa H, et al. Palatal augmentation prosthesis with alternative palatal vaults for speech and swallowing: A clinical report. J Prosthet Dent 1998;80:1–3.

Siegel RL, Miller KD, Jemal A. Cancer Statistics 2020. CA Cancer J Clin 2020 Jan;70(1):7–30.

Simó R, French G. The use of prophylactic antibiotics in head and neck oncological surgery. Curr Opin Otolaryngol Head Neck Surg 2006;14:55–61.

Singare S, Dichen L, Bingheng L, et al. Design and fabrication of custom mandible titanium tray based on rapid prototyping. Medical Engineering and Physics 2004;26:671–676.

Skelly M, Spector DJ, Donaldson RC, et al. Compensatory physiologic phonetics for the glossectomy patient. J Speech Hear Dis 1971;36:101–114.

Slaughter DP, Southwick HW, Smejkal W. Field cancerization in oral stratified squamous epithelium; clinical implications of multicentric origin. Cancer 1953 Sep;6(5):963–968.

Smeele LE, Kostense PJ, van der Waal I, et al. Effect of chemotherapy on survival of craniofacial osteosarcoma: A systematic review of 201 patients. J Clin Oncol 1997;15:363–367.

Smith RB, Apostolakis LW, Karnell LH, et al. National Cancer Data Base report on osteosarcoma of the head and neck. Cancer 2003;98:1670–1680.

Sonies CB. Considerations in evaluating and treating the oral stage of swallowing. Perspectives on Swallowing and Swallowing Disorders (Dysphagia) 2003;12(1):13–15.

Sparano A, Weinstein G, Chalian A, et al. Multivariate predictors of occult neck metastasis in early oral tongue cancer. Otolaryngol Head Neck Surg 2004;131:472–476.

Speksnijder CM, van der Bilt A, van der Glas HW, et al. Tongue function in patients treated for malignancies in tongue and/or floor of mouth; a one year prospective study. Int J Oral Maxillofac Surg 2011;40(12):1388–1394.

Spiro JD, Spiro RH, Shah JP, et al. Critical assessment of supraomohyoid neck dissection. Am J Surg 1988;156:286–289.

Stavness I, Hannam AG, Lloyd JE, et al. Predicting muscle patterns for hemimandibulectomy models. Comput Methods Biomech Biomed Engin 2010;13(4):483–491.

Stavness I, Nazari MA, Flynn C, et al. Coupled biomechanical modeling of the face, jaw, skull, tongue, and hyoid bone. In 3D multiscale physiological human. Ed. N Magnenat-Thalmann, O Ratib, HF Choi. London: Springer; 2014. pp. 253–274.

Steinhauser EW. Vestibuloplasty: Skin grafts. J Oral Surg 1971;29:777–785.

Stelzle F, Maier A, Nöth E, et al. Automatic quantification of speech intelligibility in patients after treatment for oral squamous cell carcinoma. J Oral Maxillofac Surg 2011 May;69(5):1493–1500. http://doi.org/10.1016/j.joms.2010.05.077. Epub 2011 Jan 8. PMID: 21216061.

Sturgis EM, Cinciripini PM. Trends in head and neck cancer incidence in relation to smoking prevalence: An emerging epidemic of human papillomavirus-associated cancers? Cancer 2007 Oct 1;110(7):1429–35.

Sturgis EM, Potter BO. Sarcomas of the head and neck region. Curr Opin Oncol 2003;15:239–252.

Su WF, Hsia YJ, Chang YC, et al. Functional comparison after reconstruction with a radial forearm free flap or a pectoralis major flap for cancer of the tongue. Otolaryngol Head Neck Surg 2003;128:412–418.

Sukato DC, Kerr R, Aghaloo T, et al. The implant-borne articulation splint in fibula free flap mandibular reconstruction: A technical note. J Craniofac Surg 2023 Oct 6.

Sun J, Weng Y, Li J, et al. Analysis of determinants on speech function after glossectomy. J Oral Maxillofac Surg 2007;65(10):1944–1950.

Sundaram K, Schwartz J, Har-El G, et al. Carcinoma of the oropharynx: Factors affecting outcome. Laryngoscope 2005;115:1536–1542.

Swisher-McClure S, Lukens JN, Aggarwal C, et al. A phase 2 trial of alternative volumes of oropharyngeal irradiation for de-intensification (Avoid): Omission of the resected primary tumor bed after transoral robotic surgery for human papilloma virus-related squamous cell carcinoma of the oropharynx. Int J Radiat Oncol Biol Phys 2020;106(4):725–732.

Swoope CC. Prosthetic management of resected edentulous mandibles. J Prosthet Dent 1969;21(2):197–202.

Tang JAL, Rieger JM, Wolfaardt JF. A review of functional outcomes related to prosthetic treatment after maxillary and mandibular reconstruction in patients with head and neck cancer. Int J Prosthodont 2008;21(4):337–354.

The International Dysphagia Diet Standardization Initiative 2019. Accessed 2022. https://iddsi.org/framework.

Thompson JA, Vakharia KT, Hatten KM. Advances in oral tongue reconstruction: A reconstructive paradigm and review of functional outcomes. Current Opinion in Otolaryngology & Head & Neck Surgery 2022;30(5):368–374.

Todd R, Donoff RB, and Wong DT. The molecular biology of oral carcinogenesis: Toward a tumor progression model. Oral Maxillofac Surg 1997 Jun;55(6): 613–623.

Togni L, Mascitti M, Vignigni A, et al. Treatment-related dysgeusia in oral and oropharyngeal cancer: A comprehensive review. Nutrients 2021;13(10):3325.

Toolson LB, Smith DE. A five-year longitudinal study of patients treated with overdentures. J Prosthet Dent 1983;49(6):749–756.

Toro C, Robiony M, Costa F, et al. Feasibility of preoperative planning using anatomical facsimile models for mandibular reconstruction. Head Face Med 2007;3:5.

Toto JM, Chang EI, Agag R, et al. Improved operative efficiency of free fibula flap mandible reconstruction with patient-specific, computer-guided preoperative planning. Head Neck 2015;37:1660–1664.

Trauner R. Alveoloplasty with ridge extensions on the lingual side of the lower jaw to solve the problem of a lower dental prosthesis. Oral Surg Oral Med Oral Pathol 1952;5(4):340–346.

Tso TV, Hurwitz M, Margalit DN, et al. Radiation dose enhancement associated with contemporary dental materials. J Prosthet Dent 2019;121(4):703–707.

Tsuchiya S, Nakatsuka T, Sakuraba M, et al. Clinical factors associated with postoperative complications and the functional outcome in mandibular reconstruction. Microsurgery 2013 Jul;33(5):337–341. http://doi.org/10.1002/micr.22090. Epub 2013 Apr 9. PMID: 23568609.

Ueda K, Tajima S, Oba S, et al. Mandibular contour reconstruction with three-dimensional computer-assisted models. Ann Plast Surg 2001;46(4):387–393.

United States Census Bureau. "Population." Accessed 22 Nov 2023. https://www.census.gov/topics/population.html.

Urist MR. Surface-decalcified allogeneic bone (SDAB) implants. A preliminary report of 10 cases and 25 comparable operations with undecalcified lyophilized bone implants. Clin Orthop Relat Res 1968;56:37–50.

Urken ML, Buchbinder D, Constantino PD, et al. Oromandibular reconstruction using composite flaps: Report of 210 cases. Arch Otolaryngol Head Neck Surg 1998;124:46–55.

Urken ML, Buchbinder D, Weinberg H, et al. Functional evaluation following microvascular oromandibular reconstruction of the oral cancer patient: A comparative study of reconstructed and nonreconstructed patients. Laryngoscope 1991a;101(9):935–950.

Urken ML, Weinberg H, Vickery C, et al. Oromandibular reconstruction using microvascular composite free flaps. Report of 71 cases and a new classification scheme for bony, soft-tissue, and neurologic defects. Arch Otolaryngol Head Neck Surg 1991b;117(7):733–744.

Usman S, Jamal A, Teh MT, et al. Major molecular signaling pathways in oral cancer associated with therapeutic resistance. Frontiers in Oral Health 2021 Jan 25;1:603160.

Uwiera T, Seikaly H, Rieger J, et al. Functional outcomes after hemiglossectomy and reconstruction with a bilobed radial forearm free flap. Journal of Otolaryngology 2004;33(6):356.

Vainshtein JM, Samuels S, Tao Y, et al. Impact of xerostomia on dysphagia after chemotherapy-intensity-modulated radiotherapy for oropharyngeal cancer: Prospective longitudinal study. Head Neck 2016;38(Suppl 1):E1605–1612.

van Eijden TM, Koolstra JH, Brugman P. Architecture of the human pterygoid muscles. J Dent Res 1995;74(8):1489–1495.

van Es RJ, Keus RB, van der Waal I, et al. Osteosarcoma of the jaw bones. Long-term follow up of 48 cases. Int J Oral Maxillofac Surg 1997;26:191–197.

Vandenbrouck C, Sancho-Garneir H, Chassagne D, et al. Elective versus therapeutic radical neck dissection in epidermoid carcinoma of the oral cavity: Results of a randomized clinical trial. Cancer 1980;46:386–390.

Verneuil A, Sapp P, Huang C, et al. Malignant ameloblastoma: Classification, diagnostic, and therapeutic challenges. Am J Otolaryngol 2002;23:44–48.

Vickers RA, Shapiro BL. The incidence of oral malignant neoplasia in an adult population of Minnesota. A report of results in oral cancer detection abstract 486. Washington, DC: Program of Abstracts and Papers, 45th General Meeting of the International Association for Dental Research; 16–19 Mar 1967.

Villa A, Vollemans M, De Moraes A, et al. Concordance of the WHO, RTOG, and CTCAE v4.0 grading scales for the evaluation of oral mucositis associated with chemoradiation therapy for the treatment of oral and oropharyngeal cancers. Support Care Cancer 2021;29(10):6061–6068.

Wald RM Jr, Calcaterra TC. Lower alveolar carcinoma. Segmental v marginal resection. Arch Otolaryngol Head Neck Surg 1983;109:578–582.

Walker TW, Modayil PC, Cascarini L, et al. Retrospective review of donor site complications after harvest of cancellous bone from the anteriomedial tibia. Br J Oral Maxillofac Surg 2009;47:20–22.

Wang L, Liu K, Shao Z, et al. Individual design of the anterolateral thigh flap for functional reconstruction after hemiglossectomy: Experience with 238 patients. Int J Oral Maxillofac Surg 2016 Jun;45(6):726–730. http://doi.org/10.1016/j.ijom.2015.11.020. Epub 2016 Jan 27. PMID: 26826782.

Wang TW, Gentzke AS, Creamer MR, et al. Tobacco product use and associated factors among middle and high school students—United States, 2019. MMWR Surveill Summ 2019;68(SS-12):1–22. http://doi.org/10.15585/mmwr.ss6812a1.

Wangsa D, Ryott M, Avall-Lundqvist E, et al. Ki-67 expression predicts locoregional recurrence in stage I oral tongue carcinoma. Br J Cancer 2008 Oct 7;99(7):1121–1128.

Watters AL, Cope S, Keller MN, et al. Prevalence of trismus in patients with head and neck cancer: A systematic review with meta-analysis. Head Neck 2019;41(9):3408–3421.

Weitz J, Bauer FJ, Hapfelmeier A, et al. Accuracy of mandibular reconstruction by three-dimensional guided vascularised fibular free flap after segmental mandibulectomy. Br J Oral Maxillofac Surg 2016;54:506–510.

Westra WH, Lewis JS. Update from the 4th edition of the World Health Organization classification of head and neck tumours: Oropharynx. Head and Neck Pathology 2017;11(1):41–47.

Wheeler RL, Logemann JA, Rosen MS. Maxillary reshaping prostheses: Effectiveness in improving speech and swallowing of postsurgical oral cancer patients. J Prosthet Dent 1980;43:313–319.

Whitehill TL, Ciocca V, Chan JC, et al. Acoustic analysis of vowels following glossectomy. Clin Linguist Phon 2006;20:135–140.

Wildt J, Bundgaard T, Bentzen SM. Delay in the diagnosis of oral squamous cell carcinoma. Clin Otolaryngol Allied Sci 1995;20:21–25.

Willen R, Nathenson A, Moberger G, et al. Squamous cell carcinoma of the gingiva. Histological classification and grading of malignancy. Acta Otolaryngol 1975;79:146–154.

Wołącewicz M, Becht R, Grywalska E, et al. Herpesviruses in Head and Neck Cancers. Viruses 2020 Feb 3;12(2):172. CDC 2008.

Wong RK, Poon ES, Woo CY, et al. Speech outcomes in Cantonese patients after glossectomy. Head Neck 2007;29:758–764.

World Health Organization WHO Report on the Global Tobacco Epidemic, 2017. https://www.who.int/publications.

Wu B, Abduo J, Lyons K, et al. Implant biomechanics, screw mechanics, and occlusal concepts for implant patients. In Fundamentals of implant dentistry: Prosthodontic principles. Ed. J Beumer, R Faulkner, K Shah, et al. Chicago: Quintessence; 2022a.

Wu J, Sun J, Shen SG, et al. Computer-assisted navigation: Its role in intraoperatively accurate mandibular reconstruction. Oral Surg Oral Med Oral Pathol Oral Radiol 2016;122(2):134–142.

Wu TJ, Saggi S, Badran KW, et al. Radial forearm free flap reconstruction of glossectomy defects without tracheostomy. Ann Otol Rhinol Laryngol 2022b;131(6):655–661.

Wu YQ, Huang W, Zhang ZY, et al. Clinical outcome of dental implants placed in fibula-free flaps for orofacial reconstruction. Clin Med J (Engl) 2008;121:1861–1865.

Wushou A, Wang M, Yibulayin F, et al. Patients with cT1N0M0 oral squamous cell carcinoma benefit from elective neck dissection: A SEER-based study. J Natl Compr Canc Netw 2021a;19(4):385–392.

Wushou A, Yibulayin F, Sheng L, et al. Elective neck dissection improves the survival of patients with T2N0M0 oral squamous cell carcinoma: A study of the SEER database. BMC Cancer 2021b;21(1):1309.

Yanai C, Kikutani T, Adachi M, et al. Functional outcome after total and subtotal glossectomy with free flap reconstruction. Head & Neck 2008;30(7):909–918.

Yang R, Tang Y, Zhang X, et al. Recurrence factors in pediatric ameloblastoma: Clinical features and a new classifcation system. Head Neck 2019;41(10):3491–3498.

Yerit KC, Posch M, Seemann M, et al. Implant survival in mandibles of irradiated oral cancer patients. Clin Oral Implants Res 2006;17(3):337–344.

Youmans SR, Stierwalt JA. Measures of tongue function related to normal swallowing. Dysphagia 2006;21(2):102–111.

Yuen PW, Lam KY, Chan AC, et al. Clinicopathological analysis of local spread of carcinoma of the tongue. Am J Surg 1998;175:242–244.

Yun IS, Lee DW, Lee WJ, et al. Correlation of Neotongue volume changes with functional outcomes after long-term follow-up of total glossectomy. Journal of Craniofacial Surgery 2010;21(1):111–116.

Zarbo RJ, Marunick MT, Johns R. Malignant ameloblastoma, spindle cell variant. Arch Path Lab Med 2003;127:352–355.

Zhang N, Liu S, Hu Z, et al. Accuracy of virtual surgical planning in two-jaw orthognathic surgery: Comparison of planned and actual results. Oral Surg Oral Med Oral Path Oral Radiol 2016;122:143–151.

Zhen W, Karnell LH, Hoffman HT, et al. The National Cancer Data Base report of squamous cell carcinoma of the base of tongue. Head Neck 2004;26:660–674.

Zheng GS, Su YX, Liao GQ, et al. Mandibular reconstruction assisted by preoperative simulation and accurate transferring templates: Preliminary report of clinical application. J Oral Maxillofac Surg 2013;71:1613–1618.

Chapter 3

Rehabilitation of Acquired Maxillary Defects

John Beumer III, Jay Jayanetti, Doke Buurman, Chris Butterworth, Suresh Nayar, Denny S. Chao, Mary Jue Xu, Patrick K. Ha

A rewarding area of prosthodontics is the rehabilitation of patients with acquired maxillary defects. The maxillofacial prosthodontist contributes to all facets of patient care, from diagnosis, planning, and treatment to rehabilitation. In many circumstances, the prosthetic prognosis is quite favorable and patients are pleased upon completion of rehabilitation. In dentulous patients with a reasonable distribution of healthy dentition and favorable defects, speech and swallowing are restored to normal, and masticatory performance is largely unaffected. However, in edentulous patients, and those dentate patients whose dentitions have been compromised or the defects extend across the midline, the outcomes with conventional obturator prostheses have been suboptimal. During the last 15 years, several new methods have evolved and have been refined in attempts to improve patient outcomes in such patients, including the use of zygomatic implants and removable overlay prostheses, restoring the defect with osteocutaneous flaps and implant-supported dental prostheses, and zygomatic implants and subperiosteal implants in combination with soft tissue vascularized flaps. The purpose of this chapter is to present the options available for the various patient groups and provide perspectives that will permit the clinician to make choices that best serve the needs of their patients.

It should not be forgotten that rehabilitation of such defects should be prosthodontically driven if ideal outcomes are to be achieved. Today, most implants are placed using either fully guided or semiguided implant surgery using surgical templates. Moreover, most surgical reconstructions are planned using CT scans and virtual surgical planning (VSP). When an oncologic defect is to be reconstructed primarily or implants are to be placed during surgical ablation, the prosthodontist, in collaboration with the oncologic surgeon and the reconstructive surgeon, identifies the most efficacious implant sites available following the anticipated surgical resection; determines the numbers, lengths, and diameter of implants required; and designs the surgical templates that are used to place the implants and for making osteotomy cuts of grafted bone segments.

Anatomy of the Palate and Paranasal Sinuses

Almost all acquired palatal defects are precipitated by resection of neoplasms of the palate and paranasal sinuses. The extent of the resection is dependent on the size, location, and potential behavior of the tumor. In general, malignant tumors require aggressive resection whereas benign neoplasms demand less extensive surgery. Most of the malignant tumors of this region are quite late to metastasize. Hence radical neck dissections are employed only when palpable nodal disease in the neck is detectable clinically or by radiologic studies. The pathogenesis and behavior of these tumors are best understood if the practitioner has appropriate knowledge and appreciation of the anatomy of the palate and paranasal sinuses.

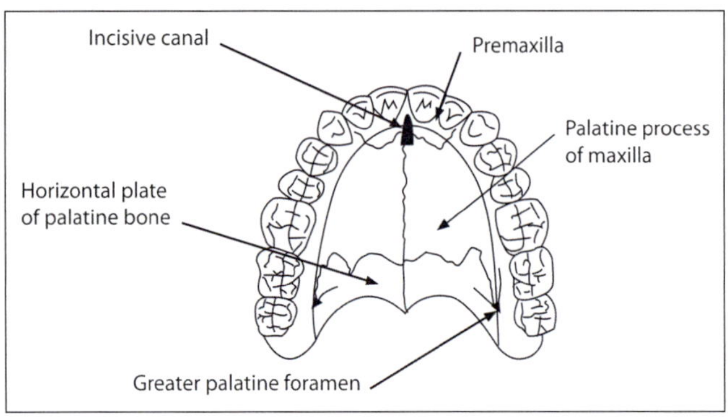

Figure 3-1 Bony anatomy of the palate.

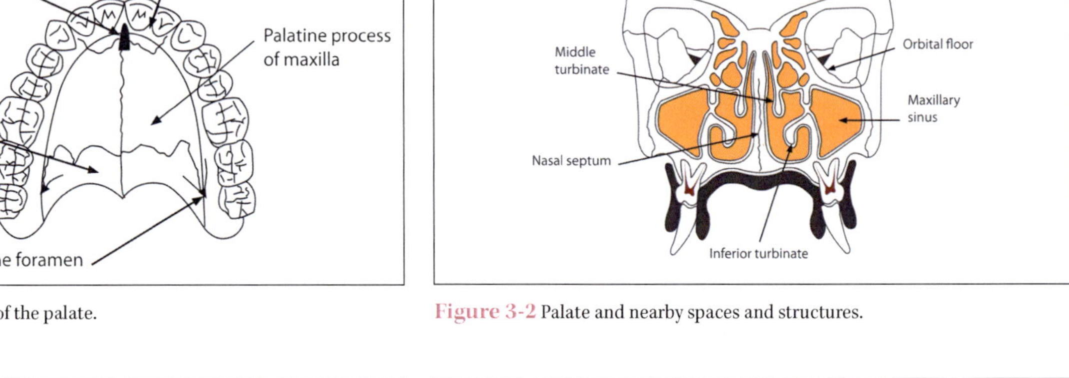

Figure 3-2 Palate and nearby spaces and structures.

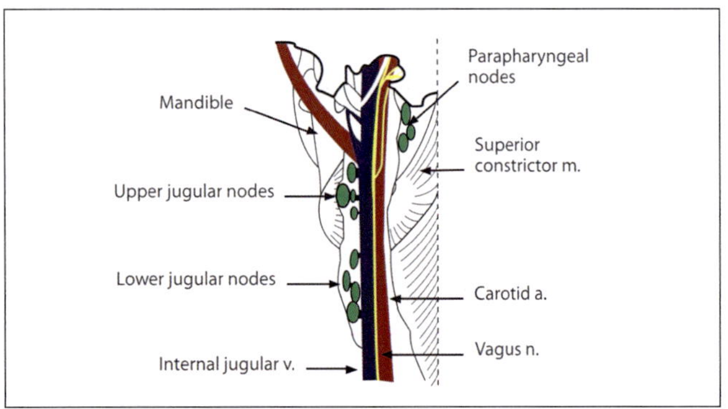

Figure 3-3 Lymphatic drainage from the palate.

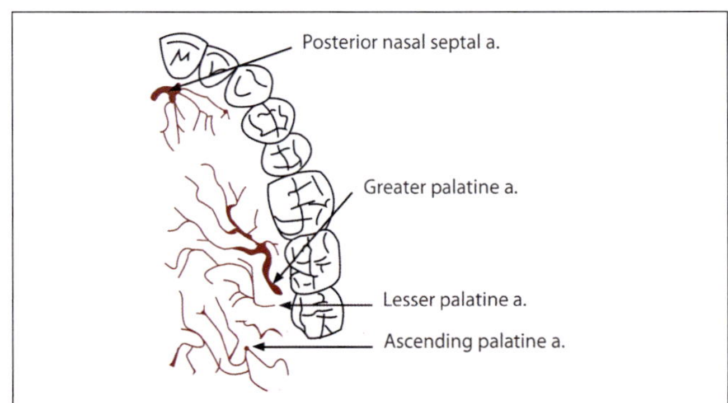

Figure 3-4 Blood supply to the palate.

The palate is composed of the maxillary and palatine bony plates. Anteriorly, the medial nasal process (anterior maxilla) carries the incisors, while, laterally, the maxillary alveolar processes bear the remaining maxillary teeth. A longitudinal suture divides the maxillary and palatine processes at the midline and a transverse suture separates the palatine bones from the maxillary processes of the palate (Fig 3-1). Blood vessels, nerves, and lymphatics traverse the palatine foramina and are located laterally and posteriorly.

The soft palate attaches to the posterior rim of the hard palate and has a posteromedial extension, the uvula. The soft palate contains a series of muscles that aid in the closure of the velopharyngeal complex during deglutition and speech and aid in opening of the eustachian tubes. The mucosa of the soft and hard palates is lined with stratified squamous epithelium and contains numerous minor salivary glands and some lymphatic tissue.

Except for the anterior maxilla, the palate arises from lateral palatine processes that fuse in the midline. Because of this embryologic feature, vascular, lymphatic, and neural elements are divided at the midline. This phenomenon explains why unilateral palatal and paranasal sinus tumors rarely demonstrate contralateral lymphatic spread (Fig 3-2). The midline may also serve as an effective anatomical barrier for resistance of local tumor extension and often serves as the medial surgical margin in resection of palatal and paranasal sinus tumors.

The lymphatics of the anterior maxillary alveolar ridge and anterior palate drain to the submandibular lymph nodes. The remaining bony palate drains to the superior jugular chain nodes. The soft palate drains posteriorly and laterally to the retropharyngeal and deep cervical nodes. The nasopharyngeal aspect of the soft palate, posterior nasal cavities, paranasal sinuses, and nasopharynx drain initially to the retropharyngeal nodes and later may extend to the deep cervical nodes or possibly directly to the deep cervical nodes. The lymphoid tissue within the adenoid pad comprising the Waldeyer ring drains to the superior deep cervical nodes (Fig 3-3).

Ohngren (1933) topographically classified the clinical behavior of sinonasal and palatal tumors based on their location. He postulated that more benign tumors tend to have an anteroinferior position, while more aggressive tumors tend to have a posterosuperior position. Although this generalized statement cannot be accurately applied in the absence of a pathologic diagnosis, it does have relevance with respect to the lymphatic drainage system of this region. The Ohngren line is an imaginary line between the medial canthus and the angle of the mandible. Tumors inferior to this line tend to drain to the submandibular and facial lymph nodes, whereas tumors superior to this line drain to the retropharyngeal nodes, resulting in a poorer ultimate outcome (Ohngren, 1933).

The vascular supply is of particular importance with regard to the control of bleeding, wound healing, wound closure, and reconstruction. The hard palate is supplied anteriorly by the posterior septal nasal artery, which enters via the incisive foramen in the midline, and the greater and lesser palatine arteries, which enter via the greater and lesser palatine foramina posterolaterally. The greater palatine artery supplies most of the hard palate. The lesser palatine artery supplies the junction of the soft and hard palates, whereas the ascending palatine artery supplies the soft palate. These vessels have rich anastomoses in the palate and deliver blood from a variety of sources (Fig 3-4). There are few anastomoses across the midline of the hard palate. In general, venous drainage parallels the arterial supply in the palate and finally drains through the external and deep facial veins to the external and internal jugular veins.

In general, foramina, lymphatics, blood vessels, nerves, and bone marrow spaces facilitate the spread of tumors, whereas periosteum, bone, and fascia can act as restrictive barriers. Once a tumor spreads into a space it tends to expand to fill it. For example, extension of a tumor along the palatine nerves can lead to tumor invasion through the pterygopalatine canal and into the pterygopalatine fossa. From here, the tumor may extend to the base of the brain via one of the foramina of the base of the skull or the inferior orbital fissure. Notably, perineural spread is especially prominent in adenoid cystic carcinoma.

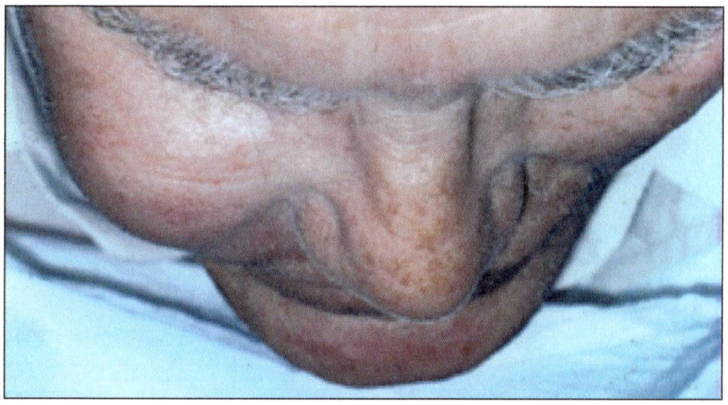

Figure 3-5 Swelling caused by a malignant tumor of the right maxillary sinus.

Neoplasms Resulting in Maxillary Defects

Neoplastic disease resulting in maxillary defects can originate from both the sinonasal and oral cavities. While this section will focus on these two anatomic subsites, it is noted that oropharyngeal malignancies can also result in soft palate defects that can be addressed with prostheses (see Chapter 4).

Sinonasal neoplasms

Sinonasal malignancies compose about 5% of all head and neck cancers (Dulguerov et al., 2001; Muir and Nantou, 1980). Among sinonasal cavity subsites, the most commonly involved are the maxillary sinus (50% to 70%) and the nasal cavity (15% to 20%) (Gotte et al., 2004). Risk factors for multiple histopathological types of malignancies include exposure to wood dust, leather, and textiles and aluminum occupational exposures (Hernberg et al., 1983; Luce et al., 1997; Demers et al., 1995). Aflatoxin, chromium, nickel, arsenic, and food industry chemical exposures have also been associated with squamous cell carcinoma of the sinonasal cavity (Leclerc et al., 1997). Furthermore, human papillomavirus (HPV) strains 6 and 11 are associated with inverted papilloma, a benign growth of the sinuses that has a 10% rate of conversion into squamous cell carcinoma, with higher risk conversion noted in patients who smoke tobacco (Kim et al., 2012; Durucu et al., 2009; Hong et al., 2013).

An estimated 76% of sinonasal malignancies present as late-stage (T3–4) disease (Bhattacharyya, 2003a, 2003b). Given their discrete location, patients often present with initially nonspecific nasal symptoms including nasal congestion, postnasal drip, facial pain and pressure, epistaxis, and facial swelling (Fig 3-5). With oral cavity involvement, patients may report dental pain and malocclusion; furthermore, trismus may be a clue that the pterygoid muscles are involved. Finally, orbital involvement may present with changes in vision and facial numbness from invasion of or pressure on the infraorbital nerve.

In terms of histopathologic classification, the World Health Organization divides sinonasal neoplasms into categories (Box 3-1; World Health Organization, 2005, 2017). Analyses of the United States Surveillance, Epidemiology, and End Results (SEER) database demonstrate that the most common sinonasal neoplasm is squamous cell carcinoma (SCC; Bhattacharyya, 2003a). In addition to SCC, common pathologies include adenoid cystic carcinoma, adenocarcinoma, sarcoma, mucosal melanoma, mucoepidermoid carcinoma, and undifferentiated carcinoma (Bhattacharyya, 2003a, 2003b). Lymphomas are rarer but can also present as sinonasal masses (Adwani et al., 2013; Dos Anjos Ramos et al., 2019). Lastly, tumors of the sinonasal cavity can also result from metastases from breast, kidney, and prostate cancers (Austin et al., 1995; Shome et al., 2007).

Oral cavity neoplasms

In addition to sinonasal malignancies, neoplasms of the oral cavity, specifically the hard palate and the retromolar trigone, can result in maxillary defects following resection. Among oral cavity malignant lesions, carcinomas of hard palate and the retromolar trigone make up 2.2% and 7.4% of all oral cavity lesions, respectively (Farhood et al., 2019). Tobacco and alcohol use are well-established, synergistic risk factors (Blot et al., 1988). Additional risk factors include betel nut chewing, Fanconi anemia, and immunosuppression such as HIV/AIDS (Birkeland et al., 2011; Butt et al., 2012).

Patients present with masses of the hard palate or retromolar trigone that can extend up to the hard palate or upper alveolar ridge (Fig 3-6). These lesions can be associated with bleeding and pain; additionally, trismus can indicate that the pterygoid muscles are involved. Given that benign and malignant lesions share similar presentations, biopsy is critical to ensure proper diagnosis (Kim et al., 2020).

Given the presence of minor salivary glands, any salivary pathology is included in the differential for oral cavity lesions. Benign lesions most commonly include pleomorphic adenomas and ameloblastomas. Pleomorphic adenomas are the most common benign salivary tumors with a low but increased risk of malignant transformation over time—1.5% over the first 5 years with an increase to 9.5% over 15 years (Kim et al., 2020; Seifert, 1992; Pires et al., 2007). Ameloblastomas are also benign lesions with the potential for mass effect as they grow and are managed with resection. Necrotizing sialometaplasia is an additional benign lesion that often appears as an ulcerative lesion that mimics squamous cell carcinoma or mucoepidermoid carcinoma; this lesion is thought to be reactive and self-resolves (Carlson, 2009). Common malignant

Box 3-1 World Health Organization classification of nasal cavity and paranasal sinus tumors

Carcinomas

- Keratinizing squamous cell carcinoma
- Nonkeratinizing squamous cell carcinoma
- Spindle cell (sarcomatoid) squamous cell carcinoma
- Lymphoepithelial carcinoma
- Sinonasal undifferentiated carcinoma
- NUT carcinoma
- Neuroendocrine carcinoma
- Adenocarcinoma
  - Intestinal-type adenocarcinoma
  - Non-intestinal-type adenocarcinoma

Teratocarcinosarcoma

Sinonasal papillomas

- Inverted papilloma
- Oncocytic papilloma
- Exophytic papilloma

Respiratory epithelial lesions

- Respiratory epithelial adenomatoid hamartoma
- Seromucinous hamartoma

Salivary gland tumors

Malignant	*Benign*
Adenoid cystic	Pleomorphic adenoma
Acinic cell	Myoepithelioma
Mucoepidermoid	Oncocytoma
Epithelial-myoepithelial	
Clear cell	
Myoepithelial	
Polymorphous adenocarcinoma	
Carcinoma ex-pleomorphic adenoma	

Soft tissue tumors

Malignant	*Borderline and low malignant potential*	*Benign*
Fibrosarcoma	Desmoid-type fibromatosis	Leiomyoma
Undifferentiated pleomorphic sarcoma	Sinonasal glomangiopericytoma	Hemangioma
Leiomyosarcoma	Solitary fibrous tumor	Schwannoma
Rhabdomyosarcoma	Epithelioid haemangioendothelioma	Neurofibroma
Angiosarcoma		
Malignant peripheral nerve sheath tumor		
Biphenotypic sinonasal sarcoma		
Synovial sarcoma		

Haematolymphoid tumors

- Extra nodal NK/T-cell lymphoma
- Extraosseous plasmacytoma

Neuroectodermal/melanocytic tumors

- Ewing sarcoma / primitive neuroectodermal tumors
- Olfactory neuroblastoma
- Mucosal melanoma

Other tumors

- Meningioma
- Sinonasal ameloblastoma
- Chondromesenchymal hamartoma

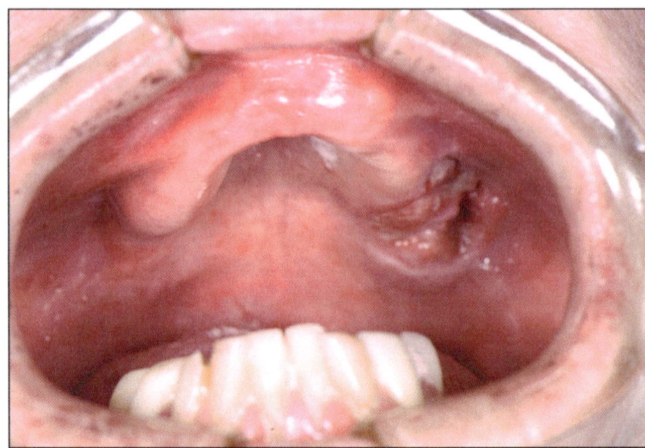

Figure 3-6 Typical squamous cell carcinoma arising from the palatal mucosa associated with leukoplakia.

lesions, similar to sinonasal malignancies, include squamous cell carcinoma, adenoid cystic carcinoma, mucoepidermoid carcinoma, adenocarcinoma, carcinoma ex-pleomorphic adenoma, and polymorphous adenocarcinoma (Kim et al., 2020; Moore et al., 2008; Buchner et al., 2007). Additionally, less common malignant lesions include acinic cell carcinoma and clear cell carcinoma (Buchner et al., 2007). Though rarer, lymphomas can also present as hard palate lesions (Nambiear et al., 2017).

Similar to the histopathologic classification of sinonasal neoplasms, the World Health Organization also classifies oral cavity neoplasms (Box 3-2; World Health Organization, 2005, 2017). These classifications emphasize the need for accurate pathology review.

Tumor behavior

The treatment, the resulting defect, and the prognosis for recurrence are dependent on the location, size, extension, and histologic characteristics of the lesion. Although many benign salivary gland and mesenchymal tumors appear well encapsulated, careful examination will often show invasion of soft tissue and even bone. For example, histopathologic studies have demonstrated that almost all pleomorphic adenomas have focally thin capsules, and one-fourth of pleomorphic adenomas demonstrate satellite nodules or pseudopodia extending beyond the capsule (Stennert et al., 2001). Therefore, the surgeon should be concerned about the existence of residual tumor after primary resection when review of the pathologic specimen does not suggest an intact capsule.

Malignant lesions, in addition to exhibiting aggressive local invasion, may extend along cranial nerves and marrow spaces and may metastasize to regional lymphatics as well as to distant sites. The extension of palatal tumors to the buccal mucosa, nasal cavity, paranasal sinuses, nasopharynx, pterygoid plates, or cranial foramina affects the prognosis adversely (Konrad et al., 1978).

A few prominent pathologies resulting in acquired or surgical maxillary defects require special attention. Squamous cell carcinoma spreads not only locally but along the regional lymphatics. The upper jugular digastric, nodes posterior to the sternocleidomastoid muscle, and parapharyngeal lymph nodes can also be involved. When tumors cross the midline of the palate, bilateral nodal involvement can occur. Tumors larger than 3 cm, extension to neighboring structures, and contralateral or bilateral lymph node metastases are associated with decreased survival (Konrad et al., 1978). When tumor thickness is greater than or equal to 3 mm, palpable adenopathy may be present (Baredes et al., 1993).

Adenoid cystic carcinomas are slower-growing malignancies. However, extended follow-up reveals that the prognosis for curing

Box 3-2 World Health Organization classification of tumors of the oral cavity

Malignant surface epithelial tumors

Squamous cell carcinoma

Oral potentially malignant disorders and oral epithelial dysplasia

Oral potentially malignant disorders
Oral epithelial dysplasia
Proliferative verrucous leukoplakia

Papillomas

Squamous cell papilloma
Condyloma acuminatum
Squamous cell papilloma
Condyloma acuminatum

Tumors of uncertain histogenesis

Congenital granular cell epulis
Ectomesenchymal chondromyxoid tumor

Soft tissue and neural tumors

Granular cell tumor
Rhabdomyosarcoma
Lymphangioma
Hemangioma
Schwannoma and neurofibroma
Kaposi sarcoma
Myofibroblastic sarcoma

Oral mucosal melanoma

Salivary type tumors

Malignant	*Benign*
Adenoid cystic	Pleomorphic adenoma
Acinic cell	Myoepithelioma
Mucoepidermoid	Oncocytoma
Epithelial-myoepithelial	
Clear cell	
Myoepithelial	
Polymorphous adenocarcinoma	
Carcinoma ex-pleomorphic adenoma	

Haematolymphoid tumors

CD30-positive T-cell lymphoproliferative disorder
Plasmablastic lymphoma
Langerhans cell histiocytosis
Extramedullary myeloid sarcoma

these lesions is poor. Perineural spread is common, both by direct extension and by discontinuous or "skip" metastasis, and it is believed that this tumor has neurotropic factors. Regional cervical metastases are uncommon. However, late distant metastases occur, predominantly in the lung and bones. These tumors require aggressive local resection with liberal margins (Fig 3-7).

Diagnostic evaluation

Diagnostic imaging defines the extent of disease and, in some cases, ought to precede biopsy. Computed tomography (CT) without contrast is critical to assess bony hard palate or skull base involvement for oral cavity and sinonasal lesions, respectively. CT imaging with intravenous contrast can further delineate the extent of soft tissue disease in neoplasms with increased vasculature and demonstrate concerning metastatic lymph node disease in the retropharyngeal, parapharyngeal, and cervical regions.

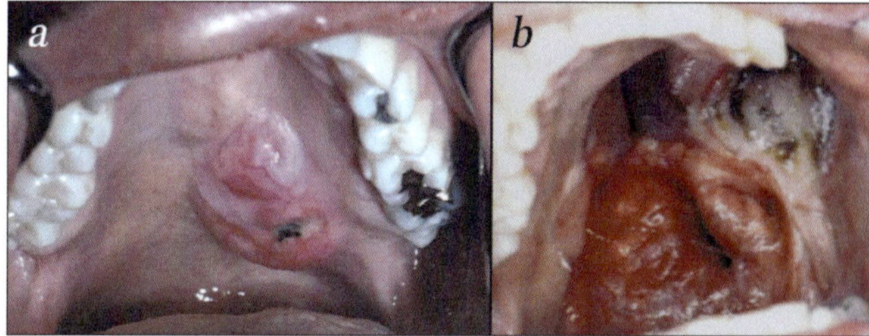

Figure 3-7 *(a)* Adenoid cystic carcinoma. These tumors require generous resection margins. *(b)* Large defect secondary to the resection of tumor shown in "a." The resection substantially crosses the midline and includes the soft palate.

Magnetic resonance imaging (MRI) is particularly valuable in cases of salivary malignancies; T1-weighted sequences with and without contrast, T2-weighted, and fat-suppressed sequences more clearly define the extent of soft tissue involvement compared to CT imaging. For malignancies with concern of neural invasion, enhancement along the nerve can be seen on MRI T1 postcontrast sequences (Loevner and Sonners, 2004). Finally, for sinonasal lesions, MRI should be used to identify encephaloceles prior to biopsy to prevent inadvertent cerebrospinal fluid leaks when sampling lesions.

In conjunction with imaging, tissue biopsy is the gold standard to confirm diagnosis and direct management. For sinonasal lesions, after an encephalocele has been excluded, biopsies can be performed in either the clinic or the operating room. Some clinicians prefer the operating room where patients are more comfortable, while larger amounts of tissue can be removed for pathology and more instruments are available for management of bleeding. Some sinonasal tumors that are not readily accessible may be more amenable to CT-guided biopsy. For oral cavity lesions, an incisional or punch biopsy is needed to assess for invasion of the basement membrane and depth of invasion, the latter of which has been incorporated in the latest American Joint Committee on Cancer (AJCC) staging system and associated with regional lymph node metastases (Lydiatt et al., 2017).

Following diagnostic evaluation, staging malignant tumors should be performed using the latest AJCC staging system.

Treatment

Management of patients with head and neck malignancies is interdisciplinary. Discussion at an interdisciplinary tumor board is recommended given the involvement of specialties including surgery (ablative and reconstructive), prosthodontics, radiation oncology, medical oncology, and speech-language pathology for rehabilitation. Any adjuvant treatment is recommended to initiate within six weeks following surgery (Network NCC, 2020). Expedited coordination of care is critical as delays in initiating adjuvant treatment have consistently been associated with poorer survival (Graboyes et al., 2019).

Surgical resection

Surgical resection of palate or sinonasal neoplasms require a spatial understanding of the maxilla and midface. The maxillary bone has been described as a hexahedron, a cube with faces of varying sizes with the hard palate sharing the same bony division as the floor of the maxillary sinus and nasal cavity (Cordeiro and Santamaria, 2000). Surgical resection needs to be performed with an adequate margin of normal tissue, leaving negative margins at the resection site. Given the function and anatomy of the oral cavity and paranasal sinuses, the width of clear margins depends on pathology and anatomic limits.

Importantly, before any surgical resection, which may result in a maxillary defect or involve dentition, it is critical for patients to receive surgical, dental, and prosthodontic consultations to discuss the best approach to rehabilitation and allow time for the creation of immediate surgical obturators if indicated.

Surgical resection can range from a limited palatectomy to various versions of maxillectomies. While there are many terms to describe approaches and resection of lesions involving the maxilla, the approach and reconstruction are always tailored to the lesion. Terms are briefly reviewed below.

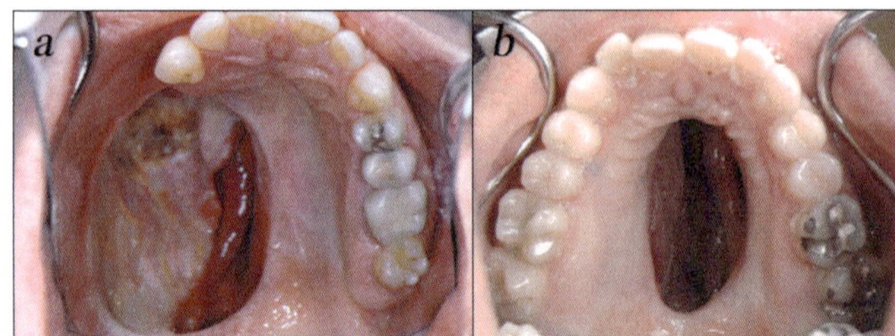

Figure 3-8 *(a and b)* Typical defects secondary to palatectomy for resection of benign tumors.

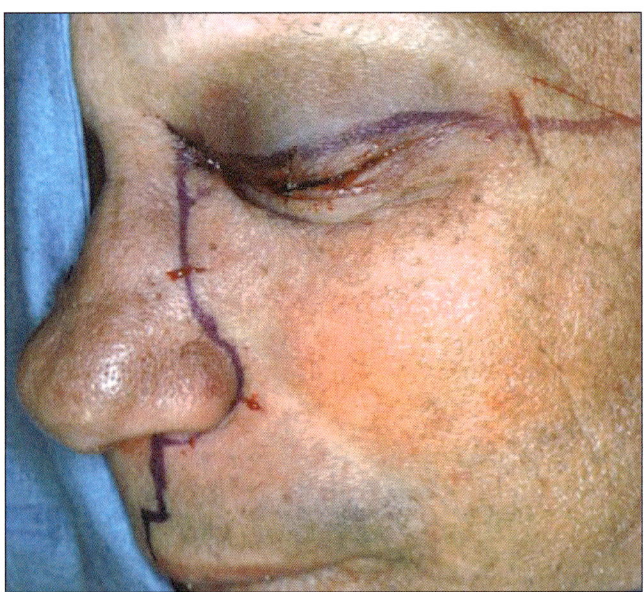

Figure 3-9 Skin incisions for maxillectomy (Weber-Ferguson incisions and exposure). Because the orbital contents were invaded by the tumor, the incision extends to the upper lid.

Palatectomy

Limited lesions of the palate are suited for a palatectomy (Fig 3-8). Preoperative appointments with the prosthodontist support patients by discussing dental rehabilitation options and allow time for design of immediate surgical obturators.

For resection, mucosal incisions are carried down to the periosteum. Surrounding tissue lateral to the lesion is elevated and may be used to cover exposed bone. Then using an osteotome or powered saw, bone cuts are made. Remnant mucosal flaps are laid down to promote healing. Additionally, any exposed tissue surfaces should be covered in split-thickness skin graft to promote epithelialization of raw surfaces. Without a skin graft, surgical sites can heal secondarily but the process may be prolonged and increased tissue contracture may occur. Iodine-impregnated gauze is packed into the site to prevent dead space and either a bolster or an obturator holds the packing in place for about one week. Obturators can be secured either to remaining dentition or with screws to stable, remaining hard palate bone (see section below entitled "Surgical obturation").

Maxillectomy

Approaches and exposure. Maxillectomies can be performed either open or endoscopically. Open approaches often require facial incisions for access. Common approaches include lateral rhinotomy, Weber-Ferguson, and the modifications to the Weber-Ferguson approach (Fig 3-9) (Shah et al., 2019). These incisions can be combined with sublabial and midface degloving approaches.

Types of maxillectomies. Maxillectomies are classified with varying nuances. Broadly, types of resections include medial maxillectomy; subtotal maxillectomy, which includes inferior maxillectomies; total maxillectomy with and without orbital exenteration; and maxillectomy with craniofacial resection (Gupta et al., 2020; Hanna, 2011).

Medial maxillectomies involve removal of the medial maxillary sinus wall, often including removal of the inferior turbinate, sphenoid, and ethmoid sinuses. This can be performed endoscopically or via an open approach with a lateral rhinotomy or midface degloving approach, the latter performed if bilateral maxillectomies are required. Medial maxillectomy can disrupt the vertical, medial maxillary buttress but leaves the remaining midface buttresses intact, thereby leaving midface volume and height intact (Hopper et al., 2006).

Infrastructure maxillectomies are suited for lesions of the alveolar ridge or hard palate that spare the maxillary antrostomy, orbital floor, and ethmoid sinuses. The orbital floor is left intact. These procedures often involve resection beginning with a sublabial or midface degloving incision. Following exposure, the infraorbital nerve is identified and preserved with resection inferior to this landmark. Incisions through the alveolar ridge should be made in the middle of tooth sockets to account for bone resorption at the osteotomy sites. Once the specimen has been removed and hemostasis obtained, tissue is repositioned over exposed bone, and a split-thickness skin graft can be placed over exposed tissue to prevent soft tissue contracture. Similar to a palatectomy as previously mentioned, iodine-impregnated gauze and an obturator or bolster help secure the surgical site during postoperative healing.

Suprastructure maxillectomies involve the orbital floor and upper portion of the maxilla, leaving the palate intact. Exposure can be similar to the above. However, the contents of the orbit are elevated subperiosteally for exposure of the inferior orbital floor and to keep the orbital fat contained and away from the resection site. Retraction and manipulation of the orbit must be done with careful attention.

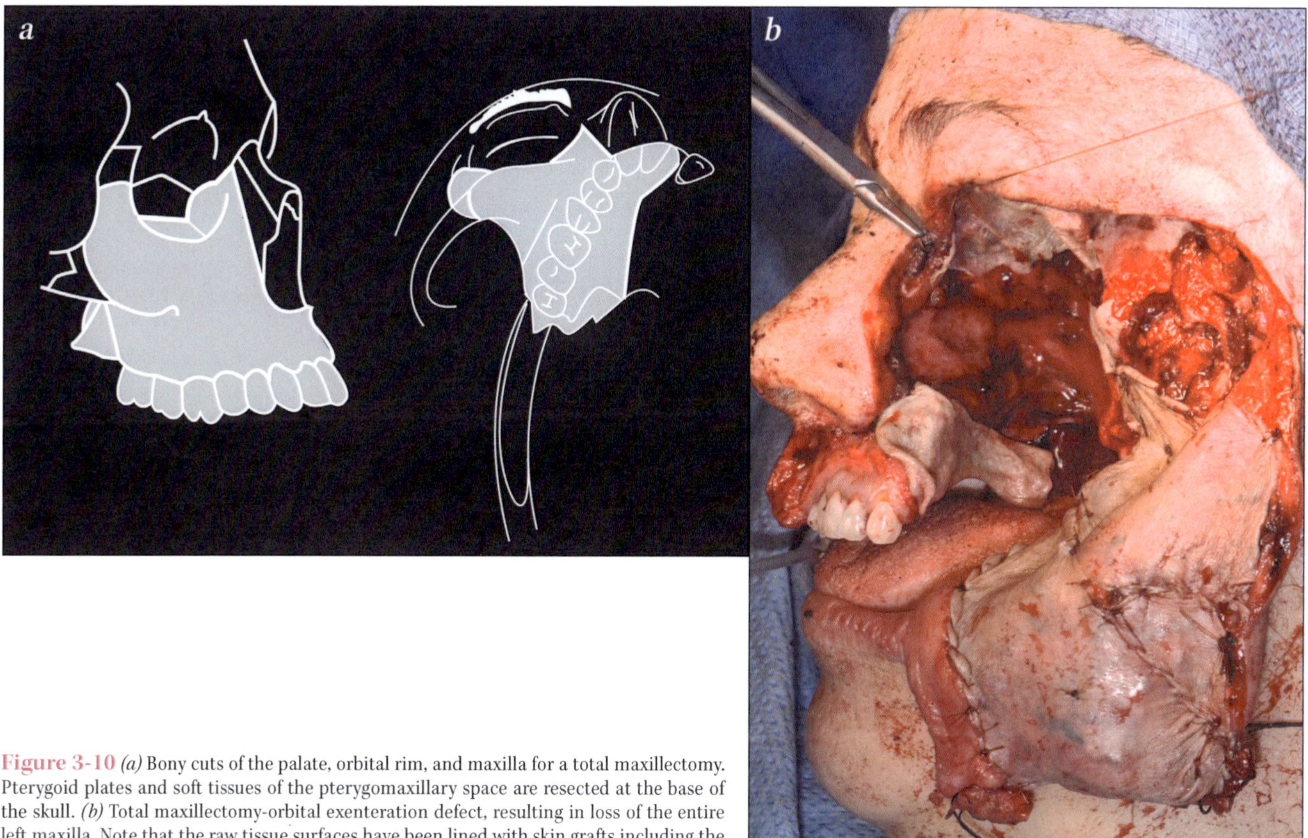

Figure 3-10 *(a)* Bony cuts of the palate, orbital rim, and maxilla for a total maxillectomy. Pterygoid plates and soft tissues of the pterygomaxillary space are resected at the base of the skull. *(b)* Total maxillectomy-orbital exenteration defect, resulting in loss of the entire left maxilla. Note that the raw tissue surfaces have been lined with skin grafts including the midpalatal bony cut.

Subtotal maxillectomies involve additional removal of the maxillary bone and often a combination of infrastructure and suprastructure maxillectomies.

Total maxillectomies involve complete resection of the maxillary bone (Fig 3-10). External incisions can involve lateral rhinotomy or Weber-Ferguson incisions with various modifications; incisions are combined with gingivobuccal and palate incisions as in the case of inferior maxillectomies. Orbital exenteration is indicated if there is gross invasion of the periorbital fat, extraocular muscles, or optic nerve but should only be included if this will impart a survival benefit (Gupta et al., 2020; Hanna, 2011).

Finally, craniofacial resections involve larger ablations for tumors that extend to the anterior cranial skull base, involving the cribriform plate or fovea ethmoidalis. Tumors such as esthesioneuroblastoma or olfactory neuroblastomas may require these resections. These surgical defects often require large, surgical osteocutaneous reconstruction with microvascular free flaps (Gupta et al., 2020).

Management of neck disease

Therapeutic neck dissections are indicated for clinically and radiologically detected neck disease and elective neck dissections are indicated when risk of occult metastases is greater than 15–20% of a given neck level (Ferlito et al., 2006).

For sinonasal malignancies, rates of occult metastases ranged from 12% to 25% (Dulguerov et al., 2001). In a recent study using the National Cancer Database to identify patients with T3/T4 sinonasal malignancy who had clinically undetectable neck disease and were surgically treated, Crawford et al. (2020) found that 19.6% of these patients underwent elective neck dissections with an occult neck metastasis rate of 12.7%. Furthermore, elective neck dissection did not impart a survival advantage (Crawford et al., 2020). In the context of these findings, each case still ought to be discussed at an interdisciplinary tumor board given the nuances of each tumor and the need for more research to better define treatment for each tumor subsite and pathology.

For oral cavity squamous cell carcinomas, elective neck dissections are further indicated when the depth of invasion of the lesion reaches a 3–4 mm threshold, at which the rate of occult neck disease is greater than 15–20% (D'Cruz et al., 2015). This threshold of depth of invasion has been studied largely in the context of oral tongue cancers but not as thoroughly in other oral cavity subsites. In a recent analysis of the National Cancer Database, 23% of patients with hard palate and upper gingival tumors and clinically node-negative neck disease underwent elective neck dissections, with 14% of these patients harboring occult neck metastases; while patients who underwent the elective neck dissections had improved survival, no variables in the study's analysis were predictive of occult metastases (Obayemi et al., 2019).

Adjuvant therapy

In terms of adjuvant therapy, commonly accepted indications for adjuvant radiation include close or positive margins, lymph node

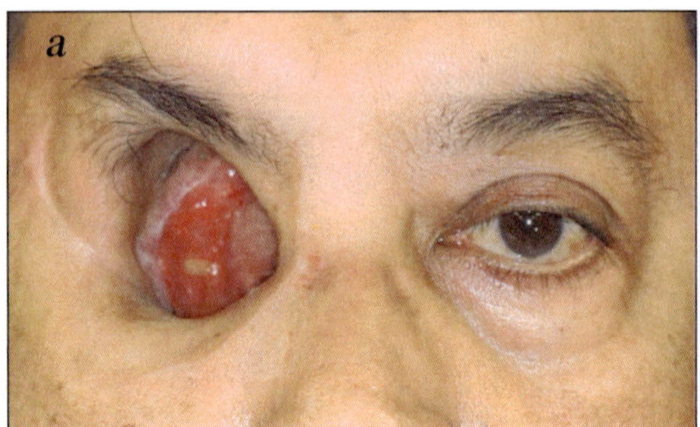

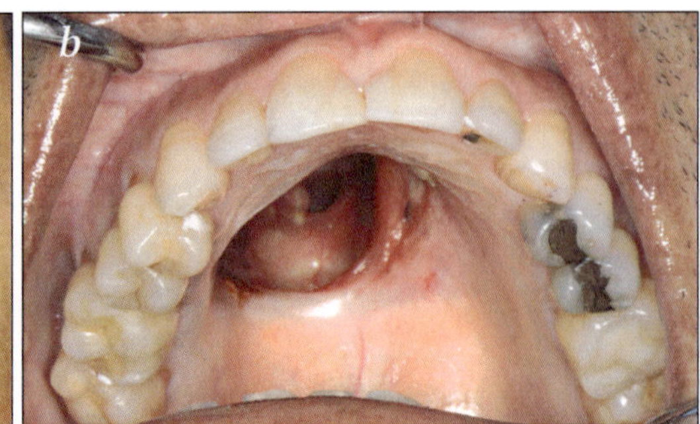

Figure 3-11 *(a and b)* Orbital and palatal defects were secondary to mucormycosis.

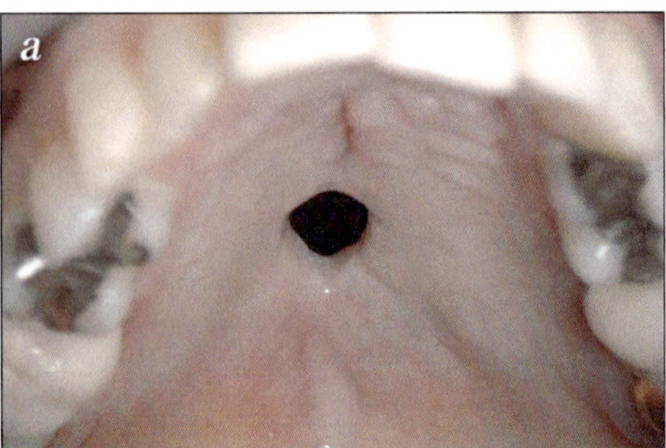

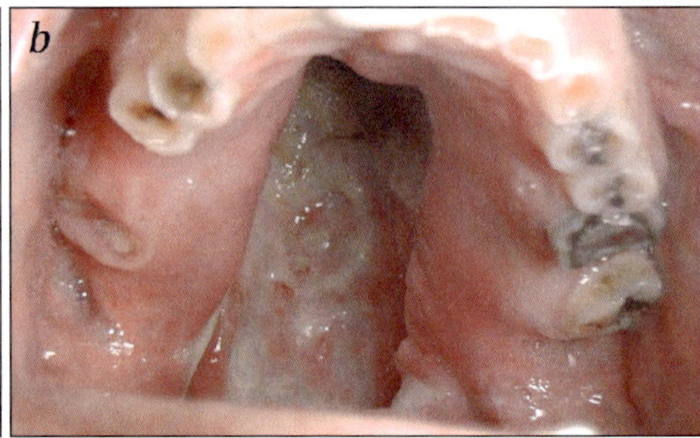

Figure 3-12 Palatal defects secondary to long-term cocaine use range from small perforations of the hard palate *(a)* to extensive defects *(b)*.

extracapsular extension, two or more positive lymph nodes, lymphovascular invasion, and perineural invasion (Network NCC, 2020). Indications for adjuvant chemotherapy include positive margins and extracapsular extension (Bernier et al., 2005). Given the heterogeneous nature of the patient populations in these studies, discussion at an interdisciplinary tumor board is again critical to personalize care for the patient and their specific disease process.

Outcomes

Survival from both sinonasal and oral cavity malignancies depends on tumor staging and varies by histopathology. Overall prognosis for sinonasal malignancies is estimated at 50% five-year survival with a 5–20% rate of neck metastases and a 17–25% rate of distant metastases (Gupta et al., 2020). The most aggressive neoplasms include mucosal melanomas with five-year overall survival of 10% to 42% (McLean et al., 2008; Shuman et al., 2011; Mihajlovic et al., 2012). SCC tends to be aggressive as well, with a five-year survival of 50–60%. Adenoid cystic carcinomas are slow-growing tumors with a high potential for local recurrence, but because of their slow growth rate, have a five-year survival of 73–90% (Lloyd et al., 2011). For oral cavity cancers, five-year overall survival is 50%, with slightly better survival for the retromolar trigone subsite compared to the hard palate (Farhood et al., 2019). Similar to sinonasal malignancies, survival depends on factors including stage and histopathology.

Other Causes of Palatal Defects

Midline granuloma and Wegener granulomatosis cause defects of the hard palate. These are rare lesions consisting of vasculitis and round cell infiltration that eventually lead to necrosis, usually of mucosa and bone of the midpalatal area. The use of cyclophosphamide, methotrexate, azathioprine, steroids, and radiation therapy has resulted in many long-term remissions in this previously rapidly fatal disease, making these patients candidates for rehabilitation of their palatal defect.

Mucormycosis and aspergillosis fungal infections can occur in patients with diabetes mellitus, in patients with major immune deficiencies, and in patients who take immunosuppressive medications. The infection usually involves the nasal cavity, maxilla, paranasal sinuses, and orbits. The organisms cause ascending venous thrombosis, resulting in necrosis of the involved structures.

Treatment may require extensive resection of the palate, maxilla, and facial tissues to remove the extent of necrosis. If the patient survives, the resulting defects often require prosthetic rehabilitation (Kurrasch et al., 1981; Barrak, 2007). These defects are more difficult to restore because they are generally lined with respiratory mucosa and poorly keratinized squamous epithelium, making it more difficult for the patient to tolerate the prosthesis (see Fig 3-11).

Persistent, long-term cocaine abuse can result in defects of the palate (Trimarchi et al., 2017; Fig 3-12). They vary from small perforations of the hard palate to large defects involving both the hard and soft palates.

Avulsive wounds of the maxilla may result in large defects that pose unique prosthodontic challenges (Fig 3-13). They differ from acquired maxillary defects in many important ways. Most of these defects are irregularly shaped and lined with poor-quality mucosa. There usually is significant scarring of tissues adjacent to the defect, and frequently, remaining maxillary segments are not secured to the cranial base. In addition, because many of these defects are self-inflicted these patients present with significant psychosocial challenges. A more detailed discussion of the prosthetic restoration of trauma-induced defects is found in Chapter 7.

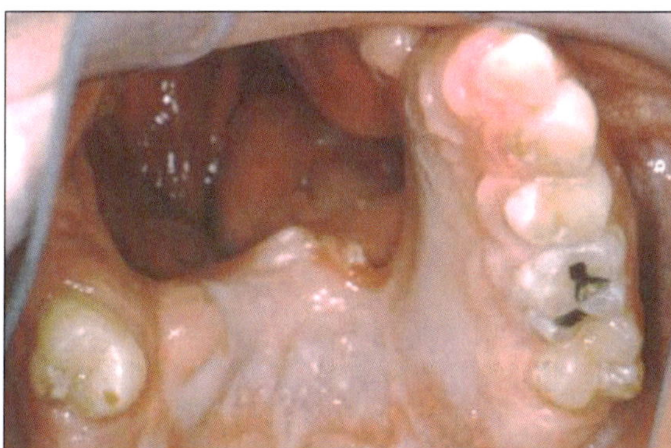

Figure 3-13 Large avulsive defect of the maxilla. These defects are usually irregular and lined with poor-quality mucosa.

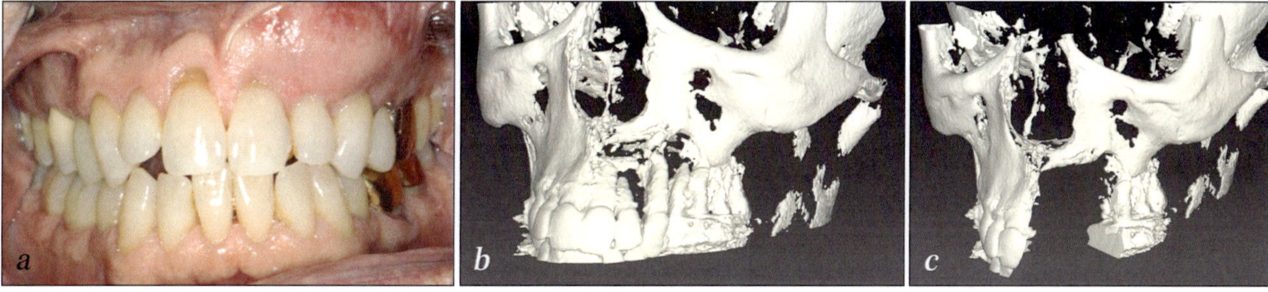

Figure 3-14 *(a)* Patient presents with an ameloblastoma of the palate. *(b)* 3D representation of the upper jaw showing the bone loss associated with the tumor. *(c)* A virtual surgical resection. With this information the prosthodontist can design the immediate surgical obturator and plan for the placement of implants at the time of tumor ablation.

Surgical Procedures during Tumor Ablation to Enhance the Prosthetic Prognosis

The goals of prosthetic rehabilitation are to restore the partition between the nasal and oral cavity, reestablish palatal contours and maintain the tongue space, replace the missing dentition, and restore midfacial contours. If the defect extends into the velopharyngeal area, access to the residual velopharyngeal musculature must be maintained so that the prosthesis can be molded to interact with the residual musculature to restore speech and swallowing. These goals can almost always be realized when good communication exists between prosthodontic and surgical colleagues. The result will be a surgical defect that is better suited for a prosthesis without compromising the resection of the tumor or the health of residual dentition and supporting structures. A well-designed defect will enhance the retention of, the stability of, and the support provided for the obturator prosthesis. To accomplish these goals, several issues and procedures during surgical resection of the tumor should be considered (Beumer et al., 1995).

This requires that a conference between surgeon and prosthodontist be conducted prior to surgery. Today with imaging and 3D reconstruction software, this conference can be conducted online. A virtual resection of the tumor can be carried out prior to surgery, identifying potential structures (teeth, implant sites) that can be retained and used to enhance the functional outcome achieved with the future obturator prosthesis (Fig 3-14).

In this chapter, the terms *total maxillectomy* and *partial maxillectomy* will be used instead of the term *radical maxillectomy*, often used by surgeons for almost any resection of the maxillae, because the former terms are more descriptive. Because the upper jaw contains two bones, or maxillae, a *total maxillectomy* is the complete resection of one of the two maxillae or resection to the midline. A *partial maxillectomy* is a bony resection that encompasses less than a total maxillectomy.

Management of the hard palate

An attempt should be made to save as much of the alveolar ridge and palatal vault as possible consistent with tumor control. Presurgical scans (CT scans, CBCT scans, and MRI) enable the surgeon to outline the extent of the tumor accurately and in three dimensions (Fig 3-14). Significant portions of the maxilla, particularly the anterior maxilla on the tumor side, can often be identified as being free of disease. In both dentulous and edentulous patients, retention of the anterior maxilla improves the prosthodontic prognosis immeasurably by enhancing the stability and support of the prosthesis (Fig 3-15). In dentate patients, partial denture designs are biomechanically more favorable, and in edentulous patients, stability and support are dramatically improved for the complete-denture-obturator prosthesis. Retention of portions of the anterior maxilla on the side of the tumor is particularly helpful in patients with tapering arches.

In edentulous patients, the anterior maxilla is a desirable site for implant placement. If more of this segment can be retained, then a

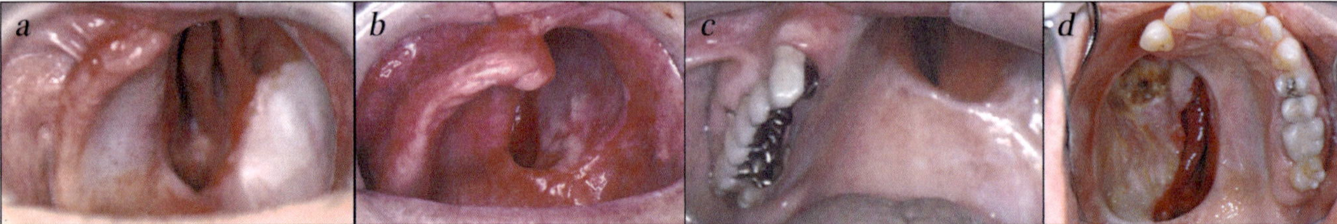

Figure 3-15 Benefits of retaining the anterior maxilla. *(a)* Tapering arch with resection to the midline. Stability and support for prosthesis would be enhanced if the anterior maxillary segment on the defect side could have been retained. *(b)* Ovoid arch with resection to the midline. The potential for stability and support for a prosthesis is greater than it is with the tapering arch because the palatal shelf area is larger. *(c)* Resection of the entire anterior maxillary segment, resulting in a linear arrangement of the remaining teeth. Indirect retention becomes impossible and retention and stability are compromised. *(d)* Defect that will have minimal impact on retention, stability, and support. The removable dental prosthesis (RDP) may be designed in a more conventional manner.

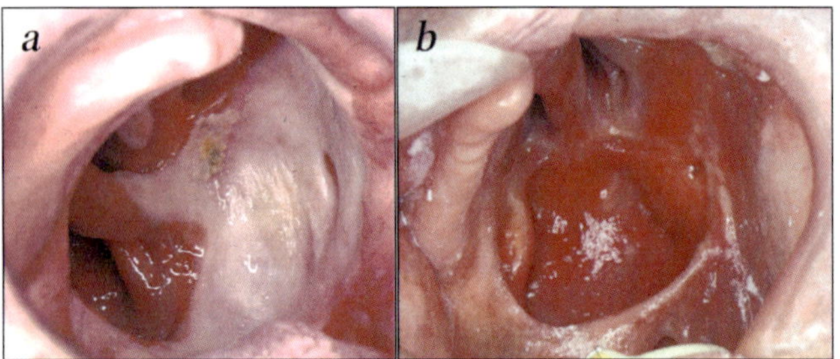

Figure 3-16 Benefits of skin grafting. *(a)* Defect lined with skin. These surfaces can be aggressively engaged prosthodontically, enhancing stability, retention, and support. *(b)* Defect lined with poorly keratinized squamous epithelium and respiratory epithelium. These surfaces are ill-suited to resist the abrasion associated with obturator use.

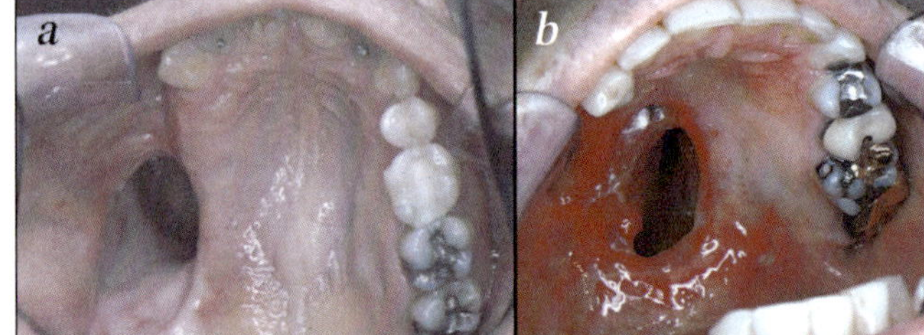

Figure 3-17 Difference in outcomes in two patients who underwent similar resections. *(a)* Skin graft was used to line the defect. *(b)* The wound was allowed to epithelialize spontaneously. The skin-lined defect can be used to help support, stabilize, and retain an obturator prosthesis, whereas the defect without a skin lining cannot be so utilized.

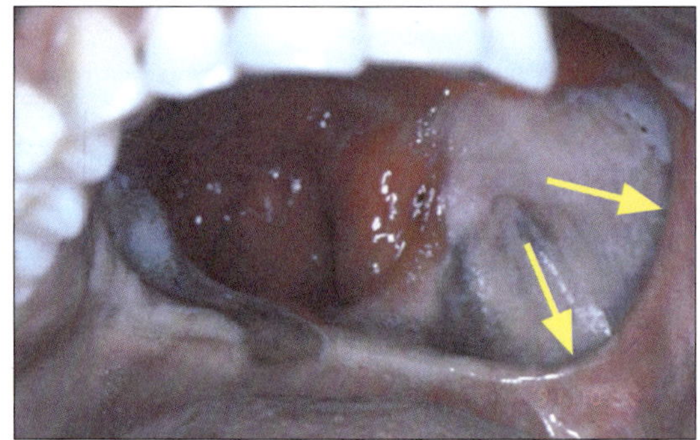

Figure 3-18 Left maxillectomy defect with a skin graft lining the buccal surface. Note the scar band *(arrows)* at the skin graft–mucosa junction.

greater number of implants can be placed. In addition, the increased anterior-posterior spread of the implants will allow them to better withstand the forces produced during mastication and improve the retention of the obturator prosthesis.

Skin grafting

In maxillectomy defects, the surgeon improves the tolerance and retention of the obturator if the raw tissue surfaces are lined with a split-thickness skin graft (Figs 3-16a and 3-17a). If the raw tissues resulting from the resection are not lined with a skin graft, these areas will granulate and eventually surface with either pseudostratified columnar or poorly keratinized squamous epithelium (Figs 3-16b and 3-17b). Highly keratinized skin-lined surfaces are more resistant to abrasion than these mucosal surfaces and therefore are a more suitable denture-bearing surface. The patient better tolerates the obturator prosthesis and the prosthesis can be designed to engage the defect more effectively, thereby improving retention, stability, and sometimes support for the obturator prosthesis, and more effectively sealing the oral cavity from the nasal cavities. The skin graft also limits scar contracture and increases the flexibility of the cheek. This enables the prosthodontist to displace the cheek on the resected side more readily and achieve better midfacial symmetry.

Additional benefits are derived from the scar band formed at the skin graft–mucosa junction. As this area contracts longitudinally during healing, it does so like a purse string, often creating a sizable lateral undercut superior to the scar band. This scar band is most prominent posterolaterally and tends to blend with the normal oral mucosa anteriorly and posteriorly (Beumer et al., 1995; Desjardins, 1978; Fig 3-18). Engaging the scar band superiorly and inferiorly with the prosthesis enhances its stability and retention.

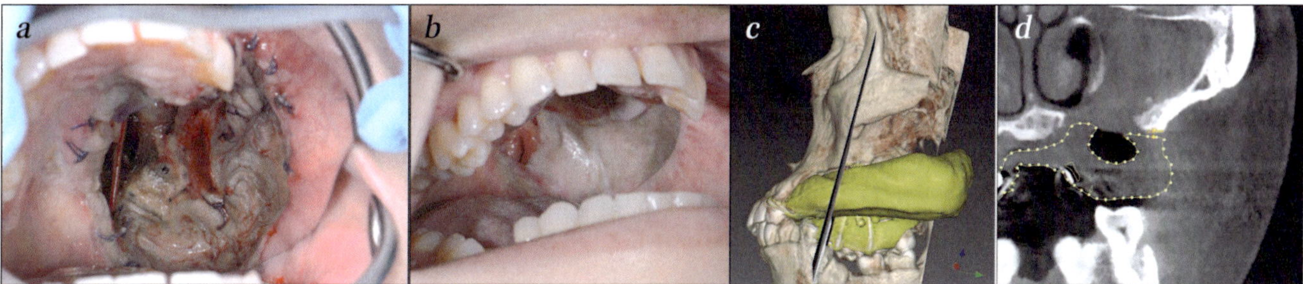

Figure 3-19 *(a)* The zygomaticoalveolar crest area has been lined with a split-thickness skin following a partial maxillectomy. *(b)* The healed site. *(c and d)* CBCT scan of the interim obturator prosthesis in position. These skin-lined areas provide valuable support on the defect side for the obturator prosthesis.

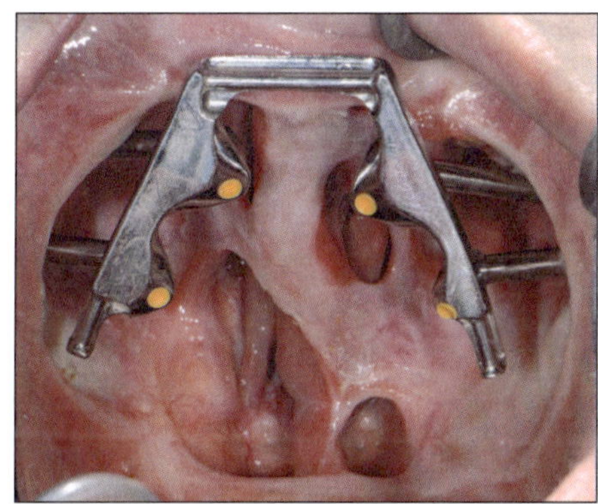

Figure 3-20 A total palatectomy defect restored with 4 zygomatic implants. The skin-lined soft tissues of the defect *minimize tissue contracture*, thereby maintaining prosthetic space and facilitating hygiene access for the zygomatic implants.

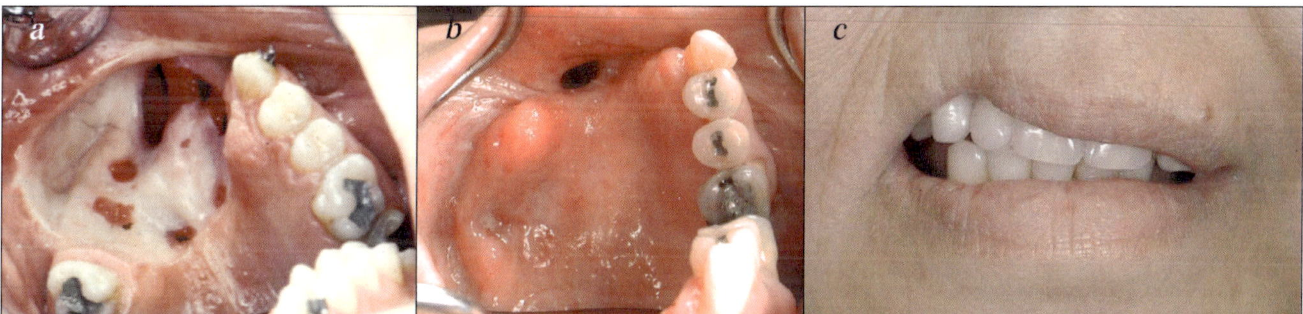

Figure 3-21 *(a)* Skin-lined defect. *(b and c)* A defect allowed to granulate and epithelialize spontaneously. Note the scarring and lip retraction in the defect that did not receive a skin graft.

If the surgeon is planning a maxillectomy, consideration should be given to stripping the nasal mucosa from the sinus side of the floor of the orbit laterally and lining this area with a skin graft. If oral access permits, engaging this surface with the prosthesis will provide support for the prosthesis on the side of the defect. However, in some patients, postsurgical trismus may preclude superior extension of the prosthesis into this area.

On some occasions, when a partial maxillectomy or palatectomy is performed, there remains a platform of bone associated with the residual zygomaticoalveolar crest (Fig 3-19). A modified vestibuloplasty can be accomplished by reflecting soft tissue laterally along the zygomaticoalveolar crest toward the body of the zygoma, laying a skin graft, and bolstering the graft with xeroform gauze. The bolster is held in position during healing with an immediate surgical obturator. This skin-lined area can then be engaged with the obturator prosthesis providing bony support on the defect side.

Skin grafting of the raw tissue surfaces secondary to tumor ablation is particularly critical to the prosthetic rehabilitation of total palatectomy defects. The placement of zygomatic implants does not obviate the need to line raw tissue surfaces secondary to the tumor ablation with skin grafts. They reduce soft tissue contracture, and skin-lined surfaces can be more aggressively engaged with the obturator extensions, thus achieving a better seal around the defect as well as improving lip and cheek contours (Fig 3-20). In addition, the prosthetic space is preserved and hygiene access around the bar and implants is enhanced (see section below entitled "Total palatectomy defects"). Skin grafting of anterior defects is equally desirable (Fig 3-21a). Skin grafting prevents undesirable contraction of the upper lip (Fig 3-21b and c) enabling the anterior extension of the prosthesis to provide more normal lip contours (see Figs 3-157 and 3-158).

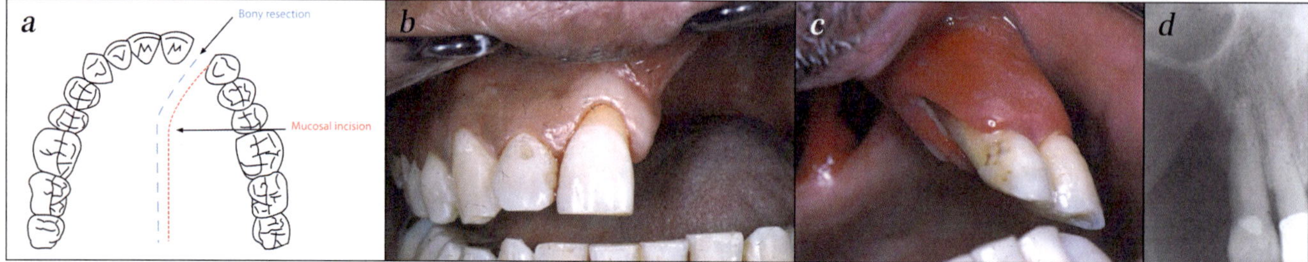

Figure 3-22 Benefits of tooth retention. *(a)* Resection planned for a left total maxillectomy. The left lateral incisor is extracted and a bony cut is made through the center of the socket. As the wound organizes and heals, ample bony support should remain for the left central incisor. Note the incision through the oral mucosa, lateral to the proposed medial resection of the bony palate. This mucosa is reflected and used to cover the medial margin of the defect after bony resection is completed. *(b)* The central incisor adjacent to defect retains ample bone and gingiva on the mesial aspect and can be used as a partial denture abutment. *(c)* During resection the bony cut was made too close to the root of this tooth, resulting in significant loss of bony support. *(d)* Radiograph showing the lack of bone on the mesial side of this tooth.

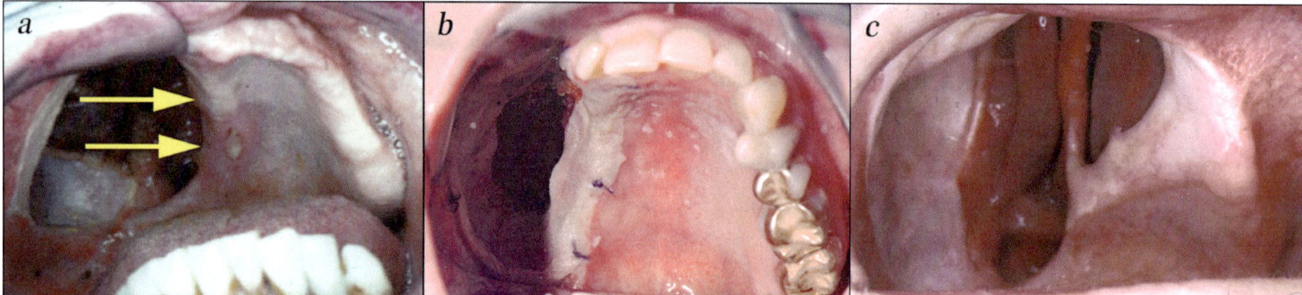

Figure 3-23 *(a)* Palatal mucosa used to cover the midpalatal bony resection *(arrows)*. *(b)* A skin graft has been used to resurface the medial portion as well as the lateral portion of the defect. *(c)* Skin graft lining the anterior wall of the maxillary sinus. Engaging these highly keratinized surfaces will enhance the stability of the prosthesis.

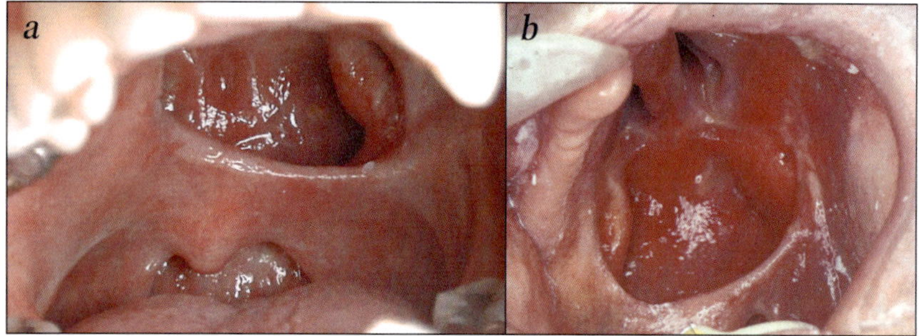

Figure 3-24 *(a)* The posterior third of the soft palate remains postsurgically. The remaining portion of the soft palate was nonfunctional and contracted superiorly, blocking access of the prosthesis to the posterolateral pharyngeal wall during movement. *(b)* The posterior third of the soft palate was maintained for this edentulous patient to aid retention of the obturator prosthesis by extending it superiorly over the nasal surface of the residual soft palate.

Retention of teeth adjacent to the defect

Transalveolar resections should be made as distant as feasible from the tooth adjacent to the resection. The next distal tooth should be extracted and the transalveolar cut made through the distal portion of this socket. This will result in the retention of more bony support and extend the clinical usefulness of the tooth adjacent to the resection (Fig 3-22a and b), making it a more effective abutment for the future RDP-obturator prosthesis.

The tooth adjacent to the resection will soon be lost if the resection is made through the transseptal bone approximating the tooth that borders the proposed defect (Fig 3-22c and d). Such teeth become mobile and/or symptomatic, often necessitating endodontic therapy, amputation at the gingival margin, or extraction. The canine is of particular importance to the prosthodontist because of its long root and greater bony support compared to its immediate neighbors.

Management of the palatal mucosa

If the surgeon can save some of the palatal mucosa normally included in the resection and reflect this tissue during the bony resection of the palate, it can be used later to cover the medial bony margin of the palatal bones (Fig 3-23a). This bony margin should be carefully rounded before it is covered with the palatal mucosa. In edentulous patients, the palatal margin of the defect often is the fulcrum around which the prosthesis rotates during function. If this margin is allowed to granulate and epithelialize spontaneously, it usually will be lined with poorly keratinized squamous epithelium or sometimes pseudostratified columnar epithelium. These types of epithelial linings are poor denture-bearing surfaces. If the palatal margin of the defect is covered with keratinized mucosa, the prosthesis may aggressively engage this surface, thus facilitating the lateral stability of the obturator prosthesis. If an adequate amount of palatal oral mucosa is not available because of the extent of the

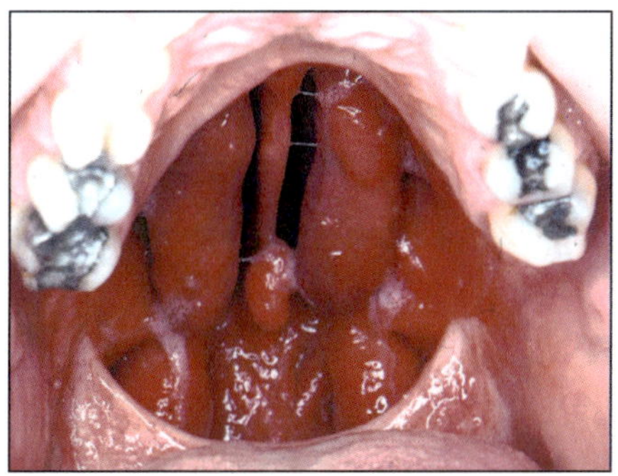

Figure 3-25 Residual turbinates restrict access to the defect and may distort the palatal contours of the prosthesis and impair the tongue space.

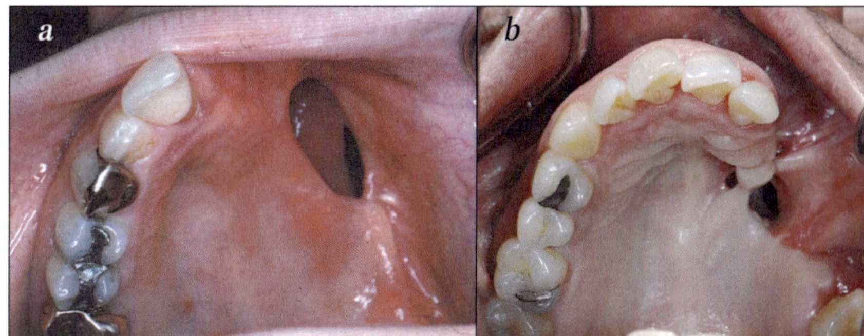

Figure 3-26 Limitations imposed by restricted access to the defect. *(a and b)* Attempts were made to close both these defects with local flaps. As a result, access is limited and the defect cannot be used to facilitate retention, support, and stability of the prosthesis.

tumor, placement of a split-thickness skin graft to cover the cut medial surface should be considered (Fig 3-23b and c).

Management of the soft palate

It is important that the remaining portion of the soft palate and associated pharyngeal wall musculature be able to properly interact with the obturator extension in order to retain the ability to affect velopharyngeal closure during speech and swallowing. With a maxillectomy or palatectomy that involves a significant portion of the soft palate or with resection of tumors primarily confined to the soft palate, the remaining portion of the soft palate must not block access to the residual velopharyngeal musculature, or speech and swallowing may be compromised.

The levator veli palatini muscle, which elevates the soft palate, is located in the middle third of the soft palate; if the resection extends posteriorly to involve the middle third of the soft palate, a posterior, narrow, nonfunctional band of intact soft palate may remain postsurgically (Fig 3-24a). This remnant will lack innervation and the capacity for normal elevation and these bands of residual soft palate often retract superiorly, preventing access for the obturator prosthesis to the posterolateral pharyngeal wall musculature still capable of contracting during speech and swallowing. As a result, the obturator will not be able to properly interact with the residual velopharyngeal musculature, resulting in hypernasal speech and leakage of fluids into the nasal cavity during swallowing.

Therefore, if one-third or less of the posterior aspect of the soft palate is to remain postsurgically on the resected side, the entire soft palate on that side should be removed. An exception can be made for the edentulous patient undergoing a total maxillectomy when the use of implants is precluded. Retention of the obturator prosthesis is always difficult in this situation and the extension of the obturator prosthesis to the nasal side of the residual soft palate is an advantage that outweighs the possible speech and leakage problems previously mentioned (Fig 3-24b).

Management of access to the defect

The surgeon should provide access to the superior and lateral aspects of the defect for the prosthodontist. Extension of the obturator up the lateral wall of the defect enhances the retention and stability of the prosthesis, and engagement of the lateral nasal side of the orbital floor or zygomaticoalveolar crest area provides support for the obturator prosthesis.

Moreover, structures such as the turbinates and bands of oral mucosa may prevent the prosthesis from engaging key areas of the defect, dramatically compromising function (Fig 3-25). If the postsurgical defect is large, these structures provide little benefit to the patient and severely limit the ability of the prosthodontist to seal the defect and provide proper obturation. Furthermore, the turbinates may enlarge because of changes in the normal nasal environment and from the leakage of food and liquids into the nasal cavity, which irritates these delicate structures. Edematous turbinates may extend inferiorly below normal palatal contours, distorting the contour of the palatal portion of the prosthesis and consequently limiting the tongue space and impairing tongue function and, with it, speech and swallowing. Consequently, these structures should be considered for resection during surgery. This suggestion may not apply to small midline defects of the hard palate–soft palate junction because significant extension superiorly into the defect is not as critical.

In most patients, closure of large maxillectomy defects with local flaps is discouraged (Fig 3-26). Lacking access to the defect, the stability, retention, and support for the obturator prosthesis will be compromised. Closure with vascularized soft tissue flaps is generally not advised unless zygomatic implants are placed into the zygoma and perforate the flap (see section below entitled "Zygomatic implant perforated (ZIP) technique").

Reconstruction of total maxillectomy defects with free vascularized soft tissue flaps is possible but undesirable from many perspectives. In noncompliant patients, mucus accumulates on the nasal cavity side of the defect. Lacking the usual ciliary network, these secretions pool, dry out, and become adherent to the nasal side of the flap, causing local infections and a strong, unpleasant odor. In addition, patients with total maxillectomy defects that have been closed with soft tissue flaps will likely present with compromised lip, cheek, and midfacial contours, which cannot be restored with a conventional RDP or complete denture. Moreover, frequently, these flaps distort the palatal contours and limit the tongue space, adversely affecting speech articulation. As a result, linguodental, linguoalveolar, linguopalatal, and velar consonant speech sounds are compromised (Matsui et al., 1995). The oral phase of swallowing may

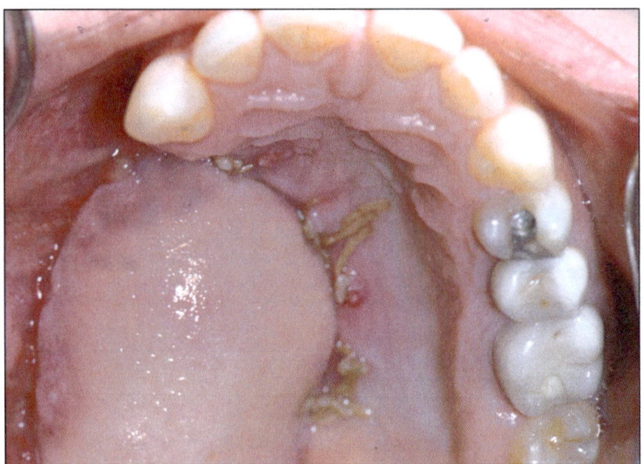

Figure 3-27 Radial forearm flap has been used to close the defect. The palatal contours are distorted and the tongue space is impaired. Moreover, prosthetic space is lacking for the placement of teeth.

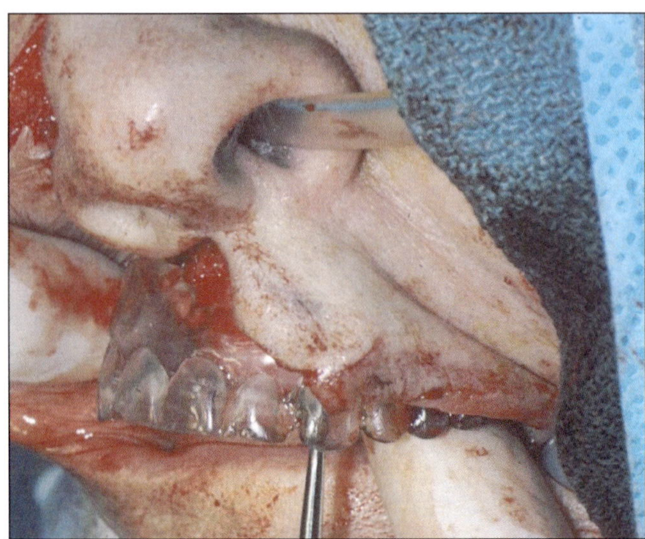

Figure 3-28 Dental implants are being placed immediately after tumor resection. Use of a surgical template ensures proper implant positioning.

also be impaired. In addition, prosthetic space may be lacking for the placement of denture teeth (Fig 3-27).

Vascularized osteocutaneous flaps, however, can be used to reconstruct large palatectomy defects. Debilitated, uncooperative patients (for example, individuals with Alzheimer's disease or mental disabilities) who are otherwise systemically healthy and could benefit from extensive resection of the maxilla or palate but would never tolerate fabrication or use of an obturator are also candidates for free flap reconstruction of their defects. However, given the high success rates seen with the use of tilted and zygomatic implants and the speed with which rehabilitation can be completed with implant-supported overlay prostheses, surgical reconstruction is often considered the less favored option by some clinicians (Sharma and Beumer, 2005).

Placement of implants

Placement of dental implants at the time of tumor resection should be considered for edentulous patients or for dentate patients when the prognosis for the remaining dentition is poor, when the defect crosses the midline or extends to the posterior pharyngeal wall, or where the residual dentition is insufficient to properly retain and stabilize and support an obturator prosthesis (Fig 3-28). Intradefect implant placement should be considered in all such patients. Providing implant support on the side of the defect prevents the obturator prosthesis from being impacted into the defect during function, improves seal, and permits bilateral mastication. Implant placement requires little additional operating time and saves the patient from undergoing an additional surgical procedure posttumor ablation. It also speeds up the process of rehabilitation. Implant success rates are comparable to that achieved with deferred placement (Wetzels et al., 2016; Wetzels et al., 2017; Butterworth, 2019; Butterworth et al., 2022; Buurman et al., 2020a; Alberga et al., 2021).

Contemporary titanium implants are well suited to this purpose. The original titanium dental implants developed by Professor Brånemark and his colleagues were prepared with a machined surface. They were predictable in bone sites of favorable quantity and quality, such as the mandibular symphysis region, but were problematic in poor-quality bone sites. Since then, numerous surface treatments (e.g., sandblasting, acid etching, titanium grit blasting, electrolytic processes, etc.) designed to change the microtopography of the implant surface have evolved that have significantly improved the osteoconductivity of titanium implants, accelerating the biologic processes associated with osseointegration and making these implants highly predictable in less favorable sites such as the posterior maxilla. In addition to the remaining anterior maxillary ridges, sites such as the pyramidal process of the palatal bone, the residual bone associated with the pyriform rim, the nasal crest, and the zygomatic arches have been employed and proven to be predictable.

If the patient is to receive postoperative radiation, the authors still prefer that the implants be placed at the time of tumor ablation. Radiation treatment following tumor surgery is usually delayed for five to six weeks to allow the surgical wounds to heal. This is sufficient time for implants with microrough implant surfaces to become osseointegrated because as mentioned above, such surfaces accelerate the pertinent biologic processes associated with osseointegration. At six weeks the bone-implant contact will be on average about 60% (Ogawa and Nishimura, 2003, 2006). It is true that the backscatter from the postoperative radiation will raise the radiation dose to the bone anchoring the implants by an additional 15% to 18%, further compromising the vasculature of the anchoring bone and its viability (Schwartz et al., 1979; Mian et al., 1987; Tso et al., 2019). However, it should be remembered that at doses above 60 Gy, implant anchorage is primarily mechanical as opposed to biologic (Nishimura, 1995). Consequently, if implants were to be placed in these same sites after radiation, lacking the normal processes associated with osseointegration, and the anchorage being primarily mechanical, the level of implant bone contact achieved would be considerably less than if they were placed prior to radiation. In these situations, implant anchorage using self-taping tapered implants with variable thread designs will improve initial anchorage and, in combination with the use of the tilted implant concept, will yield the best results (see section below entitled "Use of Dental Implants"). Also, when implants are placed prior to radiation, frequently the dose to some of the implant sites can be reduced when intensity-modulated radiation therapy is used.

Prosthetic Rehabilitation

Presurgical prosthetic planning

If the defect is to be restored prosthetically, prior to surgery the prosthodontist should examine the patient thoroughly, make impressions for diagnostic casts, mount these casts on a suitable articulator with a jaw relation record, and obtain appropriate dental radiographs. Some compromises may be necessary because of the immediacy of surgery and the distance the patient may have to travel. If time permits, a routine prophylaxis can be performed, salvageable teeth with large carious lesions can be restored, and arrangements can be made for extraction of unsalvageable teeth at surgery.

During this appointment, the plan for rehabilitation is discussed with the patient. Most patients will be unfamiliar with both the term *prosthodontist* and the services a prosthodontist can provide. The benefits, limitations, and sequence of prosthetic care should be explained to the patient. A few patients will have many questions, whereas others will prefer not to receive extensive information because discussion of the subject will evoke further anxiety. With the diagnostic aids obtained, the prosthodontist is prepared to consult with the surgeon and discuss the myriad factors related to prosthetic rehabilitation.

When appropriate, the data from the CT scans should be obtained and reviewed. From this data visual representations of the mandible, maxilla, paranasal sinuses, and adjacent structures can be created in three dimensions. Virtual surgical resections of the tumor can then be performed. This is especially valuable when implants are to be placed at the time the tumor is resected. Potential implant sites can be visualized (see Fig 3-14), implant placement planned, and when appropriate, surgical templates designed and fabricated to facilitate their placement (also see section below entitled "Use of Dental Implants").

Phases of treatment

Prosthodontic therapy for patients with acquired surgical defects of the maxilla can be arbitrarily divided into three phases of treatment, each having different objectives. The initial phase is called *surgical obturation* and entails the placement of a prosthesis at surgery. The primary objective of immediate surgical obturation is to restore and maintain oral functions at reasonable levels during the initial postoperative period.

The second phase of postsurgical prosthodontic treatment is called *interim obturation*. The objective of this phase is to provide the patient with a comfortable and functional prosthesis until healing is complete. The interim obturator phase begins when the surgical obturator and packing are removed. This phase may not be necessary if the defect is small and the patient is functioning well with the ISO. However, variations between the extent of actual surgery and presurgical estimates, rapid tissue changes immediately following surgery, and extensive surgical defects may necessitate either fabrication of a new interim prosthesis or major modifications to the surgical obturator.

Generally, four to six months after surgery, the surgical site is well healed and stable dimensionally. Completion of healing permits *definitive obturation*, or the third phase of prosthodontic therapy.

Surgical obturation

Surgical obturation has been accomplished with a variety of restorations and materials, including sponges (James and Raines, 1995), gutta-percha (Hammond, 1966), and inflatable bulbs (Payne and Welton, 1965). We prefer the use of an acrylic resin prosthesis. In most instances this prosthesis is initially limited to the restoration of palatal integrity, the reproduction of palatal contours, and in select cases the replacement of anterior teeth. Surgical packing is used to occlude the defect. In some instances (particularly in total palatectomy defects) the acrylic resin prosthesis is readapted at surgery with a temporary denture reliner to hold a skin graft in position during the first 7–10 days following surgery. Immediate surgical obturation is indicated for almost all patients (Gulbransen, 1995).

Immediate surgical obturation is well suited for either edentulous or dentate patients requiring a partial or total maxillectomy and partial or total palatectomy. The advantages of immediate surgical obturators (ISO) are as follows:

- The prosthesis provides a matrix on which the surgical packing can be placed. On closure of the wound, the obturator maintains the packing in position, thus ensuring close adaptation of the split-thickness skin graft to the raw surfaces of the cheek flap during the initial phase of healing.
- The prosthesis reduces oral contamination of the wound during the immediate postsurgical period and thus may reduce the incidence of local infection.
- The prosthesis enables the patient to speak more effectively immediately postoperatively by replacing anterior teeth as necessary, reproducing normal palatal contours, and covering the defect.
- The prosthesis permits deglutition, thus eliminating the need for a nasogastric tube for some patients or allowing its earlier removal for others.
- The prosthesis lessens the psychological impact of surgery by making the postoperative period easier to bear. The patient is reassured that rehabilitation has begun.
- The prosthesis reduces the period of hospitalization (Nakamoto, 1971). Most patients can be discharged from the hospital three to five days after surgery.

ISOs are fabricated on a maxillary cast obtained prior to surgery. If the extent of surgery is in question, it may be necessary to fabricate two or more prostheses presurgically to be prepared for most eventualities. The surgical prosthesis should be left in place for at least six days postsurgically. Retention from the wire clasp retainers is not sufficient to accomplish this objective, and the prosthesis must be ligated to the remaining teeth, wired or secured to the palate with screws, or wired to the zygoma.

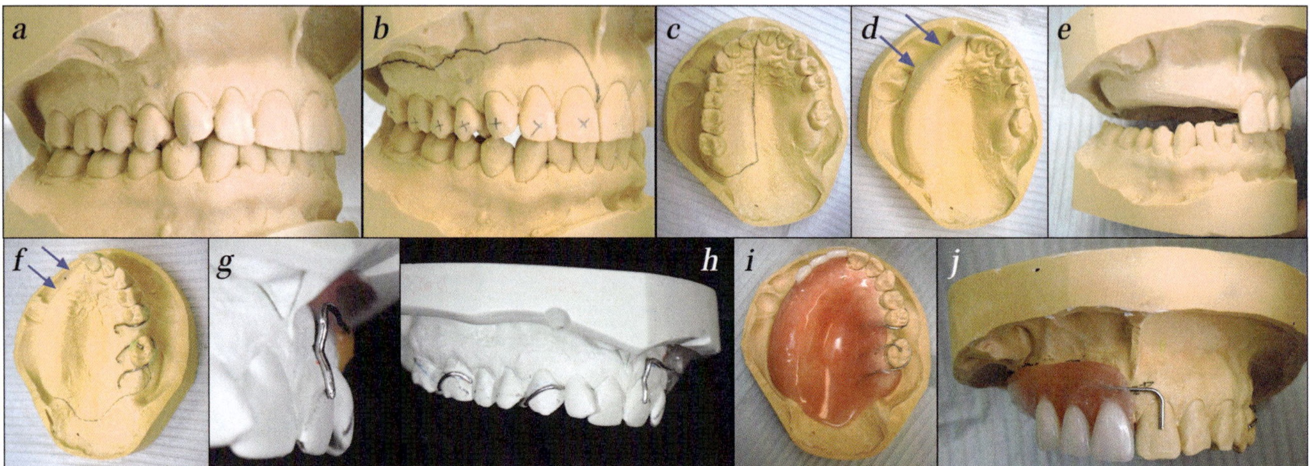

Figure 3-29 Design and fabrication of ISOs. *(a)* Prepared and mounted casts. *(b and c)* Margins of the proposed surgical resection outlined on the presurgical maxillary cast. *(d to f)* Teeth removed and anterior-labial portion of the alveolus trimmed *(arrows)*. Note the occlusal clearance. *(g and h)* The wire retainers should engage 0.10 undercuts and the I bar, free of the attached gingiva. *(i and j)* ISO with anterior teeth added.

There are several principles of design for ISOs that the prosthodontist should consider:

- The obturator should initially terminate short of the skin graft–mucosa junction. As soon as the surgical packing is removed, the ISO may be extended into the defect with a temporary denture reliner.
- The prosthesis should be kept simple and lightweight. Round 18-gauge wrought gold or stainless-steel wire retainers are sufficient for dentulous patients. The retainers and rests can also be designed digitally and milled of titanium.
- The prosthesis for dentulous patients should be perforated with a small dental bur at the interproximal extensions to allow the prosthesis to be wired to the teeth at the time of surgery.
- Normal palatal contours should be reproduced to facilitate postoperative speech and deglutition.
- If the disease process has distorted palatal contours, normal palatal contours should be reestablished on the cast. If palatal tori are evident, arrangements should be made for their removal during surgery and normal contours should be established on the presurgical cast.
- Posterior occlusion should not be established on the defect side until the surgical wound is well organized. However, if the patient is scheduled for a total maxillectomy with resection to the midline, the three maxillary anterior teeth included in the resection may be added to the prosthesis to improve aesthetics.

The surgical obturator for edentulous patients should be fabricated much like a record base, without replacement teeth, with the exception that the prosthesis is extended onto the soft palate. The prosthesis is wired to the zygoma or residual alveolar ridge or pinned or screwed to the palate for retention at the time of surgery. After 6 to 10 days, the surgical obturator is removed and discarded, and the patient's conventional maxillary complete denture may be converted into an interim prosthesis with a temporary denture reline material.

In some patients, the existing complete or partial prosthesis may be adapted for use as an ISO. However, the buccal flange of the prosthesis corresponding to the proposed defect requires reduction, and the posterior denture teeth on the defect side should be removed prior to surgery. Interim lining materials may be added to the revised prosthesis at the time of surgery to improve adaptation and to extend the prosthesis posteriorly to cover the soft palate.

Surgical resections involving the maxillae may include variable amounts of soft palate on the affected side. Therefore, standard maxillary impression trays must be extended posteriorly with waxes or impression compound to record the desired portion of the soft palate in the impression. The patient should be placed in an upright position so that the soft palate assumes a relatively normal and relaxed position. If the patient has an active gag reflex, topical anesthetics and rapid setting irreversible hydrocolloid impression material are useful.

It is important to make an accurate impression of the vestibular depth on the resected side so that the approximate position of the skin graft–mucosa junction can be determined. The adapted wire retainers should engage sufficient numbers of teeth to ensure adequate retention of the prosthesis after the initial means of retention have been removed. Minimal tooth preparation may be required for these retainers, but provision must be made for occlusal clearance. Occlusal interference is difficult to identify in the operating room and can result in unnecessary discomfort during the immediate postoperative period. If the patient has fixed partial dentures or splinted teeth, and if the proposed surgical margin will bisect these fixed units, it may be necessary to remove or segment selected fixed units prior to surgery.

After the maxillary and mandibular impressions are made and the casts are retrieved, the casts are mounted on a suitable articulator with the aid of a jaw relation record (Fig 3-29a). The surgeon and prosthodontist should discuss the surgery together and outline the proposed surgical margins on the maxillary cast (Fig 3-29b and c). This task can also be accomplished remotely by viewing a three-dimensional representation of the palate and adjacent structures with the planned virtual resection (see Fig 3-14). The lateral boundary is usually the labial and buccal vestibules and the medial boundary is the midline of the palate. The most questionable extensions are the anterior and posterior margins.

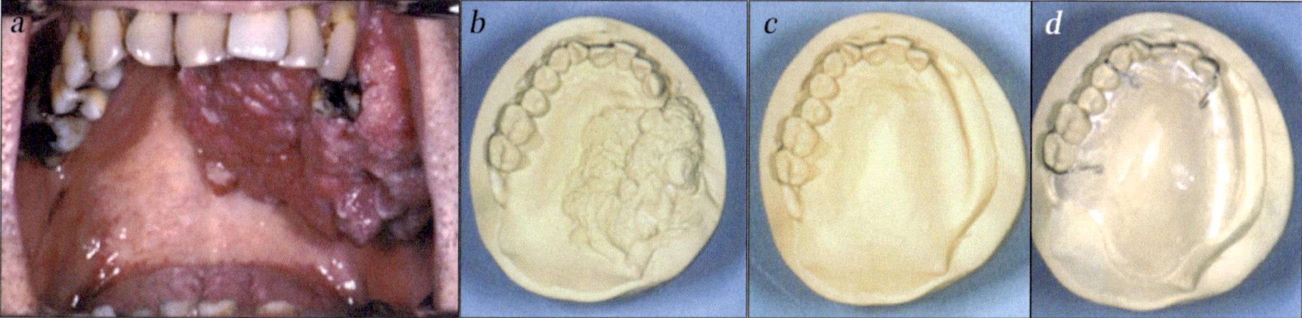

Figure 3-30 Restoration of normal palatal contours. *(a and b)* Tumor-distorted palatal contours. *(c)* Cast altered to restore palatal contours. *(d)* Completed ISO on cast (courtesy of Michael Hamada).

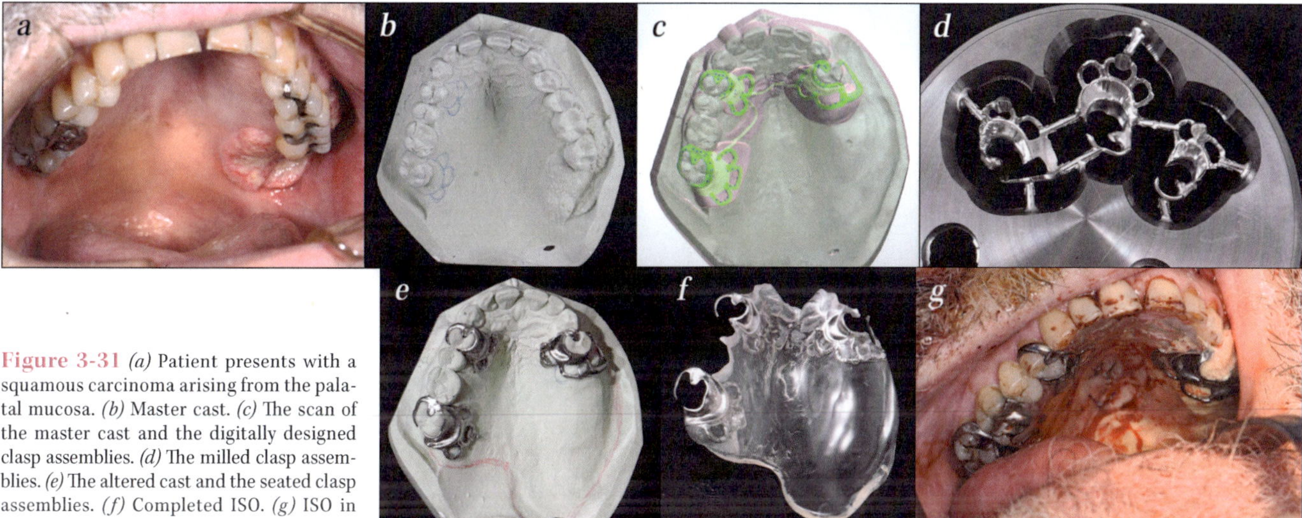

Figure 3-31 *(a)* Patient presents with a squamous carcinoma arising from the palatal mucosa. *(b)* Master cast. *(c)* The scan of the master cast and the digitally designed clasp assemblies. *(d)* The milled clasp assemblies. *(e)* The altered cast and the seated clasp assemblies. *(f)* Completed ISO. *(g)* ISO in position at surgery.

The maxillary cast is altered to conform to the proposed surgical resection. Teeth to be included in the resection are removed from the cast. The occlusal portion of the alveolar ridge must be reduced by 2–3 mm so that his portion of the ISO will not be in contact with opposing dentition during the immediate postsurgical period (see Fig 3-29e and f). The labial projection of the residual alveolar ridge is trimmed in the anterior region to reduce the tension on the skin and lip closure (Fig 3-29d–f). If the tumor or tori have distorted palatal contours, the cast must be altered to establish normal contours (Fig 3-30). In patients with excessive vertical overlap, the obturator extension anteriorly must be thinned to avoid occlusal interference with mandibular anterior teeth.

Extension of the prosthesis lateral to the pterygoid hamulus should be avoided. If the pterygoid hamulus is removed during the maxillectomy procedure, the attachment and/or function of the tensor veli palatini, buccinator, and superior constrictor muscles can be compromised resulting in the medial collapse of the distolateral portion of the defect (Gulbransen, 1995). A prosthesis overextended laterally in this area will cause tissue irritation and significant patient discomfort. If this situation is anticipated, the cast should be reduced by 2 to 3 mm medially in this area (see Figs 3-29f and i and 3-30c and d).

After the cast is altered, the wire retainers are adapted and the prosthesis is waxed, invested, and processed in autopolymerizing acrylic resin and finished and polished in the customary manner (see Figs 3-29i and j and 3-30d). Care should be taken to engage undercut areas with the wire retainers (Fig 3-29g and h) and avoid proximal extension that may interfere with the occlusion. If interocclusal space is lacking, proximal areas should be avoided or prepared prior to surgery. The I bar retainer engaging the abutment tooth adjacent to the defect should be free of the attached gingiva (Fig 3-29g). The retainers and rests can also be designed digitally and milled of titanium. However, given the physical properties of titanium, the clasps should be designed with slightly more bulk than usual to prevent inadvertent fracture (Fig 3-31). Some clinicians prefer the use of clear resin so that the overextensions and possible pressure areas can be more easily visualized at surgery and adjusted. In select patients, anterior teeth can be added for aesthetics.

During resection of unilateral tumors, often the prosthodontist is not required in the operating room for placement of the prosthesis. However, during resection of bilateral tumors or if alterations of the prosthesis are anticipated, appropriate instrumentation must be available. The armamentarium needed at surgery will vary with each clinician, but the following items are suggested: autopolymerizing acrylic resin, intermediate denture reline materials, tissue conditioning materials, suitable dental burs, clasp adjusting pliers, and a vulcanite scraper. Most head and neck operating rooms possess air-driven or electric handpieces or similar devices that accept

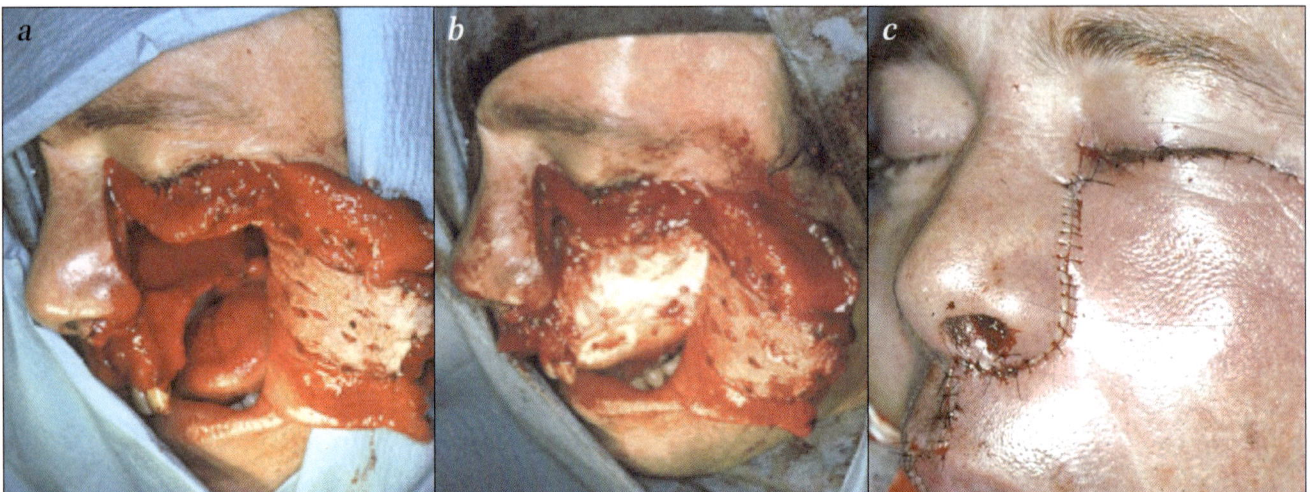

Figure 3-32 Placement of an ISO. *(a)* Total maxillectomy defect. Weber-Fergusson surgical exposure is utilized. Tension on the cheek flap is adjusted before the prosthesis is placed and the defect is packed with gauze. *(b)* The prosthesis serves as a platform for placement of surgical packing. *(c)* When the wound is closed, facial contours are nearly normal.

dental burs. Scissors, scalpels, marking pens, hemostats, and so on are always available in the operating room if needed.

Operating room protocol will vary by hospital and surgeon. However, strict conformity to operating room procedures must be observed; the prosthodontist must be scrubbed, gowned, and gloved. The required instruments and the prosthesis should be delivered to the surgical area the afternoon prior to surgery. The instruments are autoclaved, the dental materials are sterilized, and the prosthesis is immersed in a disinfectant. If the prosthodontist performs this procedure routinely, the required instruments can be assembled and stored in the surgical area.

In most instances the ISO is easily fitted and secured (Fig 3-32). If necessary, the lateral extension of the obturator should be adjusted so that it is short of the skin graft–mucosal junction. The anterior extension of the prosthesis may need to be reduced or thinned to avoid excessive tension on the lip closure. The surgical packing will compensate for most discrepancies. If the surgery was more extensive than planned, it is often preferable to add an intermediate denture reline material to the prosthesis. When the material becomes moldable, it is added to the deficient areas. The prosthesis is inserted; if the material sags or is displaced, it is manipulated into position with a wet, gloved finger. Adverse tissue reactions have not been reported with these materials. If the surgery has proceeded as planned, the application of lining materials is rarely required.

If a Weber-Fergusson exposure is used, the prosthesis should be inserted prior to closure of the cheek flap, because tension on the flap can be judged more accurately while the prosthesis is in place. When positioned, the prosthesis can be used as a platform for placement of the surgical packing. After the prosthesis is secured, the defect is packed with gauze, and the cheek flap is closed (Fig 3-32c). In dentulous patients, retention can be obtained by wiring the prosthesis to existing teeth or screwing it to the residual palate. In edentulous patients, the prosthesis is wired or screwed to the alveolar ridge, palate, zygomatic arches, and/or anterior nasal spine (Fig 3-33). If a transoral surgical approach is used, the surgeon will pack the defect prior to inserting the prosthesis.

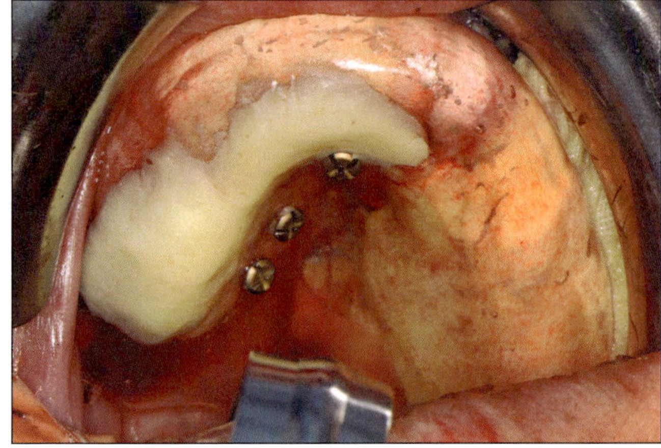

Figure 3-33 The ISO was secured with bone screws into the palate in this edentulous patient.

In patients with planned large defects that are not candidates for free flap reconstruction, the buccal inlay technique has been used to create favorable defects that possess skin-lined and strategically located undercuts. The ISO is fabricated in the usual manner, except a wire is embedded into the ISO at a level just occlusal to the vestibular extension. Following the resection, a suitable intermediate denture reline material is used to obtain a border-molded impression of the defect; the ISO is used as a carrier for the reline material. The skin graft is adhered to the border-molded ISO with a biodegradable adhesive and secured in position with wires, usually suspended from the zygomatic arches. After the border-molded appliance is secured in position, the mucosal margin is sutured to this wire.

This technique will maximize the undercut superior to the skin graft–mucosa junction, which can be used to help retain the prosthesis in position (Fig 3-34). The ISO is left wired in position for a longer period (two to three weeks) to minimize contraction of the tissues associated with the defect. Following initial removal, the appliance is readapted to the changing tissues of the defect in the manner described earlier, and anterior teeth and occlusal rims are added.

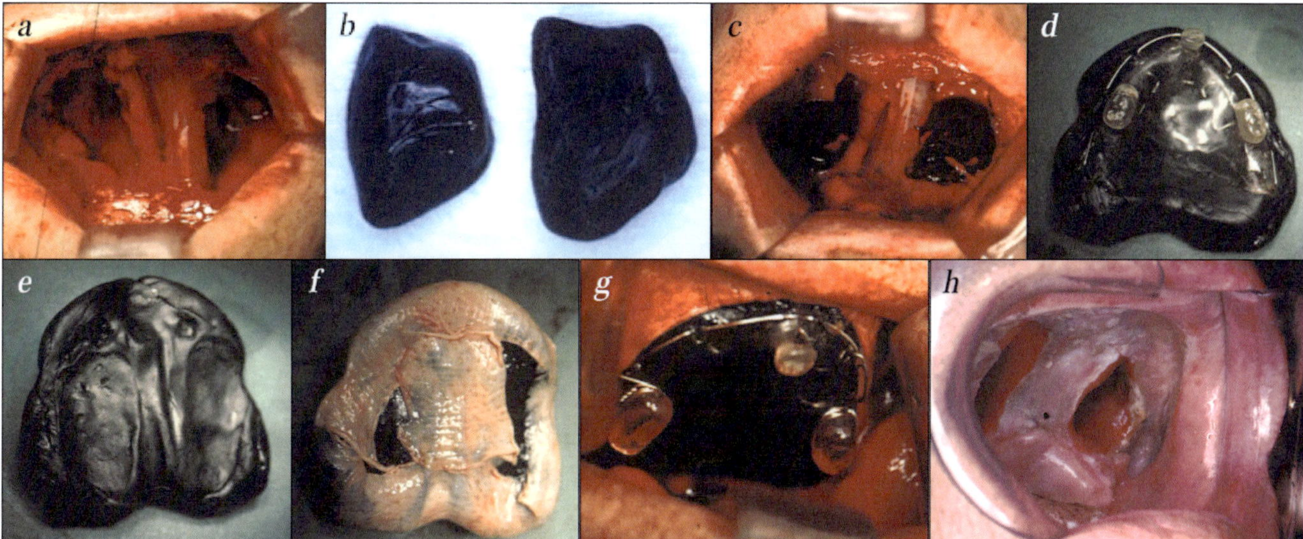

Figure 3-34 Buccal inlay technique for placement of a skin graft and ISO. *(a)* Total palatectomy defect. *(b and c)* The maxillary sinus is occluded. *(d and e)* The ISO is carefully border molded. *(f)* A skin graft is adapted to the border-molded ISO and held in place with biodegradable adhesive. *(g)* The ISO is secured in position with circumzygomatic wires *(arrows)*. The mucosal margin is sutured to wire embedded in the ISO. *(h)* Grafted defect three months postsurgery.

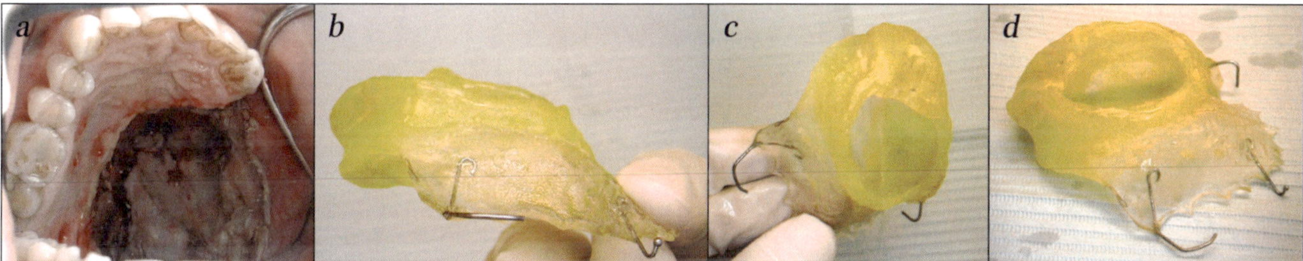

Figure 3-35 Relining the ISO to improve adaptation. *(a)* Defect after removal of the ISO. Note the appearance of the skin graft. *(b to d)* On removal of the surgical packing, the ISO is extended into the defect with a temporary denture reliner.

As healing progresses in the nonirradiated patient, trismus usually abates, which allows extension of the prosthesis further into the defect, improving seal and retention. If the patient is to receive postoperative radiation or chemoradiation, immediately postsurgery the patient should *immediately begin a physical therapy exercise program to maximize jaw opening*. Dynamic bite openers are well suited for this task (see Chapter 1) but are less effective if they are employed after radiotherapy because of posttreatment fibrosis and scarring.

Excessive trismus is a significant morbidity, and if maximum jaw opening is reduced to 15 mm or less, the superolateral extension of the obturator may be limited, compromising seal and making entry of the bolus of food difficult. Every effort should be made to maximize the patient's jaw opening prior to commencement of radiation therapy because additional scarring of the muscles of mastication following radiation therapy makes it very difficult for the patient to achieve greater jaw-opening measurements after radiation has been completed.

The prosthesis and packing are removed 7 to 10 days postsurgically. The prosthesis is cleansed and adjustments are made. Occasionally, minor occlusal discrepancies or retentive deficiencies associated with the wire retainers require attention. A new application of intermediate denture reline material will improve adaptation, seal, and comfort (Fig 3-35). The lateral extension into the defect can be developed in a way that is consistent with easy insertion and removal of the prosthesis. We prefer intermediate denture relining materials to tissue conditioning materials because the latter only have limited life spans (one week or less; Elsemann et al., 2008). In addition, the intermediate denture reline materials can be border molded and polished.

Instructions on the care of the prosthesis are given to the patient, who is scheduled for another appointment in one week. The prosthesis should be cleaned with a mild soap and water and a soft brush after every meal. Thereafter, the patient is usually examined every one to two weeks, and the prosthesis is relined to account for tissue changes secondary to healing. During the early stages of healing, we recommend that the prosthesis be worn at night, because rapid contraction of the surgical wound during these early stages may make reinsertion of the prosthesis the following morning both painful and difficult.

Instructions are also provided regarding the irrigation and cleansing of the surgical defect. Crusting of dried mucus occurs frequently. Their removal may be difficult and may trigger discomfort. Mucus and/or crusting can be removed with 2×2 or 4×4 gauze pads soaked in warm water. As the defect heals, mineral oil may be used to soften and remove the dried mucus. Oral hygiene instructions are

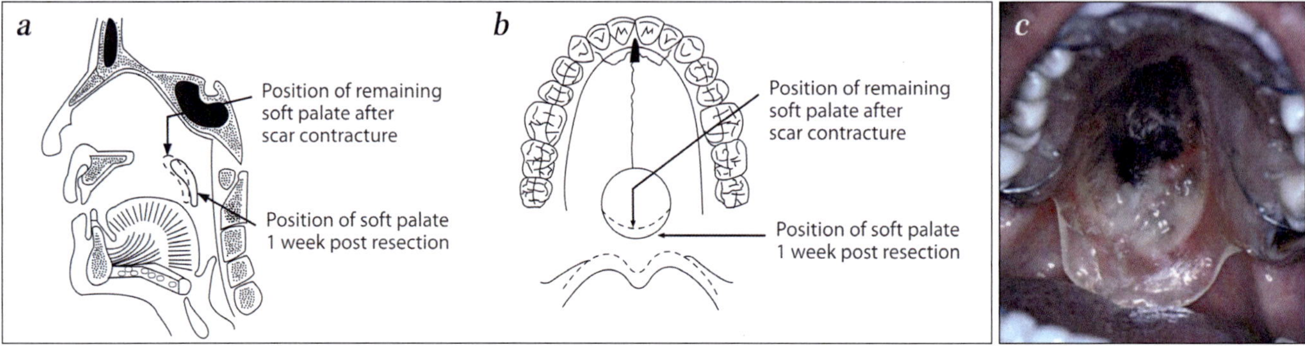

Figure 3-36 *(a and b)* Typical border defect. More frequent adjustments are expected. *(c)* The soft palate margin of the resection is subject to rapid contraction anteriorly and superiorly during the first three weeks following surgery. On rare occasions, velopharyngeal closure can be compromised secondary to this contracture.

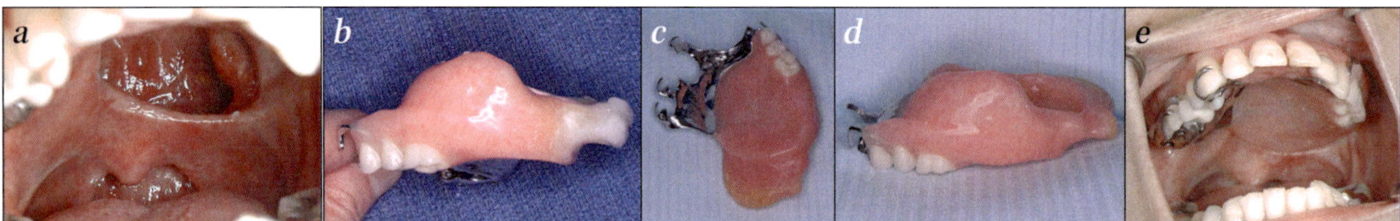

Figure 3-37 *(a)* Partial maxillectomy defect extending to the middle third of the soft palate. During elevation, the soft palate does not contact the pharyngeal wall. *(b)* Border-molded segment extending to the lateral and posterior pharyngeal walls. *(c and d)* Obturator prosthesis. *(e)* Prosthesis extending posteriorly through the palatal defect to engage the musculature of the posterior and lateral pharyngeal walls. However, the obturator could not be extended to engage the right lateral pharyngeal wall due to lack of access. As a result, speech was hypernasal. Eventually the residual soft palate remnant was removed and the obturator prosthesis extended to engage the right lateral pharyngeal wall, enabling the patient to control nasal emission during speech (see Chapter 4, Fig 4-43).

best reviewed in the presence of a family member because often the patient is not capable either physically or emotionally of cleansing the defect properly during the immediate postsurgical period. A pulsating stream irrigator is useful in some patients.

If the surgical resection included the anterior portion of the soft palate, more frequent adjustments are usually required (see Fig 3-36a and b). As healing progresses, the remaining posterior portion of the soft palate will be elevated superiorly and pulled anteriorly because of scar contracture. Such patients need to be examined more often in the immediate postoperative period to keep up with these rapid tissue changes (Fig 3-36c).

In an occasional patient, the soft palate is permanently scarred in the anterior position and is unable to contact the posterior pharyngeal wall during elevation. To allow successful obturation of such a defect, either the remaining portion of the soft palate must be resected and the prosthesis extended to the posterior pharyngeal area to interface with the residual velopharyngeal musculature still present in the pharyngeal walls (superior constrictor and levator palati), or the prosthesis must be extended posteriorly through the palatal opening to interact with these structures. This extension should be kept below the torus tubarius to avoid blockage of the eustachian tube and to effectively interface with the residual levator palatine muscle housed in the posterolateral portion of the nasopharynx (Fig 3-37).

In palatal defects that extend to the pharyngeal wall, as edema and discomfort subside, increased movement of the residual pharyngeal musculature may be noted and extensions of the prosthesis into this region must be adjusted accordingly. The obturator must maintain functional contact with these dynamic pharyngeal tissues if speech and swallowing are to be optimized. In large posterolateral defects, it is usually necessary to correct for eccentric mandibular movements because the anteromedial surface of the mandible will move forward and limit the posterolateral contours of the prosthesis in defects extending posterolaterally.

Interim obturation

The objective of the immediate surgical obturator is to serve the patient through the immediate postoperative period—usually 6–10 days. A definitive prosthesis is not indicated until the surgical site is healed and dimensionally stable and the patient is prepared physically and emotionally for the restorative care that may be necessary. The interim obturator prosthesis bridges the gap between the ISO and the definitive prosthesis.

For some patients, particularly those with large defects, appropriate function and comfort cannot be sustained without construction of a new prosthesis or a significant modification of the immediate or delayed surgical obturator. There are several reasons for constructing a new interim prosthesis. First, the periodic addition of interim lining materials increases the bulk and weight of the prosthesis, and these temporary materials tend to become rough and unhygienic with time. Second, if teeth were included in the resection, the addition of anterior, and possibly posterior, denture teeth to the obturator can be of great psychologic benefit to the patient. Third, if retention and stability are inadequate, reestablishment of occlusal contact on the defect side may improve these aspects. Fourth, a well-made interim obturator can serve as a backup prosthesis and may be useful when the definitive prosthesis has to be repaired, relined, or rebased.

In many instances, the surgical obturator can be utilized to fabricate the new interim prosthesis (Jacob and Martin, 1985). If the

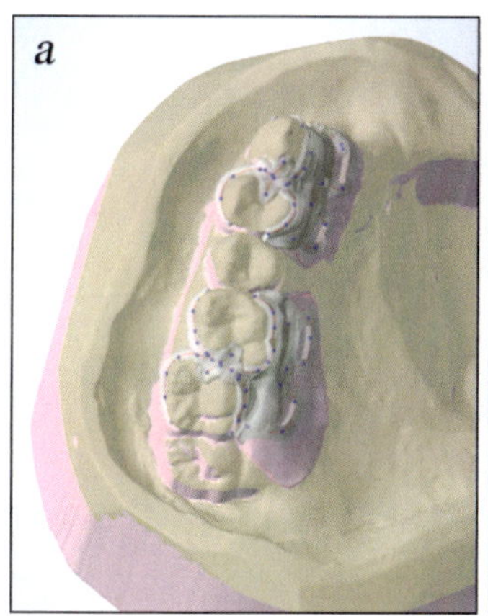
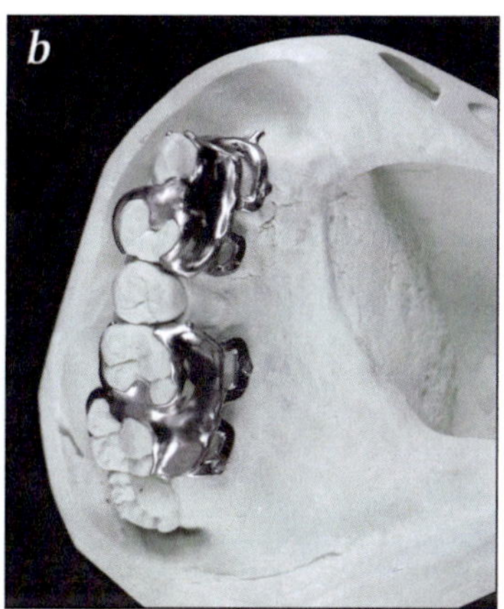

Figure 3-38 *(a and b)* Retainers and rests were designed digitally and milled of titanium.

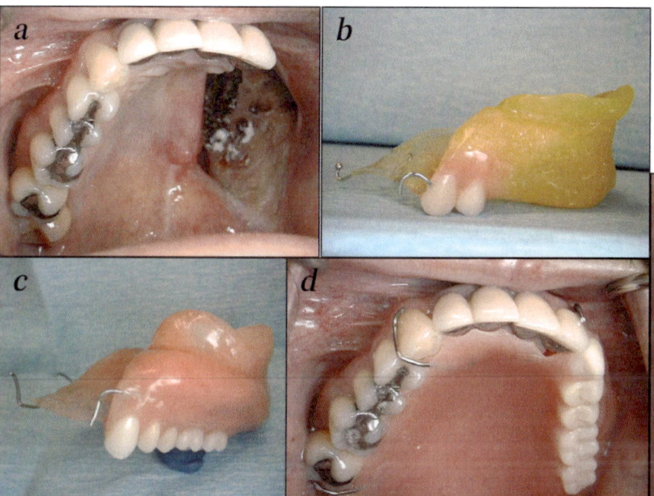
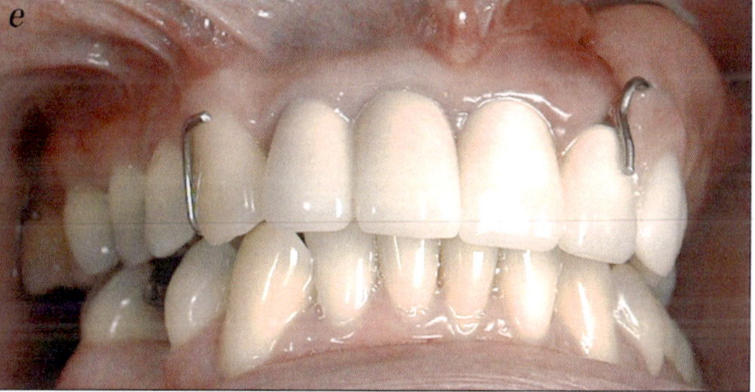

Figure 3-39 Interim obturator fabricated from a surgical obturator. *(a)* Maxillectomy defect one month postsurgery. *(b and c)* After the centric relation record has been made, posterior teeth are added and the prosthesis is relined and rebased. *(d and e)* Prosthesis in position.

patient is dentulous, a new application of interim lining material is placed over the tissue surface and the prosthesis is seated firmly to maintain correct relationships. As the material begins to polymerize, the lips and cheek are manipulated and the patient is instructed to perform eccentric mandibular movements. When the material has set, the prosthesis is removed and any excess material is trimmed from inappropriate areas.

The prosthesis is reinserted and the patient is asked to speak and to swallow fluids to test the effectiveness of the seal. If these tests confirm that the prosthesis has adequate extension and adaptation, a jaw relation record is obtained. An irreversible hydrocolloid impression is made over the prosthesis and remaining teeth. The impression is poured with dental stone and the maxillary cast, with the prosthesis in place, is related to the mandibular cast with the jaw relation record and mounted on a suitable articulator.

The prosthesis may be rebased or entirely rewaxed. Anterior and posterior teeth may be added as appropriate. If necessary new clasp assemblies can be designed digitally and milled from titanium (Fig 3-38). The laboratory procedures should be completed quickly, and the old prosthesis should be returned to the patient. A new application of temporary denture reline material may be required prior to dismissal of the patient as the interim lining material may tear or distort with retrieval of the cast.

The new obturator is processed and hollowed (Fig 3-39). The new prosthesis is relined periodically with an intermediate reline material as necessary. Follow-up care continues as previously described.

In edentulous patients, it is preferable to use the patient's existing maxillary complete denture as an interim obturator. The existing prosthesis should be inspected carefully to ensure that the occlusion is acceptable. *The labial flanges of the complete denture must be shortened aggressively on the side of the defect, especially in the anterior region.* It is usually necessary to extend the prosthesis with autopolymerizing acrylic resin to cover the margin of resection on the soft palate. After the denture is adjusted, it is relined with an intermediate reline material (Fig 3-40).

There are several clinical applications for the use of visible light-cured resins in maxillofacial prosthetics, primarily when there are time constraints. It is not unusual for an out-of-town patient to require a surgical obturator for the following day. Many times, additions to prostheses or conversion of a surgical obturator into an interim prosthesis must be completed within a few hours because the patient cannot function without a suitable prosthesis. Light-cured resin technology facilitates these changes and can minimize the time the patient is without a prosthesis (Fischman, 1989; Caputo et al., 1989; Shifman, 1990).

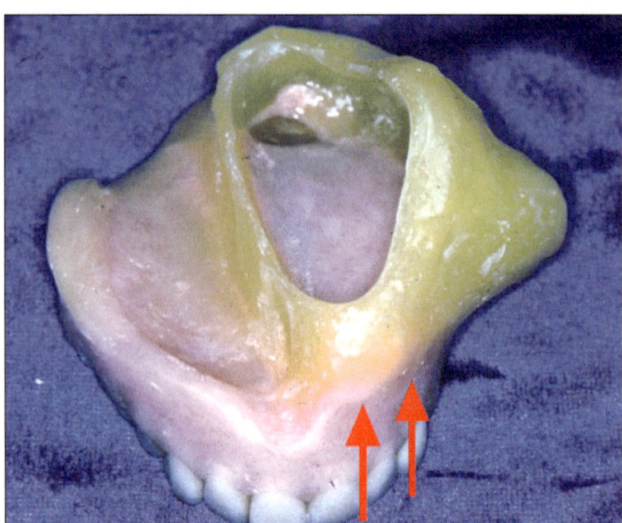

Figure 3-40 The existing denture, with modifications, may be used as an interim obturator. Labial and buccal extensions of the preexisting complete denture on the defect side are reduced prior to addition of the intermediate reline material *(arrows)*.

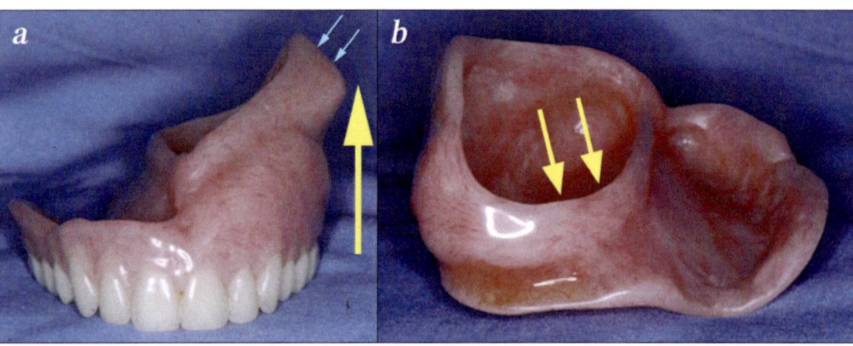

Figure 3-41 *(a)* Extension up the lateral wall of the defect improves retention and stability *(arrow)*. In some patients, support can be enhanced by engaging the superolateral portion of the orbital floor *(blue arrows)*. *(b)* The posteromedial extension must extend vertically about 1 cm to minimize leakage *(arrows)*.

Definitive obturation: Treatment concepts

The construction of a definitive obturator prosthesis may be considered three to four months after surgery. The timing will depend on the size of the defect, the progress of healing, the prognosis for tumor control, the use and timing of postsurgical radiation or chemoradiation, the effectiveness of the present obturator, and the presence or absence of teeth. For edentulous patients, the defect must be engaged more aggressively to maximize support, retention, and stability. Therefore, the recovery period is often extended for these patients before definitive treatment is begun.

As with conventional immediate dentures, changes associated with healing and remodeling will continue to occur in the border areas of the defect for at least one year. However, in contrast with patients who are receiving conventional immediate dentures, patients who have undergone tumor resection undergo dimensional changes that are primarily related to the peripheral soft tissues rather than to bony support areas.

Three to four months after surgery, the mental outlook of most patients will have improved. They realize that speech, mastication, and deglutition will not be compromised significantly. Most dentulous patients are prepared physically and emotionally for the extensive restorative procedures that may be required prior to the construction of a definitive obturator.

In addition to treatment planning associated with a standard prosthodontic evaluation, the clinician should elicit information relative to the prognosis for tumor control and the general health and desires of the patient. A patient's poor prognosis or poor health does not preclude the construction of a definitive obturator prosthesis, but the treatment plan should reflect the possible altered needs of such a patient. Mounted diagnostic casts are essential, and new radiographs of questionable teeth should be obtained. The evaluation should include opinions from the surgeon, the radiation oncologist, the medical oncologist, and the clinical social worker. Most patients will be functioning well with their interim prosthesis, so the treatment plan may be developed systematically and thoroughly. Several concepts need to be considered when designing a plan of treatment for a patient with a large palatal defect that will be prosthodontically restored.

Movement of the prosthesis

The prosthesis will move significantly during function if the maxillary alveolar ridge and teeth are involved in the resection (as is the case with most maxillary surgical procedures). Unless implant support is provided in the defect, the obturator will be displaced superiorly into the defect with the force of mastication and swallowing and will tend to drop without occlusal contact. In dentate patients the degree of movement will vary with the number and position of teeth or implants (if any) that are available, the amount of palatal shelf area remaining, as well as with the size and configuration of the defect.

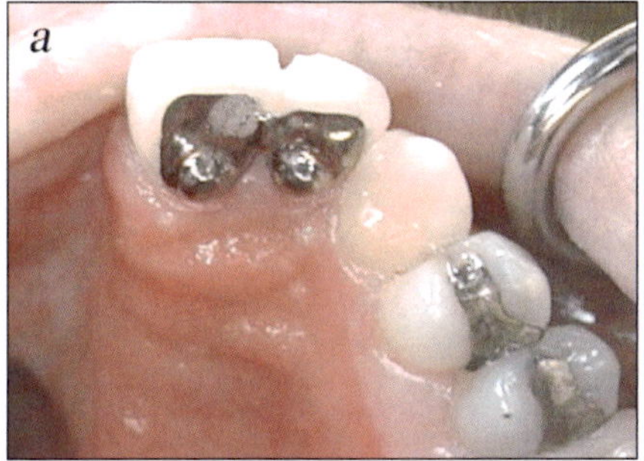
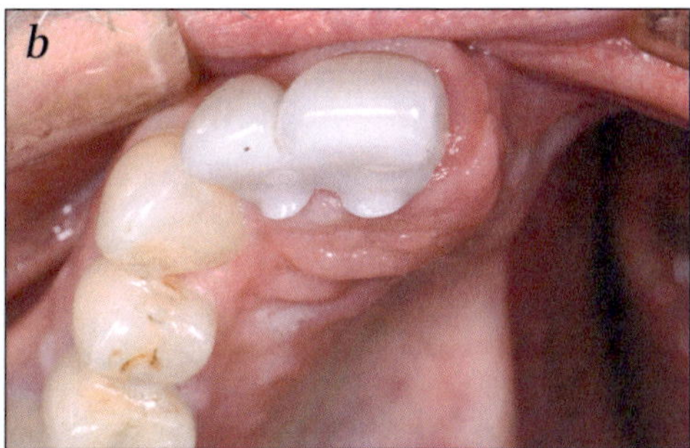

Figure 3-42 Teeth adjacent to the defect are splinted together to enhance their load-bearing capacity. *(a)* Metal-ceramic crowns. *(b)* Digitally designed and milled monolithic zirconia crowns. Note the positive cingulum rests incorporated within these crowns.

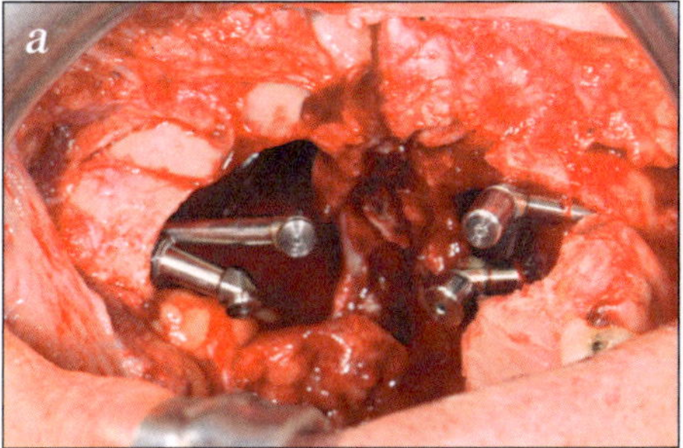
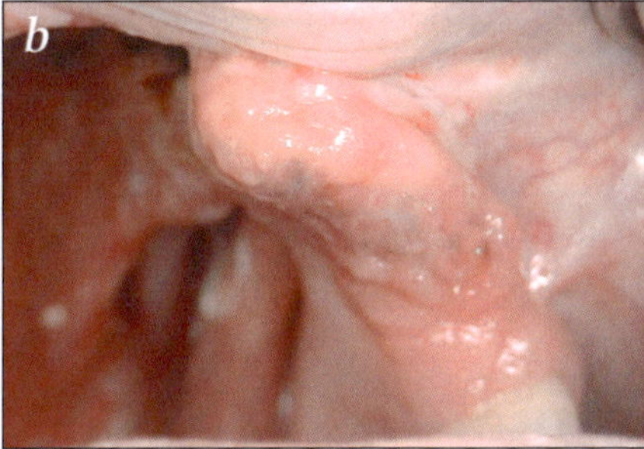
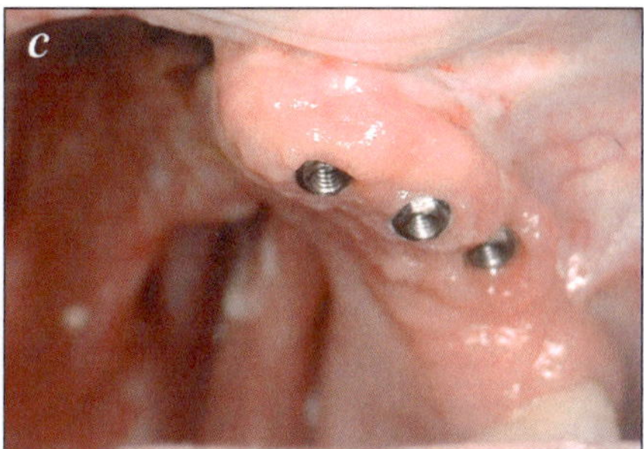

Figure 3-43 Implants can be inserted *(a)* at the time of tumor resection or *(b and c)* at some time thereafter. Note that the zygomatic implants in "a" have smooth necks (see section below entitled "Implant selection criteria").

Tissue changes

Dimensional changes will continue to occur for a least one year secondary to scar contracture and further organization of the wound, particularly in defects that extend to include portions of the soft palate. Movement of the prosthesis during function may in itself contribute to tissue changes.

Oral-nasal partition

Obturators for acquired defects of the maxillae are basically covering prostheses serving primarily to reestablish the oral-nasal partition. The obturator prosthesis is *extended into the defect to enhance its retention, stability, and support.* The contours of most defects are relatively static during function, aside from the movement of the soft tissues displaced by the movement of the coronoid process and the anterior border of the ramus of the mandible, the slight movement of the lips and cheek, and (in some patients) the elevation of the residual soft palate. In contrast, obturators that restore velopharyngeal competency must function in concert with the residual velopharyngeal musculature during speech and swallowing (see Chapter 4).

Extension into the defect

The degree of extension into the defect is dependent on the need to provide retention, stability, and support for the obturator prosthesis. In most patients, the defect must be used to improve these qualities. In addition, the extension of the prosthesis into the defect will vary according to the configuration of the defect and the character of its lining tissue. A significant extension of the prosthesis superiorly along the nasal septum offers little mechanical advantage and *may impair nasal airflow on this side.* In addition, the ciliated pseudostratified columnar epithelium lining the nasal septum and other nasal structures will tolerate little stress.

In contrast, extension superiorly along the posterior and lateral margins of the defect will enhance retention, stability, and support (Fig 3-41a). Stress is well tolerated by the skin graft and oral mucosa lining the cheek surface of the defect. In a conventional total maxillectomy defect, the vertical extension in the posteromedial region of the defect must be carefully designed to minimize leakage (Fig 3-41b).

Teeth

As with all maxillofacial prostheses, the presence of teeth enhances the prosthetic prognosis. Every effort should be made to maintain and enhance the longevity of teeth or even roots of teeth to assist with the retention, stability, and support of the prosthesis. In some instances, teeth adjacent to the defect are splinted together to enhance their load-bearing capacity (Lyons et al., 2005; Fig 3-42). Anterior teeth adjacent to the defects must be designed with cingulum rests (Fig 3-42).

Implants

The placement of implants will dramatically improve the function of the obturator prosthesis, particularly for edentulous patients (Garrett, 2008; Buurman et al., 2020b). Implants can be placed at the time of tumor resection or at some appropriate time thereafter. The most common locations suitable for the placement of implants are the residual alveolar ridge, the pyramidal process of the palatal bone, the pyriform rim region, and the zygomatic arches (Fig 3-43; see section below entitled "Use of Dental Implants").

Weight and design

Bulky areas of the obturator should be hollowed to reduce weight so that teeth and supporting tissues are not stressed unnecessarily (Minsley et al., 1986) (Fig 3-44). Wu and Schaaf (1989) reported that

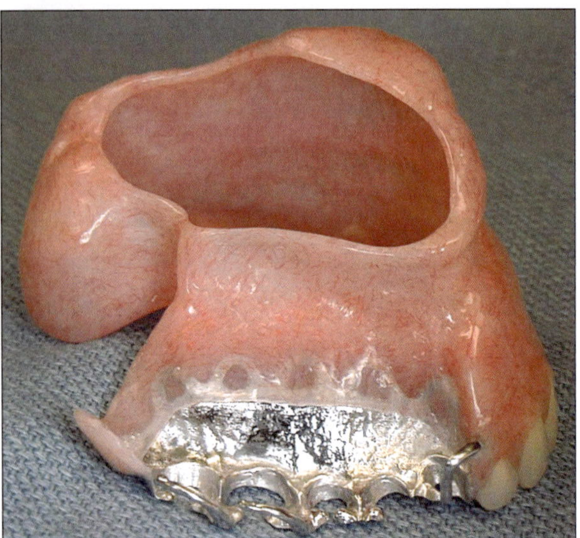

Figure 3-44 Obturator prosthesis hollowed to reduce weight.

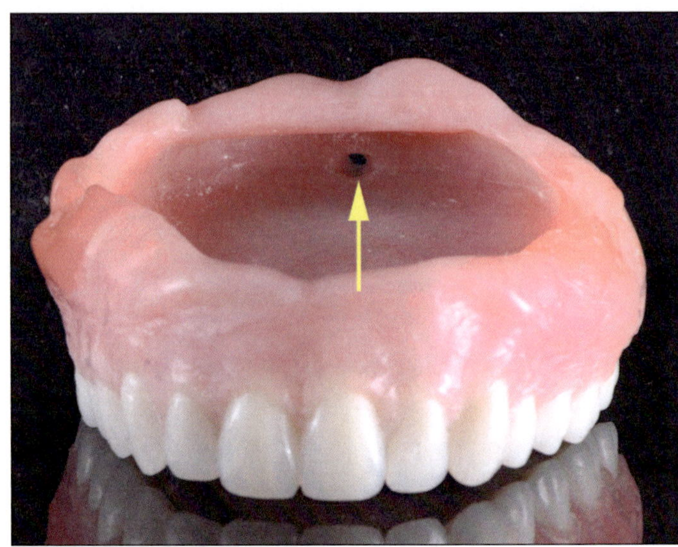

Figure 3-45 A small hole is placed posteriorly to allow secretions to drain out of the obturator *(arrow)*.

a hollow maxillary obturator prosthesis reduced the weight of the prosthesis by 7% to 33%, depending on the size of the maxillary defect. Several techniques for minimizing the weight of the obturator prosthesis have been described (Oh and Roumanas, 2008). Digitally designing and printing the intaglio surface of the obturator prosthesis out of PMMA offers a new approach that will minimize the weight of the prosthesis if the thickness of the PMMA puck is sufficient to capture the extensions of the obturator prosthesis. This option is particularly attractive in edentulous patients because adaptation to the defect is enhanced and it can be used as a record base (see section below entitled "Records").

The superior surface can be left open or can be closed. Clinicians who prefer the closed-top design maintain that nasal secretions accumulate if the obturator is left open, leading to odor and added weight. We have observed that the accumulation of secretions with an open obturator is not significant for most patients, particularly those who have previously been irradiated.

Oral et al. (1979) compared the speech of 10 patients with maxillary obturator prostheses with both open and closed superior configurations. All 10 patients had normal velopharyngeal mechanisms. Initially, an open obturator was fabricated with a lengthy superior extension along the lateral and posterolateral aspect of the defect but only a limited extension medially. After speech was recorded, a lid was added to create a hollow, closed obturator. Speech was recorded again, the speech samples were randomized and evaluated by 5 speech pathologists. Of the 50 evaluations (5 speech pathologists and 10 patient evaluations), 32 rated the open configuration best, while 18 favored the closed hollow obturator.

After the speech study was completed, the 10 obturators were left open and the patients were followed for one year. Two patients complained of leakage and/or the accumulation of fluids within the obturator well. For one patient this condition was corrected by improving the lateral seal of the obturator, while the second patient required conversion of the open obturator to a closed hollow bulb (Oral et al., 1979).

It is interesting to speculate as to the reason for the small differences in speech produced by the two obturator configurations. Lengthy superior extension along the lateral and distolateral aspect of the defect is essential for stability, support, and retention of the prosthesis. If a lid is added to the hollow obturator, a significant portion of the nasal and maxillary sinus cavities is now occupied by the closed obturator bulb. This may negatively affect the configuration, resonance balance, and airflow characteristics of the nasal cavity. The open obturator design may be less obtrusive and permit more normal airflow and nasal resonance and, therefore, more normal speech.

It is not necessary for the obturator to occupy the entire defect superiorly for effective obturation (Parel and Drane, 1976; Oral et al., 1979). We prefer the open-top design because of its simplicity, lighter weight, and ease of adjustment. Our experiences with the open top are similar to those reported by Oral et al. (1979). An occasional patient will require obturator modification and/or conversion to a closed-top hollow obturator bulb. If secretions tend to accumulate, a small, opening may be made between the posterior floor of the open-top obturator and the surface in contact with the local tissues for drainage. The mucosa will close against the opening, so seal is not compromised (Fig 3-45). The patient is advised to use a pipe cleaner to clean and maintain the patency of this drainage channel (Zaki, 1980).

The treatment of sinonasal neoplasms often requires tumoricidal doses of radiation therapy. In these patients, the minor salivary glands found in the adjacent mucosal lining exhibit a vastly reduced output of secretions. The skin graft lining the cheek surface has no secretory potential. Therefore, in such patients, nasal secretions are minimal and an open top is acceptable. However, sealing the top of the obturator may be an advantage if the patient demonstrates normal secretory output or complains of accumulation of secretions in the obturator bulb.

The technique suggested by Birnbach and Barnhard (1989) for adding a lid works well. If the clinician desires a closed-top hollow obturator bulb at the initial placement, the techniques described by Chalian and Barnett (1972), Matalon and LaFuente (1976), or Parel and LaFuente (1978) are recommended. In general, leakage of the hollow obturator bulb is less likely to occur if the hollow bulb is processed initially as a complete unit rather than if a lid is added after

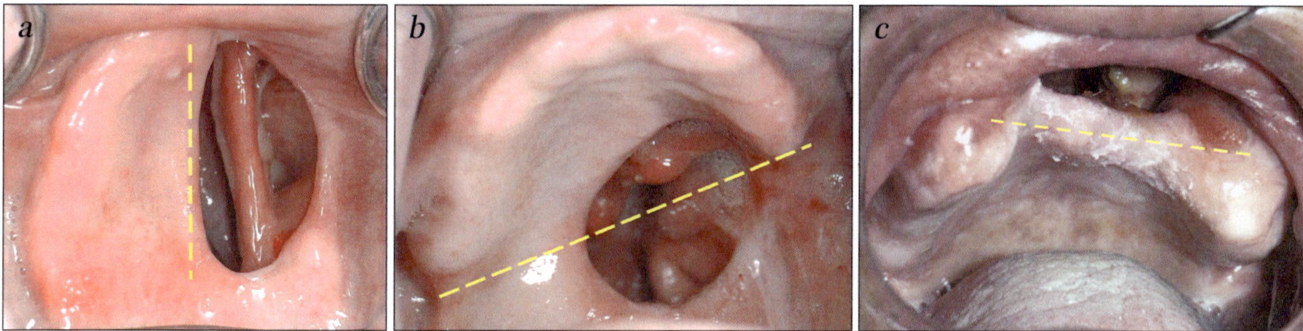

Figure 3-46 Axes of rotation of obturator prostheses. *(a)* Edentulous patient with a total maxillectomy defect. The axis of rotation *(dotted line)* of the prosthesis is along the medial margin of the defect. *(b)* Edentulous patient with a partial maxillectomy defect. When more of the hard palate remains, more stable prostheses can be fabricated, because the axis of rotation *(dotted line)* moves posteriorly. *(c)* Anterior defect. The axis of rotation *(dotted line)* of the prosthesis is located along the posterior margin of the defect.

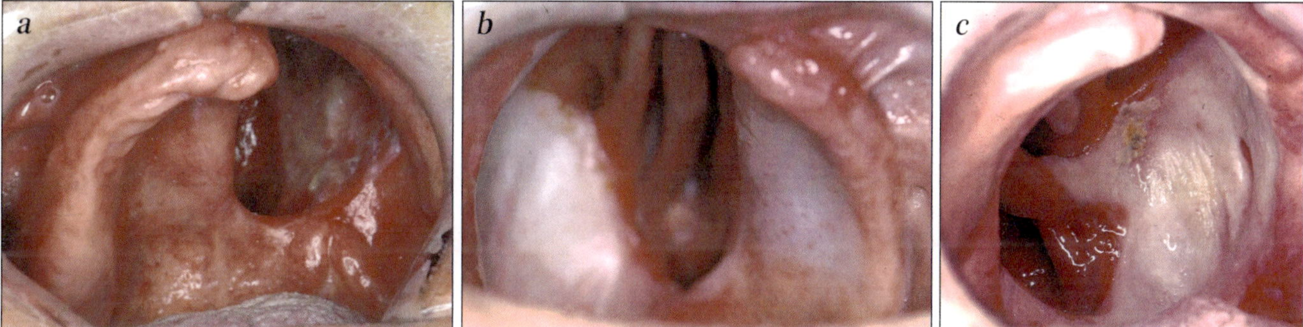

Figure 3-47 *(a)* Patient with ovoid arch form and excellent alveolar ridge contours following total maxillectomy. Note the amount and angulation of the palatal shelf area. *(b)* A tapering arch provides much less support because of the reduced palatal shelf area. Implants will be necessary to provide support for mastication. *(c)* Lacking palatal shelf, the obturator prosthesis will be easily impacted into the defect during mastication and swallowing.

processing. Another alternative is to fabricate a removable superior lid, which provides the patient with both alternatives along with access to cleaning. The lid is vacuum formed with mouthguard material but must be replaced periodically (Phankosol and Martin, 1985).

Definitive obturators for edentulous patients

Prognostic factors

Fabrication of an obturator prosthesis for an edentulous patient with a large maxillary defect will challenge the skill of even the most experienced clinician. With any sizable palatal perforation, retention in the classic sense of a complete denture prosthesis is impossible. Air leakage, poor stability and support, and reduced denture-bearing surfaces will compromise adhesion and cohesion, and therefore achievement of peripheral seal is not possible in almost all patients. Therefore, the contours of the defect must be used to maximize the retention, stability, and support of the prosthesis. The surgical defect should be well healed prior to the fabrication of the definitive obturator prosthesis.

Degree of movement. Maxillary obturator prostheses for edentulous patients will exhibit varying degrees of movement, depending on the support areas that can be engaged within and peripheral to the defect. The more movement the prosthesis exhibits during function, the more compromised the prosthodontic prognosis and the clinical outcome. In general, the less palatal shelf available, the more movement of the prosthesis during function (Fig 3-46). In some patients, the movement is of such a magnitude as to preclude any semblance of mastication and may make swallowing and speech problematic. In such instances, the placement of implants is essential if mastication, speech, and swallowing are to be returned to near-normal range.

During swallowing and mastication, the prosthesis will be impacted superiorly into the defect. With the release of occlusal pressure, the prosthesis drops in the opposite direction. In the edentulous patient with a total maxillectomy defect, the axis of rotation is located along the medial palatal margin of the defect (Fig 3-46a). The portion of the obturator at right angles and most distant from this axis will exhibit the greatest degree of motion. In a posterior maxillary defect, where the anterior maxillary segment is retained, the axis of rotation moves posteriorly (Fig 3-46b). With these smaller defects, the degree of movement during function is considerably less because additional maxillary structures remain for support and stability. With anterior resections of the maxillae, the axis of rotation is located along the anterior margin of the defect. The anterior lip margin of the prosthesis will exhibit the greatest potential for movement (Fig 3-46c).

Support. *Support* is defined as the resistance of the prosthesis to vertical forces during mastication. Support for the obturator prosthesis is primarily dependent on the amount of palatal shelf remaining and the alveolar ridge contours. The residual palatal shelf is often located perpendicular to the direction of occlusal

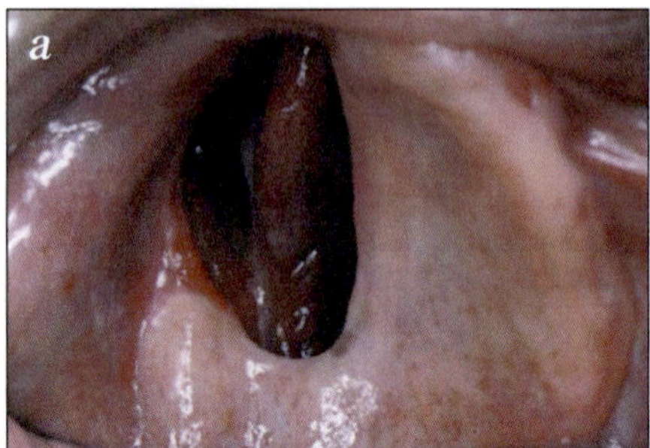

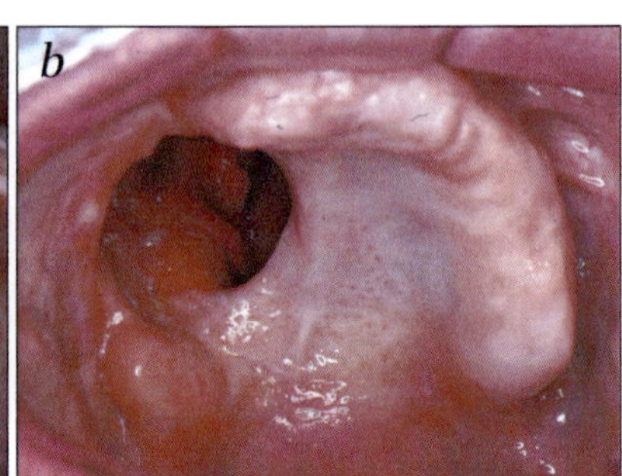

Figure 3-48 *(a and b)* The presence of a tuberosity on the side of the defect dramatically increases support and reduces movement. It is also a possible implant site. These defects are relatively static, i.e., they change little dimensionally during function.

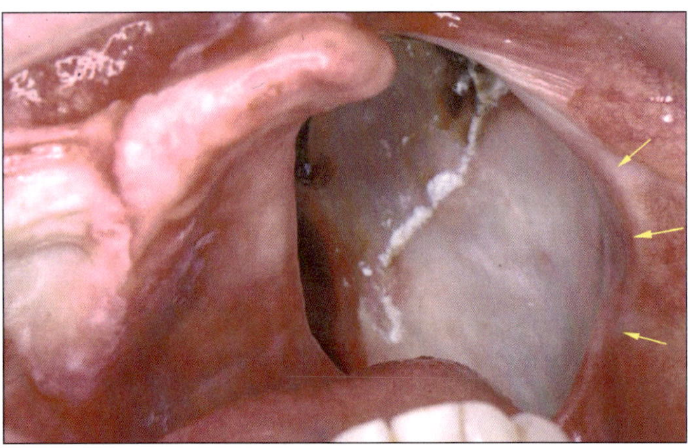

Figure 3-49 Lateral cheek surface of a total maxillectomy defect with a split-thickness skin graft lining the raw surface of the cheek. A scar band has formed at the skin graft–mucosa junction *(arrows)*.

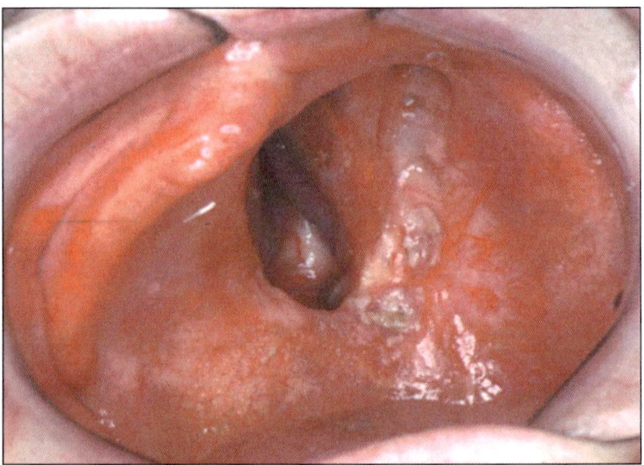

Figure 3-50 Defect allowed to granulate and epithelialize spontaneously, resulting in a defect with unfavorable mucosal lining and contours.

force and can provide considerable support during function. The patients shown in Fig 3-47 illustrate the importance of support provided by the residual palatal shelf. A square or ovoid arch will exhibit more palatal shelf area and alveolar ridge following a total maxillectomy (Fig 3-47a). In contrast, the reduced surface area available and undesirable angulation of the palatal shelf found in tapering arches provide little support for the prosthesis during mastication (Fig 3-47b). In the patients shown in Fig 3-47b and c, much of the palatal shelf has been resected. In such patients, consideration should be given to placement of zygomatic implants on the defect side combined with implants on the unresected side. Otherwise, the clinical outcome will be substantially suboptimal. In contrast, the clinical outcome achieved with a conventional complete-denture-obturator prosthesis in the patient seen in Fig 3-47a can be quite acceptable even if implants are not used. Denture adhesive can be applied to the intaglio surfaces of the prosthesis on the unresected side and combined with the retention achieved by engaging the skin-lined lateral wall of the defect, speech, swallowing, and mastication can be effectively restored.

Palatal tori should be removed at the time of surgery. If the tori are not removed less palatal shelf surface area is available for support and the thin mucosa lining the tori will likely be irritated by the movement of the obturator prosthesis.

A healthy, well-formed edentulous alveolar ridge will enhance support. If a partial maxillectomy is performed, the increased amount of hard palate and alveolar ridge on the side of the defect will dramatically enhance the support for the prosthesis. On the resected side the base of the skull, the lateral portion of the orbital floor, and the zygomaticoalveolar crest can also be engaged to enhance support when these surfaces are lined with skin. The presence of a tuberosity on the resected side will also enhance support (Fig 3-48) and is an excellent site for an implant (see section below entitled "Pyramidal process of the palatal bone").

Retention. *Retention* is defined as the ability of the prosthesis to resist the vertical forces of dislodgment. As explained previously, retention in the classic sense (peripheral seal) is not possible, but acceptable retention can usually be obtained by engaging key areas within the defect. Nevertheless, edentulous patients should be informed that their prosthesis will exhibit considerable movement during function. Most patients will be aware of any retentive deficiencies because of their experience with the immediate surgical and interim obturator prostheses. However, it is advisable to reemphasize this deficiency prior to the fabrication of the definitive prosthesis so that patients will have realistic expectations.

In large defects, retention is supplemented by the undercuts in the defect. Engagement of the skin graft and the scar band formed at the skin graft–mucosa junction will improve retention significantly. As this scar band organizes, it contracts linearly in the manner of a purse string, thus creating an undercut superiorly and a concavity inferiorly (Fig 3-49; see also Figs 3-16, 3-18, 3-19, and 3-21). This band is most prominent laterally and posterolaterally and tends to blend with the oral and nasal mucosa more anteriorly. The scar band is flexible and will permit the prosthesis to be inserted but will tend to resist dislodging forces. The skin graft above the scar band will

Figure 3-51 *(a)* Peripheral extension of the obturator against the lateral wall of the defect. In a total maxillectomy defect, this peripheral extension will exhibit greatest range of motion. *(b)* Enlargement showing appropriate obturator-tissue contact *(circle)*.

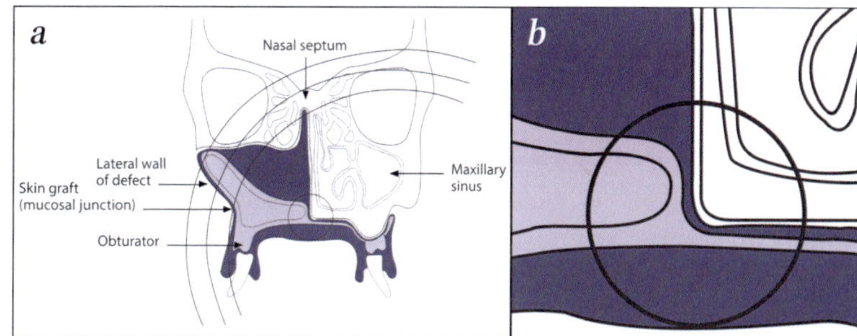

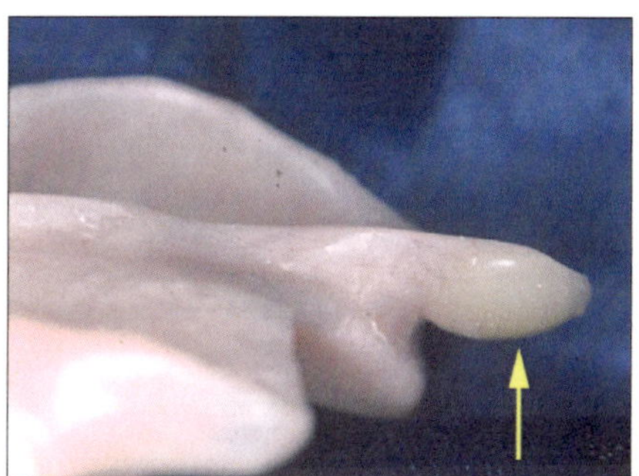

Figure 3-52 Engaging the nasal side of the soft palate *(arrow)* will improve retention.

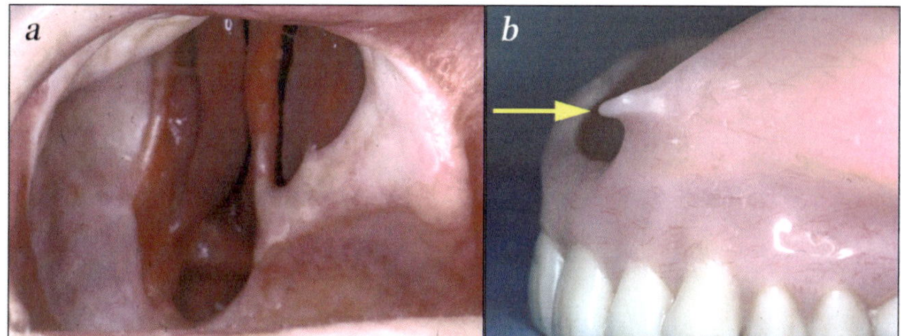

Figure 3-53 *(a)* When the premaxillary segment is removed it may be possible to *(b)* extend the prosthesis into the skin-lined nasal aperture *(arrow)*.

tend to stretch, so modest pressure exerted by the prosthesis against the skin graft laterally will enhance retention of the prosthesis. If the raw cheek surface is allowed to granulate and epithelialize spontaneously, this scar band will not form, resulting in a less favorably shaped defect (Fig 3-50). Since the lateral portion of the obturator exhibits the greatest degree of movement, retention is improved by the establishment of appropriate obturator-tissue contact superior-laterally even in the absence of a substantial undercut (Brown, 1968) (Fig 3-51). Additional retention may be gained by extending the prosthesis along the nasal surface of the soft palate (Fig 3-52). If the premaxillary segment was removed at surgery, the nasal aperture can also be engaged (3-53).

Flexible silicone materials have been used to engage undercuts associated with the defect but exhibit significant limitations, such as short length of service secondary to fungal contamination, poor wettability, and poor adjustability. However, these materials permit engagement of bony undercuts more profoundly and may be useful for some edentulous patients (Parr, 1979; Schaaf, 1977).

Denture adhesives can be effective in patients with partial maxillectomy or partial palatectomy defects but usually are not effective when the resections are more aggressive, such as total maxillectomy defects, unless the defect contains useful skin-lined undercuts areas in the defect that can be effectively engaged. The combination of adhesive, applied to the prosthesis on the unresected side, and engagement of the undercuts in the defect is usually sufficient to retain the prosthesis during speech and swallowing. Denture adhesives should only be used on the areas of the prosthesis that engage the residual denture-bearing surfaces.

Stability. *Stability* is defined as the ability of the prosthesis to withstand the horizontal forces of dislodgment. The height and contour of the residual alveolar ridge and the depth of the sulci are important considerations. In a patient with a total maxillectomy, a healthy, well-formed edentulous ridge with deep sulci on the unresected side will enhance stability (see Fig 3-47a). If a partial maxillectomy is performed and the anterior palatal segment is retained, the increased curvature of the alveolar ridge on the side of the defect will enhance the stability of the prosthesis (see Fig 3-46b).

Stability is also enhanced if the prosthesis engages the superior-lateral portion of the defect when it is skin lined and the medial margin of the defect when it is lined with palatal mucosa or skin (see Figs 3-41a and 3-23a and b). If the lateral portion of the orbital floor, the zygomaticoalveolar crest area, or the base of the skull has been resurfaced with a skin graft, engagement of these areas will also significantly improve stability.

Static defects versus dynamic defects. If the posterior margin of the defect does not extend beyond the junction of the hard and soft palates, the defect will be relatively static; it will not significantly change its shape during speech, swallowing, or movement of the mandible (see Figs 3-46a, 3-47a, and 3-48). Larger defects especially extending posteriorly beyond this junction are more dynamic; the shape of the defect changes considerably during speech, swallowing, and movement of the mandible secondary to mastication (see Fig 3-47c). Dynamic defects present a greater challenge to the clinician, and prostheses fabricated to restore them move so much that they often are difficult for the patient to control, and therefore implants are strongly recommended for such patients, especially intradefect implants. A prosthesis restoring a total palatectomy defect that extends posteriorly to the posterior pharyngeal wall will require implant retention and support if speech, swallowing, and mastication are to be restored to near-normal levels.

Status of the opposing arch. If the opposing mandible is edentulous and the patient presents with severe resorption, a retruded tongue position, and/or an unfavorable floor of the mouth posture, the patient's difficulties are compounded. Such patients are

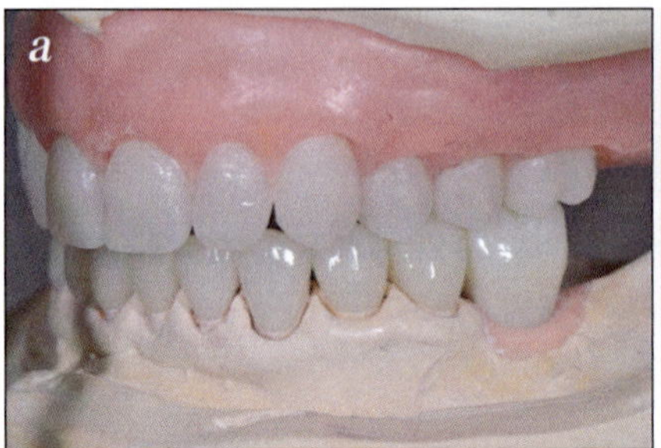
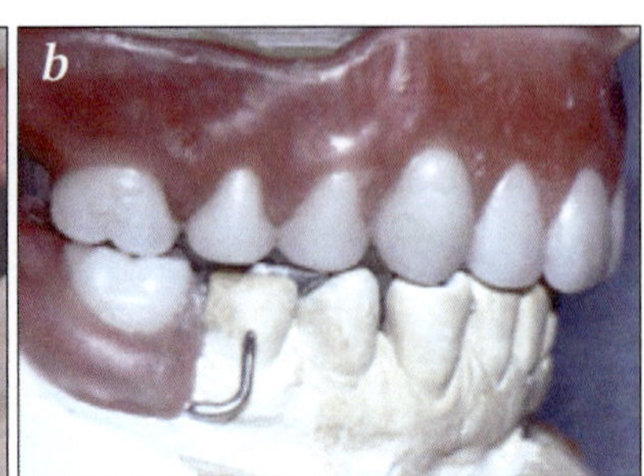

Figure 3-54 *(a)* The occlusal plane, incisal angle, compensating curve, and morphology of the posterior dentition have been idealized by individual restorations in the mandible. *(b)* Ribbon rests associated with the removable dental prosthesis were used to correct the occlusal plane discrepancy (reprinted from Beumer et al., 2022b, with permission).

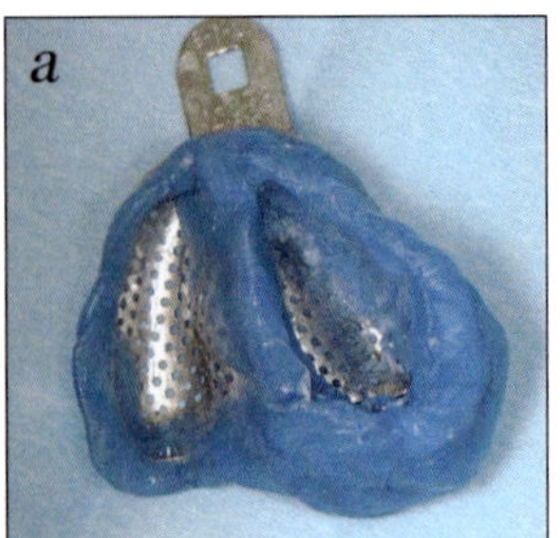
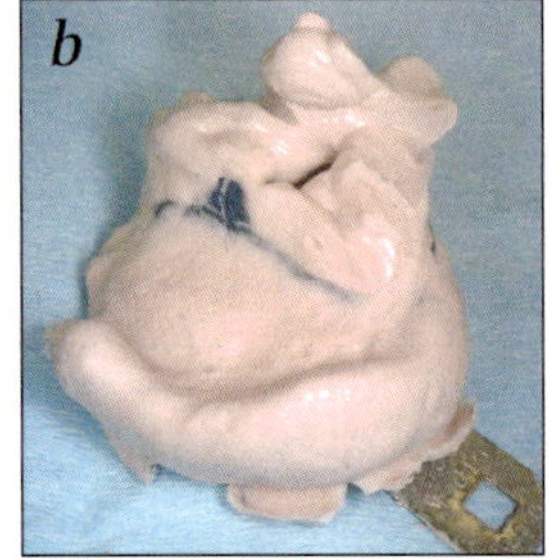
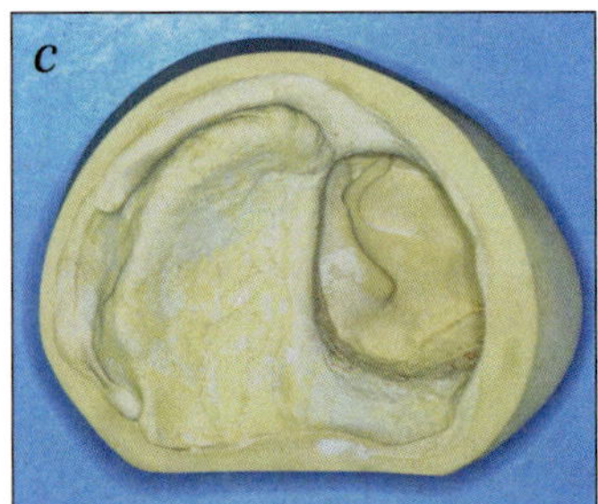

Figure 3-55 *(a)* Stock tray modified with periphery wax. Note that the wax is extended to engage the lateral wall of the defect. *(b)* Preliminary impression. *(c)* Preliminary cast.

forced to contend with unstable and poorly retained prostheses for both arches, and osseointegrated implants should be considered in both arches.

If the opposing mandible is partially or fully dentate, the plane of occlusion and occlusal contours of the mandibular teeth must be carefully scrutinized. Significant aberrations in either should be addressed by recontouring the occlusal surfaces of individual teeth, fixed dental prostheses, or removable dental prostheses (Fig 3-54).

Neuromuscular control. Maxillary obturator prostheses exhibit varying degrees of movement; if the patient is to employ the prosthesis successfully, he or she must be capable of controlling the prosthesis with the tongue, lips, and cheek musculature. Patients who are experienced successful denture wearers are generally more successful than others in this endeavor. However, a sizable number of edentulous patients are unable to manipulate their obturator prosthesis sufficiently well to perform oral functions effectively. Osseointegrated implants should be considered for those who fall into this category.

Clinical procedures

Impressions. Prior to making the preliminary impression, the clinician should ensure the defect is clean and free of dried crusts of mucus. If these crusts are not removed, the irreversible hydrocolloid impression material will remove at least some of them during withdrawal of the impression. If they are not removed from the impression surface of the defect, these crusts will transfer to the cast.

The objective of the preliminary impression is to record the remaining maxillary structures and the useful portions of the defect. An edentulous stock tray is selected according to the configuration of the remaining maxilla. Periphery wax is added to the periphery on the unresected side and extended up the lateral wall of the defect. Before the impression is made, the medial and anterior undercuts are blocked out with gauze lubricated with petrolatum, because these undercuts are seldom engaged by the prosthesis. Sensitive areas should be similarly blocked out. The lubricated gauze can also be used to prevent the impaction of the impression material into undesirable areas of the defect. If an orbital exenteration has been performed, the patch covering the orbit can be removed and direct observations made regarding the fitting and insertion of the tray.

Adhesive is applied to the tray and wax. The irreversible hydrocolloid impression material is mixed and loaded in the tray. Care must be taken to place impression material laterally to record the lateral configuration of the defect. Before the tray is seated, impression material is wiped or injected in posterior and lateral undercuts. The impression is removed and a preliminary cast is made (Fig 3-55). An accurate diagnostic cast that reproduces the usable undercuts will help the clinician evaluate the degree of retention, stability, and support provided by the defect.

The undesirable undercuts recorded in the cast are blocked out with a suitable wax prior to construction of the custom tray. Relief of one thickness of baseplate wax is provided for the skin graft–mucosa junction and the superolateral aspect of the defect. The residual palatal structures are relieved in the customary way and the tray is fabricated with acrylic tray resin (Fig 3-56). It may be necessary to section the cast to retrieve the tray. The tray must extend to the full height of the lateral wall of the defect and about 10 mm onto the oral side of the soft palate. The extension up the medial wall of the defect should be minimal. The tray can also be fabricated by duplicating the provisional either by conventional means or by scanning the provisional and printing a 3D duplicate. The duplicated provisional is then adjusted as necessary to create space for impression material and a handle is added. Some clinicians configure the handle like a bite fork so that a facebow transfer record can be made after the impression is completed (Fig 3-56c).

Extensions of the tray are verified in the mouth. Inaccessible areas can be checked with disclosing wax for overextension or excessive contour. Conventional border molding techniques using impression compound are advocated. Low-fusing compounds provide more working time and are recommended. It is suggested

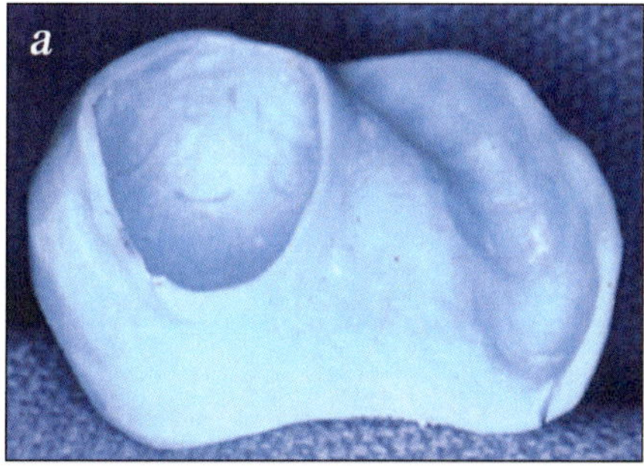
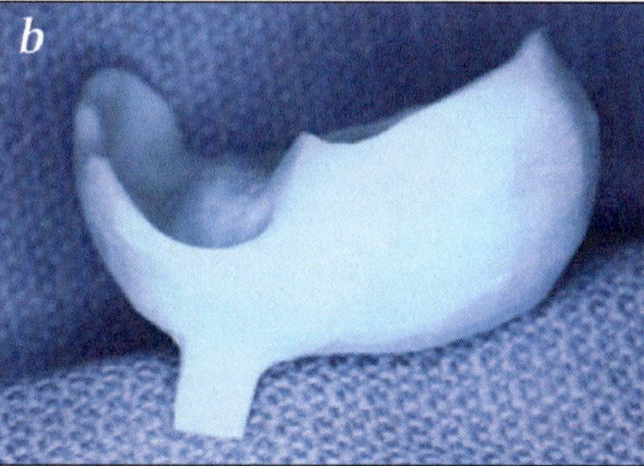
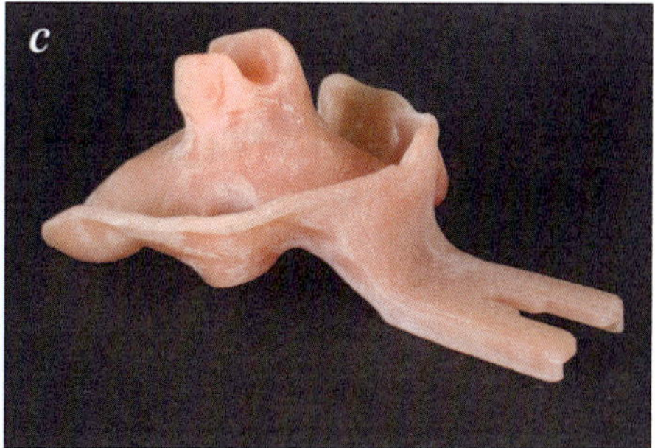

Figure 3-56 *(a and b)* Master impression tray. The defect area of the preliminary cast was blocked out with one thickness of base plate wax before making the tray. *(c)* A digitally designed and fabricated master impression tray with a handle configured like a bite fork allowing a facebow transfer record to be made along with the master impression.

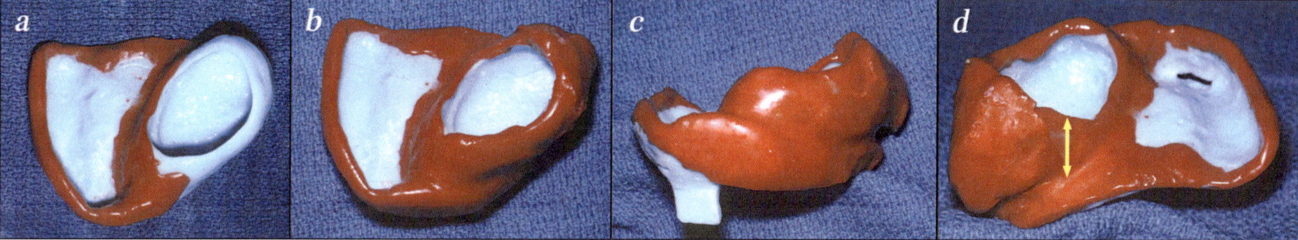

Figure 3-57 Impression for an edentulous patient. *(a)* Border molding of the nondefect side. *(b and c)* Completed border molding. Note the border molding of the lateral aspect of the defect and the indentation created by the lateral scar band. *(d)* Posterior view of the border molding. The posterior medial portion should be developed vertically about 1 cm or in some instances overlap onto the nasal side of the soft palate. A proper extension in this area will minimize the risk of nasal leakage during swallowing *(arrow)*.

that border molding be completed initially on the unresected side, including the medial margin of the defect, because this stabilizes and orients the tray to the defect (Fig 3-57a).

The superior height of the medial extension should terminate at the junction of the oral and respiratory mucosa or at the level of the nasal floor. *Further superomedial extension will only impede nasal airflow and will not contribute to retention or stability.* This is especially important if a Weber-Fergusson procedure is performed. Following this surgery, the nostril on the defective side may collapse somewhat, leading to the potential loss of airflow through the affected nostril.

Next, the soft palate extension is border molded. The impression should extend about 1 cm onto the oral surface of the residual soft palate. The extent of movement of the soft palate postsurgically will depend not only on the amount of soft palate resected but also on the amount of bony attachment remaining for the residual soft palate. If the soft palate exhibits significant elevation during function, this area may require refinement later with a thermoplastic wax. At this point, the tray should be relatively stable. Stability is a key factor in obtaining an accurate reproduction of the lateral, anterior, and posterior borders of the defect.

The lateral, posterior, and anterior aspects of the defect are recorded sequentially in two sections. First, the area below the skin graft–mucosa junction (lined with oral mucosa) is molded. Care should be taken to avoid overextension of the modeling compound in the anterior portion of the defect (Fig 3-57b and c). These tissues are heavily scarred and, if displaced during impression making, may develop painful ulcerations upon delivery of the definitive prosthesis.

Next, the lateral, posterior, and anterior aspects above the scar band are developed (Fig 3-57b–d). As mentioned previously, modest pressure should be developed laterally above the scar band because the skin graft does tend to stretch. As the posterolateral aspect (both above and below the scar band) is molded, the patient should be instructed to perform eccentric mandibular movements to account for the movement of the anterior border of the ramus and the coronoid process of the mandible. The lateral extension is developed superiorly as far as is feasible, engaging the lateral portion of the orbital floor, pterygoid plates, and base of skull when appropriate. However, the clinician must make sure that the length of this extension is compatible with insertion and removal of the tray.

Special care is taken to develop proper contours and extensions of the posterior-medial portion. This portion should be developed vertically about 1 cm or in some instances overlap onto the nasal side of the soft palate. A proper extension in this area will minimize the risk of nasal leakage during swallowing (Fig 3-57d).

The impression is completed with an elastomeric impression material. Polysulfide impression material is generally preferred for the corrected impression. Thermoplastic wax is generally not indicated for edentulous patients because of the difficulty in obtaining occlusal stops with the tray. Thermoplastic waxes are useful for making reline impressions for edentulous maxillectomy patients or when altered cast impressions are made with the aid of an RDP framework or a framework retained by osseointegrated implants.

The impression compound is relieved approximately 0.5 to 1.0 mm in all the areas before the master impression is made (Fig 3-58a). Several perforations are made to allow escape of the impression material; at least three perforations are made along the medial palatal margin. Impression material can be trapped in this location, preventing correct orientation and seating of the tray.

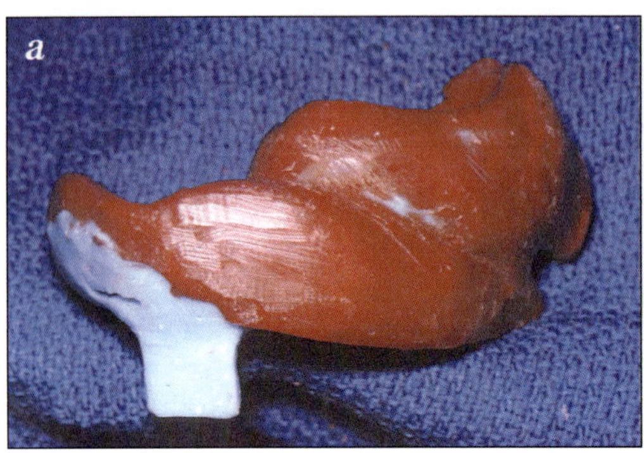

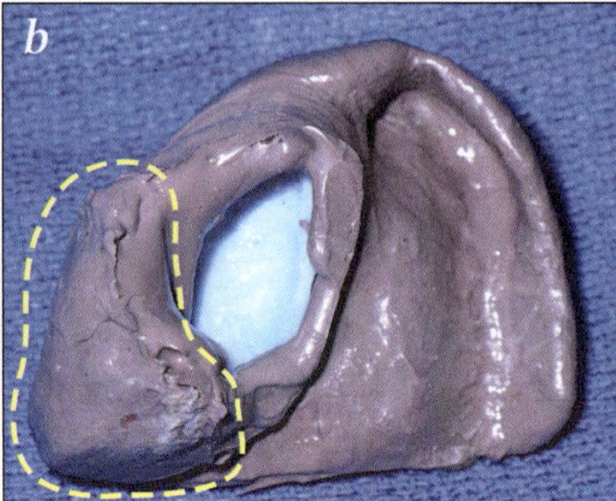

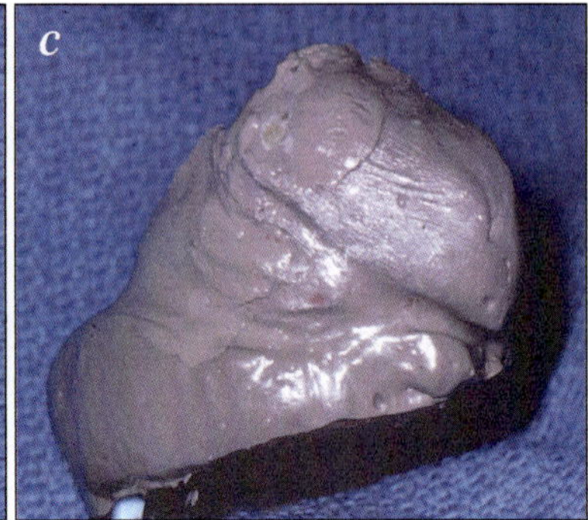

Figure 3-58 *(a)* Relief of the impression compound. The compound is cut back approximately 0.5 to 1.0 mm prior to refining the impression with an elastomeric impression material. *(b and c)* The completed impression. Note the posterior superior extension *(dotted line)* into the defect. This extension will provide considerable support for the prosthesis on the side of the defect.

The tray and impression compound are painted with adhesive. The elastic impression material is prepared by the assistant, while the clinician removes excess secretions. While the prosthodontist loads the tray with light-bodied material, the dental assistant loads a large-barreled syringe with the medium-bodied impression material. The medium-bodied material is injected into desirable undercut areas and the impression tray is seated in position. The lips and cheek are manipulated, and the patient is instructed to perform eccentric movements of the mandible.

After the material has set, the impression is removed with a gentle teasing action and inspected (Fig 3-58b and c). The impression may be difficult to remove because of the extension of the elastomeric impression material into multiple undercuts in the defect. If so, the lateral portion of the impression should be released initially because the flexibility of the scar band will enhance this maneuver.

If the anterior margin of the soft palate exhibits considerable elevation during speech and swallowing or if the defect extends all the way to the pharyngeal wall, occlusal stops are added in compound, and the portion of the impression that engages these regions is cut away with a scalpel and a functional impression of this area is made with thermoplastic wax. To reinsert the impression, it may be necessary to trim the impression material that has engaged undesirable undercuts, particularly those along the medial margin of the defect. It may be more effective to mold this area on delivery of the prosthesis and selectively reline this area.

If the patient exhibits extreme trismus, border molding can be a difficult and frustrating experience for both the prosthodontist and the patient. Therefore, an alternative impression technique using the interim prosthesis is suggested for edentulous patients. By the time the patient is ready for a definitive prosthesis, the interim prosthesis is usually well adapted and properly extended, and the effectiveness of obturation can be ascertained. If the prosthesis is acceptable, a new application of tissue conditioner (or impression material) is made and this impression is used as the master impression.

Records. Several methods can be used to fabricate record bases. If the defect is large and stability and support are difficult to obtain with a conventional record base, the prosthodontist should consider processing the definitive base from the master cast (Oh and Roumanas, 2008) (Fig 3-59). When there is minimal extension of the defect superiorly, a record base can also be fabricated by scanning the master cast, digitally designing the record base, and printing it from a PMMA puck. The record base can also be designed digitally and milled out of pucks of PMMA if the thickness of the puck permits capture of the full extent of the obturator prosthesis into the defect. These record bases are used to obtain jaw relation records and the denture teeth are added at a later date. If stability and support appear to be adequate, a conventional autopolymerizing acrylic resin record base can be constructed after all undercuts and the rugae area are blocked out for protection of the master cast (Fig 3-60).

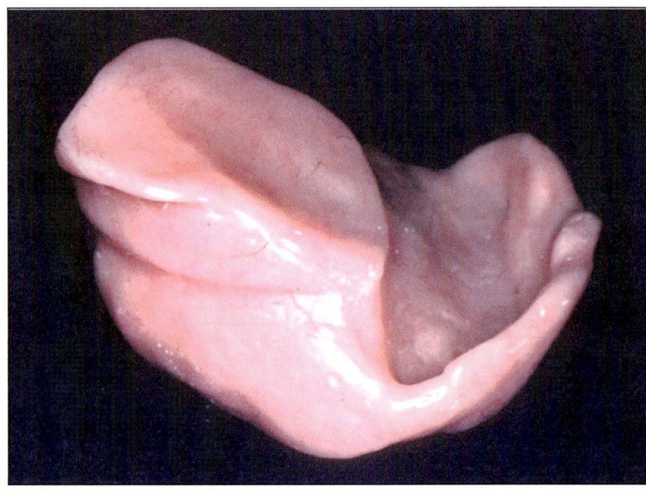

Figure 3-59 Definitive record base processed from the master cast and used to obtain centric relation records. Teeth are attached later.

The occlusal vertical dimension (OVD) is established in the customary manner with wax rims on the record bases. Conventional methods of determination and identification of the proper vertical dimension can be followed if the patient does not exhibit excessive trismus. Trismus is usually most evident in patients who have received preoperative or postoperative radiation therapy, particularly chemoradiation; whose surgical resection has resulted in edema or scarring of the muscles of mastication; or whose pterygoid plates or adjacent musculature are involved in the resection. If trismus is extreme (less than 20 mm of interridge distance), the occlusal vertical dimension should be reduced to ease the passage of bolus of food between the anterior denture teeth.

Occasionally, trismus may be so severe that it limits the superolateral extension of a conventional maxillary obturator prosthesis. The flexibility of the cheek on the defect side will often be of help

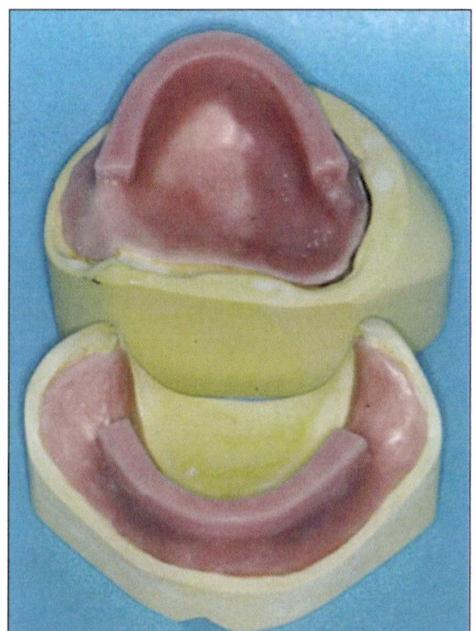

Figure 3-60 Master casts with conventional record base and wax rims. Undercuts are blocked out impacting the adaptation of the record bases making it more challenging to obtain accurate centric relation records.

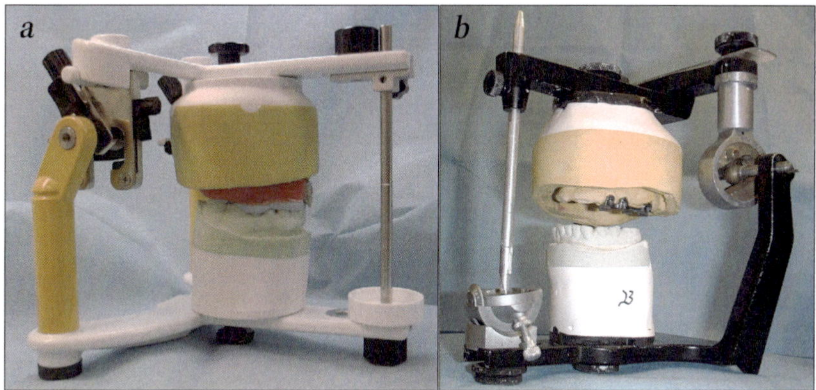

Figure 3-61 *(a)* Articulator capable of receiving large casts. *(b)* Articulator modified to accept large maxillary casts.

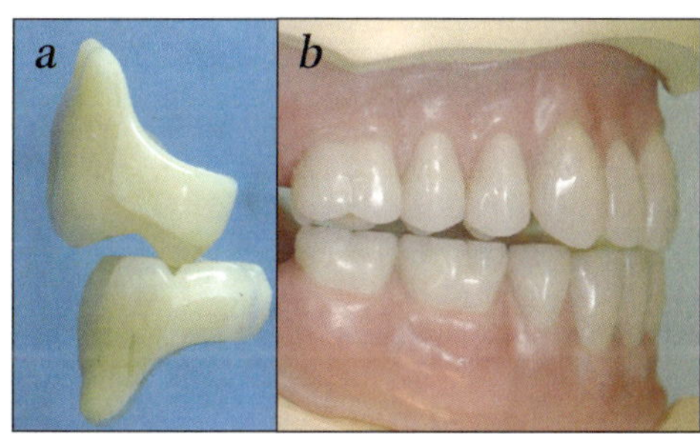

Figure 3-62 *(a)* Maxillary lingualized teeth opposing nonanatomic mandibular teeth. *(b)* Denture setup. Note the absence of vertical overlap of the anterior teeth.

when inserting and removing the prosthesis, especially if the cheek flap was lined with a skin graft during the surgical procedure. For removal, the normal side is displaced first and the obturator portion rotated out of the defect. For insertion, the obturator portion is positioned first, followed by the unresected side. If the depth of the residual palatal vault on the nondefect side is greater than the interridge or intertooth distance, the resin prosthesis cannot be inserted or removed, and adaptation to the palatal vault will be compromised.

The wax rims are reduced to the proper level, an arbitrary facebow transfer record is obtained, and centric relation is recorded with the recording medium of choice. Care must be exercised to ensure that the maxillary record base is not displaced during the registration. This may be difficult in patients with large defects.

Inaccuracies associated with jaw relation records are most evident when record bases are unstable and maxillomandibular relationships are abnormal. These conditions exist in many intraoral maxillofacial defects, particularly in edentulous patients following a total maxillectomy. As a result, reproducible centric relation records may be difficult to obtain for edentulous patients, because the prosthodontist must manage two relatively unstable record bases (Curtis et al., 1975). In patients presenting with large defects, graphic-centric relation records produced by intraoral or extraoral tracing devices are not possible.

Although a maxillary record base may exhibit acceptable stability, pressure on the defect side will result in some displacement superiorly into the defect and compromise the accuracy of the recording. We prefer soft wax, registration paste, or silicone as the recording medium. Accurate lateral records are usually not useful for the reason mentioned previously, but at times a protrusive record can be obtained, especially if the bases are relatively stable.

Because the maxillary cast is enlarged by the superior and posterior extensions of the defect, use of a high-post articulator is suggested (Fig 3-61a). However, the large cast may preclude proper maxillary cast mounting with a facebow and/or the use of a third point of reference. An acceptable alternative is lengthening of the articulator posts of conventional articulators, as suggested by Hadeed and Sprigg (1980) and Marunick and Ma (1983) to accommodate these casts (Fig 3-61b). With these altered articulators, large and thick maxillary casts can be mounted in their appropriate position with the aid of a facebow record.

Occlusal scheme and the aesthetic display of the anterior teeth. The teeth are set to contours established by the wax rims and conventional anatomical landmarks. In edentulous patients, nonanatomical and/or functional posterior teeth are arranged according to neutrocentric or modified lingualized occlusal concepts (Devan, 1956; Lang and Razoog, 1983). The authors prefer lingualized maxillary teeth opposing nonanatomic teeth in the mandible (Fig 3-62). The anterior teeth are positioned with no vertical overlap. These concepts minimize lateral forces and deflective occlusal contacts and thus improve prosthesis stability. For patients with a retracted upper lip on the defect side, the lateral incisors and/or canines may be elevated from the occlusal plane to better follow the lip line and enhance aesthetics (Fig 3-63).

The trial dentures are tried in the mouth and changes are made to accommodate the aesthetic desires of the patient. At this time, centric relation and the occlusal vertical dimension are verified. In most instances, it is advisable to reinsert the trial dentures and fabricate a remount record to refine the occlusion during the delivery appointment.

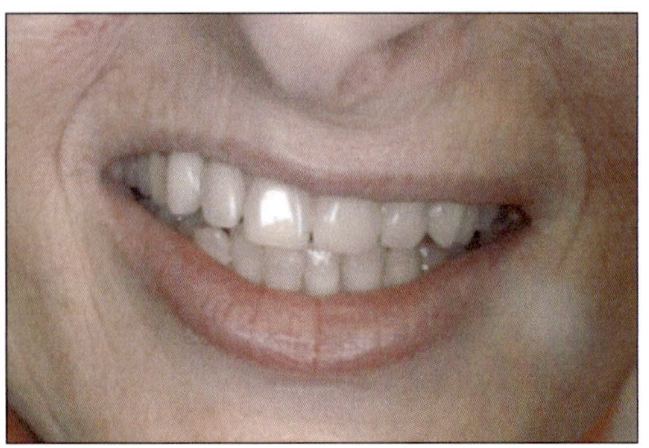

Figure 3-63 The right canine, lateral incisor, and central incisor have been elevated above the occlusal plane to create a more pleasing smile line compatible with the lip line.

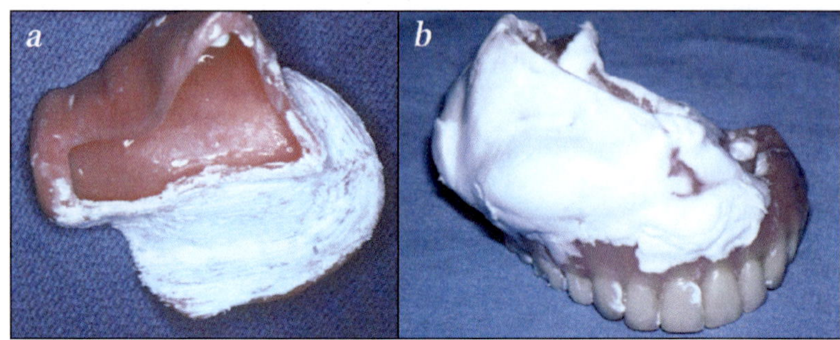

Figure 3-64 Delivery and adjustment of the obturator. *(a)* Pressure indicator paste is useful to delineate areas of excessive tissue displacement on the unresected site. *(b)* Disclosing wax is useful in checking extension areas or monitoring tissue displacement in the defect and skin-lined areas or where access is difficult. Note the displacement anteriorly.

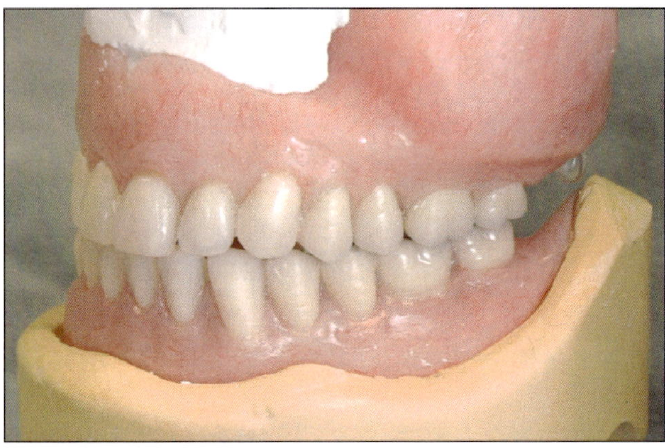

Figure 3-65 Prostheses remounted with new maxillomandibular records and equilibrated prior to delivery.

Processing, delivery, and follow-up. The dentures are processed in a standard manner with heat-cured polymethyl methacrylate. Various methods to create a hollow obturator with and without a lid have been described in the literature (Knapp, 1984). For large defects, if more profound retention is necessary, consideration can be given to using a soft silicone material for the obturator segment of the prosthesis (Schaaf, 1977; Parr, 1979; Taicher et al., 1983). This soft material allows the prosthesis to engage undercuts more aggressively. The obturator segment may be attached to the maxillary denture with a snap-on stud type of connection or magnetic attachments. The silicone obturator snaps into undercuts in the protruding studs so that the obturator segment may be replaced as required without disturbing the tissue surface of the denture. However, because of the well-known limitations of silicone, we prefer methyl methacrylate if adequate retention, stability, and support can be achieved with this material.

In waxing the obturator, the clinician must remember that the master impression may extend further superiorly, medially, or laterally into the defect areas than is consistent with insertion, removal, and function. On delivery, the resin extensions into undercut areas or the height of the superior surface may require considerable relief to permit seating of the prosthesis. We have found it easier to make these alterations after the prosthesis is processed. Those areas that may require considerable reduction should be waxed accordingly to permit these contour changes without perforation of the hollow obturator if the hollow, closed design is used.

If a closed-top design is used, the superior surface of the obturator should be well polished, have a slightly convex contour, and slope medially and posteriorly to help direct nasal secretions into the oral pharynx. Sharp projections on the lateral surfaces of the obturator should be rounded. The superolateral extension is considered a polished surface like a denture flange extension and therefore should be lightly polished with fine pumice. Polishing improves cleansibility and results in less friction at the prosthesis–soft tissue interface during functional movements. Gross overextensions into undercut areas may have to be reduced prior to delivery, but the final adjustment of these areas must be determined during delivery of the prosthesis.

Delivery and adjustment are performed in a conventional manner. Pressure indicator paste is used to delineate areas of excessive tissue displacement on the unresected side (Fig 3-64a). Disclosing wax is useful for checking peripheral extensions or for monitoring tissue displacement in skin-lined areas or where access is difficult (Fig 3-64b). With the aid of these materials, the least desirable undercuts are reduced until the prosthesis is seated appropriately. Rarely is it necessary to reduce the undercuts located along the lateral and posterolateral surfaces that are so vital for retention, stability, and support. We prefer to remount the prostheses with a new maxillomandibular record to idealize the occlusion (Fig 3-65). Home care instructions are reviewed and recall appointments are arranged. Most maxillary obturator prostheses require relining within the first year of delivery

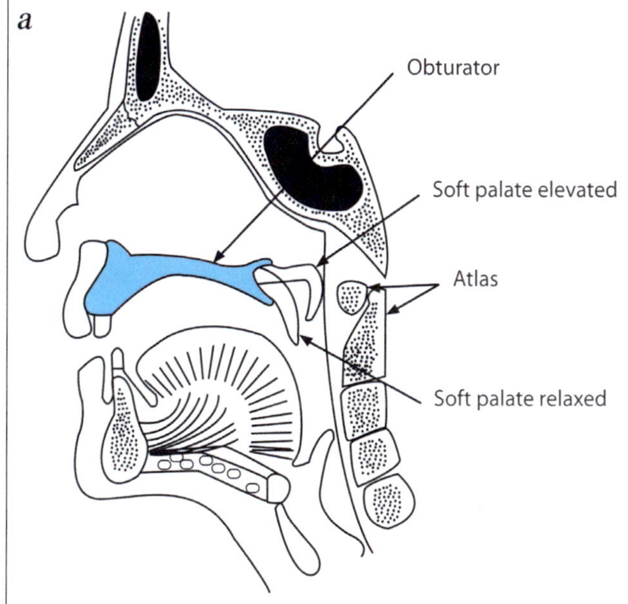

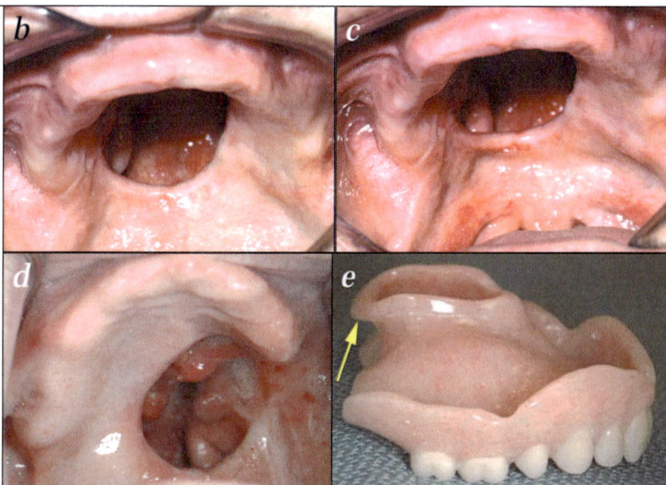

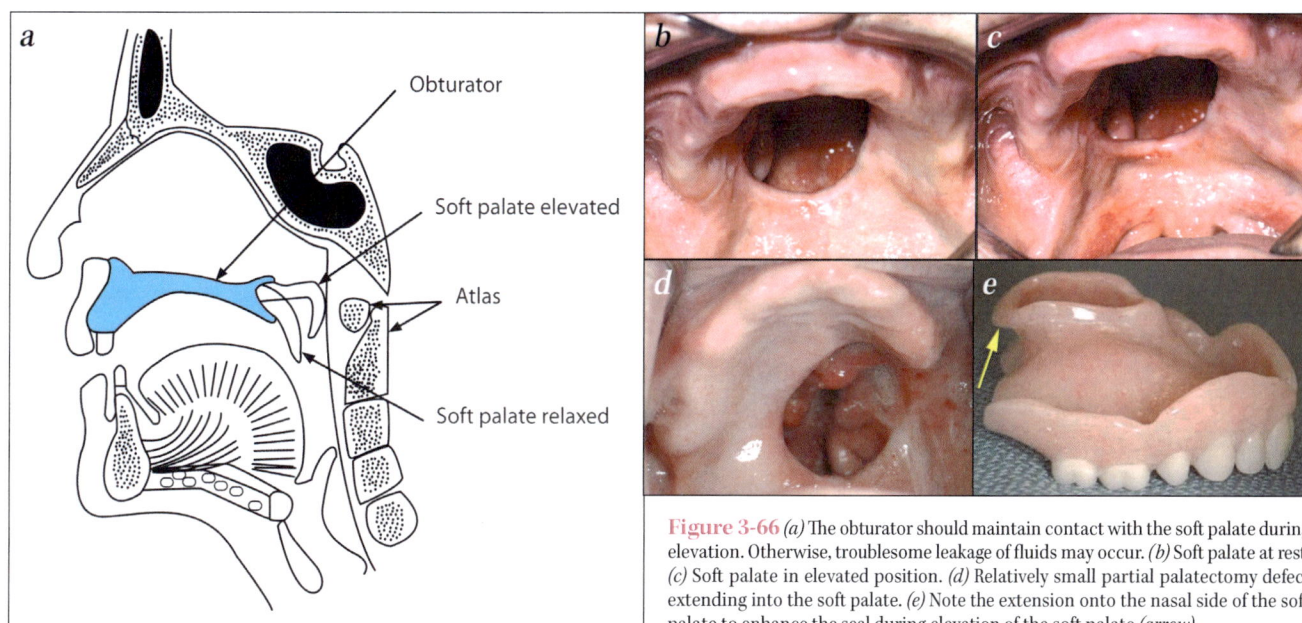

Figure 3-66 *(a)* The obturator should maintain contact with the soft palate during elevation. Otherwise, troublesome leakage of fluids may occur. *(b)* Soft palate at rest. *(c)* Soft palate in elevated position. *(d)* Relatively small partial palatectomy defect extending into the soft palate. *(e)* Note the extension onto the nasal side of the soft palate to enhance the seal during elevation of the soft palate *(arrow)*.

because of continued organization of the defect and subsequent dimensional changes.

Defects extending onto the mobile, middle third of the soft palate

Fabrication of definitive obturator prostheses for resections of the edentulous maxillae extending onto the movable middle third of the soft palates presents unique challenges. Special care must be taken to extend the prosthesis onto the nasal side of the soft palate (Fig 3-66). Otherwise, troublesome leakage will occur.

Small palatectomy defects

In smaller palatectomy defects, more of the hard palate remains and consequently the prosthesis has more stability and support. However, retention may be compromised because access to and use of the defect for retention may be impaired. Frequently these small defects are not skin lined, so it is difficult to engage the defect effectively. Implants are especially useful for this group of patients because the anterior maxillary segment on the defect side is likely to be available for implant placement. With a smaller defect, many of the prosthetic procedures are more easily accomplished. The delivery and follow-up care should follow the same sequence as described previously. However, relining may not be necessary as frequently.

Definitive obturators for dentulous patients with extensive palatal defects

It is self-evident that the prognosis improves with the availability of teeth to assist with the retention, support, and stability of the RDP-obturator prosthesis. This concept certainly applies to patients with acquired defects of the maxillae.

Treatment concepts

Several concepts that are unique to this group of dentulous patients must be considered by the prosthodontist.

Location of the defect. Invariably, the surgical resection includes the distal portion of the maxilla, and rarely does a distal abutment tooth remain following surgery. The extent of the surgical resection anteriorly varies considerably. Therefore, a Kennedy Class II partial denture with an extensive lever arm is required for most patients.

Length of the lever arm. In conventional prosthodontics, the most common Class II removable dental prosthesis involves an edentulous area distal to the canine. Considerably longer lever arms are encountered in patients with intraoral surgical defects. It is not uncommon for the defect to extend from the midline to the soft palate area or to the pharyngeal wall (Fig 3-67).

Movement of the prosthesis. In conventional prosthodontics, the degree of displacement of a Class II partial denture is dependent on the quality of the edentulous alveolar ridge and palate and the ability of the prosthodontist to balance the support available from both the edentulous segment and the remaining teeth. With resection of portions of the palate, the mucosal and bony support is compromised or may be lacking completely. Hence, the defect must be engaged to minimize the movement of the prosthesis and reduce the stress on the abutment teeth. In most defects, if forceful mastication occurs on the defect side, the prosthesis will be displaced significantly into the defect and has the potential to expose abutment teeth to damaging bending moments (lateral torquing forces).

Arch form, palatal shelf area, and support. As mentioned previously, square or ovoid arch forms possess more palatal denture-bearing surface perpendicular to occlusal stress. This provides for a more stable prosthesis during function and indirect retention can be more effectively employed to help retain the RDP-obturator prosthesis (see section below entitled "Indirect retention"). This support area must be accurately engaged in the same manner as the buccal shelf area used for support of mandibular partial prostheses. Tapering arch forms provide less palatal shelf area, and indirect

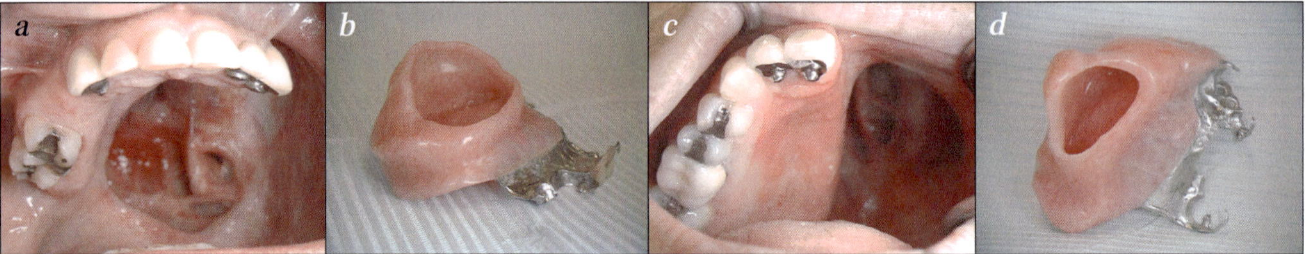

Figure 3-67 *(a)* Large maxillary defect extending posteriorly to the middle third of the soft palate. *(b)* Obturator for the defect in *(a)*. *(c)* Maxillectomy defect extending to the posterior pharyngeal wall. Note that the incisors have been splinted. *(d)* Obturator for the defect in *(c)* Note the long lever arms of both prostheses.

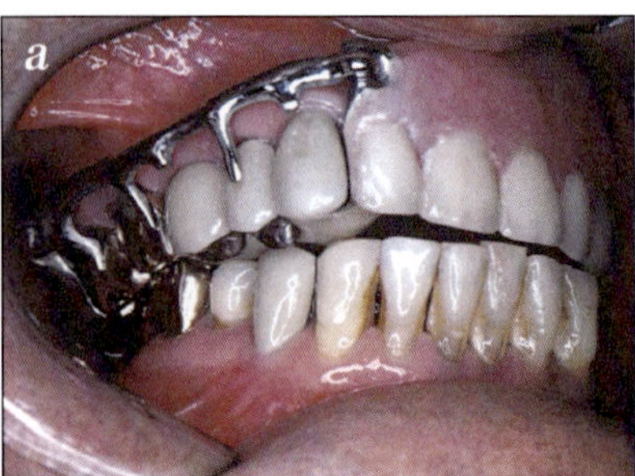

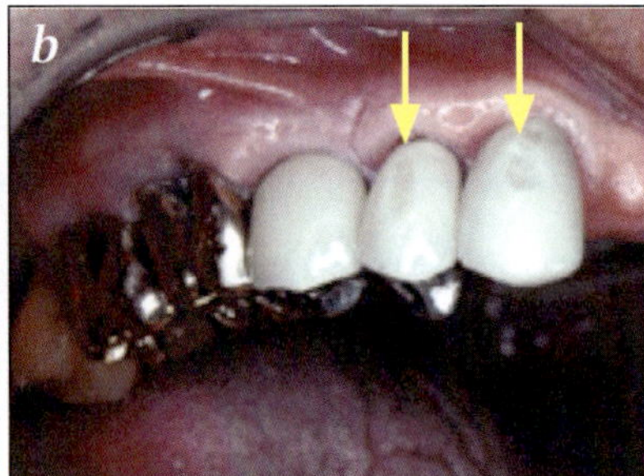

Figure 3-68 *(a)* Swing-lock design used to retain an obturator prosthesis. *(b)* Note the fractured retainers and the wear on the buccal and labial surfaces of the teeth *(arrows)*.

retention is much less effective. Therefore, support is compromised, which may lead to significant rotation and subsequent movement of the prosthesis into the defect during mastication.

Linear versus curvilinear arrangements of teeth. In prosthodontics, the preservation of that which remains (teeth and supporting structures) is the ultimate objective along with function, comfort, and aesthetics. Preservation of the remaining teeth is of particular importance because a prosthesis fashioned for an edentulous patient is far less retentive and stable. Therefore, it is strongly advised that partial denture designs anticipate and accommodate the principal movements of the prosthesis during function and minimize pathologic stresses on the abutment teeth. This is possible when the canine is retained on the side of the defect resulting in a curvilinear arrangement, but only when using the RPI or RPA concept of RDP designs (Kratochvil, 1963; Eliason, 1983; Kratochvil, 1988; Chang et al., 2019). However, there may be occasions when partial denture designs cannot be created without exposing the remaining dentition to significant pathological stresses, and as their periodontal support is compromised, the loss of these teeth may be anticipated at some future date. The placement of intradefect implants provides support on the defect side and will significantly reduce these stresses and should be considered if the defect crosses the midline and only a linear arrangement of dentition remains (see Fig 3-81).

Partial denture design concepts for maxillary defects

The basic principles of partial denture design should be followed; namely, major connectors should be rigid, rests should be positive and should direct occlusal forces along the long axis of the teeth, guiding planes should be designed to facilitate stability and bracing, retention should be within the physiologic limits of the periodontal ligament, and maximum support and stability should be gained from the residual soft tissue denture-bearing surfaces including the defect. The authors prefer to use variations of the I bar mesial rest (Kratochvil, 1963, 1988; Chang et al., 2019) or RPA (Eliason, 1983) concepts of RDP design.

The principal difference between conventional patients with extension base defects and patients with maxillectomy defects is the need for additional ***bracing*** from the RDP framework. As the defect becomes larger and less favorable and the remaining dentition arranged in a more linear fashion, more resistance to displacement in the horizontal plane must be provided. This is best accomplished by plating the lingual surfaces of the remaining dentition.

The use of partial denture designs that lock onto remaining dentition, such as the swing-lock type, is discouraged. Retention can be excellent with these designs, but they resist rotation of the prosthesis during function. This leads to several outcomes, all of which will compromise the function of the RDP-obturator prosthesis—overloading of the abutment teeth leading to their premature loss, advanced wear of the facial surfaces of the teeth engaged by the gate, or fracture of the retainers associated with the gate so as to accommodate rotation of the prosthesis during function (Fig 3-68).

As one can appreciate, developing partial denture designs that do not compromise the health of the abutment teeth and their supporting structures represents a unique challenge for prosthodontists. The compromised support, stability, and retention; the lack of cross-arch stabilization in many maxillary defects; the long lever arms and the resultant increase in load; the multiple axes of rotation that may have to be accommodated; and the increased impact of the forces of gravity in large defects present significant design challenges. It may not be possible to design an RDP-obturator prosthesis with the desired retention and stability needed to restore speech and swallowing and mastication without subjecting abutment teeth to damaging bending moments. As a result, given the predictability

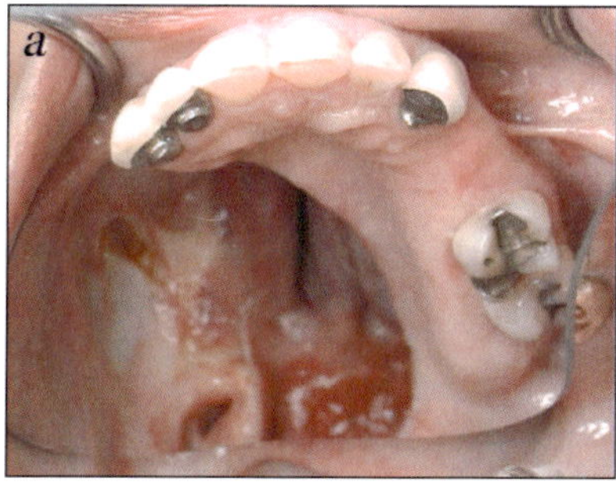
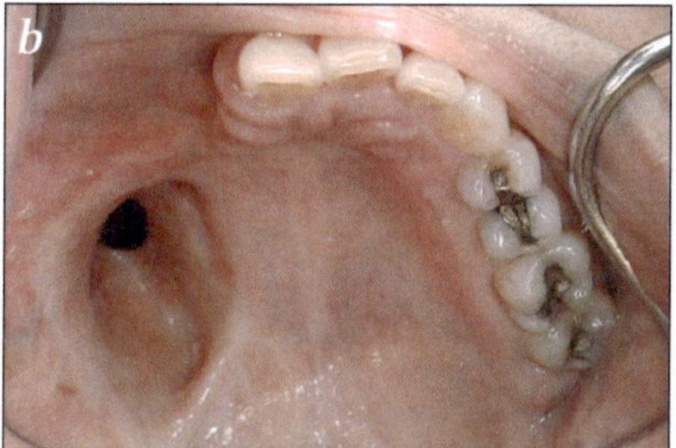
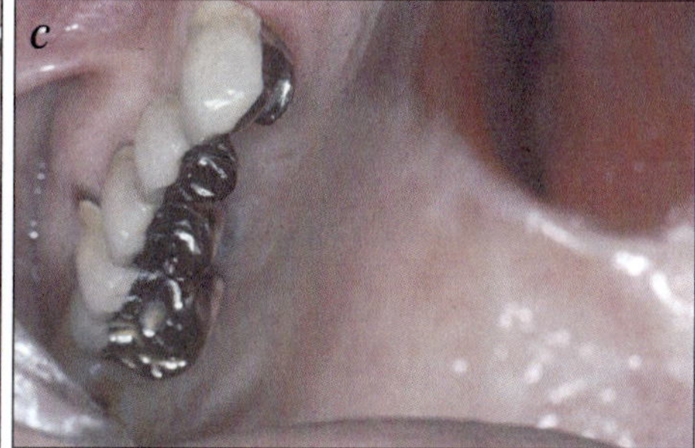

Figure 3-69 Palatal defects vary widely. The RDP design for "a" will be rather conventional. However, the designs used for "b" and "c" will require much more bracing from the residual dentition because of the loss of cross-arch stabilization secondary to the surgical resection. Zygomatic implant support on the defect side is recommended for patients such as shown in "c."

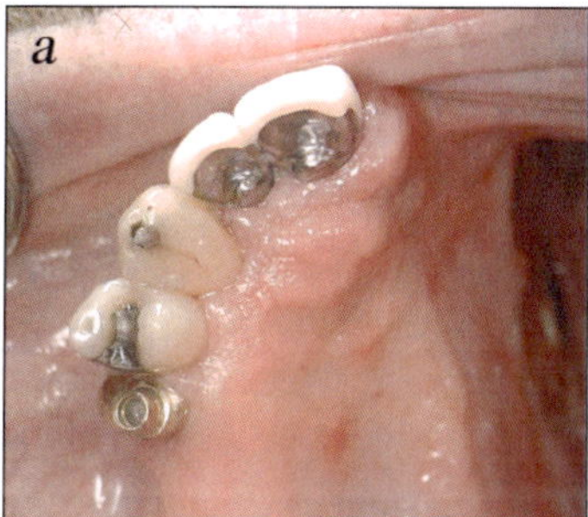
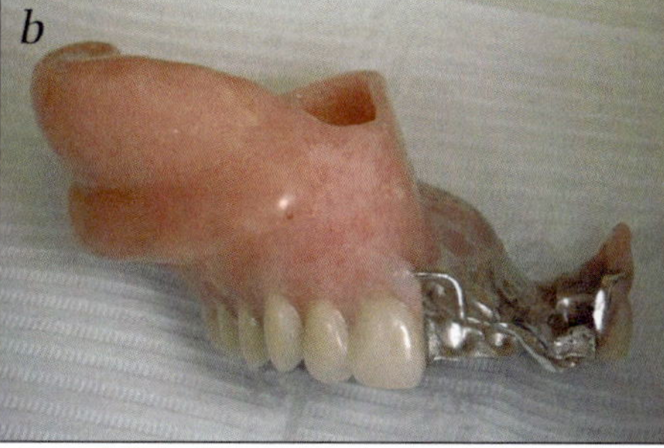
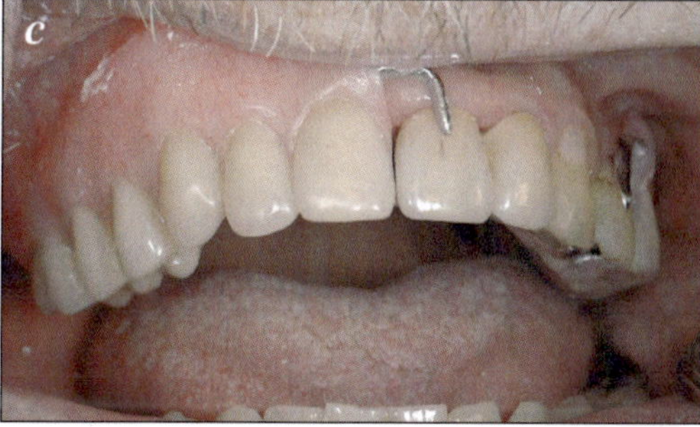

Figure 3-70 *(a)* On anterior teeth, the rest should be positioned at the junction of the gingival and middle thirds. *(b and c)* The retainer should be positioned on the tooth so that it disengages or rotates when an incising force is applied on the side of the defect.

of zygomatic implants, we suggest that when the defect is large and especially when teeth are arranged in a linear fashion, consideration should be given to providing implant support on the side of the defect (see Fig 3-81).

When a patient undergoes a partial resection of the hard palate resulting in a direct communication with the paranasal sinuses, unless the defect is effectively obturated with a prosthesis, the patient will exhibit hypernasal speech, and food and liquids will escape through the nose during swallowing. The prime objective of the clinician is to design and fabricate a prosthesis that seals the defect with sufficient retention to restore speech and swallowing. The level of mastication efficiency restored will be dependent upon the number and arrangement of teeth remaining in the unresected portion of the maxilla. As mentioned above, the authors prefer to use design concepts based on the I bar mesial rest (Kratochvil, 1963, 1988; Chang et al., 2019) or RPA (Eliason, 1983) philosophies of RDP design.

Several factors complicate RDP design in patients presenting with these defects. The most obvious is the compromised support resulting from the loss of a portion of the hard palate and associated dentition (Fig 3-69). The arrangement of the remaining dentition presents with less curvature than that seen in normal patients and in some cases offers an almost linear configuration limiting the effect of indirect retention and resulting in the loss of the value provided by cross-arch stabilization to distribute lateral forces. In addition, long lever arms are created from the necessary extension into the defect. As a result, the RDP-obturator prosthesis will be exposed to lateral forces of increased magnitude, secondary to displacement of the prosthesis associated with velopharyngeal function, excursive movements of the mandible, or contracture of the muscles of facial expression. The abutment teeth will therefore be exposed to significant levels of lateral forces, and these forces must be taken into account when designing the RDP framework.

As with conventional patients, the diagnostic casts should be surveyed carefully for location of undercuts, location and contour of potential guide planes, and selection of the path of insertion. Often a compound path of insertion must be employed to adequately use the undercuts available in the defect. For example, if the lateral and posterior undercuts in the defect are to be engaged properly, the obturator portion of the prosthesis first must be inserted into the defect and then rotated up into position to engage the teeth.

Multiple rests are suggested in order to improve stability and support for the prostheses. The rest seats should be rounded and polished so the rests on the partial denture framework can rotate without torquing abutment teeth. Surveyed crowns on selected teeth may be required to establish ideal contours for retention, guiding planes, and occlusal or cingulum rests. In defects extending to or beyond the midline, additional ***bracing*** is necessary to distribute the increased lateral forces more widely among the remaining dentition.

Abutments adjacent to the defect require special consideration. Teeth adjacent to the defect require special consideration. *These teeth must have a positive rest and be engaged by a retainer and a proximal plate* if the bone anchorage of these teeth is to be sustained long term and if adequate retention is to be achieved for the obturator prosthesis (Figs 3-70 and 3-71). This anterior retainer and rest also ensure proper orientation of the prosthesis. If this concept is not employed, the prosthesis will tend to rotate out of retentive areas posteriorly and be displaced lingually during function.

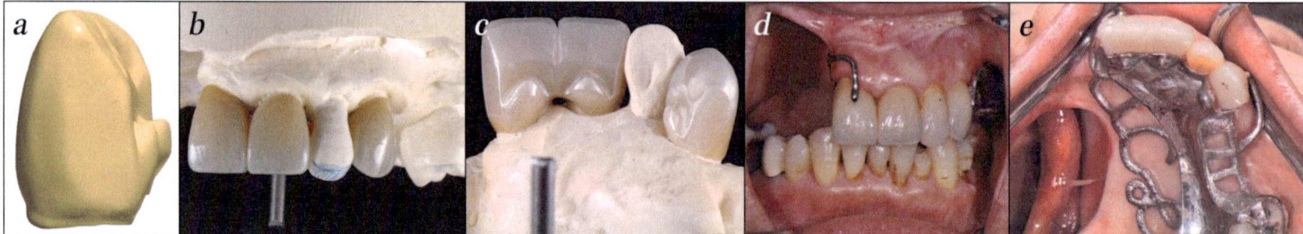

Figure 3-71 Surveyed crowns have been designed digitally and milled of zirconia for teeth #8, #9, and #11. *(a)* Digital design of the incisor crowns. *(b and c)* Incisors adjacent to the defect were splinted together to distribute stresses more broadly. Note the positive cingulum rests. *(d and e)* The framework seated. The I bars engaging #8 and #11 should be positioned in a 0.10 undercut and on the point of greatest mesial-distal curvature.

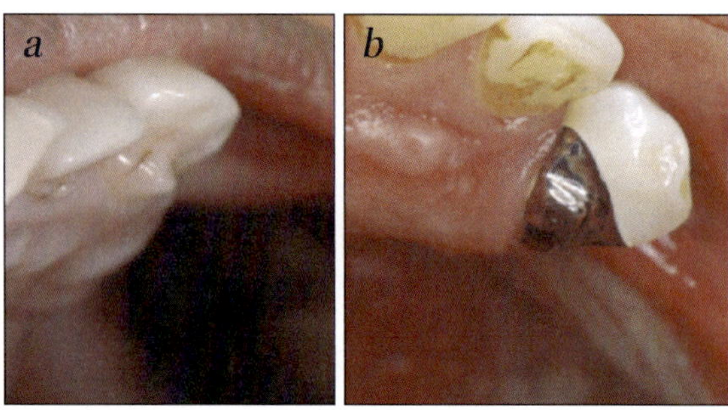

Figure 3-72 Canines are adjacent to both defects. In "a" the cingulum has been recontoured to create a positive rest. In "b" a full-coverage metal-ceramic crown was necessary to create a positive cingulum rest.

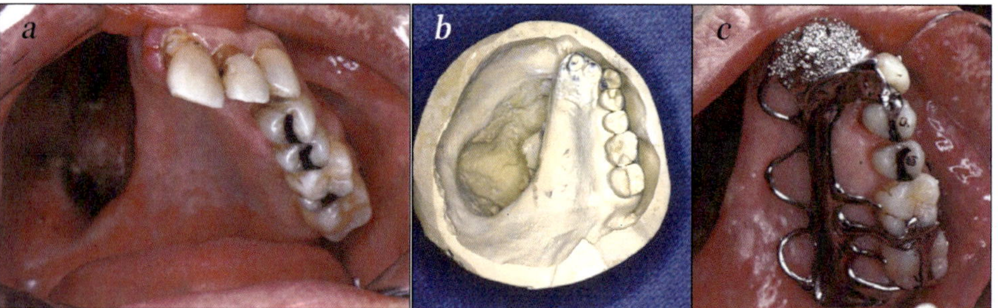

Figure 3-73 *(a)* The central incisors are adjacent to a defect with compromised periodontal bone support. *(b)* The teeth have been treated endodontically and converted to overdenture abutments. *(c)* The RDP is designed to overlay the abutments.

These abutments are subject to greater vertical and lateral forces (Schwartzman et al., 1985, 1990) and are more frequently lost than abutments in other positions. This is due to a number of factors. First, the extension area immediately adjacent to this abutment, which is basically the defect, provides little or no support. Second, the lever arms can become quite long, amplifying the forces delivered to the abutment. *Therefore, the placement of a positive rest on this tooth is critical to its long-term survival.* Anterior teeth adjacent to a maxillary defect must have positive cingulum or pothole rests so that occlusal forces are directed along the long axis of the abutment. If incisors are adjacent to the defect consideration should be given to splinting them with complete crowns and incorporating cingulum or pothole rests (Figs 3-70 and 3-71) (Lyons et al., 2005). If a canine is adjacent to the defect, cingulum rests can be created by recontouring the cingulum area or by fabricating a three-quarter or complete-coverage crown (Fig 3-72). Bonded cingulum rests hold much promise (Brudvik and Taylor, 2000), but long-term clinical studies are not yet available to assess their longevity in this group of patients.

Often, compromised bony support for the tooth adjacent to the defect does not permit its use as a partial denture abutment. Consequently, the next tooth or other adjacent teeth must be used for this purpose. Frequently, these compromised abutment teeth can be treated endodontically. The crown is then amputated and the root will serve as an overdenture abutment (Fig 3-73). Moreover, the alveolar bone and attached gingiva of these teeth will be retained improving the prospects of the implant placement into these sites at some future date. In some patients, it may be advantageous to remove such a tooth immediately and place an implant into this site (Fig 3-74).

Fulcrum lines are dynamic. The fulcrum line or axis of rotation of the partial-denture-obturator prosthesis for patients with acquired defects of the maxilla is influenced by the position of the rests, the size and configuration of the defect, and the magnitude and location of masticatory forces. The fulcrum line for the RDP restoring such defects is dynamic in that it shifts or changes during mastication relative to the size and configuration of the defect, the position of the bolus, and the masticatory force employed to penetrate it. Thus, there may be multiple axes or fulcrum lines, including the classical defined fulcrum line related to the rests on the teeth adjacent to the defect. The defect depicted in Fig 3-75 has both a surgical defect secondary to resection of a tumor and an edentulous extension area on the nonsurgical side. When an occlusal load is applied to the extension area #1, the prosthesis will rotate around axis AB. When a load is applied in the anterior section on the defect

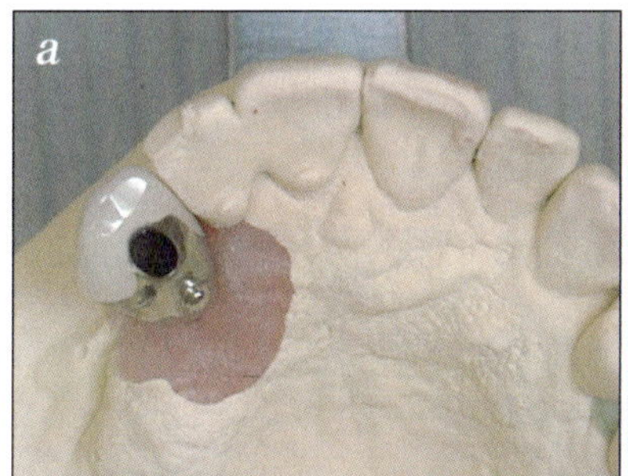

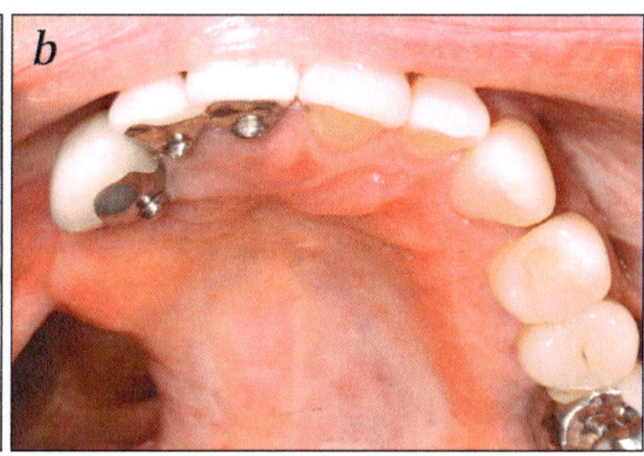

Figure 3-74 *(a and b)* The canine adjacent to the defect was lost after serving as the terminal abutment for the obturator prosthesis for 31 years. The site was grafted and an implant placed. Rather than use a resilient attachment the implant was fitted with a metal-ceramic crown with a cingulum rest. An I bar retainer engaged the labial surface. Completed prosthesis shown in Fig 3-153.

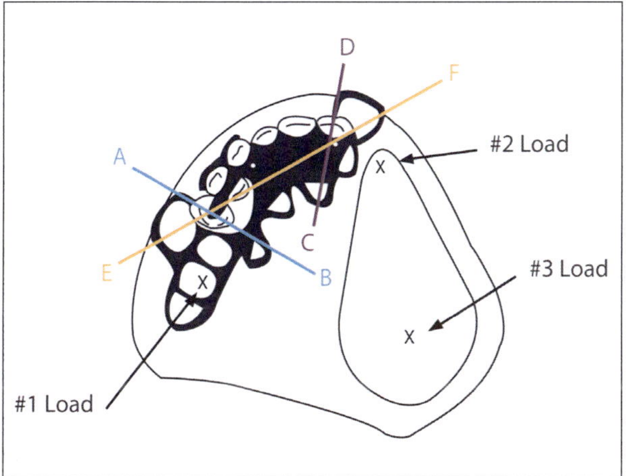

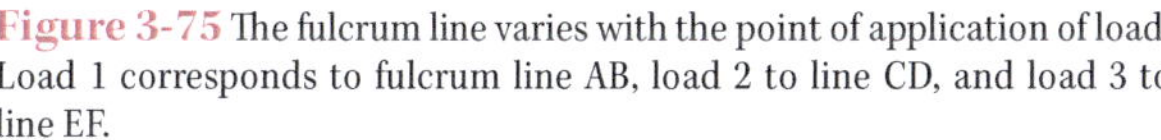
Figure 3-75 The fulcrum line varies with the point of application of load. Load 1 corresponds to fulcrum line AB, load 2 to line CD, and load 3 to line EF.

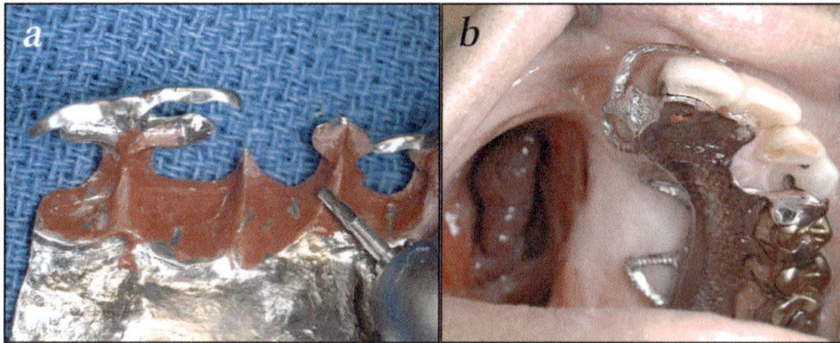

Figure 3-76 *(a and b)* The RDP framework is physiologically adjusted with chloroform and rouge or other suitable indicator.

side (#2) the prosthesis rotates around axis CD. However, when the load is applied at point #3, the axis of rotation shifts to EF. Since patients with such a defect are instructed to masticate on the dentate nonresected side partial denture designs must consider only those axes that are generated when the bolus is incised (load point #2) or when placed in the posterior extension area on the unresected side (load point #1).

Dentate patients with total maxillectomy defects learn quickly to masticate primarily on the nondefect side, as instructed. However, the food bolus may extend onto the anterior teeth of the resected side during the act of incising, and as a result, the axis of rotation shifts. The farther posteriorly the bolus and the forces are applied on the defect side, the farther posteriorly the fulcrum line shifts (see above, Fig 3-75), and the more unstable the prosthesis.

The dimensions of the defect exert some influence on the dynamics of the fulcrum line. A typical total maxillectomy defect will extend from the midline anteriorly to at least the anterior border of the soft palate posteriorly. However, it is not uncommon for a portion of the soft palate to require resection or for the resection to include more of the bony palate so that less of the remaining palatal shelf is available for support. Thus, the bulkier prosthesis is both heavier and less stable and will usually exhibit more movement when subjected to the forces of mastication on the defect side. Gravitational forces are also more of a concern because of the weight of the prosthesis.

Degree of movement. Maxillary obturator prostheses tend to rotate up into the defect with occlusal pressure on the defect side. When the pressure is released, the prosthesis will return to its former static position under the influence of weight and gravity. The degree of movement will vary but, even under the best of circumstances, will always be significantly greater than that exhibited by a similar Class II partial denture for a nonsurgical patient. If the contours of the defect cannot be used effectively to enhance stability and support of the prosthesis, then the degree of movement will be even more extensive.

The size of the defect is an important indicator of the degree of movement of the prosthesis during function; the larger the defect the greater the potential for movement. The partial denture framework must be designed to anticipate these movements and be physiologically adjusted to allow for these rotations (Fig 3-76). Otherwise, the abutment teeth will be subject to damaging bending moments (lateral torquing forces). When the resection crosses the midline and only a linear configuration of the dentition remains, the prosthesis will be very unstable, and displacement in and out of the defect may be quite significant and disconcerting to the patient. Under these circumstances, the placement of two implants into the residual zygomatic arch should be considered so as to provide support on the side of the defect. This approach limits the bending moments applied to the abutment teeth, prolonging their life span and providing implant support on the defect side with the resultant improvement in mastication.

Influence of defect and residual structures. Any Class II maxillary RDP-obturator prosthesis must be effectively retained to

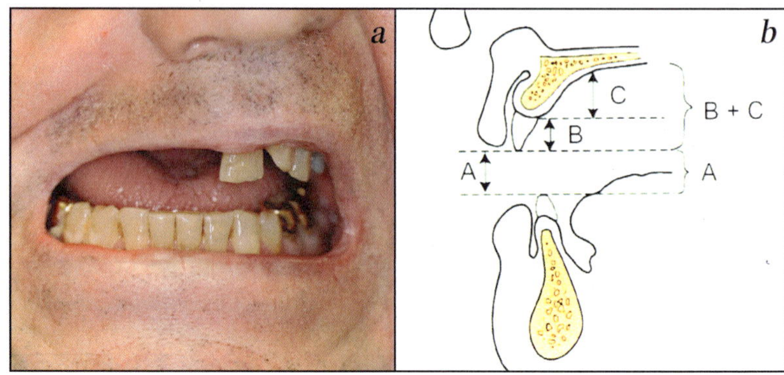

Figure 3-77 Influence of the depth of the palate on RDP design. *(a)* Posttreatment total maxillectomy patient with significant trismus. *(b)* If the sum of palatal depth (C) plus the length of any replacement teeth and partial denture components on the nondefect side (B) is greater than the distance between the maxillary and mandibular incisors at maximum opening (A), extension into the depth of the palate and defect must be compromised and an RDP cannot be removed or inserted.

achieve its functional objectives. Support and stability are important cofactors as they help maintain the correct retainer-to-tooth relationships so that the retainers serve primarily as a rescue force to compensate for dislodgment or gravitational forces. If the support, stability, and retention for the resection prosthesis can be enhanced by engaging selected areas within and peripheral to the defect, the retention, stability, and support available for the partial denture will be enhanced, and retainer-to-tooth relationships will be maintained. Thus, fewer retainers will be required in this situation than when a defect lacks these important physical characteristics.

When stability and support are limited because defect contours are less than ideal, the palatal shelf is limited, or the arch is tapered, the teeth may be used to improve these aspects. Multiple, well-prepared, and well-spaced rest seats, especially on posterior teeth, will enhance support. Stability is enhanced with the use of lingual plating, widened minor connectors, and widening guiding planes when appropriate. The horizontal bracing associated with these partial denture components will enhance the overall stability of the prosthesis, especially if retention and support are adequate.

Buccal versus lingual retention. Some clinicians have suggested the addition of lingual retentive clasp arms with buccal reciprocating arms so that, as the prosthesis is displaced superiorly, the lingual retentive arms will disengage from the teeth (Firtell and Grisius, 1980). Disengagement is an asset, but clinical experience indicates that these designs exhibit greater motion around the fulcrum line, which decreases retention. The effectiveness of lingual retention will depend on the angulation of the abutment teeth relative to the occlusal plane. Because there is no cross-arch reciprocation for either buccal or lingual retention, a partial denture framework for a patient with a total maxillectomy must be viewed in the same light as a unilateral RDP, with the important exception that the framework is supporting a large outrigger. For this reason, both buccal and lingual retentive arms may be considered to obtain cross-tooth retention and reciprocation.

This design principle is especially relevant if the remaining dentition exhibits a linear alignment pattern, as found in patients with tapering arches. In this situation the fulcrum line closely approximates the teeth and the indirect retainers will be close to or on this fulcrum line and thus less effective. Therefore, this particular prosthesis will have the potential for more movement around the fulcrum line. Multiple circumferential retainers may be necessary for proper retention and stability with the use of both buccal and lingual retention. If multiple buccal and lingual undercuts are available, some clasp assemblies should employ buccal retention and others should use lingual retention, but the net effect should be to keep the prosthesis from rotating out of position on either side of the fulcrum line.

Effect of trismus. Extreme trismus can be a very frustrating experience for both the partially edentulous patient and the clinician and may influence the design of the palatal major connector. Many maxillectomy patients receive both surgical and radiation therapy sometime during the treatment of their disease. In recent times, chemoradiation has been employed. Patients subjected to these treatment modalities, especially those treated with chemoradiation postsurgery, can develop significant trismus. It is not uncommon for patients to have a maximum opening of 10 mm or less between the incisors when the resection extends to the midline and incisors remain (Fig 3-77).

If a dynamic bite opener is not effective (see Chapter 1), the RDP design will be compromised, and the depth of the palate may influence the design of the RDP, especially for patients with tapering arches. Clinically, tapering arches tend to exhibit greater palatal depth than either square or ovoid arches. If the depth of the palate plus the sum of any replacement teeth or partial denture components on the nondefect side is greater than the maximum opening distance between the incisors, the prosthesis cannot be inserted. Moreover, the prosthesis may not be readily rotated out of the mouth on the defect side because the width of the obturator may be greater than the distance from the lip commissure to the remaining maxillary central incisor.

An alternative is to record as much of the palatal surface, teeth, and defect as possible with the master impression for the RDP framework. Many times, a sufficient amount of palate and teeth will have been recorded to accommodate an anterior strap palatal major connector. Although this type of major connector is not the major connector of choice because of its flexibility, it may be the only viable alternative.

After the partial denture framework is fitted and physiologically relieved, the defect is recorded with an altered cast impression. In these circumstances, trismus will also limit the extension into the defect, especially along the lateral wall. However, the flexibility of the lateral cheek and skin graft will often permit the prosthesis to be rotated out of the defect and the mouth with lateral displacement of the cheek. In addition, the patient should be warned that leakage will be a possibility because of the limited extensions into the defect, especially along the posteromedial margin.

Indirect retention. Cummer (1942) first introduced the concept of indirect retention. This concept is particularly useful in

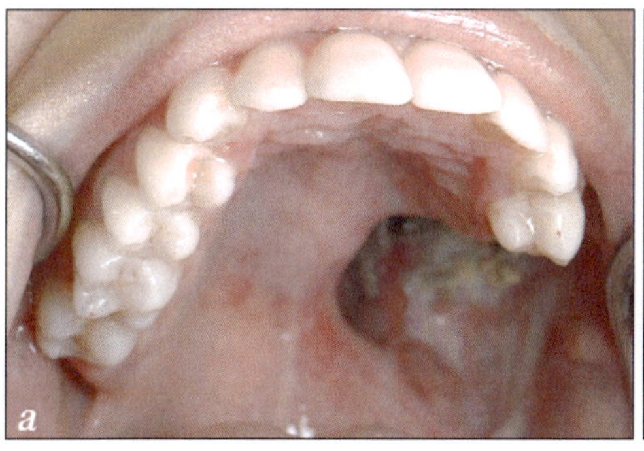

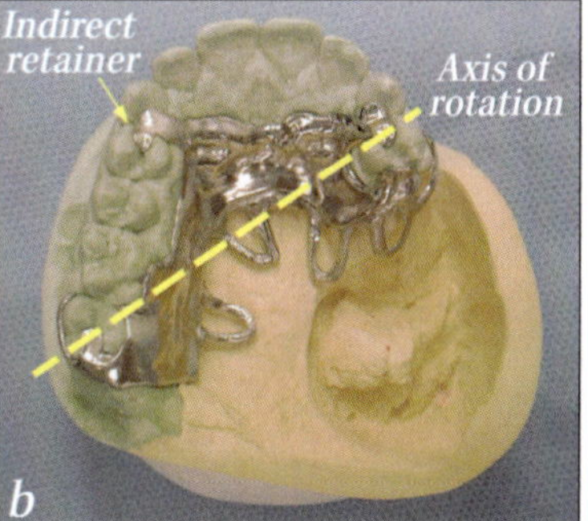

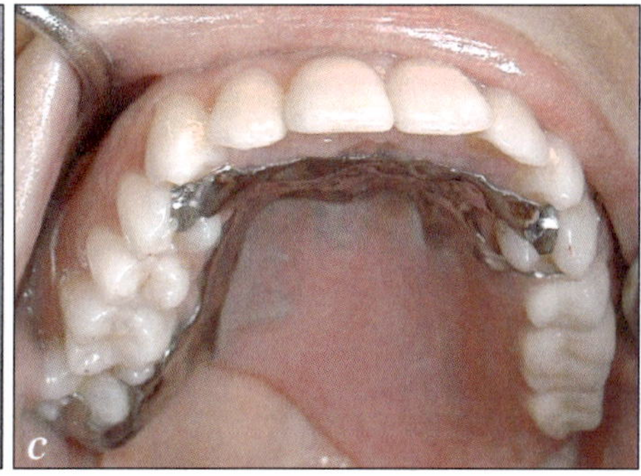

Figure 3-78 *(a, b, and c)* This is a patient with a left partial inferior maxillectomy defect. The mesial rest on the right maxillary premolar *(arrow)* acts as an indirect retainer. The forces of gravity tend to displace the obturator portion of the prosthesis, down and out of the defect. The indirect retainer resists this displacement. Reciprocation for the retainer engaging the molar is provided by the proximal plate and the lingual plate. Reciprocation for the retainer engaging the left premolar is provided by the proximal plate and the minor connector.

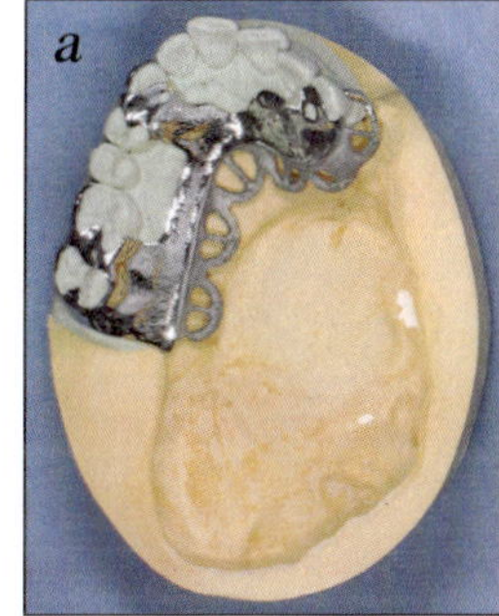

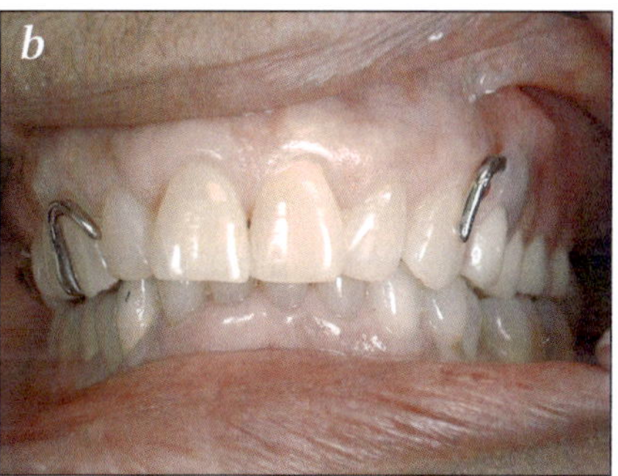

Figure 3-79 *(a and b)* Although the defect extends to include the soft palate, the RDP design differs little from that shown in Fig 3-78. The main difference is the additional retainer on the right canine.

partial palatectomy defects where the anterior portion of the palate is retained. Unlike direct retainers, indirect retainers are always placed anterior to the axis of rotation for distal extension removable dental prosthesis. In such defects, a positive rest placed on the dentate side of the axis of rotation counteracts the forces of gravity associated with the obturator extension.

The rests designed to function as indirect retainers are ideally placed perpendicular to a point in the center of the fulcrum line. This rest position allows it to be farthest from the axis of rotation and centered along the arc of rotation (Fig 3-78). The effectiveness of the indirect retainer is increased the farther it is located from the fulcrum line because the mechanical advantage increases proportionately. The direct retainers must effectively engage retentive areas if the indirect retainer is to function when the denture rotates. In the patient shown in Fig 3-78, only two direct retainers were used—an I bar engaging the first premolar and a circumferential clasp engaging the second molar on the opposite side. Given the arch form of this patient, this was quite sufficient to retain the obturator prosthesis.

Sample RDP designs

The nature of the defect and the residual palatal shelf available are the most important factors to consider when designing an RDP framework for these defects. If the premaxillary segment has been retained and the canine or a premolar along with it, the RDP design follows conventional guidelines (Fig 3-79; see also Fig 3-78). When the defect is skin lined, selected areas within and peripheral to the defect can be engaged enhancing the retention, stability, and support. There will be little movement of the prosthesis in and out of the defect. Under these circumstances, indirect retention becomes more effective, and fewer direct retainers and less bracing will be required as compared to the patient with a defect lacking these important physical characteristics. Even if the defect extends posteriorly to involve the soft palate, if the premaxillary segment is retained and the canine is present, the RDP design can be relatively conventional. In the patient in Fig 3-79, the presence of the canine on the side of the defect brings with it the benefit of cross-arch stabilization and more palatal shelf for support for the prosthesis. Therefore, little additional bracing is necessary, and the main difference between the RDP defect seen in Fig 3-78 is the additional retainer engaging the right canine.

Contrast these designs to the design shown in Fig 3-80. When the resection crosses the midline, the residual dentition is configured in a linear fashion and little palatal shelf is available to provide support for the prosthesis. When occlusal forces are applied on the defect side, the fulcrum line will essentially be identical to the tooth alignment. Patients with linear tooth and arch arrangements with large defects will tend to exhibit more movement around the fulcrum line. Such configurations of the dentition require more occlusal rests for support and additional bracing so as to distribute lateral forces as widely as possible among the remaining dentition (Fig 3-80). In such configurations, the placement of two zygomatic oncologic implants in both zygomas and exiting in the defect will dramatically improve the function of the obturator prosthesis (Fig 3-81). Cross-arch splinting of the zygomatic oncologic implants is advised so that the lever arm moment on the long and remotely anchored fixtures in zygoma in the defect is countered. In some cases, this is achieved

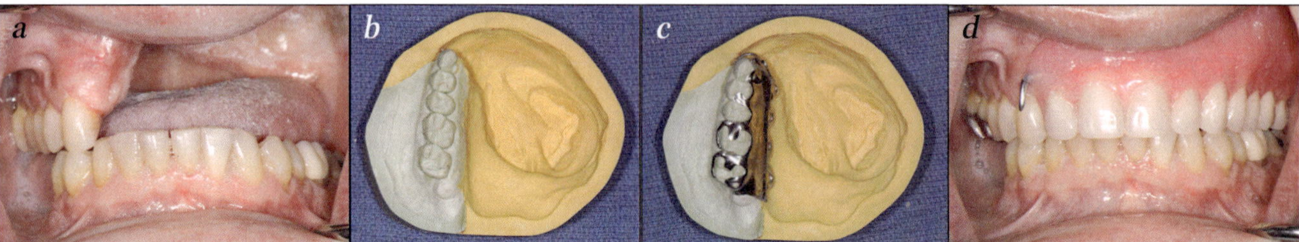

Figure 3-80 RDP design for linear configuration. *(a)* Large resection that crossed the midline. *(b)* Altered master cast. Note the cingulum rest incorporated created in the canine. *(c)* RDP design. Indirect retainers are less effective because the fulcrum line follows tooth alignment. Considerably more bracing is required with linear configurations. *(d)* Definitive prosthesis (courtesy of Dr. Scott Recksiedler).

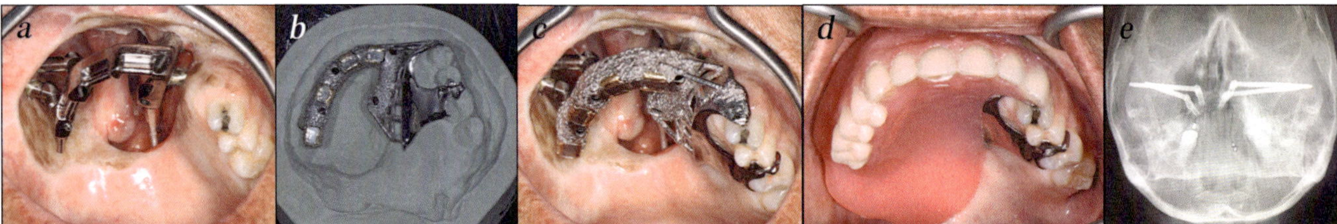

Figure 3-81 When the resection crosses the midline, implant support is recommended on the defect side. In this patient four zygomatic implants have been placed, two in each zygoma. *(a)* The implant-connecting bar in position. "Hader" bar segments are used for retention. *(b)* The overlay RDP framework. It was digitally designed and made with selective laser melting. *(c)* The RDP framework in position. *(d)* The completed prosthesis in position. *(e)* Radiograph of the implants in position.

with a conventional implant positioned in the residual alveolus along with the two zygomatic oncologic implants on the defect side. If sites are lacking for conventional implants on the unresected side, a single zygomatic oncologic implant positioned to emerge mesial and apical to the terminal abutment would be sufficient (Fig 3-82). When implants are placed in the zygoma on the unresected side, the inferior turbinate, if still present following the tumor ablation, is removed to allow access to the zygoma for oral hygiene access.

As previously mentioned, we favor using the I bar mesial rest or the "RPA" philosophy of partial denture design. We suggest that I bar retainers be used on the abutment tooth adjacent to the defect and/or the extension areas. When the I bar is positioned properly on these teeth, when occlusal forces are applied to these areas, it will disengage and rotate farther into the undercut, thus avoiding the delivery of torquing forces to the abutment in question.

This type of retainer is more aesthetic and exerts less stress on the abutment when occlusal forces are applied in the adjacent extension areas. We favor circumferential retainers in the molar region because of the improved bracing this design provides. When there is a posterior edentulous extension area on the unresected side or the potential for developing one because of the potential loss of a posterior tooth support, we favor the use of either an I bar retainer or a circumferential retainer whose suprabulge section has been relieved (the so-called RPA design concept). Some additional bracing is always required. The maxillary molars are favored and bracing can be enhanced by engaging these teeth with circumferential retainers positioned lingually at and above the height of contour or with lingual plating. Lingual plating is favored because this design tends to trap less food and debris. Presently, we suggest that RDPs be designed digitally and printed with selective laser welding. In our experience, these methodologies consistently produce more precise RDP frameworks. Moreover, it is possible to have greater interaction, via the internet, with the lab before a final design is consummated and the framework printed. Such a design and framework are shown in Fig 3-83.

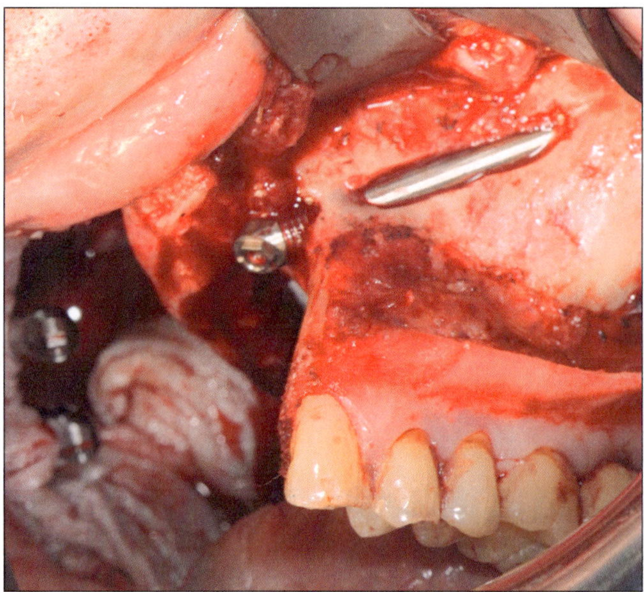

Figure 3-82 An additional zygomatic implant has been positioned on the non-resected side.

Finishing lines of the cast metal framework should be established on palatal mucosa short of the palatal shelf in order to record this area with the altered cast impression (see Fig 3-83). The retention loops for the obturator portion should extend well across the palate, and in some instances into the defect, and should be located approximately 0.5 to 1.0 mm superior to normal palatal contour. The retention should not be placed high in the defect because it becomes more difficult to hollow the obturator sufficiently without compromising the retention of the resin portion of the prosthesis.

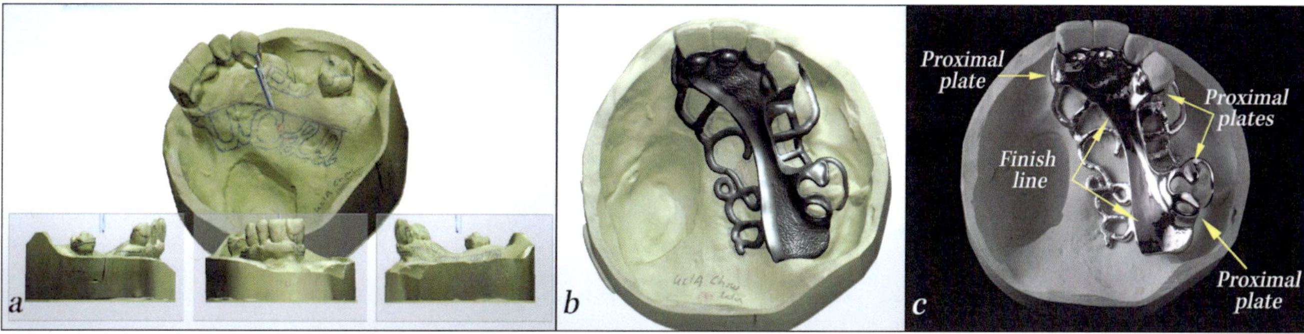

Figure 3-83 *(a, b, and c)* A typical RDP design for a total maxillectomy defect. Surveyed crowns with cingulum rests have been fabricated for teeth #8, #9, and #11 and the guide planes designed to be parallel with that on the mesial surface of the molar. I bar retainers engage abutment teeth #8 and #11. A circumferential retainer was used on the maxillary molar. Lingual plating was employed to provide additional bracing. An I bar was used on tooth "11" in the event the maxillary molar was lost. With this design, the RDP framework could be altered and still function consistent with the "RPI" concepts of RDP design. The finish line is short of the palatal vault to enable an altered cast impression of this area. Note the proximal plates. They should be physiologically adjusted with a suitable indicator.

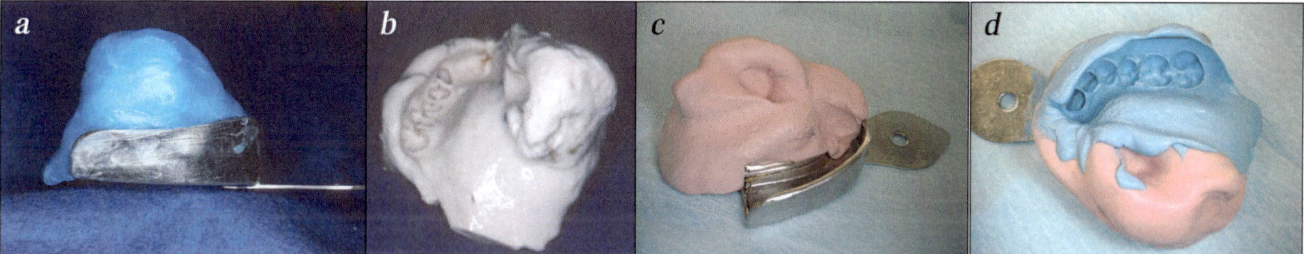

Figure 3-84 Impressions for the RDP framework. *(a)* Stock tray. *(b)* Irreversible hydrocolloid impression. *(c)* Defect recorded with silicone putty. *(d)* Impression completed with a medium-body polysiloxane.

Clinical procedures

Impressions for the RDP framework. Conventional impression materials are still the standard. Oral scanners have not proven to be sufficiently accurate for making impressions that are necessary for the fabrication of RDP frameworks. As mentioned in the implant section, there are several reasons why digital impressions are not appropriate for these RDP frameworks. First, it may be difficult to position the scanning head (scanning wand) in some patients to accurately record the guiding surfaces, particularly in patients with trismus. Also, errors are introduced because the distance between the scanner and the object (the dentition) may vary when making the scan. Moreover, only small areas can be scanned at one time, and as a consequence, the data must be stitched together to create a scan of the remaining dentition. The process has the potential to introduce angular and distance errors, especially when a significant portion of the dental arch remains (Ahlholm et al., 2018; Rutkunas et al., 2017). In addition, key areas of the defect need to be impressed and a suitable cast made in preparation for an altered cast impression of the defect. This may be problematic when using the digital method.

After the plan of treatment has been agreed to and the required restorative procedures completed, rests and guide planes are created on the remaining teeth as needed. During the restorative phase, it may be necessary to make minor changes to the interim obturator prosthesis to compensate for tooth contour changes resulting from restorative procedures.

Either irreversible hydrocolloids or polyvinyl siloxanes can be used. Before the framework impression is made, the medial palatal undercut in the defect, if present, should be blocked out with gauze lubricated with petrolatum. If not, when irreversible hydrocolloid is used and the impression removed, the palatal portion of the impression may be distorted. If silicones are used, the defect portion is first developed with silicone putty. Later the dentition is recorded with the impression material. The lateral portion of the defect should be recorded with this impression because these contours will be necessary to fabricate the tray for the future altered cast impression (Fig 3-84). *If a polyvinyl siloxane impression material is chosen, it is very important to block out bony undercuts in and adjacent to the defect because the impression can become locked into these undercuts and be very difficult to remove.*

Altered cast impressions of the defect. The RDP framework is physiologically adjusted through the use of an appropriate disclosing medium. We prefer rouge and chloroform. The framework is seated and is rotated along the predicted axes of rotation. Proximal plates, lingual plates, and minor connectors are relieved as necessary so as to prevent them from binding on the dentition during function (see Fig 3-76).

When the framework seats properly and has been physiologically adjusted, the undesirable undercuts within the defect are blocked out on the cast with baseplate wax. Relief is also placed over the scar band and lateral wall, as described in the section devoted to prostheses for edentulous patients. Tray resin is molded to the framework and the defect in preparation for the altered cast impression (Fig 3-85a).

The prosthesis is placed in the mouth and the tray is examined for extension and proximity to the tissues. Impression compound is added to the tray material, as described previously, until the desired extensions have been achieved (Fig 3-85b and c).

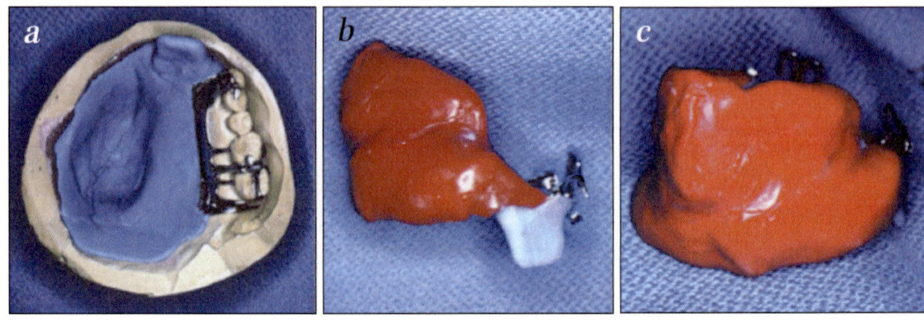

Figure 3-85 Altered cast impression. *(a)* Tray resin attached to the partial denture framework. *(b and c)* Border molding completed with impression compound.

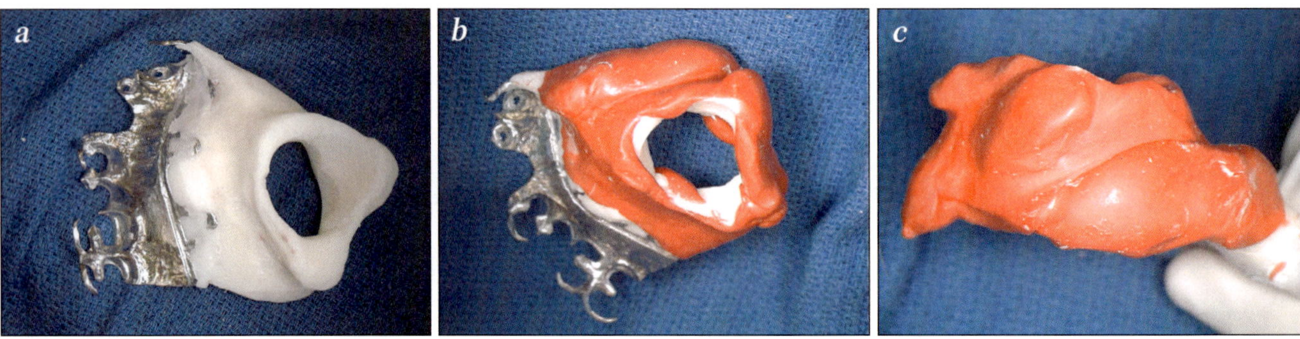

Figure 3-86 *(a–c)* Hole placed through the tray to facilitate manipulation of modeling compound up the lateral wall of the defect.

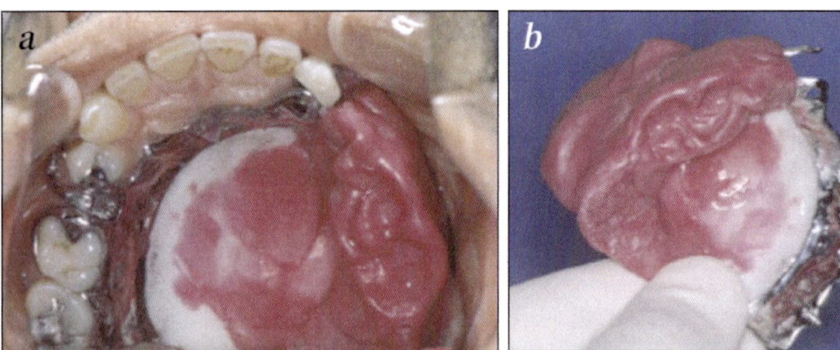

Figure 3-87 *(a and b)* Extension of impression compound to the opposing occlusion so that the impression will be stable during refinement with impression wax.

The retention, stability, and seal of the prosthesis are checked. If they are inadequate, further extension into an undercut and refinement of the portion interfacing with the soft palate may be indicated to improve these features. Recognition of the dual path of insertion required to fully engage the lateral wall of the defect and final seating of the framework can be helpful. When access to the lateral wall of the defect is impaired, making it difficult to record the undercut in this area, it is advantageous to place a hole in the tray and manipulate the compound digitally through the hole (Parel and Drane, 1976) (Fig 3-86).

As noted previously, special care is taken to develop proper contours and extensions of the posteromedial portion of the impression. The posteromedial extension must be carefully developed to minimize leakage of food and liquids, particularly when the defect extends onto the movable portion of the soft palate. This portion should be extended about 1.5–2.0 cm vertically or in some instances overlap the nasal side of the soft palate (Fig 3-86c; see also 3-66e and 3-67b). A proper extension in this area will minimize the risk of nasal leakage during swallowing. Excessive extension in this region beyond this amount, however, will impair nasal airflow on the defect side.

If desired, the impression can be extended to the level of the occlusal plane on the defect side and an occlusal index can be made (Fig 3-87). This practice also ensures that the finished prosthesis, including replacement teeth, will not be oversized. The impression compound is then relieved (Fig 3-88).

If an elastomeric impression material is used to complete the impression, escape holes are placed along the medial palatal finish line to permit the escape of wash material. A suitable adhesive is applied to the border-molded impression and up to the finish line but not to the major connector. Among the elastomeric impression materials, we prefer polysulfide, because it is less likely to displace tissues in the defect and this material is less likely to flow into undesirable areas. Before the framework is seated, medium-bodied polysulfide material is injected into the undercuts that are to be recorded.

The tray is loaded with the light-bodied material and seated. When the tray is loaded, the placement of excessive amounts of material close to the finishing line should be avoided. After the casting is seated, the patient is directed to make eccentric mandibular movements. Because of the prolonged setting time of this material, these movements should be repeated several times. The impression

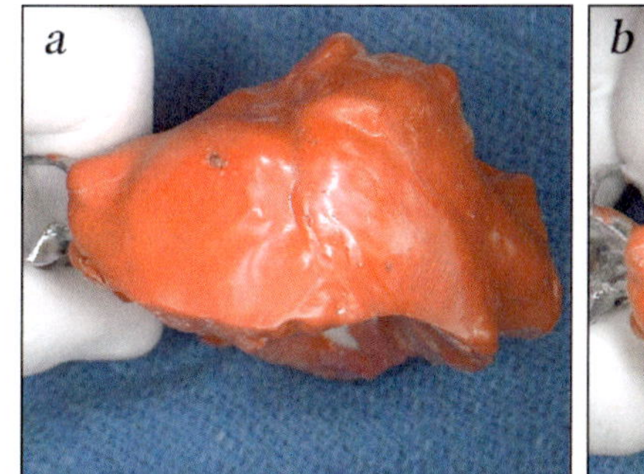
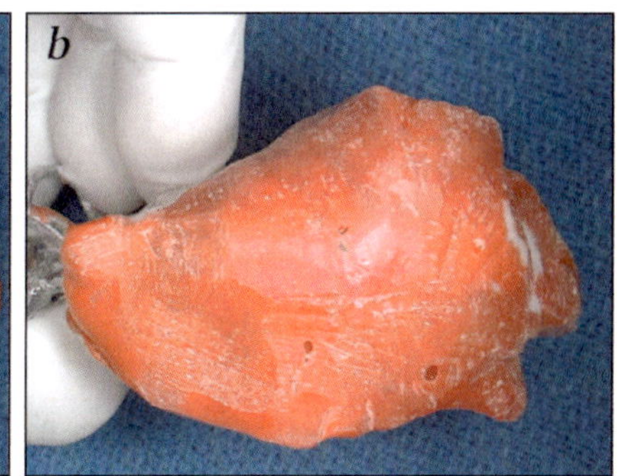

Figure 3-88 *(a and b)* Relief of impression compound prior to completion of the corrected impression. If polysulfide is used to make the corrected impression, the finish line must be liberally perforated.

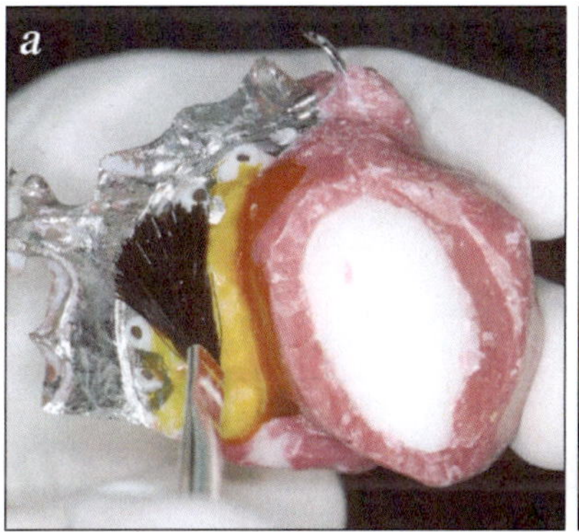
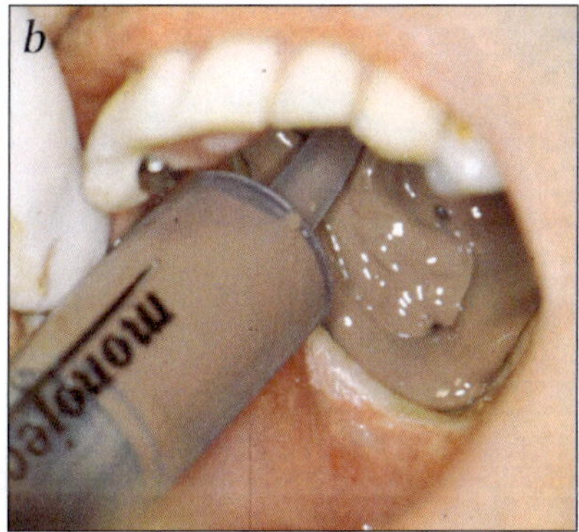

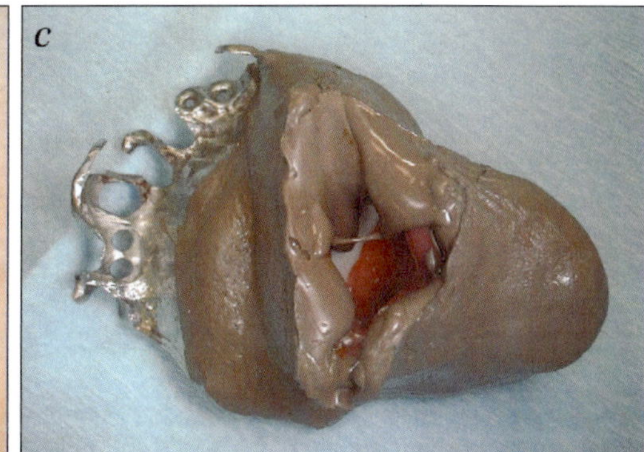

Figure 3-89 Altered cast impression with polysulfide. *(a)* Tray adhesive is applied just up to the finish line. *(b)* Injection of medium body material into the undercut before insertion of the loaded tray. *(c)* Completed impression.

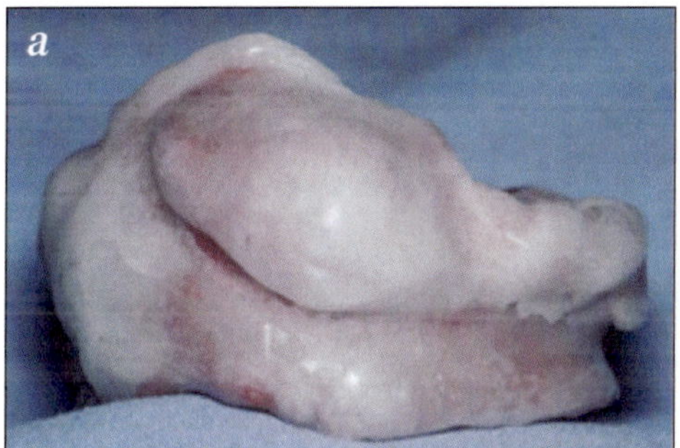
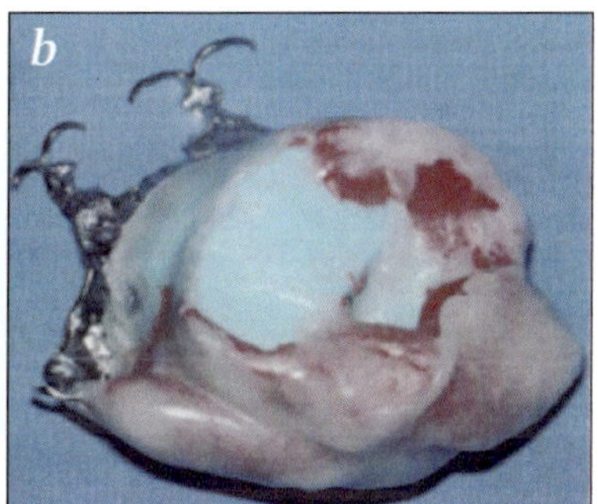

Figure 3-90 *(a and b)* Altered cast impressions with impression wax.

is removed and examined for tissue adaptation, proper extension, and excessive displacement of tissue (Fig 3-89).

Thermoplastic wax, used alone or in combination with an elastomeric impression material, can also be used to complete the impression (Fig 3-90). Impression compound is used as previously described to develop the contours of the impression that extend into the defect or to establish the extensions of other edentulous areas. When a thermoplastic wax is used to refine the impression, it is necessary to extend the impression compound to the level of the occlusal plane and develop an occlusal index (see Fig 3-87). This will ensure that the impression remains properly seated during the molding of the impression wax. The impression compound that forms the obturator is then cut back 1 to 2 mm, and the entire impression is covered with a thermoplastic wax.

The impression is inserted and refined with the border molding maneuvers previously described. It may take several insertions and removals and further cutbacks before the impression is suitably covered with a proper thickness of wax (1 to 2 mm). The patient is allowed to wear the prosthesis for 60 to 90 minutes. It is then removed, inspected, and chilled. Next, the altered cast impression is boxed and poured, and the cast is mounted on the articulator using the occlusal index (Fig 3-91). When preparing the impression for pouring, precautionary measures should be undertaken to avoid injury to the tentative centric relation record. To maintain the integrity of the occlusal index, the cast must be trimmed and mounted on the articulator prior to separating the impression from the master cast.

Elastomeric impression materials are favored for smaller static defects or when there are large undercuts that must be recorded. Thermoplastic wax is preferred for large or dynamic defects where the obturator approximates mobile border tissues or extends into the velopharyngeal complex (see section below entitled "Maxillectomy defects extending to the posterior pharyngeal wall"). A significant advantage of using this technique is that chair time during insertion will be significantly reduced when the obturator portion is refined in a thermoplastic material.

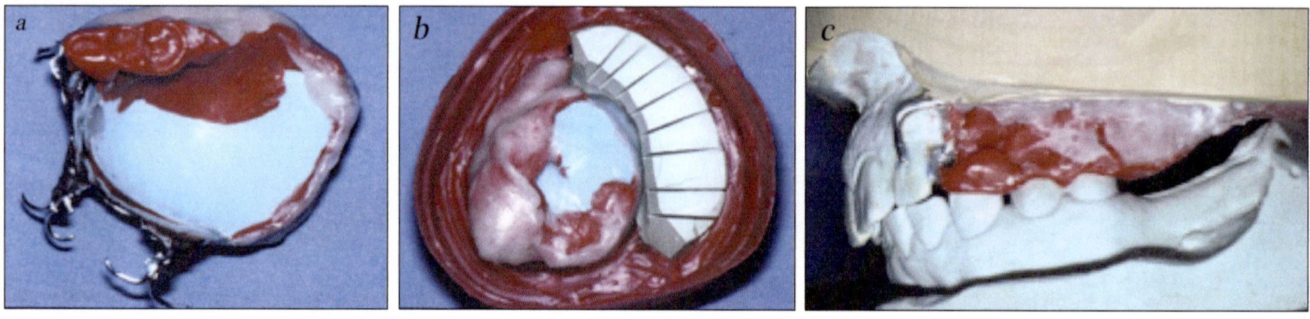

Figure 3-91 *(a)* Occlusal stops established with impression compound. *(b)* Preparation for pouring of the altered cast. *(c)* Casts mounted on the articulator.

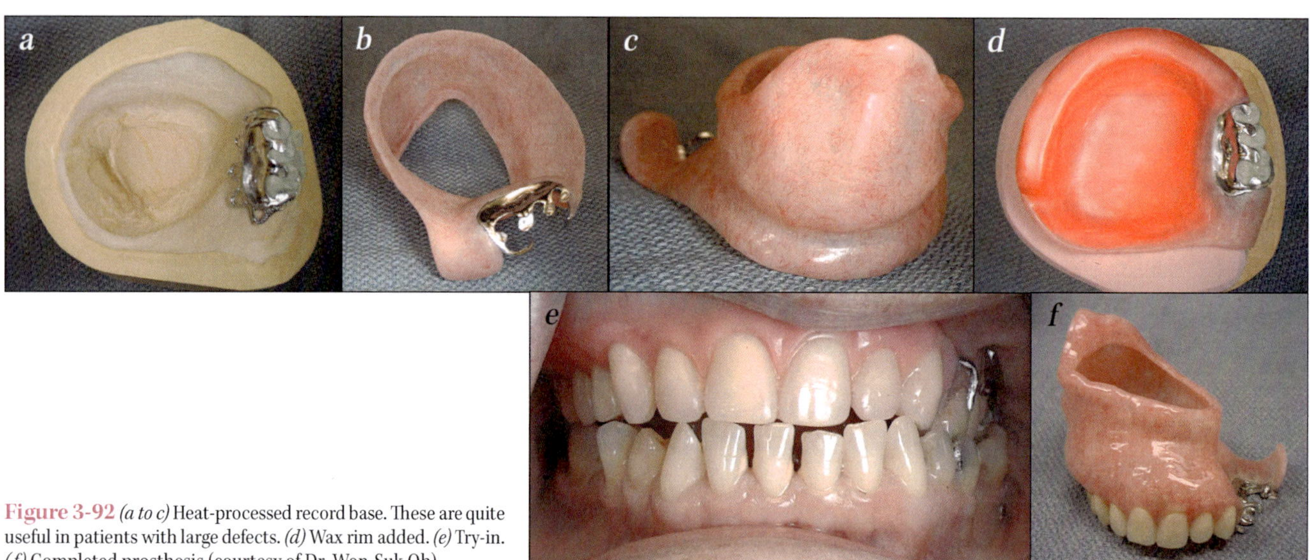

Figure 3-92 *(a to c)* Heat-processed record base. These are quite useful in patients with large defects. *(d)* Wax rim added. *(e)* Try-in. *(f)* Completed prosthesis (courtesy of Dr. Won-Suk Oh).

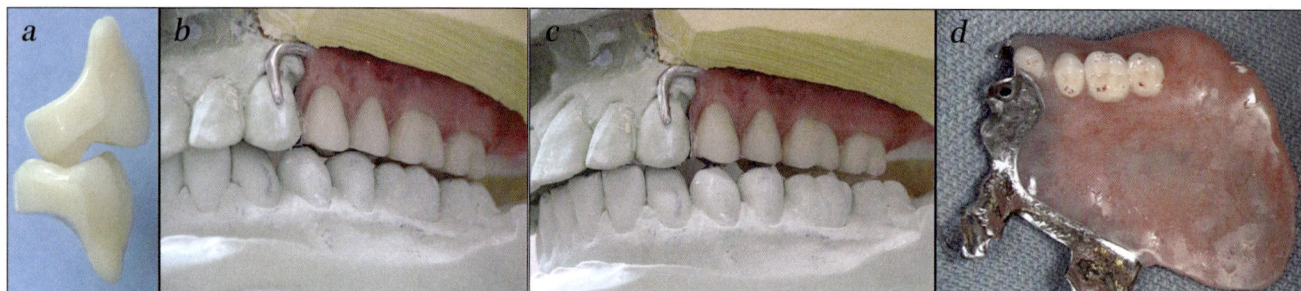

Figure 3-93 *(a to d)* Centric-only occlusion is preferred on the defect side. A lingualized scheme is shown. Guidance on the defect side during lateral excursion is provided by the residual anterior teeth.

Centric relation records. We prefer to make tentative centric relation registrations simultaneously with the altered cast impression of the defect (see Figs 3-87 and 3-91). These registrations are then verified at the time of trial denture insertion. We prefer this method because of the improved retention, stability, and support provided by the altered cast impression while making the record.

Another method is to make a record base on the blocked-out master cast resulting from the altered cast impression. A centric registration is then made with this record base in the usual fashion. An alternative method employs a processed record base (Oh and Roumanas, 2008). With this technique, the record base is processed into heat-activated acrylic resin using the altered master cast, and the denture teeth are attached at a later date (Fig 3-92). This technique is particularly advantageous for patients with large or unfavorable defects.

Occlusion. We prefer to lingualize the occlusion (Fig 3-93). In the posterior region, centric-only contact is preferred on the defect side. If possible, all guidance should be off the remaining natural teeth on the defect side. If the defect extends to the anterior region, the incisal guidance should be flattened to avoid anterior guidance on the defect side. This can be accomplished by raising the anterior teeth on the side of the defect or setting them slightly labially. Retraction of the upper lip and the usual postsurgical contours generally permit these alterations.

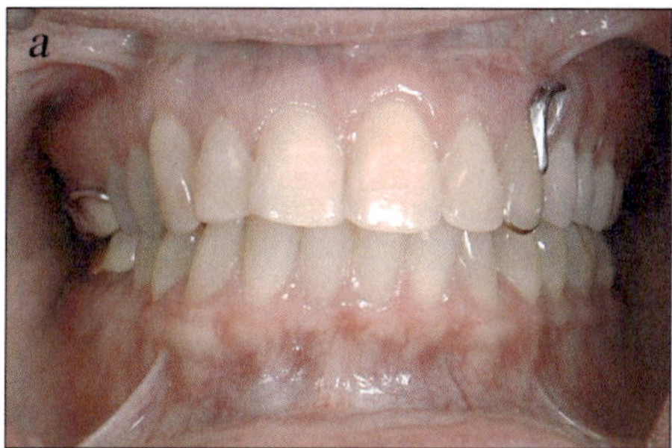
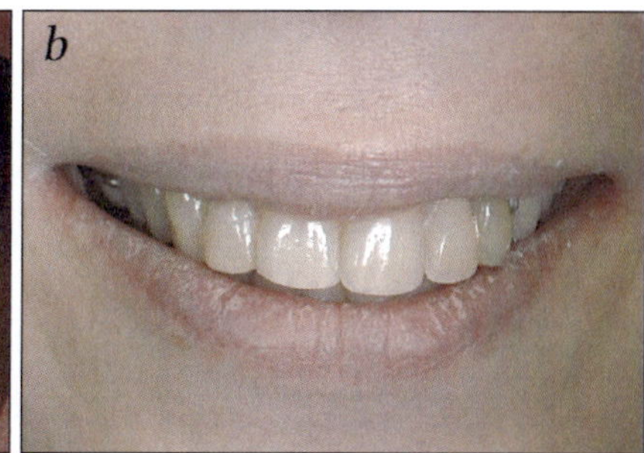

Figure 3-94 *(a and b)* Examples of an I-bar retainer on an anterior abutment.

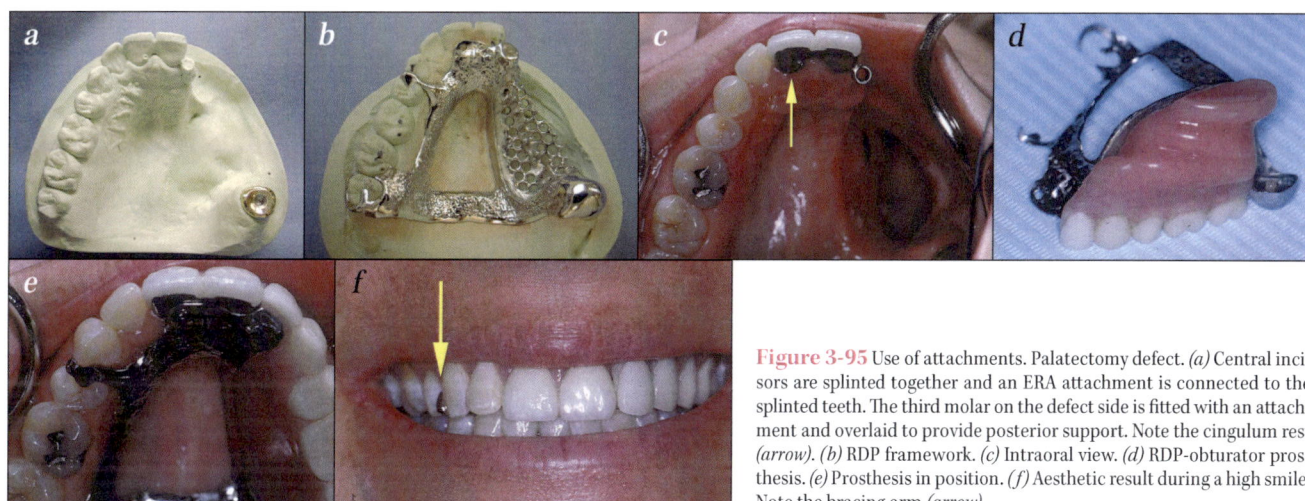

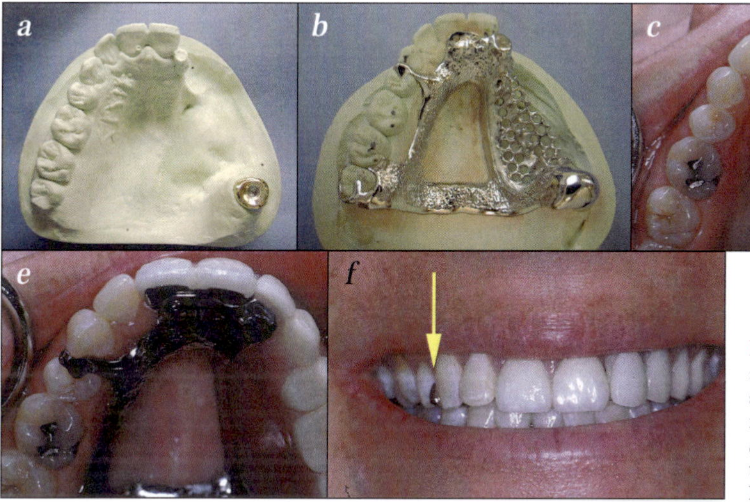

Figure 3-95 Use of attachments. Palatectomy defect. *(a)* Central incisors are splinted together and an ERA attachment is connected to the splinted teeth. The third molar on the defect side is fitted with an attachment and overlaid to provide posterior support. Note the cingulum rest *(arrow)*. *(b)* RDP framework. *(c)* Intraoral view. *(d)* RDP-obturator prosthesis. *(e)* Prosthesis in position. *(f)* Aesthetic result during a high smile. Note the bracing arm *(arrow)*.

Aesthetics. Most resections of paranasal sinus neoplasms affect the anterior region. As stated previously, to properly retain the RDP-obturator prosthesis in position, the tooth adjacent to the defect should be engaged with a positive rest and a retainer. The I bar is preferred; in most patients, just the tip of the retainer is visible during a high smile (Fig 3-94). Moreover, the I bar, when used on the abutment tooth adjacent to the extension area or the defect, can be positioned such that when occlusal forces are applied to these areas, it will disengage and rotate farther into the undercut, thus avoiding the delivery of torquing forces to this abutment.

For patients in whom the resection terminates short of the second or third molar, the use of attachments can be considered. A typical case is shown in Fig 3-95. In this patient the two central incisors were splinted together, a cingulum rest was placed on the maxillary right central incisor and an ERA attachment incorporated within the RPD framework. Following endodontic treatment, the maxillary right third molar was restored with a gold coping, and an attachment was incorporated within it. A bracing arm was placed between the premolar and the canine on the unresected side to ensure that the RDP framework remains properly seated on the occlusal and cingulum rests during function. This prosthesis lasted 20 years until the third molar on the resected side was lost secondary to a root fracture. It was replaced with an implant, and a new RDP obturator was fabricated using a similar design.

Anterior tooth arrangements influence the aesthetic result. In many maxillectomy patients, the lip is often shortened on the side of the defect, adjacent to the lip incision. If the incisal edge of the central incisor is tapered and the lateral incisor and canine are elevated, a more pleasing lip and smile line is developed (see Fig 3-63). Lip plumpers are occasionally useful in selected maxillectomy patients when facial nerve weakness or injury results in drooping of the corner of the mouth on the side of the defect.

Processing and delivery. Conventional prosthodontic methods are followed to complete the RDP-obturator prosthesis. The obturator portion is processed in a hollow configuration, as previously suggested. The lateral and posterolateral extensions are polished. Delivery and adjustments are accomplished in accordance with acceptable prosthodontic guidelines.

Slight pressure against the skin graft and cheek mucosa is desirable to ensure maximal retention, stability, and support. Disclosing wax is preferred over pressure indicator paste to identify areas of excessive tissue displacement in the defect (Fig 3-96a and b). Pressure indicator paste tends to stick to the skin graft or other dry surfaces in the defect. In addition, pressure indicator paste will be displaced or distorted when the prosthesis is seated in undercut areas. The anterior and posterolateral portions of the defect are most susceptible to displacement during impression making and must be checked carefully. Following these adjustments, the lateral and posterolateral extensions are polished (Fig 3-96c).

The patient is scheduled for recall appointments in a manner designed to gradually extend the interval between appointments. After the adjustment phase is completed, the patient is enrolled in a recall system, often one that coordinates prosthodontic recall appointments with visits to the surgeon and radiation oncologist.

Double-processing method. Oh and Roumanas (2008) have suggested that a double-processing method be used for large

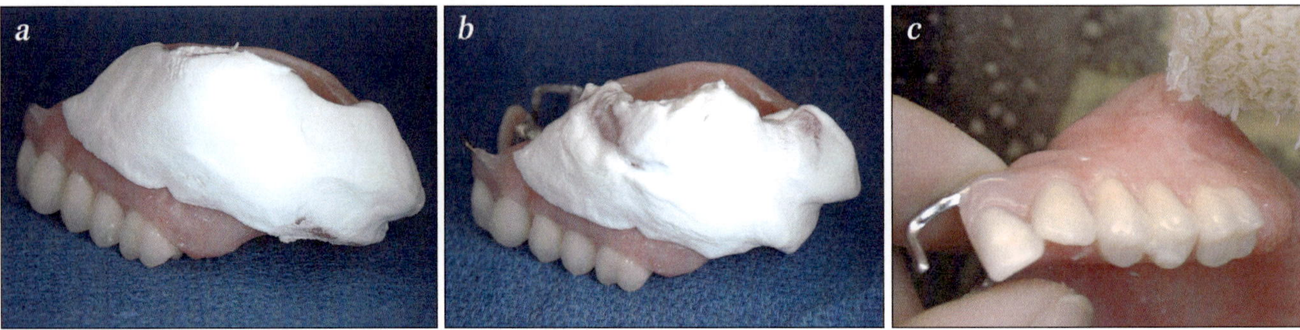

Figure 3-96 *(a and b)* The most common areas of inappropriate tissue displacement, as indicated by disclosing wax, are anterolateral and posterolateral portions of the defect. *(c)* Following adjustments, the lateral and posterolateral portions of the obturator are polished.

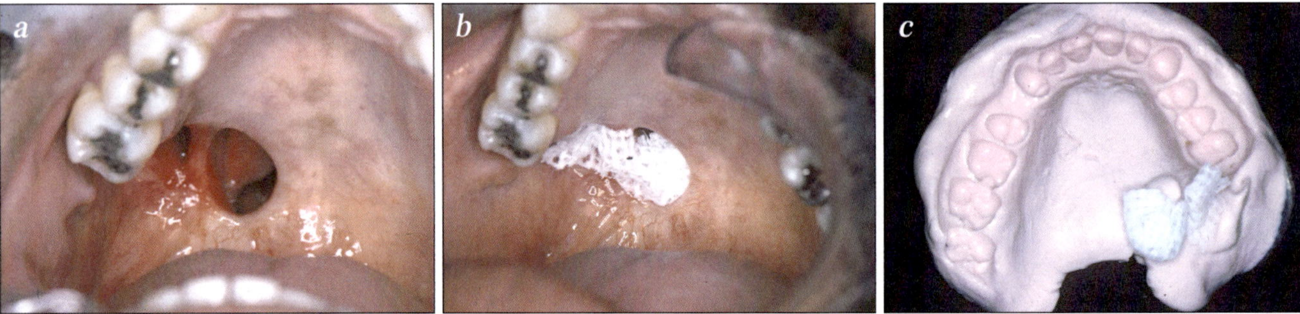

Figure 3-97 *(a)* Small defect. *(b)* Gauze packing used to prevent impression material from entering the nasal passages. *(c)* Gauze packing still embedded in the impression.

obturator prostheses. After the altered cast impression is poured, one layer of baseplate wax is adapted to the master cast. Additional wax may be added to eliminate undercuts to facilitate trial packing. The wax should extend to join the finish line of the metal RDP framework. Flasking and packing are conducted in the usual manner.

Following polymerization, the record base is divested and finished. The record base is then refined intraorally with pressure indicator paste and disclosing wax. Wax rims are added and records are made and transferred to the articulator (see Fig 3-92d). Teeth are arranged, and the aesthetics and the centric relation record are verified in the usual manner (see Fig 3-92e). The record-base trial denture is flasked, and the second processing in heat-activated acrylic resin is conducted at 138°F for 12 hours. Distortion associated with double processing is negligible because a lower temperature and a longer processing cycle are employed.

This technique has two advantages. First, it ensures an even thickness of the obturator and minimizes its weight. Second, the processed record base allows maximum extension into the defect, idealizing the support, retention, and stability of the record base when records are made. More accurate centric records are the result.

Special considerations for dentulous patients with small defects

The prosthodontic considerations for the dentulous partial maxillectomy patient are similar to those for the total maxillectomy patient, except that the prosthetic prognosis improves as the anterior margin of the resection moves posteriorly. When the maxillary canine on the defect side remains, the prosthetic prognosis improves dramatically.

The fulcrum line is dependent on the placement of occlusal rests. As more teeth are retained on the defect side, the fulcrum line shifts posteriorly. When both canines remain, the fulcrum line will be similar to that of a conventional Kennedy Class II partial denture.

As the fulcrum line shifts posteriorly, the superior distolateral extension of the obturator should be lengthened; extension into this area offers the greatest mechanical advantage because it will be at a right angle and most distant from the fulcrum line. Indirect retainers should be placed as far anteriorly as feasible from the fulcrum line. As with total maxillectomy patients, a retainer and rest placed on the tooth closely adjacent to the defect increases stability and retention.

The construction and fitting of the prosthesis are carried out as described for prostheses fabricated for total maxillectomy patients. Small defects should be blocked with gauze before impressions are made (Fig 3-97) to prevent escape of impression material into the paranasal sinuses. Occasionally edematous turbinates extend into the oral cavity, preventing restoration of normal palatal contours. If so, the offending turbinates should be removed surgically.

Use of Dental Implants

Placement of dental implants can have a dramatic impact on the function of an obturator prosthesis for both edentulous and partially edentulous patients with large palatal defects. Implants

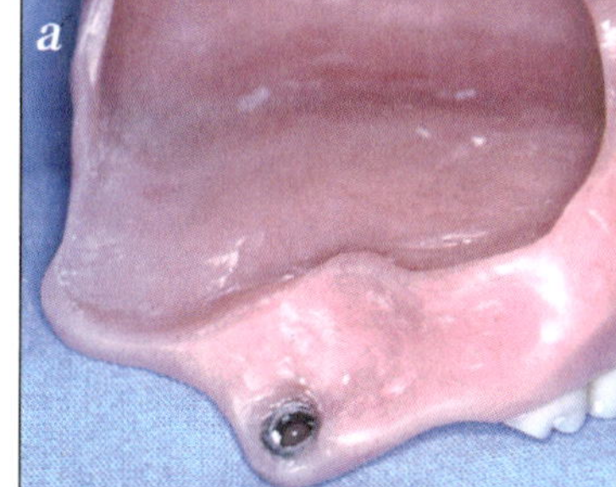

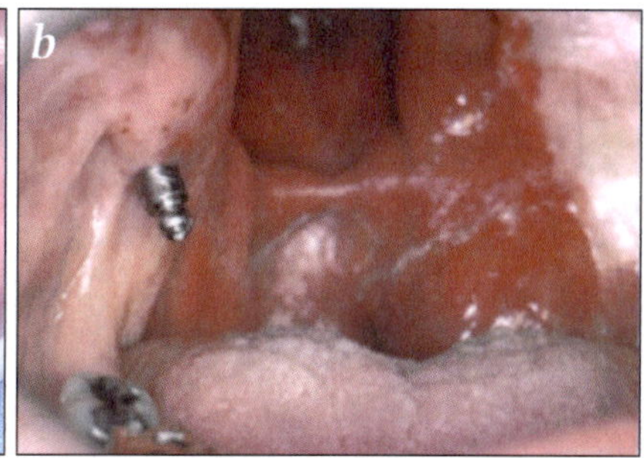

Figure 3-98 *(a and b)* Solitary implant placed in the pyramidal process of the palatal bone with an O-ring attachment used to help retain a large obturator restoring most of the hard and soft palate and extending to the posterior pharyngeal walls. The O-ring allows the prosthesis to rotate around multiple axes. Retention on the left is provided by engagement of the undercut associated with the skin-lined lateral wall of the defect. Retention on the right side is provided by the implant. The prosthesis is first rotated into the defect, engaging the undercut in the lateral wall, and then secured to the implant. The implant survived 10 years without appreciable bone loss.

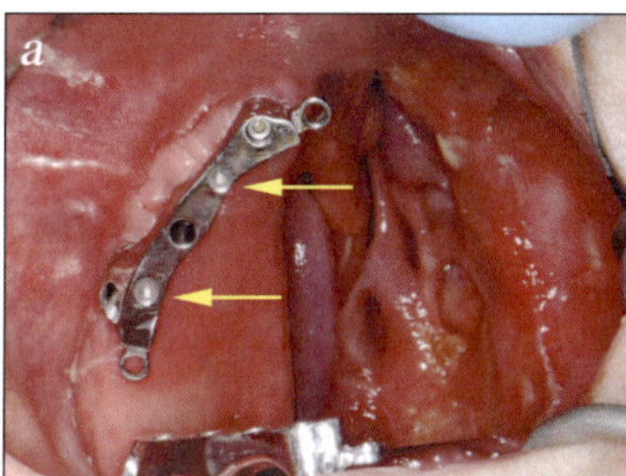

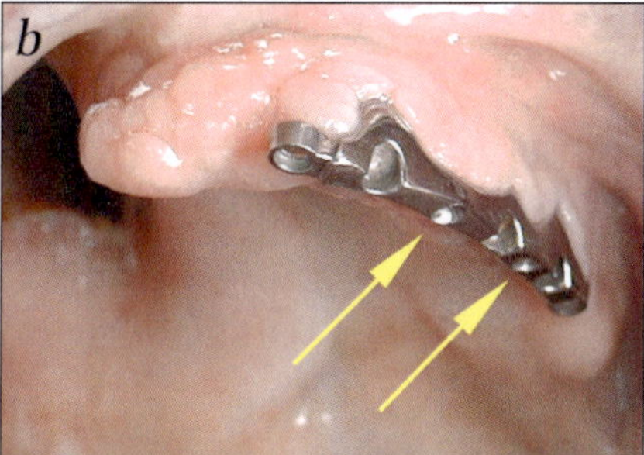

Figure 3-99 *(a)* Implants were positioned in the anterior maxilla. *(b)* Implants were placed in the posterior alveolar ridge. In both examples, the implants were splinted together with an implant-assisted connecting bar. Note the occlusal rests on both bars *(arrows)*.

provide retention and support and improve the stability of the prosthesis. Mastication performance in the edentulous may be restored to presurgical levels in some patients (Garrett, 2008; Buurman et al., 2020b), particularly when intradefect implant support is provided. Furthermore, with improved retention of the obturator prosthesis, speech and swallowing are made near normal, and the patient adapts to the prosthesis more quickly. In the presence of a well-crafted, skin-lined defect with retentive qualities, even a solitary implant in the residual alveolar ridge with an O-ring-type attachment can make a substantial difference in the quality of speech and swallowing (Fig 3-98).

Our initial experience with implants in patients with palatal defects was somewhat mixed (Roumanas et al., 1997). In the initial cases machine surface, straight-wall implants were used, and the site most often employed was the residual alveolar ridges. Since then, several innovations in implant design and implant placement have been introduced, such as microrough surface implants, tapered self-tapping implants, the zygomatic oncologic implant, the use of tilted implant placement, and most recently digitally designed patient-specific subperiosteal implants, all of which hold out the prospect of improved success rates in patients with large palatal defects. Recent reports appear to support this assumption (Butterworth, 2019, 2022; Buurman et al., 2020b). Microrough implant surfaces are osteoconductive, resulting in improved bone-implant contact. Moreover, since the process of osseointegration is accelerated by these surfaces, the implants can be placed at the time of surgical resection in patients scheduled to receive postoperative radiation therapy. By the time the radiotherapy is scheduled to begin (approximately five to six weeks postsurgery), these implants should be reasonably well osseointegrated. Furthermore, tapered, self-tapping implants dramatically improve initial implant stability, which was always a challenge when placing straight-wall implants in poor-quality bone sites such as the posterior maxilla. Also, the success of tilted implant positioning in patients with intact palates has demonstrated the value of sites such as the zygoma, the pyriform rim, and the pyramidal process of the palatal bone.

Potential implant sites

Implants placed in residual alveolar processes with axial angulation

In the past, the most commonly used site for implants for most edentulous patients with large palatal defects was the residual anterior maxillary segment (Fig 3-99a). This site is ideal biomechanically because following a total maxillectomy, the anterior maxillary alveolar ridge is directly opposite the most retentive portion of the defect, generally located along its posterior-lateral wall. In addition, frequently satisfactory bone volume and density are found in the anterior alveolar ridge.

The posterior alveolar process is an alternative site if at least 10 mm of bone is available beneath the maxillary sinus (Fig 3-99b). If insufficient bone is present and the patient has not been irradiated, the sinus membrane can be elevated and a bone graft placed to augment the site (Fig 3-100). This technique has become a popular and predictable option for treating unresected partially dentate patients, but in unresected edentulous patients, it is being supplanted by the use of tilted implants. It is likely that this will also be the case in patients presenting with palatal defects as more clinicians come to appreciate the value of tilted implants.

Previous studies have reported considerably lower success rates for implants placed in the residual alveolar ridges used to retain obturator prostheses compared to patients with intact palates (Roumanas et al., 1997; Nimi et al., 1993; Huang et al., 2014). The Roumanas study (1997) was especially revealing because it not only

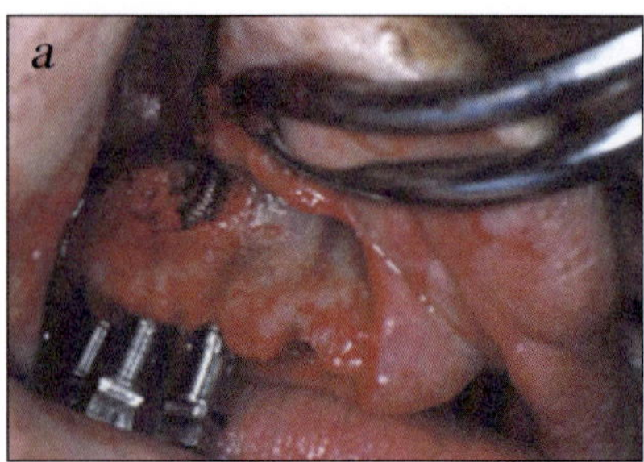
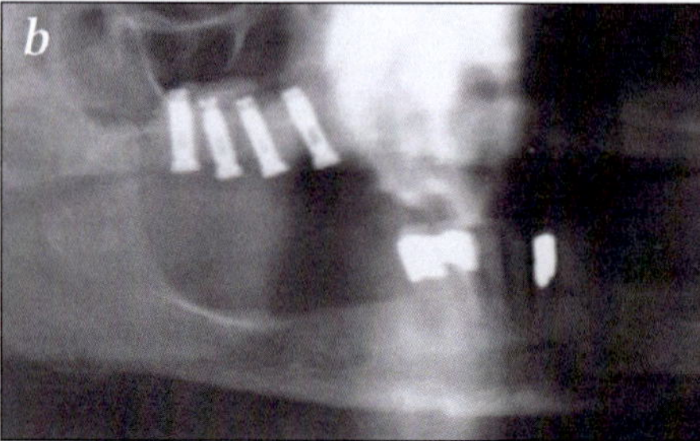
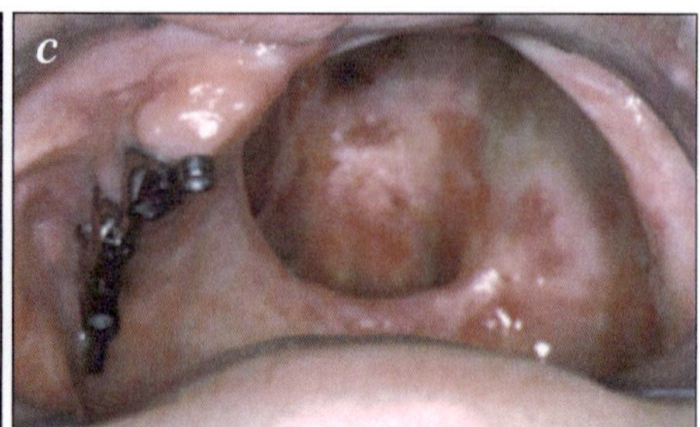

Figure 3-100 *(a, b, and c)* Sinus lift and graft used to augment the posterior alveolar ridge after total maxillectomy.

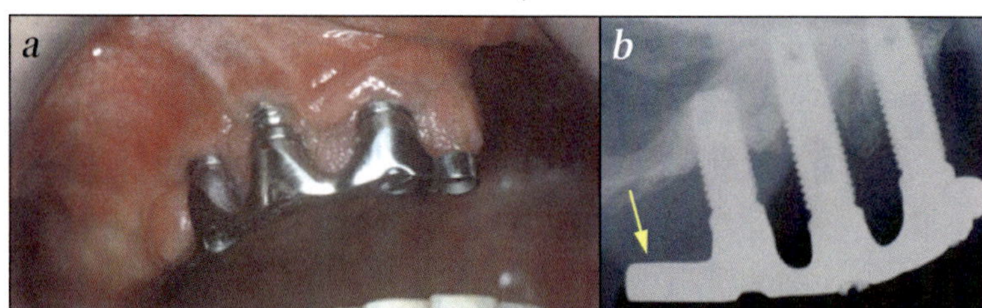

Figure 3-101 *(a)* Implant-connecting bar initially used at UCLA. The Hader bar attached posteriorly *(arrow)*, given its orientation, did not permit the prosthesis to rotate into the edentulous denture-bearing surfaces. This exposed the implants, and particularly the posterior implant, to significant bending moments during mastication of the bolus of food. *(b)* Significant bone loss is visible around all implants after 18 months.

reported success-failure rates but also recorded the pattern of bone loss around the implants that were placed into function. One hundred and two implants were placed in 26 patients with acquired maxillary defects secondary to resection of palatal and sinonasal tumors. Six patients with 19 implants were not available for follow-up because the patient either died prior to stage-two surgery or developed recurrence of the tumor. Of the 83 remaining implants, 4 were buried and 1 was in a patient who had not undergone stage-two surgery, leaving 78 implants available for study.

The implant survival rate for these 78 implants was 69.2%. The implant survival rates were 63.6% for the irradiated patients (67.0% before radiation and 50.0% after radiation) and 82.6% for nonirradiated patients. The irradiated implant sites were subjected to a mean dose of 50 Gy.

A pattern of failure and bone loss was detected around implants placed in each of the three most common sites. Failures were grouped into two categories: *(1) early*, when the implants failed to achieve osseointegration or within six months following the stage-two surgery, and *(2) late*, when implants failed after being subjected to clinical function for one year or more. Bone loss was divided into three categories: *(1) minimum*, defined as bone loss limited to one or two threads; *(2) moderate*, bone loss of three or four threads; and *(3) severe*, bone loss of more than four threads.

In the anterior maxilla, the late failures were secondary to progressive bone loss around the implants, and almost one-half of the implants in the anterior maxilla currently in function demonstrated severe bone loss. In contrast, in the maxillary tuberosity, where the bone quality and implant anchorage are generally poorer, virtually all of the implant failures were early, or prior to functional loading. However, once osseointegration was achieved and the implants were placed in function, bone levels did not appear to deteriorate over time (a typical example is shown in Fig 3-98).

The implant-connecting bar design used in the patients enrolled in the Roumanas study was an implant-supported design (almost all the forces of occlusion were borne by the implants). The implant-connecting bar attachment system had a Hader bar extension extending posteriorly on the unresected side (Fig 3-101). This implant-connecting bar design did not permit the prosthesis to rotate into the posterior edentulous denture-bearing surfaces when the bolus was being masticated, and thus was implant supported. In total maxillectomy patients, because of the limited support provided by the obturator prosthesis in the defect, the bolus of food is typically positioned posteriorly on the unresected side in the edentulous extension area. As a result, excessive bending moments were applied to the implants, leading to microfractures of bone anchoring the implants, especially the distal implant, because of the load magnification secondary to the cantilevering effect. This was most probably the primary reason why so many implants used with this design demonstrated advanced bone loss and indeed it is now well accepted that bone around implants that are subjected to excessive forces undergoes a resorption remodeling response leading to loss of bone (Hoshaw et al., 1994; Stanford and Brand, 1999; Brunski et al., 2000; Miyata et al., 1998, 2000, 2002; Miyamoto et al., 2008; Nagasawa et al., 2013).

In this report in defects where only solitary implants were available—for example, large defects where implants were placed in the tuberosity region—O-ring attachments were used to retain the prosthesis (see Figs 3-98 and 3-151). The O-ring permitted multiple axes of rotation and so the implants were used almost entirely for retention rather than to provide support for or enhance the stability of the prosthesis. As a result, the bending moments applied to these solitary implants were minimized. This may explain why such implants suffered less bone loss compared to those implants placed in the residual alveolar ridges in the anterior region and where an implant-supported implant-connecting bar design was employed.

In hindsight, the Roumanas (1997) report highlighted several issues that helped explain why UCLA's initial experience with this group of patients did not meet expectations. From these initial experiences, new solutions evolved and presently our expectation is that the success rates of implants used to retain and support maxillary obturators will approach the levels seen in normal unresected patients. For the most part, these issues have been addressed with new implant designs and configurations.

- *The difficulty in obtaining initial anchorage with the machine surface straight-wall implants.* This problem has been effectively addressed with new implant designs such as the tapered, self-tapping, variable thread designs of modern implants, dramatically improving initial implant anchorage and largely eliminating the risk of early implant failures.
- *The biomechanical deficiencies of the initial implant-connecting bar design used at the time, which exposed the implants to significant bending moments.* All the initial designs were implant supported and frequently lacked the numbers of implants and A-P spread necessary to withstand occlusal loading over sustained periods. This issue has been largely addressed by the use of implant-assisted designs when the numbers are inadequate or the implant configuration is not sufficient to support an implant-supported connecting bar design. The introduction of tilted implant concepts and the success of zygomatic implants have provided intradefect implant support that permits the predictable use of implant-supported designs.
- *The rather poor osteoconductivity of machine surface implants.* These implants were predictable in bone sites of favorable quantity and quality, such as the mandibular symphysis region, but were problematic when placed in bone sites of poor density. Since then, numerous surface treatments (sandblasting, acid etching, titanium grit blasting, electrolytic processes) designed to change the microtopography of the implant surface have evolved that have significantly improved the osteoconductivity of titanium implants, significantly improving bone anchorage, making these implants considerably more predictable in less favorable sites.
- *Moreover, the biologic events associated with the osseointegration process have been accelerated by the microrough surfaces,* enabling the practice of placing implants at the time of tumor ablation. The interval between surgery and postoperative radiation (generally five to six weeks, if it is administered) is sufficient for the modern implants to become reasonably well osseointegrated.

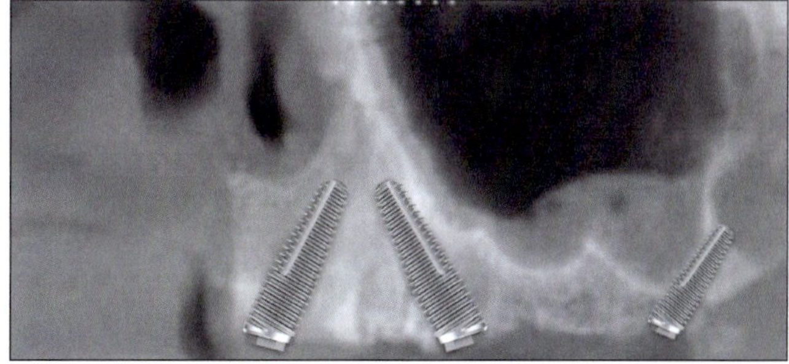

Figure 3-102 A CT scan of a patient with a total maxillectomy defect with the resection made down the midline. Tilting the implants and engaging the pyriform rim, the pyramidal process of the palatal bone permits the use of longer implants and improves initial implant stabilization. In addition, the biomechanics of the implant configuration thus created are more favorable.

Sites based on the use of tilted implants

Tilted implants offer a promising solution for patients with large palatal defects. If sufficient numbers of tilted implants are placed bilaterally and are osseointegrated, with favorable distribution patterns, implant-supported type prostheses can be fabricated, wherein all the forces of occlusion are borne by the implants. In some instances, early loading has been employed with success (see section below entitled "Immediate and early loading") (Butterworth and Rogers, 2017; Jayanetti and Fortmann, 2018; Butterworth et al., 2022).

Based on the success of tilted implants in patients with intact palates, sites such as the pyramidal process of the palatal bone, the pyriform rim region, the nasal crest, and the zygoma have emerged as potentially important sites for implant placement in patients with large palatal defects (Figs 3-102–3-108) (Wang et al., 2017; Jayanetti and Fortmann, 2018; Buurman et al., 2020a). The application of these concepts and the use of these sites appear to have special significance in patients with large palatal defects. In some patients, the residual alveolar ridges are resorbed and not of satisfactory volume or density to receive implants of sufficient length and diameter to retain large obturator prostheses over a sustained period. Moreover, initial anchorage was often difficult to achieve in such patients, especially with the original straight-wall implant designs, because of the poor density of the bone sites. Tilting implants that are placed in the anterior portion of the alveolar ridge allow the use of longer implants and permit the tips of the implants to be anchored in the cortical bone of the pyriform rim region. The use of the pyramidal process of the palatal bone adds an additional implant site. The result is that the biomechanics of the implant configurations created become more favorable. These sites and concepts combined with intradefect zygomatic implants would therefore appear to offer predictable long-term implant anchorage that previously was not obtainable in many of our patients with large palatal defects.

Pyramidal process of the palatal bone. During the 1980s and 1990s, machined-surface, straight-wall implants placed in the tuberosity region generally had a relatively low success rate, primarily because the poor-quality bone in this region made initial stabilization of implants difficult to achieve. In addition, they frequently were not angled to properly engage the pyramidal process of the palatal bone wherein lies the most bone volume. Failures before loading approached 50% (Roumanas et al., 1997). However, using tapered implants with variable thread designs, angled anteriorly to properly engage the pyramidal process of the palatal bone (Figs 3-103 and 3-104), results in improved initial implant anchorage, and the success rates at this site now approach 90% (Peñarrocha et al., 2009; Candel et al., 2012). The innovations in implant macrodesign, plus the fact that today's implants are prepared with microrough surfaces that are more osteoconductive, make this an especially attractive site for edentulous patients with large defects. Although success rates have been favorable in patients with intact palates (Peñarrocha et al., 2009; Candel et al., 2012), data reporting the outcomes in this site in patients with palatal defects is not yet available. An angled abutment or an off-axis implant needs to be employed when implants are placed into this site in order to account for the anterior tilt of the implant (see section below entitled "Implant selection criteria").

Pyriform rim region. Implants placed in this site are tilted at a 30°–45° angle posteriorly and placed just anterior to the maxillary sinus wall and engage the cortical bone associated with the pyriform rim region (Fig 3-105). If the surgeon is using a freehand approach a window should be created on the buccal wall and the sinus membrane reflected to identify the anterior sinus wall. This approach allows the surgeon to fully visualize the osteotomy site as it is being prepared. However, the semi-/fully guided approach

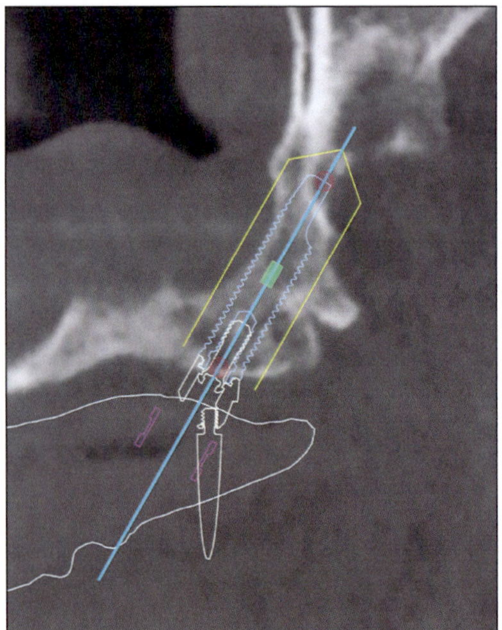

Figure 3-103 The pyramidal process of the palatal bone should be carefully considered as an implant site in patients with large palatal defects. Note the angulation. An off-angled implant or an angled abutment must be used to offset the anterior tilt of the implant (from Beumer et al., 2022b, with permission).

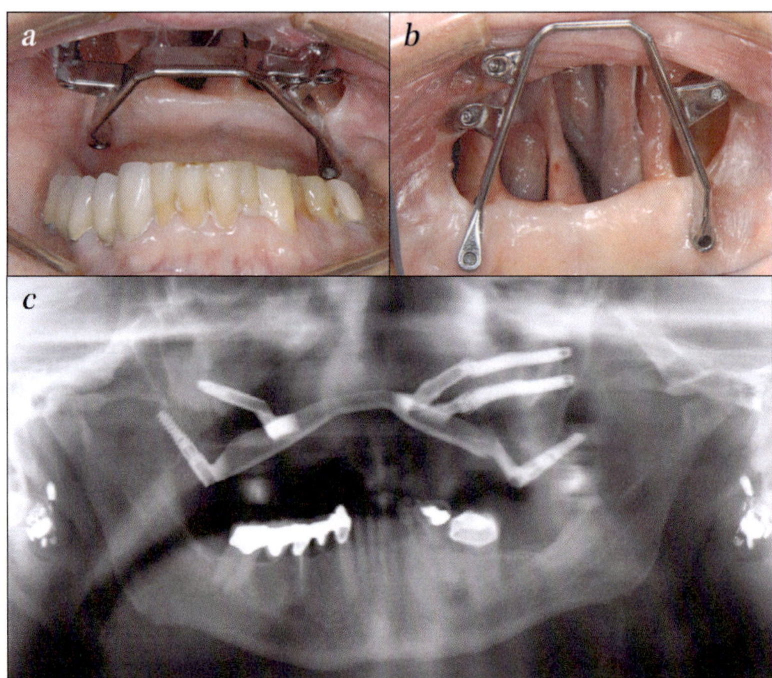

Figure 3-104 *(a, b, and c)* Implants have been placed in the pyramidal process of the palatal bones bilaterally combined with three zygomatic implants. The distribution pattern achieved permits an implant-supported implant-connecting bar design.

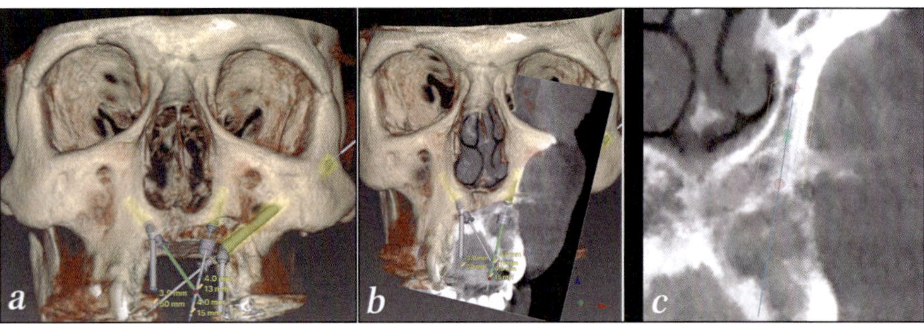

Figure 3-105 *(a)* The pyriform rim is an excellent bone site for implants and often is used in combination with zygomatic implants. *(b and c)* The left pyriform rim area appears to be a suitable site in this patient with an anticipated anterior defect.

using precise surgical drill guides is recommended for placement of implants in this region because this method allows more accurate implant placement, ensuring that the implant does indeed engage the cortical bone associated with the anterior wall of the sinus and the cortical bone associated with the pyriform rim. In addition, semi/fully guided surgical placement does not require such an aggressive dissection and exposure and as a result, the vasculature of the site is left relatively undisturbed, and postoperative morbidity is reduced. With all tilted implants, an angled abutment or an off-axis implant (see section below entitled "Implant selection criteria") needs to be employed in order to account for the angulation of the implant. Implants placed in the anterior alveolar process in the incisor region can also be tipped to engage the pyriform rim region. This permits the use of longer implants and improves initial implant anchorage.

This site can also be used in total palatectomy defects in combination with zygomatic implants. Often there remains a pyramidal-shaped segment of bone in the pyriform region after tumor ablation and occasionally it is of sufficient volume to house an implant of at least 10 mm in length and sometimes longer (see Fig 3-162c).

Nasal crest. If the anterior portion of the alveolar ridge has been retained, another site to consider is the bone associated with the nasal crest (Jensen et al., 2012). When implants are placed in the nasal crest the apical portion of the implants are tipped toward the midline (Fig 3-106). Engagement of the nasal crest allows the use of implants longer than could otherwise be employed in this region and the tips of the implants will engage cortical bone. With CBCT scans, it is now possible to determine whether patients are good candidates for this option. When this site is chosen, fabrication of a surgical drill guide (template) is suggested that permits implant placement into this challenging site with either semi-guided or fully guided surgery. It should be noted that frequently the alveolar mucosa in the premaxilla is excessively thick, particularly in those patients with moderate to severe resorption of the alveolar ridge secondary to combination syndrome or long-term denture use, and so a submucosal resection is often necessary to thin the tissues (to 4–5 mm), through which the implants will eventually emerge. This is a necessary procedure if the health of the peri-implant mucosa is to be maintained.

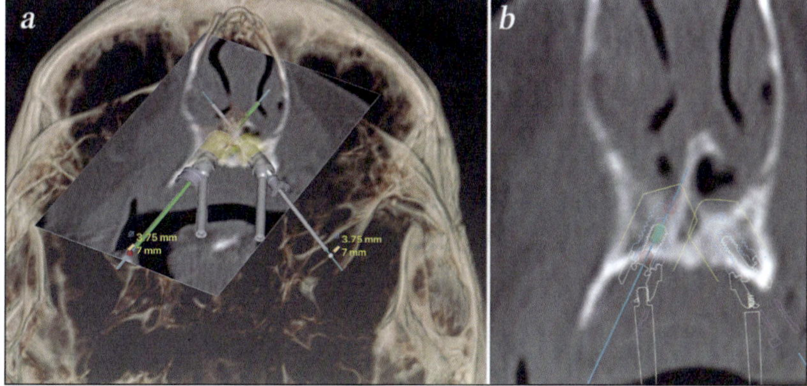

Figure 3-106 *(a and b)* When the anterior portion of the alveolar ridge has been retained, the nasal crest is an alternative site for the placement of implants in patients with palatal defects.

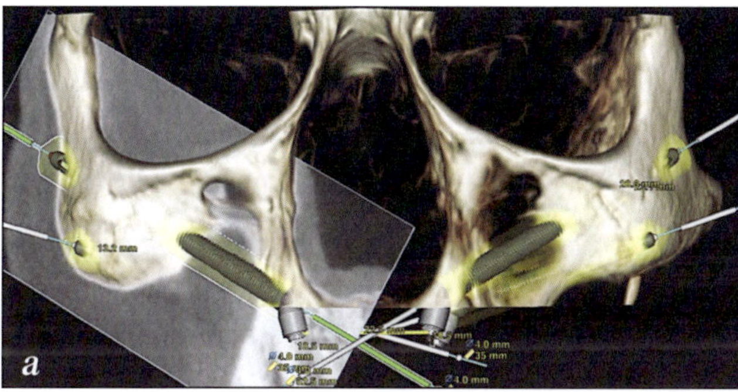

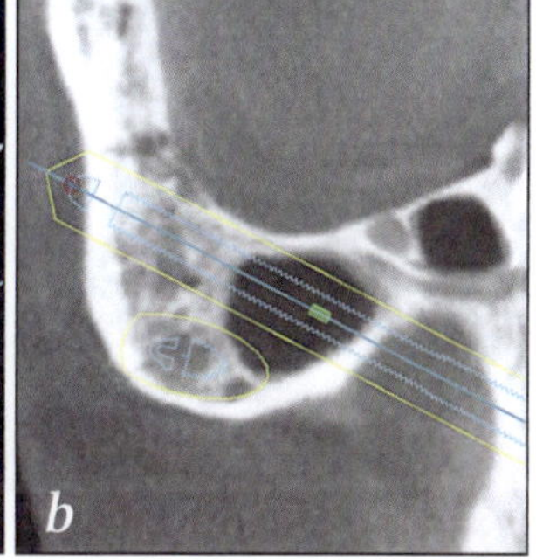

Figure 3-107 *(a and b)* Two implants are planned for placement in each of the zygomas of patients who are about to undergo a total palatectomy.

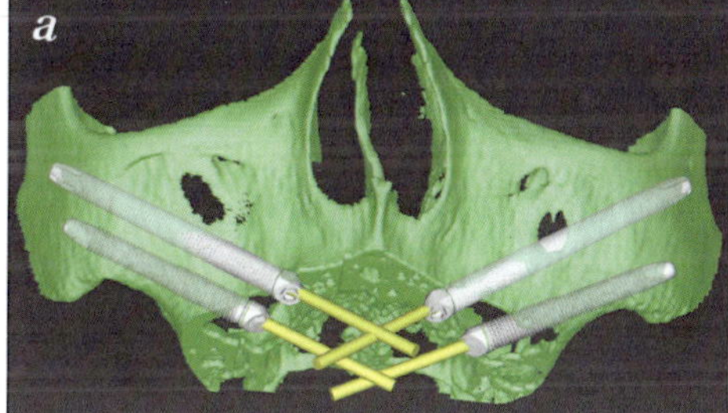

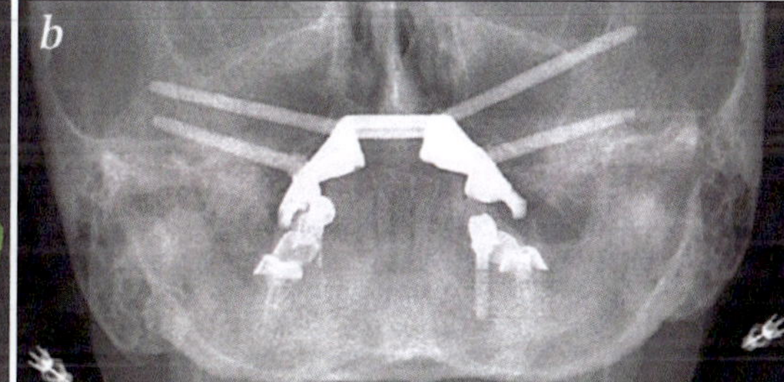

Figure 3-108 *(a)* Four zygomatic implants are planned for the total palatectomy defect. A proper implant arrangement and initial stabilization will permit early loading and fabrication of an implant-supported prosthesis if sufficient initial anchorage has been achieved with each implant. *(b)* A "Waters" view of the implants and the implant-connecting bar.

Zygoma. The zygoma has emerged as a prime site for implants used to retain large obturator prostheses (Fig 3-107). This site is composed of dense trabecular bone with thick cortices and is usually of sufficient volume to accept two implants following most maxillary resections. In some situations, the zygoma on the side opposite the defect can also be used (see Fig 3-109). The zygomatic implant was introduced by Brånemark (2004) and has frequently been employed in unresected patients as an alternative to bone grafting in those presenting with extensive sinus pneumatization and moderate to severe resorption of the edentulous maxillae. In recent years it has undergone a number of design changes, which make it better suited for patients with large palatal defects secondary to tumor ablation or unrepaired cleft palate (Southern Implants, Irene, RSA). The modern versions of these implants are designed with extended smooth areas (the so-called zygomatic oncology implant), as opposed to being threaded along its entire length, in order to minimize plaque accumulations and enhance plaque removal along the exposed area of the implant as it makes it way from the point of anchorage to the oral cavity. In addition, the neck of the implant, which accepts the abutment screw, has been augmented to reduce the risk of fracture in this region (see Fig 3-125). The angulation of the implant platform has been changed to 55° in order to accommodate the fact that as the implants enter the prosthetic space, they are almost parallel to the occlusal plane.

In most patients with large bilateral palatal defects, two implants are placed into each zygoma (Fig 3-108). *Note that the implants are planned to engage the outer layer of cortical bone in order to maximize initial anchorage.* Zygomatic implants are often combined with conventional-length implants placed in bone sites available in the defect such as the pyriform rim region (see Figs 3-105 and 3-158), the residual alveolar processes (see Fig 3-123), and the pyramidal process of the palatal bone (see Fig 3-103). The zygomatic implants are 30–60 mm in length in order to span the distance between the anchorage sites in the zygoma and the oral cavity and are designed with angulated platforms in order to account for the severe angulation of the implants (Southern Implants, Irene, RSA). Early loading can be considered when the implant distribution pattern is favorable and when the initial stabilization of the implants exceeds

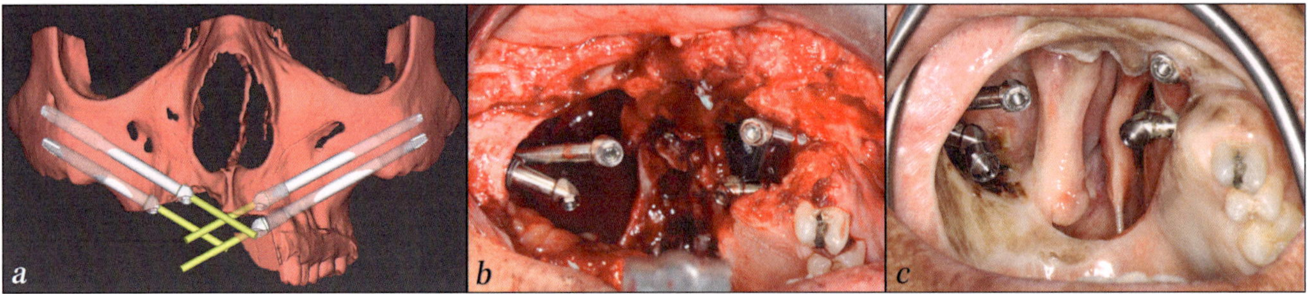

Figure 3-109 *(a)* Three-dimensional representations of potential implant sites following virtual resections of palatal tumors can be made with scans and the use of appropriate software. Implants are being considered for the zygoma. *(b)* Ultimately, four zygomatic were placed to provide implant support on the side of the defect. *(c)* The defect following healing. Note the skin grafted surfaces. They prevent undue contracture of the defect permitting appropriate extension of the prosthesis to provide support for the lip and cheek. Hygiene access is also enhanced.

30 Ncm or 60 ISQ (see section below entitled "Immediate and early loading"). Implant-supported designs can be used for the definitive implant-connecting bars when the distribution pattern is favorable and each of the implants is anchored in a reasonable volume of bone (see section below entitled "Implant-supported bar designs").

Zygomatic implants are being employed with increased frequency in partially edentulous patients with maxillectomy/palatectomy defects to provide intradefect implant support (Fig 3-109). Implant support on the defect side dramatically improves patient function and reduces the stresses on the residual dentition, potentially prolonging their life span. In a classical total maxillectomy defect, there usually will be access to both zygomas, so it is possible to provide sufficient numbers of implants with an appropriate distribution pattern biomechanically to provide implant support on the side of the defect (Fig 3-109). Likewise, in anterior defects, zygomatic implants, frequently in combination with implants placed in the pyriform rim, can be used to provide implant support in the defect (see Figs 3-105 and 3-113).

Complications are rare but can be significant and include oroantral fistula formation when used on the unresected side, perforation of the skin over the zygoma, postoperative maxillary sinusitis, periorbital hematoma formation and facial swelling, and penetration into the orbit. Surgical placement is demanding and requires specialized training.

The clinical follow-up data, although retrospective is encouraging (Schmidt et al., 2004; Aparicio et al., 2014). In a systematic review, the cumulative survival rate of zygomatic implants was above 97% (Wang et al., 2015). In one study, 28 zygomatic implants were placed in 9 patients with large maxillary defects (Schmidt et al., 2004). Six implants failed (most in irradiated patients), and 5 of the patients were eventually restored with an implant-retained obturator prosthesis. For rehabilitation of total palatectomy defects, these clinicians recommended that 2 implants be placed in each residual zygoma and that all 4 be splinted together with an implant-connecting bar.

From 2015 to 2020, Butterworth et al. (2022) employed 117 zygomatic implants in the zygoma in combination with vascularized soft tissue flaps in 33 patients (so-called ZIP flap technique) placed immediately following maxillectomies in 33 patients. Nineteen conventional implants were also used, some in extraction sites and others in healed edentulous sites. Eighteen of the 33 patients received adjuvant radiotherapy. All patients were restored with fixed prostheses. Zygomatic implant survival is 98.7% to date. Mean follow-up is 25 months (range 2–60 months).

Landes et al. (2009) reported the use of 36 zygomatic implants in 15 patients, 9 of whom were edentulous. In addition, 24 conventional implants were placed in oral sites in these patients. Of the 15 patients, 12 presented after resection of large tumors of the maxilla, and 3 presented with congenital defects. Six of the 12 oncology patients received chemotherapy and 7 received radiation therapy during the course of their treatments. Radiation doses ranged from 45 to 61 Gy. The prostheses were retained with telescopic crowns associated with, when necessary, angled abutments. Follow-up ranged from 13 to 102 months. During that period, 3 zygomatic implants were lost secondary to overloading and/or chronic infection, and 5 others were removed secondary to resection of recurrent disease (Landes et al., 2009).

Zygomatic implants have been used successfully in irradiated sites although it appears the rates of success will be reduced. Schmidt and colleagues reported (2004) a lower rate of success (slightly less than 80%) in their series of patients and they attributed the reduced success rate to the fact that most of the implant sites in their patient population were irradiated.

Implants placed during ablative surgery versus deferred implant placement

As mentioned previously, some clinicians advocate placing implants during ablative surgery as opposed to deferred placement (Wetzels et al., 2016, 2017; Butterworth, 2019; Alberga et al., 2021; Butterworth et al., 2022). The authors support this approach, especially in patients with little or no dentition available to retain an obturator prosthesis (Figs 3-109 and 3-111). Implant retention and support, particularly when provided on the side of the defect, dramatically improve mastication performance and quality of life for most maxillectomy patients compared to conventional obturator prostheses (Butterworth, 2019; Buurman et al., 2020b; Butterworth et al., 2022). This is especially true in those patients with large defects that cross the midline (Fig 3-109), those defects that extend to the posterior pharyngeal wall and extend to include the residual velopharyngeal musculature, and almost all edentulous patients. This approach saves the patient an additional implant surgery while also reducing the cost of treatment. Moreover, implant success rates appear to be comparable to those achieved with deferred placement in this group of patients (Wetzels et al., 2017; Butterworth, 2019; Butterworth et al., 2022).

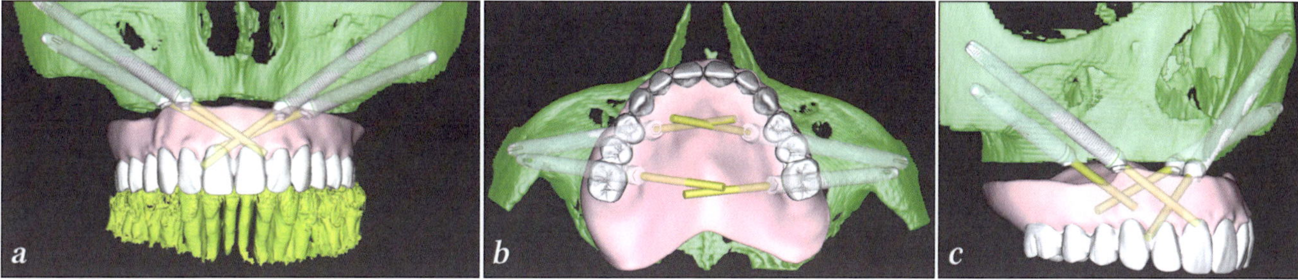

Figure 3-110 A patient scheduled to undergo a total palatectomy. *(a, b, and c)* The lengths, angulation, and position of the implants must be such that an implant-connecting bar and metal substructure can be fabricated that is compatible with the prosthetic space and so that the contours of the palatal vault are faithfully reproduced and the denture teeth can be properly positioned. Once these issues have been addressed a surgical template can be designed to aid the surgeon during implant placement.

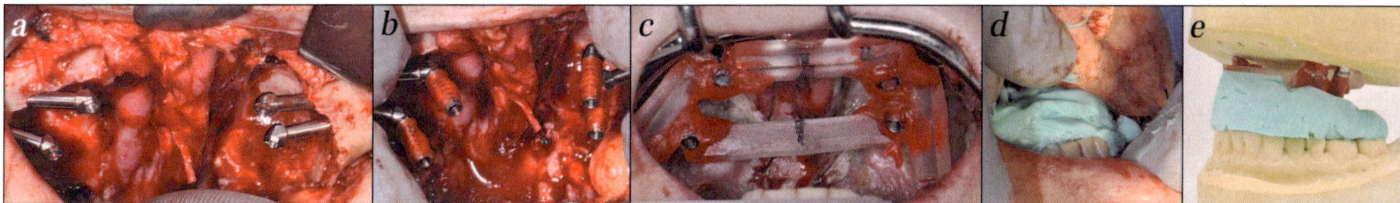

Figure 3-111 *(a)* Following the resection the implants are positioned. Note these implants have smooth necks. *(b)* Temporary abutment cylinders coated with pattern resin are secured to the implants. *(c)* Resin struts are secured to the implants with pattern resin. *(d)* A silicone recording medium is used to pick up the pattern resin assembly and an arbitrary CR record is made that allows the cast to be *(e)* mounted on an articulator.

Digital technologies have made this approach easier and more predictable. When implant placement is anticipated in concert with surgical tumor ablation, scans of the patient are obtained and the probable surgical resection can be simulated (see Fig 3-15). The possible bone sites can then be carefully evaluated and plans made for placing implants immediately upon tumor resection (Figs 3-109 and 3-111). The selection of implant sites, implant lengths, and angulations are based on the proposed prosthetic design, the prosthetic space available, and the anatomic configuration of the resected defect. Ideally, implants are positioned to permit implant-supported designs (all forces of occlusion are borne by the implants), which under most circumstances will require intradefect implant placement. The implant platforms and their abutments should be positioned so that the resulting implant-connecting bar and metal substructure allow the overlay obturator prosthesis to faithfully restore the contours of the palatal vault and properly position the prosthetic teeth (Fig 3-110).

Immediate and early loading

Immediate loading as defined by Pozzi and colleagues (2016) is the placement of the prosthesis onto implants that have just been placed or within 24 hours of placement. By definition, the immediate load prosthesis is designed to be in occlusal contact with the dentition of the opposing arch. This concept has been employed successfully in patients with intact palates and several authors have reported favorable results with the use of only four zygomatic implants when the anterior-posterior spread exceeds 20 mm (Wang et al., 2015; Tuminelli et al., 2017). Although theoretically possible, based on studies using human cadavers and 3D-designed and -printed drill guides, fully guided surgical placement of zygomatic implants (Vosselman et al., 2021), this approach has not been well documented in patients with maxillary defects and we have not attempted immediate loading in such patients at UCLA or UCSF.

However, early loading has been attempted in patients with large palatal defects (Butterworth and Rogers, 2017; Jayanetti and Fortmann, 2018; Butterworth et al., 2022). Early loading as defined by Pozzi and colleagues (2016) is securing the prosthesis to the implant(s) and placing it into occlusal function before a conventional period of healing has been completed. The healing period for microrough surface implants is six to eight weeks, so any prosthesis in occlusion with the opposing dentition—that is, delivered prior to this period—would be considered early loading.

Early loading must be undertaken with caution and several factors are taken into account before considering this option on any particular patient. The implant sites must be ideal (at least 10 mm of vertical bone volume available relative to the long axis of the implant) and the implant configuration favorable (at least two implants be positioned on each side with a favorable distribution pattern for edentulous patients). After the surgical packing is removed and before teeth are added to the prosthesis, the authors prefer that the implants be splinted together with a provisional implant-connecting bar. Splinting is recommended regardless of whether early loading is contemplated in order to ensure the implants remain immobilized during the healing period. The bar serves as an external rigid fixation device that splints the implants together during healing (Vosselman et al., 2021). This practice minimizes the risk of inadvertently exposing individual implants to bending moments that would mobilize them. The initial anchorage of each implant must be sufficient (30–40 Ncm or 60–70 ISQ) before early loading is considered (Pozzi et al., 2016). Otherwise, it is prudent to delay adding teeth to the interim obturator and the

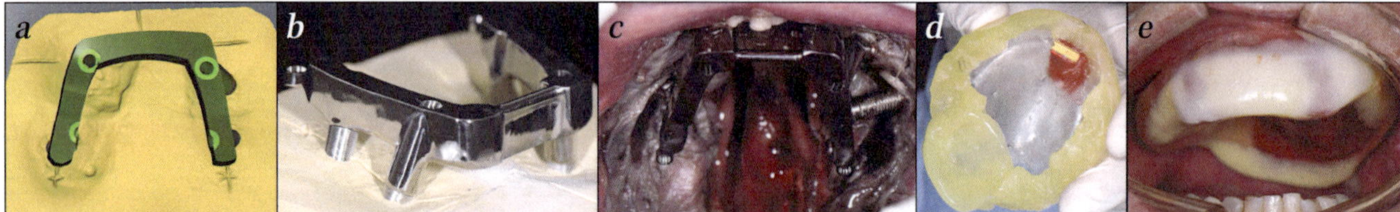

Figure 3-112 *(a)* The cast is scanned and an implant-supported implant-connecting bar is designed. *(b)* The bar was milled of titanium. *(c)* Upon removal of the ISO, the implant bar is secured to the implants. *(d)* The ISO is adapted to the defect and the velopharyngeal area with a temporary denture reliner. Note that only two clips have been used for retention. *(e)* The ISO from a patient with a similar resection secured to the provisional implant-connecting bar. Note the absence of dentition at this stage. Teeth will not be added until four to six weeks post-implant placement.

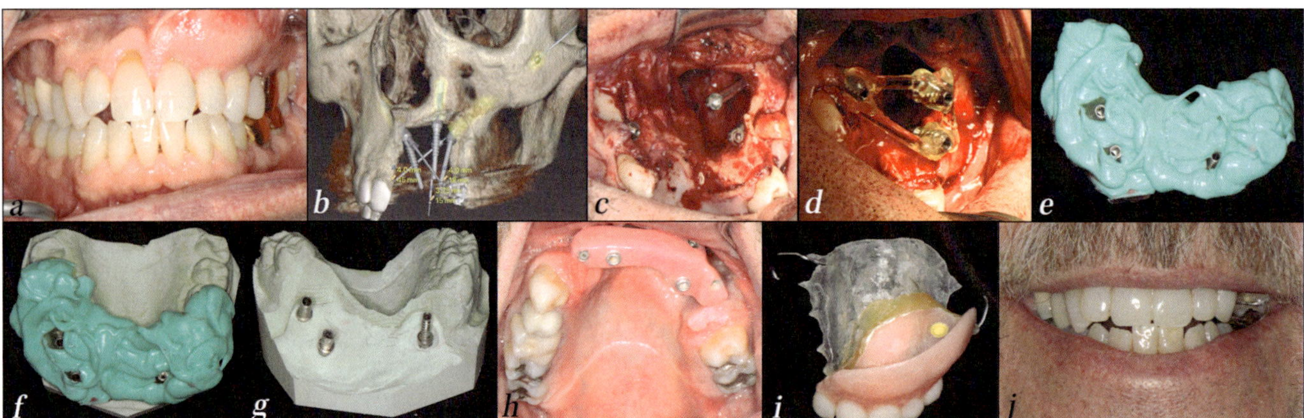

Figure 3-113 An early load prosthesis. *(a)* Patient presented with an ameloblastoma arising from anterior maxilla. *(b)* 3D representation of the maxillae and adjacent structures. A virtual resection is performed and possible implant positions are evaluated. *(c)* Three implants have been placed; two in the left zygomatic arch and one in the right pyriform region. *(d and e)* An impression is made and the *(f and g)* original cast is altered. *(h)* A provisional implant-connecting bar was designed and fabricated of acrylic resin. *(i and j)* Anterior teeth are added to the ISO, a centric occlusion record is made, the ISO is adapted to the defect, and the matrix portion of the attachments picked up and secured to the prosthesis transforming the ISO into an interim obturator.

prosthesis placed in occlusion until a normal period of healing has elapsed (six to eight weeks following implant placement).

Patients with a history of significant parafunctional activities (bruxism or clenching) are poor candidates for early loading especially if the opposing mandible is dentate. A smoking habit (Bain and Moy, 1993; Moy et al., 2005), plus radiotherapy adds an additional level of risk. If postoperative radiation therapy is anticipated the authors prefer not to employ early loading and teeth are not added to the interim prosthesis until after radiation treatments are completed and the radiation mucositis has subsided. However, some clinicians have reported good success in patients who have received postoperative radiation (Butterworth and Rogers, 2017; Butterworth et al., 2022). The patient must be compliant and religiously follow postoperative instructions because if not, success is problematic. It should be noted that the initial anchorage achieved at implant placement will steadily diminish during the first 7–10 days following surgery before it begins to improve as bone is steadily deposited on the surface of the implant. As a result, the provisional implant-connecting bar will be secured to the implants during a period (9–12 days following surgical ablation and when the surgical packing is removed) when there is risk of mobilizing the implants; hence, this procedure must be performed with great care so as not to mobilize any of the implants.

The UCLA group has attempted early loading primarily in patients who have had their implants inserted at the time of tumor resection (Jayanetti and Fortmann, 2018). An index/impression is made at the time of implant placement to record the position of the implants before the immediate surgical obturator is secured in position (Figs 3-111 and 3-113). The ISO is designed without prosthetic teeth and used merely to obturate the defect and hold the surgical packing in position during the immediate postsurgical period. If the patient is partially edentulous, the original cast from which the ISO was fabricated can be altered to accept the impression of the implants, much like an altered cast impression is used to relate edentulous extension areas to the residual dentition when fabricating removable dental prosthesis (Fig 3-113). This altered cast now represents the positions of the implants in relation to the residual dentition. In the case of a total palatectomy, the impression of the implant positions is made, and a cast is prepared and eventually scanned (Fig 3-112). The occlusal vertical dimension is determined arbitrarily based on presurgical clinical evaluations, a centric relation record is a made, and this record is used to mount the cast on an articulator (Fig 3-111e). The provisional implant-connecting bar is designed to permit restoration of palatal contours and eventually, the placement of prosthetic teeth. The ISO and the surgical packing are removed, usually about 9–12 days postsurgical ablation, and the implant-connecting bar is secured at this time. This bar can be designed and fabricated with conventional methods or by the use of CAD-CAM programs. The bar shown in Fig 3-112 was designed digitally and milled of titanium. The bar used in the patient depicted in Fig 3-113 was designed and fabricated conventionally and made of methyl methacrylate.

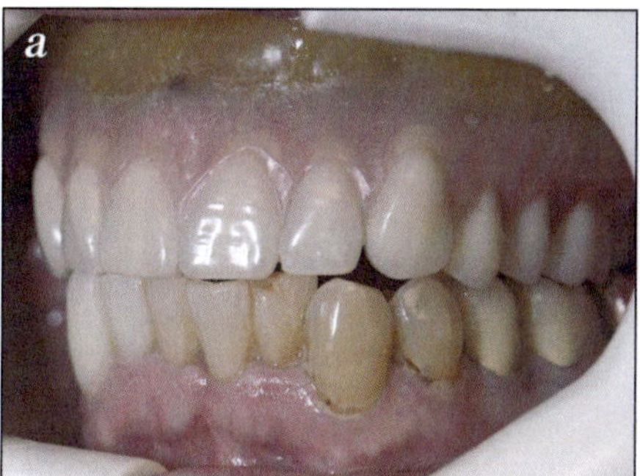

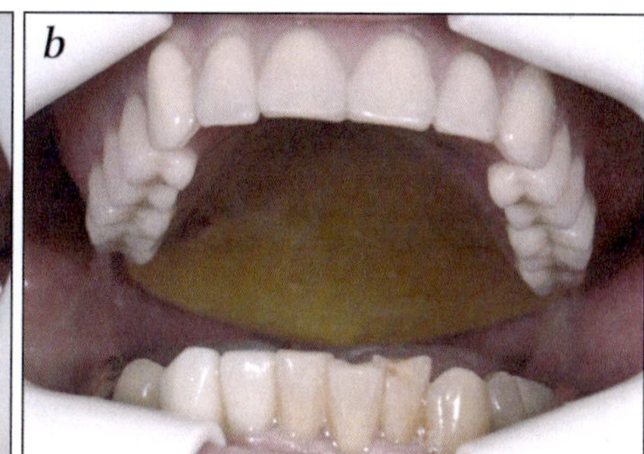

Figure 3-114 *(a and b)* A patient with a total palatectomy defect (also shown in Figs 3-112, 3-146, and 3-162). A centric relation record is made and teeth are added to the interim obturator prosthesis four to six weeks after the tumor ablation. The interim obturator prosthesis in position. The patient is placed on a liquid diet for the first three weeks and a soft diet for the following three weeks.

The provisional implant-connecting bar should be designed to minimize bending moments applied to the implants. For example, in a patient scheduled for a total palatectomy, and when titanium is used, a Hader segment is positioned anteriorly, which is perpendicular to the midline and parallel to the plane of occlusion. When the tongue elevates and presses against the palatal portion of the ISO during bolus manipulation and swallowing, the ISO will rotate around this portion of the bar. Only two clips are used for retention (Fig 3-112d).

Resin is preferred when the initial anchorage of the implants is suboptimal—for example, when an osteotomy site is overprepared and/or if the poor quality of the bone site results in a so-called spinner. Under these circumstances, the implant(s) in question may assume a slightly different position upon osseointegration. A resin bar can be quickly sectioned and corrected at chairside to create a precision fit, whereas a titanium bar, following sectioning, must be sent to the dental lab for laser welding to reunite the bar segments. However, when using resin, the bar must be bulkier so as to ensure that it is sufficiently rigid and this may compromise hygiene access. Another factor favoring the use of resin is the length of time it takes the dental laboratory to design and fabricate a titanium bar and transport it to the clinician. This may be excessive, for the ISO must be removed within 9–12 days in order to remove the surgical packing. Moreover, the use of resin is considerably less costly. As a result of these factors, currently, the authors use titanium only when the quality of the initial implant anchorage is unquestioned. Furthermore, the provisional titanium bar can often be used as the definitive implant-connecting bar if it is designed to be implant supported.

After the bar is connected to the implants, the ISO is readapted to the defect with a temporary denture reliner, and attachments are secured to transform the ISO into an interim obturator prosthesis retained by the provisional implant-connecting bar. Three to four weeks later teeth are added (Fig 3-114). As mentioned above, if the patient is to receive postoperative radiotherapy, the teeth are added three to four weeks after the completion of radiation or after the radiation mucositis has subsided. The screws securing the bar should be torqued to 15–20 Ncm but no more. Hand tightening will minimize the risk of overtorquing the screws, which generally limits screw tightening to 15–20 Ncm. Hand tightening is recommended, since mechanical torque drivers are notoriously inaccurate (Standlee and Caputo, 1999; Standlee et al., 2002; McCracken et al., 2010).

The patient is placed on a liquid diet for the first three weeks and a mechanical soft diet for the following three weeks while osseointegration is progressing. It is vital that the patient conform to these postoperative instructions because if an implant is mobilized during healing it will fail to osseointegrate (Maniatopolous et al., 1986; Szmuckler-Moncler et al., 2000). The occlusion should be verified and refined with a clinical remount record. When the opposing arch is dentate, group function is employed. Bilateral balance is used if the prosthesis opposes a complete denture.

This approach has now been employed on 25 patients by the UCLA group with total and subtotal maxillary defects. Ninety-two implants have been placed in several sites including the zygoma (84 implants), the pyriform rim (2 implants), the pyramidal process of the palatal bone (2 implants), and the residual edentulous ridge (4 implants). The median follow-up is 30 months with a range of 4–72 months. Of the 84 zygomatic implants placed, 73 are still in function as well as all 8 of the conventional-length implants placed in alternative sites. Implant losses have been concentrated in four irradiated patients, three who were irradiated prior to implant placement and one who was irradiated after implant placement. Only one of the 25 patients required a complete remake of their prosthesis.

Butterworth and colleagues (2022) have used early loading in a similar population using zygomatic implants, with the exception that the defect is obturated with a soft tissue vascularized free flap as opposed to an obturator prosthesis, and the implants perforate the flap (so-called ZIP flap). Implants are placed upon tumor ablation, an impression is made, and a tentative centric relation record is obtained in a manner similar to that described above. A provisional fixed dental prosthesis composed of denture teeth and acrylic resin is fabricated and delivered four to six weeks following tumor ablation. This delay permits proper monitoring of the vascularized flap during the initial stages of healing. The provisional prosthesis is eventually replaced with a fixed hybrid prosthesis with a metal substructure. This approach has been successfully employed in 34 patients Zygomatic implant survival is 98.4%, and only 1 prosthesis has been lost to date (mean follow-up is 25 months; Butterworth et al., 2022).

Implants placed in patients to receive postoperative radiotherapy

Definitive doses of radiation therapy dramatically impair the osseointegration process (see Chapter 1, section entitled "Dental Implants in Irradiated Tissues"). At doses in excess of 60 Gy, the biologic processes associated with osseointegration are severely compromised and anchorage in bone is most likely mechanical and secondary to the density of the bone site as opposed to biologic

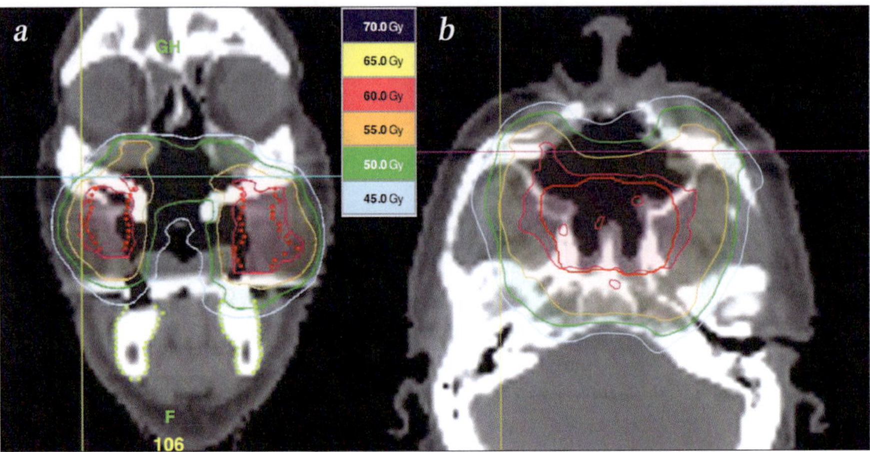

Figure 3-115 Implants were placed immediately following tumor ablation and the patient scheduled for postoperative radiation therapy. *(a and b)* The dosimetry was manipulated to limit the dosage delivered to the implant sites.

processes. As mentioned previously in most patients, postoperative radiation does not begin until four to six weeks following tumor resection, and this is sufficient time to allow microrough surface implants to become reasonably well osseointegrated. In addition, the dosimetry can be controlled so as to limit the dose to the implant sites without compromising the dosage delivered to the proposed tumor volume (Fig 3-115). Moreover, after surgical ablation and postoperative radiation therapy, many patients undergoing maxillectomy present with trismus limiting access to the desired implant sites and making implant placement problematic. For these reasons, the authors prefer, when possible, to place implants at the time of tumor ablation (see above) and prior to radiation therapy, especially when the dose to the implant sites is likely to exceed 60 Gy.

Clinical procedures

Workup

The size and extent of the defect, the state of the remaining dentition, the available implant sites, and the nature of the opposing mandibular dentition are the primary factors to consider when contemplating the use of implants in patients with palatal defects. Moreover, if the opposing arch is dentate, it deserves careful scrutiny. Significant occlusal plane discrepancies should be addressed and corrected as needed. Teeth that are rotated or supraerupted may need to be recontoured in order to idealize the plane of occlusion and idealize cusp fossa relationships. This can be accomplished with either a removable dental prosthesis in the form of ribbon rests or complete-coverage crowns and fixed dental prostheses (see Fig 3-54) (Chang et al., 2019).

Implant site selection and design and fabrication of surgical templates

Conventional method. The conventional approach requires fabrication of a radiographic guide. The existing maxillary complete denture/obturator or the interim complete denture/obturator is duplicated in autopolymerizing acrylic resin, and gutta-percha cylinders are inserted into each of the tooth sites (Fig 3-116a). Tin foil is adapted to the facial surfaces of the prosthetic dentition to indicate the facial surfaces of the proposed prosthetic teeth of the future obturator prosthesis. A CT scan is obtained while the patient wears the guide. The resulting scans are evaluated to assess the bone volume available at the possible implant sites (Fig 3-116b and c). This data and that obtained from the clinical evaluation are used to determine implant positions and angulations. The radiographic guide can then be transformed into a surgical guide and freehand surgery is used to place the implants (Fig 3-116d). Palatal support should be maintained to allow proper positioning of the surgical template during surgery. Alternative implant sites are typically prepared in the surgical guide to aid the surgeon in case a potential implant site is found to be less than ideal upon surgical exposure. With this method, acceptable positioning and angulation of implants can be achieved in the hands of an experienced surgeon. This method remains suitable and is still employed when implants are to be placed in the residual alveolar ridge with conventional angulation.

Digital method. However, if the zygoma, pyriform rim, nasal crest, or pyramidal process of the palatal bone is considered, CBCT scans with the associated software are recommended in order to assess the possible implant sites in three dimensions. When these sites are considered, implant positioning is more challenging, and alignment must be more precise, and therefore freehand drilling is rapidly being supplanted by semiguided or fully guided implant placement using sophisticated surgical templates fabricated with computer-aided design and manufacturing techniques (CAD-CAM).

Computer-guided planning tools are rapidly becoming the standard of care for patients with large palatal defects. The precision that can be achieved with these methods represents a sophisticated treatment planning tool that ensures that implant placement is directed by the demands of the prosthesis while taking maximum advantage of the bone sites available. Moreover, these methods are rapidly becoming cost effective. CBCT scans allow visualization of the bone contours of the potential bony implant sites and adjacent structures in three dimensions. The lengths, diameter, position, and probable angulation of the implants can be determined prior to implant placement.

The radiographic guide is made by duplicating the obturator prosthesis and creating fiducial markers with gutta-percha (Fig 3-117) or by applying adhesive removable radiographic fiducial markers to the existing prosthesis or its duplicate (Fig 3-118). The radiographic guide is worn while the scan is being performed.

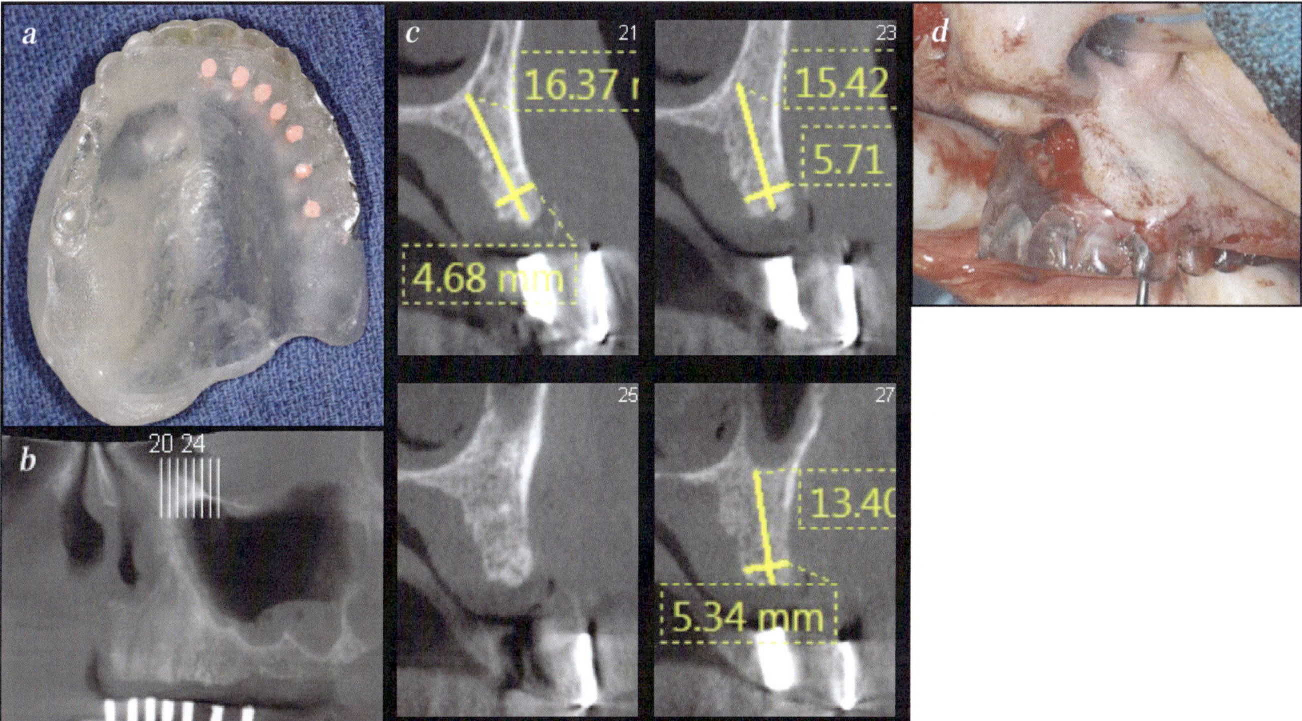

Figure 3-116 *(a)* Obturator prosthesis duplicated in acrylic resin. Potential implant positions are represented by gutta-percha cylinders. *(b)* The radiographic stent is positioned intraorally and a conventional CT scan has been obtained. *(c)* Cross sections of the possible implant sites can be visualized in two dimensions. *(d)* The radiographic guide has been transformed into a surgical drill guide designed for freehand surgery.

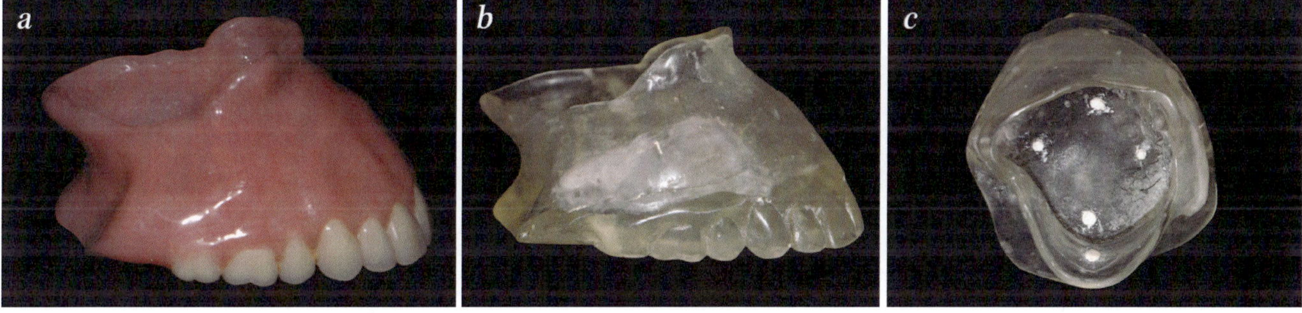

Figure 3-117 *(a, b, and c)* The obturator prosthesis is duplicated and *(c)* fiducial markers, in the form of gutta-percha cylinders are created within the body of the prosthesis in strategic locations. The radiographic guide is worn while making the CT scan.

The prosthesis must not move during the study and if necessary, it can be immobilized with a silicone occlusal index. A separate scan of the radiographic guide allows the digital rendering of the prosthesis and the DICOM data from the patient scan to be merged, permitting the denture teeth and the contours of the proposed prosthesis to be superimposed onto the bony contours of the intended implant sites (Fig 3-119). Implant size, position, and angulation can be predetermined, and a surgical template can be designed and fabricated that permits semiguided or fully guided controlled directional drilling, ensuring maximum accuracy of implant placement and alignment.

Surgical templates designed to permit semiguided controlled directional drilling. Design and manufacture of surgical templates used for semiguided surgery employ the same treatment planning software programs as for those used in fully guided surgery, but the surgical drill sleeves incorporated within the surgical templates are designed to accommodate twist drills and *control only the position and angulation* of the initial osteotomy sites. This type of surgical template is particularly well suited for placement of zygomatic implants (Fig 3-120). Note the inspection windows. These help the surgeon determine proper seating of the template and also allow the surgeon to visualize the twist drills so as to maintain the proper trajectory of the drills during the preparation of the osteotomy sites. These surgical templates are removable to permit the surgeon to alter the site as needed, such as enhancing the site with grafting or altering the apicocoronal position of the implant, and to change the rotational alignment of the implant platform. They can be keyed to existing bony structures or the residual dentition (Fig 3-121) or a combination of the two. They are generally held in place by a surgical assistant but when convenient can be

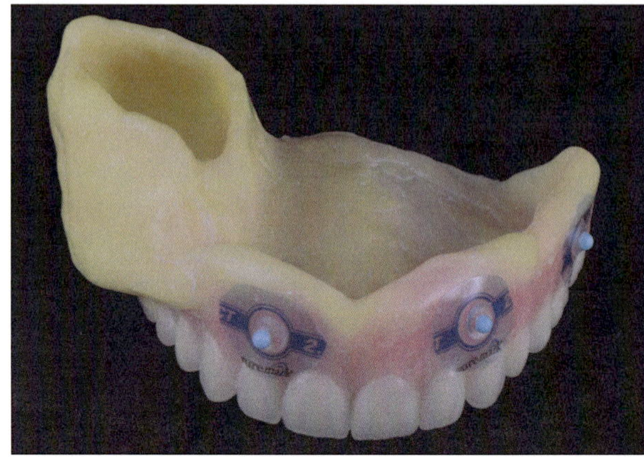

Figure 3-118 Radiographic markers can also be attached to an existing prosthesis. The markers can then be removed after the scan without altering the prosthesis. The radiographic guide is worn while making the CT scan.

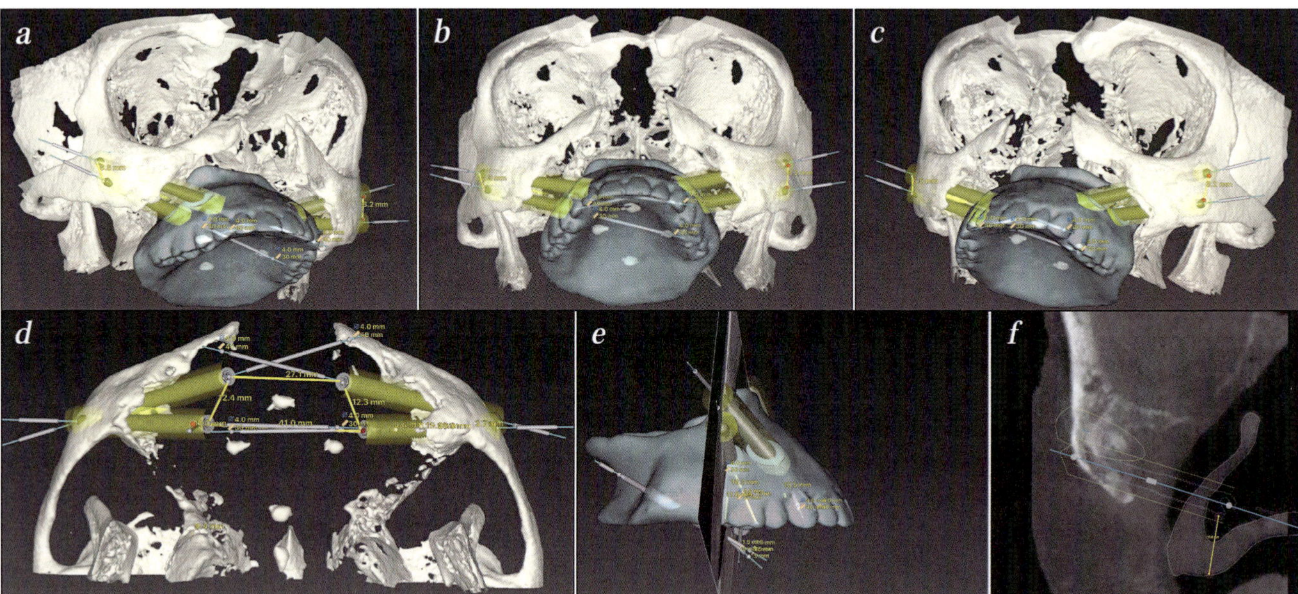

Figure 3-119 *(a, b, c, and d)* CBCT scans and the associated software programs allow digital rendering of the prosthesis superimposed onto the underlying bone contours and permit the clinician to properly position the implants consistent with the prosthetic design. *(d and e)* The software allows each of the potential implant sites to be closely scrutinized. Once positions and angulations of the implants have been determined, a semiguided surgical drill guide can then be designed to aid in development of the implant sites and placement of the implants.

secured with bone screws while the implant osteotomies are being prepared. When bone screws are used to secure the template, it is advisable to design several points of anchorage in order to account for the possible variations encountered during the oncologic resection. The final preparation of the sites and seating of the implants are completed freehand and after the surgical template has been removed. Note that the zygomatic implants are planned to engage the outer cortex of the zygoma.

Several issues arise when designing such templates for placement of implants during surgical ablation. Most importantly, *the virtual surgical ablation should be underestimated.* Otherwise, the surgical template will not seat properly and require significant adjustment in the operating room or, worse, render the template unusable. When the placement of zygomatic implants is anticipated, the length of the surgical sleeves should be extended to at least 10 mm. However, given the extended length of these implants, it is highly desirable to incorporate multiple drill sleeves within the template to maximize accuracy. In addition, possible drilling impediments should be identified and eliminated. This step can be performed virtually with the software programs currently available (Fig 3-122).

Surgical templates can be designed either as one piece or with multiple segments that fit precisely together. They allow the surgeon a bit more flexibility to perform adjunctive procedures such as bone and soft tissue grafts. Moreover, they may be necessary to avoid drilling impediments.

Surgical templates designed to permit fully guided controlled directional drilling. Fully guided surgery implies that the surgical template, with drill sleeves incorporated (bushings), controls the position, angulation, and diameter *as well as the depth* of the implant osteotomy site. These surgical templates are used when precise control of angulation, location in the arch, and apical-coronal depth are critical to achieve ideal engagement of the bone of the implant site. This approach is especially useful when tilted implants are to be placed in the residual alveolar ridge to

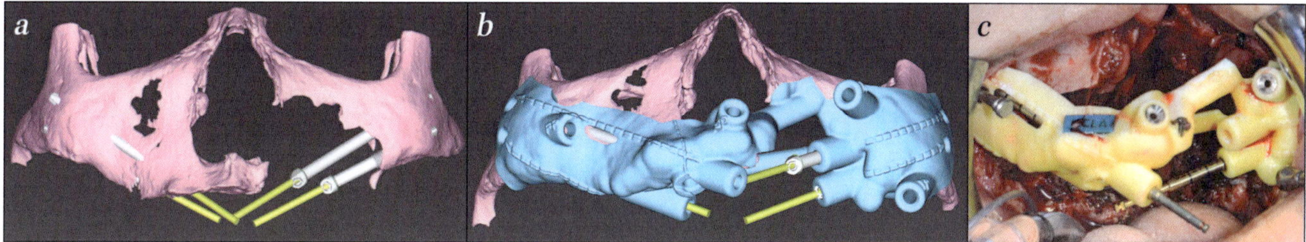

Figure 3-120 *(a)* Virtual surgical resection and estimated number, position, and angulation of zygomatic implants. *(b)* Design of surgical template. Possible impediments to the proper positioning of the handpiece and implant instrumentation should be identified and appropriate changes made. Inspection windows are helpful in determining proper seating of the template during surgery and also help the surgeon visualize the trajectory of the twist drills. Several bone screw channels were incorporated in order to secure the drill guide. *(c)* Surgical guide in position.

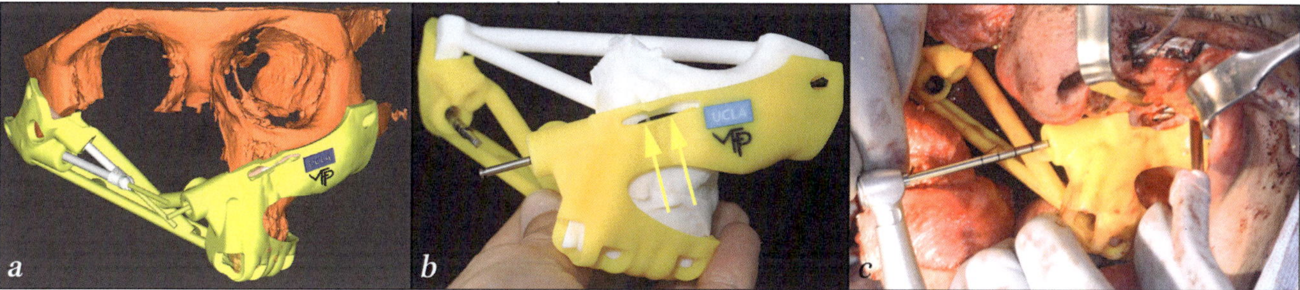

Figure 3-121 *(a)* Design of a semiguided implant surgical guide designed for placement of zygomatic implants in a patient scheduled for a total maxillectomy. *(b)* The printed surgical guide. Note the inspection window *(arrows)*. *(c)* The surgical template in position. Note that it engages the residual dentition.

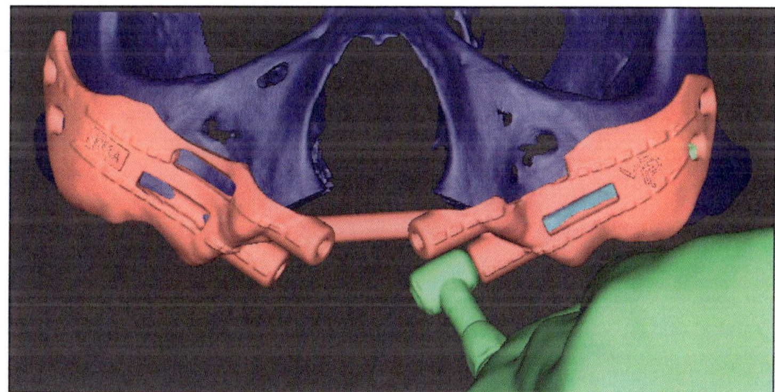

Figure 3-122 In some instances, the drill sleeves must be repositioned apically to eliminate drilling impediments. Note the large inspection windows in this design.

engage the pyriform rim region, the pyramidal process of the palatal bone, or the nasal crest, because the length and angulation of the implants and the angle correction of the abutments employed can be predetermined. In edentulous patients, these surgical templates are positioned intraorally by means of a silicone template engaging the opposing arch and then secured to the site with bone screws (Fig 3-123). In partially edentulous patients, the residual dentition can be used to retain and stabilize the template.

The surgical template is designed based on the virtually positioned implants. The data are then sent to the biomedical modeling center or dental laboratory for fabrication. Most are printed in a resin material. Drill sleeves (bushings) made of metal or zirconia are embedded within the template to aid in preparation of the osteotomy sites and insertion of the implants. Surgical drill guide keys are used to control the alignment, diameter, and depth of the osteotomy sites. These keys engage the bushings (drill sleeves) and allow the surgeon to prepare the sites with fully guided controlled directional drilling. Recently, keyless systems have been introduced and achieved wide acceptance. Once the osteotomy sites are prepared, the implants are placed through the surgical template.

Clinicians should be aware that when using these programs, discrepancies can arise when transferring the data from the 3D virtual planning program into manufacturing the actual surgical template. Deviations in all three-dimensional planes have been reported between virtual planning and the final intraoral implant position (Van Assche et al., 2007, 2012; Vasak et al., 2011; Pettersson et al., 2012; Arisan et al., 2013). Therefore, clinicians should be familiar with the software program they are using in order to plan implant placement procedures with an adequate margin of safety.

Dynamic navigation implant placement

Dynamic navigation (Fig 3-124) allows the surgeon to visualize in real time the preparation of the implant site. Many patients present

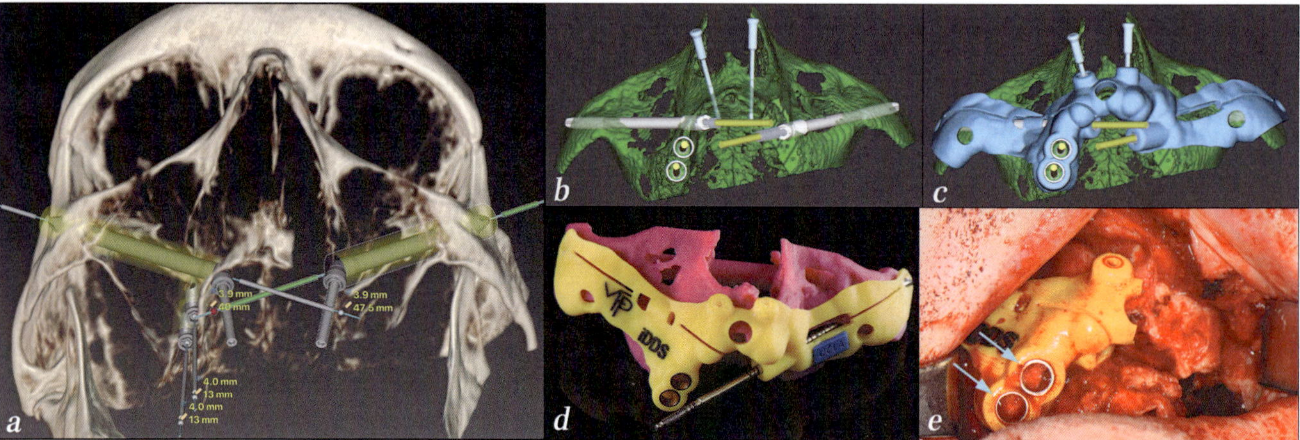

Figure 3-123 *(a)* Implants are planned for the residual alveolar ridge and both zygomas. The implant to be placed in the right zygoma will have a threaded neck to engage the alveolar process as well as the zygoma (see below, Fig 3-128). *(b)* Occlusal view of implant position and angulation. *(c)* Digital design of the surgical template. Note that bone screws will be used to secure the template to the alveolar ridge anteriorly. *(d)* The printed surgical template. Note the bushings (drill sleeves; *arrows*) incorporated for fully guided implant placement of the implants to be positioned into the alveolar ridge and the inspection windows. *(e)* The guide has been split down the middle to allow easier seating of each segment. A bone screw will be used to secure the template. Note the metal bushings incorporated with the surgical template.

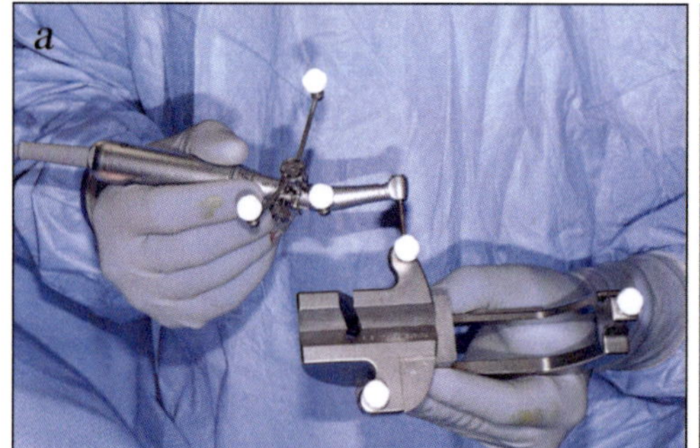

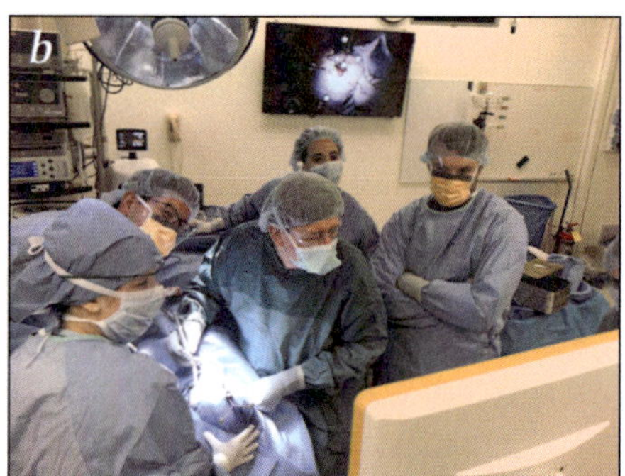

Figure 3-124 Navigation can be used to prepare implant osteotomy sites. *(a)* Sensors are attached to the handpiece and the patient. *(b)* This site is being prepared to receive a zygomatic implant (reprinted from Beumer et al., 2022, with permission).

with severe trismus following a radical maxillectomy, especially when they receive postoperative radiation. This limited access makes it difficult to properly visualize the proposed implant sites. Furthermore, the trismus often seen in this group of patients can make accurate implant placement problematic. Moreover, in some patients, it may be difficult to design and fabricate surgical drill guides that are sufficiently stable and well retained to permit precise implant placement. Under these circumstances, dynamic navigation permits the surgeon to prepare the osteotomy sites and place the implants with great precision. Prior to surgery, a CBCT scan is obtained to allow for virtual implant planning using special software. Patients can be scanned and surgical planning accomplished the same day as implant surgery. It also allows a flapless approach that will reduce postoperative morbidity and result in less disruption of the local vasculature.

Implant selection criteria

Several new implant designs have been introduced that broaden the application and improve implant success rates in patients with large palatal defects. As mentioned above, in recent years the zygomatic implant has undergone a number of design changes, which are tailored for patients with large palatal defects associated with tumor resection or an unrepaired cleft palate. They are designed with extended smooth areas in order to mitigate plague accumulations and enhance oral hygiene procedures (Southern Implants, Irene, RSA) (Figs 3-125a and 3-126). Some implants retain the threads and microrough surface around the neck of the implant. These are used when the zygomatic implant engages both the zygoma and the residual bone of the alveolus (Figs 3-125b and 3-128). The microrough surfaces accelerate the process of osseointegration by upregulating and accelerating the expression of genes of the differentiating osteoblasts associated with the osseointegration process (Ogawa and Nishimura, 2006). An additional benefit is that this leads to a different combination of collagenous and noncollagenous proteins making up the bone deposited on the microrough surfaces as compared with the bone deposited on machined-surface topographies. As a result, bone that matures on implant surfaces with microrough surface topography is harder and stiffer than bone deposited on machined surfaces (Butz et al., 2006).

These implants are also self-tapping, which results in better initial primary stability. In recent times there has been increased use of tapered, self-tapping implant designs with variable thread patterns (Fig 3-127a). These are used primarily in poor-quality bone sites, such as the posterior maxilla, and were designed for immediate loading. With these design changes, during insertion of the implant, the trabecular bone of the implant site is compressed around the implant improving the initial mechanical anchorage of the implant.

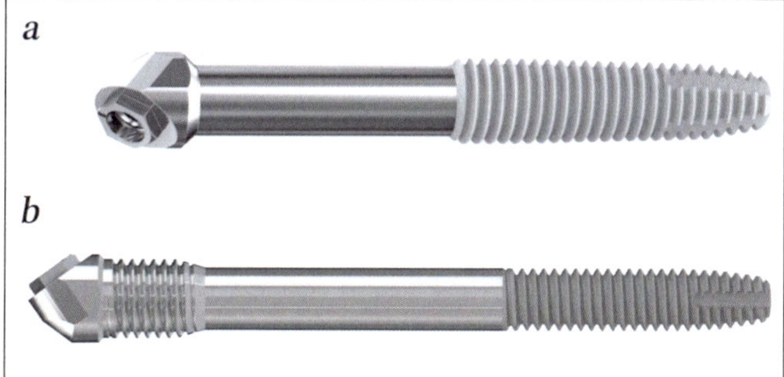

Figure 3-125 *(a)* A zygomatic implant designed for large palatal defects. That portion transiting from the zygoma to the oral cavity and implant-connecting bar is smooth (see Fig 3-124). *(b)* A zygomatic implant designed to engage the residual alveolar ridge as well as the zygoma (see Fig 3-128). Note that it is considerably longer than the implant designed for large palatal defects. The threaded portions of both implants are prepared with a microrough surface and are self-tapping (courtesy of Southern Implants, Irene, RSA).

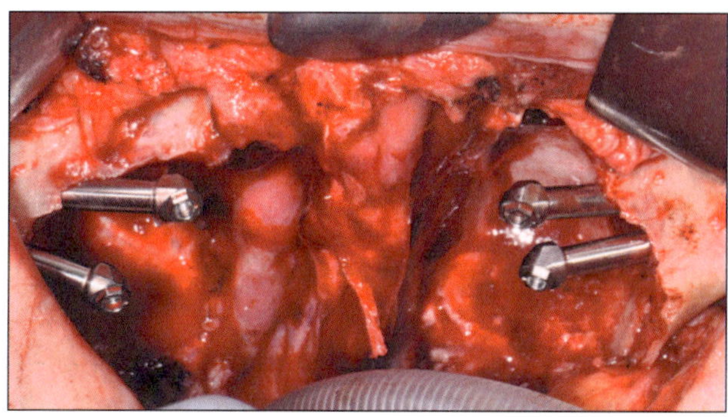

Figure 3-126 Zygomatic implants with smooth surfaces were used in this patient.

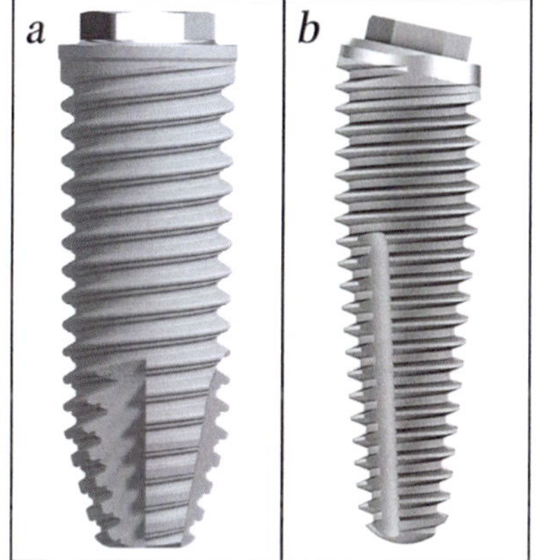

Figure 3-127 *(a)* Tapered self-tapping implants with a variable thread pattern and microthreads. *(b)* Off-axis implant design. They are available in several different angulations ("b" courtesy of Southern Implants, Irene, RSA).

Off-axis designs

With the off-axis implant design (Southern Implants, Irene, RSA), the head of the implant is machined at an angle to the long axis of the implant so that the implant platform emerges with more a favorable angulation (Howes, 2004; Fig 3-127b). When used in the alveolar ridge, these implants permit subgingival angulation correction as opposed to the supragingival correction attained with angulated abutments. As such they may save several millimeters of prosthetic space, which is especially valuable when fabricating overlay prostheses in the maxilla. They are particularly well suited for the so-called tilted implant approach when implants transit through the residual alveolar ridges and engage the pyramidal process of the palatal bone, the pyriform rim region, or the nasal crest. They are available in 12°, 24°, and 36° of angle correction.

Implants with external hex platforms are preferred since most implants will not be parallel to one another. Under these circumstances, it is easier to accommodate the various angulations encountered, particularly when tilted implants are employed (Fig 3-128).

Impressions of the implants, tentative centric relation records, and trial denture setups

Implant positions can be recorded either with conventional methods or digitally, but the authors still prefer conventional methods when recording implant positions in such large defects. The scanning strategies used to make full arch impressions, even in conventional patients, are problematic and technique sensitive. For example, when scanning in between implants, it may be difficult to position the scanning head (scanning wand) so as to accurately record the surfaces of the scanning bodies. In addition, errors may be introduced because the distance between the scanner and the objects may vary when making the scan. Moreover, only selected arch segments can be scanned at one time, and as a consequence, the data must be stitched together to create a full arch scan. This process has the potential to introduce angular and distance errors when making full arch digital impressions (Ahlholm et al., 2018; Rutkunas et al., 2017). These issues are amplified when implants are widely dispersed as is frequently the case in patients with large palatal defects. Moreover, frequently the impression is used to make a tentative centric relation record and this is not possible with the intraoral scanners used to make digital impressions.

Nonengaging pickup-type impression copings are secured to the implants and are connected to one another by means of resin struts and pattern resin. When the span between implants is excessive as was the case in the patient shown in Fig 3-129, it is prudent to add additional struts to supplement the rigidity of the impression apparatus. A preliminary impression of the defect is made with heavy and light-body elastic impression material. This impression both records the implant positions and defines the contours of the defect. These contours will be redefined with a corrected impression at a later date.

In concert with making the impression a facebow transfer record is obtained and a tentative centric relation is made. The impression serves as the "record base" for making the centric relation record (Fig 3-129c, d, and e). This method is frequently used in patients with

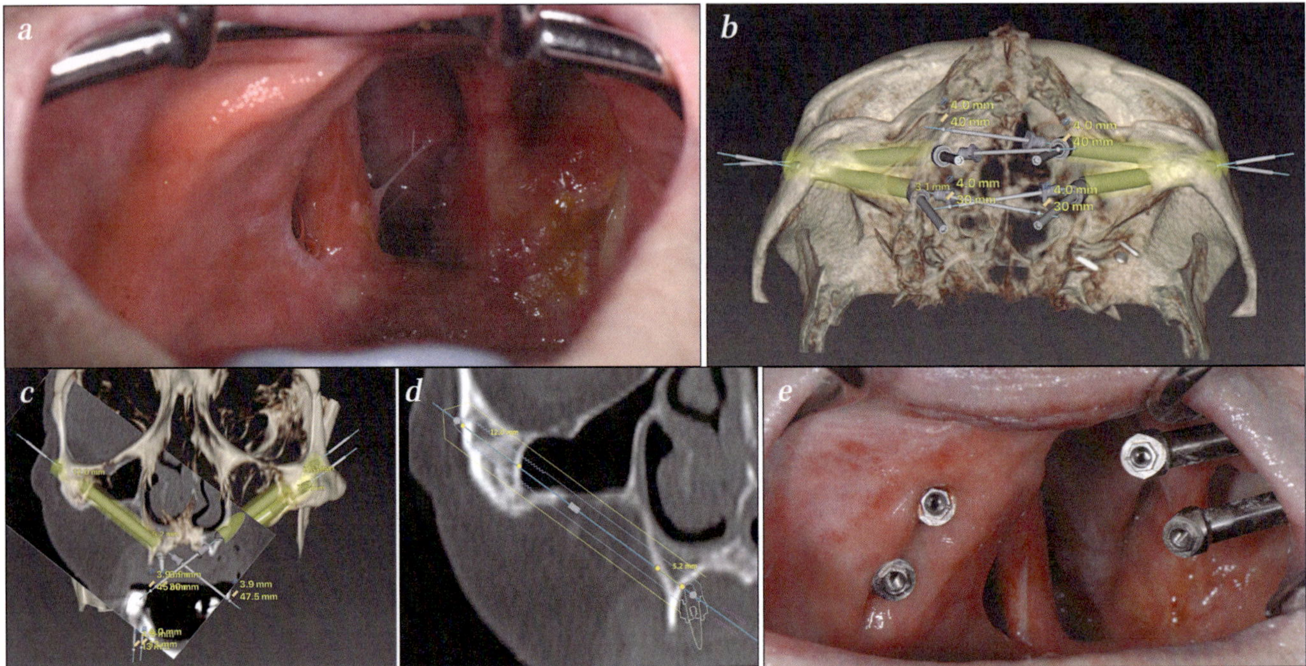

Figure 3-128 *(a)* Edentulous patient with a total maxillectomy defect. *(b, c, and d)* Four zygomatic implants are planned. The two emerging from the defect have smooth necks. The two exiting the alveolar ridge engage both the zygoma and the alveolar ridge and so implants with threaded necks were employed. *(e)* The implants in position.

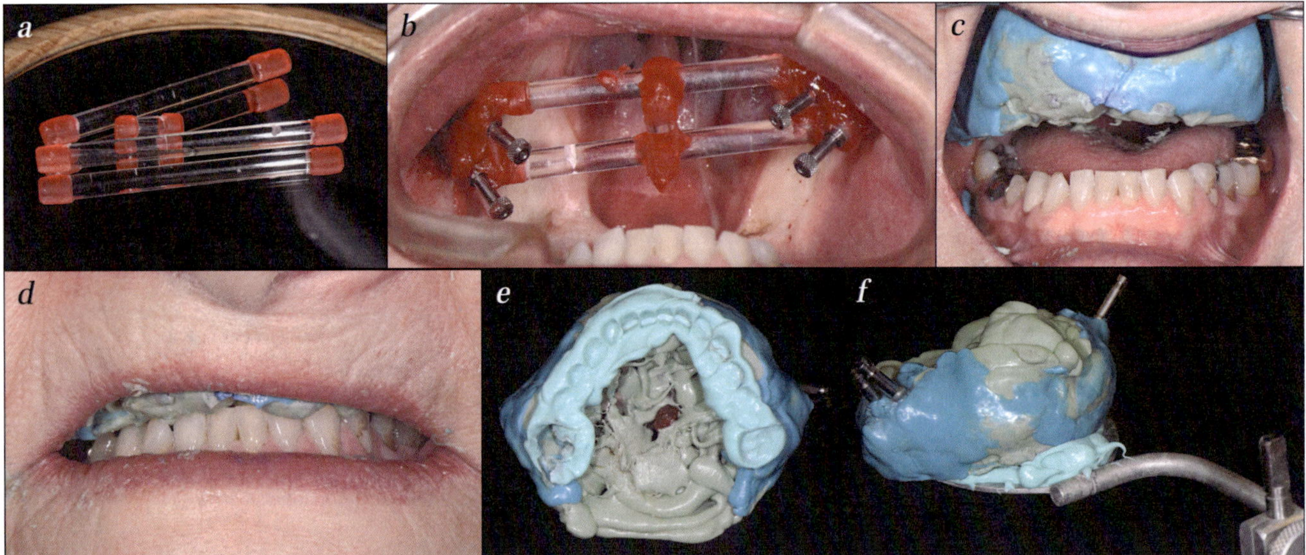

Figure 3-129 *(a)* Resin struts are *(b)* connected to pickup-type implant impression copings and united together with pattern resin. *(c, d, and e)* In concert with making the impression, a tentative centric relation is made. The impression serves as the "record base." *(f)* The maxillary cast is mounted on the articular with a facebow transfer record.

large defects, such as a patient presenting with a total palatectomy, since this initial impression is intimately adapted to the defect. This technique is also used frequently when obtaining records in partially dentate patients with large palatectomy/maxillectomy defects (see section above entitled "Definitive Obturators for Patients with Unique Palatal Defects").

Implant/abutment analogs are secured to the impression copings embedded within the impression, and the impression is boxed and poured being careful to preserve the tentative centric relation record. The maxillary cast is mounted on the articulator with a facebow transfer record and the tentative centric relation record, obtained while making the impression, is used to mount the opposing cast.

In situations where the distance between implants is significant, it is prudent to verify the implant impression with a provisional implant-connecting bar fabricated out of resin struts and pattern resin (Fig 3-130a, b, and c). This bar can also be used to retain a record base-trial denture setup. The trial denture setup is required so that the

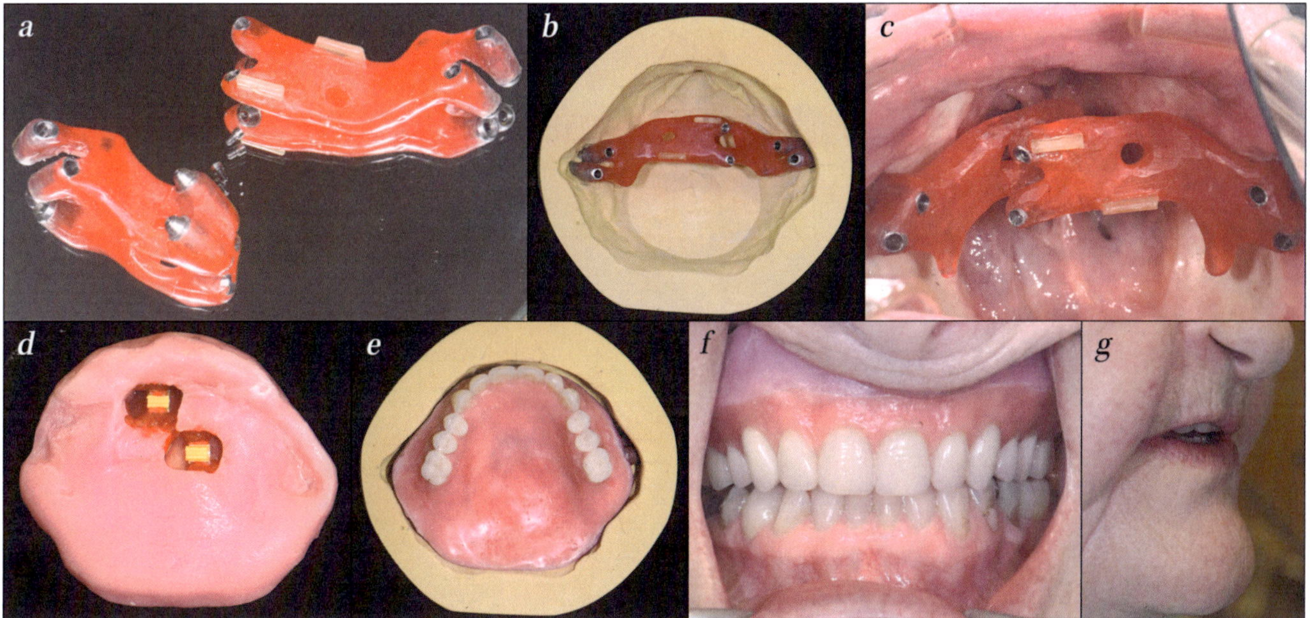

Figure 3-130 *(a)* A two-piece provisional implant bar made of pattern resin. It will be used to retain the trial denture setup. *(b)* The bar assembled on the cast. *(c)* The provisional bar secured to the implants intraorally. *(d)* Intaglio surfaces of the trial denture with "Hader" clips embedded to engage the "Hader" bar castable pattern segments incorporated within the resin bar. *(e)* The trial denture setup. *(f and g)* With retention provided by the resin provisional implant bar, the centric relation record can be confirmed, the occlusal vertical dimension determined, and the aesthetic display of the anterior teeth finalized.

bar design will permit the proper positioning of the denture teeth and the development of suitable palatal contours and tongue space. In large defects, such as total palatectomy defects, it may be problematic to reconfirm these records without implant retention, and so this technique is a useful adjunct. With the record base/trial denture effectively retained, the proper occlusal vertical dimension is determined, and the centric relation record is proven or redone as necessary before making the definitive implant-connecting bar.

Design of implant-connecting bars

The case for splinting. As mentioned previously when multiple implants are placed at the time of tumor ablation, provisional implant-connecting bars are used to splint them together during the healing period. The purpose of this practice is to minimize the risk of mobilizing one or another of the implants before they become reasonably well osseointegrated.

When designing the definitive retention apparatus involving multiple implants, the authors also prefer to splint them together when possible. Often, the bone sites available in patients with palatal defects are suboptimal (minimal bone volume, irradiated sites, etc.), and the implants are anchored in bone of less than 10 mm and placed at unusual angles. Splinted designs distribute occlusal loads more widely and effectively than nonsplinted designs, particularly off-axis loads (bending moments) (Gunter et al., 2000, 2002; Wang et al., 2002; Lemos et al., 2018). In normal patients, higher success rates are achieved with splinted designs as compared to nonsplinted designs (de Souza Batista et al., 2019), especially when the implants are shorter than 10 mm in length (Mendonca et al., 2014). Splinted designs reduce the degree of freedom that each implant can move thereby reducing the risk of mechanical overload relative to rotation, tipping, and translation (Yoda et al., 2013). Mechanical overload triggers microdelaminations and minifractures within the bone anchoring the implant, which, in turn, initiates a resorptive remodeling response, leading to bone loss around the implant (Hoshaw et al., 1994; Stanford and Brand, 1999; Brunski et al., 2000; Miyata et al., 1998, 2000, 2002; Miyamoto et al., 2008; Nagasawa et al., 2013). Splinted designs reduce the risk of implant overload.

Splinting is especially necessary when the implant sites have been irradiated, since at doses above 60 Gy (Nishimura et al., 1995), implant anchorage is primarily mechanical and directly related to the preexisting density of the local bone site, as opposed to the biologic anchorage achieved in normal vascularized bone. Only when there is a single solitary implant available do the authors resort to the use of individual attachments (see section below entitled "Solitary implants").

Implant-supported bar designs. The design of the attachment apparatus—implant-assisted (the forces of occlusion are divided between the implants and the edentulous denture foundation areas) versus implant-supported (all the forces of occlusion are borne by the implants)—is dependent upon a number of factors. These factors have been reasonably well worked out in edentulous patients with intact palates when implant-supported designs are considered. When the concept of tilted implants is employed, two implants placed on each side with *at least 2 cm of A-P spread* appear sustainable over long periods in most patients (Tealdo et al., 2014; Jensen et al., 2012, 2015a, 2015b). Implants are added posteriorly to engage the pyramidal process of the palatal bone in patients presenting with extenuating circumstances, such as a history of parafunctional activity and when the opposing arch is dentate or restored with an implant-supported prosthesis (Pozzi et al., 2016). Lacking at least two implants bilaterally, appropriate A-P spread, or sufficient bone anchorage of the implants, the clinician is advised to defer to an implant-assisted design.

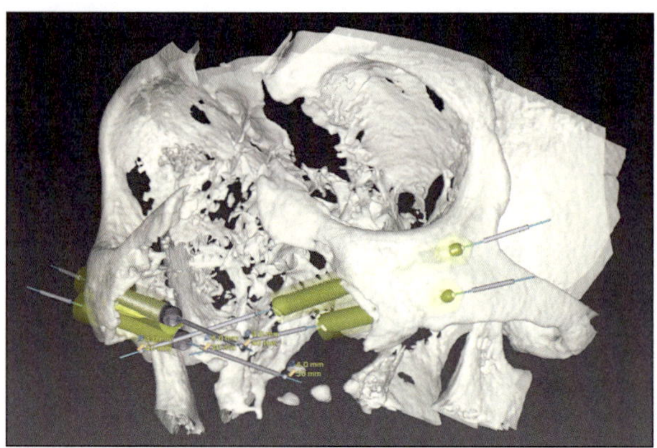

Figure 3-131 When implants are positioned in the zygoma they are somewhat "stacked" atop one another in relation to the plane of occlusion. The biomechanics of this arrangement and its suitability for implant-supported designs require further study.

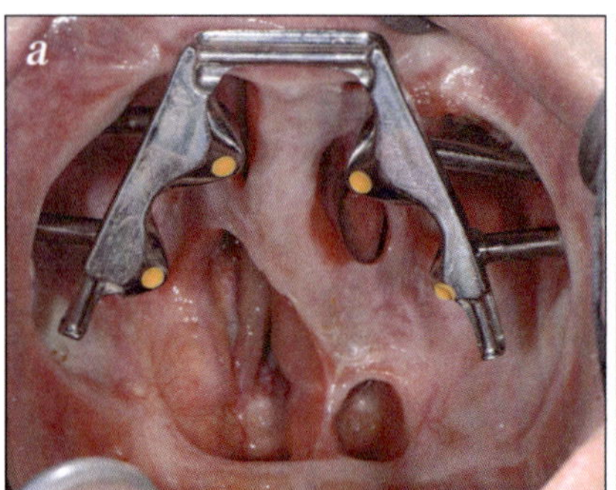

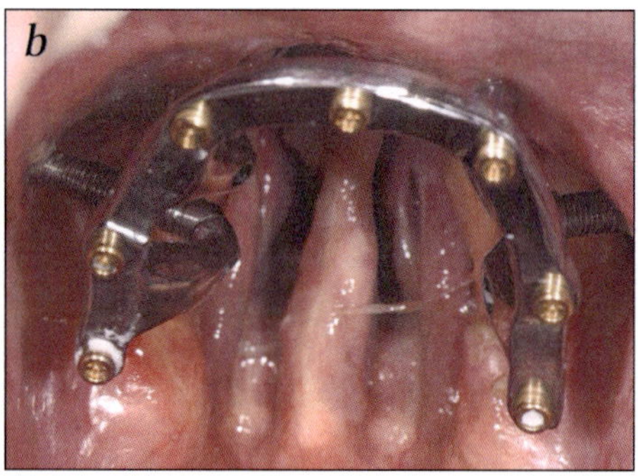

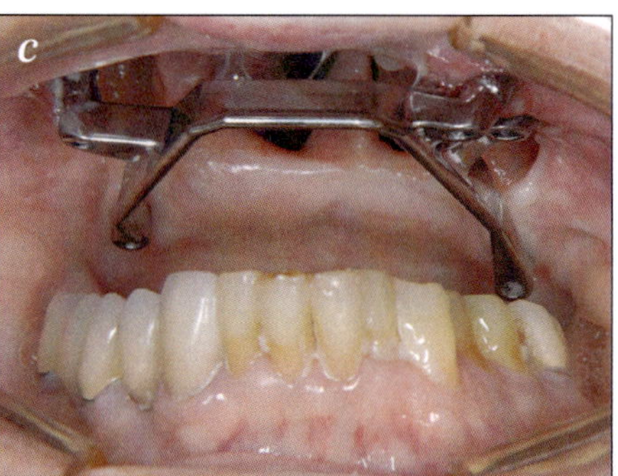

Figure 3-132 Implant-connecting bars for total palatectomy defects. All designs are implant supported. *(a)* This bar was supported by four zygomatic implants. *(b)* In this patient, three zygomatic implants were employed plus a single implant in the residual pyriform rim region. *(c)* Three zygomatic implants were combined with two implants placed in the pyramidal process of the palatal bone.

In a patient with an intact palate, and when bone is lacking in the alveolar ridges for even tilted implant placement, two zygomatic implants placed on each side appear to provide sufficient bone anchorage to enable fabrication of an implant-supported prosthesis (so-called quad-four arrangement; Stievenart et al., 2010). In these patients, the primary implant anchorage is achieved by engaging the zygoma, but in most patients, 3–5 mm of bone of the residual alveolar ridges is also engaged. This factor becomes important when considering how to best utilize zygomatic implants emerging from the zygoma into a maxillary defect because they do not enjoy multilayered bone anchorage. The critical question is whether the bone anchorage of implants placed in the zygoma in patients with large palatal defects can be sustained over prolonged periods when an implant-supported implant-connecting bar design is employed to retain an obturator prosthesis. Finite element analysis studies imply that the bone-anchoring zygomatic implants employed in such a fashion will be sustained (Miyamoto et al., 2020). However, this question remains unanswered because there are few published studies available for review that specifically address this question and our clinical experience is relatively short term and limited to only a few patients.

Nonetheless, the authors have employed implant-supported implant-connecting bar designs in most of our total palatectomy defects knowing full well that the implants are exposed to significant bending mements. To date we have observed few failures. This may be due to the fact that the bone quality of the zygoma is quite favorable and appears to be almost equivalent to that seen in the mandible. Also, when two implants are positioned in each zygoma, they are "stacked" in relation to each other, and perhaps this arrangement is more resistant to the bending moments as they are transferred through the implants into the anchoring bone (Fig 3-131). However, this arrangement requires further study with regard to its suitability for implant-connecting bar designs. In most total palatectomy defects restored at UCLA, only zygomatic implants were employed (Fig 3-132a), but on occasion, they were supplemented by implants placed in the pyriform rim (Fig 3-132b) and the pyramidal process of the palatal bone (Fig 3-132c).

The implant-connecting bars are best designed and manufactured digitally, generally with a 3° taper. Retention is achieved by means of strategically positioned "Hader" bar segments (Fig 3-132a and c) or individual attachments secured to or incorporated within the design of the bar (see Fig 3-132b). Since the prosthesis does not rotate or move during function, wear of the bar is not an issue, and so these types of bars can be milled of titanium in contrast to bars with implant-assisted designs, which should be milled or printed of a harder metal, preferably, cobalt-chromium.

If the bone sites are suboptimal (less than 10 mm of vertical bone volume available relative to the long axis of the implant) or the patient exhibits evidence of significant parafunctional activity and/or the opposing arch is dentate or restored with an implant-supported prosthesis, it is prudent to use an implant-assisted design, especially if there are potential skin-lined denture-bearing surfaces available to engage. However, in most total palatectomy defects, skin-lined denture-bearing surfaces supported by bone are

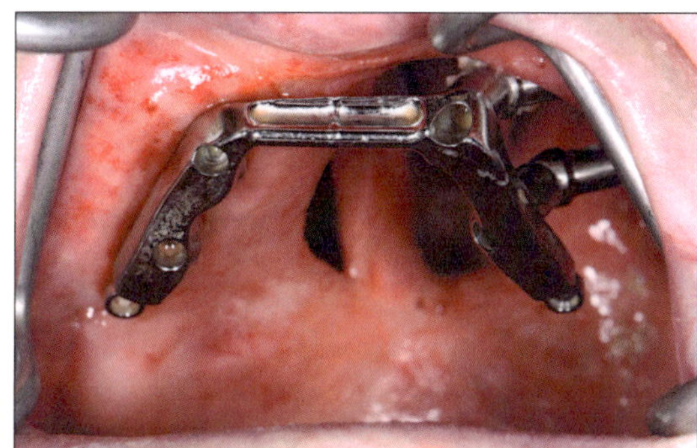

Figure 3-133 Implant-assisted connecting bar. Four zygomatic implants were used. Anchorage of the implants was considered suboptimal and so an implant-assisted design was employed.

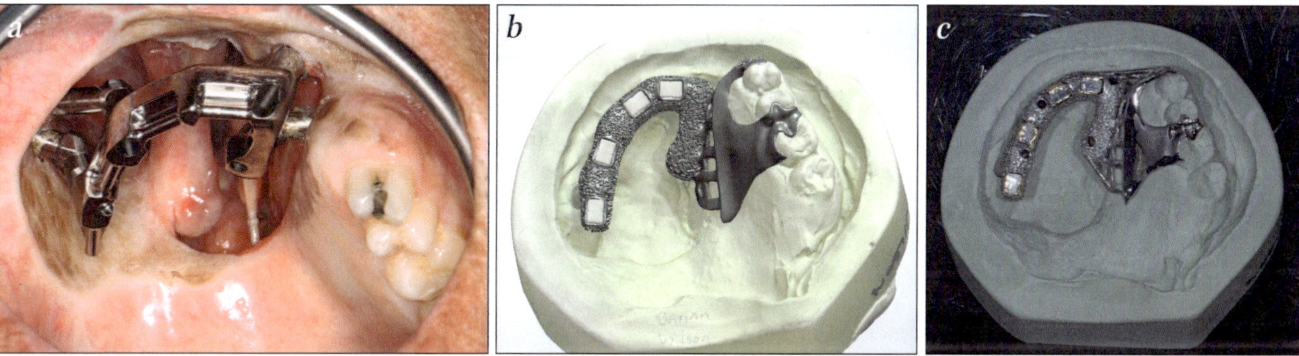

Figure 3-134 *(a–c)* A total maxillectomy defect that crosses the midline. Four zygomatic implants have been arranged to provide support on the defect side. The RDP was printed with selective laser melting.

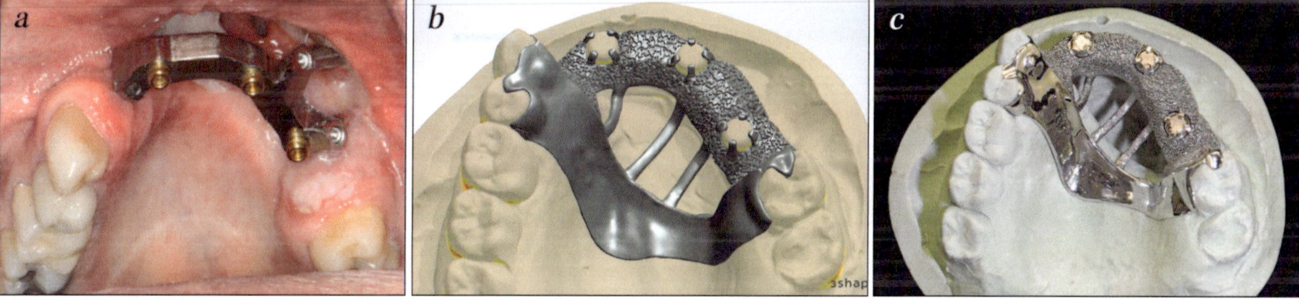

Figure 3-135 *(a–c)* An anterior palatal defect. Two zygomatic implants were combined with one implant placed in the pyriform rim region. The overlay RDP-obturator derives its support from the implants and the dentition adjacent to the defect. The RDP framework was printed with selective laser melting.

not available or accessible, so one can expect little additional support provided by such surfaces.

If an edentulous patient has undergone a classical total maxillectomy, an implant-supported implant-connecting bar design would require that two implants be placed in the residual zygoma on the resected side in concert with multiple implants positioned on the unresected side. A tilted arrangement is suggested on the unresected side, and if possible, an implant should be placed in the pyramidal process of the palatal bone. Zygomatic implants placed on the unresected side and engaging the residual alveolar ridge on the unresected side can also be employed (see Fig 3-133). However, if the quality of implant anchorage of any of the implants is questioned or compromised, or if any of the key implants are anchored by less than 10 mm of bone, implant-assisted designs are suggested, even if the numbers of implants and their distribution pattern were otherwise favorable (Fig 3-133).

Partially edentulous patients with palatectomy/maxillectomy defects may also be restored with implant-supported designs. Implants from both zygomatic arches or residual bone in the pyriform region can be used in combination with the residual dentition, to provide support. The implant-connecting bar shown in Fig 3-134 demonstrate the use of this concept. The resection of the patient shown in Fig 3-134 crossed the midline and so had two zygomatic implants placed in each zygoma, and all four of their implant platforms emerged in the defect. When implants are positioned into the zygoma on the unresected side, drainage for secretions must be maintained; otherwise, secretions may become trapped leading to local infections. In addition, the implant arrangement must be carefully planned so that all four implant platforms do not impinge upon the palatal vault or the positioning of the denture teeth. Note that in Fig 3-135, the two implants placed in the left zygoma were combined with one in the right pyriform rim region The overlay RDP of

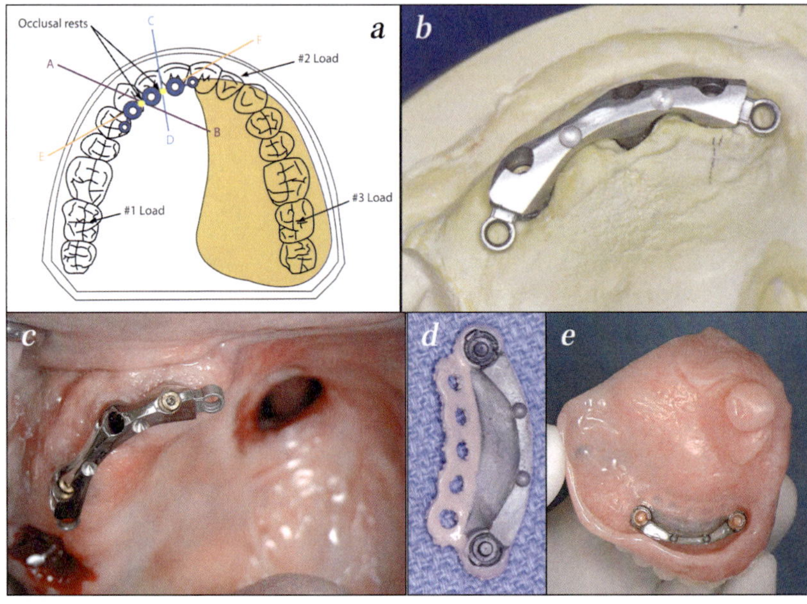

Figure 3-136 Function of resilient attachments. *(a)* Vertical compression of the prosthesis and occlusal rests improve the distribution of stresses. When load #1 is applied, the prosthesis will rotate around the new axis, AB, which passes through the distal occlusal rest. Load #2 results in fulcrum CD and load 3 results in fulcrum EF. *(b)* ERA attachments are attached to each side of the bar and occlusal rests *(arrows)* are created on top of the bar. *(c to e)* Rests on the metal framework control the axis of rotation and allow the ERA attachments to function as designed.

both frameworks engages the residual dentition with positive rests and lingual plating, providing additional support and bracing (resistance to lateral displacement) for the overlay RDP. The implant-connecting bars for both patients were designed with a 3° taper.

Implant-assisted bar designs for edentulous patients with midline resections when implants are positioned in the anterior alveolar ridge. When implants are placed unilaterally on the unresected side, implant-assisted designs are employed unless implants are available on the side of the defect. The implants are used to enhance the retention and stability of the obturator prosthesis but do not serve as the primary means of posterior support. In edentulous patients with classical, skin-lined maxillectomy defects, retention on the resected side is achieved by engaging soft tissue undercuts in the defect and using a dual path of insertion while inserting and seating the prosthesis to engage the implant attachment apparatus on the unresected side. As long as the obturator prosthesis is retained on the unresected side, it will not rotate out of the defect, providing the prosthesis properly engages the lateral wall and any available undercuts. Based on the studies conducted by Davis and colleagues (1995) and our own clinical experience, we recommend the implant-assisted bar design shown in Fig 3-136, or variations thereof. With these designs, when occlusal forces are applied on the unresected side, support is shared between the implants and the residual denture-bearing surfaces. When occlusal forces are applied on the resected side, it is not possible to prevent the implants from exposure to excessive bending moments with the resilient attachments currently available, and so the patient must be instructed to avoid chewing on the resected side.

Given these instructions to the patient, the forces that are potentially most damaging to implants result from occlusal loading in the posterior region on the unresected side; therefore, ideally, the design of the implant-connecting bar attachment apparatus should allow this portion of the prosthesis to be impacted into the residual edentulous extension areas when these forces are applied. The implant-connecting bars along with their attachments, should be designed to minimize bending moments and direct these posterior occlusal forces along the long axis of the implants. When designing the bar, the axis of rotation (resulting from the generation of posterior occlusal forces on the unresected side) should be anticipated and the bar, rests, and attachments be positioned and designed to permit rotation of the prosthesis around this axis (Fig 3-136; see also Figs 3-99a and b).

Gravitational forces secondary to the obturator extension are much less of a concern and can be somewhat mitigated on the defect side by aggressive engagement of the undercuts associated with the skin-lined lateral wall of the defect. Forces generated during the incision of the bolus are one-quarter to one-fifth of those generated posteriorly during mastication and are less of a concern. For large defects extending across the midline, lateral bending moments applied to the implants secondary to lateral displacement of a large obturator prosthesis, for example, during lateral movements of the mandible or contracture of the muscles of facial expression, also need to be taken into account by extending the prosthesis into areas that resist these forces (for example, the medial wall of the defect that is covered with skin or palatal mucosa). The clinician should not forget that with these implant configurations, cross-arch stabilization is lacking, so resistance to these lateral forces should be enhanced by the appropriate extension of the denture flanges and obturator extensions and adaptation to the denture-bearing surfaces in the defect and the unresected side (see section above entitled "Stability").

Numerous factors complicate the design of the bar and affect the distribution of occlusal forces for classical total maxillectomy defects. Occlusal loads produce multiple axes of rotation of the obturator prosthesis. These axes are dependent on the position of the implants and the point of load application (position of the bolus) on the prosthesis during mastication. When implants are only present unilaterally, the two key factors in the design that has evolved at UCLA are the placement of occlusal type rests on the bar in between the implants and the use of resilient attachments on either end of the bar (see Figs 3-99a and b and 3-136).

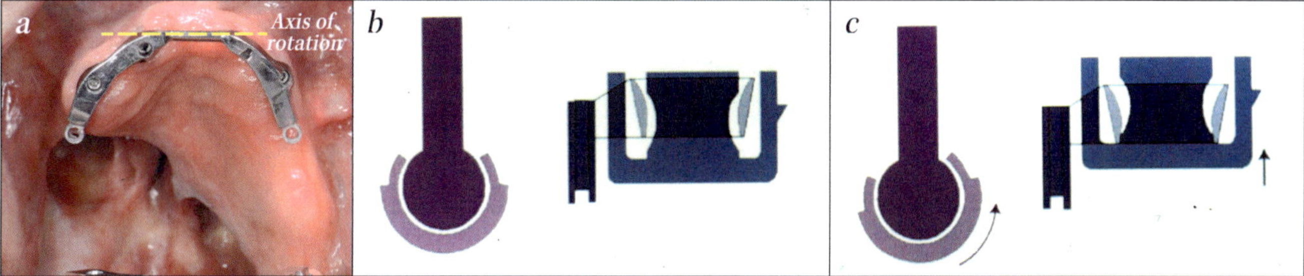

Figure 3-137 *(a)* When the anterior maxilla remains, four implants are placed and a conventional implant-assisted implant-connecting bar design using a combination of a Hader bar and ERA attachments is suggested. *(b and c)* ERA attachments are positioned adjacent to the distal implants and a "Hader" bar used to connect the two anterior implants. The bar provides retention and serves as the axis of rotation. When posterior occlusal forces are applied to the prosthesis, the ERA attachments permit the prosthesis to rotate around the bar and engage the primary denture support areas thereby minimizing the bending moments applied to the distal implants.

The design that evolved at UCLA was based in part, upon the experiments conducted by Davis et al. (1995). Using a photoelastic model, she sought to determine the most favorable implant-connecting bar attachment designs when three implants were placed in the residual anterior maxilla following a classical total maxillectomy down the midline. Photoelastic materials were used to simulate the bone around the implants and the bone along the medial and lateral aspects of the defect. The implants were positioned in the simulated anterior alveolus on the unresected side to mimic a common clinical situation, and bar attachment designs were fabricated with a gold alloy. Several designs were tested, including the following:

- An implant-connecting bar with Hader clips placed mesial to the anterior implant and distal to the posterior implant. *This is an implant-supported design.*
- An implant-connecting a bar with ERA attachments placed mesial to the anterior implant and distal to the posterior implants and occlusal rests between each of the implants. *This is an implant-assisted design.*
- An implant-connecting bar with O-ring attachments placed between the implants. *This is an implant-assisted design.*
- An implant-connecting bar with an ERA attachment placed mesial to the anterior implant and a Hader segment placed distal to the posterior implant and parallel to the alveolar ridge. *This is an implant-supported design,* particularly when occlusal forces are applied posteriorly on the unresected side because of the orientation of the "Hader" bar segment.
- An implant-connecting bar with an OSO attachment placed on the anterior and posterior implants. *This is an implant-assisted design.*

An acrylic resin obturator extension base was fabricated to extend into the defect to transmit occlusal forces to the cast. The loading regions selected for testing were anterior and posterior to the implants. Each loading zone had a ramp so that a force of 12 lb could be applied in both vertical and lateral directions at each location. The photoelastic cast was firmly fixed to the base of the stage of a straining frame. A force of 90 g was applied to the acrylic resin extension base to correspond to the weight of the obturator.

Circularly polarized light was used to illuminate the cast. To compare the stress patterns developed by the different designs, the designs were placed on the cast without any type of external load exerted. The resulting stresses were observed and recorded with a camera that had an appropriately oriented set of polarized and quarter-waved plates affixed to the lens.

The most pertinent conclusions of the study were as follows (Davis et al., 1995):

- The "Hader" *implant-supported* design showed the most unfavorable stress distribution patterns around the implants.
- The addition of occlusal rests on the bars between the implants improved the stability of the prostheses and mitigated bending moments delivered to the implants by directing the occlusal forces more along the long axis of the implants, especially when a posterior force on the unresected side was applied.
- The bar with the O-ring attachment resulted in the most favorable stress distribution patterns. However, the O-ring designs were not as retentive as the *implant-assisted* design using ERA attachments.

Based on this work and our clinical experience (Roumanas et al., 1997), we propose that implant-assisted designs be employed when implants are placed in the anterior portion of the residual alveolar processes of an edentulous patient with a total maxillectomy defect, with strategically positioned rests, and retention provided by resilient attachments (Fig 3-136b–e). Properly positioned and contoured rests serve to direct occlusal forces along the long axis of the implants, while the use of a resilient attachment such as the ERA permits the prosthesis to rotate around an axis determined by the position of the rests when an occlusal force is applied to the posterior edentulous extension area of the prosthesis on the unresected side. The principle is similar to the biomechanics of the I bar mesial rest concept of removable dental prosthesis design developed by Kratochvil (1988; Chang et al., 2019). However, it is important to note that when using this design concept for extension-based RDPs, the RDP framework must be "physiologically adjusted" to ensure that the RDP rotates around the rest as intended during function. Likewise, the metal implant substructure, like the RDP framework, must be similarly adjusted to allow the prosthesis to rotate around the rests when occlusal forces are applied. As shown in Fig 3-136a, when a load is applied to point 1, the prosthesis will rotate around axis AB, which passes through the distal occlusal rest. This is similar to the manner in which rests control the axis of rotation of RDPs for total maxillectomy defects where teeth are retained anteriorly (see Fig 3-75; see also section above entitled "Partial denture design

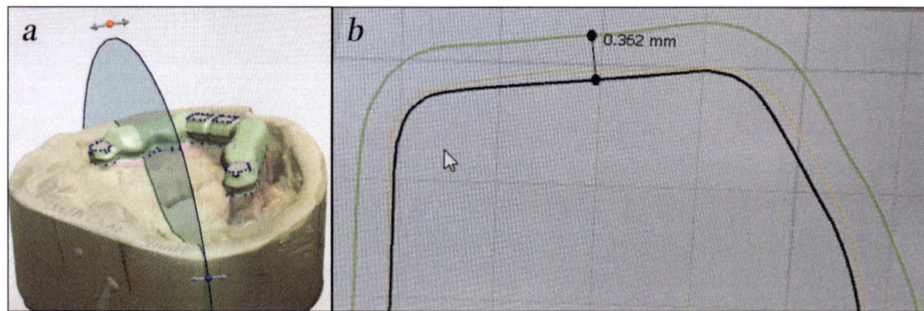

Figure 3-138 *(a)* Cross-section evaluation of an assisted implant bar overlay framework. *(b)* Note the relief space over the occlusal surface of the implant bar.

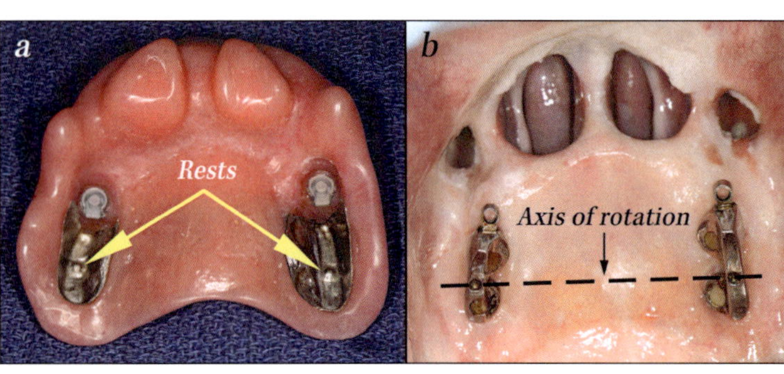

Figure 3-139 *(a and b)* The rests *(arrows)* on the bar control of the axis of rotation *(dotted line)* and direct occlusal forces along the long axis of the implants. The appliance is adjusted in the laboratory prior to delivery to ensure that the prosthesis rotates freely as intended around the rests on the implant-connecting bars.

concepts for maxillary defects"). In both scenarios, most of the occlusal load is absorbed by the residual denture-bearing surfaces posteriorly when an occlusal force is applied in the posterior edentulous extension area, and these forces are directed more favorably along the long axis of the implants/abutment teeth. The concave rest, contoured as a half sphere, is milled into the occlusal surface of the bar. Without the rests, the attachments on either side of the bar would serve as rotation points, leading to rapid wear of the attachments and exposing the implants to significant bending moments. This design allows the prosthesis to rotate around these rests, reduces wear on the attachments, and directs most of the occlusal forces along the long axes of the implants.

The patient should be advised against applying occlusal forces on the defect side (Fig 3-136a, load points #2 and #3) because little support is available in the defect to counteract these forces. Forceful occlusion on the defect side will result in rapid wear of the attachments, and since the ERA only allows 0.4 mm vertical movement of the attachment before bottoming out, the resulting application of bending moments to the implants may trigger a resorption remodeling of bone anchoring the implants, especially the bone anchoring the implant adjacent to the defect. With these designs the ERA attachments need to be replaced every six months.

Implant-assisted bar designs for edentulous patients with the anterior premaxilla intact. If the entire anterior maxilla remains, the number of implants, their distribution, and the design of the retention bar follow more conventional prosthodontic guidelines (Beumer et al., 2022b). If possible, we prefer that four implants be placed and suggest the implant-assisted design shown in Fig 3-137. Tilted implant arrangements are favored because more A-P spread can be attained, longer implants can be employed, and better bone anchorage can be achieved. In this implant-assisted design, support is provided posteriorly by the residual denture-bearing surfaces (the palatal vault and the residual alveolar ridges) and anteriorly by the implants. This design is particularly well suited for edentulous patients with defects bordering the hard and soft palate. The "Hader" bar spanning the two anterior implants provides retention and serves as the axis of rotation. These two implants should be positioned at least 20 mm apart to accommodate two "Hader" clips. The resilient attachments (ERA) connected to the distal portion of the bar allow for compression of the distal-extension area of the prosthesis into the denture-bearing surfaces without applying excess bending moments to the implants. For this design to function as planned, the paths of insertion of the Hader bar segment and the two ERA attachments should be identical and compatible with the path of insertion of the prosthesis. In addition, the Hader bar segment should be parallel to the plane of occlusion and perpendicular to the midline. This will ensure a relatively pure rotation around the Hader bar when occlusal forces are applied in the posterior region and will minimize the wear of the clips and prolong their life span. Often the prosthetic space over the bar is limited, so it is advisable to cover the bar with a metal substructure to prevent the acrylic resin overlying the bar from crazing and fracture (Beumer et al., 2022b). With this design, attachments need to be replaced every 6–12 months depending on the resilience of the posterior denture-bearing surfaces.

When using an attachment that allows hinging or vertical resiliency, it is important to design relief between the overlay framework and the occlusal surface of the bar. This can be accomplished when fabricating this framework with CAD-CAM (Fig 3-138) or by traditional blockout techniques when conventional means are employed (Beumer et al., 2022b). In the example shown (Fig 3-137), a fulcrum line is created by the two Hader clips. The incorporated gap over the occlusal surface of the bar allows the prosthesis to hinge on the Hader attachments and depress posteriorly into the *external resilient attachments* (ERAs). Because the ERAs provide 0.4 mm of vertical resiliency, the relief space over the implant bar can be digitally designed for the same height.

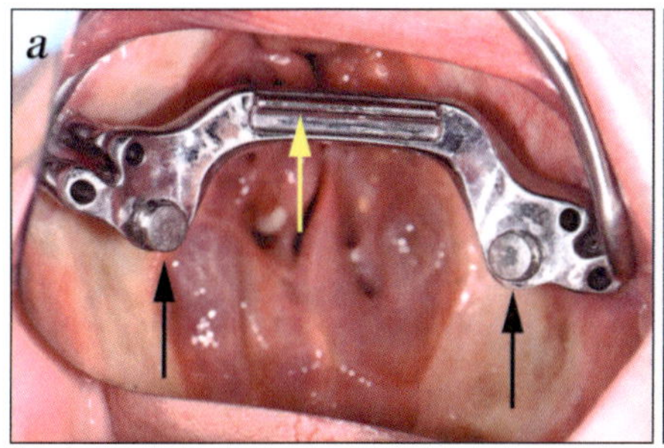

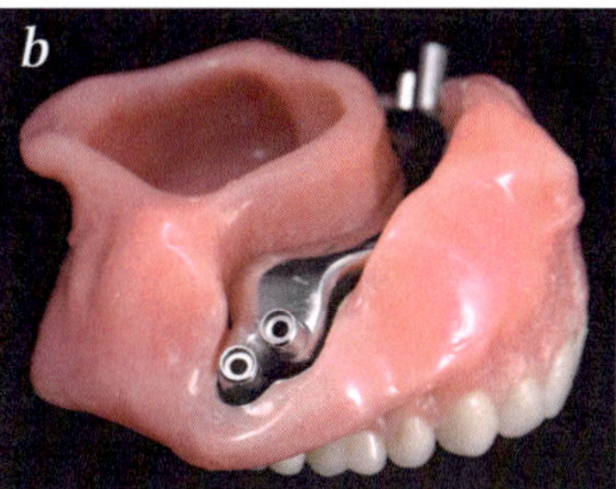

Figure 3-140 *(a)* An implant-assisted bar design. *(b)* Note that most of the prosthetic dentition is anterior to the bar. The implant-connecting bar splints four zygomatic implants together. During occlusal function, the prosthesis rotates around the "Hader" bar *(arrow)*. The magnetic attachments *(black arrows)* permit this rotation but enable the prosthesis to return to its fully seated position after the force is withdrawn.

Implant-assisted bar designs for edentulous patients with large anterior resection defects. On rare occasions, resections involve the anterior portion of the palate bilaterally, and multiple implants are placed in each of the residual posterior alveolar ridge remnants. In such defects, the prosthesis must extend a substantial distance anteriorly to restore the missing dentition and provide support for the upper lip. Lacking bone-supported denture foundation areas anteriorly or implant support for the obturator prosthesis, implant-assisted designs should be employed and anticipate and permit the prosthesis to rotate around the anticipated axis of rotation during occlusal function. In the implant-connecting bar design shown, rests are placed in between the implants, and resilient attachments are placed on the anterior section of each bar (Fig 3-139). Note the axis of rotation when an occlusal force is applied anteriorly. When an occlusal force is applied via the prosthetic dentition anterior to the implants, the prosthesis is impacted into the defect, and the resilient attachments permit the prosthesis to rotate around the rests, directing these forces down the long axis of the implants. The ERA is designed with a vertical resiliency, so it is advantageous to position the rest some distance from the attachment. The anterior extension of the obturator prosthesis should be carefully adapted to the tissues in the defect to limit its impaction into the defect during function. Ideally, the surfaces of these tissues should be skin lined. The metal substructure must be "physiologically adjusted" to allow the prosthesis to freely rotate around the rests as intended. With this design, the ERA attachments need to be replaced every three to six months depending on the support available anteriorly and the degree of rotation of the prosthesis during function.

Implant-assisted bar designs for total palatectomy defects. Another implant-assisted design is presented in the patient in Fig 3-140 with a total palatectomy defect. Four implants were placed in the residual zygomas, two in each arch, but the bone anchorage and implant configuration were not sufficient to permit the fabrication of an implant supported design. All four implants are splinted together. The prosthesis is retained with a Hader bar positioned anteriorly and magnetic attachments situated posteriorly. The prosthesis is retained with a Hader bar positioned anteriorly and magnetic attachments situated posteriorly.

When an occlusal force is applied via the prosthetic dentition anteriorly, the prosthesis rotates around the "Hader" bar segment, and the magnetic attachments disengage. When the occlusal force ceases, the magnetic attachments reengage. With such a design, bending moments to the implants are minimized. The clips engaging the "Hader" bar need replacement every six months.

Fabrication of the bar and substructure

If the implant-connecting bar is to be designed and fabricated with CAD-CAM, the cast and trial denture setup are both scanned. The two digital files are merged with the virtual design software. CAD software is then used by the clinician/laboratory technician to complete the initial design of the implant-connecting bar. A trial denture setup with the proposed palatal vault contours is scanned and the data merged with that of the scanned master cast. Sample designs are shown in (Fig 3-141). The design should conform to the principles described below. Implant-supported implant-connecting bars are best milled to a 3° taper. The attachment system selected is determined by the nature of the prosthetic space. The authors favor "Hader" and "Locator" type attachments for implant-supported bars and "ERA" type attachments for implant-assisted implant-connecting bars. Several examples of implant attachment bars for total palatectomy (Fig 3-141a–d) and palatectomy/maxillectomy defects (Fig 3-141e–j) are shown.

Conventional methods can also be used to fabricate the bar. A silicone or stone index, keyed to the cast, is created to relate the position of the denture teeth to the cast (Fig 3-142a). An alternative method for recording the position of the denture teeth is to make an occlusal index in plaster (similar to a facebow remount jig). The index is mounted on the lower member of the articulator, and the denture teeth are transferred and luted to the plaster index with sticky wax. The position of the denture teeth in relation to the master cast and, while waxing the implant-connecting bar, its position and contour can be evaluated simply by opening and closing the articulator (Fig 3-142b). Fabrication of the implant-connecting bar can now proceed, and it can be designed so that its contours and position are compatible with the predetermined position of the denture teeth and the contours of the palatal vault.

Whatever the method used to design and fabricate the implant-connecting bar, when portions of the bar overlay the residual alveolar ridges, the design should conform to basic principles previously developed for normal patients (Beumer et al., 2022). The bar must be rigid and allow for appropriate hygiene access between the implants and on the tissue side of the bar. The undersurface of the bar should be rounded and smoothed, and the bar and attachments connected to the terminal ends should be located 1 to 2 mm above the tissues. The bar must be positioned and contoured so that there is ample room for the denture teeth, the denture resin, and the metal substructure or metal framework.

The terminal path of insertion of the obturator prosthesis as it engages the implant-connecting bar and the attachments should be

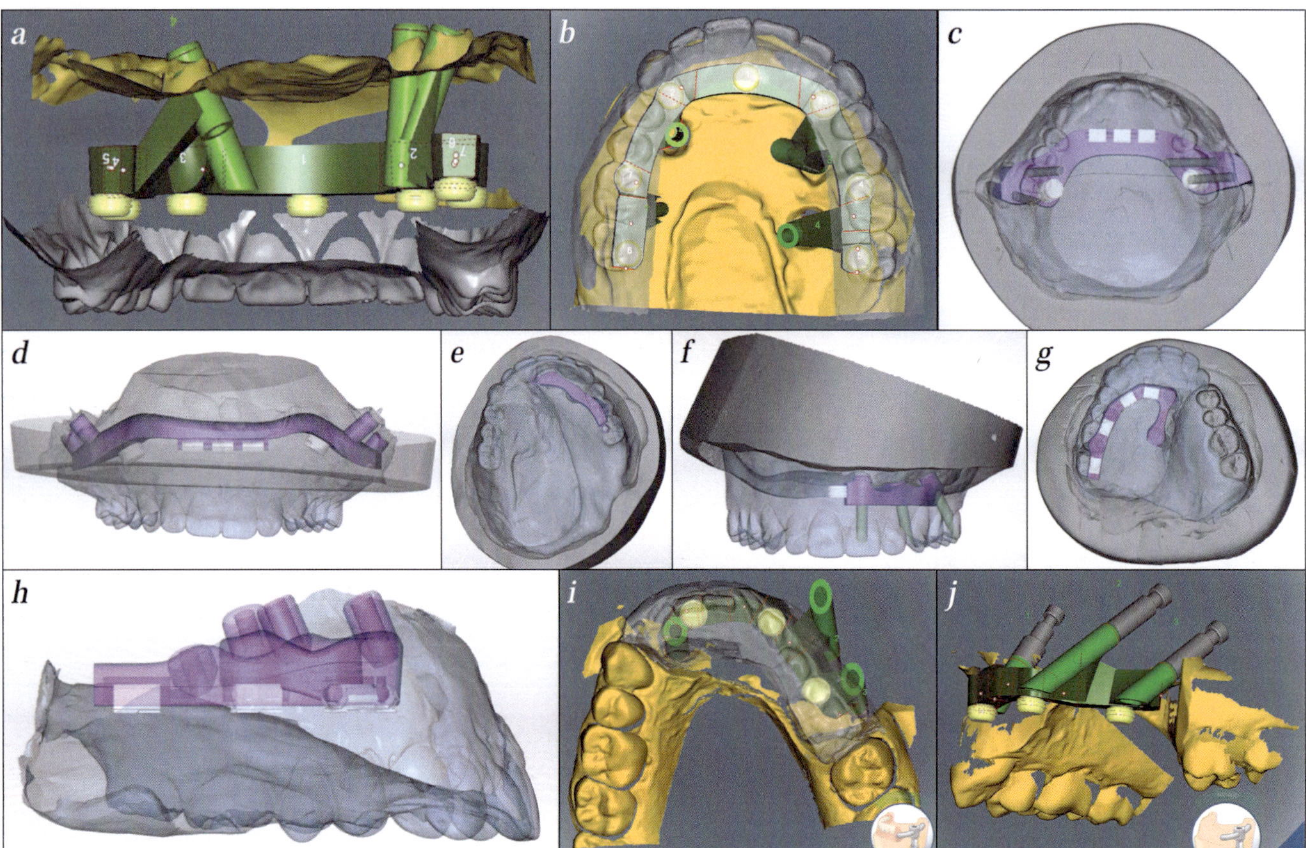

Figure 3-141 Implant-connecting bars can be designed digitally. These bars must fit within the confines of the proposed prosthesis and permit proper positioning of denture teeth and the development of appropriate palatal shelf contours and tongue space. *(a and b)* An implant-supported bar for a total palatectomy defect. The bar is milled to a 3° taper, and "locator"-type attachments are used for retention. *(c and d)* An implant-assisted bar for a total palatectomy defect. A combination of "Hader" and magnetic attachments permits the prosthesis to rotate around the bar when an anterior force is applied. *(e and f)* An implant-assisted bar for a total maxillectomy with ERA attachments incorporated. The implants were placed in the residual alveolar ridge. The rests will be milled into the bar after milling and placed between the implants. *(g and h)* An implant-supported bar design with Hader attachments for a total maxillectomy defect in a partially edentulous patient, supported by four zygomatic implants. *(i and j)* An implant-supported bar with locator-type attachments for a partially edentulous patient with an anterior palatectomy defect supported by two zygomatic implants and one implant placed in the pyriform rim region.

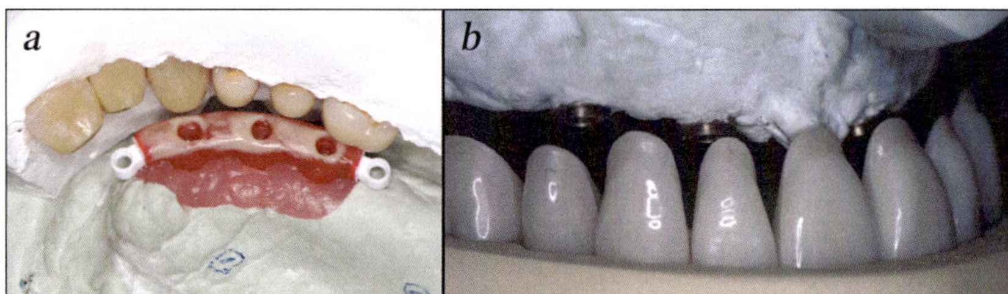

Figure 3-142 Conventional methods of relating tooth positions to the master cast while developing the contours and position of the implant-connecting bar. *(a)* A plaster index with the denture teeth secured with wax that is keyed to the master cast. *(b)* An alternative method for relating the position of the denture teeth to the defect is to make an occlusal index of plaster or stone. The index is mounted on the lower member of the articulator. The denture teeth are removed from the record base and attached to the index with sticky wax ("b" reprinted from Beumer et al., 2022).

on the same plane. However, frequently a dual path of insertion for the obturator prosthesis must be employed because of the undercuts in the defect. During insertion, this portion of the prosthesis is inserted first, and the prosthesis is then rotated into position to engage the bar. During removal by the patient, the opposite is true: the prosthesis is disengaged from the bar and then rotated out of the defect. The bar must be positioned and contoured so that there is ample room to house and retain denture teeth with sufficient volume of denture resin to retain them.

When designed digitally, it may not be possible because of the limitations of the software and/or the milling/printing apparatus to incorporate all the necessary design features into the implant-connecting bar. After milling/printing, the edges of the tissue surface of the bar may need to be rounded, or portions of the bar engaging the implants must be slightly recontoured to facilitate the removal of plaque and debris from the bar and between the implants (Fig 3-143). Rests need to be milled into the bar after printing/milling (Fig 3-143c).

Implant-assisted bars should be milled or printed from a wear-resistant metal. Titanium should not be used for such bars because the constant movement and rotation of the overdenture-obturator prosthesis during function will result in rapid wear of the bar,

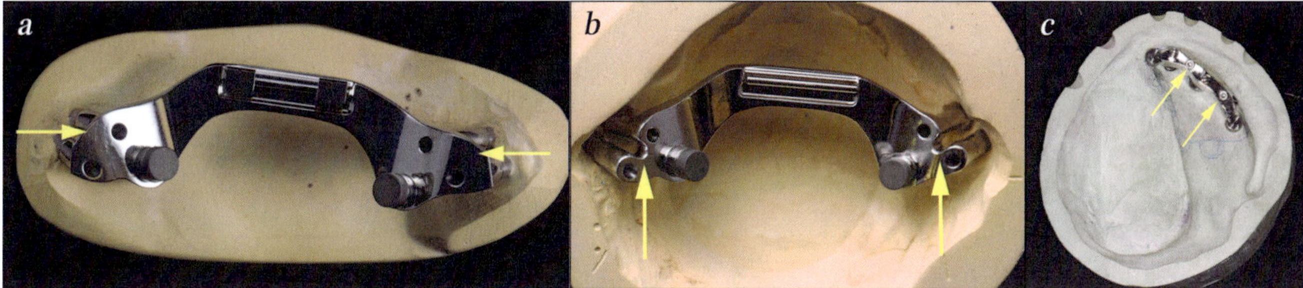

Figure 3-143 Because of the limitations of the software and manufacturing equipment, digitally designed implant-connecting bars often must be altered after milling/printing. *(a)* The printed bar. Note the lack of hygiene access between the implants *(arrows)*. *(b)* Note that the bar has been altered to enhance hygiene access between the implants *(arrows)*. *(c)* Rests *(arrows)* have been milled with a No. 8 round burr into this milled implant-assisted bar designed to retain a complete denture-obturator for a maxillectomy defect.

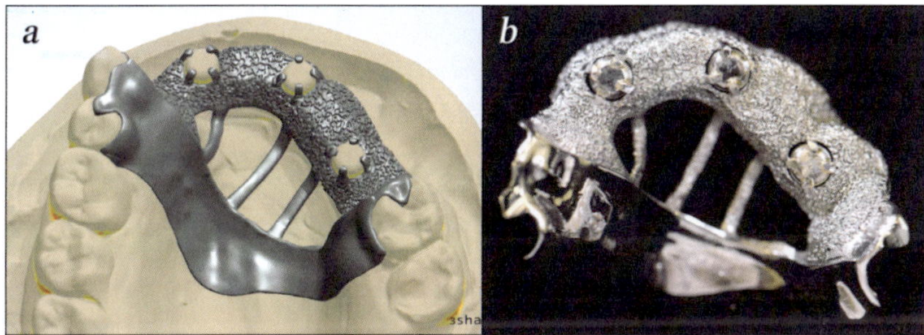

Figure 3-144 This RDP and incorporated substructure has been designed and fabricated with CAD-CAM. *(a)* The digital design of the RDP and substructure engaging the bar and the attachments incorporated within the bar. *(b)* Note that the metal substructure is designed around the metal attachment housings. The RDP framework. The metal housings are laser welded to the framework.

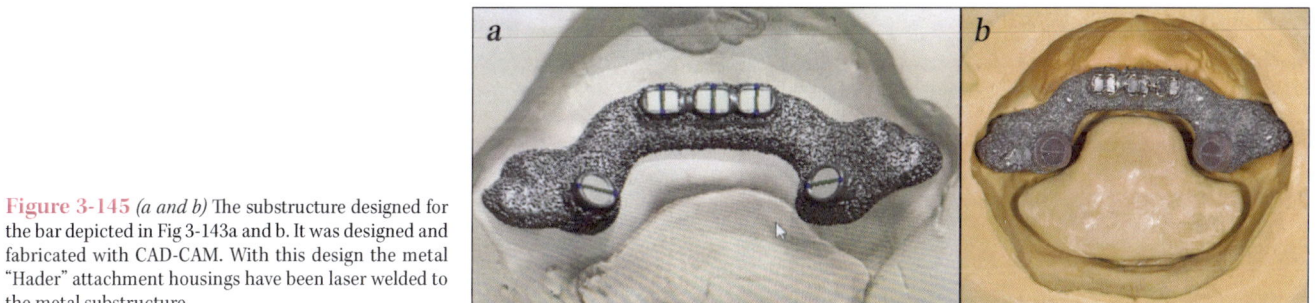

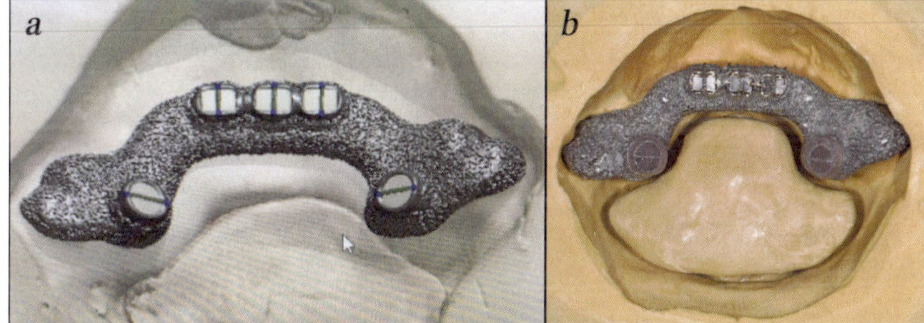

Figure 3-145 *(a and b)* The substructure designed for the bar depicted in Fig 3-143a and b. It was designed and fabricated with CAD-CAM. With this design the metal "Hader" attachment housings have been laser welded to the metal substructure.

rendering the obturator prosthesis nonretentive within just a couple of years. Cobalt-chromium is the material of choice for implant-assisted implant-connecting bars. Bars of this material can be either milled or printed. Selective laser melting is a new technology that has emerged as the preferred method of printing implant-connecting bars of cobalt-chrome alloys as well as RDP frameworks. The precision achieved with this technique surpasses that achieved with conventional casting technologies.

As mentioned previously, implant-supported connecting bars are usually milled of titanium. There is little risk of wear of such bars because the prosthesis does not move or rotate during occlusal function.

All bars must be confirmed intraorally. If the precision of fit is unsatisfactory and they are fabricated of cobalt chrome, they can be sectioned and laser welded. If made of titanium, a new impression must be made and a new bar designed and fabricated; hence the need to reaffirm the accuracy of the initial impression of the implants when using this material for the implant-connecting bar.

It is advantageous to design the substructure or that portion of the RDP overlay framework that engages the implant-connecting bar, with receptacles for the metal housings of the attachments to be used. Note the designs for such in Figs 3-144 and 3-145. These designs allow the metal attachment housings to be retained by the denture base acrylic resin. The metal housings can also be laser welded to the metal substructure. As mentioned previously, if the bar is implant-assisted, *the substructure must be "physiologically adjusted" to enable the prosthesis to rotate around the implant-connecting bar as intended when occlusal forces are generated.*

Remaining prosthodontic procedures

When the defect extends to the posterior pharyngeal wall, a new border-molded impression is required to precisely record the extension into the velopharyngeal region and this extension is best refined with a thermoplastic wax. Such impression trays are designed to be retained by the implant-connecting bar, must have normal contours

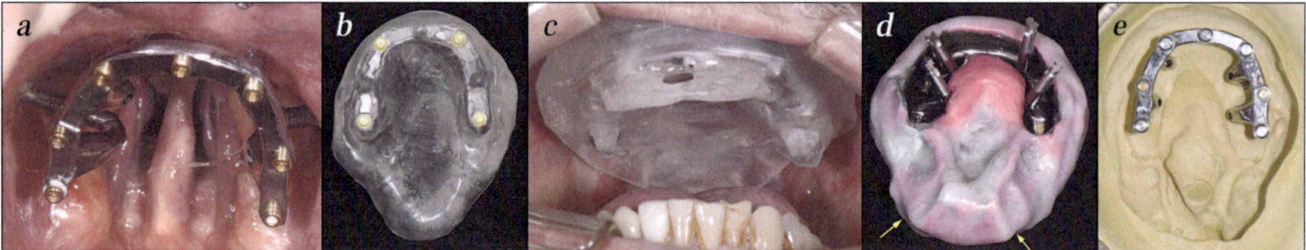

Figure 3-146 *(a)* Milled bar of titanium with locator attachments. *(b)* Impression tray with attachments embedded to secure the tray in position. Note that occlusal stops have been incorporated at the desired occlusal vertical dimension to help stabilize the tray while correcting the impression with thermoplastic wax. *(c)* Tray secured to the bar. *(d)* Border-molded impressions. Note that the obturator extends to the posterior pharyngeal wall to engage the residual velopharyngeal musculature *(arrows)*. *(e)* Mater cast with bar secured.

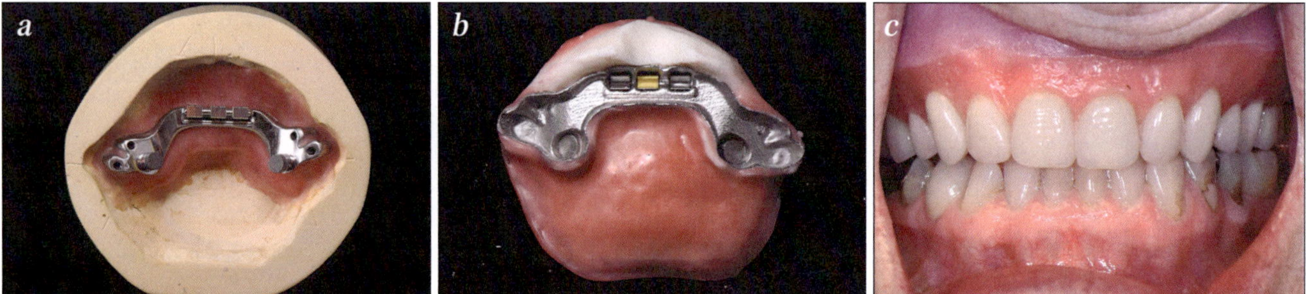

Figure 3-147 *(a and b)* The master cast is blocked out as necessary, a new record base is fabricated with the substructure attached. *(c)* The teeth are arranged, and a clinical try-in is performed in the usual manner.

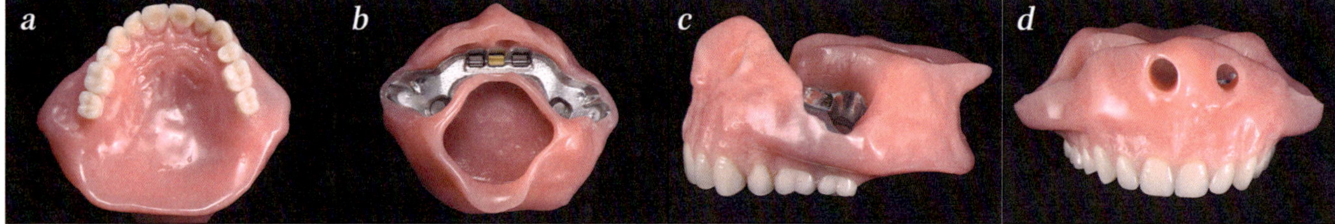

Figure 3-148 *(a)* An obturator prosthesis restoring a total palatectomy defect seen in Figure 3-140. Completed implant-assisted overlay obturator prosthesis. *(b)* Tissue side of the prosthesis. *(c)* Lateral view of the prosthesis. Note that this prosthesis extends onto the nasal side of the soft palate to enhance seal and prevent liquids from escaping into the nasal passage. *(d)* Anterior view. The orifices maintain the nasal airway.

of the palatal vault, and must have occlusal stops in order to keep the tray completely seated during the refinement of the impression with the thermoplastic wax. These design features will also allow the patient to be able to speak and swallow in a relatively normal manner while molding this extension. Note that the tray handle, if present, must not prematurely contact the opposing dentition in centric at the established occlusal vertical dimension.

Once the bar is verified, a border-molded impression is made to engage all residual edentulous extensions and bearing surfaces as well as those of the defect (Fig 3-146). Care must be taken to take maximum advantage of the defect to enhance the stability, retention, and support of the prosthesis. This is especially important when the implant-connecting bar/attachment apparatus is designed to be implant-assisted.

A new record base with the metal substructure incorporated is fabricated in order to perform the final try-in (Fig 3-147). During this appointment, the aesthetics, phonetics, occlusal vertical dimension, and centric relation record should be verified.

The occlusion should be designed with either balanced articulation when an implant-assisted bar is employed or group function when an implant-supported bar is used to retain the prosthesis. A comprehensive discussion of occlusal design concepts used for implant retained overdentures is found in Wu et al. (2022). The prosthesis is processed (Fig 3-148) and delivered in the usual fashion using PIP and disclosing wax to refine extensions and tissue adaptation (see Figs 3-64 and 3-96). A clinical remount record (Fig 3-149) is made, the occlusion is refined as needed, and the prosthesis is delivered (Fig 3-150).

Proper use of hygiene aids is demonstrated to the patient. Special aids and brushes may be needed especially in large defects restored with zygomatic implants. Initially, when the entire length of zygomatic implants was threaded and before the introduction of the modern designs with extended smooth surfaces, it was not possible for most patients to keep the portions of the implants that traversed the defect to the implant-connecting bar free of plaque. This burden has been partially mitigated by the new designs with extended

Figure 3-149 During the delivery appointment a clinical remount record is made and the occlusion is refined.

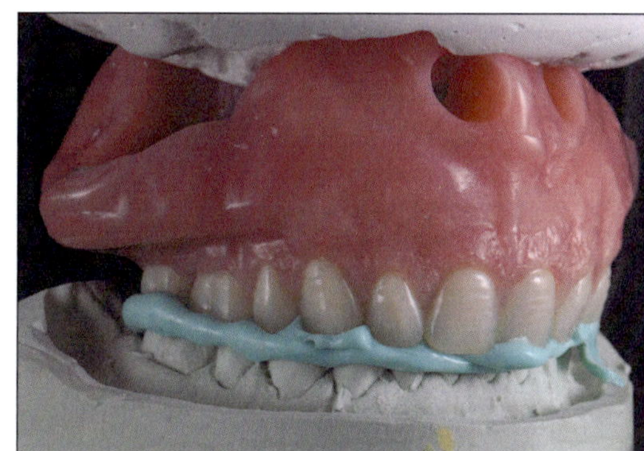

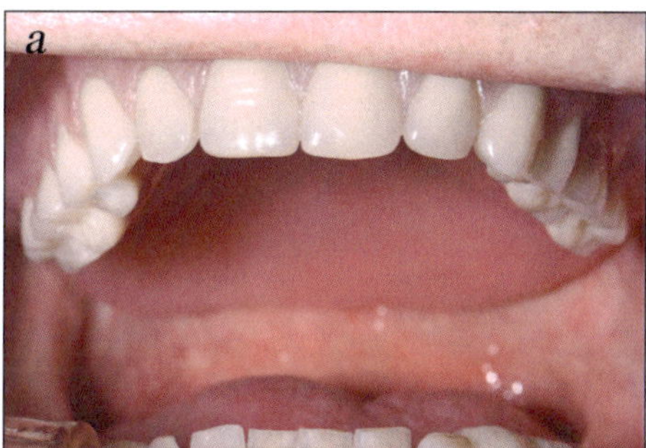

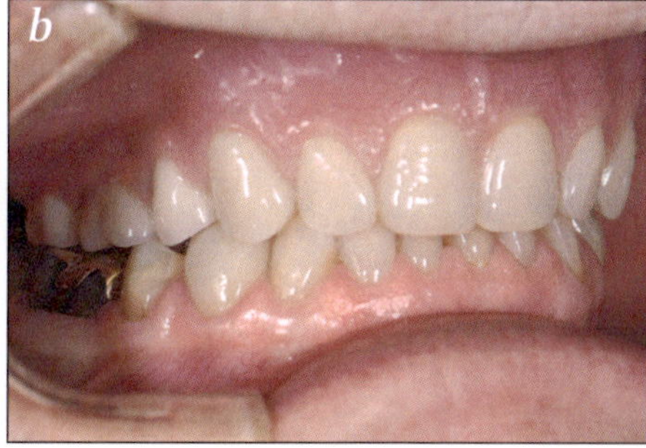

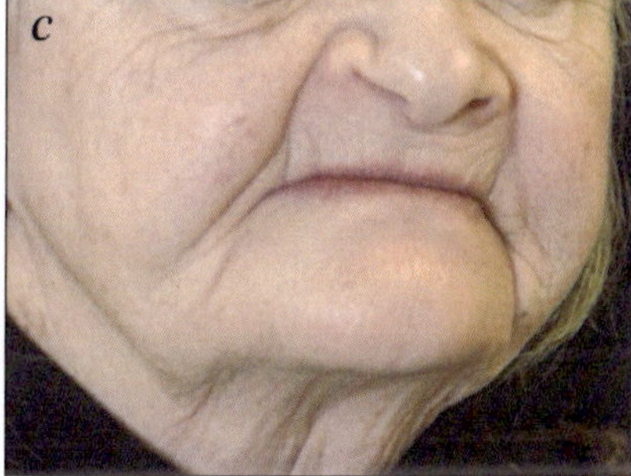

Figure 3-150 *(a and b)* The definitive prosthesis for a total palatectomy defect in position. *(c)* The contours of the upper lip are reasonably restored.

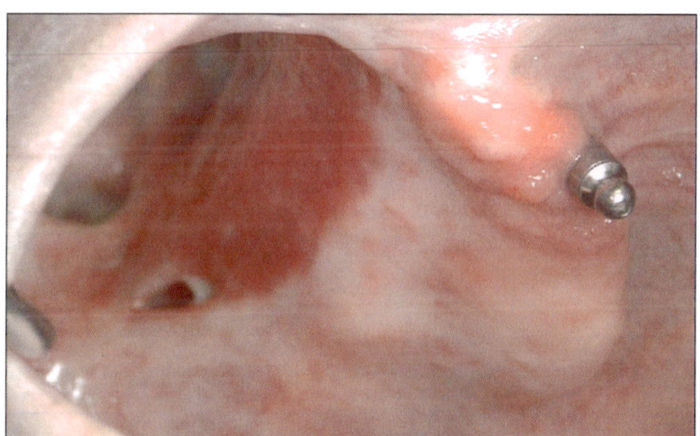

Figure 3-151 The implant placed in the canine region has been fitted with a large O-ring-type attachment. Retention on the defect side was accomplished by engaging the skin-lined divergent lateral wall of the defect. A dual path of insertion is used to position the prosthesis.

smooth surfaces. Nevertheless, these implants traverse significant distances before they engage the implant-connecting bar and require special attention by the patient, especially as the implants emerge from the bone anchorage points.

In patients with more conventional implant-connecting bars that are secured to implants emerging from the residual alveolar ridges, it is critically important that the patient keep the implant/abutment surfaces emerging through the peri-implant tissues free of plaque and debris as well as the undersurfaces of an implant-connecting bar. Otherwise, inflammatory fibrous hyperplasia of the peri-implant tissues, peri-implantitis, and hyperplasia of the mucosal tissues underneath the bar will be the inevitable result. Implant patients should be followed every three months in the first year. This period may be extended depending on the hygiene compliance of the patient. Attachments are replaced as needed and primarily depend on the movement of the prosthesis during function. Attachments associated with an implant-supported connecting bar need to be replaced only every two to three years, but those associated with implant-assisted implant-connecting bars require replacement every three to six months.

Solitary implants

Solitary implants can effectively retain a large obturator prosthesis when the defect is skin lined with undercuts and/or is divergent. Large O-ring attachments are preferred because they allow the prosthesis to rotate in multiple planes when an occlusal load is delivered or when the prosthesis drops as a result of gravity or is displaced in the horizontal plane by the movement of the mandible or contracture of the facial musculature (Fig 3-151; see also Fig 3-98). This

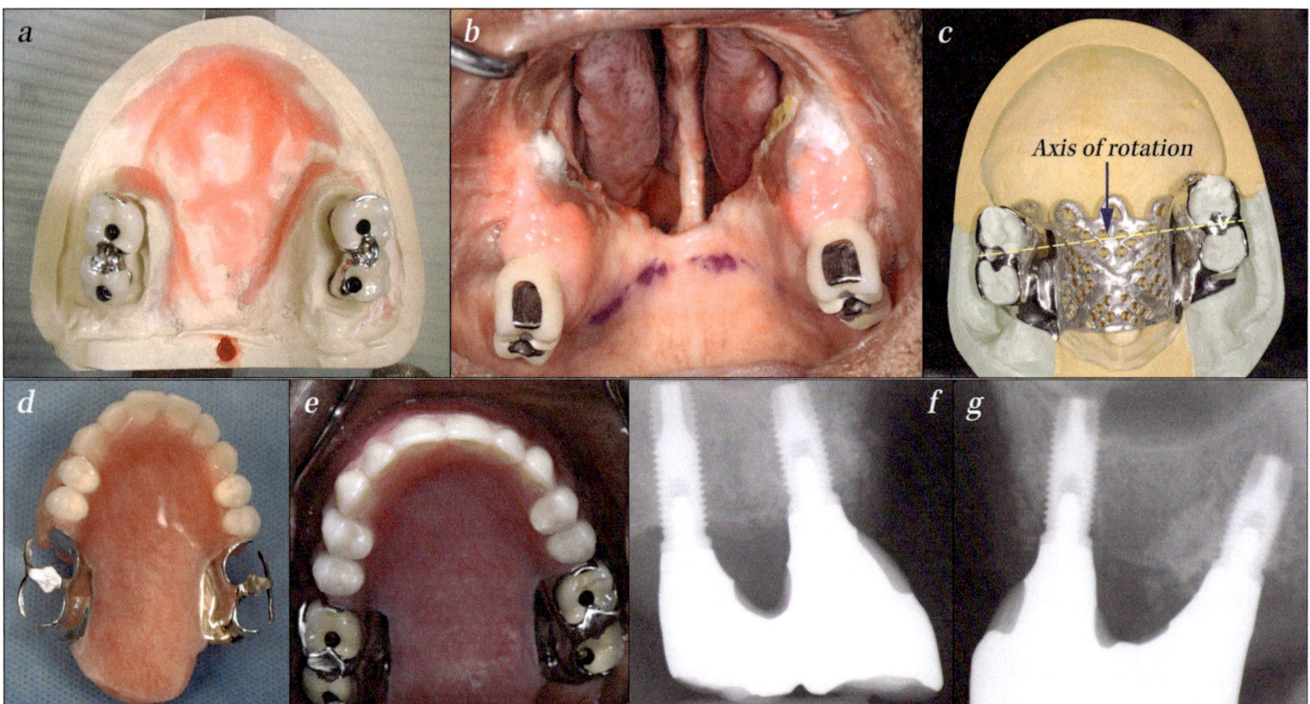

Figure 3-152 *(a and b)* Surveyed implant crowns. *(c)* Altered cast and the RDP framework. The RPA system of RDP design was employed. Only the tips of the anterior retainers engage undercuts and the portion of the clasps above the height of contour of the implant crowns has been relieved to allow rotation of the prosthesis. The posterior retainers terminate at the height of contour of the surveyed implant crowns. When an occlusal force is applied anterior to the implant crowns, the prosthesis rotates around the axis of rotation, and the tips of the anterior retainers disengage. *(d)* The RDP-obturator prosthesis. *(e)* The prosthesis in position. *(f and g)* Radiographs of the implants eight years post insertion.

property minimizes the magnitude of bending moments applied to the implant. Engagement of the lateral wall provides retention on the side of the defect and the O-ring provides retention on the normal side. This combination will result in effective retention of the prosthesis. The Roumanas et al. (1997) report indicates bone levels can be reasonably stable over the long term by the use of such attachments when only a solitary implant is available. Because of the constant movement of the prosthesis, the rubber O-rings wear rapidly and must be replaced every three to four months.

Surveyed implant crowns and RDP obturators

Another approach is to fabricate surveyed implant crowns, splint them together when appropriate, and fabricate an RDP obturator. When the I bar mesial rest philosophy of RDP design or RPA system is properly applied, RDP designs can be developed that will minimize the bending moments applied to the implants. In most instances, from the perspective of biomechanics, the outcomes are comparable to what can be achieved with implant-assisted connecting bars and individual attachments.

The principal advantage is that this approach simplifies follow-up appointments, compared to the use of implant-assisted implant-connecting bars using resilient attachments for retention. Obturator prostheses lacking support in the defect demonstrate a greater range of movement than removable prostheses fabricated for unresected patients with intact palates. The attachments incorporated within the substructure of the obturator prosthesis are therefore subject to a more rapid rate of wear. They require frequent replacement adding significant costs to maintenance and follow-up. When the implants are employed as RDP abutments it is relatively easy to restore retention by simply adjusting the retainers during a regular follow-up appointment. However, if this concept is employed, we strongly advise that the RDP frameworks be designed consistent with the I bar mesial rest (Kratochvil, 1963, 1988; Chang et al., 2019) or the "RPA" concept (Eliason, 1983) (Figs 3-152 and 3-153) because these designs will limit the bending moments applied to the implants. Furthermore, this method may be the only option when there is limited prosthetic space available for an implant-connecting bar and metal substructure.

In the anterior resection defect, shown in Fig 3-152, embrasure rests incorporated within the implant crowns serve as the axis of rotation. The buccal surfaces of the anterior crowns are designed and contoured with retentive areas, which will be engaged by the tips of the retainers. Parallel guide planes are incorporated to facilitate bracing by the proximal plates of the RDP. The RDP framework is designed such that the posterior "Akers" type retainers terminate at the height of contour whereas the tips of the anterior retainers engage a .010″ undercut. The posterior retainers add to the bracing provided by the guide planes and lingual plate (resistance to lateral displacement), while the anterior retainers provide retention for the RDP-obturator prosthesis. The RDP framework must be carefully "physiologically adjusted" to permit its free, unencumbered rotation around the rests, so as to minimize bending moments applied to the implants when occlusal forces are applied. When using this type of retainer for retention, it is important that the portion of the retainer above the height of the contour be relieved so

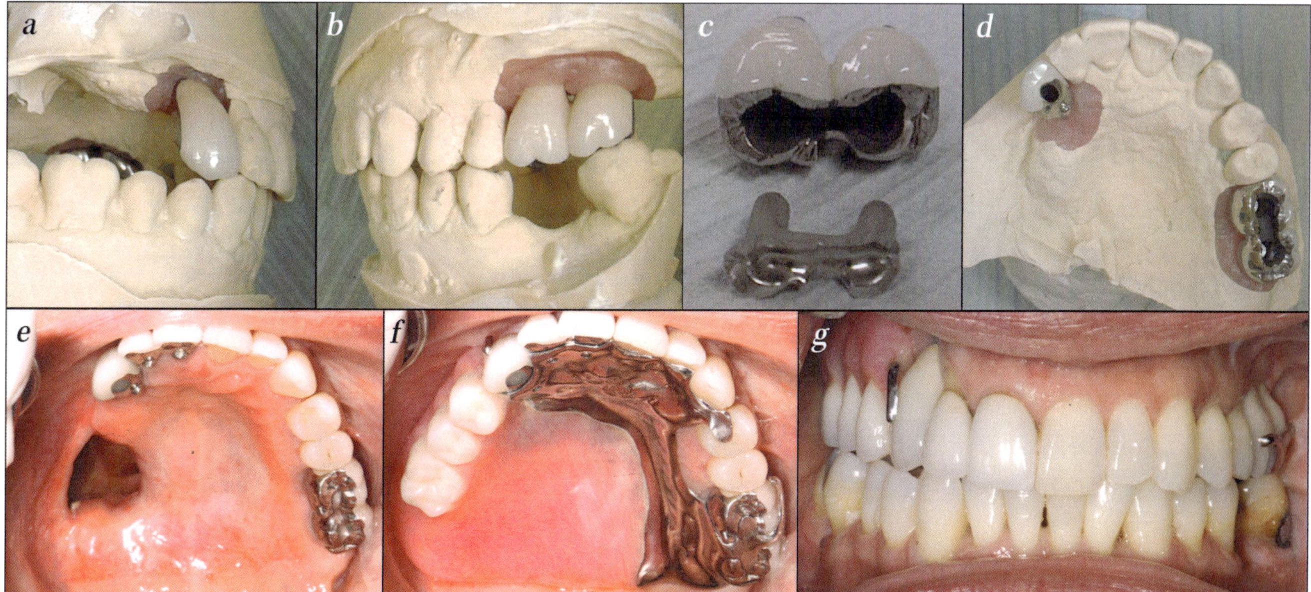

Figure 3-153 *(a, b, c, and d)* Implant crowns restored the right canine and the left maxillary molars. The right central and lateral incisors were also fitted with metal-ceramic crowns and splinted. Note the cingulum rests incorporated within the crowns. *(e, f, and g)* The RDP-obturator prosthesis in position. Guidance during right working is provided by teeth #7 and #8, which are splinted together. The solitary implant crown and the posterior denture teeth on the defect side are designed with centric-only contact. The implant crowns restoring the maxillary molars are also designed for centric-only contact (e, f, and g from Beumer et al., 2022, with permission).

as to permit proper rotation around the rests (Chang et al., 2019). This can be accomplished in the laboratory or during the physiologic adjustment appointment. When occlusal forces are applied anterior to the implant crowns, the prosthesis rotates around the embrasure rests, and the retainers rotate farther into the undercuts created on the implant crowns and are impacted into the defect, thus directing the preponderance of the occlusal forces along the long axis of the implants. In this way, an implant-assisted design is created where the forces are shared between the implants and the available denture-bearing surfaces.

Fig 3-153 demonstrates the use of surveyed implant crowns used to help retain an RDP-obturator prosthesis for a partial maxillectomy defect. This approach is especially useful when there is healthy, adjacent dentition remaining. This patient was originally restored with an RDP obturator retained by the residual dentition. However, the key abutment teeth used to retain the RDP-obturator prosthesis were lost secondary to chronic periodontitis, after 30 years of retaining the prosthesis. These teeth were removed, the canine extraction site grafted, the molar sites grafted, a sinus augmentation procedure performed subsequently on the unresected side, and eventually, implants inserted into these sites. The implant crowns were designed to share the occlusal loads with the adjacent residual dentition and available denture-bearing surfaces. The implant crowns were contoured to establish a precise path of insertion, with parallel guiding surfaces, positive rests, and facial contours that can be properly engaged by retainers. Rests were contoured and positioned such that occlusal forces were directed along the long axis of the implants. The I bar mesial rest (Kratochvil, 1963, 1988) concept of removable dental prosthesis design was employed so as to minimize the magnitude of bending moments applied to the implants, especially the implant restoring the canine, and direct occlusal forces axially onto the natural tooth and implant abutments.

The occlusion designed in the patient shown in Fig 3-153 is also noteworthy. The solitary implant restoring the canine adjacent to the defect is designed with centric-only contact to minimize bending moments applied to the implant during excursions (Wu et al., 2022). The posterior denture teeth on the defect side have been lingualized and positioned for centric-only contact as well (Wu et al., 2022). Guidance on the defect side is provided by right lateral and central incisors, which have been splinted and provided with cingulum rests. Guidance on the nondefect side is provided by the residual dentition. Further splinting action is provided by the lingual plate terminating in the mesial rest on the natural premolar. The implant crowns restoring the maxillary molars have been splinted and designed with centric-only contact.

Definitive Obturators for Patients with Unique Palatal Defects

Defects bordering the hard and soft palates

A majority of patients with benign neoplasms of the palatal mucosa or the nasal and paranasal sinuses will undergo transoral resection with a subtotal or partial maxillectomy. However, resection of some tumors will result in other types of defects. For example, pleomorphic adenomas and small, well-localized squamous cell carcinomas may require a limited surgical resection at the junction of the hard and soft palates. Often the alveolar ridge and teeth are only minimally involved in the resection.

Construction of an obturator for this type of defect is more difficult than it appears because the obturator must maintain contact

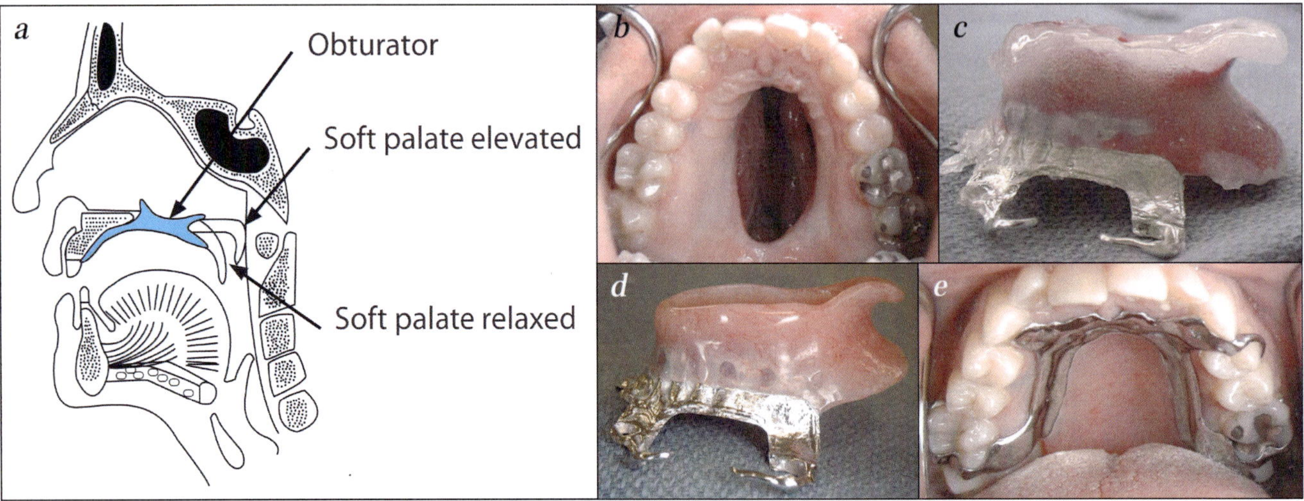

Figure 3-154 *(a)* Movement of the anterior margin of the soft palate during palatal elevation. *(b)* Patient with a defect of the hard and soft palates, with the soft palate at rest. *(c)* Border-molded impression of the defect with compound and a thermoplastic wax. Contact between the soft palate and obturator should be maintained during elevation to minimize leakage. *(d)* Processes prosthesis. *(e)* Prosthesis in position.

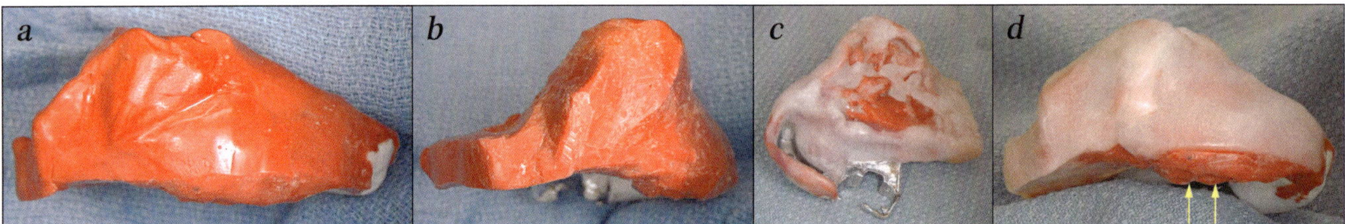

Figure 3-155 *(a)* Border-molded impression extending to the posterior pharyngeal wall. *(b)* Cutback. *(c and d)* Corrected impression with impression wax. The occlusal index, recorded with impression compound *(arrows)*, serves as a tentative centric relation record and stabilizes the impression while refining it with a thermoplastic wax.

posteriorly and laterally during soft palate elevation (Fig 3-154). Thermoplastic waxes are used to record the functional movements of the tissues bordering the defect.

Speech will be normal after delivery of the prosthesis. Occasionally, however, the patient will note excess nasal leakage when swallowing. To prevent this problem, a 5- to 10-mm extension with positive pressure is created across the intact oral side of the soft palate. The soft palate will lift from this extension in function, but this shield will serve to direct liquids and food into the oral pharynx. Leakage will be minimized without interfering with tongue function. Extension into the defect that allows for contact with the nasal side of the soft palate during elevation also is suggested (see Fig 3-154c and d).

Maxillectomy defects extending to the posterior pharyngeal wall

Occasionally a maxillectomy defect will extend posteriorly to the pharyngeal wall. This prosthesis, although very large, can be designed and fabricated to restore speech and swallowing to normal levels, if retention is adequate. The masticatory performance will depend on the presence and location of teeth and/or implants. It may be useful to place implants into the zygomatic arch on the resected side to stabilize the prosthesis and provide additional support. If implants have not been placed on the defect side, as previously described for total maxillectomy defects, the midlateral portion of the prosthesis should be extended superiorly and aggressively to engage the skin-lined lateral wall of the defect. This will provide the obturator prosthesis with additional stability, retention, and support. The velopharyngeal extension must interact with the residual velopharyngeal musculature. To do so effectively it must be properly molded and be positioned precisely within the zone of residual velopharyngeal muscular contraction. The vertical height of this extension should not exceed 10–15 mm (Figs 3-155 and 3-156) (see Chapter 4, section entitled "Total soft palate defects: Method of fabrication"). If a nonfunctional band of soft palate remains, access to the pharyngeal musculature sometimes can be gained through the defect over the nasal side of the soft palate (see Fig 3-37). If this band impairs access to the residual velopharyngeal musculature, it should be removed.

Impressions are made in the usual way. We prefer a one-step impression method that records the palatal and velopharyngeal portions during the same appointment. After border molding is completed with a low-fusing impression compound (Fig 3-155a), an occlusal index is made to stabilize the impression while the velopharyngeal portion is being refined.

Following a suitable cutback, the entire impression is refined with a thermoplastic wax (Fig 3-155b, c, and d). The prosthesis is then completed in the customary fashion (Fig 3-156). With good retention combined with adequate movement of the residual velopharyngeal musculature and precise placement of the velopharyngeal extension, speech and swallowing are restored to normal.

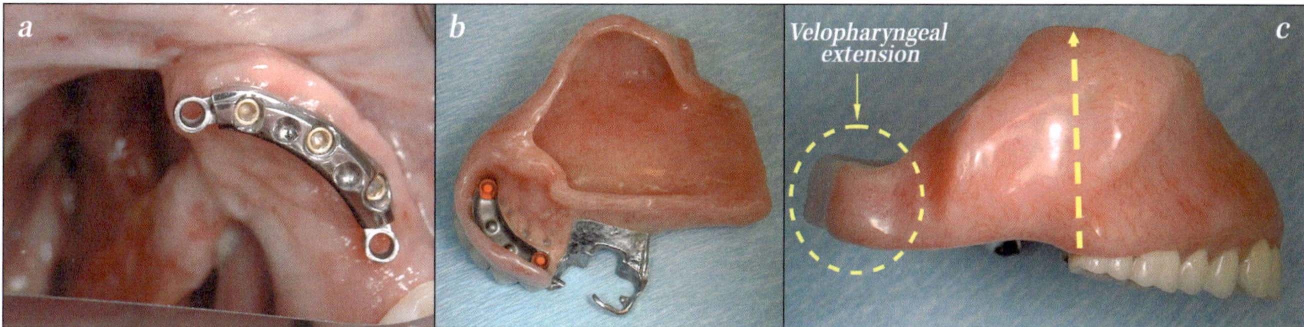

Figure 3-156 Total maxillectomy defect extending to the pharyngeal wall. The entire soft palate has been resected. *(a)* Implants added in the anterior maxilla to facilitate retention. *(b and c)* Obturator with aggressive extension superiorly into the area of hard palate resection *(arrow)*. The velopharyngeal extension is designed to interface with the velopharyngeal musculature and therefore limited to 10 to 12 mm in vertical height.

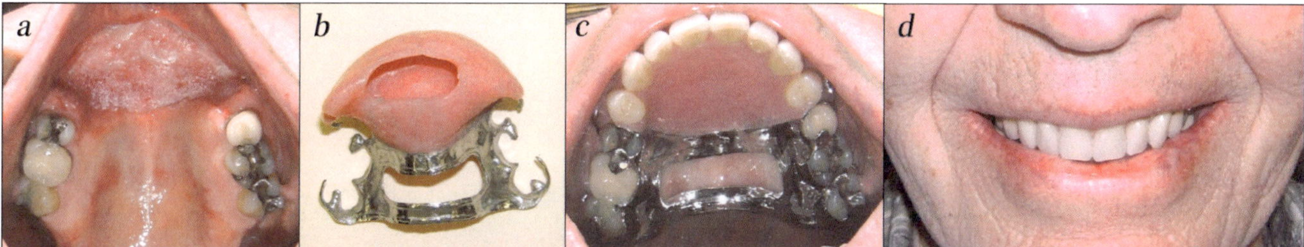

Figure 3-157 *(a)* Defect resulting from resection of squamous cell carcinoma. *(b)* Obturator prosthesis. *(c)* Prosthesis in position. *(d)* Acceptable aesthetics resulting from the prosthesis, which provides good lip support.

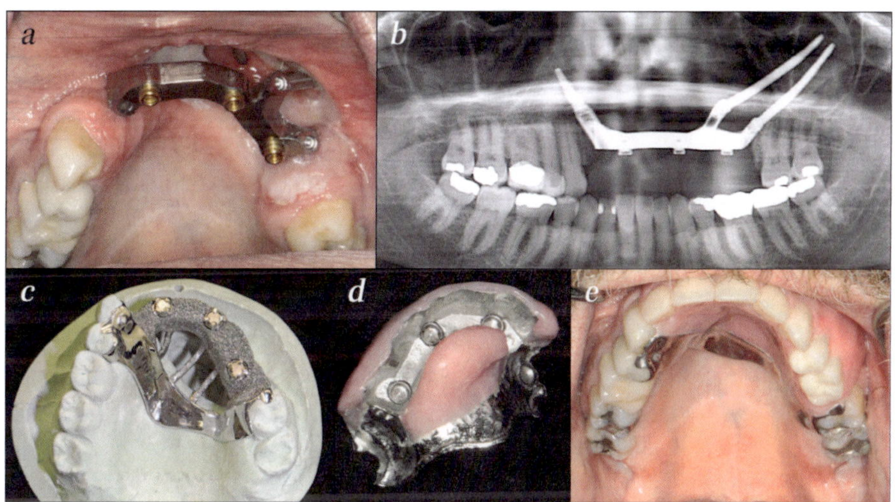

Figure 3-158 The patient depicted in Fig 3-14. Three implants have been placed to support this RDP-obturator, one in the residual bone of the pyriform rim and two in the left zygomatic arch. The defect was skin grafted to avoid undue contraction of the upper lip. *(a)* An implant-connecting bar of titanium with a 3-degree taper was designed and milled with CAD-CAM. The milled titanium bar in position. Note that the zygomatic implant surfaces extending through the soft tissues are polished. *(b)* A panoramic radiograph of the implant and bar. *(c)* The RDP framework. The rests and lingual plating provide additional support and stability. *(d)* Intaglio surface of the overlay RDP. *(e)* The definitive RDP in position.

Anterior defects

Occasionally, an anterior resection of the maxilla is required. If the defect is not skin grafted, significant scarring and contracture of the lip may occur (see Fig 3-21b and c). If a skin graft is placed, scarring and retraction of the lip are minimized, the prosthesis can be extended into the defect to support the lip, and an acceptable aesthetic result can be achieved (Fig 3-157). Note the RDP design is consistent with the I bar mesial rest concept in that the occlusal rests on the premolars are positioned on the distal side of these teeth (Chang et al., 2019). In defects such as these, the nature of the defect anteriorly may limit anterosuperior extension of the prosthesis. However, the prosthodontist should try to extend the anterior surface of the prosthesis as far superiorly as possible without interfering with nasal physiology.

Prostheses of this type lack anterior support, so the placement of implants is suggested. Frequently there is sufficient bone remaining in the pyriform rim region. If necessary zygomatic implants can be used to supplement implant support (Fig 3-158). Compare the aesthetic outcomes achieved in these two patients where the defects were grafted with skin grafts with that achieved in the patient in Fig 3-21b and c, where the defect was not grafted. Tissue contracture in this patient led to significant elevation and distortion of the upper lip, dramatically compromising the aesthetic outcome.

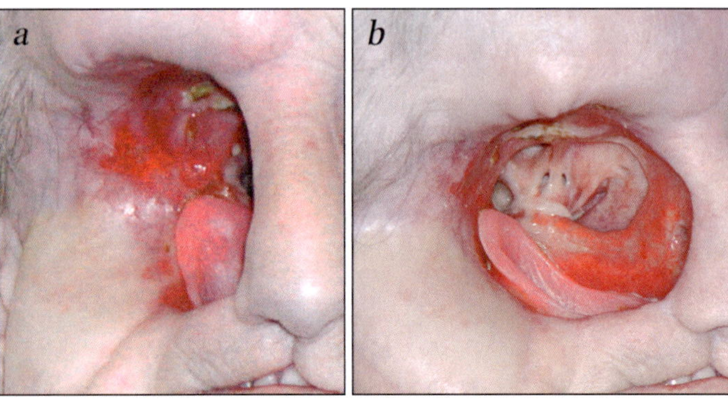

Figure 3-159 *(a and b)* The posterior extension is aggressive but the lateral extension is short of the height of contour between the oral cavity and the cheek.

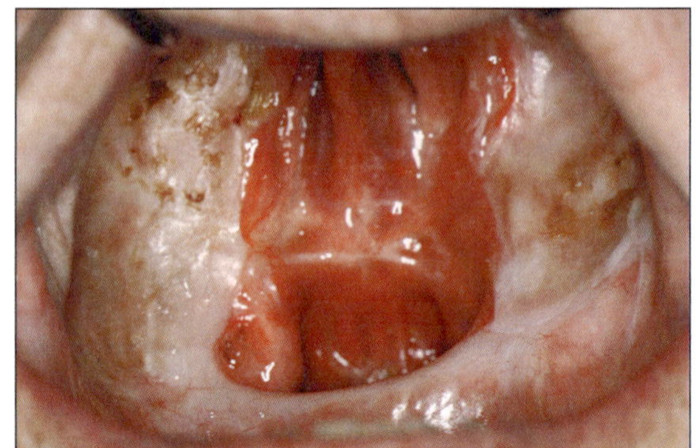

Figure 3-160 A typical total palatectomy defect. The defect has been lined with split-thickness skin grafts. The soft palate is intact.

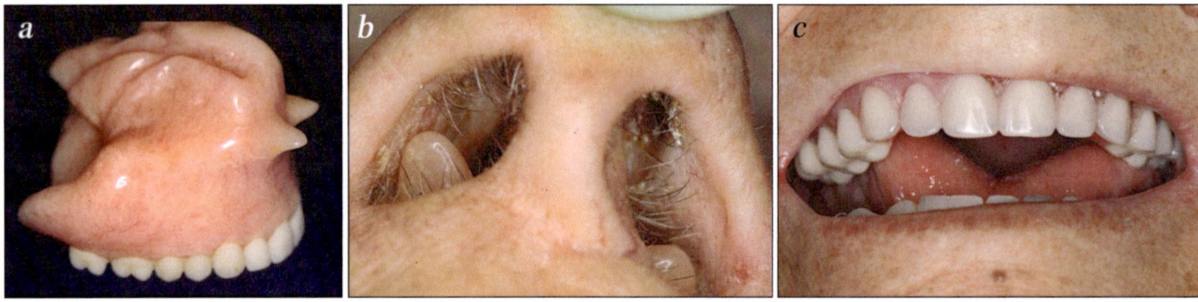

Figure 3-161 *(a)* A typical prosthesis for a total palatectomy defect. Note the nasal aperture extensions and the extension to the nasal side of the soft palate. *(b)* Prosthesis in position. Note the nasal aperture extensions. *(c)* Because of the poor retention achieved with conventional prostheses, the patient is forced to hold the prosthesis in position with the dorsum of the tongue. Such prostheses serve only to restore speech and facilitate swallowing.

Maxillectomy combined with large orbital exenteration defects that extend down onto the cheek

A significant number of patients undergoing total maxillectomy also require orbital exenteration. If the orbital defect is unusually large, the lateral extension of the obturator prosthesis should be short of the height of contour between the oral defect and the skin side of the orbital defect (Fig 3-159). *Otherwise, saliva will leak onto the skin by capillary action.* Often it is advantageous to connect the orbital prosthesis to the obturator prosthesis because this will enhance the retention of the orbital prosthesis and the support, stability, and retention of the intraoral prosthesis (see Chapter 5, section entitled "Connection of a Facial Prosthesis to an Oral Prosthesis," Fig 5-143).

Total palatectomy defects

Total palatectomy defects do not occur frequently (Fig 3-160). Formerly and before the introduction of the zygomatic implant, when the entire hard palate had been excised, the prosthetic prognosis was quite guarded. Prostheses constructed for these patients were primarily intended to improve speech and aesthetics. Surprisingly, given the poor retention of such prostheses, they restored these functions reasonably well if the patient was able to control the prosthesis with the dorsum of the tongue. Patients with excellent neuromuscular control were able to balance the prosthesis with their tongue and at the same time articulate speech sounds and manipulate the bolus in preparation for swallowing. Lacking support, however, mastication performance was dramatically degraded.

Not all patients were able to perform these tasks efficiently and with no means of direct retention the prosthesis was quite mobile. In past years these defects were skin grafted and soft tissue undercuts created. Retention was provided by engaging these soft tissue undercuts and extending the prosthesis onto the nasal side of the soft palate (if present) and into the nasal apertures (Fig 3-161a and b). However, the patient was still forced to hold the prosthesis in position with the dorsum of the tongue (Fig 3-161c). Such prostheses served only to restore speech and facilitate swallowing.

Implants have changed the clinical outcomes, even if the resection is extended to include the soft palate, and when they are effectively employed, speech, swallowing, and mastication often are restored to presurgical levels or to a level typical unresected patients achieve with conventional complete dentures (Garrett, 2008; Buurman et al., 2020b) (Fig 3-162). The most common sites employed are the residual zygomas; however, on occasion, some bone remains for implant placement in the pyriform rim region and the pyramidal process of the palatal bone to supplement them (Fig 3-162c). Implants do not obviate the need for skin grafting the raw tissues of the defect. They reduce soft tissue contracture and skin-lined surfaces can be more aggressively engaged with the obturator extensions, thus achieving a better seal around the defect (see Fig 3-132a). In addition, the prosthetic space is preserved and hygiene access around the bar and implants is enhanced. Note the number of attachments incorporated within the on bar. However, only two on each side were necessary to retain the prosthesis.

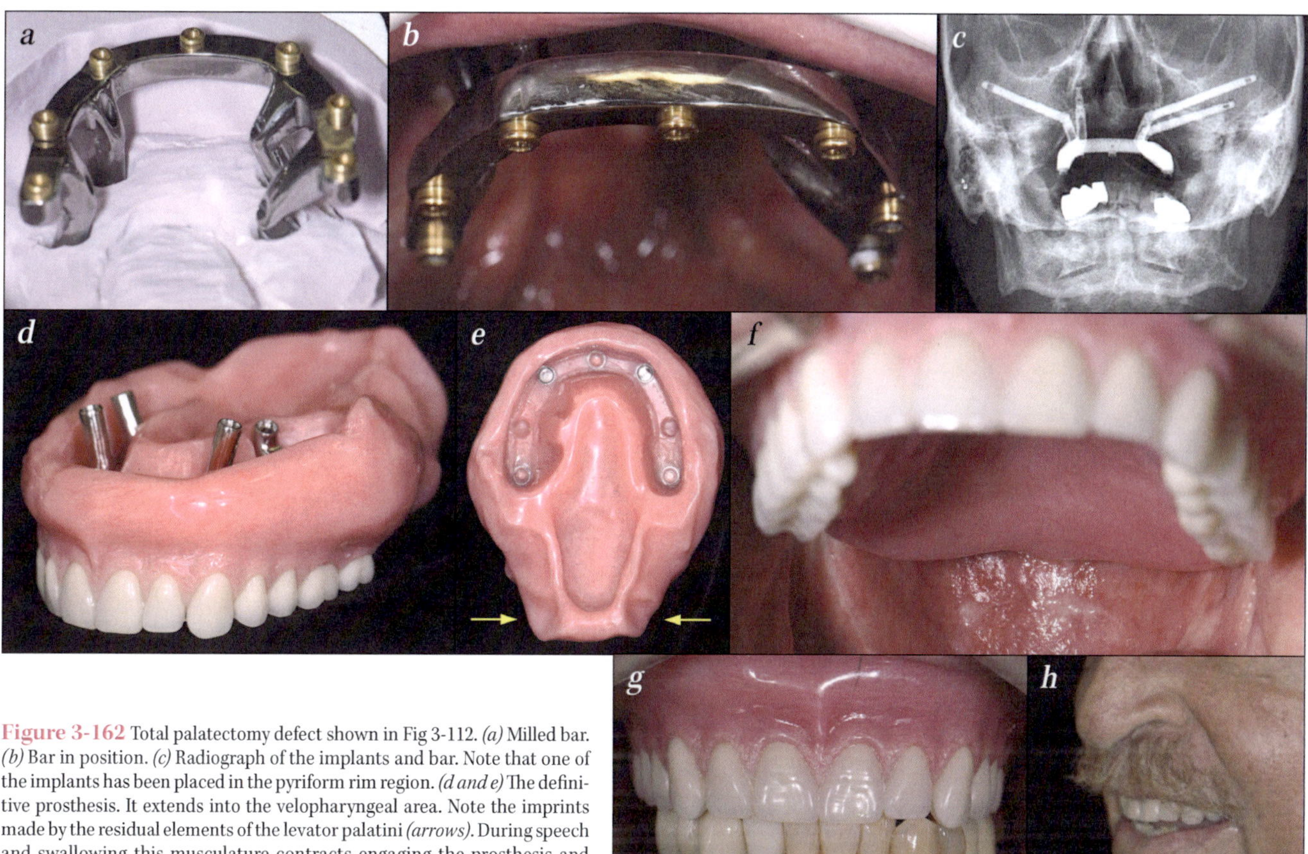

Figure 3-162 Total palatectomy defect shown in Fig 3-112. *(a)* Milled bar. *(b)* Bar in position. *(c)* Radiograph of the implants and bar. Note that one of the implants has been placed in the pyriform rim region. *(d and e)* The definitive prosthesis. It extends into the velopharyngeal area. Note the imprints made by the residual elements of the levator palatini *(arrows)*. During speech and swallowing this musculature contracts engaging the prosthesis and restoring velopharyngeal function. *(f)* The prosthesis in position. The posterior extension engages the functional musculature remaining in the posterior and lateral pharyngeal wall. *(g and h)* The aesthetic outcome.

Relining of obturator prostheses

Relining is required more often for patients with maxillary defects than for patients without such defects. In large defects, much of the support, retention, and stability for the obturator prosthesis is derived from the soft tissues of the defect, and these tissues are subject to change. The cheek surface and scar band at the junction of the skin graft and oral mucosa tend to stretch with time. The posterior margin of the defect is also subject to change if it extends into the area of velopharyngeal function. In addition, the medial bony margin of the defect remodels and becomes rounded. These changes are most noticeable during the first 18 months following surgery.

The reline must be performed with care and precision so that centric relation and the occlusal vertical dimension are maintained. Undercut areas of the obturator portion are removed. Acrylic resin adjacent to the finish line of the major connector is reduced, and this zone is perforated in several regions with a No. 4 round bur. The contours of the prosthesis are redeveloped with impression compound, as described earlier in this chapter. When border molding is completed, the impression compound is reduced by 1 to 2 mm, and either a thermoplastic wax or elastomeric impression material is used to refine the impression (Fig 3-163). We prefer thermoplastic wax when the defect is large and exhibits mobile peripheral tissues.

On completion, the impression is boxed and poured as described earlier. A reline jig is used so that all relationships are maintained. The reline jig is disassembled, the impression material is removed, the residual acrylic resin is reduced where necessary, and the reline is completed with autopolymerizing acrylic resin. The relined obturator prosthesis is delivered as described earlier. Pressure indicator paste and disclosing wax are used to verify that the prosthesis is properly adapted and extended into the defect. A clinical remount will ensure that occlusal relationships are maintained.

Vascularized Flaps and Osseointegrated Implants

Several techniques have been introduced combining the use of vascularized flaps with osseointegrated implants. The flaps are employed to obturate the defect, and the implants provide the means of retention, stability, and support for the prosthesis that replaces the dentition and adjacent structures. Both fixed and overlay removable designs have been used for the definitive prosthesis.

Rohner (2000, 2003, 2013) and colleagues (Jacquiery et al., 2004) popularized the use of vascularized osteomyocutaneous flaps combined with conventional dental implants. Variations of this approach have achieved widespread use. A number of different types of flaps have been used including flaps based on the fibula

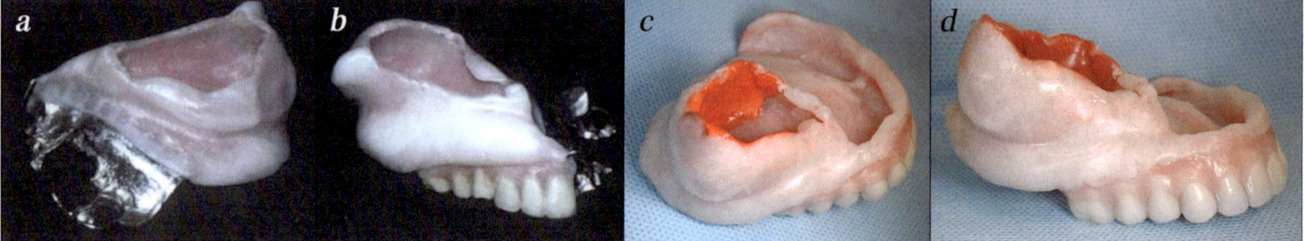

Figure 3-163 *(a and b)* Reline impression of a partially edentulous patient. These impressions were made with thermoplastic wax. *(c and d)* Wax reline of an edentulous patient.

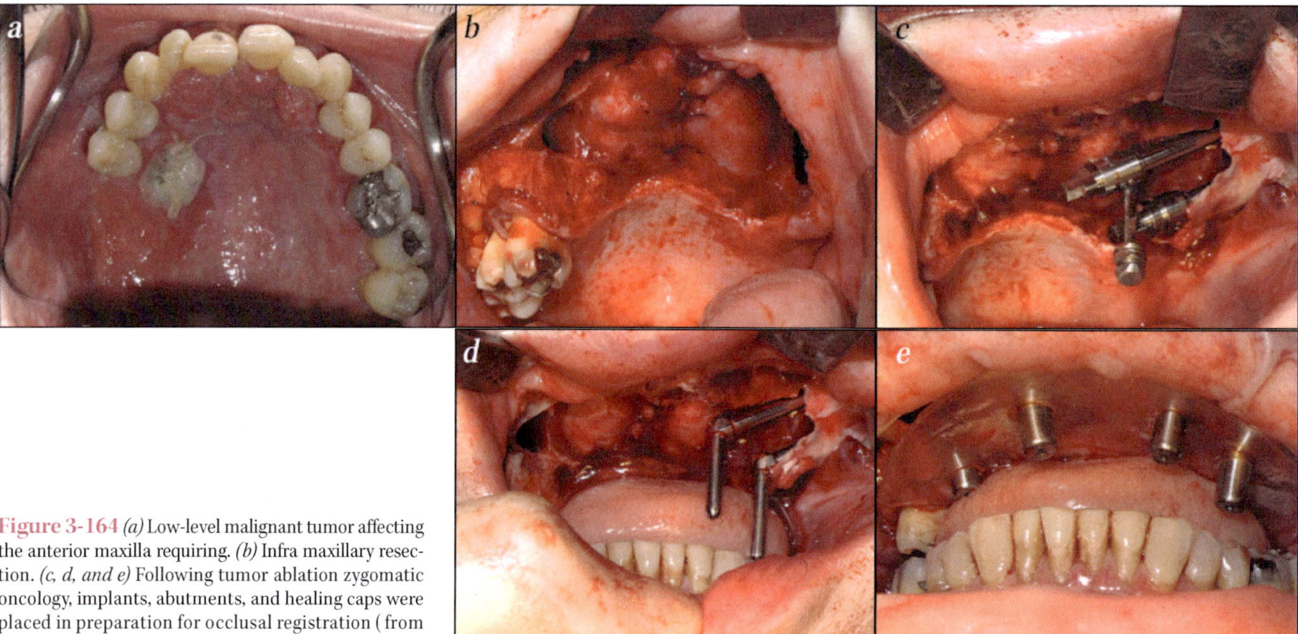

Figure 3-164 *(a)* Low-level malignant tumor affecting the anterior maxilla requiring. *(b)* Infra maxillary resection. *(c, d, and e)* Following tumor ablation zygomatic oncology, implants, abutments, and healing caps were placed in preparation for occlusal registration (from Butterworth and Rogers, 2017, with permission).

and the scapula and an iliac crest based on the deep circumflex iliac artery. Recently, Butterworth and colleagues (2017, 2019, 2022) introduced a new concept using zygomatic oncologic implants combined with vascularized soft tissue flaps (so-called ZIP flap technique). Korn and colleagues (2021) have used a similar approach where soft tissue flaps are used in combination with patient-specific digitally designed and manufactured subperiosteal implants.

Zygomatic implant perforated (ZIP) technique

Butterworth and colleagues (2017, 2019, 2021) have developed a novel technique utilizing zygomatic oncology implants and vascularized soft tissue flaps for the management of low-level tumors of the maxilla (Fig 3-164a). Following resection of the tumor (Fig 3-164b), the defect is measured to permit the harvesting of a slightly oversized fasci-cutaneous flap. The flap is oversized to account for contraction during healing and/or postoperative radiation therapy. Radial forearm flaps are most often employed (including composite radial forearm flaps to provide a strut of bone for additional facial support where deemed appropriate), but flaps from the lateral thigh have also been used.

Two zygomatic oncology implants are positioned into the zygoma on the resected side wherever possible. Implants are placed on the contralateral side as needed. The trajectory and spacing of the implants are similar to that recommended when the defect is left open and the implants are used to retain an obturator prosthesis (see Figs 3-117–3-121). The implant platforms should be angulated slightly anteriorly to provide adequate access postoperatively depending on the patient's mouth opening and the nature of the proposed prosthesis. When compromised teeth on the contralateral side occupy potential implant sites, they are removed, and zygomatic implants are placed immediately through the extraction socket. Implant abutments of at least 5 mm in length are secured to the zygomatic implants in order to ensure that they will perforate the flap (Fig 3-164e). Abutment-level impression copings are secured and an impression is made of the implant positions using a technique similar to that described previously (Fig 3-165a and b). Upon removal of the impression, abutment protection caps are secured to the abutments and a tentative centric relation record is made (Fig 3 165c).

The flap is carefully perforated over the zygomatic healing abutments using a small incision just through the skin layer, followed by blunt dissection to allow the abutment and cap to perforate the flap while ensuring a tight adaptation of the flap around the abutment (Fig 3-166). The flap anastomosis is then completed in the usual manner and the flap is secured into place.

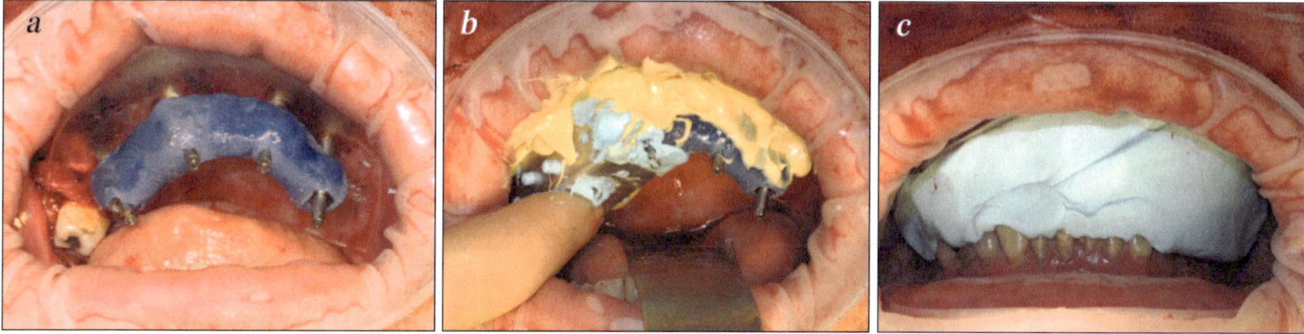

Figure 3-165 *(a and b)* Impression copings are secured, they are united with an autopolymerizing resin, and an impression is made. *(c)* Following removal of the impression a tentative centric relation is made at the estimated occlusal vertical dimension (from Butterworth and Rogers, 2017, with permission).

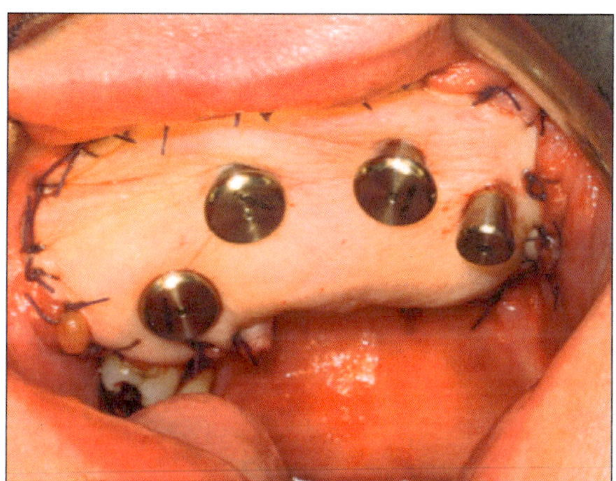

Figure 3-166 A radial forearm flap was inset and perforated to allow for penetration of the abutment healing caps (from Butterworth and Rogers, 2017, with permission).

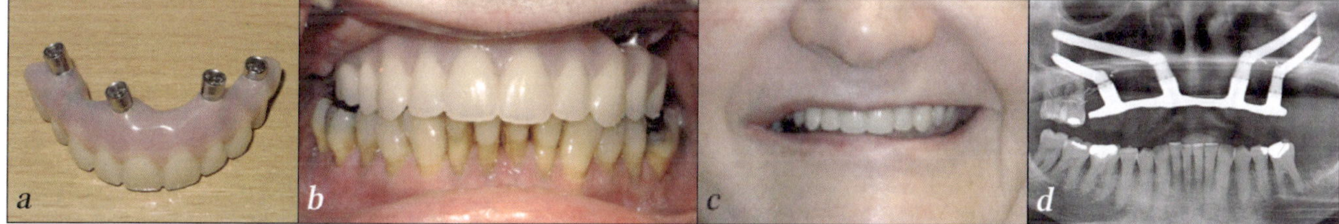

Figure 3-167 *(a)* Definitive metal-acrylic hybrid prosthesis. *(b)* Prosthesis in position three months following treatment. *(c)* Posttreatment aesthetic outcome. *(d)* Posttreatment panoramic radiograph showing implant distribution (from Butterworth and Rogers, 2017 with permission).

Three to four weeks later, after ensuring that the flap is viable, the healing caps are removed, and the prosthesis is tried by utilizing a metal framework as the substructure. In some instances, the flap will overgrow the healing caps and it may be necessary to make small incisions to expose them. The occlusal vertical dimension and centric relation record are verified, and changes are made as necessary. One week later, the definitive metal-acrylic prosthesis is delivered (Fig 3-167) and patients are fully restored prior to starting adjuvant radiotherapy if this is required for disease control. The patients are monitored and the prosthesis can be relined and/or rebased as the tissues settle and if the space beneath the prosthesis becomes problematic.

This technique has been employed primarily on patients undergoing so-called low-level maxillectomy. These resections preserve the orbital floor, the zygomatic prominence, and some bony support for the nose. As a result, midfacial contours are not dramatically affected by such resections (Fig 3-167c). All the prostheses are designed as fixed and screw-retained and are designed to replace the dentition and provide appropriate support for the lip.

In 2022, Butterworth et al. (2022) reported on the use of this approach on 35 patients following low-level maxillectomy. Thirty-four of these patients received zygomatic implants at the time of tumor ablation surgery and microvascular free flap reconstruction. One patient was treated 10 years following surgery and postoperative radiotherapy. The radial forearm flap was used in 27 patients, the composite radial forearm flap was used in 4 patients, and the anterolateral thigh flap was used in 4 patients. A total of 125 zygomatic implants were placed and supplemented by 19 conventional dental implants, although the majority of patients were treated with a "quad zygomatic" approach. All patients were restored with

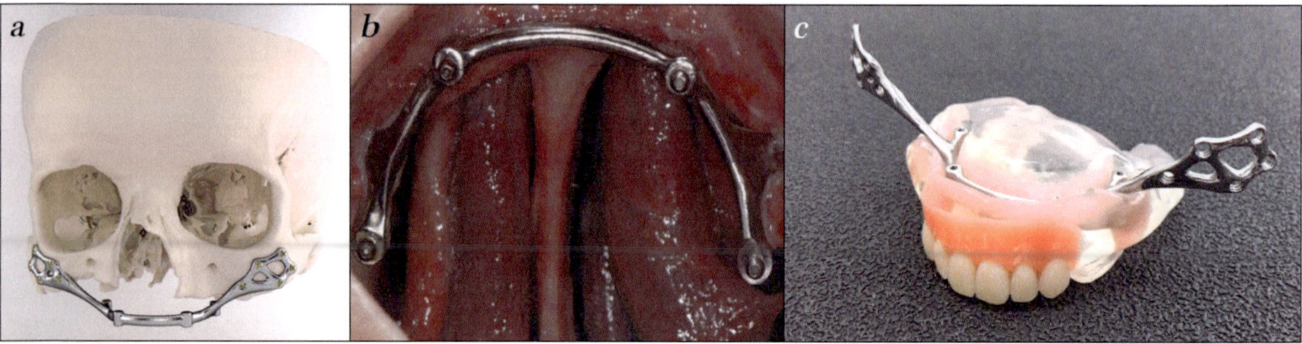

Figure 3-168. A patient-specific digitally designed subperiosteal implant for a patient with a bilateral subtotal inferior maxillectomy defect (Images Provided by Dr. Nathalie Vosselman, Groningen, Netherlands).

definitive implant-supported fixed metal-acrylic hybrid prostheses with the median time to restoration being 29 days (IQR 21–37 days) postoperatively. Patients are definitively restored even if adjuvant radiotherapy is required for disease control.

The mean patient follow-up period was 25 months with a range of 2–60 months. One patient, three months following radiotherapy, lost one zygomatic and one conventional implant. One soft tissue flap broke down following radiotherapy and the patient was fitted with an obturator prosthesis. Another patient, two years postsurgery, presented with a small fistula in close proximity to where a zygomatic implant perforated the soft tissue flap. This fistula was reclosed surgically. The overall reported zygomatic implant survival was 98.4% with a prosthesis survival of 97%. The overall quality of life was highly scored, with 19 patients reporting that their overall quality of life was excellent, very good, or good following the procedure (see section below entitled "Quality of life: Obturator prostheses and flaps combined with implants").

The peri-implant soft tissues are usually thick and mobile and as a result are susceptible to inflammation and hypertrophy. Because of the above, oral hygiene must be meticulous and the patient placed on close follow-up.

Patient-specific digitally designed and manufactured subperiosteal implants

Subperiosteal implants were first introduced in the 1940s and were most often employed in patients with severely atrophic mandibles that were unable to accommodate a conventional complete mandibular denture. They were most often fabricated of cobalt-chrome alloys. A two-stage surgical procedure was required. Initially, the bony foundation area was exposed, an impression of these areas was made, and the wound closed. At a subsequent appointment, the site was reexposed, and the implant was secured in position with two to three screws. In the 1980s, use of CT scans and the fabrication of stereolithographic models eliminated the necessity for the first surgical session. Occlusal forces were offset by the formation of fibrous slings around multiple struts of the implants that were positioned parallel to the occlusal plane. Results were mixed and most implants did not survive for extended periods. Their demise was predictable because cobalt-chrome was subject to corrosion. Corrosion, with the release of metallic ions into the surrounding tissue, triggered both acute and chronic inflammatory responses resulting in encapsulation of the implant in fibrous connective tissue. Subsequent epithelial migration, and with it, the development of extended peri-implant pockets and the associated chronic infection, ultimately led to the loss of the implant.

Contemporary subperiosteal implants are made of titanium and are digitally designed and manufactured. Titanium is not subject to corrosion, so the aforementioned fibrous encapsulation and epithelial migration associated with implants of cobalt-chrome presumably do not occur. A radiographic guide is made by duplicating the existing removable prosthesis and creating fiducial markers with gutta-percha or by applying adhesive removable radiographic fiducial markers to the existing prosthesis or its duplicate. The radiographic guide is worn while the CBCT scan is being performed. A separate scan of the radiographic guide allows the digital rendering of the prosthesis and the DICOM data from the patient scan to be merged, permitting the teeth and the contours of the proposed prosthesis to be superimposed onto the bony contours of the intended implant site. The implant is then designed and subsequently manufactured with selective laser melting. Clinical outcomes have been favorable. A recent retrospective report assessed the outcomes of 70 patients with pronounced bone atrophy, restored with fixed ceramo-metal restorations. After two years of follow-up, only three implants were lost, all due to recurrent infections. The complication rate was relatively low and comparable to the rates seen with the use of conventional osseointegrated titanium implants (Cerea and Dolcini, 2018).

This approach has recently been applied to the restoration of large maxillary defects (Vosselman et al., 2019; Korn et al., 2021; Fig 3-168). The implant framework is designed with two to four posts depending on the size and extent of the defect. It is designed to embrace the load-bearing paranasal and lateral facial buttresses but may be extended onto the residual portion of the zygomatic arch when appropriate. Implant anchorage is accomplished multivectorially with screws 1.2 to 1.5 mm in diameter and 2 mm in length The authors prefer to place at least 20 screws when the local bone sites are available. This approach is best utilized where the tumor resection is limited to a palatectomy or inferior maxillectomy. Removable prostheses using implant-connecting bar attachment systems have been used to restore the defect and replace the dentition. The defect may be reconstructed with a fasciocutaneous vascularized flap or local flaps prior to placement of the implant.

The report by Korn et al. (2021) retrospectively described their experience with 19 patients. Five of the 19 patients had been irradiated prior to implant placement. Fifteen of the 19 patients were reconstructed with free tissue transfers prior to implant placement. At follow-up, all implants were judged to be stable and there were no implant failures. Recurrent inflammation and hypertrophy of the soft tissues through which the implant posts extended and exposure of implant frameworks were reported, but these phenomena have not led to implant loss at the time of publication. An undisclosed number of the irradiated patients presented with abscesses or dehiscence, requiring additional microvascular tissue transfer. The average follow-up period was 26 months.

Long-term follow-up data for this method is lacking but it does offer a solution for patients lacking bone volume for the placement of endosseous titanium implants. Since these implants are fabricated of titanium, the tissue side effects of the aforementioned corrosion associated with cobalt-chrome implants are mitigated. However, the reported recurrent soft tissue inflammation and hypertrophy of the mucosa circumscribing the implant posts represent significant posttreatment morbidity. Moreover, the clinical significance of exposure of the implant framework is yet to be determined.

Osteomyocutaneous flaps and conventional implants

With the increasing sophistication of CAD-CAM technologies and the pioneering work of Rohner and his colleagues, new surgical methods have evolved, which when properly executed in an interdisciplinary environment, allow surgical reconstruction of large maxillary defects and provide patients with implant-retained prostheses that predictably restore form and function. Using these techniques, the surgical reconstruction and placement of implants are preplanned based on the occlusion and dental configuration of the opposing mandible (Rohner et al., 2000, 2003, 2013; Jacquéry, 2004). Digital planning and the use of surgical templates and resection guides enable accurate positioning of the osseous portion of the vascularized free flap and permit precise positioning of the dental implants. Using a two-stage surgical procedure, *the graft is preprepared* by placing implants into the donor bone and creating new peri-implant tissues by placing a split-thickness skin graft around these implants, thus creating immobile, attached, and keratinized peri-implant soft tissues. Six to eight weeks later, after the implants have osseointegrated and the split-thickness skin graft has been revascularized, the osteomyocutaneous flap is harvested, and the bone is osteotomized as preplanned and secured to a preprepared prosthesis or implant-connecting bar. The flap is then secured to the residual maxilla and skull base with miniplates to create a neomaxilla. The remaining palatal defect is closed with the soft tissues associated with the flap (Fig 3-169). The blood vessels are passed through a tunnel between the buccal surface of the mandible and the soft tissues of the cheek down into the neck and the matched vessels of the neck are identified for the anastomoses. In most instances, the facial, lingual, or maxillary artery is used as arterial inflow, whereas branches of the internal jugular vein or the internal jugular vein itself are used as venous outflow. With the help of the microscope, the vessels are anastomosed.

This method permits large maxillary defects to be surgically obturated and restored with implant-retained prostheses, which in many patients can be fixed. The main disadvantage of this innovative approach was the time required for the implants to osseointegrate and the skin graft to revascularize, rendering the procedure impractical for patients undergoing resection of malignant neoplasms (Chuka et al., 2017). In response to this shortcoming, several centers developed an alternative approach (Sharaf et al., 2010; Antony et al., 2011; Berrone et al., 2014; Kim et al., 2016; Seikaly et al., 2019; Patel et al., 2019). With this method, the implants are placed simultaneously with the harvesting of the osteomyocutaneous flap and reconstruction, significantly reducing treatment time. As was the case with the method developed by Rohner and his colleagues, the configuration of the flap and the positioning are based on the occlusion and dental configuration of the opposing mandible. The orientation and position of dental implants and the bone of the flap are preplanned based on the anticipated position of the prosthesis in the three-dimensional virtual surgical environment.

At many centers, after resection of the dentate jaw, microvascular reconstruction often is based on intraoperative intuitive decision-making. This creates a spatial design challenge when using osseointegrated implants for oral rehabilitation. The reconstructions at these centers are based on a bone-driven approach that generally includes the anterior surface of the maxilla as the templates for reconstruction, since these contours are deemed critical to the eventual cosmetic outcomes. Moreover, the position and angulation of the implants, frequently are not "prosthodontically driven." The patient is then referred to a prosthodontist for oral rehabilitation. As a result, in many patients, the functional occlusal reconstruction is suboptimal because the arrangement of the bony portions of the flap and the positioning of implants is not ideal. Moreover, with this approach, some clinicians have reported that up to a quarter of the implants could not be used because of malpositioning or improper angulation, even though they were osseointegrated (Hundepool et al., 2008; Fenlon et al., 2012).

Presurgical planning based on the occlusion and the dental configuration of the opposing arch represents a significant advance. This type of occlusal and functional reconstruction starts with VSP by developing the occlusion for the proposed prosthesis. Based on the existing dentition or a trial prosthesis, the prosthodontists can determine the most ideal positions for the dental implants. Once the implant positions are determined, the 3D location of the reconstruction bone can be finalized. The VSP reconstruction is then converted into a physical plan and implemented in the operating room using various surgical templates and resection guides.

The case for an interdisciplinary approach

Treatment and rehabilitation of jaw resection and reconstruction are highly specialized, and an interdisciplinary team with specialists across various disciplines is essential for achieving a successful outcome (Berrone et al., 2014; El Saghir et al., 2014; Patel et al., 2019; Pfister et al., 2020). This collaborative planning is crucial in the various aspects of the workflow. The surgeons are responsible for planning the soft and hard tissue resection margins, the type of defect reconstruction, the flap donor site, the length of the bone reconstruction segment(s), the positioning of the bony segment(s) within the soft tissue envelop, the access to vascular structures for the microvascular anastomoses, the effect of dental implant placement on the surgery and adjunctive treatment, and the type of plating systems used to name a few. The prosthodontist needs to consider the

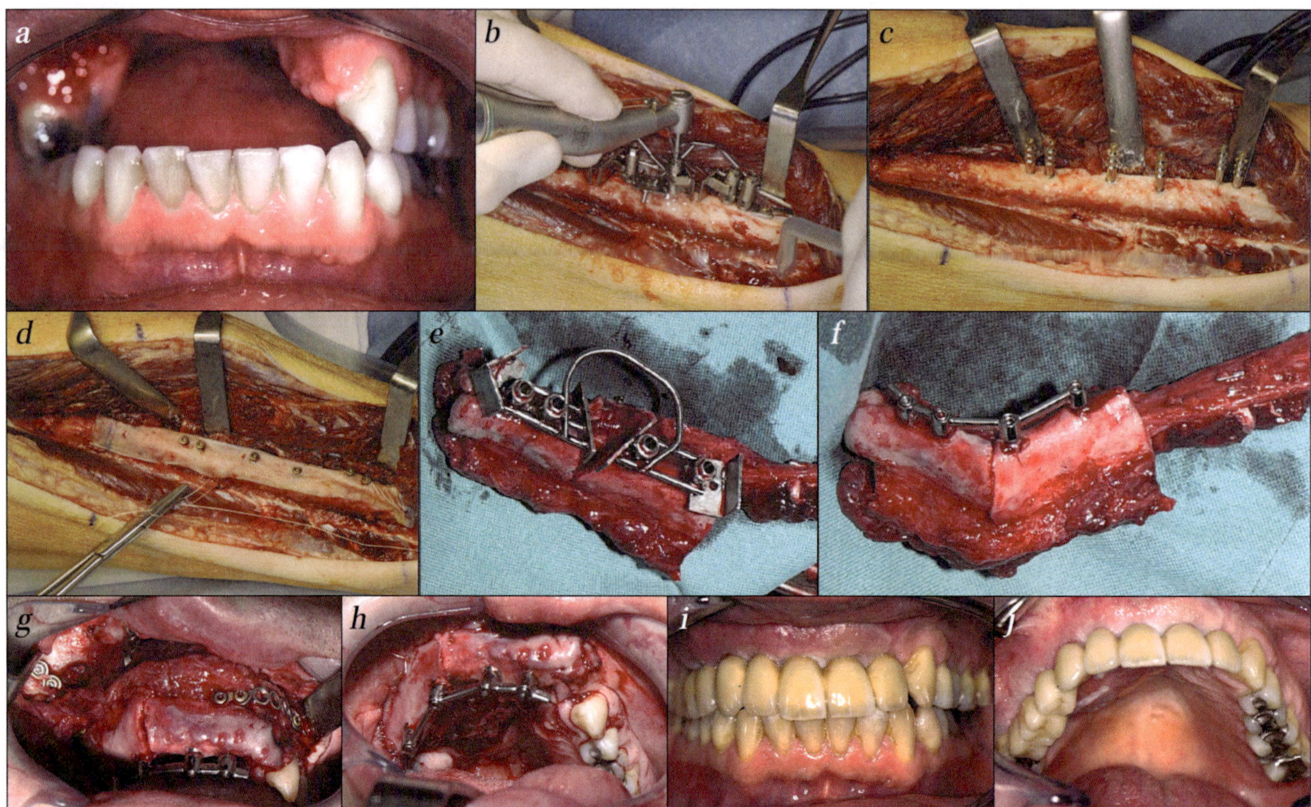

Figure 3-169 The "Rohner" technique based on occlusally driven reconstruction. *(a)* Surgical defect. *(b)* A digitally designed resection and drill guide is used to place implants into the fibula in the desired locations. *(c)* The implants in position. *(d)* A split-thickness skin graft is applied to the fibular designed to circumscribe the implants. The wound is closed, and the implants are allowed to osseointegrate. *(e and f)* Six to eight weeks later the fibula is reexposed, the drill/osteotomy guide resecured, and the osteotomies completed. Note that the implants emerge through the skin-lined fibula. An implant-connecting bar is used to stabilize the fibula. *(g and h)* The fibula is secured in position with miniplates. *(i and j)* Completed prosthesis. Note palatal contours are near normal (courtesy of Dr. D. Rohner).

Box 3-3 Five levels of approach to jaw reconstruction

Increasing levels of accuracy and sophistication	V	Navigation and robotics—no need for physical models as digital planning and robot will assist surgeon in resection and reconstruction
	IV	Planned functional reconstruction—fully guided and occlusion based—3D printed models, resection guides, occlusal transfer templates—all planned based on occlusion
	III	Guided anatomical reconstruction—digitally planned and guided—use of 3D printed models, resection guides
	II	Planned anatomical reconstruction—digitally planned but unguided—use of 3D printed models
	I	Anatomical reconstruction—intraoperative intuitive surgery

Courtesy of Dr. John Wolfaardt.

edentulous defect, propose oral rehabilitation, identify the position of the dentition, and determine the position, angulation, and number of the implants and their spacing; the prosthetic space needed for the future prosthesis; mouth opening and access issues; the 3D positioning of the reconstruction bone segments; and how that will affect the prosthodontic outcome, among other things.

The most reliable functional and occlusal reconstructions in patients with jaw defects are obtained with occlusion-based reconstruction with 3D printed models, resection guides, flap osteotomy guides, implant guides, articulation splints, and miniplates or custom midfacial plates (level IV in Box 3-3). This can be achieved using different approaches that require VSP.

Surgical factors

The main requirement for achieving a consistent functional outcome is to place the bony reconstruction in the correct three-dimensional spatial position based on the occlusion (Patel et al., 2019; Seikaly et al., 2019). The use of VSP has increased over the past decade. VSP-assisted reconstructions provide superior outcomes in terms of maintaining and restoring three-dimensional spatial relationships of the reconstruction (Okay et al., 2013; Toro et al., 2007; Antony et al., 2011; Ueda et al., 2013; Zheng et al., 2013), have been shown to be more accurate (Weitz et al., 2016; Wu et al., 2016; Ochi et al., 2013; Zhang et al., 2016), and also result in a decrease in surgical time (Weitz et al., 2016; Seruya et al., 2013; Hanasono et al., 2008; Toto et al., 2015) when compared to intraoperative surgical design or analog planning. Studies suggest that there is no increase in rates of surgical complications (Weitz et al., 2016; Toto et al., 2015), morbidity, flap survival (Seruya et al., 2013; Toto et al., 2015), and aesthetic outcomes (Toro et al., 2007; Antony et al., 2011; Ueda et al., 2013; Zheng et al., 2013) in patients treated with VSP-guided reconstructive surgery as compared to those treated with conventional intuitive intraoperative reconstruction design. VSP-assisted reconstructions provide superior outcomes in terms of maintaining and restoring three-dimensional spatial relationships of the reconstruction (Okay et al., 2013; Toro et al., 2007; Antony et al., 2011; Ueda et al., 2013; Zheng et al., 2013).

Limits

A potential disadvantage of these protocols is the uncertainty in planning resection margins preoperatively in oncologic cases. However, in instances where the resection margins must be extended beyond the virtual planning, the relevant parts of the plan can still be used and augmented with classical reconstructive techniques. In spite of careful presurgical resection planning, one can never definitively predict the nature of the disease and how rapidly it can spread, and in those instances, a return to classical resection and reconstructive techniques is warranted.

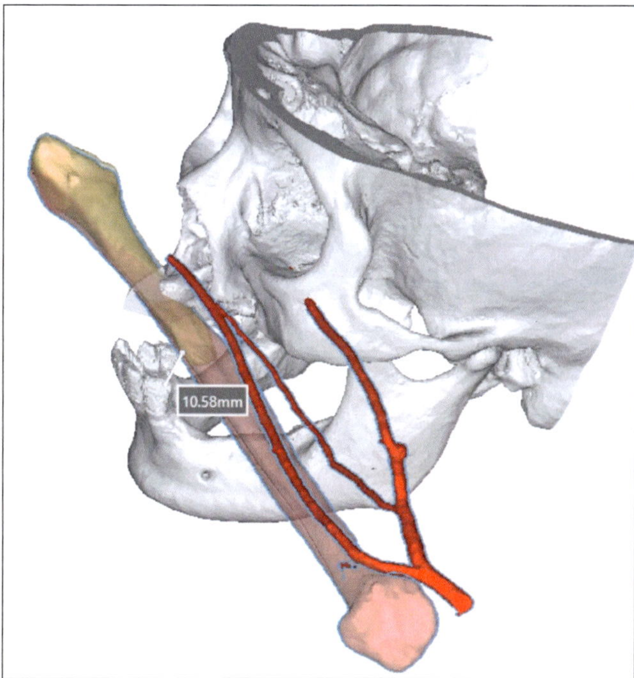

Figure 3-170. Fibula superimposed on a proposed palatal defect. The blood vessels are passed through a tunnel between the buccal surface of the mandible and the soft tissues of the cheek down into the neck and the matched vessels of the neck are identified for the anastomoses.

Indications and contraindications

Patients without significant medical comorbidities who can undergo a lengthy microvascular reconstructive surgery are good candidates for reconstruction. The jawbone defect must be a minimum of 2 cm in size. The procedure is contraindicated in patients who are not able to tolerate prolonged surgery, have poor or abnormal vascularity of the proposed donor sites, or are not motivated or whose treatment plan includes prosthetic obturation. The only absolute contraindication of microvascular reconstruction is hypercoagulability such as factor V Leiden thrombophilia, protein C or S deficiency, antiphospholipid syndrome, etc.

Choice of reconstruction flap

Several potential microvascular options exist, including the fibula-free flap (FFF), the deep circumflex iliac artery (DCIA) flap, and the scapula-free flap. The fibula-free flap is the most common microsurgical choice for maxillary reconstruction and is preferred by most clinicians (Seikaly et al., 2003; Ide et al., 2015; Patel et al., 2019). The fibula has a long bone (up to 25 cm) that can be osteotomized into multiple segments to re-create the maxillary and alveolar ridge contour (Fig 3-170). It also has sufficient bony width to accommodate dental implants of 4–5 mm in diameter. Its thick and dense cortical bone enables excellent primary stability of implants, especially with bicortical engagement. Moreover, its long pedicle can easily reach the cervical or temporal vessels for primary microvascular anastomosis without undue tension (Hayden et al., 2012). The distant surgical site allows a simultaneous two-team approach minimizing operating room time and cost. Its skin paddle is used to obturate the maxillary defect. The paranasal/zygomatic buttresses and pterygoid plates when preserved assist in vertical and horizontal stabilization of the fibula (Kim et al., 2016). The bone stock can be further augmented with a mixture of autogenous bone or allograft and mesenchymal stem cells (Barber et al., 2016; Dziegielewski et al., 2014; Kim et al., 2016).

An alternative is the DCIA flap, which provides ample bone stock for implant placement. The internal oblique muscle is often harvested with this flap to close the soft tissue defect and mucosalized to provide an adequate intraoral lining. The main limitations of this flap include a relatively short pedicle length and a higher rate of donor-site morbidity. In addition, the natural curvature of the iliac crest bone makes re-creation of the maxillary contour with osteotomies more complicated (Kim et al., 2016).

The scapula-free flap also offers adequate soft and hard tissue for maxillary reconstruction. Multiple independent skin paddles, muscle, and bone based on the subscapular system can be harvested to reconstruct complex maxillary defects involving both hard and soft tissue with minimal donor-site morbidity. This flap is less affected by atherosclerotic disease and may be the best option for patients with moderate to severe peripheral vascular disease. A significant disadvantage of this flap is the inability to perform a simultaneous two-team approach (Kim et al., 2016). Additionally, the shape of the bone, overlaying muscle, and juxtaposition of the perforator vessels make seating of the cutting guide less accurate and primary implant placement challenging.

Insetting the reconstruction flap

The flap is usually anchored to the maxillary buttress or zygoma posteriorly and the premaxilla or maxillary nasal buttress anteriorly. The pterygoid plates do not provide a stable platform for fixation and usually result in a nonideal lingual positioning of the bone. Reconstruction of high maxillectomy defects involving the orbital floor/rim with the fibula-free flap is difficult with the need for multiple osteotomies and complex orientation of the skin paddle. High maxillectomy defects with paranasal facial collapse require the use of paranasal strut bone grafts from discarded fibula segments or double-barreling of the fibula flap. When a hybrid-type fixed

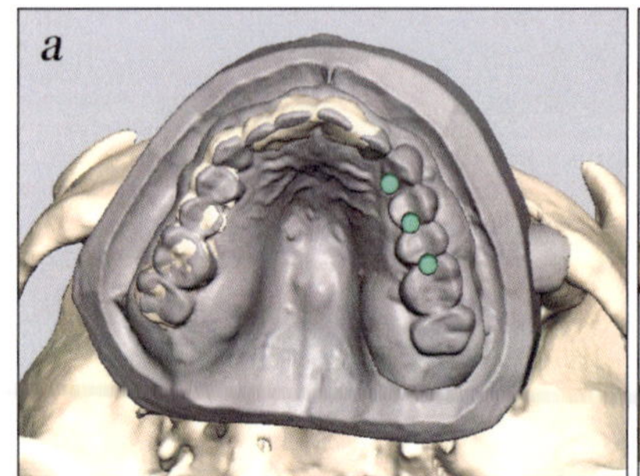
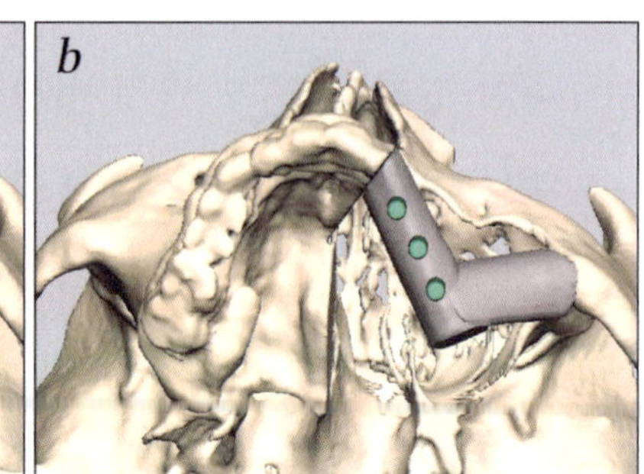

Figure 3-171 *(a and b)* Implant sites are "prosthodontically driven." When implants are arranged in a linear configuration, at least 3 implants should be placed.

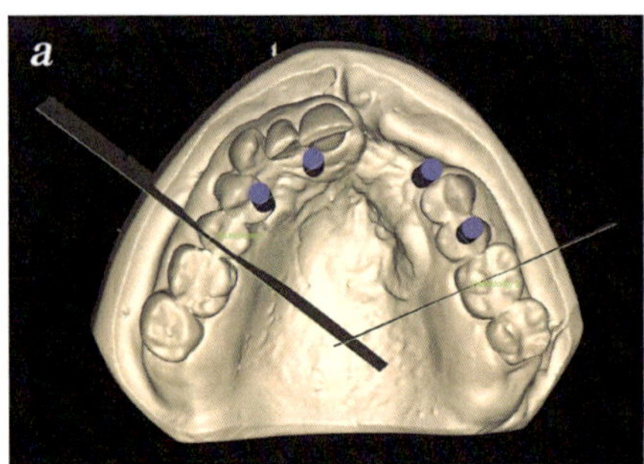
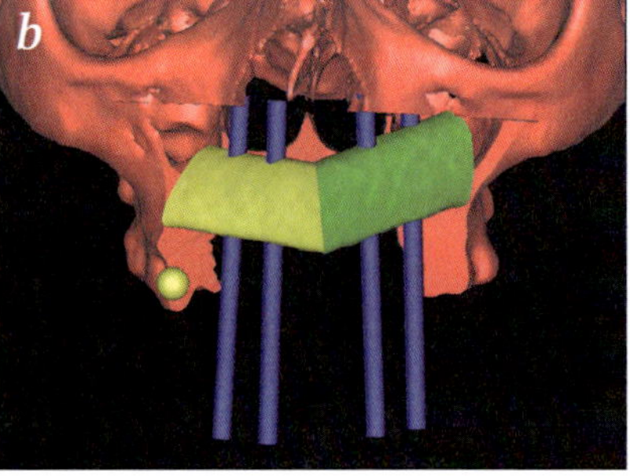

Figure 3-172 The defect will encompass the anterior curvature of the maxillary alveolar ridge. Implant distribution should idealize the A-P spread.

prosthesis is planned, and when a fibula is used, the lower surface of the fibula bone restoring the alveolar ridge should be placed at least 15 mm above the occlusal plane to provide sufficient prosthetic space when the soft tissue defect is minimal and primary closure of gingival tissues is possible in benign osseous neoplasms. However, when a skin flap is needed for closure for a palatal defect, additional prosthetic space is advised. This amount of prosthetic space is more difficult to account for in the maxilla as compared to the mandible lest you encroach into the nasal cavity by placing the bony graft superiorly. The skin flap is configured to restore the soft tissue defect and to account for tissue contracture during healing and is sutured to the mucosal margins of the defect.

Implant selection and position

Macro design. The use of tapered self-tapping implants should be avoided when the fibula has been used to reconstruct the maxillary defect. When tapered, self-tapping implants are inserted, the stresses can be excessive and, in some cases, trigger cracks in the fibula adjacent to the implant osteotomy sites, which can lead to fractures of the fibula. Implants with parallel walls are preferred, and the osteotomy sites are prepared in the usual way and tapped prior to inserting the implants.

Length. When the fibula is used, bicortical stabilization of the implants is desired. Parallel wall implants have a taper at the apical end and will not effectively engage the apical cortex, so the length of the implant selected needs to be slightly longer than the thickness of the fibula in order to achieve effective bicortical engagement. As a result, they will protrude slightly apically (see Fig 3-187), but this protrusion is inconsequential, as it will be covered by soft tissue associated with the flap or local tissues.

Diameter. Wide-diameter implants should not be used when the fibula is used to reconstruct the maxillary defect. Creating a large osteotomy in the fibula and engaging both the facial and the palatal sides of the cortices weaken the fibula, predisposing to cracks and fracture and leading to resorption of bone around the implant. Therefore, implants of 4 mm in diameter are recommended depending on the width of the bone stock. If most of the implants are less than 4 mm in diameter, when the fibular is narrow, the definitive prosthesis should be implant-assisted.

Spacing, numbers, angulation, and distribution pattern. Implants placed in native normal bone are generally positioned at least 3 mm apart. However, to avoid stressing the fibula during preparation of the osteotomy sites, and to mitigate the impact of microfractures adjacent to the osteotomy sites, a minimum of 5 mm of spacing is recommended. Additionally, because peri-implantitis is prevalent when implants emerge through skin the additional spacing facilitates hygiene access and treatment resolution (see section below entitled "Stage II implant surgery"). Lastly, 5 mm of interimplant spacing allows for the placement of plate fixation screws if a customized reconstruction plate is used to secure the fibula in position and stabilize the osteotomy sections.

When the implants are arranged in a linear configuration, at least three should be considered. The addition of a third implant dramatically improves the biomechanics of the restoration (Rangert et al., 1997; Wu et al., 2022) and the clinical outcomes (Lekholm et al., 1994; Gunne et al., 1994) (Fig 3-171). When the defect extends anteriorly to encompass the curvature of the maxillary arch, additional implants are needed. In addition, every effort should be made to optimize the A-P spread so as to idealize biomechanics and enhance the effects of cross-arch stabilization (Wu et al., 2022) (Fig 3-172).

Implants restoring the posterior dentition should be angled such that occlusal forces are directed along their long axis and compatible with the curve of Wilson and the curve of Spee. This is particularly important when the implants are aligned in a linear configuration where cross-arch stabilization is not possible (Fig 3-173).

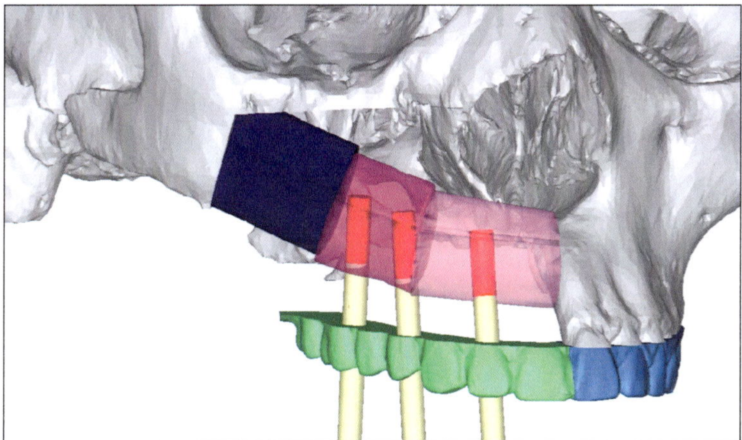

Figure 3-173 Implants restoring posterior teeth should be aligned compatible with the curve of Spee and the curve of Wilson so that posterior occlusal forces will be directed along their long axis. The prosthetic space can be determined during the virtual planning stage. Notice that to allow adequate prosthetic space, the fibula is inset partly into the nasal cavity.

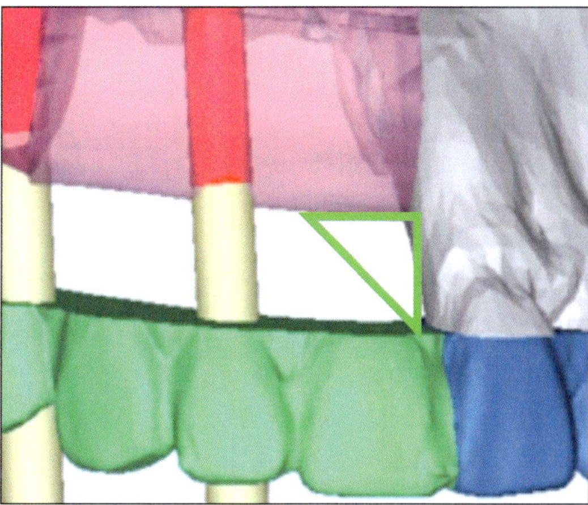

Figure 3-174 The Implant adjacent to a vertical alveolar defect should be positioned outside the right isosceles triangle formed by the height of the vertical bony wall and the fibula crest.

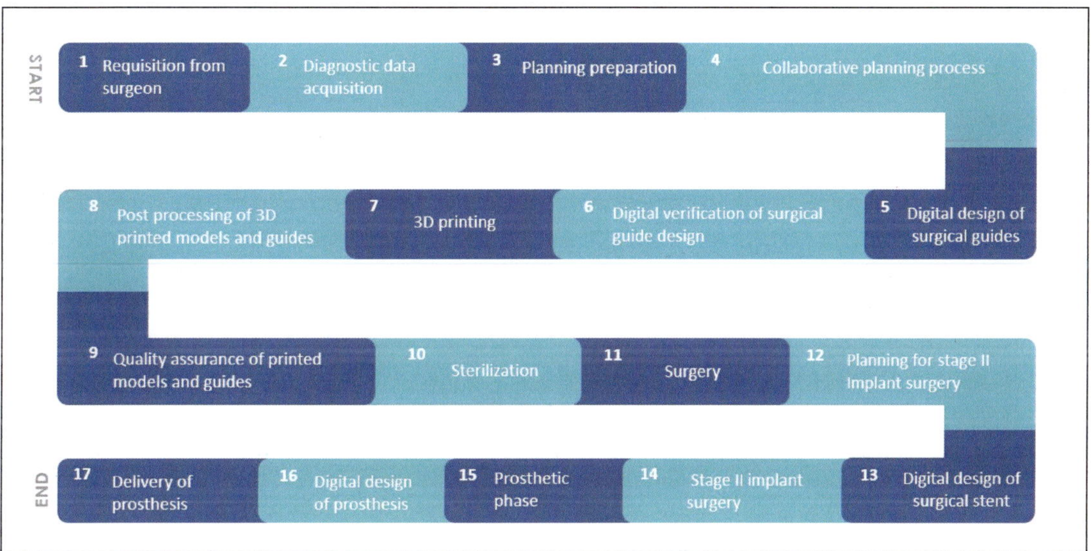

Figure 3-175 Digital workflow used in the reconstruction of a maxillary defect.

The distance of the implant osteotomy to the cut edge of a fibula segment should be no less than 4 mm. Additional spacing is also advised between the first implant adjacent to the alveolar margin. In the example depicted in Fig 3-174, the vertical bony cut was made adjacent to the left central incisor. The bony drop-off from the alveolar crest adjacent to this tooth to the fibula crest will have a tendency to tent the soft tissue such that the implants in this zone will have excessively deep peri-implant tissues. Therefore, we advise that no implant be planned within the base of a right isosceles triangle measured from the alveolar crest adjacent to the terminal tooth and the fibula. In other words, if the vertical drop-off is 6 mm, then the first implant should be planned 6 mm away from the defect margin (Fig 3-174).

Prosthetic space

The vertical positioning of the reconstructed fibula segment can be altered based on prosthodontic needs (Figs 3-173 and 3-174). As measured from the fibula crest to the occlusal plane, this equates to 16–18 mm. This practice will ensure appropriate hygiene access for the future prosthesis. When implants emerge through skin flaps, the additional thickness of the soft tissues overlying the bone stock needs to be thinned. Patients who receive postoperative radiation or chemoradiation warrant special consideration to avoid devascularizing the osteomyocutaneous flap (see section below entitled "Stage II implant surgery").

Digital design procedures

With the evolution of VSP, an optimal pathway has been created for a digital workflow in the surgical-prosthodontic continuum for head and neck cancer patients. The digital workflow, as elaborated in Fig 3-175, provides a general overview of the process.

The first step is for the surgical team to prescribe a head CT scan and a donor-site CT scan angiogram to check for congenital

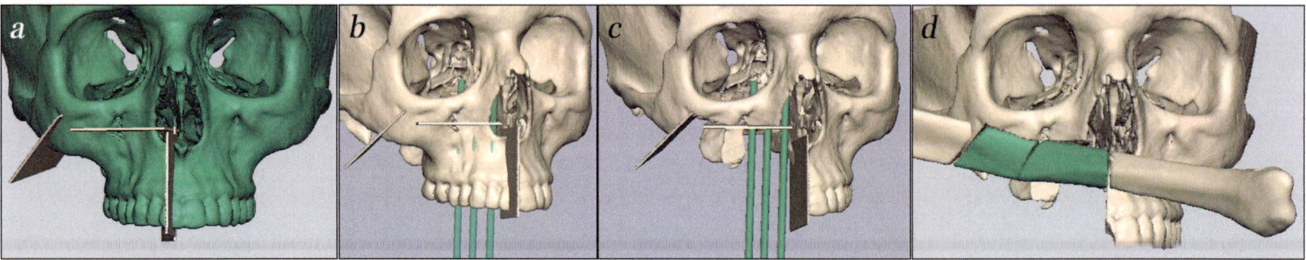

Figure 3-176 *(a, b, and c)* Three rectangular planes represent proposed resection margins for patient presenting with a tumor of the maxilla. *(b and c)* Proposed implant positions with the simulated subtotal right maxillectomy resected portion of the maxilla removed. *(d)* The osteotomized left fibula overlayed as the proposed bony reconstruction.

vascular anomalies and peripheral vascular disease. The prosthodontist makes impressions of the dental arches. If the area to be reconstructed is partially or completely edentulous, then either a digital or an analog wax-up of the missing teeth is needed for subsequent planning of implant positions. In the case of complete edentulism, a trial complete denture needs to be verified and worn during the head CT scan after radiographic markers (fiducial makers) are added. The trial denture is also scanned and later merged with the head CT scan. It is critical for the accuracy of any tooth-borne guides that digitized data of dental casts or intraoral scans are provided, since CT scan data of teeth can be riddled with dental artifacts.

Ahead of the planning session, the biomedical engineer merges the dental data with the CT scan data. The prosthodontist, the reconstructive surgeon(s), and the biomedical engineers meet to discuss and plan the jaw resection and the occlusion-based reconstruction. The biomedical engineer has been trained in the use of advanced digital software, has a working knowledge of the surgical anatomy, and assists with using the digital design software in the planning process. The surgeon finalizes resection margins and the size and contour of the bone segments used in the reconstruction. The prosthodontist determines the planned oral rehabilitation and the position and angulation of the dental implants. The position of the osseous reconstruction is collaboratively finalized between the prosthodontist and surgeon.

Resection. The first step is to identify the surgical resection margins, which are determined by the ablative surgeon. In the example shown in Fig 3-176, notice how three rectangular planes of specific dimensions were maneuvered to simulate the anterior, superior, and posterior en bloc resection. The 1 mm thickness is just wider than the width of the oscillating saw blade used in the procedure. The 3 cm length of the rectangle matches the slit length of the future guides. The same anterior and posterior planes will direct the software to make the distal and proximal fibula osteotomies (Fig 3-176a and d). Once the surgical defect is known, the reconstruction follows.

Osseous reconstruction. The osseous reconstruction considers facial symmetry, tooth positions, avoiding sharp turns, and avoiding fibula segments smaller than 2 cm. The dental implants are positioned next, and lastly the positions and angulations of both the fibula and the implants are finalized.

The left leg is the default donor side for anyone who drives and who is right-footed. The biomedical engineer is asked to "toggle on" to the donor fibula and the teeth or trial tooth arrangement to orient the reconstruction. The proximal fibula is oriented toward the side of the recipient neck vessels, ipsilateral toward the defect. For bilateral defects, either neck may be an option. In the right maxillectomy example shown in Fig 3-176, the proximal fibula is positioned toward the zygoma and the distal fibula toward the anterior alveolar margin. The fibula is situated with the anterior border in an occlusal direction and the lateral border facially. Because these two borders will have only periosteum and no muscle, artery, or vein overlaying them, they are the most ideal for the placement of dental implants and plating (Fig 3-177).

Palatofacially, the graft is positioned within the defect to restore facial symmetry while encompassing the roots of the ipsilateral dentition, which are "toggled on" during virtual insetting. As long as the graft encompasses the tooth roots by at least one millimeter, it will allow for the subsequent planning of dental implants.

The osseous spine found in the anterior border of the middle fibula can be thin enough to complicate dental implant placement. The reconstructive surgeon and prosthodontist must determine how to best address this situation. Five options are available. The first three are the best-case scenarios. The latter two options carry additional risk to the perforator vessels and periosteal blood supply to the fibula.

1. Rotating the fibula on its axis to direct the spine either in the direction of the implant axis or deliberately away so as to have the implant emerge more from the lateral border of the fibula.
2. Using a narrower implant (3.5 mm) instead of 4 mm. This is the simplest alternative when the spine is moderately thin (5.5 mm) with 1 mm on either side of the implant assuming the guide is very well fitting.
3. Using a subcrestal implant and countersinking the implant. This option may also be combined with the placement of a 3.5 mm–wide implant. It is critical to use a countersink drill to develop an appropriate emergence to allow abutment connection.
4. Switching to the contralateral leg and rotating the fibula on its axis so that the dental implant enters the broader posterior border of the fibula. This requires a modification of the combination fibula-implant surgical guide (see Fig 3-184c).
5. Osteoplasty of the spine, as is done on a thin resorbed alveolar ridge until a wide enough platform is prepared. Because this technique reduces the periosteal blood supply to the fibula segment, its benefit must be weighed against the increased risk to the flap survival. If this option is selected a reduction guide is needed and the implant length is selected based on the reduced intercortex width of the fibula. Ide et al. (2015) investigated the anatomical characteristics and available fibula bone volume for installing implants. They concluded that the cross section of the middle part of the fibula is triangular in shape and will require osteoplasty to flatten the surface to create a platform for implant placement.

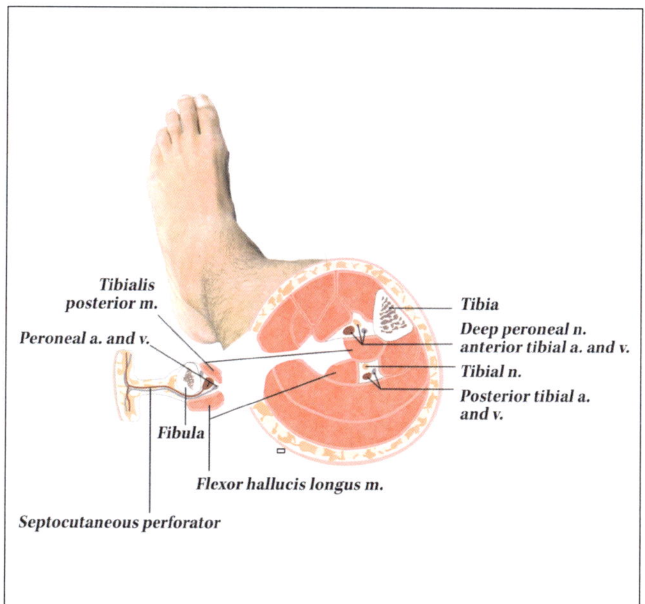

Figure 3-177 This axial cut through the lower leg shows the harvested osteomyocutaneous fibula flap. Note that the superior-lateral borders are free of vessels and muscle. The medial (deep) and posterior borders are closely associated with the peroneal artery, vein septocutaneous perforator artery, vein and tibialis poster, and flexor hallucis longis muscle.

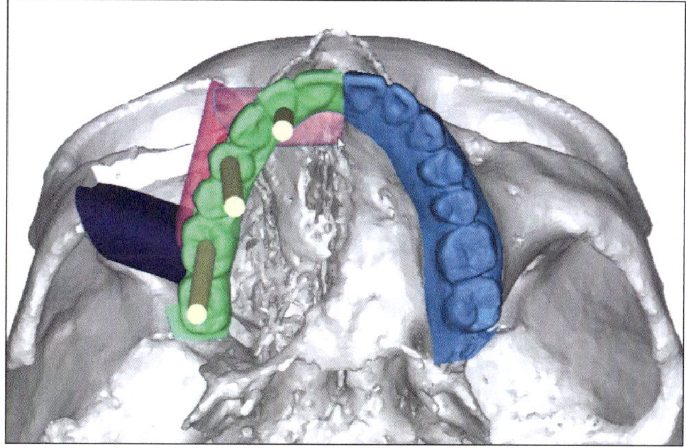

Figure 3-178 Midline maxillectomy reconstructed with a three-piece fibula. Cylinders representing the implants are positioned along the long axis of the first molar, second premolar, and lateral incisor. Note that the second molar site, since its position is posterior to the fibula.

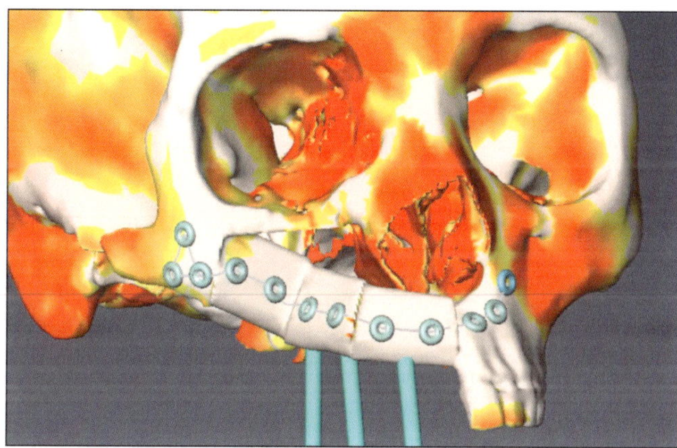

Figure 3-179 Custom reconstruction midfacial plate. Fixation screw holes are positioned two per fibula segment and three on either end for the residual facial bones. In this example, there are three on the zygoma and three along the piriform rim avoiding the tooth roots.

Once the fibula axis rotation and whether or not to flatten the thin spine are determined, the software uses the rectangular plane used for the maxillary alveolus resection (Fig 3-176a, b, and c) to make the first fibula cut (Fig 3-176d). About 6–8 cm of distal fibula is preserved to maintain the stability of the ankle. The subsequent fibula cuts are made as wedge osteotomies to produce the desired angle between fibula segments. The final and most proximal fibula cut is made with the same rectangular plane determined for the posterior maxillectomy margin; Fig 3-176 shows an example where the posterior maxillectomy margin is midway through the body of the right zygoma.

Positioning the implants. The prosthodontist can then develop the plans for oral rehabilitation. The biomedical engineer is asked to toggle on the dentition within the maxillectomy defect and to import cylinders of the same width as the proposed implants but longer so that the angulation and screw access can be appreciated (Figs 3-173 and 3-178). The prosthodontist directs the engineer to superimpose the cylinders over the native dentition following the long axis of the tooth and tooth roots.

When we take into account the recommended interimplant spacing, implant to osteotomy distance, spacing from the alveolar margin, and minimum fibula segment length, it may become necessary to modify the previously positioned fibula segments. Fig 3-178 illustrates why placement of an implant in the second molar site can be impossible. Either the fibula extends to the pterygoid plates, which are often too medial relative to the molar sites, or an acute angle is formed between the lateral and zygoma segments. Note also that the implants are placed along the long axis of the tooth following the occlusal curves of Spee and Wilson, which means some acceptable divergence of the dental implants.

Designing custom reconstruction plates. The fibula can be secured with either miniplates or customized milled titanium reconstruction plates. Fixation screw holes are positioned two per fibula segment and three on either end for the residual facial bones (Fig 3-179).

Designing maxillectomy, fibula osteotomy, and dental implant guides. After completing the surgical plan and before closing the collaborative planning session, a list of the 3D printed models and guides is prescribed: preoperative skull, the reconstructed maxilla, surgical guides, and the articulation splint.

Tooth-supported maxillectomy guide. Tooth-supported guides require either a direct intraoral scan of the dentition or a desktop scan of a cast. Once provided with this data, the biomedical engineer should merge and align the surface scan of the dentition with the CT scan of the head. The maxillectomy guide is designed to index all available teeth as they present prior to resection. The rectangular plane used to simulate the anterior maxillectomy cut during the planning session is toggled on and is used to orient a digital model of a metal cutting sleeve. The actual metal sleeve will be cemented or press-fitted postprocessing to the printed nylon or resin guide. Fig 3-180 shows the final CAD of a tooth-supported anterior

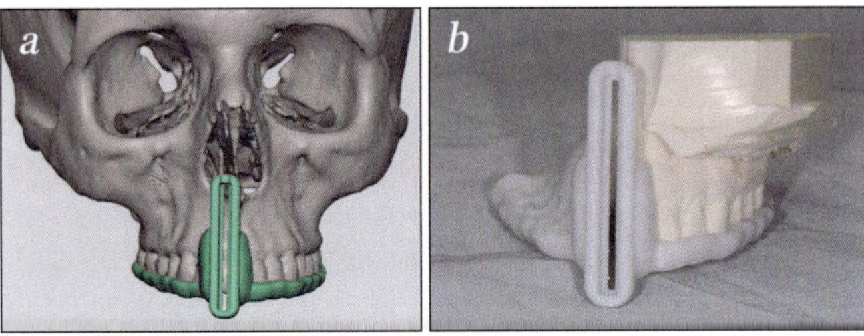

Figure 3-180 *(a)* Digital design of the maxillary resection guide. *(b)* The printed resection guide verified on the cast.

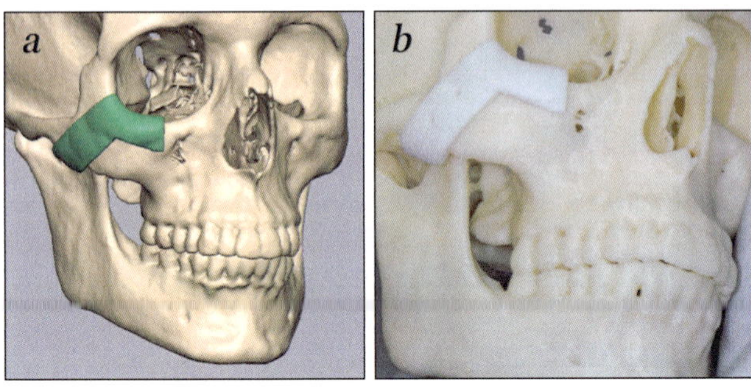

Figure 3-181 *(a)* CAD of the bone-supported zygomatic resection guide. *(b)* The printed zygomatic resection guide seated on a printed model of the skull.

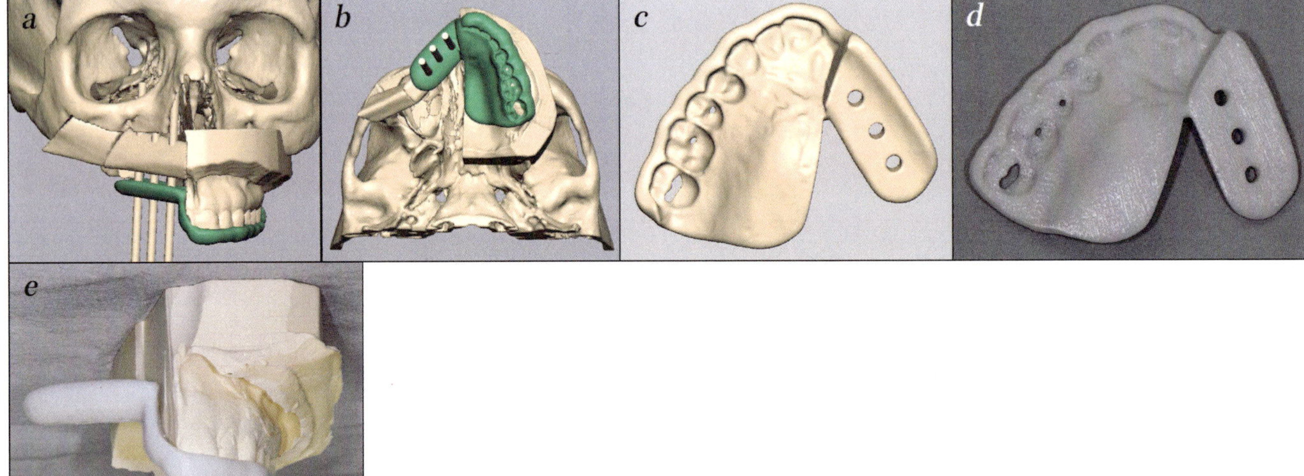

Figure 3-182 *(a–b)* The IBAS with interocclusal extension designed. *(c)* Intaglio surface of the IBAS. *(d)* The printed splint. *(e)* The printed IBAS seated on an altered cast representing the residual dentition following the resection.

maxillary osteotomy guide and the printed guide prior to cementation of the metal sleeve. Once printed, the tooth-supported guide is verified on a maxillary cast (Fig 3-180b) or printed model. Even one periodontally stable tooth can improve indexing for an osteotomy guide. In the edentulous patient, however, or for cuts distant to the dentition, a bone-supported guide is designed (Fig 3-181).

Bone-supported maxillectomy guide. When tooth support is not possible due to location or edentulism, a bone-supported surgical template is prescribed. The rectangular planes used in the planning session to simulate the superior and posterior margins of the maxillectomy (Fig 3-176a) are toggled on and used to create 5 mm–tall edges. Unlike a metal sleeve, which works well when access is unhindered, cuts at the zygoma are restricted by the facial skin, unless a transfacial, Weber-Ferguson approach is employed. The guide is designed to index over the interior orbital rim and under the zygomatic arch after raising a full-thickness flap. The software should automatically eliminate any undercuts with virtual parallel block out. Retention of the guide is achieved with fixation screws (Fig 3-181b). If a custom reconstruction plate will be designed, then the fixation screws for the zygoma cutting guide can be made to correspond with the position of screw holes of the custom plate also called "predictive holes." Once printed, the guide is positioned on the printed preoperative patient skull model and verified for fit (Fig 3-181b).

Articulation splint. As discussed in Chapter 2, during insetting, an implant-borne-articulation-splint (IBAS) is helpful to orient the osteotomized fibula that houses the dental implants. Fig 3-182 shows an articulation splint that is tooth and implant-borne. The portion that extends over the fibula is designed with a soft tissue gap to account for an estimated thickness of the periosteum that should not be raised off the fibula. Channels aligned with the position of the dental implants are generated by subtracting the "Boolean" difference of the cylinders used to generate the implant positions: think of the channels as an occlusal extension of the implant osteotomies. Intraoperatively, once the articulation splint is clamped onto the dental implants with healing abutments, the fibula-IBAS complex is articulated to the residual maxillary dentition while the reconstructive surgeon fixates the fibula segment(s) with either a customized reconstruction plate or miniplates.

Combination fibula-implant guide. The final guide to be designed is the combination fibula-implant osteotomy guide. There are four components to this surgical guide: indexing, securing, guiding the fibula, and implant osteotomies.

1. Indexing. The guide saddles the fibula barrel on the two surfaces where the soft tissues are thinnest: the anterior and lateral fibula borders (Figs 3-183c,d and 3-184). By contrast, the peroneal vascular bundle runs adjacent to the medial fibula border, as does the

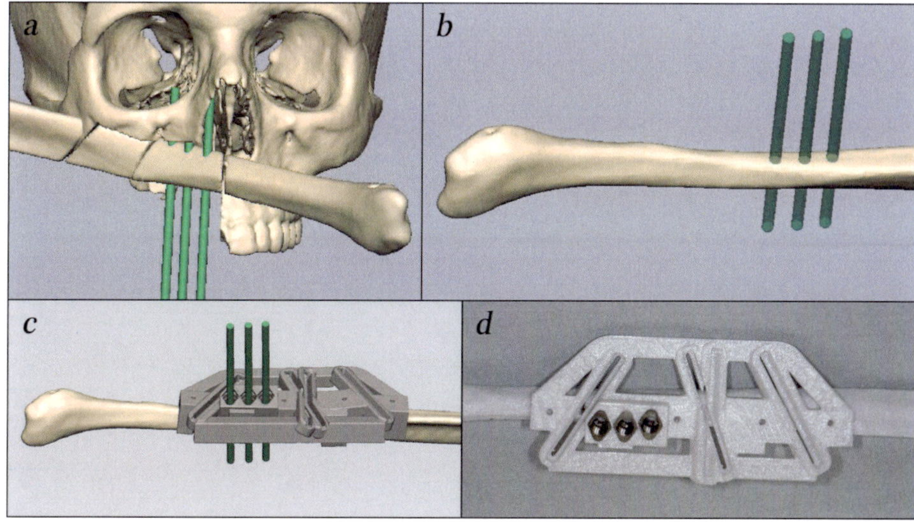

Figure 3-183 *(a and b)* The proposed implant positions superimposed on the fibula. *(c and d)* implant osteotomy and fibula sectioning guide is digitally designed and printed.

dissected tibialis posterior muscle. The posterior border is where the septocutaneous perforator vessels are found and where the flexor hallucis muscle is located (see Fig 3-177). Once the guide is finalized, it is helpful to measure the distance from the distal-most portion of the guide to the lateral malleolus of the fibula so that intraoperatively the landmark will help situate the guide along the correct length of the fibula. On that same note, because the position of the perforator vessels is identified intraoperatively with an arterial doppler, a microvascular surgeon may require the freedom to slide the guide proximally or distally so that the perforator vessels and associated skin island is best positioned over the fibula graft. Because the cross-sectional geometry of the fibula changes considerably along its length (Ide et al., 2015), becoming more triangular toward the knee, moving the guide from the planned position, specifically moving it proximally, may result in dental implants entering the thin spine as discussed earlier. This change may lead to implant thread fenestration. Large, cross-arch palatal defects that require more fibula length present the challenge of having to place implants into the thin anterior border spine of the fibula. Indexing the guide in these cases becomes particularly important to prevent rotation of the barrel. To this, the level of indexing intimacy of the guide to the fibula is balanced between the need to slide the guide along the fibula length and keeping the guide correctly rotated so as to optimize the dental implant in the planned fibula cross section. Fig 3-184a and b shows two levels of indexing intimacy. The "anatomic" option is the most intimate and offers the best precision. The generic option is "L" shaped and offers the microvascular surgeon the most freedom to slide the guide along the length of the fibula. A third "hybrid" option may be prescribed that offers an intermediate level of indexing.

2. Securing. Once the position along the length of the fibula and barrel rotation is indexed, the guide must be secured. This is achieved with bone screws. At least three fixation screws are needed and guide holes are distributed to prevent movement or unseating of the guide during instrumentation. The better indexed the saddle of the guide, the less reliant on screws the guide needs to be.
3. Guiding the fibula. The plane cuts determined in the planning session are merged to the fibula and "toggled" on. These planes are used to orient digital models of the cutting inserts as was done for the tooth-supported maxillectomy guides. Once printed the metal inserts are cemented or friction-fitted to the guide. If selective laser melting technology is used to print metal guides, then no separate inserts are needed. Metal guides have the advantage of rigidity, which allows for a lower profile guide. Notice that Figs 3-183 and 3-184 are two-piece fibula guides, which require four plane cuts: the distal fibula cut, two for a wedge osteotomy between the two fibula segments, and a proximal cut.
4. Implant osteotomies. The planned position of the dental implants, indicated by the positioned cylinders, is used to align the implant drill sleeves. Digital sleeve models specific to the implant system chosen are imported for the final design. If the guide is printed in nylon then the outer diameter of a metal sleeve is designed for post-processing cementation of the sleeve (Fig 3-183c and d). "Boolean" difference also allows subtracting the implant cylinders from the fibula model so that when it is printed the chamber corresponds to a prepared implant osteotomy. Fig 3-184c is an example of a guide where the implant drill sleeves are oriented over the posterior fibula surface. Because the guide sits on different surfaces from where the implants enter, extension bases are designed to house the drill sleeves over the posterior fibula. Additionally, as previously explained the posterior border is where the septocutaneous perforators and flexor hallucis muscle are located (Fig 3-177), and so a larger soft tissue gap is prescribed. The increased distance from the top of the drill sleeve to the fibula cortex is noted so the appropriate length twist drills are available in the operating room.

The completed digital designs are forwarded to the prosthodontist and surgeons for final verification and approval prior to the digital files being prepared for printing. This involves converting into an appropriate file format for the 3D printer to read and carry on with the 3D printing process. The manufacturer's instructions for postprocessing of the 3D printer and materials used are followed, and the 3D printed models and guides are completed. Quality assurance is carried out by assessing fit and accuracy by the biomedical engineer, surgeon, and prosthodontist. Once the printed surgical guides and models are verified for fit, they are sterilized for use in the operating room.

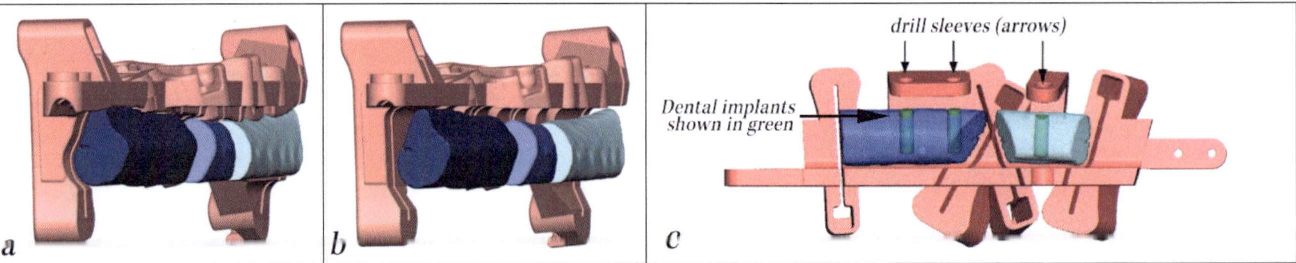

Figure 3-184 *(a and b)* For the same case compare the adaptation of the inner surface of the combination fibula-implant guide, to the graft. *(a)* An "anatomic" fit is patient specific and offers the best indexing. *(b)* A "generic" "L"-shaped inner surface to allow the microvascular surgeon maximum freedom to slide the guide along the length of the fibula. *(c)* A design for a fibula cutting guide and placement of implants. Note the incorporation of implant drill sleeves that enable fully guided implant placement. The guide can be printed in nylon or titanium (see Chapter 2). Note that the implants for this case will enter the posterior fibula border. Therefore, a bigger soft tissue gap is planned ("c" reprinted from Moy et al., 2016, with permission).

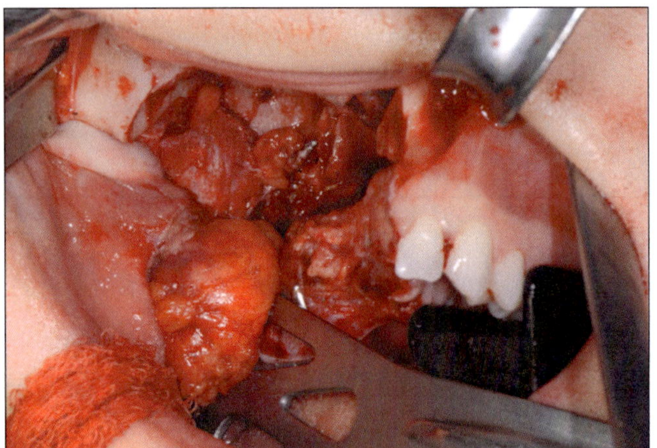

Figure 3-185 Status post inferior maxillectomy.

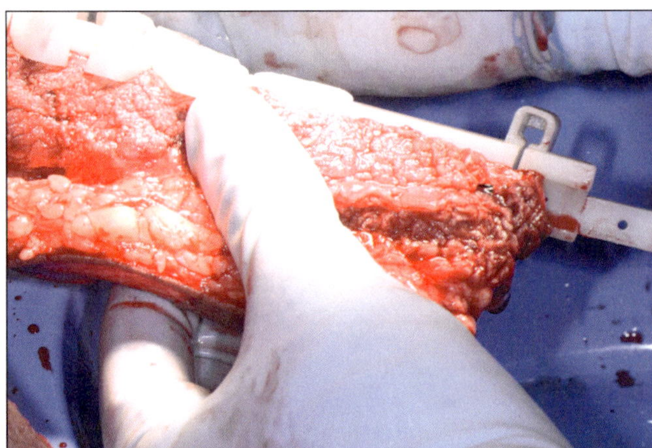

Figure 3-186 Fibula raised with a small skin paddle. The cutting guide is applied to the fibula and osteotomy sites prepared.

Surgical phase

The sterilized models, guides, and articulation splint are then transferred to the operating room. The tooth-borne anterior resection guide is seated and the mucosa is marked for the initial incision. A full-thickness flap is raised to expose the zygoma and allow seating of the posterior-superior bone-supported zygomatic cutting guide. Fixation is achieved with monocortical bone screws. If "predictive holes" were planned, then these same screw osteotomies are later used to align and secure a custom printed or milled midfacial reconstruction plate, with slightly wider fixation screws. If "predictive" holes are not used, then new screw osteotomies are made when plating. Because the palatectomy margins don't affect the seating of the osteotomized graft, this resection is done freehand while respecting the necessary oncologic margin (Fig 3-185). While the ablative surgeon resects the lesion, the reconstruction team raises the osteomyocutaneous flap. When a fibula is employed, it allows the teams to work simultaneously. Before seating the combination fibula-implant osteotomy guide, an arterial doppler is used to auscultate and locate the perforator vessels at the posterior border of the fibula. Because bicortical osteotomies are prepared for the implants, it is important that the twist drills do not damage this/these vessel(s), especially when a skin paddle will be used to close a soft tissue palatal defect. In situations where the implant osteotomies are initiated at the posterior border (Fig 3-184c), the auscultation of the perforators is even more critical. The combination fibula-implant osteotomy guide is secured to the fibula, using a predetermined measurement from the lateral malleolus for orientation. Once the guide is oriented and seated to the anterolateral border of the fibula, it is secured with bone screws. Using the implant drill sleeves, the sequential implant osteotomies are performed followed by implant installation in a fully guided fashion (Fig 3-186).

The implant osteotomy begins with a 2 mm twist drill to place the first pilot osteotomy using the implant osteotomy guide secured on the fibula. The drill will perforate both fibula cortices for bicortical stabilization. Wider osteotomy drills are used sequentially until the implant osteotomy diameter is near the planned implant width. Then a screw tap of the same width as the planned implant is used to the full depth engaging both the cortices (Fig 3-187). This is followed by the use of a countersink to widen the crestal area of the fibula to allow passive seating of the implant head and subsequently the abutment. Of note, the tactile feedback of placing an implant into the prepared fibula osteotomy is different from alveolar bone, since the fibula has a hollow marrow space. The surgeon must pay extra attention to the implant direction as the implant apex enters the second fibular cortex. It is possible that a slight misangulation will result in the implant apex missing the second cortex by tilting within the marrow space.

With the guide still secured, the reconstructive surgeon proceeds to section the fibula with an oscillating saw. Because a guide

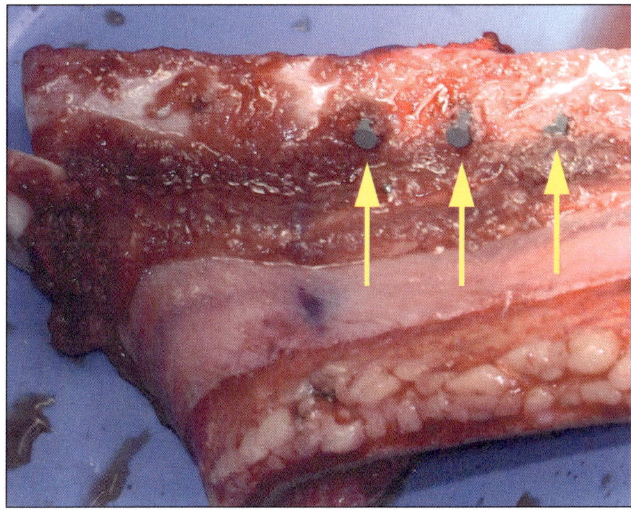

Figure 3-187 Effective bicortical engagement of the fibula requires perforating the inferior cortex. Notice the tips of the implants *(arrows)* on this fibula prior to wedge osteotomies.

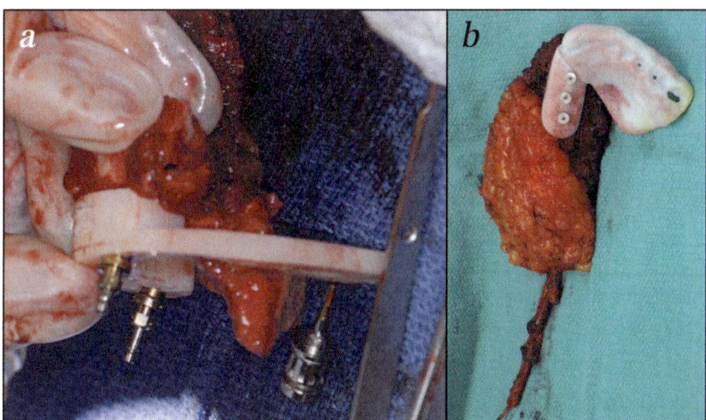

Figure 3-188 Two examples of Fibula-IBAS's complexes ready to articulate with the residual maxillary dentition for insetting the osteomyocutaneous free flap. *(a)* In this example, implant mounts are used to secure the IBAS to the implants in the fibula. *(b)* The second example shows healing abutments used to secure the IBAS to the fibula ("a" reprinted from Moy et al., 2016, with permission).

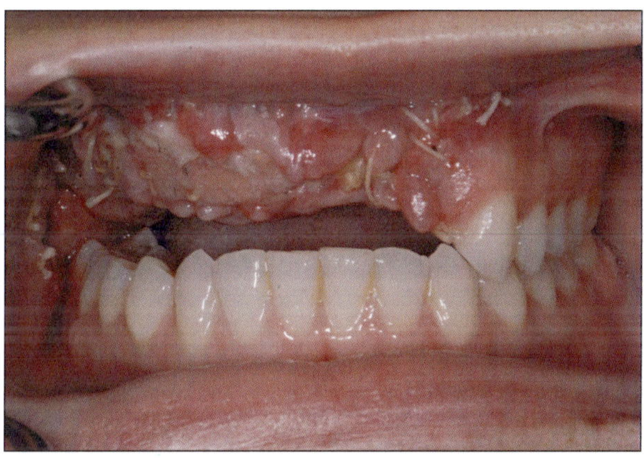

Figure 3-189 One week after surgery of the patient shown in Figure 3-178 following reconstruction of a large maxillary defect with a fibula flap (reprinted from Moy et al., 2016, with permission).

diminishes the tactile feedback perceived when the saw blade completes the cut, particularly when both sides of the cut are secured to a rigid guide, great care is needed to avoid damaging the peroneal vessels. Some surgeons may prefer to perform two-thirds of each osteotomy guided, then remove the guide and complete the osteotomies freehand. While this can incur some inaccuracy in the cut, it provides full tactile feedback. Next the intersegment wedges are dissected out.

The prosthodontist articulates the IBAS to the implants with abutment screws (shown in Chapter 2) or with healing abutments (Fig 3-188). The entire composite flap with the articulation splint is then transferred to the oral cavity defect and articulated to the remaining maxillary dentition. Once the prosthodontist verifies the fidelity of the articulation, the microvascular surgeon completes the insetting to the native bone using a midfacial plate or mini bone plates. The IBAS is removed, and cover screws, multiunit abutments, or low-profile healing abutments are seated. The choice of using a multiunit/healing abutment over a cover screw is that it is more easily palpated through the skin paddle during stage II implant surgery. The microvascular surgeon proceeds to complete the anastomosis before completing soft tissue closure.

The patient is reviewed with the surgeon two to three weeks postoperatively (Fig 3-189), and the necessary adjunctive treatments are arranged.

Stage II implant surgery

Once all necessary treatments are completed and the patient is ready for stage II implant surgery, a postoperative CT scan is obtained to start the planning process for the design and fabrication of the surgical stent used during stage II surgery. The postoperative CT scan data are imported into CAD software for the design of the stage II surgery surgical stent (Kincade et al., 2021). After completion of the design of the surgical stent, it can be conventionally fabricated or 3D printed. The stent is sterilized and sent to the operating room for use at stage II implant surgery.

During second-stage surgery when the implants are uncovered, the soft tissues overlying the implants are thinned and modified as needed. The subcutaneous resection is extended down to the periosteum overlying the fibula, and a surgical stent secured to the implants is used to ensure that the lining epithelium remains adherent to the underlying periosteum during healing (Fig 3-190). The

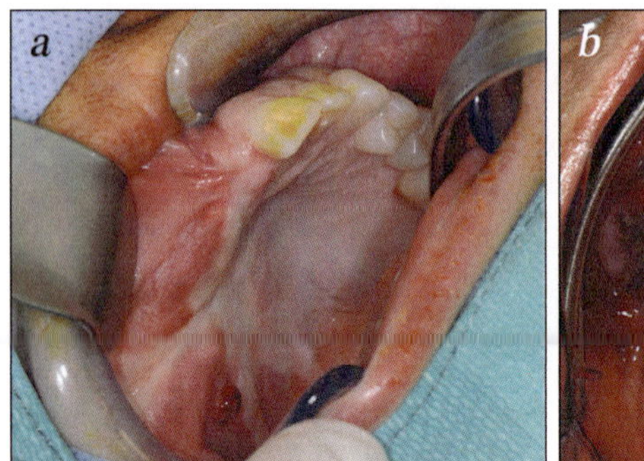
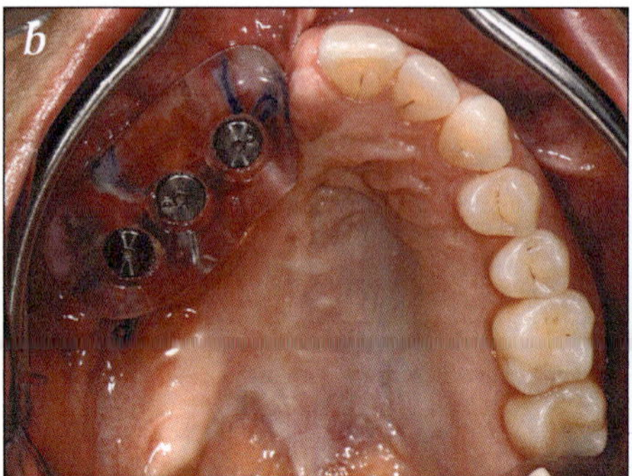
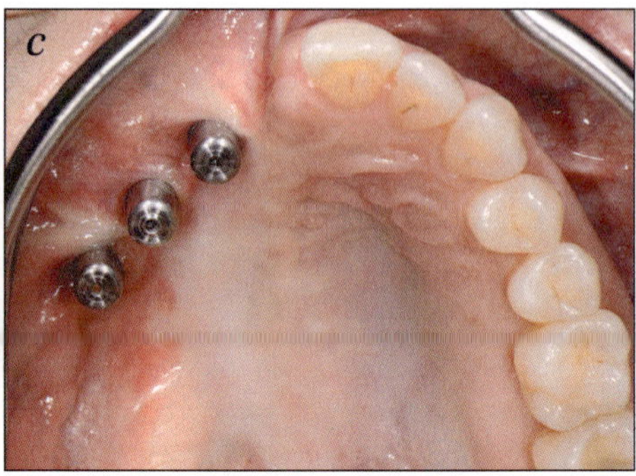

Figure 3-190 *(a)* Several months postreconstruction of a maxillary defect with a fibula flap. *(b)* The implants have been exposed, the overlying tissues thinned, healing abutments attached and a stent secured to hold the peri-implant soft tissues in position during healing. *(c)* Several weeks following second-stage surgery. The peri-implant tissues are nicely healed.

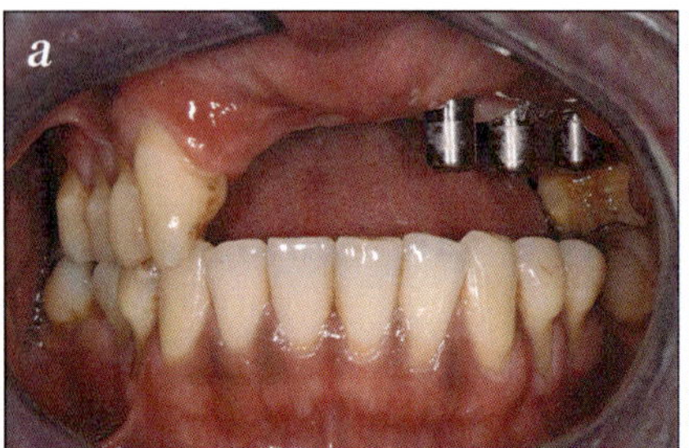
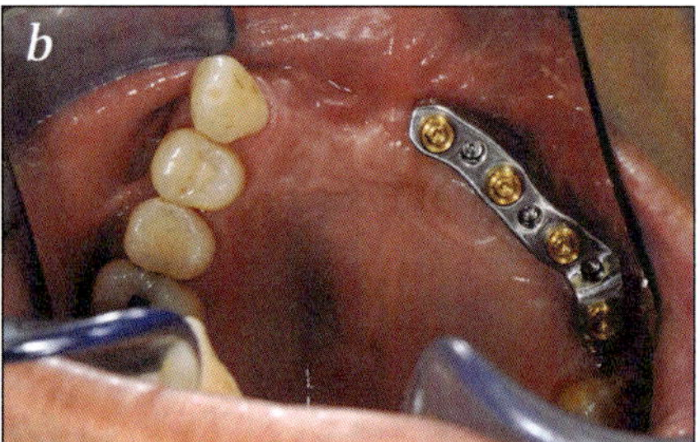
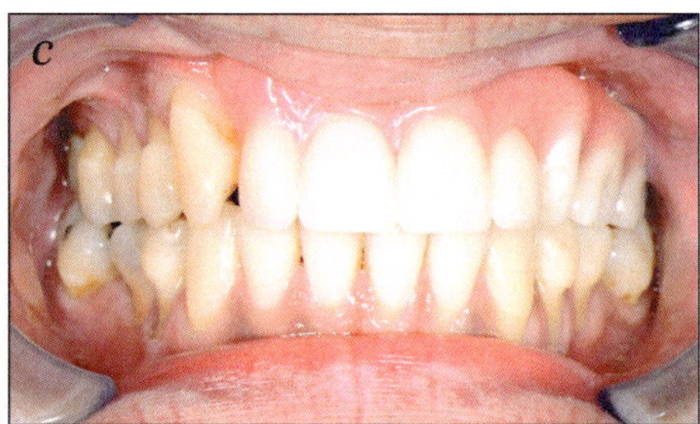

Figure 3-191 *(a)* The anterior implant failed to osseointegrate. As a result, there was a significant distance between the most anterior implant and the dentition, which would have resulted in a significant cantilever had a fixed prosthesis been utilized. *(b)* Implant-connecting bar. *(c)* The completed removable overlay prosthesis.

objective is to create attached, immobile keratinized peri-implant soft tissues of minimal thickness (3–5 mm). After a suitable period of healing (two to three weeks), the stent is removed, and healing abutments of sufficient length that extend above the soft tissue margins are positioned.

If the patient has undergone postoperative radiation or chemoradiation, the tissues overlying the implants should be carefully manipulated during the second-stage surgery and exposure of the implants. Inadvertent exposure of the bony portion of the flap and postoperative soft tissue breakdown in this patient population is a significant concern and, if it occurs, can lead to infection and necrosis of the bony portion of the flap. However, the clinician should realize that failure to thin the peri-implant soft tissues will predispose to a higher risk of inflammation and hypertrophy of the peri-implant soft tissues. In such patients, soft tissue healing can be enhanced with hyperbaric oxygen (HBO) treatments (Dauwe et al., 2014; Hoggan and Cameron, 2014).

Prosthesis fabrication

Once the peri-implant soft tissues heal and stabilize (Fig 3-190c), conventional implant prosthodontic procedures commence. Impressions are made, a master cast is retrieved, maxillomandibular records are obtained, and the maxillary and mandibular casts are mounted on a semiadjustable articulator.

Prosthesis design

Fixed versus removable. In maxillary reconstruction, prosthodontic planning is usually geared toward provision of a fixed prosthesis. Based on the oral rehabilitation needs and implant biomechanics (Wu et al., 2022), the number of implants and their distribution pattern can be planned and subsequently restored with the appropriate fixed prosthesis. However, there are times when implants fail. Under these circumstances, there may be an insufficient number of implants to support the forces of occlusion with an implant-supported fixed prosthesis, and as a result, a removable prosthesis whose support is supplemented by the existing dentition and denture-bearing surfaces is warranted. Moreover, the overlay prosthesis retained by the implant-connecting bar or individual attachments can be designed to provide lip support as needed. Additional bracing (resistance to lateral forces) and support for the prosthesis can be obtained by incorporating a removable dental prosthesis framework within the overlay removable prosthesis that engages the residual dentition with positive rests, guide planes, and lingual plating (see Fig 3-81). In addition, since the prosthesis is removable, oral hygiene procedures are more easily accomplished by the patient because of improved access (Fig 3-191).

Interim versus definitive prostheses. Although functional outcomes such as mastication, swallowing, and speech are the objective indicators of success of oral rehabilitation for oncology patients, oral rehabilitation also provides dignity to these patients. Replacement of teeth is often seen as an aesthetic need and is frequently equated with vanity! However, this is far from the truth in almost all situations and certainly not the case with head and neck oncology patients. To be able to provide oral rehabilitation is to provide dignity to these unfortunate individuals. To that end, replacement teeth need to provide the patient with the dignity

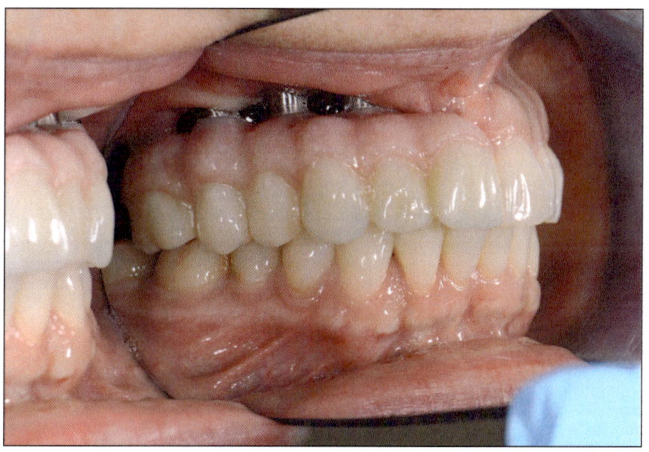

Figure 3-192 A fixed implant–supported prosthesis restoring a large maxillary defect. The defect was reconstructed with a fibula-free flap. Note the high water design and hygiene access.

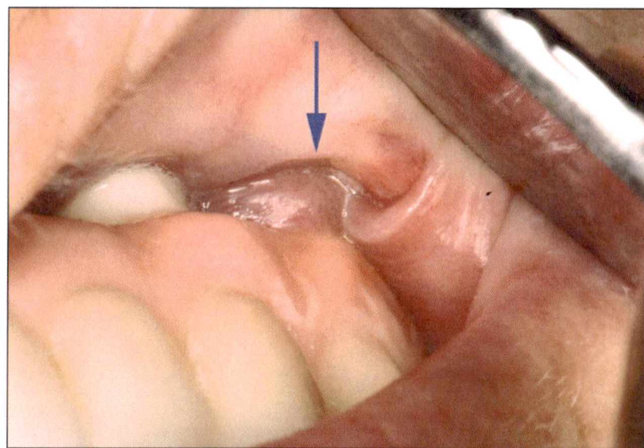

Figure 3-193 Implants emerging through the skin of a fibula flap tend to trigger inflammatory hypertrophic tissue reactions *(arrow)*.

and confidence to face the world. There are many variables in the replacement of teeth, especially in the maxillary arch, including smile lines, buccal corridors, and so on. Additionally, one must also consider the soft tissue healing around the surgical site. Given this, it is advised to provide the patient with an interim prosthesis. This is usually made of acrylic resin, but with the improvement in milling and additive manufacturing technologies and materials, long-term interim prostheses can be fabricated out of pucks of PMMA (polymethylmethacrylate). The decision to consider a definitive prosthesis is up to the individual prosthodontist in consultation with the patient.

Hygiene access. As has been mentioned previously in the prosthetic space segment, the prosthodontic plan must incorporate appropriate hygiene space under the fixed prosthesis or the implant-connecting bar. When fixed is employed, the authors prefer a high-water design (Fig 3-192). Failure to incorporate the space under the prosthesis for hygiene access invariably leads to peri-implant tissue inflammation, hypertrophy, and eventually peri-implantitis. It must be kept in mind that many of these patients would have undergone radiotherapy as part of their oncology management, and hence inflammation or infection to the peri-implant soft and hard tissues could culminate in tissue breakdown, loss of implants, and even loss of the vascularized flap.

Remaining prosthodontic procedures. The prosthesis is completed in the usual fashion. If removable, conventional techniques are used. If the prosthesis is fixed, either conventional analog or CAD-CAM procedures can be employed (Davodi et al., 2022). The patient is given oral hygiene instruction and placed on follow-up.

It is preferable to place the patient on a three-month follow-up schedule the first year following delivery of the prosthesis. Machined/microrough surface titanium implants and/or abutment surfaces retain dental plaque tenaciously, and if they perforate the skin of an osteomyocutaneous flap in the oral cavity, there is an increased risk of precipitating inflammatory and hypertrophic tissue reactions (Fig 3-193). Likewise, if the peri-implant soft tissues are thick and mobile, they will be susceptible to inflammation and hypertrophy. These soft tissue responses are relatively common but may be minimized by the use of customized, highly polished abutments or by using a ceramic material to interface with the peri-implant tissues between the implant platform and the prosthesis, such as metal-ceramic or monolithic zirconia (Beumer et al., 2011). Because of the above, oral hygiene must be meticulous and the patient placed on close follow-up.

Evaluation of Treatment Outcomes: Maxillary Defects

Numerous treatment options are available, ranging from conventional obturator prostheses to fixed implant-supported prostheses combined with surgical reconstruction of the defect. With respect to prosthetic obturation, several issues affect the quality of life of the patient including aesthetics, speech, leakage of fluid and air into the nasal cavity, and mastication performance. In partially dentate patients, strict plaque control will be required to maintain the health of the residual dentition. However, significant difficulty may be encountered when the patient attempts to perform the appropriate oral hygiene measures and these are often compounded in irradiated patients by postradiation trismus and xerostomia. If implants were used, whether to help retain an obturator prosthesis or in combination with a vascularized flap, maintenance of peri-implant tissue health is very challenging. The poor quality of tissue often circumscribing these implants combined with difficult access makes chronic inflammation and hypertrophy of the peri-implant soft tissues a perpetual concern. The necessary oral hygiene procedures can be very difficult to perform by such patients and are especially challenging for the elderly patient who presents with compromised visual acuity and manual dexterity. All these factors affect the quality of life of the patient. In the following section, the authors will attempt to bring some of these issues into perspective. Each of these additional aspects will be discussed from the perspective of recent studies, because a clinical evaluation alone may not reliably determine the adequacy of obturation.

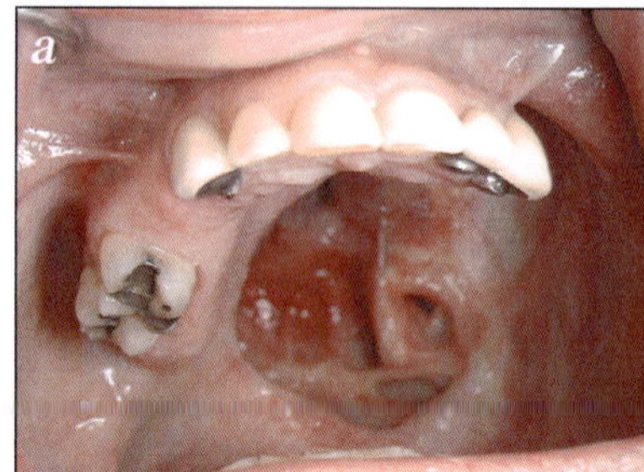

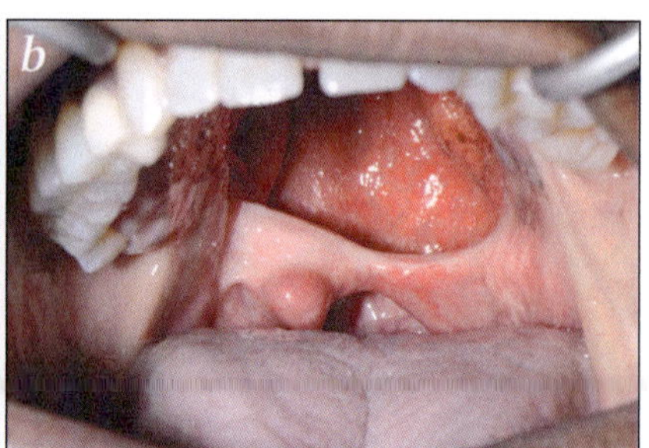

Figure 3-194 *(a)* A large maxillectomy defect that crosses the midline and extends to the mobile, middle third of the soft palate. *(b)* The resection has encompassed the middle third of the soft palate leaving a nonfunctional posterior remnant. Effective obturation cannot be achieved in such a defect. This remnant should be removed in order to permit the engagement of the residual functioning velopharyngeal musculature with the obturator extension.

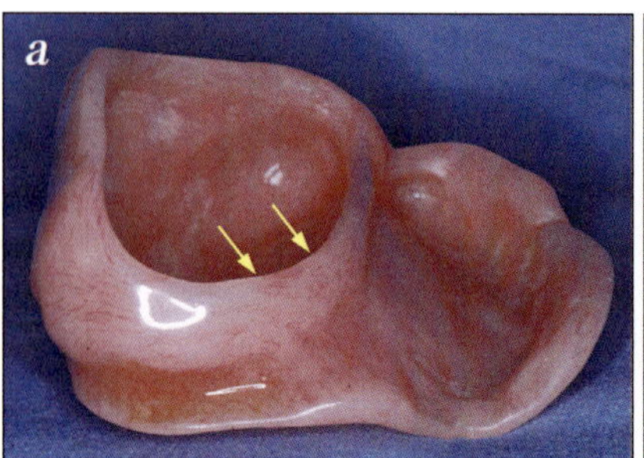

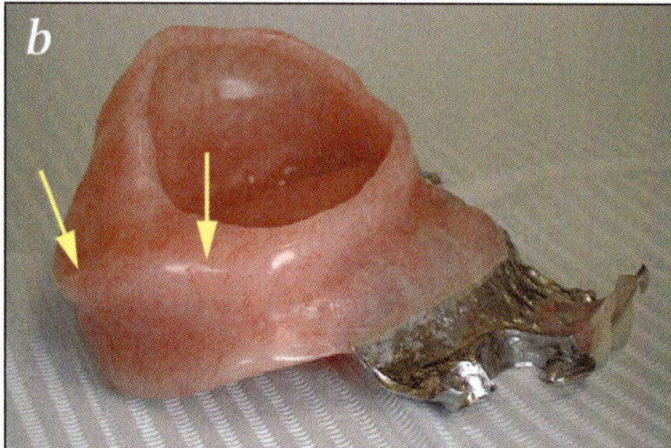

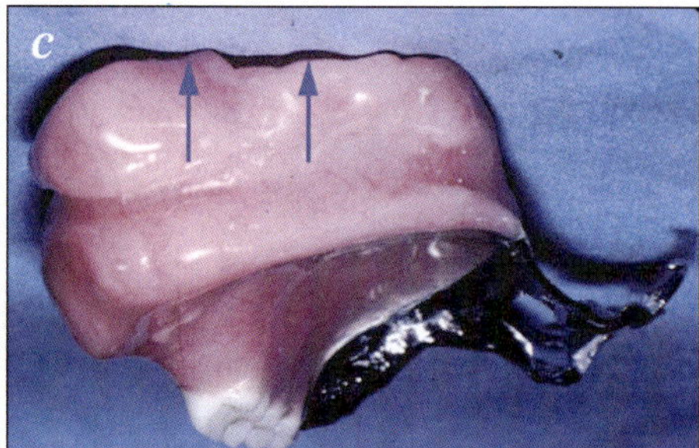

Figure 3-195 *(a, b, and c)* With proper posterior extension vertically into the defect, the patient will experience virtually no leakage. As the defect extends posteriorly onto the mobile middle third of the soft palate, the posterior-medial extension must be extended approximately one cm above the level of the nasal side of the soft palate if the leakage is to be eliminated *(arrows)*. It is also beneficial to slightly overlap onto the nasal side of the soft palate posteriorly.

Fluid leakage around obturator prostheses

Upon delivery of a new obturator prosthesis, patients occasionally complain of varying amounts of fluid leakage around the periphery of the obturator and into the nasal cavity. Leakage may occur posteriorly during swallowing due to the elevation of the soft palate. Posterolaterally, the functional movements of the medial surfaces of the mandible may contribute to leakage. During mandibular movements, the coronoid process and the anterior border of the ramus of the mandible displace the soft tissues along the distolateral aspect of the defect, just as these structures influence the width and lateral contours of the buccal pouch area of a maxillary complete denture.

Leakage during swallowing is rarely seen with static defects confined to the hard palate. However, leakage can occur when the defect is dynamic—that is, the defect extends onto the mobile middle third of the soft palate (Fig 3-194). In such patients, most leakage occurs around the medial posterior extension of the obturator prosthesis. During swallowing, the soft palate uplifts and the dorsum of the tongue elevates forcefully against the hard and soft palates. When the defect extends into the mobile, middle third of the soft palate a space is often created between the obturator prosthesis and the soft palate and the pressure created by tongue elevation superiorly may force fluids around the obturator bulb and into the nasal cavity. If the prosthesis is underextended in this area and not properly contoured and extended, leakage will occur.

The posterior surfaces of the obturator prostheses that extend into these areas require careful molding and development of proper extensions. At the midline of the defect and where the prosthesis engages the soft palate, the prosthesis should cover at least one cm of the oral side of the soft palate and also be extended at least 1 cm *above the level of the nasal side of the soft palate* and, if possible, should overlap the soft palate in this region (Fig 3-195). Developing these contours is best accomplished with thermoplastic materials such as impression wax (see Figs 3-90a and 3-154c).

When a nonfunctional posterior remnant of the soft palate remains (Fig 3-194b), leakage during swallowing is common because the obturator extension is unable to properly engage the residual functioning velopharyngeal musculature residing in the posterolateral pharyngeal wall. Under these circumstances, the residual soft palate can be split and the nonfunctional remnant removed to facilitate access to the residual portions of the levator palati muscles in lateral pharyngeal walls that contract during swallowing and speech (see Chapter 4, Fig 4-43).

Patients often experience difficulty identifying the exact site of the leakage because of the sensory deficits associated with the surgical resection and the altered and compromised innervation arising from skin graft linings in the defect. Disclosing wax is the most practical method of identifying the area where leakage occurs. The wax is applied selectively to specific areas, starting first with the posterior-medial extension and progressing laterally. After each application, the patient is given liquids to swallow and leakage is assessed. Obturator extension areas found to be deficient in contour or extension can then be remolded using a thermoplastic material and the area selectively relined with autopolymerizing acrylic resin.

Direct visualization of the interface between the peripheral soft tissues and the obturator bulb during swallowing is possible in some patients. Occasionally, the contents of the orbital cavity must be exenterated in continuity with the maxillary resection for control of the disease, thus permitting direct visualization of the superior surface of the obturator through the orbit. Oral endoscopy and nasoendoscopy (Beery et al., 1983, 1985) with a fiber-optic light source also permit direct visualization.

Excessive leakage can occur when the soft palate is included in the resection such that the hard palate defect extends to the

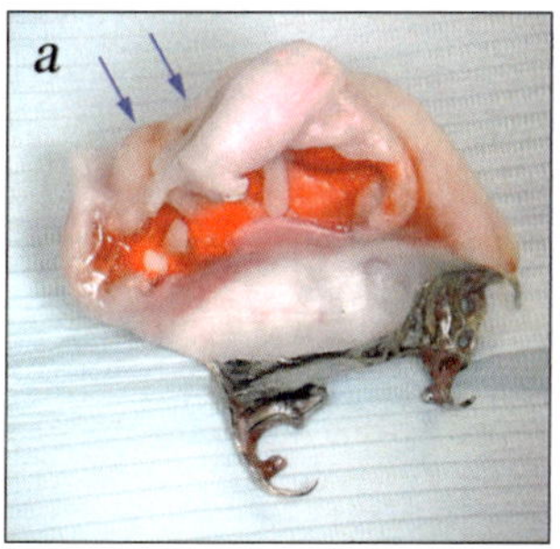

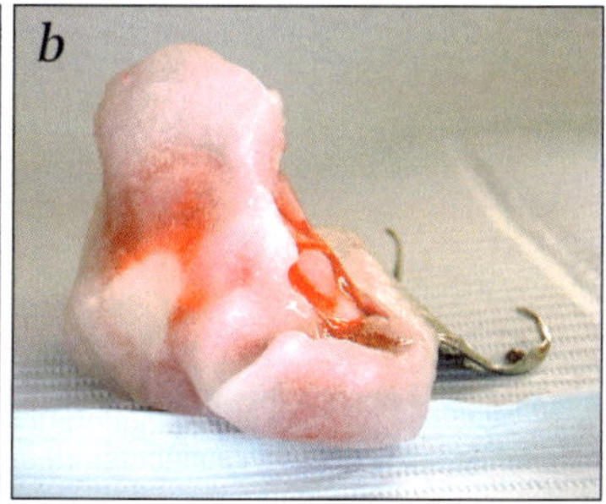

Figure 3-196 *(a and b)* Impression extending to the velopharyngeal zone posteriorly. The superior extension engaging the hard palate defect is maximized to enhance the retention and stability support of the prosthesis. Note the imprint made by the medial surface of the mandible *(arrows)*. As the prosthesis approaches the velopharyngeal area, the prosthesis tapers down to about 10 mm in vertical height so as to interact with residual levator muscle remnants still present in the pharyngeal wall.

posterior pharyngeal wall. Three factors are key to prevention of leakage around obturator prostheses in such patients. The first is the presence of functioning contracting remnants of the levator palati muscle still present in the posterolateral pharyngeal walls. Second, there must be access to these muscle remnants with the obturator prosthesis. Third, the posterior extension of the obturator must be contoured with great care and positioned precisely and retained effectively to properly interact with these residual velopharyngeal muscle remnants (Fig 3-196). Such extensions can only be developed functionally and with a thermoplastic material. The vertical height of this extension should not exceed 10–15 mm or contact the pharyngeal wall above or below the zone of levator contracture. Otherwise, the patient will not be able to breathe through the nose, and speech will be hyponasal (see Chapter 4, section entitled "Definitive obturation," Fig 4-29). During swallowing the residual velopharyngeal wall musculature contracts around the obturator extension in this area in a sphincteric manner. Such large prostheses must also be effectively retained. If retention is suboptimal because the patient either is edentulous or lacks sufficient dentition, consideration should be given to providing intradefect implant support and retention. This is best accomplished with zygomatic oncologic implants. It should be noted that when the defect extends to the posterior pharyngeal wall and the patient is fitted with a properly extended and contoured obturator prosthesis, leakage cannot be prevented unless the patient maintains their head in a relatively upright position during swallowing. If the patient flexes their neck during swallowing, the spatial relationships between the obturator extension in the residual velopharyngeal musculature are altered.

Air Leakage around Obturator Prostheses and Speech Outcomes

Surgical removal of portions of the maxillae can affect speech in several ways. First, the oral-nasal resonance balance is distorted because the patient cannot confine oral emissions within the oral cavity, which leads to hypernasal speech. Second, 17 of the 25 consonant phonemes used in the English language require labiodental, linguodental, and linguo-palatal contacts. With the loss of palatal tissues, correct tongue-palate contacts are impossible and articulation is compromised (Bloomer and Hawk, 1973). Third, the loss of anterior teeth further compromises the articulation of speech.

Several investigators have reported that patients exhibited normal speech after placement of obturator prostheses for acquired surgical defects of the maxillae (Warren, 1970; Bloomer and Hawk, 1973; Bradley, 1971; Arigbede et al., 2006; Rieger et al., 2011; Dalkiz and Dalkiz, 2018; Dholam et al., 2020). Kipfmueller and Lang (1973) recorded the speech of six patients who were to undergo maxillectomy procedures for the control of neoplastic disease. After surgery, the patients recorded the same speech sequence at intervals up to nine months postsurgically both with and without the use of the prosthesis. Three of the patients were edentulous and three had teeth remaining for retention and support of the prosthesis. The results of this study demonstrated that speech following the placement of the prosthesis may not always be "normal." Two of the dentulous patients demonstrated improved speech compared to presurgical recordings. Of the remaining four patients, three demonstrated a slight loss (up to 14%) of intelligibility when speaking with the prosthesis compared to the presurgical recordings.

Plank et al. (1981) studied the speech of eight patients, both dentate and edentulous, rehabilitated with a maxillary obturator prosthesis following surgical resection of various segments of the maxillae. A speech sample was recorded presurgically while the patient wore the ISO and following placement of the definitive prosthesis. The speech samples were randomized and evaluated by 10 untrained listeners following a period of instruction. The average intelligibility of all subjects was 98.8% correct presurgically, 92.1% correct with their ISOs, and 97.3% correct with their definitive prosthesis.

Acoustic and aerodynamic patterns of speech can provide a better understanding of the basis for the effect of obturation on speech intelligibility. Tobey and Lincks (1989) examined the acoustic speech patterns of five patients before and after prosthodontic rehabilitation to determine the effectiveness of maxillary obturator prostheses in eliminating or reducing nasal resonance. In two patients the resection was confined to the anterior maxillae, while in the other three, the resections included the posterior maxillae and varying portions of the anterior soft palate. A digital sonograph with a 30 Hz filter was used to record speech samples presurgically and after prosthodontic rehabilitation. Vowels were primarily studied because these phonemes are particularly sensitive to changes in nasal resonance and their production requires different areas of tongue-palate approximation. Excess nasal energy was found in the speech of all five patients, but there was proportionally less nasal resonance in the two patients with prosthodontic rehabilitation of the more anterior resections.

Similar results were found by Rieger et al. (2002), who used more advanced nasalance measures and size estimates of the opening between the oral and nasal cavities. Evaluations of 12 maxillectomy patients were made prior to surgery, postsurgically without obturation, and postsurgically with obturation. Defects were categorized as greater than half of the hard palate, half of the hard palate or less, and combined hard and soft palate. For the total sample, average speech with obturation was not significantly different than the preoperative speech. Speech was significantly impaired without obturation.

Minsley et al. (1987) studied four patients with maxillary obturator prostheses using the methodology based on airflow, pressure, velopharyngeal orifice size, and respiratory volumes, as suggested by Warren et al. (1964, 1964, 1967, 1969, 1970; see Chapter 4 for a more complete discussion of these and other related studies). The theory developed by Warren and coworkers involves a modification of hydraulic principles and assumes that the smallest cross-sectional area of a structure can be determined if the differential pressure across this opening is measured simultaneously with the rate of airflow through it. Of the four patients studied by Minsley et al. (1987), two required partial maxillectomies, one required the complete resection of both maxillae, and the fourth required the complete resection of the soft palate. Oral pressures and respiratory volumes were recorded during the production of consonant sounds both prior to and during each phase of prosthodontic treatment, both while the patients were wearing their prostheses and while they were not.

The respiratory volume increased approximately threefold as a compensatory mechanism while the patients were speaking without the prosthesis. When the prostheses were inserted, the respiratory effort and the oral pressure returned to nearly normal. The oral opening around the definitive obturators was less than 0.05 mm, which did not significantly impact speech but might lead to the percolation of fluids into the nasal cavity during swallowing (Minsley et al., 1987). Reisberg and Smith (1985) confirmed the efficacy of this methodology by reporting the data of three patients requiring maxillary maxillofacial prostheses.

To summarize, when the maxillectomy is confined to the bony palate, speech following the placement of a prosthesis is usually within normal limits. Rarely is velopharyngeal function affected (either directly or indirectly) through scar contracture, loss of bony attachment for the soft palate, or denervation. However, it is not uncommon for slight articulatory deficiencies to be associated with speech following placement of the definitive prosthesis. Errors in articulation tend to diminish as the patient uses the prosthesis, but speech therapy is sometimes required for patients who experience difficulty in adaptation (Kipfmueller and Lang, 1972). Resonance balance usually is normal. In a few patients, distortions in resonance will be noted, and these distortions are most often associated with more extensive resections of the maxillae that involve significant portions of the soft palate, particularly when the patient is treated with high-dose radiotherapy. In the latter group of patients, especially if chemoradiation is used, the residual velopharyngeal musculature is often rendered fibrotic, impairing its sphincteric muscular contraction around or against an obturator prosthesis. Under these circumstances, a properly molded obturator that engages the residual velopharyngeal musculature and speech is likely to exhibit mixed nasality (see Chapter 4, Fig 4-2). In edentulous patients, the primary issue is retention of the obturator prosthesis, and if it is suboptimal, the placement of implants should be considered.

Speech following surgical reconstruction with vascularized flaps and implant-retained prostheses

This issue has not been well studied. Resonance of speech is not an issue following reconstruction of defects confined to the hard palate with a vascularized flap, since the flap closes the defect, but speech articulation may be impaired. Dentition can be restored with fixed or removable prostheses retained by zygomatic oncologic implants or subperiosteal implants perforating a vascularized soft tissue flap or by inserting conventional-length implants into the bony segments of an osteomyocutaneous flap and using the implants to retain the prosthesis. However, articulation can be impaired if palatal contours have been distorted and the tongue space limited by an excessively bulky flap (Ohashi et al., 2021). As is the case when fitting the patient with a new denture or a new obturator prosthesis, errors in articulation tend to diminish over time as the patient adjusts to the new palatal contours.

Mastication performance: Obturator prostheses and flaps combined with implants

Studies have indicated that edentulous patients with maxillary obturator prostheses do not masticate as effectively as conventional complete denture patients unless osseointegrated implants are available to facilitate retention, stability, and support of the obturator prosthesis (Garrett, 2008; Buurman, 2020b). Edentulous patients historically have fared poorly and before the introduction of implants, a complete-denture-obturator prosthesis primarily served to restore speech and swallowing. Except in rare instances, masticatory performance was close to zero (Garrett, 2008) because the patient was forced to contend with unstable and poorly retained prostheses in both arches.

The capability of bilateral chewing and effective neuromuscular control are important cofactors that allow the effective use of conventional complete dentures. A patient with a maxillary resection prosthesis is compromised in both areas because of the defect and surrounding sensory deficits. The added movement of the edentulous maxillary resection prosthesis into the defect and the compromised support accentuate this functional disparity. Moreover, retention in the classic sense of complete dentures is unobtainable because the surgical opening permits the leakage of air beneath the prosthesis and eliminates the retentive contribution of atmospheric pressure.

While both dentate and edentulous maxillectomy patients may learn to confine most of their mastication to the nondefect side, mastication comparatively is much more effective in dentate patients. The size and location of the resection, the contours of the remaining alveolar ridge and palate, and the potential for retention, stability, and support within the defect will influence the level of function of both dentate and edentulous patients.

Mastication performance is affected by a number of factors including bite force, the presence of dentition and the proprioception derived from their presence, and neuromuscular control. In edentulous patients, the retention, stability, and support of the prosthesis are obviously important factors as well.

Shipman (1987) studied 10 edentulous patients with maxillary resection obturator prostheses. A gnathodynamometer was attached to each prosthesis. The maximum bite force recorded was approximately 50% of the forces reported for conventional complete denture patients and had little relationship to the size of the maxillary defect. Denture adhesives increased bite force by approximately 12%. However, there was considerable variation in the forces recorded between patients, and the individual standard deviations were high. These results could indicate that defect contours and neuromuscular control may be important cofactors in the performance of patients with obturator prostheses; however, factors including sensation and motor coordination are critical to masticatory function.

Relying on only force as a surrogate may be misleading. In fact, Matsuyama et al. (2006) found that bite force was a poor predictor of masticatory performance in maxillectomy patients treated with a conventional obturator, at least when residual dentition remained in the maxilla. Maxillectomy patients treated with a conventional obturator, most of whom had residual dentition for obturator support and chewing, were found to perform at levels similar to dentate controls. Although bite force was significantly reduced in the maxillectomy group, the presence of the critical residual dentition, combined with the obturator, resulted in masticatory performance that was not significantly different from dentate controls. The presence of remaining dentition is clearly an important factor in the restoration of masticatory function. Similar results were reported by Koyama et al. (2005) who found that the remaining maxillary teeth had a strong relationship to patients' perceptions of masticatory function.

When the retention, stability, and support of the obturator are improved with implants, significant improvements in masticatory performance may be obtained for select patients, particularly those with natural dentition in the mandible. These improvements in performance may approach the level of a conventional edentulous patient restored with implant-retained overdentures. However, the performance levels achieved remain considerably impaired relative to those of "normal" dentate individuals (Garrett, 2008).

The report by Buurman and colleagues (2020b) nicely documents the value of implant retention and support for large obturator prostheses fabricated for edentulous maxillectomy patients. Nineteen edentulous patients with large palatal defects participated in the study. Nine patients were restored with implant retained and supported obturator prostheses. Ten patients were restored with conventional maxillary obturator prostheses. In general, the implant group presented with more extensive defects. Implant sites included the residual alveolar ridge, the zygoma, the pyriform rim region, and the pyramidal process of the palatal bone. The opposing mandible in both groups presented with a variety of configurations—some were edentulous but were fitted with implant-retained overdentures, some wore conventional complete dentures, while others were either fully or partially dentate. Masticatory performance was measured objectively by the mixing ability test (MAT) and subjectively by three OHRQoL questionnaires: (1) the Oral Health Impact Profile for Edentulous people (OHIP-EDENT), (2) the Obturator Function Scale (OFS), and (3) the Dutch Liverpool Oral Rehabilitation Questionnaire version 3 (LORQv3-NL). The independent *t* test and the Mann–Whitney *U* test were used to test for differences in outcomes of patients with and without implant retention of their obturator prostheses. The implant group was able to achieve a level of masticatory efficiency equivalent to that of dentate obturator patients, which in turn was equal to the performance recorded in healthy complete denture patients.

In an international cooperative endeavor, Buurman and colleagues at Maastricht University Medical Centre, Maastricht, the Netherlands, in collaboration with their contemporaries at the University of Alberta, Edmonton, Canada, compared the masticatory performance of patients restored with implant retained and supported obturator prostheses to those reconstructed with osteocutaneous vascularized flaps where the dentition was restored with implant retained prostheses. Eleven surgically reconstructed maxillectomy patients from the University of Alberta were compared with nine implant-supported obturator patients restored at Maastricht University Medical Centre. The mixing ability test (MAT) was also used to measure masticatory performance. The results indicated that patients with reconstructed maxillae and patients with implant-supported obturator prostheses had similar mean mixing ability indices (18.20 ±2.38 resp. 18.66 ±1.37; $p = 0.614$). Moreover, the seven oral health-related quality of life (OHRQoL) questions administered, showed no differences in masticatory ability between the two groups (Buurman et al., 2020a).

When maxillary defects are restored with flaps and implants, the mastication performance of edentulous patients restored with flaps and implants mastication performance is dramatically improved. However, when compared to dentate patients restored with RDP-obturator prostheses, mastication performance parameters of patients reconstructed with flaps and implants are improved only marginally if at all (de Groot et al., 2020; Ohashi et al., 2021).

Quality of life: Obturator prostheses and flaps combined with implants

As expected, the functional and aesthetic impairments triggered by a maxillectomy can have a negative impact on the psychological state of the patient and their perceived quality of life (QOL). The psychological effects of developing a life-threatening disease, compromised oral functions (speech, swallowing mastication, saliva control, etc.), and cosmetic disfigurement, plus the significant challenge of executing appropriate oral hygiene procedures when implants are used, all contribute.

A key factor influencing the quality of life of these patients is the impact of the aftereffects of radiation therapy (Riaz and Warriach, 2010; Kreeft et al., 2012; Chigurupati et al., 2013; Chen et al., 2016a, 2016b). High doses of radiation, especially in combination with concomitant chemotherapy, result in xerostomia, significant fibrosis, and foreshortening of the muscles of mastication and velopharyngeal closure predisposing to trismus (Wetzels et al., 2014) as well as velopharyngeal incompetence. Trismus can be so severe as to prevent easy entrance of the bolus of food. It also compromises the extensions of the obturator in the defect, adversely affecting the seal and leading to leakage of fluids into the nasal cavity during swallowing. Atrophy of the muscles associated with velopharyngeal closure can be so significant as to result in velopharyngeal incompetence in even normal unresected patients.

Prior to the use of implants to retain and support obturator prostheses and the introduction of vascularized flaps to surgically reconstruct the palate, QOL was dramatically impacted in edentulous patients. In edentulous patients, the size of the defect was an important factor as well as the extension of the defect into the velopharyngeal region (Kornblith et al., 1996; Rogers et al., 2003; Artopoulou et al., 2017). Although speech and swallowing were restored with the prosthesis, rarely were these patients able to masticate with any degree of efficiency, and as a result, QOL levels remained suboptimal. QOL was less affected in dentate patients fitted with RDP-obturator prostheses.

The effective employment of dental implants to provide retention and support for obturator prostheses has had a significant impact on QOL especially when intradefect implant support is provided. Buurman and associates (2020b) have shown significant improvements in QOL in edentulous maxillectomy patients with implant-retained and -supported obturator prostheses compared to conventional obturator prostheses. Recently, Buurman and colleagues (2020a) and others (Breeze et al., 2016; Wang et al., 2017; Ohashi et al., 2021) have also shown that the QOL achieved with implant retained and supported prosthesis is equivalent to that achieved by reconstructing the defect with osteocutaneous flaps, accompanied by implant placement and fabrication of implant retained dental prostheses. In the report by Buurman and colleagues (2020a), the overall quality of life reported was excellent with 83% (19/23) reporting that their QOL was good, excellent, or outstanding following treatment. Key functional performance indicators of rehabilitation following maxillectomy such as speech, chewing, and swallowing proved to be highly rated, especially the chewing domain. The surgery plus radiotherapy group reported slightly worse QOL outcomes generally, which is well recognized.

Butterworth et al. (2022) reported the results of the quality-of-life assessment of their patients that were reconstructed with the "ZIP flap" technique (see section above entitled "Zygomatic implant perforated (ZIP) technique"). Twenty-three patients completed quality-of-life questionnaires (University of Washington QOL v4; Liverpool Oral Rehabilitation Questionnaire v3) at 12 months post-treatment demonstrating high levels of acceptance of the technique especially for the chewing domain. Overall quality of life was highly scored, with 19 patients reporting that their overall quality of life was excellent, very good, or good following the procedure.

It should be noted that studies assessing the quality of life of patients undergoing maxillary resections secondary to tumor ablation and subsequently rehabilitated with obturator prostheses or surgical reconstruction have relatively small sample sizes. This is because such tumors are relatively rare and mortality rates are high. Hence comparisons between studies are difficult. Moreover, there is no universally accepted instrument for measuring head and neck cancer patients' quality of life following maxillary resection and rehabilitation. In addition, variables such as the quality of the prosthesis, and the nature of the prosthetic design are difficult to measure objectively. Consequently, the results of such studies will be open to question, especially when several treatment options are compared with one another.

Closing Thoughts: Guidelines for Determining the Method Best Suited for the Patient

Several different approaches are now available for the rehabilitation of defects of the hard palate. Until recent times obturation with a prosthesis was the only method. However, with the advent of vascularized flaps, several new options are now available, especially in combination with the use of implants. The purpose of this segment is to provide insight into how to determine which method best serves any patient.

Several factors are considered when determining the best mode of rehabilitation for any patient. They include but are not limited to the etiology and size of the defect, the cost and complexity of treatment, the overall health of the patient, treatment time, and whether the patient has sufficient healthy dentition to effectively retain, stabilize, and support an obturator prosthesis. Experience in wearing a removable prosthesis is also an important factor. Another important factor, particularly with regard to surgical reconstruction and implant placement, is the availability of an experienced team with the appropriate skill set and access to the digital technologies necessary for planning the resection in combination with a *prosthodontically driven* surgical reconstruction and implant placement.

It should be noted at the beginning of this discussion, notwithstanding the availability of tools such as PET scans for follow-up to monitor recurrence, many surgical oncologists prefer to monitor the surgical site directly and not to reconstruct such defects primarily with vascularized flaps, particularly following resection of malignant tumors. Even following the resection of benign tumors, negative margins from frozen sections are a minimal requirement for surgical reconstruction of a palatal defect. However, all too often, negative margins based on frozen sections cannot be called following resection of such tumors and this determination must await processing of permanent sections. Closure of the defect could make the subsequent surgery for persistent tumors more problematic and may result in greater loss of tissue for the patient.

The goal of rehabilitation is to restore speech, swallowing, mastication, and aesthetics. Conventional prosthodontic treatment successfully addresses these issues in dentate patients if the anterior maxillary segment has been retained after the resection and the canine on the side of the resection is preserved along with its bony support. In such defects there will be little movement of the prosthesis in and out of the defect during function and as a result, an RDP-obturator will effectively seal the defect and restore speech, swallowing, and mastication, especially when a positive cingulum rest is incorporated within the aforementioned canine (Fig 3-197). A similar result is achieved when a posterior abutment is retained on the resected side (Fig 3-198) even if the resection extends to the midline. Unless the patient requires extensive restorative work, the cost of treatment is minimal, and definitive treatment can be completed within six to eight months following tumor ablation. In such patients closing the defect and the placement of implants within the defect offer little or no improvement in function or aesthetics. Furthermore, the defect is open for inspection by the surgical and/or radiation oncologist. Oral hygiene compliance is crucial, however, because the health of the residual natural dentition, especially the key abutments, is essential for sustainable treatment outcomes. The primary disadvantage of this approach is that the patient has to manage a removable prosthesis. Based on these factors, in patients presenting with such defect configurations, RDP-obturator prostheses are preferred.

However, conventional RDP-obturator prostheses become less effective, even in dentate patients when the surgical resections are more aggressive, especially when they cross the midline. In such defects, the obturator prosthesis moves considerably in and out of the defect during function, even when retained by residual

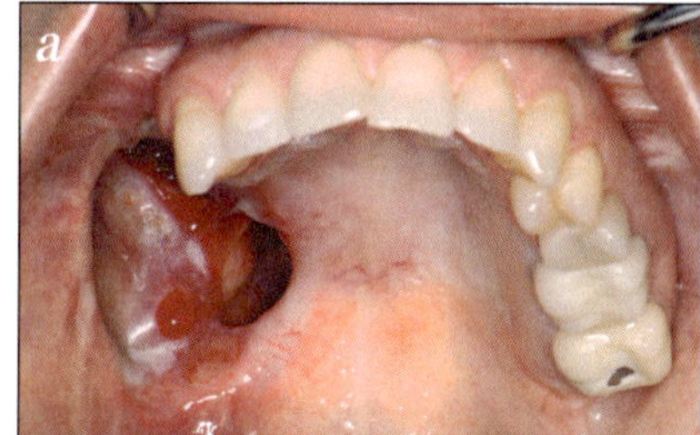

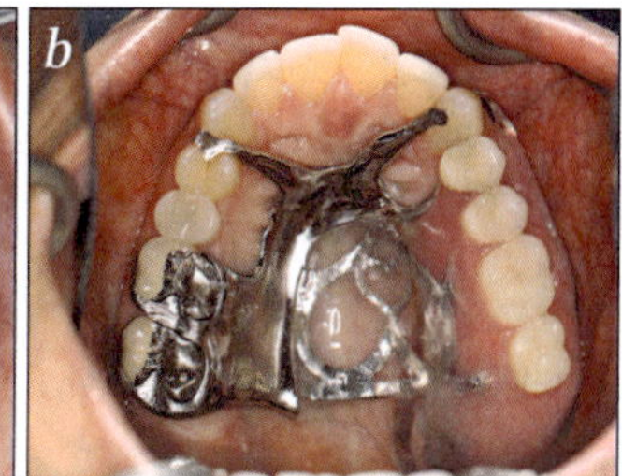

Figure 3-197 *(a)* A patient with an inframaxillectomy. The defect is skin lined. *(b)* Following completion of surveyed crowns and preparation of a cingulum rest on the canine adjacent to the defect, the definitive prosthesis was fabricated.

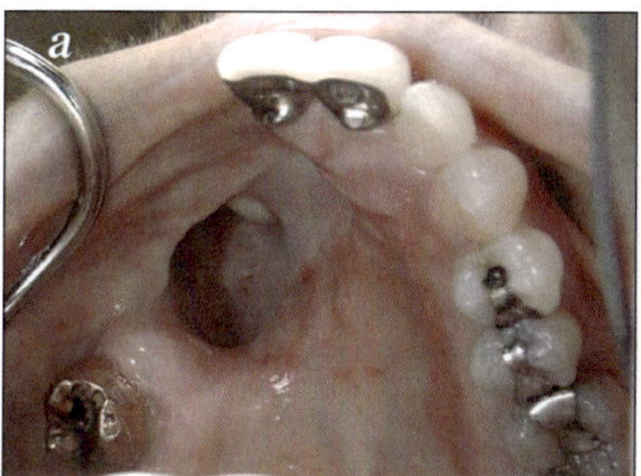

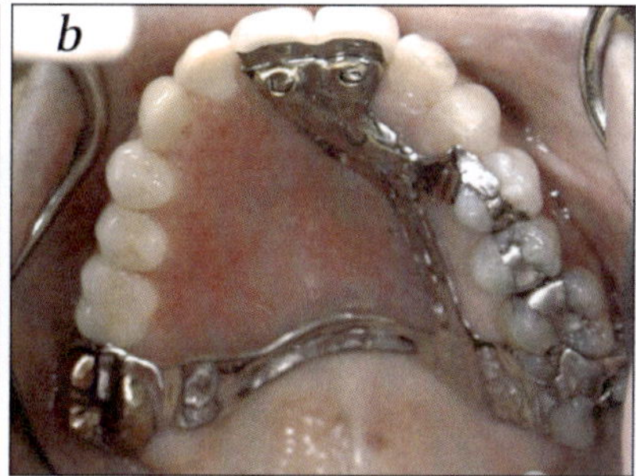

Figure 3-198 *(a and b)* A posterior abutment significantly improves the prosthetic prognosis of an RDP-obturator prosthesis. This is an 11-year follow-up photo.

dentition. Speech and swallowing are effectively restored with the RDP-obturator prosthesis but occasional leakage occurs, mastication performance is impaired and the patient has to deal with the management of a large removable prosthesis. In addition, the biomechanics of the RDP designs employed are usually unfavorable, and as a result, these large prostheses inflict significant wear and tear on the residual dentition, often leading to their premature loss. Edentulous patients with such defects will have even greater difficulty, and although speech and swallowing are restored with a complete-denture-obturator prosthesis, mastication may not be possible particularly when the opposing mandible is also edentulous.

A key factor in restoring mastication for patients with such large defects is to provide implant support on the side of the defect and bilaterally when needed (as would be the case in an edentulous patient). Two approaches have evolved in the restoration of such maxillary defects, whether the patient presents dentate or edentulous. The first and more traditional approach leaves the defect open. Implants are placed within the available bone volume (either zygomatic oncologic or conventional) in the defect and if needed on the unresected side, and the defect is restored with an implant-connecting bar and an overlay obturator prosthesis combined with a complete denture (CD) or RDP. The second involves closing the defect with either an osteomyocutaneous or a fasciocutaneous vascularized flap and using implants to help retain the prosthesis replacing the dentition and missing structures. When a fasciocutaneous vascularized fap is used to close the defect, either zygomatic oncologic implants or subperiosteal implants are placed, which perforate the flap. When an osteomyocutaneous vascularized flap is used to close the defect, conventional endosseous implants are placed into the bony portion of the flap.

Leaving the defect open and placing zygomatic oncologic implants have become the method of choice at many centers. These implants have made an appreciable impact on the way we rehabilitate these defects, even in patients with residual dentition, since they provide implant support on the side of the defect (Fig 3-199). Moreover, they can be placed at the time of tumor ablation. They are used in combination with the residual dentition in dentate patients or with conventional endosseous implants placed in the unresected portions of the palate in edentulous patients. The bilaterally supported obturator prosthesis is stable and virtually immobile during function and as a result, the defect can be sealed effectively, restoring speech and swallowing. In addition, mastication performance is restored to reasonable levels. Unless the patient requires extensive restorative work on the residual dentition, in addition to the usual surveyed crown on the tooth adjacent to the defect, the cost of treatment is within reasonable limits and definitive treatment can be completed within six to eight months following tumor ablation. Moreover, the defect is open for inspection by the surgical and/or radiation oncologist. However, given the nature of these defects and the difficult hygiene access, a major challenge for such patients is sustaining the health of the peri-implant tissues and preventing peri-implantitis and, with it, loss of bone anchoring the implants and the subsequent loss of implants. The primary disadvantage of this approach is that the patient has to manage a large removable prosthesis.

Surgical reconstruction with osteomyocutaneous flaps and placement of implants into these flaps that are used to retain a prosthesis has become the method of choice at some centers for such large defects (Fig 3-200). If the numbers are sufficient (at least three implants) and the implant distribution pattern is favorable, an implant-supported fixed prosthesis can be fabricated. If the number of implants is insufficient or the implant distribution pattern is unfavorable, a removable overlay prosthesis, retained by an implant-connecting bar, can be fabricated and designed to engage the residual dentition with an RDP framework. Mastication performance and quality-of-life outcomes are similar to that achieved with obturator prostheses retained and supported with zygomatic implants. Speech, swallowing, and mastication are maintained at near-normal levels and if the prosthesis is fixed, the patient does not have to deal with a large removable prosthesis. The main challenge

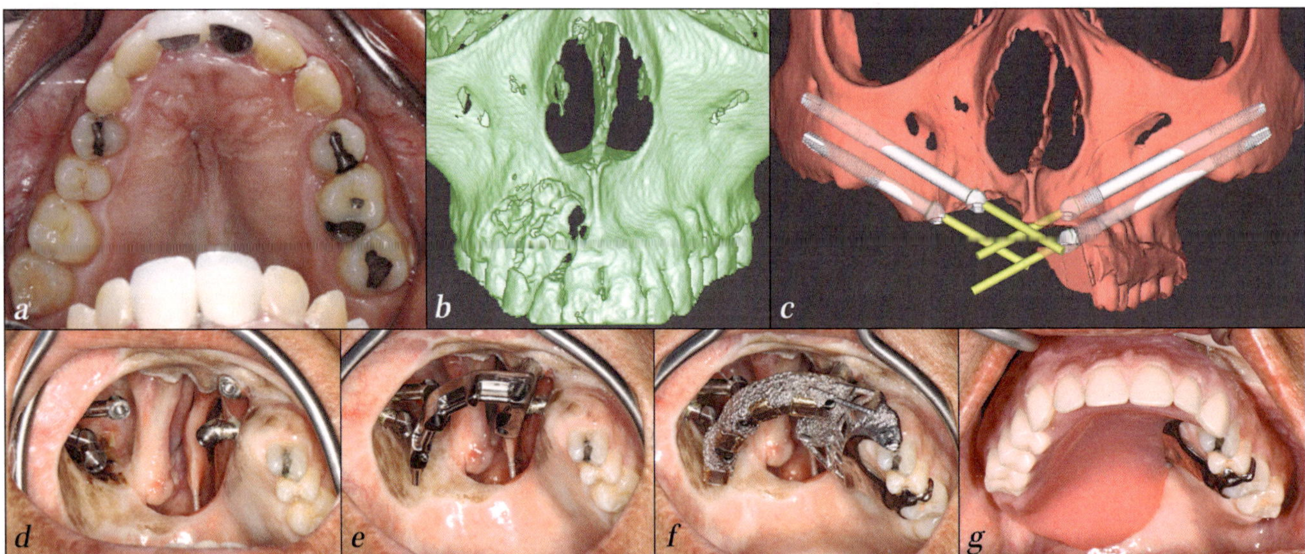

Figure 3-199 *(a and b)* A large ameloblastoma extending anteriorly crossing the midline. *(c)* VSP was accomplished with the appropriate software and 4 zygomatic implants were planned. A surgical template was designed and fabricated and the implant inserted using semiguided implant surgery. *(d)* The implants in position. Note that a skin graft was used to resurface the raw tissue surfaces in the defect. The skin graft accelerates healing and minimizes contraction of the wound, helping to maintain the prosthetic space. *(e)* The implant-supported implant-connecting bar. *(f)* The RDP framework that engages the bar and the residual dentition. The portion engaging the dentition provides additional bracing and support for the prosthesis. *(g)* The definitive prosthesis in position.

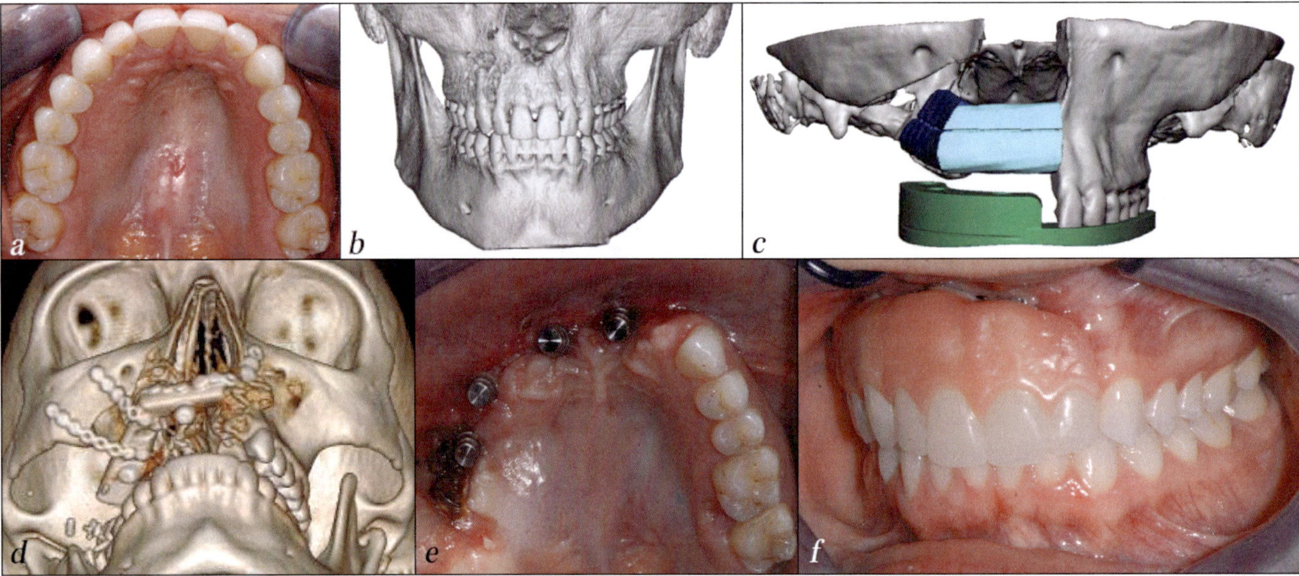

Figure 3-200 *(a and b)* A 25 y/o female presented with a recurrent keratocyst of the right maxilla. The lesion was scheduled to be removed with a maxillectomy. *(c)* Following VSP a fibula was fashioned to restore the defect. A fibula-positioning guide was designed based on the patient's mandibular dentition and proposed dental implant positions. *(d)* Immediate postoperative CT revealing position and angulation of the fibula and implants. *(e)* Soft tissue healing completed. *(f)* Definitive fixed hybrid prosthesis (from Moy et al., 2016 with permission).

for the patient, as is the case with zygomatic oncologic implants, is to maintain peri-implant soft tissue health. Such implants frequently are circumscribed by poorly keratinized and mobile mucosa or skin, making oral hygiene difficult for the patient and predisposing to the development of peri-implantitis and subsequent loss of implants. Donor-site morbidity and the disruptions of flow patterns of mucous and accumulation of secretions within the altered configurations of the paranasal sinuses are additional concerns. Moreover, if the patient has been treated with postoperative radiotherapy, it is very difficult to properly thin the tissues overlaying the implants without exposing the bone and triggering an osteoradionecrosis of the bony portion of the flap. Fear of this outcome often results in excessively thick peri-implant tissues further increasing the risk of peri-implantitis. Moreover, hygiene access is also difficult when large fixed implant-supported restorations are employed, particularly if the implants and/or the bony portions of the flap are not ideally positioned, requiring extensive ridge laps. The main disadvantages of the latter option are the high cost of treatment, prolonged hospital stays, number of surgical procedures, several years to complete treatment, and the availability of a well-trained interdisciplinary team that can execute a *prosthodontically driven* treatment plan. Furthermore, unless the bony portion of the flap is properly configured and the implants are suitably positioned, it is not possible to fabricate a fixed implant-supported prosthesis that is sustainable.

Several clinicians have reported successful outcomes closing the defect with a fasciocutaneous vascularized flap combined with the placement of implants (either zygomatic oncologic osseointegrated implants or a patient-specific digitally designed subperiosteal implant; Butterworth et al., 2022; Korn et al., 2021). The zygomatic oncologic implants or the implant posts from the subperiosteal implant are configured to perforate the flap. Either fixed prostheses or removable overlay prostheses retained by an implant-connecting bar have been used to restore the dentition and the residual tissue deficit. In most instances, definitive prosthodontic treatment is completed within six months of the tumor ablation. Maintenance of peri-implant soft tissue health is a major challenge because these implants are circumscribed by either skin or poorly keratinized mucosa predisposing to peri-implant soft tissue inflammation and hypertrophy. Donor-site morbidity and the disruptions of flow patterns of mucous and accumulation of secretions within the altered configurations of the paranasal sinuses are additional concerns. However, these two methods offer several advantages; treatment is usually completed within six months with fewer surgeries reducing cost. Flap survival has been acceptable as well as short-term implant survival. However, long-term follow-up data regarding implant survival is still not available.

In large defects, the key to restoring mastication performance to reasonable levels is bilateral support (Wang et al., 2017; Buurman et al., 2020b). This can be achieved solely with implants in edentulous patients or with a combination of implants and natural dentition in dentate patients. The key challenge for the approaches outlined in this segment is to sustain the implants over a prolonged period. For this to occur the health of the peri-implant tissues must be maintained. The clinical examples of the two patients shown (Figs 3-199 and 3-200) with similar defects help us differentiate between the two approaches and the advantages and disadvantages of each. Given similar treatment outcomes, the choices made at any particular treatment center depend on the training and expertise of the treatment teams, the availability of the necessary digital technologies, and the wishes and expectations of the patient.

An issue yet to be resolved with respect to each of these three options is the role biomechanics plays and the risk of implant overload given the implant configurations employed. As mentioned previously in this chapter, with respect to the use of zygomatic oncologic implants, these factors have been reasonably well worked out in edentulous patients with intact palates when implant-supported designs are employed (Jensen et al., 2012, 2015a, 2015b). A significant difference however is that zygomatic implants in normal patients are anchored in both the zygoma and the alveolar ridge. Zygomatic oncologic implants used to support obturator prostheses are anchored solely in the zygoma. However, these implants are "stacked" in relation to one another (see Fig 3-133), and perhaps this arrangement, when rigidly splinted across the arch, is resistant to the bending moments that are transferred through the implants into the anchoring bone. However, this assumption has yet to be challenged by either theoretical or long-term clinical studies. The biomechanics of implants placed in osteomyocutaneous flaps used to reconstruct palatal defects is also open to question. Frequently the implant configuration is primarily linear and if a fixed prosthesis is used these implants lack the benefits of cross-arch stabilization and may be subject to implant overload.

The impact of postoperative radiotherapy on the long-term survival of either zygomatic oncologic implants or conventional implants positioned within vascularized osteomyocutaneous flaps has yet to be determined. However, if the clinician is guided by the experiences gained in other irradiated sites, there is cause for concern with regard to their long-term survivability. One report involving 71 patients and 316 implants is especially revealing (Yeret et al., 2006). When implants were placed in intact but irradiated mandibles, where doses were limited to 50 Gy, implant loss rates approached 30% at the end of an eight-year follow-up period. Reports from other long-term studies assessing other sites show a similar pattern of implant loss over time (Roumanas et al., 2002). In a report by Buurman et al. (2020b), implant survival in irradiated sites currently stands at 82.6%. In the UCLA series, implant survival at irradiated sites is 76.36%: 93.1% of implants placed prior to radiation treatment and 57.69% when implants were placed in previously irradiated sites.

It is logical to assume that a similar loss rate would be seen when the implants and their anchoring bone are exposed to postoperative radiation and when those housed within osteomyocutaneous flaps would seem to be particularly vulnerable. The postoperative dose varies anywhere from 50 to 70 Gy and is determined by a number of factors, including the diagnosis, close or positive margins, lymph node extracapsular extension, two or more positive lymph nodes, lymphovascular invasion, and perineural invasion. When the dose to the bone anchoring the implants exceeds 60 Gy, the biologic phenomenon associated with osseointegration and the remodeling apparatus are shut down, and as a result, anchorage becomes primarily mechanical as opposed to biologic (Nishimura, 1995). When postoperative radiation is employed and implants are already in position, the dose enhancement effect secondary to backscatter will increase the dose substantially to the bone anchoring the implants. As a result, the dose to the bone anchoring the implants often exceeds the 60 Gy threshold. When postoperative radiotherapy is employed in a patient that has been reconstructed with an osteocutaneous flap and dental implants, the entire flap will be within the radiation clinical treatment volume and receive the tumor dose, whereas when zygomatic implants are placed in the zygoma and the defect is not reconstructed with a flap, IMRT can be used to reduce the dose delivered to select implant sites.

Nonetheless, the issue of long-term implant survival in irradiated patients may be somewhat moot given that most patients who develop malignancies in the region are age 60 and above and are generally afflicted with significant comorbidities, which in addition to their tumor diagnosis may impact their life span. Moreover, the loss of a single implant may not necessarily lead to the loss of the prosthesis or preclude the fabrication of a new prosthesis based on the status of the remaining implants, their distribution pattern, and their available dentition.

Another concern is that many authors have described the use of fixed restorations fabricated of acrylic resin with a metal core provided for strength and rigidity. Unfortunately, acrylic resin, particularly the autopolymerizing form, is quite porous and when in constant contact with the underlying tissues becomes infested with oral fungal organisms. Over time this can trigger a form of what is commonly referred to as denture stomatitis (i.e., chronic candidiasis), which in many patients leads to inflammation and hypertrophy of the affected tissues. In addition, these restorations are secured to the implants via abutments with machined surfaces and these surfaces accumulate plaque rapidly and retain it tenaciously, further contributing to the peri-implant tissue inflammation. If fixed is desired, it would seem prudent to select other materials such as monolithic zirconia for the prosthesis or to design the metal framework used to reinforce the resin to contact the intaglio surfaces per the original Branemark design. For these and other reasons, such as the need to provide proper support for the lip and midfacial area consistent with oral hygiene access, many authors prefer the use of implant-connecting bars and overlay prostheses.

In summary, many new treatment options have evolved during the last several years that have significantly improved oral function for patients undergoing aggressive resection of the palate and adjacent structures. However, these new therapies are not available uniformly throughout the world, and if not prosthodontically driven, clinical outcomes may not be acceptable or sustainable. In edentulous patients, a complete-denture-obturator prosthesis remains a viable option if the primary objectives are to restore speech and swallowing. If the patient is dentate and retains periodontally sound abutment teeth on the side of the resection, speech and swallowing are restored and mastication performance is maintained close to presurgical resection levels with a properly designed and crafted RDP-obturator prosthesis. However, if the resection extends across the midline, only by providing intradefect implant support in concert with either implant or dental support on the unresected side can functional outcomes be idealized.

Summary

Dentulous patients with a reasonable distribution of dentition and favorable defects of the hard palate are very effectively restored with an RDP-obturator prosthesis. Speech and swallowing are restored and mastication is accomplished with the residual maxillary dentition. The challenge clinicians face is to create favorable defects that can be used to facilitate the retention, support, and stability of the prosthesis to minimize the stress and strain exerted on key abutments; this goal is best accomplished when there is close interaction between the oncologic surgeon and the maxillofacial prosthodontist prior to tumor resection.

RDP designs require more bracing when defects are dynamic or unfavorable or when the remaining dentition is arranged in a linear fashion. Fulcrum lines for these RDPs are usually multiple and depend on where the bolus is incised or masticated in relation to the appropriate rests.

When the patient is edentulous, the defect must be engaged more aggressively to retain, support, and stabilize the complete-denture-obturator prosthesis; consequently, more attention should be paid during resection of the tumor to create more favorable defects (skin grafting of the defect, preservation of the anterior maxillary segment, maintenance of access to the defect, etc.). For these patients, speech and swallowing can be restored, but mastication is generally ineffective unless retention and stability are facilitated by the placement of osseointegrated implants. When multiple implants are placed in the residual bone in edentulous patients, the tilted concept of implant position and angulation are suggested. When implants are employed, we recommend that they be splinted together. In edentulous patients where implants are solely positioned on the unresected side, implant-assisted tissue bar designs must be employed. When implants are placed both within the defect and into the unoperated side, an implant-supported type implant-connecting bar can be considered. The addition of implants restores mastication to presurgical levels in most patients. Success rates are lower for implants in irradiated sites than for those in nonirradiated sites.

Large maxillary defects can be restored with free vascularized osteomyocutaneous flaps and osseointegrated implants. Occlusion-based protocols combined with digital workup, design, and manufacturing techniques are suggested. Another option is to place zygomatic implants or a subperiosteal implant within the defect at the surgical resection of the tumor and close the defect with a fasciocutaneous flap, with the implants extending through the flap. A prosthesis is then fabricated to restore the missing dentition and adjacent tissues.

References

Adwani DG, Arora RS, Bhattacharya A, et al. Non-Hodgkin's lymphoma of maxillary sinus: An unusual presentation. Ann Maxillofac Surg 2013;3:95–97.

Ahlholm P, Sipila K, Vallittu P, et al. Digital versus conventional impressions in fixed prosthodontics: A review. J Prosthodont 2018;27:35–41.

Alberga JM, Vosselman N, Korfage A, et al. What is the optimal timing for implant placement in oral cancer patients? A scoping literature review. Oral Dis 2021 Jan;27(1):94–110. http://doi.org/10.1111/odi.13312. Epub 2020 Mar 19.

Antony AK, Chen WF, Kolokythas A, et al. Use of virtual surgery and stereolithography-guided osteotomy for mandibular reconstruction with the free fibula. Plast Reconstr Surg 2011;128(5):1080–1084.

Aparicio C, Manresa C, Francisco K, et al. Zygomatic implants: Indications, techniques and outcomes, and the zygomatic success code. Periodontol 2000 2014;66:41–58.

Arigbede AO, Dosumu OO, Shaba OP, et al. Evaluation of speech in patients with partial surgically acquired defects: Pre and post prosthetic obturation. J Contemp Dent Prac 2006;15:89–96.

Arisan V, Karabuda CZ, Mumcu E, et al. Implant positioning errors in freehand and computer-aided placement methods: A single-blind clinical comparative study. Int J Oral Maxillofac Implants 2013;28:190–204.

Artopoulou II, Kardemas E, Papadogeogakis N, et al. Effects of sociodemographic, treatment variables, and medical characteristics on quality of life of patients with maxillectomy restored with obturator prostheses. J Prosthet Dent 2017;118:783–789.

Austin JR, Kershiznek MM, McGill D, et al. Breast carcinoma metastatic to paranasal sinuses. Head Neck 1995;17(2):161–165.

Bain C, Moy PK. The association between the failure of dental implants and cigarette smoking. Int J Oral Maxillofac Implants 1993;8:609–615.

Barber BR, Dziegelewski PT, Chuka R, et al. Bone-impacted fibular free flap: Long-term dental implant success and complications compared to traditional fibular free tissue transfer. Head Neck 2016;38(suppl 1):E1783–E1787.

Baredes S, Leeman DJ, Chen TS, et al. Significance of tumor thickness in soft palate carcinoma. Laryngoscope 1993;103:389–393.

Barrak HA. Hard palate perforation due to Mucormycosis: Report of 4 cases. J Laryngol Otol 2007;121:1099–102.

Beery QC, Aramany MA, Katzenberg B. Oral endoscopy in prosthodontic management of the soft palate defect. J Prosthet Dent 1985;54:241–244.

Beery QC, Rood SR, Schramm VL Jr. Pharyngeal wall motion in prosthetically managed cleft palate adults. Cleft Palate J 1983;20:7–17.

Bernier J, Cooper JS, Pajak TF, et al. Defining risk levels in locally advanced head and neck cancers: A comparative analysis of concurrent postoperative radiation plus chemotherapy trials of the EORTC (#22931) and RTOG (#9501). Head Neck 2005;27(10):843–850.

Berrone M, Crosetti E, Succo G. Repositioning template for mandibular reconstruction with fibular free flap: An alternative technique to pre-plating and virtual surgical planning. Acta Otorhinolaryngol Ital 2014;34:278–282.

Beumer J, Faulkner RF, Lyons KM, et al. Restoration of the edentulous maxilla with implant retained overdentures. In Fundamentals of implant dentistry—prosthodontic principles. 2nd ed. Ed. J Beumer, R Faulkner, K Shah, et al. Chicago: Quintessence; 2022a. pp. 202–243.

Beumer J, Lyons K, Kahensa N, et al. Implants in irradiated tissues, patients with osteoporosis and patients treated with bisphosphonates. In Fundamentals of implant dentistry—prosthodontic principles. 2nd ed. Ed. J Beumer, R Faulkner, K Shah, et al. Chicago: Quintessence; 2022b. pp. 498–515.

Beumer J, Marunick M, Silverman SS, et al. Rehabilitation of tongue-mandibular defects. In Maxillofacial rehabilitation: Prosthodontic and surgical management of cancer related, acquired, and congenital defects. 3rd ed. Chicago: Quintessence; 2011. pp. 61–154.

Beumer J, Nishimura R, Roumanas E. Maxillary defects: Alterations at surgery which enhance the prosthetic prognosis. In Proceedings of the First International Congress on Maxillofacial Prosthetics. Ed. I Zlotolow, S Esposito, J Beumer. New York: Memorial Sloan-Kettering Cancer Center; 1995. pp. 22–26.

Bhattacharyya N. Factors affecting survival in maxillary sinus cancer. J Oral Maxillofac Surg 2003a;61:1016–1021.

Bhattacharyya N. Survival and staging characteristics for non-squamous cell malignancies of the maxillary sinus. Arch Otolaryngol Head Neck Sur 2003b;129:334–337.

Birkeland AC, Auerbach AD, Sanborn E, et al. Postoperative clinical radiosensitivity in patients with fanconi anemia and head and neck squamous cell carcinoma. Arch Otolaryngol Head Neck Surg 2011;137:930–934.

Birnbach S, Barnhard B. Direct conversion of a solid obturator to a hollow obturator prosthesis. J Prosthet Dent 1989;62:58–60.

Bloomer HH, Hawk AM. Speech disorders associated with ablative approaches to learning. In ASHA Reports 8: Orofacial anomalies: Clinical and research implications. Washington, DC: American Speech-Language-Hearing Association; 1973. p. 42.

Blot WJ, McLaughlin JK, Winn DM, et al. Smoking and drinking in relation to oral and pharyngeal cancer. Cancer Res 1988;48:3282–3287.

Bradley DD. Congenital and acquired palatopharyngeal insufficiency. In Cleft lip and palate. Ed. WC Grabb, S Rosenstein, KR Bzoch. Boston: Little, Brown; 1971.

Brånemark PI, Gröndahl K, Ohrnell LO, et al. Zygoma fixture in the management of advanced atrophy of the maxilla: Technique and long-term results. Scand J Plast Reconstr Surg Hand Surg 2004;38:70–85.

Breeze J, Rennie A, Morrison A, et al. Health-related quality of life after maxillectomy: Obturator rehabilitation compared with flap reconstruction. British J Oral Maxillofac Surg 2016;54:857–862.

Brown KE. Peripheral consideration in improving obturator retention. J Prosthet Dent 1968;20:176–181.

Brudvik J, Taylor T. Resin bonding for maxillofacial prostheses. In Clinical maxillofacial prosthetics. Ed. T Taylor. Chicago: Quintessence; 2000. pp. 53–62.

Brunski JB, Puleo DA, Nance A. Biomaterials and biomechanics of osseointegrated implants: Current status and future developments. Int J Oral Maxillofac Implants 2000;15:15–46.

Buchner A, Merrell PW, Carpenter WM. Relative frequency of intra-oral minor salivary gland tumors: A study of 380 cases from northern California and comparison to reports from other parts of the world. J Oral Pathol Med 2007;36:207–214.

Butt FM, Chindia ML, Rana F. Oral squamous cell carcinoma in human immunodeficiency virus positive patients: Clinicopathological audit. J Laryngol Otol 2012;126:276–278.

Butterworth CJ. Primary vs secondary zygomatic implant placement in patients with head and neck cancer—a 10-year prospective study. Head Neck 2019;1–9. http://doi.org/10.1002/hed.25645.

Butterworth CJ, Lowe D, Rogers SN. The zygomatic implant perforated (ZIP) flap reconstructive technique for the management of low-level maxillary malignancy—clinical & patient related outcomes on 35 consecutively treated patients. Head Neck 2022;44:345–358.

Butterworth CJ, Rogers SN. The zygomatic implant perforated ZIP flap: A new technique for combined surgical reconstruction and rapid fixed dental rehabilitation following low-level maxillary. Int J Implant Dent 2017;3:37. http://doi.org/10.1186/s40729-017-0100-8.

Butz F, Aita H, Wang CC, et al. Harder and stiffer osseointegrated bone to roughened titanium. J Dent Res 2006;85:560–565.

Buurman DJM, Speksnijder CM, de Groot RJ, et al. Mastication in maxillectomy patients: A comparison between reconstructed maxillae and implant supported obturators: A cross-sectional study. J Oral Rehabil 2020a Jul 2. http://doi.org/10.1111/joor.13043.

Buurman DJM, Speksnijder CM, de Groot RJ, et al. Masticatory performance and oral health-related quality of life in edentulous maxillectomy patients: A cross-sectional study to compare implant-supported obturators and conventional obturators. Clin Oral Implants Res 2020b;31:405–416.

Candel E, Peñarrocha D, Peñarrocha M. Rehabilitation of the atrophic posterior maxilla with pterygoid implants: A review. J Oral Implantol 2012;38(spec no.):461–466.

Caputo TL, Ryan JE. An easy fast technique for making immediate surgical obturators. J Prosthet Dent 1989;61:473–475.

Carlson DL. Necrotizing sialometaplasia: A practical approach to the diagnosis. Arch Pathol Lab Med 2009;133:692–698.

Cerea M, Dolcini GA. Custom-made direct metal laser sintering titanium subperiosteal implants: A retrospective clinical study on 70 patients. Biomed Res Int 2018 May 28;2018:5420391. http://doi.org/10.1155/2018/5420391. eCollection 2018.

Chalian VA, Barnett MO. A new technique for constructing a one-piece hollow obturator after partial maxillectomy. J Prosthet Dent 1972;28:448–453.

Chang TL, Orellana D, Beumer J. Kratochvil's fundamentals of removal partial dentures. Chicago: Quintessence; 2019.

Chen C, Ren W, Gao L. Function of obturator prosthesis after maxillectomy and prosthetic obturator rehabilitation. Brazil J Otorhinolaryngol 2016;82:177–183.

Chen C, Ren WH, Huang RZ, et al. Quality of life in patients after maxillectomy and placement of prosthetic obturator. Int J Prosthodont 2016;29:363–368.

Chigurupati R, Aloor N, Salas R, et al. Quality of life after maxillectomy and prosthetic obturator rehabilitation. J Oral Maxillofac Surg 2013;71:1471–1478.

Chuka R, Abdullah W, Rieger J, et al. Implant utilization and time to prosthetic rehabilitation in conventional and advanced fibular free flap reconstruction of the maxilla and mandible. Int J Prosthodont 2017;30:289–294.

Cordeiro PG, Santamaria E. A classification system and algorithm for reconstruction of maxillectomy and midfacial defects. Plast Reconstr Surg 2000;105:2332–2346.

Crawford KL, Jafari A, Qualliotine JR, et al. Elective neck dissection for T3/T4 cN0 sinonasal squamous cell carcinoma. Head Neck 2020;42:3655–3662.

Cummer WE. Partial denture service. In The American textbook of prosthetic dentistry in contributions by eminent authorities. 7th ed. Ed. LP Anthony. Philadelphia: Lea and Febiger; 1942. p. 753.

Curtis TA, Taylor RC, Rositano SA. Physical problems in obtaining records of the maxillofacial patient. J Prosthet Dent 1975;34:539–554.

Dalkiz M, Dalkiz AS. The effect of immediate obturator reconstruction after radical maxillary resections on speech and other functions. Dent J (Basel) 2018 Sep;6(3):22. Published online 2018 Jun 21. http://doi.org/10.3390/dj6030022.

Dauwe PB, Pulikkottil BJ, Lavery L, et al. Does hyperbaric oxygen therapy work in facilitating acute wound healing: A systematic review. Plast Reconstr Surg 2014;133(2):208e–215e.

Davis B, Roumanas E, Hong S, et al. Stress distributions of implants used for retention of maxillary obturators. In Proceedings of the First International Congress on Maxillofacial Prosthetics. Ed. I Zlotolow, S Esposito, J Beumer. New York: Memorial Sloan-Kettering Cancer Center; 1995. pp. 204–208.

Davodi A, Beumer J, Faulkner RF, et al. Restoration of edentulous maxillae with fixed prostheses. In Fundamentals of implant dentistry—prosthodontic principles. Ed. J Beumer, R Faulkner, K Shah, et al. 2nd ed. Chicago: Quintessence; 2022. pp. 244–295.

D'Cruz AK, Vaish R, Kapre N, et al. Elective versus therapeutic neck dissection in node-negative oral cancer. N Engl J Med 2015;373:521–529.

de Groot RJ, Rieger JM, Rosenberg AJ, et al. A pilot study of masticatory function after maxillectomy comparing rehabilitation with an obturator prosthesis and reconstruction with a digitally planned, prefabricated, free, vascularized fibula flap. J Prosthet Dent 2020;124:616–622.

Demers PA, Kogevinas M, Boffetta P, et al. Wood dust and sino-nasal cancer: Pooled reanalysis of twelve case-control studies. Am J Ind Med 1995;28:151–166.

Desjardins RP. Obturator prosthesis design for acquired maxillary defects. J Prosthet Dent 1978;39:424–435.

de Souza Batista VE, Verri FR, Lemos CA, et al. Should the restoration adjacent implants be splinted or nonsplinted? A systematic review and meta-analysis. J Prosthet Dent 2019;121:41–51.

Devan MM. The prosthetic problem: Its formulation and suggestions for its solution. J Prosthet Dent 1956;6:291–301.

Dholam KP, Bachhcr G, Gurav SV. Changes in the quality of life and acoustic speech parameters of patients in various stages of prosthetic rehabilitation with an obturator after maxillectomy. J Prosthet Dent 2020;123:355–363.

Dos Anjos Ramos EA, Munhoz L, Milani BA, et al. Maxillary sinus natural killer / T-cell extranodal lymphoma mimicking a dentoalveolar abscess. Case Rep Dent 2019;2019:6701783.

Dulguerov P, Jacobsen MS, Allal AS, et al. Nasal and paranasal sinus carcinoma: Are we making progress? A series of 220 patients and a systematic review. Cancer 2001;92:3012–3029.

Durucu C, Baglam T, Karatas E, et al. Surgical treatment of inverted papilloma. J Craniofac Surg 2009;20:1985–1988.

Dziegielewski PT, Mlynarek AM, Harris JR, et al. Bone impacted fibular free flap: A novel technique to increase bone density for dental implantation in osseous reconstruction. Head Neck 2014;36:1648–1653.

El Saghir NS, Keating NL, Carlson RW, et al. Tumor boards: Optimizing the structure and improving efficiency of multidisciplinary management of patients with cancer worldwide. American Society of Clinical Oncology educational book. American Society of Clinical Oncology Meeting 2014:e461–e466.

Eliason C. RPA clasp design for distal-extension removable partial dentures. J Prosthet Dent 1983;49:25–27.

Elsemann RB, Cosme DC, Souto AA, et al. Degradation of tissue conditioners in complete dentures: An in situ study. Int J Prosthodont 2008;21:486–488.

Farhood Z, Simpson M, Ward GM, et al. Does anatomic subsite influence oral cavity cancer mortality? A SEER database analysis. Laryngoscope 2019;129:1400–1406.

Fenlon MR, Lyons A, Farrell S, et al. Factors affecting survival and usefulness of implants placed in vascularized free composite grafts used in post-head and neck cancer reconstruction. Clin Implant Dent Relat Res 2012;14(2):266–272.

Ferlito A, Rinaldo A, Silver CE, et al. Elective and therapeutic selective neck dissection. Oral Oncol 2006;42:14–25.

Firtell D, Grisius R. Retention of obturator-removable partial dentures: A comparison of buccal and lingual retention. J Prosthet Dent 1980;43:212–217.

Fischman B. The use of light-cured material for immediate hollow obturator prosthesis. J Prosthet Dent 1989;61:215–216.

Garrett N. Outcomes of maxillectomies with conventional and implant restorations. Presented at the International Congress on Maxillofacial Rehabilitation, Bangkok, Thailand, 24–27 Sep 2008.

Gotte K, Hormann K. Sinonasal malignancy: What's new? ORL J Otorhinolaryngol Relat Spec 2004;66:85–97.

Graboyes EM, Kompelli AR, Neskey DM, et al. Association of treatment delays with survival for patients with head and neck cancer: A systematic review. JAMA Otolaryngol Head Neck Surg 2019;145:166–177.

Guichet DL, Yoshinobu D, Caputo A. Effect of splinting and interproximal contact tightness on load transfer by implant restorations. J Prosthet Dent 2002;87:528–535.

Gulbransen H. Immediate surgical obturators. In Proceedings of the First International Congress on Maxillofacial Prosthetics. Ed. I Zlotolow, S Esposito, J Beumer. New York: Memorial Sloan-Kettering Cancer Center; 1995. pp. 144–151.

Gunne J, Jemt T, Linden B. Implant treatment in partially edentulous patients: A report on prostheses after 3 years. Int J Prosthodont 1994;7:143–148.

Gunter T, Merz B, Meriscske-Stern R, et al. Testing dental implants with an in vivo finite element model [in German]. Biomed Tech (Berl) 2000;45:272–276.

Gupta P, Zanation AM, Ganly I. Malignancies of the paranasal sinus. In Cummings otolaryngology head and neck surgery. 7th ed. Ed. P Flint, B Haughey, V Lund, et al. New York: Elsevier; 2020. pp. 1363–1390.

Hadeed G, Sprigg R. Articulator modification for maxillofacial prosthesis. J Prosthet Dent 1980;44:209–210.

Hammond J. Dental care of the edentulous patient after resection of the maxilla. Br Dent J 1966;120:591–594.

Hanasono MM, Weinstock YE, Yu P. Reconstruction of extensive head and neck defects with multiple simultaneous free flaps. Plast Reconstr Surg 2008;122:1739–1746.

Hanna E. Maxillectomy. In Atlas of head and neck surgery. Ed. GL Clayman, JI Cohen. New York: Elsevier Health Sciences; 2011. pp. 419–426.

Hayden RE, Mullin DP, Patel AK. Reconstruction of the segmental mandibular defect: Current state of the art. Curr Opin Otolaryngol Head and Neck Surg 2012;20:231–236.

Hernberg S, Westerholm P, Schultz-Larsen K, et al. Nasal and sinonasal cancer: Connection with occupational exposures in Denmark, Finland and Sweden. Scand J Work Environ Health 1983;9:315–326.

Hoggan BL, Cameron AL. Systematic review of hyperbaric oxygen therapy for the treatment of non-neurological soft tissue radiation-related injuries. Support Care Cancer 2014;22:1715–1726.

Hong SL, Kim BH, Lee JH, et al. Smoking and malignancy in sinonasal inverted papilloma. Laryngoscope 2013;123:1087–1091.

Hopper RA, Salemy S, Sze RW. Diagnosis of midface fractures with CT: What the surgeon needs to know. Radiographics 2006;26:783–793.

Hoshaw SJ, Brunski JB, Cochran GVB. Mechanical loading of Brånemark implants affects interfacial bone modeling and remodeling. J Oral Maxillofac Implants 1994;9:345–360.

Howes DG, Boyes-Varley JG, Blackbeard GA. An angulated implant for the maxilla: Development and evaluation. Presented at the Thirteenth Annual Scientific Meeting of the European Association for Osseointegration, Paris, 16–18 Sep 2004.

Huang W, Wu Y, Zou D, et al. Long-term results for maxillary rehabilitation with dental implants after tumor resection. Clin Implant Dent Relat Res 2014;16:282–291.

Hundepool AC, Dumans AG, Hofer SO, et al. Rehabilitation after mandibular reconstruction with fibula free-flap: Clinical outcome and quality of life assessment. Int J Oral Maxillofac Surg 2008;37:1009–1013.

Ide Y, Matsunaga S, Harris J, et al. Anatomical examination of the fibula: Digital imaging study for osseointegrated implant installation. J Otolaryngol Head Neck Surg 2015 Feb 3;44(1):1. http://doi.org/10.1186/s40463-015-0055-9.

Jacob R, Martin J, King G. Modification of surgical obturators to interim prostheses. J Prosthet Dent 1985;54:93–95.

Jacquiéry C, Rohner D, Kunz C, et al. Reconstruction of maxillary and mandibular defects using prefabricated microvascular fibular grafts and osseointegrated dental implants: A prospective study. Clin Oral Implants Res 2004;15:598–606.

James AG, Raines DR. The management of cancer of the maxillary antrum. Surg Gynecol Obstet 1995;101:395–400.

Jayanetti J, Fortmann C. Early implant loading for palatal defects: The UCLA experience with zygomatic implants. Presented at the Annual Meeting of the American Academy of Maxillofacial Prosthetics, Baltimore, MD, 2018 Oct.

Jensen OT, Adams MW. Angled (tilted) implants. In Fundamentals of implant dentistry: Prosthodontic principles. Ed. J Beumer, R Faulkner, K Shah. Chicago: Quintessence; 2015. pp. 88–94.

Jensen OT, Adams MW, Butura C, et al. Maxillary V-4: Four implant treatment for maxillary atrophy with dental implants fixed apically at the vomer-nasal crest, lateral pyriform rim, and zygoma for immediate function: Report on 44 patients followed from 1 to 3 years. J Prosthet Dent 2015;114:810–817.

Jensen OT, Cottam JR, Ringeman JL, et al. Angled dental implant placement into the vomer/nasal crest of atrophic maxillae for all-on-four immediate function: A 2-year clinical study of 100 consecutive patients. Oral Craniofac Tissue Eng 2012;2:66–71.

Kim BB, Zaid W, Spagnoli D, et al. Reconstruction of major maxillary and mandibular defects with implants. In Fundamentals of implant dentistry—surgical principles. Ed. PK Moy, A Pozzi, J Beumer. Chicago: Quintessence; 2016. pp. 259–289.

Kim DY, Hong SL, Lee CH, et al. Inverted papilloma of the nasal cavity and paranasal sinuses: A Korean multicenter study. Laryngoscope 2012;122:487–494.

Kim HY, Jung EK, Lee DH, et al. Clinical difference between benign and malignant tumors of the hard palate. Eur Arch Otorhinolaryngol 2020;277:903–907.

Kincade C, Karimi-Boushehri F, Osswald M, et al. Use of digital technologies in fabrication of a custom healing stent after stage II implant surgery for advanced jaw reconstruction. J Prosthetic Dent 2021;125:545–550.

Kipfmueller LJ, Lang BR. Presurgical maxillary prosthesis: An analysis of speech intelligibility. J Prosthet Dent 1972;28:620–625.

Knapp JG. A simplified approach to the fabrication of a hollow obturator prosthesis. J Prosthet Dent 1984;51:67–69.

Konrad HR, Canalis RF, Calcaterra TC. Epidermoid carcinoma of the palate. Arch Otolaryngol 1978;104:208–212.

Korn P, Gellrich NC, Jehn P, et al. A new strategy for patient-specific implant bone dental rehabilitation in patient with extended maxillary defects. Front Oncol 2021 Dec 10;11:718872. http://doi.org/10.3389/fonc.2021.718872. eCollection 2021.

Kornblith AB, Zlotolow IM, Gooen J, et al. Quality of life of maxillectomy patients using an obturator prosthesis. Head Neck 1996;18:323–334.

Koyama S, Sasaki K, Inai T, et al. Effects of defect configuration, size, and remaining teeth on masticatory function in post-maxillectomy patients. J Oral Rehabil 2005;32:635–641.

Kratochvil FJ. Influence of occlusal rest position and clasp design on movement of abutment teeth. J Prosthet Dent 1963;13:114–124.

Kratochvil FJ. Partial removable prosthodontics. Philadelphia: WB Saunders; 1988.

Kreeft AM, Krap M, Wismeijer D, et al. Oral function after maxillectomy and reconstruction with an obturator. Int J Oral Maxillofac Surg 2012;41:1387–1392.

Kurrasch M, Beumer J, Kagawa T. Mucormycosis: Oral and prosthodontic implications. J Prosthet Dent 1981;47:422–429.

Landes CA, Paffrath C, Koehler C, et al. Zygoma implants for midfacial prosthetic rehabilitation using telescopes: 9-year follow-up. Int J Prosthodont 2009;22:20–32.

Lang BR, Razoog ME. A practical approach to restoring occlusion for edentulous patients: 2. Arranging the functional and rational mold combination. J Prosthet Dent 1983;50:599–606.

Leclerc A, Luce D, Demers PA, et al. Sinonasal cancer and occupation: Results from the reanalysis of twelve case-control studies. Am J Ind Med 1997;31:153–165.

Lekholm U, Gunne J, Henry P, et al. Survival of the Brånemark implant in partially edentulous jaws: A 10-year prospective multicenter study. Int J Oral Maxillofac Implants 1999;14:639–645.

Lemos CA, Verri FR, Santiago JF Jr, et al. Splinted and nonsplinted crowns with different implant lengths in the posterior maxilla by three-dimensional finite element analysis. J Health Eng 2018 Sep 3;2018:3163096. http://doi.org/10.1155/2018/3163096. eCollection.

Lloyd S, Yu JB, Wilson LD, et al. Determinants and patterns of survival in adenoid cystic carcinoma of the head and neck, including an analysis of adjuvant radiation therapy. Am J Clin Oncol 2011;34:76–81.

Loevner LA, Sonners AI. Imaging of neoplasms of the paranasal sinuses. Neuroimaging Clin N Am 2004;14:625–646.

Luce D, Gerin M, Morcet JF, et al. Sinonasal cancer and occupational exposure to textile dust. Am J Ind Med 1997;32:205–210.

Lydiatt WM, Patel SG, O'Sullivan B, et al. Head and Neck cancers-major changes in the American Joint Committee on cancer eighth edition cancer staging manual. CA Cancer J Clin 2017;67:122–137.

Lyons KM, Beumer J, Caputo A. Abutment load transfer by removable partial denture obturator frameworks in different acquired maxillary defects. J Prosthet Dent 2005;94:281–288.

Maniatopoulos C, Pillar RM, Smith DC. Threaded vs porous-surfaced designs for implant stabilization in bone-endodontic implant model. J Biomed Mater Res 1986;20:1309–1333.

Marunick MT, Ma T. Articulator modification for maxillofacial prosthetics. J Prosthet Dent 1983;49:685–686.

Matalon V, LaFuente H. A simplified method for making a hollow obturator. J Prosthet Dent 1976;36:580–582.

Matsui Y, Ohno K, Shirota T, et al. Speech function following maxillectomy reconstructed by rectus abdominis myocutaneous flap. J Craniomaxillofac Surg 1995;23:160–164.

Matsuyama M, Tsukiyama Y, Tomioka M, et al. Clinical assessment of chewing function of obturator prostheses wearers by objective measurement of masticatory performance and maximum bite force. Int J Prosthodont 2006;19:253–257.

McCracken MS, Mitchell L, Hegde R, et al. Variability of mechanical torque-limiting devices in clinical service at a US dental school. J Prosthodont 2010;19:20–24.

McLean N, Tighiouart M, Miller S. Primary mucosal melanoma of the head and neck: Comparison of clinical presentation and histopathologic features of oral and sinonasal melanoma. Oral Oncol 2008;44:1039–1046.

Mendonca JA, Franischone CE, Senna PM, et al. A retrospective evaluation of the survival rates of splinted and non-splinted short dental implants posterior partially edentulous jaws. J Periodontol 2014;85:787–794.

Mian TA, Van Putten MC, Kramer DC, et al. Backscatter radiation at bone-titanium interface from high-energy X and gamma rays. Int J Radiat Oncol Biol Phys 1987;13:1943–1947.

Mihajlovic M, Vlajkovic S, Jovanovic P, et al. Primary mucosal melanomas: A comprehensive review. Int J Clin Exp Pathol 2012;5:739–753.

Minsley G, Nelson D, Rothenberger S. An alternative method for fabrication of a closed hollow obturator. J Prosthet Dent 1986;55:485–490.

Minsley G, Warren DW, Hinton V. Physiologic responses to maxillary resection and subsequent obturation. J Prosthet Dent 1987;57:338–344.

Miyamoto S, Ujigawa K, Kizu Y, et al. Biomechanical three-dimensional finite-element analysis of maxillary prostheses with implants: Design of number and position of implants for maxillary prostheses after hemimaxillectomy. Int J Oral Maxillofac Surg 2010;39:1120–1126.

Miyamoto Y, Koretake K, Hirata M, et al. Influence of static overload on the bony interface around implants in dogs. Int J Prosthodont 2008;21:437–444.

Miyata T, Kobayashi Y, Araki T, et al. The influence of controlled occlusal overload on peri-implant tissue: A histologic study in monkeys. Int J Oral Maxillofac Implants 1998;13:677–683.

Miyata T, Kobayashi Y, Araki T, et al. The influence of controlled occlusal overload on peri-implant tissue: 3. A histologic study in monkeys. Int J Oral Maxillofac Implants 2000;15:425–431.

Miyata T, Kobayashi Y, Araki T, et al. The influence of controlled occlusal overload on peri-implant tissue: 4. A histologic study in monkeys. Int J Oral Maxillofac Implants 2002;17:384–390.

Moore BA, Burkey BB, Netterville JL, et al. Surgical management of minor salivary gland neoplasms of the palate. Ochsner J 2008;8:172–180.

Moy PK, Medina D, Shetty V, et al. Dental implant failure rates and associated risk factors. Int J Oral Maxillofacial Implants 2005;20:569–567.

Moy PK, Pozzi A, Beumer J. Fundamentals of implant dentistry—surgical principles. Chicago: Quintessence; 2016.

Muir CS, Nectoux J. Descriptive epidemiology of malignant neoplasms of nose, nasal cavities, middle ear and accessory sinuses. Clin Otolaryngol Allied Sci 1980;5:195–211.

Nagasawa M, Takano R, Maeda T, et al. Observation of the bone surrounding an overloaded implant in a novel rat model. Int J Oral Maxillofac Implants 2013;28:109–116.

Nakamoto R. Use of immediate obturators in maxillary resections. Res Rep No. 20. Houston: MD Anderson Hospital and Tumor Institute; 1971.

Nambiar R, Narayanan G, Soman LV, et al. Lymphoblastic lymphoma of the palate. Proc (Bayl Univ Med Cent) 2017;30:445–446.

Network NCC. Head and neck cancers version 1.2021. Published 2020. Accessed 29 Nov 2020. https://www.nccn.org/professionals/physician_gls/pdf/head-and-neck.pdf.

Nimi A, Ueda M, Kaneda T. Maxillary obturator supported by osseointegrated implants placed in irradiated bone: Report of cases. J Oral Maxillofac Surg 1993;51:804–809.

Nishimura R, Roumanas E, Shimizu K. Implants in irradiated bone. In Proceedings of the First International Congress on Maxillofacial Prosthetics, 27–30 Apr 1994. Ed. I Zlotolow, S Esposito, J Beumer. Indian Wells, CA: Memorial Sloan-Kettering Cancer Center; 1995. pp. 199–203.

Obayemi A Jr, Cracchiolo JR, Migliacci JC, et al. Elective neck dissection (END) and cN0 hard palate and upper gingival cancers: A National Cancer Database analysis of factors predictive of END and impact on survival. J Surg Oncol 2019;120(7):1259–1265.

Ochi M, Kanazawa M, Sato D, et al. Factors affecting accuracy of implant placement with mucosa-supported stereolithographic surgical guides in edentulous mandibles. Comput Biol Med 2013;43:1653–1660.

Ogawa T, Nishimura I. Different bone integration profiles of turned and acid-etched implants associated with modulated expression of extracellular matrix genes. Int J Oral Maxillofac Implants 2003;18:200–210.

Ogawa T, Nishimura I. Genes differentially expressed in titanium healing. J Dent Res 2006;85:566–570.

Oh WS, Roumanas E. Optimization of maxillary obturator thickness using a double-processing technique. J Prosthodont 2008;17:60–63.

Ohashi Y, Shiga K, Katagiri K, et al. Evaluation and comparison of oral function after resection of cancer of the upper gingiva in patients who underwent reconstruction surgery versus those treated with a prosthesis. BMC Oral Health 21:347. Published online 2021 Jul 15. http://doi.org/10.1186/s12903-021-01709-7.

Ohngren LG. Malignant tumors of the maxilloethmoidal region. Acta Otolaryngol 1933;19:1–476.

Okay DJ, Buchbinder D, Urken M, et al. Computer-assisted implant rehabilitation of maxillomandibular defects reconstructed with vascularized bone free flaps. JAMA Otolaryngol Head Neck Surg 2013;139:371–381.

Oral K, Aramany MA, McWilliams BJ. Speech intelligibility with the buccal flange obturator. J Prosthet Dent 1979;41:323–328.

Parel SM, Drane JB. Reproducing the vertical-lateral defect space in obturator construction. J Prosthet Dent 1976;35:314–318.

Parel SM, LaFuente H. Single-visit hollow obturators for edentulous patients. J Prosthet Dent 1978;40:426–429.

Parr GR. A combination obturator. J Prosthet Dent 1979;41:329–330.

Patel A, Harrison P, Cheng A, et al. Fibular reconstruction of the maxilla and mandible with immediate implant-supported prosthetic rehabilitation: Jaw in a day. Oral Maxillofac Clin North Am 2019;31:369–386.

Payne AG, Welton WG. An inflatable obturator for use following maxillectomy. J Prosthet Dent 1965;15:759–763.

Peñarrocha M, Carrillo C, Boronat A, et al. Retrospective study of 68 implants placed in the pterygomaxillary region using drills and osteotomes. Int J Oral Maxillofac Implants 2009;24:720–726.

Pettersson A, Komiyama A, Hultin M, et al. Accuracy of virtually planned and template guided implant surgery on edentate patients. Clin Implant Dent Relat Res 2012;14:527–537.

Pfister DG, Spencer S, Adelstein D, et al. Head and neck cancers, version 2. NCCN Clinical Practice Guidelines in Oncology 2020;18(7):873.

Phankosol P, Martin J. Hollow obturator with removable lid. J Prosthet Dent 1985;54:98–100.

Pires FR, Pringle GA, de Almeida OP, et al. Intra-oral minor salivary gland tumors: A clinicopathological study of 546 cases. Oral Oncol 2007;43(5):463–470.

Plank D, Weinberg B, Chalian V. Evaluation of speech following prosthetic obturation of surgically acquired maxillary defects. J Prosthet Dent 1981;45:626–638.

Pozzi A, Beumer J, Moy P. Loading principles: Immediate loading, immediate provisionalization and delayed loading. In Fundamentals of implant dentistry—surgical principles. Ed. P Moy, A Pozzi, J Beumer. Chicago: Quintessence; 2016. pp. 333–374.

Rangert BR, Sullivan RM, Jemt TM. Load factor control for implants in the posterior partially edentulous segment. Int J Oral Maxillofac Implants 1997;12:360–370.

Reisberg D, Smith B. Aerodynamic assessment of prosthetic speech aids. J Prosthet Dent 1985;54P:686–690.

Riaz N, Warriach RA. Quality of life in patients with obturator prostheses. J Ayub Med Coll Abbottabad 2020;22:121–125.

Rieger J, Wolfaardt J, Seikaly HJ, et al. Speech outcomes in patients rehabilitated with maxillary obturator prostheses after maxillectomy: A prospective study. Int J Prosthodont 2002;15:139–144.

Rieger JM, Tang JA, Wolfaardt J, et al. Comparison of speech and aesthetic outcomes in patients with maxillary reconstruction versus maxillary obturators after maxillectomy. J Otolaryngol Head Neck Surg 2011;40:40–47.

Rogers SN, Lowe D, McNally D, et al. Health related quality of life after maxillectomy: A comparison between prosthetic obturation and free flap. J Oral Maxillofac Surg 2003;61:174–181.

Rohner D, Bucher P, Hammer B. Prefabricated fibula flaps for reconstruction of defects of the maxillofacial skeleton: Planning, technique, and long-term experience. Int J Oral Maxillofac Implant 2013;28:e221–e229. http://doi.org/10.11607/jomi.te01.

Rohner D, Jacquiéry C, Kunz C, et al. Maxillofacial reconstruction with prefabricated osseous free flaps: A 3-year experience with 24 patients. Plast Reconstruct Surg 2003;112:748–757.

Rohner D, Kunz C, Bucher P, et al. New technique for reconstruction of jaw defects with a prelaminated fibula flap and dental implants. Mund Kiefer Gesichtschir 2000;4:365–372.

Roumanas E, Nishimura R, Davis B, et al. Clinical evaluation of implants retaining maxillary obturator prosthesis. J Prosthet Dent 1997;77:184–190.

Rutkunas V, Geciaukaite A, Jegelevicius D, et al. Accuracy of digital implant impressions with intraoral scanners: A systematic review. Eur J Oral Implantol 2017;10(suppl 1):101–120.

Schaaf NG. Obturators on complete dentures. Dental Clin North Am 1977;21:395–401.

Schmidt BL, Pogrel MA, Young MA, et al. Reconstruction of extensive maxillary defects using zygomaticus implants. J Oral Maxillofac Surg 2004;62:82–89.

Schwartz H, Wollin M, Leake D, et al. Interface radiation dosimetry in mandibular reconstruction. Arch Otolaryngol 1979;105:293–295.

Schwartzman B, Caputo A, Beumer J. Gravity induced stresses by an obturator prosthesis. J Prosthet Dent 1990;64:466–468.

Schwartzman B, Caputo A, Beumer J. Occlusal force transfer by removable partial denture designs for a radical maxillectomy. J Prosthet Dent 1985;54:397–403.

Seifert G. Histopathology of malignant salivary gland tumours. Eur J Cancer B Oral Oncol 1992;28:49–56.

Seikaly H, Chau J, Li F, et al. Bone that best matches the properties of the mandible. J Otolaryngol 2003;32:262–265.

Seikaly H, Idris S, Chuka R, et al. The Alberta reconstruction technique: An occlusion-driven and digitally based jaw reconstruction. Laryngoscope 2019;129(suppl 4):S1–S14. http://doi.org/10.1002/lary.28064. Epub 2019 Jun 26.

Seruya M, Fisher M, Rodriguez ED. Computer-assisted versus conventional free fibula flap technique for craniofacial reconstruction: An outcomes comparison. Plast Reconstr Surg 2013;132:1219–1228.

Shah JP, Patel SG, Singh B. Nasal cavity and paranasal sinuses. In Jatin Shah's head and neck surgery and oncology. Eds. Shah JP et al. Philadelphia: Elsevier; 2019.

Sharaf B, Levine JP, Hirsch DL, et al. Importance of computer-aided design and manufacturing technology in the multidisciplinary approach to head and neck reconstruction. J Craniofac Surg 2010;21:1277–1280.

Sharma A, Beumer J. Reconstruction of maxillary defects: The case for prosthetic rehabilitation. J Oral Maxillofac Surg 2005;63:1770–1773.

Shifman A. Clinical applications of visible-light cured resin in maxillofacial prosthetics: 1. Denture base and reline material. J Prosthet Dent 1990;64:578–582.

Shipman B. Evaluation of occlusal force in patients with obturator defects. J Prosthet Dent 1987;57:81–84.

Shome D, Honavar SG, Gupta P, et al. Metastasis to the eye and orbit from renal cell carcinoma—a report of three cases and review of literature. Surv Ophthalmol 2007;5:213–223.

Shuman AG, Light E, Olsen SH, et al. Mucosal melanoma of the head and neck: Predictors of prognosis. Arch Otolaryngol Head Neck Surg 2011;137:331–337.

Standlee J, Caputo AA. Accuracy of an electronic torque-limiting device for implants. Int J Oral Maxillofac Implants 1999;14:278–281.

Standlee J, Caputo AA, Chwu MY, et al. Accuracy of mechanical torque-limiting devices for implants. Int J Oral Maxillofac Implants 2002;17:220–224.

Stanford CM, Brand RA. Toward an understanding of implant occlusion and strain adaptive bone modeling and remodeling. J Prosthet Dent 1999;81:553–556.

Stennert E, Guintinas-Lichius O, Klussman JP, et al. Histopathology of pleomorphic adenoma in the parotid gland: A prospective unselected series of 100 cases. Laryngoscope 2001;111:2195–2200.

Sullivan M, Gaebler C, Beukelman D, et al. Impact of palatal prosthodontic intervention on communication performance of patients' maxillectomy defects: A multilevel outcome study. Head Neck 2002;24:530–538.

Szmuckler-Moncler S, Piatelli A, Favero GA, et al. Considerations preliminary to the application of early and immediate loading protocols in dental implantology. Clin Oral Implants Res 2000;11:12–25.

Taicher S, Rosen A, Arbree N, et al. A technique for fabrication of polydimethylsiloxane-acrylic resin obturators. J Prosthet Dent 1983;50:65–68.

Tealdo T, Menini M, Bevilacqua M, et al. Immediate versus delayed loading of dental implants in edentulous patients' maxillae: A 6-year prospective study. Int J Prosthodont 2014;27:207–214.

Tobey E, Lincks J. Acoustic analysis of speech changes after maxillectomy and prosthodontic management. J Prosthet Dent 1989;62:449–455.

Toro C, Robiony M, Costa F, et al. Feasibility of preoperative planning using anatomical facsimile models for mandibular reconstruction. Head Face Med 2007;3:5. http://doi.org/10.1186/1746-160X-3-5. PMID: 17224060; PMCID: PMC1783647.

Toto JM, Chang EI, Agag R, et al. Improved operative efficiency of free fibula flap mandible reconstruction with patient-specific, computer-guided preoperative planning. Head Neck 2015;37:1660–1664.

Trimarchi M, Bondi S, Della Torre E, et al. Palate perforation differentiates cocaine-induced midline destructive lesions from granulomatosis with polyangiitis. Acta Otorhinolaryngol Ital 2017;37:281–285.

Tso TV, Hurwitz M, Margalit DN, et al. Radiation dose enhancement associated with contemporary dental materials. J Prosthet Dent 2019;121:703–707.

Tuminelli FJ, Walter LR, Neugarten J, et al. Immediate loading of zygomatic implants: A systematic review of implant survival, prosthesis survival and potential complications. Eur J Oral Implantol 2017;10(suppl 1):79–87.

Ueda K, Tajima S, Oba S, et al. Mandibular contour reconstruction with three-dimensional computer-assisted models. Ann Plast Surg 2001;46:387–393.

Van Assche N, van Steenberghe D, Guerrero ME, et al. Accuracy of implant placement based on pre-surgical planning of three-dimensional cone-beam images: A pilot study. J Clin Periodontol 2007;34:816–821.

Van Assche N1, Vercruyssen M, Coucke W, et al. Accuracy of computer-aided implant placement. Clin Oral Implants Res 2012;23:112–123.

Vasak C, Watzak G, Gahleitner A, et al. Computed tomography-based evaluation of template (NobelGuide™)-guided implant positions: A prospective radiological study. Clin Oral Implants Res 2011;22:1157–1163.

Vosselman HH, Glas HH, de Visscher SAHJ, et al. Immediate implant-retained prosthetic obturation after maxillectomy based on zygomatic implant placement by 3D-guided surgery: A cadaver study. Int J Implant Dent 2021 Jun 14;7(1):54. http://doi.org/10.1186/s40729-021-00335-w.

Vosselman N, Merema BJ, Schepman KP, et al. Patient-specific sub-periosteal zygoma implant for prosthetic rehabilitation of large maxillary defects after oncological resection. Int J Oral Maxillofac Surg 2019;48:115–117.

Wang F, Huang W, Zhang C, et al. Functional outcome and quality of life after a maxillectomy: A comparison between an implant supported obturator and implant supported fixed prostheses in a free vascularized flap. Clin Oral Implants Res 2017;28:137–143.

Wang F, Monje A, Lin GH, et al. Reliability of four zygomatic implant-supported prostheses for the rehabilitation of the atrophic maxilla: A systematic review. Int J Oral Maxillofacial Implants 2015;30:293–298.

Wang TM, Leu LJ, Wang J, et al. Effects of prosthesis materials and prosthesis splinting on peri-implant bone stress around implants in poor quality bone: A numeric analysis. Int J Oral Maxillofac Implants 2002;17:231–237.

Warren DW. Nasal emission of air and velopharyngeal function. Cleft Palate J 1967;4:148–155.

Warren DW. A physiologic approach to cleft palate prosthesis. J Prosthet Dent 1965;15:770–778.

Warren DW. Restorative treatment of the dentofacial complex. In ASHA Reports 5: Speech and the dentofacial complex: The state of the art. Ed. RT Wertz. Washington, DC: American Speech-Language-Hearing Association; 1970. pp. 132–145.

Warren DW. Velopharyngeal orifice size and upper pharyngeal pressure-flow patterns in cleft palate speech: A preliminary study. Plast Reconstr Surg 1964;34:15–26.

Warren DW, Wood MT, Bradley DP. Respiratory volumes in normal and cleft palate speech. Cleft Palate J 1969;6:449–460.

Weitz J, Bauer FJ, Hapfelmeier A, et al. Accuracy of mandibular reconstruction by three-dimensional guided vascularised fibular free flap after segmental mandibulectomy. Br J Oral Maxillofac Surg 2016;54:506–510.

Wetzels JW, Koole R, Meijer GJ, et al. Functional benefits of implants placed during ablative surgery: A 5-year prospective study on the prosthodontic rehabilitation of 56 edentulous oral cancer patients. Head Neck 2016 Apr;38(suppl 1):E2103–E2111. http://doi.org/10.1002/hed.24389. Epub 2016 Feb 13.

Wetzels JW, Meijer GJ, Koole R, et al. Costs and clinical outcomes of implant placement during ablative surgery and postponed implant placement in curative oral oncology: A five-year retrospective cohort study. Clin Oral Implants Res 2017;28:1433–1442.

Wetzels JW, Merkx MAW, de Haan AF, et al. Maximum mouth opening and trismus in 143 patients treated for oral cancer: A 1-year prospective study. Head Neck 2014;36:1754–1762.

World Health Organization. Classification of head and neck tumours. Vol 9. 4th ed. Lyon: International Agency for Research on Cancer; 2017.

World Health Organization. Classification of tumours: Head and neck tumours. 3rd ed. Lyon: International Agency for Research on Cancer; 2005.

Wu B, Abduo J, Lyons K, et al. Implant biomechanics, screw mechanics, and occlusal concepts for implant patients. In Fundamentals of implant dentistry: Prosthodontic principles. Ed. J Beumer, R Faulkner, K Shah, et al. Chicago: Quintessence; 2022.

Wu J, Sun J, Shen SG, et al. Computer-assisted navigation: Its role in intraoperatively accurate mandibular reconstruction. Oral Surg Oral Med Oral Pathol Oral Radiol 2016;122(2):134–142.

Wu Y, Schaaf NG. Comparison of weight reduction in different designs of solid and hollow obturator prostheses. J Prosthet Dent 1989;62:214–217.

Yoda N, Gunji Y, Ogawa T, et al. In vivo load measurement for evaluating the splinting effects of implant-supported superstructures: A pilot study. Int J Prosthodont 2013;26:143–146.

Zaki HS. Modified bypass in maxillary hollow bulb obturators. J Prosthet Dent 1980;43:320–321.

Zhang N, Liu S, Hu Z, et al. Accuracy of virtual surgical planning in two-jaw orthognathic surgery: Comparison of planned and actual results. Oral Surg Oral Med Oral Path Oral Radiol 2016;122:143–151.

Zheng GS, Su YX, Liao GQ, et al. Mandibular reconstruction assisted by preoperative simulation and accurate transferring templates: Preliminary report of clinical application. J Oral Maxillofac Surg 2013;71:1613–1618.

Chapter 4

Rehabilitation of Soft Palate Defects

John Beumer III, Arun Sharma, Jana Rieger

The maxillofacial prosthodontist may be called upon to reestablish velopharyngeal integrity in order to provide the potential for normal speech. This additional dimension of prosthetic therapy requires a basic understanding of the speech mechanism. Therefore, the objectives of this chapter are to describe the components of speech, to explore the anatomy and physiology of the velopharyngeal complex, and to relate this information to the rehabilitation of patients with defects or deficiencies of the soft palate and pharyngeal walls.

Speech

Speech, as formulated, executed, perceived, and decoded, is unique to humans. From an evolutionary perspective, speech developed as a learned process that took advantage of the anatomical structures designed primarily for respiration, mastication, and deglutition (MacNeilage, 1998). The production of speech requires the selective modification and control of an outgoing airstream (Huntington, 1968) through the complex and skilled coordination of more than 100 muscles within the respiratory, laryngeal, velopharyngeal, and oral mechanisms (Levelt, 1994). This intricate process begins within the central nervous system, where formulation of speech relies on intact central nervous system components. Following formulation, execution of speech relies not only on intact central nervous system components but also on peripheral nervous system components, such as the cranial nerves that supply the head and neck region and the spinal nerves that power the respiratory system. An intact auditory system is required in the speaker to monitor and adjust speech output, as needed, and in the listener to perceive and decode the speech signal. Disturbance of any one of the speech mechanisms or neural systems–through injury, ablative surgery, or congenital malformation–can lead to a speech disorder.

Components of speech

Kantner and West (1941) divided speech into five components: *(1)* respiration, *(2)* phonation, *(3)* resonation, *(4)* articulation, and *(5)* neural integration. Chierici and Lawson (1973) added *(6)* audition, or the ability to hear sounds, to this list. The successful performance of these functions is necessary for the production of acceptable speech.

Respiration

The primary function of the respiratory system is to provide the body with a gas exchange system necessary for sustaining life. During respiration for life preservation purposes, inhalation and exhalation are approximately equal in duration and the airflow is regular and repetitive. During speech, however, the process begins with a relatively brief inspiration followed by an extended expiration during which pulmonary air interacts with resonating tubes and chambers in the throat, mouth, nose, and cranium to produce an audible speech signal.

The muscles primarily responsible for inspiration to support speech are the diaphragm and the external intercostals. When inspiration of a greater volume of air is necessary (such as for long or loud utterances), accessory muscles such as the sternocleidomastoid, scalenes, subclavius, pectoralis major and minor, and the latissimus dorsi may become active. The inspiratory muscles enlarge the thorax and consequently decrease alveolar pressure to create a pressure gradient that will favor the inward flow of air.

For speech to be produced, alveolar pressure must exceed atmospheric pressure so that an outward flow of air will occur. Exhalation is regulated by passive mechanical and/or muscle forces depending on the air supply necessary for the desired sentence length during connected speech. At higher lung volumes, alveolar pressure is high and the outward flow of air occurs passively as a function of compression of the chest wall in response to the recoil forces of the lungs and thorax, gravity, and torque. The external intercostal muscles may be active during expiration at higher lung volumes to "brake" the compression of the chest wall, thereby counteracting the passive forces imposed on the respiratory system and preventing expiratory air from rushing out of the lungs.

When the demands for speech exceed the alveolar pressure produced by passive compression of the chest wall, active expiration must take place. The muscles primarily responsible for active expiration during speech production are those of the rib cage (e.g., internal intercostals, transversus thoracis, and subcostals) and the abdomen (e.g., rectus abdominus, external and internal oblique, and transversus abdominus). These muscles contract to further decrease the size of the thorax so that the alveolar pressure necessary for speech is maintained. Poor projection of the voice may be due in part to the reduced volume and pressure of the expired air.

Phonation

The primary function of the laryngeal structures is to protect the upper and lower airways from inhalation of particulate matter. Through the process of evolution, the laryngeal structures, in particular the vocal folds and their associated laryngeal musculature, developed a vital role in the process of speech production. The outward flow of air from the lungs during expiration is the power supply for speech. For unvoiced sounds, air from the lungs passes through an open larynx and is modified by downstream articulatory structures to produce speech sounds that are periodic in nature. For voiced sounds, air from the lungs sets adducted vocal folds into vibration, which creates a periodic sound wave that is selectively resonated and filtered within the vocal tract.

As has been described by others (Jiang et al., 2000; Hillman et al., 1989), the vibration of the vocal folds requires the development of pressure beneath the adducted vocal folds (i.e., subglottal pressure) to drive them apart and then elastic restoring forces and the Bernoulli effect to bring them back together. This cycle is repeated very rapidly during phonation, resulting in the creation of a series of sound waves in the tract above the vocal folds by the pulses of air that escaped while the vocal folds were displaced. During voice production, this cycle of vocal fold opening and closure occurs approximately 110 times per second in an average male voice and approximately 200 times per second in an average female voice (Jiang et al., 2000; Boone and McFarland, 1988).

The mass, tension, and stiffness of the vocal folds will determine the pitch of the phonated sound. In the production of low-pitched sounds, the vocal folds are relatively thick and flaccid. In high-pitched sounds, the margins of the approximated folds are thin and tense.

Certain pathologic conditions may produce changes in the normal vibratory patterns of the vocal folds, which in turn, may eventually affect the behavior of the respiratory system. If the larynx is resected, the patient must learn to use the esophagus or a substitute mechanical device (e.g., electrolarynx or voice prosthesis) as an alternative vibrating source. Because alternative vibrating systems may produce a constant tone, speech after laryngectomy often lacks the modulations and inflections of normal speech. Neurologic disorders and pathologic conditions affecting the vocal folds, such as carcinoma, papilloma, or contact ulcers, also can produce phonatory defects of varying degrees.

Resonation

The sound produced at the level of the vocal folds is not the final acoustic signal that is perceived as speech (Chierci and Lawson, 1973). This sound is augmented and modified by the chambers and structures above the level of the glottis. The pharynx, oral cavity, and nasal cavity act as resonating chambers by selectively filtering some frequencies and damping others, thus refining tonal quality.

The pharynx, being a muscular tube, serves as an excellent resonating chamber. This tube is formed by three closely associated muscles: the inferior, middle, and superior constrictor muscles. These muscles are unique in that they have a common insertion (the medial pharyngeal raphe) but different anterior origins. Also, it appears that each constrictor as well as portions of each muscle can contract selectively (Cole, 1971). The dimensional changes imparted by this muscular action influence the resonant characteristics of the pulsating airstream as it emerges from the larynx.

The soft palate, which achieves separation of the oral and nasal cavities in concert with the pharynx, achieves elevation primarily by the levator veli palatini. The velopharyngeal mechanism proportions the sound and/or airstream between the oral and nasal cavities and influences the resonant quality of the speech signal or the basic sound that is perceived by the listener.

All English vowels and most consonants use the oropharynx and the oral cavity as the primary resonating chambers. However, three nasal consonants (*/m/*, */n/*, and */ng/*) use the nasal cavity as the primary resonating chamber. All speech sounds require at least a small amount of nasal resonance, as evidenced by the distortions in voice quality exhibited by individuals with severe nasal congestion. The balance of sound emanating from the mouth versus the nose influences the speech quality that is perceived by the listener. If velopharyngeal closure is compromised, or if the structural integrity or relative size of the oral, pharyngeal, or nasal cavities has been altered, resonance can be compromised.

Articulation

For English sounds, articulation occurs when resonated sound reaches the oral cavity. There, the sound waves are formed into meaningful speech by the action of the moveable articulators, including the mandible, tongue, lips, and soft palate, against the immoveable articulatory structures, including the hard palate, alveolar ridge, and teeth (Fig 4-1).

The tongue is considered to be the single most important articulator of speech because of its ability to affect rapid changes in movement and shape. The extrinsic tongue muscles, including the genioglossus, hyoglossus, styloglossus, and palatoglossus, are responsible for general postural adjustments of the tongue. The intrinsic tongue muscles (transversus, verticalis, and inferior and

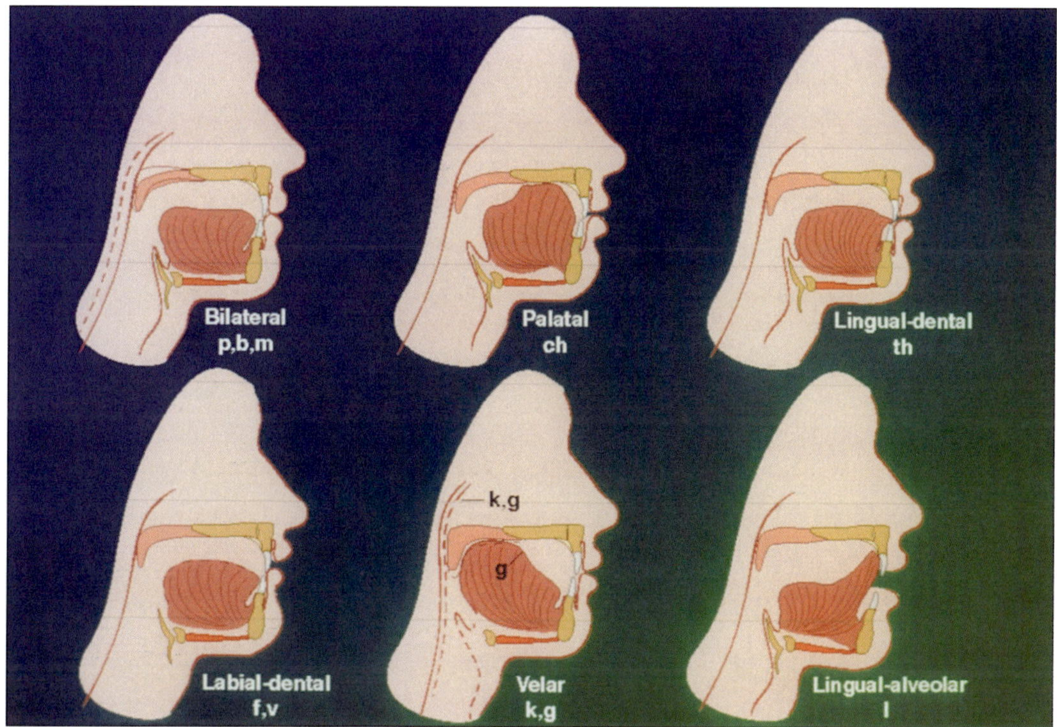

Figure 4-1 Static structures are important in establishing the route air takes during connected speech. Dynamic structures control and direct exhaled air to form appropriate speech sounds (courtesy of Dr. S. Esposito).

superior longitudinal) are required for more discrete and rapid movements that change the shape of the tongue. In modifying the shape of the oral cavity, the tongue affects the resonant characteristics of the produced speech signal. The tongue may impede, selectively restrict, and channel the airstream with precise contact against the teeth and palatal areas, thus articulating the basic laryngeal sound or the nonphonated airstream into recognizable speech.

If oral structures such as the tongue, adjacent soft tissues, jaws, or lips are altered surgically and/or neurologically, articulation may be compromised. Structural alterations in the oral cavity that allow air to leak from what should be a closed system, whether the leak is artificially induced or results from an anatomical defect, induce compensatory respiratory responses to maintain adequate oral air pressures for speech (Warren et al., 1981, 1984, 1989, 1992; Putnam et al., 1986; Warren, 1986; Dalston et al., 1990; Laine et al., 1988a, 1988b; Moon et al., 1993). The compensatory regulation/control phenomenon is likely related to the existence of mechanoreceptors for pressure in the vocal tract that act as a detection system (Warren, 1986, Putnam et al., 1986; Warren et al., 1992b). Feedback from the detection mechanism leads to a relevant change in the respiratory system to maintain the pressure levels in the vocal tract necessary for voice and speech (Moon et al., 1993; Putnam et al., 1986; Warren et al., 1984, 1992b; Warren, 1986).

This phenomenon is commonly observed when patients' palatopharyngeal system is compromised. Patients often compensate for a loss of air pressure in the oral cavity, which results from the inappropriate coupling of the oral and nasal cavities, by increasing respiratory drive. Such patients often will complain of feeling breathless and tiring easily when speaking.

Neural integration

Speech is integrated by the central nervous system at both the peripheral and the central levels. The sequential and simultaneous movements required throughout the speech complex demand precise coordination. MacNeilage and DeClerk (1969) noted that at least 17,000 different motor patterns are required during speech.

Neurologic impairments may compromise a specific component of the speech mechanism, such as the vocal folds, soft palate, or tongue, or it may indirectly affect the entire speech system. A cerebrovascular accident may compromise the ability of the patient to comprehend and/or formulate meaningful speech even though all structures used to produce speech are anatomically within normal limits. In addition, a neurologic impairment may produce a specific type of speech disorder. For example, the loss of motor innervation to the soft palate may compromise elevation and velopharyngeal closure.

Audition

Audition, or the ability to receive acoustic signals, is vital for normal speech. Hearing permits the reception and interpretation of acoustic signals and allows the speaker to monitor and control speech output. It has been hypothesized that the speech system acts as a servomechanism (i.e., a self-regulating machine) by using auditory feedback to regulate and control the subsequent speech output (Attanasio, 1987; Borden et al., 1984; Fairbanks, 1955; Fucci, 1977; Hood, 1998; Larson, 1998; Ludlow and Cikoja, 1998; Hain et al., 2001). The speech system is a closed-loop servomechanism in which information is sent back to the control mechanism to adjust for errors in performance that are detected (Hood, 1998).

Multiple closed-loop systems act on the speech system. One of them is an auditory loop that allows the speaker to monitor the accuracy of the intended speech targets; another allows the speaker to monitor the reception of a spoken message by a listener. With respect to the first type of closed-loop system, research suggests that auditory feedback provides a speaker with a mechanism for online adjustments to the speech system when the acoustic output does not meet the acoustic target that is stored in the speaker's brain (Houde, 1998).

With the second type of closed-loop system, appropriate corrections will be made to a message generated by a speaker if the reaction of the listener indicates that there is a problem with the message. Experimental support for this can be found in studies that have examined the changes that an individual makes in order to be understood when speaking (Helfer, 1997; Picheny et al., 1989; Uchanski, 1996). Evidence from studies of "clear speech" (Kangathoran et al., 2021) has suggested that speakers will adjust their articulation to make their speech clearer by inserting extra acoustic information and by increasing the duration of sounds such as vowels, voiced plosives, unvoiced fricatives, and semivowels. Experimental evidence such as this suggests that the closed-loop speech monitoring system can detect inaccuracies in listener perception and that the speech production system responds to that feedback by altering the manner in which sounds are produced.

Compromised hearing can preclude accurate feedback and hence affect speech, especially nasal resonance (Kim et al., 2012; Baudonck et al., 2015; Zamani et al., 2021).

Speech and maxillofacial prosthetics

Of the six components of speech, resonance and articulation are most readily influenced by maxillofacial prosthodontic rehabilitation. These two components of speech are intimately related. Patients with acquired defects or congenital malformations of the soft palate may exhibit excessive nasal resonance because they are unable to control and divert sufficient acoustic energy into the oral cavity without surgical and/or prosthodontic intervention. Although the degree of velopharyngeal closure remains the major determinant of resonance balance, other factors, such as tongue position relative to velar elevation (Subtelny et al., 1966b; Shelton et al., 1971a, 1971b) and structural resistance within the nasal cavity (Warren and Ryon, 1967), influence the perceived oral-nasal resonance balance.

Resonance disturbances manifest in four basic forms: *(1) hypernasality*, where there is too much nasal resonance; *(2) hyponasality*, where there is too little nasal resonance; *(3) mixed nasality*, where there is variation between too much and too little nasal resonance; and *(4) cul-de-sac resonance*, where acoustic energy is resonated in the pharynx, behind a more anterior constriction, instead of flowing freely through the oral cavity. With hypernasality, excessive acoustic energy flows into the nasal cavity and the patient sounds as though he or she were "speaking through the nose." In contrast, patients with hyponasality exhibit insufficient acoustic flow through the nasal cavities. Prostheses used for velopharyngeal incompetence or velopharyngeal insufficiency (VPI) can create hyponasality if they excessively occlude the velopharyngeal port (Minsley et al., 1991). More often, however, the prosthodontist is challenged to provide sufficient obturation to avoid hypernasality and yet maintain patency for nasal breathing and the proper production of nasal consonant sounds. Attempts to restore balance between occlusion of the velopharynx for speech and patency for breathing have led investigators to trial obturators with soft membranes (Bou et al., 2018; Naveau et al., 2022).

Mixed nasality (hypernasality and hyponasality) can be experienced by patients with a pharyngeal obturator when there is little or no muscular movement available around the prosthesis to assist with closure of the velopharynx for speech; however, nasal patency for breathing is often compromised in such cases (Fig 4-2). Thus, an opening often is created between the obturator and the lateral pharyngeal walls to provide patency for nasal breathing, which also results in a certain degree of hypernasality. From time to time, this opening can become occluded by nasal secretions, which may be thick and viscous, especially in irradiated head and neck cancer patients, resulting in hyponasality.

Altered resonance can be the result of any structural alteration that blocks the normal flow of acoustic energy into the oral cavity, such as a bulky flap in the base of the tongue area or an ill-fitting prosthesis that encourages the patient to use the posterior aspect of the tongue to stabilize it.

Articulation deficiencies are primarily heard in patients with acquired defects of the mandible and tongue (see Chapter 2). In conjunction with the resections of portions of the mandible, adjacent soft tissues may be sacrificed, or sensory and motor innervation of the lower lip, tongue, and cheeks may be compromised. The misshaped oral cavity may produce changes in oral resonance, but even more challenging are the speech distortions related to impaired articulation in these patients.

Patients with cleft lip and cleft palate may exhibit distortions in both articulation and resonance. Errors in articulation may be classified as either obligatory or compensatory (Kummer, 2018). Obligatory errors of articulation include weakened consonants and nasal air emission. Weakened consonants are a direct result of the inability to achieve adequate intraoral air pressure because of inappropriate coupling of the oral and nasal cavities. Nasal air emission is usually associated with high-pressure sounds, such as /*s*/ and /*sh*/, and may result in a distorted speech signal. Compensatory errors are exhibited when the patient makes an effort to produce a sound before it reaches an inappropriate palatopharyngeal opening, thereby averting an inappropriate flow of air through the nasal cavity. For example, many children with cleft palate will substitute glottal stops (i.e., a stop produced by abruptly approximating the vocal folds and then releasing the air) for anterior stops such as /*t*/ and /*d*/ to avoid the inappropriate airflow into the nasal cavity that occurs with normal tongue placement for those sounds in the context of a deficient velopharynx. Children with cleft palate also may display other sound distortions or even sound omissions.

When hypernasality and articulation deficiencies coexist, these components of speech are intimately related and may be difficult to separate into distinct entities without formal testing of the speech system (Brandt and Morris, 1968; Barnes, 1967).

Speech phonemes

Classification and description

American English contains 44 different speech sounds, or *phonemes*, which are classified as *vowels*, *voiceless consonants*, and *voiced*

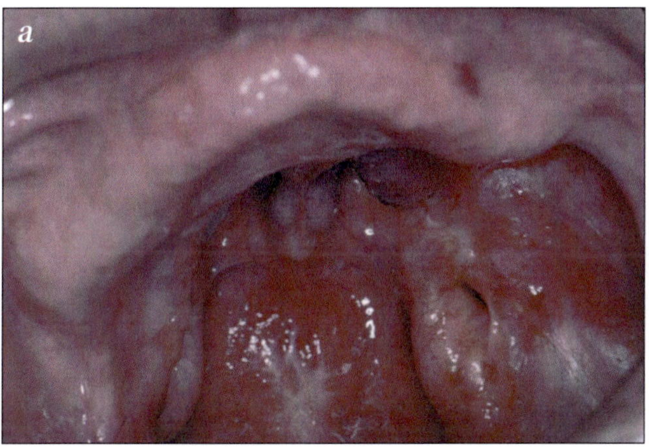

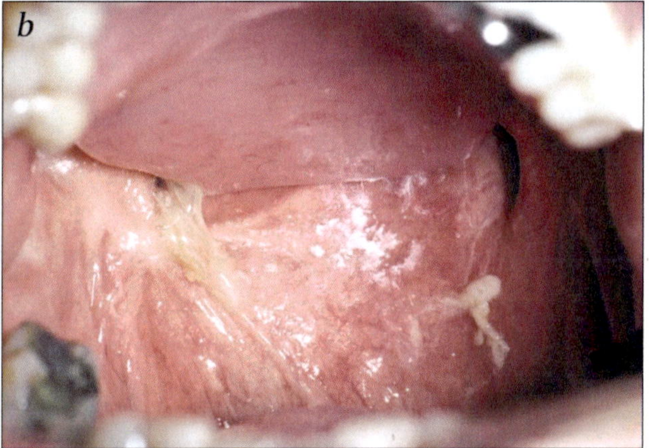

Figure 4-2 Mixed nasality. *(a)* The entire velopharyngeal mechanism has been resected and rendered nonfunctional. Examination revealed no appreciable movement of the lateral pharyngeal walls. Therefore, proper resonance balance cannot be achieved with a prosthesis. *(b)* Another patient with a similar presentation. There was no movement of the lateral and posterior pharyngeal walls. Obturator prosthesis in position. After proper adjustment, the best speech result that can be achieved is speech with mixed nasality.

consonants. Phonemes vary in terms of the frequency, intensity, and duration of the sound produced.

Vowels are voiced sounds that are produced via a series of air puffs that are released into the vocal tract as air passes from the lungs through the vibrating vocal folds. Vowels are associated with a relatively open vocal tract and little pressure buildup within the oral cavity. Each vowel has a unique harmonic spectrum with peaks of energy at particular frequencies, known as *formant frequencies*. The positions of the tongue, the jaw, and the lips all play a part in determining the formant frequencies. Vowel combinations, such as /ie/, are called *diphthongs*.

Voiceless consonants, such as /p/, /t/, /f/, and /s/, are formed with a column of air (without laryngeal phonation) that, when restricted within the oral cavity, produces sounds of moderately high frequency and low intensity. Voiced consonants, such as /b/, /d/, and /g/, combine laryngeal phonation plus airflow with variable frequencies and intensities. Consonants (voiced or unvoiced) can be further divided by the duration of the sound, the principal resonating chamber utilized to produce the sound, and the articulators used to form the sound (Table 4-1). Some consonants, such as /sh/ and /s/, are prolonged, while other consonants, such as /p/ and /t/, are called *stop-plosives* because the air-sound volume is contained and suddenly released.

Table 4-1 Place and manner classification of American English consonants*

	Manner of production				
Place	*Plosive*	*Fricative*	*Affricative*	*Semivowel*	*Nasal*
Bilabial	p b (pole) (bowl)			w (watt)	m (sum)
Labial dental		f v (fat) (vat)			
Lingual dental		0 alpha (thigh) (thy)			
Lingual alveolar	t d (toll) (dole)	s z (seal) (zeal)	l (lot)	n (sun)	
Palatal		j z (ash) (azure)	ch (choke)		
Velar	k g (coal) (goat)			ng (sing)	

* Reprinted from Esposito (1995) with permission.

Speech phonemes and maxillofacial prosthetics

The articulation of individual or groups of phonemes is beyond the scope of this review; however, the articulation of fricative and sibilant consonant phonemes will be described because these sounds are often utilized as guides for verification of the position of anterior denture teeth. Fricative sounds, such as /f/ and /v/, are formed by constricting the airflow in a friction-like manner. Classically, these sounds are produced by the approximation of the wet-dry line of the vermilion border of the lower lip with the maxillary incisors. Since the lips are flexible, some accommodation to aesthetic demands is possible without phonemic distortion (McNulty et al., 1968). However, if the maxillary or mandibular incisor denture teeth are positioned beyond the range of lip accommodation or fail to provide proper lip support, fricative sounds can be distorted.

Sibilant sounds such as /s/ and /sh/ are produced in a friction-like manner, resulting in a hissing sound. An acceptable /s/ is produced in several ways. Most individuals will elevate the tongue tip against the hard palate, forming a median furrow that directs the airstream between the incisal edges of the maxillary and mandibular incisors. Other individuals will depress the tongue tip so that it rests behind the mandibular incisors. In either case, the mandibular incisors are positioned slightly lingual to and approximately 1 mm from the maxillary incisors. This is the *closest speaking space* referred to by Silverman (1967) and is used by many clinicians to verify anterior tooth position (Fig 4-3) (Pound, 1966; Pound, 1977). This evaluation is simplified because sibilant sounds are prolonged.

Fricative and sibilant sounds, along with continuous speech, can be used to evaluate the vertical dimension of occlusion. Premature

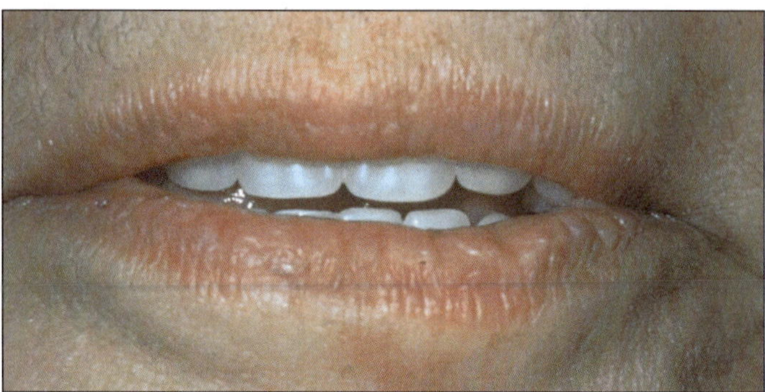

Figure 4-3 The closest speaking space is used by many clinicians to verify anterior tooth position and the occlusal vertical dimension when fabricating complete dentures.

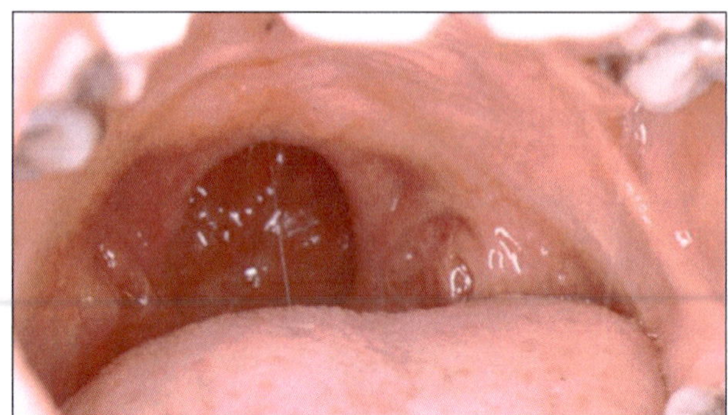

Figure 4-4 Palatal insufficiency after repair of a cleft of the hard and soft palate. The soft palate is of insufficient length to reach the posterior pharyngeal wall during velopharyngeal closure.

tooth contact during articulation may indicate that the appropriate vertical dimension of occlusion has been exceeded (Silverman, 1952; Silverman, 1967). Conversely, if the space between the anterior and posterior denture teeth during continuous speech is excessive, the vertical dimension of occlusion may have to be increased.

Some caution should be expressed regarding the use of sibilant sounds as a diagnostic aid during the construction of prostheses. The phoneme /*sh*/ is an unvoiced linguoalveolar fricative and is the sixth most common consonant used in general American English. Fairbanks and Lintner (1951) noted that approximately 90% of all speakers with defective articulation have difficulty with /*sh*/.

Pound (1966) believed that the mandible (dentulous or edentulous) is carried anteriorly and superiorly to a precise position during the production of /*s*/ and that this position is as definitive as the terminal hinge position of the condyles. Although he noted some exceptions to this statement, the literature does not support the premise of a reproducible /*s*/ position. For example, Benediktsson (1957) used cephalometric radiographs to study the position and movements of the tongue and mandible during the production of /*s*/ in 246 subjects with normal and abnormal incisor relationships. This study revealed a variety of incisor, tongue, and lip approximations during the production of /*s*/ in both normal and abnormal speakers.

Subtelny et al. (1964) compared 31 subjects with a Class II, division 1 malocclusion and normal speech and 20 subjects with a similar malocclusion and defective speech. Excessive protrusion of the mandible to approximate the incisors was not found to be a generalized compensatory adjustment to extreme maxillary variations. Only one normal speaker demonstrated the extensive mandibular protrusion necessary to attain incisor approximation during speech. The lower lip often created the restriction with the maxillary incisors for /*s*/ production in these Class II patients.

In addition, mandibular movements during speech and /*s*/ production are not always precise. Gibbs and Messerman (1972) found that mandibular movements during speech are quite limited compared to the envelope of motion displayed by the mandible during mastication. Silverman (1972) noted that movements of the mandible during the production of /*s*/ are skeletal and are required to enhance the precise movements of the tongue.

Speech pathologists and maxillofacial prosthodontists now recognize that considerable positional variation can occur during articulation without causing phonemic distortion. In addition, sounds produced in isolation are more likely to be correct than these same sounds produced during spontaneous and continuous speech. Therefore, the clinician must consider the dynamics of the speech mechanism (Martone, 1962). Speech can and should be used as one of the guidelines for placement of the denture teeth, yet judgments regarding tooth position and jaw relationships based solely on speech should be used with the understanding that there are many exceptions from the norm.

Velopharyngeal Function

Hypernasality and poor intelligibility of speech may result from congenital or acquired defects of the velopharyngeal mechanism. Velopharyngeal deficits may result from congenital malformations such as cleft palate, developmental aberrations such as a short hard or soft palate or deep nasopharynx, acquired neurologic deficits, or following the surgical resection of neoplastic disease.

Classification and etiology

Velopharyngeal deficiencies may be classified on the basis of physiology and/or structural integrity. Palatal insufficiency and palatal incompetency are often used to define velopharyngeal deficits. These terms are often used interchangeably, but there are subtle differences. *Palatal insufficiency* occurs when the hard and/or soft palate is of inadequate length to affect velopharyngeal closure but the movement of the remaining tissues is within normal physiologic limits (Fig 4-4). The defect is secondary to a structural limitation. Patients with congenital and developmental aberrations and acquired soft palate defects would fall into this classification. *Palatal incompetence* occurs when velopharyngeal structures are essentially normal, but the intact mechanism is unable to affect velopharyngeal closure. Patients with neurologic diseases such as bulbar poliomyelitis or myasthenia gravis or neurologic deficits secondary to cerebrovascular accidents or closed head injuries are included in this category.

The largest group of patients with soft palate defects are those with congenital clefts of the palate (see Chapter 6). However, in most patients, velopharyngeal function can be restored by surgical

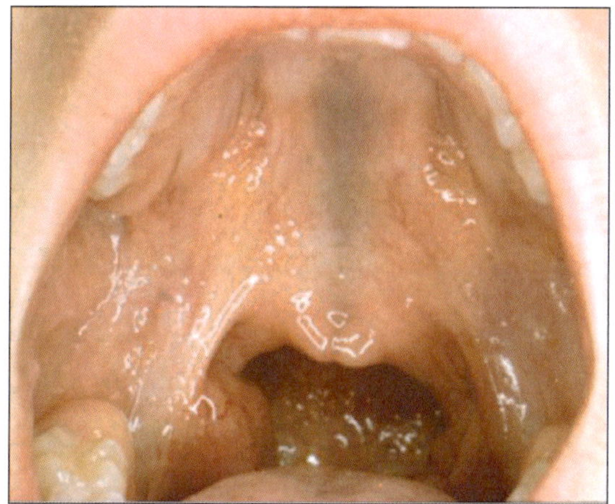

Figure 4-5 Patient with a submucous cleft that is unable to achieve velopharyngeal closure.

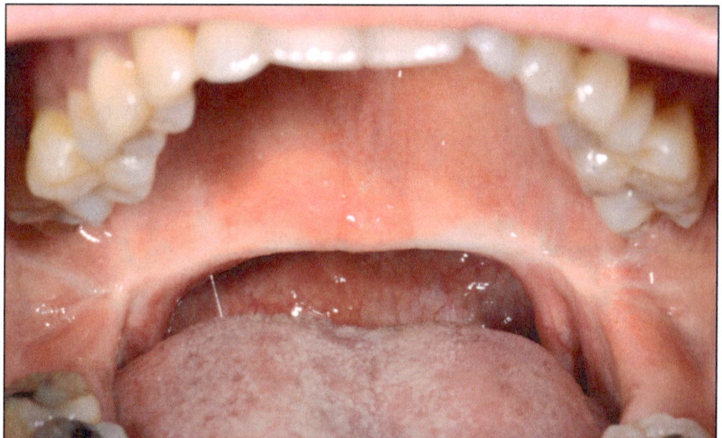

Figure 4-6 This patient underwent an uvulopalatopharyngoplasty for obstructive sleep apnea. The soft palate has been shortened and scarred leading to velopharyngeal insufficiency.

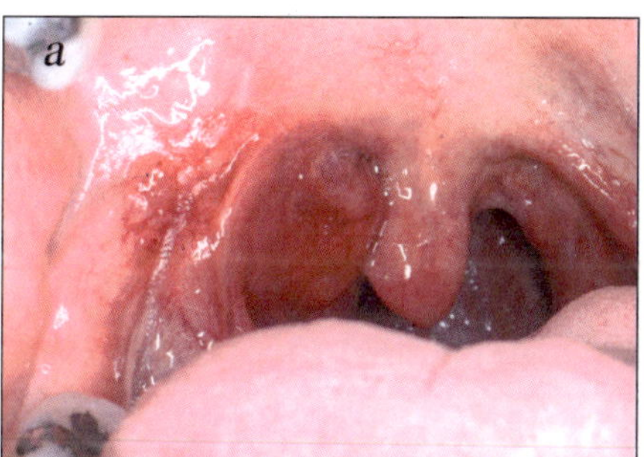

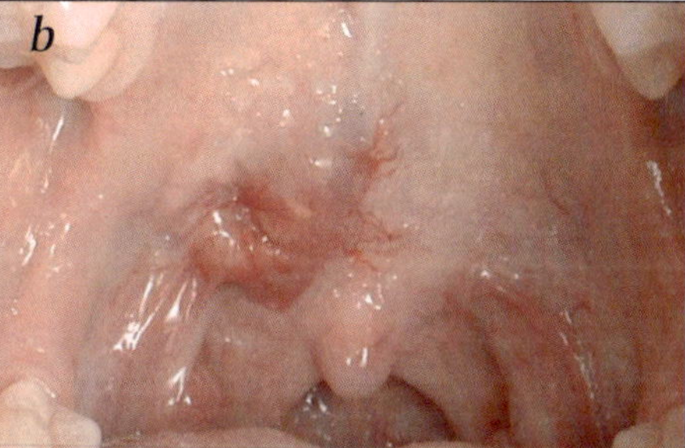

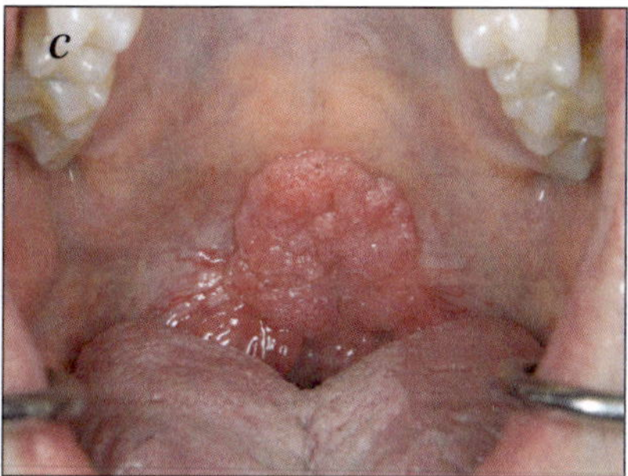

Figure 4-7 Neoplastic disease. *(a)* Squamous cell carcinoma of the tonsil. *(b)* Low-grade mucoepidermoid of the soft palate. In both patients, significant portions of the soft palate were removed. *(c)* A verrucous carcinoma of the soft palate. Surgical resection resulted in a posterior border defect.

reconstruction. When surgical treatment outcomes fall short of expectations or when these services are unavailable, these patients will benefit from placement of either an obturator prosthesis or a palatal lift prosthesis. With some developmental deficiencies, such as those with a short hard and/or soft palate with a deep nasopharynx or those with an occult submucous cleft palate (Fig 4-5), structural integrity may appear adequate, but the velopharyngeal mechanism is unable to affect closure. Palatal surgery is almost always the treatment of choice (Jefferson et al., 2021).

Occasionally, patients undergoing uvulopalatopharyngoplasty for obstructive sleep apnea will present with velopharyngeal insufficiency triggered by excessive tissue reduction and/or scarring (Varendh et al., 2012; Tang et al., 2017) (Fig 4-6). When the surgical resection is excessively aggressive, the residual soft palate is of insufficient length to reach the posterior pharyngeal wall during velopharyngeal closure. In addition, scarring may impair elevation of the residual soft palate. Long-term follow-up indicates that following this procedure, 10–15% of the patients demonstrate signs of velopharyngeal disfunction as evidenced by nasal regurgitation and change in voice quality.

Most acquired soft palate defects result from surgical resection for neoplastic disease (Fig 4-7). In the past, reconstructive surgery generally was not indicated for patients with acquired defects because tissue loss was excessive. In addition, reconstruction of the soft palate was thought to be contraindicated because of the need to monitor the tumor site for recurrent disease. However, with new imaging technologies, concern about monitoring the defect area visually has been somewhat attenuated.

Previous reports of surgical reconstruction of extensive acquired surgical defects of the soft palate indicated that the procedures resulted in deficient, nonfunctioning velopharyngeal mechanisms that compromised subsequent prosthetic intervention (Seikaly, 2003). More recent reports of innovative soft palate reconstructive procedures have achieved functional results in select patients (Rieger and Zalmanowitz, 2008; Seikaly et al., 2008; Rieger et al., 2009; Melan et al., 2021) (Fig 4-8). However, many surgical teams do not possess the resources and expertise to reconstruct soft palate defects, and this procedure is particularly challenging and problematic when more than half of the soft palate is resected. When surgical reconstruction is ineffective, excessive scarring and impaired movement of and limited access to the residual velopharyngeal mechanism may preclude successful obturation with a prosthesis (Fig 4-9). In particular, postoperative radiation can lead to excessive scarring of the flap and impair movement of the residual velopharyngeal musculature, particularly the levator remnant in the lateral pharyngeal wall.

When a soft palate defect is properly prepared following tumor ablation, restoration of velopharyngeal function is highly predictable and the treatment of choice. In the patient shown in Fig 4-10, following tumor ablation, the lateral wall of the pharynx was resurfaced with a free flap, and the soft palate was allowed to hang free. Consequently, movement of the residual velopharyngeal mechanism was

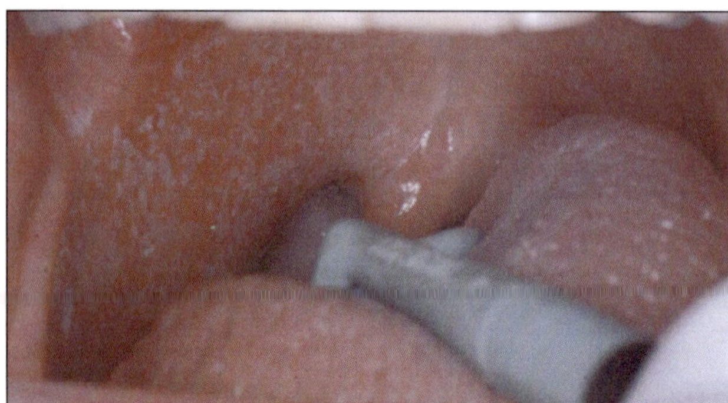

Figure 4-8 Resection that falls short of the uvula. The soft palate defect has been effectively reconstructed with a free flap. If resection extends across the midline, the defect is best restored with an obturator prosthesis.

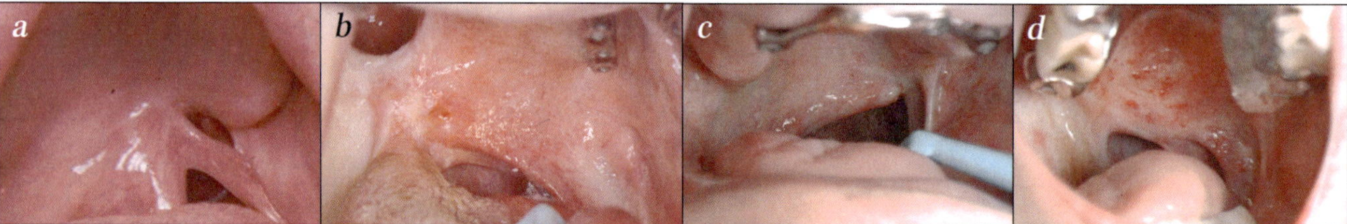

Figure 4-9 Failed attempts at surgical reconstruction of the soft palate. *(a)* Patient with posterolateral border defect following resection of squamous cell carcinoma. Attempts were made to reconstruct the defect surgically. Breakdown of the flap and scar contracture has compromised soft palate elevation, closure, and subsequent prosthodontic therapy. *(b)* Surgical closure was attempted primarily. The procedure tethered the soft palate in an inferior position. A prosthesis was fabricated, but the patient could not tolerate it because of its low position in the oropharynx. *(c and d)* In these two patients, the residual soft palate was tethered to a flap. Scarring, limited movement of the residual velopharyngeal mechanism, and difficult access preclude successful obturation with a prosthesis in these two patients.

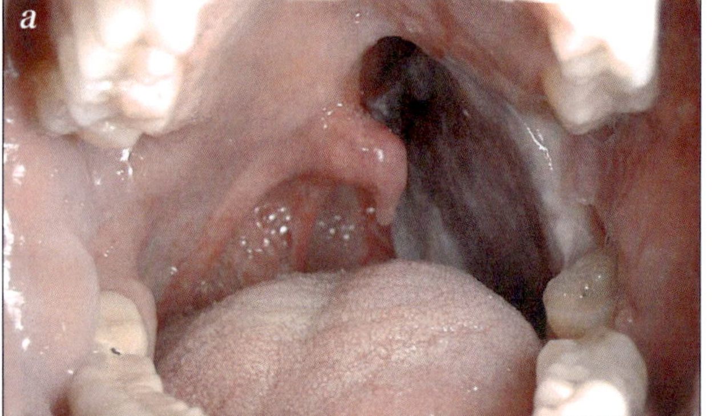

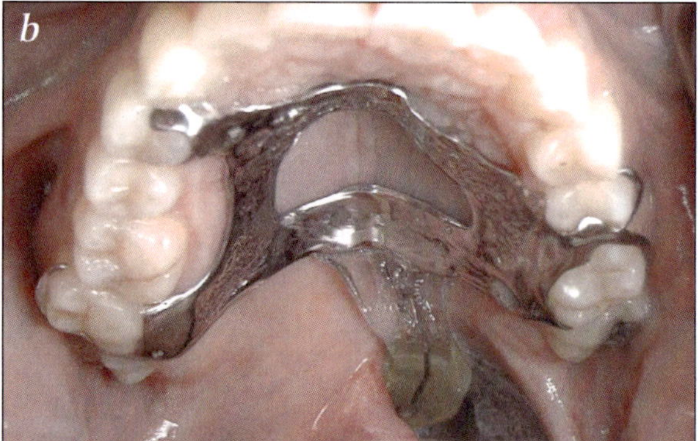

Figure 4-10 Soft palate defect. *(a)* The lateral wall of the pharynx has been resurfaced with a radial forearm flap. *(b)* The obturator prosthesis extends around and behind the residual soft palate to engage the still functional right pharyngeal wall and the residual portion of the soft palate. Velopharyngeal function is restored to normal.

retained, and these areas were accessible to the obturator prosthesis. As a result, velopharyngeal function was restored to normal limits.

Soft palate defects also can result from other diseases and from trauma. Patients with neurologic deficiencies that impair motor control of the velopharyngeal mechanism often benefit from prosthodontic therapy (Wolfaardt et al., 1993). Palatal lift prostheses are often indicated for these patients (see section below entitled "Palatal lift prostheses").

General considerations

Early investigations of the velopharyngeal mechanism centered on anatomical dissection. The information gleaned from these dissections was applied to the physiology of velopharyngeal closure. These early investigators believed that a simple elevation of the soft palate accounted for velopharyngeal closure. Although Gustov Passavant described a forward movement of the posterior pharyngeal wall and the medial movement of the lateral pharyngeal walls in patients with a cleft palate (Passavant, 1869), his descriptions received little attention.

The velopharyngeal mechanism is a precisely coordinated valve formed by several muscle groups. At rest, the soft palate drapes downward so that the oropharynx and nasopharynx are open and coupled to allow normal breathing through the nasal passages. When velopharyngeal closure is required for speech, individuals with normal velopharyngeal physiology may display one of four typical patterns of closure, described by Skolnick et al. (1973).

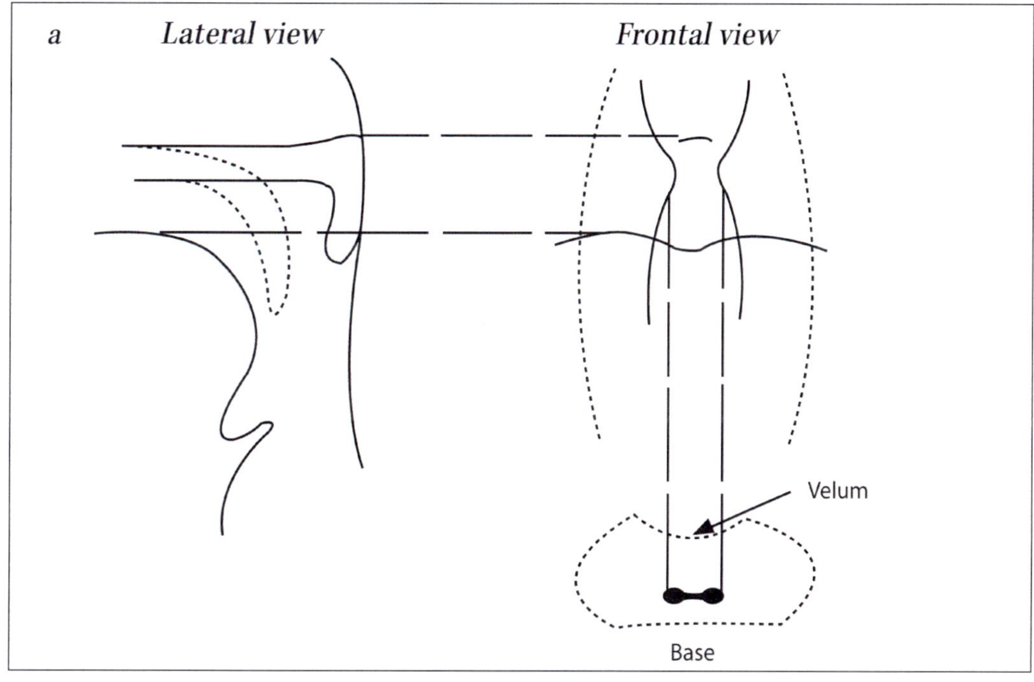

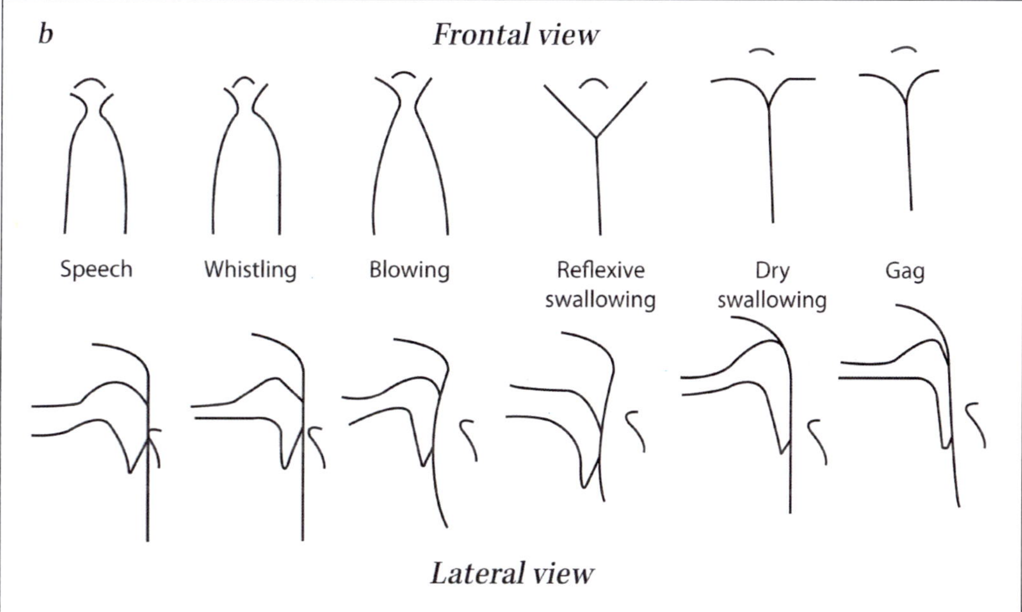

Figure 4-11 *(a)* Pharynx of a normal subject showing the sphincteric mechanism of velopharyngeal closure from lateral, frontal, and base radiographic projections. Dotted lines represent the positions of the soft palate and pharyngeal walls at rest; solid lines represent the same structures during velopharyngeal closure (adapted from Skolnick et al., 1973, with permission). *(b)* Tracings of frontal and lateral views of a normal subject during various activities requiring velopharyngeal closure. Speech, whistling, and blowing are often described as pneumatic activities, whereas swallowing and gagging are nonpneumatic functions. Note the variation in closure patterns during various activities (adapted from Sphrintzen et al., 1974, with permission).

- In the *coronal pattern of closure*, the middle third of the soft palate arcs upward and backward to contact the posterior pharyngeal wall at or above the level of the palatal plane (Fig 4-11a). In individuals with normal velopharyngeal mechanisms, this is the most commonly observed pattern of closure.
- The next most common pattern is *circular closure*. The lateral pharyngeal walls move medially to contact the margins of the elevated soft palate at or slightly below the level of the torus tubarius. Contributions from the lateral walls and the soft palate are relatively equal, but the posterior pharyngeal wall contributes little to this type of closure.
- The third type of closure is *circular closure with the Passavant ridge*. Closure follows the circular pattern and, in addition, the Passavant ridge moves anteriorly to facilitate contact with the elevated soft palate and medially displaced lateral pharyngeal walls.

- The last and least common pattern is *sagittal closure*, in which the lateral walls move medially to approximate one another and the soft palate elevates to abut the medially displaced lateral walls.

Velopharyngeal closure patterns vary depending on the desired function performed (Fig 4-11b). Closure is much more profound during dry swallowing and gagging than it is during swallowing. If gagging occurs or if the patient is asked to perform a dry swallow during border molding, the prosthesis will be underextended. The patient should be instructed to speak and to perform reflex swallowing with ample liquids during molding of the prosthesis to produce the desired contours.

Complete velopharyngeal closure is required for normal deglutition and the production of oral consonants. In contrast, the velopharyngeal port will be open during the production of nasal consonants. For vowels produced in isolation, the velopharyngeal port will be closed and may demonstrate differing closure patterns, depending on the vowel produced (Matsuya et al., 1974). When vowels precede or follow nasal consonants in connected speech, the velopharyngeal port may be open slightly during the vowel production, resulting in a normal occurrence known as *assimilation nasality*.

Methods of evaluation

Previous methods

Wardill (1928) and Dorrance (1930) were the first to propose that normal velopharyngeal closure involved the synchronous movement of selected portions of the pharyngeal musculature. Since that time, numerous methods have been developed to observe and assess the function and structures that constitute the velopharyngeal system. Among these investigations are aerodynamic and airflow studies (Warren et al., 1965, 1969; Subtelny et al., 1968; Minsley et al., 1991); lateral and frontal plane radiographic analyses (Ashley et al., 1961; Griffith et al., 1968; Denegri et al., 2021); lateral, frontal, and base radiographic analysis (Skolnick et al., 1969, 1970, 1973); spectrographic and coordination analyses (Chierci and Lawson, 1973; Fletcher and Frost, 1974); direct observation through large facial defects (Wardill, 1928; Bloomer, 1953); instrumentation for direct oral observation (Taub, 1966); videofluoroscopic and nasal endoscopic studies (Pigott et al., 1969a, 1969b; Miyazaki et al., 1975; Croft et al., 1981; Witzel and Posnick, 1989a); anatomical dissections (Dickson, 1972; Dickson and Dickson, 1972; Fara and Dvorak, 1970); electromyographic analysis (Fritzell, 1969; Bell-Berti, 1976); and neurologic innervation (Nishio et al., 1976a, 1976b). These studies demonstrate that velopharyngeal closure is complex, especially when altered developmentally, anatomically, physiologically, or neurologically, and that there should be consideration of the relative ratios between the depth of the nasopharynx and the length of the soft palate (Denegri et al., 2021).

Current methods

Currently, a wide range of velopharyngeal evaluation methods are available to study the physiology of the velopharyngeal complex during speech and nonspeech functions. These include multiview videofluoroscopic assessment (Witt et al., 2000; Seagle et al., 2002; Beer et al., 2004; Dudas et al., 2006; Kummer et al., 2003; Rowe and D'Antonio, 2005), nasopharyngoscopic evaluation (Ngim et al., 1988; Witt et al., 2000; Sie et al., 2001; Seagle et al., 2002; Eblen and Sie, 2002; Kummer et al., 2003; Rowe and D'Antonio, 2005; Lam et al., 2006; Rieger et al., 2006), magnetic resonance imaging (MRI; Witt et al., 2000; Beer et al., 2004; Ehmer and Broll, 1992; Li and Fu, 1998; Sakamoto et al., 1999; Zarrinkelk et al., 1996), aerodynamic measurement (Reisberg and Smith, 1985; Sharp et al., 1999; Devani et al., 1999; Seikaly et al., 2008), nasometric measurement (Van Lierde et al., 2002; Seikaly et al., 2003; Trindade et al., 2003; Van Lierde et al., 2004), and perceptual appraisals (Rohrich et al., 1996; Tonz et al., 2002; McKinstry and Perry, 2003; Nicoletti et al., 2004). These methodologies allow evaluations to be conducted with little or no impact on the physiology of the region. These testing methods will be described and their major contributions noted.

Multiview videofluoroscopy

A series of classic studies employed three-dimensional videofluoroscopy to examine the velopharyngeal mechanism in the frontal, sagittal, and base views simultaneously (Skolnick et al., 1973; Shprintzen et al., 1974). From these recordings, researchers were able to trace the movements of the soft palate, lateral pharyngeal walls, and the posterior pharyngeal wall from rest to complete closure during speech and nonspeech tasks. They confirmed that the character of velopharyngeal closure during speech is different from that during swallowing and other nonspeech functions (Bloomer, 1953; Bzoch et al., 1959; Moll, 1965; Skolnick et al., 1970; Dickson and Dickson, 1973). This is not surprising, because swallowing is a primary physiologic function (Bosma and Fletcher, 1962; Shprintzen et al., 1974), while speech is a learned function.

In speech, the superior fibers of the superior constrictor muscle only appear to be involved during closure. The pharynx is more forcefully involved in closure during swallowing than during speech (Bloomer, 1953; Moll, 1965). Shprintzen et al. (1974) surmised that the superior, middle, and inferior constrictors fire in overlapping sequence during swallowing and that contact of the soft palate with the posterior and lateral pharyngeal walls is more extensive and at a lower level than it is during speech.

As discussed previously, Skolnick et al. (1973) noted that, while closure is always sphincteric, it occurs in four distinct patterns, depending on the range of movement and the manner of approximation of the soft palate and the lateral and posterior pharyngeal walls. These investigators delineated these closure patterns, coronal, sagittal, circular, and circular with the Passavant ridge, based on their appearance in base view videofluoroscopy during closure.

Nasoendoscopy

Nasoendoscopy (also known as *nasal endoscopy* and *nasopharyngoscopy*) became a primary and important diagnostic and research tool in the 1980s, superseding the use of multiview videofluoroscopy in many circumstances (Lewin et al., 1980; Croft et al., 1991; Witzel and Posnick, 1989a). The flexible nasal endoscope has the advantage of visualization of the velopharyngeal sphincter from above in the nasopharynx without interference with the speech mechanism or exposing the patient to radiation, unlike videofluoroscopic techniques. For children who are not cooperative with nasoendoscopy, multiview videofluoroscopy may still be the evaluation method of choice (Ysunza et al., 2008).

The flexible tube and tip are inserted through the nostril, passed through the middle meatus, if possible, and into the nasopharynx above the level of velopharyngeal closure. In this position, the angle

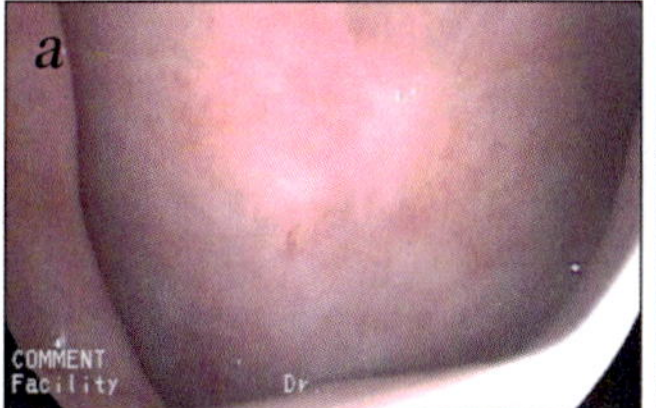

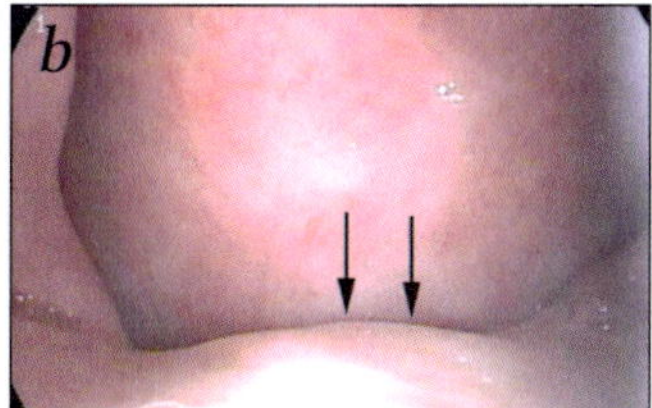

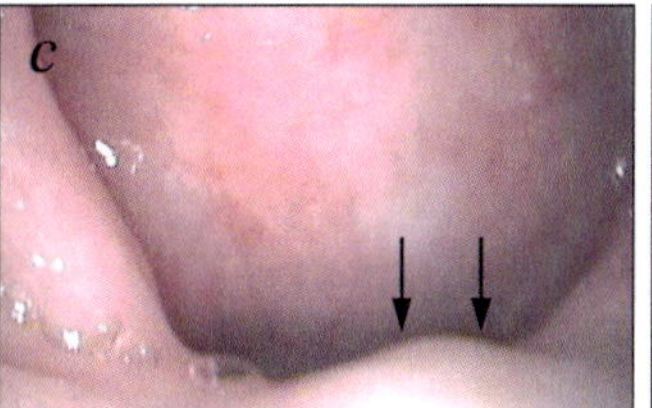

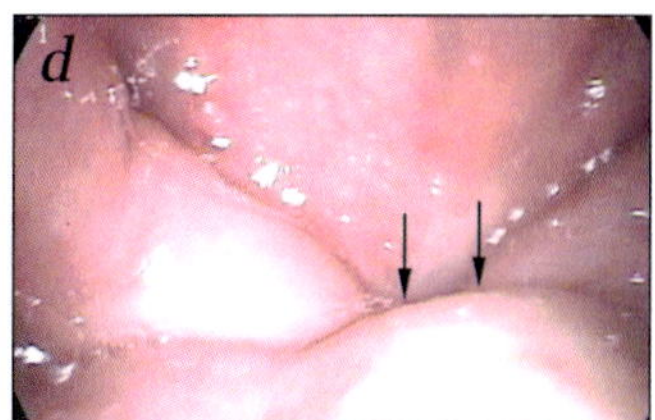

Figure 4-12 Nasal endoscopic view of velopharyngeal closure of a patient with and without a palatal lift in position. *(a)* Velopharyngeal mechanism at rest without a palatal lift prosthesis. *(b)* Lift in position. Note the bulge of the soft palate created by the presence of the lift *(arrows)*. *(c)* Lift in position during a partial closure. Note the space between the soft palate and the lateral and posterior pharyngeal walls. *(d)* Lift in position during a complete closure.

of the tip can be adjusted to obtain the best view of this sphincteric mechanism. The fiber-optic xenon light source provides sufficient illumination for direct viewing and digital videorecording during speech (Fig 4-12).

It appears that multiview videofluoroscopy and nasoendoscopy complement each other (Stringer and Witzel, 1989; Henningsson and Isberg, 1991). Although fluoroscopy may delineate lateral wall motion more clearly, nasal endoscopy is more likely to reveal hypoplasia of the musculus uvulae, the position and the contribution to the closure of the adenoids, and gaps or leakage around an obturator prosthesis (Karnell et al., 1987; Walter, 1990; Turner and Williams, 1992; Rieger et al., 2006).

The value of nasoendoscopy is evident from several studies that have addressed its usefulness in resolving misdiagnoses, facilitating prosthetic intervention, and refining the knowledge of patterns of velopharyngeal closure. In a study by Lewin and colleagues (Lewin et al., 1980), 29 of 131 patients with VPI without cleft palate had palates that appeared normal when viewed orally, both in appearance and in the range of motion of the soft palate. These 29 patients were classified as having congenital palatal insufficiency resulting from a short soft and/or hard palate. The group included patients with the following referral diagnoses: 10 with palatal paresis; 9 with congenital palatal insufficiency; 7 with congenital short palate; 2 with idiopathic palatal insufficiency; and 1 with hysterical conversion reaction.

The researchers found that 26 of the patients had undergone tonsillectomies and adenoidectomies. In 19 patients, the symptoms became apparent after the operation; in 7 patients, the symptoms were preexisting and the tonsillectomies and adenoidectomies were performed to correct the condition. Subsequent nasal endoscopic evaluation in the clinic revealed that the correct diagnosis for all 29 patients should have been occult submucous cleft palate with midline gaps in the nasal surface that resulted from the absence or severe hypoplasia of the musculus uvulae.

The value of nasoendoscopy to improve functional outcomes in patients undergoing prosthetic management of velopharyngeal dysfunction was demonstrated by Rieger et al. (2006). In that study, treatment with a prosthesis designed via conventional functional impression technique resulted in substandard acoustic and aeromechanical speech outcomes. After nasoendoscopy was used to guide adjustment of the impression wax–derived prosthesis, both forms of speech measurement were within normal limits for all patients.

Patterns of velopharyngeal closure

Nasoendoscopy provides a perspective from above the velopharyngeal portal, which has led to refinement of the four velopharyngeal closure patterns initially described by Skolnick et al. (1973) from base view videofluoroscopy. For example, Siegel-Sadewitz and Shprintzen (1982) described the four closure patterns as viewed with nasoendoscopy as follows (Fig 4-13):

- **Coronal pattern:** The majority of the valving is palatal, and the full width of the soft palate contacts the posterior wall. The lateral walls exhibit limited movement to contact the lateral margins of the velum. There is no posterior pharyngeal wall movement.
- **Sagittal pattern:** The majority of the valving is pharyngeal. The lateral walls move extensively to the midline and approximate each other. The velum does not contact the posterior pharyngeal wall but elevates to contact the approximated lateral pharyngeal walls. The posterior pharyngeal wall does not contribute to closure.
- **Circular pattern:** Participation of the soft palate and the lateral pharyngeal walls is essentially equal, and the contracting musculus uvulae acts as a focal point. The lateral walls contact the musculus uvulae as it contracts and contacts the immobile posterior pharyngeal wall.
- **Circular pattern with the Passavant ridge:** The same as the circular closure pattern except that the posterior pharyngeal wall (Passavant ridge) moves forward to complete the closure pattern around the musculus uvulae posteriorly.

How often do these four individual closure patterns occur? Two studies have addressed this question. Croft et al. (1981) used both multiview videofluoroscopic and nasal endoscopic examinations to study 80 patients with normal speech and 500 patients with VPI. The VPI patients included 360 patients with repaired cleft palate and 140 patients with unrepaired submucous clefts of the palate. While the majority of participants exhibited a coronal pattern closure (56% of normal population and 45% of patient population), patients were more likely than the control group to exhibit a circular pattern of closure (29% versus 10%, respectively).

Witzel and Posnick (1989a) reviewed 246 consecutive nasopharyngoscopy studies of patients with VPI. The types of closure observed in that study are listed in Table 4-2. Gaps were found in 181 patients. Of these, 121 were considered centrally located and resulted from hyperplasia of the musculus uvulae. The other gaps were variable and sometimes attributed to the shape of the adenoids or to the anatomy or function of the posterior border of the soft palate.

In both studies, the most common pattern of closure was coronal. Witzel and Posnick (1989a) found proportionally more atypical valving associated with a coronal pattern of closure.

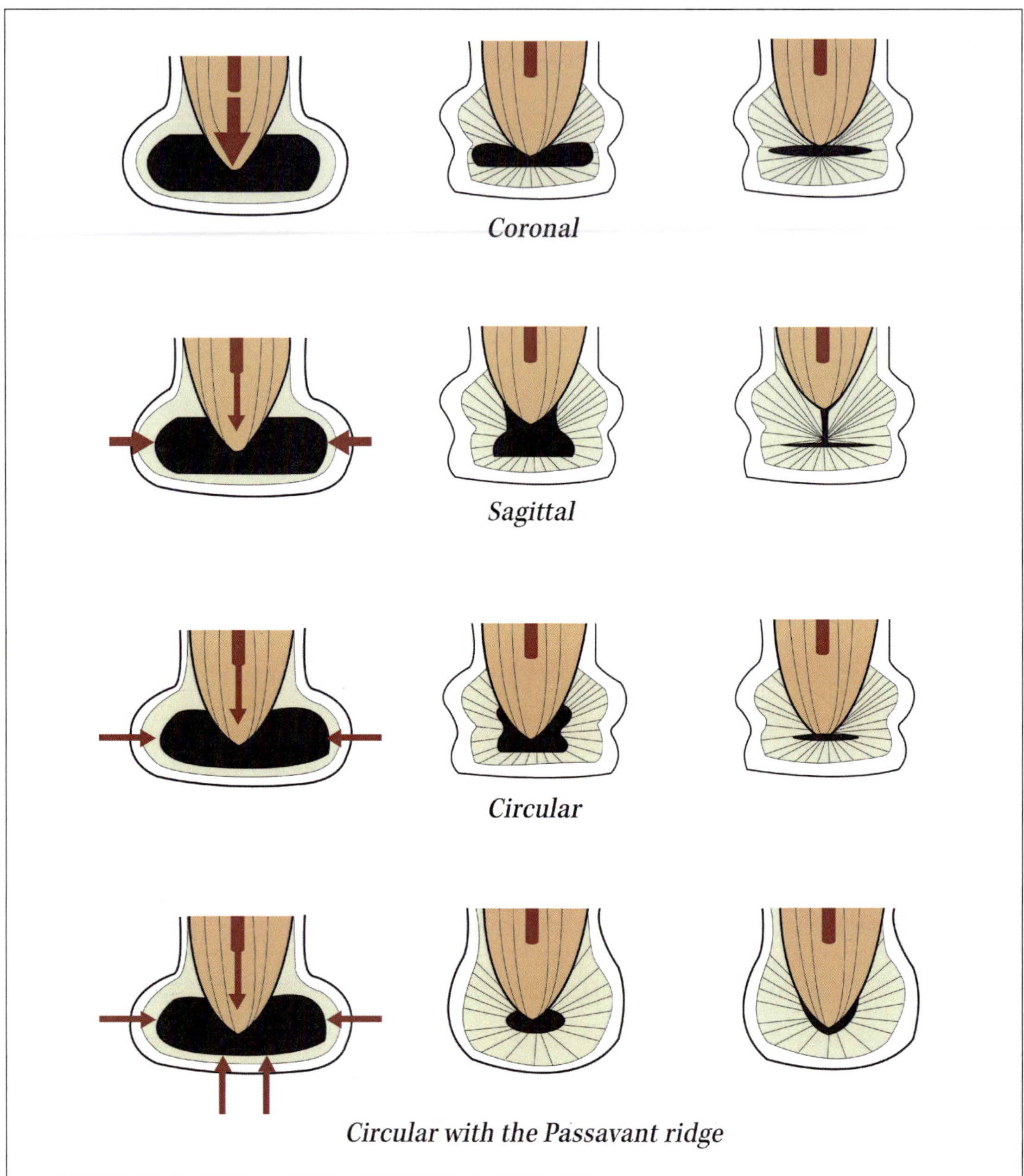

Figure 4-13 Four patterns of velopharyngeal valving. See text for description (adapted from Siegel-Sadewitz and Shprintzen, 1982, with permission).

What determines the pattern of closure? Croft et al. (1981) hypothesized that the type of pattern in the normal population is influenced by many factors, such as learning capability and slight anatomical variations. Are individuals able to change their closure pattern to compensate for anatomical changes such as surgery to a portion of the velopharyngeal complex? Some authors believe that the development of a Passavant ridge should be classified as a compensatory mechanism developed by some patients in response to VPI (Carpenter and Morris, 1968; Casey and Emrich, 1988; Isberg and Henningsson, 1990). Warren believed that the Passavant ridge may be an airway response to the loss of nasal pathway resistance, including velopharyngeal dysfunction (Warren, 1986).

Table 4-2 Patterns of VP valving in patients with complete VP closure or VPI[*]

Closure pattern	VP closure		VPI		Total	
	No.	%	No.	%	No.	%
Coronal	45	69	122	67	167	68
Circular	15	23	42	23	57	23
Circular with Passavant's ridge	3	5	10	6	13	5
Sagittal	2	3	7	4	9	4

[*] Reprinted from Witzel and Posnick (1989a) with permission.

Because the Passavant ridge is only associated with a circular closing pattern, are humans able to change from a coronal or sagittal pattern to a circular pattern if the need arises? These and other related questions are impossible to answer at the present time, but two interesting studies seem apropos to this speculative discussion. Siegel-Sadewitz and Shprintzen (1982) explored the possibility of using biofeedback to see if a normal subject (the first author) could change her closure pattern. The examinations were performed so that the subject could see a video monitor and her circular pattern. During the course of six 20-minute biofeedback sessions, the subject was able to change from a circular to a sagittal pattern and to use both patterns interchangeably in continuous speech without the aid of the monitor.

Witzel et al. (1989b) used a biofeedback monitoring technique during speech therapy for three adult cleft palate patients. All three subjects had recently undergone a pharyngeal flap surgical procedure, but residual hypernasality and articulation errors remained. With the combination of biofeedback and speech therapy, two patients developed normal speech, while the third patient demonstrated marked improvement. The authors cautioned, however, that the biofeedback technique is expensive and requires the patient to be both motivated and compliant.

One final consideration about nasoendoscopy is its subjective nature. Perceptual evaluation of velopharyngeal function through nasoendoscopy relies on the judgment of the viewer. Clinicians have used rating systems to describe closure patterns in an attempt to assess velopharyngeal closure more objectively. These rating systems have increased the objectivity of assessments of velopharyngeal function that are made via nasoendoscopy; however, issues with interrater reliability are still evident, especially when velopharyngeal gap size and lateral wall movements are determined (Sie et al., 2008). It may be that, in the future, machine-learning techniques that are currently being applied to radiographic analysis and MRI of the pharynx could also be applied to nasendoscopic recordings (Liu et al., 2021; Shahid et al., 2021).

Magnetic resonance imaging

The use of MRI to evaluate velopharyngeal function recently has become popular. In a study comparing MRI to videofluoroscopy, results revealed that the pattern of closure depicted by both technologies was consistent for all subjects (Beer et al., 2004). The benefit of using MRI instead of videofluoroscopy is the lack of ionizing radiation when MRI is used.

Other research into the use of MRI holds exciting possibilities for assessing a three-dimensional representation of velopharyngeal anatomy, with the addition of a time dimension so that movement of the three-dimensional structure can be observed (i.e., four-dimensional representation). Kane and colleagues (2002) used gated MRI to assess velopharyngeal function during repetitive utterances in a population of adults with no history of speech problems and two patients with a history of cleft lip and palate. A portion of each utterance was acquired to build a full image over multiple utterance cycles. These researchers then used four-dimensional visualization methods to reveal real-time visualization of velopharyngeal anatomy during its entire range of motion. The authors also were able to image anatomical differences in the subjects with cleft lip and cleft palate.

In an excellent review of the evaluation of velopharyngeal dysfunction, Rowe and D'Antonio (2005) noted that, while MRI has several advantages, such as the lack of ionizing radiation and the ability to follow muscle fibers from origin to insertion, there are still several obstacles to overcome. First, many young children will not tolerate an MRI evaluation and may have to be sedated for the procedure. This prohibits a dynamic functional speech assessment. Recent research has focused on novel ways to assess children without the need for sedation (Kollara et al., 2017; Kotare et al., 2021). Rowe and D'Antonio (2005) also pointed to the cost of MRI, suggesting that it may prohibit routine use of this technology. Another factor to consider is that the patient must be in the prone position during the MRI, altering velopharyngeal dynamics from those of an upright sitting position. Finally, the technology is not yet fast enough to acquire images in a sequence that is sufficient for connected speech, although dynamic protocols are being developed and show promise (Perry et al., 2014; Bae et al., 2011). Thus, multiple sequences have to be overlaid on one another to fill in the missing information, as was the case in the study by Kane et al. (2002).

Pressure-flow studies

The third noteworthy methodology for evaluating patients with various velopharyngeal dysfunction was developed by Warren and coworkers at the University of North Carolina (Hairfield et al., 1987; Dalston et al., 1988, 1990; Laine et al., 1988a, 1988b; Minsley et al., 1991). While this methodology has been useful as a diagnostic aid, the primary contribution of these pressure-flow studies has been to the understanding of the physiology of the speech complex. These aerodynamic studies are based on a modification of a theoretical hydraulic principle that was first reported by Warren and DuBois (1964). It assumes that the smallest cross-sectional area of a structure can be determined if the differential pressure across the structure is measured simultaneously with the rate of airflow through it. This principle has been verified by other independent investigators (Smith and Weinberg, 1980, 1982).

Prior to this body of research, it was known that complete separation of the oral and nasal cavities was not essential for acceptable speech (Subtelny et al., 1961; Blackfield et al., 1962; Carney and Morris, 1971). Researchers also knew that the degree of inadequacy and the severity of the resultant speech disorder do not appear to be linear (Brandt and Morris, 1965; Warren et al., 1985). Pressure-flow studies have provided some insight into these complex interrelationships.

Velopharyngeal orifice size

Warren (1965), using these hydraulic principles to compute velopharyngeal orifice size, found that this opening should be less than 20 mm^2 during the production of plosive and fricative sounds. Normal velopharyngeal orifice opening values range between 0 and 5 mm^2 during oral consonant production. Hence, surgical reconstruction or prosthetic obturation need not be perfect to enable the patient to function normally.

If the velopharyngeal opening is greater than 20 mm^2, the respiratory effort must be increased to compensate for velopharyngeal inadequacy and improve the oral pressure available for speech (Warren, 1986; Laine et al., 1988a, 1988b; Warren et al., 1990a, 1990b). Individuals with velopharyngeal deficiencies have the capability of doubling their respiratory volume depending on the degree of velopharyngeal incompetence and the amount of resistance to airflow within the nasal cavity (Warren, 1986). Oral pressures greater than 3 cm H_2O were considered adequate to provide the aerodynamic capability for plosive and fricative phonemes. In studying 267 cleft palate subjects with various levels of speech proficiency, Dalston et al. (1988) found that 87% of these patients were able to produce pressures greater than 3 cm H_2O. This adaptive capacity occurred even though speech was considered borderline or inadequate in 86 of these patients.

Warren (1986) suggested that this adaptation may be a regulation/control phenomenon and thus may have both beneficial and adverse effects. For example, an increase in oral pressure along with velopharyngeal inadequacy may improve articulation but increase nasal airflow, which, in turn, may increase the perceived level of nasality.

Four categories of velopharyngeal adequacy based on orifice area have been developed (Warren, 1979): *(1) adequate closure* is 0 to 4.99 mm^2; *(2) borderline adequate closure* is 5 to 9.99 mm^2; *(3) borderline inadequate closure* is 10 to 19.99 mm^2; and, *(4) inadequate closure* is greater than 20 mm^2. In studies of listener perception, velopharyngeal orifice areas between 10 and 20 mm^2 result in air pressure and flow patterns similar to those associated with velopharyngeal impairment, leading listeners to judge the speech to be hypernasal during nonnasal consonant production (Warren, 1979; Warren et al., 1994).

Nasal resistance

It is now known that resistance to nasal airflow may increase oral pressure and, consequently, improve the effectiveness of speech for patients with larger velopharyngeal orifices. It is the sum of the resistance provided by the velopharyngeal mechanism, nasal resistance, and the increase in respiratory effort that determines the oral pressure available for the proper articulation of speech.

An analog model was used by Warren and Ryon (1967) to demonstrate that, even in patients with slight to moderate velopharyngeal incompetence (0.2 to 0.4 cm), nasal resistance can account for as much as 30% to 90% of the recorded oral pressure amplitude. Warren et al. (1969) compared the nasal resistance to airflow of 25 cleft lip and/or palate patients with that of an unaffected control group. The cleft group had significantly greater nasal resistance to airflow.

Resistance within the nasal cavity may be created by maxillary surgery for neoplastic disease or cleft lip and cleft palate repair, enlarged turbinates, vomerine spurs, atresia of the nostrils, or deviation of the septum. Clefts of the lip and palate produce deformities that tend to reduce the size and patency of the nasal airway (Warren et al., 1992a). Interestingly, patients with repaired bilateral cleft lips and palates have larger airways and less nasal resistance, and thus poorer articulation of speech, than do patients with unilateral cleft lips and palates (Dalston et al., 1992). Therefore, a nose that is "good" for breathing may be "bad" for speech under these circumstances.

Nasal valve

Laine et al. (1988a, 1988b) introduced the concept of the nasal valve. The valve is considered the area between the upper and lower lateral cartilages, the pyriform aperture, and the anterior terminus of the inferior turbinates. In physiologic terms, the nasal valve is considered to be the regulator with the smallest cross-sectional area within the nasal cavity based on anatomical and flow-resistive characteristics. Laine et al. (1988a, 1988b) used pressure-flow studies to measure the cross-sectional area of the nasal valve during both inspiration and expiration. The nasal valve dilates during inspiration and both active and passive flattening occur during expiration. The authors concluded that the nasal airway is an active participant in the breathing process rather than a passive conduit for airflow.

The nasal valve concept may explain the reason for facial grimaces in patients with velopharyngeal dysfunction. Clinically we have observed facial grimaces associated with some surgically repaired cleft lip and cleft palate patients who exhibit hypernasality during speech production. Facial grimaces may be a physiologic adaptive process used to enhance the breaking potential of the nasal valve to improve intraoral pressure for speech (Hairfield et al., 1987). The aerodigestive tract contains a number of valves or restrictive braking mechanisms, such as the larynx, velopharyngeal mechanism, tongue-oral approximations, and the lips, that prolong expiration and, in turn, enhance speech and the interchange of gases in the lungs. It appears the nasal valve should be added to this list.

A study by Dalston et al. (1992) disclosed the relationship between the patency of the nasal airway and articulation capabilities. These investigators noticed that children with bilateral cleft lip and palate were nearly twice as likely to exhibit compensatory articulation errors as similarly aged children with either unilateral cleft lip and palate or cleft palate only. When subjects were grouped according to speech performance, pressure-airflow evaluations suggested that children with compensatory articulation patterns had nasal cross-sectional areas that were significantly larger than those of children without compensatory articulation. These larger airways were more likely to occur in children with bilateral cleft lip and palate. This reduced level of nasal resistance was not as effective in improving oral pressure for articulation.

Oral versus nasal breathing

Restrictions within the nasal cavity may lead patients with repaired cleft lip and cleft palate to favor oral rather than nasal breathing. Warren et al. (1990b), in a study of 50 randomly selected cleft palate patients, found the average nasal valve area was reduced to 0.38 cm and these individuals were predominantly oral breathers. Ricketts (1968) and Warren and coworkers (Warren et al., 1988) believed that individuals with nasal valve areas of less than 0.40 cm should be considered to have impaired nasal airways and will be predominately mouth breathers with the potential to alter the dentofacial complex.

Minsley et al. (1991) cautioned that the patency of the nasal airway must be considered when obturators are fabricated for cleft palate patients. They measured the nasal cross-sectional area of eight cleft palate patients with obturator prostheses. Four of these patients had nasal airways that measured less than 0.40 cm when their prosthesis was in place and thus were classified as mandatory oral breathers. Consideration of nasal patency also would apply to other patients who are rehabilitated with a prosthesis, such as those who have undergone ablative surgery of the palatopharyngeal structures or those with palatal dysfunction secondary to a neurologic injury.

Timing of velopharyngeal closure

The timing of velopharyngeal closure in relationship to the phoneme being articulated has been studied using pressure-flow techniques (Warren et al., 1985). In this study, the experimental group included 10 patients with normal velopharyngeal function, 20 patients with cleft palate and adequate velopharyngeal closure (0 to 9.99 mm^2), 20 patients with borderline inadequate closure (10 to 19.99 mm^2), and 20 patients with inadequate closure (≥ 20 mm^2). The word *hamper* was used in this and in most of these pressure-airflow studies conducted by these researchers. The nasal-plosive blend /*mp*/ in *hamper* tests the velopharyngeal complex during an open-to-closed maneuver. The isthmus must be open for the nasal phoneme /*m*/ and closed for the stop-plosive /*p*/. Airflow and pressure curves were recorded simultaneously. This permitted the investigators to note the timing of closure to prepare for the articulation of /*p*/ and the amount of nasal airflow or perceived nasality during the formulation of /*p*/. The findings revealed that patients with borderline inadequate or inadequate closure had peak oral pressure and nasal airflow that overlapped almost in entirety whereas those with adequate closure or those in the control group demonstrated traces where nasal airflow ceased before the pressure peak for /*p*/ was reached. Thus, the timing errors noted in this study seemed to compound the problems known to be associated with velopharyngeal inadequacy.

In another study, 209 noncleft adults with normal speech and 26 adults with repaired cleft palates and normal speech were studied aerodynamically (Dalston et al., 1990). While subjects in both groups achieved velopharyngeal closure, the cleft group produced speech with significantly less nasal airflow. In addition, the intraoral pressure curve shifted forward, indicating that the cleft group had to make certain compensatory adjustments to produce closure because of differences in the potential movement of the velopharyngeal complex. As mentioned previously, there is not a direct linear relationship between velopharyngeal orifice size and the level of perceived nasality. This is understandable because of the number of variables, including nasal resistance and timing, that can influence the aerodynamic characteristics of the speech mechanism.

Nasometrics

Early studies of listeners' ability to judge disorders of resonance revealed that factors such as articulatory proficiency (McWilliams, 1954; Van Hattum, 1958), vocal pitch and intensity (Hess, 1959; Spriestersbach, 1955), and type of speech stimulus (Counihan et al., 1970; Lintz and Sherman, 1961; Sherman, 1954) can influence judgments of nasality. The Nasometer (Kay Pentax), introduced in the 1980s, made it possible to supplement perceptual judgments with an objective measure of nasal resonance. The Nasometer is a computer-based tool used in the measurement of *nasalance*, which is the ratio of nasal acoustic energy (N) to nasal-plus-oral acoustic energy (N + O) expressed as a percentage [(N)/(N + O) x 100]. Nasalance has been found to be a correlate of human perception of resonance (Hardin et al., 1992; Dalston et al., 1991b, 1991c). The Nasometer is useful, therefore, in complementing clinical judgments of resonance disorders (Hardin et al., 1992; Dalston et al., 1991b, 1991c, 1993).

Its many clinical applications include identification of nasal obstruction (Dalston et al., 1991a, 1991b); assessment of nasality both before and after velopharyngeal surgery (Andreassen et al., 1990; Clendaniel et al., 1990; Nellis et al., 1992); identification of individuals with velopharyngeal impairment (Dalston et al., 1991a); assessment of velopharyngeal impairment in patients with head and neck cancer (Seikaly et al., 2003; Rieger et al., 2008); assessment in conjunction with fitting palatal lifts and obturators for those individuals with compromised palatopharyngeal function (Wolfaardt et al., 1993; Clendaniel, 1990; Rieger et al., 2002, 2003; Molt, 1990); assessment of individuals with cleft palate (Van Lierde et al., 2004; Persson et al., 2006; Chanchareonsook et al., 2007); assessment of endoscopic sinus surgery (Jiang and Huang, 2006); assessment after uvulopalatoplasty (Van Lierde et al., 2004); and use as a visual biofeedback tool in training individuals to reduce mild hypernasality (Goldstein, 1990).

Clinicians in North America have collaborated on the development of a database for nasalance using standardized testing procedures, instrumentation, and comparable spoken materials. As information from several studies has accumulated, differences in nasalance have emerged for speakers' native languages, regional dialects within the same language, sex, and age (Dalston et al., 1993; Anderson, 1996; Kavanagh et al., 1994; Leeper et al., 1992; Nichols, 1999; Rochet et al., 1998; Seaver et al., 1991). The between- and within-language differences are now well-documented. The validity of the male-female differences in nasalance scores remains questionable until sample sizes are sufficient to analyze such differences with confidence. There also has been a noticeable trend toward an increase in nasalance with age (Rochet et al., 1998). Preliminary impressions reported by Seaver and colleagues (1991) revealed that older subjects tended to obtain higher nasalance scores than younger subjects when reading nonnasal passages. Leeper et al. (1992) also reported significant age differences in nasometric values between younger age groups (7 to 19 years) and older age groups (65 years and older) of the same dialect. Hutchinson et al. (1978) investigated patterns of nasalance in a sample of 60 normal gerontologic participants using Tonar II, a prototype of the Nasometer. Their results revealed that older participants exhibited noticeably higher nasalance values while reading than did young adults studied in other investigations (Hutchinson et al., 1978).

Explanations for age differences include possible changes in physiology and structure. Physiologic changes associated with advancing age may alter neuromuscular control capabilities. Structural changes in the resonating chambers of the head may influence the acoustic impedance characteristics of intrinsic sound barriers such as the bony hard palate and resonating cavities such as the mouth, nose, and sinuses. Any one or a combination of these explanations may be pertinent to the increased nasality detected in older individuals.

Slower speaking rates also have been cited to explain higher nasalance with advancing age (Hutchinson et al., 1978). Reduction in the speaking rate of elderly individuals, a well-documented phenomenon (Hartman, 1976; Ramig, 1972; Ryan, 1972), has been hypothesized to result in discontinuity of velopharyngeal closure, thereby contributing to increased nasalance by providing an opportunity for normally nonnasalized speech sounds to become nasalized (Hutchinson et al., 1978; Colton and Cooker, 1968). Discontinuity of velopharyngeal closure is more likely to occur just before and after inspiratory pauses within a stream of connected speech. Speaking at a slower rate restricts the number of words that can be produced in one breath group, thereby increasing the number of breath groups occurring within a passage. This, in turn, will increase the occurrence of pauses within a selected passage and increase the opportunity for discontinuity of velopharyngeal closure and thus increased nasalance on voiced segments around such junctures.

Perceptual evaluation

Frequently, assessment of disordered resonance and management outcomes is based on perceptual judgments via the auditory system of listeners; that is, does the patient sound hypernasal, or hyponasal, or does he or she present with a normal resonance balance? The difficulty with these types of judgments is that there is a continuum of severity that can be associated with nasal resonance disorders, especially hypernasality. Commonly, a patient's speech will be rated as mildly, moderately, or severely hypernasal.

Four-point equal-appearing interval scales are quite commonly reported (Redenbaugh and Reich, 1985; Reich and Redenbaugh, 1985; Bressmann et al., 2000). It is unlikely that scales such as these can adequately represent the continuum of severity of velopharyngeal dysfunction. In fact, equal-appearing interval scales have been criticized as being unreliable and invalid for rating hypernasality of speech (Zraick and Liss, 2000).

As an alternative, direct magnitude estimation has been suggested as a more reliable and valid method of completing perceptual ratings of nasality (Zraick and Liss, 2000; Whitehill et al., 2002). The process of direct magnitude estimation usually requires that listeners be calibrated to a modulus, which is a standard stimulus to which other listening tokens are compared and judged (Lee et al., 2009).

Prosthesis evaluation

Unfortunately, almost all of the speech evaluation methods discussed—that is, multiview videofluoroscopy, nasoendoscopy, and pressure-airflow aerodynamic assessment equipment—are usually found only in the more established craniofacial rehabilitation centers where a prosthodontist and speech pathologist are included among the professional staff. Rarely would a prosthodontist or a speech pathologist have this equipment in the private sector.

Both nasoendoscopy and pressure-airflow equipment have been used as an aid during prosthetic treatment (see Fig 4-12). Karnell et al. (1987), Walter (1990), and Turner and Williams (1991) discussed the use of nasal videoendoscopy during prosthodontic treatment. Rieger et al. (2006) presented data that revealed that better speech outcomes could be achieved when prosthetic rehabilitation of velopharyngeal dysfunction occurred with the aid of nasal videoendoscopy. La Velle and Hardy (1979), Reisberg and Smith (1985), and Minsley et al. (1991) used oronasal airflow data to compute the velopharyngeal orifice and nasal valve areas as guidelines during obturator fabrication and adjustment.

Riski et al. (1989) demonstrated the advantages of employing both pressure-flow and nasal endoscopic assessments in the successful revision of existing obturator prostheses. These evaluations revealed that the obturator for one patient required sequential additions, while the speech of a second patient was judged to be hyponasal, which necessitated sequential reduction of the obturator laterally to enhance nasal airflow and subsequent speech improvement. Wolfaardt et al. (1993) monitored 32 patients with palatal lift prostheses prior to, during, and after treatment using nasoendoscopy, pressure-flow equipment, and a Nasometer. With continued monitoring with this equipment, these investigators were able to eliminate the lift prosthesis for 14 patients by reassuring them that they had now developed the aerodynamic capabilities for normal speech without the need for their lift prosthesis.

Anatomy and Physiology

The anatomy and physiology of the velopharyngeal mechanism will be described by dividing the descriptions into the following anatomical components: the soft palate, the posterior pharyngeal wall, and the lateral pharyngeal walls. This is an arbitrary division for descriptive purposes in that closure is usually achieved with synchronous and sphincteric movements of this entire muscular complex.

Soft palate

The soft palate runs continuously from the hard palate and ends posteriorly in a free margin, which forms an arch with the palatoglossus and palatopharyngeal folds on each side. Its framework is formed by a strong, thin fibrous sheet, the palatine aponeurosis, which is primarily tensor veli palatine tendon. The muscles that make up the soft palate complex are the levator veli palatini, the tensor veli palatini, the musculus uvulae, the palatoglossus, and the palatopharyngeus.

Position and movement

The position and movement of the soft palate in relation to the pharynx change with age (Aram and Subtelny, 1959; Fletcher, 1970). At birth and shortly thereafter, the soft palate at rest is roughly parallel to the roof of the pharynx so that the upper nasopharynx is only a narrow slot. Closure of the velopharyngeal mechanism is accomplished essentially by a superior-inferior movement of the soft palate. As growth occurs in the pharyngeal area and as the adenoidal tissues regress, the movement of the soft palate takes on the characteristic anteroposterior elevation displayed by most adults. When the adenoidal tissues are removed, the soft palate shifts to an anteroposterior movement very abruptly (Aram and Subtelny, 1959). Velopharyngeal closure is slightly below the level of the palatal plane up to eight years of age and is consistently above the level of the palatal plane thereafter (Fig 4-14) (Aram and Subtelny, 1959; Fletcher, 1970).

The extent of the closure of the soft palate with the posterior pharyngeal wall varies with head position. An extended head position results in a deeper nasopharynx than is found when the head is held in the Frankfort plane (Lloyd et al., 1957). McWilliams et al. (1968), in a radiographic study of 101 children with repaired cleft palates, found that the inferosuperior length of contact of the soft palate with the posterior pharyngeal wall was reduced significantly when the head was in an extended position (Fig 4-15).

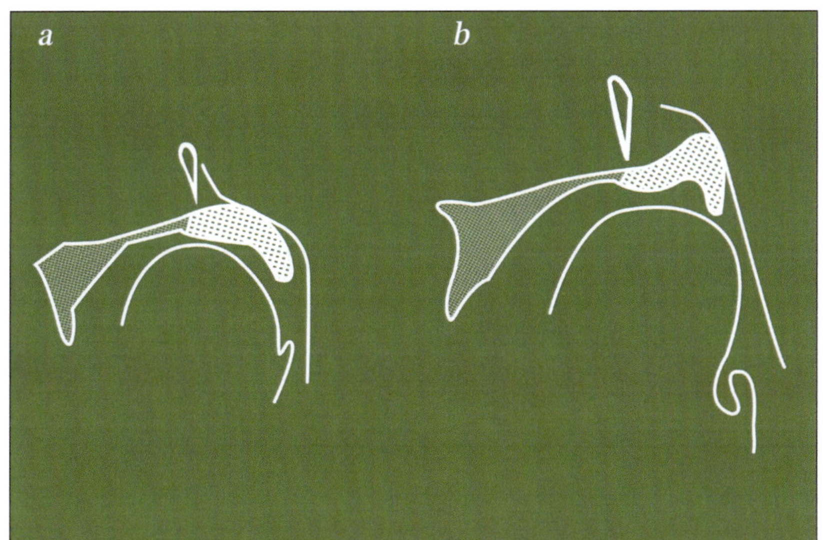

Figure 4-14 Velopharyngeal closure. *(a)* Closure in a 5-year-old child. Closure is obtained with superoinferior movement of the soft palate at a level below the palatal plane. *(b)* Closure in an 18-year-old individual. At this age, velopharyngeal closure is characteristically above the palatal plane, with an anteroposterior movement of the soft palate (adapted from Aram and Subtelny, 1959, with permission).

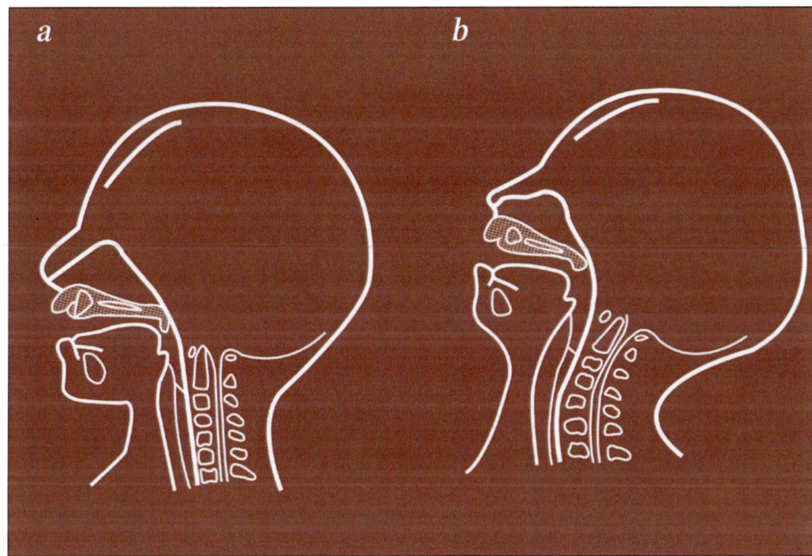

Figure 4-15 Tracings of velopharyngeal closure in a patient with a repaired cleft palate. *(a)* Velopharyngeal closure is achieved when the patient is in an upright position. *(b)* The nasopharynx is deepened when the patient is in an extended head position, so closure is not achieved (adapted from McWilliams et al., 1968, with permission).

The pattern of soft palate movement varies between men and women (McKerns and Bzoch, 1970). The soft palate is longer, the elevation is greater, the amount of contact with the posterior pharyngeal wall is less, and the inferior point of contact with the posterior pharyngeal wall is consistently higher in men than in women.

Velar eminence and musculus uvulae

While the entire soft palate increases in length during closure (Bzoch et al., 1959; Pruzansky and Mason, 1969), the posterior two-thirds demonstrates a greater degree of lengthening and a significant thickening (Simpson and Austin, 1972). Several investigators have noted a central longitudinal thickening or elevation of the nasal surface of the soft palate that has been termed the *velar eminence* (Bloomer, 1953; Pigott, 1969a, 1969b; Croft, 1978). Pigott (1969a), in his nasal endoscopic observations of 25 normal subjects, described the velar eminence as a large ridge occupying the central third of the nasal surface of the soft palate and rising to a height almost equal to its width. He believed that the velar eminence is an essential component of velopharyngeal closure.

Croft (1978) confirmed these observations. He examined 20 patients, aged 4 to 36 years, who demonstrated hypernasal speech, small central gaps on velopharyngeal closure as determined from multiview videofluoroscopy, and normal palatal morphology on oral examination. This triad of conditions is known as *occult submucous cleft palate* (see Chapter 6). These patients were reexamined with direct-view nasoendoscopy during speech production. This examination confirmed the presence of central gaps along the nasal surface that were associated with the lack of a velar eminence in all 20 patients.

It is now understood that the musculus uvulae is responsible for the velar eminence, contributes to velar stretch, and is essential for normal velopharyngeal closure (Croft, 1978; Azzam and Kuehn, 1977; Kuehn et al., 1988). This paired muscle is the only intrinsic muscle of the soft palate. Because it lacks an attachment outside the velum, its contribution to velopharyngeal closure previously was considered minimal. However, its importance may be related more to its size and position rather than its physiologic contribution. Each of the two bundles of the musculus uvulae has its origin from the tendinous palatal aponeurosis posterior to the hard palate and anterior to the insertion of the levator veli palatini muscle. The bundles converge above and at right angles to the sling of the levator veli palatini and redivide and insert into the basement membrane and connective tissue of the uvula. The bulk of the uvula consists of glandular tissue interspersed with muscle fibers.

In a cadaver study, the anatomy of the musculus uvulae was found to be quite variable (Kuehn and Moon, 2005). In general, the pendulous uvula was found to contain little muscle tissue, and both paired and unpaired samples of the muscle were found. Kuehn and Moon (2005) thought this was of little significance to the biomechanical function of this muscle and that its presence would add bulk to the region on contraction as long as it is located dorsally above the levator sling.

Kuehn et al. (1988) studied three normal adults with electromyography. They found that the electromyographic activity of the levator veli palatini and the musculus uvulae were synchronous during speech in all three subjects, but this synergistic activity was not always present during nonspeech activities. Thus, the levator supplies the force with contraction and elevates the soft palate. At the same time, the musculus uvulae contracts to fill the central gap between the soft palate, the lateral pharyngeal walls, and the posterior pharyngeal wall along the central third of the nasal surface of the soft palate. The contraction of the musculus uvulae is considered essential for those individuals with any circular pattern of closure (Siegel-Sadewitz and Shprintzen, 1982).

Although the entire soft palate increases in length during closure (Bzoch et al., 1959; Pruzansky and Mason, 1969; Simpson and Chin, 1981), the central and posterior portions demonstrate a proportionally greater degree of lengthening along with thickening. This lengthening during closure has been termed *velar stretch*. Simpson and Austin (1972) reported a 20.6% increase in length, or stretch, from rest to the production of the /s/ sound in normal adult subjects.

Later evidence confirmed these early findings, suggesting that the velum can stretch anywhere from 13% to 28% with an average stretch of 19% from rest (Ettema et al., 2002). The amount of velar stretch seems related to the task and/or anatomical or functional variables associated with the structures involved in closure (Simpson and Chin, 1981). These authors developed a "need ratio" by dividing the pharyngeal depth (posterior nasal spine to the posterior pharyngeal wall) by the velar length (posterior nasal spine to the tip of the uvula along the nasal surface) at rest as measured from lateral cephalometric radiographs. Larger need ratios indicated the need for greater velar stretch to achieve closure. More recently, Denegri and colleagues have described the relationship between velar length and thickness and the depth of the nasopharynx in children with cleft palate. Their findings revealed that children who demonstrated hypernasality and nasal air emission were characterized as having a shorter, thinner velum along with a deeper nasopharynx and that depth-to-length ratios larger than 0.93 were always associated with signs of velopharyngeal dysfunction (Denegri et al., 2021).

Neiman and Simpson (1975) studied children with normal speech with lateral cephalometric radiographs prior to and following adenoidectomies. Because the soft palate could no longer close against the protruding adenoidal pads, velar stretch increased from 12.7% to 27.8% postsurgically to maintain normal closure patterns.

Histology

Kuehn and Kahane (1990) studied the soft palates of 10 normal human adult cadavers and found some interesting correlations at the cellular level. The soft palates were resected and divided equally into 10 sections anteroposteriorly, and 300 representative slides were prepared and examined histologically. The nasal mucosa consisted of typical pseudostratified, ciliated columnar epithelium anteriorly but stratified squamous epithelium posteriorly. This more posterior mucosa appeared to be well supplied with underlying mucous glands. Because the nasal mucosal surface contacting the posterior pharyngeal wall was lined with stratified squamous epithelium, it seemed well adapted for the stress of repeated closures. The oral mucosa surface of the soft palate consisted of stratified squamous epithelium with a basement membrane that was well endowed with a dense meshwork of elastic fibers. The underlying seromucous glands would have served to create a lubricated surface for the passage of a bolus, while the large deposits of adipose tissue located laterally primarily would provide protection from the pressure generated during the propulsion of the bolus.

In a follow-up study, Kuehn and Moon (2005) aimed to describe the tissue composition and structure of the central portion of the soft palate (i.e., that which exists between the faucial pillars). They replicated the finding that the layers from oral to nasal epithelium were fairly uniform across the 12 cadavers that they studied. They also confirmed the cellular composition and glandular tissue of the anterior velum to be consistent with the previous findings. Kuehn and Moon (2005) also found that the tensor tendon, located in the anterior portion of the velum, diminished in bulk as it coursed in a posterior direction. At the same time, the velar muscles began to increase in bulk, increasing markedly in the middle third of the velum. Furthermore, the posterior portion of the velum was noted to be more anatomically variable.

Stål and Lindman (2000) used postmortem specimens to study the fiber types of the soft palate muscles. These authors reported that the type of muscle fibers found in the palatopharyngeus and musculus uvulae suggest that these muscles are functionally involved in quick movements. The fiber types found in the levator and tensor veli palatini muscles suggest that they are involved in slower and more continuous contractions. The authors also found a high aerobic capacity and the rich capillarization of the palate muscles, which suggests that they are relatively fatigue resistant. No ordinary muscle spindles were found in the palatal muscles, which may suggest that the soft palate muscles are governed by a special proprioceptive control system.

Levator veli palatini and other muscles

Although opinions regarding the specific muscles responsible for lateral and posterior pharyngeal wall movements are almost as numerous as the authors who discuss them, there is general agreement that the levator veli palatini muscles are the most important muscles of palatal elevation (Dickson et al., 1974; Kuehn et al., 2005). Evidence suggests that the tensor veli palatini contributes little to the form and function of the soft palate and that its primary function

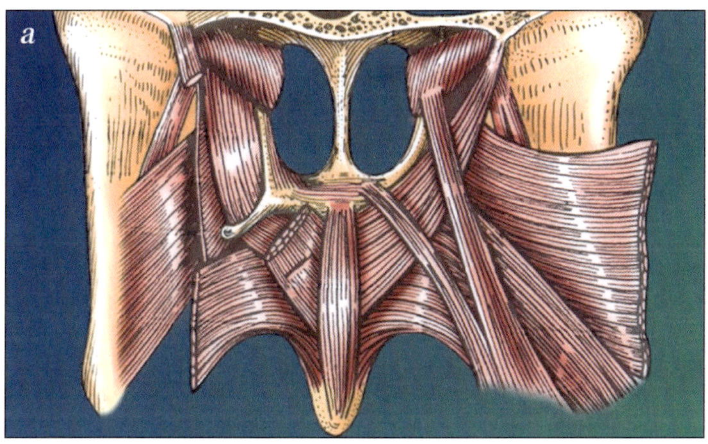

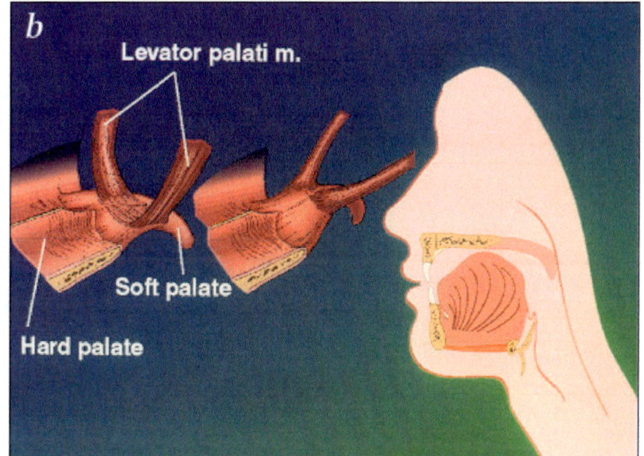

Figure 4-16 Muscles directly involved with velopharyngeal closure. *(a)* Uvulus (U) and levator veli palatini (L) muscles, viewed from behind. *(b)* The levator veli palatini elevates the soft palate and pulls it posteriorly (courtesy of Dr. S. Esposito).

is the dilation of the eustachian tubes (Dickson and Dickson, 1972; Bluestone et al., 1972; Huang et al., 1997; Takasaki et al., 2002).

The levator veli palatini muscle has its origin lateral to the torus tubarius without attachment to the eustachian tube. The levator courses downward, forward, and medially and inserts into the middle third of the soft palate (Fig 4-16). Although the levator veli palatini muscles supply the force for palatal elevation, the finite positioning of the soft palate may be under the control of several other muscles acting in a reciprocal manner with the levator.

Kuehn et al. (1982) studied the relationship between muscle activity and velar position in five normal subjects. Hooked-wire electrodes were placed transnasally in the levator veli palatini, palatoglossus, palatopharyngeus, and the superior constrictor muscles, and their electromyographic activity was measured during speech. A consistent interaction among the levator, the palatoglossus, and the palatopharyngeus muscles was observed. If the levator contracted forcefully, the palatoglossus and the palatopharyngeus also contracted forcefully. The reverse scenario was also true. It was surmised that the palatoglossus and the palatopharyngeus create a downward pull on the soft palate and oppose the upward contraction of the levator.

In an anatomical dissection study, however, Kuehn and Moon (2005) discovered a lack of palatoglossus muscle fibers that crossed or even approached midline. This prompted these authors to question the contribution of the palatoglossus muscle in creating an antagonistic sling in opposition to the levator sling. They found, instead, that the important fibers in the middle third of the palate consisted of the levator veli palatini muscle fibers that cross the midline, the longitudinal fibers of the musculus uvulae, and the palatopharyngeus.

The reciprocal muscular relationships that do exist help explain the interrelationship between tongue position or velopharyngeal closure and speech. Tongue posture and movement may differ in individuals with velopharyngeal incompetence or VPI. These patients often have a more posterior and superior tongue position during speech (Moll, 1965; Graber et al., 1958, 1959; Powers, 1962; Brooks et al., 1965, 1966; Lawrence et al., 1975). Warren (1986) believed that a high tongue carriage would increase vocal tract resistance for patients with a velopharyngeal deficiency. These investigators thought that this compensatory tongue posture assisted with soft palate elevation but contributed to the faulty articulation reported for these patients. For example, the tongue contacted the soft palate during speech in 13 of 28 cleft palate patients, whereas in a matched control group of patients without cleft palate, this contact was not observed (Brooks et al., 1965).

Kuehn (1976) studied the timing and speed of palatal movements relative to articulatory activity with cineradiography and reported that soft palate movements are generally slower than tongue movements.

Posterior pharyngeal wall

In 1863 and 1869, Gustof Passavant described a horizontal "cross roll" on the posterior pharyngeal wall that occurred during speech and swallowing in cleft palate patients (Calnan, 1957). This forward bulging, corresponding to the level of the atlas, has been termed the *Passavant ridge* or *pad*. This cross roll may vary from a slight forward bulging of the posterior pharyngeal wall to a very distinct roll that extends horizontally across the posterior pharyngeal wall to blend with the mediolateral movement of the lateral pharyngeal walls. In its prominent form, the Passavant ridge may extend forward and superiorly as much as 5 mm in both directions. The Passavant ridge serves as a guide for proper placement of the soft palate obturator prosthesis (Fig 4-17).

The relative importance of any forward movement of the posterior pharyngeal wall and its contribution to velopharyngeal closure is subject to debate among many knowledgeable investigators. There are several reasons for this controversy. For example, most normal speakers do not exhibit any detectable forward movement of the posterior pharyngeal wall during velopharyngeal closure (Bzoch et al., 1959; Croft et al., 1981). However, in patients with velopharyngeal incompetence or VPI, the degree of posterior wall movement, the Passavant ridge, or both are more likely to be observed (Calnin, 1957; Nylen, 1961; Skolnick et al., 1973; Croft et al., 1981; Casey and Emrich, 1988) and thus may be compensatory in nature (Carpenter, 1968). Yet many individuals with obvious hypernasal speech patterns and observable velopharyngeal deficiencies do not exhibit any compensatory forward movement of the posterior pharyngeal wall during attempts at velopharyngeal closure.

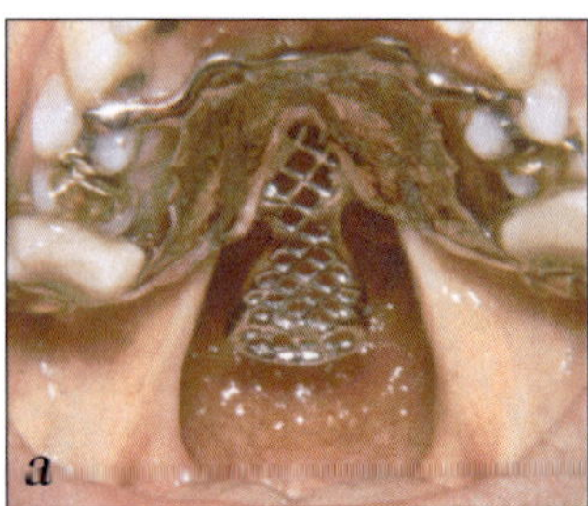

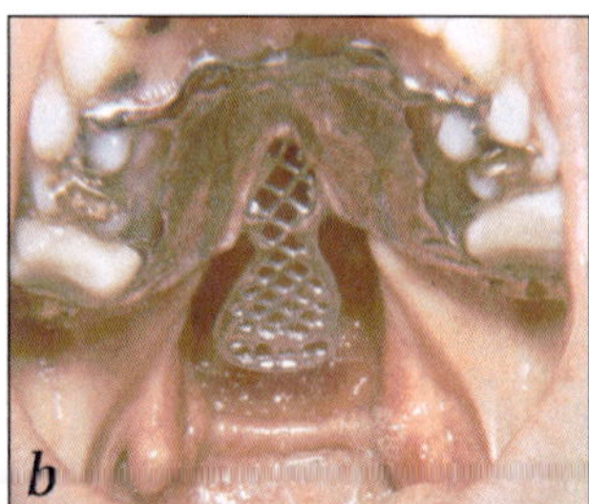

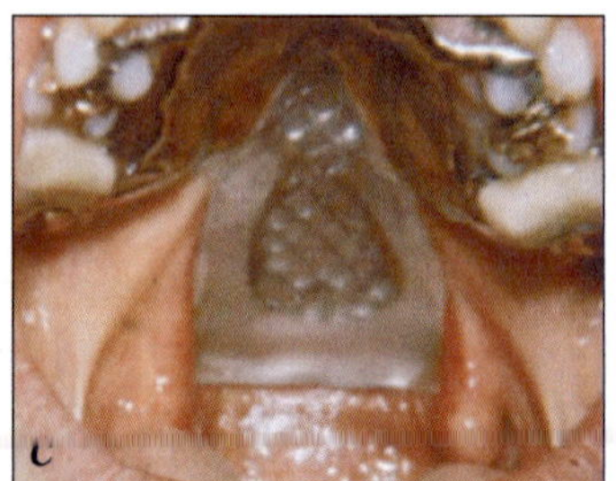

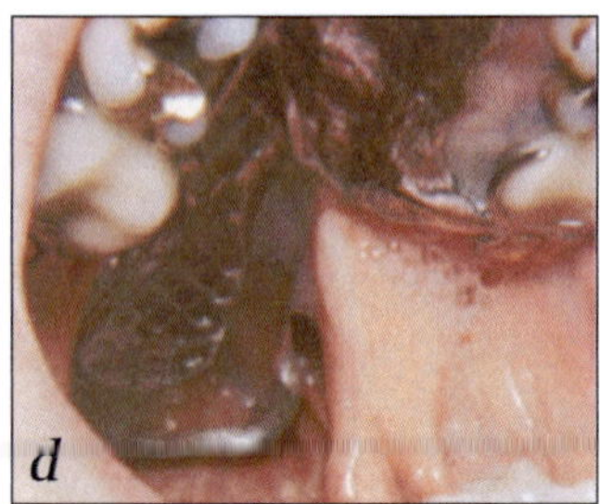

Figure 4-17 Patient with unrepaired cleft palate demonstrating a definitive Passavant ridge. *(a)* RDP framework in position with the V-P muscular complex at rest. *(b)* The V-P mechanism in a contracted state. *(c)* Definitive obturator prosthesis in position. The VP musculature embraces the prosthesis during speech and swallowing. *(d)* When the V-P musculature is at rest, that is space between the surface of the obturator and the lateral and pharyngeal walls permitting normal nasal breathing and the production of nasal consonants.

Kuehn et al. (1982) found that the level of electromyographic activity in the superior constrictor in five subjects was inconsistent and variable and not in harmony with the activity level of the other three palatal muscles (i.e., palatoglossus, palatopharyngeus, and levator veli palatini). It was observed that speech segments requiring essentially complete velopharyngeal closure could be produced with dramatically different levels of electromyographic activity from the superior constrictor among the five subjects. Although activity was found in all subjects during velar elevation, the specific role of the superior constrictor needs further investigation. Because the most superior fibers of the superior constrictor insert into the soft palate (Nylen, 1961), Kuehn et al. (1982) speculated that these muscle fibers may assist the musculus uvulae to draw or stretch the velum posteriorly.

Although the degree of movement, if present, of the posterior pharyngeal wall is limited in comparison to the range of movement demonstrated by the soft palate and the lateral pharyngeal walls, any movement of these structures lateral and peripheral to the soft palate and functioning in concert with the velum during closure is important. Both the surgical prognosis for a pharyngeal flap procedure and the prosthetic prognosis for an obturator prosthesis are enhanced if the patient has any movement of the posterior as well as the lateral pharyngeal walls (Casey, 1983; Casey and Emrich, 1988). In part, it is this peripheral movement that permits the patient to control airflow and the degree of nasal resonance by the required intermittent approximation of these structures with the pharyngeal flap or obturator prosthesis.

The incidence of the Passavant ridge has been reported by several investigators. Calnan (1957) found that 32% of 105 patients with inadequate velopharyngeal closure displayed considerable forward movement of the posterior pharyngeal wall. Nylen (1961) reported that the Passavant ridge was present in 11 of 27 cleft palate patients with hypernasality. Skolnick et al. (1973) reported that 17 of 62 patients with inadequate velopharyngeal closure displayed evidence of the Passavant ridge, whereas only 1 of 23 normal patients showed similar movement.

Croft et al. (1981) examined 500 cleft palate patients with videofluoroscopic and nasal endoscopic examinations and found the Passavant ridge in 24% of this group. Using the same methods, they found the ridge in 17% of 80 individuals without cleft palate. Casey and Emrich (1988) examined 29 patients with an oral panendoscope following resection of varying amounts of the posterior soft palate for oral cancer. They found that the Passavant ridge was present in 83% of these patients postsurgically.

To what extent does the Passavant ridge contribute to velopharyngeal closure? This point continues to be a matter of debate. Calnan (1957) reported that the Passavant ridge varied in location, tended to be located below the level of palatal closure, contracted slowly and in an uncoordinated manner, and tended to fatigue easily. He concluded that it contributed little to velopharyngeal closure. However, Carpenter and Morris (1968) selected six patients who exhibited hypernasality and a detectable Passavant ridge. Cinefluorographic films demonstrated that, in four patients, the Passavant ridge was located at or above the level of the palatal plane, contributed to closure during speech, and did not fatigue with sustained discourse.

Glaser et al. (1979) studied 43 patients with a discernible Passavant ridge using multiview videofluoroscopy in conjunction with simultaneous speech recordings. These investigators found that the Passavant ridge corresponded to the level of normal velopharyngeal closure 88% of the time, while the ridge was located too low for closure in 12% of the patients. In 37% of all patients, it was the primary structure that closed or locally narrowed the velopharyngeal portal. The Passavant ridge was most prominent with active lateral pharyngeal wall motion and was consistently synchronous with velar movements.

Is the presence of a Passavant ridge primarily a compensatory mechanism in response to altered velopharyngeal function? Walter (1981, 1990) found that the Passavant ridge was present in 10% of speakers without cleft palate but in 57% of patients with unrepaired cleft palate. He believed that evidence was lacking to suggest that the presence of this entity was a compensatory factor associated with cleft palate. Walter (1981, 1990) thought that the Passavant ridge was more likely a feature of a syndrome arising from altered muscle attachment and function. Warren (1986) speculated that Passavant ridge may be a compensatory response to inadequate velopharyngeal closure or reduced nasal resistance to airflow during speech. Recently, Lin and colleagues found that in a sample of 91 patients with velopharyngeal insufficiency who received an obturator prosthesis, 79% demonstrated a Passavant's ridge during phonation, and 91% demonstrated it during gagging (Lin et al., 2019).

Casey and Emrich (1988) examined 29 partial and total soft palatectomy patients with an oral panendoscope following surgical resections for oral carcinoma. Twelve of the patients had total palatectomies, and 17 had partial soft palate resections. They found that 24 of 29 patients (83%) demonstrated a Passavant ridge. The results of this study confirmed our clinical impression that the incidence of a Passavant ridge may be higher in patients with acquired

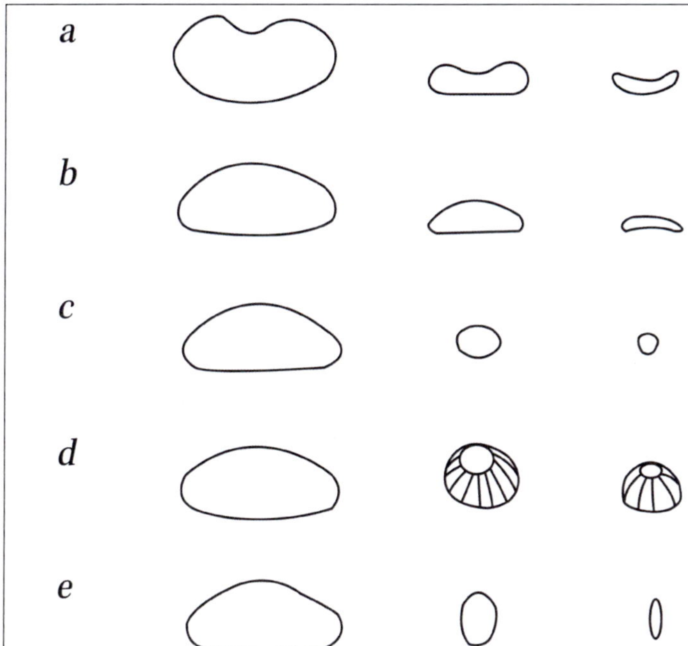

Figure 4-18 Various closure patterns shown in base projection. The left column represents the contour of velopharyngeal portal at rest, the middle column shows partial closure, and the right column shows full closure. *(a)* Normal subject. Note the convex projection of the uvula portion of the soft palate into the velopharyngeal portal at rest. *(b)* Subject with repaired cleft palate. Note the absence of a uvula muscular bulge at rest. *(c)* Subject with a repaired cleft palate and a circular closure pattern. *(d)* Subject with a repaired cleft palate, a circular closure pattern, and a Passavant ridge *(shaded areas)*. *(e)* Patient with a repaired cleft palate and a sagittal closure pattern (adapted from Skolnick et al., 1973, with permission).

soft palate defects than in patients with surgically repaired cleft palates. Most postsurgical cancer patients will have a detectable Passavant ridge if the posterior pharyngeal wall is not altered during the surgical resection, and this forward movement may improve the prosthetic prognosis considerably.

Isberg and Henningsson (1990) examined 80 patients with hypernasal speech for the Passavant ridge by means of videofluoroscopy and nasoendoscopy. The patients were divided into three groups: those with repaired cleft palates, those with submucous or occult submucous cleft palates, and those with velopharyngeal disproportion. Twenty-four of the 80 hypernasal patients exhibited a Passavant ridge, and the incidence was divided evenly among the three groups. The researchers found that the ridge tended to disappear when complete velopharyngeal closure was accomplished. Therefore, they believed that the Passavant ridge is compensatory and does contribute to velopharyngeal closure. Shprintzen (1990), in his commentary on this study, disagreed. He believed that the presence or absence of the Passavant ridge is related to other factors, such as the method of closure exhibited by the patient.

The Passavant ridge is associated only with a circular pattern of closure (Fig 4-18). Croft et al. (1981) studied 80 patients with normal velopharyngeal structures and 500 patients with VPI with a nasal endoscope. They found that 19% of the normal group exhibited a circular closure pattern with a Passavant ridge, whereas 24% of the VPI group displayed the same configuration. These investigators found the circular closure pattern was more common in individuals with a discernible Passavant ridge than in those without it.

In contrast, Witzel and Posnick (1989a) reported that 23% of 64 patients with normal structures and 23% of 179 VPI patients examined with a nasal endoscope had a circular closure pattern without a visible Passavant ridge. Approximately 5% of both groups exhibited a circular closure pattern and a ridge.

Many unanswered questions remain. Why do some patients with VPI and a circular closure pattern have the capacity to develop a Passavant ridge while other VPI patients with the same closure pattern do not? Do some patients with VPI, such as patients with recent surgical resections of the soft palate for cancer, have the adaptive capacity to change to a circular closure pattern and thus have the potential to develop a Passavant ridge?

What muscles are responsible for posterior pharyngeal wall movement? This point, too, is debatable. The lateral and posterior walls of the oral and nasopharynx are composed of muscle fibers of the fan-shaped superior constrictor muscle. It has its origin along the pterygomandibular raphae and the tuberosities of the maxilla and its fibers course posteriorly and horizontally to insert and anastomose with its counterpart into the aponeurosis in the midline of the posterior pharyngeal wall of both the oral and the nasopharynx.

The anatomical components of the Passavant ridge have been debated because fibers of the pharyngopalatinus muscle were found to intermingle with those of the superior constrictor (Calnan, 1957). Calnan (1957) speculated that it was the pharyngopalatinus muscle that forms the Passavant ridge. Others believe that fibers of the superior constrictor form this unusual configuration and are responsible for the anterior movement displayed by the posterior pharyngeal wall (Siegel-Sadewitz and Shprintzen, 1982).

Lateral pharyngeal walls

Lateral pharyngeal wall movement is very important if normal speech is to be achieved with either prosthetic obturation or surgical reconstruction. Lateral pharyngeal wall motion is difficult to assess because the drape of the soft palate precludes direct oral observation, and lateral radiographic projections will not disclose lateral pharyngeal wall motion unless the head is extended posteriorly while the patient is in a supine position (Isshiki et al., 1969). Nasoendoscopy may provide better visualization of lateral wall movement; however, the reliability of rating this movement has been shown to be variable (Sie et al., 2008).

Lateral pharyngeal wall motion has been assessed by different methods of evaluation. Bloomer (1953) observed and photographed the velopharyngeal mechanism of two patients through large facial defects. He traced lateral wall movements during speech and swallowing from motion picture films and concluded that lateral wall movements are an essential component of closure. Kelsey et al. (1972) studied 67 cleft palate patients with inadequate velopharyngeal closure during speech. These patients were tested with an ultrasound apparatus that permitted monitoring of lateral wall motion prior to and after pharyngeal flap surgical procedures. Kelsey et al. (1972) noted that the patients with the best postoperative result had acceptable lateral pharyngeal wall movement prior to surgery.

Following placement of an obturator or a pharyngeal flap procedure, the adjacent pharyngeal tissues demonstrate increased motion (Rosen and Bzock, 1958; Bzock, 1964; Blakeley, 1964; Hagerty et al., 1968). The physiologic basis for this phenomenon has not been explained completely. Rosen and Bzoch (1958) found that a number of patients require reduction of the obturator soon after placement of the prosthesis. Bzoch (1964) reported that 53 of 163 cleft palate patients require a significant reduction of the obturator because of increased muscle activity.

Wong and Weiss (1972) have employed this phenomenon to improve lateral wall movements and the prognosis for pharyngeal flap procedures by serially reducing the obturator. They reported a significant increase in lateral wall motion to the point where the obturator prosthesis was eliminated for a few patients. However, these results have been questioned by other clinicians who have not been able to achieve similar results (Shelton et al., 1968, 1969). In a preoperative and postoperative videofluoroscopic study of 28 subjects with a pharyngeal flap for treatment of VPI, Liedman-Boshko et al. (2005) found that lateral pharyngeal wall movement increased in some patients after pharyngeal flap surgery, whereas it decreased in others.

Wolfaardt et al. (1993) conducted a well-documented study of 32 patients with palatal lift prostheses. All patients were evaluated with nasoendoscopy, pressure-flow equipment (palatal efficiency rating computed instantaneously [PERCI]), and a Nasometer prior to, during, and following treatment. The researchers selected 21 of the patients for a time reduction program after the prosthesis was in use for 6 to 12 months. The prosthesis was not reduced, per se, but the amount of time the prosthesis was used was gradually reduced until its use was completely eliminated in 14 of 21 patients. During the reduction program, the patients were continuously monitored with the 3 evaluation methods so that the patients could be reassured that they retained the capability for normal speech without their palatal lift prosthesis. The authors believed that the continuous use of the prosthesis for 6 to 12 months helped the patients learn the sound of normal speech so that they could continue to function at this level when the prosthesis was provisionally discarded.

Other forms of stimulation of the velopharyngeal mechanism, such as muscle exercises (Morley, 1966; Massengill et al., 1968), speech therapy (Shelton et al., 1969), and electrical stimulation (Weber et al., 1970), have not been effective in demonstrating a sustained increase in pharyngeal movements that leads to improved speech.

Velopharyngeal closure tends to be sphincteric (Skolnick, 1970; Shprintzen et al., 1975, 1977; see Fig 4-18). Movement of the posterior pharyngeal wall blends with the movements of the lateral pharyngeal walls and elevation of the soft palate. The level of closure is at or slightly below the level of the tori tubari (the medial bulging of the pharyngeal terminus of the eustachian tube). Different patterns of closure are present; variability is the rule rather than the exception. Shprintzen et al. (1977), in a study of five patients with palatopharyngeal insufficiency or incompetency, found that the type of closure and the amount of lateral pharyngeal wall motion vary considerably. This study implied that the patients' speech deficiencies could be traced to either inadequate soft palate elevation or inadequate lateral wall motion. In addition, lateral wall motion is not necessarily similar on both sides of the pharynx (Isshiki et al., 1969; Kelsey et al., 1972).

The muscles contributing to the movement of the lateral pharyngeal walls, the direction of lateral wall movement, and the level laterally of velopharyngeal closure remain points of contention. As mentioned previously, the levator veli palatini muscle has its origin lateral to the torus tubarius without attachment to the eustachian tube. Because of its position lateral to the torus tubarius, Dickson (1972) and Maue-Dickson (1979) postulated that lateral wall motion is achieved solely by the contraction of the levator muscles. As the levator sling contracts, it moves the torus tubarius and lateral pharyngeal walls in a medial and sometimes in a posterior direction to engage the lateral margins of the soft palate at the level of the torus tubarius. Both researchers believed that, from a biomechanical point of view, the superior constrictor could not contribute to this vector of movement (Dickson, 1972; Maue-Dickson, 1979). Electromyographic studies by Bell-Berti (1976) supported this theory.

In a cadaveric study, Mehendale (2004) found that the levator divides into two parts immediately before it enters the velum. An anterolateral bundle of muscle fibers runs anteriorly, close to the lateral pharyngeal wall, and inserts via a number of tendons into the palatine aponeurosis. These fibers do not enter the medial part of the velum. The remaining bulk of the levator muscle runs medially into the velum, fanning out and joining the contralateral levator to form the levator sling. These findings may support the notion that the levator contributes to lateral wall movement.

However, Skolnick et al. (1973) and Shprintzen et al. (1974, 1975, 1977) speculated that lateral pharyngeal wall movements might have a two-muscle model because the incongruous movements of the lateral pharyngeal walls noted in these and other studies would be difficult to account for solely with levator contraction. They postulated that the superior constrictor muscle is responsible to some degree for lateral pharyngeal wall motion. The electromyographic studies of Fritzell (1969) and Kuehn et al. (1982) support this observation.

The level of velopharyngeal closure laterally has been questioned. Several authors believed that velopharyngeal closure occurs at the level of the tori tubarius (Bell-Berti, 1976; Maue-Dickson, 1979). However, Croft et al. (1981) examined 80 normal adult subjects with multiview videofluoroscopy and nasoendoscopy. They found that the level of closure generally is approximately 1 cm below the torus tubarius or about the level of the palatal plane. These investigators found that lateral wall movement during closure occurs primarily in a medial direction. A posteromedial movement is found primarily with circular closure patterns. The researchers suggested that their results were consistent with the hypothesis that the superior constrictor muscle contributes to lateral pharyngeal wall movement in patients with a circular closure pattern.

Why are there such diverse opinions regarding lateral wall movements? Several authors have provided some thoughts and information regarding this question. Shprintzen et al. (1983) cautioned that the velopharyngeal valve is three-dimensional, with height, width, and depth. Therefore, muscle movements and valving may occur at more than one level in the velopharyngeal tube. Many times, the 4 different closure patterns are not distinct entities. Walter (1990) used nasoendoscopy to examine 30 unrepaired cleft palate subjects without their prosthesis and described 10 different closure patterns.

Berry et al. (1983) used nasoendoscopy to examine five adult cleft palate patients who had worn an obturator prosthesis for more than 20 years. They found that lateral wall motion is variable but always below the torus tubarius. Siegel-Sadewitz and Shprintzen (1986) reported that it is not uncommon for children with large adenoids to have velopharyngeal valving at more than one vertical and horizontal location, both with different closure patterns.

Witzel and Posnick (1989a) reviewed 246 consecutive nasal endoscopic studies for patients suspected of having velopharyngeal dysfunction. Velopharyngeal gaps were found in 181 of these patients. Of these gaps, 121 were considered typical; that is, they were centrally located and resulted from hypoplasia of the musculus uvulae. In 28 patients, the gaps were located laterally. In the remaining 32 patients, the gaps were attributed to the shape of the adenoids and/or to the anatomy or function of the posterior border of the soft palate.

Henningsson and Isberg (1991) compared the results of multiview videofluoroscopy and nasoendoscopy in 80 subjects with hypernasal speech. They believed that multiview videofluoroscopy provided more conclusive information regarding lateral wall motion, while nasoendoscopy was best for viewing the levator eminence and movements of the posterior pharyngeal wall.

Because of these variations, it is best to employ multiple diagnostic procedures. Stringer and Witzel (1989) examined 25 subjects with hypernasal speech with multiview videofluoroscopic projections (lateral, Towne, and base views) and nasal endoscopic studies. Each author separately rated the degree of velopharyngeal closure (adequate, inadequate, or uncertain) for each view with each type of evaluation. The Towne view with videofluoroscopy and nasoendoscopy had the closest agreement (Table 4-3).

The salpingopharyngeus muscle, which has been reported to have some responsibility for lateral wall motion (Bloomer, 1953; Sharry, 1974), does not contribute to closure. Dickson and Dickson (1972) and Bluestone et al. (1972) found the salpingopharyngeus muscle to be extremely inconsistent or absent and, when present, rarely of substantial size. Likewise, the salpingopharyngeal fold was found to be primarily glandular and not muscular.

It had been thought that the palatopharyngeus muscle contributed little to the medial and posterior movement of the lateral pharyngeal walls. Its primary function was thought to be to mobilize the larynx and narrow the pharynx in speech and swallowing (Kuehn and Folkins, 1982). Dickson et al. (1973) believed that in the adult the fibers of the palatopharyngeus are so intertwined with the superior constrictor that the function and boundaries of the palatopharyngeus are difficult to delineate. Recent cadaveric research using microcomputed tomography has been able to delineate these boundaries and has shown that the palatopharyngeus may play a greater role in velopharyngeal closure than originally thought. Di and colleagues (2021) surmised that the palatopharyngeus works to elevate the pharynx and move the lateral pharyngeal walls medially in concert with the superior constrictor of the pharynx. The authors also describe its role in elevating the soft palate and controlling and stabilizing the levator veli palatini.

Table 4-3 Ratings of velopharyngeal closure in subjects on multiview videofluoroscopy and nasopharyngoscopy*

	Closure			
View	*Adequate*	*Inadequate*	*Uncertain*	*Total*
Lateral view	12	13	0	25
Towne view	3	20	2	25
Basal view	2	13	7	22
Nasopharyngoscopy	2	21	2	25

* Reprinted from Stringer and Witzel (1989b) with permission.

The palatoglossus muscle, which forms the anterior tonsillar pillar, acts as an antagonist for the levator veli palatini by elevating the tongue and lowering the soft palate but plays no role in velopharyngeal closure. Because both the palatopharyngeus and the palatoglossus muscles narrow and bulge in their central portion during contraction, the imprint of both muscles can be noted during waxing procedures for construction of the obturator prosthesis for patients with extensive soft palate defects.

Considering the multiple variations and the different patterns of velopharyngeal closure with varying levels of participation of the soft palate, lateral pharyngeal walls, and the posterior pharyngeal wall, it is difficult to conceive that contraction of the levator veli palatini only could produce all these variations.

Innervation

Previous descriptions have reported the innervation of the velopharyngeal mechanism to derive from the pharyngeal plexus. Although the innervation to this plexus was not completely understood, most researchers believed it was supplied by the glossopharyngeal and vagus nerves. An exception is the tensor veli palatini muscle, which is innervated by the trigeminal nerve. However, studies by Nishio et al. (1976a, 1976b) have indicated that the facial nerve also innervates this complex.

These early observations have been confirmed in more recent studies. According to Shimokawa et al. (2004), the levator veli palatini is innervated by nerve branches of the pharyngeal plexus, which can be classified into three groups according to their origins: *(1)* supplying branches originating from the pharyngeal branch of cranial nerve IX (type I); *(2)* branches originating from the communicating branch between the pharyngeal branches of cranial nerves IX and X (type II); and *(3)* branches originating from the pharyngeal branch of cranial nerve X (type III). The superior constrictor also was found to be innervated by branches of the pharyngeal plexus. The facial nerve (VII) does contribute to the innervation of soft palate muscles through the lesser palatine nerve, which provides motor innervation to the levator veli palatini, the medial strand of the palatopharyngeus, and the musculus uvulae (Shimokawa et al., 2005). The pharyngeal plexus was found to innervate most of the superior part of the levator veli palatini, and the facial nerve only

Table 4-4 Obturator prostheses for soft palate and other palatopharyngeal defects

Type of defects	Structures involved	Cause
Total soft palate defects		
Total soft palate defects	Entire soft palate	Surgical excision of neoplastic disease Unoperated cleft palate
		Surgically redivided soft palate
Posterior border defects		
Posteromedial border defects	Posterior half of palate	Surgical excision of neoplastic disease
		Postsurgical cleft palate with insufficient length
Posterolateral border defects	Lateral half of soft palate and often the pharyngeal wall	Surgical excision of neoplastic disease
Special obturator prostheses		
Palatal lift	All structures intact	Neurological diseases
	Posterior border of soft palate	Postsurgical cleft palate with insufficient length and movement

innervated a small portion of the inferior part of the muscle through the lesser palatine nerve (Shimokawa et al., 2005).

Prosthodontic Rehabilitation

Obturator is derived from the Latin verb *obturare*, which means to close or to shut off. This definition provides an appropriate description of the objective of obturation in patients with velopharyngeal incompetence or velopharyngeal insufficiency. A prosthesis placed following resection of portions of the bony maxillae and adjacent structures (see Chapter 3) is basically a covering prosthesis to reestablish the oral-nasal partition. The extension superiorly of the obturator into the defect improves the retention, stability, and support for the prosthesis. There is only very little movement of the tissues bordering these defects during speech and swallowing. In contrast, obturators constructed for patients with soft palate defects must function in concert with peripheral tissues that display considerable movement during speech and swallowing.

Obturator prostheses fabricated for patients with velopharyngeal deficits vary with the location and nature of the defect or deficiency (Table 4-4). There are differences between obturator prostheses constructed for patients with developmental or congenital malformations of the soft palate and those constructed for patients with acquired defects. However, the objectives of obturation are identical—that is, to provide the patient with the capability to control nasal emission during speech and to prevent the leakage of material into the nasal passage during deglutition. The rehabilitation of cleft lip and cleft palate patients is discussed in Chapter 6, but the fabrication of all types of obturator prostheses will be discussed in this chapter.

Table 4-4 implies that resections for control of neoplastic disease of the soft palate can be categorized into homogenous groups with a well-defined pattern of prosthetic treatment for each category (Fig 4-19). However, resections for malignant neoplasms confined solely to a portion or all of the soft palate are quite rare (Zlotolow et al., 1995). Most soft palate defects originate from the resection of tumors in adjacent structures, such as the tonsillar pillars, the retromolar trigone, the base of the tongue, the oropharynx, or the nasopharynx. The velopharyngeal mechanism will be affected to varying degrees, depending on the extent of the initial resection and the method of surgical closure. Most raw surfaces of these surgical defects are lined with free flaps; the radial forearm being the preferred donor site. Therefore, the prosthesis must engage portions of a velopharyngeal defect that may be nonfunctional. *However, if the opposite lateral pharyngeal wall exhibits a normal range of movement and access enables the obturator to engage these areas, velopharyngeal function, and therefore speech and swallowing, can be restored to normal limits.*

If the residual velopharyngeal musculature peripheral to the defect does not display appreciable movement, rarely will speech be normal, either with an obturator prosthesis or with surgical reconstruction (see Fig 4-2). The speech produced will be a mixture of hyponasality and hypernasality (mixed nasality) and there will be some leakage during swallowing (see section below entitled "Inadequate mobility of the residual velopharyngeal mechanism"). Movement of at least one lateral pharyngeal wall is essential for either method of rehabilitation. Likewise, if the residual velopharyngeal musculature is rendered nonfunctional secondary to chemoradiation and the soft palate is shortened by fibrosis and atrophy, speech with a prosthesis will be of mixed nasality (see section below entitled "Chemoradiation and velopharyngeal dysfunction"; see also Fig 4-46).

Surgical obturation

If resection of portions of the velopharyngeal mechanism is contemplated for the control of neoplastic disease, the placement of an immediate surgical obturator may be indicated in select patients. Immediate surgical obturation is most useful for patients in whom significant portions of the soft palate are resected in combination with a partial maxillectomy (Fig 4-20). The principal advantage of immediate surgical obturators (ISO) for such defects is to provide support for the surgical packing used to support the split-thickness skin graft lining the lateral wall of the maxillectomy defect during the initial stages of healing (see Chapter 3). The obturation of the

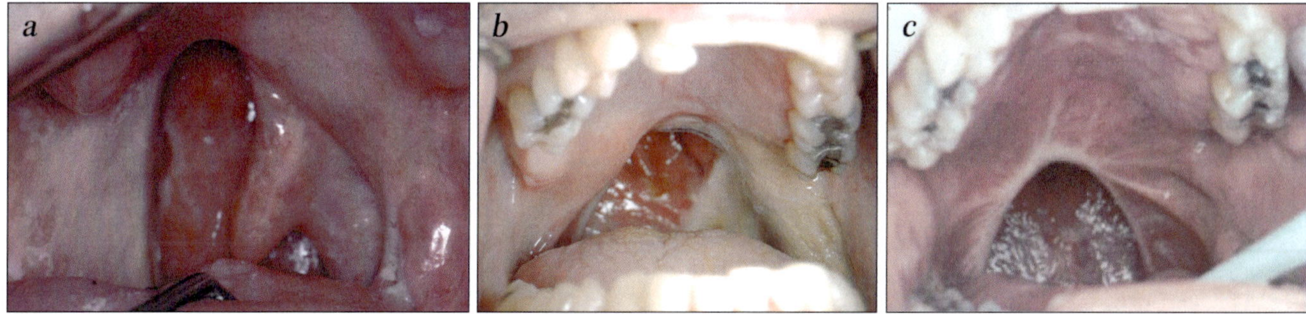

Figure 4-19 Alteration of velopharyngeal function. *(a)* The right side of the soft palate and the right lateral pharyngeal wall were resected. The defect was lined with a myocutaneous flap. The right reconstructed lateral pharyngeal wall does not have movement potential. The obturator prosthesis must be extended behind the residual soft palate to engage the posterior and left lateral pharyngeal walls. However, normal resonance balance can be achieved with the prosthesis. *(b)* The entire soft palate was resected and the left lateral pharyngeal wall was lined with a radial forearm free flap. Examination revealed excellent movement of the right lateral pharyngeal wall. Normal resonance balance can be achieved with the prosthesis. *(c)* A posterior border defect. The scarring from surgery has somewhat immobilized the residual soft palate, but there was still acceptable movement of the lateral pharyngeal walls that enabled reestablishment of normal resonance balance with a prosthesis.

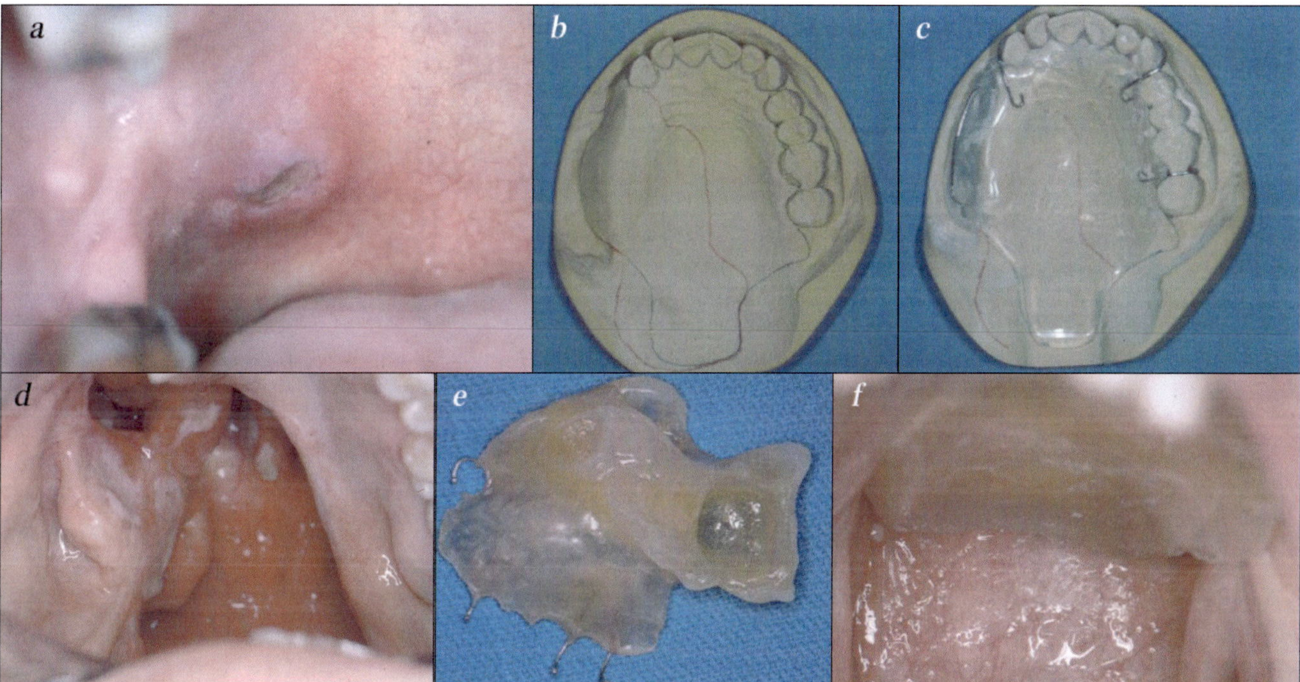

Figure 4-20 Immediate surgical obturation of a combined hard and soft palate defect. *(a)* Adenoid cystic carcinoma of the right lateral region of the soft palate. *(b)* Cast altered for the prosthesis. The tumor extended further anteriorly than it appeared in *(a)*. *(c)* Immediate surgical obturator on the cast. The posterior extension should be short of the posterior pharyngeal wall. *(d)* Defect two months postoperatively. *(e)* Prosthesis with a lining of tissue conditioning material. *(f)* Prosthesis in position.

hard palate portion of the defect with an ISO offers several other advantages as well, and these are listed in detail in Chapter 3 (see section entitled "Surgical obturation").

The ISO is primarily used to obturate the hard palate defect. The soft palate component of an ISO constructed presurgically is approximated with regard to the level of placement and the contours of the lateral and posterior margins. The guesswork can be minimized if an extended impression of the soft palate is obtained. The soft palate portion should be underextended with regard to the lateral and posterior pharyngeal walls and mimic those of a palatal lift (see section below entitled "Palatal lift prostheses"). After the cast is retrieved, it is altered to correspond to the proposed defect (Fig 4-20a, b, and c). The superior-inferior level of the obturator that extends into the velopharyngeal area is determined by the plane of the hard palate. This portion of the cast is altered to extend the prosthesis along the palatal plane to within 2 to 3 mm of the estimated position of the posterior pharyngeal wall. The width of the soft palate extension of the obturator is determined by the nature of the resection and the width of the soft palate. These guidelines will usually produce a prosthesis that will not be overextended. However, adjustments at surgery may be necessary to avoid potential contact with the lateral or posterior pharyngeal walls and to provide space for a nasogastric tube. Adaptation need not be precise because the surgical packing will correct minor discrepancies during the immediate postoperative period.

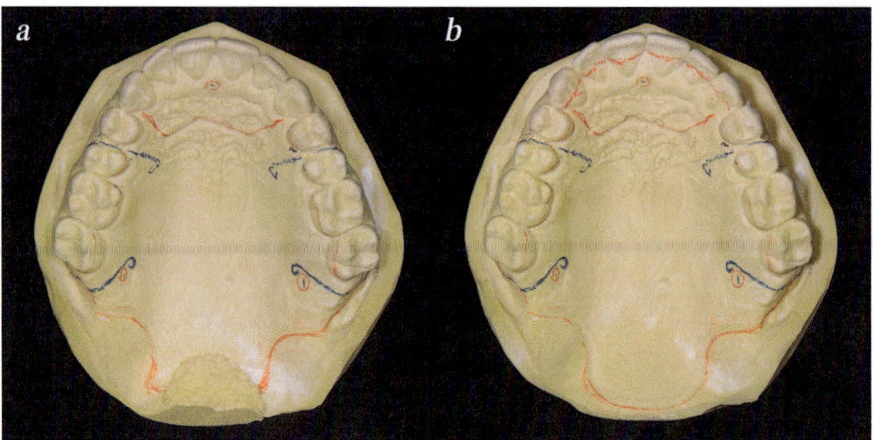

Figure 4-21 *(a)* A cast of the patient depicted in Fig 4-7c being prepared for a delayed surgical obturator. Note that the impression was extended across the soft palate to the anterior margin of the tumor. *(b)* The cast has been altered for the extension across the soft palate to the proposed defect.

Approximately 7 to 10 days postsurgically, the prosthesis and the surgical packing are removed (Fig 4-20d). Appropriate corrections are made to the ISO, and a tissue conditioner or temporary denture reliner is used to develop the appropriate extensions and tissue adaptation. The extension restoring the soft palate portion of the defect is refined separately and after the extension into the hard palate portion has been completed. When the material becomes moldable, the prosthesis is inserted, and the patient is instructed to swallow, speak, and flex the neck to activate the velopharyngeal complex and mold the lining material (see section below entitled "Total soft palate defects: Method of fabrication").

In the immediate postsurgical period, frequently patients are reluctant or unable to activate the remaining velopharyngeal musculature because of discomfort, edema, or possible neurologic deficits. Hence, speech in the immediate postoperative period can be muffled and hyponasal, as lateral pharyngeal wall movements are necessary to control nasal emissions and establish proper resonance balance. As healing progresses and the peripheral tissues display a greater range of movement, trimming and reapplication of a suitable liner will be necessary (Fig 4-20e and f). As edema abates and movement of the velopharyngeal musculature improves, speech will improve. During this period, the patient is monitored regularly during sequential appointments, and the prosthesis is modified or remade as necessary.

Delayed surgical obturation is reserved for patients scheduled to undergo posteromedial or posterolateral border resections of the soft palate where a only small portion of the hard palate is resected or where the resection is confined to the soft palate. For example, in a patient scheduled to lose the lateral half of the soft palate secondary to the resection of a tumor originating in the tonsillar bed, delayed obturation is preferred. There are several reasons we favor this approach. First, the drape of the intact soft palate precludes the clinician from obtaining an impression of the nasopharynx where normal velopharyngeal closure occurs and where the surgical obturator should be positioned. Second, functional movements of the lateral wall portion of the velopharyngeal mechanism cannot be recorded prosthetically either prior to or at the time of surgery. Conscious control by the patient is necessary to initiate contracture of the muscles associated with velopharyngeal closure.

In dentate patients, an impression is made prior to surgery, and a palatal stent or treatment RDP is fabricated of autopolymerizing acrylic resin. The cast is altered as necessary, and stainless-steel wire retainers are adapted to key teeth in the usual manner (Fig 4-21). The patient returns after discharge from the hospital, the palatal stent is tried, and the palatal extension is adjusted as necessary. The portion engaging the velopharyngeal defect is molded with a temporary denture reliner (Fig 4-22). For edentulous patients, the delayed surgical obturator is attached to the existing maxillary complete denture (Fig 4-23).

Interim obturation

In dentulous patients, an interim obturation is necessary during the postsurgical phase of treatment. As soft tissue healing occurs, modification of the surgical prosthesis becomes more difficult. The periodic additions and corrections of the surgical obturator often leave it heavy and uncomfortable. In addition, if a tissue conditioner is used initially, it becomes contaminated with oral microflora, which will adversely affect tissue adaptation and its physical properties. In addition, the biofilms that form on the surface of these materials can cause tissue irritations. These phenomena frequently require the fabrication of a new so-called interim obturator. An irreversible hydrocolloid impression is made that records the residual dentition and that extends posteriorly to record the posterior and lateral margins of the resection defect. An autopolymerizing methyl methacrylate palatal retainer with appropriate retention is fabricated, and a moldable temporary denture reliner is used to mold the velopharyngeal extension. This type of prosthesis enables more precise engagement of the residual velopharyngeal musculature and bridges the gap between the surgical obturator and the definitive prosthesis (Fig 4-22). In edentulous patients, the preexisting complete denture can be employed for the same purpose (see Fig 4-23).

This prosthesis can also be used to develop the initial contours of the definitive obturator prosthesis. Following fabrication of the removable dental prosthesis framework, the interim obturator prosthesis is seated on the master cast. Silicone putty is adapted to the obturator extension. The interim prosthesis is removed, the removable dental prosthesis framework is positioned on the master cast, and autopolymerizing acrylic resin is poured in the silicone pattern. These resin patterns can then be modified as needed, border molded with a low-fusing modeling compound, and refined

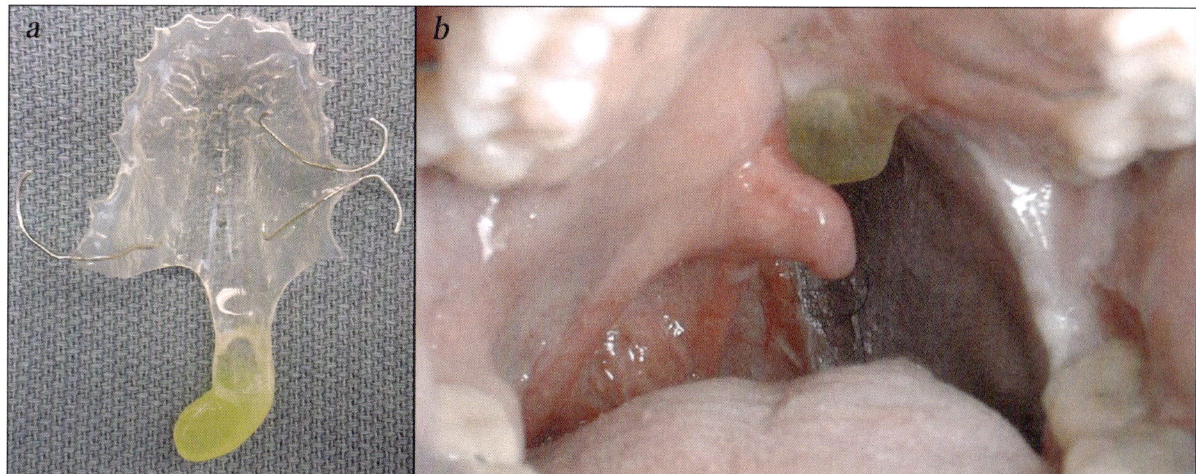

Figure 4-22 Delayed surgical obturation. *(a)* Obturator extension developed with a temporary denture reliner that can be adjusted and polished. This prosthesis can also serve as the interim obturator. *(b)* Prosthesis in position.

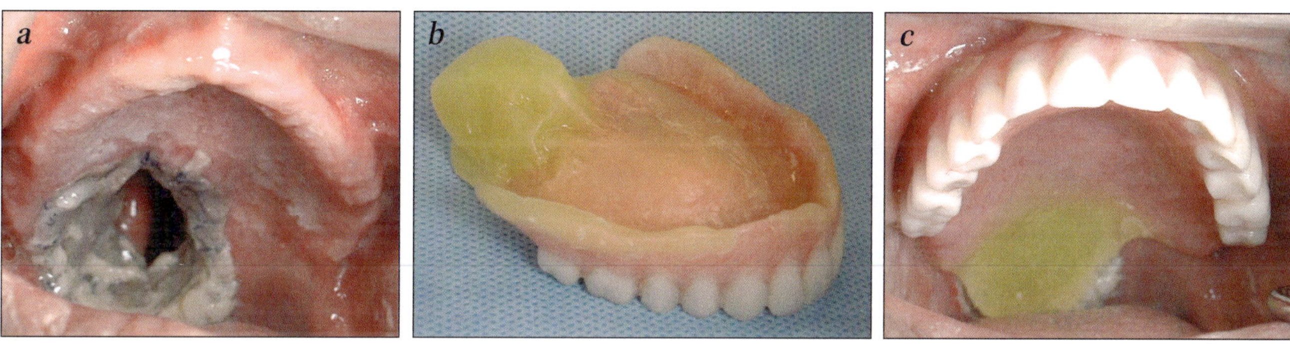

Figure 4-23 Delayed surgical obturation. *(a)* Soft palate defect secondary to surgical resection. *(b)* Obturator extension developed with a temporary denture reliner that can be adjusted and polished. This prosthesis can serve as the interim obturator. *(c)* Prosthesis in position.

with a thermoplastic wax (Fig 4-24). This technique will save considerable chair time during border molding of soft palate obturator prostheses.

Definitive obturation

General concepts

Patients exhibiting reasonable movement of the residual velopharyngeal complex during function have an excellent prognosis for achieving normal speech and swallowing with a prosthesis. Movement of the lateral and posterior pharyngeal walls is essential for the control of nasal emission. If the patient has little or no movement of the remaining velopharyngeal mechanism, he or she will not be able to achieve completely normal speech with an obturator prosthesis (see Figs 4-2 and 4-46). Under these circumstances, the best that can be achieved is mixed nasality (see the section below entitled "Chemoradiation and velopharyngeal dysfunction").

The obturator is attached to a conventional prosthesis. If the patient is dentulous, a chrome-cobalt partial denture framework retains the obturator. For edentulous patients, a new complete denture is generally indicated to allow the prosthodontist to idealize its retention and stability. For edentulous patients, if the posterior palatal seal areas have been compromised by either surgical resection or radiotherapy, it may be necessary to place osseointegrated implants in order to achieve sufficient retention to accurately position the obturator extension so it can properly engage the residual velopharyngeal musculature (see section below entitled "Use of implants"). This is particularly true in irradiated patients, since the diminution of saliva and the fibrosis of the posterior palatine salivary glands will render peripheral seal impossible, dramatically compromising retention of the complete denture-obturator prosthesis.

The obturator should be rigid and should not attempt to duplicate the movements of the soft palate. It is a fixed platform of acrylic resin that engages the remaining musculature of the velopharyngeal mechanism during function (Fig 4-25a). If the lateral and posterior pharyngeal walls exhibit normal movement, a space will exist between these structures and the obturator when these tissues are at rest. The surrounding space permits breathing through the nasal cavity and the production of nasal consonant phonemes (Fig 4-25b).

The level of optimal obturator placement in the nasopharynx is determined by the level in the nasopharynx of contracture of the

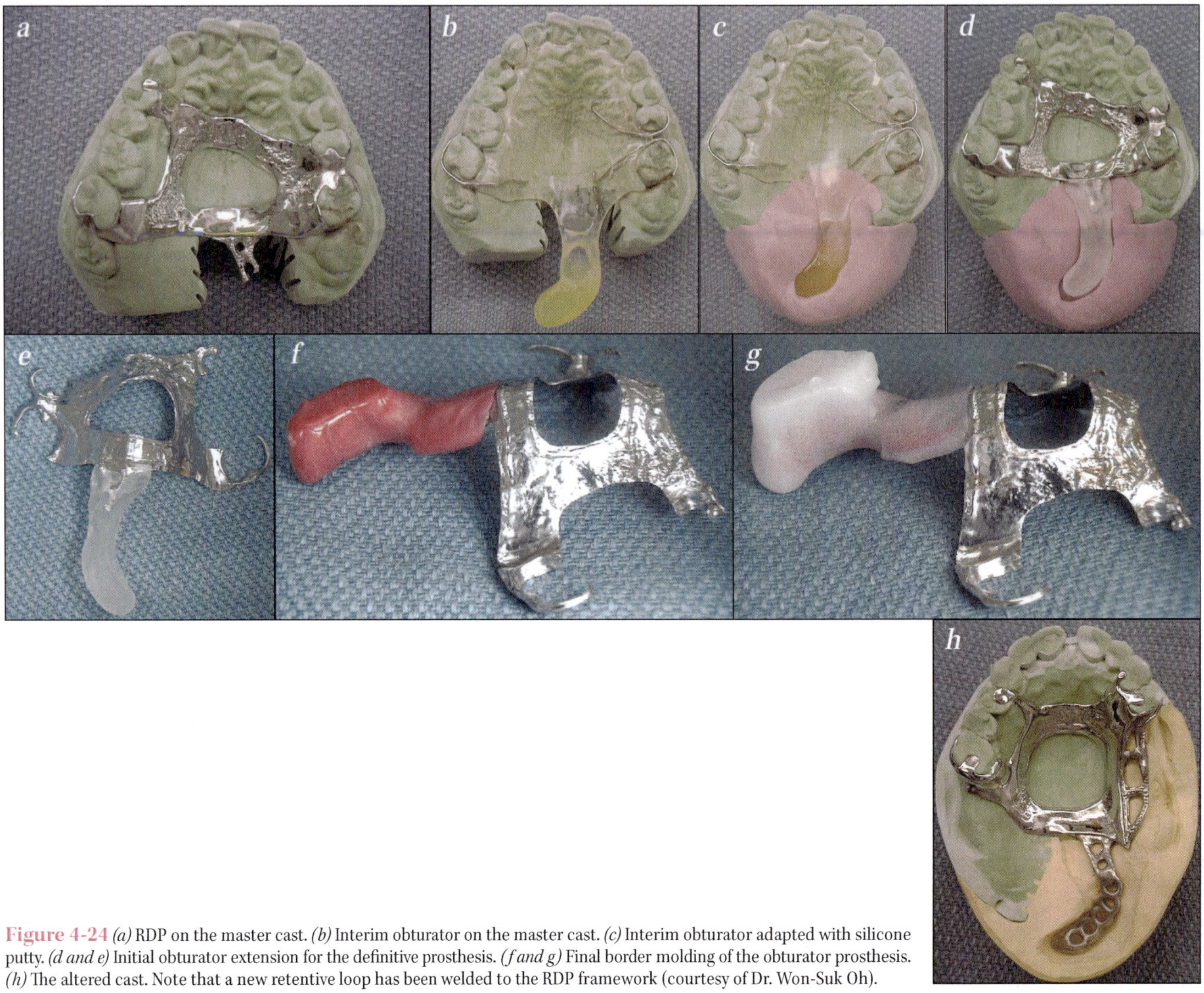

Figure 4-24 *(a)* RDP on the master cast. *(b)* Interim obturator on the master cast. *(c)* Interim obturator adapted with silicone putty. *(d and e)* Initial obturator extension for the definitive prosthesis. *(f and g)* Final border molding of the obturator prosthesis. *(h)* The altered cast. Note that a new retentive loop has been welded to the RDP framework (courtesy of Dr. Won-Suk Oh).

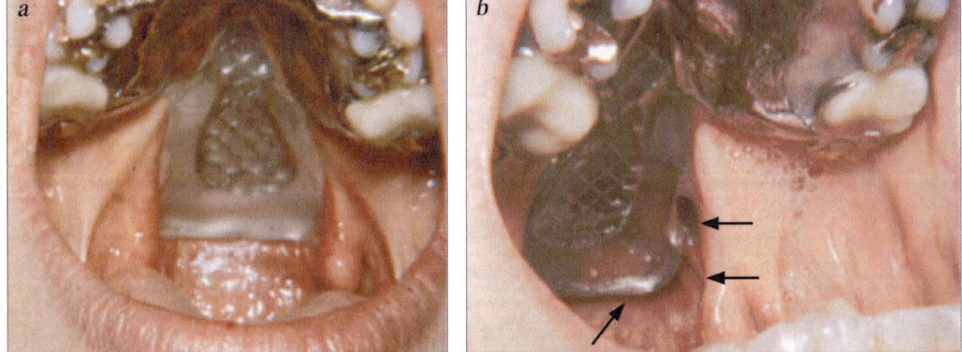

Figure 4-25 Obturator prosthesis for 27-year-old woman with an unrepaired cleft palate. *(a)* The patient is saying ah. Note the approximation of the lateral and posterior pharyngeal walls with the obturator. *(b)* Obturator prosthesis in position with tissues at rest. A space now exists between the obturator and the lateral and posterior pharyngeal walls to permit normal nasal breathing and production of nasal consonant phonemes *(arrows)*.

residual velopharyngeal musculature (Rosen and Bzock, 1958; Rahn and Boucher, 1970; Mazaheri and Millard, 1964; Harkins et al., 1960; Terkla and Laney, 1963). The Passavant ridge and the anterior tubercle of the atlas can vary in location in relation to normal velopharyngeal closure (Aram and Subtelny, 1959; Glaser et al., 1979; Rahn and Boucher, 1970). Therefore, definite landmarks regarding obturator placement are somewhat difficult to delineate. As a general rule, the prosthodontist should consider the following guidelines for the location of the obturator segment of the prosthesis:

- The obturator for an adult patient should be located in the nasopharynx at the level of normal velopharyngeal closure.
- The inferior margin of the obturator should not extend below the lower level of muscular activity exhibited by the residual velopharyngeal complex.
- The superior margin of the obturator should not extend above the level of muscular activity.
- The inferior extension of the obturator will usually be an extension of the palatal plane, as extended to the posterior pharyngeal wall.

Total soft palate defects: Method of fabrication

Construction of obturators for all soft palate deficiencies begins with the fabrication of the conventional prosthesis. When impressions are obtained for diagnostic casts, the palatal portion of the stock tray should be extended with wax or impression compound so that some of the defect will be recorded (Fig 4-26a and b). Irreversible hydrocolloid is the material of choice (Fig 4-26c). The residual velopharyngeal musculature will contract when contact is made with the impression material, resulting in some distortion. Care is taken to avoid displacing impression material onto the dorsum of the tongue because this will trigger the gag reflex. This can be avoided by preparing a thicker mix of the material.

Conventional impressions have remained the most cost-effective and accurate means of obtaining a full arch master cast, although this method may also be displaced with intraoral scanners in the not-too-distant future. The challenge will be to record the extensions into the velopharyngeal defect so that the retentive loop can be properly extended and situated within the velopharyngeal defect.

Partial denture designs for patients with defects or functional deficiencies of the soft palate and contiguous tissues are similar to partial denture designs for nonsurgical patients and are primarily driven by existing edentulous extension areas. The authors prefer to use the I bar mesial rest design concept proposed by Kratochvil (1988; Chang et al., 2019). However, the prosthodontist must also consider the long lever arm created by the posterior extension of the obturator. This extension is not within the confines of the bony palate and teeth, and the additional weight and length increase the effect of gravitational forces and the potential for rotation around the most posterior retainers where they engage the tooth surfaces. The effect of this extension will be most significant for patients requiring a Kennedy Class I or Class II partial denture and minimal for patients with Class III or Class IV partial dentures. Fortunately, the forces directed against the obturator are minimal. If the obturator is positioned properly in the nasopharynx, it need not be bulky, and thus weight and the effects of gravity will not be significant.

Placement of rests anteriorly, bilaterally positioned, serve as indirect retainers, provides resistance to the downward displacement of the obturator, and improves the stability of the prosthesis (Fig 4-26d and e). For patients with an anterior edentulous area, consideration should be given to the placement of surveyed crowns with positive rests on the abutment teeth adjacent to the anterior edentulous extension area. These rests act as indirect retainers and enhance the stability and retention of the obturator extension.

A retention loop for the obturator prosthesis should extend into the middle of the defect. Tray resin is added to the cast retention loops to approximate the area of the defect, and the metal framework is inserted (Fig 4-26f). The tray resin is adjusted so that contact does not occur with the lateral and posterior walls as the patient says *ah* (Fig 4-26g). There should be a 2–3 mm gap between the tray extension and the contracting velopharyngeal musculature. Disclosing wax is valuable in checking these extensions.

The low-fusing impression compound is added to the tray resin. We prefer to start border molding at the immobile anterior margins of the defect before proceeding posterolaterally (Fig 4-26h). After the tempered impression compound is placed in the mouth, the patient is instructed to move his or her head in a circular manner from side to side and to flex the neck so that the chin contacts the chest. The latter maneuver will bring the anterior tubercle of the atlas anteriorly and ensure that the prosthesis will not be overextended in this area. This is followed by connected speech and the swallowing of liquids. Speech passages with plosive sounds are suggested. These maneuvers activate the residual velopharyngeal musculature and mold the impression compound. As described previously, velopharyngeal closure varies with head position and activity (speech and swallowing).

Dry swallowing (without liquids) should not be used to develop the obturator bulb physiologically, because the velopharyngeal musculature contracts more forcefully, and this contraction extends over a greater area than during swallowing with liquids or speech (Walter, 1981; Karnell et al., 1987). This will lead to an underextended bulb, especially posterolaterally, where the potential for the most extensive velopharyngeal motion exists. However, some have suggested that underextension of the prosthesis initially is preferred to overextension, particularly when it is anticipated that potential compensatory function may develop (Berry et al., 1985).

Minsley et al. (1991) warned that a soft palate obturator prosthesis may compromise nasal breathing in some cleft palate patients. These investigators computed the nasal cross-sectional area for eight cleft palate patients with obturator prostheses during both inspiration and expiration using pressure-airflow recording equipment. The results showed that 50% of this sample had nasal cross-sectional areas of less than 0.40 cm with concomitant impairment in nasal respiration. Patients with airways of less than 0.40 cm are considered obligatory mouth breathers. On the basis of this data, the authors cautioned that the prosthodontist must consider the patency of the nasal airway when developing the contours and extension of a soft palate obturator prosthesis. This factor is particularly pertinent in patients where the defect is created via an oncologic resection combined with aggressive radiation treatment because in some of these patients, there may be minimal movement of the residual velopharyngeal mechanism.

A proper balance between oral and nasal resonance is always necessary for the production of normal speech. A speech pathologist can be particularly helpful in this regard. Nasoendoscopy can also be used to judge the nature of velopharyngeal closure achieved with the prosthesis. In the past, the emphasis and challenge have been to provide velopharyngeal obturation that will generate sufficient

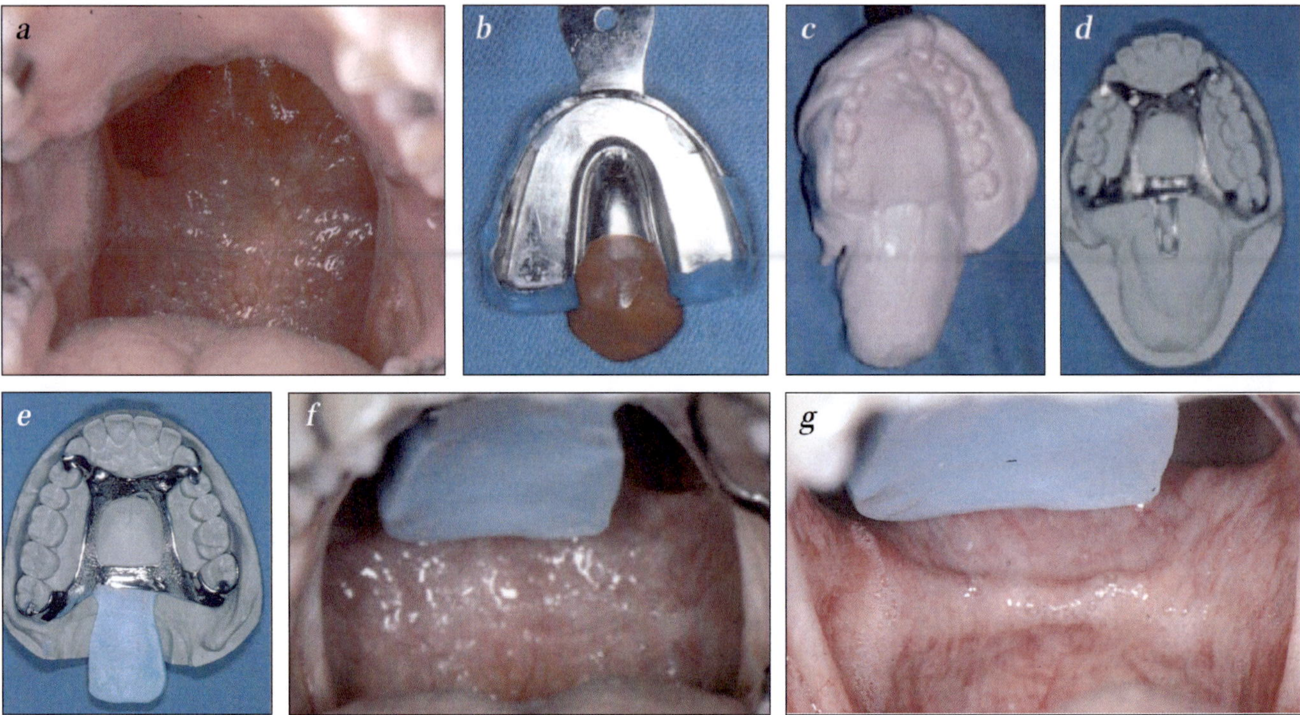

Figure 4-26 Fabrication of an obturator for a total soft palate defect. *(a)* Large soft palate defect. Clinical exam indicates significant movement of the residual velopharyngeal musculature. *(b)* Stock impression tray extended with impression compound. Adhesive is applied to both the tray and the impression compound prior to impression. *(c)* Impression for RDP framework. *(d)* Removable dental prosthesis framework. Rests on the premolars provide needed indirect retention. *(e)* Tray resin attached to the framework in preparation for altered cast impression. *(f)* The framework inserted and the patient at "rest." Note the space between the posterolateral pharyngeal walls and the tray extension. *(g)* The patient is instructed to say "ah." Note that on the right side, there is little space between the pharyngeal walls and the tray extension. This area was relieved prior to making the final impression.

oral pressure for the oral components of speech and oral resonance. However, nasal resonance must not be ignored. An adequate nasal airway is always necessary for the production of nasal phonemes, proper nasal resonance, and nasal breathing. The range of tissue movement of the lateral and posterior pharyngeal walls represents the potential space between the obturator and these tissues at rest. If there is limited space around the obturator prosthesis, when the velopharyngeal musculature is at rest, nasal breathing will be impaired and speech will be hyponasal.

Good movement of the lateral and/or posterior pharyngeal walls is essential for proper oronasal airflow. If the remaining peripheral structures forming the residual velopharyngeal complex do not display some movement, the prognosis for normal speech following pharyngeal flap reconstruction (in the case of a patient with a repaired cleft of the soft palate) or prosthetic obturation will be compromised. In such circumstances, speech will demonstrate mixed nasality.

Some patients present with anatomical and/or postsurgical limitations that compromise the nasal airway and subsequent speech production. Thus, an ideal oral-nasal resonance balance may not be attainable with either surgical or prosthetic rehabilitation. Any patient with a surgically repaired cleft palate or who has undergone velar resection for cancer has the potential for this type of resonance imbalance. If the patency of the nasal airway is already compromised at the level of the nasal valve, aggressive obturation at the level of the velopharyngeal port will further compromise nasal breathing.

If the obturator extends inferiorly below or superiorly above the level of velopharyngeal muscle contracture and is in contact with these static tissues, the prosthesis will compromise the patency of the nasal airway and speech will be hyponasal. Therefore, the prosthodontist must position the obturator to engage the zone of residual velopharyngeal muscular contracture.

Swallowing liquids during the physiologic molding is performed at the end of the sequence during molding with modeling compound. Note that the molding of the obturator segment with impression compound is analogous to an altered cast impression in that the modeling process is in essence refinement of the extension of the tray. However, because the velopharyngeal musculature exhibits limited force during closure, finite functional contours are best perfected and recorded with a thermoplastic material.

As molding of the impression compound continues, the prosthodontist may be able to identify the indentations made by adjacent structures such as the tori tubari. The impression compound must be trimmed so that the prosthesis does not extend superiorly to engage this structure; otherwise, the nasal airway will be impaired and speech will be hyponasal. Indentations of the Passavant ridge (if present), the anterior tubercle of the atlas, and the residual levator muscle remnants in the posterolateral pharyngeal walls should also be identified and indicate a properly extended impression. Shiny areas indicate a lack of tissue contact. During the molding of the speech appliance, the impression compound is often displaced superiorly and inferiorly beyond the velopharyngeal contraction zone. As mentioned previously, these areas must be reduced so that the molded pattern is centered within the zone of velopharyngeal muscle contraction (Fig 4-26i

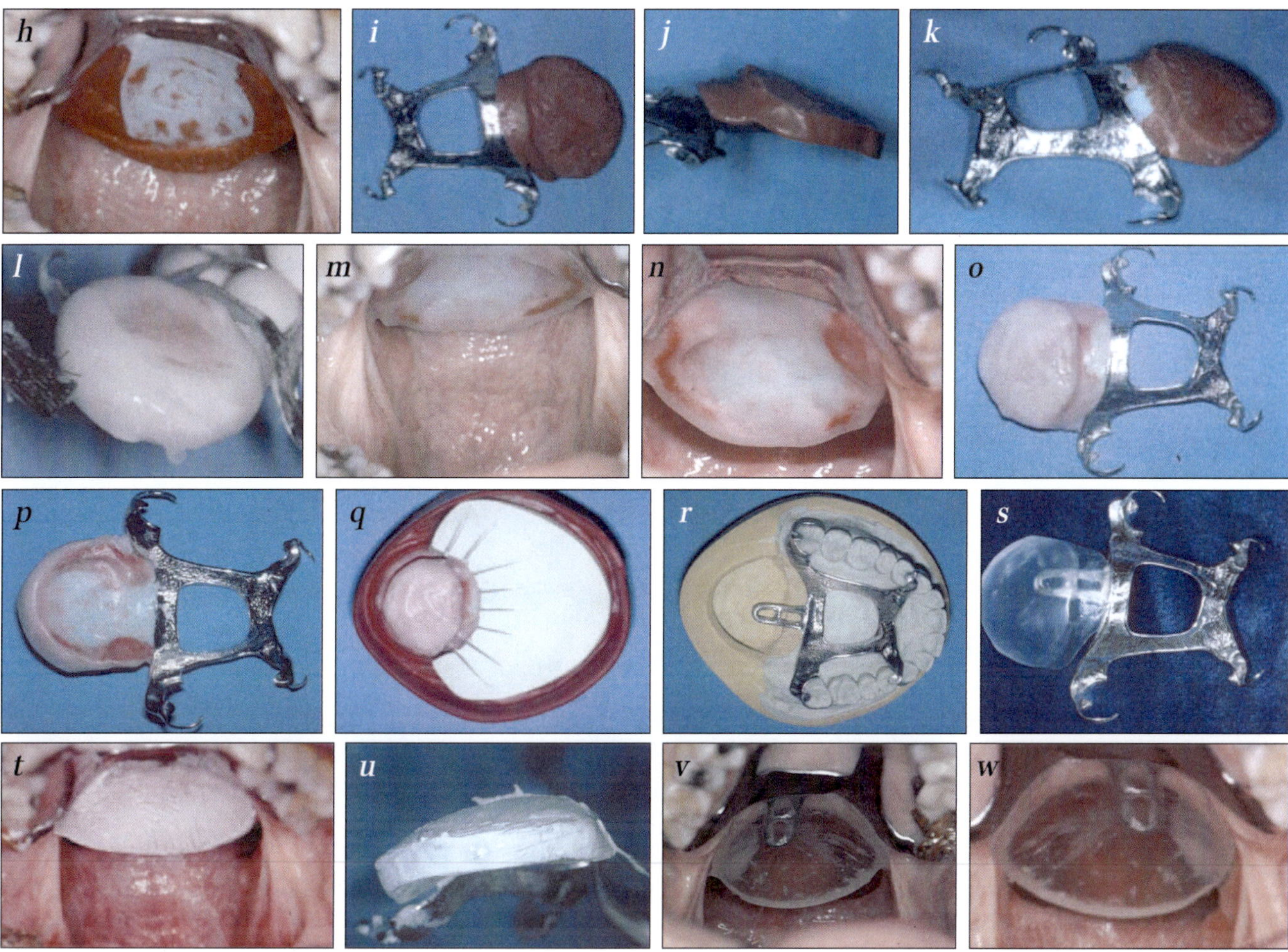

Figure 4-26 (*continued*) *(h)* The initial contours of the prosthesis are developed with impression compound *(i and j)* Completed molding process. The impression compound is trimmed to ensure the pattern is confined within the zone of velopharyngeal muscle movement. *(k)* Cutback in preparation for the addition of thermoplastic wax. *(l)* Addition of thermoplastic wax. *(m and n)* The prosthesis is being refined. Note that *(m)* during a forceful contraction of the residual VP musculature, the posterolateral surfaces of the molded prosthesis are engaged. *(m)* Completed impression in the mouth with velopharyngeal tissues at rest. Tissues will approximate the obturator bulb during function, but space permits normal breathing through the nasal cavity when tissues are at rest. *(o)* Completed impression. The convex contour of the superior surface directs nasal secretions posteriorly. Contours will be refined after processing. *(p)* Completed impression of the inferior surface. The concave contours provide ample space for the tongue. *(q)* Boxing for pouring the altered cast impression. *(r)* Altered cast ready for processing in clear acrylic resin. *(s)* Completed prosthesis. *(t)* Pressure indicator paste added to the obturator and the patient asked to speak and swallow. Note the light contact of the tongue on oral side of the defect as indicated by the PIP pattern. Usually, only minimal adjustment is necessary at this time. *(u)* An appropriate PIP pattern. The bush marks have been eliminated but the PIP has not been displaced. *(v)* Completed prosthesis with the patient at rest. Note the space around the posterolateral surfaces of the prosthesis. *(w)* Prosthesis in position during the initial stages of contraction of the VP musculature. During a plosive sound, these spaces will be eliminated.

and j). In most patients, this zone spans 10–12 mm. Obturator prostheses that extend inferiorly will disrupt swallowing patterns, induce abnormal tongue movements, and precipitate gagging. The impression compound should be as warm as the patient can tolerate because pharyngeal tissues do not contract forcefully except in swallowing. For this reason, lower-fusing impression compounds are favored.

When the molding process is completed, the patient is asked to speak, swallow, and breathe through the nostrils to test the effectiveness of the formed obturator. When the position and contours of the obturator are satisfactory, the lateral and posterior extensions of the molded impression compound are reduced by approximately 1 to 2 mm with a sharp scalpel (Fig 4-26k).

A mouth-temperature thermoplastic material is then added to the molded impression compound. The authors prefer Iowa wax. The wax is heated in a ladle, and when it begins to thicken and congeal, it is applied to the impression compound with a brush. Note that if the wax is applied too hot, it will distort the impression compound. The wax-compound impression is then tempered in a water bath and placed in the mouth (Fig 4-26l). The functions that activate the velopharyngeal musculature, such as head movement, speech, and swallowing, are repeated to reestablish the contours of the obturator. The use of thermoplastic wax prevents overextension of the obturator that may be created with the impression compound, especially anteriorly adjacent to the anterior and posterior tonsillar pillars. Adequate areas of tissue contact demonstrate a dull, stippled appearance, while a shiny surface indicates a lack of contact. The obturator prosthesis is left in the mouth for approximately five minutes to allow for adequate shaping of the impression wax by the previously described functions, which are repeated several times. When molding is complete, the contracted residual velopharyngeal musculature will lightly engage the obturator extension (Fig 4-26m), enabling the production of oral sounds. However, when the musculature is at rest, there should be space around the obturator prosthesis, enabling the production of nasal sounds, normal nasal resonance, and normal nasal breathing (Fig 4-26n).

The prosthesis is removed and chilled with cold water (Fig 4-26o and p). Gross excesses of the thermoplastic wax are trimmed away with a scalpel. Overextended areas can be identified where the wax is displaced, exposing the impression compound (Fig 4-27). These areas are trimmed and additional wax is applied. The wax is tempered in a water bath and the prosthesis is reinserted and functional movements are repeated.

When speech and swallowing are normal and the contour of the obturator appears adequate, the prosthesis is tempered in a water bath and replaced in the mouth for an extended period (60 to 90 minutes). The patient is instructed to wear the prosthesis without removal and is encouraged to speak, swallow, and perform the head movements previously described.

Prior to removal of the prosthesis, the patient is given a glass of cold water and instructed to gargle to chill the thermoplastic wax. The prosthesis is removed and further chilled in cold water. At this point, the thermoplastic material should not be trimmed because it is easily distorted. Contour modifications are safer to perform prior to delivery, when the obturator has been converted into acrylic resin. The altered cast impression is boxed and the altered master cast is completed (Fig 4-26q and r).

The obturator is processed in a customary manner with heat-activated methyl methacrylate. Following processing, gross excesses are removed. The superior surface should be *convex* and well polished to facilitate the deflection of nasal secretions into the oropharynx (Fig 4-26s). The tongue-surface side of the prosthesis should be slightly *concave*, and during swallowing, there should be only light contact between the prosthesis and the tongue (Fig 4-26t). As mentioned previously, if the obturator bulb is bulky and weight is a problem, the obturator should be hollowed (see Chapter 3, Fig 3-156). All surfaces of the obturator are polished to a mat finish so that PIP and disclosing wax will stick to the surfaces during the delivery appointment.

The final position and contour of the obturator are best determined while the prosthesis is positioned in the mouth. Pressure indicator paste and disclosing wax are helpful aids in identifying areas of overextension (see Fig 4-26t and u). The material is placed on the lateral and oral surfaces of the obturator, and the patient is instructed to repeat the movements used to fabricate the prosthesis. The contour and the level of placement are reaffirmed, and areas of excessive pressure are relieved. As mentioned above, at rest, there should be space around the prosthesis in the zone of muscle contraction (Fig 4-26v). When the patient activates the velopharyngeal musculature, these areas will engage the surface of the prosthesis (Fig 4-26w). However, if the obturator extends into an area of the pharyngeal wall that has been reconstructed with a flap or otherwise immobilized, light contact should be constantly maintained with the surface of these tissues. All surfaces of the obturator are then highly polished, and the patient is scheduled for follow-up appointments.

Several clinicians have reported increased movement of the residual velopharyngeal complex following obturation (Fig 4-28). This suggests that the prosthesis acts as a stimulus for increased muscle activity. Indeed, many obturators for soft palate defects require reduction after delivery. If the patient complains of soreness, pressure, stuffiness, hyponasal speech, or difficulty in breathing or swallowing, the obturator should be checked with PIP and/or disclosing wax and adjusted accordingly. If this maneuver is unsuccessful in alleviating these symptoms, the posterolateral aspects are reduced judiciously over two to three sequential visits. If these tissues exhibit some mobility, they will often compensate with time by increasing their range of movement. At the same time, the nasal airway is enlarged when the residual velopharyngeal musculature is in a relaxed state.

If hyponasal speech and breathing difficulties persist, the level of the obturator in the nasopharynx should be reevaluated. A common error is the extension of the obturator superiorly above the level of muscular activity. Continuous contact of these immobile tissues with the posterolateral border of the obturator prevents the patient from controlling nasal airflow and creates hyponasality and breathing problems.

Size and position of the obturator

What are the ideal dimensions of the obturator in the nasopharynx? The superior extension need not be extensive if the obturator is positioned correctly in the nasopharynx. The lateral dimensions of the obturator are determined by lateral and posterior pharyngeal wall movement. The position and length of the superior extension of the obturator are controlled by the prosthodontist. If the obturator is positioned correctly at the level of greatest lateral and posterior pharyngeal wall movement, the prosthesis need be no more than approximately 10–12 mm thick (Fig 4-26u; see also Chapter 3, Fig 3-156c). The most common errors detected in obturator prostheses constructed by inexperienced clinicians are related to position (too low), superior extension (too extensive), and lateral extension (underextended), especially of the posterolateral aspect (Fig 4-29).

Several factors should be considered relative to the position and the superior extension of the obturator. As reported previously, several investigators have noted that closure of the soft palate against the posterior pharyngeal wall normally extends approximately 5 to 7 mm in vertical height and that closure occurs at or above the level of the palatal plane (Aram and Subtelny, 1959; Moll, 1965; McKerns and Bzoch, 1970). Therefore, the superior extension need not be extensive to duplicate the normal contact area with the lateral and posterior pharyngeal walls.

Furthermore, the pharynx is a conical tube that has its widest dimension superiorly in the nasopharynx, so further superior extension of the obturator may add additional width and extra weight (see Fig 4-29c). As mentioned previously, extension and continuous tissue contact superior to the level of pharyngeal wall movement will also occlude the nasopharynx, resulting in difficulty with nasal breathing and hyponasal speech. Conversely, if the obturator is placed too low in the oropharynx, tongue function will be disrupted and gagging may be precipitated. This is important to understand because the gag reflex is primarily triggered when the dorsal surface of the tongue contacts an obtrusive portion of the prosthesis (see Fig 4-29a).

Two studies are relevant with regard to the position and size of the obturator. Mazaheri and Millard (1964) studied 10 young, adult, cleft palate patients with socially acceptable speech who were using an obturator prosthesis. The level of placement and the vertical extension of the obturators were studied with regard to their effect on speech. Three positions were tested with interchangeable

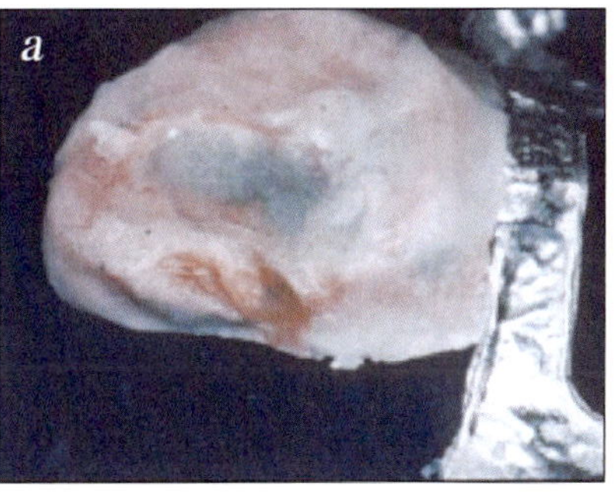

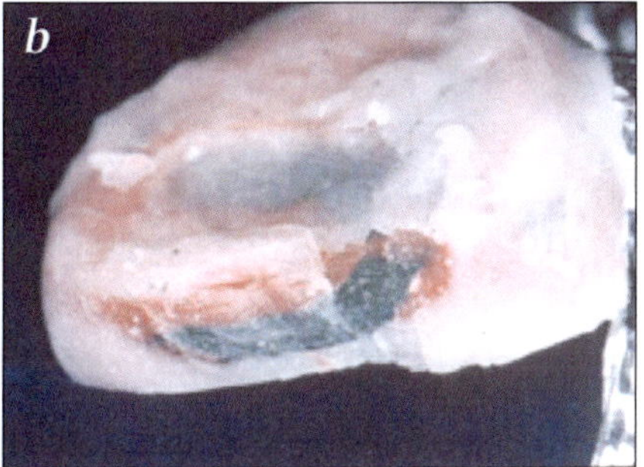

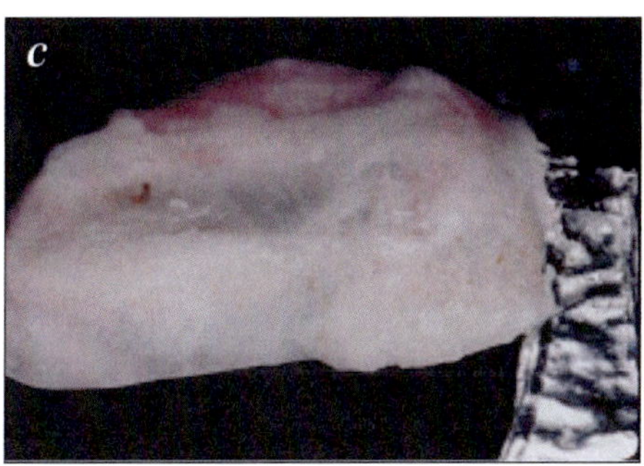

Figure 4-27 Functionally formed obturator. *(a)* During functional molding of the obturator bulb, thermoplastic wax was displaced so that impression compound was visible, indicating tissue displacement. *(b)* impression compound is cut back and thermoplastic wax is reapplied. *(c)* The impression compound is no longer visible. Note the change in contours (indentation) in this area.

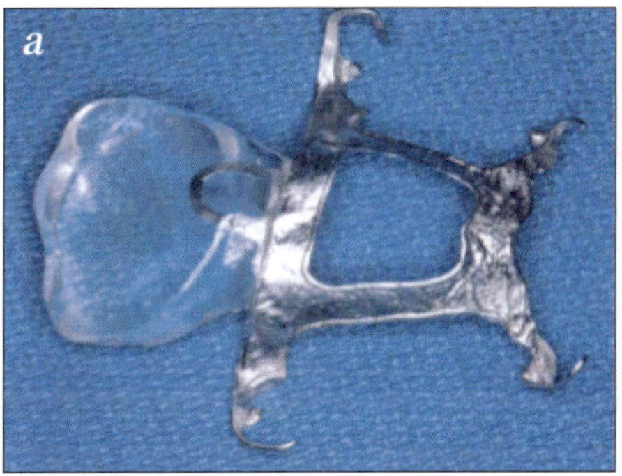

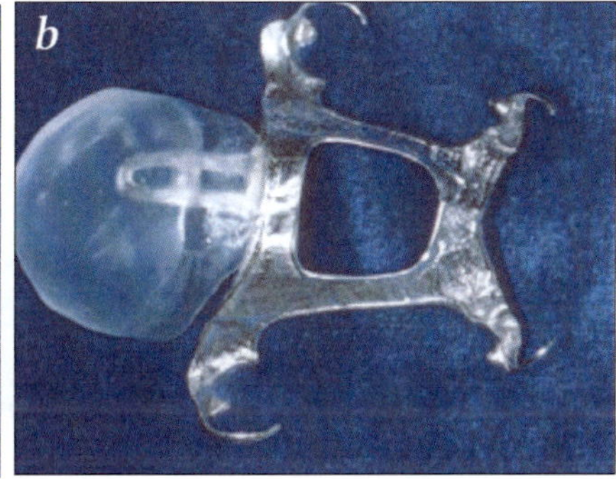

Figure 4-28 Changes in obturator dimensions over a 7-year interval. *(a)* Initial prosthesis. *(b)* Replacement prosthesis fabricated seven years later. The obturator is significantly smaller in all dimensions and there are considerable contour changes in the extension that engage the posterior and lateral pharyngeal walls.

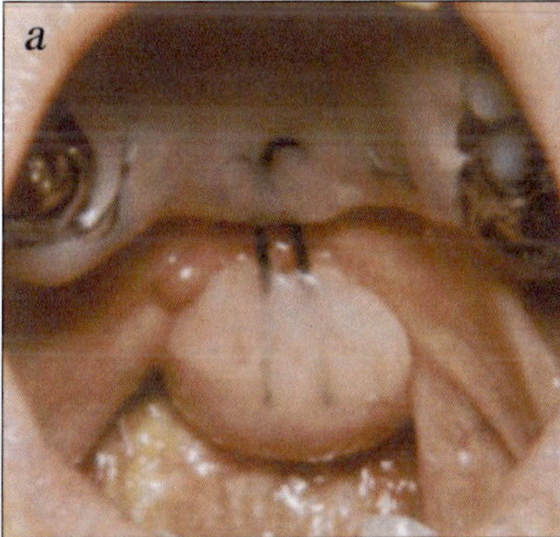

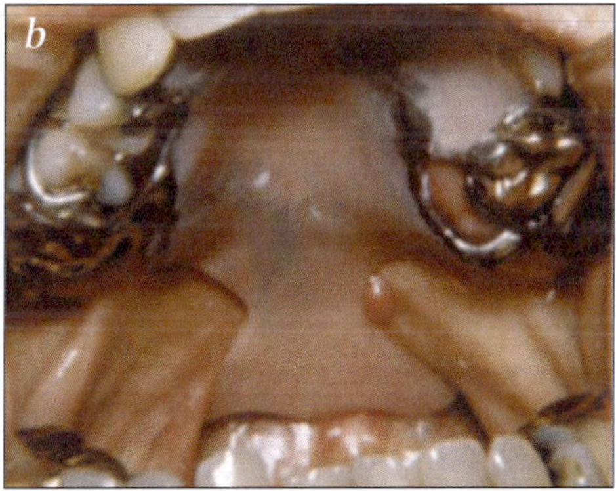

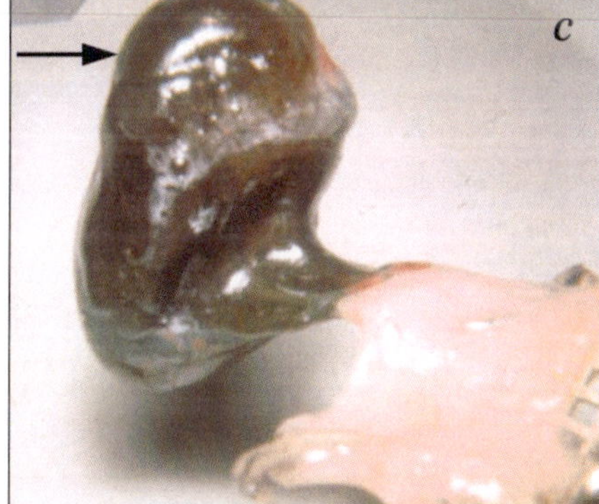

Figure 4-29 Obturation errors. *(a)* Inappropriately contoured obturator. The oral surface has a convex contour that may interfere with tongue function and the obturator is underextended laterally. *(b)* Properly contoured obturator for the same patient. The concave contours of the oral surface allow space for the tongue. *(c)* Obturator bulb molded with a thermoplastic material. Note the displacement of the material superiorly. Because the pharynx is a conical tube with its widest dimension located superiorly, extension above the level of velopharyngeal motion *(arrow)* creates continuous contact, predisposing the patient to hyponasal speech.

obturators: high (above posterior pharyngeal wall activity), medium (at pharyngeal wall activity), and low (below pharyngeal wall activity). Each obturator was adjusted for five weeks before speech recordings were made. This investigation disclosed that the middle position resulted in the best speech for most patients. The superior-inferior dimension of the original medium obturator for these subjects varied from 13 to 19 mm (mean of 13.09 mm). Each obturator was reduced inferiorly and/or superiorly to an average of only 3 mm in superior-inferior extension with no effect on speech.

Subtelny et al. (1966a) studied the speech of 23 adult and adolescent cleft palate speakers with obturator prostheses. They reported a wide variation in obturator position and size. The position of the obturator varied from 20 mm below the palatal plane to 6 mm above the plane. The vertical extension varied from 11 to 35 mm. The best speech results were obtained with the higher placement of the obturator or at the level of the palatal plane, which corresponded to the zone of contraction of the velopharyngeal musculature. Where deficiencies were noted clinically regarding tissue approximation, the lateral dimension was most commonly found to be deficient in extension.

Speech evaluation and therapy

After the initial adjustment period is completed, cleft palate patients will benefit from the services of a speech pathologist to

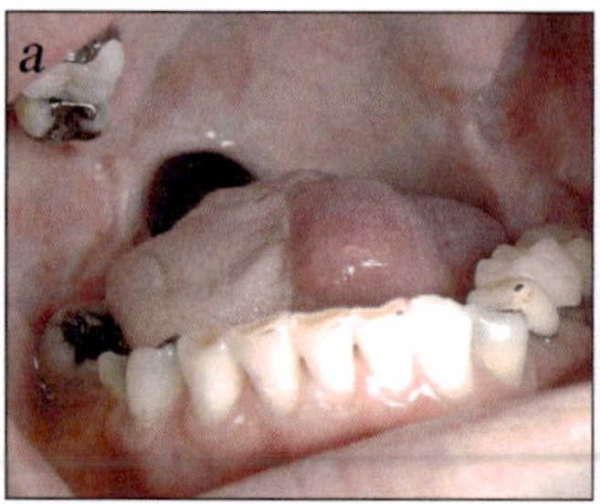
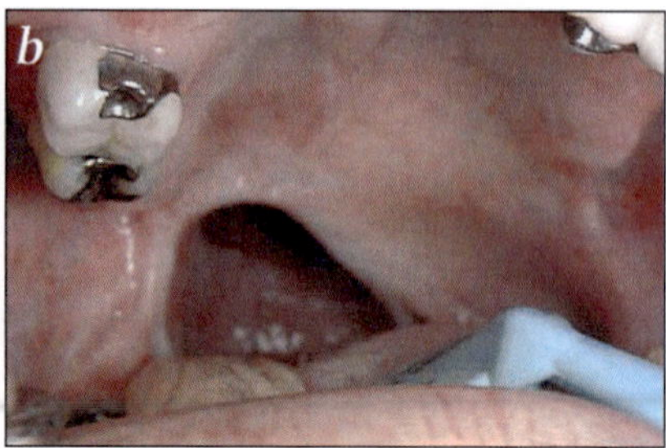
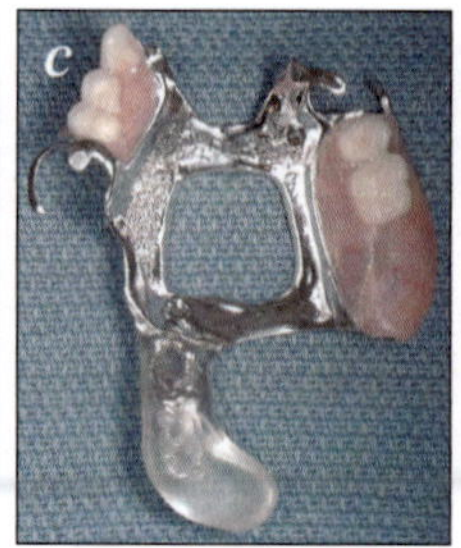
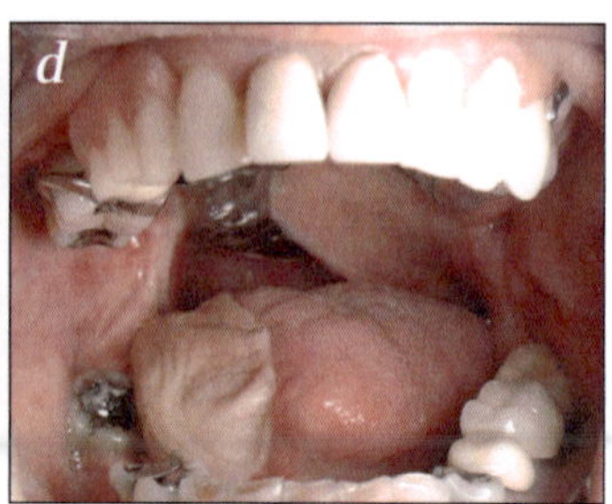

Figure 4-30 *(a and b)* Tumor ablation required removal of a significant portion of the tongue, the tonsillar area, the soft palate, and the lateral pharyngeal wall. The pharyngeal wall was resurfaced and the resected portion of the tongue was reconstructed with a vascularized free flap. *(c and d)* The velopharyngeal deficit was restored with an obturator prosthesis. However, speech articulation deficits are best addressed with speech therapy.

assist them in using their obturator prosthesis more effectively. Some cleft palate patients may have faulty articulatory patterns along with various degrees of hypernasality and may have never developed normal speech patterns. Many cleft palate patients will invariably require speech therapy to use their obturator prosthesis more effectively in order to break some of the compensatory habit patterns developed and ingrained before prosthetic treatment. In contrast, patients with obturators for acquired defects confined to the soft palate usually do not need speech therapy.

However, some patients with soft palate defects secondary to tumor ablation will also benefit from speech therapy following delivery of the prosthesis but for a different reason. Frequently a tonsillar or retromolar trigone lesion will require resection of substantial portions of the tongue as well as the pharyngeal wall and soft palate (see Fig 4-30). The velopharyngeal deficit is restored with an obturator prosthesis. However, the articulation errors resulting from resection and reconstruction of the tongue need to be addressed with speech therapy (see Chapter 2, section entitled "Speech").

The prosthodontist may require the assistance of a speech pathologist to evaluate articulation errors and inappropriate oral-nasal resonance balance following obturator placement. The articulation test in Table 4-5 or the Iowa Pressure Articulation Test (Morris et al., 1961) can be administered by the prosthodontist, but definitive judgments concerning articulatory deficiencies should be reserved for the speech pathologist.

The obturator is adjusted to the point where the patient can produce a clear /*p*/ and a sustained /*if*/ or /*is*/ sound without emission of air through the nose and can produce understandable nasal consonant sounds such as /*m*/ (Rosen and Bzoch, 1958). Several authors have suggested that the sustained pressure required for the /*s*/ phoneme may also be a reliable method of evaluating the effectiveness of the obturator (Rosen and Bzoch, 1958; Lubker and Schweiger, 1969). Whereas greater intraoral pressure may be required for stop-plosives such as /*p*/, the sustained pressure required for /*is*/ mitigates the compensatory elevation of the tongue to assist with closure.

The evaluation tests discussed previously, such as comparative oral and nasal airflow measurements, and nasoendoscopy, will aid in assessing the perceived resonance balance. Nasoendoscopy, especially, can be very helpful because this instrument does not interfere with speech. Larger openings can be visualized through the scope, while the bubbling of mucus may indicate smaller openings that require correction (Fig 4-31) (Karnell et al., 1987).

Soft palate posterior border defects: Method of fabrication

Most patients in this category have undergone surgical resections of the posterior portion of the soft palate for control of neoplastic disease. Still other patients present with a shortened soft palate secondary to an overly aggressive uvulopalatopharyngoplasty (see Fig 4-6) or in cleft palate patients presenting with an inadequate repair of the soft palate (Fig 4-32). They exhibit a variety of defects, but the anterior portion of the soft palate remains intact with its attachment to the posterior border of the palatine bones. The obturation of two prototype defects will be discussed: *(1)* posteromedial border defects that occur following the surgical resection of lesions of the uvula and the posterior soft palate and *(2)* posterolateral border defects that occur following the resection of lesions of the anterior tonsillar pillar and the retromolar trigone. In both instances, the velopharyngeal mechanism may be compromised and prosthetic obturation is usually the treatment of choice.

The objectives for the obturation of these defects are similar to those previously described for the obturation of total soft palate defects. However, the prosthetic approach differs because the remaining intact portion of the soft palate must be slightly elevated and circumvented so that the obturator can be placed at the proper level in the nasopharynx and engage the residual velopharyngeal musculature. The characteristics of the remaining portion of the soft palate will determine the best approach for the patient. A short, taut soft palate may be circumvented easily by the extension from the basic prosthesis (Fig 4-32).

Circumventing lengthy, immobile soft palates can be difficult and affect the clinical outcome. In this instance, if the soft palate is circumvented without displacement, the prosthesis must extend across the soft palate into the oropharynx and may interfere with tongue movements. Under these circumstances, it may be desirable to lift the palate with a narrower version of a palatal lift as the prosthesis is extended into the defect area (Fig 4-33).

A study by Subtelny et al. (1966a) sheds light on this phenomenon. In their study of 23 prosthetically managed cleft palate patients, they reported that patients with the poorest speech after prosthetic treatment were those with long, immobile soft palates in whom the soft palate was circumvented without displacement. The lengthy, immobile soft palate compromised the superior extension of the obturator into the nasopharynx and resulted in an obturator position that was lower than the position in patients who achieved better speech. In these situations, presumably, the obturator

Table 4-5 Test sentences for evaluation of articulatory factors involved in consonant sounds*

Phoneme	Contract	Test sentence
p, b, m	Bilabial contact	Bobby popped a balloon.
k, g, ng	Linguo-velar contact	Go get the coat and bring it back.
t, d, n	Linguo-alveolar contact	Tom did not do it.
f, v	Labio-dental contact	Father found some coffee.
th	Linguo-dental contact	They thought there were three.
j, ch	Linguo-palatal contact	Jack jumped by the children.
L	Lateral lingual aperture	The little lamp was lit in school.
r	Central lingual aperture	Roy Rogers's horse was Trigger.
w	Widening labial aperture	Will you go with William?
y	Widening lingual aperture	You and your young sister will go next year.
s, z	Linguo-alveolar contact	Six sisters saw the zebra in the zoo.
sh, zh	Linguo-palatal contact and wide air blade	She will wash the dish in the garage.

* Reprinted from Chierici and Lawson L (1973) with permission.

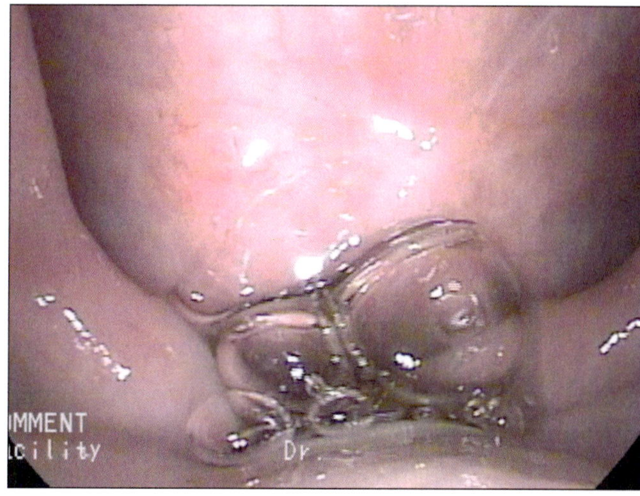

Figure 4-31 Patient fitted with a palatal lift. Bubbling of mucous indicates incomplete velopharyngeal closure. The lift was adjusted and the bubbling was eliminated (see Fig 4-12).

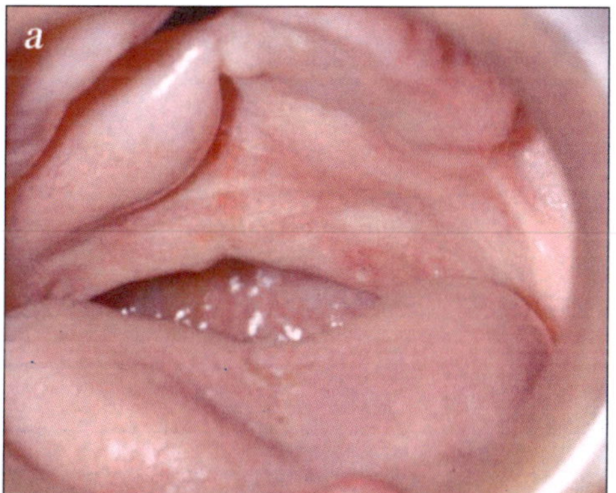

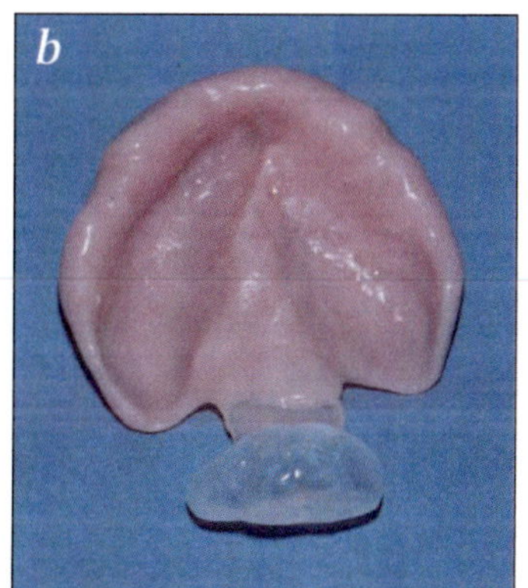

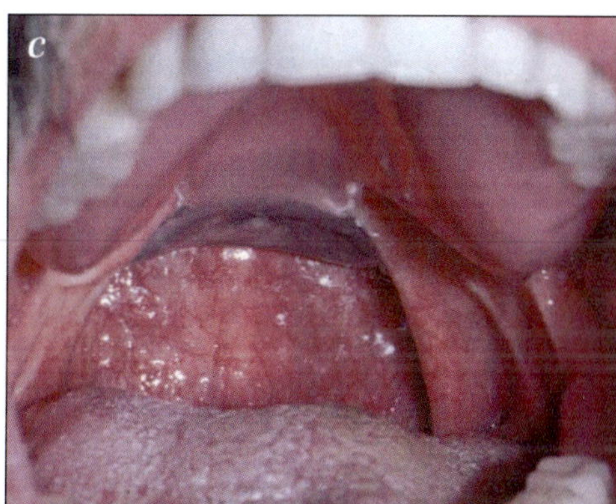

Figure 4-32 Congenital posteromedial border defect. *(a)* Edentulous patient with a short, immobile soft palate. *(b)* Prosthesis. The extension across the intact residual soft palate is intended to position the obturator properly in the nasopharynx. A circumvented soft palate was included in the altered cast impression and made quite thin. *(c)* Prosthesis in position. The inferior surface has a slightly concave contour.

extension was insufficient superiorly to engage the velopharyngeal musculature up and behind the drape of the residual soft palate during function. These findings support the view that in patients with considerable amounts of soft palate remaining, it is desirable to lift the soft palate with the transpalatal extension in combination with the obturator prosthesis.

Many clinicians have reported that they have been able to reduce the overall dimensions of the obturator over time because of perceived compensatory muscle activity (see Fig 4-28). One group of investigators, however, extended this argument to a population of young children with repaired clefts but with residual velopharyngeal incompetence and/or insufficiency. Following the use of an obturator prosthesis, they reported increased lateral wall movement to such a degree that resulted in the complete removal of the obturator without any change in speech quality (Weiss, 1971). This study was conducted in children during a period when some cleft palate teams deferred pharyngeal flaps until the age of 12–13. These results have been questioned and have not been reproduced by others. We have observed changes in obturator size but have never observed a patient where the prosthesis was slowly reduced to the point where the prosthesis could be removed without affecting speech quality.

Posteromedial border defects: Method of fabrication

In past years and before the surgical repair of soft palate defects of cleft palate patients was refined and mastered, many patients presented with repaired soft palates exhibiting insufficient length or movement to effect velopharyngeal closure and required prosthetic obturation (see Fig 4-32). In recent times, similar anatomic deficiencies have been seen postuvulopalatopharyngoplasty (see Fig 4-6). Neoplastic disease of the uvula and posterior soft palate is rare. Small, well-localized lesions usually can be controlled with radiation therapy. However, lesions that fail to respond to radiation or more extensive lesions may require surgical resection, resulting in this type of defect (Fig 4-35a).

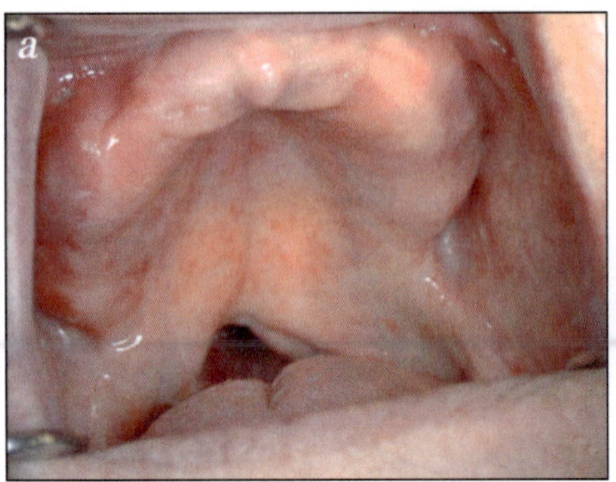

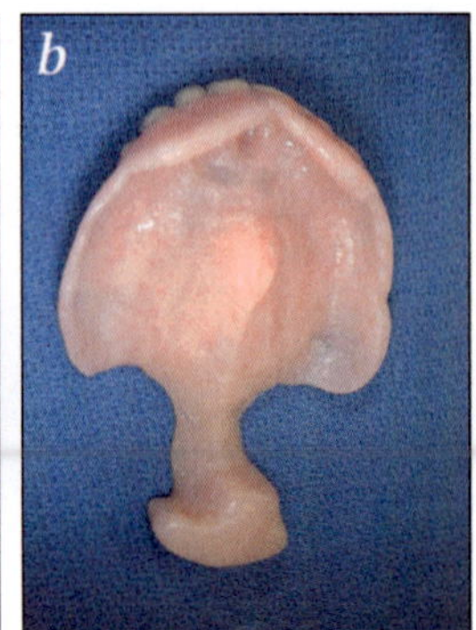

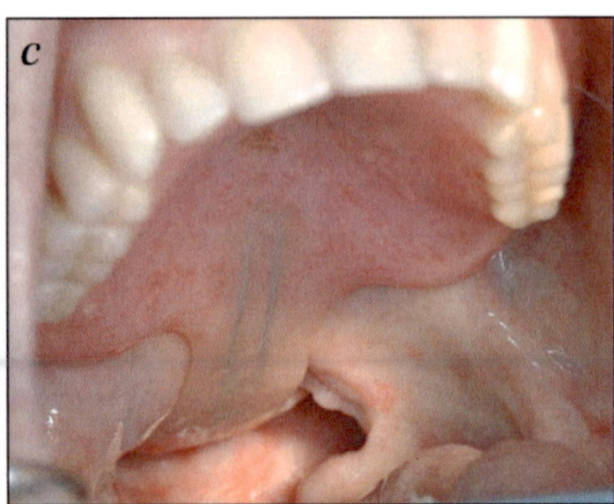

Figure 4-33 Acquired posteromedial border defects. *(a)* Edentulous patient with a posteromedial border defect. *(b)* The complete denture with the obturator extension. *(c)* The prosthesis in position.

The basic prosthesis is completed as described earlier. The presence of teeth or implants enhances the prognosis for all types of soft palate defects because improved retention permits accurate positioning of the obturator. Obturators restoring soft palate defects attached to complete maxillary dentures may adversely affect their retention because of the additional weight and the long, cantilevered lever arm necessary for obturator positioning. The preliminary impression should include the residual soft palate and at least the posterior margin of the soft palate. The diagnostic cast retrieved from this impression will have distortions secondary to displacement and contraction of the soft palate during the impression procedure, but the length of the residual soft palate will be approximately correct.

In edentulous patients, the complete denture is fabricated. The usual procedures conducted during the delivery appointment are completed, including verifying tissue adaptation with pressure indicating paste, checking peripheral extensions with disclosing wax, and executing a clinical remount procedure to refine the occlusion. A wire loop is attached to the complete denture and extended into the defect to retain tray resin and the impression material during molding of the obturator. The loop should be adjusted so that 1 mm of space exists between the wire retention and the soft palate at rest. After tray resin is added to the wire loop, the impression compound is added for border molding. The portion traversing the residual soft palate should displace the residual soft palate as necessary and be 1–1.5 cm wide depending on the size of the velopharyngeal deficit. This extension should be kept as thin as possible to preclude interference with tongue function.

In dentate patients, an RDP framework is obtained in the usual manner. The impression for the RDP framework should traverse the existing soft palate and extend into the defect. The RDP design is primarily driven by the nature of the edentulous extension areas (Chang et al., 2019), although as mentioned above, provision of indirect retention in the form of positive rests positioned on anterior abutments is recommended. A retaining loop that traverses the soft palate and extends into the defect is designed to be connected to the posterior palatal strap. This loop may need to be changed later because while making the impression of the residual soft palate for the RDP, its contour may be distorted (Fig 4-34). In addition, in most patients, it is desirable to lift the soft palate with the extension that traverses it.

The factors determining the level of placement of the obturator are the same as those for patients with a total soft palate defect. However, direct visualization of the area of normal velopharyngeal closure may not be possible except with an oral mirror or nasal endoscope. As a result of the presence of significant portions of the soft palate, a lengthy superior extension will be necessary to reach the level of normal closure and engage the residual velopharyngeal musculature.

If the posterior border of the resected soft palate is scarred and exhibits little motion, it may be feasible to extend the obturator across the nasal surface of the soft palate for a short distance. This extension provides some retention for the obturator and is especially helpful for edentulous patients when implants are not utilized. The margin of the soft palate must be slightly displaceable and a compound path of insertion must be used to engage this undercut. This extension may contact nasal mucosa; consequently, it must be molded carefully to avoid excessive displacement of tissue as well as to permit any residual elevation of the residual soft palate.

After the extension across the soft palate has been recorded, tray resin is added to the retention loop in the area of the defect. The resin must be 3 to 4 mm short of the adjacent tissues at their maximum level of contraction. Impression compound is then added and the patient is instructed to conduct the maneuvers to mold the obturator as previously described (head rotation and neck flexure, speech, swallowing). After molding procedures are completed, all tissue-contacting surfaces of the impression compound are trimmed back (Fig 4-35b and c) by approximately 1–2 mm with a sharp instrument. A thermoplastic material is added to the obturator and the molding procedures are repeated (Fig 4-35d). In posterior border defects, the most common mistake made is for the oral side of the prosthesis to be situated too low in the nasopharynx, resulting in premature contact with the tongue during speech and swallowing, triggering the gag reflex.

Frequently, the retention loop used to retain the obturator is not in the most advantageous position. An ideal time to replace the retention loop is after the prosthesis has been flasked, the flasks separated, and the mold cleansed of wax prior to processing with resin (Fig 4-34a and b). At this point, all structures will have been recorded in their correct relationship, so the adaptation of a new retention loop is facilitated. The new loop is laser welded to the RDP framework, and the obturator is processed with heat-polymerizing methyl methacrylate.

After processing and prior to insertion, the superior surface of the obturator is trimmed and rounded slightly to form a convex surface, and the extension of resin across the soft palate is thinned

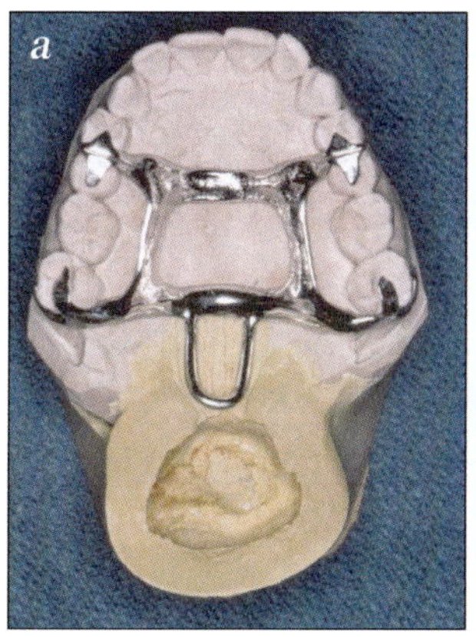
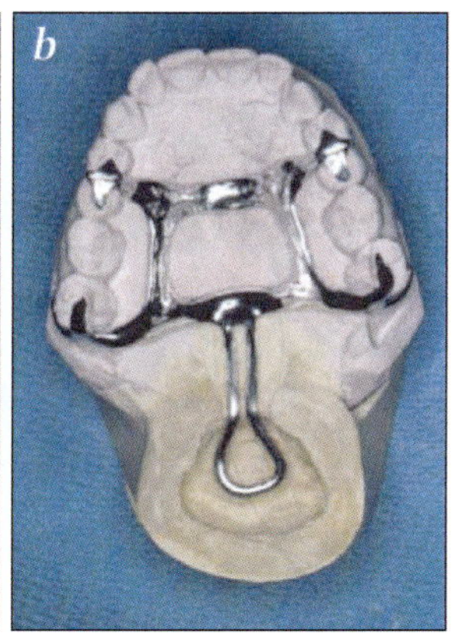

Figure 4-34 *(a and b)* Frequently, the retentive loop must be altered and extended. This is done after the altered cast impression is made.

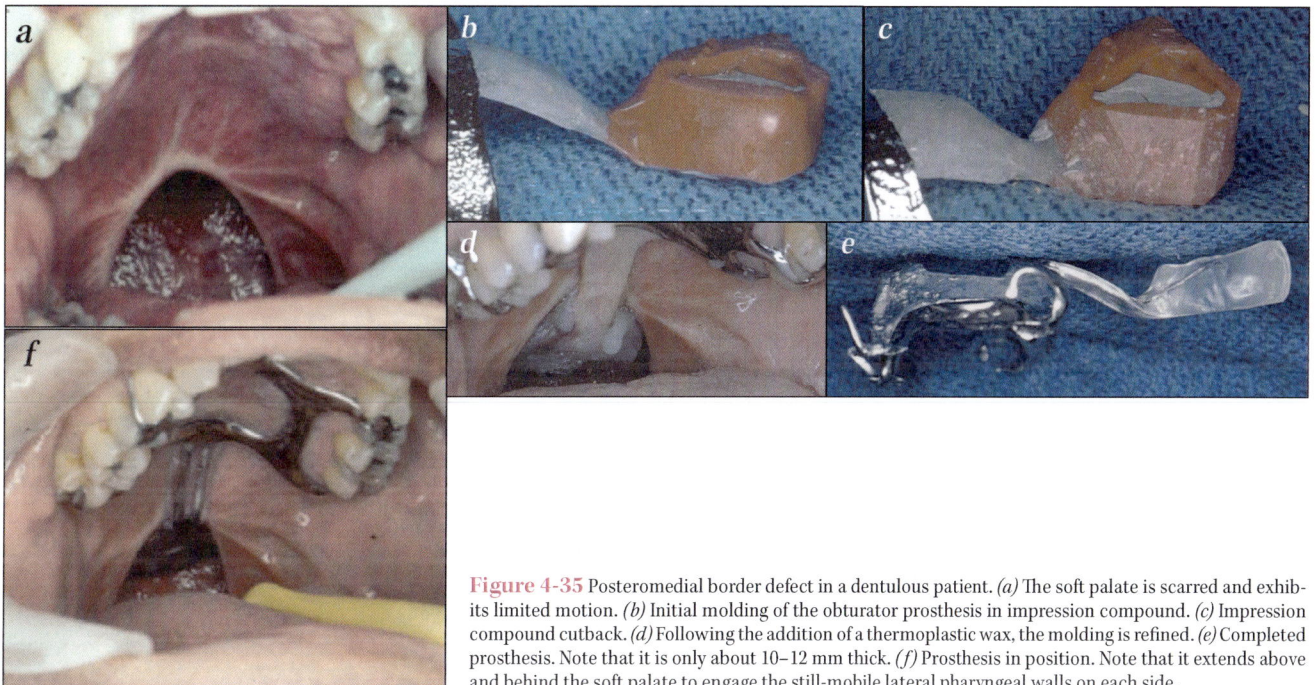

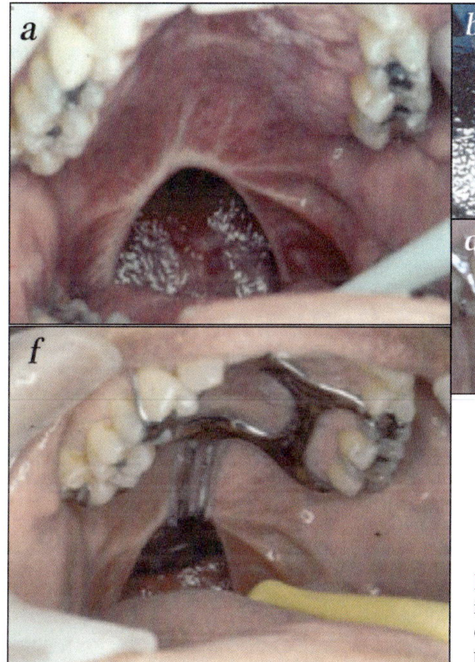
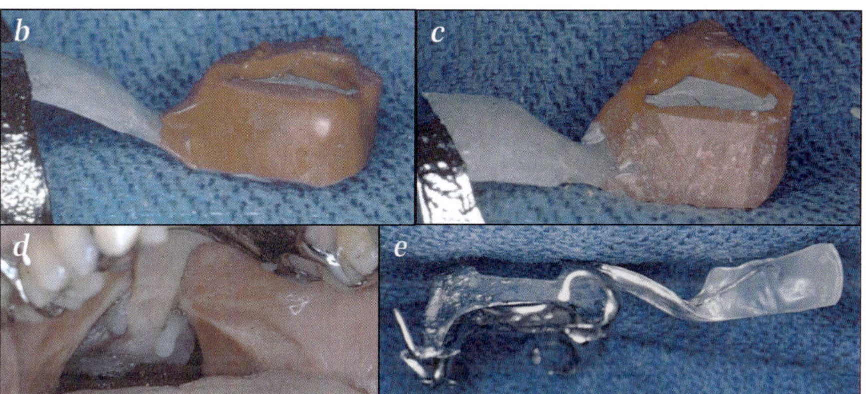

Figure 4-35 Posteromedial border defect in a dentulous patient. *(a)* The soft palate is scarred and exhibits limited motion. *(b)* Initial molding of the obturator prosthesis in impression compound. *(c)* Impression compound cutback. *(d)* Following the addition of a thermoplastic wax, the molding is refined. *(e)* Completed prosthesis. Note that it is only about 10–12 mm thick. *(f)* Prosthesis in position. Note that it extends above and behind the soft palate to engage the still-mobile lateral pharyngeal walls on each side.

as much as possible This extension will be approximately 10–15 mm wide and 2 to 3 mm thick. Usually, this width will not interfere with tongue function, but excessive thickness of resin can be bothersome.

If the obturator was extended superiorly along the nasal surface of the soft palate, the length of this particular extension may require reduction to allow the patient to insert the prosthesis comfortably. Pressure indicator paste or disclosing wax is applied to the surfaces of the obturator that will contact velopharyngeal tissues. If the PIP is rubbed off during insertion because of difficult access to the defect, disclosing wax is recommended. After the prosthesis is inserted, the patient is instructed to repeat all head and swallowing movements. Areas of displacement are noted and relieved. Several trial insertions may be necessary until the prosthesis will seat comfortably. When disclosing wax is used for this purpose, care must be taken to temper it before insertion into the defect. If the level of normal velopharyngeal closure is considerably above the posterior border of the soft palate, it is advisable to reduce the inferior surface of the obturator. This bulk is not necessary for obturation and its removal will provide more space for tongue function (Fig 4-35f). The patient is given instructions in the care of the prosthesis and a sequence of recall visits is established.

Posterolateral border defects: Method of fabrication

These defects result from the surgical resection of neoplasms arising from the tonsillar tissues, retromolar trigone, or posterolateral tongue (Fig 4-36a). Often the surgery includes a partial resection of the mandible and tongue as well as resection of the lateral oropharynx and soft palate in continuity with a neck dissection. Flaps are often used to reconstruct the mandible and resurface the lateral portions of the surgical defect, resulting in an immobile lateral pharyngeal wall (Fig 4-36b). In some patients, the residual soft palate is tethered to the pharyngeal wall or the flap used to resurface the pharyngeal wall, compromising its elevation (see Fig 4-9). This practice is discouraged because it limits the elevation of the residual

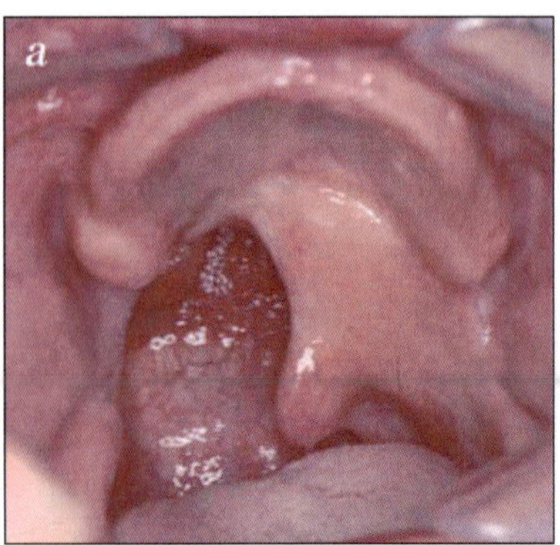
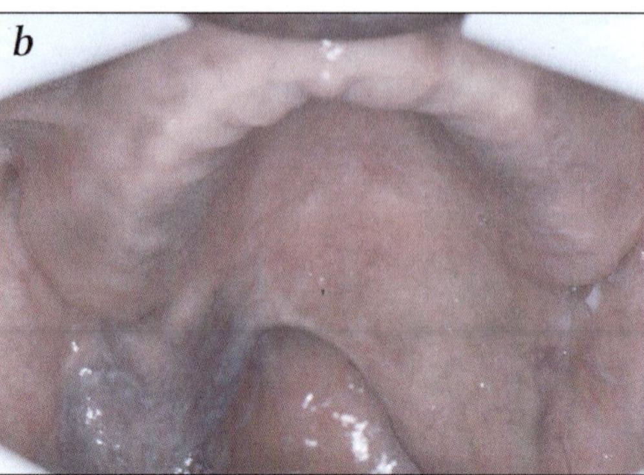

Figure 4-36 Posterolateral border defects. *(a)* Right posterolateral border defect. The resection and defect are confined to the lateral aspect of the soft palate. A rare defect with an excellent prognosis because of movement of peripheral tissues. *(b)* Right posterolateral border defect. The right lateral wall has been restored with a radial forearm flap. The residual soft palate and left pharyngeal wall exhibit excellent movement during function, so the prognosis for normal speech with the prosthesis is excellent. The challenge in these two patients will be retention of the CD-obturator prosthesis, since the posterior palatal seal area in both are compromised. Both would be prime candidates for osseointegrated implants.

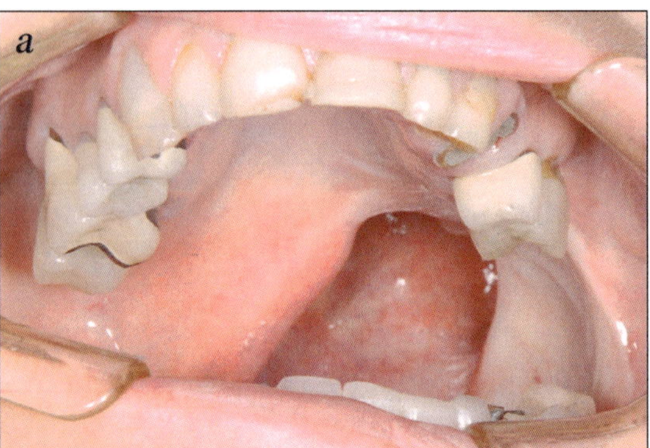
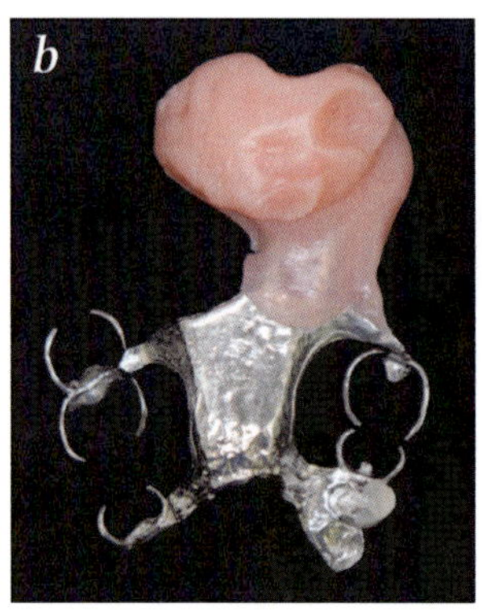
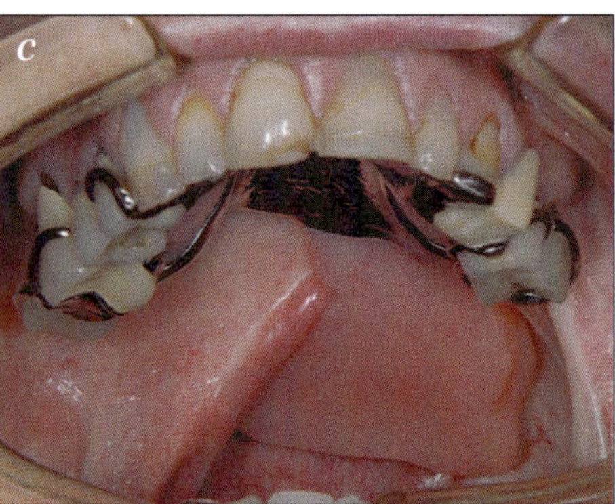

Figure 4-37 *(a, b, and c)* A typical obturator prosthesis for a posterolateral border defect. Note how the prosthesis enters the defect on the resected side. It curves around the residual soft palate and engages the active residual velopharyngeal musculature on the opposite unresected side.

portion of the soft palate and compromises access to the residual lateral pharyngeal wall on the unresected side.

Whatever the method of closure, the prosthesis must engage the opposite and still functional lateral pharyngeal wall behind the residual soft palate to permit the patient to achieve velopharyngeal closure (Fig 4-37). In patients with tongue dysfunction associated with the combined tongue-mandible-tonsil resection, the velopharyngeal deficits may appear inconsequential, yet these patients will derive considerable benefit from obturation, especially if the tongue is reconstructed and its bulk restored with a vascularized flap (Fig 4-38a). Under these circumstances, the obturator prosthesis restores velopharyngeal function, and the reconstructed tongue enables reasonable movement of the residual tongue (Fig 4-38a). With speech therapy, many of the articulation errors associated with tongue dysfunction can be mitigated. With the combined effects of effective obturation and restoration of the tongue bulk with a vascularized flap, speech will approach near normal in select patients.

As with all types of soft palate defects, a complete or partial prosthesis must be constructed before the obturator can be fabricated. In dentate patients, the RDP design is primarily driven by the nature of the edentulous extension areas (Kratochvil, 1988; Chang et al., 2019), although as mentioned above, provision of indirect retention in the form of positive rests positioned on anterior abutments is suggested (Fig 4-39). A retaining loop that traverses the soft palate and extends into the defect is designed to be connected to the posterior palatal strap. As mentioned previously, this loop may need to be changed later, because while making the impression of the residual soft palate for the RDP, its contour may be distorted.

The clinician should observe the configuration of the defect and the degree and direction of movement of the tissues bordering the defect prior to molding the obturator. In contrast to the tissues associated with defects confined to the soft palate, the tissues bordering lateral defects can exhibit variable movements. In most instances, the residual soft palate and lateral pharyngeal wall on the defect side will display little movement. If the residual soft palate is tethered on the defect side, it will be relatively immobile during velopharyngeal function. Frequently, almost all of the movement of the velopharyngeal complex is confined to the contralateral lateral pharyngeal wall. Consequently, to effect velopharyngeal closure, the prosthesis must extend from the defect side superiorly behind the soft palate, along the posterior pharyngeal wall, to engage the residual velopharyngeal musculature in the contralateral lateral pharyngeal wall.

The obturator is fabricated as previously described using impression compound and thermoplastic materials. The objective is to record the tissues bordering the defect during functional movements. There must be adequate movement of the residual velopharyngeal mechanism to control nasal airflow and nasal resonance.

In defects with limited mobility of the residual velopharyngeal musculature, there will be insufficient space between these tissues and the obturator, both at rest and during function. This will result in an inadequate nasal airway and hyponasal speech. Under these circumstances, it is usually necessary to reduce the size of the obturator to permit nasal breathing. However, doing so will result in mixed nasality, and this must be explained to the patient. It is best to affect these adjustments after the obturator has been fabricated.

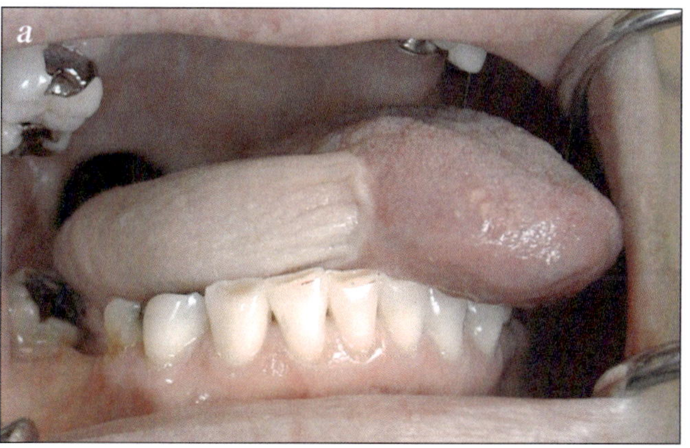

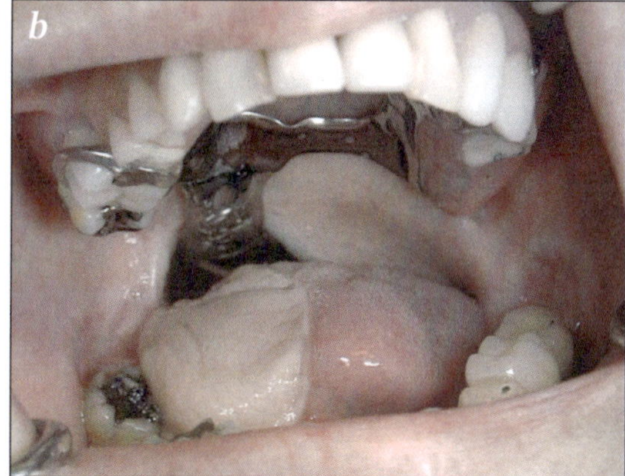

Figure 4-38 *(a)* Tumor ablation required removal of a significant portion of the tongue, the tonsillar area, the soft palate, and the lateral pharyngeal wall. The pharyngeal wall was resurfaced and the resected portion of the tongue was reconstructed with a vascularized free flap. Note the mobility of the reconstructed tongue. *(b)* Obturator prosthesis in position.

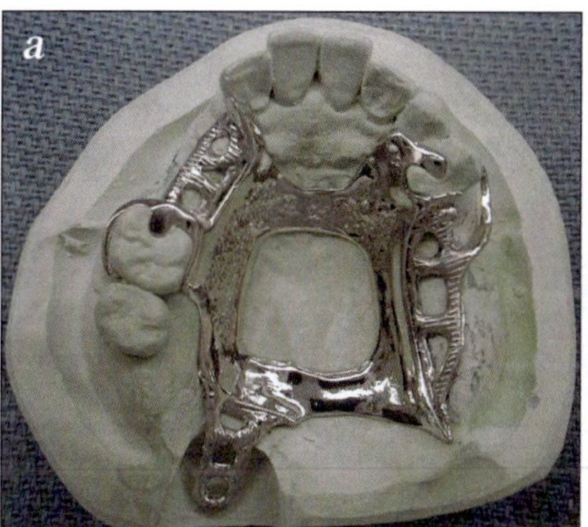

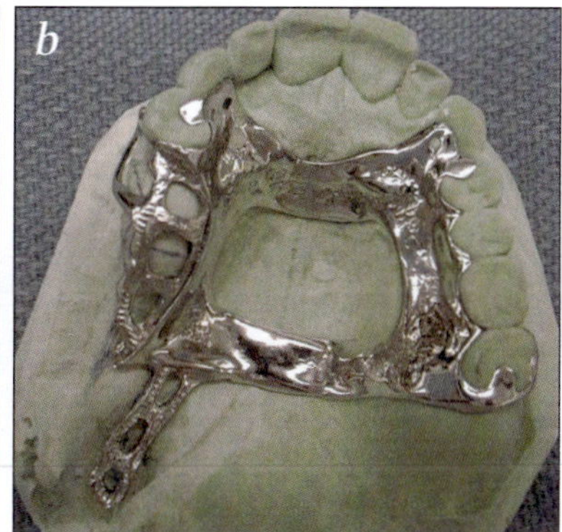

Figure 4-39 *(a and b)* RDP designs for patients with posterolateral border defects. The I bar mesial rest design concept has been used in these two patients.

The lateral extensions of the obturator are reduced gradually until nasal breathing is acceptable. Sequential monitoring appointments are essential following the delivery of these prostheses.

Use of implants

Obturators restoring defects of the soft palate and pharyngeal wall must be accurately positioned and securely retained in the nasopharynx if speech and swallowing are to be restored. This may be difficult to accomplish when the residual maxilla is edentulous because the residual edentulous arch, whether congenital or acquired, may be compromised, predisposing to inadequate retention of the complete denture-obturator prostheses. The posterior palatal seal area may be altered and scarred (see Figs 4-32, 4-33, and 4-36), making it difficult to obtain and maintain peripheral seal. Retention may also be compromised, as previously described, by posterior extension of the obturator into the nasopharynx. In other patients, a portion of the hard palate may be resected making it impossible to obtain peripheral seal. Also, patients with radiation-induced xerostomia lack the saliva to retain their dentures via peripheral seal. In all such patients, osseointegrated implants provide a reliable means of retention.

Osseointegrated implants enable the design and fabrication of overlay complete denture-obturator prostheses with retentive capacities similar to that achieved with RDP frameworks in dentulous patients. In most patients four or more implants should be placed (Figs 4-40 and 4-41). The design of the implant connecting bar is dictated by the implant distribution and the apparent anchorage of each of the implants. Under most circumstances, it is preferred to place adequate numbers with sufficient A-P spread to permit an implant-supported connecting bar design, especially when the opposing arch is fully or partially dentate (Fig 4-40). However, this may not be possible in all patients, and when adequate numbers (minimum four implants) cannot be placed and sufficient A-P spread (2 cm) cannot be achieved, an implant-assisted design is required. In large defects that involve a substantial portion of the hard palate, the use of an implant-supported design may require the placement of zygomatic implants on the side of the defect. If one or more of the implant sites has been heavily irradiated (dose in excess of 6,000 cGy; see Chapter 1, section entitled "Dental Implants in Irradiated Tissues"), implant-assisted bar designs are preferred. In such cases, maximum use should be made of the residual primary support areas.

When an implant-assisted design is employed, the design in Figure 4-41 is suggested. This design consists of a Hader bar positioned between the two anterior implants and ERA attachments secured to the posterior side of the distal implants. The ERA attachments are resilient. With this design, the support is shared between the implants anteriorly and the denture-bearing surfaces

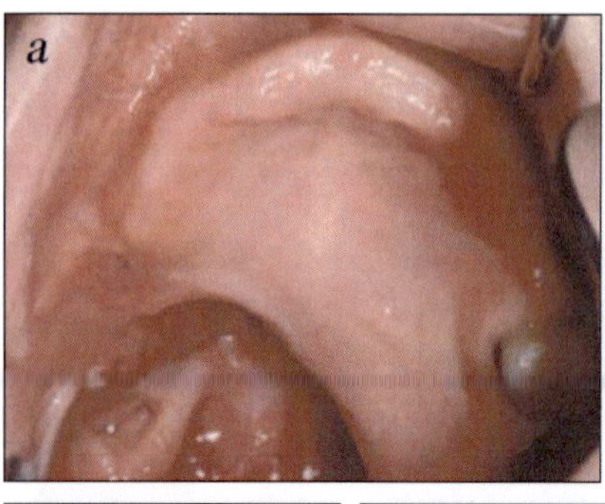
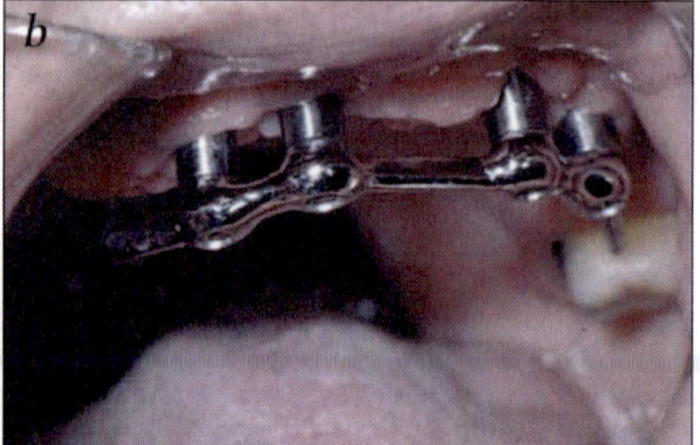
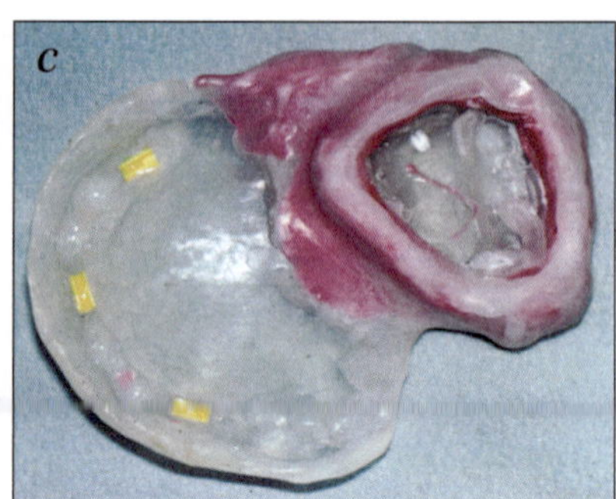
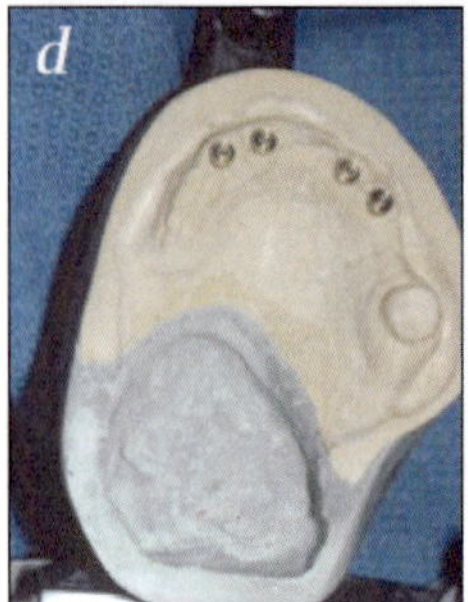
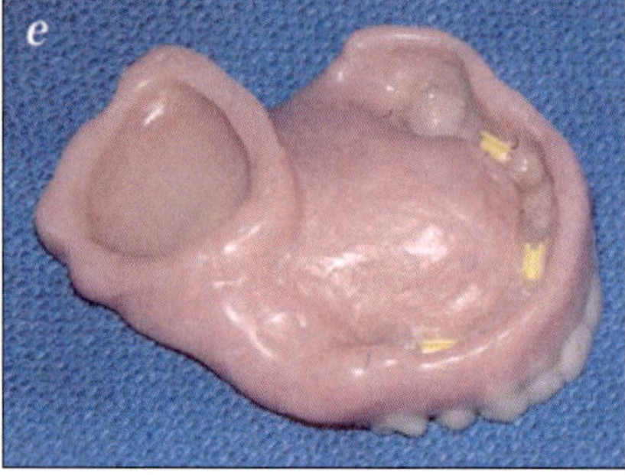

Figure 4-40 Overlay denture with obturator. *(a)* Large right posterolateral border defect that extends anteriorly into the right lateral hard palate. The remaining tooth was overlaid. *(b)* Four implants and a bar, positioned in the anterior maxillary segment. *(c)* Altered cast impression of the defect. *(d)* Altered cast. *(e)* Prosthesis with clips.

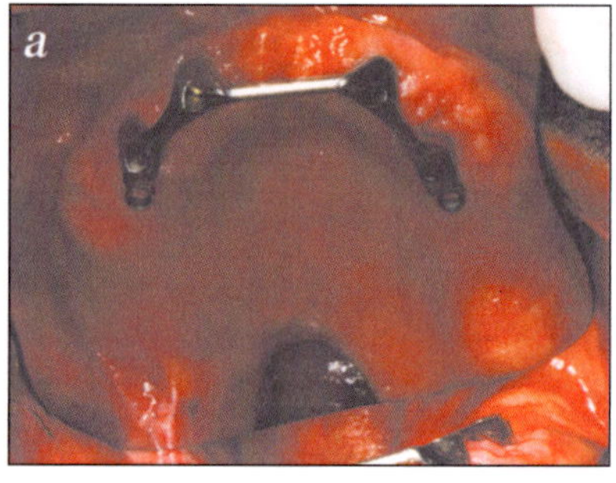
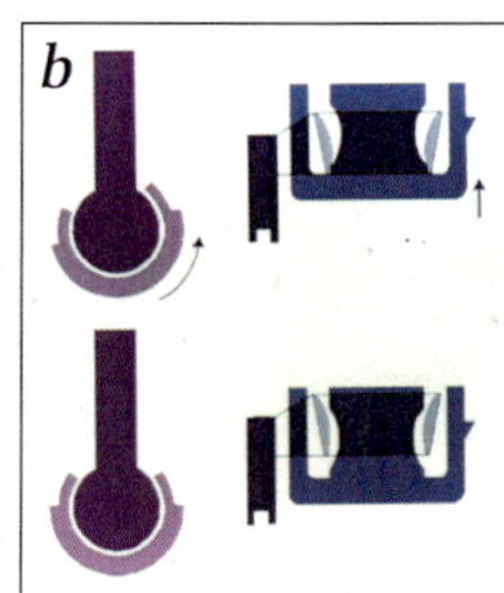

Figure 4-41 Implant-assisted connecting bar design used to retain overlay denture with a soft palate obturator extension. *(a)* The anterior-posterior (A-P) spread of the implants should be maximized. Resilient attachments provide retention and the anterior segment of the bar provides indirect retention. *(b)* During mastication, the anterior segment of the tissue bar serves as the axis of rotation and resilient attachments allow the posterior denture-bearing areas to support occlusal forces. The ERA attachments permit the extension base to be compressed into denture-bearing tissues up to 0.4 mm.

posteriorly. When occlusal forces are applied posteriorly, the denture is designed to rotate around the Hader segment anteriorly. The ERA attachments provide retention but permit a vertical displacement of up to 0.4 mm at the attachment before bottoming out. The mucoperiosteum of the posterior maxilla compresses less than this amount when an occlusal force is applied; therefore, when these denture-bearing surfaces are covered by a well-extended denture base, the distal implants are at little or no risk of exposure to cantilever forces. This allows the posterior denture-bearing surfaces to absorb the posterior occlusal loads. The retention provided by the implants will be enhanced if the implants can be positioned in a quadrilateral design.

Potential implant sites

In most oncologic patients, sufficient amounts of the alveolar ridge will be available because the premaxilla is rarely affected by the surgical resection. In larger defects, particularly those patients with large unrepaired clefts of the hard and soft palate, in patients undergoing radical maxillectomy in association with resection of the soft palate, the zygomatic arches may be considered (see Chapters 3 and 6).

When implants are placed in the residual alveolar ridges, the tilted concept of implant placement is highly recommended (see Chapter 3, section entitled "Sites based on the use of tilted implants"). This concept increases the anterior-posterior spread of the implants and allows for the use of longer implants. Moreover, the initial anchorage of the implants will be enhanced since the tips of the implants engage the cortical bone associated with the pyriform rim (Jensen et al., 2015).

Implants placed during ablative surgery versus deferred implant placement

As mentioned in Chapter 3, in edentulous patients, or those patients with insufficient dentition to properly retain the obturator prosthesis, the authors advocate placing implants during ablative surgery as opposed to deferred placement. This approach saves the patient an additional implant surgery and reduces treatment time. Moreover, implant success rates appear to be comparable to those achieved with deferred placement (Wetzels et al., 2017; Butterworth, 2019; Butterworth and Rogers, 2022).

Digital technologies and CBCT scans make this approach easier and predictable. When implant placement is anticipated in concert with surgical tumor ablation, scans of the patient are obtained, and when portions of the hard palate are to be included in the resection, the probable surgical resection can be simulated and the possible bone sites can then be carefully evaluated. The selection of implant sites, implant lengths, and angulations are based on the proposed design of the implant connecting bar and overlay complete-denture-obturator prosthesis. Ideally, as mentioned above, implants are positioned to permit implant-supported designs (all forces of occlusion are borne by the implants). In addition, the implant platforms and their abutments should be positioned to allow for sufficient space for the implant connecting bar and metal substructure.

Workup

The conventional approach entails the fabrication of a radiographic guide with an accurate duplication of the idealized artificial tooth setup or the existing denture in autopolymerizing acrylic resin. A CT scan is obtained while the patient wears the radiographic guide. The resulting data are evaluated to ensure that adequate bone volume and contours are available at the proposed implant sites. The number, location, and trajectory of implants can be determined with careful radiographic analysis (see Chapter 3).

Digital planning tools are rapidly replacing conventional methods. As stated in Chapter 3, the precision that can be achieved with these methods represents a sophisticated treatment planning tool and has become more cost effective. CBCT scans allow visualization of the bone contours of the maxilla in three dimensions as well as adjacent structures such as the bony walls of the paranasal sinuses, the floor of the nose, and the nasal crest region. A separate scan of the radiographic guide allows the digital rendering of the prosthesis and the DICOM data from the scan to be merged, permitting the contours of the proposed prosthesis to be superimposed onto the bony contours of the intended implant sites. When tilted implants are to be placed, these planning programs are invaluable. Implant sites are selected based on an analysis of the three-dimensional bone contours and the probable tooth positions of the overlay complete denture obturator prosthesis. Positions and angulation of the implants can be determined and a surgical template designed and fabricated that permits either semiguided or fully guided controlled directional drilling, ensuring maximum accuracy of implant placement and alignment. The methodology is quite simple and has been detailed in Chapter 3.

Implant selection criteria

Several new implant designs have been introduced that broaden the application and improve the implant success rates. As mentioned in Chapter 3, in recent years the zygomatic implant has undergone a number of design changes, which are tailored for patients with large palatal defects associated with tumor resection or unrepaired clefts of the hard and soft palates. They are designed with extended smooth areas in order to mitigate plague accumulations and enhance oral hygiene procedures (see Chapter 3, Fig 3-125a and b and 3-26). Some implants retain the threads around the neck of the implant and these are used when the zygomatic implant engages both the zygoma and the residual bone of the alveolus.

Contemporary implants are prepared with microrough surfaces. These microrough surface topographies accelerate the process of osseointegration by upregulating and accelerating the expression of genes of the differentiating mesenchymal stem cells associated with the osseointegration process (Ogawa and Nishimura, 2006) and lead to bone that is harder and stiffer than bone anchoring machined-surface implants (Butz et al., 2006; Takeuchi et al., 2005). Tapered, self-tapping implant designs with variable thread patterns are favored because during insertion of the implant, the trabecular bone of the implant site is compressed around the implant improving its initial mechanical anchorage. The expected result should be an increase in implant survival, even in sites that have been heavily irradiated.

Implants with an off-axis design (Southern Implants, Irene, RSA) are particularly well suited for the so-called tilted implant approach when implants are placed along the anterior wall of the maxillary sinus and transit through the residual alveolar ridge and engage the pyriform rim or when an implant is positioned to engage the pyramidal process of the palatal bone (Fig 4-42). They are available in 12°, 24°, and 36° of angle correction.

Factors affecting restoration of normal speech with an obturator prosthesis

Most if not all patients with repaired clefts demonstrate excellent movement of the velopharyngeal mechanism during function. However, timing, regulation, and control, along with compensatory habit patterns, may contribute to oral-nasal resonance imbalance in these patients (Warren et al., 1985, 1986). In patients undergoing tumor resection, the prognosis for the restoration of speech to normal with an obturator prosthesis depends on the mobility of the residual velopharyngeal mechanism, access to these areas of movement, and the quality of retention available for the obturator prosthesis.

Compensatory habit patterns and outcomes of prosthetic obturation

Some adolescent cleft palate patients with poorly repaired or partially repaired clefts develop faulty articulatory patterns along with various degrees of hypernasality. They have never developed normal speech patterns. Improvements in velopharyngeal competence provided by either surgical or prosthetic means do not automatically translate into improved or normal speech. These patients often exhibit facial grimaces to partially occlude the nostrils and the nasal valve or abnormal tongue postures as a compensatory adjustment to reduce nasal emission. These compensations develop over many years and may persist after improved obturation.

Sell and Grunwell (1990) illustrated this point nicely when they studied the speech following late palatal surgery for 18 Sri Lankan adolescents with previously untreated cleft palates. Speech was recorded prior to palatal surgery and 8 and 12 months postsurgically. Speech was very distorted prior to surgery, but there was minimal spontaneous improvement postsurgically or following a limited amount of speech therapy. Ortiz-Monasterio et al. (1974) reported that speech therapy will help those youngsters who are operated before they are 12 years old but will have little effect on teenagers or adults with well-ingrained and abnormal speech patterns. Based on the authors' experiences, similar outcomes are to be expected if such patients are managed prosthetically and fitted with an obturator prosthesis after the compensatory speech mechanisms have become ingrained.

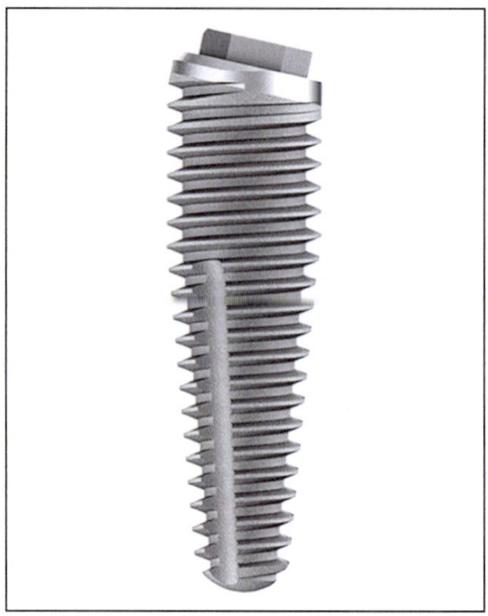

Figure 4-42 Off-axis implant design. They are available in several different angulations and are especially useful when the tilted implant concept is used (courtesy of Southern Implants, Irene, RSA).

In contrast, patients with acquired defects will usually achieve acceptable speech almost immediately after insertion of the prosthesis if a functional portion of the peripheral velopharyngeal complex remains essentially undisturbed by the surgical resection.

Inadequate mobility of the residual velopharyngeal mechanism

A reasonable amount of movement of residual velopharyngeal musculature is necessary if the speech outcomes are to be ideal. If lateral pharyngeal wall motion is minimal or absent the clinician will not be able to achieve appropriate resonance balance with the prosthesis. This phenomenon is seen primarily in patients treated aggressively with chemoradiation combined with surgical resection. When the obturator is molded in the usual manner, there will be little or no space between the surface of the obturator and velopharyngeal complex. As a result, normal nasal breathing is impaired and speech will be hyponasal. Under these circumstances, the authors prefer to reduce portions of the prosthesis that engage the *lateral pharyngeal walls* to the point where normal nasal breathing is permitted. Nonetheless, even with these adjustments, the space around the prosthesis at rest will still be insufficient to produce normal nasal consonant sounds (*/m/*, */n/*, and */ng/*), hence speech will be hyponasal. Moreover, the lack of the ability to engage the prosthesis by contracture of the residual velopharyngeal musculature leads to hypernasal speech. The overall result is speech with so-called mixed nasality.

Access to residual velopharyngeal musculature

The prosthesis must be able to precisely interact with the residual velopharyngeal musculature if normal velopharyngeal function is to be restored. The patients with the defects shown in Figure 4-9b, c, and d were dentate, and the lateral wall musculature on the contralateral side was functional, but tethering of the residual soft palate limited access to these areas of the defect. As a result, although hypernasality was partially mitigated with a prosthesis, normal nasal resonance could not be restored.

Defects that border the hard and soft palate where the resection extends to the posterior third of the soft palate and where the levator veli palatini aponeurosis is resected create a similar problem. The levator veli palatini muscle, which elevates the soft palate, is located in the middle third of the soft palate; if the resection extends posteriorly to involve the middle third of the soft palate, a posterior, narrow, nonfunctional band of intact soft palate may remain postsurgically (Fig 4-43a). This remnant will lack innervation and the capacity for normal elevation and these bands of residual soft palate often retract superiorly, preventing access for the obturator prosthesis to the posterolateral pharyngeal wall musculature still capable of contracting during speech and swallowing. As a result, the obturator will not be able to properly interact with the residual velopharyngeal musculature, resulting in hypernasal speech and leakage of fluids into the nasal cavity during swallowing. If normal resonance balance is to be restored consideration should be given to separating the soft palate in two and providing access to the still functional posterolateral pharyngeal walls (Fig 4-43d).

Quality of retention available for the obturator prosthesis

As mentioned on several occasions, the quality of the retention will impact the effectiveness of the obturator prosthesis. Prior to the introduction of osseointegrated implants, this was a significant problem for edentulous patients because in most cancer patients, the posterior palatal seal area is compromised by surgical resection or high-dose radiation. In other patients, significant portions of the hard palate are resected in combination with the soft palate. Under these circumstances, the patient is forced to retain the prosthesis in position with the dorsum of the tongue during speech, which impairs their ability to make the maneuvers required for normal speech articulation. Therefore, the authors recommend that unless a peripheral seal for the complete denture-obturator prosthesis can be established and maintained during speech and swallowing, implants should be placed to retain the prosthesis.

Surgical issues

It is extremely important for the prosthodontist to be an integral part of the presurgical team. The surgical management of the patient presenting with a soft palate neoplasm can dramatically affect the short and long-term prosthetic prognosis. Whenever possible there should be presurgical dialogue between the prosthodontist and the surgeon. With regard to resection of tumors extending to the soft palate, we recommend the following:

- If the proposed resection extends posteriorly to include the middle third of the soft palate (the area occupied by the levator veli palatini) the resection should be extended to include the remaining third. When the posterior third is left, this small strip of mucosa is nonfunctional and prevents proper extension of the obturator into the functional velopharyngeal area (Fig 4-43a, b,

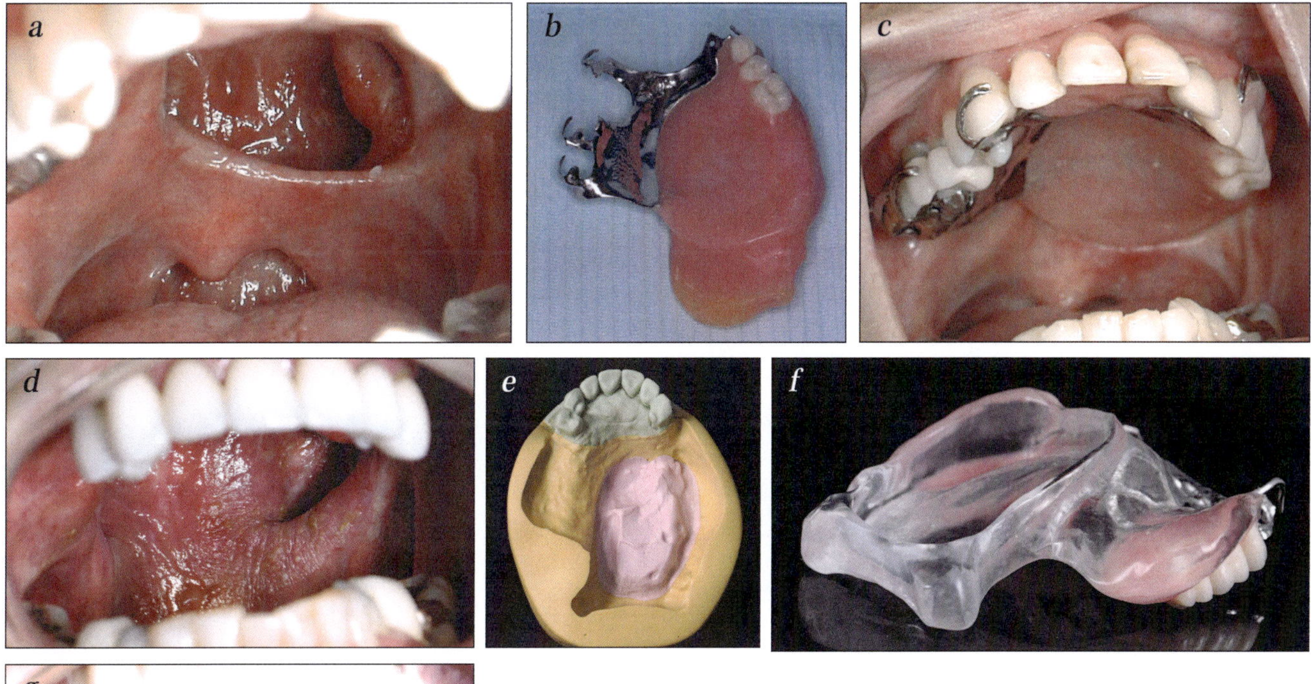

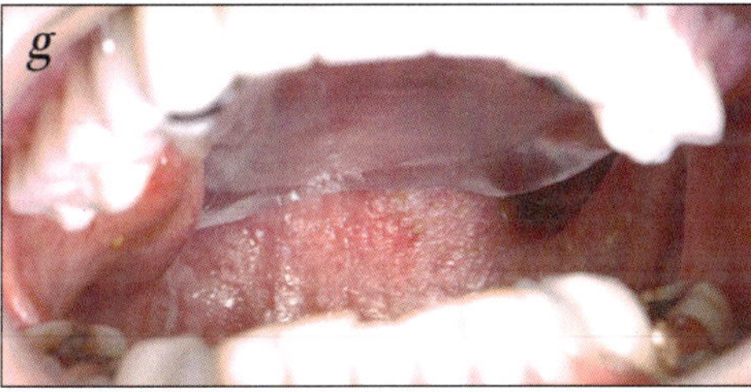

Figure 4-43 *(a)* The nonfunctional posterior third of the soft palate has been retained and prevents proper positioning of the soft palate portion of the obturator. *(b and c)* The soft palate portion of the obturator could not be extended to engage the right lateral pharyngeal wall due to lack of access. As a result, speech was hypernasal. *(d)* The nonfunctional portion of the soft palate has been split in two. *(e, f, and g)* As a result the soft palate portion of the prosthesis could be extended to engage both lateral pharyngeal walls permitting velopharyngeal closure. The extension on the left side has remained largely unchanged, but the extension onto the right lateral pharyngeal wall has been expanded significantly.

and c). If necessary, the residual soft palate can be split to facilitate access to the still functional lateral pharyngeal walls.

- It is possible to reconstruct unilateral soft palate defects with free vascularized flaps if the resection stops short of the midline (see Fig 4-8). However, if the resection approaches the midline, the residual portion should not be tethered to the free flap (Fig 4-44). In our experience, if such defects are reconstructed with a free flap and velopharyngeal closure is compromised leading to hypernasal speech and leakage of bolus into the nasal passage, access to the residual velopharyngeal mechanism is usually not possible with an obturator prosthesis.

The patient shown in Fig 4-44 provides a good example. A radial forearm flap was used to reconstruct a retromolar trigone and soft palate defect following tumor ablation. A radical maxillectomy had been performed previously to resect another primary lesion. The contralateral lateral pharyngeal wall was still functional but inaccessible. The hard palate portion of the defect was easily restored with an implant-retained overlay obturator prosthesis. However, because the residual soft palate was tethered to the flap and the still functional contralateral pharyngeal wall was inaccessible, it was impossible to restore oral-nasal resonance.

For these patients, it is best to use the flap to resurface the lateral pharyngeal wall, let the residual soft palate hang free, and obturate the defect with a prosthesis. Hard palate defects involving the soft palate and extending to the posterior pharyngeal wall are easily restored prosthetically as long as sufficient retention is provided for the prosthesis (see Chapter 3, section entitled "Maxillectomy defects extending to the posterior pharyngeal wall," Fig 3-156).

- The soft palate should not be tethered to the residual hard palate or the lateral pharyngeal wall. Tethering limits the movement of the residual remnants of the levator muscle and impairs access to the lateral pharyngeal wall on the contralateral side (Fig 4-45). The residual portion of the soft palate should be allowed to hang free. This practice allows maximum movement of the residual velopharyngeal mechanism and will not preclude access to the contralateral pharyngeal wall for the obturator prosthesis.

Chemoradiation and velopharyngeal dysfunction

Recently, as radiation doses escalate and as chemotherapy is combined with radiotherapy, an increasing number of patients are presenting with a combination of velopharyngeal insufficiency and velopharyngeal incompetence. With concomitant chemoradiation, frequently the biologically equivalent dose approaches 7,500–8,000 cGy, and when the clinical treatment volume is large and includes the entire velopharyngeal complex three to five years posttreatment, velopharyngeal functional deficits become apparent secondary to progressive scarring and muscle atrophy. Moreover, when the muscles

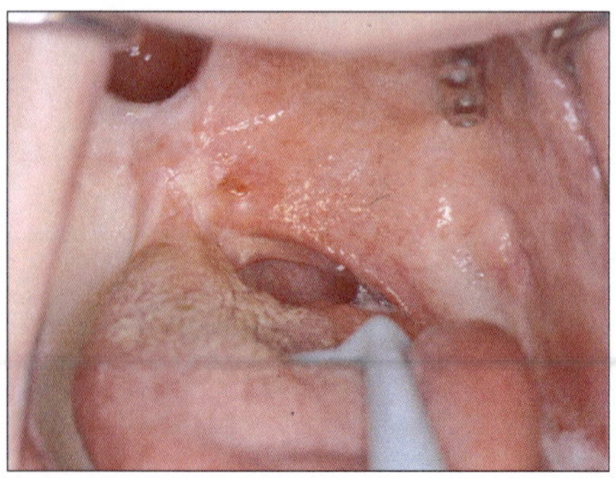

Figure 4-44 A patient who previously underwent a maxillectomy and subsequently developed another primary tumor in the retromolar trigone area. The resection extended beyond the midline of the soft palate. A flap used to reconstruct the defect was tethered to the residual soft palate inhibiting its elevation. Speech is hypernasal and prosthetic obturation of this area is impossible because the posterior and lateral pharyngeal walls on the unresected side are inaccessible.

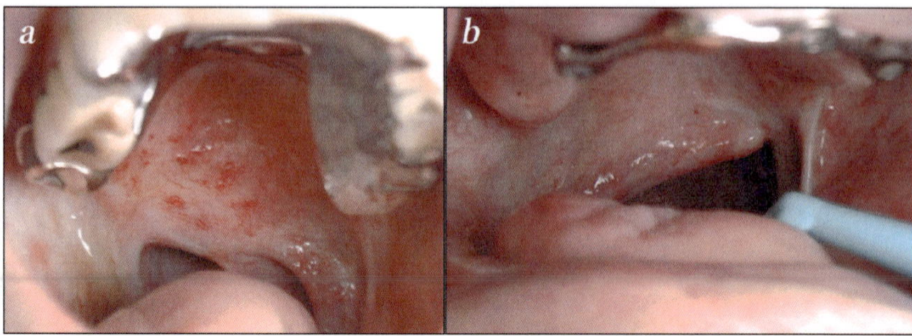

Figure 4-45 *(a and b)* Soft palate tethered to the lateral pharyngeal wall. This practice limits the movement of the residual velopharyngeal mechanism and may preclude access to the remaining functional velopharyngeal musculature present on the unresected side behind the residual soft palate.

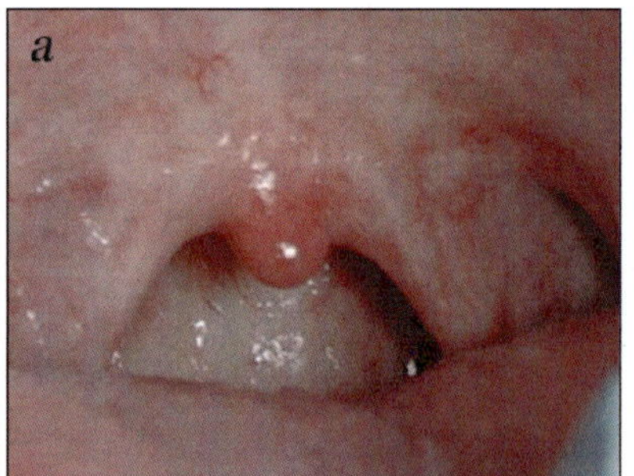

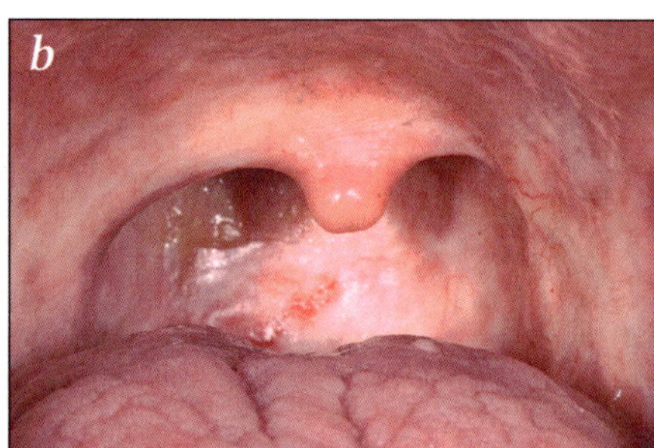

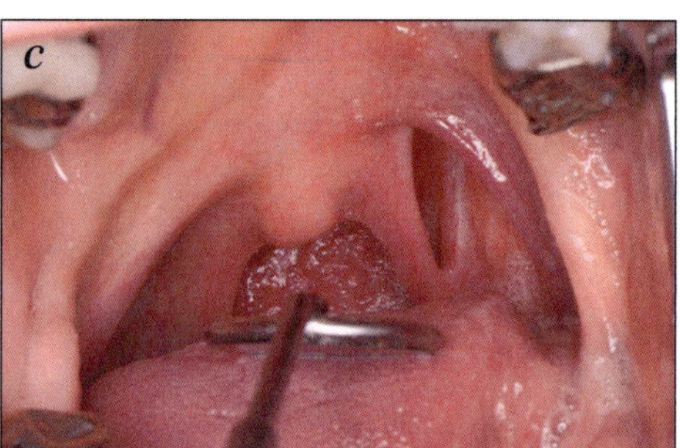

Figure 4-46 Chemoradiation and velopharyngeal insufficiency and velopharyngeal incompetence. These patients presented with hypernasal speech. *(a)* Patient received chemoradiation for a nasopharyngeal tumor. The soft palate has become short and heavily scarred. *(b)* Patient received chemoradiation for a carcinoma of the left tonsil. Following treatment, the soft palate was foreshortened and with significant scarring and fibrosis, especially in the left tonsillar fossa. *(c)* Soft palate shortened, a portion has been lost.

of mastication are within the clinical target volume, these patients also present with trismus (see Chapter 1, section entitled "Trismus, velopharyngeal incompetence, and dysphagia"). Examination usually reveals a shortened, fibrotic, heavily scarred soft palate and a lack of movement of the entire velopharyngeal complex (Figs 4-46 and 4-47a).

Prosthetic obturation is extremely challenging because of difficult access (the prosthesis must extend around and behind the residual soft palate) and trismus (Fig 4-47). Even if successful, speech will not be restored. The obturator bulb must be molded to allow nasal breathing, and because contraction of the muscles of velopharyngeal closure will be limited or absent, speech will be of a "mixed nasality" (both hypernasal and hyponasal). Moreover, these patients are not good candidates for a palatal lift even if sufficient dentition or osseointegrated implants are available to retain the prosthesis. The soft palate is usually quite short and is very difficult to lift because of fibrosis and scarring.

Palatal lift prostheses

The palatal lift prosthesis, as its name implies, displaces the soft palate superiorly and posteriorly to assist the soft palate to effect closure with the peripheral pharyngeal tissues. The popularity of the palatal lift prosthesis has increased since it was first advocated by Gibbons and Bloomer (1958). This type of prosthesis is especially useful for patients with velopharyngeal incompetence, a condition in which the velopharyngeal mechanism is anatomically intact, but the patient exhibits compromised motor control of the soft palate and related musculature. Such problems are found in patients affected by myasthenia gravis, cerebrovascular accidents, traumatic brain injuries, bulbar poliomyelitis, neuromuscular disease with bulbar symptoms, amyotrophic lateral sclerosis, cerebral palsy, injury to the soft palate (such as sequelae following adenoidectomy, tonsillectomy, or maxillary resections), cleft palate with VPI, and submucous cleft palate.

The objective of a palatal lift prosthesis is to displace the soft palate to the level of normal palatal elevation, enabling closure through the activity of the pharyngeal wall (Fig 4-48). If the length of the soft palate is insufficient to effect closure after maximal displacement, the addition of an obturator behind the displaced soft palate may be necessary (Fig 4-49). *Adequate lateral pharyngeal wall movement is necessary for the lift to be effective.* At rest, space for breathing should be present laterally between the displaced soft palate and the pharyngeal walls.

The advantages of a palatal lift prosthesis are as follows: *(1)* the gag response is minimized because of the superior position and

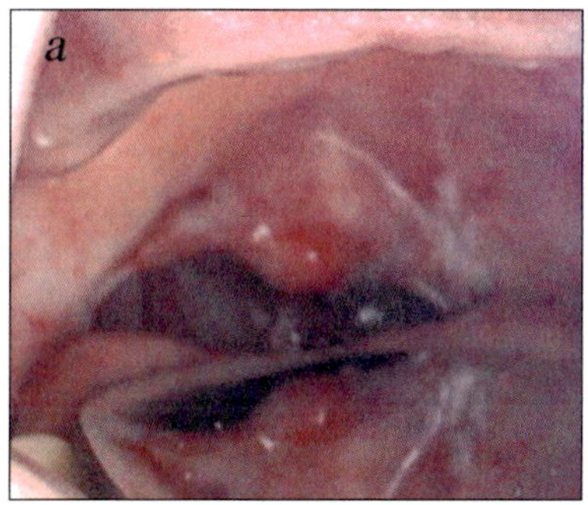

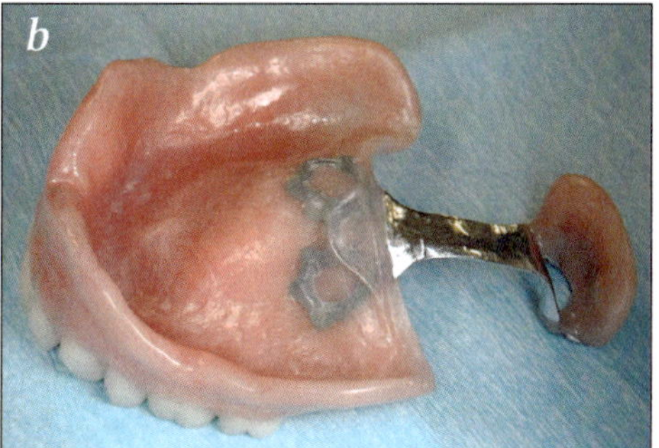

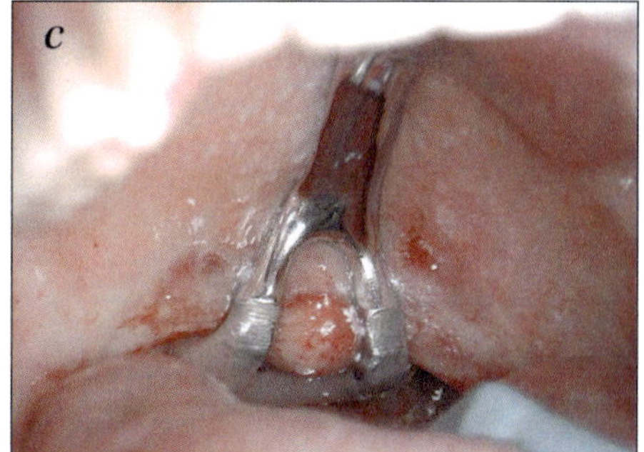

Figure 4-47 *(a)* Patient is four years postchemoradiation for a nasopharyngeal carcinoma. The soft palate is heavily fibrotic, severely scarred, and shortened. There is little movement of the velopharyngeal mechanism. *(b)* Complete denture-obturator prosthesis. *(c)* Prosthesis in position.

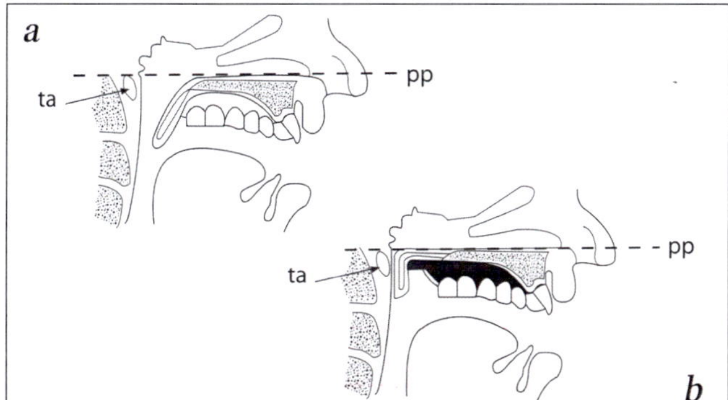

Figure 4-48 *(a)* Anatomically normal but paralyzed soft palate. *(b)* Palatal lift prosthesis in position, elevating the soft palate to produce velopharyngeal closure. PP—palatal plane; TA—median tubercle of the atlas (adapted from Gonzalez and Aronson, 1970, with permission).

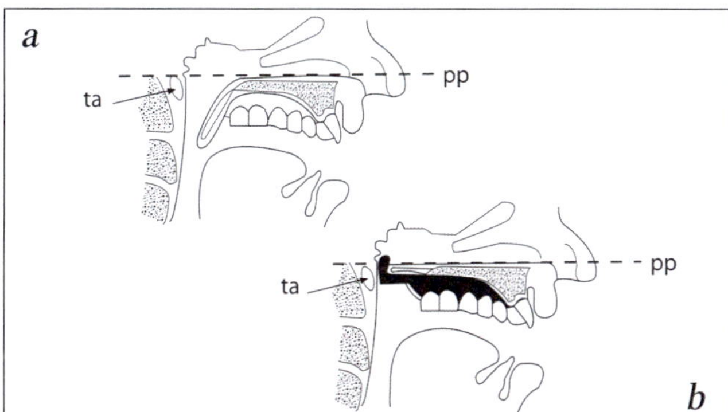

Figure 4-49 *(a)* Congenital anatomical insufficiency of velopharyngeal region. *(b)* Palatal lift plus obturator in position elevating the soft palate and obturating the velopharyngeal space. PP—palatal plane; TA—median tubercle of the atlas (adapted from Gonzalez and Aronson, 1970, with permission).

the sustained pressure of the lift portion of the prosthesis against the soft palate; *(2)* the physiology of the tongue is not compromised because of the more superior position of the palatal extension; *(3)* the access to the nasopharynx for the obturator (if necessary) is facilitated; *(4)* the lift portion may be developed sequentially to aid patient adaptation to the prosthesis; and *(5)* the lift principle has application to a diverse patient population that cannot be treated as effectively with palatal surgery or other types of obturator prostheses.

A palatal lift prosthesis is contraindicated if *(1)* adequate retention is not available for the basic prosthesis, *(2)* the palate is not displaceable, or *(3)* the patient is uncooperative. The displaceability of the soft palate can be checked by mechanical elevation of the soft palate with a mouth mirror.

The literature substantiates the effectiveness of palatal lift prostheses for neurologically handicapped patients. Lang (1967) advocated the use of lift prostheses for this group of patients but cautioned that concomitant speech therapy may be necessary for best results. Hardy et al. (1969) compared the surgical and prosthetic management of 17 children with cerebral palsy, inadequate velopharyngeal closure, and defective speech. Six children received pharyngeal flaps and 11 were treated with palatal lift prostheses. Only 3 of 6 surgical patients demonstrated improved speech, while 10 of 11 patients treated prosthetically demonstrated improved speech. Hardy et al. (1969) believed that the hyperactive gag reflex of the neuromuscularly handicapped child with an upper motor neuron lesion contraindicates the use of a conventional obturator prosthesis. In their view, palatal lift prostheses minimize the gag response and therefore are the treatment of choice. Surprisingly, these patients demonstrated sufficient lateral pharyngeal wall motion to achieve closure with the displaced soft palate and yet nasal breathing was maintained. Gonzalez and Aranson (1970), in a comprehensive study of 35 patients with palatal lift prostheses, reported that all but 3 patients exhibited improved speech and tolerated the prosthesis. The best results were obtained for patients in whom the neurologic disorder was confined to the soft palate. Patients with severe muscular paralysis of the lips, tongue, larynx, or respiratory musculature had residual articulatory defects following placement of the lift prosthesis. Several patients reported that less effort was involved in speaking. Also, the prosthesis stimulated soft palate and pharyngeal wall motion, permitting sequential reduction of the lift portion of the prosthesis.

Mazaheri and Mazaheri (1976) concurred with these observations and suggested myofunctional therapy in addition to speech therapy following delivery of the prosthesis. They reported that it was possible to stimulate the soft palate and contiguous tissues to the point where the prosthesis could be eliminated in some patients. Neither hard nor soft palate irritation nor adverse tooth movement was reported for patients using palatal lift prostheses. La Velle and Hardy (1979) studied 44 neurologically handicapped children and adults with intact but nonfunctional soft palates who were treated with palatal lift prostheses between 1972 and 1979.

Table 4-6 Number of patients with satisfactory and unsatisfactory results with palatal lift prostheses*‡

	Optimum	Successful	Desirable	Unsatisfactory	Total
Initial session	7	5	20	8	40
Last session	14	7	19	4	44

* Prostheses were made initially prior to 1972 for 4 of the 44 patients. Graph of palatopharyngeal port areas obtained while a patient was counting without a palatal lift prosthesis, after the prosthesis was first constructed, and after the last modification of the prosthesis.
‡ Reprinted from La Velle and Hardy (1970) with permission.

The molding process was monitored with oronasal airflow measurements, and the velopharyngeal port area was determined prior to, during, and after treatment was completed (Table 4-6). The authors cautioned that ideal treatment was not always possible. Every effort was made to mold the lift in one session, but some patients required additional sessions to reduce the size of the velopharyngeal portal.

Turner and Williams (1991) described the use of both multiview videofluoroscopy and nasoendoscopy for the design, placement, and modification of a palatal lift prosthesis. Wolfaardt et al. (1993) monitored 32 patients with palatal lift prostheses with nasoendoscopy, oronasal airflow measurements (PERCI), and a Nasometer prior to, during, and after treatment. It was possible to eliminate the prosthesis in 14 of 32 patients as velar function improved.

Esposito et al. (2000) reported on 25 patients with amyotrophic lateral sclerosis and bulbar symptoms. The patients presented with varying levels of dysarthria and were treated with palatal lift prostheses, regardless of their degree of debilitation. An independent speech pathologist determined that 21 of 25 (85%) demonstrated a reduction in hypernasality. The prosthesis was successfully worn by 19 of 25 patients (76%), and only two patients indicated that it was too uncomfortable to wear, even though there was speech improvement. Of the 19 who were successful, 17 felt that they personally experienced improvement, found it easier to speak (because oral air pressure was increased), and it was worth the effort to complete treatment.

Fabrication

A speech pathology consultation prior to fabrication of the prosthesis often proves helpful for the development of its extensions and contour. Video nasoendoscopy can also provide insight into the directional and volumetric demands of the appliance. A reasonably intact dentition, especially the presence of molar teeth bilaterally, is necessary for retention of the appliance. Edentulous patients can benefit from a palatal lift but require placement of osseointegrated implants (Montagner et al., 2012). The authors suggest that at least four implants be placed with a reasonable A-P spread in order to provide the necessary retention for the palatal lift. The posterior implants should be placed as far posteriorly as possible in order to reduce the length of the lever arm. For this reason, the tilted concept of implant placement is suggested, and if possible, implants should be placed in the pyramidal process of the palatal bone. For patients in whom the prospect of improvement may be difficult to predict, it is advisable to fabricate a provisional palatal lift prosthesis (Fig 4-50). The clinician may then proceed with the definitive prosthesis if it appears that meaningful improvement in speech can be achieved.

Construction of a palatal lift prosthesis begins with an impression procedure intended to record and displace the soft palate superiorly. To achieve this objective, the custom tray is extended with baseplate wax or impression compound as described previously (see Fig 4-26b). A suitable partial denture framework is fabricated and verified (Fig 4-51). A retentive loop for the lift is extended onto the soft palate as shown. It may require adjustment or replacement after the lift is molded (Fig 4-51d). RDP design concepts are similar to those employed for the fabrication of soft palate obturators. The placement of rests anteriorly, bilaterally positioned, serves as indirect retainers and provides resistance to the downward displacement of the palatal lift.

Tray resin is added to the retentive loop followed by a low-fusing impression compound until the appropriate displacement of the soft palate is achieved. It may be necessary to alter the cast in order to extend the tray along the palatal plane (Fig 4-50c and d). Appropriate displacement of the soft palate clinically is determined by speech and by monitoring nasal breathing. Nasoendoscopy can also be used to verify appropriate extensions and lifts. The posterior extension should be at or slightly posterior to the middle third of the soft palate in the area of the levator eminence. To achieve appropriate displacement of the soft palate, the width of the appliance varies according to the need to lift the palate while maintaining a nasal airway laterally (Fig 4-52). The patient's speech should be monitored for appropriate nasal resonance during the molding sequence. A thermoplastic material is used to refine the compound molded pattern.

Some patients may have difficulty adapting to the lift. In such circumstances, the lift may be extended posteriorly by sequential additions over several appointments. When complete, the appliance lifts the central portion of the palate so that it contacts the posterior pharyngeal wall but maintains space laterally for nasal breathing. The appliance can be extended behind the deficient soft palate if displacement does not achieve adequate obturation with a combination palatal lift–obturator prosthesis. Many patients present with little or no movement of the velopharyngeal musculature, so speech will have a "mixed nasality" character. Moreover, in such patients, usually the tongue has also been affected by the precipitating event (disease, trauma, CVA, etc.), so articulation errors will usually be significant. However, overall speech intelligibility will be significantly improved in these patients.

Palatal lift prostheses are usually of limited value for completely edentulous patients because of problems associated with retention of the maxillary complete denture. Loss of retention is caused by the combination of the long lever arm created by the lift extension and the downward dislodging force developed by any residual muscular tonicity of the soft palate. The desired lifting force most often must be reduced to be compatible with the amount of retention exhibited by the complete denture, defeating its purpose. As mentioned above, in such patients, placement of implants is recommended.

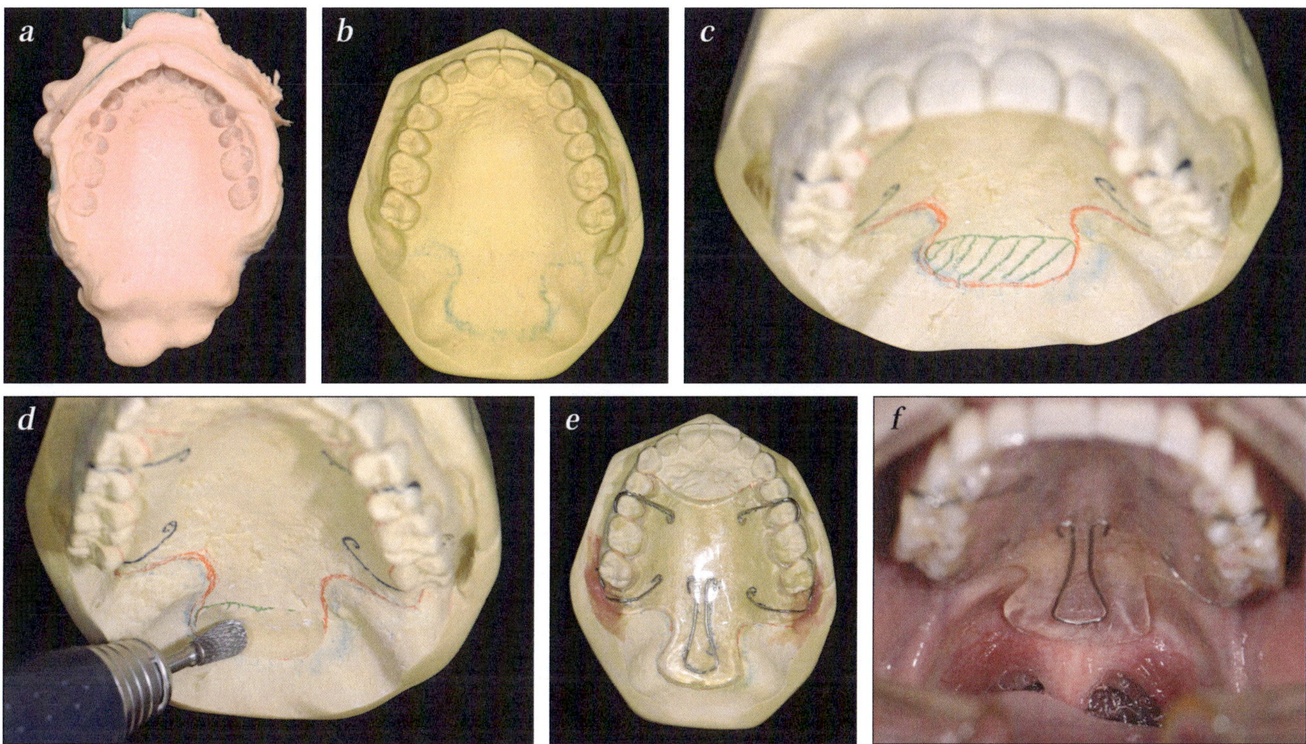

Figure 4-50 Fabrication of a provisional palatal lift. *(a)* Preliminary impression. Note that the soft palate has been displaced. *(b)* Preliminary cast. *(c and d)* The cast is altered arbitrarily. *(e)* The completed provisional palatal lift. *(f)* The provisional palatal lift in position. It is adjusted as necessary to ensure comfort and nasal breathing.

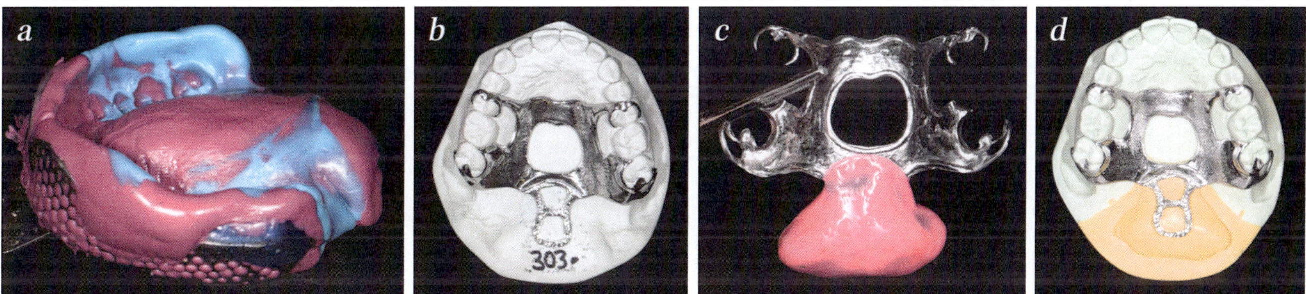

Figure 4-51 *(a)* Impression for the RDP framework. Note that the soft palate has been displaced with the impression. *(b)* RDP framework. The retentive loop is extended onto the soft palate. *(c)* Molded palatal lift. *(d)* Altered cast.

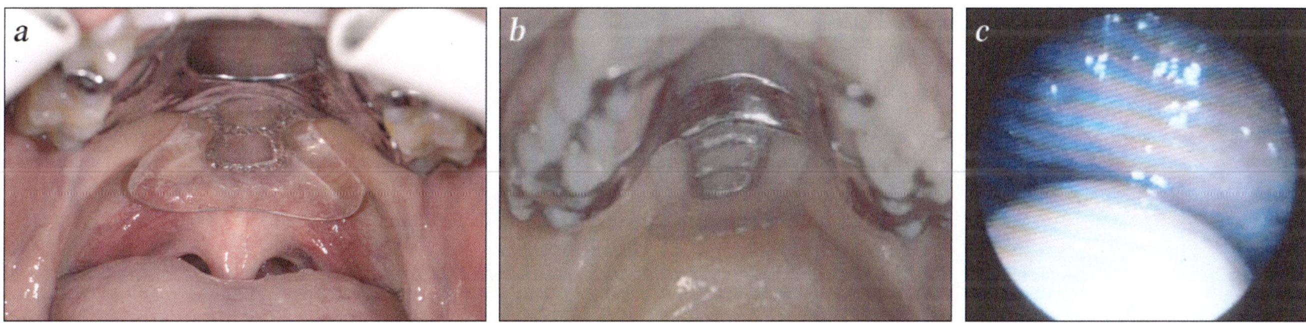

Figure 4-52 *(a and b)* Palatal lifts on two different patients. Note that the lift in "a" is wider than the lift in "b." The posterior extension and width of the lift are dependent upon the need to lift the palate to engage the posterior pharyngeal wall at the midline but still maintain a nasal airway. Upon delivery, lateral extensions are adjusted for comfort and speech. When the contours of the lift are complete it should lift the palate in the midline with space provided laterally for nasal breathing. This can be managed clinically but some clinicians *(c)* prefer to verify the degree of lift with a nasal endoscope. In this patient, the central portion of the palate has been nicely lifted while maintaining the nasal airway laterally ("c" courtesy of Dr. S. Esposito).

Occasionally, as in patients with amyotrophic lateral sclerosis and bulbar symptoms, both resonance and articulation are problematic. In these cases, a combination of a palatal lift/augmentation prosthesis can be used to improve both speech problems (Esposito et al., 2000). A similar approach has been used successfully in a patient presenting with velopharyngeal incompetency, dysarthria, and dysphagia secondary to surgical resection of a chondrosarcoma of the base of the skull (Asfar et al., 2019).

Patients with palatal lift prostheses should be monitored closely to ensure that the lifting force does not create soreness and that the force of the displaced soft palate does not have an adverse effect on the dentition retaining the appliance. It has been reported that increased soft palate and pharyngeal wall motion in some patients following delivery postinsertion have required reduction of the prosthesis (Gonzales and Aranson, 1970; Mazaheri and Mazaheri, 1976; Wolfaardt et al., 1993).

Summary

The components of speech that can be impacted by prosthodontic treatment are articulation and resonance. A thorough understanding of speech and velopharyngeal function is necessary if the prosthodontist is to achieve successful outcomes with obturator prostheses for patients with soft palate defects. Obturator prostheses can restore speech and swallowing to normal limits in patients with soft palate defects under the following circumstances: *(1)* when there is functional movement of the residual velopharyngeal musculature and *(2)* when access permits the maxillofacial prosthodontist to properly engage this musculature with the obturator prosthesis. Without access to the residual velopharyngeal mechanism, an obturator prosthesis cannot help restore speech; therefore, surgical closures that preclude access to the defect are discouraged.

Proper retention is required if the prosthesis is to be accurately and reproducibly positioned; the placement of osseointegrated implants is recommended in edentulous patients. Surgical reconstruction of soft palate defects, although possible with some defects, is risky because it often precludes the fabrication of a successful obturator prosthesis in the event of an unfavorable result. Thorough knowledge and understanding of speech and the velopharyngeal mechanism are absolutely mandatory for clinicians who seek to fabricate effective obturator prostheses for soft palate defects.

Palatal lift prostheses play an important role in the care of patients with velopharyngeal incompetence. However, the speech therapist, the maxillofacial prosthodontist, and the patient must understand the limits in functional speech improvements that can be achieved with this device.

References

Anderson R. Nasometric values for normal Spanish-speaking females: A preliminary report. Cleft Palate Craniofac J 1996;33:333–336.

Andreassen ML, Leeper HA, MacRae DL. Clinical applications of nasometry: Tonsillectomy and adenoidectomy. In Nasometer application notes: Model 6200. Pine Brook, NJ: Kay Elemetrics; 1990. pp. 2–9.

Aram A, Subtelny JD. Velopharyngeal function and cleft palate prosthesis. J Prosthet Dent 1959;9:149–158.

Asfar MM, Hutcheson KA, Won AM. Prosthetic Rehabilitation with Palatal Lift/Augmentation in a Patient with Neurologic/Motor Deficit Due To Cancer Therapy for Chondrosarcoma. J Prosthodont 2019;28:234–238.

Ashley FL, Sloan RF, Hahn E, et al. Cinefluorographic study of palatal incompetency cases during deglutition and phonation. Plast Reconstr Surg 1961;28:347–364.

Attanasio JS. Relationships between oral sensory feedback skills and adaptation to delayed auditory feedback. J Commun Disord 1987;20:391–402.

Azzam NA, Kuehn, DP. The morphology of the musculus uvulae. Cleft Palate J 1977;14:331.

Bae Y, Kuehn DP, Sutton BP, et al. Three-dimensional magnetic resonance imaging of velopharyngeal structures. J Speech Lang Hear Res 2011;54(6):1538–1545. http://doi.org/10.1044/1092-4388(2011/10-0021).

Barnes IJ. Interrelationships among oral breath pressure ratios and articulation skills for individuals with cleft palate. J Speech Hear Res 1967;10:506–514.

Baudonck N, Van Lierde K, D'haeseleer E, et al. Nasalance and nasality in children with cochlear implants and children with hearing aids. Int J Pediatr Otorhinolaryngol 2015;79(4):541–545. http://doi.org/10.1016/j.ijporl.2015.01.025.

Beer AJ, Hellerhoff P, Zimmermann A, et al. Dynamic near-real-time magnetic resonance imaging for analyzing the velopharyngeal closure in comparison with videofluoroscopy. J Magn Reson Imaging 2004;20:791–797.

Bell-Berti F. An electromyographic study of velopharyngeal function in speech. J Speech Hear Res 1976;19:225–240.

Benediktsson E. Variation in tongue and jaw positioning "S" sound production in relation to front teeth occlusion. Acta Odontol Scand 1957;15:275–301.

Berry QC, Aramany MA, Katzenberg B. Oral endoscopy in prosthodontic management of the soft palate defect. J Prosthet Dent 1985;54:241–244.

Blackfield HM, Miller ER, Owsley JQ, et al. Comparative evaluation of diagnostic techniques in patients with cleft palate speech. Plast Reconstr Surg 1962;29:153–158.

Blakeley RW. The complementary use of speech prostheses and pharyngeal flaps in palatal insufficiency. Cleft Palate J 1964;1:194–198.

Bloomer H. Observations on palato-pharyngeal movements in speech and deglutition. J Speech Hear Disord 1953;18:230–246.

Bluestone CD, Paradise JL, Beery QC, et al. Certain effects of cleft palate repair on eustachian tube function. Cleft Palate J 1972;9:183–193.

Boone DR, McFarlane SC. The voice and voice therapy. Englewood Cliffs, NJ: Prentice-Hall; 1988.

Borden GJ, Harris KS. Speech science primer: Physiology, acoustics, and perception of speech. Baltimore: Williams & Wilkins; 1984.

Bosma JF, Fletcher SG. The upper pharynx: A review: II. Physiology. Ann Otol Rhinol Laryngol 1962;71:134–157.

Bou C, Liang Fat AS, de Mones Del Pujol E, et al. A new membrane obturator prosthesis concept for soft palate defects. Int J Prosthodont 2018 Nov/Dec;31(6):584–586. http://doi.org/10.11607/ijp.5755. PMID: 30408140.

Brandt SD, Morris HL. The linearity of the relationship between articulation errors and velopharyngeal incompetence. Cleft Palate J 1965;2:176–183.

Bressmann T, Sader R, Whitehill TL, et al. Nasalance distance and ratio: Two new measures. Cleft Palate Craniofac J 2000;37:248–256.

Brooks AR, Shelton RL, Youngstrom KA. Compensatory tongue-palate posterior pharyngeal wall relationships in cleft palate. J Speech Hear Disord 1965;30:166–173.

Brooks AR, Shelton RL, Youngstrom KA. Tongue-palate contact in persons with palate defects. J Speech Hear Disord 1966;31:14–25.

Butterworth CJ, Lowe D, Rogers SN. The zygomatic implant perforated (ZIP) flap reconstructive technique for the management of low-level maxillary malignancy—clinical & patient related outcomes on 35 consecutively treated patients. Head Neck 2022;44:345–358.

Butz F, Aita H, Wang CC, et al. Harder and stiffer osseointegrated bone to roughened titanium. J Dent Res 2006;85:560–565.

Bzoch KR, Grabner TM, Aoba T. A study of normal velopharyngeal valving for speech. Cleft Palate Bull 1959;9:3–4.

Bzoch KR. Clinical studies of the efficacy of speech appliances compared to pharyngeal flap surgery. Cleft Palate J 1964;35:275–286.

Calnan JS. Modern views on Passavant's ridge. Br J Plast Surg 1957;29:89–113.

Carney PJ, Morris HL. Structural correlates of nasality. Cleft Palate J 1971;8:307–321.

Carpenter MA, Morris HL. A preliminary study of Passavant's pad. Cleft Palate J 1968;5:61–72.

Casey DM. Palatopharyngeal anatomy and physiology. J Prosthet Dent 1983;49:371–378.

Casey DM, Emrich LJ. Passavant's ridge in patients with soft palatectomy. Cleft Palate J 1988;25:72–77.

Chanchareonsook N, Whitehill TL, Samman N. Speech outcome and velopharyngeal function in cleft palate: Comparison of Le Fort I maxillary osteotomy and distraction osteogenesis—early results. Cleft Palate Craniofac J 2007;44:23–32.

Chang TL, Orellana D, Beumer J. Kratochvil's fundamentals of removal partial dentures. Chicago: Quintessence; 2019.

Chierici G, Lawson L. Clinical speech considerations in prosthodontics: Perspectives of the prosthodontist and speech pathologist. J Prosthet Dent 1973;29–39.

Clendaniel C. Three cases involving nasality. In Nasometer application notes: Model 6200. Pine Brook, NJ: Kay Elemetrics; 1990. pp. 48–53.

Cole RM. Speech. In ASHA Reports 6: Patterns of oral growth and development. Ed. RT Wertz, HL Morris. Washington, DC: American Speech-Language-Hearing Association; 1971. pp. 79–95.

Colton RH, Cooker HS. Perceived nasality in the speech of the deaf. J Speech Hear Res 1968;11:553–559.

Counihan DT, Cullinan WL. Reliability and dispersion of nasality ratings. Cleft Palate J 1970;7:261–270.

Croft CB. The occult submucous cleft palate and the musculus uvulae. Cleft Palate J 1978;15:150–154.

Croft CB, Shprintzen RJ, Rakof SJ. Patterns of velopharyngeal valving in normal and cleft palate subjects: A multiview videofluoroscopic and nasoendoscopic study. Laryngoscope 1981;91:265–271.

Dalston RM, Neiman GS, Gonzalez-Landa G. Nasometric sensitivity and specificity: A cross-dialect and cross-culture study. Cleft Palate Craniofac J 1993;30:285–291.

Dalston RM, Warren DW, Dalston E. The identification of nasal obstruction through clinical judgments of hyponasality and nasometric assessment of speech acoustics. Am J Orthod Dentofacial Orthop 1991a;100:59–65.

Dalston RM, Warren DW, Dalston E. A preliminary investigation concerning the use of nasometry in identifying patients with hyponasality and/or nasal airway impairment. J Speech Hear Res 1991b;34:11–18.

Dalston RM, Warren DW, Dalston E. Use of nasometry as a diagnostic tool for identifying patients with velopharyngeal impairment. Cleft Palate Craniofac J 1991c;28:184–189.

Dalston RM, Warren DW, Dalston ET. A preliminary study of nasal airway patency and its potential effect on speech performance. Cleft Palate Craniofac J 1992;29:330–335.

Dalston RM, Warren DW, Morr KE, et al. Intraoral pressure and its relationship to velopharyngeal inadequacy. Cleft Palate J 1988;25:210–219.

Dalston RM, Warren DW, Smith LR. The aerodynamic characteristics of speech produced by normal speakers and cleft palate speakers with adequate velopharyngeal function. Cleft Palate J 1990;27:393–401.

Denegri MA, Silva PP, Pegoraro-Krook MI, et al. Cephalometric predictors of hypernasality and nasal air emission. J Appl Oral Sci 2021;29:e20210320. http://doi.org/10.1590/1678-7757-2021-0320.

Devani P, Watts R, Markus AF. Speech outcome in children with cleft palate: Aerophonoscope assessment of nasal emission. J Craniomaxillofac Surg 1999;27:180–186.

Di W, Zhao J, Ma H, et al. Three-dimensional anatomy of the palatopharyngeus and its relation to the levator veli palatini based on micro-computed tomography. Plast Reconstr Surg 2021;148(3):389e–397e. http://doi.org/10.1097/PRS.0000000000008275.

Dickson DR. Anatomy of the normal velopharyngeal mechanism. Clin Plast Surg 1975;2:235–248.

Dickson DR. Normal and cleft palate anatomy. Cleft Palate J 1972;9:280–293.

Dickson DR, Dickson WM. Velopharyngeal anatomy. J Speech Hear Res 1972;15:372–381.

Dickson DR, Grant JC, Sicher H, et al. Status of research in cleft palate anatomy and physiology, July 1973. Cleft Palate J 1974;11:471–492.

Dorrance GM. Congenital insufficiency of the palate. Arch Surg 1930;21:185–248.

Dudas JR, Deleyiannis FW, Ford MD, et al. Diagnosis and treatment of velopharyngeal insufficiency: Clinical utility of speech evaluation and videofluoroscopy. Ann Plast Surg 2006;56:511–517.

Eblen LE, Sie KC. Perceptual and instrumental assessment of velopharyngeal insufficiency. Plast Reconstr Surg 2002;109:2589–2590.

Ehmer U, Broll P. Mandibular border movements and masticatory patterns before and after orthognathic surgery. Int J Adult Orthodont Orthognath Surg 1992;7:153–159.

Esposito S. Speech and palatopharyngeal function. In Proceedings of the First International Congress on Maxillofacial Prosthetics. Ed. I Zlotolow, S Esposito, J Beumer. New York: Memorial Sloan-Kettering Cancer Center; 1995. pp. 43–48.

Esposito S, Mitsumoto H, Shanks M. Use of palatal lift and palatal augmentation prostheses to improve dysarthria in patients with amyotrophic lateral sclerosis: A case series. J Prosthet Dent 2000;83:90–98.

Ettema SL, Kuehn DP, Perlman AL, et al. Magnetic resonance imaging of the levator veli palatini muscle during speech. Cleft Palate Craniofac J 2002;39:130–144.

Fairbanks G, Lintner MV. The study of minor organic deviations in functional disorders of articulation: 4. The teeth and hard palate. J Speech Disord 1951;16:273–279.

Fairbanks G. Selective vocal effects of delayed auditory feedback. J Speech Hear Disord 1955;20:333–346.

Fara M, Dvorak J. Abnormal anatomy of the muscles of palatopharyngeal closure in cleft palates: Anatomical and surgical considerations based on the autopsies of 18 unoperated cleft palates. Plast Reconstr Surg 1970;46:488–497.

Fletcher SG. Process and maturation of mastication and deglutition In ASHA Report 5: Speech and the dentofacial complex: The state of the art. Ed. RT Wertz. Washington, DC: American Speech-Language-Hearing Association; 1970. pp. 92–105.

Fletcher SG, Frost SD. Quantitative and graphic analysis of prosthetic treatment for nasalance in speech. J Prosthet Dent 1974;32:284–291.

Fritzell B. The velopharyngeal muscles in speech. Acta Otolaryngol 1969;suppl 250:1–81.

Fucci D, Crary M, Warren JA, et al. Interaction between auditory and oral sensory feedback in speech regulation. Percept Mot Skills 1977;45:123–129.

Gibbons P, Bloomer H. A supportive-type prosthetic speech aid. J Prosthet Dent 1958;8:362–368.

Gibbs CH, Messerman T. Jaw motion during speech. In ASHA Reports 7: Orofacial function: Clinical research in dentistry and speech pathology. Ed. RT Wertz. Washington, DC: American Speech-Language-Hearing Association; 1972. pp. 104–112.

Glaser ER, Skolnick ML, McWilliams BJ, et al. The dynamics of Passavant's ridge in subjects with and without velopharyngeal insufficiency—a multi-view videofluoroscopic study. Cleft Palate J 1979;16:24–33.

Goldstein J. Two case studies: Evaluation of hypernasality and management of cleft lip and palate. In Nasometer application notes: Model 6200. Pine Brook, NJ: Kay Elemetrics; 1990. pp. 54–56.

Gonzalez JB, Aronson AE. Palatal lift prostheses for treatment of anatomic and neurologic palatopharyngeal insufficiency. Cleft Palate J 1970;7:91–104.

Graber BH, Monroe CW, Hill BJ, et al. Motion of the lateral pharyngeal wall during velopharyngeal closure. Plast Reconstr Surg 1958;41:338–342.

Graber TM, Bzoch KR, Aoba T. A functional study of the palatal and pharyngeal structures. Angle Orthod 1959;29:30–40.

Griffith BH, Monroe CW, Hill BJ, et al. Motion of the lateral wall during velopharyngeal closure. Plast Reconstr Surg 1968;41:338–342.

Hagerty RF, Hess DA, Mylin WK. Velar motility, velopharyngeal closure and speech proficiency in cartilage pharyngeoplasty: The effect of age at surgery. Cleft Palate J 1968;5:317–326.

Hain TC, Burnett TA, Larson CR, et al. Effects of delayed auditory feedback (DAF) on the pitch-shift reflex. J Acoust Soc Am 2001;109(5 Pt 1):2146–2152. http://doi.org/10.1121/1.1366319.

Hairfield WM, Warren DW, Hinton VA, et al. Inspiratory and expiratory effects of nasal breathing. Cleft Palate J 1987;24:183–189.

Hardin MA, Van Demark DR, Morris HL, et al. Correspondence between nasalance scores and listener judgments of hypernasality and hyponasality. Cleft Palate Craniofac J 1992;29:346–351.

Hardy JC, Netsell R, Schweiger JW, et al. Management of velopharyngeal dysfunction in cerebral palsy. J Speech Hear Disord 1969;34:123–137.

Harkins CS, Harkins WR, Harkins JF. Principles of cleft palate prosthesis. New York: Columbia University; 1960.

Hartman DE, Danhauer JL. Perceptual features of speech for males in four perceived age decades. J Acoust Soc Am 1976;59:713–715.

Helfer KS. Auditory and auditory-visual perception of clear and conversational speech. J Speech Lang Hear Res 1997;40:432–443.

Henningsson G, Isberg A. Comparison between multi-view videofluoroscopy and nasendoscopy of velopharyngeal movements. Cleft Palate Craniofac J 1991;28:413–418.

Hess DA. Pitch, intensity, and cleft palate voice quality. J Speech Hear Res 1959;2:113–125.

Hillman RE, Holmberg EB, Perkell JS, et al. Objective assessment of vocal hyperfunction: An experimental framework and initial results. J Prosthet Dent 1989;32:373–392.

Hood LJ. An overview of neural function and feedback control in human communication. J Commun Disord 1998;31:461–470.

Houde JF, Jordan MI. Sensorimotor adaptation in speech production. Science 1998;279:1213–1216.

Huang MH, Lee ST, Rajendran K. A fresh cadaveric study of the paratubal muscles: Implications for eustachian tube function in cleft palate. Plast Reconstr Surg 1997;100:833–842.

Huntington DA. Anatomical and physiological bases for speech. In Cleft palate and communication. Ed. DC Spriestersbach, D Sherman. New York: Academic; 1968. pp. 1–25.

Hutchinson JM, Robinson KL, Nerbonne MA. Patterns of nasalance in a sample of normal gerontologic participants. J Commun Disord 1978;11:469–481.

Isberg AM, Henningsson GE. Intra individual change in occurrence of Passavant's ridge due to change in velopharyngeal sphincter function: A videofluoroscopic study. Cleft Palate J 1990;27:253–255.

Isshiki N, Honjow I, Morimoto M. Cineradiographic analysis of movement of the lateral pharyngeal wall. Plast Reconstr Surg 1969;44:357–363.

Jefferson ND, Willging JP. Management of noncleft velopharyngeal insufficiency. Curr Opin Otolaryngol Head Neck Surg 2021 Aug;29(4):283–288. http://doi.org/10.1097/MOO.0000000000000735.

Jensen OT, Adams MW, Butura C, et al. Maxillary V-4: Four implant treatment for maxillary atrophy with dental implants fixed apically at the vomer-nasal crest, lateral pyriform rim, and zygoma for immediate function: Report on 44 patients followed from 1 to 3 years. J Prosthet Dent 2015;114:810–817.

Jiang JJ, Lin E, Hanson DG. Vocal fold physiology. Otolaryngol Clin North Am 2000;33:699–718.

Jiang RS, Huang HT. Changes in nasal resonance after functional endoscopic sinus surgery. Am J Rhinol 2006;20:432–437.

Kane AA, Butman JA, Mullick R, et al. A new method for the study of velopharyngeal function using gated magnetic resonance imaging. Plast Reconstr Surg 2002;109:472–481.

Kangatharan J, Uther M, Gobet F. The effect of hyperarticulation on speech comprehension under adverse listening conditions. Psychol Res 2022 Jul;86(5):1535–1546. http://doi.org/10.1007/s00426-021-01595-2.

Kantner CE, West R. Phonetics. New York: Harper & Brothers; 1941.

Karnell MP, Rosenstein H, Fine L. Nasal videoendoscopy in prosthetic management of palatopharyngeal dysfunction. J Prosthet Dent 1987;58:479–484.

Kavanagh ML, Fee EJ, Kalinowski J, et al. Nasometric values for three dialectical groups within the Atlantic provinces of Canada. J Speech Lang Pathol Audiol 1994;18:7–13.

Kelsey CA, Ewanowski SJ, Crummy AB, et al. Lateral pharyngeal-wall motion as a predictor of surgical success in velopharyngeal insufficiency. New Engl J Med 1972;287:64–68.

Kim EY, Yoon MS, Kim HH, et al. Characteristics of nasal resonance and perceptual rating in prelingual hearing impaired adults. Clin Exp Otorhinolaryngol 2012;5(1):1–9. http://doi.org/10.3342/ceo.2012.5.1.1.

Kollara L, Schenck G, Jaskolka M, et al. Examining a new method to studying velopharyngeal structures in a child with 22q11.2 deletion syndrome. J Speech Lang Hear Res 2017;60(4):892–896. http://doi.org/10.1044/2016_JSLHR-S-16-0084.

Kotare KJ, Sitzman TJ, Williams JL, et al. Nonsedated magnetic resonance imaging for visualization of the velopharynx in the pediatric population. Cleft Palate Craniofac J 2023;60(2):249–252. http://doi.org/10.1177/10556656211057361.

Kratochvil FJ. Partial removable prosthodontics. Philadelphia: WB Saunders; 1988.

Kuehn DP. A cineradiograph investigation of velar movement variables in two normals. Cleft Palate J 1976;13:88–103.

Kuehn DP, Folkins JW, Cutting CB. Relationships between muscle activity and velar position. Cleft Palate J 1982;19:25–35.

Kuehn DP, Folkins JW, Linville RN. An electromyographic study of the musculus uvulae. Cleft Palate J 1988;25:348–355.

Kuehn DP, Kahane JC. Histologic study of the normal human adult soft palate. Cleft Palate J 1990;27:26–34.

Kuehn DP, Moon JB. Histologic study of intravelar structures in normal human adult specimens. Cleft Palate Craniofac J 2005;42:481–489.

Kummer AW. Cleft palate and craniofacial conditions: A comprehensive guide to clinical management. 4th ed. Burlington, MA: Jones & Bartlett; 2018.

Kummer AW, Brigs M, Lee L. The relationship between the characteristics of speech and velopharyngeal gap size. Cleft Palate Craniofac J 2003;40:590–596.

La Velle WE, Hardy JC. Palatal lift prostheses for treatment of palatopharyngeal incompetence. J Prosthet Dent 1979;42:308–315.

Laine T, Warren DW, Dalston RM, et al. Intraoral pressure, nasal pressure and airflow rate in cleft palate speech. J Speech Hear Res 1988a;31:432–437.

Laine T, Warren DW, Dalston RM, et al. Screening of velopharyngeal closure based on nasal airflow rate measurements. Cleft Palate J 1988b;25:220–225.

Lam DJ, Starr JR, Perkins JA, et al. A comparison of nasendoscopy and multiview videofluoroscopy in assessing velopharyngeal insufficiency. Otolaryngol Head Neck Surg 2006;134:394–402.

Lang B. Modification of the palatal lift speech aid. J Prosthet Dent 1967;17:620–626.

Larson CR. Cross-modality influences in speech motor control: The use of pitch shifting for the study of F0 control. J Commun Disord 1998;31:489–502.

Lawrence CW, Philips BJ. A telefluoroscopic study of lingual contacts made by persons with palatal defects. Cleft Palate J 1975;12:85–94.

Lee A, Whitehill TL, Ciocca V. Effect of listener training on perceptual judgment of hypernasality. Clin Ling Phonet 2009;23:319–334.

Leeper H, Rochet A, MacKay I. Characteristics of nasalance in Canadian speakers of English and French. Presented at the Second International Conference on Spoken Language Processing, Banff, Alberta, Canada, 13–16 Oct 1992. pp. 49–52.

Levelt WJM. Speaking: From intention to articulation. Cambridge, MA: MIT University; 1989.

Lewin ML, Croft CB, Shprintzen RJ. Velopharyngeal insufficiency due to hypoplasia of the musculus uvulae and occult submucous cleft palate. Plast Reconstr Surg 1980;65:585–591.

Li W, Lin J, Fu M. Electromyographic investigation of masticatory muscles in unilateral cleft lip and palate patients with anterior crossbite. Cleft Palate Craniofac J 1998;35:415–418.

Liedman-Boshko J, Lohmander A, Persson AL, et al. Perceptual analysis of speech and the activity in the lateral pharyngeal walls before and after velopharyngeal flap surgery. Scand J Plast Reconstr Surg Hand Surg 2005;39:22–32.

Lin HC, Cheng CH, Chen G. The prevalence of Passavant's ridge in patients with velopharyngeal insufficiency in a Taiwan Chinese population. J Dent Sci 2019;14(1):15–20. http://doi.org/10.1016/j.jds.2018.10.002.

Lintz LB, Sherman D. Phonetic elements and perception of nasality. J Speech Hear Res 1961;4:381–396.

Liu JL, Li SH, Cai YM, et al. Automated radiographic evaluation of adenoid hypertrophy based on VGG-lite. J Dent Res 2021;100(12):1337–1343. http://doi.org/10.1177/00220345211009474.

Lloyd RS, Pruzansky S, Subtelny JD. Prosthetic rehabilitation of a cleft palate patient subsequent to multiple surgical and prosthetic failures. J Prosthet Dent 1957;7:216–230.

Lubker JF, Schweiger JW. Nasal airflow as an index of success of prosthetic management of cleft palate. J Dent Res 1969;48:368–375.

Ludlow CL, Cikoja DB. Is there a self-monitoring speech perception system? J Commun Disord 1998;31:505–510.

MacNeilage PF. The frame/content theory of evolution of speech production. Behav Brain Sci 1998;21:499–511.

MacNeilage PF, DeClerk JL. On the motor control of coarticulation of CVC monosyllables. J Acoust Soc Am 1969;45:1217–1233.

Martone AL. Clinical applications of concepts of functional anatomy and speech science to complete denture prosthodontics. J Prosthet Dent 1962;12:817–834.

Massengill R Jr, Quinn GW, Pickrell KL, et al. Therapeutic exercise and velopharyngeal gap. Cleft Palate J 1968;5:44–47.

Matsuya T, Miyazaki T, Yamaoka M. Fiberscopic examination of velopharyngeal closure in normal individuals. Cleft Palate J 1974;11:286–291.

Maue-Dickson W. The craniofacial complex in cleft lip and palate: An updated review of anatomy and function. Cleft Palate J 1979;16:291–317.

Mazaheri M, Mazaheri EH. Prosthodontic aspects of palatal elevation and palatopharyngeal stimulation. J Prosthet Dent 1976;35:319–326.

Mazaheri M, Millard RT. Changes in resonance related to differences in location and dimension of speech bulbs. Cleft Palate J 1964;2:167–175.

McKerns D, Bzoch KR. Variations in velopharyngeal valving: The factor of sex. Cleft Palate J 1970;7:652–662.

McKinstry A, Perry A. Evaluation of speech in people with head and neck cancer: A pilot study. Int J Lang Commun Disord 2003;38:31–46.

McNulty EC, Lear CS, Moorrees FA. Variability in lip adaptation to changes in incisor position. J Dent Res 1968;47:537–547.

McWilliams BJ. Some factors in the intelligibility of cleft-palate speech. J Speech Hear Disord 1954;19:524–528.

McWilliams BJ, Musgrave RH, Crozier PA. The influence of head position upon velopharyngeal closure. Cleft Palate J 1968;5:117–124.

Mehendale FV. Surgical anatomy of the levator veli palatini: A previously undescribed tendinous insertion of the anterolateral fibers. Plast Reconstr Surg 2004;114:307–315.

Melan JB, Philouze P, Pradat P, et al. Functional outcomes of soft palate free flap reconstruction following oropharyngeal cancer surgery. Eur J Surg Oncol 2021 Sep;47(9):2265–2271. http://doi.org/10.1016/j.ejso.2021.04.044. Epub 2021 May 7. PMID: 33994058.

Minsley GE, Warren DW, Hairfield WM. The effect of cleft palate speech aid prostheses on the nasopharyngeal airway and breathing. J Prosthet Dent 1991;65:122–126.

Miyazaki T, Matsuya F, Yamaoka M. Fiberscopic methods for assessment of velopharyngeal closure during various activities. Cleft Palate J 1975;12:107–114.

Moll KL. A cinefluorographic study of velopharyngeal function in normals during various activities. Cleft Palate J 1965;2:112–122.

Molt LF. Use of the Nasometer in palatal prosthesis configuration adjustments. In Nasometer application notes: Model 6200. Pine Brook, NJ: Kay Elemetrics; 1990. pp. 64–67.

Montagner A, Fontoura-Frasca LC, Rivaldo EG. Implant-supported palatal lift prosthesis in a patient with velopharyngeal incompetence: A case report. Gerodontology 2012;29:1180–1184.

Moon JB, Folkins JW, Smith A, et al. Air pressure regulation during speech production. J Acoust Soc Am 1993;94:54–63.

Morley ME. Cleft palate speech. Baltimore: Williams & Wilkins; 1966.

Morris HL, Spriestersbach DC, Darley FL. An articulation test for addressing competency of velopharyngeal closure. J Speech Hear Res 1961;4:48–55.

Naveau A, Kret M, Plaire V, et al. Efficacy of a new membrane obturator prosthesis in terms of speech, swallowing, and the quality of life of patients with acquired soft palate defects: Study protocol of the VELOMEMBRANE randomized cross-over trial. Trials 2022;23:221. http://doi.org/10.1186/s13063-022-06163-6.

Neiman GS, Simpson RK. A roentgencephalometric investigation of the effect of adenoid removal upon selected measures of velopharyngeal function. Cleft Palate J 1975;12:373–389.

Nellis JL, Neiman GS, Lehman JA. Comparison of Nasometer and listener judgments of nasality in the assessment of velopharyngeal function after pharyngeal flap surgery. Cleft Palate Craniofac J 1992;29:157–163.

Ngim RC, Chua E, Lee ST. Speech and nasendoscopic evaluation of velopharyngeal incompetence (VPI) in cleft palate patients. Ann Acad Med Singapore 1988;17:380–383.

Nichols A. Nasalance statistics for two Mexican populations. Cleft Palate Craniofac J 1999;36:57–63.

Nicoletti G, Soutar DS, Jackson MS, et al. Objective assessment of speech after surgical treatment for oral cancer: Experience from 196 selected cases. Plast Reconstr Surg 2004;113:114–125.

Nishio J, Matsuya I, Machida J, et al. The motor nerve supply of the velopharyngeal muscles. Cleft Palate J 1976a;13:20–30.

Nishio J, Matsuya T, Sbuki K, et al. Roles of the facial, glossopharyngeal and vagus nerves in velopharyngeal movement. Cleft Palate J 1976b;13:201–214.

Nylen BO. Cleft palate and speech. Acta Radiol Suppl 1961;203:1–124.

Ogawa T, Nishimura I. Genes differentially expressed in titanium healing. J Dent Res 2006;85:566–570.

Ortiz-Monasterio F, Olmedo A, Trigos I, et al. Final results from the delayed treatment of patients with clefts of the lip and palate. Scand J Plast Surg 1974;8:109–115.

Passavant PG. Uber die Verschliesung des Schlunmdes beim Sprechen, (Virchows) Arch Path Anat (Berlin) Virchows 1869;1–31.

Perry JL, Sutton BP, Kuehn DP, et al. Using MRI for assessing velopharyngeal structures and function. Cleft Palate Craniofac J 2014;51(4):476–485. http://doi.org/10.1597/12-083.

Persson C, Lohmander A, Elander A. Speech in children with an isolated cleft palate: A longitudinal perspective. Cleft Palate Craniofac J 2006;43:295–309.

Picheny MA, Durlach NI, Braida LD. Speaking clearly for the hard of hearing III: An attempt to determine the contribution of speaking rate differences in intelligibility between clear and conversational speech. J Speech Hear Res 1989;32:600–603.

Pigott RW. The nasendoscopic appearance of the normal palato-pharyngeal valve. Plast Reconstr Surg 1969;43:19–24.

Pound E. Let /s/ be your guide. J Prosthet Dent 1977;38:482–489.

Pound E. The mandibular movements of speech and their seven related values. J Prosthet Dent 1966;16:835–843.

Powers GR. Cinefluorographic investigation of articulatory movements of selected individuals with cleft palates. J Speech Hear Res 1962;5:59–69.

Pruzansky S, Mason RM. The "stretch factor" in soft palate function. J Dent Res 1969;49:972.

Putnam AH, Shelton RL, Kastner CU. Intraoral air pressure and oral air flow under different bleed and bite-block conditions. J Speech Hear Res 1986;29:37–49.

Rahn AO, Boucher LJ. Maxillofacial prosthetics. Philadelphia: Saunders; 1970.

Ramig L. Effects of psychological aging on speaking and reading rates. J Commun Disord 1983;16:217–226.

Redenbaugh MA, Reich AR. Correspondence between accelerometric nasal/voice amplitude ratio and listeners' direct magnitude estimations of hypernasality. J Speech Hear Res 1985;28:273–281.

Reich AR, Redenbaugh MA. Relation between nasal/voice accelerometric values and interval estimates of hypernasality. Cleft Palate J 1985;22:237–245.

Reisberg DJ, Smith BE. Aerodynamic assessment of prosthetic speech aids. J Prosthet Dent 1985;54:686–690.

Ricketts RM. Respiratory obstruction syndrome. Am J Orthod 1968;54:495–507.

Rieger J, Bohle G III, Huryn J, et al. Surgical reconstruction versus prosthetic obturation of extensive soft palate defects: A comparison of speech outcomes. Int J Prosthodont 2009;22:566–572.

Rieger JM, Wolfaardt J, Seikaly H, et al. Maxillary obturators: The relationship between patient satisfaction and speech outcome. Head Neck 2003;25:895–903.

Rieger JM, Wolfaardt JF, Seikaly H, et al. Speech outcomes in patients rehabilitated with maxillary obturator prostheses after maxillectomy: A prospective study. Int J Prosthodont 2002;15:139–144.

Rieger JM, Zalmanowitz J, Li S, et al. Speech outcomes after soft palate reconstruction with the soft palate insufficiency repair (SPIR) procedure. Head Neck 2008;30:1439–1444.

Rieger JM, Zalmanowitz JG, Wolfaardt JF. Nasopharyngoscopy in palato-pharyngeal prosthetic rehabilitation: A preliminary report. Int J Prosthodont 2006;19:383–388.

Riski WE, Hoke JA, Dolan EA. The role of pressure flow and endoscopic assessment in successful palatal obturator revision. Cleft Palate J 1989;26:56–62.

Rochet A, Rochet BL, Sovis E, et al. Nasalance in speakers of western Canadian English and French. J Speech Lang Pathol Audiol 1998;22:94–103.

Rohrich RJ, Rowsell AR, Johns DF, et al. Timing of hard palatal closure: A critical long-term analysis. Plast Reconstr Surg 1996;98:236–246.

Rosen MS, Bzoch KR. The prosthetic speech appliance in rehabilitation of patients with cleft palate. J Am Dent Assoc 1958;57:203–210.

Rowe MR, D'Antonio LL. Velopharyngeal dysfunction: Evolving developments in evaluation. Curr Opin Otolaryngol Head Neck Surg 2005;13:366–370.

Ryan WJ. Acoustic aspects of the aging voice. J Gerontol 1972;27:265–268.

Sakamoto T, Ohtsuka K, Harazaki M, et al. An electromyogram study on mandibular movement in unilateral cleft lip and palate patients before and after orthodontic treatment. Bull Tokyo Dent Coll 1999;40:195–202.

Seagle MB, Mazaheri MK, Dixon-Wood VL, et al. Evaluation and treatment of velopharyngeal insufficiency: The University of Florida experience. Ann Plast Surg 2002;48:464–470.

Seaver EJ, Dalston RM, Leeper HA, et al. A study of nasometric values for normal nasal resonance. J Speech Hear Res 1991;34:715–721.

Seikaly H, Rieger J, Wolfaardt J, et al. Functional outcomes after primary oropharyngeal cancer resection and reconstruction with the radial forearm free flap. Laryngoscope 2003;113:897–904.

Seikaly H, Rieger J, Zalmanowitz J, et al. Functional soft palate reconstruction: A comprehensive surgical approach. Head Neck 2008;30:1615–1623.

Sell DA, Grunwell P. Speech results following late palatal surgery in previously unoperated Sri Lankan adolescents with cleft palate. Cleft Palate J 1990;27:162–168.

Shahid MLUR, Mir J, Shaukat F, et al. Classification of pharynx from MRI using a visual analysis tool to study obstructive sleep apnea. Curr Med Imaging 2021;17(5):613–622. http://doi.org/10.2174/1573405616666201118143935.

Sharp P, Kelly S, Main A, et al. An instrument for the multiparameter assessment of speech. Med Eng Phys 1999;21:661–671.

Sharry JJ. Complete denture prosthodontics. 3rd ed. New York: McGraw-Hill; 1974.

Shelton RL, Chisum L, Youngstrom KA, et al. Effect of articulation therapy on palatopharyngeal closure, movement of the pharyngeal wall, and tongue posture. Cleft Palate J 1969;6:440–448.

Shelton RL, Lindquist AF, Arndt WB, et al. An effect of speech bulb reduction on movement of the posterior wall of the pharynx and posture of the tongue. Cleft Palate J 1971a;8:10–17.

Shelton RL, Lindquist AF, Chisum L, et al. Effect of prosthetic speech bulb reduction on articulation. Cleft Palate J 1968;5:195–204.

Shelton RL, Lindquist AF, Knox AW, et al. The relationship between pharyngeal wall movements and exchangeable speech appliance sections. Cleft Palate J 1971b;8:145–158.

Sherman D. The merits of backward playing of connected speech in the scaling of voice quality disorders. J Speech Hear Disord 1954;19:312–321.

Shimokawa T, Yi SQ, Izumi A, et al. An anatomical study of the levator veli palatini and superior constrictor with special reference to their nerve supply. Surg Radiol Anat 2004;26:100–105.

Shimokawa T, Yi SQ, Tanaka S. Nerve supply to the soft palate muscles with special reference to the distribution of the lesser palatine nerve. Cleft Palate Craniofac J 2005;42:495–500.

Shprintzen RJ. Commentary on Isberg AM, Henningsson GE. Intraindividual change in the occurrence of Passavant's ridge due to change in velopharyngeal sphincter function: A videofluoroscopic study. Cleft Palate J 1990;27:255–277.

Shprintzen RJ. An invited commentary on the preceding article by Ibuki, Karnell, and Morris. Cleft Palate J 1983;20:105–107.

Shprintzen RJ, Lencione RM, McCall GN, et al. A three-dimensional cinefluoroscopic analysis of velopharyngeal closure during speech and non-speech activities in normals. Cleft Palate J 1974;11:412–428.

Shprintzen RJ, McCall GN, Skolnick ML, et al. Selective movement of the lateral aspects of the pharyngeal walls during velopharyngeal closure for speech, blowing, and whistling in normals. Cleft Palate J 1975;12:51–58.

Shprintzen RJ, Rakof SJ, Skolnick ML, et al. Incongruous movements of the velum and lateral pharyngeal walls. Cleft Palate J 1977;14:148–157.

Sie KC, Starr JR, Bloom DC, et al. Multicenter interrater and intrarater reliability in the endoscopic evaluation of velopharyngeal insufficiency. Arch Otolaryngol Head Neck Surg 2008;134:75–763.

Sie KC, Tampakopoulou DA, Sorom J, et al. Results with Furlow palatoplasty in management of velopharyngeal insufficiency. Plast Reconstr Surg 2001;108:17–25.

Siegel-Sadewitz VL, Shprintzen RJ. Changes in velopharyngeal valving with age. Int J Pediatr Otorhinolaryngol 1986;11:171–182.

Siegel-Sadewitz VL, Shprintzen RJ. Nasopharyngoscopy of the normal velopharyngeal sphincter: An experiment of biofeedback. Cleft Palate J 1982;19:194–200.

Silverman MM. Vertical dimension must not be increased. J Prosthet Dent 1952;2:188–197.

Silverman MM. The whistle and swish sounds in denture patients. J Prosthet Dent 1967;17:144–148.

Silverman SI. Degeneration of dental and orofacial structures. In ASHA Reports 7: Orofacial function: Clinical research in dentistry and speech pathology. Ed. RT Wertz. Washington, DC: American Speech-Language-Hearing Association; 1972. pp. 33–67.

Simpson RK, Austin AA. A cephalometric investigation of velar stretch. Cleft Palate J 1972;9:341–351.

Simpson RK, Chin L. Velar stretch as a function of task. Cleft Palate J 1981;18:1–9.

Skolnick ML. Videofluoroscopic examination of velopharyngeal portal during phonation in lateral and base projections. A new technique for studying the mechanics of closure. Cleft Palate J 1970;7:803–816.

Skolnick ML. Video velopharyngography in patients with nasal speech, with emphasis on pharyngeal motion in velopharyngeal closure. Radiology 1969;93:747–755.

Skolnick ML, McCall GN, Barnes M. The sphincteric mechanism of velopharyngeal closure. Cleft Palate J 1973;11:286–305.

Smith BE, Weinberg B. Prediction of modeled velopharyngeal orifice areas during steady flow conditions and during aerodynamic simulation of voiceless stop consonants. Cleft Palate J 1982;19:177–180.

Smith BE, Weinberg B. Prediction of velopharyngeal orifice area: A re-examination of modeled experimentation. Cleft Palate J 1980;17:277–282.

Spriestersbach DC. Assessing nasal quality in cleft palate speech of children. J Speech Hear Disord 1955;20:266–270.

Stål PS, Lindman R. Characterization of human soft palate muscles with respect to fibre types, myosins, and capillary supply. J Anat 2000;197:275–290.

Stringer DA, Witzel MA. Comparison of multi-view videofluoroscopy and nasopharyngoscopy in the assessment of velopharyngeal insufficiency. Cleft Palate J 1989;26:88–92.

Subtelny JD, McCormack RM, Subtelny JD, et al. Synchronous recording of speech with associated physiological and pressure-flow dynamics: Instrumentation and procedures. Cleft Palate J 1968;5:93–116.

Subtelny JD, Mestre JC, Subtelny JD. Comparative study of normal and defective articulation of /s/ as related to malocclusion and deglutition. J Speech Hear Disord 1964;29:269–285.

Subtelny JD, Sakuda M, Subtelny JD. Prosthetic treatment for palatopharyngeal incompetence: Research and clinical implications. Cleft Palate J 1966a;3:130–158.

Subtelny JD, Worth JH, Sakuda M. Intraoral pressure and rate of flow during speech. J Speech Hear Res 1966b;9:498–518.

Subtelny JS, Koepp-Baker H, Subtelny JD. Palatal function and cleft palate speech. J Speech Hear Disord 1961;26:213–224.

Takasaki K, Sando I, Balaban CD, et al. Functional anatomy of the tensor veli palatini muscle and Ostmann's fatty tissue. Ann Otol Rhinol Laryngol 2002;111:1045–1049.

Takeuchi K, Saruwatari L, Nakamura H, et al. Enhancement of biomechanical properties of mineralized tissue by osteoblasts cultured on titanium with different surface topographies. J Biomed Mater Res 2005;72A:296–305.

Tang JA, Salapatas A, Bonzelaar L, et al. Long-term incidence of velopharyngeal insufficiency and other sequelae following uvulopalatopharyngoplasty. Otolaryngol Head Neck Surg 2017 Apr;156(4):606–610.

Taub S. The Taub oral panendoscope: A new technique. Cleft Palate J 1966;3:328–346.

Terkla LC, Laney WR. Partial dentures. St Louis, MO: Mosby; 1963.

Tonz M, Schmid I, Graf M, et al. Blinded speech evaluation following pharyngeal flap surgery by speech pathologists and lay people in children with cleft palate. Folia Phoniatr Logop 2002;54:288–295.

Trindade IE, Yamashita RP, Suguimoto RM, et al. Effects of orthognathic surgery on speech and breathing of subjects with cleft lip and palate: Acoustic and aerodynamic assessment. Cleft Palate Craniofac J 2003;40:54–64.

Turner GE, Williams WN. Fluoroscopy and nasoendoscopy in designing palatal lift prostheses. J Prosthet Dent 1991;66:63–71.

Uchanski RM, Choi S, Braida LD, et al. Speaking clearly for the hard of hearing: 4. Further studies of the role of speaking rate. J Speech Hear Res 1996;39:494–509.

Van Hattum RJ. Articulation and nasality in cleft palate speakers. J Speech Hear Disord 1958;1:383–387.

Van Lierde KM, De Bodt M, Van Borsel J, et al. Effect of cleft type on overall speech intelligibility and resonance. Folia Phoniatr Logop 2002;54:158–168.

Van Lierde KM, Monstrey S, Bonte K, et al. The long-term speech outcome in Flemish young adults after two different types of palatoplasty. Int J Pediatr Otorhinolaryngol 2004;68:865–875.

Varendh M, Berg S, Andersson M. Long-term follow-up of patients operated with uvulopalatopharyngoplasty from 1985 to 1991. Respir Med 2012 Dec;106(12):1788–1793.

Walter JD. The design of prostheses used in the treatment of velopharyngeal insufficiency. Br Dent J 1981;151:338–342.

Walter JD. Palatopharyngeal activity in cleft palate subjects. J Prosthet Dent 1990;63:187–192.

Wardill WEM. Cleft palate. Br J Surg 1928;126:127–148.

Warren DW. Compensatory speech behaviors in individuals with cleft palate: A regulation/control phenomenon? Cleft Palate J 1986;23:251–260.

Warren DW. PERCI: A method for rating palatal efficiency. Cleft Palate J 1979;16:279–285.

Warren DW. A physiologic approach to cleft palate prosthesis. J Prosthet Dent 1965;15:770–778.

Warren DW, Allen G, King HA. Physiologic and perceptual effects of induced anterior open bite. Folia Phoniatr 1984;36:164–173.

Warren DW, Dalston RM, Dalston ET. Maintaining speech pressures in the presence of velopharyngeal impairment. Cleft Palate J 1990a;27:53–58.

Warren DW, Dalston RM, Mayo R. Hypernasality and velopharyngeal impairment. Cleft Palate Craniofac J 1994;31:257–262.

Warren DW, Dalston RM, Trier WC, et al. A pressure-flow technique for quantifying temporal patterns of palatopharyngeal closure. Cleft Palate J 1985;22:11–19.

Warren DW, Drake AF, Davis JV. Nasal airway in breathing and speech. Cleft Palate Craniofac J 1992a;29:511–519.

Warren DW, Duany LF, Fischer ND. Nasal pathway resistance in normal and cleft lip and palate subjects. Cleft Palate J 1969;6:134–140.

Warren DW, DuBois AB. A pressure-flow technique for measuring velopharyngeal orifice area during continuous speech. Cleft Palate J 1964;1:52–71.

Warren DW, Hairfield WM, Dalston ET. The relationship between nasal airway size and nasal-oral breathing in cleft lip and palate. Cleft Palate J 1990b;27:46–51.

Warren DW, Hairfield WM, Seaton D, et al. The relationship between size of the nasal airway and nasal-oral breathing. Am J Orthod Dentofacial Orthop 1988;93:289–293.

Warren DW, Hall D, Davis J. Oral port constriction and pressure-airflow relationships during sibilant productions. Folia Phoniatr 1981;33:380–394.

Warren DW, Morr KE, Rochet AP, et al. Respiratory system response to a decrease in velopharyngeal resistance. J Acoust Soc Am 1989;86:917–924.

Warren DW, Rochet AP, Dalston RM, et al. Controlling changes in vocal tract resistance. J Acoust Soc Am 1992b;91:2947–2953.

Warren DW, Ryon WE. Oral port constriction, nasal resistance and respiratory aspects of cleft palate speech: An analog study. Cleft Palate J 1967;4:38–46.

Weber J Jr, Jobe RP, Chase RA. Evaluation of muscle stimulation in the rehabilitation of patients with hypernasal speech. Plast Reconstr Surg 1970;46:173–174.

Weiss CE. Success of an obturator reduction program. Cleft Palate J 1971;8:291–297.

Wetzels JW, Meijer GJ, Koole R, et al. Costs and clinical outcomes of implant placement during ablative surgery and postponed implant placement in curative oral oncology: A five-year retrospective cohort study. Clin Oral Implants Res 2017;28:1433–1442.

Whitehill TL, Lee AS, Chun JC. Direct magnitude estimation and interval scaling of hypernasality. J Speech Lang Hear Res 2002;45:80–88.

Witt PD, Marsh JL, McFarland EG, et al. The evolution of velopharyngeal imaging. Ann Plast Surg 2000;45:665–673.

Witzel MA, Posnick JD. Patterns and location of velopharyngeal valving problems: Atypical findings on video nasopharyngoscopy. Cleft Palate J 1989a;26:63–67.

Witzel MA, Tobe J, Saluer KE. The use of videonasopharyngoscopy for biofeedback therapy in adults after pharyngeal flap surgery. Cleft Palate J 1989b;26:129–134.

Wolfaardt JF, Wilson FB, Rochet A, et al. An appliance based approach to the management of palatopharyngeal incompetency: A clinical pilot project. J Prosthet Dent 1993;69:186–195.

Wong LP, Weiss CE. A clinical assessment of obturator-wearing cleft palate patients. J Prosthet Dent 1972;27:632–639.

Ysunza A, Pamplona MC, Ortega JM, et al. Video fluoroscopy for evaluating adenoid hypertrophy in children. Int J Pediatr Otorhinolaryngol 2008;72:1159–1165.

Zamani P, Bayat A, Saki N, et al. Post-lingual deaf adult cochlear implant users' speech and voice characteristics: Cochlear implant turned-on versus turned-off. Acta Otolaryngol (Stockh) 2021;141(4):367–373. http://doi.org/10.1080/00016489.2020.1866778.

Zarrinkelk HM, Throckmorton GS, Ellis E, et al. Functional and morphologic changes after combined maxillary intrusion and mandibular advancement surgery. J Oral Maxillofac Surg 1996;54:828–837.

Zlotolow I. Restoration of the acquired soft palate deformity with surgical resection and reconstruction. In Proceedings of the First International Congress on Maxillofacial Prosthetics. Ed. I Zlotolow, S Esposito, J Beumer III. New York: Memorial Sloan-Kettering Cancer Center; 1995. pp. 49–55.

Zraick RI, Liss JM. A comparison of equal-appearing interval scaling and direct magnitude estimation of nasal voice quality. J Speech Lang Hear Res 2000;43:979–988.

Chapter 5

Rehabilitation of Facial Defects

John Beumer III, Jay Jayanetti, Sudarat Kiat-amnuay, Khim Hean Teoh, Zhi Hui (Janice) Tan, Henry Cherrick, Denny S. Chao

Facial defects can result from trauma, treatment of neoplasms, or congenital malformations. Facial defects referred to the prosthodontist for rehabilitation are usually the result of surgical resection of epithelial tumors (Fig 5-1). Occasionally, however, remission of a tumor mass successfully treated with radiation therapy and/or chemotherapy can result in significant facial deformity. Given the effectiveness and predictability of osseointegrated implants used to retain facial prostheses, prosthetic rehabilitation has become the method of choice at most centers. Facial congenital malformations, such as microtia, can be rehabilitated with either surgical reconstruction or prosthetically.

Rehabilitation of tumor-related facial defects is a difficult challenge for the surgeon as well as the prosthodontist. Both surgical reconstruction and prosthodontic restorations have distinct limitations. The surgeon is limited by the availability of tissue, the compromise of the local vascular bed by radiation in tumor patients, the need for periodic visual inspection of an oncologic defect, and the physical condition of the patient. The prosthodontist is limited by the properties of the materials available for facial restorations and the mobility of soft tissues surrounding the defects.

The difficulties associated with adhesive retention have largely been overcome by the success of osseointegrated implants, and as a result, acceptance of facial prostheses by patients has improved dramatically (Flood and Russell, 1998; Markt and Lemon, 2001; Chang et al., 2005; Flood and Downie, 2009; Viverberg et al., 2019). The retention provided by implants permits the margins to be made thinner and more flexible and hence more effectively camouflaged when extending into movable tissues. Acceptance by patients is enhanced because of the quality of retention, the improved aesthetics that result from accurate and repeatable positioning of the prosthesis, and the ease of maintenance compared to adhesive-retained prostheses.

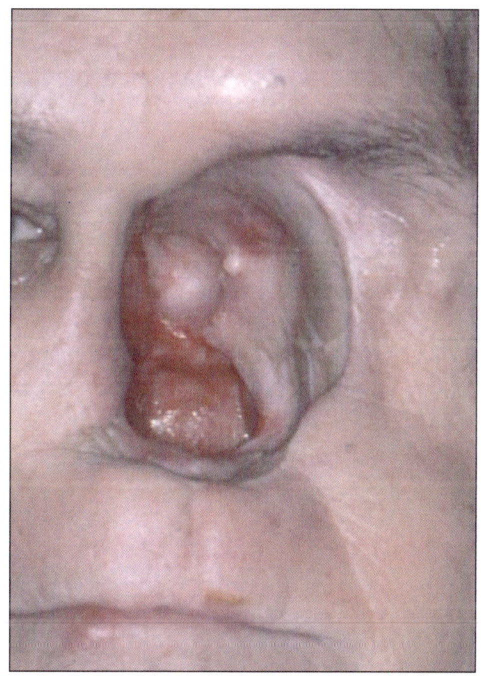

Figure 5-1 Large facial defect secondary to removal of a recurrent basal cell carcinoma.

Whatever the mode of rehabilitation, the patient should be fully informed of future problems and of the expected quality of the final outcome. For patients with extensive facial tumors requiring resection, the method of facial rehabilitation should be chosen prior to surgery.

The benefits and limitations of prosthetic rehabilitation should be carefully reviewed with the patient and their family or significant others. Success with a prosthesis is highly dependent on a sincere commitment by an informed, motivated patient. The option of wearing a patch, particularly in a patient with orbital defects, should also be included in the discussion. If the prosthetic option is selected, a successful prosthetic outcome frequently requires site-specific surgical preparation of the defect (see section below entitled "Surgical Procedures during Tumor Ablation to Enhance the Prosthetic Prognosis").

The objective of these discussions is a well-informed patient with realistic expectations. This is especially true for congenital defects, such as microtia. Osseointegrated implants create effective bone anchors that allow the prosthodontist to fabricate an auricular prosthesis that the patient will actually wear. Some of these patients may have received treatment from early childhood to adulthood, so their management must take into consideration the nature of the defect, the attitude of the patient and the patient's family, the management of ear remnants, and the overall treatment of what may be a complex congenital syndrome (Tjellström et al., 1981; Sugar and Beumer, 1994; Roumanas et al., 2002; Subramaniam et al., 2018; Viverberg et al., 2019).

Patients with craniofacial anomalies frequently present with a variety of complex facial deformities that require the expertise of many health science disciplines. Many of these deformities are best treated with surgical reconstruction. However, prosthodontic rehabilitation is a viable option for patients with microtia because of the predictability of craniofacial implants (Sugar and Beumer, 1995; Parel and Tjellström, 1991; Jacobsson et al., 1992). Fewer and less invasive surgical procedures, consistently excellent aesthetic results, and reduced cost make this option one that is chosen with increased frequency by microtia patients and their families.

The facial skin is the most common site for cutaneous cancer and many of the tumors that arise on the face require extensive surgical intervention to achieve a cure. The surgical defects that remain after tumor resection can be significant, requiring reconstructive surgery, prosthetic rehabilitation, or a combination of the two to restore adequate function and aesthetics. The malignant neoplasms that occur on the face may invade underlying structures, necessitating the excision of muscle, bone, or cartilage. When tumors invade the orbit, nose, or ear, these anatomical structures may require resection, and reconstructive surgery may not provide an acceptable aesthetic result. Therefore, a facial prosthesis constitutes a viable alternative for most patients.

The maxillofacial prosthodontist must be familiar with the pathology and natural history of tumors in this location because interaction with the head and neck surgeon and radiotherapist is an integral part of proper patient management. Also, the prosthodontist may offer valuable input on surgical treatment planning, advising the surgeon on tissue contours and skin linings that will be most retentive and receptive for a prosthesis. Moreover, it may be desirable to place osseointegrated implants at the time of tumor ablation.

Box 5-1 Common epithelial tumors of the face

Keratinocytic origin
Seborrheic keratosis
Keratoacanthoma
Basal cell carcinoma
Squamous cell carcinoma
Melanocytic origin
Nevi
Lentigo maligna and lentigo maligna melanoma
Superficial spreading melanoma
Nodular melanoma
Adnexal origin
Benign adnexal epitheliomas
Microcystic adenocarcinoma
Other malignant adnexal carcinomas
Merkel cell carcinoma

Neoplasms of the Facial Area

Classification

The neoplasms that occur on the face arise from the basilar keratinocytes of the skin, melanocytes, and skin adnexal structures, including sebaceous glands, hair follicles, and sweat glands. The most commonly encountered epithelial tumors of the face are listed in Box 5-1.

The tumors derived from keratinocytes all take their origin from basal cells because these are the germinative or dividing cells of the epithelium. Many benign growths are the consequence of human papillomavirus infection, including warts and papillomas. Other benign growths without a documented, although probable, viral origin include seborrheic keratosis and keratoacanthoma. Both are self-limited proliferations of keratinocytes that are clinically characterized by well-demarcated borders and an inability to invade underlying structures. Keratoacanthomas can be quite large and may require wide excision. If they are located on or near the ear or nose, prosthetic reconstruction may become necessary after excision.

Basal cell carcinomas also arise from basal keratinocytes; however, unlike the benign lesions, they have the potential for locally aggressive behavior, characterized by invasion of adjacent and underlying tissues. They do not typically metastasize (fewer than 1%) and should be considered locally aggressive benign neoplasms with potential for persistent growth and recurrence after removal. Conversely, squamous cell carcinomas of the skin are true malignancies with significant growth potential and a propensity to metastasize to regional lymph nodes.

Melanocytes are derived from the neural crest and migrate through the mesenchyme during embryonic life to the skin and mucous membranes. These cells then populate the lower strata of the epithelium, interposed between basilar keratinocytes. They synthesize melanin pigment, which shields and protects the basal keratinocyte from the effects of solar irradiation. In this regard, light-skinned individuals are more prone to develop carcinomas than dark-skinned people.

Benign proliferations of melanocytes, termed *nevi*, are self-limited in their growth potential. Most nevi arise in childhood from basal layer melanocytes at the junction of the epithelium and the connective tissue.

Figure 5-2 *(a)* Early basal cell. Note the elevated margins and centrally depressed area of ulceration. *(b)* An advanced basal cell carcinoma.

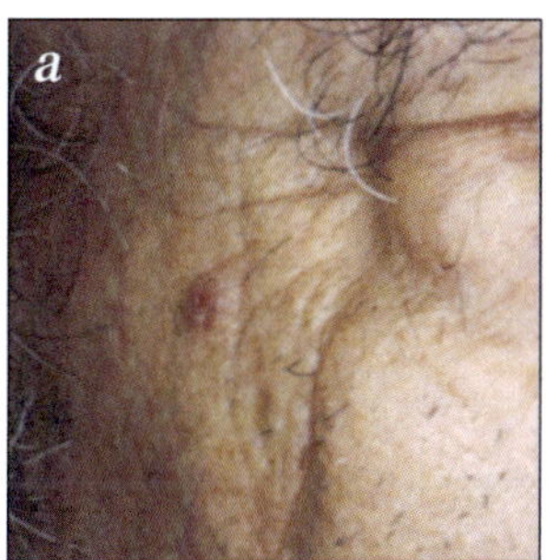

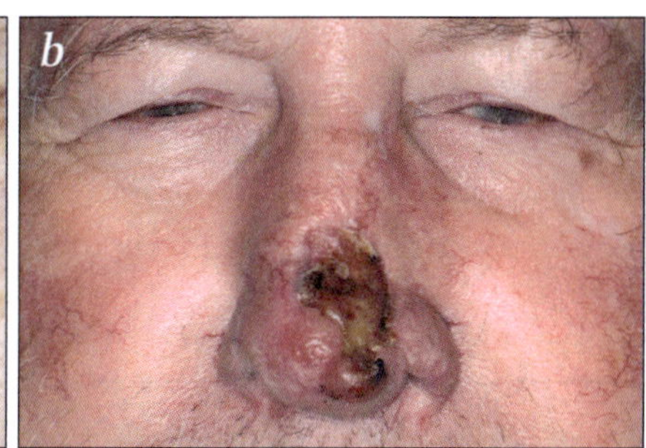

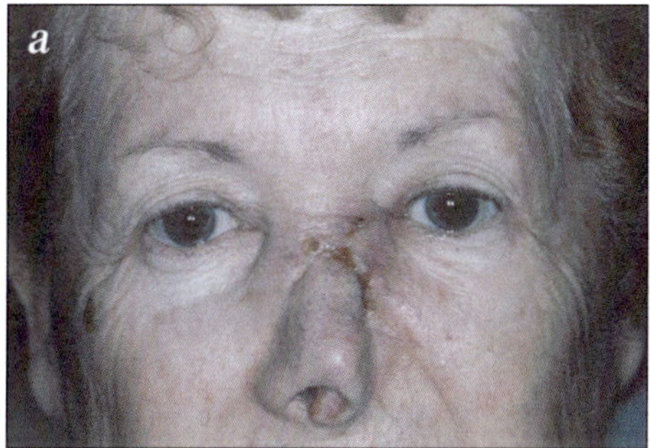

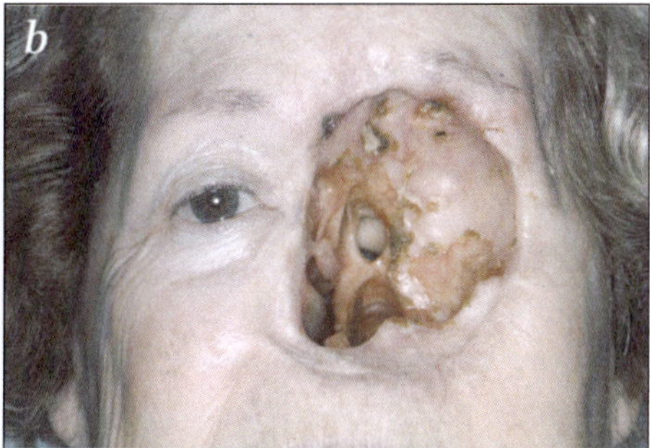

Figure 5-3 *(a)* Recurrent basal cell carcinoma. *(b)* Large postresection facial defect.

In contrast, proliferation and invasion with the potential for hematogenous spread are the classic features of malignant melanoma. The earliest change, termed *melanoma in situ*, occurs in the basal layer. The proliferating cells may then spread laterally along the basal layer or invade the connective tissue. Melanomas are highly malignant tumors and require extremely wide surgical margins.

The skin adnexa include hair follicles, sebaceous glands, and sweat glands. Tumors derived from these differentiated cells are collectively termed *adnexal tumors*. The benign lesions are usually small, grow slowly, and are often self-limited, requiring only minor surgical excision. Malignant adnexal tumors are quite rare, but they can behave in a fashion similar to squamous cell carcinoma (Misago et al., 1993; Romeu et al., 2017; Oyasiji et al., 2018).

One aggressive adnexal tumor that requires wide excision is microcystic adenocarcinoma (Mayer et al., 1989; Mills et al., 2016). Its cell of origin is not known but is probably the sweat gland duct. This aggressive tumor rarely metastasizes. Other adnexal tumors include sebaceous carcinoma, commonly found on the eyelid, and ceruminous carcinoma of the ear canal (ear wax glands).

A rare, yet highly malignant tumor of the skin is Merkel cell carcinoma. The cell of origin remains unknown. This tumor is highly invasive and has metastatic potential. It is strongly associated with advanced age and immunosuppression. The majority of MCCs are caused by the monoclonal integration of Merkel cell polyomavirus (Feng et al., 2008), and the remainder are associated with exposure to ultraviolet light (Harms et al., 2015; Goh et al., 2016; Wong et al., 2015). Merkel cell carcinomas histologically resemble other neuroendocrine round cell tumors and may be mistaken for basal cell carcinomas. Such tumors have a poor prognosis.

Only the more common skin cancers, including basal cell carcinoma, squamous cell carcinoma, and melanoma, will be described in detail in this section.

Basal cell carcinoma

Derived from basilar keratinocytes, basal cell carcinoma is the most common form of skin cancer. Actinic or solar irradiation plays an important role in the etiology of basal cell carcinoma. The tumor is far more prevalent in "sun belt" regions and has a high predilection for individuals with a light complexion. In the United States, Hawaii appears to have the highest incidence annually among whites: 576 men and 298 women per 100,000 population (Reizner et al., 1993). In Queensland, Australia, the incidence of nonmelanoma skin cancer in white men and women aged 20 to 59 years is very high: 2,389 per 100,000 and 1,908 per 100,000, respectively; the ratio of basal cell to squamous cell carcinomas is 4:1. The studies concentrated on white individuals; basal cell carcinoma is extremely rare among black persons. Chronic immunosuppression associated with organ transplants increases the risk of basal cell carcinoma (Berg et al., 2002; Euvard et al., 2003).

Clinical features. Early basal cell carcinomas may appear as small pearly white nodules of the skin and will usually show erythema or superimposed telangiectasia. A surface keratosis or scale may also be evident. These nodules soon ulcerate and become a persistent ulcer with rolled margins (Fig 5-2). The center of the ulcer is often scabbed with a crusted core.

If left untreated, they will continue to invade and enlarge circumferentially. Large and/or recurrent basal cell carcinomas have resulted in the loss of facial structures, including the lip, nose, eye, and ear (Fig 5-3; see also Fig 5-1). Untreated basal cell carcinomas have been known to invade the facial and skull bones with extension into the sinuses and even into the brain. Although it is rare, some patients have died of local disease despite the absence of metastases.

The most common facial locations for basal cell carcinomas are the forehead, nose, malar region of the cheek, and helix of the ear.

The fair-haired, light-skinned individual may be prone to develop multiple lesions of the face, and such tumors may be contiguous with cutaneous evidence of solar damage and actinic keratoses, which appear as red maculae with a fine surface scale.

Certain variants of basal cell carcinoma are known to occur and may show clinical appearances that differ from the typical crateriform ulcer. The morphea variant is often invasive without surface ulceration or rolled margins; rather, it appears yellowish or shows pallor over the surface of the skin and is indurated. This form is highly invasive and induces collagenization of the adjacent stromal connective tissues. Tumor cells may extend for a considerable distance in the dermis and subcutaneous tissues, beyond areas of palpable induration, thereby necessitating wide excision to prevent recurrence.

Treatment. Both surgery and radiation therapies have been employed successfully in the management of basal cell carcinoma. Small basal cell carcinomas are amenable to both surgical and radiation therapies, whereas large invasive tumors, particularly those invading bone and cartilage, are most appropriately managed by wide surgical excision. Basal cell carcinoma is invasive and may extend for a considerable distance both laterally and deeply beyond the clinically apparent tumor margin. Fingerlike projections of tumor islands are even more extensive in the morphea-type tumor. Incomplete excision will lead to recurrence, and each recurrence tends to become larger and more extensive. Therefore, the clinician should avoid incomplete excision by taking adequate margins both laterally and deeply.

Although electrosurgical intervention has been employed for early lesions, the adequacy of excision cannot be confirmed histologically because the effects of electrocautery on tissue obfuscate the histologic appearance of residual tumors. Complete excision is most readily confirmed by histologic examination of all margins. Examination of frozen sections during surgery is most appropriate for basal cell carcinomas. Morphea-type lesions may not always be adequately evaluated by frozen section for complete excision, requiring detailed examination of paraffin-embedded material. Despite attempts to document total excision microscopically, recurrent disease is a common complication, particularly for large lesions.

Mohs (1976) introduced a combined surgical-chemical technique for the definitive and complete excision and chemical cautery of cutaneous neoplasms. The method involves the application of zinc chloride paste, which causes necrosis and fixation of the neoplastic tissues (Mohs, 1976; Nelson et al., 1997). The chemically treated skin is excised and examined by the frozen section. Should the tumor remain, the process is repeated in an organized, mapped configuration until pathologic evidence of tumor cells is no longer evident. Although dermatologists prefer this method, it is time consuming and expensive. Its chief advantage is the preservation of uninvolved tissue.

Most head and neck surgeons usually prefer to excise the tumors with wide margins, which are examined by frozen section at the time of excision. In both approaches, the goal is to remove all tumor cells and leave tumor-free margins. Large tumors will usually require reconstructive surgical approaches with free grafts and myocutaneous skin flaps, depending on the size of the defect. Loss of the orbital contents, external nose, or external ear usually necessitates postsurgical fabrication of facial prostheses.

Radiation therapy has also proven effective in the treatment of basal cell cancers, particularly for smaller lesions; however, tumors that have invaded bone and cartilage do not respond well to irradiation. Different forms of local radiation are used, including superficial radiation therapy using low-energy photons, conventional radiation therapy with electrons, and brachytherapy. Radiation is a popular choice for those deemed poor surgical candidates and for esthetically important areas such as the nose and the eyelids. Those tumors amenable to radiation are treated over a 3- to 5-week period with an external beam dosage of 45 to 50 Gy.

Topical chemotherapy is efficacious only in very early lesions. The most commonly employed agents are 5% 5-fluorouracil ointment and imiquimod. They are applied daily for 6 to 12 weeks. Large lesions cannot be treated with these methods.

Squamous cell carcinoma

Squamous cell carcinoma of the skin has the same predisposing factors as basal cell tumors. Squamous cell cancers have metastatic potential and therefore constitute a much more serious disease (Green and Battistutta, 1990). Like basal cell tumors, squamous cell carcinomas have a propensity to involve sun-exposed skin, and light-skinned subjects are more susceptible to the disease. Although other etiologic factors such as low-dose radiation, chronic immunosuppression associated with organ transplantation (Euvard et al., 2003; Preciado et al., 2002; Lanz et al., 2019), arsenic, and cold tars have been implicated in cutaneous squamous cell cancer, solar irradiation remains the chief predisposing factor. Xeroderma pigmentosum, a genetic disease in which DNA repair mechanisms are defective, predisposes children to cutaneous squamous cell cancer.

Squamous cell carcinomas associated with chronic immunosuppression and organ transplantation behave more aggressively and frequently present at an advanced stage. These patients present with a higher rate of metastasis and do not respond as favorably to standard treatments (Kuijken and Bavinck, 2000; Lanz et al., 2019).

Clinical features. Akin to basal cell carcinomas, squamous cell carcinomas are frequently associated with actinic keratoses. The early lesion is often an erythematous plaque with a keratotic scale. Unlike basal cell tumors, squamous cell cancers usually have irregular, jagged margins. Ulceration is common and rolled, indurated borders are the rule. As the lesion enlarges, it may progress to a keratotic papillary or verrucous, warty appearance. Some lesions stay local and destroy local tissues (Fig 5-4). On palpation, squamous cell carcinomas are indurated and not clearly defined, particularly when they are large.

The skin of the forehead is a common location, as is the lower lip. Indeed, squamous cell carcinomas of the lip may be preceded by actinic cheilitis, a leukoplakia that can persist for many years before carcinoma evolves (Nuutinen and Karla, 1981). Actinic cheilitis appears as a white keratosis of the vermilion border of the lower lip among individuals who work outdoors. When these keratotic lesions begin to ulcerate and become nodular and indurated, carcinomatous transformation is likely.

Neck metastases occur in a minority of patients with facial skin squamous cell carcinomas, usually those with large extensive lesions. Metastatic nodes from facial primary tumors are usually detected along the cervical chain, whereas scalp tumors spread to posterior neck scalene nodes. The nodes are indurated and may be fixed to adjacent tissues.

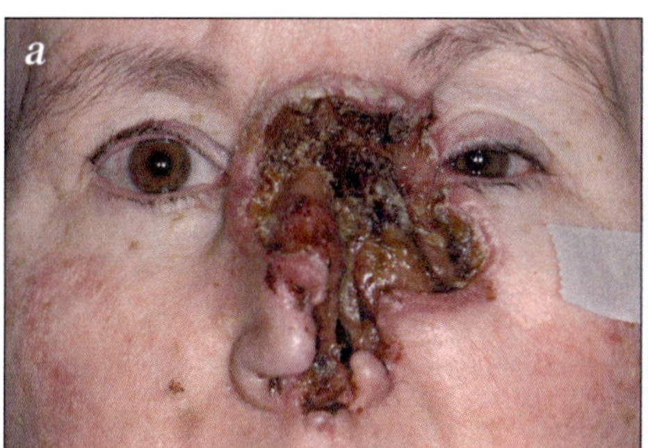

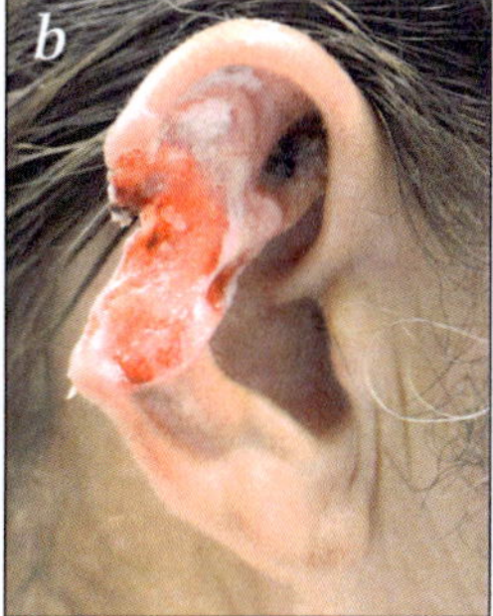

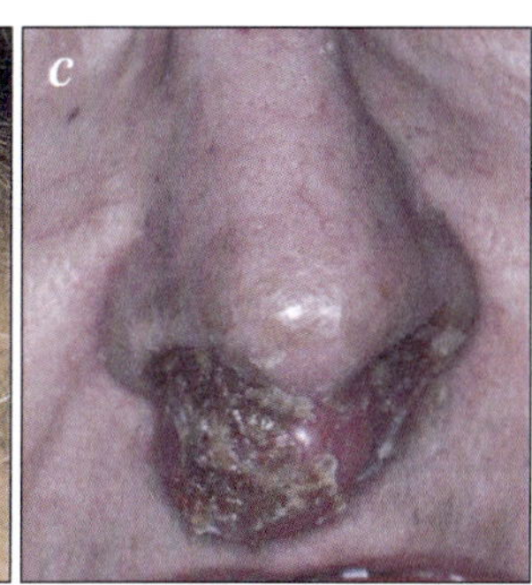

Figure 5-4 *(a and b)* Large squamous cell carcinomas arising from the skin, and *(c)* the nasal septum.

Variant forms of squamous cell carcinoma of the skin are adenoid squamous cell carcinoma and spindle cell carcinoma. The adenoid variant shows malignant squamous epithelial islands with foci of acantholysis and ductlike configurations (Banks and Cooper, 1991). Spindle cell carcinomas may be mistaken for sarcoma; however, origin from the basal layer of the surface epithelium can usually be demonstrated, and epithelial markers such as cytokeratin and epithelial membrane antigen can be employed immunohistochemically to confirm the epidermal origin of the spindle cells (Ellis and Corio, 1980). Both histologic variants behave as moderately to poorly differentiated carcinomas.

Treatment. Squamous cell carcinoma of the skin must be treated aggressively because it is infiltrative without having well-delineated margins. Surgical excision includes a wide margin of normal-appearing skin and microscopic assessment of the lateral and deep margins to ensure complete removal of malignant tumor islands and nests. Carcinomas that overlie bone often invade the periosteum, necessitating the inclusion of bone in the surgical resection. Therefore, based on the size of the initial lesion, surgical defects can vary considerably in size and the degree of disfigurement they present. Because squamous cell cancers are capable of invading lymphatic and blood vessel walls, assessment for both regional lymph node and distant metastases must be undertaken. When lymph node involvement is clinically or radiographically detectable, lymph node dissection is included along with surgical excision of the primary tumor. Loss of facial structures is unavoidable in patients with large tumors; these patients require plastic surgery, myocutaneous flaps, and/or prosthetic reconstruction (Alam et al., 2018).

Radiation therapy is also effective in the treatment of skin squamous cell carcinomas; it may be used alone for smaller lesions or in combination with surgical excision for more extensive tumors (Abbatucci et al., 1989; Alam et al., 2018). In general, a dosage of 45 to 60 Gy, delivered in fractionated doses, is effective. Radiation therapy may also be included in the treatment regimen for sterilization of the neck.

In general, the prognosis for patients with cutaneous squamous cell carcinoma is much better than that for patients with squamous cell cancers arising in the mucous membranes of the head and neck. Carcinoma of the lower lip is slow to metastasize and has a high (90%) 5-year survival rate. Carcinomas of the facial skin, forehead, ear, and nose are more prone to metastasize; however, only large lesions have a poor prognosis. Recurrence is more commonly encountered than metastasis. Metachronous lesions are also common, particularly in patients with sun-damaged skin (field cancerization). The spindle cell and adenoid variants have a greater propensity for recurrence and metastasis than ordinary squamous cell carcinomas of the face.

Malignant melanoma

Melanomas derive from melanocytes, the pigment-producing cells that embryologically migrate from the neural crest and eventually become situated above and between basal keratinocytes of the skin. Nevi, benign lesions of these cells, usually arise during childhood as focal, self-limited proliferations of melanocytes. The proliferating cells are initially confined to the basal layer at its junction with the dermis and are therefore termed *junctional nevi*. Within a few years, these cells drop off into the connective tissue and are known as *compound nevi*. By puberty, most nevus cells reside solely within the dermis as *intradermal nevi*.

New nevi do not arise in adulthood, and the occurrence of a new pigmented lesion in an adult is cause for concern. Some nevi are thought to be prone to malignant transformation into melanomas, and this trend often follows a familial pattern. Such dysplastic nevi may be numerous. About 50% of melanomas probably arise de novo, whereas the other half are thought to arise from preexisting nevi. Malignant melanoma accounts for about 2% of all cancers.

On the facial and cervical skin, solar irradiation plays a dominant role in the pathogenesis and etiology of malignant melanoma (Fisher, 1989). The malar and lateral neck skin receive maximal sun exposure and are favored sites. The disease is more common among white people than among dark-skinned people.

Clinical features. There is no sex predilection for melanoma, and most patients are elderly; the average age is 60 years. Among males, the skin of the ear auricle, neck, and scalp are most often affected whereas in women the facial skin is the most frequently affected area (Agnese et al., 2007).

The clinical appearance of cutaneous melanoma varies according to the histologic type. Nevi are common in the general population, but certain features must be encountered to raise suspicion of melanoma. First and most important is duration or onset. As mentioned previously, most nevi arise in childhood; hence, the occurrence of a new focus of pigmentation in an adult should be viewed with suspicion. Second, the configuration of the pigmented area is important. Nevi are round or oval and symmetric with smooth margins. Melanomas, in contrast, often show ragged irregular margins. A third feature is coloration. Nevi may be brown or black, yet the color of a given mole is always homogenous. Melanomas tend to be heterogenous, and varying shades of black, gray, and brown are mixed together in a single lesion (Fig 5-5).

Those lesions that are macular without tumefaction usually represent melanomas that are growing laterally or radially, superficial spreading melanoma, and have a better prognosis than raised

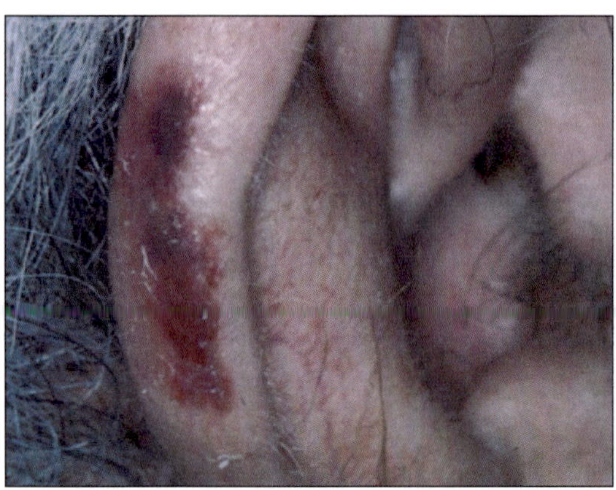

Figure 5-5 Typical superficial spreading malignant melanoma.

lesions. Lentigo maligna and lentigo maligna melanoma are also radial in their pattern of growth, yet such lesions differ from the superficial spreading type both histologically and clinically. Lentigo maligna and lentigo maligna melanoma are progressive stages of the same entity. Such lesions occur most often on the face of elderly individuals with light complexions and may persist for 20 years before any invasion occurs. They are multicolored and may show admixed foci of depigmentation, representing areas of tumor regression. Those pigmented lesions with nodular excrescences are prone to invasion of the dermis and are termed *nodular melanomas*; they are highly malignant and have a great propensity for metastasis. The propensity for metastasis dramatically escalates with increasing levels of invasion (Clark, 1969; Breslow, 1970).

Treatment. Surgical excision remains the treatment of choice and, the level of invasion dictates the prognosis (Al-Quarayshi et al., 2017; Han et al., 2019). Adjuvant immunotherapy may improve survival (Al-Quarayshi et al., 2017).

Wide excision is required along with examination of the lateral and deep margins to ensure that all melanoma cells have been excised. Lentigo maligna melanoma of the face must be deeply excised because junctional changes extend down pilosebaceous skin appendages. Superficial spreading and lentigo maligna melanomas (thin tumors) enjoy a good prognosis after wide excision, whereas invasive nodular melanomas that arise de novo or evolve from superficial spreading melanomas metastasize widely and result in death in 50% of the patients even with wide excision of the primary tumor (Agnese et al., 2007; Han et al., 2019). This is explained by the fact that invasive lesions have probably already metastasized at the time of initial surgical excision of the primary tumor.

Surgical Reconstruction versus Prosthetic Rehabilitation

The choice between surgical reconstruction and prosthetic rehabilitation of large facial defects is a difficult and complex decision and depends on the size, location, and etiology of the defect as well as on the wishes of the patient. Surgical reconstruction of small facial defects is preferable in most cases. Many patients prefer that the defect be masked with their own tissue rather than with a prosthetic restoration. However, it is difficult, if not impossible, for the surgeon to reconstruct a facial part that is as cosmetic as a well-made prosthesis. However, not everyone will accept an artificial part, and many patients would rather have a permanently reconstructed facial part than an artificial one. The application of osseointegrated implants in facial defects has, to some extent, changed patients' perceptions about facial prostheses because of the effectiveness of retention and the improved aesthetic results.

Advanced or recurrent tumors of the lips and skin of the head and neck, although often benign in behavior, may require aggressive surgical removal for control. These lesions may result in the extensive loss of facial structures, including the nose, upper lip, cheek, orbital contents, and ear. Sometimes facial defects occur in combination with resection of oral structures, such as portions of the maxilla, mandible, and buccal mucosa (see section entitled "Large Midfacial Defects Extending into the Oral Cavity"). Reconstruction of large oncologic defects is technically difficult, and the final cosmetic and functional results are usually suboptimal.

A variety of circumstances favor prosthetic rehabilitation of facial defects. When a large resection is necessary and local recurrences likely, it is advantageous to be able to monitor the surgical site closely. A prosthesis permits such observation, whereas primary surgical reconstruction makes examination and detection problematic. Furthermore, surgical reconstruction of large defects is technically difficult and requires multiple procedures and hospitalizations. Patients confronted with this type of defect are usually older and less able or willing to tolerate the multiple procedures required. Moreover, many tumors in the region are irradiated. Reduced vascularity, increased fibrosis, and scarring of the tissues bordering the defect complicate and increase the risk of complications associated with reconstruction. Even when surgical reconstruction is deemed possible, many surgeons prefer to wait at least one year after a large resection before considering surgical reconstruction of a facial defect resulting from a facial neoplasm.

In skilled hands, nasal reconstructive surgery for partial rhinectomy defects can produce acceptable results (Fig 5-6), but it is difficult to achieve consistently esthetically acceptable results with total rhinectomy defects. Bilateral symmetry is rarely achieved, and frequently the patient must be fitted with a nasal stent (Fig 5-6c) to maintain the nasal airway and improve nasal contours. In addition, both basal cell carcinoma and squamous cell carcinoma of the nasal structures are prone to reoccur, so prostheses are often suggested to the patient.

Although some surgeons have achieved reasonable results with staged ear construction for patients with congenital defects, consistently good results have not been demonstrated by surgeons. Autogenous reconstruction of congenital auricular defects often fails (Fig 5-7), and prosthetic reconstruction becomes the only viable option. In contrast, implant-retained auricular prostheses have achieved superior aesthetic results and a high degree of patient acceptance (Chang et al., 2005). Orbit exenteration defects are impossible to restore surgically. An orbital prosthesis is indicated in this instance. However, surgery to augment missing soft tissue in the malar and infraorbital areas or to close off the orbital defect from the nasal cavity may enhance the prosthetic outcome.

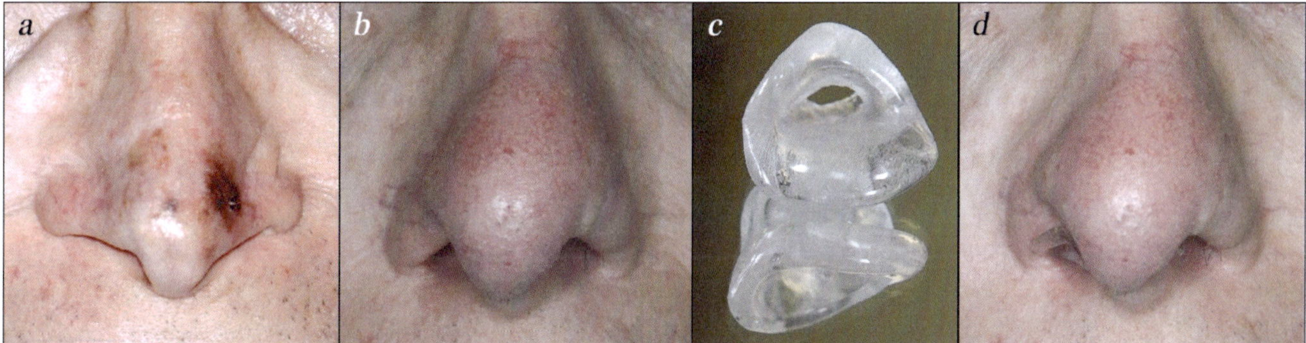

Figure 5-6 *(a)* A basal cell carcinoma associated with the tip and ala region. *(b)* Following resection, the tip and ala region have been reconstructed surgically with local flaps. *(c and d)* A nasal stent has been fabricated in order to maintain the nasal airway.

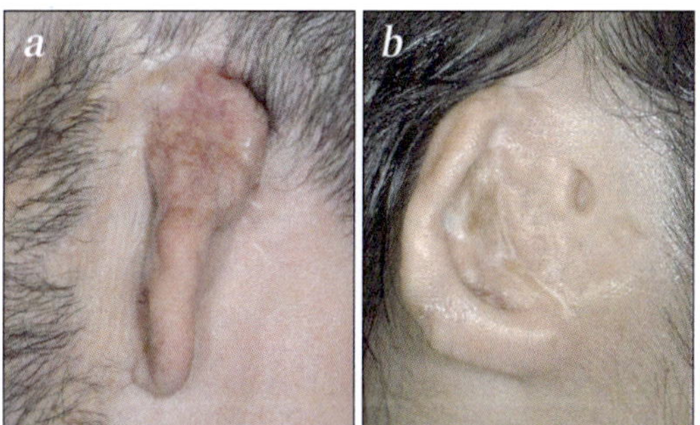

Figure 5-7 *(a and b)* After several surgical procedures, the attempt at reconstructing the auricles of these two patients has been unsuccessful.

Facial prostheses retained with osseointegrated implants have achieved wide acceptance in the surgical community for the management of both congenital and acquired defects (Flood and Russel, 1998; Tjellström et al., 1981; Jacobsson et al., 1992; Tjellström et al., 1995; Granstrom, 2005; Ethunandan et al., 2010) and have been totally embraced by the prosthodontic community. Superior aesthetic results can be achieved with this approach; it is also cost effective, and patient acceptance is high (Chang et al., 2005).

Prosthetic Materials

Successful prosthetic rehabilitation of facial defects provides pleasing aesthetic results and enables most patients to live relatively normal lives. The challenge to maxillofacial prosthodontists is to use their artistic skill sets to fabricate esthetically pleasing prostheses, but to best accomplish this goal, they also must understand the science behind the materials used. Knowledge of the evidence-based literature helps the clinician choose materials and fabrication methods that improve the aesthetic outcomes and clinical life span of the prosthesis and, with it, patient satisfaction. This section will provide a thorough literature review of the types of materials used for the fabrication of facial prostheses, their history and properties, their interaction with colorants, the effects of aging on their appearance, and the physical properties of the prostheses and will suggest future lines of research for the improvement of facial prosthetic materials.

The ideal processing characteristics and biologic properties of maxillofacial materials are listed in Boxes 5-2 and 5-3, respectively.

Box 5-2 Ideal processing characteristics of maxillofacial materials should do the following:

- Reproduce fine detail
- Be dimensionally stable during processing
- Accept intrinsic and extrinsic colorants.
- Possess high tear (edge) strength
- If a pour material,
  - Possess viscosity that is low enough to permit processing in a mold
  - Possess viscosity high enough to allow intrinsic coloration
- Be nonporous to minimize absorption of stains
- Possess sufficient working time for ease of processing
- Not release by-products
- Not possess toxic components or produce toxic by-products
- Process at room temperature
- Be free of odor
- Allow for use of reusable molds
- Permit repair without damaging the prosthesis
- Not exhibit chemical or physical changes during storage

Box 5-3 Ideal biologic properties of processed or cured maxillofacial materials should have the following:

- No irritation of supporting tissues
- No allergenic potential
- No toxic response
- No support for the growth of microorganisms

Materials that are easily processed with readily available instrumentation and technology offer distinct advantages. The blending of individual components should be easy and permit some margin for error and artistic license. The material should remain stable when exposed to microbial biofilms and environmental insults such as ultraviolet (UV) light, oxygen, fluctuating temperatures, secretions (sebaceous, perspiration, nasal, and salivary), stain, and adhesives and their solvents. Lastly, it is highly desirable that the prostheses should be durable and capable of use without significant deterioration of aesthetics and material for at least one year.

The ideal physical and mechanical properties of processed maxillofacial materials are listed in Box 5-4. The prosthesis should possess sufficient flexibility for use on movable tissue beds. The material should be dimensionally stable and lightweight and possess suitable edge strength to permit feathering of margins. Variations in temperature should not affect physical properties, and thermal conductivity should be sufficiently low to permit comfortable use in cold environments.

Ideally, the completed facial prosthesis should be unnoticeable in public, faithfully reproducing lost structures in the finest detail. The color, texture, form, and translucency of the prosthesis must duplicate those of missing structures and adjacent skin. A conspicuous prosthesis will increase patient anxiety and compromise social readjustment. The final aesthetic result and color stability are the most important factors in clinical success or failure of facial prostheses (Anderson et al., 2003, 2013). The amount of time a patient wears his/her prosthesis is indicative of treatment success (Markt et al., 2001; Chang et al., 2005).

Advancements in biomaterials research and digital technology have changed the way in which current facial prostheses can be fabricated. Since 2010, the use of 3D scanning, 3D modeling, and 3D printing to fabricate molds and/or to print the basic shape of the facial prosthesis has been reported (Unkovskiy et al., 2018; Cruz, 2020a, 2020b; Farook et al., 2020; Rodriguez et al., 2021). A detailed description of these technologies is provided below (see section below entitled "Use of digital technology").

Box 5-4 Ideal physical and mechanical properties of processed maxillofacial materials should do the following:

- Be chemically inert—that is, not have unreacted groups or residual components after processing
- Be cleansable with common soaps and disinfectants without loss of color, aesthetics, or detail at the surface or margins
- Have colorants (intrinsic and extrinsic) that do not change during normal use
- Be dimensionally stable—that is, not expand or shrink over time or with changes in temperature
- Tolerate cyclic loading with a flexibility and resistance to indentation similar to that of tissues being replaced (no tensile or compression set)
- Be stable over a range of temperatures (−40°C to 60°C; −40°F to 140°F), not stiffen in cold weather or sag in warm weather, and not readily conduct heat or cold to supporting tissues
- Not be brittle or distort when elongated or compressed
- Be resistant to wear from abrasion
- Not tear at feather edges
- Have high tensile strength to resist breakage when stretched
- Not be dissolved by solvents, primers, varnishes, or adhesives
- Be inexpensive to allow refabrication as needed
- Be lightweight
- Have low surface tension and low water sorption to resist staining
- Be odorless
- Be lifelike with controllable translucency and opacity for coloring at depth
- Have a usable life of at least one year

History

Facial prostheses were fabricated as early as 3000 BCE. Archaeologists have discovered artificial eyes, noses, and ears constructed from waxes, clay, and wood among ancient Egyptian and Chinese artifacts. Ambroise Paré (1510–1590), a French surgeon, was the first to describe facial prostheses in the medical literature. In his textbook, *Les oeuvres d'Ambroise*, published in 1575, Paré included a section on nasal, ocular, and auricular prostheses fabricated from gold, silver, paper, and linen cloth, all glued together. Tycho Brahe (1546–1601), Danish scientist and astronomer, fabricated his own adhesive-retained nasal prostheses in copper or gold and painted them with oil paint; he used them for 35 years (Ring, 1991). Pierre Fauchard (1678–1761), the father of scientific dentistry, described ingenious methods to fabricate and retain facial and oral prostheses. In 1833, Sir William Whymper published a report describing "The Gunner with the Silver Mask," credited to a French dental surgeon, Dr. Forget, who made a silver mask to replace the lost portion of the mandible of a French soldier. The silver prosthesis was painted with oil paints, and the margins of the prosthesis were covered with facial hair to make it less inconspicuous (Roberts, 1971).

By the middle of the 19th century, vulcanite rubber was being used by the dental profession for fabrication of intraoral prostheses. By the end of the century, it was adapted for use as facial prostheses. In 1901, Upham (1901) described the fabrication of nasal and auricular prostheses made from vulcanite rubber, but its rigidity posed a problem. By 1932, Kazanjian et al. (1932) described the use of celluloid paints for coloring vulcanized rubber facial prostheses. After the introduction of latex, which overcame the rigidity of vulcanized rubber, Bulbulian (1939) and Clarke (1941) described techniques for the use of prevulcanized latex with water-soluble dyes for facial prostheses.

Anna Coleman Ladd, an American sculptor, pioneered the modern era of facial prosthetics. During World War I, Ladd created the American Red Cross's Studio for Portrait-Masks in Paris, which provided facial prostheses for those who had been badly disfigured in World War I. A cast of plaster was made of the face, and the facial features to be replaced were sculpted of clay or plasticine. This sculpture was then used to construct a facial prosthesis from extremely thin galvanized copper. The metal was painted with hard enamel to resemble the recipient's skin tone. Hair was used to create eyelashes, eyebrows, and mustaches. These prostheses were generally retained with eyeglass frames or ear loops (Alexander, 2007).

Acrylic resin was introduced to the dental profession in 1937. The translucency, colorability, and ease of processing of heat-cured acrylic resin were attractive to most clinicians, and excellent cosmetic outcomes could be achieved with facial prostheses (Fig 5-8). This material is still being used today for temporary facial prostheses. Both chemically activated and heat-activated acrylic resins have been used, although heat activated was favored because it was considerably more color stable. They were processed in stone molds, and as a result, only one prosthesis could be processed since the mold was destroyed while extracting the prosthesis. Artists' acrylic paints, dissolved in either monomer or chloroform, were used for extrinsic coloration (Brasier, 1954). It was relatively easy to touch up select areas where the extrinsic coloration had become compromised. Some clinicians used a thin layer of clear acrylic resin to protect the extrinsic coloration. This material was used for definitive prostheses through the 1970s.

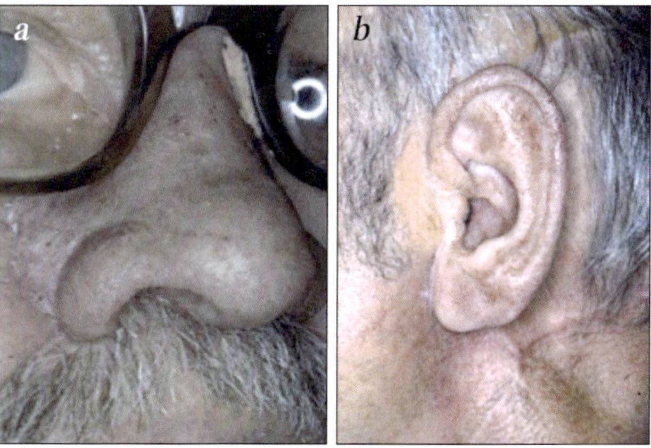

Figure 5-8 *(a and b)* Heat cure acrylic resin prostheses. Extrinsic colorants are applied with acrylic paints dissolved in chloroform.

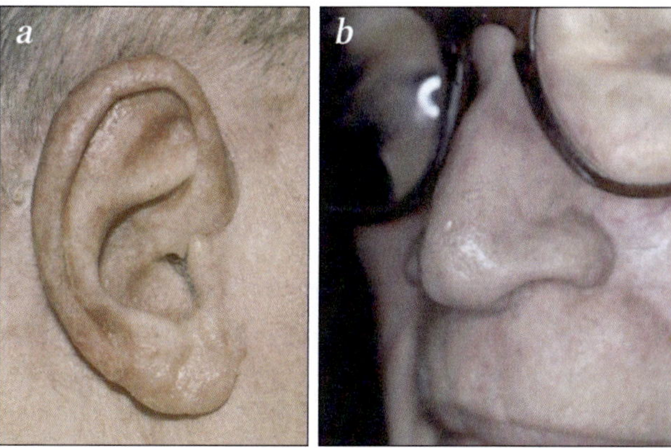

Figure 5-9 *(a and b)* Polyurethane facial prostheses. Excellent cosmetic results could be achieved because the margins of the prosthesis can be made very thin, and the translucency and coloration are close to those of human skin.

Polyvinyl chlorides (PVC) were used by many clinicians in the 1950s and 1960s. They were relatively rigid, although the addition of plasticizers mitigated this feature to some degree. Processing required high temperatures (150 degrees Centigrade) and metal molds. Moreover, they were not color stable when exposed to ultraviolet light, which limited their life span. In addition, there were concerns raised regarding the release of vinyl chloride, a carcinogen, into the local environment during processing (Guerra and Kronoveter, 1978). For these reasons and the development of silicone elastomers, this material fell into disuse by the early 1970s.

The polyurethanes, introduced in the early 1970s, provoked great interest because of their superior cosmetic outcomes, excellent edge strength, softness, and flexibility and because they could be colored both intrinsically and extrinsically (Gonzales, 1978; Gonzales et al., 1978) (Fig 5-9). Lewis and Castleberry (1980) reported the development of an aliphatic polyurethane prepolymer, isophorone, and preliminary data on its physical and mechanical properties was favorable. Turner et al. (1985a, 1985b) evaluated the mechanical properties of this material before and after 900 hours of accelerated aging and reported that it did not disintegrate and demonstrated desirable characteristics. However, polyurethanes had serious deficiencies, such as difficulty processing in humid environments, a tendency toward yellow discoloration with aging and exposure to ultraviolet light, poor adhesive compatibility, migration of extrinsic colorants, and difficulty cleaning. Typical facial prostheses of this material were serviceable for only three to four months. This material no longer became available by the early 1980s.

Barnhart (1960) was the first to use a silicone elastomer to fabricate facial prostheses by combining a silicone base material with acrylic resin polymer stains. A variety of pigment systems were employed for intrinsic and extrinsic coloration (Firtell and Bartlett, 1969; Schaaf, 1970; Fine, 1978; Fine et al., 1978). The original silicones were quite unsatisfactory. Edge strength was poor, they were difficult to color, and they appeared opaque and lifeless. However, since their introduction, significant alterations have resulted in substantial improvements in physical properties, color stability, and aesthetic outcomes achievable. They are by far the most commonly employed material used today for facial prostheses.

Advances in polymer chemistry have renewed interest in the development of alternative materials for facial prostheses. Another generation of acrylic resins was studied by Antonucci and Stansbury (1992). Gettleman (Gettleman, 1992; Gettleman and Khan, 1992) proposed using polyphosphazenes for facial prostheses (see section below entitled "Polyphosphazenes"), and May and Guerra (1978) suggested that polyethylenes be considered (see section below entitled "Chlorinated polyethylene"). Silicone block copolymers have also been studied (Tsai et al., 1992).

Table 5-1 Degradation of facial prostheses as affected by changes in physical and mechanical properties

Observed degradation	Important physical or mechanical property
Color fade or changes	Color stability (outdoor/indoor weathering)
Tearing at margins	Low tear strength, low fatigue life
Breakage when stretched	Low tensile strength
Elongation at margins	Low % elongation and increased tensile set
Stiffer or softer	Lower or increased durometer hardness
Change in surface texture	Increase in surface roughness
Lack of bonding to skin adhesives	Permit use of adhesives
Weakened margins by colorants, adhesives, solvents, or cleaners	Low absorption of offensive agents

The quest for new materials continues because the clinical performance of polymeric materials is far from ideal (Lai et al., 1999). Moreover, degradation of facial materials observed clinically is affected by various physical and mechanical phenomena, as shown in Table 5-1. The impact of these phenomena has been subject to intense scientific scrutiny since the 1970s, and research has led to substantial improvements.

Silicone elastomers

Silicone elastomers and ancillary materials, which include thixotropic additives, pigments and opacifiers, adhesives and primers, and extrinsic colorant sealants, are commonly used today. The current generation of silicone elastomers are easy to handle, are biocompatible, are chemically inert, are translucent, are strong, are durable, readily accept coloration, are flexible, bond to underlying materials, and have a full range of different softness choices for different areas of tissue.

Silicone elastomers are a combination of organic and inorganic compounds. The first step in their production is the reduction of silica (SiO_2) to elemental silicon. By various reactions, silicon is combined with methyl chloride to form dimethyldichlorosilane, which forms a polymer when reacted with water. Kipping (1904) assigned the name *silicones* based on their similarity with ketones because, in most cases, there is an average of one silicone atom, one oxygen, and two methyl groups. These polymers are translucent, white fluids whose viscosity is determined by the length of the polymer chain. Polydimethylsiloxane is the most common silicone elastomer and is made from these fluid silicone polymers (Colas and Curtis, 2004).

Most rubbery forms of silicone are compounded with fillers that provide additional strength. Additives are used to provide color, and antioxidants and vulcanizing agents are used to transform the fluid into an elastomer during processing. The long-chained polymers, when tied together at various points (cross-linked), create a stable network that can be separated only with difficulty. This network makes the silicones relatively resistant to degradation from UV light exposure. The percentage of cross-linking (Tamareselvy and Rueggeberg, 1994) and change in the extension of cross-linking caused by environmental factors (Haug et al., 1992a) are the most important factors affecting the physical and mechanical properties of silicones (Mouzakis et al., 2010). The process of cross-linking the monomers is referred to as *vulcanization*, which occurs both with and without heat, depending on the catalytic or cross-linking agents utilized. Using a chain of silica and oxygen atoms and attaching suitable side chains or organic radicals to them, a material evolves with the inertness of quartz and the flexibility of the organic plastics.

Silicones are classified into groups according to their applications:

1. *Implant grade.* These materials must undergo extensive testing and must meet or exceed USFDA requirements.
2. *Medical grade.* These materials are approved for external use only and are the materials most commonly used for the fabrication of facial prostheses.
3. *Industrial grade.* These materials are mostly used for consumer and industrial applications.
4. *Food grade.* These materials meet FDA regulations for containers holding food.

The silicone elastomers are available in two forms: *(1)* high-temperature vulcanizing (HTV) silicone and *(2)* room-temperature vulcanizing (RTV) silicone.

HTV silicones

Results from a survey of currently used materials for the fabrication of extraoral maxillofacial prostheses indicated that only 3% of maxillofacial prosthodontists and dental technicians used HTV silicone (Montgomery and Kiat-amnuay, 2010). In general, HTV silicones have more desirable physical and mechanical properties than RTV silicones. However, they are more opaque, are difficult to color intrinsically and extrinsically, and are difficult to process (Bell et al., 1985).

Silastic 4-4514 and 4-4515 (Dow Corning). Uncured HTV silicone is usually a white, opaque material with a highly viscous, puttylike consistency. They can be preformed into various shapes for alloplastic implantation or for facial prostheses. Processing of heat-cured silicones requires sophisticated instrumentation and high temperatures. They have excellent thermal stability, are color stable when exposed to UV light, and are biologically inert. However, they do not possess sufficient elasticity to function well in movable tissues, possess low edge strength and the finished prostheses appear lifeless. They do not readily accept extrinsic coloration, so the internal colorants must be incorporated in the gum stock with a milling device. Because high temperatures are required for vulcanization, metal molds are necessary. A detailed description of their use was provided by Chalian et al. (1967).

Q7-4635, Q7-4650, Q7-4735, Q-4720, and SE-4524U (Dow Corning). Succeeding generations of HTV silicones demonstrated improved physical and mechanical properties compared to the most commonly used RTV silicones (Bell et al., 1985). The processing characteristics of Q7-4635 and SE-4524U (Shincor Silicones) were particularly favorable because their one-component system had unlimited shelf life. Dos Santos et al. (2020) studied Silastic Q-4735, an enhanced tear-resistant heat-cured high-consistency silicone elastomer with intrinsic and extrinsic coloring. They showed that Q-4735's hardness and color stability were clinically acceptable after 1,008 hours of artificial aging.

TechSil S25 (Technovent). This is an HTV addition-cured platinum silicone that can be cured with heat or at room temperature under pressure. Several investigators have studied its physical properties but the results have been inconsistent and contradictory. Al-Harbi et al. (2015) found that it possessed more desirable mechanical properties and better color stability when exposed to outdoor weathering in hot and humid climatic conditions as compared to the commonly used RTV silicones. However, Eleni et al. (2009b, 2009c, 2011a, 2011b) reported that natural weathering adversely affected its mechanical properties and found that TechSil S25 becomes harder and more brittle after being exposed to outdoor weathering for one year, in contrast to M 511 (an RTV silicone) and chlorinated polyethylene (CPE). Hatamleh et al. (2011) studied the effect of porosity on color subjected to two aging conditions and found that some properties of TechSil S25 were enhanced, while others were adversely affected.

Mollomed S20, S21, S24, S27 (Detax). This is another generation of condensation-cured HTV silicones from Europe. However, Polyzois et al. (2011a) showed that color changes were visually unacceptable after outdoor and indoor aging.

RTV silicones

Results from an international survey by Cardoso et al. (2022) of maxillofacial prosthodontists and dental technicians revealed that RTV silicones were the elastomers most commonly used for fabrication of facial prostheses, confirming the results of earlier surveys (Montgomery and Kiat-amnuay, 2010; Andres, 1992; Andres et al., 1992). Commonly used silicone maxillofacial prosthetic materials from this international survey, in order of their popularity, are listed in Table 5-2.

Composition and setting reactions. The polymerization reactions are *(1)* condensation cross-linking with by-products, *(2)* silicone-to-silicone medical adhesives using acetoxy cure, and

Table 5-2 Rankings of commonly used silicone facial prosthetic materials: 2020 international survey

	First	Second	Third	Fourth	Fifth	Sixth
Intrinsic packing	MDX4-4210	MDX4-4210 and Med Adhesive A	A-2186/A-2186F	M511	VST-50	A-2000
Extrinsic layer	Med Adhesive A	MDX4-4210	A-2186/A-2186F	M511	A-2000	

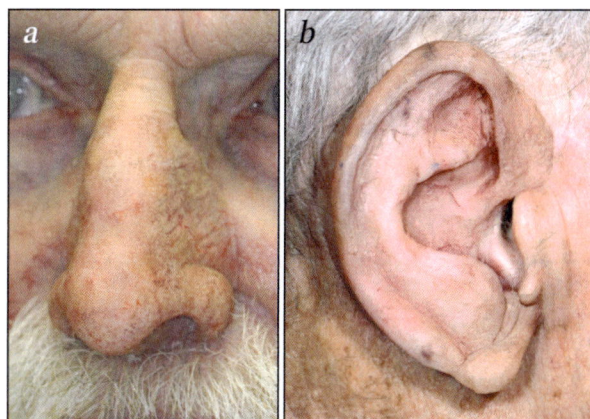

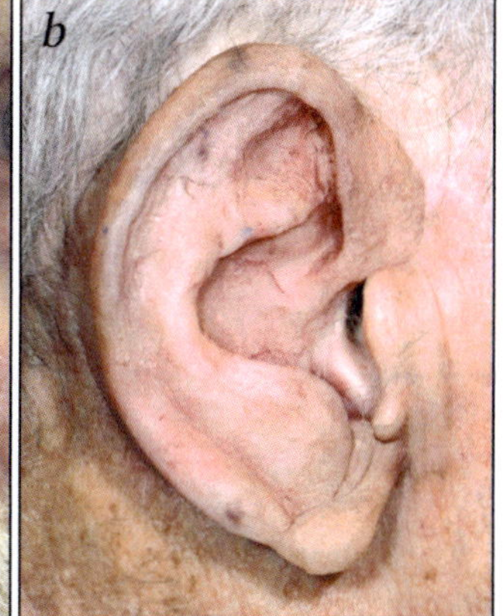

Figure 5-10 *(a and b)* Silicone (MDX4-4210) prostheses. Note the excellent color matching, surface texture reproduction, and marginal adaptation.

(3) addition cross-linking by platinum catalyst with no reaction by-products (Colas and Curtis, 2004). Modern silicones have a chloroplatinic acid catalyst and hydromethyl siloxane as cross-linking agents. Polymerization of platinum silicones is easily disturbed because the platinum is easily bonded to electron-donating substances such as organosulfur compounds or amines, resulting in the inactivation of the catalyst and inhibition of the polymerization process. *Therefore, the silicone mixture should not be exposed to organic materials such as oil, petrolatum, or clay* (Kiat-amnuay et al., 2002; Colas and Curtis, 2004; Bayer and Goldschmidt, 1991). Inhibition of polymerization of platinum-cured silicone is commonly caused by sulfur and other nitrogen-containing compounds, acidic materials, organic compounds, some RTV silicone catalysts, and latex. Therefore, it is advisable to use latex-free gloves when mixing.

After the silicone elastomer has polymerized, the platinum catalyst is mostly transformed into platinum metal nanoparticles (Stein et al., 1999; Brook, 2006). Because silicone polymers tend to stabilize platinum metal nanoparticles (Chauhan et al., 2003; Huang et al., 2004; Ramirez et al., 2004), brown or yellow hues are commonly observed in silicone elastomers, especially when the material is prepared with high concentrations of platinum (Brook, 2006).

Silastic MDX 4-4210 with catalyst A-103 (Dow Corning; 10:1 ratio of base to catalyst). MDX 4-4210 is a medium medical-grade polydimethylsiloxane with vinyl groups, introduced in the 1970s. It has been studied extensively. This silicone was the most frequently used facial prosthetic material in a 1992 survey (Andres, 1992; Andres et al., 1992) as well as surveys completed in 2008 and 2020 (Montgomery and Kiat-amnuay, 2010; Cardoso et al., 2022). Excellent aesthetic results can be achieved with this material (Fig 5-10).

Moore et al. (1977) showed that MDX 4-4210 exhibits good-quality coloration and edge strength. This material is not heavily filled, so it is translucent. The physical properties can be modified by the addition of silicone fluid. The material has been found to be nontoxic, color stable, and biologically compatible. Early clinical testing revealed cured MDX 4-4210 to be compatible with most skin adhesive systems and to exhibit reasonable tensile strength. More importantly, the increased elongation and resistance to tear compared favorably to other materials (Moore et al., 1977) and have reduced the need for reinforcement of the thin edges of the prosthesis. In addition, the surface texture and Shore A hardness values are within the range of human skin. Shade guides for intrinsic coloration have been developed. Accelerated aging tests have shown that the elastomer is reasonably color stable (Craig et al., 1978).

Extensive testing on the physical and mechanical properties of MDX 4-4210 has been conducted. Although MDX 4-4210 is not an ideal material, it has many advantages compared to earlier materials and exhibits many desirable characteristics. Processing is simple because molds of dental stone (gypsum) are acceptable (metal molds are not recommended because of the acid released by the silicone). Digitally designed molds printed out of a proprietary resin have also been used successfully. However, care should be taken to avoid contamination of the mold with petrolatum or clay residue. The prepared molds are placed in a dry heat oven at 50°C for approximately 30 minutes before use. Warming of all the mold segments assists in retaining the position of the custom colors used for intrinsic shade coloring. After appropriate surface detail has been applied, a syringe is loaded with the base material and used to fill the mold, which has recovered its viscosity after mixing. The mold is closed with finger pressure and held tightly together with a web clamp.

Flasking the mold and use of moist heat will increase the longevity of the mold. Unflasked gypsum molds in dry heat used for multiple processing will dehydrate the gypsum and cause loss of surface detail and/or cracking and disintegration of the mold. During processing air removal of the fluid silicone before packing, use of a controlled injection packing technique, and soaking of the flasked mold in slurry water before application of moist heat will result in a dense and porosity-free casting (Kent et al., 1983).

Combined Silastic MDX 4-4210/Silastic Medical Adhesive, Type A (Dow Corning). Udagama and Drane (1982) introduced the technique of combining Silastic Medical Adhesive Silicone, Type A with the base component of MDX 4-4210 for fabrication of facial prostheses. Farah et al. (1987, 1988) studied the mechanical and force-displacement properties of specimens with various ratios of MDX 4-4210 and Silastic Medical Adhesive, Type A (from 50/50 to 10/90 mix). They found that different ratios (except the 50/50 mix) showed acceptable mechanical properties and that varying these ratios could allow the production of facial prostheses that more closely simulated the properties of facial tissues.

The combination of Silastic MDX 4-4210/Medical Adhesive, Type A is the second most popular facial material, according to the 2020 international survey. According to surveys conducted in 2008 (Montgomery and Kiat-amnuay, 2010) and 2020 (Cardoso et al., 2022), 25% and 17% of respondents, respectively, were using these materials and techniques, a reduction from 52% in the 1992 survey (Andres, 1992). Unlike platinum-curing silicones, the setting of a mixture of Silastic MDX 4-4210 and Silastic Medical Adhesive, Type A, is not easily disturbed if contaminated by organic material, such as oil, petrolatum, or clay. The mixture contains a higher percentage of Silastic Medical Adhesive, Type A, mixed with a lower percentage of the MDX 4-4210 base component. This mixture has been widely used with artists' oil pigments.

Because the thin edges of the material tear relatively easily from cleaning of skin adhesives, Udagama (1987) developed a technique of bonding prostheses made of Silastic MDX 4-4210/Medical Adhesive, Type A, to a polyurethane sheet liner, by applying a primer, drying, then applying Silastic Medical Adhesive, Type A, that serves as the adhesive. Incorporating a polyurethane liner improves the tear resistance of the feathered edges of the prosthesis, separates silicone from contact with microbial organisms and biofilms (especially nasal prosthesis), and improves prosthesis-skin adhesive retention.

Silastic 891 Medical Adhesive Silicone, Type A (Dow Corning). Silastic Medical Adhesive Silicone, Type A, a dimethyl siloxane-triacetoxy–terminated silane, is cross-linked by a condensation reaction. This material is a relatively low molecular weight polymer with hydroxyl-blocked ends. It is a translucent, nonflowing paste. This material is called a *one-component RTV silicone* but actually requires moisture as a second component. The filler is typically diatomaceous earth, which is similar to that used in HTV silicones. The cross-linking agent methyl triacetoxysiloxane is easily hydrolyzed by water vapor present in air. When water contacts methyl triacetoxysiloxane, an acetic acid by-product is formed, replacing an acetoxy with a hydroxyl group. The cross-linking reaction starts once the product comes in contact with moisture and after the silicone is squeezed from the tube. Polymerization proceeds from the outer surface inward (Colas and Curtis, 2004). Although this silicone is designed for caulking and sealants in the construction industry, it has been used in medical devices as an adhesive for the adherence of materials to silicone elastomers. It is translucent and requires no mixing. Results from surveys conducted in 2008 and 2020 showed that 57% and 27% of respondents were using Silastic Medical Adhesive Silicone, Type A, for extrinsic coloring of facial prostheses (Montgomery and Kiat-amnuay, 2010; Cardoso et al., 2022). The curing temperature and time parameters followed by survey respondents varied greatly (Montgomery and Kiat-amnuay, 2010; Cardoso et al., 2022). The advantages of the material are that no catalyst is required, and it is compatible with a wide range of colorants. The material does share some of the disadvantages of other RTV silicones—namely, insufficient flexibility and less-than-ideal edge strength.

A-2186 and A-2186F (Factor II; 10:1 ratio of base to catalyst). A lower-cost platinum-cured RTV silicone elastomer was introduced and became commercially available in 1986 as an alternative silicone to MDX4-4210. A-2186 ranked sixth, first, and fourth in preferred maxillofacial material according to the 1992 (Andres, 1992; Andres et al., 1992), 2008 (Montgomery and Kiat-amnuay, 2010), and 2020 (Cardoso et al., 2022) surveys, respectively. Many research studies on A-2186 material have been reported (Haug et al., 1992a, 1992b, 1999a, 1999c; Sanchez et al., 1992; Dootz et al., 1994; Polyzois et al., 1994; Waters et al., 1997, 1999; Lai and Hodges, 1999; Lai et al., 2002; Aziz et al., 2003a, 2003b; Han et al., 2007, 2008, 2010a, 2010b; Haider et al., 2019; Nobrega et al., 2019; Babu et al., 2018; Meran et al., 2018; Willett and Beatty, 2015; Al-Harbi et al., 2015; Hungerford et al., 2013; Mount et al., 2018; Atay et al., 2013; Liska et al., 2009; Xiao-na, 2007; Zheng, 2003). Some claim that A-2186 has better physical and mechanical properties than MDX 4-4210 (Sanchez et al., 1992). However, Haug et al. (1992a, 1992b) reported that, when subjected to environmental variables, A-2186 did not retain its physical and mechanical properties. Willett and Beatty (2015) studied unpigmented A-2186 specimens after 3,000 hours of outdoor aging and found small changes in color, tensile properties, and durometer hardness with time. However, the results may not be clinically significant since facial prostheses must be colored to match skin shade. Most recently, Haider and colleagues (2019) reported that reinforcement of A-2186 with 5% polyester powder significantly improved overall mechanical properties.

Additional color stability studies by several investigators have shown that some dry earth pigments and opacifiers mixed with A-2186 undergo significant color degradation over time rendering the clinical outcomes unacceptable (Kiat-amnuay et al., 2002; Beatty et al., 1995, 1999; Gary et al., 2001; Kiat-amnuay et al., 2005). Because this silicone is commonly used, Kiat-amnuay et al. studied A-2186 mixed with silicone intrinsic pigments and opacifier; the results were satisfactory for both color stability and mechanical properties (see Table 5-7). It should be noted that clinicians should use silicone pigments designed only for A-2186 until further clinically acceptable research with other types of pigments is conducted.

A-2186F, introduced in 1987, is a rapid-polymerizing version of A-2186 with higher platinum content. It is not as popular as A-2186, according to surveys (Andres, 1992; Andres et al., 1992; Montgomery and Kiat-amnuay, 2010; Cardoso et al., 2022). As stated earlier, high platinum concentrations in silicone elastomers are associated with the development of brown or yellow hues after polymerization (Brook, 2006). Atay et al. (2013) evaluated the adherence of *Candida albicans* to the surface of various maxillofacial silicones. They found that A-2186F had the lowest *C. albicans* accumulation. This was due in part to the material being more hydrophobic (highest surface contact angle) when compared to A-2006 and VST-50. Based on this data, A-2186F may be a useful material for nasal prostheses.

Cosmesil (Cosmedica; base with drops of flexibilizer/cross-linker/catalyst). Cosmesil is an RTV "tin-cured" silicone. Introduced in 1982, it can be processed to varying degrees of hardness by varying the amount of flexibilizer/cross-linker/catalyst to the base, as described in 1985 by Wolfaardt et al. (1985). The material was shown to have higher tear strength at failure than MDX 4-4210. Several research studies on this material have been reported (Wolfaardt et al., 1985; Polyzois and Andreopoulos, 1993; Polyzois, 1995, 1999; Dootz et al., 1994; Mohite et al., 1994; Waters et al., 1997, 1999; Aziz et al., 2003a, 2003b; Veres et al., 1990a, 1990b, 1990c; Kiat-amnuay et al., 2002; Polyzois et al., 1993; Murata et al., 2003). Cosmesil was popular in Europe but this tin-cured silicone version is no longer available.

M511 (Technovent) and A-588 (Factor II). A "platinum-cured" RTV silicone elastomer (10:1 ratio of base to catalyst), M511 is the European version of US Factor II's A-588. These translucent silicones are designed to produce softer and more lifelike prostheses (with shore A of 14±2) and were specially developed for implant-retained prostheses, not for adhesive-retained, due to fewer desirable physical and mechanical properties. They bond well to the acrylic resin substructures enclosed within implant-retained silicone facial prostheses that retain the attachment housings.

Aziz et al. (2003b) and Bellamy et al. (2003) of the same research group developed M511, an improved polymeric material, and showed this material to have high tear strength (22.2 ± 1.6 N/mm). Bates et al. (2021) evaluated color stability and mechanical properties of A-2000 and M511 silicone elastomers mixed with e-Skin and Reality Series pigment/opacifier systems before and after artificial aging. They found similar tear strength of 23.2–27.7 N/mm but Shore A hardness Increased to 40–45, which is considered to be stiff (see Table 5-7). Several research studies on M511 material have been reported (Aziz et al., 2003a; Bellamy et al., 2003; Güngör et al., 2020; Sonnahalli et al., 2019; Babu et al., 2018; Farah et al., 2018; Karakoca et al., 2018; Bibars et al., 2018; Mehta and Nandeeshwar, 2017; Cifter et al., 2017; Kosor et al., 2015; Akash and Guttal, 2014; Bangera and Guttal, 2014; Bankoglu et al., 2016; Kheur et al., 2012; Hatamleh et al., 2010a; Eleni et al., 2009b, 2011a, 2011b; Bates et al., 2021).

A-2000, A-2006, A-2009 (Factor II), and Z2004 (Technovent; 1:1 ratio of base to catalyst). A-2000, A-2006, and A-2009 are platinum-cured RTV silicones, introduced in 2000, 2006, and 2009, respectively. A-2000 is the first generation of a 1:1 mixture of silicone modified from A-588 (10:1 mixture) with the same chemistry. The control of the properties is more consistent with a 1:1 ratio than a 10:1 ratio mixture. A-2006 is a lower durometer version of A-2000, whereas A-2009 is a basic flesh-tone pigmented version of A-2006. A-2006 and A-2009 bond well to acrylic resin when implant-retained facial prostheses are fabricated using A-330-G primer.

Numerous research studies have been conducted on A-2000 (Kurtoglu et al., 2009; Bishal et al., 2019; Chamaria et al., 2019; Akay et al., 2018; Bibars et al., 2018; Bennie et al., 2018; Cevik et al., 2017; Hu et al., 2009a, 2009b, 2011, 2014; Mohammad et al., 2010; Kiat-amnuay et al., 2009), A-2006 (Akay et al., 2018; Artopoulou et al., 2016a, 2016b; Atay et al., 2013; Mount et al., 2018; Liska et al., 2009), and Z2004 (Güngör et al., 2020; Mulcare et al., 2019; Bibars et al., 2018; Kheur et al., 2017; Mehta et al., 2017; Kheur et al., 2012; Hatamleh et al., 2010). In a comprehensive research effort, Kiat-amnuay and her team (2009) at the John M. Powers Houston Center for Biomaterials and Biomimetics found that A-2000, when mixed with intrinsic silicone pigments and opacifier, exhibited excellent color stability and very favorable mechanical properties (Table 5-7).

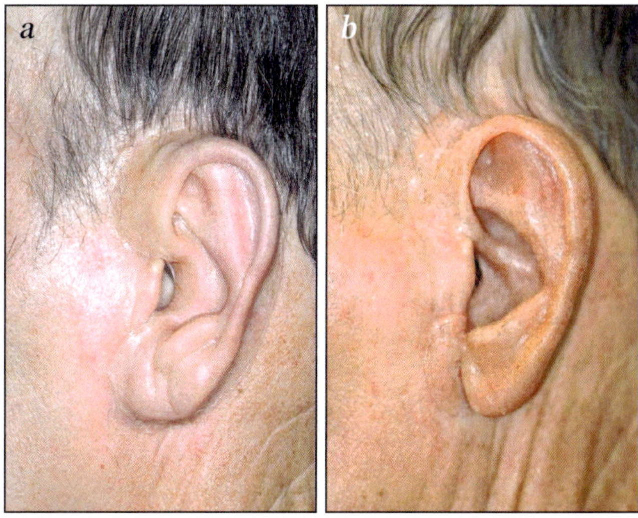

Figure 5-11 *(a)* Silicone prosthesis (MDX 4-4210/Silastic Medical Adhesive, Type A) delivered in 1999. *(b)* CPE prosthesis delivered in 2005 to the same patient (reprinted from Kiat-amnuay et al., 2010, with permission).

Table 5-3 Composition of GSRI-CPE 726/19-15 for facial prostheses

Component	Amount
Dow CPE 3614A (Tyrin CM0136),* now Sundow Wellpren, CPE	100.0 grams powder
Calcium stearate lubricant (Mallinckrodt)	1.5 grams powder
Low-density polyethylene (Dow 991)	6.0 grams powder
Irganox 1010 antioxidant (CIPA-Geigy)	0.2 grams powder
Tinuvin 327W stabilizer (CIBA-Geigy)	0.2 grams powder
Chlorinated paraffin (Dow Chemical, Chlorowax 40)	35.0 mL liquid

Other polymers

Chlorinated polyethylene

In the late 1970s, thermoplastic chlorinated polyethylene (CPE) was proposed for use as a facial prosthetic material (May and Guerra, 1978). Gettleman (1992) evaluated a variation of CPE (CPE 3614, now Tyrin CPE CM0136, Dow Chemical), a 36% chlorinated material with a molecular weight of ~200,000 Da, as an alternative material. The formula and properties are listed in Table 5-3. It is an inexpensive industrial-grade thermoplastic rubber, available in granulated form. Lewis and Castleberry (1980) tested chlorinated polyethylene elastomer (CPE), which is similar to modified polyvinyl chloride (PVC) in both physical properties and chemical composition (May and Guerra, 1978; May et al., 1981). Various shades are prepared for facial prostheses on a heated rubber mill with pigments. A phase II clinical trial suggested few differences between the silicone and the less expensive CPE (Gettleman et al., 1987; Lemon et al., 2005).

The matching skin-colored blankets of CPE elastomer are artistically laid up to simulate natural skin color at depth in gypsum molds in a regular denture or giant bronze flask (Kiat-amnuay et al., 2010) or metal molds (Guerra and Canada, 1976). The processing technique involves placing the clamped flask in a domestic pressure cooker or steam autoclave, heated to 110°–115° (60 kPa or 10 psi) for 10 minutes (Kiat-amnuay et al., 2008, 2010). Repeated molding is possible until the prosthesis is free of voids with minimal flash because the material is thermoplastic (no chemical reactions). Extrinsic coloring is done with the patient present by mixing the pigments, using a special flexible varnish with methyl ethyl ketone (MEK) as a carrier solvent that penetrates the CPE and then evaporates. A thin layer of clear and/or flocked CPE is then laid over the final molded prosthesis to encase the pigmentation under a protective laminate. Further extrinsic coloring can be painted on the prosthesis using the MEK carrier.

Clinical trials of this material, used with extrinsic colorants and colored rayon flocking, have been conducted (Kiat-amnuay et al., 2010) (Figs 5-11 and 5-12). The randomized controlled, single-crossover, double-blind multicenter phase III clinical trial, tested the noninferiority of CPE to silicone rubber (Silastic MDX 4-4210/ Medical Adhesive, Type A) for fabricating prostheses. Overall, patients rated the silicone prosthesis higher than the CPE

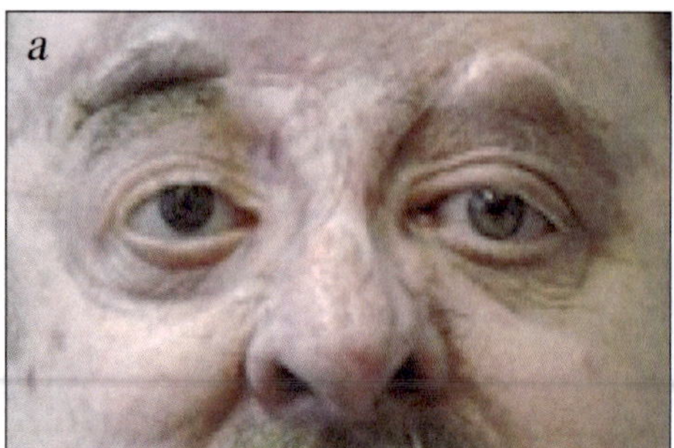

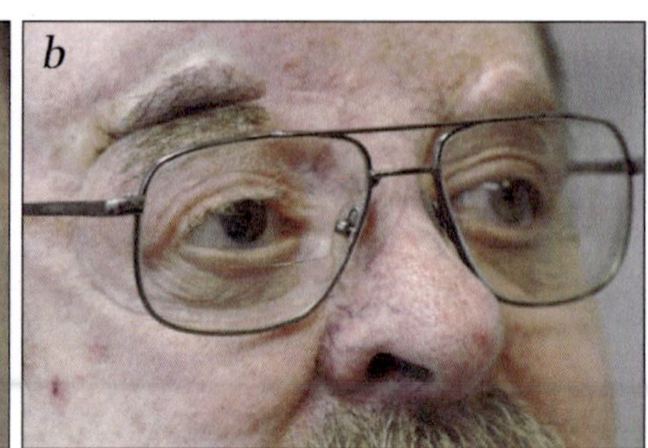

Figure 5-12 *(a and b)* CPE orbital prosthesis restoring the right orbit, characterized by threads and flocking.

prosthesis. Patients with prior experience with silicone prostheses had a stronger preference for silicone, while new users (no prior experience) rated the two materials similarly.

Because there is no curing chemical reaction, CPE is less toxic than silicone elastomers (Autian, 1977; Gettleman et al., 1982). It is not carcinogenic (Gettleman et al., 1992), is less irritating to mucosa than silicone, and is well tolerated by patients (Gettleman et al., 1958, 1985). It is easy to grind and adjust, is repairable by remolding in the flask or with a hot spatula, has an indefinite working time, is resistant to the growth of microorganisms, and is much less expensive. However, CPE is stiffer and less comfortable for the patient, uses a different molding technique, and is less color stable than silicone (Kiat-amnuay et al., 2010).

Research studies comparing CPE with silicone elastomers are continuing (Kiat-amnuay et al., 2010; Eleni et al., 2009b, 2011a, 2013a; Cevik et al., 2022). Kiat-amnuay et al. (2008) performed an in-vivo trial of the Epithane-3 and Secure[2] medical adhesives applied to CPE and urethane-lined Silastic MDX4-4210/Medical Adhesive, Type A strips to the skin of human subjects. The adhesive bond strengths of all materials were not significantly different. Cevik et al. (2022) evaluated outdoor and artificial weathering on the color stability of CPE, A-2186, and Silastic MDX4-4210/Medical Adhesive Type A. They found that CPE specimens had the most color changes when compared to A-2186 and Silastic MDX4-4210/Medical Adhesive Type A silicone elastomer specimens after being subjected to one-year outdoor weathering and 450 kJ/m^2 of artificial aging. Eleni et al. (2009a, 2009b, 2011a, 2011b, 2011c) reported that CPE and M511 became softer and more ductile after outdoor weathering.

Polyphosphazenes

Polyphosphazene fluoroelastomer (PNF) is a semiorganic polymer with a phosphorus and nitrogen backbone and fluorocarbon pendant groups. When compounded (Table 5-4) with pigment, originally it was developed for use as a resilient denture liner (U.S. Patent No. 4,661,065; May and Guerra, 1978; May et al., 1981; Gettleman et al., 1985, 1987, 1989a, 1989b) and marketed as Novus (Hygenic) until 1994, when the source of the raw material became unavailable. It was reintroduced to the market by Lang Dental in 2010 and now is distributed by White Square Chemical. Novus, as compounded, has a durometer hardness (Shore A) H_{DA} of 35, tensile strength of 1.65 MPa, elongation of 18%, bond strength to PMMA of 3.4 kN/m^2, and tan δ of 1.4 (Gettleman, 2004).

A variety of physical properties can be achieved by *(1)* altering the ratio of interpenetrating acrylic resins to the fluoroalkoxy-substituted polyphosphazene rubber (Shore A hardness values of 10 to 90; Gettleman, 1999), *(2)* substituting longer or shorter side groups during polymer synthesis, *(3)* changing the cross-linking functionality during polymer synthesis, and *(4)* changing fillers. Standard skin shades and stiffnesses (to simulate cartilage) can be layered during trial packing to simulate deep cartilage and coloring, then covered by more superficial translucent and softer layers for adaptation to a feather edge. It can be cured in hot water in gypsum molds.

Table 5-4 Proposed composition of polyphosphazene fluoroelastomer for facial prostheses

Chemical name	Function	phr	Grams
Polyphosphazene fluoroelastomer	Gum rubber	100	50
Trimethanolpropane trimethacrylate	Trifunctional cross-linker	18	9
PMMA beads	Polymer filler	10	7.5
Ethylene glycol dimethacrylate	Difunctional cross-linker	2	1
Benzoyl peroxide	Initiator	1	0.5

Compared to silicones, polyphosphazenes have higher edge and tensile strengths, are easy to adjust with rotary instruments, have an indefinite shelf life and working time if refrigerated, chemically bond to acrylic resins, are biocompatible, are stable, and are permanently soft (no plasticizers). They are compatible with skin adhesives and are more resistant to the growth of microorganisms than silicone rubber (Gettleman et al., 1982, 1985, 1987, 1989a, 1989b, 1992, 1999; May and Guerra, 1978). This elastomer has the potential for use as an alternative facial prosthetic material, but further studies are needed.

Regardless of the type of materials used in the fabrication of facial prostheses, the service life of a facial prosthesis is limited. A survey by Chen et al. (1981) indicated that the average wearing time of a facial prosthesis was 10 months. In the recent survey by Cardoso et al. (2022), the average wearing time was one to two years.

Colorants

The results from the 2020 survey (Cardoso et al., 2022) indicated that the pigments most used as intrinsic (base) color and extrinsic color of facial prostheses were silicone Functional Intrinsic pigments, followed, in order, by oil pigments and dry earth pigments. Also, clinicians frequently employed rayon flocking fibers for intrinsic coloring and extrinsic coloring. Fewer respondents used the Spectromatch Reality Series, or the e-Skin coloration system (Table 5-5).

Table 5-5 Most commonly used pigments for silicone facial prosthetic materials

	First	Second	Third	Fourth	Fifth	Sixth
Intrinsic colorants	Silicone	Oil	Dry earth	e-Skin	Reality	No colorants used
Extrinsic colorants	Silicone	Oil	Dry earth	Reality	e-Skin	No colorants used

Cardoso et al., 2022.

From the same survey, the top five materials used for extrinsic coloring of prostheses were Silastic Medical Adhesive, Type A; Silastic MDX4-4210; A-2186; M5111; and A-2000 (Table 5-2). About half (52%) of clinicians did not apply any extrinsic coating, and 48% of respondents applied a combination of Factor II A-564, TS-564, MD-564, TS-564-NFS, MD-564-NF, and/or Technovent P799 extrinsic sealant.

Some colorants may be incompatible with the base elastomer and adversely affect its physical and mechanical properties (Turner et al., 1985a, 1985b). For example, artist's oils were found to interfere with the setting reaction of platinum-cured silicone elastomers (Kiat-amnuay et al., 2002; Colas and Curtis, 2004; Bayer and Goldschmidt, 1991); therefore, oil pigments should only be used with Silastic MDX4-4210/ Medical Adhesive, Type A.

Silicone "intrinsic" colorants (Factor II) were introduced in 1996 to be used with platinum-cured silicones. They were formulated with dimethyl fluid, which at the time was the industry standard. Food, dye, and cosmetic (FD&C) pigments were milled into a dimethyl polymer but settling introduced a fluid that could alter the physical properties of the silicone if used in excess. In 1999, a fluid that was more compatible with the addition of silicone elastomers was introduced. Use of the same FD&C pigments in a cross-linking fluid maintained the viscosity and allowed the user to dispense it drop by drop. With the addition of more pigment to the cross-linking fluid, silicone "extrinsic" colorants (Factor II) were introduced using the same pigments and fluid as extrinsic colorants but with increased intensity.

Coloration techniques can be divided into three groups: *(1)* extrinsic, *(2)* intrinsic, or *(3)* a combination of both. The combination technique is widely used because it produces prostheses with a more lifelike appearance. The color match of the prosthesis depends on the skill of the clinician, the color acuity of the individual, and the light source under which the color-matching procedure is performed.

Color matching and color formulation

Color matching of prostheses to human skin has long been a challenge for maxillofacial prosthodontists. Human skin is a multilayered structure, composed of epidermis, dermis, hypodermis, and subcutaneous tissue. Each layer differs in thickness, histologic components, and pigments (melanin, hemoglobin, and beta-carotene). The color effect of human skin is a result of combinations of light that are reflected, refracted, and scattered directly or diffusely by this multilayered structure. Since the introduction of more color-stable facial elastomers and colorants, there has been an emphasis on research toward developing methods for color matching of facial prostheses to human skin (Box 5-5).

Many techniques have been developed to achieve accurate skin matching. Gillman (1950) made an early attempt at objectifying skin color matching. Firtell and Bartlett (1969) attempted to quantitively record the number of colorants used for the custom formulation of the base shade and extrinsic characterization. It was the beginning of the color formulation idea. Custom facial skin shade guides for facial prostheses have been described using a trial-and-error method (Godoy et al., 1992; Over et al., 1998). These clinicians focused only on facial skin shades for Caucasian patients.

Cantor and colleagues (1969) were the first to report using a reflectance spectrophotometer to evaluate the color of human skin and select silicone elastomers used for facial prostheses. They suggested that the study of the reflectance characteristics of human skin might lead to the development of an isometric pigment for coloring facial prostheses. Spectral measurements of human skin have been reported by both Cantor et al. (1969) and Koran et al. (1981). Since then, color, optical density, and reflectance spectrophotometry have been used to evaluate the color of facial prosthetic materials (Koran et al., 1979a, 1979b; Haug et al., 1992a, 1992b, 1999a, 1999b, 1999c; Beatty et al., 1995, 1999; Han et al., 2008; Kiat-amnuay et al., 2002, 2005, 2006a, 2006b; Gozalo-Diaz et al., 2007; Coward et al., 2008; Lemon et al., 1995; Bryant et al., 1994; Hulterstrom et al., 1999; Johnston et al., 1996; Johnston and Kao, 1989; Paul et al., 2002; Wang et al., 2016; Kurt et al., 2021; Seelaus et al., 2011; Wee et al., 2006, 2013; Douglas et al., 2007; Kim et al., 2008; Hungerford et al., 2013; Hu and Johnston, 2010, 2009a, 2009b; Nemli et al., 2018).

Contact-measuring instruments, including colorimeters and spectrophotometers, have been used to provide more reliable, consistent, and quantitative assessments of skin color and facial prosthetic measurements under controlled conditions (Haug et al., 1992a; Han et al., 2008; Kiat-amnuay et al., 2002, 2005, 2006a, 2006b; Koran et al., 1981; Johnston and Kao, 1989; Paul et al., 2002). However, edge loss has been reported when using contact reflectance instruments while measuring translucent materials (Johnston et al., 1996). Edge loss occurs when incident light enters into a translucent object such as elastomers used for facial prostheses or human skin, and some light is scattered beyond the contact aperture edges of the measuring instrument without being absorbed, with the result that this scattered light is not measured by the instrument (Hu, 2010).

Coward et al. (2008) conducted a pilot study on the effectiveness of a computerized color formulation system and spectrophotometry to predict pigment formulas of pigmented silicone elastomers to match the skin color of 19 African-Canadian subjects. These systems provided an objective method for the color-matching procedure for facial prostheses as opposed to the subjective methods currently employed. The authors suggested that further study was needed to establish a precise and repeatable color-matching system that would predict required colorants and control of metamerism. In a follow-up study, the same group of researchers (Seelaus et al., 2011) explored the relationship between an objective computer measurement and subjective clinical evaluation of color match between silicone samples and skin. They concluded that spectrophotometry and computerized color formulation technology offer enhanced color matching; however, a reasonable correlation existed between the subjective and objective assessments of color matching.

Noncontact color measuring systems using a spectroradiometer have shown benefits in obtaining more accurate color information of translucent prosthetic materials by eliminating edge loss (Bolt et al., 1994). Gozalo-Diaz et al. (2007) described a lighting setup for noncontact measurements with a spectroradiometer that avoided shadowing in order to achieve the most accurate color measurement of vital craniofacial structures. They found that the spectral reflectance could be measured with acceptable validity and test-retest reliability using a noncontacting 45/0-degree optical configuration. Therefore, they recommended this configuration as a viable alternative to obtain CIELAB color values for shade replication in facial prosthetic rehabilitation (Gozalo-Diaz et al., 2007; Wee et al., 2006). This system has also been utilized in many research studies for color matching in dentistry (Douglas et al., 2007; Kim et al., 2008).

Wee and colleagues (2013) proposed a shade guide for human facial skin and lips for fabrication of silicone facial prostheses. They measured facial skin in a sample human population, stratified by age (five age groups), gender, and race (four racial/ethnic groups). Reflectance measurements were made by using a spectroradiometer and xenon arc lamp with a 45/0 optical configuration. They identified five shade tabs that permit a selection of base pigments. This facial shade guide may reduce the time needed to obtain an acceptable shade match for the fabrication of silicone facial prostheses. The methodology used in this study appears to provide a more reliable, consistent, and quantitative assessment of skin color.

Hungerford et al. (2013) measured L*a*b* values of 11 skin tone pigments combined at 0.1%, 1%, and 10% by weight of Factor II Functional Intrinsic silicone pigments with A-2186 elastomer. They found that silicone pigments and A-2186 elastomer appeared to be too white and not sufficiently red to adequately match the skin tones of the subject population. This study suggested that adjustments must be made to the existing pigmenting system in order to provide an adequate match of facial prostheses. *(Authors' note: Reflectance spectrophotometry is used to evaluate the color changes of aged materials. The CIELAB system has been widely used by investigators in this field to assess color change [ΔE] and has been used to evaluate the color stability of silicone elastomers subjected to artificial aging. The L*a*b* coordinates can be used to calculate color differences or color changes, by using the CIELAB color-difference equation ΔE* = [(ΔL*)2 + (Δa*)2 + (Δb*)2]1/2. Values that exceed ΔE of 3 are considered clinically unacceptable.)*

Hu and Johnston (2010) compared noncontact and four-contact color measuring instruments in accuracy and precision on measurements of pigmented maxillofacial elastomer specimens. They concluded that the contact-measuring devices performed differently in accuracy, possibly due to edge loss, but performed comparably in precision with the noncontact measuring instrument, the spectroradiometer. Although a noncontact device is recommended for color measurement of maxillofacial prosthetic materials, improvements are needed due to measurement time, lack of portability, and potential sensitivity to surface features of the object.

Hu and Johnston (2009a, 2009b) measured specimens at different thicknesses of each of the 19 shades of skin-colored maxillofacial elastomers using the interfacial reflection corrections for Kubelka–Munk (K–M) theory on each of three backings. They concluded that the reflectance measurements using a 45°/0° noncontact measuring system provide higher accuracy on maxillofacial elastomers over the more important visible wavelengths for translucent materials. The significance of this study was that the color and translucency of maxillofacial elastomers can now be predicted using corrected K-M theory. In addition, they found that the complete second-order regression model performed accurately in determining the concentration additivity of pigmented maxillofacial elastomer mixtures. This regression model was recommended as an alternative for colorant formulation applications based on a corrected K–M model for improving color matching of pigmented maxillofacial prostheses to human skin.

Hu et al. (2011) compared a method of laser light diffusing area and color difference due to edge loss in measuring the accuracy of translucency estimations of thick pigmented prosthetic facial elastomers. They found that the laser-light-diffusing method, a noncontact and nondestructive method, appeared to be highly reliable for the estimation of translucency of maxillofacial elastomers and human skin and could further be incorporated into the appearance matching of facial prostheses to human skin.

E-Skin (Spectromatch) is a moderate-cost handheld contact spectrocolorimeter designed for shade matching facial prostheses. This device collects reflectance data for two sets of illuminants, natural daylight (D65) and tungsten (A), with a 10-degree observer angle. The device has a measuring area that can be adjusted for 4 or 8 mm and an independent tridirectional 25 light-emitting diode (LED) source. The software in the device converts the colorimeter data to values that correspond with spectrophotometric data previously collected by the company. The device uses these values to find the closest color match in a database of 22,000 skin shades. Each color in the database corresponds with an available formula for skin shade fabrication (Bulbulian, 1939). One possible major issue with this device is loss of accuracy due to the edge loss that occurs from applying pressure to the skin during readings.

Nemli et al. (2018) evaluated the accuracy of e-Skin in color and translucency matching of 28 different skin colors fabricated from M511 silicone and Technovent pigments. Although they found that the mean CIELAB ΔE* for all 28 shade tabs was 3.83, considered clinically unacceptable according to Paravina et al. (2009), they concluded that e-Skin was found to be reliable to determine color and translucency matching of human skin.

Wang et al. (2016) compared spectral curves of skin shade tabs fabricated from the e-Skin handheld colorimeter formula and a traditional anaplastology mixing method against noncontact spectroradiometer measurements of human skin at the same position. They also clinically evaluated both methods of shade reproduction in terms of color match to human subjects using blinded clinical evaluators. Results from a "spectroradiometer" showed that the e-Skin formulation and pigment system resulted in a closer color match to the human subject than the traditional method using commonly used pigments by an anaplastologist. The "clinical evaluation" found that a clinically acceptable match was shown with both methods, but a closer color match was found using e-Skin two-thirds of the time. The e-Skin proved to be helpful with the color matching and replication process in addition to saving time and helpful for recordkeeping purposes. However, it is much costlier than the commonly used trial-and-error silicone and coloring method.

Kurt et al. (2021) determined the acceptable color match of light- and dark-skin silicone replicas fabricated with the use of two handheld contact computerized color-matching systems, a spectrophotometer and colorimeter (e-Skin). Silicone skin tabs for participants were produced from the color formulations provided by the online calculator tool of both systems. They also clinically evaluated both methods of shade reproduction in terms of color match to human subjects using blinded clinical evaluators. Similar to Wang et al. (2016), the clinical evaluation showed that a clinically acceptable match was found with the e-Skin system.

Mulcare et al. (2019) were the first to compare the trueness and precision of the RGB Colorimeter mobile phone noncontact colorimeter application (White Marten UG) installed on a smartphone (iPhone 5s) and the e-Skin handheld colorimeter contact device, measuring 10 silicone elastomer swatches mimicking a range of human skin tones at a distance of 25, 30, and 35 mm from the test instruments. They found that the trueness of both devices varied depending on the distance. For "absolute trueness and relative trueness," the overall mean ΔE values were greater than the clinical acceptability threshold, whereas "absolute precision and relative precision" were well within the clinical acceptability threshold. They concluded that the mobile phone colorimeter applications have the potential to provide affordable and accessible skin-color measurements. However, future study assessing image calibration to improve trueness and the control of measuring distance, background noise, and uniformity of illumination is required.

Scientific color matching involves quantitatively describing the optical properties of colorants and applying them to a mathematical model that simulates the multilayered optical characteristics of human skin. Currently, there has been no randomized controlled clinical trial evaluating color matching of facial prosthetic materials (Ranabhatt, 2017). Facial skin shade guides and color formulations that cover various ethnic groups must be developed.

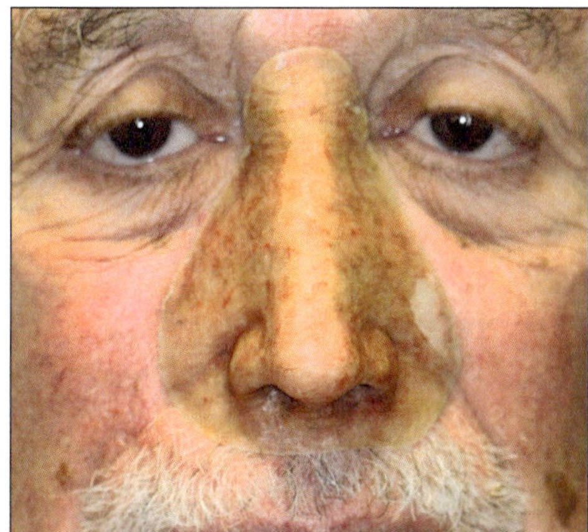

Figure 5-13 This prosthesis has been in service for over two years and has yellowed and darkened, and some of the extrinsic coloration has worn off the left edge.

Table 5-6 Suggested desirable performance characteristics of mechanical properties of elastomer base with "no" pigments/opacifiers

Mechanical properties	Desirable property values	Silicone MDX4-4210	CPE
Tensile strength (MPa) psi	6.9–13.8 1,000–2,000	3.2 470	8.3 1,200
Tear strength kN/m. PPI	5.3–17.5 60–100	21 120	18.4 105
Elongation %	400–800	410	950–1,350
Hardness (Shore A)	25–35	18	42–45

Lewis and Castleberry, 1980; May and Guerra, 1978.

Color stability and mechanical property studies following artificial aging

The color stability and mechanical properties of maxillofacial prostheses in a service environment have been a major concern (Fig 5-13). According to the 2020 international survey (Cardoso et al., 2022), 63% of respondents reported that "color fading" was the most common reason for remaking facial prostheses, followed by "margin tears" (26%). The remaining 12% cited "microorganism growth," "liner debonding," "tissue change," and "prosthesis became harder," respectively. In addition, most respondents (68%) reported remaking a facial prosthesis for a patient within one to two years, 20% after two years, and 10% within six months. Since the 1970s, these issues have directed most investigations (Box 5-5).

Lewis and Castleberry (1980) suggested desirable performance characteristics of mechanical properties of elastomer base with "no" pigments/opacifiers (Table 5-6). All elastomeric manufacturing companies reported mechanical and physical property information for each silicone tested with no colorant, opacifier, UV light protection, or thixotropic agent added but without subjecting the material to aging conditions.

To date, there have only been a few research groups that combine testing of color stability and mechanical properties on the same silicone/pigments/opacifiers.

The University of Michigan team published numerous articles regarding color stability and physical properties of various materials used for facial prostheses subjected to artificial aging. The color stability of six maxillofacial elastomers was evaluated using reflectance spectrophotometry during 900 hours of accelerated aging in a Weather-Ometer (Craig et al., 1978). The silicone elastomers evaluated in the study, especially Silastic 4-4210 (now MDX4-4210), demonstrated good color stability. Because the color of the "base" silicone elastomer was largely unaffected by "accelerated aging," they suggested that the discoloration of a facial prosthesis observed clinically might be the result of the colorants used. The investigators then studied the color stability of 11 dry mineral earth pigments under accelerated aging of the same Silastic 4-4210. Quantitative color analysis showed that 4 of 11 pigments showed small but statistically significant color changes (Koran et al., 1979).

After verifying 4-4210's color and physical property stability, the team investigated the ultimate tensile strength, shear strength, maximum elongation percentage, Shore A hardness, and permanent deformation of intrinsically colored Silastic 4-4210 after 900 hours of accelerated aging (Yu et al., 1980a). They found that pigment incorporation of 0.2% by weight can alter the physical and mechanical properties of the "base" elastomer. However, accelerated aging had no effect on the physical properties of the pigment and elastomer combinations.

A team at the Houston Center for Biomaterials and Biomimetics has conducted several investigations on color stability and mechanical properties of various silicone elastomers, opacifier types, and

Table 5-7 Mean (SD) values of commonly used pigmented silicone elastomers subjected to 450 kJ/m² of artificial aging studied at HCBB

Silicone	Pigment	Opacifier	CIELAB	Tensile strength (MPa)	Tear strength (kN/m)	% elongation	Hardness Shore A
MDX4-4210 (10:1)	Silicone	Silicone	0.3 (0.1)	1.0 (0.2)	11.8 (2.0)	245 (36)	23 (0.9)
MDX4-4210/Type A	Oil	Titanium dry earth	1.1 (0.2)	1.4 (0.0)	12.7 (2.3)	454 (71)	20 (0.7)
MDX4-4210/Type A	Oil	Oil	1.2 (0.2)*	2.0 (0.1)	9.5 (0.1)	462 (43)	19 (0.7)
MDX4-4210/Type A	Silicone	Silicone	0.9 (0.1)	1.2 (0.3)	8.6 (2.0)	481 (32)	18 (1.7)
A-2186 (10:1)	Cosmetic dry earth	Titanium dry earth	2.4 (0.1)*	Not recommended			
A-2186 (10:1)	Silicone	Silicone	0.8 (0.1)	1.6 (0.2)	21.3 (3.7)	232 (12)	31 (1.6)
VST-50 (10:1)	Silicone	Silicone	1.0 (0.1)	2.1 (0.3)	22.8 (3.2)	447 (68)	25 (1.3)
M511 (10:1)	e-Skin	e-Skin	0.5 (0.04)	1.7 (0.2)	27.7 (6.4)	189 (19)	39 (1.0)
M511 (10:1)	Reality	Reality	0.4 (0.2)	1.9 (0.3)	23.2 (3.4)	184 (28)	45 (0.3)
A-2000 (1:1)	Silicone	Silicone	0.8 (0.1)	1.8 (0.5)	17.4 (4.6)	294 (70)	28 (1.1)
A-2000 (1:1)	e-Skin	e-Skin	0.3 (0.2)	1.9 (0.3)	23.5 (6.0)	202 (37)	40 (1.5)

* Above the clinical perceptibility threshold

percentages of various pigments commonly used by maxillofacial prosthodontists, anaplastologists, and clinicians. Their studies were triggered by the data obtained from two surveys, one conducted in 2008 (Montgomery and Kiat-amnuay, 2008) and the other conducted in 2020 (Cardoso et al., 2022). The results of their work are shown in Table 5-7.

Initially, their team evaluated perceptibility and acceptability thresholds for color differences of light- and dark-skin-colored facial elastomers (Paravina et al., 2009). Color match or mismatch and acceptable or unacceptable mismatch of each pair of facial silicone specimens were visually evaluated by 45 evaluators under controlled conditions. A spectrophotometer was used to assess before and after aging CIELAB/CIEDE 2000 50:50% perceptibility and acceptability thresholds were 1.1/0.7 and 3.0/2.1, respectively, for light specimens and 1.6/1.2 and 4.4/3.1, respectively, for dark specimens.

Subsequently, they published a two-part study emphasizing the importance of studying both the color stability (part 1) and the mechanical properties (part 2) of the same experimental materials, in the same laboratory, and using the same artificial aging conditions for pigmented silicone elastomers (Han et al., 2013; Nguyen et al., 2013). They reported that Sunforgettable UV light absorber (a commercially available sunscreen), used as an opacifier at 5%, 10%, and 15%, protected commonly used pigmented (primary colors [red, yellow, blue] mixture of primary colors, and no colors) silicone MDX4-4210/Type A from color degradation after aging. However, the mechanical properties of the elastomer were degraded significantly, and therefore, the use of this material as an opacifier was not recommended.

The team also evaluated the color stability and the mechanical properties of A-2000 and M511 silicone elastomers mixed with the e-Skin and Reality Series pigment/opacifier systems before and after artificial aging (Bates et al., 2021). They found that artificial aging affected color stability and the mechanical properties of the pigmented silicone elastomers with added opacifier. Overall, A-2000 mixed with the e-Skin group displayed the most color stability, with its mechanical properties being the least affected by artificial aging. Artificial aging significantly increased hardness for all silicone groups beyond the ideal range for facial prostheses in addition to lowering the elongation percentage.

Their research group also studied the color stability and mechanical properties of A-2186, A-2000, VST-50, and MDX4-4210 (10:1) mixed with Functional Intrinsic pigments subjected to artificial aging at 450 kJ/m² (Mount et al., 2018). They concluded that aging significantly affected the mechanical properties of A-2186 the most and MDX4-4210 and VST-50 the least. A-2000 showed the most improvement in mechanical properties. For the color stability study, MDX4-4210 was the most color-stable silicone after aging.

Tables 5-7 and 5-8 report mean (SD) values of commonly used pigmented silicone elastomers subjected to 450 kJ/m² of artificial aging (Kiat-amnuay et al., 2002, 2009; Kiat-amnuay, 2006a, 2006b; Bates et al., 2021). The team published data on color stability and mechanical properties and shared results with Factor II (no conflict of interest, since no funding/compensation was received from the company). The company used the data provided to improve its materials. The data shown in Table 5-7 is the most current, and some of the experimental protocols were repeated after improvements were made. Overall, most pigmented silicones are color stable after 450 kJ/m² artificial aging within CIELAB 50:50% perceptibility (<1.1) and acceptability (<3.0) thresholds. When tear strength increased, Shore A hardness also increased.

With these long-term data, the author suggests color stability thresholds and desirable performance characteristics of mechanical properties of silicone mixed with pigments/opacifiers (Table 5-9). These studies, in their aggregate, have shown that these combinations result in long-term color stability with retention of mechanical properties (Table 5-10).

Similar studies conducted by other laboratories

Stathi and colleagues (2010) studied the effect of UV protection (Tinuvin 770 from Ciba) with dry earth (Principality Medical Ltd.) and functional pigments (Technovent Ltd.) on mechanical properties and color stability of MDX4-4210 silicone elastomers after

Table 5-8 Experimental and company information of materials studied as listed in Table 5-6

Silicone	Base: cross-linker/catalyst	Company information
MDX4-4210/Type A	1:3 ratio or 25:75%	Dow Corning Corp. or Factor II Inc.
MDX4-4210	10:1 ratio	Dow Corning Corp. or Factor II Inc.
A-2186	10:1 ratio	Factor II Inc. or Technovent Ltd.
VST-50	10:1 ratio	Factor II Inc. or Technovent Ltd.
A-2186	10:1 ratio	Factor II Inc. or Technovent Ltd.
A-2000	1:1 ratio	Factor II Inc. or Technovent Ltd.
M511	10:1 ratio	Technovent Ltd. or Factor II Inc.
Pigments/opacifiers (white)	**Primary color (0.01 each of Red + Yellow + Blue)**	**Company information**
Titanium dry earth	10% opacifier by volume	Factor II Inc.
Cosmetic dry earth	0.03 g pigment and 10% opacifier by volume	Factor II Inc.
Silicone functional intrinsic	0.03 ml pigment and 10% opacifier by volume	Factor II Inc.
Oil	0.03 cc pigment and 10% opacifier by volume	M. Grumbacher Inc.
e-Skin	0.03 g pigment and 10% opacifier by volume	Spectromatch Ltd. or Factor II Inc.
Reality	0.03 g pigment and 10% opacifier by volume	Spectromatch Ltd. or Technovent Ltd.

Table 5-9 Suggested color stability thresholds and desirable performance characteristics of mechanical properties of silicone mixed with pigments/opacifiers

Mechanical properties	Current materials (Tables 5-6 and 5-10)		Desirable property values	
Tensile strength (MPa) psi	1–8 145–1160		>1.0 >145	
Tear strength kN/m PPI	8–28 46–160		>10 >57	
Elongation %	180–950		>200	
Hardness (Shore A)	18–45		<45	
Color stability threshold185	**CIELAB**		**CIEDE 2000**	
	Light shade	*Dark shade*	*Light shade*	*Dark shade*
50% perceptibility	1.1	1.6	0.7	1.2
50% acceptability	3.0	4.4	2.1	3.1

Table 5-10 Recommended silicone/colorant combination for extraoral maxillofacial prostheses with overall best performance on color stability and mechanical properties testing

Silicone	Pigment	Opacifier
MDX4-4210/Type A	Oil	Titanium dry earth
MDX4-4210 (10:1)	Silicone	Silicone
A-2186 (10:1)	Silicone	Silicone
VST-50 (10:1)	Silicone	Silicone
A-2000 (1:1)	Silicone	Silicone
A-2000 (1:1)	e-Skin	e-Skin

875 hours of artificial accelerated aging. The results showed that the mechanical properties (tensile strength, modulus of elasticity, and % strain at break) were not affected. However, for color stability, the yellow and green dry earth pigments used in the study "severely" affected the MDX4-4210 silicone adversely with a ΔE* value >59.6 in the yellow group and >47.7 in the green group (clinical acceptability threshold <3.0); therefore, it is not recommended for use clinically. For functional pigments, yellow (ΔE* value = 10.8) and blue (ΔE* value = 8.1) showed better results than dry earth pigments, but significant color changes were still noted, exceeding the clinically acceptable threshold ΔE* value of 3.0. Tinuvin UV light absorber did not protect silicone from color degradation when mixed with dry earth pigments and is not recommended for clinical use.

Al-Harbi et al. (2015) examined the effects of outdoor weathering in a hot and humid climate on the mechanical properties and color stability of TechSil S25 (HTV silicone) and two commonly used RTV silicones, MDX4-4210 and A-2186. They found that outdoor weathering adversely affected the properties of all silicones, but heat-polymerized TechSil S25 showed better mechanical durability and color stability; it can be used as an alternative silicone for the fabrication of facial prostheses for patients living in a hot and humid environment.

Photooxidation and degradation of facial prosthetic materials and research tools used to determine color stability

Facial prostheses are subject to mechanical and chemical degradation that affects their appearance and physical properties. The degradation of a polymer surface due to the combined action of light and oxygen in polymer chemistry is called photooxidation or oxidative photodegradation (Weifel et al., 2009). Silicone facial prostheses are especially subject to photooxidation. The general process for photooxidation can be divided into several stages, which can all occur simultaneously (Rabek, 1992):

- Initiation: The process of formation of the first free chemical radicals
- Propagation: The conversion of one active radical to another, resulting in chain scissions (the degradation of a polymer main chain)
- Chain branching: Steps that end with more than one active radical being produced
- Termination: Steps in which active radicals react with one another, often creating cross-links between the chains

Susceptibility to photooxidation varies depending on the elastomer's chemical structure. In addition to photooxidation, continuous cross-linking and polymerization can lead to color changes. In general, organic pigments are more susceptible to color changes than inorganic pigments due to their larger particle size and their ability to migrate and separate from the polymer matrix more readily (dos Santos et al., 2010; Cruz et al., 2020). Many pigments and dyes also affect the rate of photooxidation due to their ability to absorb UV-energy and, in doing so, protect the polymer. However, UV absorption could cause the dyes to enter an excited state where they may attack the elastomer. Interactions may become even more complicated when other additives, such as thixotropic agents, and radiopaque additives are present (Allen et al., 1989). Silicones are considered to have good color stability compared to many other materials including polyethylene. The majority of the 2020 survey respondents, however, reported that color fading was the most common reason for remaking facial prostheses (Cardoso et al., 2022). Photooxidation and thermal degradation can occur simultaneously and accelerate each other.

Color stability can be investigated by either natural (outdoor) or artificial (accelerated weather) testing (Jacques et al., 2020). Such testing is important in determining the expected service life of facial prostheses. For artificial (accelerated weather) testing, the external environment to which facial prostheses are exposed is not constrained to the conditions set by an aging chamber. For example, prostheses are typically not exposed to a constantly wet environment as in artificial aging. Aging at an accelerated rate could produce greater changes than routine use or natural aging of prostheses (Lemon et al., 1995; Tran et al., 2004; Bates et al., 2021). Artificial accelerated aging is a method of correlating the color stability of materials exposed to natural aging. Calculation of the correlation or acceleration of artificial aging in comparison to natural aging in different climate conditions is complicated (Weathering Testing Guidebook, 2001). Researchers must be cautious in comparing real-time data. Inconsistencies in lighting hours for different types of cycles and machines suggest the reporting of kJ/m^2 instead of total hours of artificial aging (Weathering Testing Guidebook, 2001). The artificial aging method is highly valuable for assessing color stability and mechanical properties of materials used in dentistry.

Color stability of "intrinsic" coloration

Colorants and opacifiers are added to create lifelike color and translucency to facial prostheses. Several studies have been conducted to assess the impact of these factors on the long-term color stability and clinical life span of facial prostheses. What follows is a summary of the most pertinent investigations of the commonly used materials combined with various colorants and opacifiers.

Silastic MDX 4-4210 with catalyst A-103 (Dow Corning)

Dos Santos et al (2011) studied ceramic powder and oil paint and barium sulfate opacifier on color stability of MDX4-4210 submitted to accelerated aging at 1,008 hours. Similar to previous studies (Haug et al., 1999; Kiat-amnuay et al., 2006b; Han et al., 2010), they showed that opacifier and oil pigment (with and without opacifier) protect Silastic MDX4-4210/Medical Adhesive Type A against color degradation. The same group of investigators (Pesqueira et al., 2011) studied color stability of ceramic powder (inorganic) and a makeup powder (organic pigment), both from Brazil, of MDX4-4210 silicone submitted to disinfection and accelerated aging at 1,008 hours. They found that ceramic pigment showed greater color stability regardless of period and disinfection and the makeup pigment exhibited the highest values of chromatic alteration. In 2012, dos Santos et al. studied color stability of MDX4-4210 submitted to natural weathering in Brazil for 90 and 180 days. Both colorless ($\Delta E^* > 3.5$) and pigmented ($\Delta E^* > 8.8$) MDX4-4210 showed color changes greater than the clinical acceptability threshold. Results from outdoor aging of the ceramic powder group were not consistent with artificial aging as reported.

The use of microencapsulated thermochromic (color-changing) leuco dyes pigment in MDX4-4210 silicone elastomer was first investigated by Kantola et al. (2013). They also added thixotropic agents to the silicone mixture with functional silicone intrinsic pigments and 0.2 and 0.6 wt% of thermochromic pigments. They concluded that the addition of 0.2 wt% thermochromic pigments gives rise to color changes when the temperature decreases and could be used to compensate for a change in the color of the facial tissue in colder temperatures. Future research focusing on color stability and mechanical properties under aging and environmental studies of thermochromic pigments is needed.

Combined MDX 4-4210 / Silastic Medical Adhesive, Type A: 25:75 mix

An extensive research study done by Kiat-amnuay and her team at the HCBB laboratory found that MD4-4210/Type A, when mixed with oil, silicone, and/or dry earth pigments and opacifiers, exhibited satisfactory results for color stability and mechanical properties (Table 5-7). They measured the effects of six different opacifiers (5%, 10%, and 15% each) on the color stability of intrinsically pigmented maxillofacial MDX 4-4210/Silastic Medical Adhesive, Type A, after it was subjected to artificial aging. Silicone pigments (primary colors: red, yellow ochre, blue, and a mixture of all three colors) mixed with 5% titanium white oil, 15% Artskin white dry earth, or 15% dry pigment titanium white remained the most color stable over time, and pigments mixed with 10% calcined dry earth kaolin had the most color changes. Yellow ochre had a significant effect on all opacifiers (ΔE^* values increased from 0.6 to 5.9 after 450 kJ/m^2; Kiat-amnuay et al., 2004b).

Results from a color stability study (Kiat-amnuay et al., 2006) showed that oil pigments mixed with five different types of opacifiers (5%, 10%, and 15% concentrations) helped protect the MDX 4-4210/Silastic Medical Adhesive, Type A, combination from color degradation over time (artificial aging at 450 kJ/m^2) with color changes (ΔE^*) of less than 1.54 for all groups. A delta E (ΔE^*) of less than 3.0 is considered to be a clinically acceptable color change. Titanium white opacifier remained the most color stable over time, followed in order by calcined kaolin powder, Georgia kaolin, Artskin white, and titanium white artists' oil pigment.

Han et al. (2010a) investigated the color stability of oil-pigmented maxillofacial silicone MDX4-4210/Type A with different opacifiers, subjected to 10 years of dark storage and artificial aging. Five widely used dry earth and oil opacifiers were evaluated at 5%, 10%, and 15% concentrations. Five pigment conditions were chosen: no pigment, cadmium-barium red deep, yellow ochre, burnt sienna, and a mixture of the three. Pigments were mixed with MDX4-4210/Type A silicone and subjected to 450 kJ/m^2 exposure of artificial weathering in the HCBB laboratory. The CIE L*a*b* values of all specimens were measured by a spectrophotometer before and after artificial aging in 1999. Then all specimens were placed in dark storage for 10 years, and CIE L*a*b* values were measured again in 2009. The specimens were then placed once again in an artificial aging chamber for another 450 kJ/m^2 exposure, and CIE L*a*b* values were measured. The data from baseline reading in 1999 were also compared with the final reading after artificial aging in 2009 as overall color changes. They concluded that, overall, after 10 years of dark storage and 900 kJ/m^2 of artificial aging, dry pigment titanium white opacifier provided the highest protection to oil-pigmented MDX4-4210/ Type A silicone elastomer from color degradation over time (change in ΔE* value of only 1.0 after 10 years in dark storage), followed by calcined kaolin (ΔE* value of 1.8), Georgia kaolin (ΔE* value of 2.4), Artskin (ΔE* value of 4.7, clinically unacceptable), and titanium white oil pigment (ΔE* value of 5.2, clinically unacceptable).

A-2186

Beatty et al. (1995, 1999) investigated color changes in dry-pigmented and oil-pigmented maxillofacial silicone elastomers after exposure to UV light. Five dry rare-earth pigments were mixed with A-2186. Cosmetic red and cadmium yellow pigments underwent significant color degradation after 400 hours of UV light exposure. Cosmetic yellow ochre and Mars violet remained color stable after 1,800 hours of exposure.

Five oil pigments were mixed with A-2186 and Silastic Medical Adhesive, Type A, intrinsically. The intrinsic (base) colors of cadmium red, cadmium yellow, and yellow ochre underwent the greatest color changes (ΔE* values of 7.1 to 9.4) after 1,800 hours of UV exposure. Overall, neither dry earth nor oil pigments mixed with A-2186 in these studies were color stable after UV light exposure (ΔE* greater than the perceptibility and acceptability thresholds of 1.1 and 3.0, respectively; Paravina et al., 2009).

Gary et al. (2001) evaluated color changes of A-2186 silicone elastomer mixed with three pigments (a natural inorganic dry earth pigment and two synthesized organic pigments) and subjected to sunlight natural weathering exposure in Miami (1,305.7 MJ/m^2) and Phoenix (1,310.2 MJ/m^2). Mean color changes were greater in Phoenix (ΔE* of 3.5 for controls and ΔE* of 6.0 to 9.3 for pigmented specimens) than in Miami (ΔE* of 1.1 for controls and ΔE* of 7.3 to 8.9 for pigmented specimens). None of the pigments mixed with A-2186 was color stable after natural weathering.

Kiat-amnuay et al. (2002) studied the effects of four different opacifiers (5%, 10%, and 15% concentrations) on the color stability of cosmetic dry earth–pigmented maxillofacial silicone A-2186 when it was subjected to artificial aging. They also found that mixing inorganic dry earth cosmetic pigments (red, yellow, burnt sienna, and a mix of all three colors) with opacifiers did not protect silicone A-2186 from color degradation over time, especially in the case of red pigment (ΔE* values of 16.6 to 49.6 after 450 kJ/m^2). Yellow ochre remained the most color stable over time. The group in which pigments were mixed with 10% Artskin white had the smallest color changes over time, followed, in order, by pigments mixed with 10% titanium white dry pigment, 10% calcined kaolin powder, and 5% Georgia kaolin.

Han and colleagues (2010b) were the first to introduce nano-oxides as alternative opacifiers to silicones. TiO_2, ZnO, and CeO_2 at 1%, 2%, and 2.5% were mixed with silicone intrinsic pigments to A-2186 and subjected to 450 kJ/m^2 exposure of artificial weathering at the HCBB laboratory. Overall, ΔE* values of the mixed groups of TiO_2, ZnO, and CeO_2 were below the 50:50% acceptability threshold (ΔE* = 1.2–2.3; below 3.0 is clinically acceptable) except 2% CeO_2 (ΔE* = 4.2, clinically unacceptable). Of all nano-oxides, yellow silicone pigment significantly affected the color stability of A-2186 (increased ΔE* values significantly from 3.7 up to 8.4, clinically unacceptable) and should be used with caution. TiO_2 and ZnO at 1–2.5% could be used safely as opacifiers for A-2186 silicone. Akay et al. (2018) evaluated the cytotoxicity of nanoparticles of TiO_2, fumed silica, and silanated silica added to A-2000 and A-2006 silicone elastomers and found that they are nontoxic.

A-2000

Kiat-amnuay and colleagues (2006a, 2006b, 2009) investigated the effects of five different opacifiers (5%, 10%, and 15% each) on the color stability of silicone functional intrinsic pigments (red, yellow ochre, burnt sienna, and a mix of all three colors) in A-2000 silicone maxillofacial elastomer when subjected to 450 kJ/m^2 of artificial aging at the HCBB laboratory. Color changes (ΔE*) in all groups were less than 3.0 and were clinically acceptable. Yellow ochre had a significant effect on all opacifiers (ΔE* values of 2.1 to 10.3 after 450 kJ/m^2). They concluded that functional intrinsic silicone pigments mixed with all five opacifiers tested protected silicone A-2000 from color degradation over time.

Bishal et al. (2019) assessed the ability of TiO_2 nanocoating to prevent color degradation of functional intrinsic pigmented A-2000 maxillofacial silicone elastomers after being exposed to artificial aging for 120 hours at 450 kJ/m^2. Changes in the color were measured before and after the atomic layer deposition coating and before and after aging. They found that the specimens with TiO_2 nanocoated surface showed the least color change (ΔE* values of = 1.4 ±0.6). Nanocoating remained on the surface when subjected to artificial aging, and the change was significantly lower than the established acceptability threshold of 3.0. Therefore, the TiO_2 nanocoating was shown to be effective in reducing the color degradation of A-2000 silicone elastomer over time similar to the other opacifiers used (Kiat-amnuay et al., 2009).

Bates et al. (2021) evaluated the color stability and mechanical properties of A-2000 and M5111 mixed with e-Skin and Reality Series pigment and opacifier systems subjected to 450 kJ/m^2 of artificial aging at the HCBB. They found that A-2000 mixed with e-Skin group pigments displayed the most favorable color stability and mechanical properties. All A-2000 and M5111 groups showed ΔE* values <0.9, which are below the clinical perceptibility level.

M511

Akash and Guttal (2014) studied the effect of incorporating TiO_2 and ZnO on the color stability of intrinsically colored M511 silicone elastomer, subjected to outdoor weathering. They also incorporated an antislump agent. The authors suggested that the incorporation of nano-oxides as an opacifier improved the color stability of M511 and that ZnO showed minimal or no color change and proved to be the most color stable after being subjected to six-month outdoor weathering.

Bangera et al. (2014) evaluated the degree of ultraviolet (UV) protection after incorporating 0.5%, 1.0%, 1.5%, 2.0%, and 2.5% by weight of TiO_2 and ZnO in M511 silicone elastomer. There were no pigments added. All specimens were subjected to UV A and B radiation and the percentage transmission was measured with a UV spectrophotometer. They found that Zn nano-oxides in lesser concentrations provided more significant and consistent UV protection in M511 elastomer, compared to TiO_2 at higher concentrations.

Bankoglu et al. (2013) measured color changes of Technovent pigmented M511, M522, and Multisil-Epithetic after storage for one year in a dark environment at ambient room temperature. After storage for one year in a black box, the color changes were considered clinically unacceptable in all groups (ΔE* > 3.0, range from 4.7 to 21.6) except white color (opacifier groups, ΔE* = 1.3 and 1.8) of M511 and Multisil-Epithetic. Therefore, pigments and silicone combinations used in this study should be used with caution.

Farah et al. (2018) evaluated the color stability of nonpigmented and Spectromatch Pro colorants in pigmented M511 when stored in darkness and exposed to artificial accelerated aging and natural outdoor weathering (1,500 hours or about two months). All pigmented M511 specimens demonstrated clinically acceptable color stability. The greatest color changes were observed for all specimens exposed to artificial aging for 1,500 hours and were considered clinically unacceptable.

Sethi et al. (2015) compared the change in color of pigmented M511 packed in three commonly used investing materials: orange die stone (gypsum), white stone, and green dental stone coated with three separating media—Unifol (alginate-based medium), Dove soap solution, and Yeti resin-based die hardening material. Control group samples were made by packing pigmented elastomer in stainless-steel molds. Orange die stone showed clinically unacceptable color changes in the silicone. The best combination found in this investigation was a green dental stone and alginate-based separating medium. Similar results were reported by Cifter et al. (2017). Five different colors (white, blue, yellow, green, and reddish-brown) of dental stones were used to fabricate M511 specimens at 25°C and 100°C. Reddish-brown dental stones vulcanized at 100°C caused the most color changes. Like the Sethi et al. study, green dental stone with the silicone vulcanized at 25°C showed the best color stability outcomes. Blue dental stone was the second best and presented clinically acceptable color changes when the silicone was vulcanized at 25°C.

Various silicone elastomers

Haug et al. (1992a, 1992b) investigated the color changes in six nonpigmented elastomers (MDX4-4210, Silastic 4-4515, A-2186, Medical Adhesive A, A-102, and Epithane-3) subjected to natural weathering for six months. All specimens showed acceptable color changes (ΔE*), close to 1.0. Haug and colleagues (1999c) proceeded to evaluate the color stability and color effect of six colorants (no colorant, artists' oil pigment, dry earth pigments, kaolin, liquid cosmetic, and rayon fiber flocking) on three silicone elastomers (MDX 4-4210, A-2186, and Medical Adhesive Type A) that were subjected to three conditions (control, time passage, and natural weathering). The results supported the concept that the color degradation of silicone elastomers may be prevented by the use of an opacifier.

Haug et al. (1999a, 1999c) also evaluated the color stability of commonly used colorant-elastomers (MDX4-4210, A-2186, Medical Adhesive Type A) combinations. The time passage group was sealed in glass containers and kept in the dark for six months before testing. They found that pigments tended to protect the silicones from weathering and that silicones were not as stable as had been assumed. Color changes occurred not only in the pigmented but also in the unpigmented (control) specimens over time, even though specimens were kept in sealed containers and in unlighted conditions without exposure to weathering.

Mount et al. (2018) studied the color stability of A-2000, VST-50, A-2186, and MDX4-4210 (10:1) mixed with Functional Silicone Intrinsic pigments subjected to artificial aging at 450 kJ/m^2. They found that, after aging, mixed pigmented MDX4-4210 (ΔE* = 0.34) was the most color-stable elastomer by a significant margin, followed in order by A-2000 (ΔE* = 0.77), A-2186 (ΔE* = 0.82), and VST-50 (ΔE* = 1.02). All functional intrinsic pigmented A-2000, VST-50, A-2186, and MDX4-4210 were very color stable and had color changes after aging below the ΔE* perceptibility threshold.

Color stability of extrinsic coloring

Beatty et al. (1999) measured base colorants (intrinsic) or surface tints (extrinsic) color changes caused by 400, 600, and 1,800 hours of ultraviolet radiation of oil-pigmented A-2186 and Medical Adhesive Type A. They concluded that oil-pigmented extrinsic coloring may protect color change, provided that a sufficient amount of pigment is present.

Liska et al. (2009) measured the effects of six "extrinsic" coloring techniques on the color stability of MDX4-4210/Type A, A-2186F, A-2000, and A-2006 silicones. Extrinsic coloring was applied on one side of the specimen, which was eight times stronger than the intrinsic color. Color readings were done on both sides of the specimen to measure the effects of color degradation of both intrinsic and extrinsic coloring, and specimens were artificially aged at 150 kJ/m^2. They concluded that all silicone elastomers and intrinsic and extrinsic coloring techniques tested showed clinically acceptable color stability (ΔE* < 3.0) after artificial aging.

Environmental staining

Koran et al. (1979) evaluated the resistance of one polyvinyl chloride and three silicone elastomers (including Silastic MDX4-4210) to staining by tea, lipstick, and disclosing solution. The changes in color caused by staining measured by reflectance spectrophotometry were much greater than the color instability of base elastomers or pigments that had been reported.

The use of cleansers to remove environmental staining may cause discoloration of prostheses. Yu et al. (1981a, 1981b) evaluated the effects of superficial stain removal from intrinsically pigmented Silastic MDX4-4210. They tested four organic solvents (toluene, benzene, *n*-hexane, and 1,1,1-trichloroethane) and found that the solvents were effective in stain removal and did not affect the color of either the pigments or the base elastomer. Yu et al. (1983) also studied the effects of cigarette staining on Silastic 4-4210 and subsequent stain removal with 1,1,1-trichloroethane. The solvent was effective in removing cigarette stains without affecting the color of the base elastomer.

Effect of mixing methods on color

Hatamleh and Watts (2011) investigated pore numbers, volumes, and percentages of pigmented and unpigmented TechSil S25 silicone mixed by two mixing techniques (manual and mechanical under vacuum) subjected to two aging conditions (stored in simulated sebum for six months and exposed to accelerated daylight aging for 360 hours). Pore numbers, volumes, and percentages were calculated using X-ray microfocus computerized tomography (Micro-CT). Color changes (ΔE^*) were measured at the start and end of aging. They concluded that mechanical mixing under vacuum reduced pore numbers and porosity percentages more than manual mixing within silicone elastomer, whether pigmented or not. However, the effect of pores on silicone elastomer color stability varies with the presence of pigmentation and aging methods. Color changes of almost all (seven groups) but one group (manual unpigmented sebum) after aging showed clinically unacceptable values of ΔE^*, ranging from 3.48 to 10.48.

Nobrega et al. (2019) investigated the influence of three mixing methods (conventional, mechanical, and industrial) on color change, dimensional stability, and detail reproduction of the pigmented MDX4-4210 and A-2186 silicones after being subjected to 1,008 hours of artificial aging. They concluded that mechanical and industrial methods produced better results, although all three methods generated acceptable dimensional and color stability of both silicones, regardless of the pigment and aging conditions. In addition, the detailed reproduction of both A-2186 and MDX4-4210 silicones was satisfactory after aging periods in all cases of this study.

Effect of UV light absorbers

The addition of a UV light absorber was evaluated for its potential to protect against color changes in silicone elastomers. Bryant et al. (1994) studied the effect of three UV-absorbing agents (Coppertone [Schering-Plough], Native Tan [Tropical Seas], and Photoplex [Herbert Laboratories], all with a sun protection factor of 15) as well as para-aminobenzoic acid on the color stability of MDX 4-4210 silicone elastomer. None of the sunscreens provided any protection to silicone against UV radiation, and para-aminobenzoic acid caused significant color degradation. Similar results were found by Lemon et al. (1995). A UV-absorbing agent, UV-5411 (American Cyanamid), did not protect combined MDX 4-4210/Silastic Medical Adhesive, Type A, from color degradation after exposure to either artificial or outdoor weathering.

Tran et al. (2004) studied the effect of a UV light absorber (Tinuvin 213, Ciba Specialty Chemicals) and hindered amine light stabilizer (Tinuvin 123) on the color stability of A-2186 silicone elastomer mixed with three pigments (a natural inorganic dry earth pigment and two synthesized organic pigments). The elastomer was subjected to natural weathering exposure in Miami and Phoenix. Both products retarded color changes in some of the pigments mixed with A-2186 silicone elastomer.

As mentioned above, Han et al. (2013) reported that Sunforgettable UV light absorber (a commercially available sunscreen), used as an opacifier at 5%, 10%, and 15%, significantly protected commonly used materials from color degradation after artificial aging at 450 kJ/m^2. They also noted that the mechanical properties of the elastomer were degraded significantly. Nguyen et al. (2013) evaluated the same Sunforgettable UV light absorber on the mechanical properties of pigmented silicone MDX4-4210/Type A and also reported that the mechanical properties were significantly degraded. Therefore, the use of this material as an opacifier is not recommended.

Mechanical properties

Skin is an organ consisting mainly of connective tissues and is a highly nonlinear, viscoelastic, anisotropic, and more or less incompressible material. The tensile stress-strain behavior for skin is representative of the mechanical behavior of many (collagenous) soft connective tissues. Mechanical characteristics of soft tissues present properties that have different values when measured in different directions because of their fibers. Microscopically, soft tissues are nonhomogeneous materials because of their composition. Tensile strength of soft tissue depends on the strain rate, and the tensile response is nonlinear stiffening. Soft tissues may undergo large deformations and some show viscoelastic behavior such as relaxation and/or creep, which has been associated with the shear interaction of collagen with the matrix of proteoglycans (Minns et al., 1973). The intramolecular cross-link of collagen fibrils gives the strength to connective tissues and varies with age, genetics, sex, presence of pathology, and so on (Holzapfel, 2000). The table below shows the mechanical properties of soft connective tissues of human skin (Holzapfel, 2000; Fung, 1993; Ní Annaidh et al., 2012).

In the past decades, there has been a significant increase in the number of publications assessing the mechanical properties of maxillofacial prosthetic elastomers in the hope of creating materials compatible with the mobile tissue beds. The majority of researchers study tensile strength (ASTM D-412, ISO 37 Type 2), tear strength (ASTM D624, ISO 24 Type 1, and D1938), elongation percentage (Lf – Lo / Lo, where Lf is the distance between the grips at specimen rupture and Lo is the initial distance between the grips), and durometer shore A hardness (ASTM D-2240, ASTM D-1415, and BS 903; Hatamleh et al., 2016; Bates et al., 2021). From the most recent survey (Cardoso et al., 2022), mechanical properties (margin integrity / high edge strength / durability) were the third most important characteristic of facial prosthetic materials, after nontoxic/nonallergic properties and color stability. Of the mechanical properties assessed, tear strength, from a clinical perspective, is the most important.

In 1972, Sweeney and colleagues (1972) were the first to test the mechanical properties of silicone elastomers using the Weather-Ometer as an artificial aging method to stress the material. Since then, many investigators reported using artificial aging (Turner et al., 1975a, 1975b; Yu et al., 1980a, 1980b; Polyzois and Andreopoulus, 1993; Dootz et al., 1994; Mohite et al., 1994; Eleni et al., 2007; Yu and Koran, 1979; Eleni et al., 2009; Goiato et al., 2012; Nguyen et al., 2013; Wang et al., 2014; Bates et al., 2021; Mount et al., 2018) and natural indoor and outdoor aging (Haug et al., 1992a, 1992b, 1999a, 1999c; Eleni et al., 2009b, 2011; Hatamleh et al., 2011; Kheur et al., 2012; Al-Harbi et al., 2015; Willett and Beatty, 2015; Guiotti et al., 2010; Hatamleh et al., 2011; Polyzois et al., 2011a, 2011b).

Yu et al. (1980) led the first investigation of the effect of intrinsic colorant and accelerated aging on the mechanical properties

Table 5-11 Mechanical properties of soft connective tissues

	Ultimate tensile strength (MPa)	Ultimate tensile strain (%)	Ultimate tensile stress (MPa)	Elastic modulus (E) (Low stretch ratio)	Elastic modulus (E) (High stretch ratio)
Human skin	1-20	30-70	13-30	0.3-2.0	27-31
Articular cartilage	9-40	60-120			

Holzapfel, 2000; Fung, 1993; Ní Annaidh et al., 2011.

of a silicone elastomer. Research continued in the 1990s with new silicone elastomers assessing the impact of simulated extraoral aging conditions on mechanical properties (Haug et al., 1992; Sanchez et al., 1992; Polyzois and Andreopoulos, 1993; Polyzois, 1995; Mohite et al., 1994; Lai and Hodges, 1999; Polyzois, 1999; Polyzois and Pettersen, 1998). During the first two decades of the 21st century, continued research efforts have been made to find new and improved silicone properties in addition to testing materials under aging conditions and to investigate the interaction of materials mixed into the silicone base (Lai et al., 2002; Aziz et al., 2003b; Eleni et al., 2007; Maxwell et al., 2003; Xiao-na et al., 2007; Han et al., 2007; Hatamleh et al., 2010, 2011; Goiato et al., 2009, 2010; Eleni et al., 2009, 2011b, 2011c, 2013b; Polyzois et al., 2011b; Al-Harbi et al., 2015; Nguyen et al., 2013; Taylor et al., 2003; Han, 2008; Hu et al., 2014; Mouzakis et al., 2010; Bellamy et al., 2003; Liu et al., 2013). Han et al. (2008) pioneered the evaluation of the addition of TiO_2, ZnO, or CeO_2 nanosized oxides and found that 2.0% and 2.5% nano-oxides improved the overall mechanical properties of silicone A-2186. Similarly, Wang et al. (2014) found that 2% TiO_2 improved the mechanical properties of MDX4-4210 silicone.

In 1980, Lewis and Castleberry (1980) suggested the desirable performance characteristics and mechanical properties of an elastomer base, with "no" pigments/opacifiers (Table 5-6). In 2021, Kiat-amnuay and Powers suggested color stability thresholds and desirable mechanical properties for silicones mixed with pigments/opacifiers (Table 5-9), based on their studies (Tables 5-7 and 5-8). Due to various experimental factors and several silicone elastomers tested within the same study, a summary of mechanical property data in the past half century is combined in Table 5-12. Please note that although ASTM and ISO standards are used, different laboratories performed their experiments at different locations and with different protocols, materials, and equipment; therefore, results may not be directly or accurately compared. Only studies that tested at least two mechanical properties are listed.

These mechanical property data can be used as a guideline when selecting appropriate facial prosthetic materials. But clinicians should take into consideration the effect of different materials added to the mix that could adversely affect the mechanical properties of prostheses, such as a thixotropic agent found in a study by Kurtoglu et al. (2009) and a UV light absorber found in the Nguyen et al. (2013) study. It is critically important to review data from studies that include the mixture of colorants (to mimic the patient's final facial prosthesis) and aging conditions (to represent long-term usage of the prosthesis). In addition to mechanical properties, clinicians should also take into consideration the importance of color stability. Knowledge of all properties will help the clinician choose the best combination of materials that provide the longest-lasting prosthesis. Clinicians should note that research studies on mechanical properties in the field date back to 1969 and have continued until recently, but many do not include aging conditions (Bell et al., 1985; Koran and Craig, 1975; Abdelnnabi et al., 1984; Kouyoumdjian et al., 1985; Moore et al., 1977; Wolfaardt et al., 1985; Polyzois et al., 1994; Aziz et al., 2003b; Polyzois et al., 1999; Firtell, 1976; Han, 2008; Hatamleh and Watts, 2010a, 2010b; Begum et al., 2011; Liu et al., 2013; Abdullah and Abdul-Ameer, 2018), and many studies used no colorants.

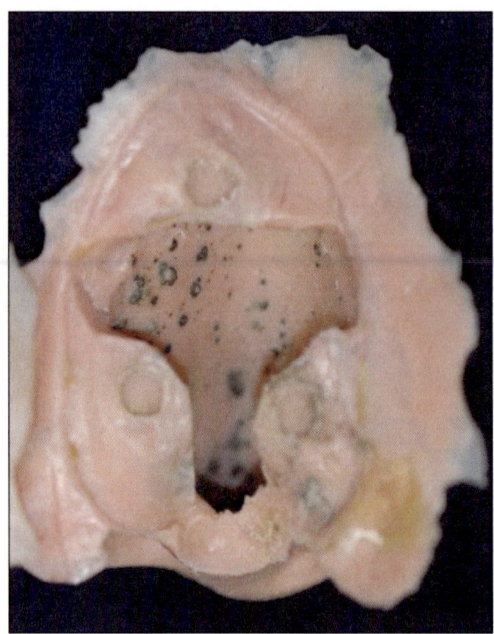

Figure 5-14 Nasal prostheses are especially prone to degradation and discoloration secondary to the formation of fungal and bacterial biofilms.

Microbial adhesion and biofilms on facial prostheses

Bacterial and fungal biofilms form on the surfaces of implanted medical devices such as voice prostheses, catheters, prosthetic cardiac valves, denture liners, and so on (Del Pozo, 2008; Neu et al., 1993; Lyons et al., 2020). Biofilms also form on the surface of facial prostheses by microbial colonization (Fig 5-14) and can cause skin or mucosal irritation (Morris-Jones et al., 2002). Santhaveesuk et al. (2022b) demonstrated the capacity of skin and respiratory pathogens to form in vitro biofilms with densities as high as 4×10^8 per square inch of material. Scanning electron microscopy has revealed that biofilm microorganisms penetrate silicone facial prostheses (Ariani, 2012) and contribute to material degradation.

Table 5-12 Summary of mechanical property data testing of facial prosthetic materials

Authors	Pigment	Opacifier	Aging	Tensile (MPa)	Tear (kN/m)	% elongation	Hardness shore A
MDX4-4210 (10:1)							
Moore et al., 1977						390 (28)	27 (1.2)
Lewis and Castleberry, 1980				3.2	21	410	18
Abdelnnabi et al., 1984				2.6 (0.3)		305 (30)	26 (0.9)
Kouyoumdjian et al., 1985				4.6 (0.8)		499 (50)	31 (0.9)
Wolfaardt et al., 1985						394 (46)	30 (0.8)
Sanchz et al., 1992				2.2 (0.2)		330 (31)	28 (0.7)
Haug et al., 1992				2.5 (0.2)	5.2 (0.5)	356 (61)	29 (0.5)
Mount et al.,* 2018				0.7 (0.1)	8.4 (2.8)	246 (31)	22 (0.7)
Mount et al.,* 2018			Artificial 450 kJ/m^2	0.7 (0.3)	11.6 (2.0)	241 (39)	26 (0.9)
Mount et al.,* 2018	Silicone	Silicone		0.7 (0.3)	10.7 (4.1)	240 (69)	23 (0.7)
Mount et al.,* 2018	Silicone	Silicone	Artificial 450 kJ/m^2	1.0 (0.2)	11.8 (2.0)	245 (36)	23 (0.9)
Dootz et al., 1994				4.0		438	24
Dootz et al., 1994			Artificial (900 hrs)	3.6		408	25
Yu et al., 1980			Artificial (900 hrs)	4.5 (0.1)		457 (8)	33 (0.7)
Yu et al., 1980	Dry earth	Dry earth	Artificial (900 hrs)	3.8 (0.1)–4.5 (0.2)		438 (16)–471 (20)	22 (0.8)–31 (0.6)
Wang et al., 2014			Artificial	2.7 (0.1)		203 (31)	25 (1.1)
Wang et al., 2014		Nano-TiO_2	Artificial	2.8 (0.3)–3.3 (0.4)		142 (15)–254 (20)	29 (0.8)–32 (1.7)
Haug et al., 1992			Outdoor (6 months)	2.2 (0.5)	4.8 (0.7)	218 (55)	31 (0.4)
Al-Harbi et al., 2015				3.0 (0.2)	5.4 (0.4)	564 (51)	
Al-Harbi et al., 2015			Outdoor (6 months)	2.6 (0.2)	4.7 (0.5)	500 (57)	
Authors	Pigment	Opacifier	Aging	Tensile (MPa)	Tear (kN/m)	% elongation	Hardness shore A
MDX4-4210/Type A (25%/75%)							
Nguyen et al.,* 2013				1.4 (0.3)	10.8 (1.8)	369 (88)	27 (0.9)
Nguyen et al.,* 2013			Artificial 450 kJ/m^2	1.4 (0.2)	10.7 (2.4)	330 (92)	24 (0.9)
Nguyen et al.,* 2013	Oil	Silicone		1.2 (0.4)	9.5 (2.6)	425 (84)	20 (1.3)
Nguyen et al.,* 2013	Oil	Silicone	Artificial 450 kJ/m^2	1.2 (0.3)	8.6 (2.0)	481 (32)	18 (1.7)
Nguyen et al.,* 2013	Oil	Titanium dry earth		1.6 (0.2)	11.8 (2.1)	539 (95)	22 (0.5)
Nguyen et al.,* 2013	Oil	Titanium dry earth	Artificial 450 kJ/m^2	1.4 (0.0)	12.7 (2.3)	454 (71)	20 (0.7)
Nguyen et al.,* 2013	Oil	UV light absorber		1.4 (0.1)	12.8 (1.7)	505 (78)	21 (3.2)
Nguyen et al.,* 2013	Oil	UV light absorber	Artificial 450 kJ/m^2	0.5 (0.0)	5.1 (0.9)	221 (29)	15 (1.8)
Kiat-amnuay et al. HCBB data	Oil	Oil		2.0 (0.1)	9.5 (0.1)	462 (43)	19 (0.7)
Kiat-amnuay et al. HCBB data	Silicone	Silicone		1.8 (0.1)	6.7 (0.7)	459 (19)	19 (0.5)
Authors	Pigment	Opacifier	Aging/	Tensile (MPa)	Tear (kN/m)	% elongation	Hardness shore A
A-2186 (10:1)							
Sanchez et al., 1992				3.5 (0.4)		391 (25)	20 (0.6)
Aziz et al., 2003				4.2 (0.4)	17.6 (2.2)	651 (41)	16.3 (2.5)
Polyzois et al., 1994				3.8 (0.1)	15.4 (2.1)	321 (7)	21 (1.2)
Haug et al., 1992				4.8 (0.7)	36 (5.1)	488 (75)	23 (0.4)
Dootz et al., 1994				5.0		480	25
Dootz et al., 1994			Artificial (900 hrs)	5.1		418	30
Mount et al.,* 2018				2.0 (0.3)	27.7 (4.6)	255 (42)	37 (1.4)

continued

Table 5-12 Summary of mechanical property data testing of facial prosthetic materials (*continued*)

Authors	Pigment	Opacifier	Aging	Tensile (MPa)	Tear (kN/m)	% elongation	Hardness shore A
Mount et al.,* 2018			Artificial 450 kJ/m²	2.0 (0.2)	20.3 (5.9)	214 (15)	41 (0.3)
Mount et al.,* 2018	Silicone	Silicone		1.9 (0.3)	18.1 (6.0)	266 (38)	31 (1.7)
Mount et al.,* 2018	Silicone	Silicone	Artificial 450 kJ/m²	1.6 (0.2)	21.3 (3.7)	232 (12)	31 (1.6)
Al-Harbi et al., 2015				4.5 (0.4)	6.4 (0.3)	646 (17)	
Al-Harbi et al., 2015			Outdoor (6 months)	4.5 (1.0)	4.7 (0.3)	592 (40)	
Haug et al., 1992			Outdoor (6 months)	5.6 (1.2)	17.3 (4.8)	332 (63)	29 (0.3)
Willett and Beatty 2015			Outdoor (3,000 hrs)	3.7 (0.2)			30 (1.6)
Kurtoglu et al.,* 2009			No thixo	3.0 (0.2)	8.1 (0.7)	507 (31)	30 (0.9)
Kurtoglu et al.,* 2009			Thixo 1 drop 10 g silicone	1.2 (0.2)	10.9 (2.1)	376 (81)	27 (0.7)
Kurtoglu et al.,* 2009			Thixo 2 drop 10 g silicone	3.2 (0.5)	18.9 (3.3)	326 (68)	27 (1.1)
Authors	**Pigment**	**Opacifier**	**Aging/thixo**	**Tensile (MPa)**	**Tear (kN/m)**	**% elongation**	**Hardness shore A**
VST-50 (10:1)							
Tukmachi et al., 2021				3.3 (0.1)	15.8 (0.5)	314 (4.3)	30 (0.3)
Tukmachi et al., 2021		Nano-ZrO		3.8 (0.1)–4.2 (0.1)	16.4 (0.4)–18.7 (0.4)	293 (5.5)–314 (4.3)	33 (0.4)–37 (0.3)
Mount et al.,* 2018				2.3(0.2)	28.8 (2.1)	446(65)	30 (0.5)
Mount et al.,* 2018			Artificial 450 kJ/m²	2.4 (0.2)	27.2 (4.3)	462 (79)	32 (0.8)
Mount et al.,* 2018	Silicone	Silicone		2.0 (0.3)	24.1 (3.1)	447 (90)	26 (3.8)
Mount et al.,* 2018	Silicone	Silicone	Artificial 450 kJ/m²	2.1 (0.3)	22.8 (3.2)	447 (68)	27 (2.8)
Kurtoglu et al.,* 2009			No thixo	5.1 (0.1)	32.4 (1.4)	542 (34)	21 (0.9)
Kurtoglu et al.,* 2009			Thixo 1 drop 10 g silicone	1.5 (0.2)	15.9 (5.6)	282 (57)	16 (1.3)
Kurtoglu et al.,* 2009			Thixo 2 drop 10 g silicone	2.8 (0.5)	15.6 (2.3)	390 (120)	14 (0.5)
Authors	**Pigment**	**Opacifier**	**Aging**	**Tensile (MPa)**	**Tear (kN/m)**	**% elongation**	**Hardness shore A**
M-511 (10:1)							
Hatamleh and Watts, 2010				1.9 (0.2)	6.5 (1.8)	581 (48)	13 (1.8)
Bates et al.,* 2021				1.4 (0.2)	20.0 (2.2)	340 (37)	24 (1.0)
Bates et al.,* 2021			Artificial 450 kJ/m²	1.8 (0.2)	30.2 (6.2)	172 (22)	43 (0.4)
Bates et al.,* 2021	e-Skin	e-Skin		1.4 (0.2)	20.1 (2.6)	346 (30)	24 (0.6)
Bates et al.,* 2021	e-Skin	e-Skin	Artificial 450 kJ/m²	1.7 (0.2)	27.7 (6.4)	189 (19)	39 (1.0)
Bates et al.,* 2021	Reality	Reality		1.4 (0.2)	16.5 (2.5)	369 (38)	27 (0.7)
Bates et al.,* 2021	Reality	Reality	Artificial 450 kJ/m²	1.9 (0.3)	23.2 (3.4)	184 (28)	45 (0.3)
Bibars et al., 2018	Silicone		No thixo	2.7 (0.7)		195 (33)	34 (1.1)
Bibars et al., 2018	Silicone		Thixo 0.02 g 10 g silicone	2.4 (0.5)		174 (46)	34 (1.4)
Authors	**Pigment**	**Opacifier**	**Aging**	**Tensile (MPa)**	**Tear (kN/m)**	**% elongation**	**Hardness shore A**
TechSil S25 (9:1)							
Hatamleh and Watts, 2010				4.9 (0.4)	6.6 (1.7)	941 (94)	25 (0.5)
Hatemleh et al., 2011			Sebum (6 months)	3.9 (0.5)	4.8 (1.2)	712 (112)	21 (1.4)
Hatemleh et al., 2011			Acidic perspiration (6 months)	4.2 (0.8)	4.5 (1.4)	620 (73)	29 (1.0)
Hatemleh et al., 2011			Light aging (360 hrs)	4.6 (0.8)	6.0 (0.9)	997 (127)	28 (1.4)
Hatemleh et al., 2011			Cleaning solution (30 hrs)	4.8 (0.7)	4.2 (1.0)	1092 (133)	25 (0.7)
Hatemleh et al., 2011			Light and sebum (360 hrs)	3.7 (0.7)	3.2 (1.4)	784 (151)	20 (0.7)

Table 5-12 Summary of mechanical property data testing of facial prosthetic materials (*continued*)

Authors	Pigment	Opacifier	Aging	Tensile (MPa)	Tear (kN/m)	% elongation	Hardness shore A
Hatemleh et al., 2011			Outdoor (6 months)	4.3 (0.7)	5.5 (1.1)	891 (113)	27 (0.5)
Al-Harbi et al., 2015				6.1 (0.3)	6.5 (0.1)	937 (8)	
Al-Harbi et al., 2015			Outdoor (6 months)	5.7 (0.3)	5.7 (0.3)	871 (14)	
Authors	**Pigment**	**Opacifier**	**Aging/thixo**	**Tensile (MPa)**	**Tear (kN/m)**	**% elongation**	**Hardness shore A**
A-2000 (1:1)							
Bates et al.,* 2021				1.5 (0.1)	17.6 (2.7)	306 (44)	25 (0.6)
Bates et al.,* 2021			Artificial 450 kJ/m²	2.0 (0.5)	23.6 (3.3)	182 (50)	40 (2.2)
Bates et al.,* 2021	e-Skin	e-Skin		1.4 (0.2)	19.3 (5.9)	297 (63)	32 (0.5)
Bates et al.,* 2021	e-Skin	e-Skin	Artificial 450 kJ/m²	1.9 (0.3)	23.5 (6.0)	202 (37)	40 (1.5)
Mount et al.,* 2018			Artificial 450 kJ/m²	2.2 (0.5)	19.8 (1.5)	218 (32)	39 (1.2)
Mount et al.,* 2018	Silicone	Silicone		1.0 (0.2)	15.8 (3.4)	225 (32)	25 (0.7)
Mount et al.,* 2018	Silicone	Silicone	Artificial 450 kJ/m²	1.8 (0.5)	17.4 (4.6)	294 (70)	28 (1.1)
Kurtoglu et al.,* 2009			No thixo	5.3 (0.2)	28.5 (1.8)	550 (31)	27 (0.8)
Kurtoglu et al.,* 2009			Thixo 1 drop 10 g silicone	1.6 (0.3)	10.7 (1.2)	275 (44)	30 (0.8)
Kurtoglu et al.,* 2009			Thixo 2 drop 10 g silicone	3.0 (0.6)	15.9 (4.6)	363 (78)	31 (1.0)
Bibars et al., 2018	Silicone		No thixo	4.2 (0.7)		107 (24)	43 (1.7)
Bibars et al., 2018	Silicone		Thixo 0.02 g 10 g silicone	3.9 (0.6)		77 (13)	37 (2.1)
Authors	**Pigment**	**Opacifier**	**Aging**	**Tensile (MPa)**	**Tear (kN/m)**	**% elongation**	**Hardness shore A**
Z004 (1:1)							
Hatamleh and Watts, 2010				3.9 (0.4)	7.0 (2.2)	609 (38)	36 (1.8)
Bibars et al., 2018	Silicone		No thixo	6.3 (0.9)		171 (31)	40 (0.7)
Bibars et al., 2018	Silicone		Thixo 0.02 g 10 g silicone	6.1 (0.7)		150 (18)	35 (4.4)
Authors	**Pigment**	**Opacifier**	**Aging**	**Tensile (MPa)**	**Tear (kN/m)**	**% elongation**	**Hardness shore A**
Chlorinated polyethylene (CPE)							
May and Guerra, 1978				8.3	18.4	950–1,350	42–45

* Values below Kiat-amnuay's suggested desirable performance characteristics of mechanical properties of silicone mixed with pigments/opacifiers
Studies highlighted in gray are considered more clinically relevant.

Biofilms are notoriously difficult to remove, and a general cleaning regimen suggested to patients cannot be expected to remove all biofilms from the porous and rough surfaces of a silicone prosthesis (Goiato, 2010). Nikawa et al. (2001) studied Candida albicans growth on thermal-cycled maxillofacial prosthesis materials. They found that the biological fluids of the host and the aging of the materials increased fungal growth on the prostheses. They also suggested that the thermocycling process reduced the unpolymerized components of the materials, which helped with the antifungal effects.

Kurtulmus and colleagues (2010) studied the effect of polymerization exposure and duration of simulated nasal secretion and saliva of *C. albicans* adherence on silicone elastomers. They found that in both saliva and nasal secretions, VST-50 (12-hour overnight) had the lowest *C. albicans* adherence, followed by VST-50F (6-hour); VST-30 (20-minute) had the most. Atay et al. (2013) found a close relationship between *C. albicans* and the surface contact angle of silicone elastomers studied, VST-50, A-2186F, and A-2006. The highest quantity of *C. albicans* adherence was found on A-2006 specimens due to its low surface angle values.

The smoother the surface of the silicone elastomer the less likely the surfaces will be colonized by fungal and microbial organisms (Khalaf et al., 2015, 2017). Also, it has been shown that applying a silver nanoparticle coating to the surfaces of silicone elastomers imparts some antifungal activity (Meran et al., 2018). The best means of creating smooth tissue surfaces of facial prostheses and the impact of silver nanoparticle coating on color stability and mechanical properties of silicone elastomers require further study.

Disinfection of facial prostheses

Goldschmidt et al. (1993) showed that microwave irradiation at 700 watts for six minutes was a safe and effective means of home disinfection for contaminated silicone nasal prostheses. Santhaveesuk et al. (2022b) validated the antimicrobial efficacy of microwaves on biofilms of *S. aureus*, *S. epidermidis*, and *K. pnemoniae* isolated from the nasal passages of patients and as well as the prostheses. However, exposure of the prosthesis to eight minutes or longer of microwave energy may damage the silicone surface and reduce tensile strength (Kotha et al., 2016).

Kiat-amnuay and colleagues (2005) have studied the long-term use of microwave disinfection (700 watts at six minutes) on the color stability of commonly used pigments and silicone elastomers. Silicone or oil pigments in combination with silicone or titanium dry earth opacifiers used with Silastic MDX4-4210/Medical Adhesive Type A, A-2186, A-2000, VST-50A, and VST-20A are safe to be disinfected using 700 watts of household microwave at six minutes. Color stability is not affected, with overall ΔE* values below 0.4 even after 18 months of disinfection simulation. However, cosmetic dry earth–pigmented A-2186 and MDX4-4210/Medical Adhesive Type A underwent significant color changes after microwave disinfection. The red dry earth pigment group had the most significant color changes after 18 months of exposure to microwave energy, similar to that observed with artificial aging studies (Kiat-amnuay et al., 2002; Beatty et al., 1995, 1999).

Santhaveesuk et al. (2022a) studied the long-term use of microwave disinfection (660 watts at six minutes) on the mechanical properties of commonly used pigments and silicone elastomers, Silastic MDX4-4210/Medical Adhesive Type A, Silastic MDX4-4210, A-2186, A-2000, VST-50A, and M511. These studies indicated that most silicones are safe to be disinfected using 660 watts of household microwave for six minutes once a month for 12 months.

Guiotti et al. (2015) compared conventional (water, neutral soap, and 4% chlorhexidine) and plant-extract disinfectant solutions (*Cymbopogon nardus* and *Hydrastis canadensis*) on specimens of MDX4-4210 contaminated with *C. albicans* and *S. aureus* biofilms. They found these disinfectant solutions produced a significant reduction in both biofilms. Washing with neutral soap and water was the most effective protocol against both microorganisms. However, immersion in 4% chlorhexidine altered the surface of the elastomer. In a follow-up study (Guiotti et al., 2016), they found that after 30 days of disinfection using the same solutions in the previous study, specimens of MDX4-4210 underwent major color degradation (ΔE* ranged from 3.9–10.6) and were considered clinically unacceptable.

Cevik and Yildirim-Bicer (2018) studied color stability and hardness of silicone A-2000 elastomer mixed with silicone intrinsic (red, tan, and brown) pigments after being subjected to five disinfectant solutions (neutral soap, effervescent tablet, 0.2% chlorhexidine, 4% chlorhexidine, sodium hypochlorite) after 48 hours of disinfection and 1,008 hours of artificial aging. They found the 0.2% chlorohexidine oral rinse to be the most suitable agent for disinfection of facial prostheses. Washing with neutral soap caused pigment loss on the surfaces. Sodium hypochlorite degraded the color of silicone specimens the most, like studies by Eleni et al. (2013a) or the JAOS study, and therefore is not recommended.

Chamaria et al. (2019) evaluated the color stability of silicone A-2000 elastomer mixed with silicone intrinsic cream pigments after being subjected to five disinfectant solutions (antibacterial soap and 2% chlorhexidine) 6 times/day for 60 days to simulate 1 year of usage. They found that the color stability of all groups was affected, especially by antibacterial soap, which produced clinically unacceptable results (ΔE* value 3.9–4.9). The color stability of 2% chlorhexidine exceeded the perceptibility threshold (ΔE* value 2.42–2.63) but was clinically acceptable and could be used as a disinfecting solution.

Thixotropic agents

Thixotropic agents are designed to produce a buttery consistency within seconds of addition to the silicone elastomer and raise the viscosity of the uncured silicone while filling the mold. The increased viscosity helps create sufficient pressure inside the mold to reduce air bubbles and can be used as an alternative to vacuum de-airing. One to two drops of thixotropic agent added per 10 grams of silicone are recommended.

A recent survey (Cardoso et al., 2022) indicated that 58% of clinicians used a thixotropic agent with 54% reporting using one to two drops per 10 grams of silicone and 4% reporting using greater than two drops per 10 grams. However, the addition of one to five drops of thixotropic agent can adversely affect the mechanical properties of VST-50 and A-2000 silicone elastomers (Kurtoglu et al., 2009). Similarly, when as little as 0.06 grams of a thixotropic agent are mixed with 30 g of M511, A-2000, and Z004 (with 0.12 grams of Technovent P402 silicone pigment), the thixotropic agent reduces tear strength and elongation percentage of all silicones (Bibars et al., 2018). Clinicians must therefore exercise extra caution when adding thixotropic agents, as they adversely affect properties of commonly used silicones, especially A-2000, M511, Z004, and VST-50. The exception is A-2186. Two to five drops of a thixotropic agent improved the tensile and tear strengths of silicone A-2186 and made this silicone softer.

Adhesives

Implant-retained facial prostheses have been shown to have a longer life span than adhesive-retained prostheses (Hatamleh et al., 2016). However, some patients are not candidates for implants, and so many patients are forced to rely on skin adhesives to retain their facial prosthesis. A recent survey indicated that about half of facial prostheses are retained with adhesives (Cardoso et al., 2022). The ideal characteristics of adhesives for maxillofacial prostheses are shown in Box 5-5. The choice of adhesive is subjective, depending on individual preference, skin condition, and the prosthetic materials and design.

Most cured silicones, because of their low solubility and low surface energy, will not adhere well to conventional tissue adhesives. A number are available, and selection depends on the patient's tolerance, the ease of application and removal, and the compatibility of the adhesive with the material used for the facial prosthesis. Unfortunately, the formulations of most commercial medical adhesives are unknown.

A variety of adhesive systems have been employed to retain facial prostheses. They are commonly classified by the method with which they are dispensed: spray-on adhesives, pastes, double-sided tapes, and liquid emulsions. Spray-on adhesives contain an inert silicone base in a propellant. Paste (latex-based) adhesives or

Box 5-5 Ideal properties of adhesives for facial prostheses

The adhesive must be biocompatible, nontoxic, and nonirritating.
The material should be odorless and moisture repellent.
The dried adhesive should be porous and absorbent to allow passage of secretions.
The patient should find it easy to apply.
The material should work quickly.
The bond should hold the prosthesis in place for at least 12 hours.
The adhesive must be easy to remove without injuring the skin or damaging the prosthesis.
The adhesive should be available in a travel-sized package.

Roberts, 1971; Bulbulian, 1973.

surgical cements have an odor and are not as popular because they are difficult to remove and accumulate on the prosthesis and the skin. Double-sided tape is commonly used because of its ease of application, removal, and maintenance. It is primarily used to retain prostheses that engage tissues with little or no movement. However, the poor flexibility of double-sided tape limits its usefulness, and it must be changed frequently due to loss of adhesion (Bulbulian, 1973). Liquid adhesive (spirit gum adhesive) is one of the most commonly used adhesives. It consists of mastic gum dissolved in a fast-evaporating solvent (ether or an ether-alcohol combination).

The type of adhesive and the cleaning solution should be carefully chosen. Adhesives and their solvents can have adverse effects on the physical and optical properties of facial elastomers (Haug et al., 1992b). A recent survey reported that Epithane-3 (Daro) water-based adhesive was used the most by respondents (52%), followed in order by Secure Medical Adhesive (SMA, silicone-based, 24%), adhesive tape (4%), Hollister adhesive spray (4%), and others (16%; Cardoso et al., 2022).

Kiat-amnuay et al. (2000) evaluated the in-vivo adhesive retention (peel test) of two skin adhesives against MDX 4-4210/Silastic Medical Adhesive, Type A, as affected using skin dressing (Skin-Prep, Smith & Nephew) and its solvent remover (Uni-Solve, Smith & Nephew). They studied the materials in 20 human participants and found that the skin dressing created a barrier that improved the adhesion of both adhesives by 15% to 27%. Solvent remover had no effect on adhesive retention. Secure II Medical Adhesive (SMA), a silicone-based adhesive, was three to five times more retentive than Epithane-3 (Daro), a water-based adhesive. After removal, SMA remained on the prosthesis and Daro remained on the skin. In a follow-up study, the effects of time and reapplication were evaluated in 21 human participants (Kiat-amnuay et al., 2001). Bond strength decreased during the course of the day and the application of a second coat of adhesive enhanced retention.

Another clinical study by Kiat-amnuay et al. (2004) investigated the effect of single- and multiadhesive layering of Daro and SMA on the retention of facial silicone elastomer strips adhered to the skin of 30 human forearms using a peel test. The multiadhesive sandwich combination of SMA to skin / Daro to silicone had the highest adhesion, followed in order by SMA alone, Daro to skin / SMA to silicone, and Daro alone. Kiat-amnuay et al. (2008), in another study that included 26 human participants, found that the adhesive bond strengths of SMA and Daro adhesives to urethane-lined MDX 4-4210 / Silastic Medical Adhesive, Type A, and to chlorinated polyethylene (CPE) were not significantly different, regardless of whether Skin-Prep was used.

Primers

Primers bonding urethane sheets to silicone elastomers

As mentioned previously, Udagama (1987) pioneered the concept of bonding urethane-lined silicone prosthesis using Silastic MDX4-4210 combined with Silastic Medical Adhesive, Type A. He studied the use of two primers to bond the silicone to urethane sheets in 88 patients—1205 primer (Dow Corning) and S-2260 primer (Dow Corning). Follow-up times ranged from 12 to 60 months, and S-2260 primer was found to be clinically the most effective primer of the two tested.

Singer and colleagues (1988) evaluated the bond strength of combined MDX 4-4210 (50% base only) and Silastic Medical Adhesive, Type A (50%), to polyurethane sheets when three commercial primers were used. The primers were A-4040 (Dow Corning), S-2260, and 1205. Laboratory adhesion-in-peel tests were performed, showing that S-2260 and A-4040 primers formed the strongest bonds between the polyurethane sheet and the silicone mixture. Wang et al. (1994) studied two primers, three polymerization methods, and seven different reaction times to find the optimum adhesive bond strength. Using T-peel strength (ASTM Standard D1876) as the evaluation parameter, they found, in contrast to Singer and colleagues, that 1205 primer resulted in greater bond strength than S2260 between the polyurethane sheet and a mixture of MDX 4-4210 (40% base only) and Silastic Medical Adhesive, Type A (60%).

Deng et al. (2004) investigated the bond strength of silicone to a polyurethane sheet after soaking in hot or room-temperature soapy water in a simulation of a one-year (five minutes a day) cleaning cycle. They used A-222 PSE-70 platinum-cured silicone with primer A-330 Beige (Factor II) in a T-peel test. The soaked specimens had significantly lower bond strengths than control specimens (no soaking), so they recommended that patients be informed not to soak their prosthesis in either hot or room-temperature soapy water.

Primers used to bond acrylic resin substructures housing attachments to silicone elastomers

The incorporation of osseointegrated implants in retentive schemes for facial prostheses creates additional demands on maxillofacial prosthetic materials. The incorporation of retentive elements (bar-clip or magnetic attachments) within the prosthesis requires the fabrication of a rigid substructure that retains the attachment housings (Fig 5-15). An adhesive joint between the substructure and the facial prosthetic material is desirable in order to prevent separation between the two surfaces during routine placement and removal of the prosthesis. Mechanical retention between the framework and the facial prosthetic material is also needed to mitigate this phenomenon. Bond strength is dependent on several factors, such as primer type, rigidity of the substrate, surface treatment, airing time, humidity, and compatibility of the silicone elastomer and the primer (Polyzois and Frangou, 2002; Frangou et al., 2003).

The substructure is usually fabricated from light-curing, heat-polymerizing, or autopolymerizing acrylic resin. Primer is used to enhance the bond between the silicone and the retentive matrix.

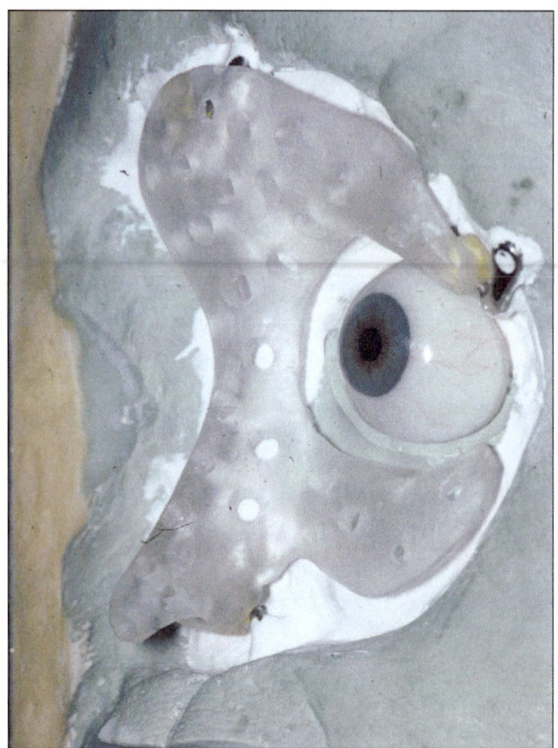

Figure 5-15 This large orbital nasal prosthesis was retained with implants. The metal housings for the clips are mechanically retained within the acrylic resin matrix. Note the numerous perforations. This combined with a primer will secure the resin substructure to the silicone elastomer.

McMordie and King (1989) evaluated the bond strength of Silastic 891 (Dow Corning) to denture base resin (Lucitone 199, Dentsply) using three primers: A-4040, S-2260, and 1200 (Dow Corning). The results indicated that the A-4040 primer had the greatest bond strength. Polyzois et al. (1991) evaluated the bond strength of either Silskin II (DePuy) or Cosmesil SM4 (Principality) silicone elastomer to a light-activated resin (Triad VLC, Dentsply) using three different primers (Triad VLC bonding agent, Z-6032 [Dow Corning], and Z-6076 [Dow Corning]). Primer Z-6032 produced the highest bond strength between the resin and both silicone elastomers. Taft et al. (1996) found that 1205 primer had significantly higher peel bond force than S-2260 primer, regardless of the type of resin or surface preparations used.

Hatamleh and Watts (2010) studied the effect of three primers (611, A304, A330-G) on shear and peel bond strengths of TechSil S25, M511, and Z004 silicone elastomers against an acrylic resin after 360 hours of accelerated daylight aging. The optimum bonding achieved in a shear test was Cosmesil Z004 with any primer and M511 with A304 and 330-G primers. Bonding was achieved for both TechSil S25 and Cosmesil Z004 using A330-G primer.

Bonatto et al. (2017) performed an in-vitro analysis of the biocompatibility of primers and an adhesive used for implant-retained silicone prostheses. They found that acrylic resin bonded to Silastic Medical Adhesive, Type A, and MDX4-4210 was the most biocompatible. They also found that when DC 1205 primer was not used with Medical Adhesive, Type A, an inflammatory process occurred in patients.

The effect of surface treatments on the peel bond strength of two acrylic resins (autopolymerizing Paladent RR and Triad VLC light-curing urethane dimethacrylate denture base resin; Güngör et al., 2020). These resins were bonded to M5111 and Z004 silicones using G611 platinum primer with and without thermocycling. Six different surface treatments were tested (polished, ground, polished + argon plasma, polished + oxygen plasma, ground + argon plasma, and ground + oxygen plasma). They concluded that argon and oxygen plasma and polishing were effective in improving the bond strength between acrylic resin and silicone elastomers. Polished specimens showed higher peel bond strength than ground specimens.

Primers for fiber-reinforced silicone prostheses

Hatamleh and Watts (2010a, 2010b) studied the effect of three primers (G611, A-330-Gold, and A-304) on the bending strength of impregnated glass fibers and their bond strength to M511 silicone elastomer. They found that the A-330-G primer produced the highest bond strength for M511 at baseline for the silicone-glass fiber. Bond strength degraded significantly after 360 hours of accelerated daylight aging. Still, sufficient bonding between M511 silicone and fibers existed when A-330-G was compared to other primers.

Primers for bonding titanium-encapsulated magnets to silicone elastomers

Delamination of titanium-encapsulated magnets from silicone elastomers shortens the life span of implant-retained facial prostheses. Artopoulou et al. (2016a) investigated the interfacial microleakage patterns of MDX4-4210 and A-2006, retained by commercially pure titanium-encapsulated magnets when three metal primers (A-304, A-320, and Super-Bond C&B monomer) and cyanoacrylate (Super Glue) were tested. They found that A-2006 combined with three metal primers showed the least microleakage. Cyanoacrylate (Super Glue) was not recommended for bonding titanium-encapsulated magnets to the silicone elastomers used in the study.

They also studied the peel strength (Artopoulou et al., 2016b) of the same silicones and titanium-encapsulated magnets against four primers (A-330-G, A-304/A-320 bonding enhancer, superbond C&B monomer, and cyanoacrylate [Super Glue]). They found the highest peel bond strength for A-2006 silicone bonded to heat-cured polymethyl methacrylate resin (PMMA) when using A-330-G primer, followed by A-2006 bonded to commercially pure titanium-encapsulated magnets using superbond C&B monomer and MDX4-4210 silicone group bonded with PMMA and A-330-G primer.

Kantola et al. (2011) investigated the adhesion of MDX4-4210 silicone elastomer to a fiber-reinforced composite resin framework using three primers (A-330-G, Softreliner, and VMS). The highest tensile bond strength was found with A-330-G, followed by Softreliner primers. A ground surface treatment enhanced the adhesion of both primers.

Materials research: Current status and future challenges

In the past half century, numerous investigations of the physical and mechanical properties of facial prosthetic materials have been conducted (see Boxes 5-4 and 5-5), since Sweeney et al. (1972) and Lewis and Castleberry (1980) defined the desirable properties of facial elastomer (see Table 5-6). A one-day conference was organized by Gettleman and Khan at the Academy of Dental Materials annual meeting at the American Dental Association in February 1992, devoted to maxillofacial prosthetic materials, and the transactions were published (Gettleman and Khan, 1992; Khan et al., 1992). Recently, the ADA Standards Committee on Dental Products Working Group No. 2.16 on Extraoral Maxillofacial Prosthetic Materials, led by Gettleman and Kiat-amnuay, has been established to write performance standards for materials currently in use and for those that may be developed in future years.

The discoloration of a facial prosthesis has both intrinsic and extrinsic components. Investigations have concentrated on the intrinsic color stability of elastomers and colorants. So far, there are only a few studies on color stability of extrinsic coloration after aging (Liska, 2009; dos Santos et al., 2020). The extrinsic discoloration of facial prostheses has another added factor: the loss of adhesion between the colorant and the facial prosthesis and the abrasion of extrinsic coloration away from the base elastomer. Investigations of materials and techniques used to bond extrinsic coloration to the base elastomer and the effects of cleansers or methods of cleansing on adhesion and color stability of extrinsic colorants to base elastomers have been limited.

In addition, other ancillary materials such as thixotropic agents commonly used in the mixture of pigmented silicone prostheses and disinfection solution/energy may contribute to the degradation of prostheses and, most importantly, to the long-term color stability and tear strength of prosthesis feather-edge margins. These two properties are the most common causes of prosthetic failure.

To date, none of the commercially available materials satisfies all the requirements of the ideal material. Each of the materials available has its strengths and weaknesses as well as its own unique physical and mechanical properties. From the most recent international 2020 survey (Cardoso et al., 2022) and review of current literature, the majority of commonly used silicone elastomers and pigments provide adequate short-term and medium-term color stability and mechanical properties for extraoral maxillofacial prostheses using conventional methods of fabrication (see Tables 5-7, 5-8, and 5-10). Advancements in research and collaboration among maxillofacial prosthodontists, anaplastologists, patients, materials scientists and researchers, and manufacturers have improved the quality of the materials used for facial prostheses. We are now at an inflection point of research to support innovations and new developments of prostheses fabricated with 3D manufacturing technology. Improving current materials and finding alternative materials are needed to provide greater quality and access to care with possible lower costs to the patients.

Extensive laboratory evaluations of physical and mechanical properties of maxillofacial elastomers have been published for conventional prosthetic fabrication but not for those fabricated with 3D printing technology. There is no doubt that laboratory testing is an important step in developing a better facial elastomer, but publications describing the long-term clinical evaluations of performance of facial prostheses are limited. It would be helpful if better correlations could be drawn between clinical performance and laboratory research data. In addition, new methods of laboratory testing should be developed that would be more predictive of clinical performance as opposed to the trial-and-error method using human subjects currently employed.

Future research should concentrate on several major goals:

- Identifying or developing long-term, color-stable coloring agents that are compatible with different elastomers with conventionally processed as well as with 3D printed facial materials
- Improving the physical and mechanical properties of commonly used materials or developing alternative materials (for both conventional and advanced 3D manufacturing) so that they will behave more like human tissue and be resistant to color fading, thin-section tearing, and biofilm formation, thereby increasing the service life of the prosthesis
- Studying properties of materials with organic and inorganic colorants (human skin shades) and ancillary materials, which include thixotropic additives, pigments, and opacifiers, mixed with the base elastomers to mimic the clinical phenomenon of color at depth, not just the bulk material alone
- Developing a scientific method and clinical methodology for color matching of human skin in the fabrication of facial prostheses
- Developing a scientific color formulation system that conforms to a color-matching tool to allow objective replication of human skin shades
- Calibrating and validating a mobile phone application with universal access for rapid 3D scanning, 3D design, color matching, and color formulation for fabrication of facial prostheses

Surgical Procedures during Tumor Ablation to Enhance the Prosthetic Prognosis

During the resection of the tumor, minor manipulations of the residual adjacent tissues and those within the defect can have a profound effect on the aesthetic outcome of the prosthesis and, ultimately, patient acceptance (Beumer et al., 1995). It is very important that these issues be thoroughly discussed with the oncologic surgeon prior to resection. For best results, the surgeon must create skin-lined defects that minimize distortions of adjacent facial structures. In some instances, it may be desirable to remove structures that are otherwise uninvolved with the tumor (for instance, the nasal bones and portions of the nasal septum in nasal defects) if ideal results are to be obtained. Sometimes it is desirable to line a defect with skin, whereas on other occasions, resurfacing with local or vascularized flaps may be more desirable. For midfacial defects (nasal, orbital, etc.), the creation of skin-lined undercuts is desirable because they can be engaged to supplement the retention and stability provided the future prostheses.

If surgical reconstruction of the auricle is not contemplated, the entire ear should be removed, leaving a flat, immobile tissue surface. The raw tissues should be lined with split-thickness skin, full-thickness skin, or a pedicle flap. Vascularized flaps are used to cover larger defects such as those associated with a temporal bone resection. Hair-bearing flaps should be avoided. The presence of hair complicates the long-term maintenance of implants because of the accumulation of sebaceous secretions on their surfaces and makes

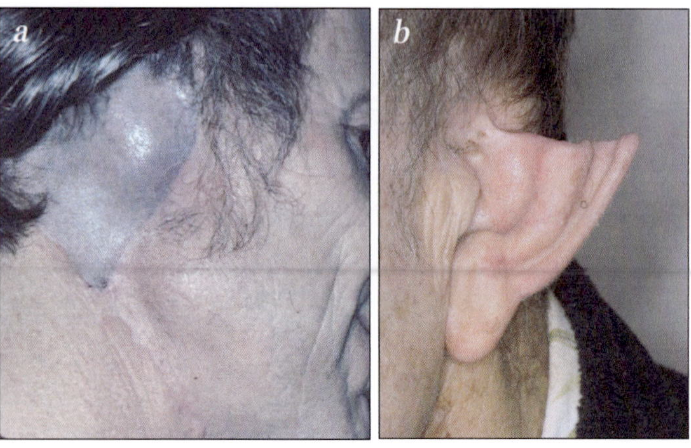

Figure 5-16 Unfavorable auriculectomy defects. *(a)* Defect resurfaced with a hair-bearing flap. *(b)* Large displaced ear fragment.

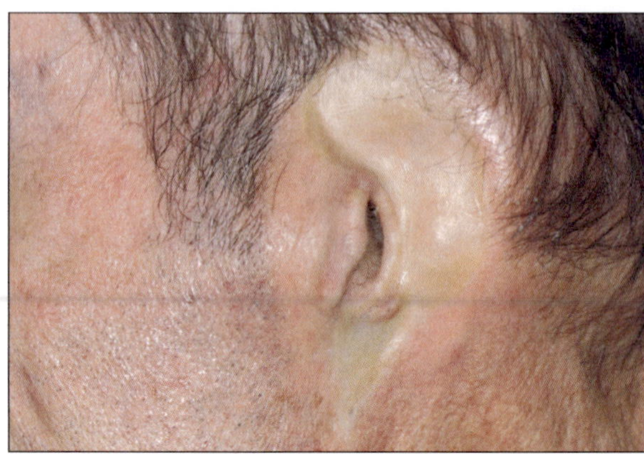

Figure 5-17 Favorable auriculectomy defect. Only the tragus remains in the surgical defect. The remaining area is flat and lined with skin graft, making it an ideal base for an ear prosthesis.

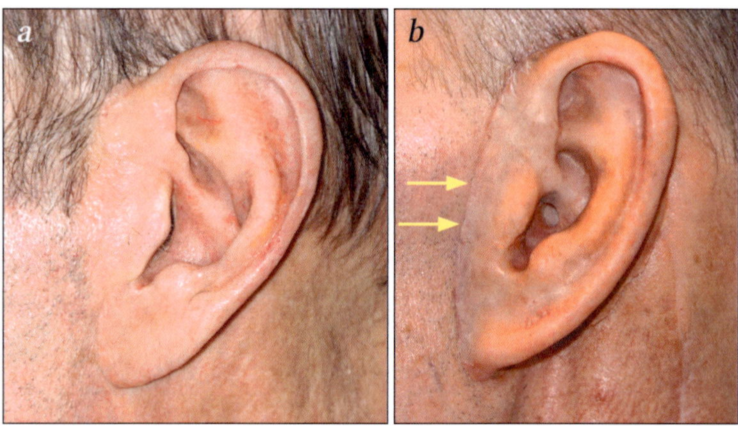

Figure 5-18 *(a)* Patient shown in Fig 5-17. Tragus retained. The anterior margin is partially hidden behind it. *(b)* Tragus removed. The anterior margin is noticeable *(arrows)*.

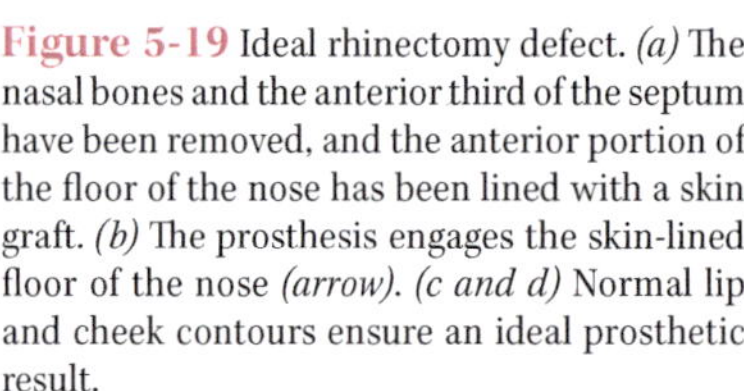

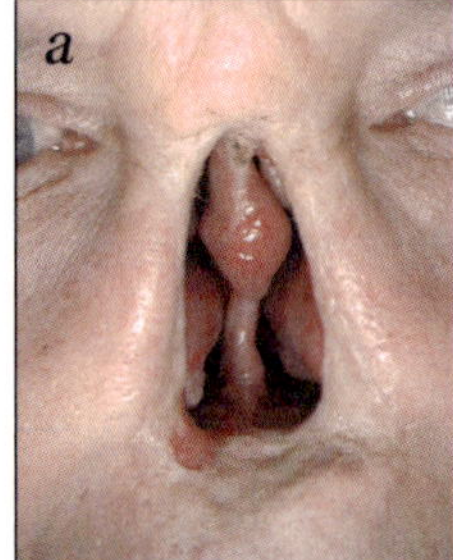

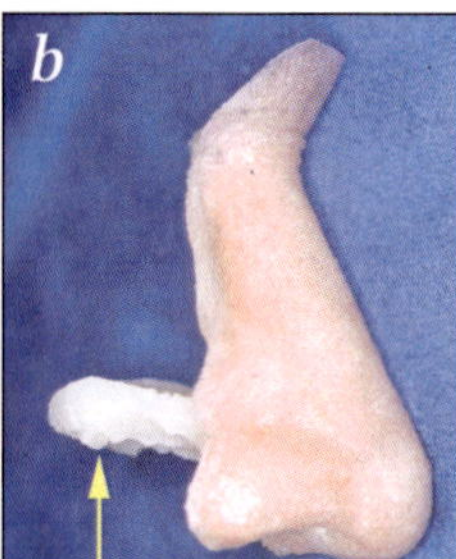

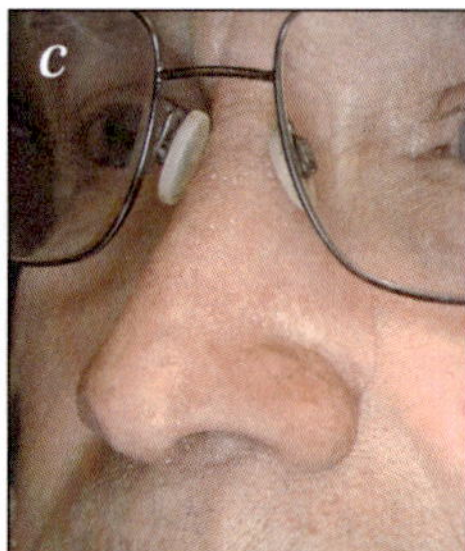

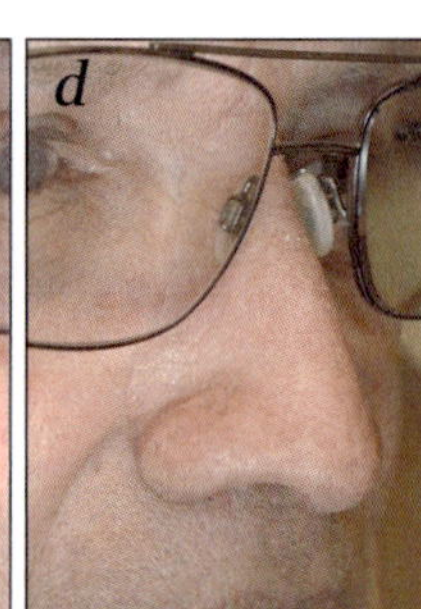

Figure 5-19 Ideal rhinectomy defect. *(a)* The nasal bones and the anterior third of the septum have been removed, and the anterior portion of the floor of the nose has been lined with a skin graft. *(b)* The prosthesis engages the skin-lined floor of the nose *(arrow)*. *(c and d)* Normal lip and cheek contours ensure an ideal prosthetic result.

it difficult to use skin adhesives (Fig 5-16a). Residual tissue tags have little or no retentive value and may become displaced and complicate sculpturing and positioning of a prosthetic ear that is symmetric with the remaining auricle (Fig 5-16b). The tragus, however, should be retained because the anterior margin of the prosthesis can be wrapped behind this structure, helping to camouflage the anterior line of juncture between the prosthesis and the skin (Figs 5-17 and 5-18). In select tumor patients, implants can be placed during the same surgical session as the resection of the tumor. Ear remnants secondary to congenital malformations should also be removed if reconstructive surgery is not contemplated. When a prosthesis is used to restore such defects, the auricular remnants can be repositioned and used to reconstruct the tragus.

Almost all rhinectomy defects are secondary to resection of neoplasms. When a total rhinectomy is contemplated, the nasal bones should be removed, even if these structures are not infiltrated with tumor (Fig 5-19). When retention of the nasal bones is combined with a foreshortened and retracted upper lip (Fig 5-20a), it is virtually impossible to fabricate a nasal prosthesis that is acceptable. If the nasal bones remain, the prosthesis must either terminate just above the superior surgical margin, exposing the prosthetic line of juncture, or extend superiorly over the nasal bridge. Extension of the prosthesis over the nasal bones permits proper margin placement but creates an overcontoured, thin prosthesis in this area that is subject to tearing. Of greater significance is that the retained nasal bones will dictate the prosthetic position and contour of the nasal tip. Nasal

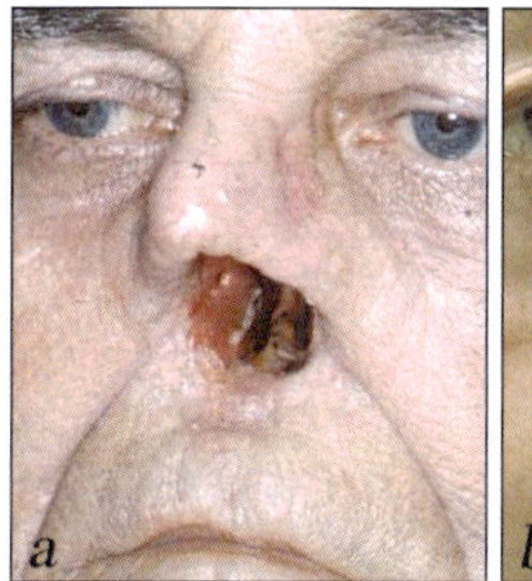
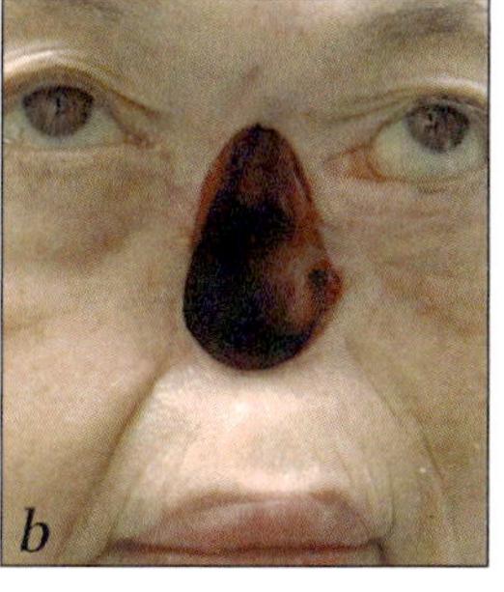

Figure 5-20 Unfavorable rhinectomy defects. *(a)* The nasal bones have been retained and the upper lip has been retracted superiorly. It will be difficult to attain acceptable contours of the nasal bridge and impossible to properly position the tip of the nose in relation to the upper lip. The problem is accentuated by retraction of the upper lip superiorly. *(b)* Primary closure of the wound has resulted in deficient lip and cheek contours and distortion of the left nasolabial fold.

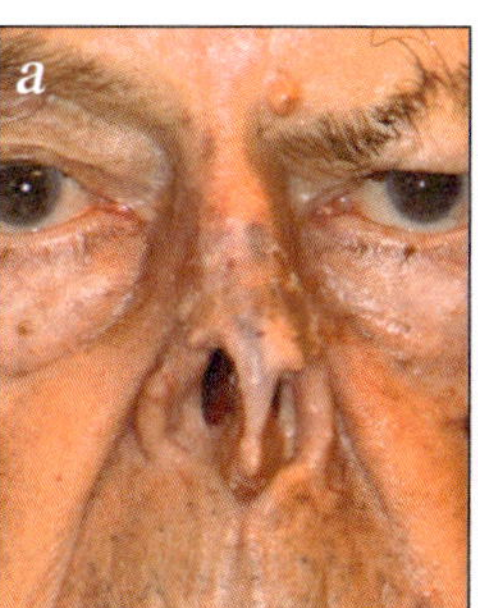
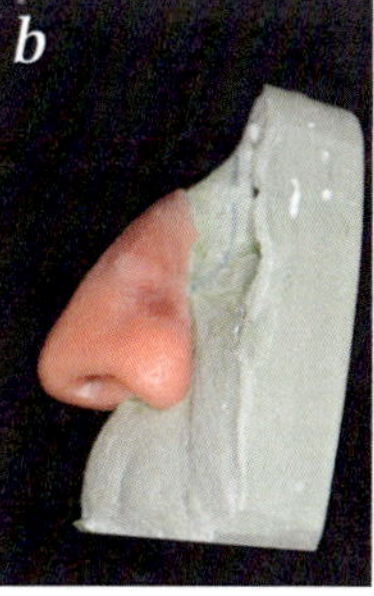
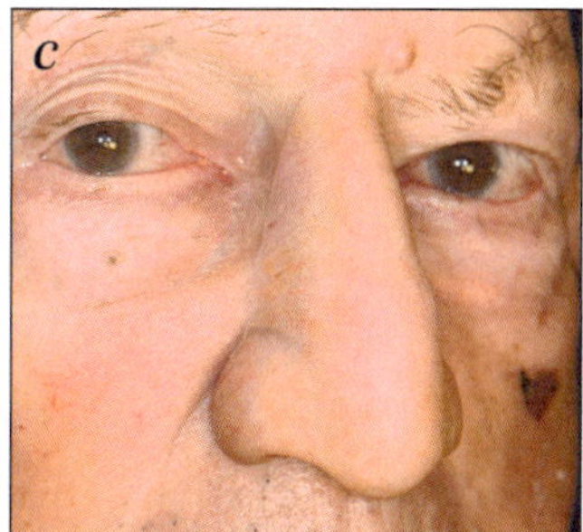

Figure 5-21 *(a)* An unfavorable defect. The nasal bones have been retained and the upper lip has been foreshortened and retracted superiorly. *(b)* The wax sculpture of the nasal prosthesis. Note the acute angle between the columella and the upper lip. *(c)* The definitive prosthesis. It appears to be disproportionately large and excessively long.

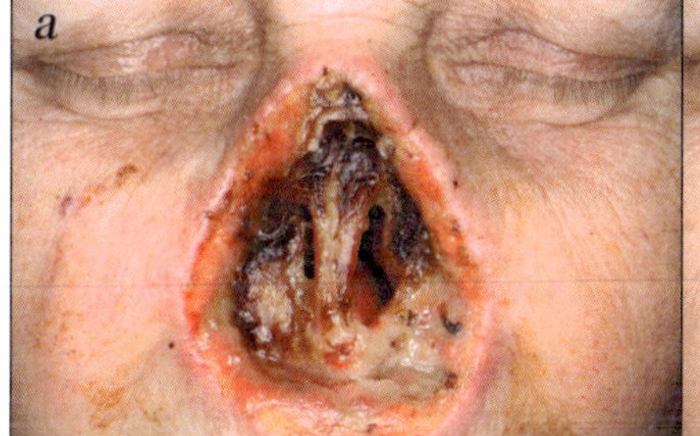
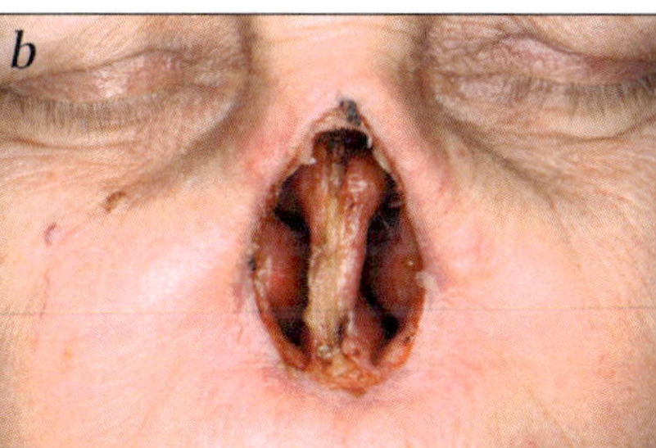
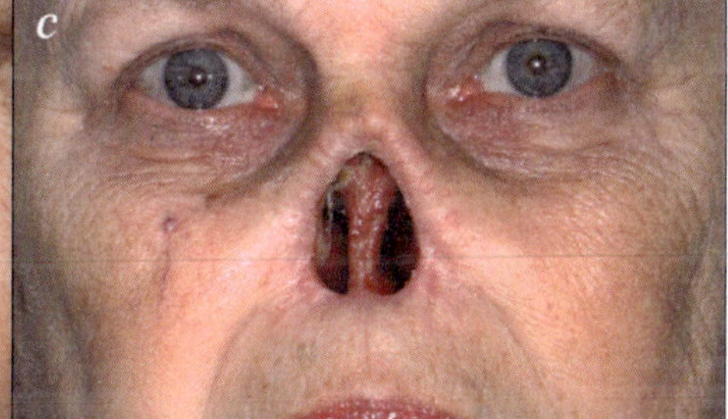

Figure 5-22 *(a, b, and c)* A total rhinectomy defect that was not skin grafted. Note the tissue contracture during healing. As the wound contracts, the lip is pulled superiorly and posteriorly and the surface contours of midfacial area adjacent to the defect become distorted.

prostheses for such defects appear disproportionately large, and the tip of the nose will appear to be unreasonably long (Fig 5-21).

Moreover, it is usually not possible to insert an implant into the thin nasal bones. The glabella appears to be a good site because of the dense nature of the bone associated with this site, but results have been inconsistent (Sugar and Beumer, 1994), presumably because in the past, very short implants (3–4 mm in length) were employed at this site. Recently, however, when longer implants designed for the oral cavity have been used, outcomes appear to have improved (see section below entitled "Nasal defects"). If this site is employed, the position and angulation of the implant must be precise; otherwise, the implant platform or abutment may adversely affect the contour of the nasal bridge of the prosthesis.

It is highly desirable to remove the anterior third of the nasal septum, strip the mucosal lining of the floor of the nose in this area, and resurface it with a split-thickness skin graft (see Fig 5-19a). As a result, the lip will retain much of its original contour and position, and this area can be then engaged to enhance the stability and support for the nasal prosthesis (see Fig 5-19b, c, and d).

Care should be taken to avoid surgical displacement and/or distortion of the upper lip during resection and closure. All raw tissue surfaces should be lined with skin to minimize tissue contracture in the region; otherwise, the upper lip will be elevated and the adjacent midfacial contours will also be distorted (see Figs 5-20b and 5-22). If the lip is retracted posteriorly, foreshortened, and displaced superiorly it is impossible to fabricate a nasal prosthesis that will faithfully reproduce presurgical facial contours, particularly from the lateral perspective (Fig 5-23). The position and contour of the tip of the nose will be compromised and an acute angle created between the columella and the upper lip (Figs 5-21b and 5-23b). Moreover, a retracted upper lip draws attention to the rhinectomy defect and makes it more difficult to conceal the margins of the prosthesis.

During surgical resection of the tumor, care should also be taken to avoid undue distortion of the cheeks and nasolabial folds (Fig 5-20b). Obliteration or displacement of the nasolabial folds adversely affects the contour and position of the nostril and columella portions of the prosthesis. Primary closure (skin to mucosa) of these defects should be avoided because it accentuates the distortion of lip and midfacial contours (Figs 5-21–5-23).

In select patients, osseointegrated implants can be placed immediately following tumor resection (Fig 5-24). The preferred site is the floor of the nose, although in select patients, it may be possible to

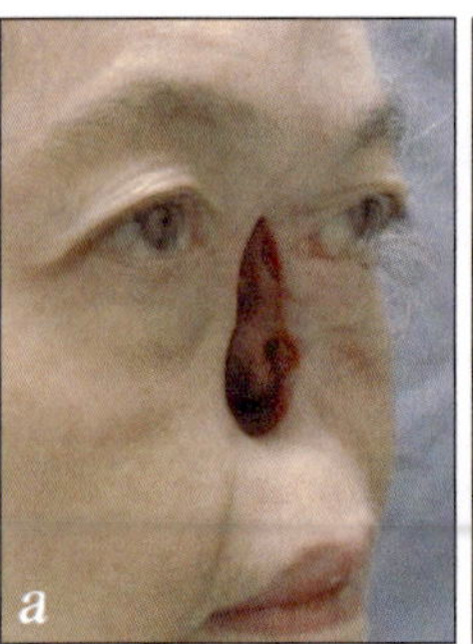
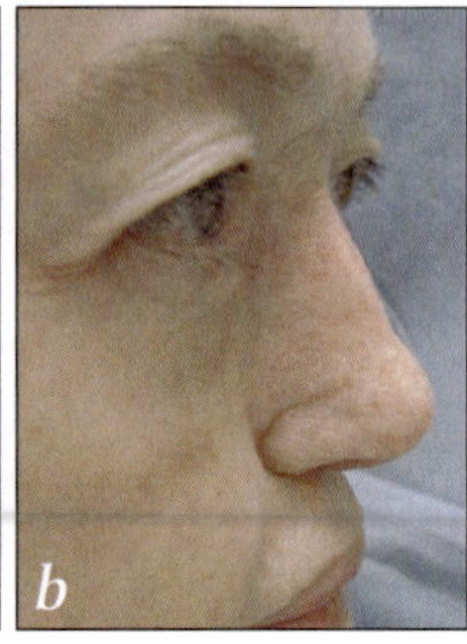
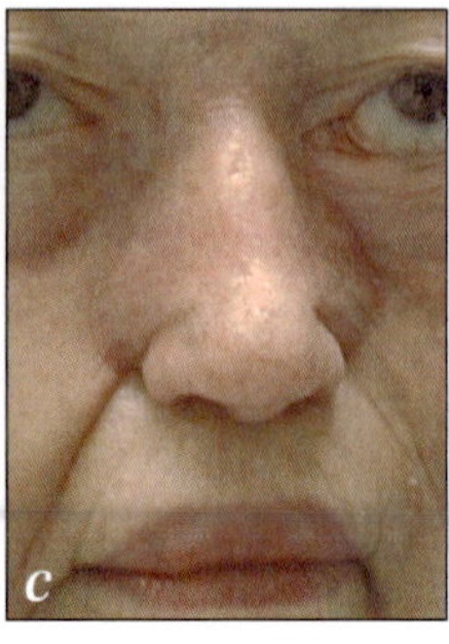

Figure 5-23 Unfavorable rhinectomy defect. *(a)* Note deficient cheek contours and superior displacement of the upper lip. *(b and c)* Because of distortion of the cheeks and retraction of the lip, the size and contours of the prosthesis are made to be compatible with existing contours and do not reproduce the patient's preresection nasal size and contour.

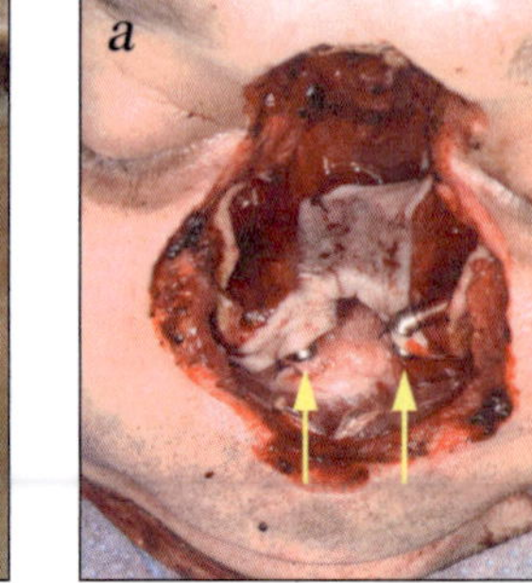
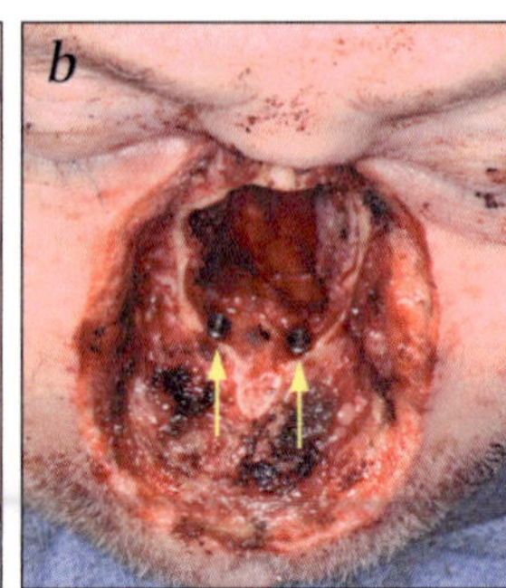

Figure 5-24 Immediate implant placement. Two defects following total rhinectomy. *(a)* Zygomatic implants *(arrows)* were placed in this large defect. *(b)* Craniofacial implants *(arrows)* were placed in the floor of the nose in this more conventional rhinectomy defect.

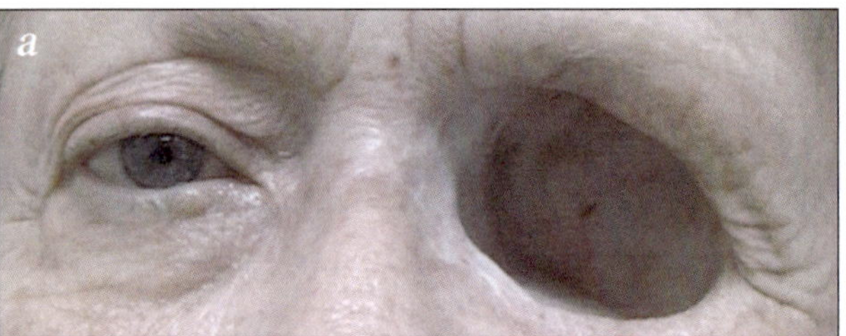
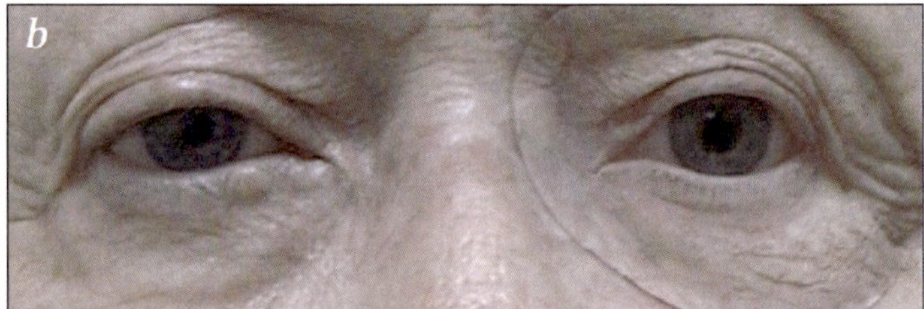

Figure 5-25 Ideal orbital exenteration defect. *(a)* The defect is lined with skin, the eyebrow is in reasonable position, and adjacent facial contours are not distorted. *(b)* Orbital prosthesis in position.

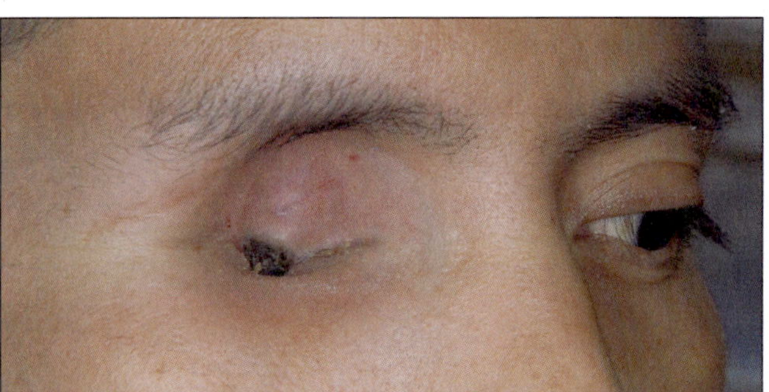

Figure 5-26 The eyelids were retained. They must be removed and sufficient space for the ocular portion of the prosthesis created if a successful outcome is to be achieved.

place implants into the zygoma, particularly when the rhinectomy defect extends laterally onto the cheek. In dentate patients, care must be taken to avoid the roots of the maxillary teeth during implant placement (see section below entitled "Nasal defects").

Following orbital exenteration, the eyelids should be removed and the orbital defect should be lined with a split-thickness skin graft (Fig 5-25). If the eyelids are retained, there may be insufficient space to properly position the ocular portion of the prosthesis at the appropriate depth within the orbital cavity (Fig 5-26). As a result, the prosthesis will appear proptotic. Care should be taken to avoid displacement of the eyebrow.

In most instances attempts should not be made to occlude the orbit with local pedicle or vascularized flaps. After such reconstructions, little room remains for placement of a suitable orbital prosthesis. In addition, recognition of recurrent tumor may be delayed because the margins of the resection are not clearly visible.

The proper use of flaps when resurfacing raw tissues adjacent to an orbit exenteration defect is shown in Fig 5-27. A vascularized flap was used to restore a lateral facial-orbital exenteration defect, but the flap was thinned in the orbital area to avoid filling the orbital cavity. As a result, sufficient space was available to properly position the ocular portion, which enabled the fabrication of a suitable orbital prosthesis.

Large midfacial defects involving the nose and orbit can be effectively restored with a prosthesis even if they involve the upper lip and extend into the oral cavity. However, the surgical resection must be carefully planned and the defect prepared to provide retention, stability, and support for the large, often multiunit prostheses that are necessary to restore these large defects. Surgical modifications that may be indicated at the time of tumor resection include the following:

- The raw tissue surfaces adjacent to the defect should be resurfaced with skin grafts to minimize their contracture and distortion. The skin-lined undercut areas can be aggressively engaged and used to help retain, stabilize, and support such large prostheses (see Fig 5-28a; see also Figs 5-1 and 5-29a).
- Osseointegrated implants should be placed at the time of tumor ablation (Fig 5-28a). Without the benefit of implants, it is not possible to retain, stabilize, and provide sufficient support for such

Figure 5-27 Proper use of a vascularized flap. *(a)* A lateral facial-orbital defect has been resurfaced with a free flap, but sufficient space has been left for an orbital prosthesis. *(b)* Orbital prosthesis in position.

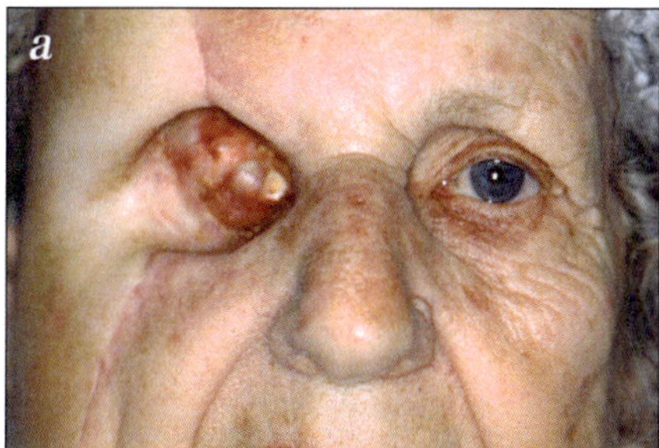

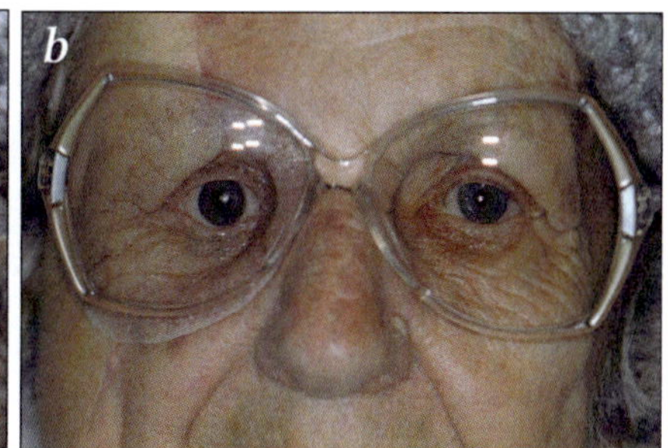

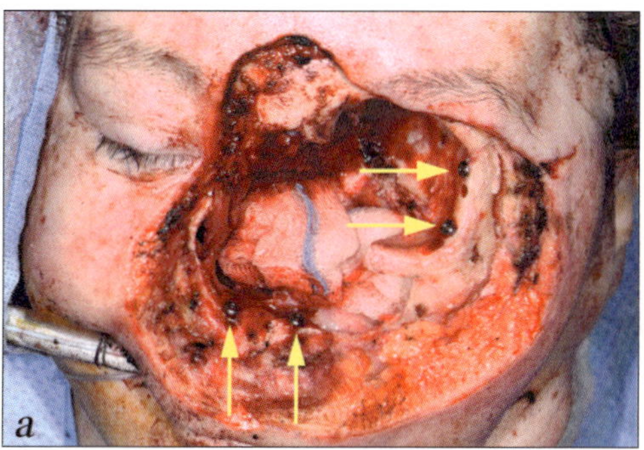

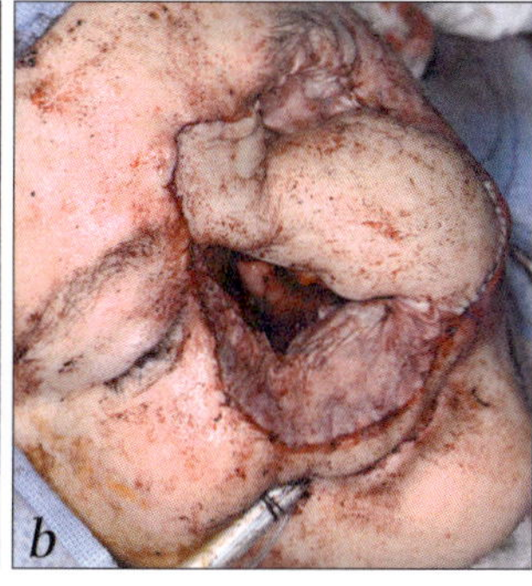

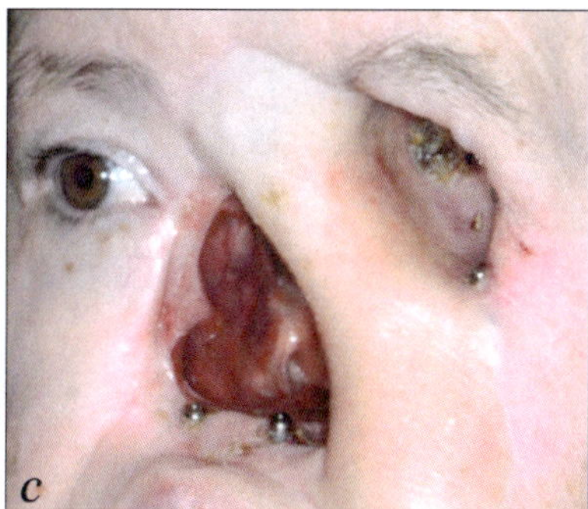

Figure 5-28 *(a)* Resection of the large squamous cell carcinoma shown in Fig 5-4a. In preparation for prosthetic rehabilitation, implants were placed in the floor of the nose and the lateral orbital rim *(arrows)*. *(b)* A vascularized flap was used to restore the lateral facial defect and split-thickness skin grafts used to resurface the remaining raw tissue surfaces. Note that the flap was tailored to avoid obliterating the orbit, thus allowing the placement of an orbital prosthesis at a later date. *(c)* Several months postoperatively the flap has contracted, the implants exposed and the patient is ready to be fitted with a prosthesis restoring the orbit, cheek area and the nose. The definitive prosthesis is shown in Figure 5-138.

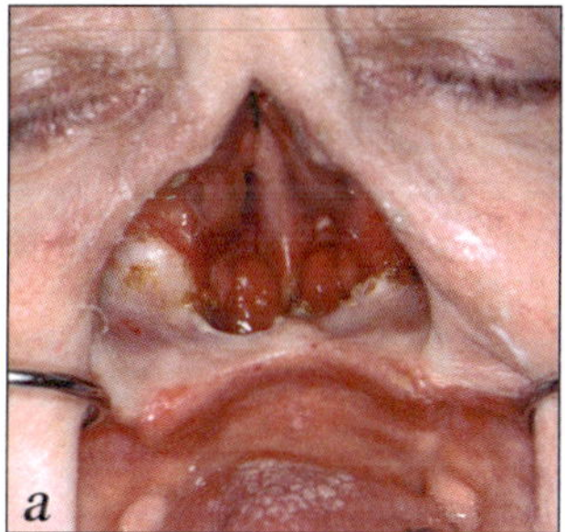

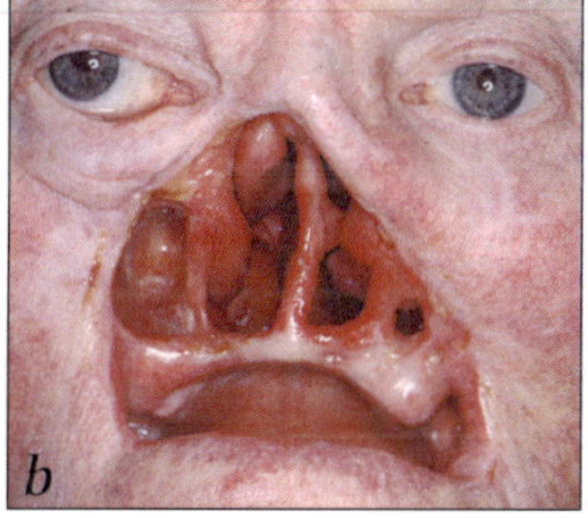

Figure 5-29 Two almost identical midfacial defects. *(a)* Conventional resection with portions of the defect lined with skin. These areas can be engaged to facilitate retention and stability provided for the prosthesis. *(b)* Secondary to resection with Moh's chemosurgery. The defect is unfavorable because it cannot be engaged to facilitate the retention and stability of the prosthesis.

large prostheses. The usual sites available are the zygoma, the glabella, the floor of the nose, and the orbital rims.

- If the defect extends into the oral cavity, teeth that can be used to support and retain the combined facial and intraoral prosthesis should be retained. Bony cuts through the alveolus should be made so as to avoid the roots of the remaining teeth and to preserve the alveolar bone anchoring these roots.
- If flaps are employed, they must be tailored and if necessary, debulked in such a way as to avoid distortion of facial contours and facilitate the fabrication of the prostheses (Fig 5-28b and c).
- If the defect extends laterally to approach the anterior border of the ramus of the mandible, this portion of the defect should be restored with a vascularized flap (Fig 5-28c).
- During the resection, closure, use of flaps, and so on, all efforts must be made to *avoid distortion of adjacent facial contours.*

Large facial defects secondary to resection of skin tumors with Mohs surgery are generally unfavorable and difficult to rehabilitate prosthetically, especially if they extend into the oral cavity. Because of the nature of the procedure, skin grafts can rarely be used, and the raw tissues are left to granulate and epithelialize spontaneously (Fig 5-29a). As a result, the defect cannot be engaged effectively, and local scarring may displace residual facial structures and create unfavorable facial contours adjacent to the defect (Fig 5-29b).

Basic Principles: Fabrication of Facial Prostheses

If the prosthesis is to be undetectable to the casual observer it must have natural contours, surface texture, sheen, color, and translucence, and it must blend well with the adjacent tissue contours. If any one of these factors is not carefully addressed, the result will be less than desirable. Restoration of symmetry may not be possible or

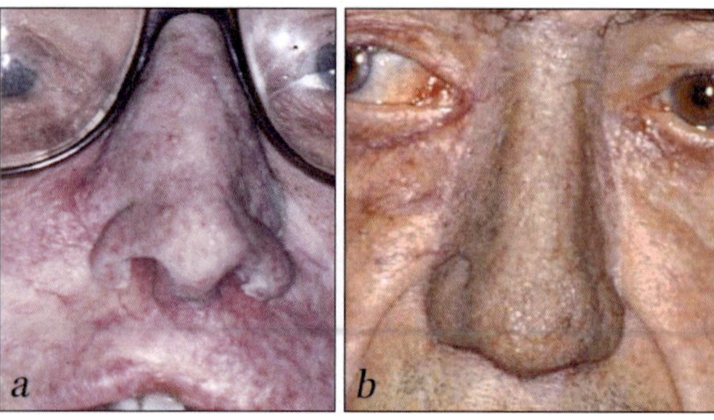

Figure 5-30 Restoration of form. *(a)* Rehabilitation of a nasal defect with significant elevation of the right side of the upper lip, which has been displaced superiorly by multiple local resections and scarring. The right ala of the nasal prosthesis has been reduced and elevated to blend better with existing lip contours. *(b)* The nasolabial fold in this patient is higher on the right than on the left. Note the difference in size of the right and left alae.

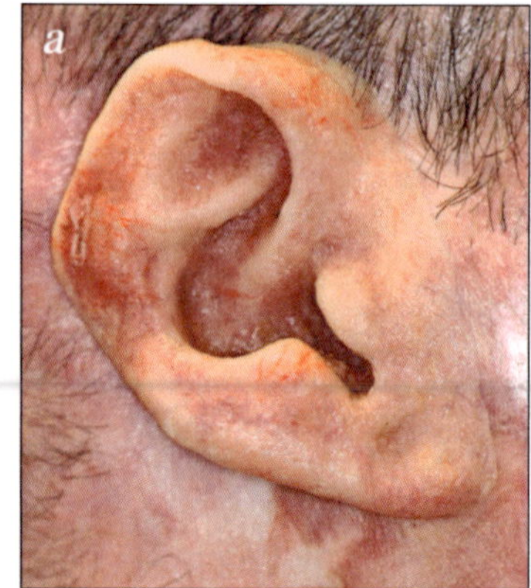

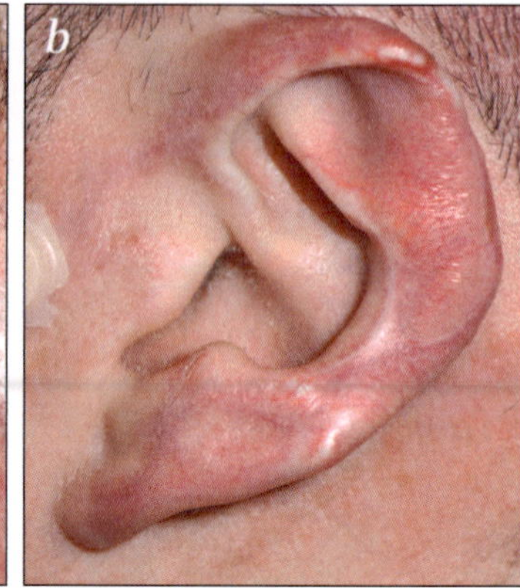

Figure 5-31 *(a)* An ear prosthesis for a burn patient. Note that the contours of the helix mimic those of the *(b)* damaged residual ear.

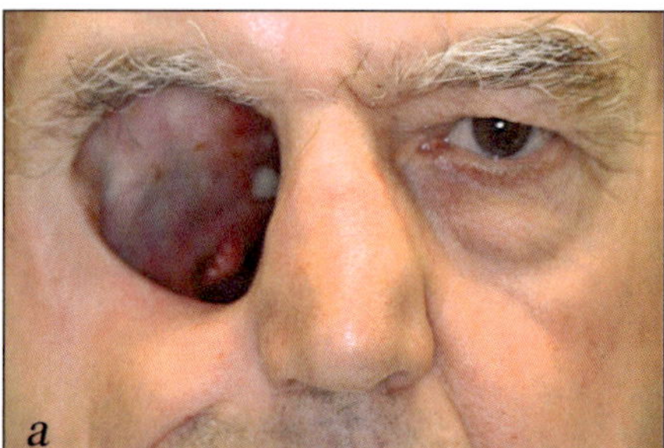

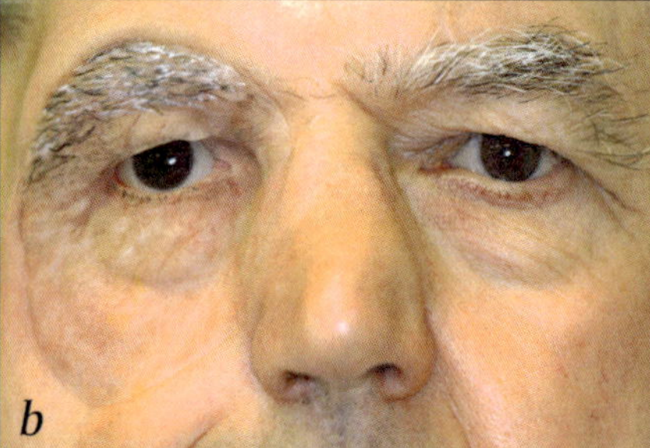

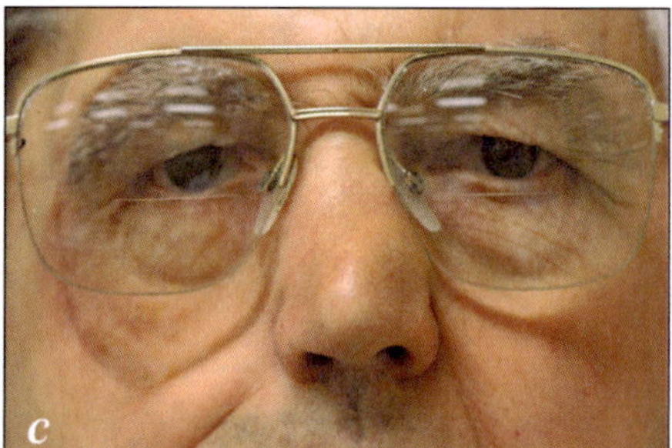

Figure 5-32 Restoration of form. *(a)* Maxillectomy-orbital exenteration defect. Note the altered cheek contours. *(b)* Orbital prosthesis in position. Symmetry is restored in the orbital region but not in the cheek. The contour of the zygomatic-malar area is not restored. The cheek portion is blended with existing cheek contours. *(c)* The eyeglass frames and the shadows cast by them help camouflage the defect.

appropriate in all patients. The prosthesis must be compatible with and blend in with the existing facial form, even if facial contours are somewhat distorted.

Form and symmetry

If the defect is ideal and the adjacent tissue contours are undisturbed by the surgical resection and closure, the size and shape of the facial prosthesis can be nearly identical to those of the structure resected. Defects of this kind, such as a simple auriculectomy, are relatively easy to rehabilitate. However, in many instances the adjacent facial contours are somewhat distorted, and the facial prosthesis must be sculpted to accommodate these contour changes. For instance, in total rhinectomy defects, one of the nasolabial folds may be slightly displaced. It therefore may be esthetically more natural to reduce the size of the ala on that side so that the alar groove of the prosthesis matches the nasolabial fold on that side rather than to fabricate a nasal prosthesis that is perfectly symmetric (Fig 5-30). The patient depicted in Fig 5-31 lost the right ear secondary to burns. The helix of the remaining left ear was also deformed by the incident. It was preferred in this patient that the helix of the prosthesis mimic the contours of the helix of the residual ear.

Perfect symmetry is not always desirable. In some orbital defects, particularly those associated with a maxillectomy, the supraorbital rim may be less prominent and the contour of the cheek may be deficient even with the obturator prosthesis in position. For combined maxillectomy and orbital exenteration defects, it is usually counterproductive to attempt to restore deficient cheek contours with the orbital prosthesis. It is best to blend in this area with the existing facial contours (Fig 5-32). Moreover, in such patients, because of contraction and thinning of the periorbital tissues, the ocular portion of the orbital prosthesis should be placed medial and posterior to the original location of the globe, or the prosthesis will appear proptotic.

Surface texture

If the prosthesis is to be effective, the surface texture of the skin must be faithfully reproduced. The texture of the skin varies considerably as a function of age and site. For example, the texture of the suborbital region is considerably different than that of the adjacent cheek. Likewise, the surface texture of the ala and the tip of the nose is quite different than that of the bridge of the nose (Fig 5-33). In many instances, a simple stippling of the sculpting with a denture cleaning brush (Fig 5-34) may be sufficient to produce appropriate skin texture for the prosthesis, but in many prostheses, this method alone is not sufficient, and the surface texture must be carved into the wax sculpting. Excellent examples of reproduction of the surface

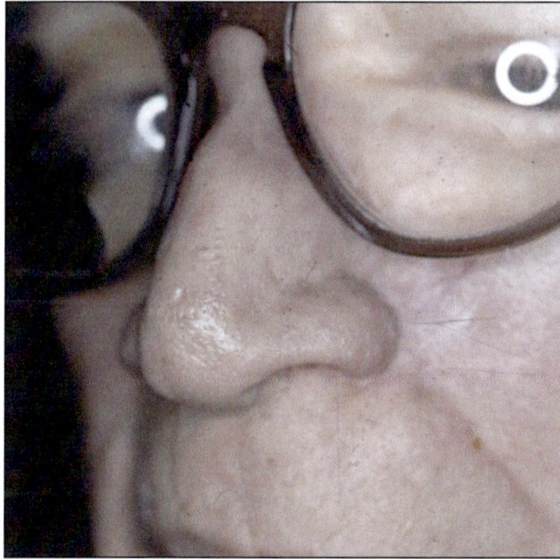

Figure 5-33 A typical nasal prosthesis restoring a total rhinectomy defect. The stipple pattern of the tip and ala is more prominent than that seen on the bridge or lateral surfaces of the nose. Note also that the surfaces of the tip and the ala are shinier than the adjacent skin, reflecting the presence of sebaceous secretions.

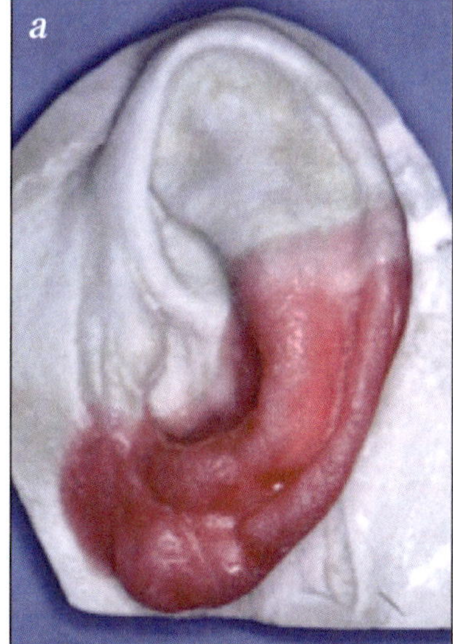

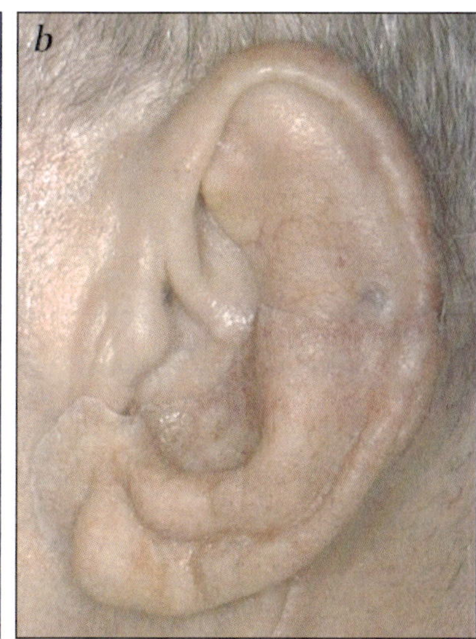

Figure 5-34 *(a and b)* A simple stipple made with a denture cleaning brush is all that is required to create surface texture in most ear prostheses.

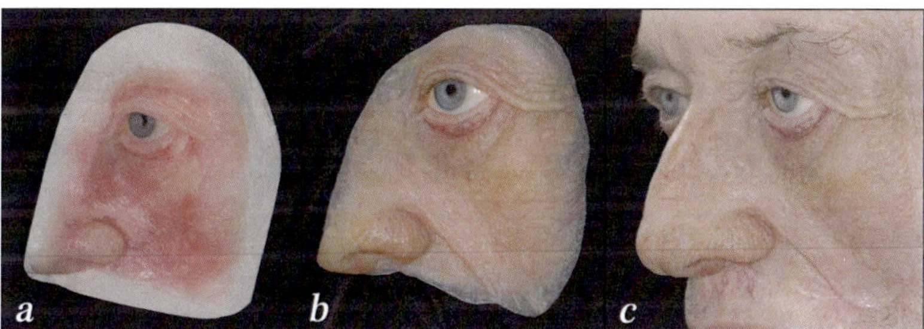

Figure 5-35 Reproduction of surface texture. *(a)* The patient underwent an orbital exenteration, and partial rhinectomy extending onto the cheek. The wax pattern. The surface texture has been created with a stipple supplemented with a wax carver. The surface texture has been carefully configured to match the patient's skin. The nasal margin extends at an angle to the bridge of the nose and is short of the midline. *(b)* The completed prosthesis. Note the surface texture of the ala and the suborbital region. *(c)* The cheek extension has been carefully blended into the surface contour of the skin. The nasolabial fold and alar groove have been painted to simulate the unaffected side. The area beneath the lower lid has been painted to simulate the coloration on the opposite side.

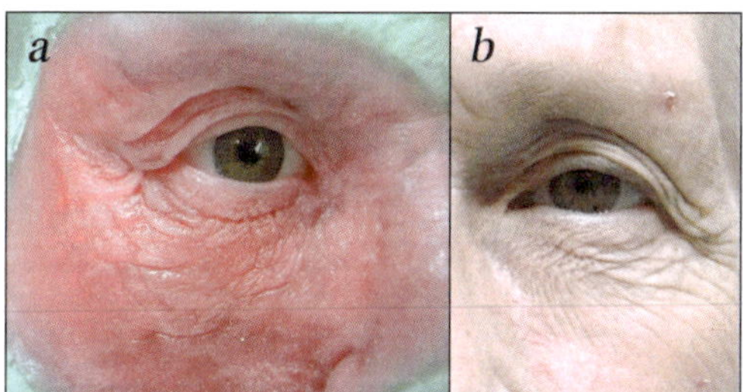

Figure 5-36 Reproduction of surface texture to rehabilitate a large orbital defect. *(a and b)* The surface texture of the suborbital area and cheek has been faithfully reproduced. The texture of the sculpting is slightly more prominent than that of skin, because some detail is lost during processing, extrinsic coloration and sealing.

texture of the skin of the orbital, cheek, and nasal areas in elderly patients are shown in Figs 5-35 and 5-36. The texture created in wax should be sharper and more prominent than that of the patient's natural skin because some of the detail is lost during processing, extrinsic coloration and sealing.

Sheen and light reflection

The sheen or gloss of the prosthetic surfaces must be carefully controlled. This is accomplished during the deglossing process (see section below entitled "Coloration"). For example, the tip and ala of the nose are shinier than the lateral surfaces of the nose due to the abundance of sebaceous glands and their secretions in these areas (see Fig 5-33). If the deglossing step is executed too aggressively, these surfaces and indeed the entire prosthesis will appear dull and lifeless (Fig 5-37).

Lines of juncture between skin and prosthesis

When possible, lines of juncture (margins) should be positioned beneath eyeglass frames or the shadows cast by them (see Figs 5-32 and 5-33) or in skin folds or creases such as the nasolabial fold (see Figs 5-19, 5-30b, and 5-33). In total auriculectomy defects, the midportion of the anterior margin is placed behind the tragus, when it has been retained (see Figs 5-18a, 5-40f, 5-46a, 5-47, and 5-48h). However, in most patients, at least a portion of the margin of the prosthesis will be exposed. In these instances, it is important that the margins be located in areas that are as inconspicuous as possible and the contours of the prosthesis blend smoothly with those of the adjacent tissues (see Figs 5-44 and 5-51). For example, when a portion of the nose is remaining and is not to be covered with the prosthesis, it is advisable to terminate the margin on either side of the midline, because this makes the margin less conspicuous (see Figs 5-53 and 5-64). The margin will be concealed far more effectively if it is placed on the slopes of the lateral wall of the nose.

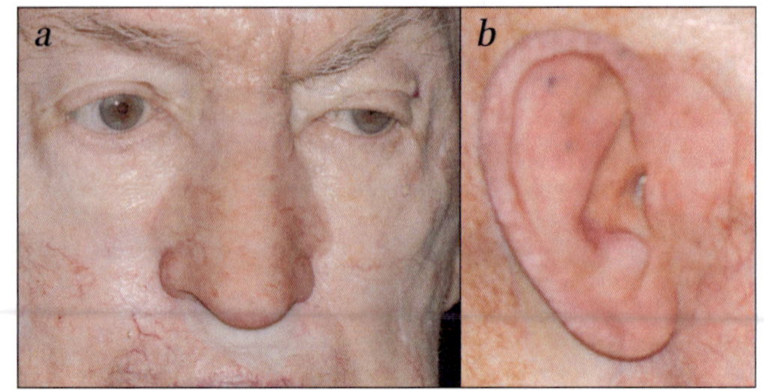

Figure 5-37 Coloration of these two prostheses is acceptable but the deglossing has been excessive and as a result the prostheses do not have the proper sheen and appears dull and lifeless.

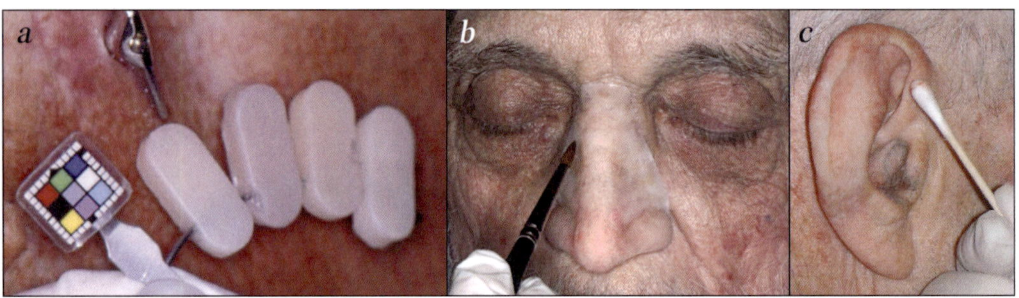

Figure 5-38 Color matching. *(a)* Shade guides will ensure consistency in the color and translucence of the base. *(b and c)* Coloration is accomplished under corrected light conditions.

Exposed margins must also be very carefully contoured to blend perfectly with the adjacent facial contours. The margin should be as thin as possible in these areas. It is almost always advantageous to score the master cast slightly when the prosthesis extends to highly displaceable tissues such as the cheek. This will ensure proper tissue contact at the margin and facilitate a smooth and aesthetic transition between the prosthesis and adjacent skin in these exposed areas.

Coloration

Best results are achieved with a combination of intrinsic and extrinsic coloration. If extrinsic coloration is the primary technique used, the prosthesis is cast in a base shade and surface details and character can be added by extrinsic coloration. Shade guides are useful and will ensure consistent, reproducible color and translucence of the base. These guides should be fabricated with care and precision to ensure reproducibility. Base shades should strike a proper balance between translucence and opacity. The base shade selected for a patient should be slightly lighter than the lightest skin tones of the patient, because as color is added the prosthesis will darken (Fig 5-38a).

Extrinsic coloration should be accomplished under corrected light conditions. Shadows must be embellished with paint because of the translucence of the materials. For the same reason, lines and skin creases must be painted to create a lifelike appearance (Fig 5-38b and c). Paints for extrinsic coloration are available commercially or prepared by mixing earth pigments with RTV silicone. We prefer to use the paints supplied by the manufacturer because much of the surface texture is lost with the older methods. In addition, the colors of the commercial preparation are more consistent, easier to apply and control, and more color stable and do not affect the physical properties of the silicone elastomer.

When painting is completed, the prosthesis is allowed to cure at room temperature for one to two days. The extrinsic coloration is then sealed with a fast-curing RTV platinum silicone and allowed to cure overnight in a dry heat oven. The addition of small amounts of fumed silicone dioxide (Cab-O-Sil, Factor II) to seal the RTV silicone will moderate some of the shine. Application of an excessive thickness of sealant should be avoided. Excessive shine can also be avoided if a dry brush is used as a blotter, because the silicone begins to cure after the initial layer of sealant is applied. This process is repeated twice at five-minute intervals on application of the silicone sealant. This technique will also maintain the original surface texture of the prosthesis.

After 20 to 30 minutes of curing, selected areas of the prosthesis are further deglossed with fumed silicone dioxide. Deglossing with Cab-O-Sil is ineffective after the sealant has completely cured. Care should be taken to avoid excessive deglossing. Some areas of the prosthesis should retain some shine, such as the ala and the tip of the nose of elderly patients with oily skin (see Fig 5-33).

After a day or two of allowing the extrinsic coloration to cure, carefully apply TS-564 with a disposable paint brush. Allow to dry for 30 min. This will prime the surface for the addition of the sealant silicone A-564. The sealant is very viscous, and care must be taken to avoid losing all surface texture. The manufacturer recommends using a brush, but we have found this impossible to spread. Instead, use clean fingers. Tap-tap on the wet silicone with a different unused and clean finger to add texture. A-564 can be diluted with TS-564. After 30 min, a matting solution is made by mixing a 5:1 ratio of A-564 with MD-564. While MD-564 is the matting agent, A-564 is needed to create the sealing medium. MD-564 separates readily in the jar and must be stirred prior to use. These elements cannot be premixed before shipping because they have a very short shelf life once mixed together. This process will create a suitable matte finish for the prosthesis.

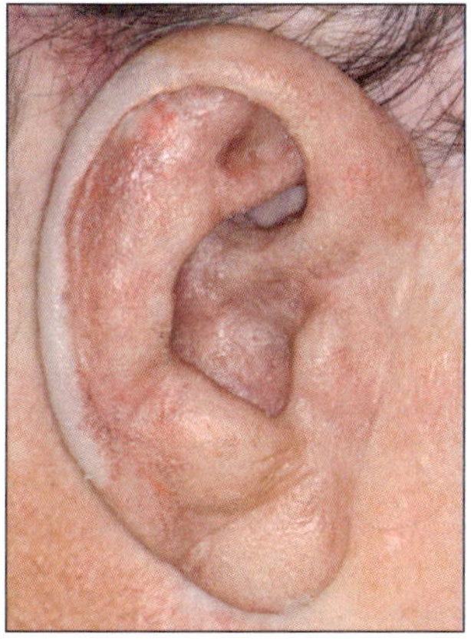

Figure 5-39 Extrinsic coloration has worn off the helix.

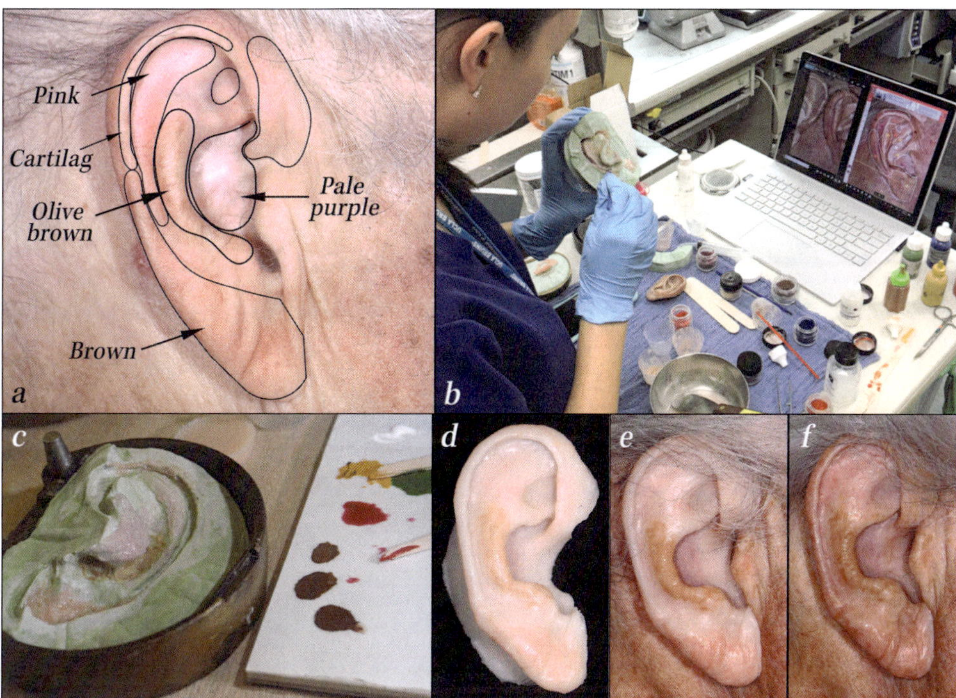

Figure 5-40 Intrinsic coloration. A three-piece mold for an auricular prosthesis is important for deflasking but also to allow easy access for application of regional coloration. *(a)* Color map. Areas of distinct colors have been outlined. Note that the conchal bowl is a pale purple and the scaphoid fossa is pink and the antihelix in olive brown populated with freckles. *(b)* Colored RTV silicone added to select areas. In the background is a laptop with a color map on the screen. *(c)* A close-up view of the cope portion with colored silicone applied to their respective areas. Areas in between will be filled with the base shade. *(d and e)* Cured prostheses with intrinsic coloration. The goal is to err on the side of less chroma. *(f)* Extrinsic characterization is applied chair side to complete coloration.

The extrinsic coloration tends to wear off (Fig 5-39), so many clinicians have resorted to extrinsic combined with intrinsic coloration (Figs 5-40 and 5-41). If intrinsic coloration is employed, a color map is created with delineated regions (Fig 5-40a). A base shade is mixed as described above. A small amount of the base shade is transferred to a separate dish and further characterized with color and flocking. Flocking has the advantage of creating texture in the color as opposed to a monochromatic mix. Red flocking simulates areas of telangiectasia and small vessels close to the surface.

The prepared molds are placed in a dry heat oven at 50°C for approximately 30 minutes before use. Warming of all the mold segments assists in retaining the position of the custom colors used for intrinsic shade coloring. A thixotropic agent is added to reduce flow and allow the application of the various tinted batches of silicone to their respective areas in the mold. Care is taken not to trap air bubbles when stroking the accelerated silicone. Once all mapped areas have their respective colors, long strands of fibers can be laid to accentuate small blood vessels close to the surface. Finally, the base shade is injected into the mold with a syringe. The mold is closed, compressed to 500 PSI, clamped to prevent rebound, and allowed to cure overnight. Curing can be accelerated and completed in two hours by placing the mold in a dry heat oven set at 163°F.

Unused portions of the various colors can be made into patient-specific shade tabs and stored in a dry cool place. These tabs serve as records of color samples for later prosthesis remakes. After complete polymerization, extrinsic coloration is added as needed (Figs 5-40 and 5-41).

Restoration of Auricular Defects

Auricular defects occur secondary to congenital malformations, burns, trauma, or surgical removal of neoplasms. Defects secondary to total resection of the auricle are easily rehabilitated prosthetically. Partial auricular defects are more difficult to rehabilitate (see section below entitled "Partial auriculectomy defects").

Preoperative consultations are extremely valuable for patients with auricular tumors requiring resection of the auricle. Besides informing the patient of the nature of the defect and the future prosthesis, preoperative impressions, photographs, or scans make construction of the postsurgical auricular prosthesis relatively simple. After surgery, the wax duplicate of the patient's ear is easily positioned, adapted to the defect, and altered as necessary. All that remains to be completed is to position the wax pattern, feather the margins, and incorporate appropriate surface detail and texture. Under some circumstances, many of these steps can be performed remotely using digital technologies (see section below entitled "Use of digital technology").

Temporary auricular prostheses

In most patients, the tissue bed is sufficiently organized four to six weeks after surgery to allow the placement of a temporary ear prosthesis. The use of heat-polymerizing acrylic resin to fabricate this

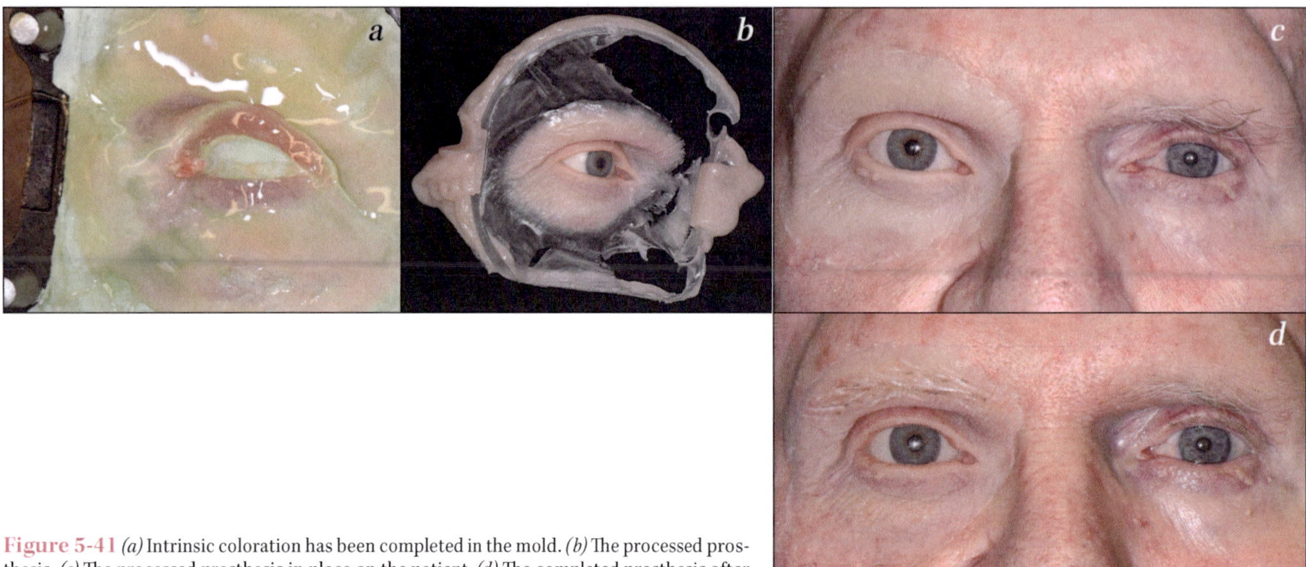

Figure 5-41 *(a)* Intrinsic coloration has been completed in the mold. *(b)* The processed prosthesis. *(c)* The processed prosthesis in place on the patient. *(d)* The completed prosthesis after extrinsic coloration.

temporary prosthesis will allow periodic adjustment and relining with a temporary denture reliner. Alternatively, a temporary prosthesis can be made from silicone elastomer. This too may be refitted with silicone rubber as healing progresses. This is a useful service to some patients as they transition to their new normal since few complications have resulted from this practice. Retention is accomplished with medical grade skin adhesives. For most patients, four to five months is a suitable period to allow for organization and contracture of the wound before fabrication of the definitive prosthesis commences.

Definitive auricular prostheses

Impressions

Unlike orbital or nasal defects, the tissues in the auricular area are not particularly displaceable, and significant distortions do not result from postural changes. However, in some patients, the jowls may be displaced by gravity if the patient is sitting back, and if so, this will lead to an open margin in the preauricular area. Hence, patients need to either sit upright or lie on their side. However, condylar movements should be noted, for this may result in mobility of the tissues adjacent to the defect, which can affect marginal placement, tissue coverage, and ultimately the retention of the prosthesis if it is retained with skin adhesives. The working cast may need to be lightly sanded in areas of soft tissue mobility to prevent gapping and allow a more intimate prosthesis fit in these areas.

Before the impression is made, a skin-marking pen or indelible marking stick is used to place orientation marks indicating the location of the external auditory meatus and the angulation of the long axis of the ear. The defect area is isolated with drapes or a fast-setting silicone paste, cotton is placed in the ear canal, and a suitable impression material is applied (Fig 5-42). Adjacent hair should be covered with tape, a water-soluble lubricant, or cold cream. Note that petroleum-based products may inhibit the polymerization of some silicones and should be used with caution.

Disposable syringes are useful for depositing impression material into areas with difficult access. A spatula is used to thin the impression material over the area to be impressed. Light-bodied polysulfide, polyvinyl siloxane, and irreversible hydrocolloid are appropriate impression materials. If irreversible hydrocolloid is used, the addition of 50% more water will improve its flow properties.

A backing of quick-setting plaster provides suitable support for the impression. The plaster backing must be applied in succeeding thin layers to avoid distorting the underlying tissues and the impression. Strips of gauze or wisps of cotton partially embedded within the setting impression material and painted with the appropriate adhesive are used to unite the impression material with the plaster backing. It is critical that the first layer of plaster be allowed to set before the subsequent layers are added.

Sculpting

If a presurgical cast of the resected ear is available, it is reproduced in wax and compared to the remaining ear. Use of a skin-colored wax rather than pink baseplate wax is preferred by some clinicians and may be helpful because it gives the patient and clinician a more realistic perspective of the future definitive prosthesis (Fig 5-43). Appropriate changes are made in the basic contours, and at the next appointment the wax ear is positioned and adapted to the defect to achieve natural symmetry in all planes with the opposite side. A water bath and flame are necessary to complete this procedure successfully. A modified facebow or a Fox occlusal plane (Dentsply Trubite) may be useful aids to verify the position of the wax ear sculpture.

If preoperative casts are not available, either the prosthesis can be sculpted from the beginning, or the "donor" technique may be employed. Sculpting an ear from the beginning is time consuming, but it may be necessary for select patients. This task is facilitated by dividing the cast of the normal ear into equal sections so that contours are more easily visualized (Fig 5-44).

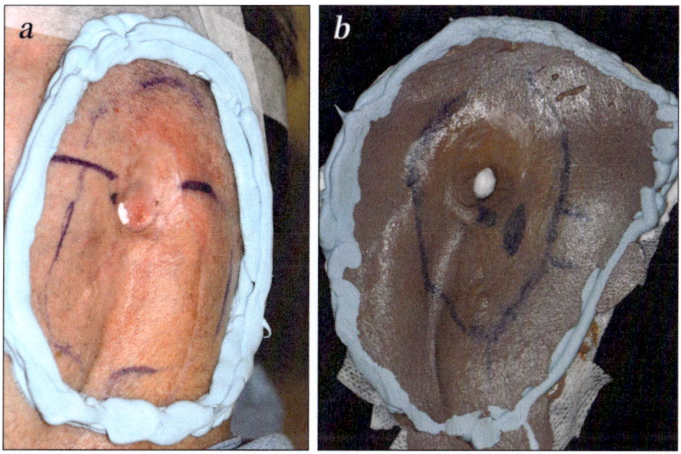

Figure 5-42 *(a)* The defect is isolated and orientation markings are drawn with indelible pencil sticks. *(b)* The impression.

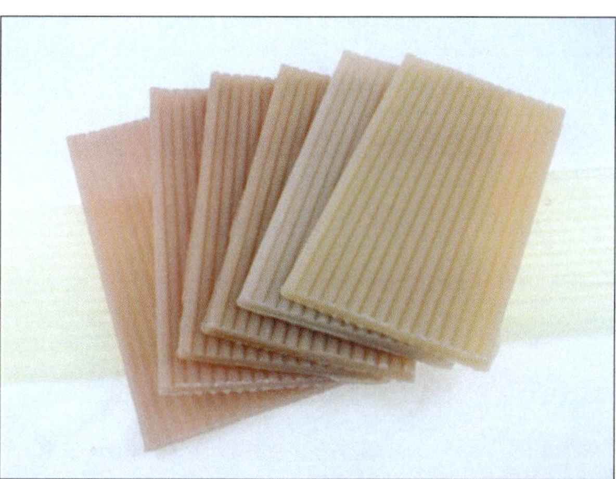

Figure 5-43 Skin colored wax is available in a number of shades (courtesy of Factor II, Scottsdale, AZ).

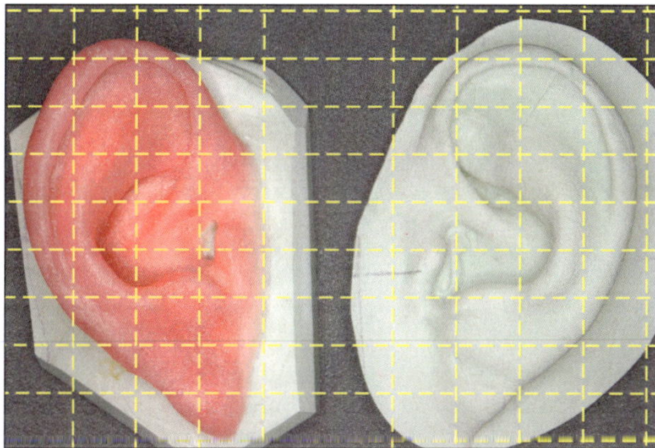

Figure 5-44 Dividing the normal ear into equal compartments with a grid will aid in sculpting. Note how the anterior margin is feathered to blend in with the adjacent skin.

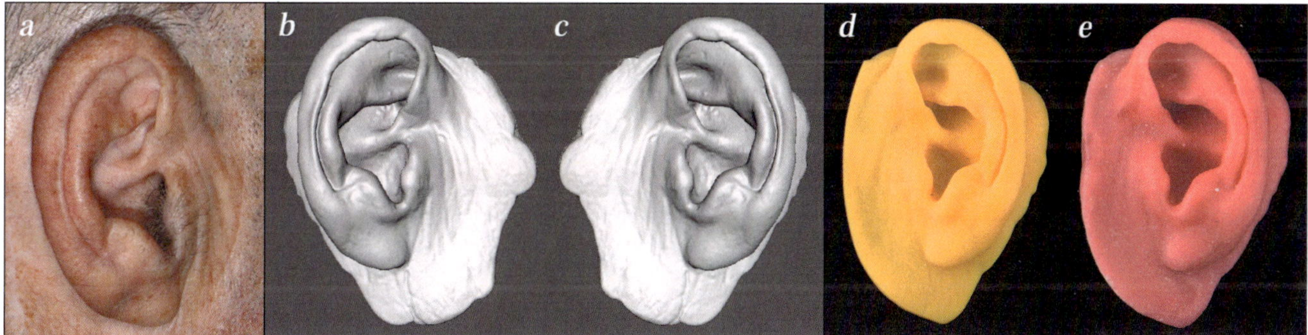

Figure 5-45 CAD-CAM techniques were used to develop this wax pattern. *(a)* Normal ear. *(b)* The scan of the normal ear. *(c)* The mirror image of the residual ear. *(d)* Printed resin ear of the mirror image. *(e)* Duplicated wax pattern.

The donor technique is an easier method. A person with ear contours that closely mimic those of the patient is selected. Often, this may be a family member. An impression of the appropriate ear of the donor is made and a wax cast is retrieved. The wax ear is adapted and recontoured as necessary. If the clinician makes wax duplicates of the ears of their auriculectomy patients, he/she soon will have a suitable donor supply and will not need to seek a donor. CAD-CAM techniques can also be employed to develop the initial wax sculpting (Fig 5-45). The ear on the opposite site is scanned and the data is manipulated to create a mirror image of the scanned normal ear. Most intraoral scanners can be used to obtain the scan. A resin duplicate is printed and this in turn can be duplicated in a suitable wax pattern. If appropriate instrumentation is available, the initial wax pattern can also be printed in wax.

When the basic contours of the wax pattern match the unresected ear, the wax sculpting is tried on the patient (Fig 5-46).

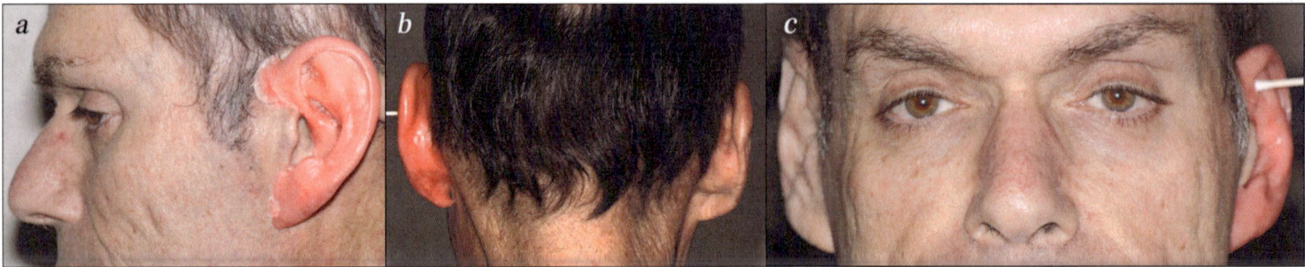

Figure 5-46 *(a, b, and c)* The wax sculpture is tried on the patient and checked for size, contour and symmetry with regards the opposite normal ear.

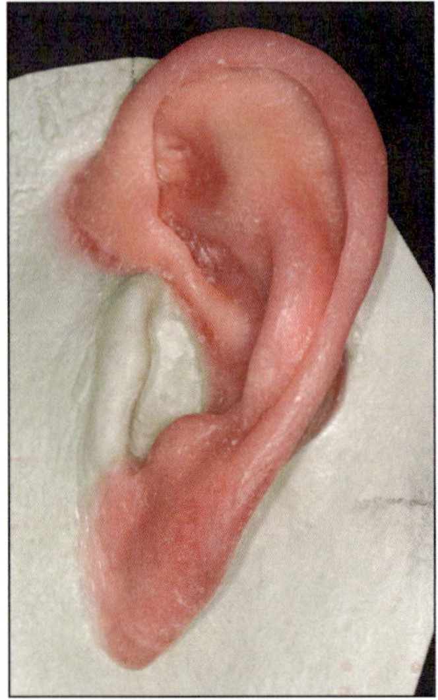

Figure 5-47 The wax sculpture Is luted to the master cast. The exposed anterior margins are feathered and blended with the adjacent skin and a surface texture created that mimics that of the normal ear.

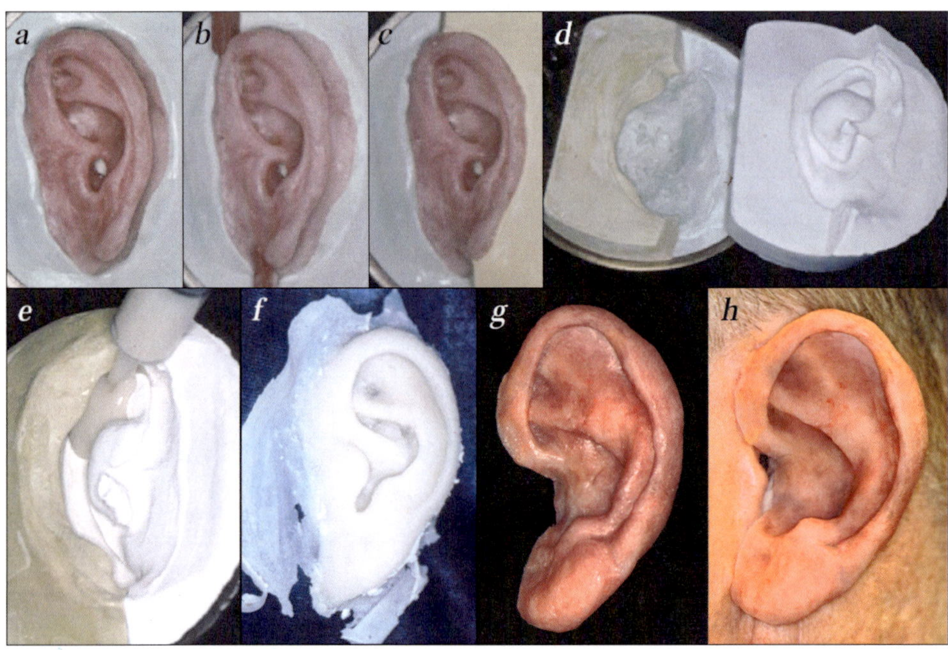

Figure 5-48 Processing of the auricular prosthesis. *(a to d)* A three-part mold is made to facilitate removal of the auricular casting without tearing. *(e)* Facial material is syringed into the mold. *(f)* The polymerized prosthesis is removed. *(g)* The prosthesis is painted to match the opposite ear and adjacent skin and allowed to cure. After curing, it is sealed. *(h)* After deglossing the definitive prosthesis is delivered.

Adjustments are made as necessary in order to create the semblance of bilateral symmetry. When the position and basic contours of the wax pattern are acceptable, the patient is dismissed and the surface details are applied. The upper portion of the anterior margin will be exposed and should be carefully blended and feathered (see Fig 5-47). The middle portion should be wrapped around the tragus, if this structure is present. The inferior margin, in most patients (particularly elderly patients), is designed to look like a crease in the skin. The entire surface must be textured to match the skin textures of the adjacent skin and opposite ear. The texture should be made a little more prominent than that of the adjacent skin, because some detail is lost during processing and painting.

Proper texture is important for several reasons. Without the proper texture, the prosthesis can never be suitably matched to adjacent skin. Moreover, without texture, extrinsic tinting becomes extremely difficult inasmuch as appropriate application, control, and distribution of paint on a smooth surface is almost impossible. Care should be taken to avoid making the stipples excessively deep, because paint has a tendency to pool in deep stipples. Proper texturing provides mechanical retention for extrinsic colorants and lengthens the period of service of the prosthesis.

Processing

The wax ear is invested in a manner to construct a three-part mold (Fig 5-48a–d). When flexible materials are used, three-part molds are necessary because they allow the casting to be removed from the mold without tearing (Fig 5-48e and f). These molds can also be designed and fabricated with CAD-CAM techniques (see Fig 5-51). The appropriate material is selected, base shades are determined, and the processing is completed. As mentioned previously, color characterization can be accomplished either intrinsically, extrinsically, or both (Fig 5-48g and h). Select areas of extrinsic coloration, regardless of the method employed, tend to rub off eventually (see Fig 5-39).

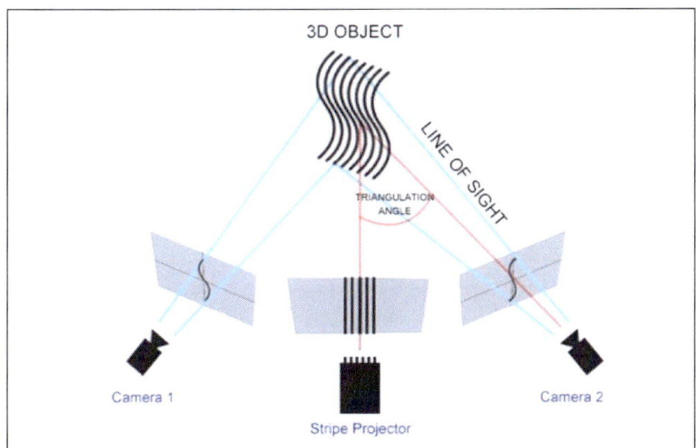

Figure 5-49 A diagrammatic representation of scanning 3D objects with structured light scanning technology.

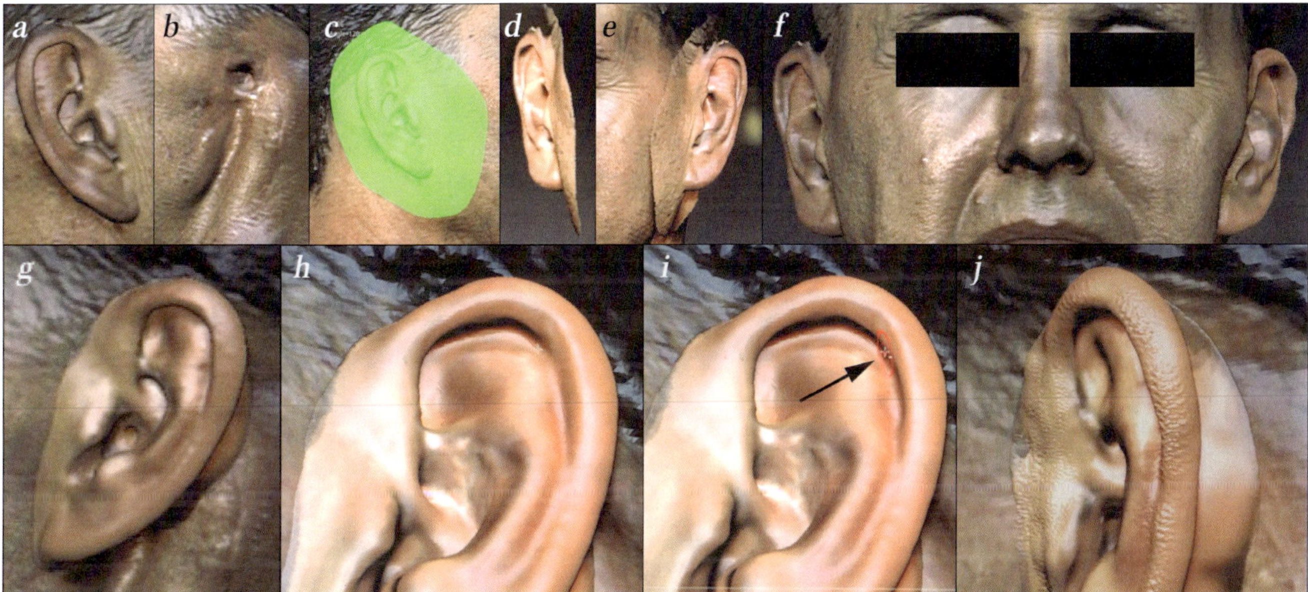

Figure 5-50 *(a, b, and c)* The defect and the patient's normal ear are scanned using phase measuring profilometry. *(d)* The data encompassing the normal ear and the surrounding tissues are "separated" and manipulated creating a mirror image of the normal ear. *(e, f, and g)* The mirror image of the normal ear is superimposed upon the defect and position and oriented to achieve a semblance of bilateral symmetry. *(h and i)* A sculpting tool can be used to deepen concavities and grooves *(arrow)*. *(j)* Another tool can be used to create the appropriate surface texture and detail.

Use of digital technology

Many of the steps can be performed digitally. The defect and the normal ear of the patient are scanned. A number of different scanning technologies have evolved including light scanning (Wu et al., 2008; Feng et al., 2010; Sun et al., 2011), 3D photography (Liacouras et al., 2011; Sabol et al., 2011), laser scanning (Chandra et al., 2005; Reichinger et al., 2013), and photogrammetry (Ross et al., 2018; Sohaib et al., 2018). In this example, the patient was scanned using structured-light-scanning technology. This method uses trigonometric triangulation and works by projecting a pattern of light onto the object of interest. One or more sensors/cameras look at the shape of the light pattern and calculate the distance of every point in the field of view to map the surface of the object being scanned (Fig 5-49). The data retrieved is used to develop three-dimensional images and print casts. There are several advantages to this technique. The working models made from these images are reasonably accurate and enable the recording of the contours of the defect with the head in an upright position. Moreover, this technique avoids distortion of displaceable tissues associated with the use of conventional impression techniques. Furthermore, the scanning time is relatively rapid, a large area can be scanned, and the technique is capable of scanning color.

The data can be manipulated so that a mirror image of the normal ear is created, and this image in turn can be digitally adapted to the defect (Fig 5-50). The image can be easily manipulated to create a prosthesis that is properly oriented and that restores shape, contour, and symmetry. The clinician can manipulate the position, the contours, and the surface texture of the prosthesis on a computer screen using an iPad Pro with a pressure-sensitive touch pad and the appropriate software (Zbrush). The finished sculpting is invested, digitally creating a three-piece mold (Fig 5-51). Each of the segments of the mold is printed, and the prosthesis is processed in a normal

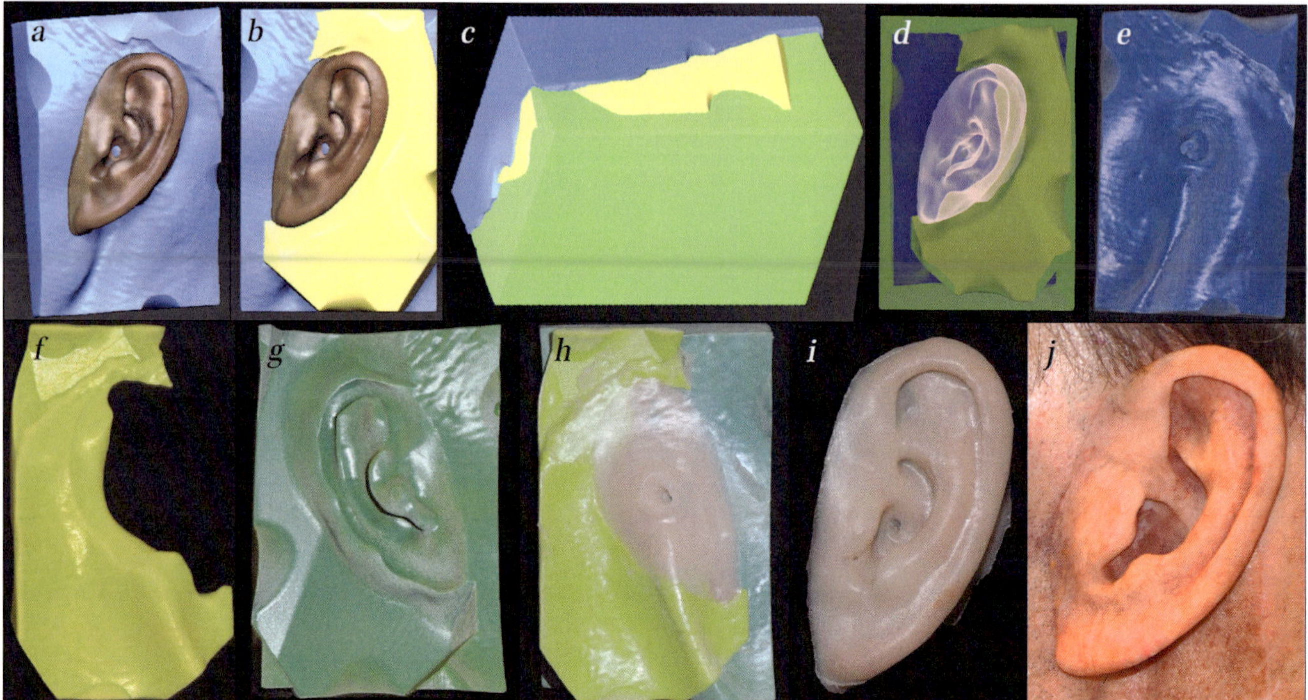

Figure 5-51 Fabricating a prosthesis with CAD/CAM. The mold is created with 3D design software. *(a)* The virtual master cast (depicted in blue) is derived from the digital scan of the patient's defect. The auricular prosthesis is oriented to the virtual master cast based on the digital design (see Fig 5-46). Depressions are added to the virtual master cast to index the subsequent pieces of the mold. *(b)* The second portion of the mold (depicted in yellow) is created by positioning a three-dimensional block engaging the undercut area at the backside of the auricular prosthesis by using the "Boolean Difference" function. This phenomenon subtracts overlapping parts of the auricular prosthesis and virtual master cast from the block, which in turn generates the mold. Note that the margin of the yellow segment of the mold contacting the auricular prosthesis is kept at or slightly below the height of contour of the helix. *(c)* The final piece of the mold (depicted in green) is designed in a similar manner. *(d)* The "Boolean Difference" function allows the operator to visualize an image of the prosthesis within the mold *(e–g)*. The three-part mold is printed with a Polyjet printer. *(h)* The auricular prosthesis is processed via conventional means. *(i)* The polymerized prosthesis is removed from the three-part mold and trimmed. *(j)* The prosthesis is painted, sealed, deglossed, and delivered.

fashion. Following the making of the initial scans of the normal ear and the defect, these steps can be accomplished remotely, including coloration, and may not require the presence of the patient.

Digital technologies have been developed to perform most clinical procedures (Fig 5-51) and to print the prosthesis in silicone (Table 5-13). However, 3D printing of silicone elastomers is still in the development stage, and the clinical outcomes at present cannot match the results achieved with analog techniques. A number of droplet-based additive manufacturing methods have been used (Brunton et al., 2015; Napadensky, 2010; Salmi et al., 2016). However, the current commercially available materials for droplet-based technologies are designed for nonfunctional models and do not meet the mechanical properties, surface finish, and biocompatibility requirements for a facial prosthesis. Moreover, there are limitations to both the strategies and the investigative materials being developed for this application. For example, facial prostheses fabricated using binder-jetting technology, where starch powder is fused together with a water-based binder and subsequently infiltrated with silicone polymer, had mechanical properties and durability limitations because of the starch powder embedded throughout the silicone prosthesis (Zardawi, 2013). Studies using silicone powder-based approaches have had problems with poor resolution (1.54 mm droplet size) as well as challenges with printing simple geometric shapes (Liravi and Vlasea, 2018). Flexible photoreactive polymers, such as urethane acrylate, offer better mechanical

Table 5-13 CAD-CAM processes for facial prostheses

3D scanning of the patient's anatomy (Chandra et al., 2005; Coward et al., 1997, 2000; Ciocca and Scotti, 2004; Ciocca et al., 2007, 2010a, 2010b, 2010c; De Crescenzio et al., 2011; Reiffel et al., 2013; Reichinger et al., 2013; Watson and Hatamleh, 2014; Wu et al., 2008; Feng et al., 2010; Sun et al., 2011, 2013; Rennesson et al., 2012; Zardawi et al., 2015b; Sabol et al., 2011; Ross et al., 2018; Sohaib et al., 2018; Subburaj et al., 2007; Zheng et al., 2009; Liacouras et al., 2011; Qiu et al., 2011; Kang, 2016; Yadav, 2017; Nuseir, 2019; Farook, 2020)
Computer 3D modeling or computer-aided design (CAD; Ciocca and Scotti, 2004; Sun, 2011; Ciocca et al., 2010c; De Crescenzio et al., 2011; Wu et al., 2008; Ciocca et al., 2010a, 2010b, 2010c; Qiu et al., 2011; Fantini et al., 2013; Sun et al., 2013)
Rapid prototyping
• *Direct 3D printing of silicone prosthesis* (Nuseir et al., 2019; Hinton, 2016; Stieghorst, 2016; Muth, 2014; LeBlanc, 2016; Jindal et al., 2016, 2017) • *Polyjet technology* (Doubrovski et al., 2015; Mohammed et al., 2017; Sitthi-Amorn et al., 2015; Alam et al., 2017; Chandra et al., 2005; Nuseir et al., 2019) • *Binder jetting or power printing* (Fereshtenejad et al., 2016; Xiao et al., 2013, 2014; Hoffman et al., 2014; Zardawi, 2015a, 2015b; Berens et al., 2016) • *Fused deposition modeling (FDM) or fused filament freeform* (Ciocca et al., 2007, 2010a, 2010b, 2010c; De Crescenzio et al., 2011; He, 2014; Crump, 1992) • *Selective laser sintering (SLS)* (Yuan et al., 2016; Sabol et al., 2011; Wu et al., 2008; Feng et al., 2010) • *Stereolithography (SLA)* (Hofmann et al., 2014; Qiu et al., 2011; Sabol et al., 2011; Sun et al., 2011; Rodriquez et al., 2021)

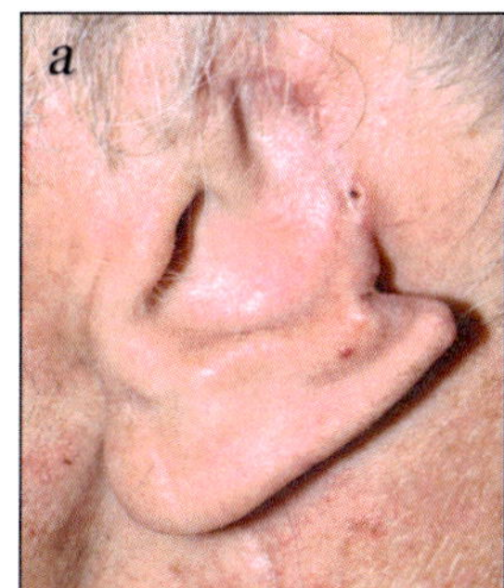

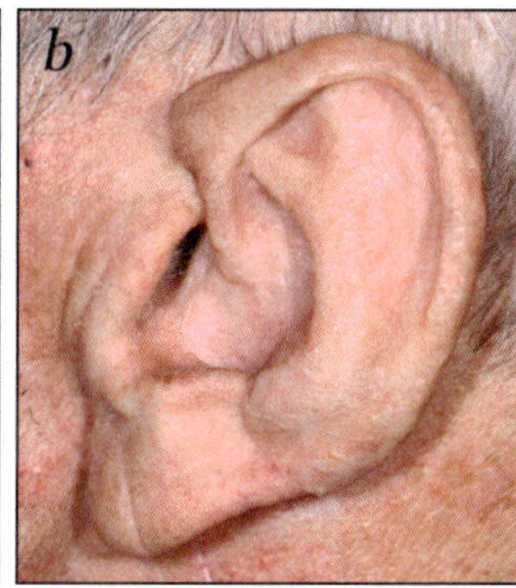

Figure 5-52 Rehabilitation after partial auriculectomy. *(a)* Small defect of the ear. *(b)* The prosthesis engages undercuts behind the ear and in the concha to facilitate the retention provided by skin adhesives. Note the slight sheen of the helix matches that of the residual ear fragment.

properties and wear resistance, but their relatively low elongation at break (Yap et al., 2016) and potential toxicity limit their potential for use as facial prostheses (Walsh et al., 2016). Direct inkjet deposition of silicone resins with high resolution remains a challenge due to the high viscosity of medical-grade silicone, which hinders stable droplet generation from printheads (Liravi and Toyserkani, 2018), which leads to poor layer deposition and a loss of detail. Another study developed UV-curable silicone resins for droplet-on-demand 3D printing with 0.6 mm print resolution (Grunewald, 2015); however, additional work is needed to eliminate the Z-step lines.

In a recent study (Lee et al., 2022), a binder-jetting 3D-printing process with polyvinyl butyral (PVB)–coated silicone powder was developed for direct 3D printing of facial prostheses. Nano-silica-treated silicone powder was spray-dried with PVB by controlling the Ohnesorge number and processing parameters. After printing, the interconnected pores were infused with silicone and hexamethyldisiloxane (HMDS) by pressure-vacuum sequential infiltration to produce the final parts. Particle size, coating composition, surface treatment, and infusion conditions influenced the mechanical properties of the 3D printed preform and of the final infiltrated structure. In addition to demonstrating the feasibility of using silicone powder-based 3D printing for facial prostheses, these results can be used to inform the modifications required to accommodate the manufacturing of other biocompatible elastomeric materials.

Delivery and retention

Additional benefits, besides the obvious cosmetic improvement, are derived from the prosthesis. The prosthesis helps support eyeglass frames and protects the ear canal from wind, dust, and other particulate matter. Hearing will also be improved and, with it, the perception of specific pitches and tones.

Retention is accomplished by means of tissue adhesives or osseointegrated implants. If an adhesive is used, selection is dependent on many factors, including the size of the prosthesis, the quality, stability, and retention of the tissue-bearing areas of the defect, the material of the prosthesis, the functional demands, and the needs of the patient to secure the prosthesis for extended periods without displacement. The clinician must consider all these factors before recommending an adhesive (see section above entitled "Adhesives"). There may be a trial period before the most desirable adhesive is identified.

The skin and prosthesis must be kept meticulously clean. The prosthesis should be removed on a daily basis to keep supporting tissues healthy and to maintain hygiene. All adhesive must be removed from the prosthesis. The prosthesis is soaked in room-temperature water to soften the adhesive and then gently rubbed with gauze or a textured cloth. Any residual adhesive can be removed with warm water.

The prosthesis can be cleaned with a mild soap and rinsed in room temperature water. If some adhesive remains on the tissue, rubbing alcohol can be used. The use of harsh solvents such as benzene or xylene on the tissues and the prosthesis should be avoided. The patient should be informed to report any areas of irritation and should be scheduled for quarterly follow-up.

Partial auriculectomy defects

Partial auriculectomy defects are more difficult to rehabilitate for several reasons: The residual auricular remnant may be displaced, making it difficult to restore facial symmetry (see Fig 5-16b). It also can be challenging to fabricate impressions without distorting the ear remnant. In addition, the lines of juncture between the skin and the prosthesis are more clearly visible. In addition, color matching between the prosthesis and the adjacent residual ear remnant is much more challenging than is the case for a total auriculectomy defect.

With small defects, there may be insufficient surface area on the tissue side of the prosthesis to achieve suitable retention. In these defects, the prosthesis must engage soft tissue anatomical undercuts to facilitate the retention provided by adhesives. However, in spite of all these difficulties, acceptable cosmetic results can be attained if the residual ear remnant has not been unduly displaced (Fig 5-52; see also Fig 5-34).

Restoration of Nasal Defects

The vast majority of nasal defects are secondary to treatment of neoplasms, although occasionally patients present with defects secondary to burns and trauma. In general, most small partial nasal defects are best rehabilitated surgically (see Fig 5-6), whereas total nasal defects are best rehabilitated with a prosthesis. The wishes of the patient, however, are paramount and must be carefully considered before the method of rehabilitation is selected.

Irrespective of whether the defect is going to be permanently or temporarily rehabilitated with a prosthesis, presurgical consultation with both the patient and the surgeon is necessary. For partial rhinectomy defects, even if the surgeon is planning a surgical reconstruction, he/she may wish to have the defect temporarily restored with a prosthesis (Fig 5-53) and embark upon surgical reconstruction

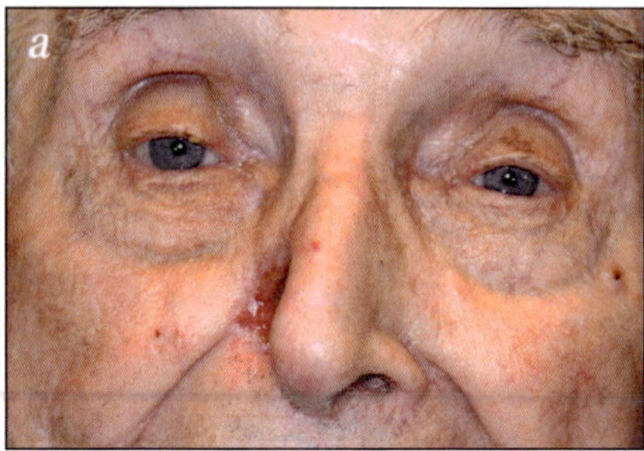

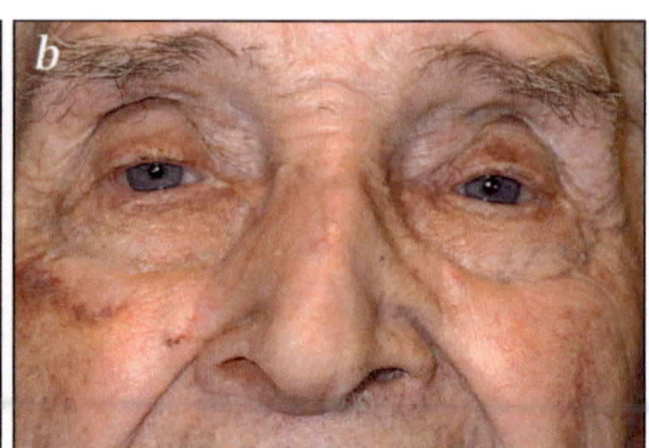

Figure 5-53 The right ala was removed. Note however that the position and contours associated with the nasolabial fold are relatively normal, allowing the alar prosthesis to blend in effectively. This defect could also be surgically reconstructed.

only after a suitable observation period has elapsed and the patient is shown to be free of tumor. These observation periods are especially important for advanced and/or recurrent basal cell carcinomas of the midfacial region, because these tumors frequently are locally invasive and infiltrative. Covering the defect with a local flap may significantly delay the discovery of recurrent tumors and ultimately result in greater tissue loss.

The patient should be informed of the benefits and limitations of the prosthesis. Photographs of patients with similar nasal defects are valuable educational aids. Some patients will benefit from a conversation with a rhinectomy patient who is wearing a nasal prosthesis. It is important that the expectations of the patient be realistic. Family members are encouraged to be present during these consultations. Psychosocial evaluations and consultations should be provided prior to the resection.

Prior to surgery, facial impressions, photographs, and scans (if the instrumentation is available) should be obtained. Facial impressions or scans are desired because they provide useful information for the clinician to fabricate the postsurgical nasal prosthesis. Before the impression is obtained, undesirable tissue undercuts should be blocked out with moist or petrolatum-covered gauze.

Temporary nasal prostheses

The prosthodontist is only occasionally called upon to correct small nasal defects. Most small defects are reconstructed surgically (see Fig 5-6). A variety of local flaps, skin, and composite auricular grafts is used to cover and repair smaller alar defects. Reconstruction of full-thickness alar defects requires the replacement of mucosal lining, cartilaginous support, and external skin coverage. As mentioned above, the disease must be controlled before reconstruction begins.

Approximately four to six weeks following surgery, the wound has usually healed sufficiently to allow placement of a temporary nasal prosthesis. While an eye patch or a longer hairstyle can camouflage an orbital or auricular defect, loss of facial profile as the result of a rhinectomy is more difficult to hide. Because a rhinectomy creates the most obvious loss of facial contour, early rehabilitation of the nasal defect is appreciated by some patients; it enables them to resume social interactions and to return to work.

Heat-polymerizing methyl methacrylate is the material preferred by some clinicians because it can be relined with a temporary denture reliner to compensate for tissue changes secondary to scar contracture and wound organization (see Fig 5-8a). A silicone elastomer may also be employed. Retention of the prosthesis is accomplished with a medical-grade skin adhesive. Prior to or in place of a temporary nasal prosthesis, a nasal conformer may be used to restore facial contour and profile. As was the case for auricular defects, four to five months is sufficient time to account for contraction and organization of the tissue bed before fabrication of the definitive prosthesis is begun.

Definitive nasal prostheses

The effectiveness of the nasal prosthesis is dependent on the nature and extent of the defect. Defects in which the lip and cheek contours are relatively normal and the nasolabial folds remain undisturbed are the easiest to rehabilitate prosthetically (Fig 5-54).

Defects with surgical margins that extend beyond the nasal area are less effective, especially those that extend to include the upper lip, and are more difficult to restore. In these patients, the upper lip is foreshortened and often displaced superiorly and posteriorly, especially if the raw tissues in this region have not been lined with a skin graft (see Fig 5-22). The angle formed between the columella of the prosthesis and the lip will be excessively acute (Fig 5-55). These two factors bring attention to the prosthesis and the defect. When the resection extends laterally onto the cheeks, the postsurgical cheek contours frequently are deficient. It is usually not appropriate to attempt to restore these contours with the prosthesis, and as a result, the prosthesis must be smaller and positioned more posteriorly than the presurgical facial configuration (see Fig 5-23). Furthermore, in such defects, the lines of juncture between the skin and the prosthesis are more exposed and may not be easily camouflaged with eyeglass frames. In males, margins that extend to the upper lip may be camouflaged by a mustache (Fig 5-56).

In most patients, the tissues bordering the lower portion of the defect are highly mobile. It is difficult to account for this mobility with impression procedures. Therefore, the prosthesis should be designed to be as flexible as possible in this region. Flexibility is enhanced if the columella portion is not connected to the base of the ala (Fig 5-57).

Impressions

Postural changes may result in distortions of the tissue bed. Therefore, it is advisable to obtain the master impression while the patient is in a relatively upright position (Fig 5-58). Elastic impression materials that possess good flow properties are suitable for this task. We prefer to use a light-bodied polysulfide material. Irreversible

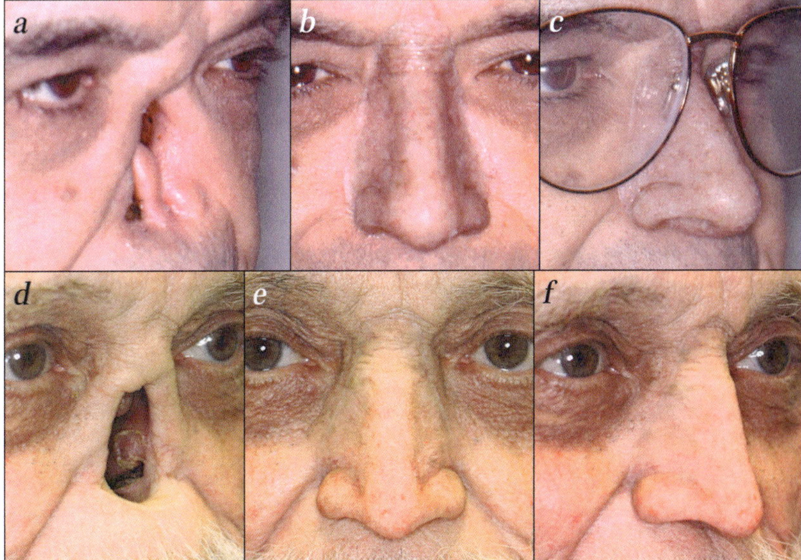

Figure 5-54 *(a to f)* Two total rhinectomy defects that are ideally suited esthetically for a prosthesis. However, note that the defect depicted in "a" retains the nasal septum whereas the defect in "d" does not. Retention of the prosthesis shown in b and c will therefore be somewhat compromised as a result.

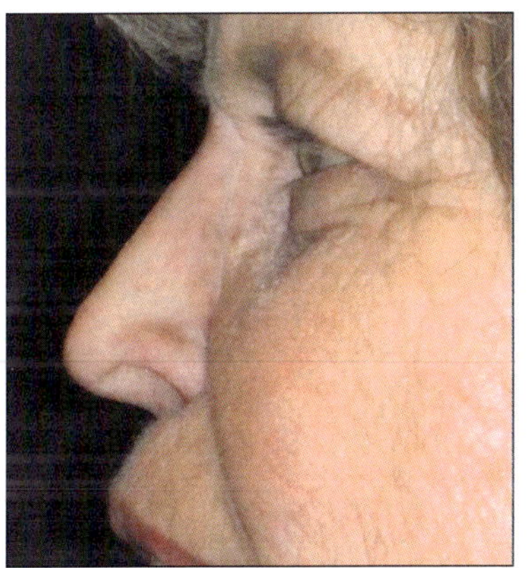

Figure 5-55 The patient depicted in Fig 5-22. Following surgery, the lip was retracted posteriorly and superiorly, making the angle between the columella and the lip excessively acute.

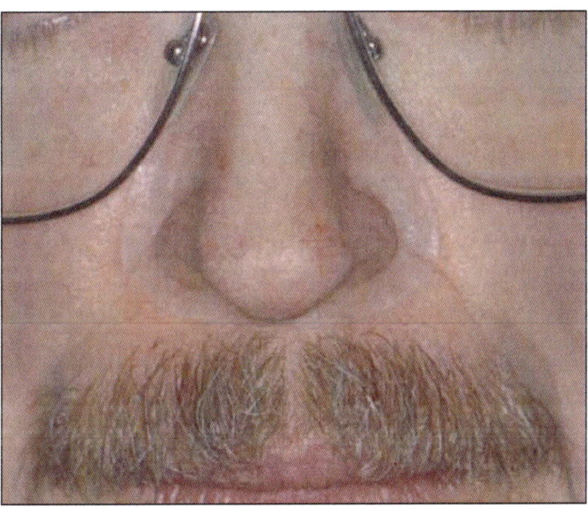

Figure 5-56 Defect that extends laterally and onto the upper lip. The mustache helps camouflage the lip margin.

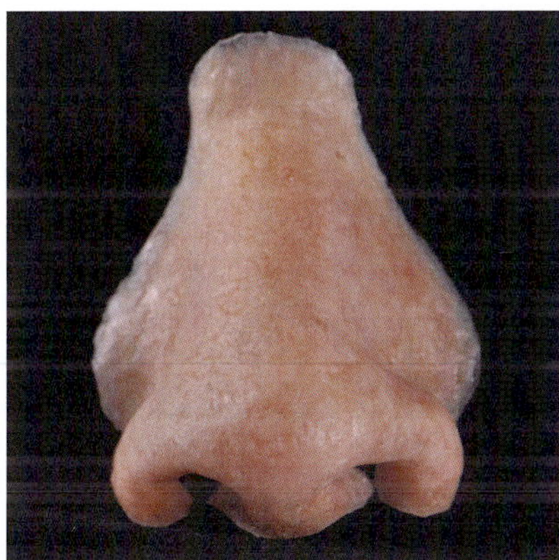

Figure 5-57 Flexibility will be enhanced if the columella portion and the base of the ala are not connected.

hydrocolloid with additional water added to the mix or a light or medium-bodied polyvinyl siloxane work equally well.

The nasal passage should be blocked with lubricated gauze to prevent entry of impression material. A syringe is used to inject impression material into skin creases, areas of difficult access, usable undercut areas, the defect, and the adjacent skin. The impression material is thinned out by a cement mixing spatula in order to prevent the weight of the material from displacing tissues associated with the defect and the adjacent skin.

Small gauze segments or wisps of cotton are embedded within the impression material as it begins to polymerize. A thin layer of adhesive is then applied to the gauze and impression material; this is followed by placement of succeeding layers of fast-setting impression plaster. The first two layers should be kept as thin as possible to avoid distortion of the thin underlying layer of impression material. The impression is removed and poured in an improved dental stone (Fig 5-58).

The defect can also be scanned and a cast printed. This allows the clinician to record the contours of the defect with the patient in an upright position and avoids compression of the easily displaced soft tissues adjacent to the defect (Fig 5-59). A number of different scanning technologies have evolved, including light scanning (Wu et al., 2008; Feng et al., 2010; Sun et al., 2011), 3D photography (Liacourad et al., 2011; Sabol et al., 2011), laser scanning (Chandra et al., 2005; Reichinger et al., 2013), and photogrammetry (Ross et al., 2018; Sohaib et al., 2018).

Sculpting

A sculpture of the proposed prosthesis can be developed digitally or with analog techniques. The clinician can use a scan obtained prior to surgical resection, adapt this image to the defect, and sculpt the image appropriately. The clinician can also choose a suitable image from a facial anatomy library and adapt it to the defect (Ciocca and Scotti, 2004; Ciocca, 2010a, 2010b, 2010c; Sun, 2011; De Crescenzio, 2011; Wu, 2008; Qiu, 2011; Fantini, 2013; Sun, 2013). Once the sculpted image is completed, a digital mold is created, and the prosthesis is processed (see section above entitled "Use of digital technology").

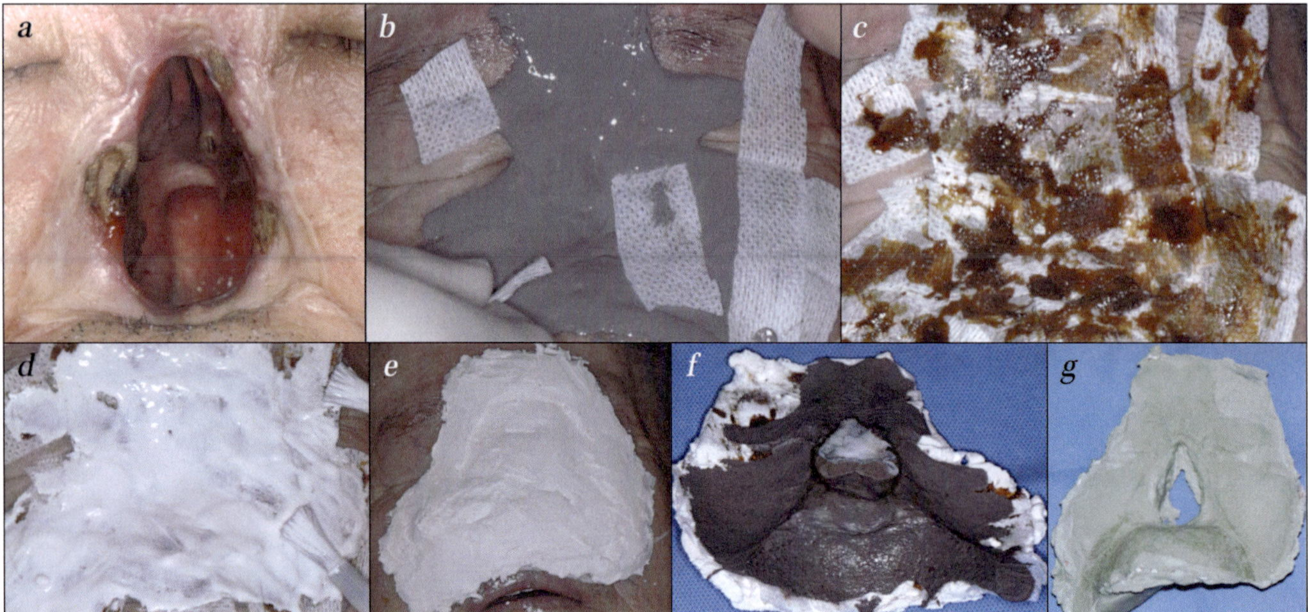

Figure 5-58 Impression procedures for a nasal prosthesis. *(a)* Nasal defect. *(b)* A thin layer of polysulfide impression material is applied. *(c)* A layer of gauze is applied. *(d)* A thin layer of quick-setting plaster is placed and followed by *(e)* placement of succeeding layers. *(f)* Completed impression. *(g)* Master cast.

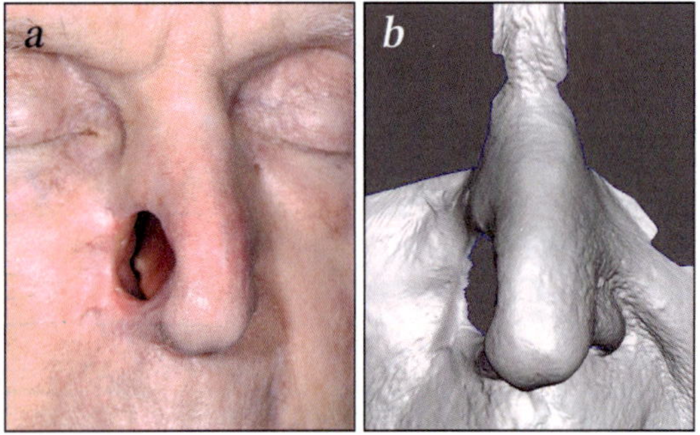

Figure 5-59 *(a and b)* Digital impressions allow for recording the contours of the defect with the patient in an upright position.

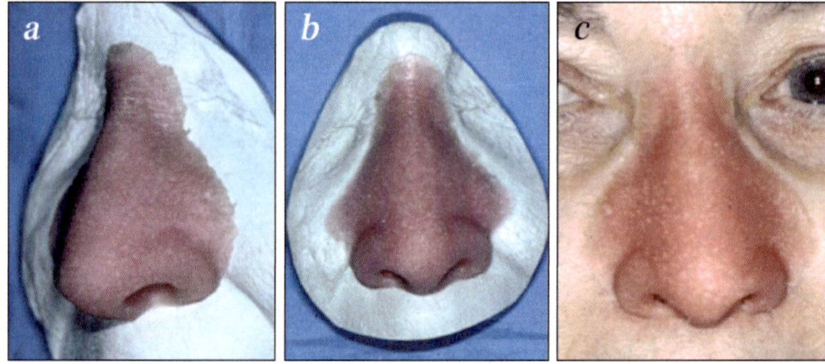

Figure 5-60 Sculpting of the nasal prosthesis. *(a)* The alar groove should be continuous with the nasolabial fold. *(b)* The alae should be tucked underneath so the prosthesis will cast a shadow on the line of juncture. Note the symmetric nasal apertures and the contour of the columella. *(c)* The wax sculpture in position. Lateral margins must blend with the contours of the cheek and be placed beneath eyeglass frames if possible.

Another approach is to use the data from the sculpted image to print a wax pattern. The pattern is then refined in the usual way and processed. The authors still prefer to use analog techniques because they remain the most cost and time effective, and superior clinical outcomes can be achieved. As mentioned above, 3D printing of silicone elastomers is still under development, and the clinical outcomes at present cannot match the results achieved with analog techniques.

To be effective, the nasal prosthesis must reproduce the contour and texture of the resected nose and be consistent with existing facial contours. These two factors may be in conflict when there is significant alteration of adjacent facial structures (see Figs 5-23 and 5-30). Another important factor is the placement and camouflage of the lines of juncture. In an ideal total rhinectomy defect, only small portions of the lines of juncture are apparent if they are positioned properly and the nasal prosthesis is properly sculpted.

If a presurgical facial cast has been fabricated, a wax duplicate of the nasal portion is adapted to the cast of the postsurgical defect. A donor cast may also be used to obtain a pattern to begin wax adaptation. If presurgical casts are not available, a mass of wax is adapted to the cast of the defect and basic contours are completed. The patient will usually have numerous facial photographs available for reference. It is always helpful to have a family member present during sculpting, because such a person may have a better perception of appropriate contours than does the patient.

The alae should be located in their appropriate position in relationship to the nasolabial folds (Fig 5-60). The lateral projection of the alae can be tucked into the nasolabial fold to make these margins inconspicuous. Care should be taken not to make the nose too wide in the alar region. Usually, this distance is no greater than the medial inner canthus distance. If possible, the nares should be symmetric and consistent with presurgical contours. However, their contours can only be made appropriate if the columella is contoured accurately.

For most patients, it is desirable to position the margin between the lip and the columella above the tip of the nose to hide this

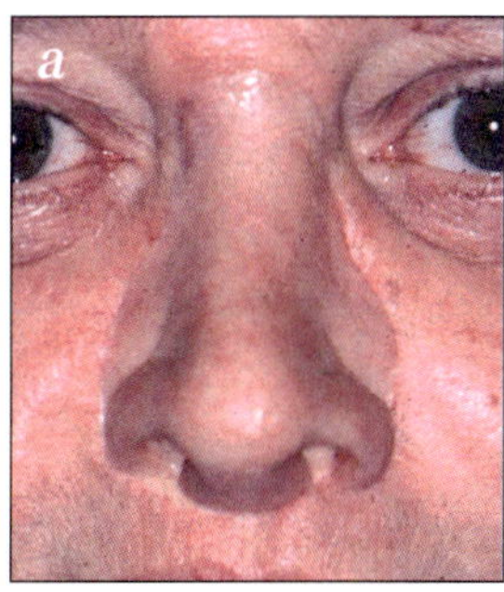
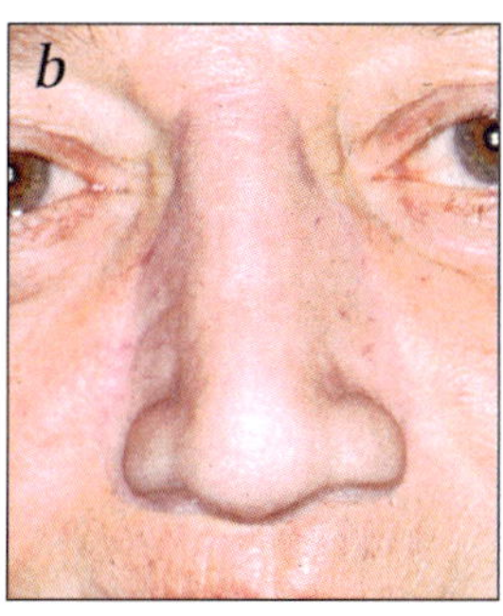

Figure 5-61 Proper contour and positioning of the columella. *(a)* The columella is improperly contoured and the margin between the columella and the lip is visible. *(b)* The columella contours are corrected and the margin is repositioned in the new prosthesis.

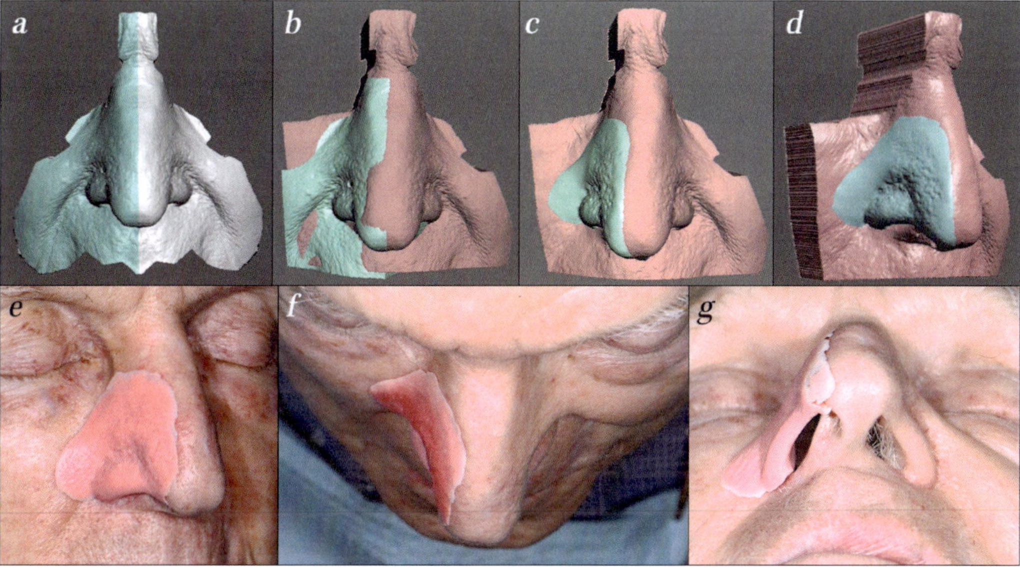

Figure 5-62 *(a, b, c, and d)* CAD is used to develop a tentative sculpting of the partial nasal prosthesis. The data encompassing the normal side and the surrounding tissues are "separated" and manipulated creating a mirror image of the normal side. The mirror image of the normal side is superimposed upon the defect and positioned and oriented to achieve a semblance of bilateral symmetry. *(e, f, and g)* The printed wax pattern in position.

margin. The juncture between columella and skin should be at a right angle or a slight acute angle. This line of juncture positioned accordingly is usually difficult to detect because of the shadow cast by the tip of the nose. The nostril portion should not be connected to the columella portion. Otherwise, the flexibility of this portion of the prosthesis will be impaired (see Fig 5-57).

In an ideal defect where the adjacent cheek and lip are of normal contour, the tip, dorsum, and bridge of the nose should be similar to presurgical contours. When midfacial contours are deficient and the upper lip is retracted superiorly and has abnormal contour where the base of the nasal prosthesis will be positioned (see Fig 5-23), it is advisable to reduce the size and anterior projection of the prosthesis. Abnormal lip contours may also have to be taken into account when the size, position, and contour of the ala are developed. Under these circumstances, a nose of perfect symmetry and equivalent to the size of the patient's original structure will be aesthetically displeasing and actually bring unwanted attention to the deformity. Care must be taken not to make the bridge too wide. Presurgical photos or casts or can be used to verify this dimension.

If eyeglass frames are worn, they improve the appearance of the prosthesis immeasurably. If possible, the lateral and superior margins of the prosthesis should be placed directly beneath the eyeglass frames. In prostheses in which lines of juncture are properly positioned, only the margins from the bottom of the eyeglass frame to the point where the alae insert into the nasolabial groove will be exposed. Care should be taken to feather this margin and develop the lateral contours of the prosthesis so that there is a smooth transition between the surface of the prosthesis and adjacent cheek contours. These lateral contours of the prosthesis are especially significant if the margin of the defect extends far beyond the eyeglass frame. In males, the presence of a moustache will camouflage the margin of the prosthesis that rests on the lip (see Fig 5-56).

When sculpting, the clinician should take into consideration the facial form of the patient, recognizing the wide variability of sizes and shapes encountered. The sculpting should be viewed from all views and must look like it belongs on the patient. Special attention should be paid to the contour and position of the columella. In most patients the columella should not be visible from the anterior projection, and this margin should be hidden behind the tip of the nose. Otherwise, the prosthesis will assume an unsightly appearance (Fig 5-61a).

Development of proper surface texture is important. The texture developed in the sculpture should be slightly more prominent than that of the adjacent skin, because some of this detail is lost during processing and painting. Stippling is usually most prominent on the tip and nostrils and must be particularly prominent in elderly patients.

Computer-aided design software can be used to develop the final sculpting. This method is particularly useful when restoring unilateral defects such as an auriculectomy (see Fig 5-50) or a partial rhinectomy where the intent is to restore perfect bilateral symmetry (Fig 5-62). The data can be manipulated such that a

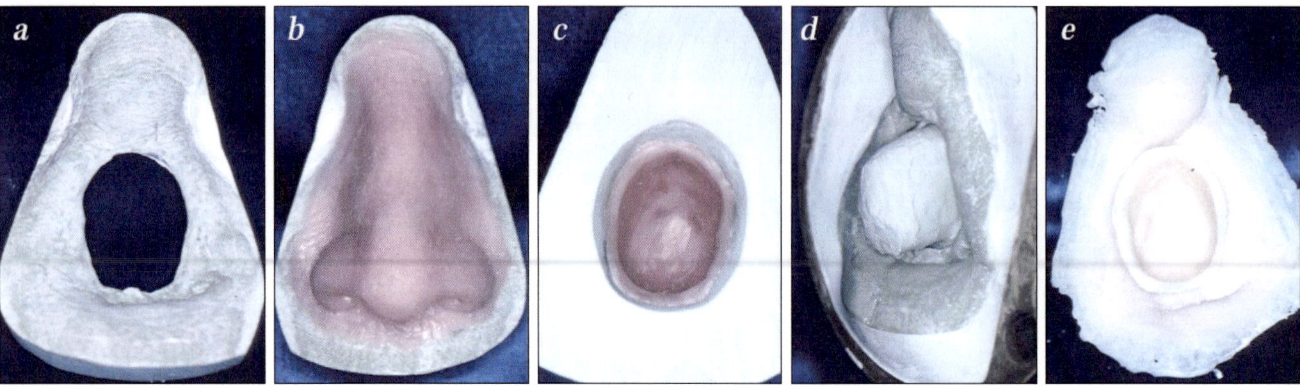

Figure 5-63 Flasking and processing of the nasal prosthesis. *(a)* A hole is placed through the master cast. *(b and c)* The wax sculpture is luted to the cast externally and from the back. *(d)* Stone is vibrated through the opening in the back of the cast. *(e)* The polymerized casting is thin and light weight.

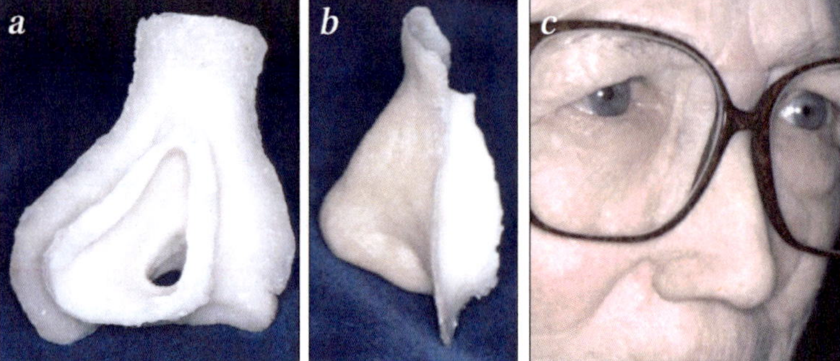

Figure 5-64 Retention of the nasal prosthesis. *(a and b)* Retention is achieved by engagement of undercuts in the nasal cavity. The posterior portion of the prosthesis is hollow to reduce weight and improve flexibility. *(c)* Adhesive is not necessary to maintain the prosthesis in position.

mirror image of the normal unresected side of the nose is created, and this image in turn can be digitally adapted to the defect (Fig 5-62a–d). The image can be easily manipulated to create a sculpting that is properly oriented and that restores shape, contour, and symmetry. The clinician can manipulate the position, the contours, and the surface texture of the sculpting on a computer screen using an iPad Pro with a pressure-sensitive touch pad and the appropriate software (Zbrush). The digital sculpting can be used to develop a virtual mold that when printed is used to process a silicone casting of the sculpting (see Fig 5-51). The digital sculpting can also be printed, tried on the patient, and altered as necessary (Fig 5-62e–g). A silicone casting of the prosthesis can then be obtained by using either conventional analog (see the section below entitled "Conventional processing") or digital techniques (see section above entitled "Use of digital technology"; Fig 5-51). This approach can also be used with total rhinectomy defects when a scan is made of the nose prior to surgical resection.

Conventional processing

The wax pattern is invested with appropriate mold material. Two-piece molds are adequate. The wax pattern should be thinned internally to reduce weight as well as to allow normal nasal airflow. A hole is placed through the master cast in the middle of the defect area, and the wax pattern is luted in position; care must be taken to extend the prosthesis onto the nasal floor and into desirable undercuts, particularly if adhesives are used for retention (Fig 5-63a–c). Stone is then poured through the hole in back of the cast to fill the air space behind the wax pattern (Fig 5-63d). When the prosthesis is processed it will be thin, flexible, and lightweight (Fig 5-63e).

The base shade of the prosthesis should closely match the lightest area of coloration in the local area. If the base shade is too dark it will not be possible to achieve an aesthetic match because as more extrinsic coloration is added, the prosthesis becomes progressively darker. Extrinsic colorations should be applied while the patient is present and under adequate lighting. Evaluation of coloration under varied light sources is also suggested. Alternatively, an intrinsic coloring technique, performed as described for auricular prostheses, may be used. However, even when the intrinsic coloring technique is used, some extrinsic coloring is usually necessary.

Delivery and retention

Retention is achieved with adhesives, engagement of undercuts (Fig 5-64), or osseointegrated implants. If adhesives are used, the patient should be warned to avoid adhesive buildup on either the skin or the prosthesis. After the initial adjustment period, the patient is placed on a follow-up schedule consistent with the life of the prosthesis. The completed prostheses in Fig 5-65 reflect the variety of facial contours encountered.

Partial nasal prostheses

Definitive partial prostheses are fabricated in the same fashion as total nasal prostheses. If the remaining portions of the nose are not displaced or distorted, acceptable aesthetic results can be attained

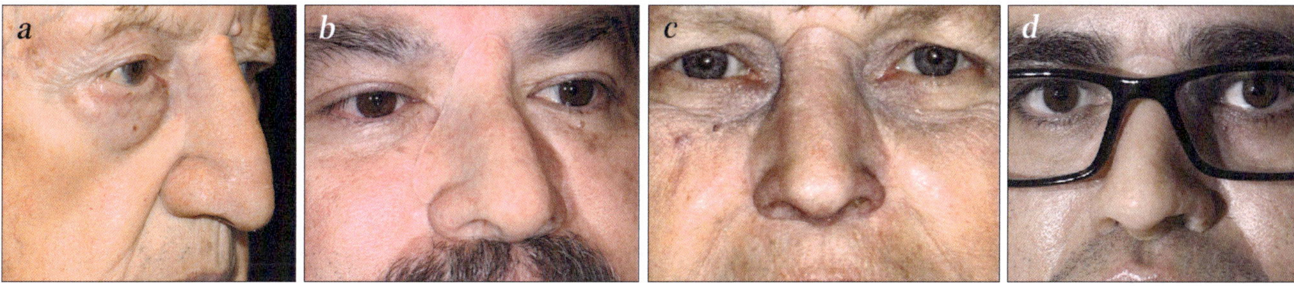

Figure 5-65 Completed nasal prostheses in a variety of sizes and shapes. *(a, b, and c)* The lateral and superior margins are exposed, but *(d)* eyeglass frames will hide these margins.

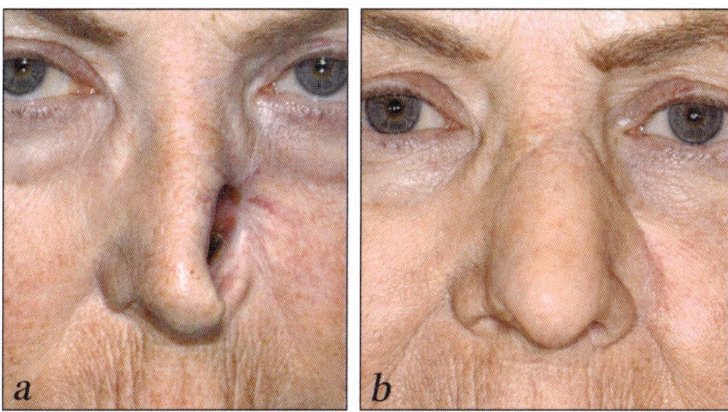

Figure 5-66 *(a)* A partial nasal defect involving the ala but short of the midline. The remaining portion of the nose has been unaffected by the resection. *(b)* The partial nasal prosthesis. Note the margin has been extended across the midline and ends on the lateral slope of the nose.

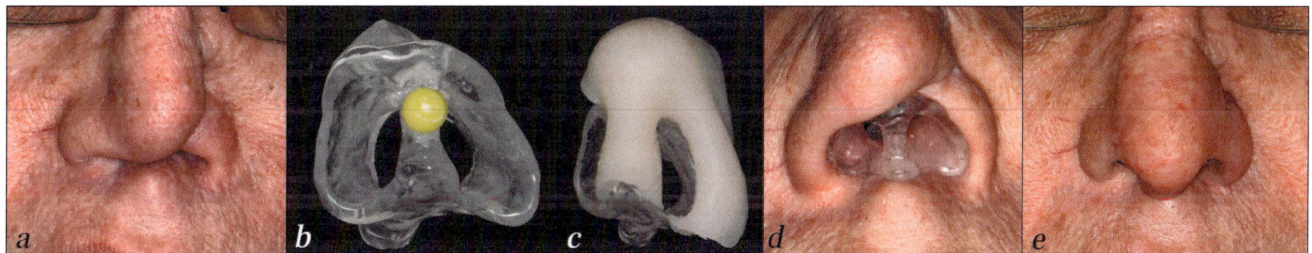

Figure 5-67 *(a)* Following resection of the columella and a portion of the ala, the nasal airway was compromised. *(b)* Nasal stent to open the airway. *(c)* Unpainted silicone prosthesis is designed to interface with the nasal stent. *(d)* The nasal stent position. *(e)* The partial nasal prosthesis in position.

(Figs 5-66 and 5-67; see also Fig 5-53). However, more of the lines of juncture between prosthesis and adjacent tissues will be exposed, because they do not fall beneath eyeglass frames. These margins should be carefully contoured, feathered, and colored to achieve an acceptable result. For defects that approach the midline, it is advisable to position margins on the lateral wall of the nose as opposed to the midline (Fig 5-66b). This practice will render this margin less apparent and will increase the surface area for the adhesive.

Sometimes, a partial resection of the alar region will result in the collapse of the nasal airway. Under these circumstances, a clear stent of acrylic resin can be fabricated and designed to increase the size of the nasal airway. The partial nasal prosthesis is then designed to engage the stent and restore the alar defect (Fig 5-67).

Nasal defects that extend onto the cheek and lip

On occasion, the resection will extend laterally onto the cheek or inferiorly to involve portions of the upper lip. These defects are difficult to camouflage with a prosthesis because of the movement of the adjacent tissues through activation of the facial musculature during changes in facial expression, speaking, and so on. Because these prostheses are larger and of greater mass, and especially because they engage moveable tissues, retention is frequently a major concern. Such defects should be carefully prepared during the surgical ablation so as to minimize the distortion of adjacent tissues. In addition, all potential undercuts and areas of the defect that can be engaged should be lined with split-thickness skin grafts. These areas can then be aggressively engaged by the prosthesis and will facilitate its retention and stability. If the resection involves significant portions of the upper lip, frequently the facial defect created extends to involve the oral cavity. As a result, the residual dentition can be used to retain both the RDP-obturator prosthesis and the facial prosthesis (Fig 5-68). Implants are obviously advantageous as well, and the most common sites employed are the floor of the nose and the zygoma (see section below entitled "Craniofacial Implants"). Nevertheless, in spite of these difficulties, effective facial prostheses can be fabricated for patients with such defects.

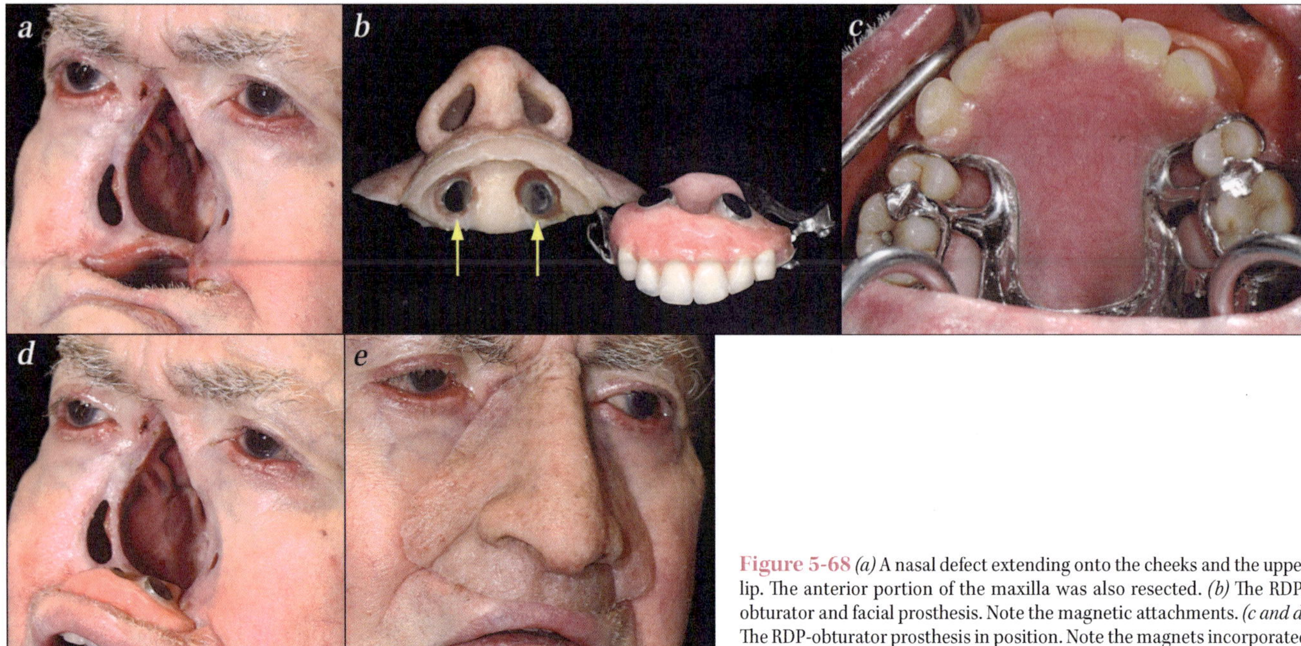

Figure 5-68 *(a)* A nasal defect extending onto the cheeks and the upper lip. The anterior portion of the maxilla was also resected. *(b)* The RDP-obturator and facial prosthesis. Note the magnetic attachments. *(c and d)* The RDP-obturator prosthesis in position. Note the magnets incorporated within each prosthesis *(arrows)*. *(e)* The facial prosthesis in position.

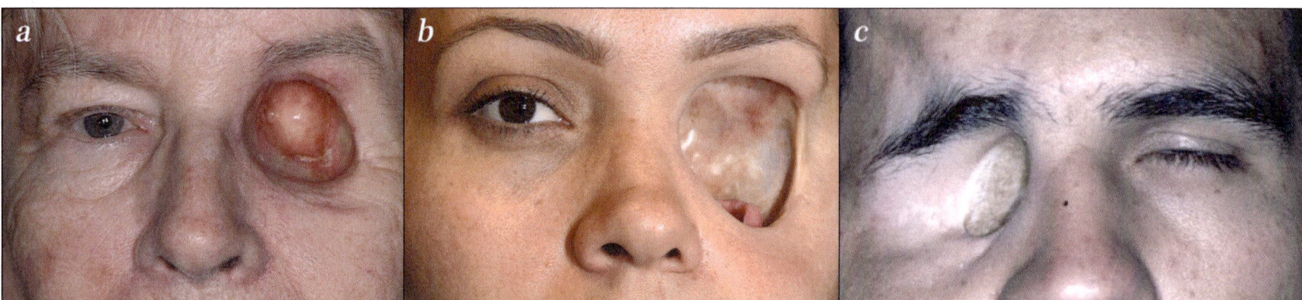

Figure 5-69 *(a)* Resections confined to the orbital contents are the easiest to rehabilitate because the contours of adjacent tissues are undisturbed. *(b and c)* Unfavorable orbital defects. *(b)* In this orbital defect combined with total maxillectomy, tissues of the middle third of the face lack support, creating significant midfacial asymmetry. The obturator prosthesis provides support and restores most but not all, contours. *(c)* In this patient the resection extended beyond the orbital area, distorting the brow and extending to mobile tissues laterally and inferiorly.

Restoration of Orbital Defects

Fabrication of orbital prostheses that are aesthetic is a difficult challenge. Because conversation with others is often initiated with eye contact, slight discrepancies in the position of the eye, lid contour, or color of the prosthesis are immediately noticed by the observer. For some patients, it may not be possible to duplicate the appearance and contour of the remaining normal eye and adjacent orbital structures. For such patients with orbital defects in particular, a simple patch is recommended because an unesthetic prosthesis brings attention to the defect and creates more psychologic trauma than no prosthesis at all.

Preoperative consultation is valuable for informing the patient of the nature of the defect and the choices available for rehabilitation. Many patients are under the impression that the prosthesis will move and function in concert with the remaining eye. Photographs of prostheses to rehabilitate similar defects are helpful in eliminating this misconception. For most patients it is not necessary to obtain preoperative photographs or impressions, because they are of little value in fabricating the postsurgical prosthesis.

Surgical resection of orbital tumors is dependent on the nature and extent of the tumor. Resections that are confined to removal of the orbital contents result in defects that are easier to rehabilitate (Fig 5-69a). As the surgical margins extend beyond the confines of the orbit, prostheses are less effective because of the inability to camouflage the lines of juncture between skin and prosthesis. Additionally, as the prosthesis extends beyond the orbit, movable tissue beds may be encountered, resulting in further exposure of the lines of juncture (Fig 5-69b and c). Those associated with a maxillectomy are likewise challenging because the contours of the midfacial area may be altered significantly (Fig 5-69b; see also Fig 5-32).

Impressions

Accurate impressions of orbital defects are difficult to obtain because the periorbital tissues are easily displaced. It is particularly

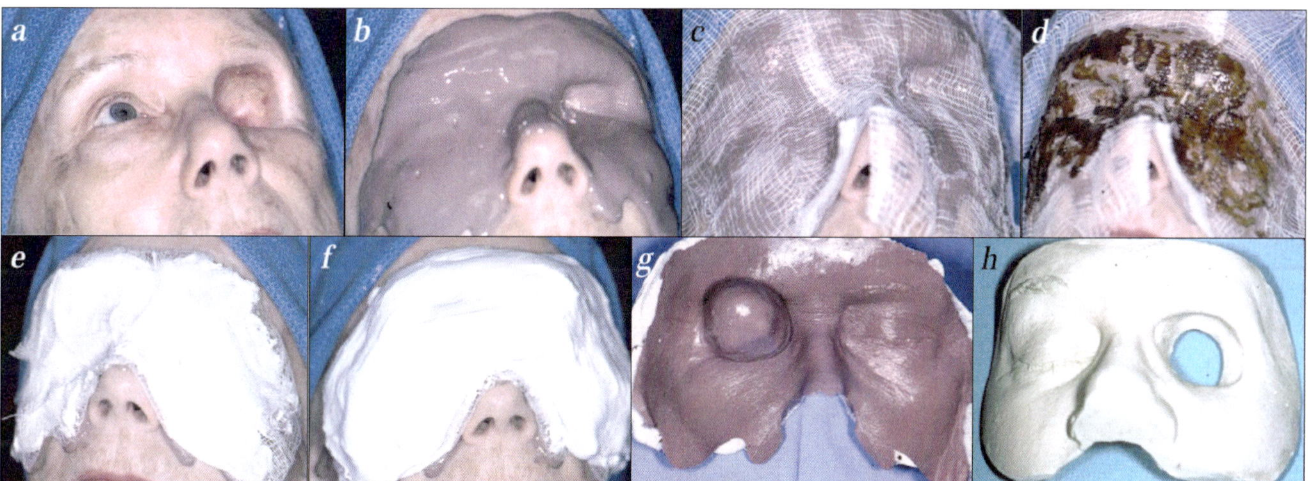

Figure 5-70 Facial impression procedures for an orbital prosthesis. *(a)* The field is isolated. *(b)* A thin layer of impression material is applied. *(c)* A layer of gauze is applied. *(d)* A layer of adhesive is placed. *(e and f)* Several layers of impression plaster are applied to support the impression material. The first layer is kept thin to avoid distortion of the impression. *(g)* Completed impression. *(h)* Master cast. Note the hole through the back of the cast. This will facilitate positioning the ocular within the wax sculpting.

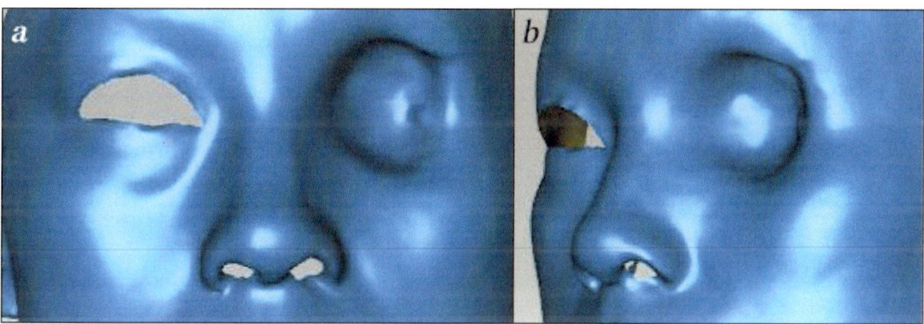

Figure 5-71 3D images from phase-measuring profilometry data (courtesy of Dr. Yi-min Zhao).

challenging to avoid tissue displacement when patients have had a total maxillectomy in conjunction with an orbital exenteration, because the zygoma is included in the resection and as a result the cheek area is no longer supported by bone. For these patients, the definitive obturator must be fabricated, appropriately contoured, and properly positioned and adjusted before impressions of the orbital area can be made.

The purpose of the facial impression is to record the orbital and periorbital tissue beds as accurately as possible. The patient must be in a semiupright position, and extreme care must be taken not to displace the periorbital tissues. Before the impression is obtained, undesirable undercut areas should be blocked out with lubricated gauze. A skin-marking pen may be used to mark the midpupillary locations.

The field is isolated, and a thin layer of light-bodied elastic impression material is applied to the defect and adjacent tissues (Fig 5-70a and b). Gauze strips are then embedded within the material, and a thin layer of adhesive is applied (Fig 5-70c and d). Several thin layers of fast-setting impression plaster are applied until sufficient support has been provided (Fig 5-70e and f). *During the procedure the patient should close the remaining eye in a relaxed manner.* This will prevent undesirable contraction of residual lid musculature on the defect side and prevent distortion of the defect. The impression is removed (Fig 5-70g). A cast is fabricated in dental stone. A hole should be drilled through the posterior orbital wall to facilitate movement and adjustment of the ocular portion of the prosthesis while positioning the globe within the wax pattern (Fig 5-70h).

As mentioned above, digital impressions overcome many of these difficulties (Fig 5-71). The working casts printed from the data from these methods are accurate, enable the recording of the contours of the defect while the patient's head is in an upright position, and avoid the distortion of displaceable tissues associated with the use of conventional impression techniques.

Sculpting

A stock ocular prosthesis that closely approximates the color and size of the iris and sclera of the remaining eye is selected. Alternatively, a custom ocular prosthesis may be fabricated. The spherical contours of the ocular prosthesis should also closely match that of the normal eye. Otherwise, it will be difficult to reproduce the proper surface area of the sclera in the final prosthesis. Usually, the ocular prosthesis must be reduced superiorly so that it will fit easily into the orbital defect in the appropriate position. An orientation arrow is ground into the back side of the stock eye to aid the technician during processing. Techniques currently under development will enable digital fabrication of the ocular portion of these prostheses with the aid of a photo of the opposite eye.

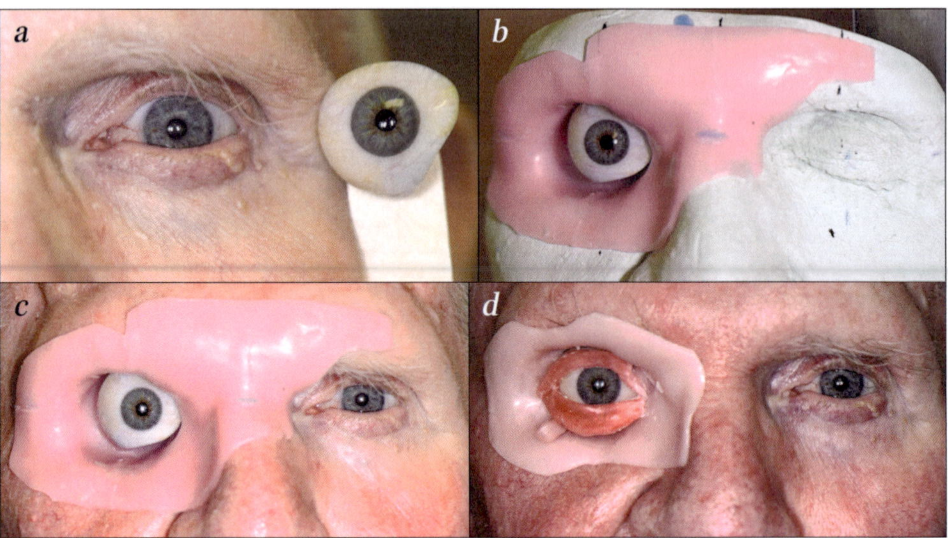

Figure 5-72 Sculpting of the orbital prosthesis. *(a)* A stock eye is reduced in size to fit within the confines of the cast. An arrow is carved on the posterior surface. *(b)* The ocular is positioned in wax on the master cast with the aid of the indelible pencil marking picked up during the impression. The wax pattern will be more stable if at this stage it is extended to cover a portion of the forehead and cheek. These portions will be removed during the development of the final contours and extensions of the prosthesis. *(c)* The wax carrier is tried on the patient and the position of the ocular is adjusted as necessary on the patient. *(d)* Assessing position is made easier by developing the initial lid contours.

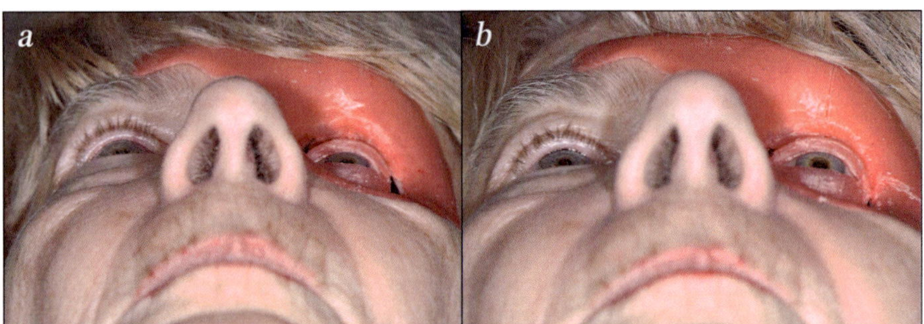

Figure 5-73 The depth of the ocular prosthesis can be checked by viewing its position inferiorly. *(a)* Initially the ocular portion was positioned too deeply in the orbital defect. *(b)* It was brought slightly forward to bring it into better symmetry with the normal eye.

Wax is used as the sculpting medium by most clinicians. The ocular prosthesis is positioned in the wax (Fig 5-72) and the entire apparatus is transferred to the patient. Skin markings to indicate the location of the pupil have been transferred to the cast and can be used to initially orient the position of the ocular portion. The patient should be standing or sitting upright in a relaxed position with the remaining eye focused on a distant point directly forward.

A colleague holds the prosthesis in place with a small dental instrument, the patient is directed to look directly forward, and the clinician evaluates ocular positioning. A reference mark is placed at the midline and either a tongue blade or a ruler can be used to verify the mediolateral position. The pupils are used as reference points in this evaluation. A flashlight can be used to evaluate the proper gaze. When the gaze is correct, the light reflected from this light source will be centered on the pupil of the ocular portion when the patient is looking directly forward with the normal eye (Fig 5-72d). For patients with orbital exenteration defects that do not affect the contours of the orbital rims or adjacent cheek, the mediolateral, anterior-posterior, and superior-inferior positioning of the ocular prosthesis should mimic the position of the normal eye if a successful prosthesis is to be fabricated. Discrepancies in gaze and in superior-inferior position must be avoided. The anterior-posterior (depth) of the ocular is carefully scrutinized. For most patients, particularly those who also have had a total maxillectomy, a better aesthetic result will be achieved if the ocular prosthesis is positioned slightly medial and posterior in relation to the position of the eye occupied prior to surgery (Fig 5-73). Otherwise, the prosthetic eye may appear proptotic. Before accepting what appears to be an appropriate ocular position, the clinician should ask local observers to verify the positioning.

At the next appointment, sculpting of the periorbital tissues is completed (Fig 5-74). To ensure that the normal eye has appropriate eyelid contour, the sculpting should be performed during the middle of the day. The patient should be rested and relaxed, because fatigue and anxiety will affect lid contours dramatically in many patients. Eyelid contours and periorbital tissues should simulate those of the normal eye as closely as possible. *At this stage of sculpting, the lid contours should be slightly more open than the lid contours of the normal eye.*

When the sculpting is completed, the previously selected synthetic eyelashes should be pressed into the underside of the upper eyelid. They will be removed prior to processing but will be reinserted following completion of the prosthesis. These lashes cast a shadow and occupy some space, and their presence will impact the perception of lid opening and lid contour. Final adjustments to lid contours can now be made. All details must be faithfully reproduced. The surface texture of the periorbital skin surface must then be carefully reproduced (Fig 5-75a; see also Figs 5-35 and 5-36).

The lines of juncture should be feathered and ended beneath the eyeglasses or the shadows cast by them. The best results are obtained in older patients with numerous lines and fissures of the periorbital tissues. If possible, the lines of juncture should not extend beyond the area covered by the eyeglass frames because such margins are difficult to camouflage. Plastic eyeglass frames are usually preferable

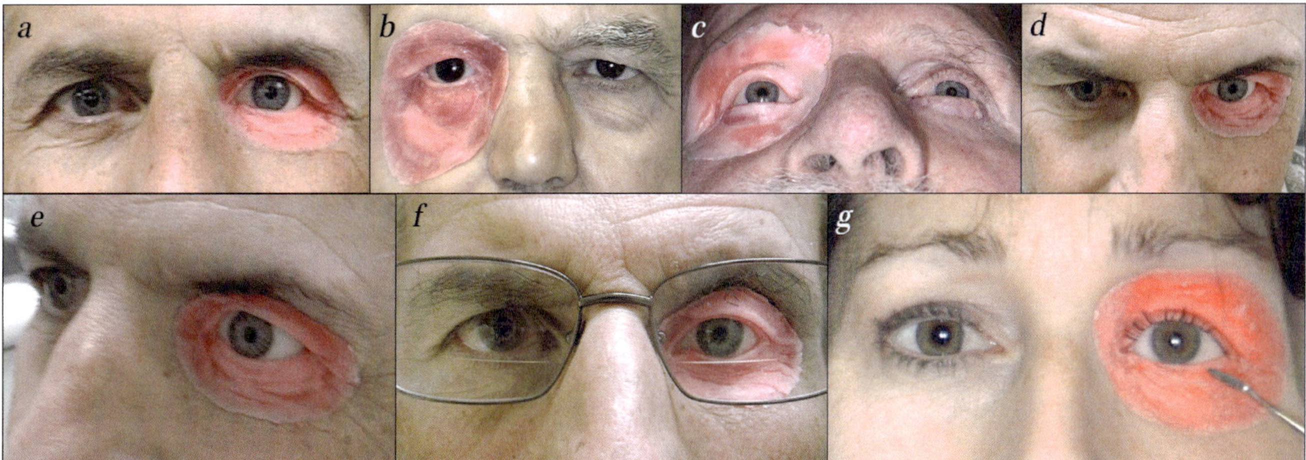

Figure 5-74 Sculpting of periorbital tissues. *(a and b)* The eyelid and surrounding tissue contours have been completed. *(c, d, and e)* The prosthesis is checked from several angles. Because of contour deficiency on the defect side, the ocular prosthesis is embedded in wax slightly posterior to the normal globe. *(f)* Lines of juncture are placed behind eyeglass frames. *(g)* Synthetic eyelashes are fitted underneath the upper lid. They are thinned out in order to match the opposite side. They are removed prior to processing.

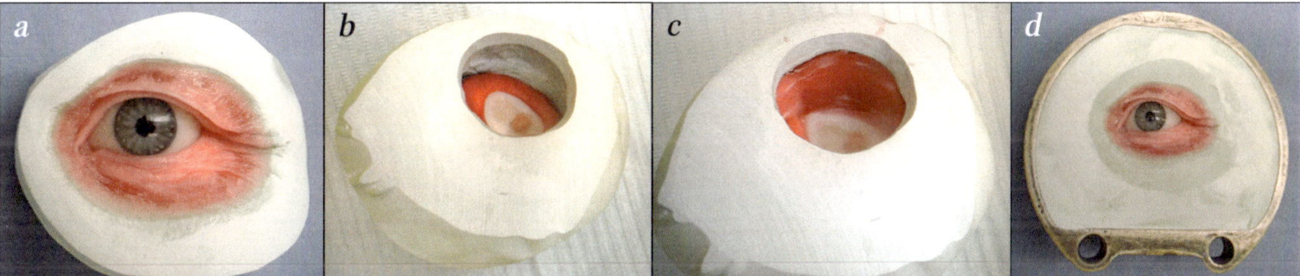

Figure 5-75 Flasking of the orbital prosthesis. *(a)* The wax pattern is sealed to master cast. *(b and c)* Wax is flowed into desired undercuts and support areas through a hole made in the back of the cast. Stone will be poured in this opening during the first stage of flasking. *(d)* The first stage of flasking is completed.

to metal frames because they cast larger shadows under which portions of the lines of juncture can be positioned.

When completed, the wax sculpting is luted at both the front and the back of the cast. Care must be taken to ensure that the wax pattern effectively engages any useful undercuts (Fig 5-75b and c).

The initial wax pattern can also be created with CAD-CAM techniques. Scans of the defect and the opposite unaffected eye are made, and the data are then manipulated to create a mirror image of the normal unaffected periorbital tissues on the side of the defect. The image is then adapted to the defect and manipulated as appropriate (see section above entitled "Use of digital technology"). The data from the mirrored image are entered into another computer to print a wax pattern of the proposed facial prosthesis. This step is accomplished with selective laser sintering utilizing a wax powder (Wu et al., 2009). The printed wax pattern is then refined as described above.

Processing

Stone is poured through the hole in the back of the cast to begin fabrication of the mold. The indicating arrow on the back side of the stock eye must be engaged. The cast is then invested in a flask in the usual fashion. When the stone has set, the flask is separated and the stock eye is secured to the index. If intrinsic coloring is to be used, the catalyzed colors are painted into the mold in layers. The base shade is injected to fill the rest of the mold. If intrinsic coloration is to be employed, the mold is heated, and the colorants are applied in select areas (see Fig 5-41a). Upon completion of this task or if only extrinsic coloring is used, the base shade of silicone or another preferred material is injected into the flask and the material is allowed to polymerize (Fig 5-76).

The prosthesis is processed in the favored material, and the extrinsic color is added as needed to the surface to complete the color characterization. When appropriate, prosthetic eyelashes are secured beneath the upper lid. Some clinicians prefer to use commercially available eyelashes rather than sew lashes into the silicone (Fig 5-77). The synthetic eyelashes are easily replaced when they become dirty or when they lose their shape. Eyelashes sewn into the prosthesis are not so easily replaced. Because the lower lashes are quite scanty, they can be simulated with a few vertical lines of extrinsic painting on the lower lid. Eyebrows, if necessary, can be simulated by painting (see Fig 5-20b), eyebrow pencil, or custom-made prosthetic eyebrows.

However, if desired, eyelashes and eyebrow hair can also be sown into a prosthesis. A foot-long strand of hair is passed through a 30-gauge dental anesthetic needle until 3 to 4 mm of the hair extends past the needle tip, leaving the rest of the strand out of the hub (Fig 5-77). Mindful of the direction the lash should emerge, the

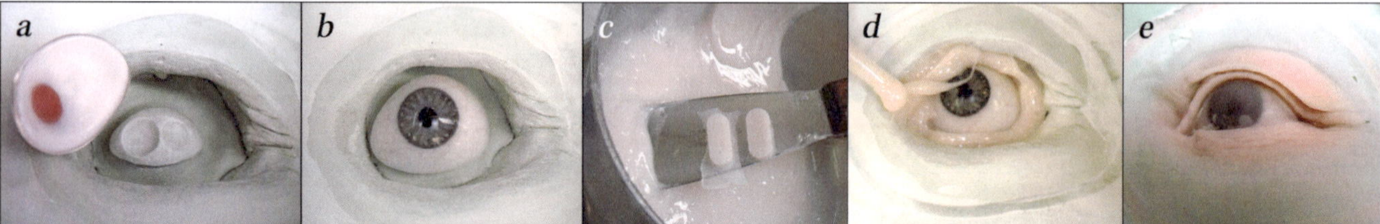

Figure 5-76 Processing of the orbital prosthesis. *(a and b)* The acrylic resin eye is secured. *(c)* Silicone is mixed to match the base shade selected, *(d)* injected into the mold, and allowed to polymerize. *(e)* The polymerized casting.

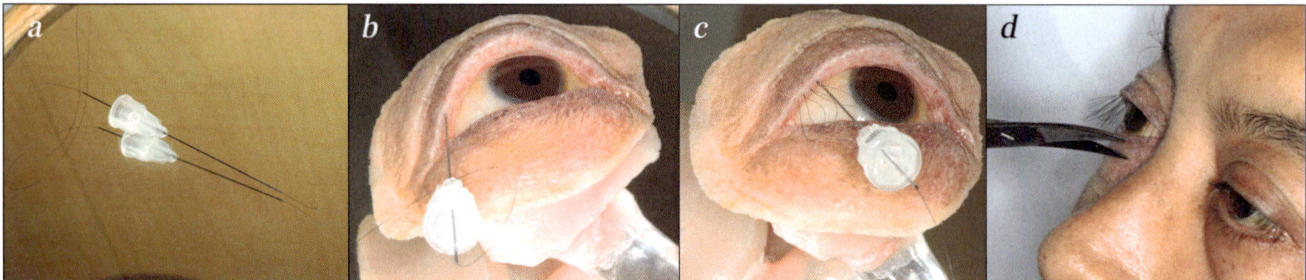

Figure 5-77 Sewing eyelashes into the prosthesis. *(a)* A 30 gauge needle with a strand of hair extending 3–4 mm beyond the tip. *(b and c)* The needle is inserted into the silicone to a depth of at least 3 mm and then withdrawn. Repeating this step several times will result in sufficient number of eyelashes. *(d)* The lashes are then trimmed to the appropriate length.

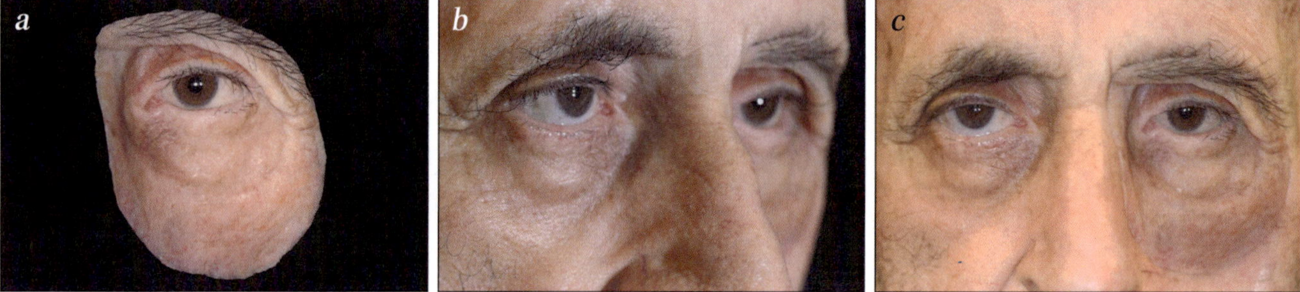

Figure 5-78 Eyebrow hair and eye lashes have been sown into the prosthesis in this patient.

needle is inserted into the silicone to a depth of at least 3 mm. This penetration depth sufficiently embeds the exposed end of the hair. As the needle is drawn back out of the silicone, the hair will remain embedded in the silicone. The needle is pulled out to allow at least twice the desired length of the lash or eyebrow hair and then reinserted into the next site. Repeating these steps will form several loops of hair, which will later be cut to the desired length, each loop becoming two lashes or eyebrows (Fig 5-77). In cases where the silicone is very thin—for example, the portion overlaying the patient's brow—retention of the individual hairs requires that a silicone adhesive be applied to lute the ends of the hairs that perforate the tissue side of the prosthesis.

Upon close observation, it may be evident that the cut-off, squared ends of the sewn hair do not faithfully replicate the tapered ends of natural eyelashes or brows. They best match the hair of a trimmed mustache. Although this detail is not noticeable from a normal conversational distance, a second technique offers a solution to the appearance created by the cut-off ends. Actual eyelashes or eyebrow hairs are secured and embedded into the prosthesis one at a time. The tool required to perform this task is a sewing needle that has been cut through the middle of its eye. This creates a two-prong fork that is used to insert the follicle end of a lash or eyebrow hair into the desired site. The tool is removed, and the hair remains embedded within the prosthesis. A disadvantage of this technique is that obtaining the needed quantity of donor eyelashes or brow hairs can be challenging. Furthermore, since a portion of the length of each eyelash or eyebrow hair is embedded in the silicone, each lash or eyebrow hair will be shorter than usual.

Completed prostheses are shown in Figs 5-78 to 5-80. Tinted lenses enhance the effectiveness of the prosthesis (Fig 5-80).

Delivery and retention

The use of tissue adhesives and/or engagement of undercuts provides suitable retention for most defects. If the resection extends to the cheek and movable tissues, the use of osseointegrated implants is preferred. In patients with concomitant maxillectomy defects, the orbital and oral prosthesis can be connected with magnetic attachments (see section below entitled "Connection of a Facial Prosthesis

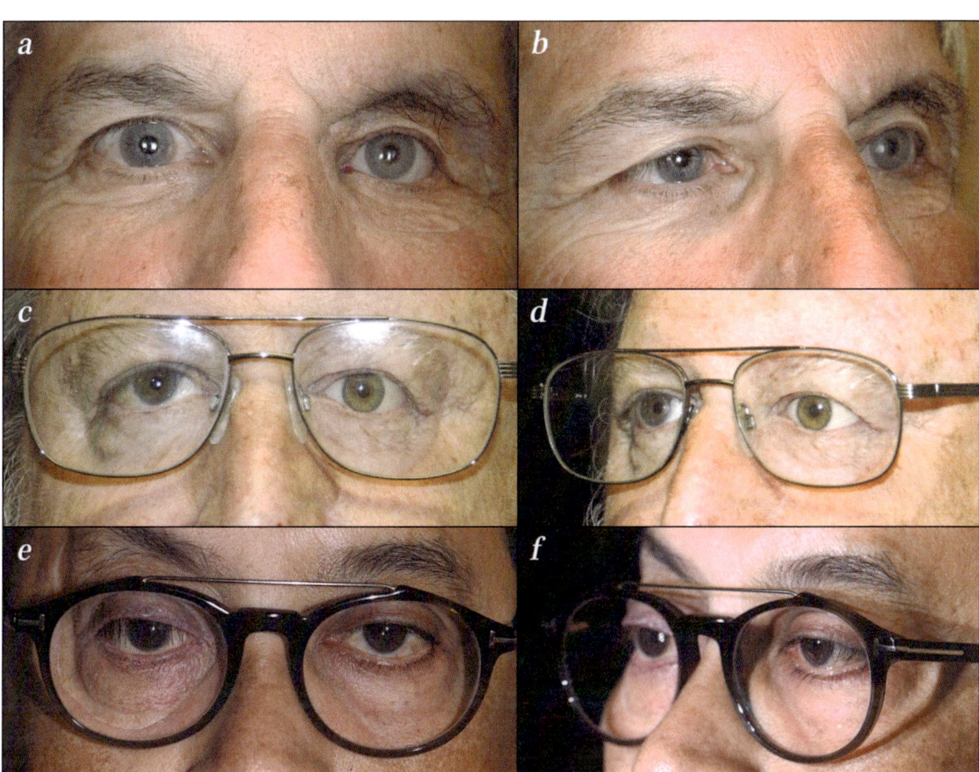

Figure 5-79 *(a–f)* Completed orbital prostheses.

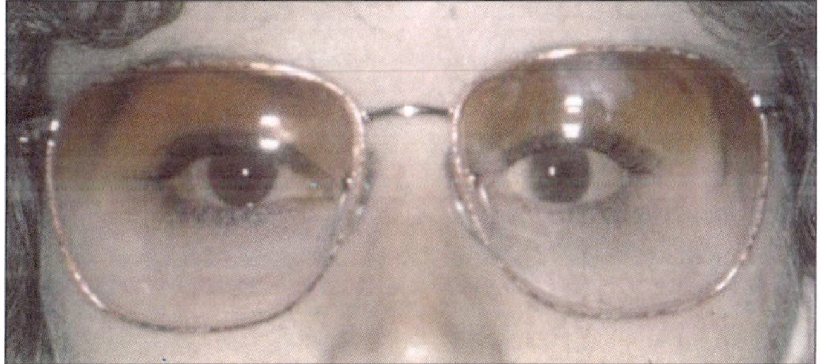

Figure 5-80 Tinted lenses help hide the margins and camouflage the prosthesis.

to an Oral Prosthesis"). When eyeglass frames are worn, the optometrist must prepare the lens over the prosthesis so that it is identical to the lens covering the normal eye, or asymmetric distortion of the prosthesis will be perceived. The patient should be instructed to turn his or her head and direct the gaze of the natural eye straight ahead rather than vary the gaze of the natural eye. In this manner, the lack of eye movement of the prosthesis will not be as noticeable.

Craniofacial Implants

In the past, prosthodontic restorations had distinct limitations because of movable tissues, inadequate retention of large prostheses, and some patients' reluctance to accept the prosthesis. The use of osseointegrated implants has eliminated some of these problems. The retention provided by implants makes it possible to fabricate large prostheses that rest on movable tissues. Patient acceptance is significantly enhanced because of the quality of the retention (Flood and Russell, 1998; Markt and Lemon, 2001; Chang et al., 2005) and is accompanied by significant improvements in the quality of life (Nemli et al., 2013). This enables the prosthodontist to concentrate on aesthetics and to fabricate thin prosthetic margins that blend more effectively with mobile peripheral tissues.

The same is true for posttraumatic and congenital defects, especially of the external ear. The use of osseointegrated implants has made it possible to produce effective bone-anchored ear prostheses that patients will accept. The prosthodontist must consider the special problems affecting patients with congenital malformations such as microtia, the attitude of the patient and the family, the management of ear remnants, and the overall treatment of what may be a complex congenital syndrome.

Benefits derived from the use of implant-retained prostheses include *(1)* improvement of the retention and stability of the prosthesis, *(2)* avoidance of the occasional skin reactions to adhesives, *(3)* improvement of the ease and accuracy of prosthesis placement, *(4)* improvement of skin hygiene and patient comfort, *(5)* elimination of the daily maintenance associated with the removal and

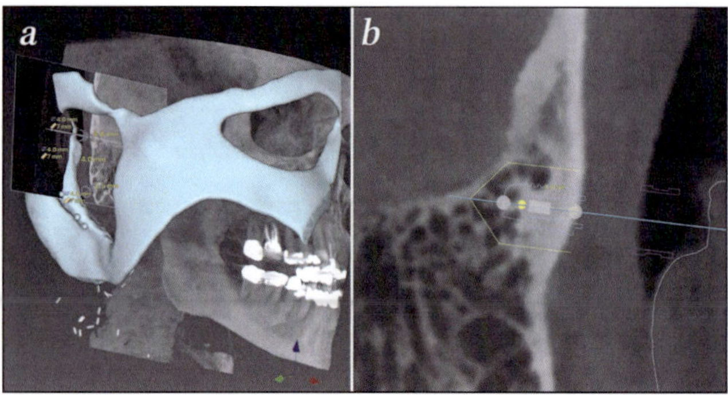

Figure 5-81 The mastoid is an excellent site for placement of implants.

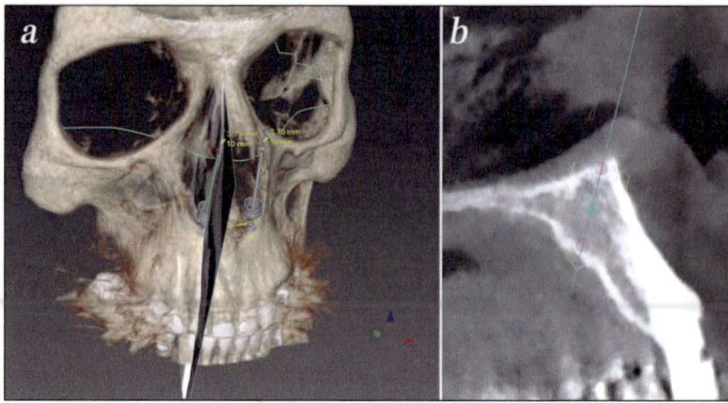

Figure 5-82 CBCT scans and associated software are used to evaluate possible implant sites in three dimensions. *(a and b)* The floor of the nose is being considered. The roots of the anterior teeth must be avoided.

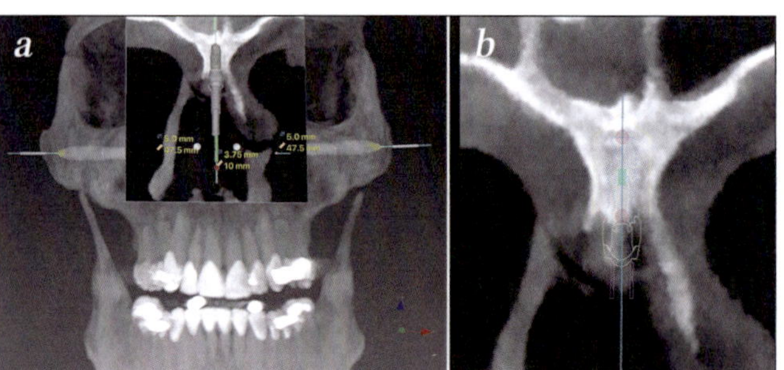

Figure 5-83 The glabella region may have sufficient bone volume to receive an implant 7–10 mm in length.

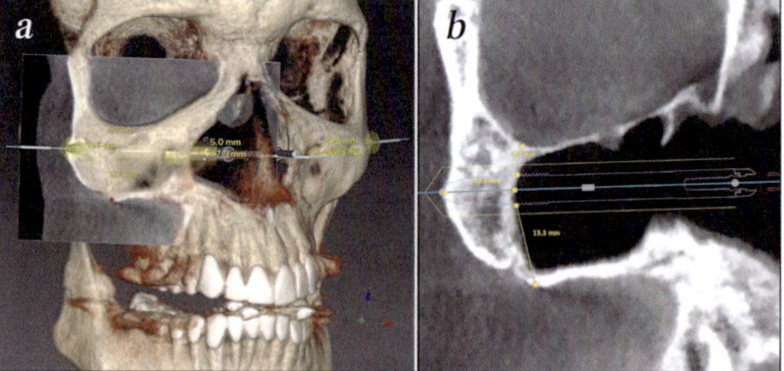

Figure 5-84 The zygomas have been used in large nasal and midfacial defects.

reapplication of skin adhesives, *(6)* enhancement of the aesthetics of the lines of juncture between the prosthesis and skin, and *(7)* an increase in the life span of the facial restoration; when skin adhesives are used for retention, they must be removed and reapplied each day, leading to loss of colorants at the margin of the prosthesis that eventually renders the prosthesis unacceptable. When an implant-borne prosthesis is fabricated, its margins can be made thinner and designed to exert positive pressure on the underlying skin. These practices will render the lines of junction less noticeable.

Implant sites

Auricular defects

These defects can be secondary to oncologic resections or congenital deformities. The mastoid area has proven to be an excellent site for craniofacial implants. There is sufficient cortical bone at this site to enable excellent initial stabilization of the implants, and the peri-implant tissues can be made to be thin and relatively immobile (Fig 5-81). Success rates have been excellent, and few complications have been encountered (Tjellström et al., 1981; Jacobsson et al., 1992; Sugar and Beumer, 1994; Roumanas et al., 2002; Visser et al., 2008; Subramaniam et al., 2018). The 20-year survival of implants placed in this region exceeded 90% in a recent report (Subramaniam et al., 2018). However, implants placed in patients with congenital ear deformities tend to have a higher success rate than those with auriculectomy defects secondary to an oncologic resection (Subramaniam et al., 2018). This difference is probably driven by the fact that most oncologic defects occur in older age groups and are frequently irradiated.

Nasal defects

Most patients in this group have undergone total rhinectomy secondary to resection of neoplasms. The floor of the nose is the site most often employed to retain nasal prostheses. Bone quality at this site is sufficient to allow initial implant stabilization, although the surgeon must take care to avoid the roots of the anterior teeth in dentate patients (Fig 5-82). The glabella region or the midline area of the frontal bone between the two orbits has sufficient bone volume to receive implants of 7–10 mm in length but has been used less frequently (Fig 5-83). Recent reports have also described the successful use of zygomatic implants placed in the zygoma to retain nasal prostheses (Fig 5-84).

The success rates of implants placed in the floor of the nose are between 75% and 85% with 3 and 4 mm implants (Jacobsson et al., 1992; Nishimura et al., 1996; Sugar and Beumer, 1994; Flood, 1998; Roumanas et al., 2002; Visser et al., 2008; Flood and Downie, 2009; Subramaniam et al., 2018). Success rates appear to be improved by the use of longer dental-type implants for this site (Flood and Downie, 2009). Success rates for implants placed in the glabella region have been mixed. There is little data on the long-term success rates of implants placed in the zygoma to retain nasal prostheses. This site is relatively inaccessible in patients with rhinectomy defects, and its use has become possible largely because of the

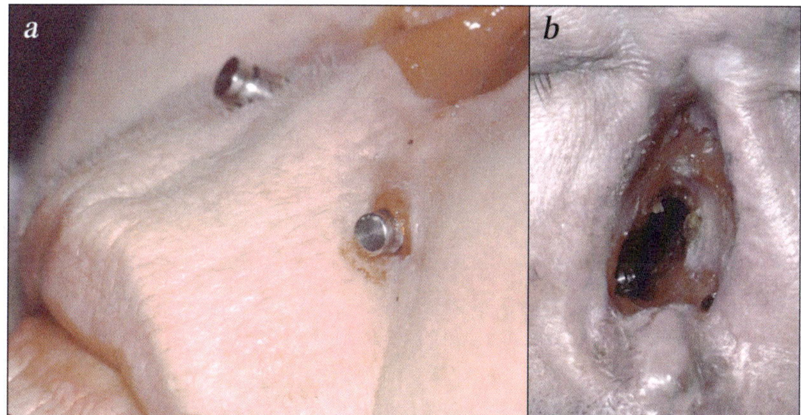

Figure 5-85 Implants should not be positioned within *(a)* the mobile tissues of the upper lip or *(b)* too far posteriorly.

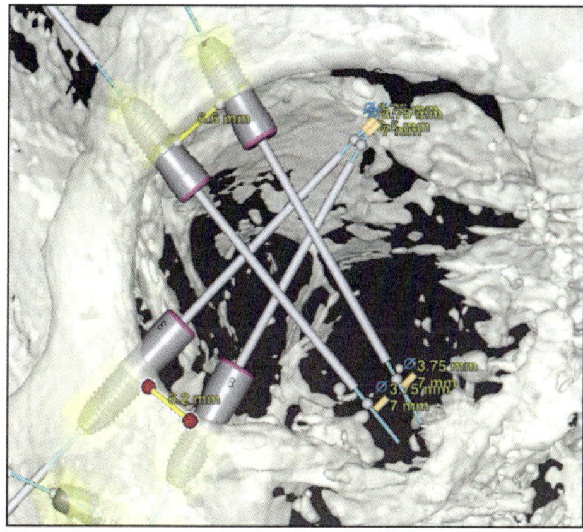

Figure 5-86 Initially most of the implants were placed in the superior-lateral portion of the orbital rim. Recently, the authors have switched to the malar body as the preferred site.

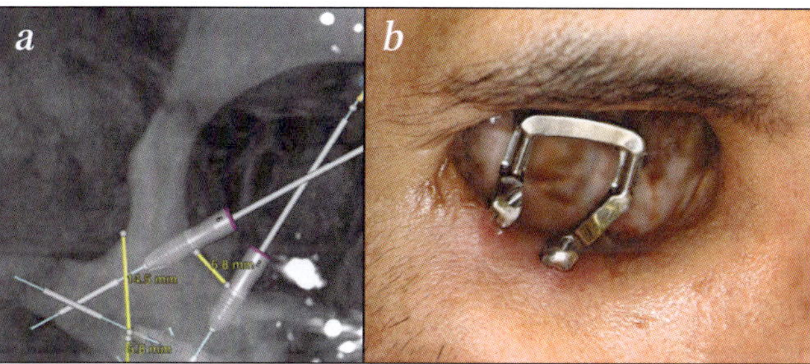

Figure 5-87 The malar body presents with sufficient bone volume to accept implant 7–10 mm in length.

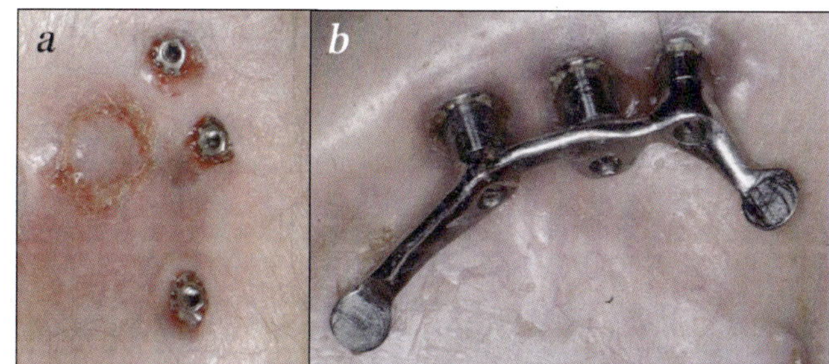

Figure 5-88 Flange exposure in irradiated sites.

recent development of dynamic navigation as a means of implant placement (see Fig 5-100).

The implants should not exit the mobile tissues of the lip or the nasolabial fold region (Fig 5-85a). The mobility of the peri-implant tissues will lead to intractable peri-implantitis and hypertrophy of the peri-implant tissues. Also, in these instances, space for the retention bar may be insufficient for good hygiene, compounding the risk of peri-implantitis. Implants placed too far posteriorly into the nasal passage will also compromise access for hygiene and predispose the patient to peri-implant soft tissue problems (Fig 5-85b).

Orbital defects

Most orbital exenteration defects are secondary to tumor ablation. In most centers, the implant site usually employed has been the lateral portion of the supraorbital rim (Fig 5-86). Initial implant anchorage is usually excellent in this site because of the dense cortical bone available. However, the success rates of implants at this site have been disappointing. Short-term follow-up studies initially revealed a relatively high success rate (Curi et al., 2012; Karakoca et al., 2008); however, long-term failure rates appear to be three to four times greater than those reported for auricular and floor-of-the-nose sites (Roumanas et al., 2002; Subramaniam et al., 2018). The 10-year survival rate of implants placed in the orbital region was 44% in a recent report (Subramaniam et al., 2018). Recently the authors have begun placing longer dental-type implants into the malar body in an attempt to increase success rates (Fig 5-87). However, long-term data is not available to assess implant success using this site.

Most failures have occurred secondary to persistent peri-implant soft tissue inflammation and pain. The orbital peri-implant soft tissues frequently are thick and mobile. It is challenging to thin these tissues with a subcutaneous resection, and this may be one of the factors responsible for the high frequency of the soft tissue problems. Furthermore, many of the patients are elderly and have compromised manual dexterity, making it difficult to manipulate hygiene aids. Moreover, their monocular vision and compromised depth perception make it difficult to visualize the implants. The high failure rate also may be related to the poor blood supply and slow remodeling of bone at this site (Roumanas et al., 2002; Granstrom, 2005; Visser et al., 2008).

Impact of radiation

The success rates are diminished if the implant sites have been irradiated previously (Granstrom, 2005), particularly for implants placed in the orbital rim (Roumanas et al., 2002) (Fig 5-88b). Definitive doses of radiation therapy dramatically impair the osseointegration process (see Chapter 1, section entitled "Dental Implants in Irradiated Tissues"). At doses in excess of 60 Gy, the biologic processes associated with osseointegration are severely compromised, and anchorage in bone is most likely mechanical

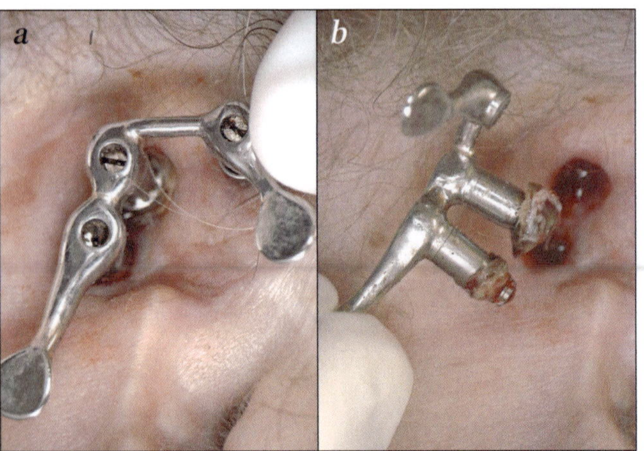

Figure 5-89 Implant failure. *(a)* Tissue bar with magnetic retention in an irradiated patient. Note the exposed flanges. *(b)* Two of three implants were lost.

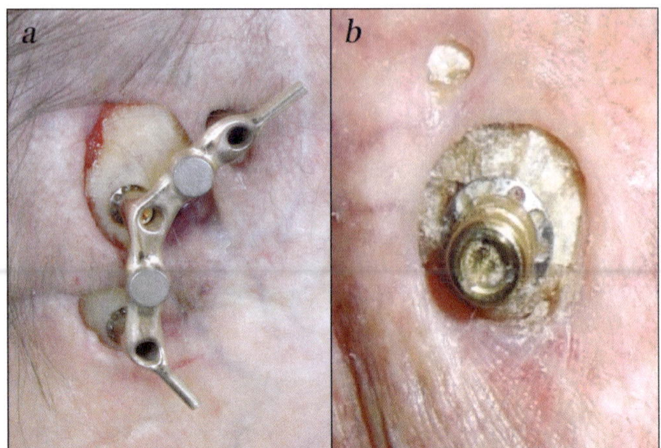

Figure 5-90 *(a and b)* ORN associated with implants in the mastoid area in two different patients. Both patients had received radiation doses in excess of 60 Gy. Following the removal of the implants, the necrotic bone sequestrated, and both lesions healed with conservative measures.

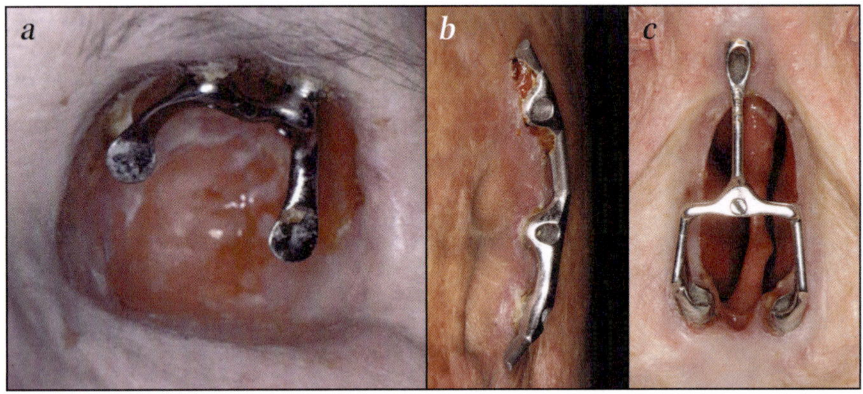

Figure 5-91 *(a and b)* Poor hygiene has led to the accumulation of keratin and debris around the abutments. Local infections eventually will lead to loss of implants. Neither of these patients were irradiated. *(c)* Implants were placed in the floor of the nose and the glabella region. Hygiene has been excellent. This is a 19-year follow-up.

and secondary to the density of the bone site as opposed to biologic processes. Long-term success rates vary widely and range from as low as 21% in the orbit to 70–80% in the temporal bone and the floor of the nose (Roumanas et al., 2002; Nishimura et al., 1996; Nishimura et al., 1998; Roumanas et al., 2002; Toljanic et al., 2005; Karakoca et al., 2008; Subramaniam et al., 2018). A factor contributing to the failure of short craniofacial implants in irradiated patients is flange exposure. When the flanges of these implants are exposed, it becomes impossible even for a compliant patient to keep this area clean, leading to persistent irritation of the peri-implant skin or mucosa and subsequent bone loss and implant failure (Figs 5-88 and 5-89). Success rates in irradiated sites appear to be improved by the use of adjuvant hyperbaric oxygen treatments (Granstrom, 2005; see Chapter 1, the section entitled "Human studies").

Osteoradionecrosis (Fig 5-90) is relatively rare, presumably because of the conservative doses employed for these tumors. In our experience, the few osteoradionecrosis we have seen were self-limiting and resolved with conservative measures.

Most of the oncologic resection patients in the series reported in the literature to date received their implants after their radiotherapy, so many clinicians are now placing implants at the time of tumor ablation. When postoperative radiation is used, it is usually commenced four to six weeks following tumor resection, and this is sufficient time to allow microrough surface implants to become reasonably well osseointegrated. It is not yet known whether this practice will impact implant survival in irradiated sites.

Peri-implant soft tissue reactions

Peri-implant soft tissue reactions include inflammation and formation of granulation tissue, hypertrophy, bleeding, and infection. If not treated successfully, these phenomena can lead to loss of the bone anchoring the implant and implant loss.

There appears to be a direct correlation between the level of hygiene compliance and soft tissue reactions at all sites (Nishimura et al., 1995, 1996, 1998; Visser et al., 2008; Balik et al., 2016; Subramaniam et al., 2018). Nishimura and colleagues (1995, 1996, 1998) reported that orbital sites were the most difficult for the patients to clean and had the highest rates of peri-implant tissue reactions (Fig 5-91a). Implants placed in the floor-of-the-nose site were the easiest to clean and had the lowest rate of soft tissue reactions (Fig 5-91c). Auricular sites were between these two extremes (Fig 5-91b). At all sites, when hygiene was improved, the inflammatory soft tissue reactions subsided or were eliminated.

Figure 5-92 *(a)* The auricle was lost secondary to severe burns. The implant-connecting bar was designed digitally and made of monolithic zirconia. *(b)* A patient suffered from persistent soft tissue irritation. All conservative measures failed, including a course of systemic antibiotics that was based on the results of culture. The addition of porcelain to the transcutaneous portion of the bar resolved the tissue irritation.

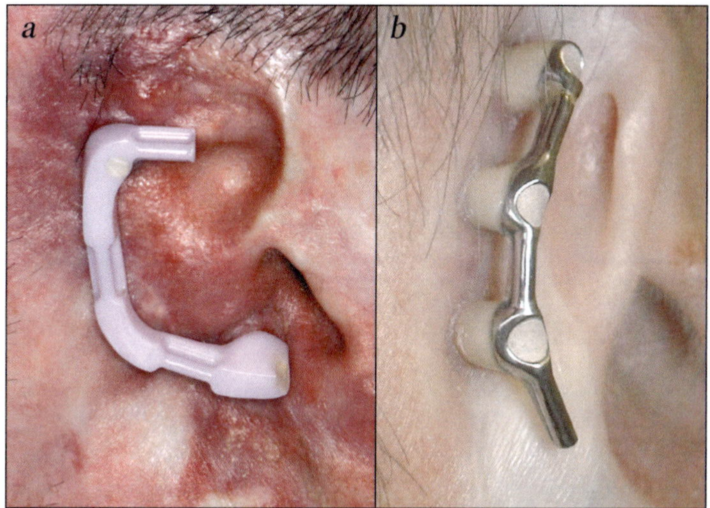

Patients with skin-penetrating implants in the facial skeleton need proper hygiene instruction and should be followed closely. Patients tend to forget the necessity for good implant and implant-connecting bar hygiene; therefore, hygiene instruction must be reinforced continually during periodic recall visits. Keratin and sebaceous secretions tend to accumulate on the abutments and the attachment apparatus, even in patients with relatively good hygiene practices, and are predisposed to peri-implantitis and should be removed during the follow-up visits. This is easily accomplished with a plastic scaler.

Minimizing the thickness of the peri-implant tissues will keep soft tissue complications to a minimum. With the exception of the orbit, the skin and overlying tissues in auricular or rhinectomy defects secondary to trauma or tumor resection usually are thin, and the overlying skin or mucosa is usually adherent to the underlying periosteum. In contrast, patients with congenital malformations of the ear region often present with thick and sometimes mobile tissues at proposed implant sites. Frequently, these patients have been subjected to multiple surgical reconstructions aimed at restoring the auricle. Careful thinning of the flap at stage-two surgery or placement of a split-thickness skin graft will result in thinner peri-tissues and will keep soft tissue complications to a minimum.

Treatment of persistent peri-implant tissue reactions consists of improved home care, local debridement, removal of hyperplastic tissue, and topical or systemic antibiotics. Inflammation and granulation tissue formation are typically treated locally with topical bacitracin ointment and chemical cautery (Hildrew et al., 2015). A three-month course of Clobetasol, a steroid cream topically applied, has also been used successfully in the treatment of hyperplastic tissue reactions around implants that emerge from the skin in the mastoid region (Falcone et al., 2008; Hildrew et al., 2015).

Use of metal-ceramic and zirconia bars

Patients for whom the defects are secondary to burns, given the compromised health status of their skin, find it difficult to maintain peri-implant soft tissue health even when they are able to keep the implants free of debris, keratin buildup, and sebaceous secretions. In other patients, peri-implant skin irritation persists even in the face of good hygiene compliance. Two solutions have emerged that appear to have successfully addressed the persistent soft tissue irritation in these patients—the use of implant-connecting bars fabricated of zirconia and metal-ceramic bars designed such that the ceramic portion of bars interfaces with the peri-implant soft tissues (Fig 5-92). These ceramic surfaces retain debris less readily, which presumably explains why soft tissue health is better maintained.

Workup

Pretreatment planning should involve all members of the treatment rehabilitation team. If the patient is scheduled to lose a facial part secondary to resection of a neoplasm, the team should consider placing implants during the same surgery as tumor resection (see Fig 5-24). This practice spares the patient an additional anesthetic and speeds the process of rehabilitation. We recommend this practice even in patients scheduled to receive a postoperative course of radiation. Radiation treatment following tumor surgery is usually delayed for about four to six weeks to allow the surgical wounds to heal. This is sufficient time for implants with microrough implant surfaces to become osseointegrated because such surfaces accelerate the pertinent biologic processes associated with osseointegration (Ogawa and Nishimura, 2006). It is true that the backscatter from the postoperative radiation will raise the radiation dose to the bone anchoring the implants by an additional 15% to 18%, further compromising the vasculature of the anchoring bone and its viability (Schwartz et al., 1979; Tso et al., 2019). However, at doses above 60 Gy, implant anchorage is primarily mechanical as opposed to biologic (Nishimura, 1996). Consequently, if implants were to be placed in these same sites after radiation, lacking the normal process of osseointegration, the anchorage being primarily mechanical, the level of implant bone contact achieved would be considerably less than if they were placed prior to radiation. However, the results of this practice have yet to be determined.

Once the facial prosthesis has been designed, the number and arrangement of the implants required to retain and stabilize the prosthesis are determined, and the possible bone sites are evaluated.

Figure 5-93 *(a)* Patient presented with microtia. *(b)* The ear remnant has been removed in preparation for placement of implants.

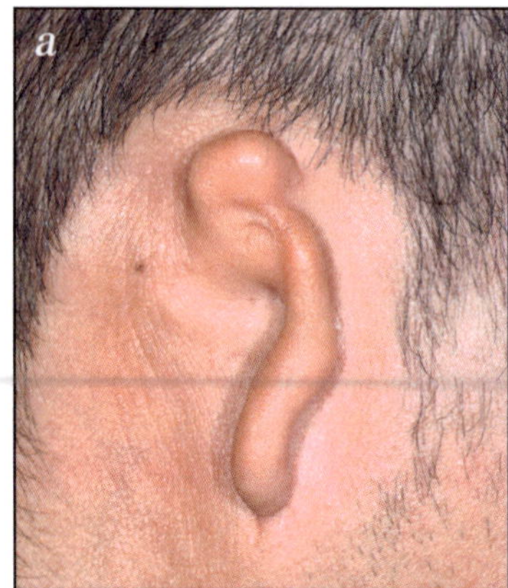

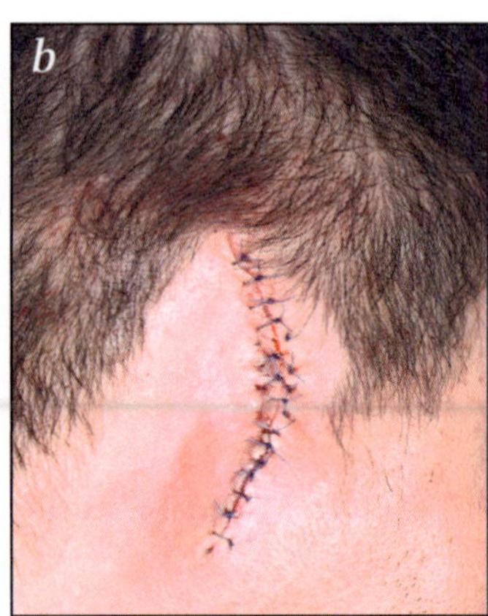

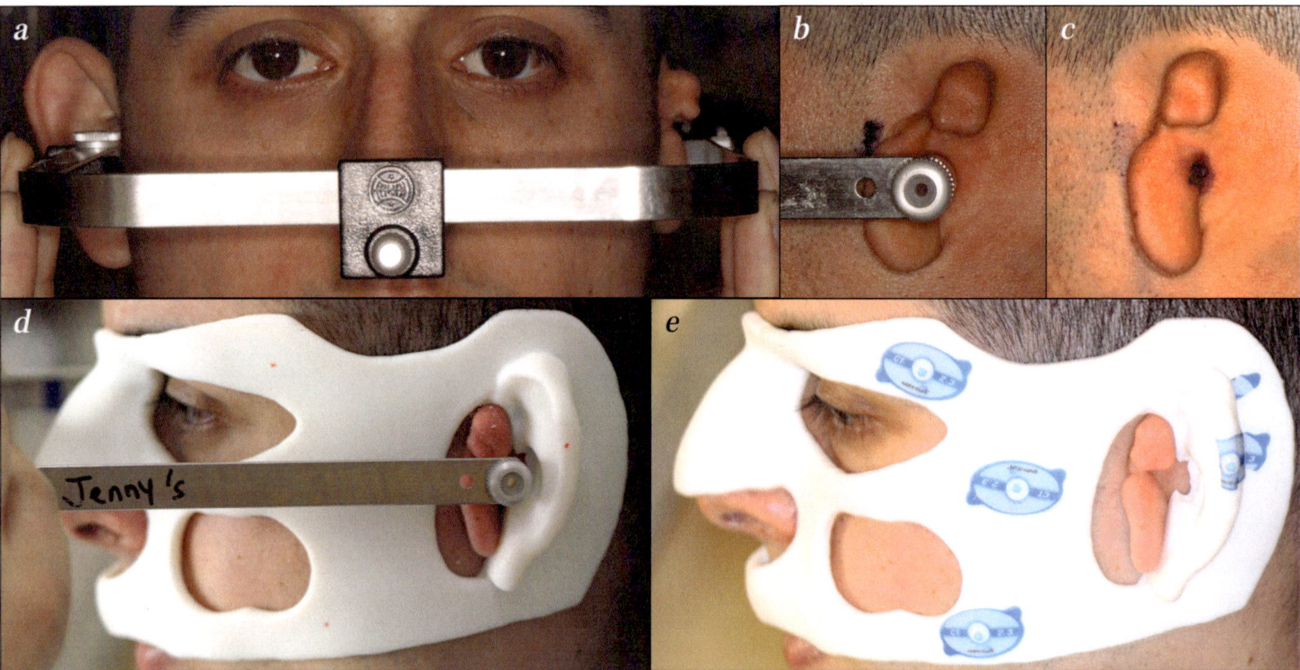

Figure 5-94 *(a)* A Facebow positioned into the intact ear and parallel to the interpupillary plane. *(b)* Once properly oriented, the left earpiece of the facebow will indicate where the missing EAC should go. *(c)* An indelible marker is used to mark the proposed EAC. *(d)* A printed template of the ear confirming the proper position. *(e)* Fiducial markers are placed on the template in preparation for a dual scan protocol.

CBCT scans with the associated software are recommended in order to assess the possible implant sites in three dimensions (see Figs 5-81–5-84). In patients with ear defects, the position of the facial nerve canal, the sigmoid sinus, the level of the middle cranial fossa, the size of the mastoid, and the configuration of the mastoid air cell system need to be determined. With rhinectomy defects, the position of the roots of the teeth can be determined radiographically in relation to the probable implant sites in the floor of the nose. Alternative sites such as the zygoma and the glabella region can also be carefully scrutinized. With orbital exenteration defects, the position and contours of the frontal sinus need to be taken into account if implants are to be placed in the supraorbital rim.

For patients with congenital ear defects such as microtia, the major issue is the fate of tissue remnants. In patients with microtia, ear remnants will vary in size, shape, and position and often need to be removed (Fig 5-93). Before these remnants are resected, all possible options for rehabilitation must be presented, explored, and discussed with the patient and the family. In some patients, it may be necessary to reconstruct the ear canal. If so, this procedure can be performed during the same surgery as implant placement. A facebow transfer apparatus can be used to identify the proper position of the auricle. The proposed contours and position of the auricle can also be developed virtually with CAD programs. In order to assess the implant sites a radiographic template is fabricated, fiducial markers are added in key positions, and a CBCT scan is obtained (Fig 5-94). The contours of the proposed facial prosthesis can now be superimposed onto the potential implant sites. Once the sites are determined, the radiographic template can be altered and used as a surgical template in order to identify the selected implant positions during surgery.

The skin and soft tissues overlying the proposed implant sites also require careful examination. As mentioned previously, the health of

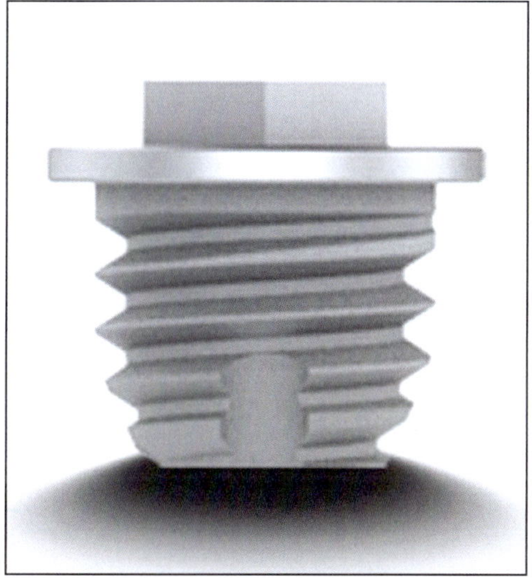

Figure 5-95 A typical craniofacial implant. It has a flange, is tapered, and is self-tapping with a microrough surface (courtesy of Southern Implants, Irene, SA).

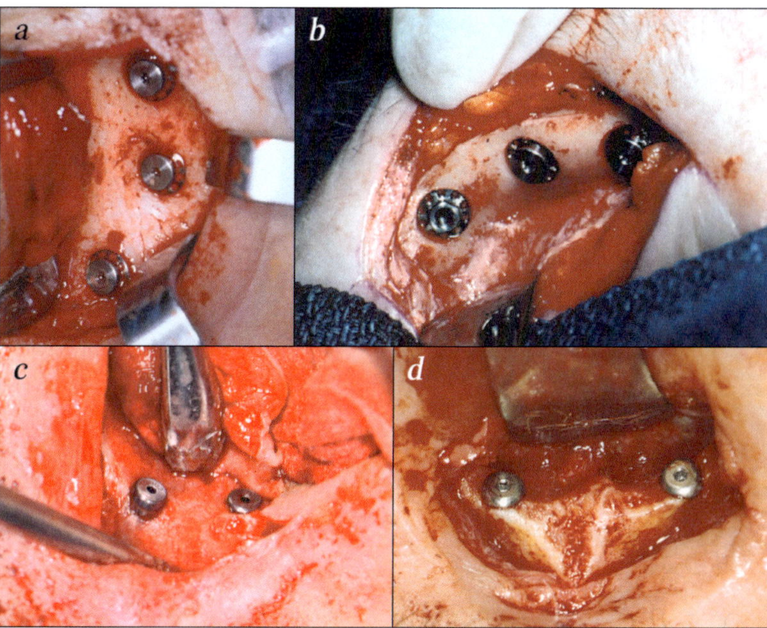

Figure 5-96 *(a)* Three craniofacial implants were placed in the mastoid. Note the flanges. *(b)* Three craniofacial implants were placed in the supraorbital rim. *(c)* Two dental implants were placed in the malar body. *(d)* Two dental implants were placed in the floor of the nose.

the soft tissues circumscribing osseointegrated implants is easier to maintain if these tissues are thin (less than 5 mm in thickness) and attached to underlying periosteum. If the skin and soft tissues overlying the implant sites contain hair follicles, scar tissue, or tissue remnants of past reconstructive procedures, these tissues should be considered for removal and replacement with a skin graft.

Implant selection

Several craniofacial implant designs have emerged in recent times, but most are cylindrical, based on the original design developed by Branemark and his colleagues (Fig 5-95). They are available from several companies (Entific, Cochlear, Strauman, Southern) and are available in lengths of 3.0 to 4.5 mm with a 5-mm-diameter flange. Most have microrough surfaces and some are tapered and self-tapping. These short lengths are designed to permit placement in areas with limited available bone. The flange facilitates initial stabilization of the implant and prevents undue penetration into interior compartments. Self-tapping designs are available and enhance the initial stabilization of the implant. The disappointing long-term success rates of the short implants in some sites (Roumanas et al., 2002; Flood and Downie, 2009; Subramaniam et al., 2018) have led clinicians to employ longer, tapered, self-tapping dental implants, particularly in locations where the bone volume is greater (e.g., glabella, malar body, nasal floor).

Implant positioning and placement

A two-stage surgical procedure is usually employed (Tjellström et al., 1981). Surgical placement can be conducted with regional anesthesia, but conditions must be sterile. A full-thickness flap is reflected and potential implant sites are scrutinized with the help of a surgical template prepared from presurgical diagnostic casts, wax-ups, and/or 3D representations of the sites from CBCT scans. The implant sites are prepared in the usual atraumatic manner. A one-stage surgical procedure has been advocated for uncomplicated ear and hearing aid implants in adults who have not been irradiated, but this requires experience and care (Tjellström and Granström, 1995). There is some risk of soft tissue necrosis when one-stage surgery is used, so prosthesis construction should be delayed for at least six weeks. This will also allow the implants to become osseointegrated.

For anchorage of an external ear prosthesis, two implants are usually sufficient, unless the site has been irradiated, is to be irradiated, or is compromised in some other fashion. The implants are usually placed in the 1-o'clock and 3-o'clock positions for the left side and 9-o'clock and 11-o'clock positions for the right side, typically 15 to 18 mm posterior to the external auditory canal (Fig 5-96a). The aim is to place the retentive implant-connecting bar beneath the antihelix portion of the prosthesis. If an additional implant is to be placed for anchorage of a bone conduction hearing processor, it is usually placed above and posterior to the area that will be occupied by the prosthesis. Direct contact between the ear prosthesis and the hearing processor should be avoided.

In the orbital area, the lateral portion of the supraorbital rim (Fig 5-96b) and the malar body (Fig 5-96c) are the preferred sites. They offer the best combination of bone volume, density, and blood supply. Short, craniofacial-type implants are used in the supraorbital rim, but it is possible to use intraoral implants 7–10 mm in length in the malar body. Two implants are sufficient to retain an orbital prosthesis, but the higher incidence of implant loss in the supraorbital rim and the high percentage of patients who will have received radiation therapy may dictate the placement of extra implants. Special care must be taken to place the implants with the proper spacing and at the correct angulation. There should be a minimum of

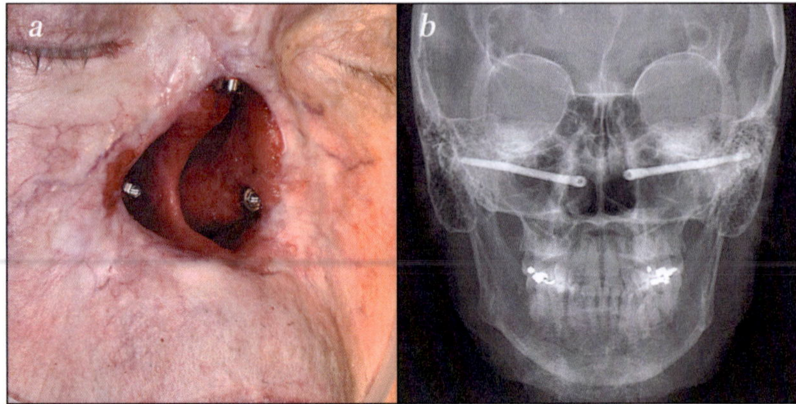

Figure 5-97 *(a)* The zygoma is a site that can be considered for the retention of nasal prostheses. *(b)* Note that the implant in the glabella region failed to osseointegrate.

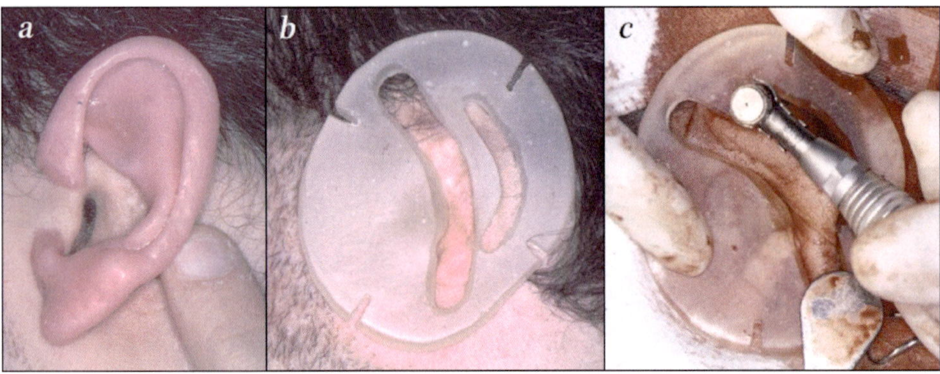

Figure 5-98 Surgical template designed for free hand surgery. *(a)* The wax sculpting is fitted to identify proper implant position. *(b)* The template is used to locate the proper implant positions. Implants should be placed beneath the antihelix. *(c)* The mastoid is exposed and sites are prepared for three implants.

7 mm between the outer surfaces of the implants to allow access for hygiene. The implants should not be angled outwardly or they may interfere with the contour of the orbital prosthesis.

For nasal prostheses, the anterior floor of the nose is the preferred site. Two are sufficient to retain most nasal prostheses. They should be placed in the anterior portion of the nasal floor about 8 to 10 mm apart (Fig 5-96d) and exit in attached, immobile tissues. As mentioned above, if implants exit through the mobile tissues of the lip, the incidence of soft tissue reactions around the implants is increased (see Fig 5-85a). If implants are placed too far posteriorly, access for hygiene is compromised (see Fig 5-85b). If the patient is edentulous in the anterior maxillary area, the bone thickness is generally sufficient for the vertical placement of the implants in the anterior nasal floor. Most clinicians prefer the longer dental implants for this site, particularly if the site has been irradiated (Flood and Downie, 2009). When roots of teeth are present, care must be taken to avoid contact between them and the implants. Alternatively, the lateral wall of the pyriform aperture can be selected for horizontal placement of one implant on each side. The zygoma (Fig 5-97; see also Fig 5-84) is also an excellent site, especially in larger defects that extend onto the cheeks, and has been employed more frequently, especially since the introduction of dynamic navigation surgery.

Placement of implants in the glabella area may be considered provided that the nasal bones have been resected, but results with craniofacial-length implants have been inconsistent (Sugar and Beumer, 1994; Roumanas et al., 2002). Some clinicians have suggested that success rates will improve if longer dental implants are placed in this site (Roumanas et al., 2002).

Surgical templates

Ideally, the implants must be positioned within the confines of the proposed facial prosthesis. However, this may not be possible in patients with acquired auriculectomy defects secondary to temporal bone resections (see Fig 5-104). For most patients, it is desirable to sculpt a reasonable facsimile of the future prosthesis, duplicate the wax pattern in acrylic resin, and modify this replica to serve as a surgical template (Fig 5-98). CAD/CAM systems can also be employed to fabricate the surgical templates (Fig 5-99). The template is sterilized and used as a guide at surgery to ensure the proper position of the implants. We suggest that the prosthodontist be present in the operating room to advise the surgical team on the location and angulation of the implants.

Freehand drilling is used for most patients with rhinectomy and orbital exenteration defects. However, when implants are to be placed in the temporal bone, implant positioning is more challenging, and alignment must be more precise; therefore, surgical templates fabricated with computer-aided design and manufacturing techniques (CAD-CAM) may be preferred. These surgical templates identify the appropriate implant sites and allow the surgeon to make the initial pilot holes (Fig 5-99). The site is then prepared with freehand surgery. These templates dictate the position but not the depth or angulation of the osteotomy sites.

Digitally designed and manufactured skin-supported drill guides used to place craniofacial implants with fully guided or semiguided implant surgery do not appear to achieve the same precision as obtained with intraoral templates. Dings and colleagues (2019)

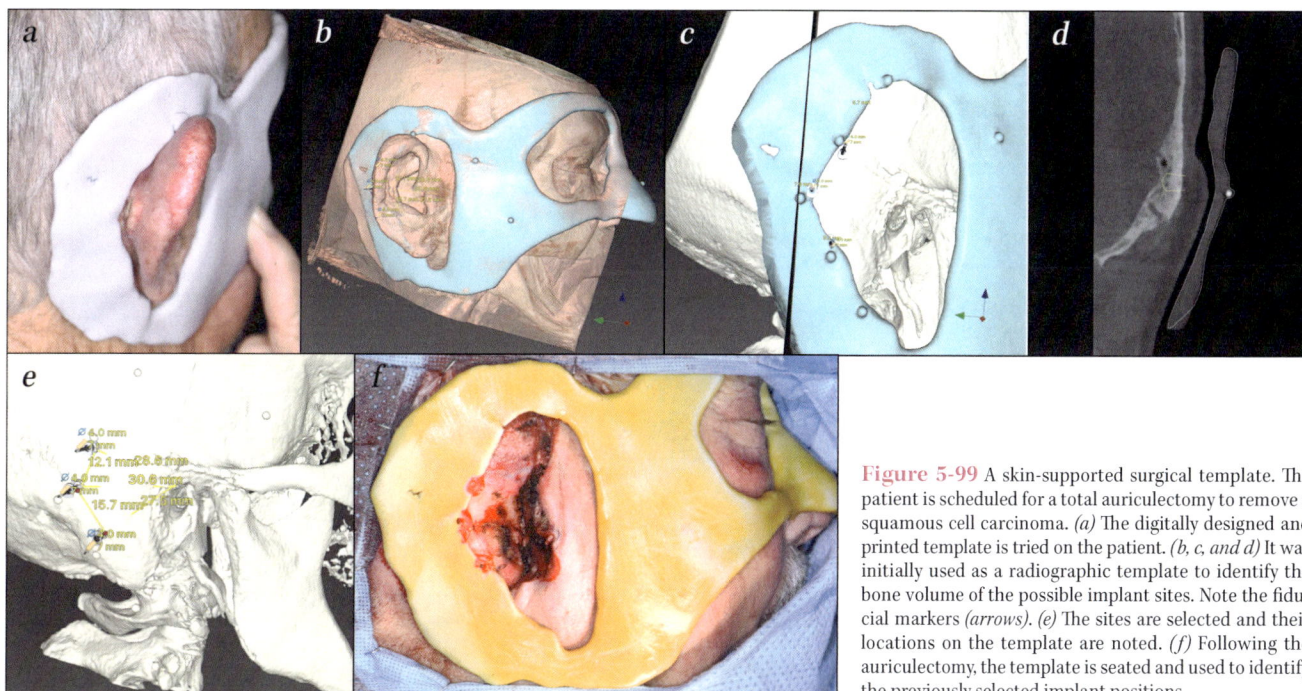

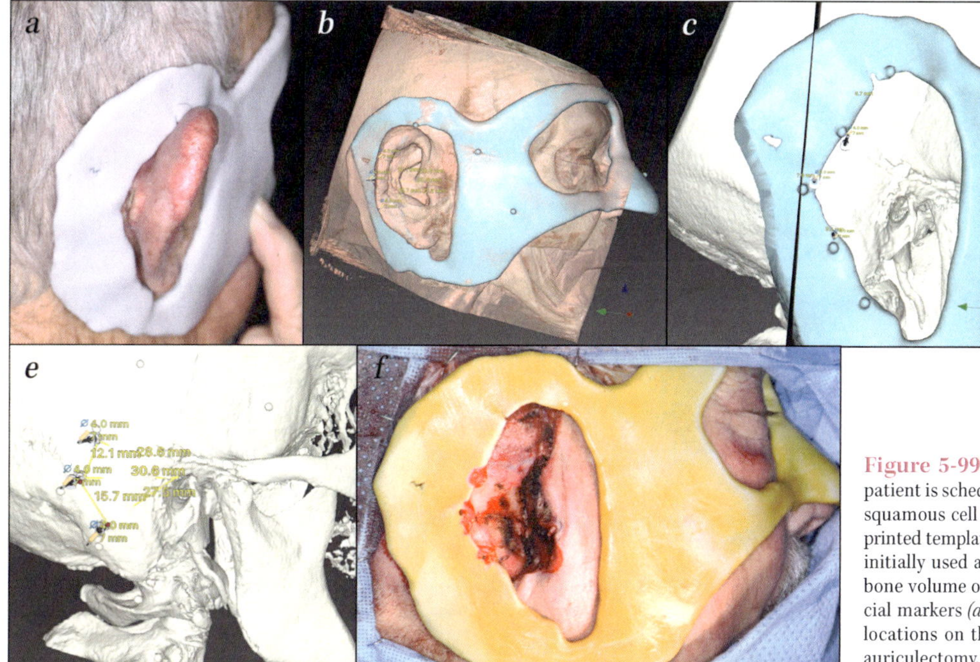

Figure 5-99 A skin-supported surgical template. The patient is scheduled for a total auriculectomy to remove a squamous cell carcinoma. *(a)* The digitally designed and printed template is tried on the patient. *(b, c, and d)* It was initially used as a radiographic template to identify the bone volume of the possible implant sites. Note the fiducial markers *(arrows)*. *(e)* The sites are selected and their locations on the template are noted. *(f)* Following the auriculectomy, the template is seated and used to identify the previously selected implant positions.

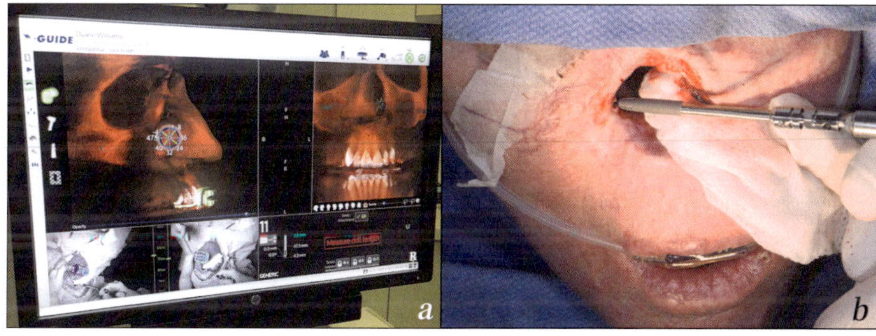

Figure 5-100 *(a and b)* Dynamic navigation permits placement of implants into locations with difficult access. In this patient zygomatic implants were to be placed to retain a nasal prosthesis.

studied the accuracy of these templates designed for guided implant placement in orbital sites and the auricular region. The surgical templates were either skin supported or held in place with bone fixation screws. The skin-supported templates were designed to permit flapless implant placement. Significant deviations were noted especially those secured with bone fixation screws. Based on this report, it appears that dynamic navigation may offer a better alternative when absolute accuracy of implant placement is required (see below).

Advantage of two-stage implant placement

As mentioned above two-stage implant placement is preferred when craniofacial implants are placed. Surgical closure over the site enables more predictable osseointegration, particularly in poor-quality bone sites or if the implant site is overprepared and initial implant immobilization is suboptimal. During the second stage, the major goal is to reduce the thickness of the overlying soft tissues to less than 5 mm as well as to create immobile tissues around the implants. This approach will lead to the formation of epithelial cuffs around the abutments and will promote healthy peri-implant soft tissues. The stage-two surgical exposure procedure is usually performed three to four months after the stage-one procedure. Healing time for osseointegration is extended to six to eight months when initial implant anchorage is judged to be suboptimal and for irradiated sites. Stage-two surgery may be performed with general anesthesia or local anesthesia with conscious sedation.

Dynamic navigation

Dynamic navigation (Fig 5-100) allows the surgeon to visualize in real time the preparation of the implant site. Many patients with rhinectomy or midfacial defects present with limited access to the proposed implant sites, particularly the zygoma, and this can make accurate implant placement problematic. Moreover, in these sites, it may be difficult to design and fabricate surgical drill guides that are sufficiently stable and well retained to permit precise implant placement. Under these circumstances, dynamic navigation permits the surgeon to prepare the osteotomy sites and place the implants with appropriate precision (Tso et al., 2021; Jorba-Garcia et al., 2021). Prior to surgery, a CBCT scan is obtained to allow for virtual implant

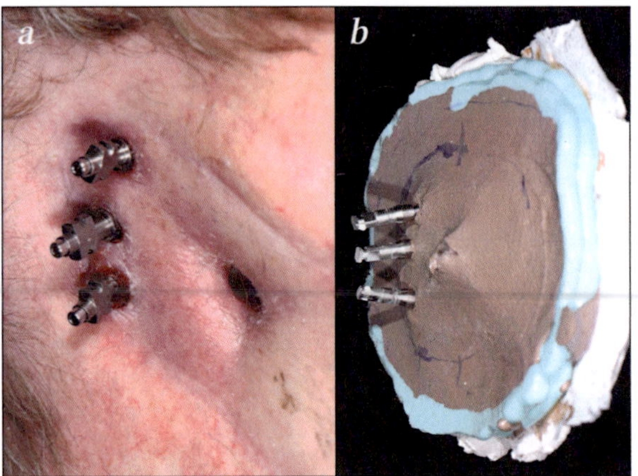

Figure 5-101 *(a)* Pickup type impression copings are secured directly to the implants. *(b)* Impression with the implant fixture analogs attached.

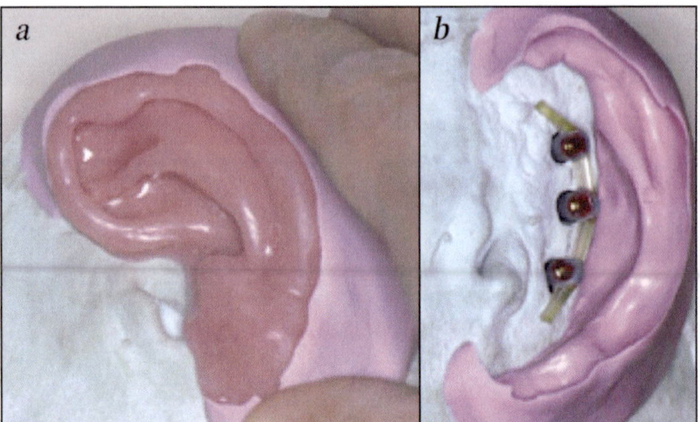

Figure 5-102 *(a)* A silicone template is fabricated as an aid to fabricate the tissue bar. *(b)* Pattern for the tissue bar.

planning using special software. Triplet reflective marker spheres on the handpiece, plus three marker spheres secured to the patient and an overhead infrared camera, position the handpiece in relation to the patient's computed tomography scan. A real-time image merging the handpiece, preoperative CBCT scan, and planned implant position is generated for use on an intraoperative computer. Patients can be scanned and surgical planning accomplished on the same day as implant surgery. Dynamic navigation also allows a flapless approach, which will reduce postoperative morbidity and result in less disruption of the local vasculature.

Prosthetic procedures

Auricular defects

Approximately six weeks are required for healing of the soft tissues following stage-two surgery. The impression site is prepared as described previously. The authors favor implant-level impressions because we prefer to connect the tissue bar directly to the implant platform. When implant-level impressions are made, impression copings are secured directly to the implants (Fig 5-101). We prefer the pickup type of impression copings, linked together with plaster, resin, or another suitable material.

When abutment-level impressions are made, the healing abutments are removed and the soft tissue depth from the implant flange to the skin surface is measured with a periodontal probe. A standard abutment that extends 1 to 2 mm above the skin surface is seated on the implant. *Given the short length of craniofacial implants, while their abutment screws are tightened, a smooth-surfaced clamp should hold the abutment in place to provide counter torque on the implant.* Impression copings are then connected to the abutments.

A thin layer of suitable elastic impression material is syringed around the impression copings and the tissues of the defect. Gauze and a thin layer of adhesive are applied followed by succeeding layers of impression plaster (described earlier) to avoid distorting the underlying soft tissues and to provide support for the impression material. Care must be taken to maintain access to the screws holding the impression copings in place, because they must be loosened to permit removal of the impression.

After the impression has been removed, implant fixture or abutment analogs are secured to the impression copings embedded within the impression. The master cast is prepared in the usual way. The manufacturer's recommendations for the water-powder ratio should be followed carefully when pouring up the impression. The wax sculpting of the prosthesis is prepared and tried on the patient to ensure that the pattern faithfully restores contour and symmetry and is properly oriented.

Several attachment systems have been used to retain facial prostheses, including bar-clip assemblies, magnets, and O-rings. The retentive apparatus must fit within the confines of the prosthesis without affecting its contour or symmetry. The authors favor the bar-clip systems for auricular defects because these systems provide superior retention. In addition, implant-connecting bars overcome misalignment and improper positioning of implants more easily than individual attachments. Moreover, from a biomechanical perspective, it is desirable to splint all the implants together with a rigid implant-connecting bar (Rangert, 1997; Mendonca et al., 2014; Yoda et al., 2013). In this way, the stresses delivered to the implants will be distributed more equitably among the implants minimizing the risk of implant overload of an individual implant.

Until recently, conventional methods using the lost-wax technique have been used to fabricate the implant-connecting bar. The wax sculpture is positioned on the master cast, and a template of silicone or other suitable material is fabricated to aid in the design of the implant-connecting bar (Fig 5-102). A wax pattern of the proposed bar is then developed that fits beneath the antihelix. Stability of the prosthesis will be enhanced if the bar is shaped in the form of an arc rather than a straight line. The pattern is invested and cast with a gold alloy. Alternatively, a round gold bar may be bent or sectioned and soldered to gold cylinders that connect to the abutments or implants.

CAD/CAM techniques can be used to design and fabricate the implant-connecting bar, and these techniques are rapidly supplanting conventional methods. If the bar is to be designed and fabricated digitally, the master cast with the wax pattern is scanned. The digital files are merged with the virtual design software. CAD software is

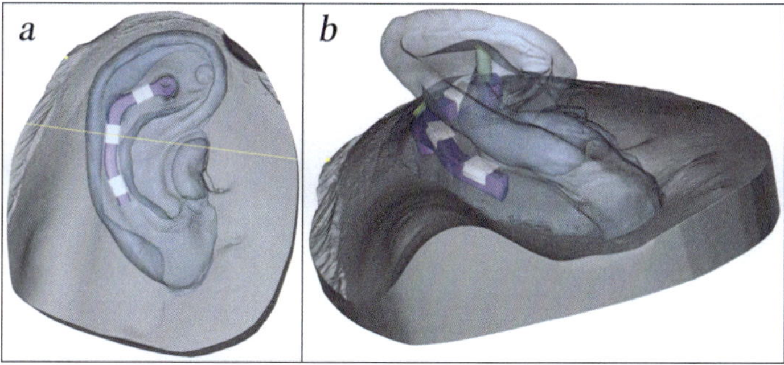

Figure 5-103 The bar can also be designed digitally.

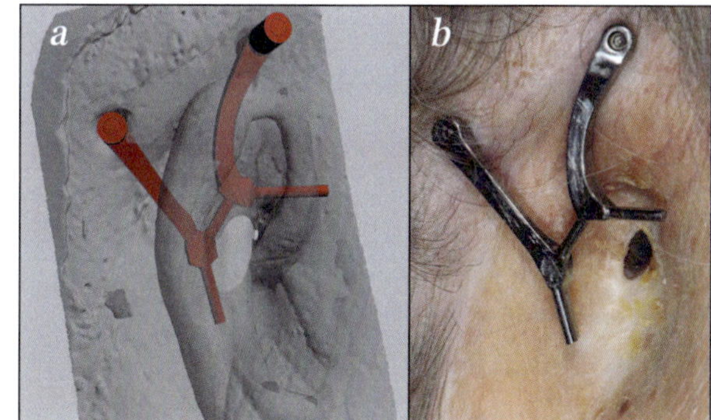

Figure 5-104 *(a and b)* A digitally designed implant-connecting bar for a patient following an auriculectomy and temporal bone resection, hence the posterior superior positioning of the implants. The retentive portion of the bar is positioned beneath the antihelix.

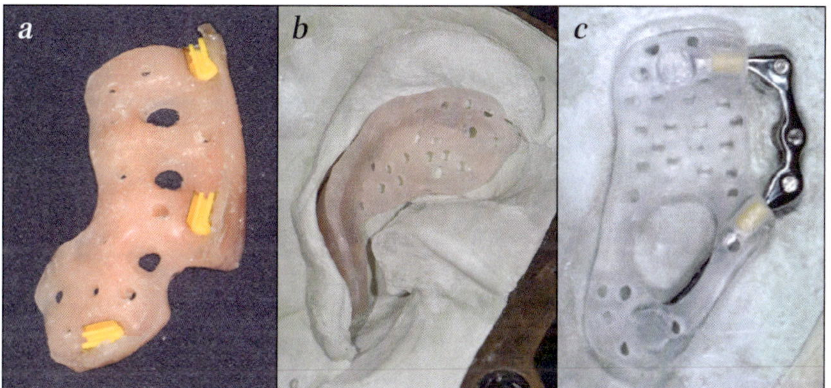

Figure 5-105 Acrylic resin retentive substructures and retentive elements designed to be embedded within the silicone prosthesis. *(a and b)* The substructure is colored to match the skin tones of the patient. *(c)* This substructure is of acrylic clear resin.

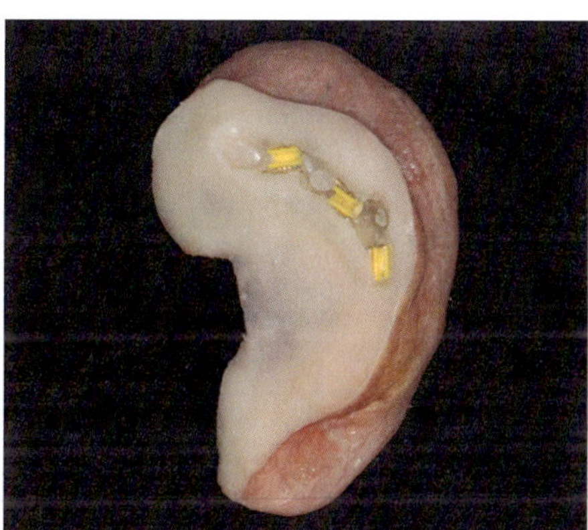

Figure 5-106 Completed ear prosthesis with the clips positioned.

then used by the clinician/laboratory technician to complete the initial design of the implant-connecting bar (Figs 5-103 and 5-104). These implant-connecting bars can be milled out of grade 5 titanium or zirconia and can be made to fit multiple implants with great precision. However, not all CAD systems allow control of the tissue side contours, and so frequently they need to be manually recontoured.

The finished implant-connecting bar is taken to the patient and attached to the implants. The undersurface of the bar should be slightly concave and highly polished to facilitate daily hygiene. If the bar does not fit passively, a solder/laser-welding relation record is made with cyanoacrylate or pattern resin. The bar is removed and embedded within a thin matrix of improved dental stone. The water-powder ratio of the stone prepared for this template must be measured carefully. The bar is soldered (gold alloy bars) or laser welded (titanium bar) as required, and the fit is verified both on the stone template and on the patient. If the bar is made of zirconia, the clinician must retake the impression and begin the design and fabrication process anew.

An acrylic resin retentive substructure housing the attachments is then designed and fabricated to fit within the confines of the silicone prosthesis. It can be made of either clear acrylic resin or a resin matching the skin tones of the patient. The retentive substructure should extend into the body of the silicone prosthesis and possess sufficient surface area so that the bond between the substructure and the silicone prosthesis will not fail during insertion or removal of the prosthesis. Multiple perforations in the retentive substructure will increase the surface area (Fig 5-105). Prior to processing a primer or bonding agent is applied to the resin substructure to enhance the bond between the silicone and the retentive substructure. Several primers have been tested when bonding acrylic resin to silicone elastomers. See section above entitled "Primers used to bond acrylic resin substructures housing attachments to silicone elastomers" for the latest research regarding the selection of the primer and which is best suited for the prosthetic material used.

The auricular wax pattern is flasked in the customary manner (see Fig 5-48). Following wax elimination, the bar and retentive substructure are attached to the master cast, facial prosthetic material is injected, and the flasks are closed and allowed to cure. Intrinsic and extrinsic coloration are applied as previously described, the attachments are secured to the acrylic resin substructure, and the prosthesis is prepared for delivery (Fig 5-106).

The patient is instructed in the proper use of appropriate hygiene aids such as orthodontic floss (e.g., Superfloss, Oral-B), proxybrushes, cotton-tipped applicators, and end-tufted brushes.

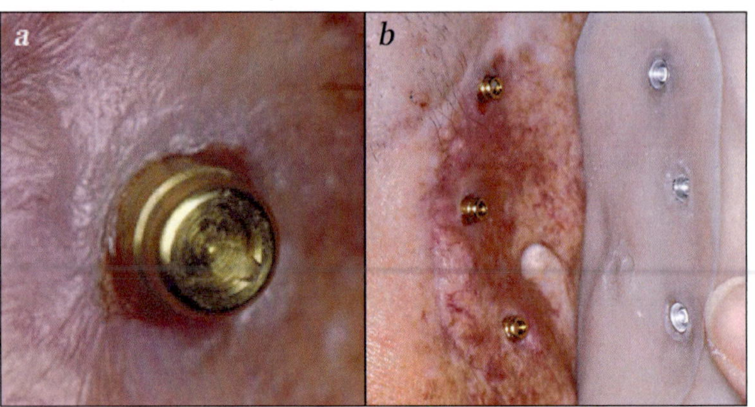

Figure 5-107 *(a)* Individual retentive attachment. *(b)* Individual attachments attached to implants used to retain an ear prosthesis.

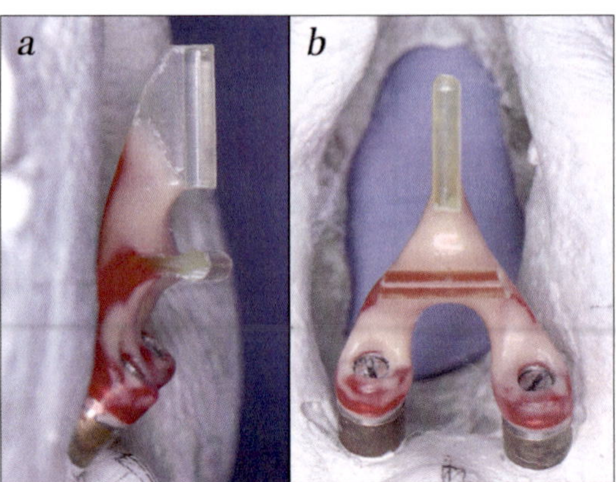

Figure 5-108 Wax pattern of an implant-connecting bar. There should be a vertical and horizontal component to idealize retention and stability. The bar should fit within the confines of the nasal prosthesis and not impair the nasal airway.

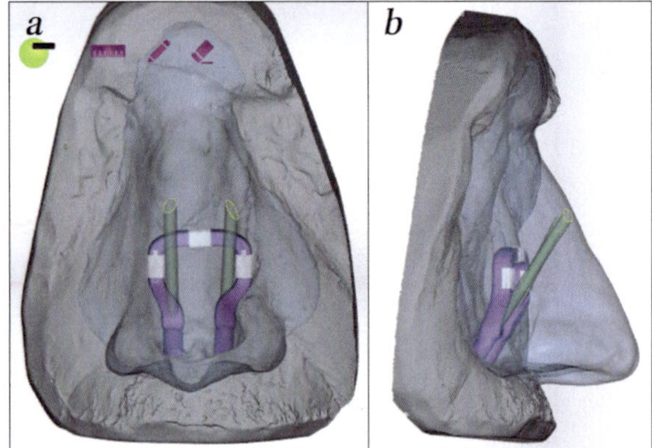

Figure 5-109 *(a and b)* Bars can also be digitally designed.

All patients should be assigned to a three-month recall schedule for the first year. At follow-up, the skin surrounding the implants may be irritated. Most skin problems are reversed after removal of accumulations of keratin, sebaceous secretions, or other debris and improvement in home care compliance (Henry, 1992). Persistent skin irritation can sometimes be resolved by the use of a metal-ceramic or zirconia implant-connecting bar (see Fig 5-92).

Individual attachments have also been used to retain ear prostheses (Fig 5-107). They are easy to use, and hygiene access is excellent, but they offer less retention and stability (de Sousa and Mattos, 2008). However, in our experience, the rate of implant loss is higher with the use of individual attachments as compared to implant-connecting bars, especially in irradiated patients. This is probably due to the biomechanical advantages gained when implants are splinted together (Wang et al., 2002; Mendonca et al., 2014; Yoda et al., 2013). As a result of our experience, we no longer employ this method of retention for auricular prostheses.

Nasal defects

Fabrication of an implant-retained nasal prosthesis is similar to fabrication of an auricular prosthesis. Impressions of the implants and adjacent facial structures are made as previously described, and a master cast is retrieved. The bar can be fabricated with conventional methods (Fig 5-108) or with CAD-CAM (Fig 5-109).

In most rhinectomy patients, sites for two implants will be available in the floor of the nose. The glabella region is considered a secondary site. Our success in this region using short craniofacial implants has been poor (Roumanas et al., 2002). The authors seldom use this site to restore rhinectomy defects, but if we do, we employ longer dental-type implants.

As with auricular defects, an implant-connecting bar and clip retentive mechanism are preferred (Fig 5-110a, b, and c), although a number of other retention designs have been described (Rubenstein, 1995). Magnetic retention is recommended when only a single implant is available. The retention achieved is satisfactory but the defect must be engaged somewhat to prevent accidental lateral displacement of the prosthesis (Fig 5-110d and e). The corrosion of the magnets seen with the early systems has largely been overcome by the use of laser-welded keepers.

The bar design should be kept simple, allowing easy access for cleaning around all areas. Because of the possibility that nasal mucous secretions will accumulate around the bar, hygiene is especially important. Our preferred design is a bar-clip design in which one bar segment is arranged vertically and another horizontally (see Figs 5-108–5-110). This design provides adequate resistance to lateral displacement and excellent retention. An acrylic resin retentive substructure housing the plastic retentive clips is designed and fabricated, and the nasal prosthesis is completed in a manner similar to that previously described for auricular prostheses (Fig 5-111).

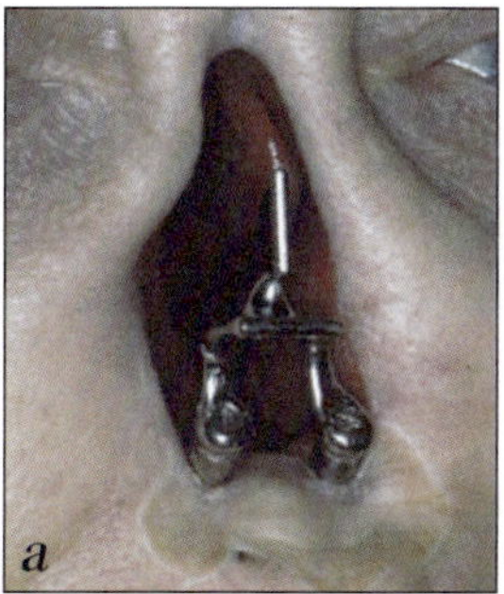
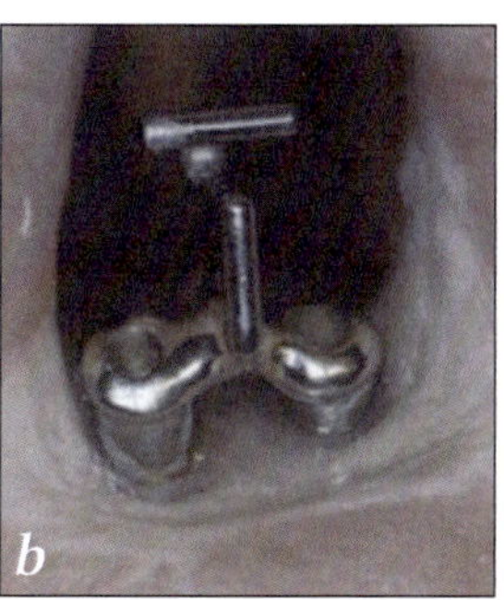
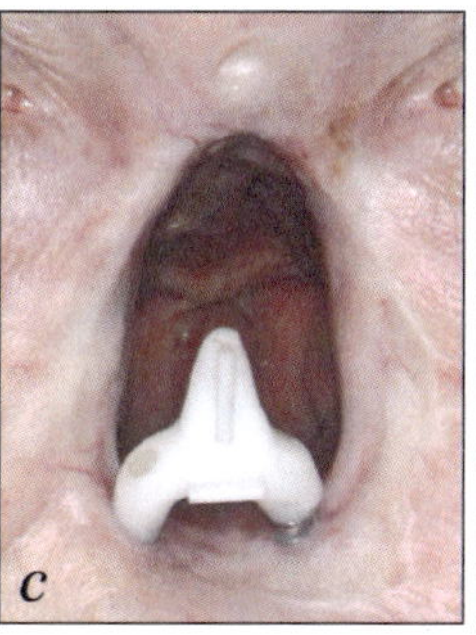
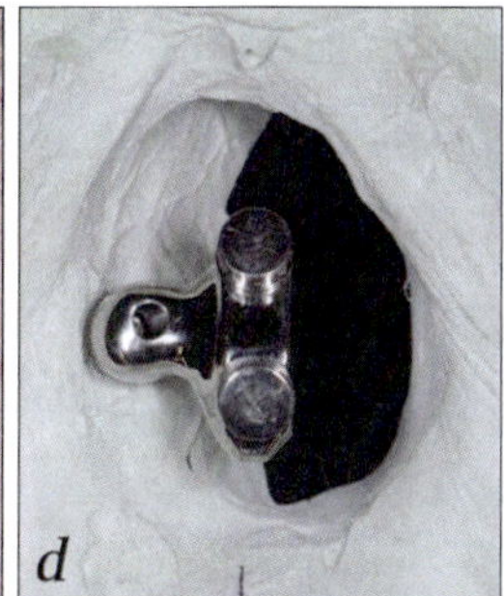
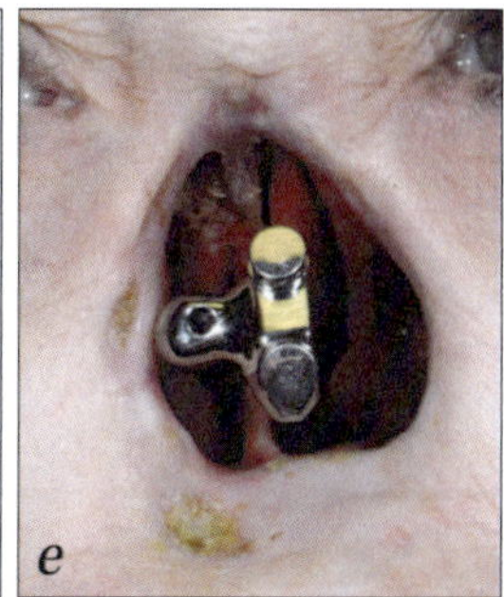

Figure 5-110 *(a, b, and c)* Bar-clip attachments with implant-connecting bar designs for use in nasal defects. The two "Hader bar" segments are perpendicular to one another. The bar depicted in "c" is milled from zirconia. *(d and e)* Magnetic attachments. The magnets should be slightly divergent to enhance the stability of the prosthesis. The attachment apparatus is designed not to interfere with nasal contours or nasal airflow.

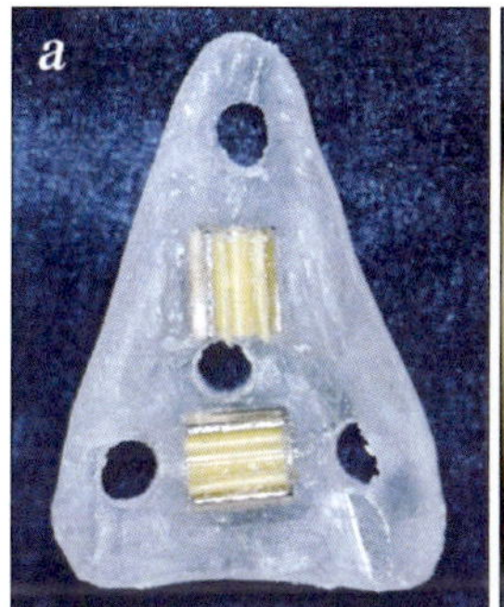
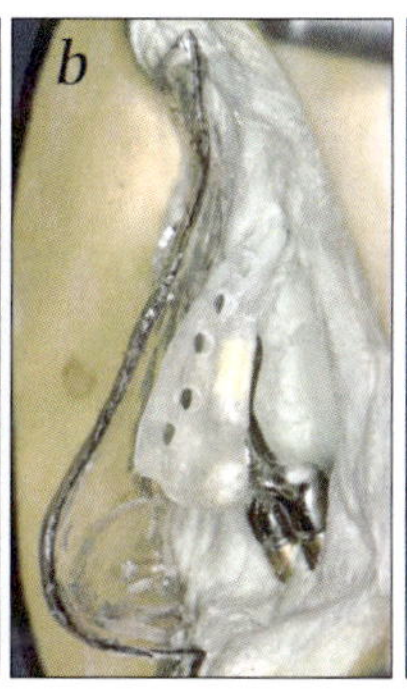
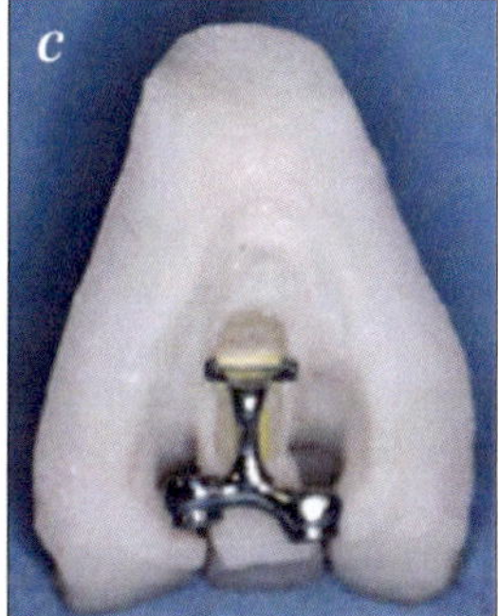
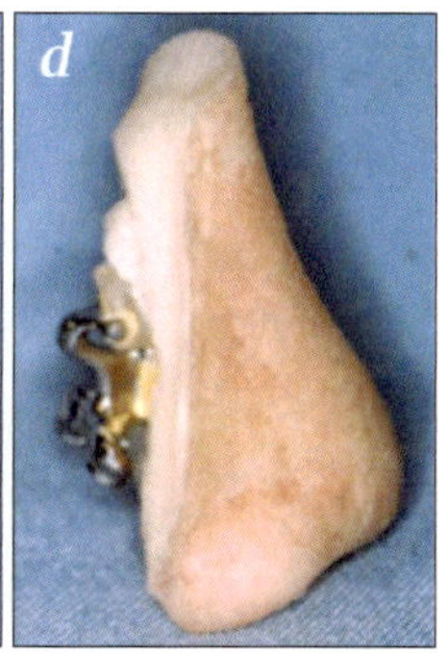

Figure 5-111 Bar-clip design for retention of a nasal prosthesis. *(a and b)* The acrylic resin retentive substructure must fit within the confines of the nasal prosthesis. *(c and d)* Finished bar and prosthesis.

When magnetic attachments are employed, two magnets with 20 degrees of divergence are suggested to enhance the stability of the nasal prosthesis. The authors prefer magnets with a 3.0-Ncm withdrawal strength. Less maintenance with magnetic attachments is expected compared with bar-clip systems. Moreover, magnetic attachments provide a degree of self-alignment, making it easier for the patient to position the prosthesis. However, increased prosthetic space is required by the magnets relative to other commonly used attachment systems. Corrosion of the magnets because of the high humidity at this site limited the life span of the previous generation of magnets. However, magnets are now available encased in laser-welded titanium, and hopefully, this innovation will address this issue. Another important consideration when using magnets is the patient's future need for magnetic resonance imaging (MRI), which may be a part of their routine cancer surveillance. Prior to a scheduled MRI, the patient would need to be seen for removal of the magnetic attachment apparatus and then again subsequently for replacement.

The prosthesis is delivered and hygiene instruction is provided. Soft tissue complications have been less frequent around implants placed in the floor of the nose, probably because the implants are more easily visualized by the patient and are more accessible for hygiene (Nishimura et al., 1996).

Orbital defects

Techniques for fabrication of implant-retained orbital prostheses are similar to those described for auricular and nasal implant-retained prostheses. Impressions are made and a master cast is retrieved. The bar can be fabricated with conventional methods or with CAD-CAM. If conventional methods are used, the wax sculpture is completed, a silicone template is constructed, and the implant-connecting bar is designed and fabricated to fit within the confines of the orbital prosthesis without distorting its contours. If the implant-connecting bar is to be designed and fabricated digitally, the master cast and the wax pattern are scanned. The two digital files are merged with the virtual design software. CAD software is then used by the clinician/laboratory technician to complete the design of the implant-connecting bar, and the bar is milled out of grade 5 titanium or zirconia (Fig 5-112).

As with the nasal prosthesis, methods of retention vary (Rubenstein, 1995). We prefer magnetic retention in conventional orbital exenteration defects, particularly in older patients who may have difficulty positioning the prosthesis with a bar-clip system. The ease of insertion of magnetically retained prosthesis in such patients outweighs the negative aspects, such as the risk of corrosion of the magnets and decreased retention. The retention bar should be designed to interface with three or four magnets arranged in a triangular or circular fashion (Figs 5-113 and 5-114).

For large defects, an acrylic resin retentive substructure that houses the magnetic attachments is prepared (Fig 5-113b and c). For small defects where space is limited, the magnetic attachments may be secured to the ocular portion of the prosthesis (Fig 5-114). In these smaller defects, consideration should be given to the use of individual magnets because they will require less space than a bar-magnet construction. The ocular portion is then embedded within the silicone prosthesis. The prosthesis should be perforated to permit aeration of the defect (Fig 5-115). Instructions for hygiene and maintenance of the prosthesis are provided at delivery.

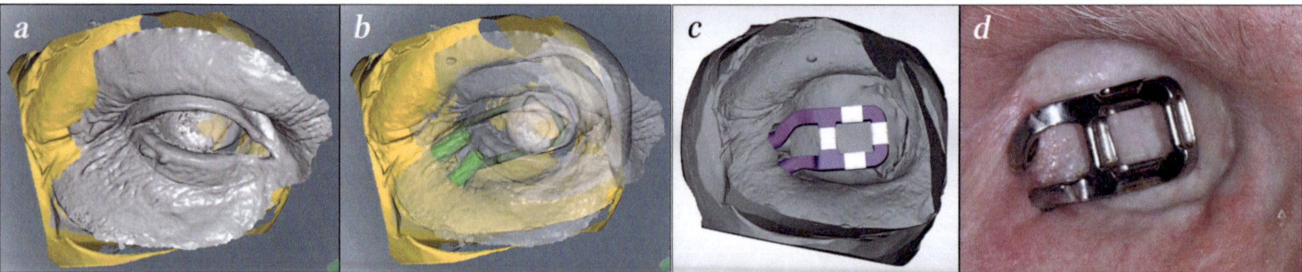

Figure 5-112 *(a and b)* The master cast and the orbital wax pattern with the ocular are scanned and the files merged. *(c)* The digital design of the implant-connecting bar. *(d)* The milled titanium bar in position.

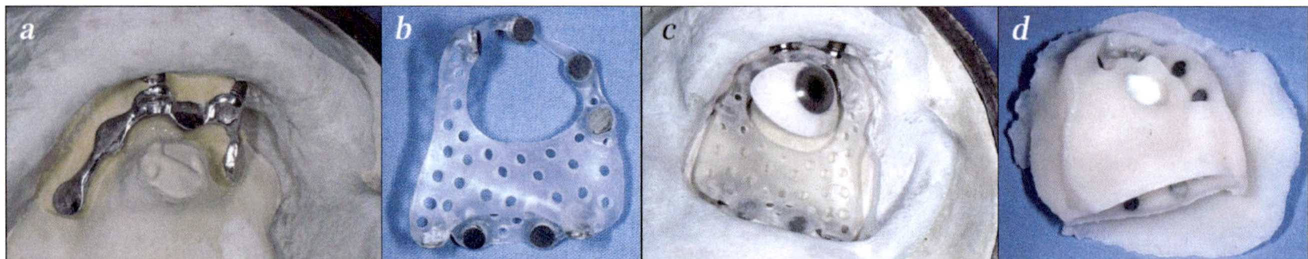

Figure 5-113 Magnetic retention for an orbital prosthesis. *(a)* The tissue bar is secured to the master cast. *(b)* Magnetic attachments are housed within the acrylic resin retentive substructure. *(c)* The retentive substructure is seated and the ocular prosthesis is secured to the plaster index. *(d and e)* Silicone casting with magnetic attachments (courtesy of Dr. Michael Hamada).

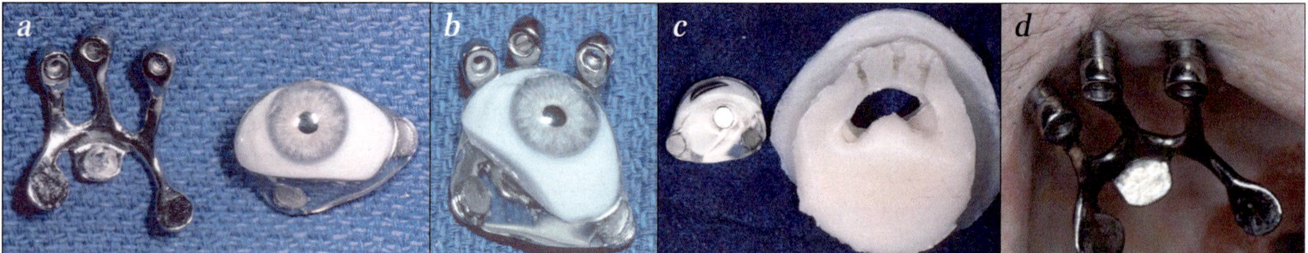

Figure 5-114 *(a and b)* The ocular prosthesis with magnets were incorporated. It is designed to *(c)* be embedded within the silicone orbital prosthesis and engage the *(d)* implant-connecting bar.

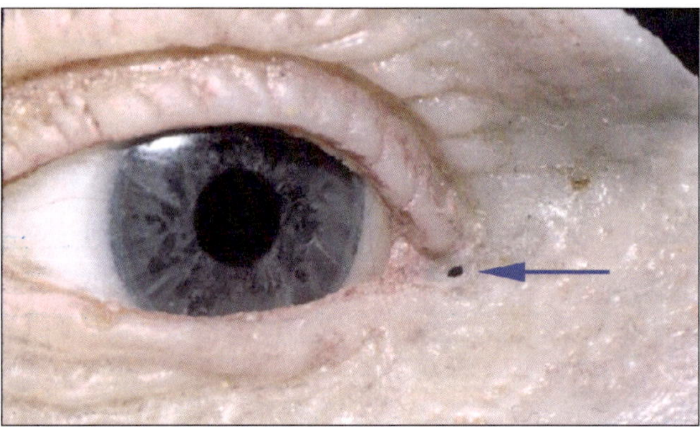

Figure 5-115 Perforation of the inner canthus *(arrow)* provides aeration for the skin around the implants.

Hygiene procedures are more difficult to perform for patients with orbital defects. Compliance suffers, so these patients demonstrate a higher rate of skin irritation around their implants (Nishimura et al., 1998). These patients have monocular vision and their compromised depth perception makes it difficult to visualize the plane of the implant bar. In addition, many of the patients are elderly and have compromised manual dexterity and may have difficulty manipulating the hygiene aids. Most elderly patients require eyeglasses for close vision and their presence overlying the defect complicates access. Therefore, it is advisable to train a patient's spouse or a friend to clean the bar and implants. These patients should be assigned to a strict three-month follow-up schedule because severe infections can result if appropriate hygiene is not maintained (see Fig 5-91a).

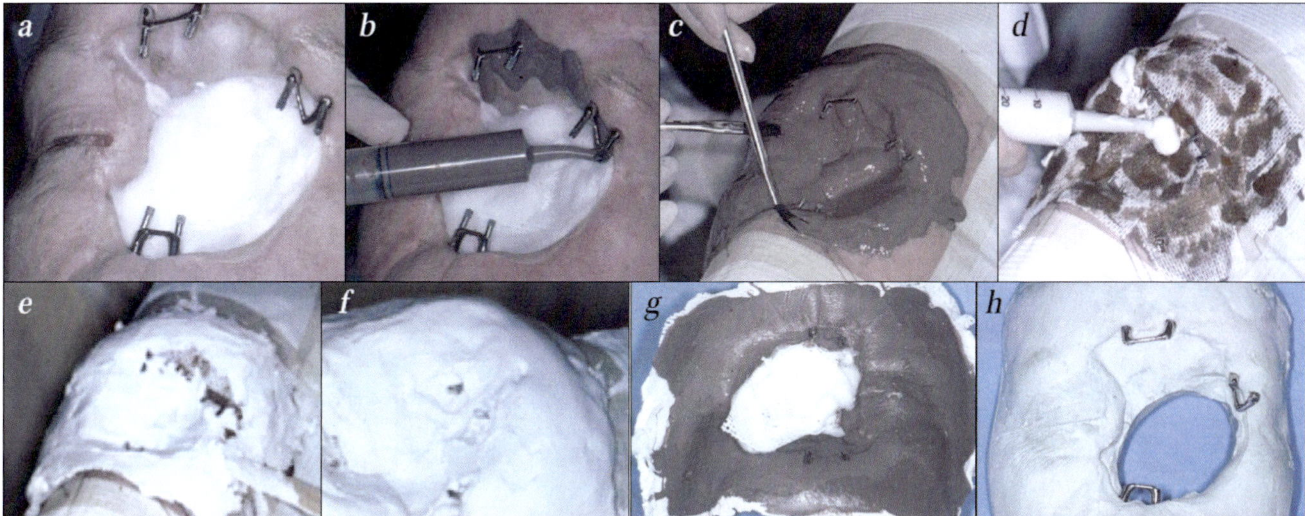

Figure 5-116 Impression procedures for an orbital-nasal-cheek prosthesis. *(a)* The patient is positioned and draped. Implant tissue bars (previously fabricated) have been secured. *(b and c)* A thin layer of polysulfide impression material is applied. *(d)* Gauze is applied with a layer of adhesive for retention of the plaster backing. *(e)* The first layer of plaster is thin. *(f)* Succeeding layers will support the impression material. *(g)* Completed impression. *(h)* The master cast has been poured in layers to minimize distortion.

Summary: Craniofacial implants

This technology has had a remarkable impact on our ability to restore facial defects with facial prostheses. The improved retention and the relatively high predictability of these implants, with the exception of the orbit, have dramatically improved patient acceptance and, combined with the aesthetic outcomes, have led to this method becoming the preferred choice of most clinical centers when restoring facial defects. However, significant challenges remain, and many are related to the limited life span of the facial prosthesis itself as opposed to the implants (Visser et al., 2008). In one report, the average life span of an implant-retained facial prosthesis averaged only 14.1 to 17.6 months depending on the site of the defect (Karakoca et al., 2010). The most common causes of prosthesis failure were discoloration of the prosthesis, tearing of the margins of the prosthesis, and loss of attachment between the acrylic resin substructure housing the attachments and the silicone of the facial prosthesis. The resolution of many of these difficulties awaits the development of improved facial materials.

Large Orbital, Nasal, and Cheek Defects

A one-piece prosthesis is usually preferred for large facial defects involving the orbital, nasal, and cheek regions that do not involve the lip or the oral cavity. In these large defects, craniofacial implants are a necessity if the prosthesis is to be retained effectively. It is extremely difficult to retain such large prostheses with adhesives or by engaging undercuts.

Accurate impressions are difficult to obtain because the skin and soft tissues bordering the defect may be quite thick and mobile and may not have an underlying bony foundation. These tissues are easily compressed by the impression material or distorted by changes in posture while making the impression. When possible, the patient should be seated in a semiupright position.

The following technique will minimize tissue distortion and compression (Fig 5-116). First, select areas in the defect that will not be engaged by the prosthesis are blocked out with gauze. A very thin layer of a suitable light-body impression material is then painted onto the tissues bordering the defect. A thin layer of gauze is embedded within the impression material before it polymerizes, and a very thin layer of adhesive is applied. It is useful to dilute the adhesive with a suitable solvent before its application. This is followed by succeeding thin layers of quick-set impression plaster. This technique will minimize compression of the skin and tissues adjacent to the defect. The impression is removed, and the cast is prepared in an improved dental stone, being careful to observe water-powder rations recommended by the manufacturer. It is poured in layers to minimize distortion.

Digital impressions of such large facial defects are theoretically possible, but as yet, the models printed from these scans do not appear to be sufficiently accurate. The most common systems use trigonometric triangulation and work by projecting a pattern of light onto the patient. One or more sensors/cameras look at the shape of the light pattern and calculate the distance of every point in the field of view to map the surface of the defect and adjacent structures. The data retrieved is used to develop three-dimensional images and print casts. This approach holds much promise, since the scans can be obtained with the patient in an upright position, precluding the risk of gravity-driven distortion of the tissues bordering the defect secondary to the postural position. Also, the distortion of the tissues secondary to the weight of the impression material is eliminated. Scanning time is relatively rapid, generally just a few seconds. As the technologies associated with the making of the scans and the printing of the casts/models become more refined, and as the cost of the armamentarium is reduced, it is expected that this technique will eventually supplant conventional impression methods.

A wax sculpture is developed on the master cast. Restoration of presurgical contours and symmetry may not be possible or desirable. In these defects, significant distortion of contour, symmetry,

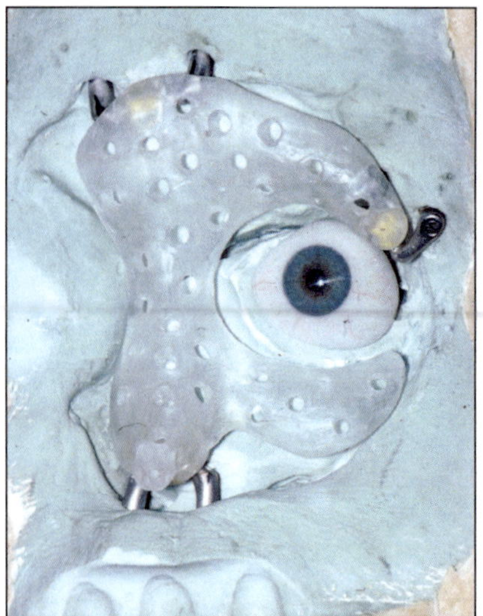

Figure 5-117. The acrylic resin retentive substructure houses the attachments and fits within the confines of the silicone prosthesis.

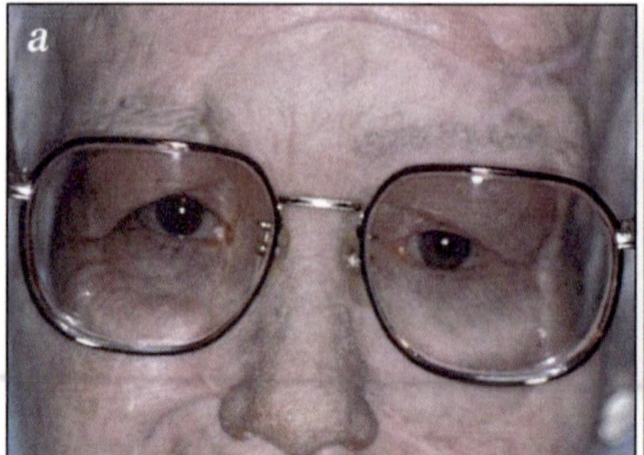

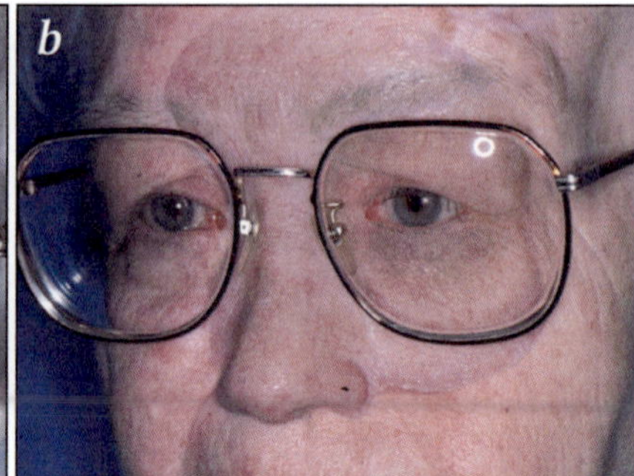

Figure 5-118 The prosthesis for the patient shown in Fig 5-116.

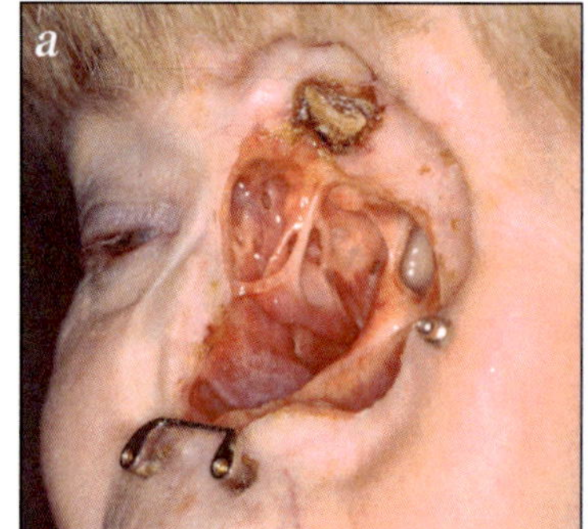

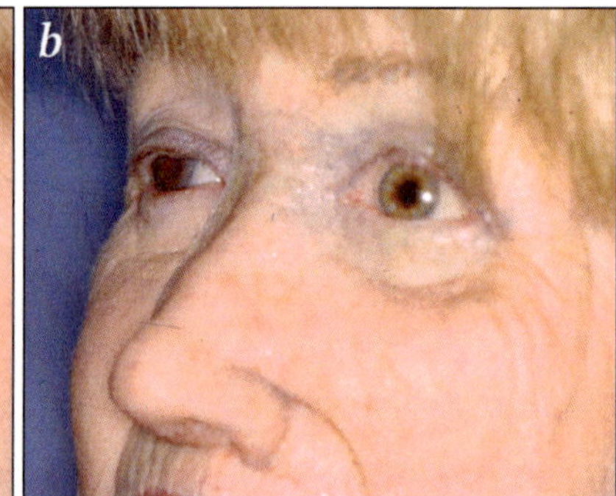

Figure 5-119 *(a)* A large orbital nasal cheek defect. Dental type implants were placed in the floor of the nose and the malar body. *(b)* Prosthesis in position.

and skin coloration may be present secondary to multiple surgeries and courses of radiation therapy. For best results, the contours, texture, and color of the prosthesis must blend with those of the patient. Matching the surface texture of the prosthesis with the existing skin is particularly important. In some areas, it may be necessary to score the cast in order to ensure proper adaptation of the margins of the prosthesis to the underlying skin.

The pattern is flasked, and an acrylic resin retentive substructure is designed and fabricated to house the attachments (Fig 5-117). It must fit within the confines of the facial prosthesis. The prosthesis is then processed in the customary way. Intrinsic and extrinsic coloration are applied as described earlier. Examples of the patient outcomes are shown in Figs 5-118 and 5-119.

Large Midfacial Defects Extending into the Oral Cavity

Advanced tumors of the midfacial region occasionally require extensive surgical removal to eradicate the disease. The resulting surgical defect may involve loss of both extraoral and intraoral structures, including portions of the nose, upper lip, cheek, and orbital contents. Segments of the maxilla, mandible, associated soft tissues, and teeth may also be involved. The functional impairment produced by such extirpative procedures is severe. Loss of the integrity of the oral cavity results in difficulty in mastication, swallowing, control of saliva, and speech production. These functional disabilities, in combination with the accompanying cosmetic disfigurement, usually have a severe psychologic impact on the patient and the family.

However, many patients with such surgical defects have been rehabilitated successfully with prosthetic restorations. Speech and swallowing may be restored to nearly normal levels, and control of saliva and mastication may be improved. The cosmetic appearance of the patient, although far from ideal, makes participation in social activities possible.

The best results are obtained when all members of the therapy and rehabilitation team have the opportunity to see and discuss the methods used in the rehabilitation of the patient prior to treatment. Pretreatment consultation gives the prosthodontist the opportunity to obtain records, such as photographs, oral and facial impressions, and scans, that will be useful during fabrication of the oral-facial prostheses. This consultation also provides the prosthodontist with the opportunity to explain to the patient the potential functional and aesthetic outcomes achieved with prosthetic rehabilitation. The patient's successful adjustment to the postsurgical defect often is dependent on his or her realistic understanding of the degree of rehabilitation afforded by the future restoration.

Surgical reconstruction is virtually impossible for large midfacial defects because of their size, extent, and complexity. Facial transplants, although theoretically possible and a viable option for some,

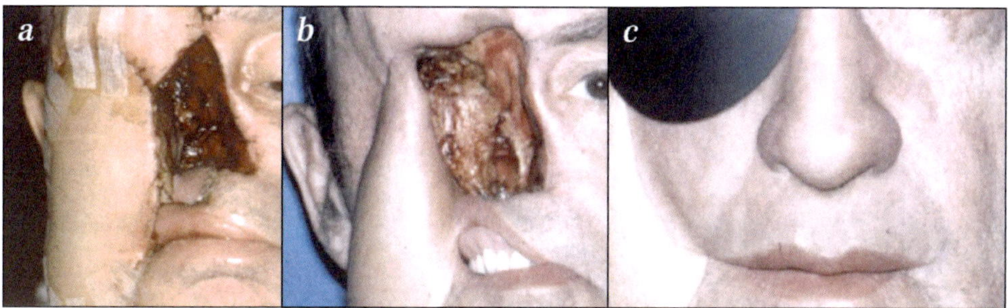

Figure 5-120 *(a)* The lateral portion of the face and the upper lip have been reconstructed. *(b)* the lip portion has retracted superiorly. *(c)* The lip is overlaid with the prosthesis to restore speech articulation and aesthetic appearance.

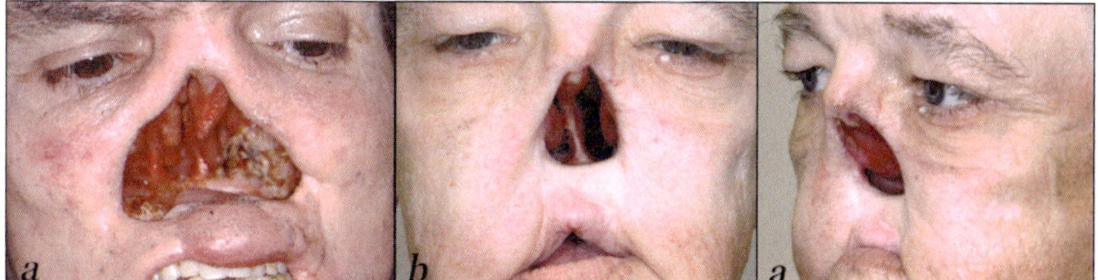

Figure 5-121 *(a, b, and c)* Most reconstructed upper lips become heavily scarred and retracted posteriorly and superiorly, restricting oral access.

are not available to most patients with such defects for a variety of technical and logistical reasons.

When the facial defect extends to the oral cavity, the prosthetic prognosis is primarily dependent on the presence and condition of the teeth, the nature of the implant sites available, the amount and contour of the remaining hard palate, the functional status of the lower lip, and the motivation and adaptability of the patient. The presence of a small strip of upper lip, if it is sensate, is of some value because secretions can be detected and more easily confined to the oral cavity. However, if the entire upper lip is resected, it is not advisable to reconstruct it surgically (Fig 5-120). These reconstructions frequently are improperly positioned, heavily scarred, and immobile. Moreover, the reconstructed commissures are relatively inflexible, and access to the oral cavity is compromised as a result. Such reconstructed lips are usually retracted posteriorly and superiorly (Fig 5-121) and must be overlayed with the facial prosthesis if normal lip valving during speech is to be restored. In addition, the poor aesthetics of the reconstructed upper lip tend to focus attention on the defect and the midfacial prosthesis. The small oral opening and the impaired flexibility of the reconstructed oral stoma make it difficult for the prosthodontist to fabricate accompanying oral prostheses and make insertion and removal of these prostheses difficult for the patient. In addition, oral hygiene procedures will be compromised by the impaired oral access, predisposing the remaining dentition to caries and periodontal disease.

Equally important to the successful tolerance of these restorations is the adaptability of the patient. Their emotional responses should be anticipated. The importance of social service counseling and consultations in the care of these patients cannot be overemphasized. In some instances, patients will not accept the restoration because of unrealistic expectations. The clinician must prepare the patient for the prosthesis and explain the level of rehabilitation achievable. Experienced denture wearers seem to do best with these prostheses. They have learned to tolerate and manipulate foreign objects within their mouths and generally have mastered the delicate balance between function and stability when wearing their prostheses (Beumer and Calcaterra, 1976; Marunick et al., 1985). These prostheses may be of great value in the care of terminally ill cancer patients (Cantor et al., 1968). Limited life expectancy should not preclude such prosthetic therapy. These restorations give the patient the opportunity to live the remainder of his or her life in a more comfortable and dignified manner.

Surgical modifications that may be indicated at the time of tumor resection include *(1)* retention of teeth that can be used to support and retain the combined facial and intraoral prosthesis; *(2)* preparation of the soft tissue bed so that undercut areas are created for retention; *(3)* placement of skin grafts to minimize tissue distortion or contraction of the adjacent facial tissues; and *(4)* placement of osseointegrated implants for retention and support of the future prosthesis (Fig 5-122).

If soft tissue undercuts are created surgically, they should be lined with split-thickness skin. Failure to do so results in excessive contracture and, in some cases, loss of the created undercut. In addition, these tissues will usually become epithelialized with nonkeratinized squamous or respiratory epithelium, thereby limiting their usefulness as a prosthesis-bearing area. Keratinized tissue at the anterior palatal margin will also increase the bearing surface available for the prosthesis. If the nasal floor of the residual hard palate is skin grafted, this surface may be used to retain and support the midfacial prosthesis.

Placement of osseointegrated implants has had a dramatic impact on the function of these large and heretofore difficult to retain midfacial prostheses. Possible sites for implants include the lateral orbital rim, the floor of the nose, the residual portions of the zygomatic bone, and the glabella region. These large facial prostheses can be effectively retained with implants. When possible, the implants should be placed at the time of the tumor resection.

The prosthetic prognosis is primarily dependent on the presence and condition of teeth, the bone volume of the implant sites available, the amount and contour of the remaining alveolar ridges and hard palate, the functional status of the lower lip, and the motivation and adaptability of the patient (Fig 5-123). Oral function can be restored to impressive levels and accompanied by an acceptable aesthetic result, but for this outcome to be achievable, there must be a solid foundation upon which to build the oral prosthesis.

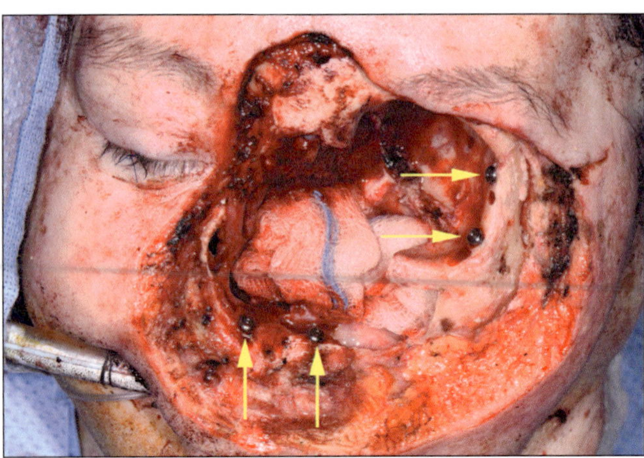

Figure 5-122 Large midfacial defect. Following resection of the tumor, osseointegrated implants *(arrows)* have been placed in the available bone sites.

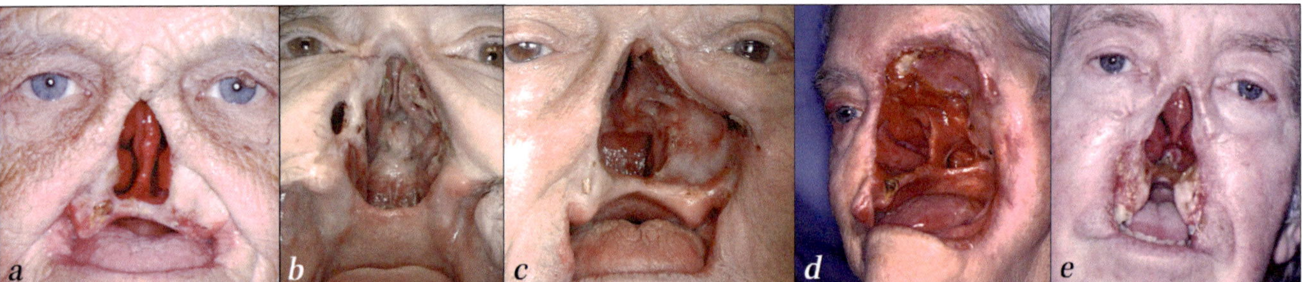

Figure 5-123 Prosthetic prognoses for midfacial defects involving the oral cavity. *(a and b)* Significant portions of the palate and/or alveolar ridges remain in these edentulous patients with large midfacial defects. There are many suitable implant sites. The prosthetic prognosis is good even without the aid of implants. *(c)* Less hard palate remains but the maxillary sinus on the left has been exposed and lined with a skin graft. This area can be engaged to facilitate the retention and stability of both the oral and the facial portions. Multiple implant sites are available and accessible and so the prosthetic prognosis is good. *(d)* The left maxilla and orbital contents have been included in this resection. Although there are several implant sites available the prosthetic prognosis was guarded because of the large size and weight of the prosthesis and the low position of the left side of the lower lip. *(e)* The presence of most of the posterior teeth dramatically improves the prosthetic prognosis for this midfacial defect.

During surgical ablation, all raw tissue surfaces should be lined with split-thickness skin grafts. It is also desirable to resurface the exposed maxillary sinuses with skin. These areas can later be engaged to provide support for and to help retain and stabilize the oral/facial prostheses. For most patients, particularly edentulous patients and those with compromised dentition, osseointegrated implants should be positioned in all available sites, and it is suggested that these implants be placed at the time of tumor ablation (see section above entitled "Surgical Procedures during Tumor Ablation to Enhance the Prosthetic Prognosis"). The malar body and the residual zygoma are favored implant sites because of their bone volume and quality and are best suited to provide additional support for the oral portion of the prosthesis. Sites such as the floor of the nose and the glabella and orbital rims are considered supplemental and are best suited to help retain the facial portion of the prosthesis as opposed to providing support for the oral portion. Potential implant sites, because of their limited bone volume, are best evaluated with CBCT scans and the associated treatment-planning software.

Temporary prostheses

A temporary restoration may aid recovery during the initial postoperative period by eliminating the need for large bandages and permitting social intercourse. A temporary facial prosthesis, constructed of autopolymerizing acrylic resin or silicone rubber and combined with an oral prosthesis, will permit swallowing, facilitate salivary control, and enable reasonable speech articulation. During this period, the probable implant sites can be carefully assessed, and a definitive treatment plan can be developed.

A two-piece prosthesis is preferred for such defects. One restores the integrity of the oral cavity and the missing dentition, and the other masks the facial defect. These prostheses restore the integrity of the oral cavity, enabling the patient to swallow more effectively and speak reasonably intelligibly, and provide the patient with an aesthetic appearance that permits social interaction with family and friends. If there is a significant portion of the posterior alveolar ridges and palatal vault remaining, the existing denture can be readapted with a temporary denture reline material and relined and extended to engage suitable portions of the defect. This will allow many patients to masticate with some degree of efficiency. In patients retaining dentition, partial dentures are fabricated with either magnets or attachments embedded designed to help retain the facial prosthesis (Fig 5-124).

At this stage of the patient's recovery, the use of the existing complete denture is preferred, as opposed to making a new one. The patient will have already adapted to its palatal contours and can use the dorsum of the tongue to help retain the temporary complete denture-facial prosthesis complex. The denture is extended to engage suitable areas

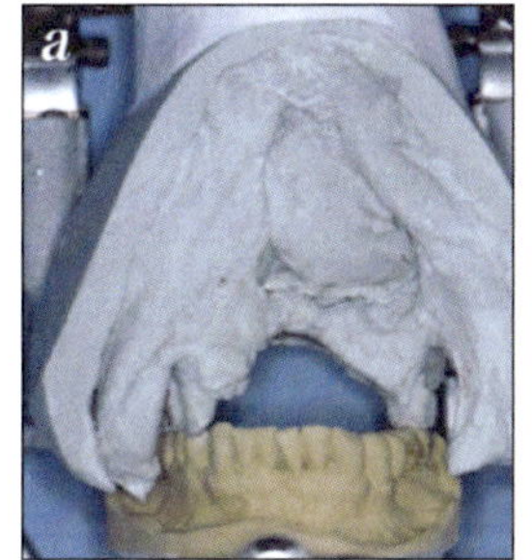
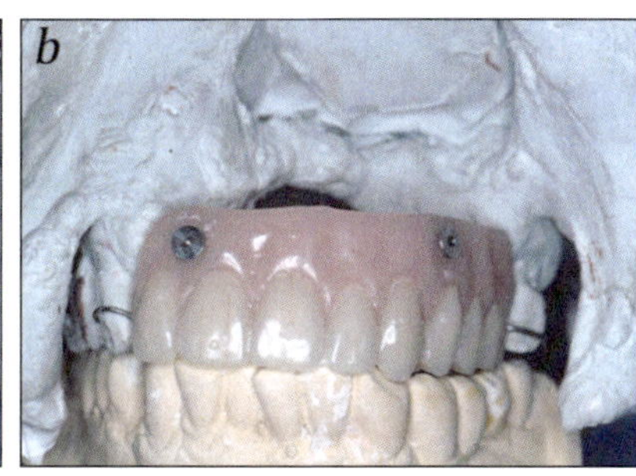

Figure 5-124 *(a)* Mounted casts of a large midfacial defect. *(b)* A treatment partial with magnetic attachments was fabricated.

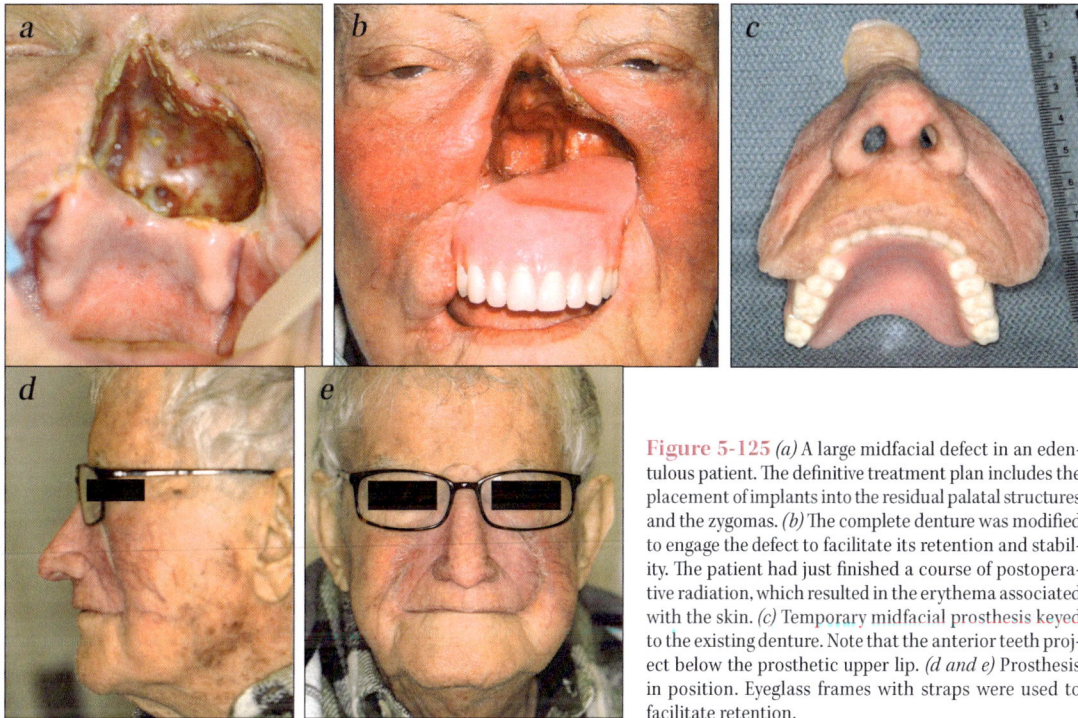

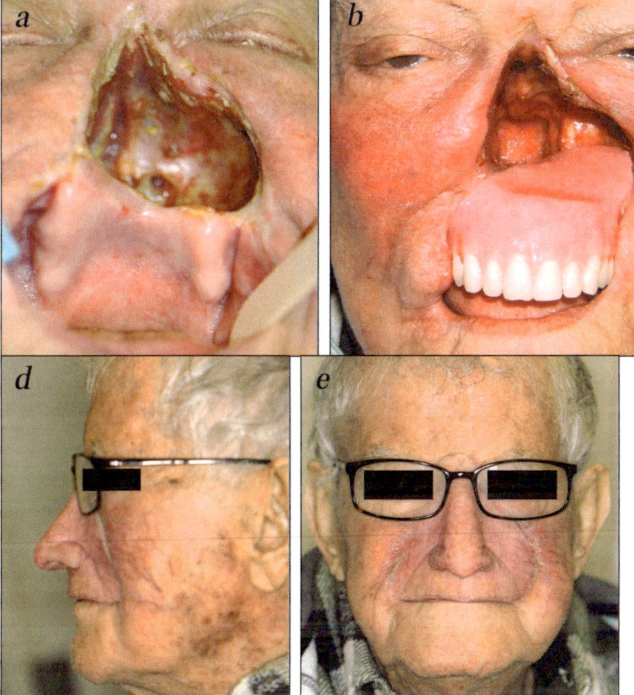
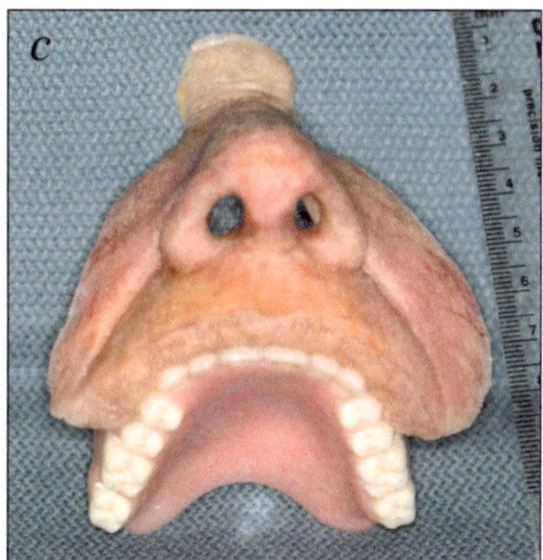

Figure 5-125 *(a)* A large midfacial defect in an edentulous patient. The definitive treatment plan includes the placement of implants into the residual palatal structures and the zygomas. *(b)* The complete denture was modified to engage the defect to facilitate its retention and stability. The patient had just finished a course of postoperative radiation, which resulted in the erythema associated with the skin. *(c)* Temporary midfacial prosthesis keyed to the existing denture. Note that the anterior teeth project below the prosthetic upper lip. *(d and e)* Prosthesis in position. Eyeglass frames with straps were used to facilitate retention.

of the defect and relined (Fig 5-125). The facial portion is fabricated after the denture has been modified. Magnets, O-rings, or similar types of attachment mechanisms can be used to connect the two.

The facial prosthesis is designed to gain most of its retention and stability from the oral prosthesis. The facial portion is usually made of silicone and should be made as light as possible. Eyeglass frames with straps can be used to facilitate retention. If the patient is edentulous, the tongue keeps the oral portion of the prosthesis seated on the residual maxillary denture-bearing surfaces, and the eyeglass frame with straps prevents the oral/facial prosthesis from being displaced anteriorly. This is usually sufficient to carry the patient through the initial healing processes until more effective means of retention, stability, and support can be created, either by engaging skin-lined undercuts or with the placement of implants (Fig 5-125).

Definitive prostheses

These prostheses are most often fabricated in two sections. Two-piece restorations are advantageous because the oral prosthesis can be designed so that the movement created during swallowing and mastication need not be transferred to the facial portion. Also, the facial portion can be designed to engage areas in the defect that have been designed and prepared specifically for that purpose, such as the extensions into skin-lined undercuts or craniofacial implants placed in areas of limited bone volume. In some defects, it is desirable to use the craniofacial implants placed in these sites exclusively for retention for the facial portion, since their limited numbers and length and bone anchorage may be insufficient to employ them as a means of support for the oral portion (see Fig 5-128). However, in other patients, it may be desirable to combine all the means of retention, stability, and support from the defect and the oral cavity, including the residual dentition and implants, in effect transforming the facial-oral prosthesis into a single functioning unit.

In most patients, whether edentulous or dentate, it is useful to place implants. The zygoma, the malar body, and the glabella region present with the most bone volume and are positioned advantageously to resist applied forces when implants are placed in these sites. Implant lengths should be maximized and take full advantage of the volume of bone available at each site. Obviously, dental and zygomatic implants are preferred, but short, craniofacial-type implants can be used for supplementation in bone sites of limited volume.

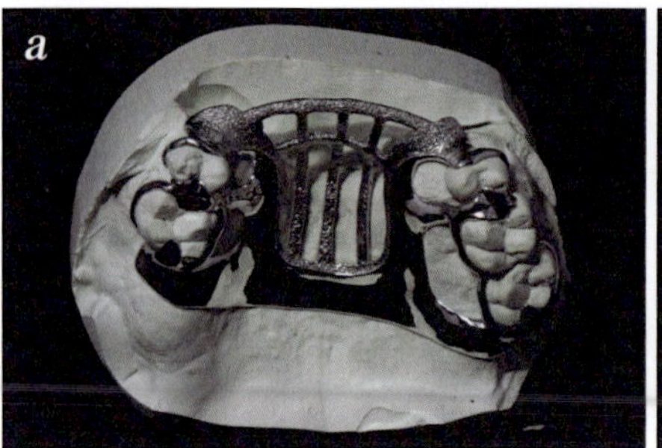
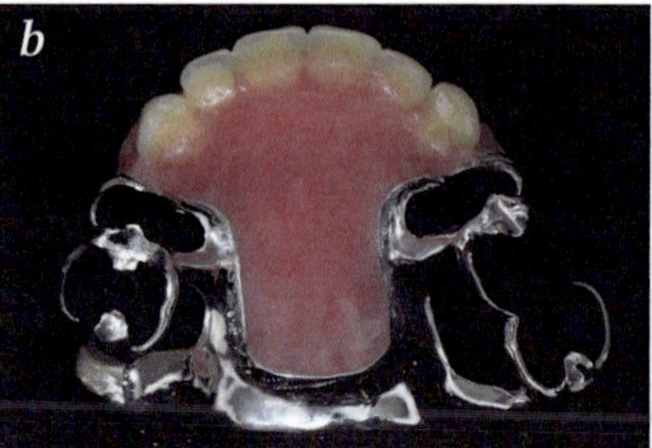
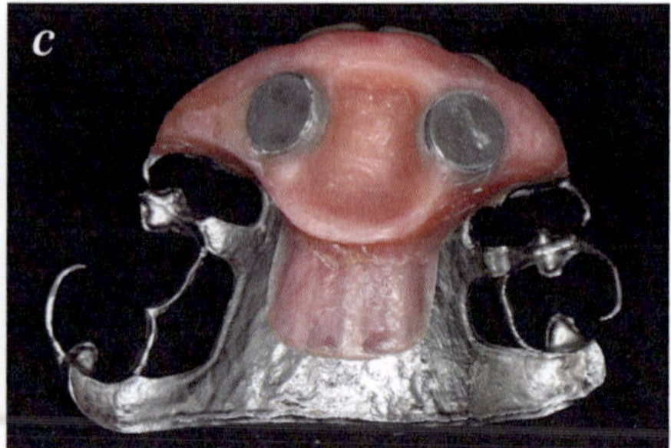

Figure 5-126 *(a)* RDP framework for a midfacial defect. The RDP design with the rests positioned on the distal side of the premolars adjacent to the defect. *(b and c)* Completed RDP. Note the magnetic attachments. These will be used to help retain the facial prosthesis that restores the upper lip and the nose.

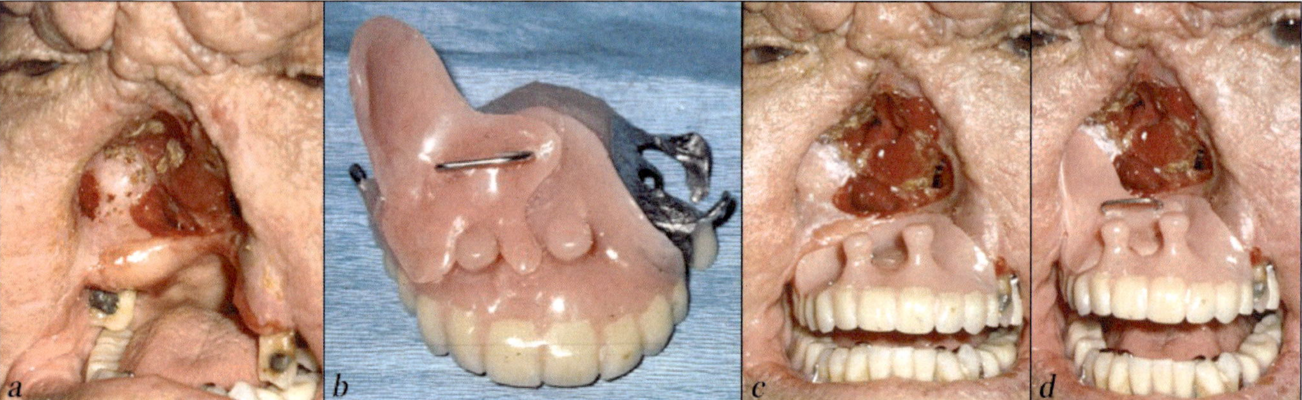

Figure 5-127 Oral prosthesis for a partially dentate patient with a large midfacial defect. *(a)* Posterior teeth remain bilaterally. *(b)* A two-piece RDP is fabricated. *(c)* One segment engages the dentition and residual palatal structures. *(d)* Another portion engages the skin-lined maxillary sinus and enhances retention.

The oral prosthesis is completed first. For dentate patients, removable dental prosthesis (RDP) designs are dictated by the nature and direction of the occlusal forces. The RDP should be designed to direct occlusal forces along the long axis of the abutment teeth (Kratochvil, 1963; Chang et al., 2019). Indirect retainers should be placed bilaterally and as far posteriorly as feasible to counteract gravitational forces from the anterior RDP extension and the attached facial prosthesis (Fig 5-126). Most defects present with an anterior extension area (Kennedy Class IV), requiring distal or cingulum rests on the anterior abutments adjacent to the defect and with properly contoured guide planes. The axis of rotation during function runs through these anterior rests, and when the food bolus is incised, the RDP will be allowed to rotate into the defect. Either the RPI (Kratochvil, 1963; Chang et al., 2019) or the RDP system (Eliason, 1983) can be used effectively. Select areas of the defect can be engaged to provide anterior support and somewhat resist this rotation, similar to the residual anterior edentulous denture-bearing surfaces in a normal patient. The path of insertion of the RDP may not be compatible with the engagement of some of the skin-lined undercuts in the midfacial defect. In these situations, two-piece prostheses can be designed in order to engage these undercuts more aggressively (Fig 5-127).

A key question that must be addressed in each patient is whether the implant-connecting bar(s) should be used as the sole means of support for the forces of mastication (so-called implant-supported design) or support should be shared by the implants and the available and accessible denture/prosthesis-bearing areas (so-called implant-assisted design). For a majority of patients, it is not advisable to use implants as the sole means of supporting the forces of occlusion. In most instances, the unfavorable implant distribution patterns, insufficient numbers, irradiated bone sites, unfavorable angulations, and often-limited volume of bone engaged by the implants preclude their use as the sole means of occlusal support. Key areas such as the walls of the maxillary sinus and the base of the skull should be lined with skin grafts, and these areas should be aggressively engaged to supplement the support provided by the implants (Figs 5-128 and 5-129).

Upon completion of the RDP framework or implant-connecting bar(s) (in some defects with residual dentition, the RDP framework unites the dentition with the implants; see Chapter 3, Figs 3-81 and 3-158), the oral prosthesis may be completed. An altered cast impression is made to maximize the engagement of potential denture/prosthesis-bearing surfaces, including those in the defect. Record bases are fabricated, the occlusal vertical dimension is determined, and a tentative centric relation record is made. In edentulous patients, this task is complicated by the lack of an upper lip, unstable record bases, compromised motor control, and altered proprioceptive patterns. Similar to the methods used when making complete dentures, swallowing and speech articulation are the most useful guides in determining the occlusal vertical dimension. It is advisable to reverify the occlusal vertical dimension and the centric relation record when the lip contours of the facial prosthesis have been completed. This can also be accomplished at try-in by adding a bulk of wax to the anterior teeth that mimic the proposed contours

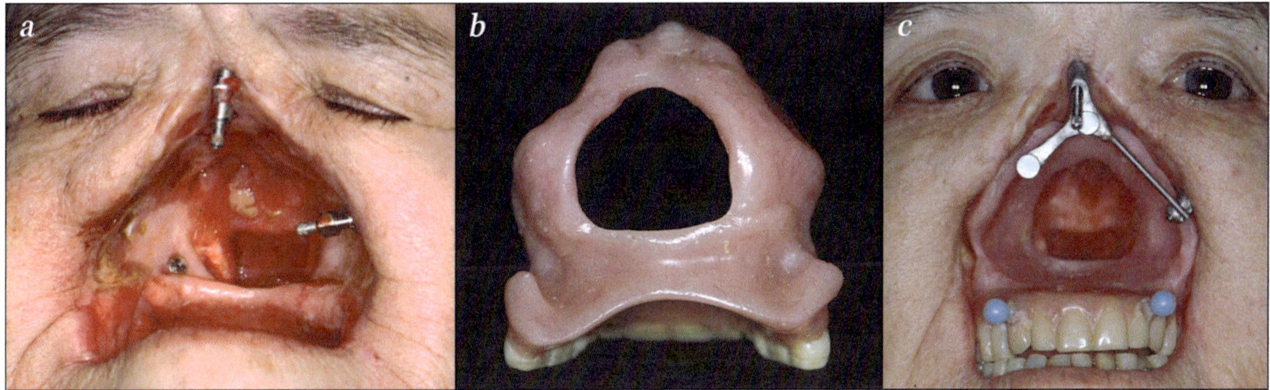

Figure 5-128 Oral prosthesis for an edentulous patient with a large midfacial defect. *(a)* Two implants have been placed, one in the glabella region and one in the malar body. The lateral and superior walls of the maxillary sinus are lined with skin grafts. *(b)* The skin-lined areas *(arrows)* are engaged by the oral prosthesis to enhance the support and stability provided by the residual oral structures. *(c)* The implant-connecting bar with its magnetic attachments is secured. The oral prosthesis derives its support and stability from the skin-lined walls of the maxillary sinuses. Implants are used to retain the facial portion (courtesy of Dr. E. Roumanas).

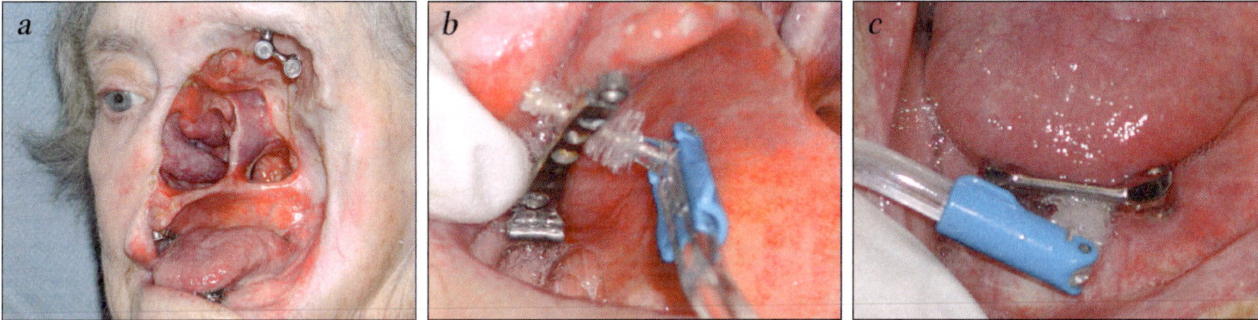

Figure 5-129 Implant retention for prostheses to rehabilitate a large combination orofacial defect. *(a)* Implants in the supraorbital rim will help retain the facial portion of the restoration. *(b and c)* Implants have been placed in the right maxilla and anterior mandible to retain and stabilize the oral prosthesis.

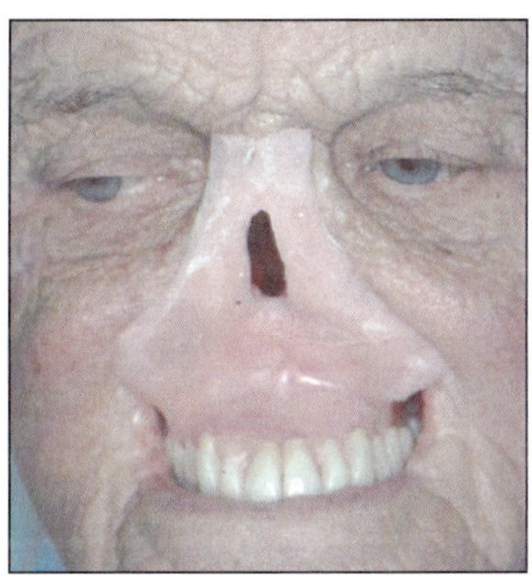

Figure 5-130 The occlusal vertical dimension and CR record are verified during the try in appointment

of the upper lip. Teeth are arranged according to the requirements of speech articulation, aesthetics, and occlusal function (Fig 5-130). The anterior teeth should extend 1 to 2 mm below the proposed margin of the upper lip to permit proper interaction between the tongue and these teeth during speech articulation (Fig 5-130).

The impression for the facial portion of the prosthesis is made after the oral prosthesis is completed (Fig 5-131). The oral prosthesis is positioned, and the impression is made. Variable degrees of movement and compressibility of tissues adjacent to the defect are encountered. The techniques used should minimize the distortion of these tissues and are similar to those employed for impressions of local facial defects (see above). The objective is to obtain an impression with minimal distortion of facial tissues adjacent to the defect. The patient should be in a semiupright position while the master impression is made to prevent distortions secondary to postural changes. The impression is made with a light-body impression material (Fig 5-132). A syringe is useful in injecting impression material into desirable undercuts or into areas of difficult access. The impression material is thinned with a cement spatula or PIP brush to minimize displacement of facial tissues. Succeeding layers of fast-setting impression plaster are added to provide support. The master cast is prepared in an improved dental stone (Fig 5-132d).

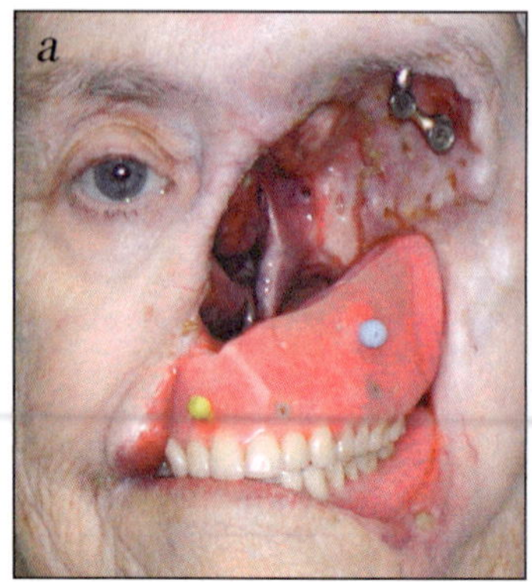

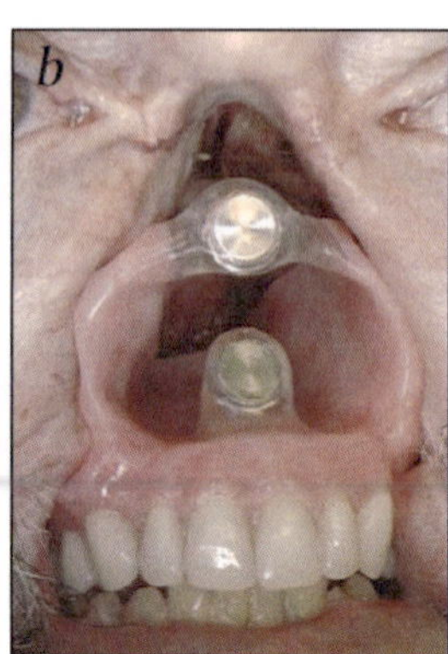

Figure 5-131 *(a)* The completed oral prostheses. The prosthesis is retained by the implants positioned in the right alveolar ridge (Fig 5-129b). It is designed to engage the facial portion with O-ring-type attachments. The prosthesis in "b" is retained by engagement of the residual oral structures and the skin lined areas in the defect. It is designed to engage the facial portion with magnetic attachments.

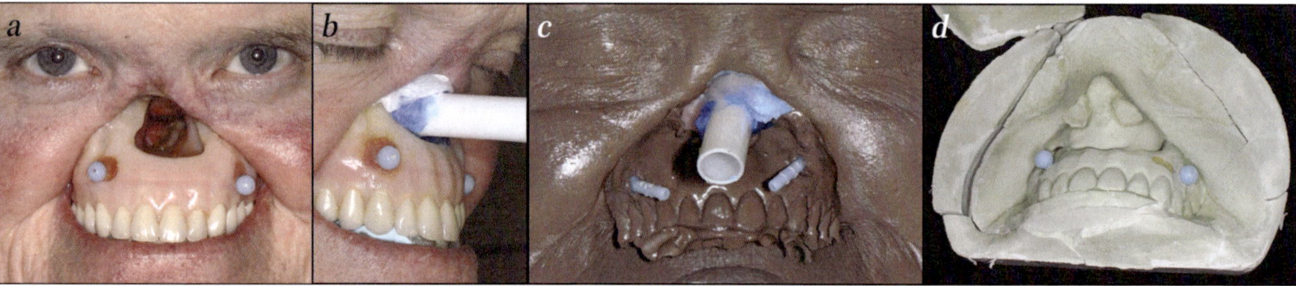

Figure 5-132 *(a)* Intraoral prosthesis in position. *(b)* A clinical remount record is made for the oral prosthesis with a silicone registration material and the defect prepared to make an impression. The airway is maintained with a large plastic tube. *(c)* The completed impression. *(d)* The master cast.

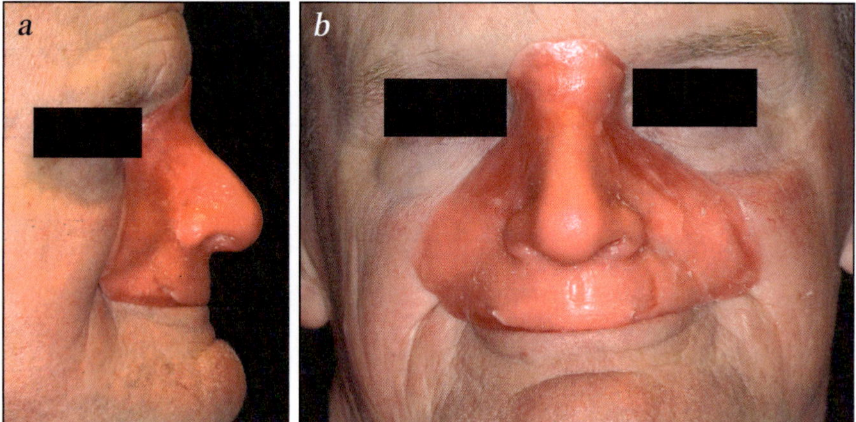

Figure 5-133 The wax pattern of the facial prosthesis is tried on. The prosthetic upper lip must be contoured to engage the lower lip and maximize the effectiveness of lip seal and the production of bilabial sounds.

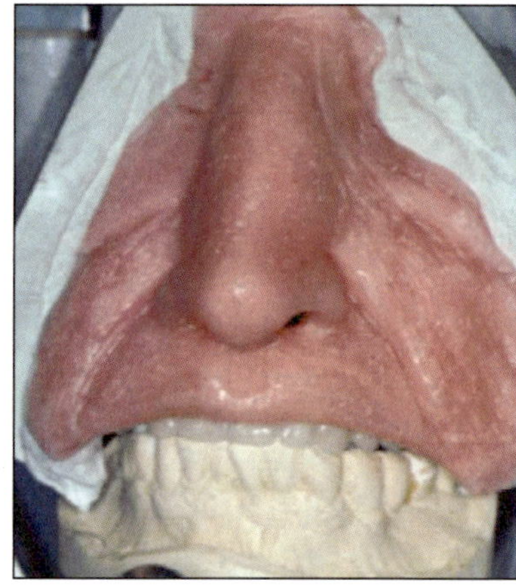

Figure 5-134 Wax sculpture of the facial prosthesis. The maxillary anterior teeth are exposed to permit articulation with the lower lip.

The facial prosthesis is completed in the usual fashion. The defect should be utilized as much as possible to facilitate stability and retention of the combined oral and facial prostheses. It is important to engage areas in the defect that will provide resistance to the forces of gravity in order to avoid exposing abutment teeth or implants to undesirable stresses.

Care must be taken to ensure that the prosthetic upper lip functionally engages the lower lip to idealize lip seal and the production of bilabial sounds (Fig 5-133). Occasionally this leads to unusual prosthetic lip contours. Often it may be necessary to slightly alter the master cast in order to idealize contours in the corner of the mouth region to accommodate tissue movement in this area. As mentioned earlier, the maxillary anterior teeth must project 1 to 2 mm below the lip to permit proper speech articulation (Fig 5-134).

Completed prostheses are shown in Fig 5-135. When appropriate the oral portion is secured to the facial portion with magnetic, O-ring, or equivalent attachments. This is especially useful when the facial portion engages skin-lined undercuts in the defect. As such, it will contribute to the overall retention, stability, and support of both prostheses. In some instances, it is desirable that the facial portion be somewhat independent of the oral portion and be primarily retained by the implants. An example of this method of retaining the facial portion independent of the oral portion is shown in Figs 5-128 and 5-135d.

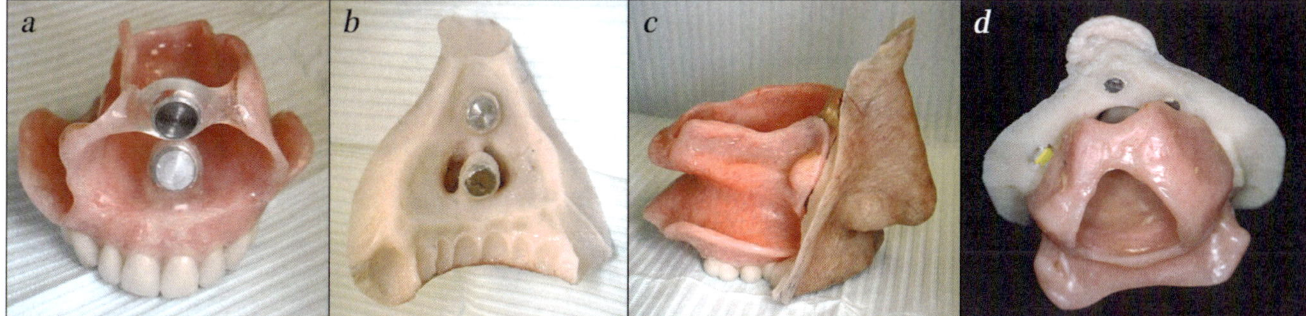

Figure 5-135 Typical midfacial prostheses. *(a, b, and c)* Magnetic attachments are incorporated within the intraoral portion of the prosthesis. *(d)* The facial portion is retained by implants. Note the "Hader" clips and the magnetic attachments. The intraoral portion engages the residual alveolar ridges and the skin lined portions of the defect.

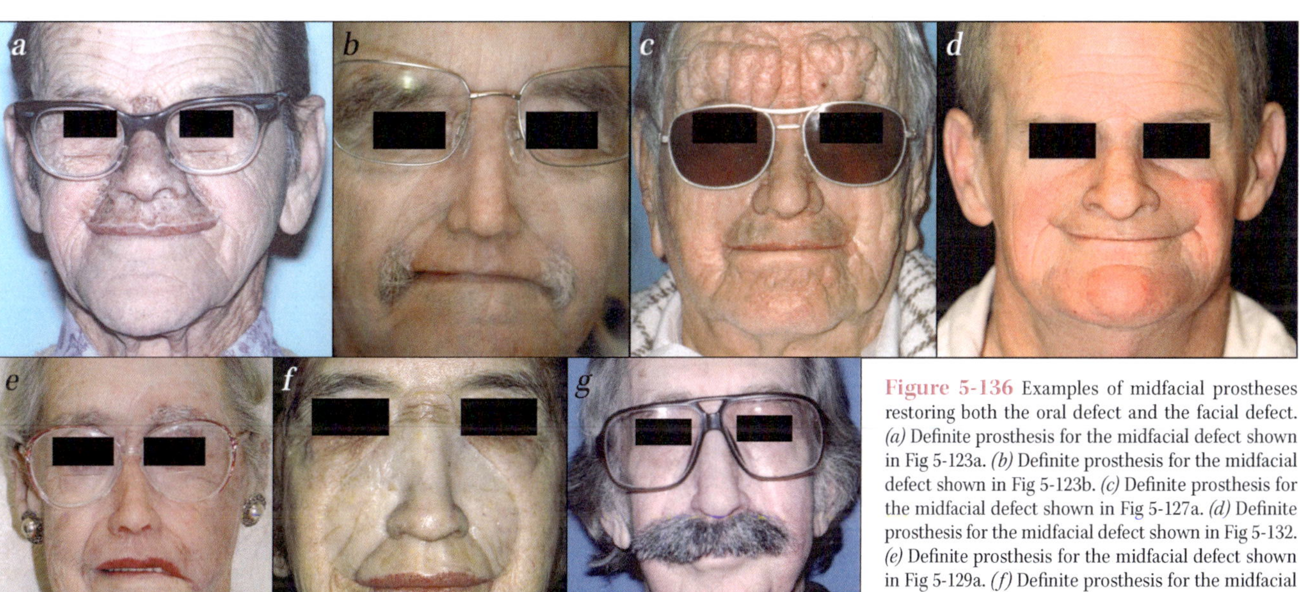

Figure 5-136 Examples of midfacial prostheses restoring both the oral defect and the facial defect. *(a)* Definite prosthesis for the midfacial defect shown in Fig 5-123a. *(b)* Definite prosthesis for the midfacial defect shown in Fig 5-123b. *(c)* Definite prosthesis for the midfacial defect shown in Fig 5-127a. *(d)* Definite prosthesis for the midfacial defect shown in Fig 5-132. *(e)* Definite prosthesis for the midfacial defect shown in Fig 5-129a. *(f)* Definite prosthesis for the midfacial defect shown in Fig 5-128a. *(g)* Definite prosthesis for the midfacial defect shown in Fig 5-123e.

Retention of the facial/oral complex may be enhanced by eyeglass frames with straps. The prosthesis is delivered in the customary fashion; areas of overextension and excessive tissue displacement of the oral portion are identified and adjusted as appropriate with pressure indicating paste and disclosing wax. A clinical remount record is made to refine the occlusion. The finished restoration usually provides the patient with an acceptable appearance, nearly normal speech articulation, and swallowing. Mastication is dependent upon the quality of the support provided by the oral portion. For men, a mustache can be attached to the upper lip to enhance aesthetics. Completed prostheses of patients with typical combined oral and midfacial defects are shown in Fig 5-136.

Lateral Facial Defects

If a midfacial defect extends significantly laterally, the lateral portion is best restored surgically with a flap (Figs 5-137 and 5-138). Tissue movement and displacement are primarily associated with movement of the mandible; as a result, conventional facial/oral prostheses are ineffective and poorly tolerated by most patients. Retention is challenging, even with osseointegrated implants. Moreover, if the defect extends below the oral commissure, oral competence cannot be restored by a prosthesis. Saliva will leak from the inferior portion of the defect, regardless of the design or fit of the prosthesis. Facial prostheses are most effective when they restore structures that are relatively immobile such as the ear, nose, and upper lip.

This approach was used successfully in the patient shown in Fig 5-137. The lateral portion of this large defect was covered with a vascularized flap. The orbital structures, midcheek area, nose, and upper lip were restored with a prosthesis. Mastication was effectively restored with a complete denture and maxillary obturator. Speech was essentially normal and the patient exhibited reasonable oral competence. The aesthetic result was quite acceptable.

Likewise, in the patient shown in Fig 5-138, the lateral portion of this large orbital, nasal, and cheek defect was restored with a vascularized flap. The orbital and nasal portions of the defect were restored with an implant-retained prosthesis.

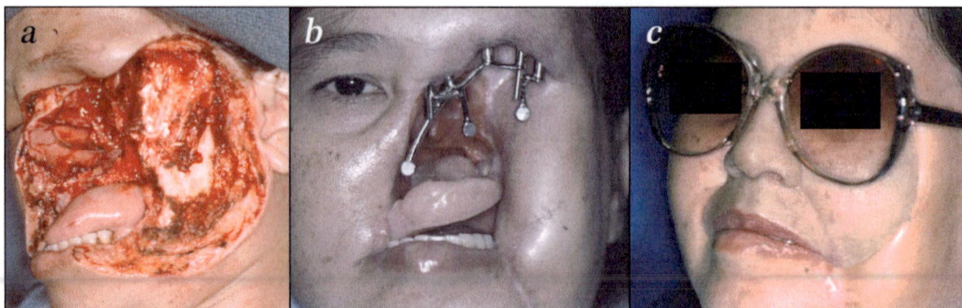

Figure 5-137 Combined surgical and prosthetic rehabilitation of a large facial defect. *(a and b)* The lateral portion of the defect is rehabilitated with a free flap. *(c)* The middle portion is rehabilitated prosthetically.

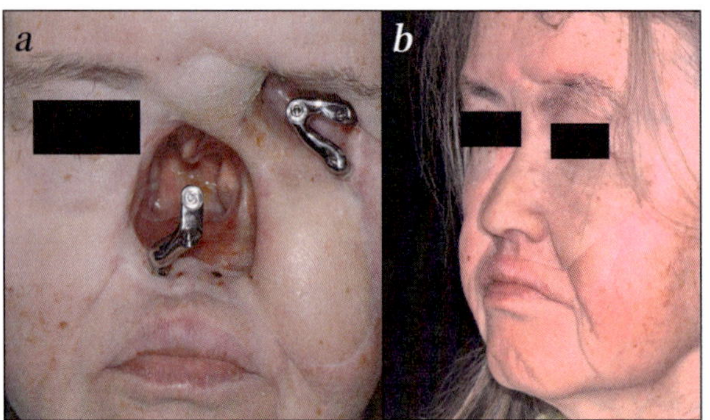

Figure 5-138 Completed midfacial prosthesis of patient shown in Figs 5-4a and 5-28a. *(a)* Implants have been placed in the lateral orbital rim and the floor of the nose. *(b)* Prosthesis in position.

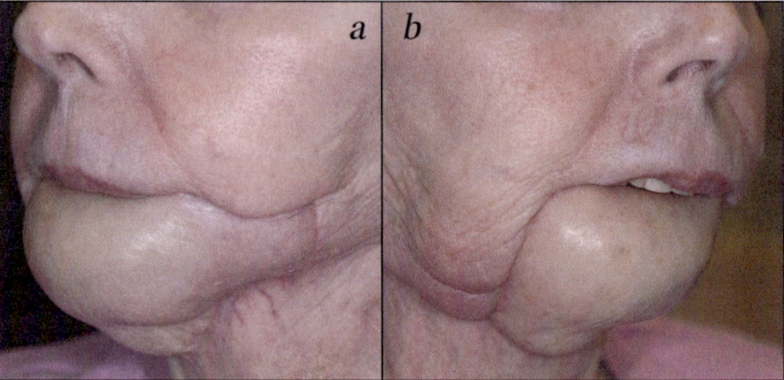

Figure 5-139 *(a and b)* The anterior mandible and the lower lip were reconstructed with a vascularized fibula flap.

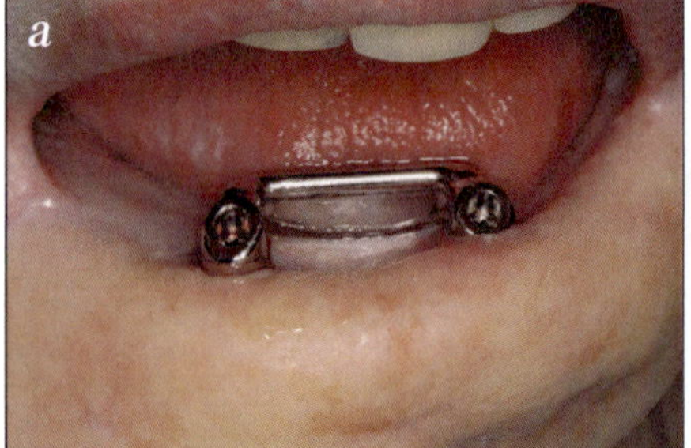

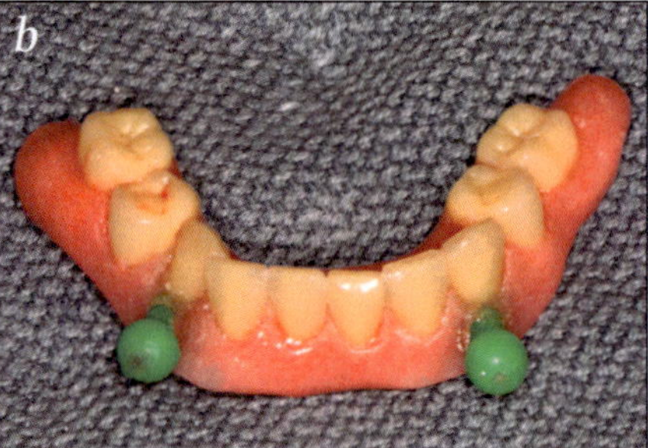

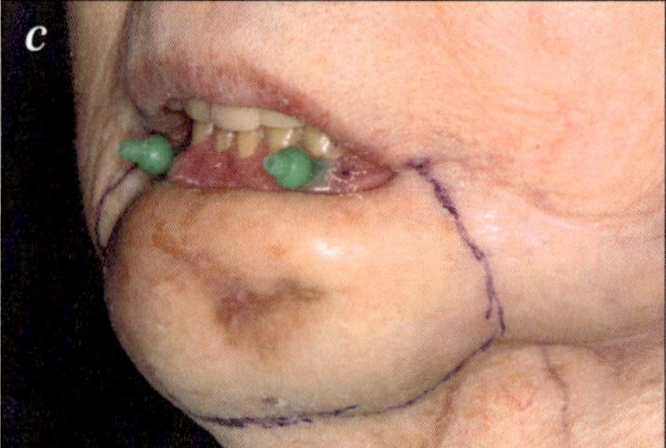

Figure 5-140 Following a tumor ablation the lower lip, chin and mandible were reconstructed with a vascularized fibula free flap. Implants were placed in the mandible and *(a)* an implant-connecting bar fabricated. *(b)* The implant retained overdenture with O-ring-type attachments embedded to retain the lower lip chin prosthesis. *(c)* The overdenture in position and without the prosthesis.

Lower Lip-Chin Prostheses

An intact lower lip plays a greater role in speech than the upper lip because of its greater potential for movement. Clinical experience confirms this observation. Patients with large midfacial defects (resection of the anterior maxilla, upper lip, and nasal structures) will usually exhibit normal speech with a prosthesis. In contrast, prosthetic replacements for the lower lip and cheek are generally less effective, and surgical reconstruction is usually the treatment of choice. However, following resection of the anterior mandible and lower lip, the reconstructed lower lip is often static, and unless the reconstruction is perfectly contoured and positioned, it is not possible for it to functionally engage the upper lip (Fig 5-139). These reconstructed lips are immobile and frequently retracted, further increasing the challenge of appropriate valving with the upper lip. Speech articulation is adversely affected, and the patient is unable to prevent a steady stream of saliva from escaping from the oral cavity.

Prosthetic lower lips can be fabricated in a way that permits reasonable valving with the upper lip. Adhesives are insufficient for retention, and either implants or the residual dentition (Zeno et al., 2013) must be employed (Fig 5-140). They can be confined to the lip (Fig 5-141) or extended to cover the entire chin in select patients (Fig 5-142). These prostheses restore lip valving and thus improve speech articulation. The cosmetic appearance can also be significantly improved—and with it, the patient's self-esteem. However, such prostheses do not prevent saliva from escaping the oral cavity. The flaps used to reconstruct the area are nonsensate, so patients cannot detect escaping saliva. In addition, saliva accumulates at the interface between the prosthesis and the underlying tissue by means of capillary action and slowly seeps out along the edges of the prosthesis.

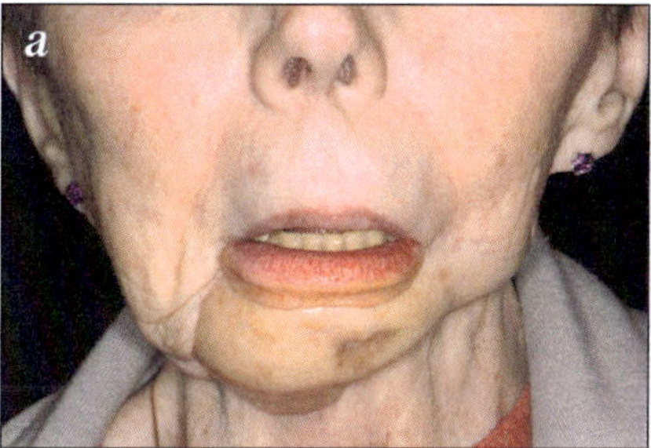
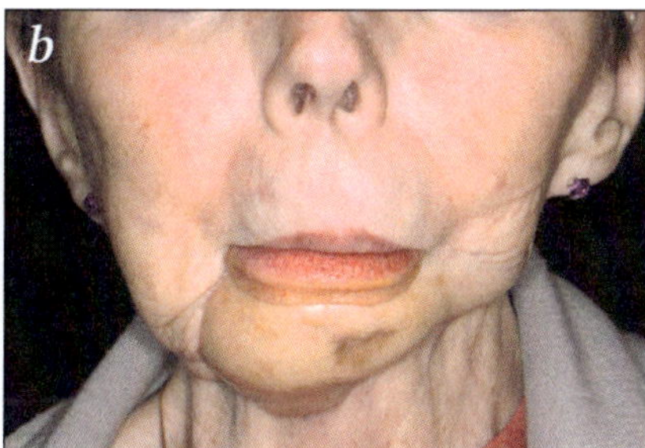

Figure 5-141 The prosthesis restores only the lower lip and is designed to permit proper valving with the upper lip during speech articulation.

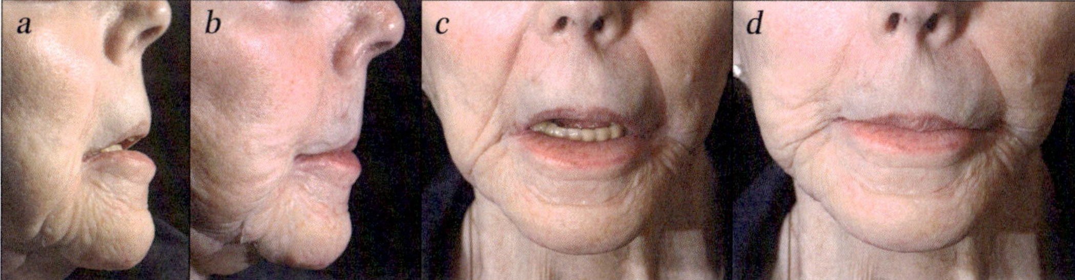

Figure 5-142 This version of the prosthesis extends to cover the chin.

Connection of a Facial Prosthesis to an Oral Prosthesis

Frequently, particularly with large nasal or orbital defects, it is advantageous to connect a facial prosthesis to the oral portion to facilitate the retention of both prostheses. This practice is most effective when the oral portion is retained by implants or residual dentition. We prefer to use magnetic attachments. These types of attachment enhance the retention of both the oral and the facial prostheses but allow some independent movement of each (Fig 5-143; see also Fig 5-68).

Restoration of Ocular Defects

Evolution of the ocular prosthesis

The use of prosthetic eyes was first recorded in Iran in 2900–2800 BCE. It was made of bitumen paste and was covered in a thin layer of gold (Pine et al., 2015; Conroy, 1993). Egyptians were also known to have used prosthetic eyes to decorate their mummies, though there were no records that they were used for medical purposes (Hita et al., 2016).

In the sixteenth century, Frenchman Ambroise Pare described the use of an artificial eye with a bent arm made of gold and silver around the head to hold it in place, while Venetian glassblowers used glass-blowing techniques to fabricate glass eyes (Pine et al., 2015). However, these techniques were largely kept as a trade secret. The war in the 17th century resulted in a decline in the prosthetic-eye glass-blowing industry. Stock glass eyes were made available in standard sizes and sold at high prices. Friedrich Phillip Ritterich set up the Leipzig Eye Institute and introduced the concept of customized ocular prostheses. Ludwig Muller-Uri developed the first artificial eye made from cryolite, which was found to be more durable than glass (Pine et al., 2015).

In the twentieth century, polymethyl methacrylate (PMMA) was introduced and was quickly adopted by dentists as an alternative material for denture base. The lack of access to German glass eyes during World War II led to the adoption of PMMA for the fabrication of ocular prostheses that were in demand for war veterans who lost their eyes during the war.

Due to the familiarity with the use of PMMA by dentists, the fabrication and provision of ocular prosthetic services shifted from the optometry profession to dentists. Dr. Arthur Perry later introduced the use of a pegged orbital implant made of hydroxyapatite. The connection between the implant and the prosthesis helped improve its overall motility.

Today, digital technologies have been adopted to facilitate designing and streamlining the manufacturing of prostheses. Development on the use of 3D technology using printed resin is still ongoing.

Anatomy of the eye

The globe is located in the orbit and is protected by the eyelids. The eyelid is made up of an external superficial layer of keratinized epithelial tissue and an inner layer of conjunctiva that contacts the globe. It consists of a fibrous framework that thickens at the margins of the lids to form the tarsal plates. The orbicularis oculi muscle is superficial to the tarsal plates (Fig 5-144).

The average size of the interpalpebral fissure is 10–11 mm in width and 30–31 mm in length (Fig 5-145). The lateral angle of the fissure tends to be more acute than the medial angle. In the primary gaze position of most individuals, the margin of the upper eyelid rests 1.5–2 mm below the superior corneal limbus, while the lower eyelid margin rests at the position of the inferior corneal limbus.

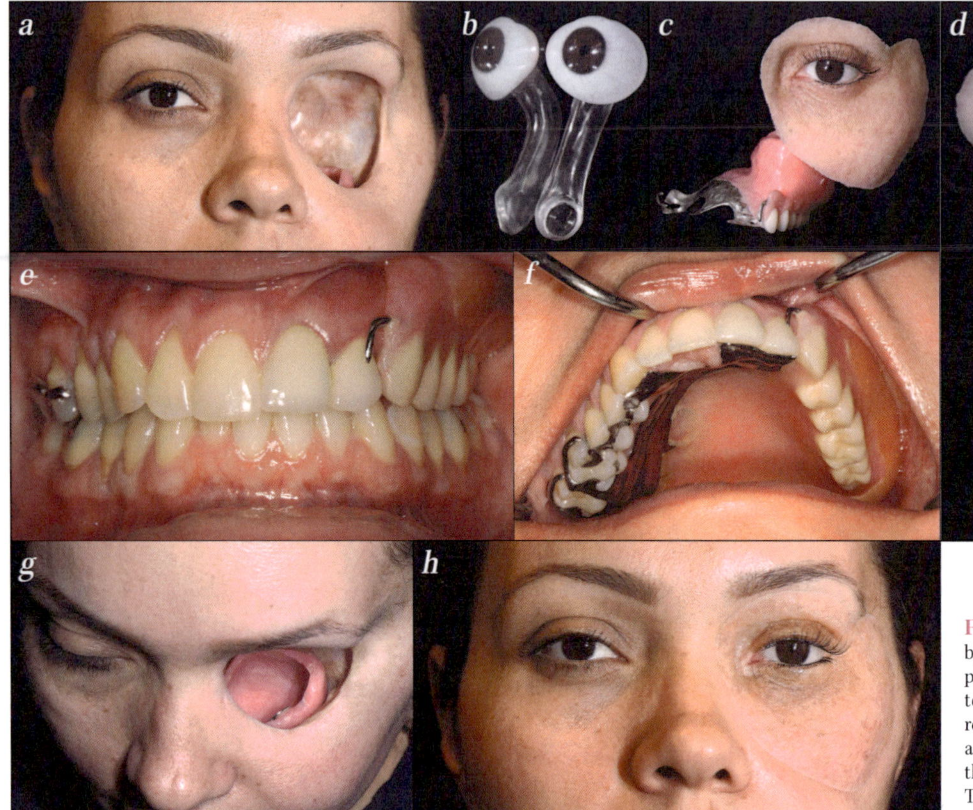
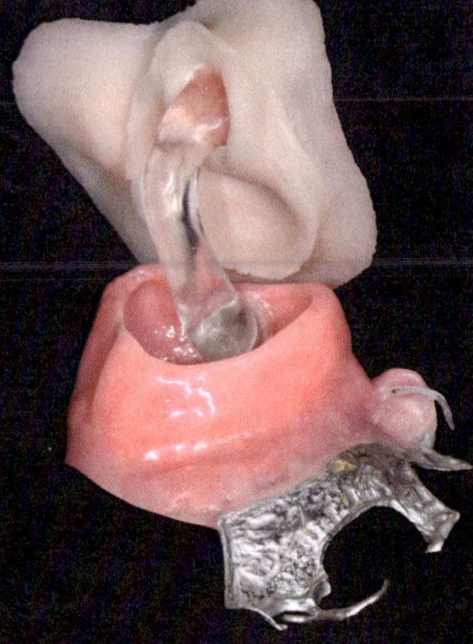

Figure 5-143 Orbital prosthesis retained by magnetic attachment to an RDP-obturator prosthesis. *(a)* Maxillectomy-orbital exenteration defect. *(b)* Ocular prosthesis with resin strut. *(c and d)* The resin strut engages a magnetic attachment incorporated within the RDP-obturator prosthesis. *(e, f, and g)* The RDP-obturator prosthesis in position. *(h)* The orbital prosthesis in position.

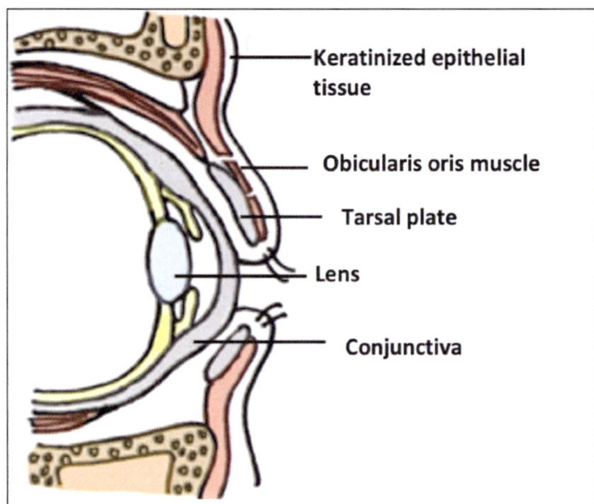

Figure 5-144 Anatomy of the eye and eyelids.

The iris is a thin disclike structure located in front of the lens and ciliary body and behind the cornea. It has an opening in the center, called the pupil. It is made up of two distinct layers, a layer of pigmented fibrovascular tissue known as the stroma and a layer of pigmented epithelial cells beneath it (Fig 5-146).

The iris consists of two major zones; the outer circumference is called the ciliary zone, and the inner circumference is called the pupillary zone. These two zones are separated by the collarette. The iris is highly pigmented with a complex series of colors ranging from brown, green, blue, gray, and hazel. The phenotypic color of the eye is determined by the quantity of melanin.

Eye loss

There are many reasons for eye loss, but they can be widely grouped into trauma, malignancy, and congenital defects. Among the various causes, trauma is the most common reason for eye loss. A study by Spraul and Grossnikalus (1997) found that 41% of the enucleation cases were due to trauma, while 24% were due to neoplastic disease. Other common causes include painful blind eye, infection, and cosmetic improvement of a disfigured eye.

Koylu et al. (2015) analyzed the indications of 123 patients who had undergone eye removal at a military hospital in Turkey and

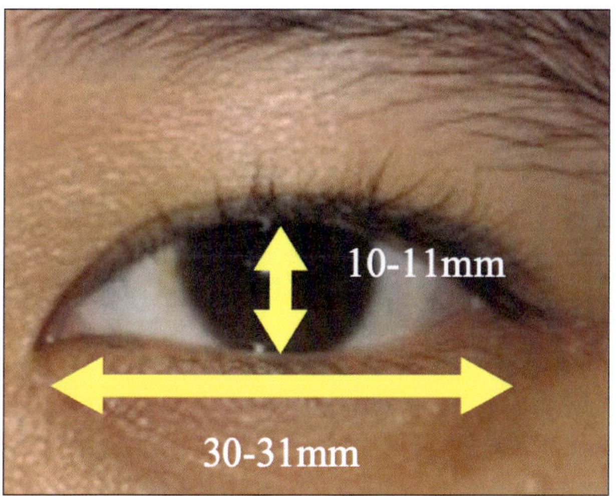

Figure 5-145 Average dimensions of the eye.

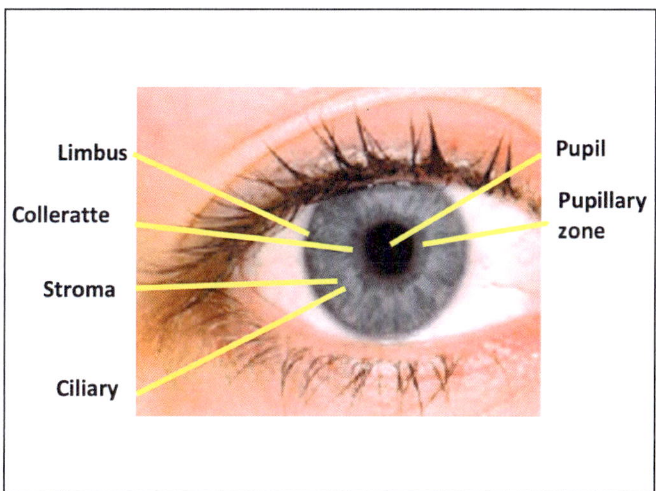

Figure 5-146 Anatomy of the iris.

found that the majority were due to trauma. The authors reviewed other studies and found a male predominance for eye loss. Evisceration was the most commonly used technique for eye removal (Table 5-14) (Koylu et al., 2015). Among the papers they reviewed, the top indication for eye removal was trauma, followed by infection and painful blind eye. Endophthalmitis is an intraocular bacterial or fungal infection involving the vitreous and/or aqueous humors (Durand, 2013). It is first treated with a course of antibiotics. Failure of resolution of the infection may require more aggressive treatment to remove the eye.

Eye removal

Removal of the eye can be performed by the following surgical procedures (Fig 5-147):

- enucleation
- evisceration
- exenteration

Evisceration refers to the removal of the contents of the globe while leaving the sclera and extraocular muscles intact (Hita et al., 2016). This allows good motility of the ocular implant. It is contraindicated when there is a presence or suspicion of intraocular malignancy. Evisceration is preferred over enucleation in the presence of endophthalmitis to reduce the chance of subarachnoid spread of intraocular infection.

Enucleation is defined as the removal of the entire eyeball from the orbit after severing the optic nerve while preserving all the other orbital structures like the extraocular muscles, allowing an implant to be placed into the enucleated socket for reconstruction. This technique is indicated for intraocular malignancies, painful blind eye, phthisis bulbi, and microphthalmia.

Exenteration is the removal of the globe as well as the soft tissues of the orbit such as the connective tissue, fat, and muscles (Fig 5-148) (Hita et al., 2016). Exenteration can be classified into subtotal, total, or radical depending on the number of orbital contents removed (Honavar and Rao, 2019). This is usually indicated when there is an invasive orbital tumor that can be cutaneous, conjunctival, or intraocular in origin (Rubin, 1993). Exenteration is also indicated when malignancies in the paranasal sinuses extend into the orbital floor.

A survey done on 896 ophthalmologists in the UK found that among the three methods of eye removal, most surgeons indicated a preference for evisceration (42%) over enucleation (27%) (Viswanathan et al., 2007). A higher incidence of evisceration (62%) was also found in a study conducted at the Jordan University Hospital over a five-year period (Ababneh et al., 2015). This was because

Table 5-14 Gender ratio, distribution of evisceration and enucleation rates, and the top indications for eye removal in various countries

Country	Study group	Male-to-female ratio	Evisceration	Enucleation	Top three common indications
USA	Yousuf et al., 2012	1.1	54	31	Trauma, painful blind eye, and glaucoma, retinal ischemia
Cameroon	Kagmeni et al., 2014	1.4	181	69	Infection, trauma, painful blind eye, and glaucoma
Palestine	Keenan et al., 2011	1.5	21	11	Trauma, infection, painful blind eye, and glaucoma
Nigeria	Etebu et al. 2013	2.6	63	15	Trauma, endophthalmitis, malignancy
Turkey	Koylu et al., 2015	2.9	95	28	Trauma, malignancy, endophthalmitis

Adapted from Koylu et al., 2014.

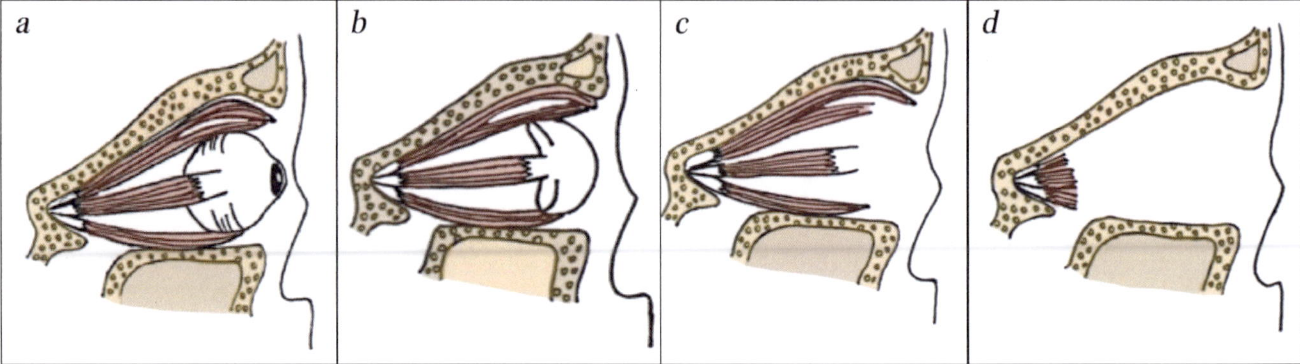

Figure 5-147 Eye removal: *(a)* normal, *(b)* evisceration, *(c)* enucleation *(d)* exenteration.

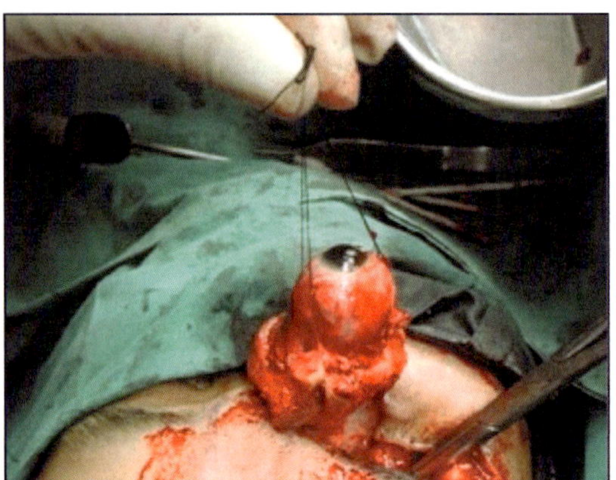

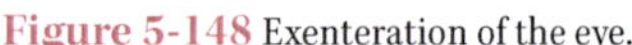
Figure 5-148 Exenteration of the eye.

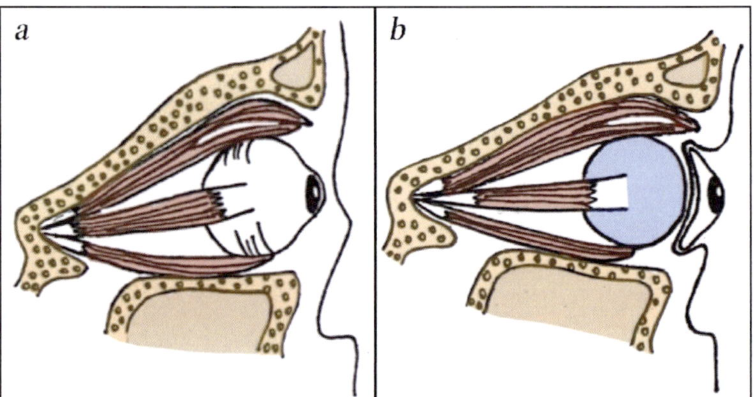

Figure 5-149 Goal of socket rehabilitation: *(a)* normal or *(b)* with an orbital implant.

evisceration was deemed to be less complicated and would cause less disruption to the anatomical structures in the orbit (Ababneh et al., 2015). This would also in turn result in fewer complications such as ptosis, implant migration, and socket contracture (Smith et al., 2011). Evisceration may be preferred due to better prosthetic motility and socket stability (Viswanathan et al., 2007).

However, in some cases, enucleation is still preferred, as it provides more space for a larger implant or prosthesis and will allow for histological diagnosis in malignancy cases (Lin and Liao, 2017).

Goal of socket rehabilitation

The goal of socket rehabilitation is to achieve a centrally located, well-covered implant with adequate volume restoration (Fig 5-149) (Rubin, 1993). The socket should be lined with healthy conjunctiva and fornices deep enough to retain an ocular prosthesis to permit horizontal and vertical excursion of an artificial eye (Fig 5-150).

The ideal outcome should consist of a comfortable and properly fitted ocular prosthesis that is in the normal position and well supported by the upper and lower eyelids. The replacement volume of the implant and the prosthesis should give a result that looks similar to the sighted contralateral globe and in the same horizontal plane. An interdisciplinary team approach consisting of the ophthalmic surgeon, prosthodontist, and/or ocularist is required to achieve a functional and aesthetic outcome (Fig 5-151).

Intraorbital implants

According to the 2002 consensus of the American Society of Ocularists and the American Academy of Ophthalmology, orbital implants can also be classified as buried, buried-integrated, and exposed-integrated (Fig 5-152) (Sami et al., 2007).

A buried implant has an uninterrupted conjunctival lining. It is usually smooth and encased in a capsule of tissue with little or no contact with the muscles. Some materials used include PMMA, glass, rubber, iron, gold, and silver (Fig 5-153).

Buried-integrated implants have rough surfaces that allow fibrovascular attachment, therefore reducing the risk of implant extrusion or migration (Hita et al., 2016; Chalasani et al., 2007). The irregular surfaces also improve translation of implant-prosthesis movement. Exposed-integrated implant involves direct coupling of the prosthesis through a peg to the implant, thereby improving implant motility.

Examples of integrated implants include hydroxyapatite (HA), polyethylene, and aluminum oxide (alumina) (Figs 5-154, 5-155, and 5-156) (Migliori, 2002). Improved vascular supply also reduces the risk of postoperative infections and promotes healing. However, due to its rough surface, the conjunctiva is easily eroded with movement of the implant. Hence they are usually covered with donor sclera to prevent implant exposure (Jordan, 2002). Wladis et al. (2018) found that the exposure rates for porous and nonporous implants are generally comparable. To date, there is no consensus

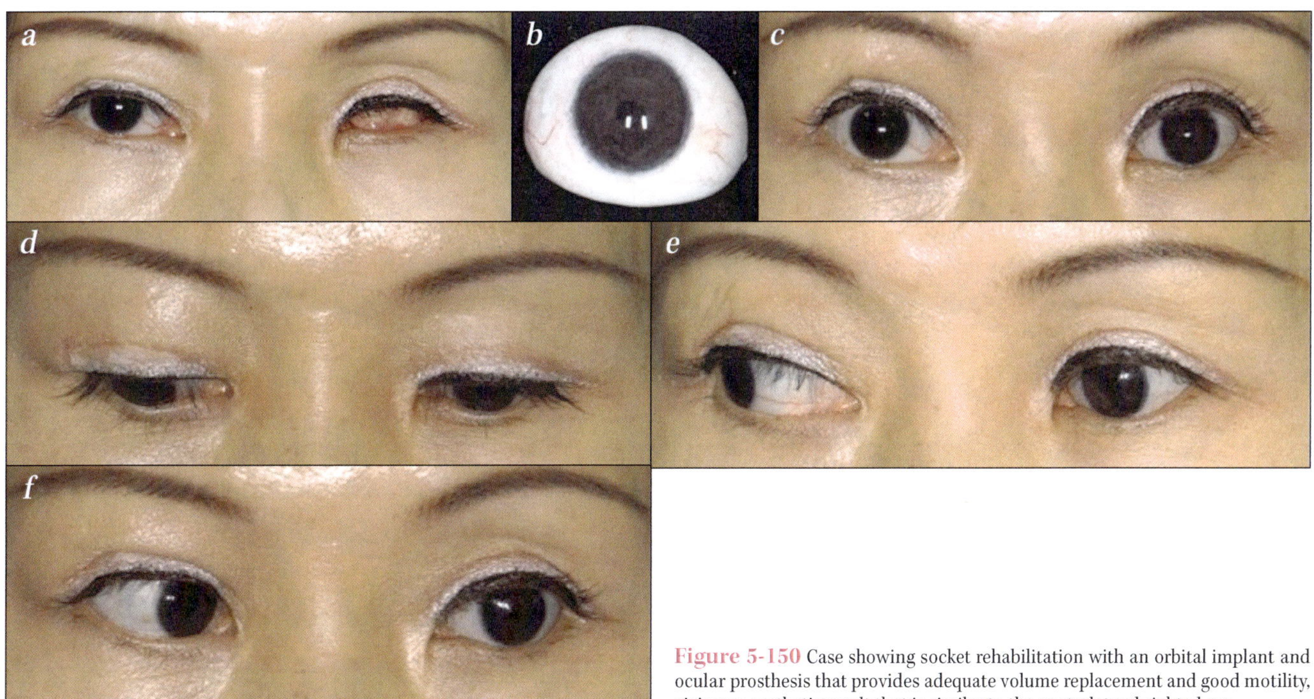

Figure 5-150 Case showing socket rehabilitation with an orbital implant and ocular prosthesis that provides adequate volume replacement and good motility, giving an aesthetic result that is similar to the contralateral sighted eye.

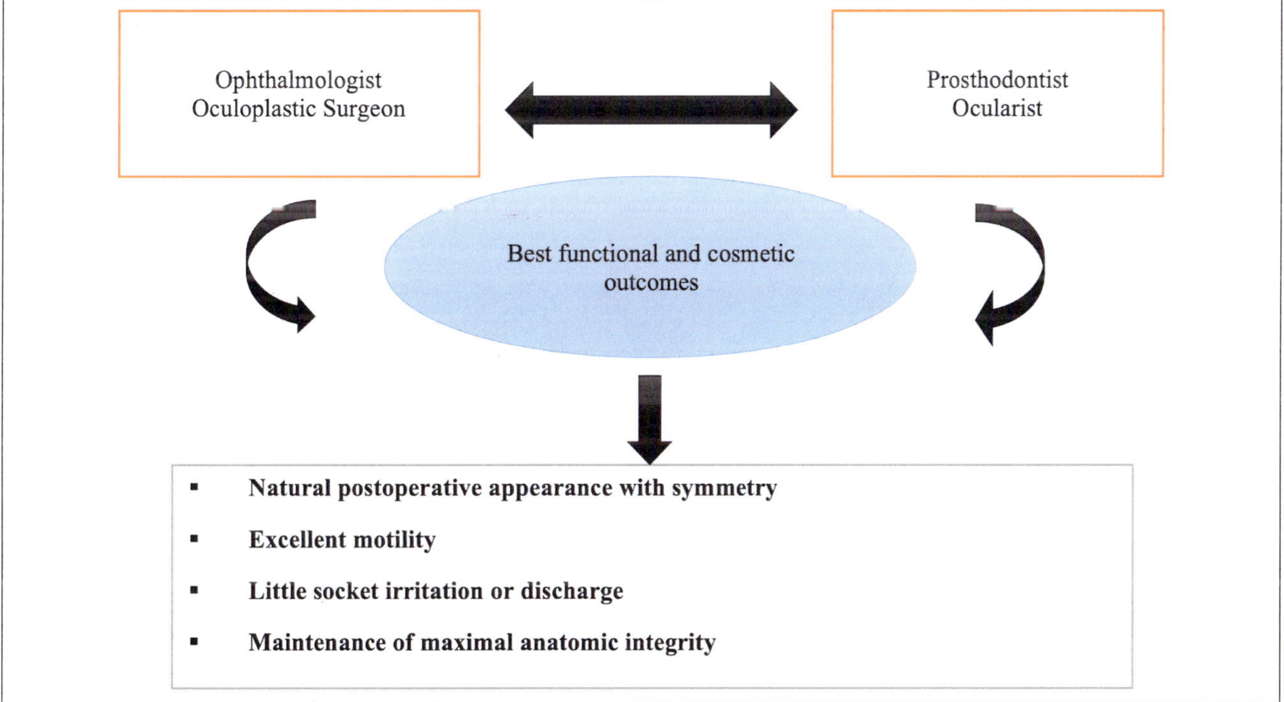

Figure 5-151 Interdisciplinary collaboration required for best functional and cosmetic outcomes.

regarding the choice of porous or nonporous implants (Chalasani et al., 2007). A survey done in the UK found that the majority of surgeons prefer the use of porous spherical implants due to their light weight, retention, cosmesis, and possible pegging (Viswanathan et al., 2007).

The size of the orbital implant should compensate for the loss of volume, allowing for the fabrication of a thinner and lighter prosthesis to reduce the weight on the lower eyelid and minimize ectropion formation and lid laxity. Implant size selection can be determined either before or during the time of surgery. The volume of an average adult-sized globe is 8 ml (Fig 5-157). Ideally, the implant should take up 70–80% of this volume (5–6 ml), while the ocular prosthesis fills the remaining 20–30% (2–3 ml) (Baino and Potestio, 2016).

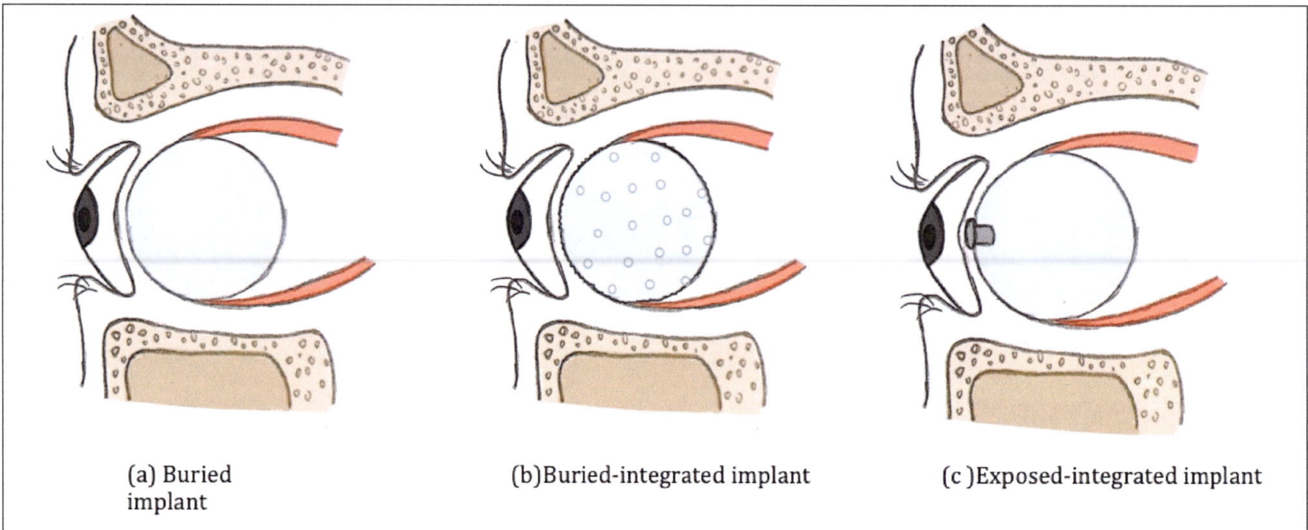

Figure 5-152 Types of Orbital implants.

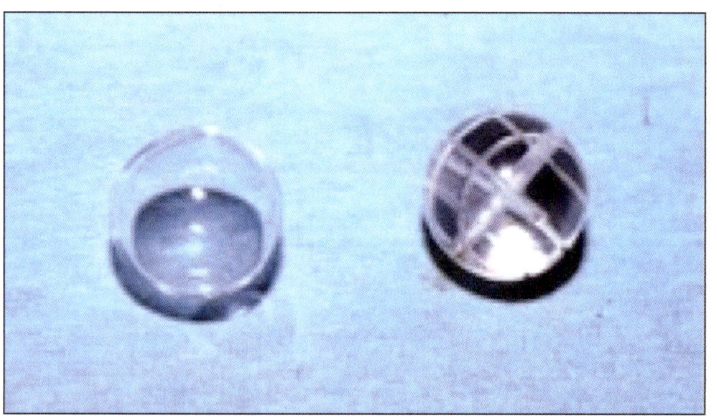

Figure 5-153 Smooth synthetic implants—silicone and polymethylmethacrylate.

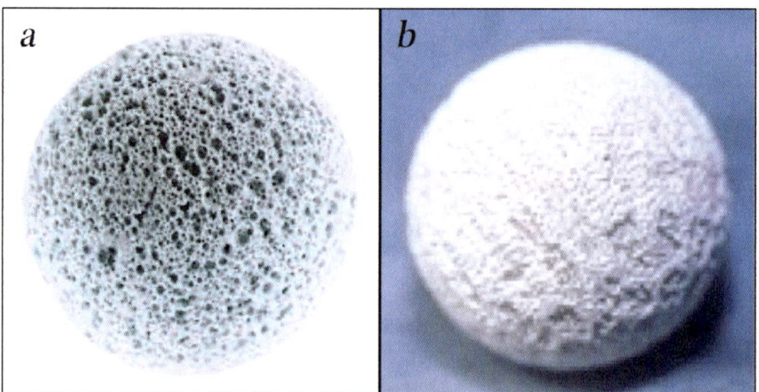

Figure 5-154 Porous implant *(a)* Hydroxyapatite. *(b)* Polyethylene.

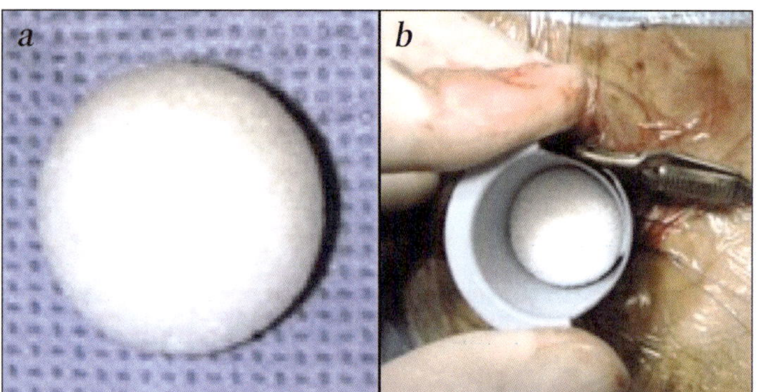

Figure 5-155 Porous implant—aluminum oxide.

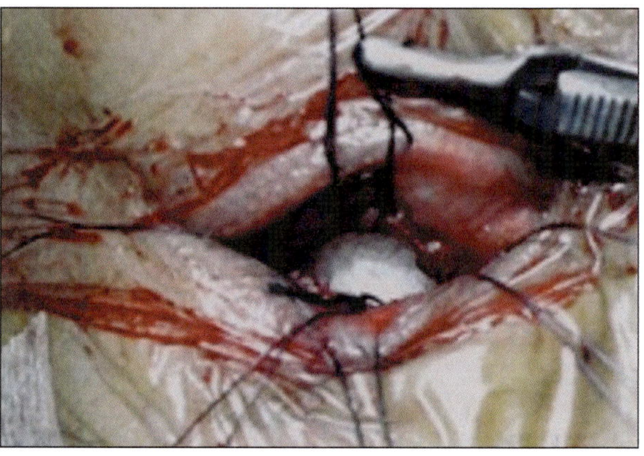

Figure 5-156 Implant placement into the anophthalmic socket.

A retrospective study by Kaltrieder et al. (2000) found no significant difference between the volume of the enucleated eye and the remaining contralateral eye. They also found that enophthalmos and superior sulcus deformity were more common in patients whose volume replacement was less than 100% of the volume of the remaining eye.

The orbital implant should also permit prosthesis motility. The motility of the ocular prosthesis refers to its movement in relation to the contralateral natural eye. Motility can be affected by preoperative eye movements, age, the contact of the prosthesis with the conjunctiva, the movement of the superior and inferior fornices, the status of the extraocular muscles, the presence of implants, and implant

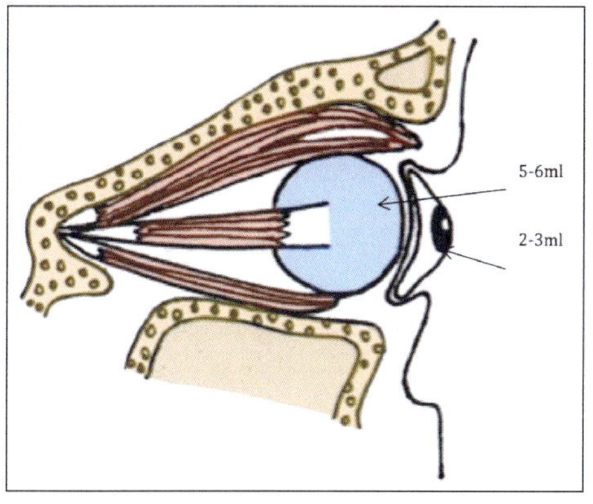

Figure 5-157 Distribution of volume to be taken up by the implant and the prosthesis.

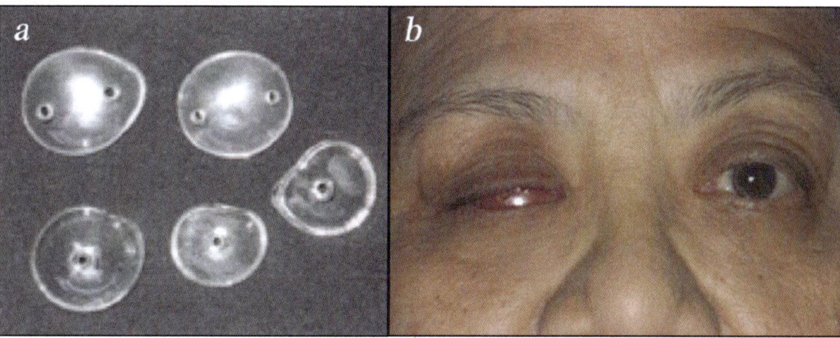

Figure 5-158 *(a and b)* Postsurgical conformer.

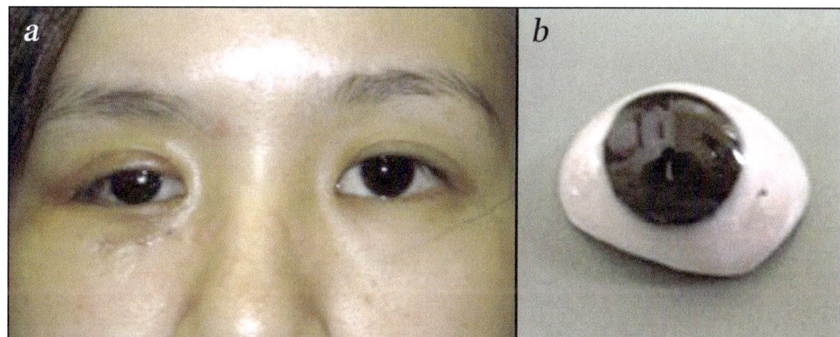

Figure 5-159 Customized aesthetic conformer.

pegging. Attachment of the extraocular muscles to the implant allows for near-normal movement of the implant. The motility of the prosthesis, however, will often still lag behind the natural eye.

Implant pegging refers to the coupling of the prosthesis to the implant with a motility peg (see Fig 5-152c). A titanium or plastic peg used with the prosthesis allows an improved range of movement (Chalasani et al., 2007; Jordan, 2018). A study by Viswanathan et al. (2007) found that only 7–8% of ophthalmologists place motility pegs in implants. This is due to the associated higher risk of complications, such as pyogenic granuloma, exposure, discharge, and peg malposition. Factors such as increased cost, requirement for additional surgeries, and satisfactory prosthetic movement without pegging also influence the decision not to peg. A report by the American Academy of Ophthalmology in 2003 also found that coupling the prosthesis with a motility peg may improve prosthetic motility, but there is little evidence to show the degree of improvement (Custer et al., 2003).

Types of ocular prostheses

There are various types of ocular prostheses available. The indications for each differ depending on the extent of replacement required after eye removal and time after removal.

Conformer shell

After the surgery, a thin acrylic shell of appropriate size and shape is placed into the socket to maintain the space (Fig 5-158). This shell is known as a conformer. The conformer allows the underlying tissue to heal, prevents adhesions, and reduces swelling (Cooper, 2010). It usually has holes on its surface to allow administration of ointments and medication. The conformer is left in place until complete healing and fabrication of the new ocular prosthesis.

Customized aesthetic conformer

Another variation is a customized aesthetic conformer (Fig 5-159). This cosmetic conformer is shaped and functions like a regular conformer. However, it has pupil, iris, and scleral coloring that help provide better aesthetics and improve self-esteem for the patient before the fitting of the definitive prosthesis. This helps reduce the downtime for patients. It also has a hole to allow drainage and administration of antibiotics.

Scleral shell

A scleral shell is a thin-fitting prosthesis that is used to cover a phthisical or eviscerated eye (Fig 5-160). Fabrication of a scleral shell is technically challenging due to the limited prosthetic space present for the prosthesis, possibly compromising the overall aesthetic outcome. The scleral shell provides good motility, often allowing synchronous movement to the contralateral normal eye.

Stock eye

The most appropriate iris size and color and scleral shape are selected from a prefabricated set of stock eyes and adjusted as

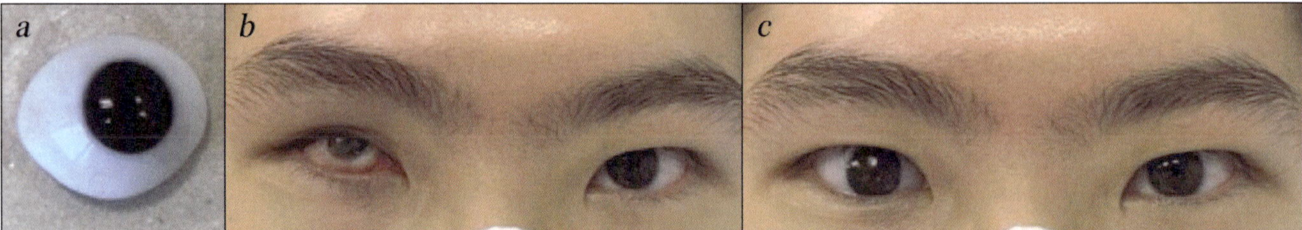

Figure 5-160 *(a)* Scleral shell. *(b)* Right phthisical eye. *(c)* After placement with a scleral shell.

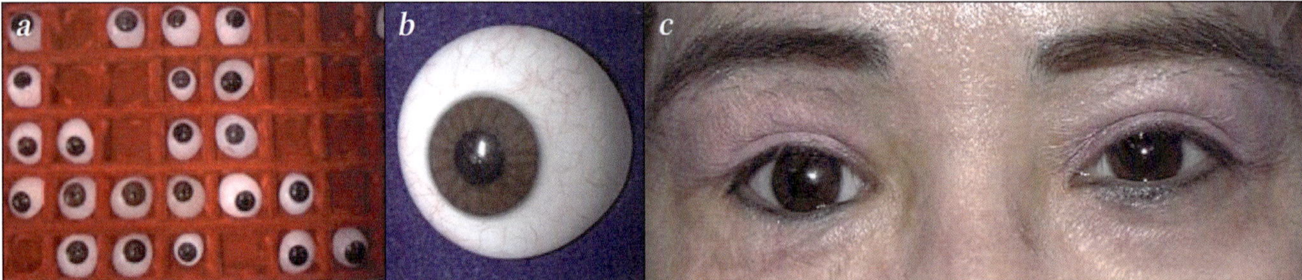

Figure 5-161 *(a)* Set of stock eyes. *(b)* Stock eye. *(c)* Patient wearing a stock eye (right).

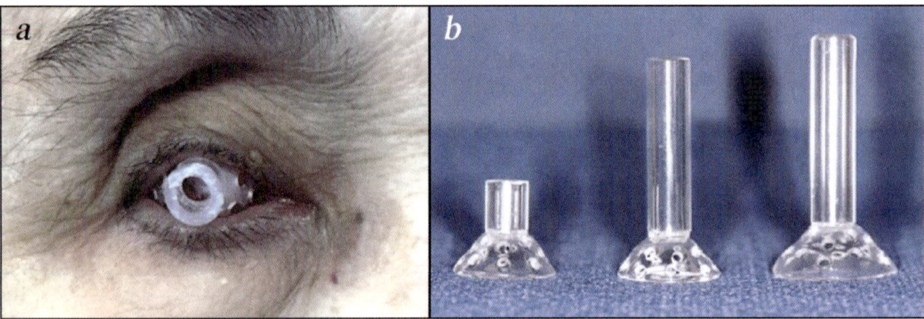

Figure 5-162 Selection of a suitable size ocular impression tray (Factor II).

necessary (Fig 5-161). Though cheaper, these are not customized, and hence the fit and aesthetics may be compromised.

Customized ocular prosthesis

The fabrication of a customized ocular prosthesis via the conventional workflow involves four clinical and laboratory stages (see Fig 5-177).

Stage I. After six to eight weeks of complete healing of the surgical site, fabrication of the ocular prosthesis can commence. The first clinical visit includes examination and diagnosis, making an impression, painting the iris disc, and determining the pupil size.

A thorough examination of the socket should be performed to ensure the absence of infection and to ascertain the position and motility of the implant. Measurements of the palpebral fissure opening and position in relation to the contralateral eye should be recorded. Examination of the margins, the position and movement of the eyelid, and the depth of the superior sulcus is essential. The socket should have adequate volume, and the fornices should be deep enough to retain the prosthesis.

An impression of the socket can be made using a suitably sized ocular impression tray (Fig 5-162). Irreversible hydrocolloid and elastomeric impression materials such as addition polymerization silicone are commonly used. The impression tray consists of a hollow handle through which impression materials can be syringed into the socket. Proper selection of the ocular impression tray size is crucial to avoid unwanted distortions of the tissues. The contralateral eye opening can be used as a guide to select the tray size. The impression should be made with the tray in a central position (Fig 5-163). Upon removal of the impression, it should be inspected for complete registration, drags, and voids (Fig 5-164).

Next, the diameter of the iris as well as the pupil should be chosen in reference to the contralateral natural iris. The appropriate size can then be selected from a range of prefabricated iris discs (Fig 5-165). The diameter of the chosen iris disc is usually 0.5 mm smaller than the contralateral eye to account for the magnifying effect of the transparent corneal curvature.

An opaque color, usually white, is first painted over the black iris disc prior to the addition of other colors (Fig 5-166). The complex coloring of the iris begins with the selection of the base color. This is usually blue, gray, green, brown, and black. This base color will act as the background color at the region between the collarette and the limbus. The limbus is the area on the outer circumference

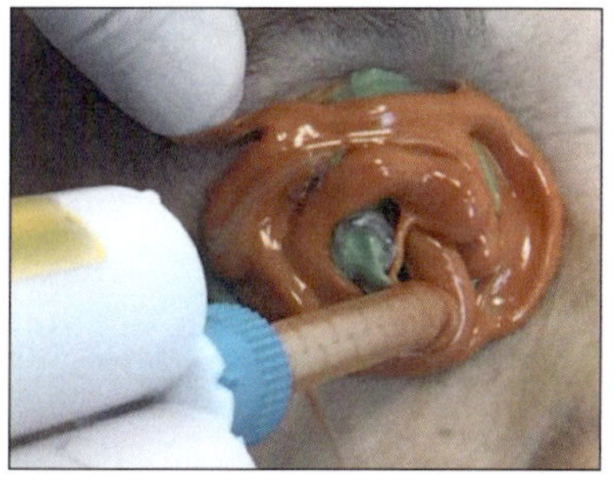

Figure 5-163 Impression making with addition polymerization silicone.

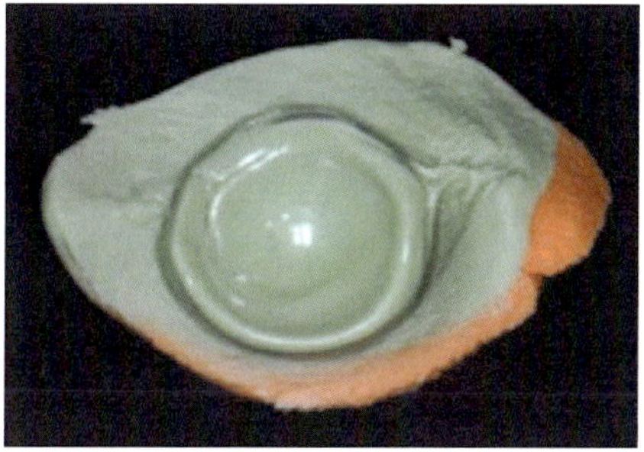

Figure 5-164 Silicone impression of an ocular defect.

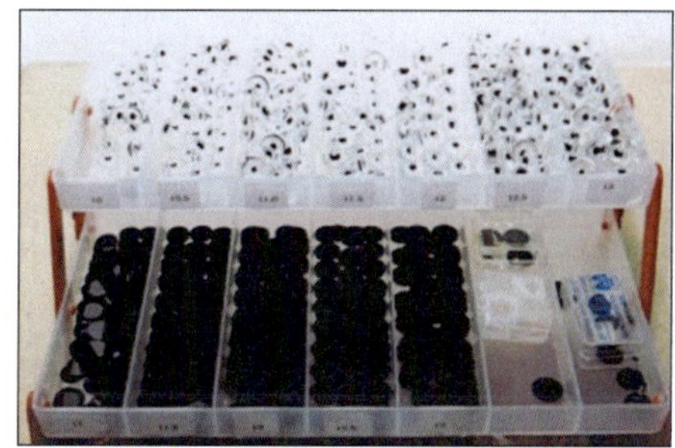

Figure 5-165 Tray of iris discs and corneal button of different sizes.

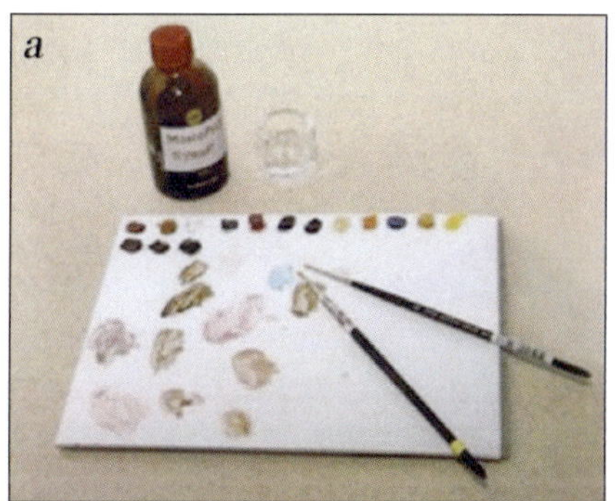

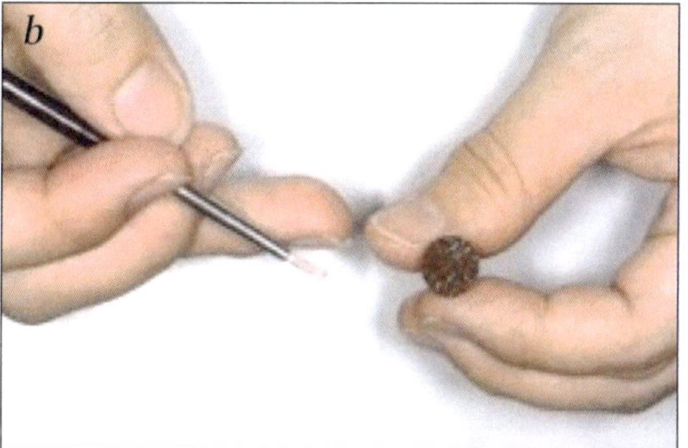

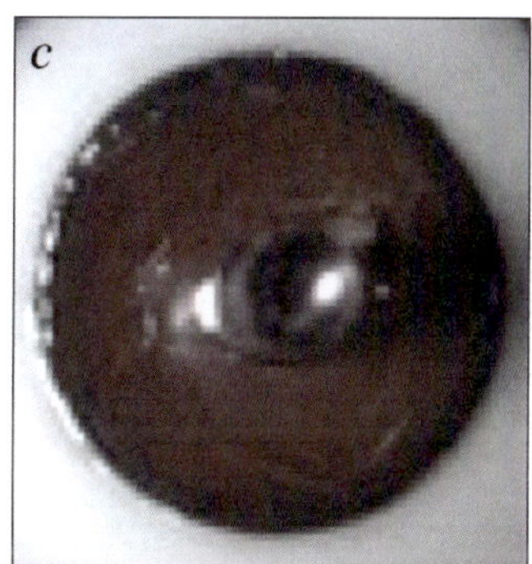

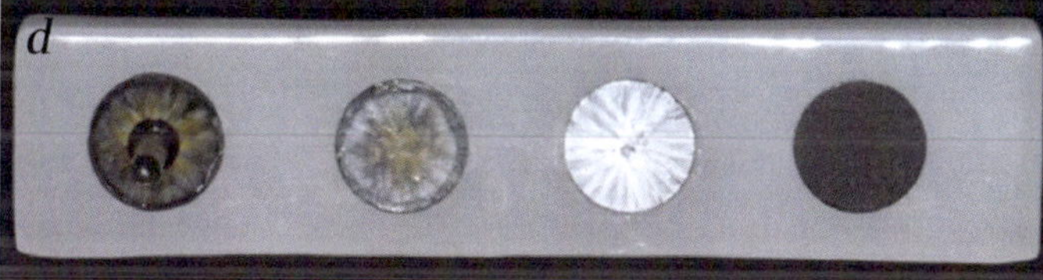

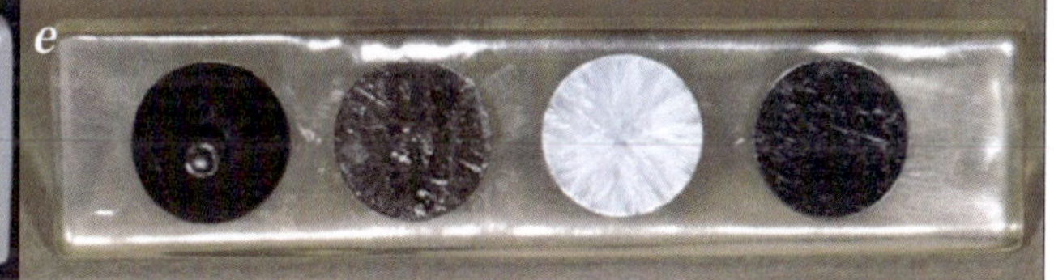

Figure 5-166 *(a–e)* Different stages of painting the iris disc.

of the iris. It is often seen as a dark ring of margin next to the sclera (see Fig 5-146). Overlapping brushstrokes of paint are used to create striations and to give depth when painting the stroma. Following this, the collarette and the limbus are painted. The collarette tends to be of a lighter shade than the stroma, but this may differ between individuals. The completed iris painting on the corneal button is compared with the contralateral iris to verify the shade matching.

Next, the painted iris disc is fixed onto the corneal button. Clear polymethyl methacrylate is flowed over the painted disc, and the corneal button is pressed down directly without trapping any air bubbles. This iris-pupil assembly is then set in a pressure pot (Fig 5-167).

The master cast is poured in Type III dental stone. The impression is poured in stages to create a two-piece master cast that can be separated and relocated (Fig 5-168). The posterior surface of the impression is first poured and allowed to set. Grooves are added for the relocation of the two halves of the master cast. A separating medium is applied. Dental stone is poured to create the second half of the master cast. The wax pattern is formed by flowing melted wax through eye aperture (Fig 5-169).

Stage II. During the second clinical visit, the wax pattern is inserted to review the contour, leveling, and projection with reference to the contralateral natural eye (Fig 5-169). Modification of the wax may be required to achieve the desired palpebral opening and eyelid support. The position of the iris-pupil assembly is determined with the patient seated upright in a primary gaze. The palpebra opening is outlined and the sclera color is selected.

The wax iris-pupil assembly is invested in two pours in a flask with dental stone (Fig 5-170). Upon complete set, the wax is boiled out, and the two halves of the flask are separated (Fig 5-171). Acrylic resin is packed into the flask and placed in a heated water bath for complete curing (Fig 5-172). After curing, the prosthesis is deflasked (Fig 5-173). A superficial cutback of the cured resin is done to allow the addition of surface characterization and a final layer of clear acrylic resin (Fig 5-174).

Stage III. During the third clinical visit, surface characterization and tinting of the ocular prosthesis are done with reference to the contralateral natural eye. Red cotton fibers may be used to mimic thin capillary vessels in the eye. The hue of the sclera is matched with the addition of small quantities of colors like blue or yellow.

Next, a layer of clear acrylic resin is packed over the prosthesis and heat cured. Upon deflasking, excess flash is removed and surface irregularities are smoothened. The prosthesis is then polished to a high shine (Fig 5-175).

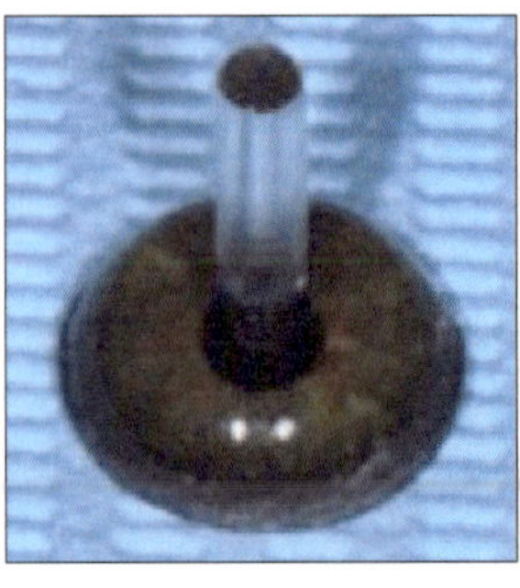

Figure 5-167 Iris-pupil assembly-corneal button sealed to the iris disc.

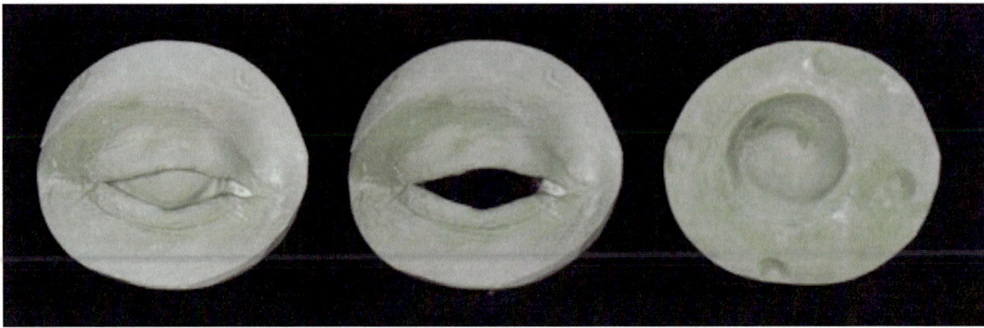

Figure 5-168 A two-piece master cast in Type III dental stone (Quickstone; Whip Mix Corp.).

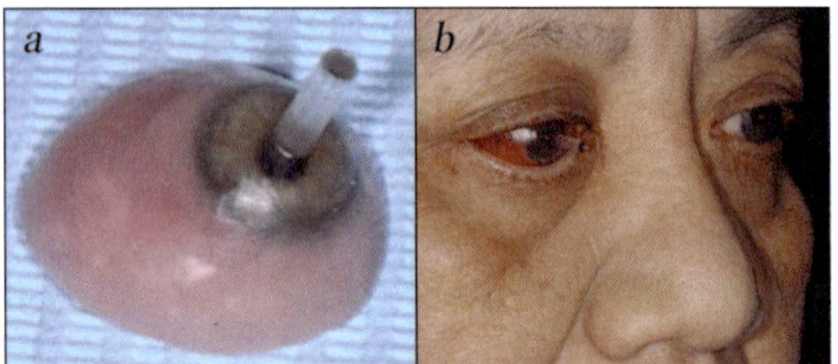

Figure 5-169 *(a)* The iris-pupil assembly is attached to the wax pattern following determination in a *(b)* primary gaze position.

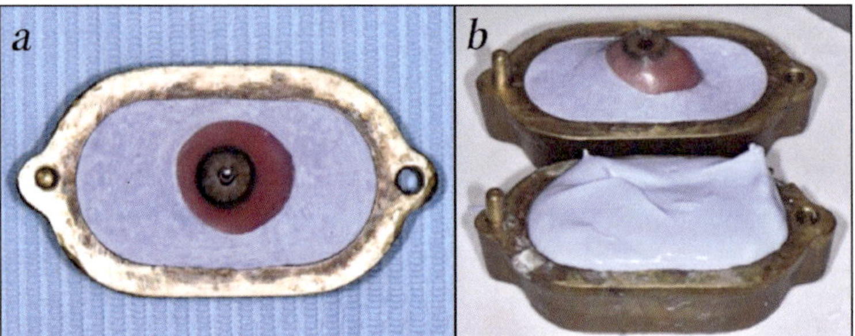

Figure 5-170 *(a and b)* Investment of the wax pattern in two pours.

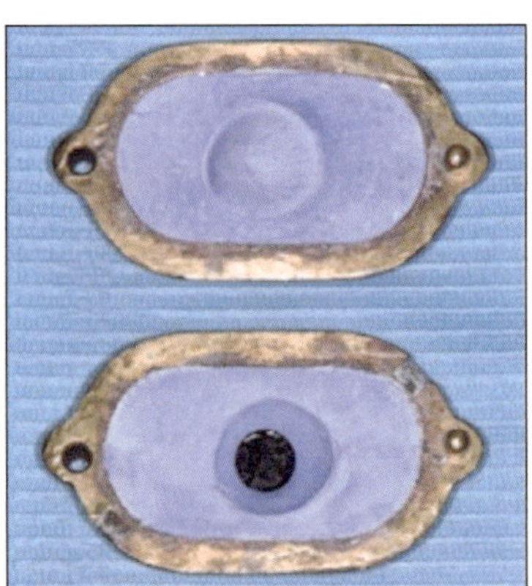

Figure 5-171 Boil out of wax from the investment.

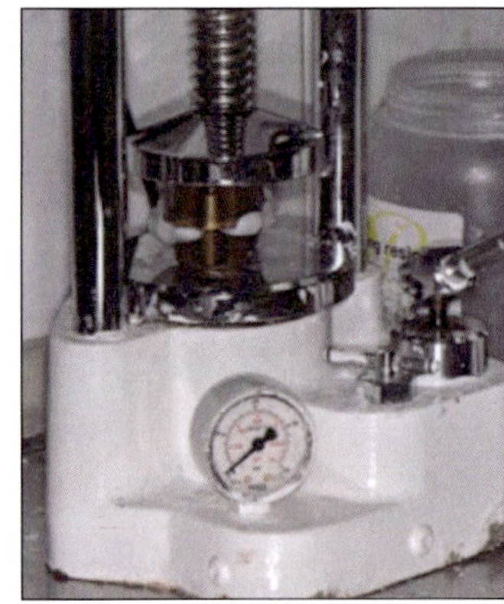

Figure 5-172 Acrylic resin (clear polymer and cross-linked monomer kit; Factor II) is packed into the flask under pressure.

Stage IV. The fourth and final clinical visit is for the delivery of the ocular prosthesis (Fig 5-176). The retention, stability, and fit of the prosthesis are evaluated, and adjustments are made as necessary. The patient is also taught how to insert and remove the prosthesis.

Maintenance. The frequency of cleaning differs between individuals, depending on the quantity of tear production. A survey of 429 prosthetic-eye wearers in New Zealand found an association between discharge frequency and cleaning regimens. Frequent cleaning results in an increase in discharge (Pine et al., 2013b). Similar findings were noted by Kashkouli et al. (2016) and Adrian et al. (2018).

The UK National Artificial Eye Service recommends that the ocular prosthesis be worn continuously with monthly removal for cleaning. Pine et al. (2013b) also found the lowest frequency of discharge with monthly cleaning. In cases with large amounts of discharge production, the frequency of cleaning may be increased.

The ocular prosthesis can be cleaned with saline or mild soap and water. The prosthesis should not be left out to dry when not in use and should be regularly inspected for scratches and deposits.

Common complications following the issue of the ocular prosthesis include dryness, discharge, and irritation of the mucosa. Dryness may occur due to the reduction in tear production over time. The use of tear supplements or lubricants may help relieve these symptoms. Foreign body reaction and constant movement of the prosthesis over the tissues may result in irritation and increased mucous production. This may be aggravated by the accumulation of debris and loss of prosthetic surface polish. The accumulation of debris between the prosthesis and the conjunctiva results in the increased production of debris and

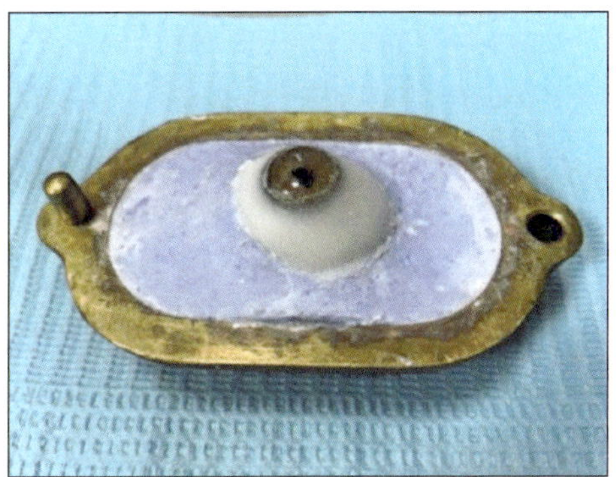
Figure 5-173 The investment is deflasked.

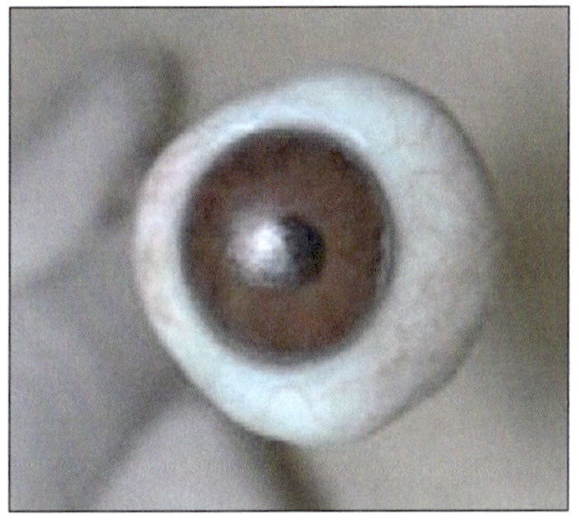
Figure 5-174 After cutback with tinting of sclera and placement of fibers to simulate vessels.

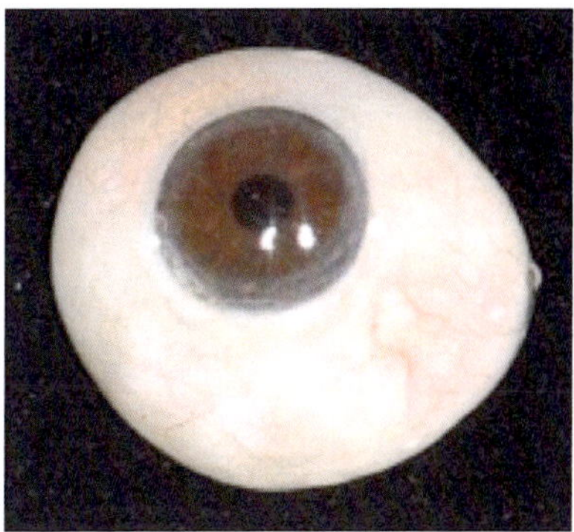
Figure 5-175 Polished ocular prosthesis ready for insertion.

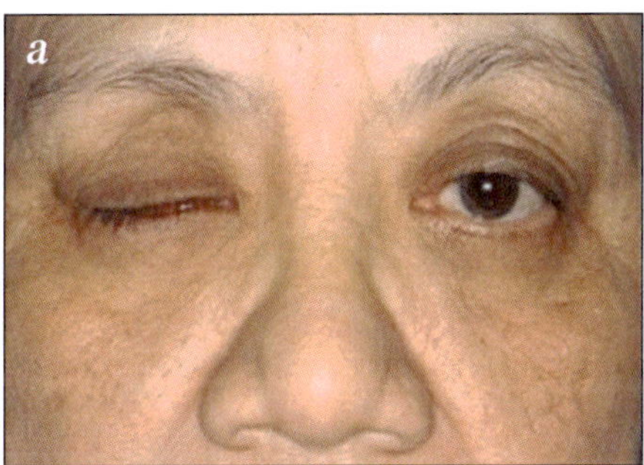

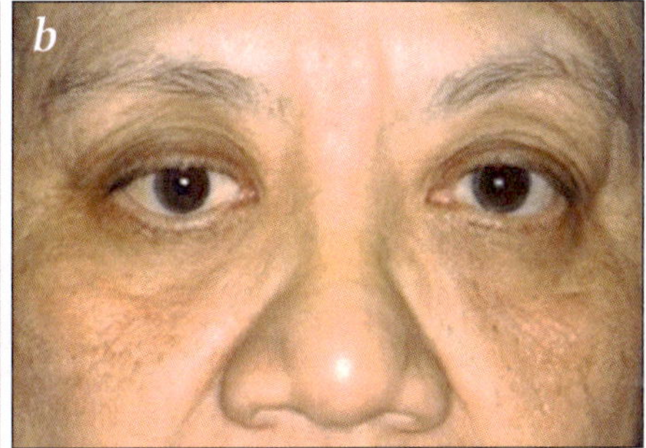

Figure 5-176 Insertion of the ocular prosthesis.

discharge. Regular annual follow-up and polishing of the prosthesis is recommended.

Incorporation of digital technologies into the ocular prosthesis workflow. Due to the technical sensitivity and complexity demands of fabricating a matching ocular prosthesis, many have adopted the use of digital technology to simplify the fabrication process.

Conventional impression making of the anophthalmic socket involves the injection of impression material into the socket, and inaccuracies from tissue and material distortion during the impression making may result in a poor fit of the prosthesis, which may cause discomfort and require additional clinical adjustments. To circumvent this, the substitution of the conventional impression techniques with digital scanning has been introduced and adopted by some.

Ruiters et al. (2016) suggested the use of cone beam computed tomography (CBCT) to digitally delineate the anophthalmic cavity. The accuracy of this impression-free geometric model made via CBCT was studied, and a mean absolute deviation of 0.28–0.37 mm was found. The 3D master model was used to design the ocular prosthesis, and a prototype was printed for chairside adjustments and verifications. It was then used to guide the conventional fabrication of the final prosthesis in polymethylmethacrylate (Ruiters et al., 2016). However, the use of CBCT to substitute the uncomfortable conventional impression-making procedure subjects the patient to additional radiation exposure, and hence its cost-to-benefit ratio will need to be weighed and considered.

The complexity of the characterization and depth of color of the iris makes matching to the contralateral natural eye a challenge. Replicating this on acrylic or glass requires years of skill, experience, and a keen eye for color. This process may be simplified by the use of digital photography. Kale et al. (2008) described a technique of taking a photograph of the contralateral iris and incorporating the printed photograph by vacuum pressing a clear copolyester sheet over the photo paper onto the prosthesis. Shah et al. (2014) recommended printing an image of the iris onto a self-adhesive glossy vinyl paper sticker before positioning it onto the scleral shell. Walshaw et al. (2018) suggested photographing nine different images of the contralateral eye in the same gaze and then merging and printing the images onto an adhesive paper prior to incorporating them into the prosthesis.

Although printed digital photographs are able to capture the general color and characterization of the iris, the depth of color via inkjet printing is still inferior to the layering and painting of colors by hand. Hence some have gone a step further to perform additional customization and color modifications to the printed photograph prior to embedding it into clear acrylic (Artopoulou et al., 2006; Lanzara et al., 2019). However, the longevity of the printed digital photograph is still unknown.

The use of 3D printing technology has also been adopted to ease the fabrication of the prosthesis. Ko et al. (2019) described the fabrication of a customized ocular prosthesis using digital technology. The impression mold of the anophthalmic socket is scanned to form a digital model. The prosthesis was then designed and printed using a biocompatible photopolymer resin. Dye sublimation transfer printing was used to transfer the photographed image of the contralateral iris and blood vessels onto the 3D-printed prosthesis (Ko et al., 2019). This described method however still requires the conventional impression-making technique to obtain a mold of the anophthalmic socket.

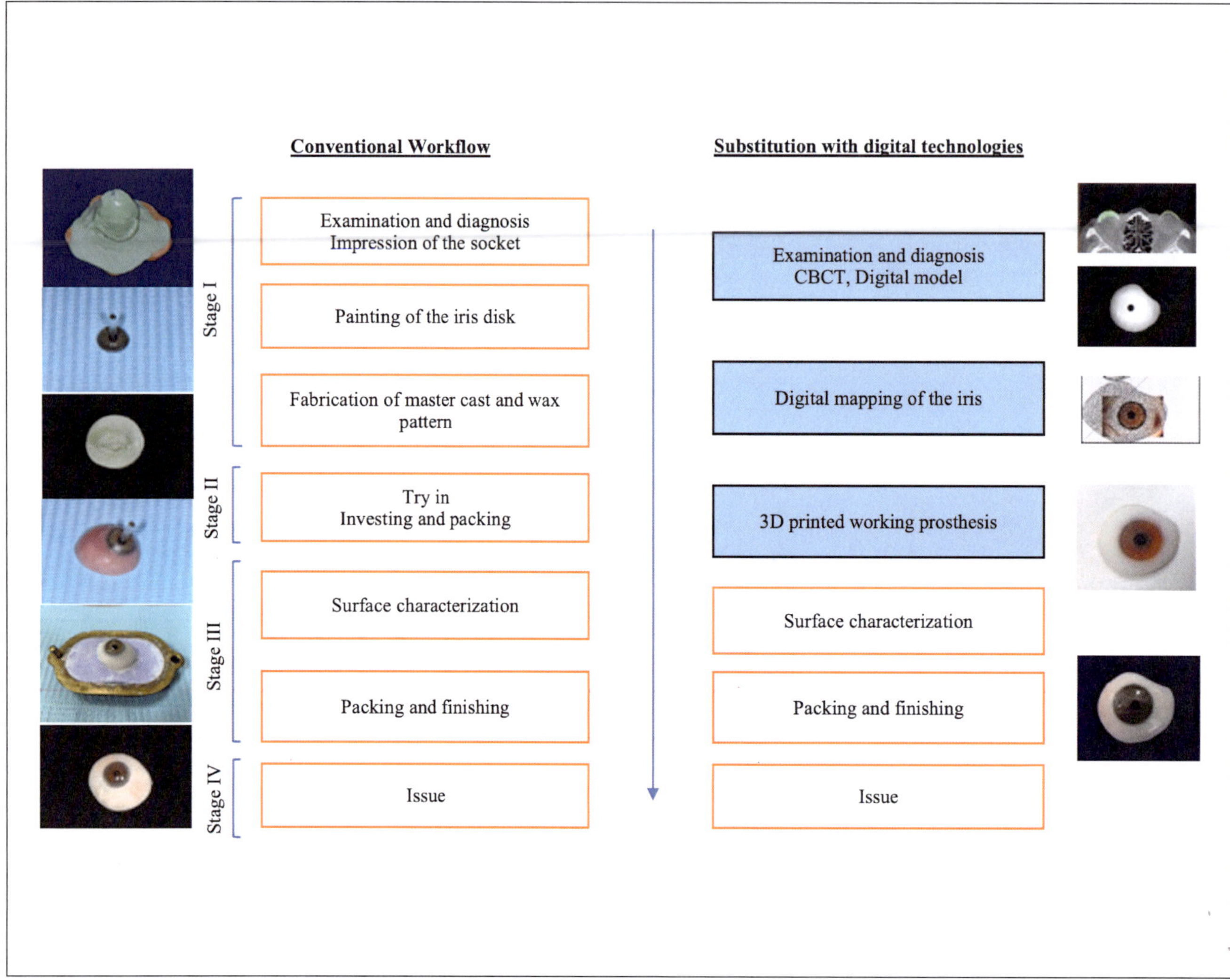

Figure 5-177 Conventional workflow and current digital advances to substitute stages.

There is currently no published literature on the end-to-end fabrication of ocular prostheses using digital technology (Fig 5-177). However, CNN recently reported that the first 3D-printed ocular prosthesis was issued to a patient in Moorfields Eye Hospital in London with details yet to be published. Progress is ongoing in digital technology to slowly substitute the conventional fabrication stages with digital techniques (Groot et al., 2021).

Outcome measurements. The outcome of ocular rehabilitation can be assessed by grading the quality of the ocular prosthesis and its impact on the patients' quality of life.

The eyes are usually the most noticeable feature on the face. Hence the loss of the eye often results in significant psychosocial impact on the patients due to facial disfigurement, loss of vision, or lower self-esteem (Goiato et al., 2013). The study by Goiato et al. (2013) evaluated the improvement in psychosocial domains of anophthalmic patients after the issue of the ocular prosthesis. The study found positive influences on personal relationship, household income, and psychosocial awareness after rehabilitation.

Ruiters et al. (2021a) developed a condition-specific questionnaire to evaluate patients' experience living with an ocular prosthesis. Vision, comfort, aesthetics, motility, and psychosocial functioning were assessed. The study found that most patients were satisfied with their physical appearance and reported adequate psychosocial functioning postocular rehabilitation. McBain et al. (2014) evaluated the patients' mood and appearance-related social anxiety and avoidance using the Hospital Anxiety and Depression Scale (HADS) and the Derriford Appearance Scale. They found an association between psychological variables and the patient's adaptation to the use of an ocular prosthesis. The successful adaptation to an artificial eye appeared to be associated with a number of underlying beliefs held by the patient rather than clinical aspects of their condition (McBain et al., 2014).

Dave et al. (2016) developed a grading scale to assess the characteristics of the limbus, vascularity, and pigmentation. Other grading scales have also been developed for the measurement of the inferior palpebral conjunctival inflammation and deposit accumulation on the ocular prosthesis (Pine et al., 2013a).

A well-fitted ocular prosthesis significantly impacts the overall emotional well-being of the patient. It is instrumental in improving the patient's self-confidence and rehabilitating them back to their normal social life.

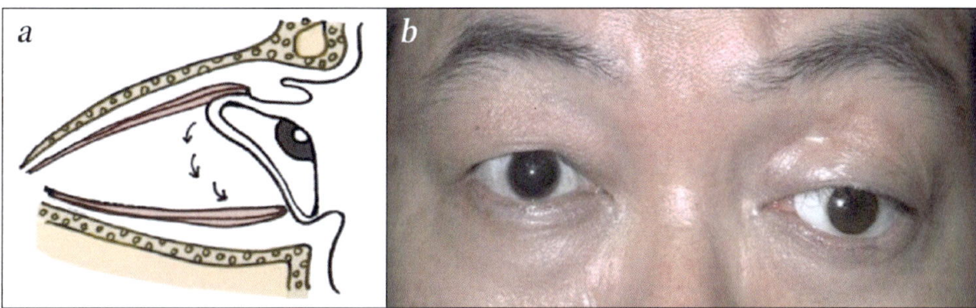

Figure 5-178 *(a and b)* Postenucleation socket syndrome.

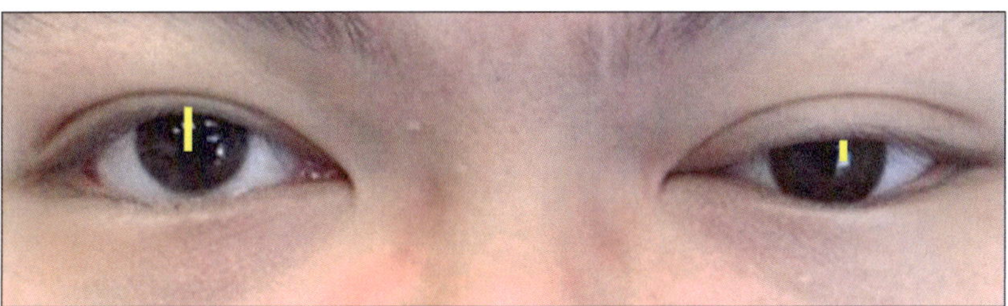

Figure 5-179 Marginal Distance (in yellow) for the right eye is normal (4.5 mm), while the left eye has ptosis (2 mm).

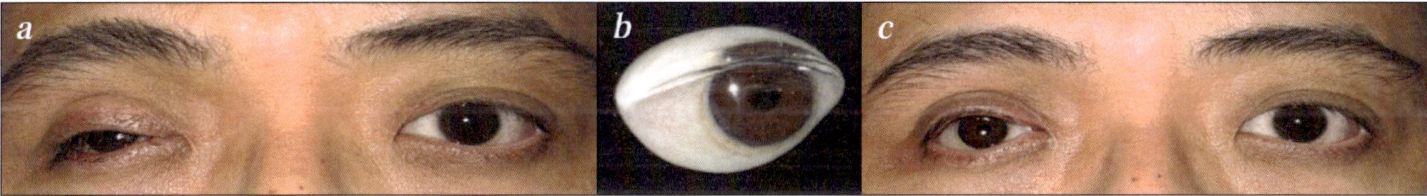

Figure 5-180 Correction of persistent ptosis. *(a and b)* Patient with upper eyelid ptosis. *(b)* Modified prosthesis with a ledge to prop up the upper eyelid. *(c)* Corrected ptosis.

Structural changes in the anophthalmic socket

After a period of wear, the weight of the prosthesis and the involutional aging changes in the eyelid may result in some structural changes. These commonly occur due to the sagging and retraction of the superior muscle complex, rotary displacement of the orbital content, and downward and forward redistribution of orbital fat (Smit et al., 1990).

In 1982, Tyers and Collins described these changes as postenucleation socket syndrome (PESS). It is characterized by clinical features such as enophthalmos, ptosis, superior sulcus deformity, lower lid laxity, and inferior positioning of the ocular prosthesis (Fig 5-178) (Tyers and Collin, 1982).

Ptosis is a clinical feature characterized by a droopy upper eyelid (Fig 5-179). Margin reflex distance (MRD) is defined as the measurement of the distance between the corneal light reflex and the upper eyelid margin. The average margin reflex distance in a healthy normal eye ranges from 4 to 5 mm. The severity of the ptosis is affected by the function of the levator muscle.

Ptosis can be classified into two categories: true ptosis and pseudoptosis. True ptosis occurs due to a lack of muscle tone and is caused by a variety of factors, such as the placement of an inadequate implant size, the migration of the orbital implant, a poorly fitted ocular prosthesis, the laxity and rotation of the orbital tissues, trauma, and the senile dehiscence of the levator aponeurosis. This may be corrected by a levator advancement surgery that shortens the muscle to reduce the droop over the prosthesis. Prosthesis volume augmentation and correction of the socket volume deficiency may be used to improve the palpebral opening (Figs 5-180 and 5-181).

Pseudoptosis occurs due to the loss of orbital volume between the implant and the eyelids after the removal of the eye. This can occur when the size of the ocular prosthesis is too small (Fig 5-182). Pseudoptosis can be managed by the fabrication of an adequately sized prosthesis that provides sufficient support to the eyelids.

Superior sulcus deformity manifests as a deep groove between the upper eyelid and superior orbital rim (Fig 5-183). This is a result of the loss of the orbital volume and sagging of the tissues.

Lower lid laxity can sometimes occur over time due to the weight of the ocular prosthesis on the lower eyelid (Fig 5-184). The disruption of the fibrous framework of the orbit may result in the rotation of the orbital contents inferiorly and anteriorly. The shallower the inferior fornix results in the tilt of the prosthesis. The inferior portion of the prosthesis pushes on the inferior eyelid while the superior portion moves posteriorly inside the orbit, deepening the superior sulcus. This may be managed by adjusting the inferior aspect of the prosthesis to reduce the pressure on the lower eyelid. Surgical intervention can also be done to tighten the lower eyelid musculature.

Other possible complications apart from PESS include implant migration, implant exposure, entropion, ectropion, and socket contracture.

Implant migration may occur with long-standing alloplastic, nonporous orbital implants. This may be caused by the poor placement of the initial implant or the lack of attachment to the extraocular

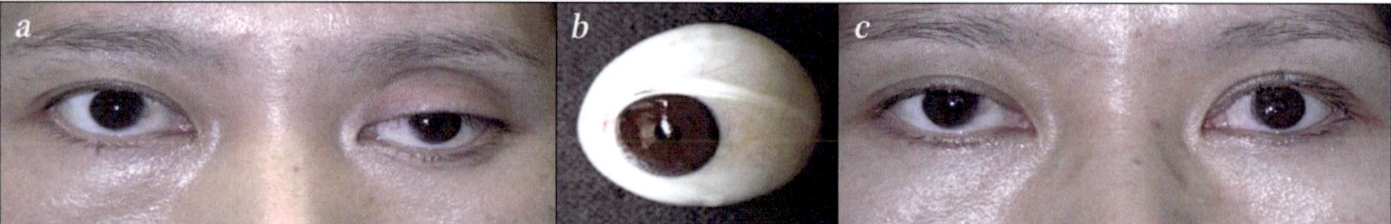

Figure 5-181 *(a)* Case of left eye ptosis that could not be corrected with modification of the prosthesis. *(b)* Modified ocular prosthesis with a ledge. *(c)* After levator advancement surgery to repair ptosis with significant improvement.

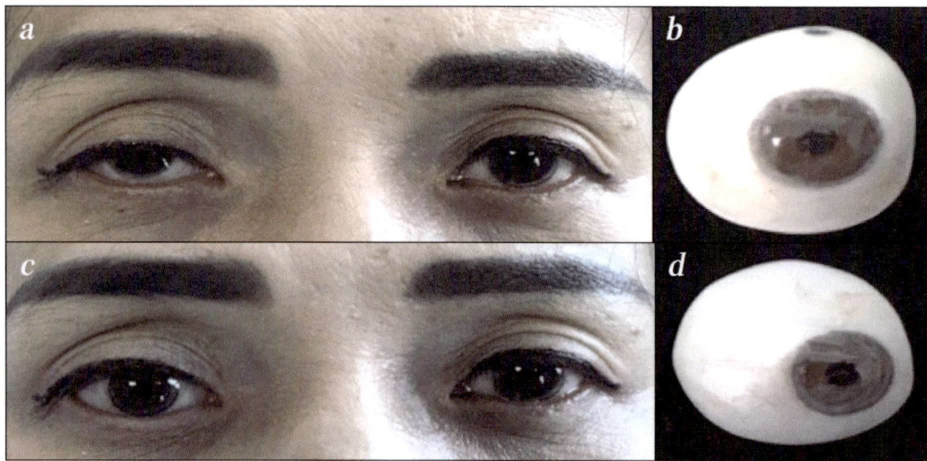

Figure 5-182 *(a)* Pseudoptosis noted on the right eye due to a poorly contoured ocular prosthesis. *(b)* Contour of ocular prosthesis. *(c)* Correction of the pseudoptosis after replacement with a new prosthesis. *(d)* Contour of the newly made ocular prosthesis.

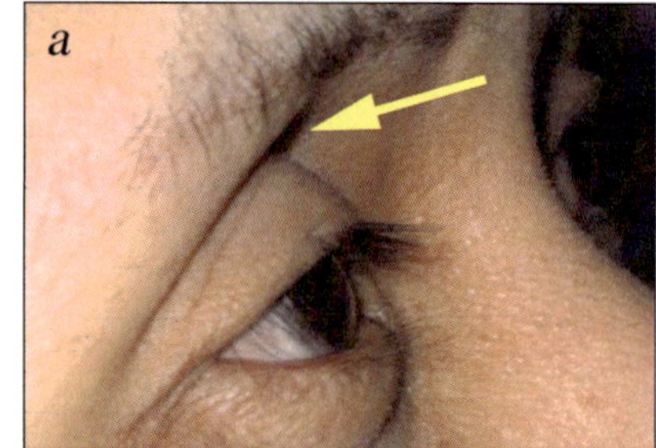

Figure 5-183 Superior sulcus deformity *(arrow)*.

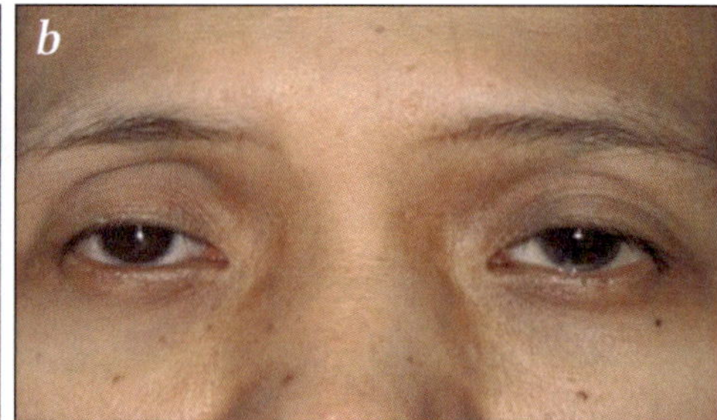

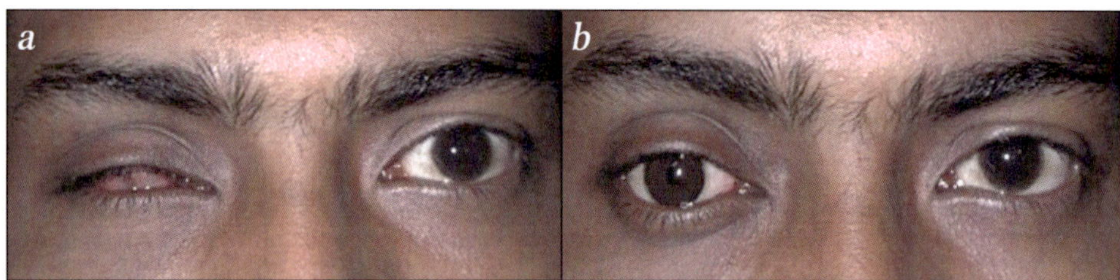

Figure 5-184 Lower lid laxity *(a)* without prosthesis and *(b)* with prosthesis in place.

muscles, resulting in poor motility and a poorly positioned prosthesis. Treatment requires removal and replacement of the implant (Fig 5-185).

Implant exposure in the socket can sometimes occur (Fig 5-186). Factors that predispose to it include closing the wound under tension, poor wound closure techniques, infection, inflammation, frictional irritation, pressure from the prosthesis, and delayed ingrowth of fibrovascular tissue with subsequent tissue breakdown. The incidence of implant exposure in patients with the use of rough porous implants was found to be higher than with nonporous implants. The highest incidence was found with the use of bovine hydroxyapatite implants (Custer and Trinkaus, 2007). A study by Lin and Liao (2017) found that eviscerated globes and pegged implants are risk factors for implant exposure. High exposure rates were also found with Medpor implants (Lin and Liao, 2017). If the exposure is small, conservative management is preferred. Vaulting of the intaglio surface of the prosthesis can be done to reduce pressure on the exposure site to prevent further breakdown of the

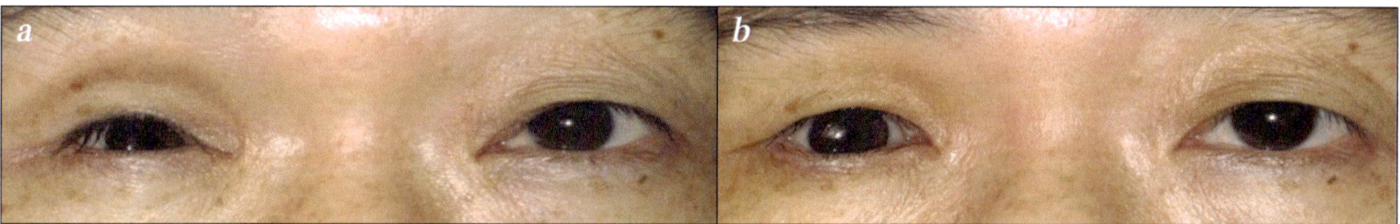

Figure 5-185 *(a)* Downward implant migration resulting in a superior tilt of the prosthesis (right). *(b)* After surgical removal of the implant and reconstruction with a dermis fat graft.

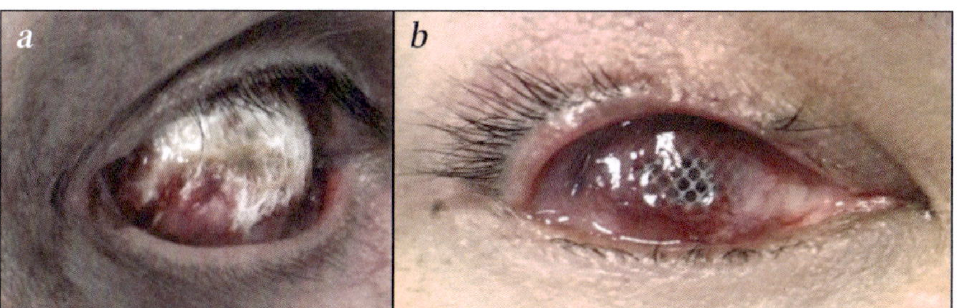

Figure 5-186 *(a and b)* Exposed orbital implants.

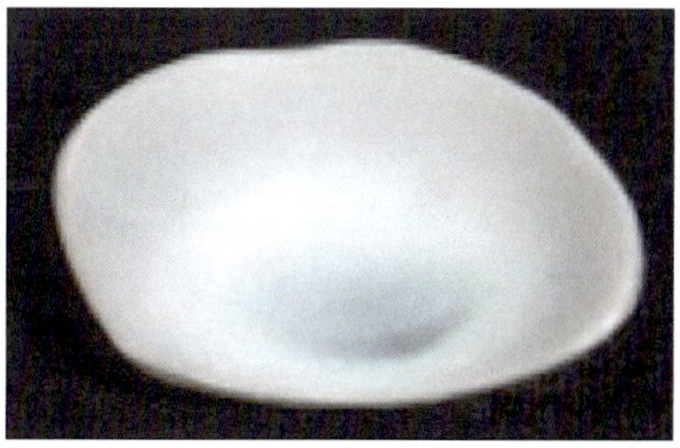

Figure 5-187 Vaulting of the intaglio surface of the prosthesis.

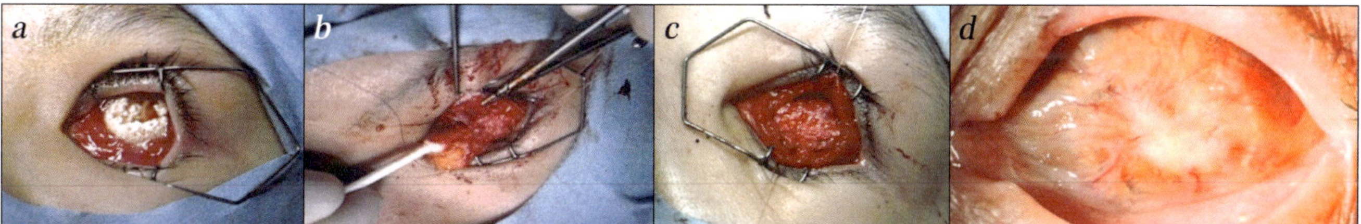

Figure 5-188 *(a–d)* Surgical coverage of an implant exposure with an autogenous tissue graft.

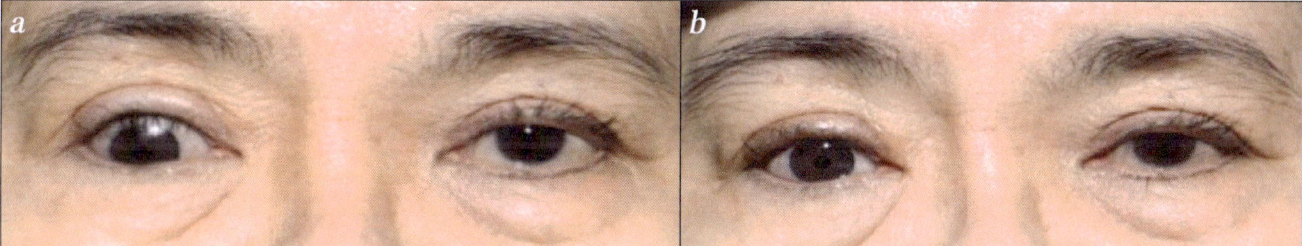

Figure 5-189 *(a)* Right eye with entropion. *(b)* After surgical correction.

tissues and to allow healing (Fig 5-187). However, if the exposure is medium or large (>3 mm), surgical intervention may be needed to cover the exposure site with an autogenous tissue graft (Fig 5-188). Burring down of the anterior implant surface can be carried out prior to coverage with a tissue graft.

Entropion refers to the inward rotation of the eyelid margin and vertically directed eyelashes (Fig 5-189). This is a result of the contracture of the inferior fornix, lower lid laxity, and dehiscence of the lower lid retractors from the inferior border of the tarsus due to chronic inflammation (Hita et al., 2016). This can be corrected surgically with a marginal tarsotomy procedure.

Ectropion is defined as a condition in which the eyelid turns outward, leaving the inner eyelid exposed and irritated (Fig 5-190). This condition is commonly associated with lower eyelid laxity, use of a heavy prosthesis, and the frequent removal of the artificial eye prosthesis. These factors contribute to the laxity of the medial and canthal tendons, resulting in horizontal lid laxity, deficient anterior lamella, or nerve palsy. Surgical management is required to correct this via a lateral tarsal strip procedure, canthoplasty, or tarsorrhaphy.

Socket contracture occurs due to the shrinkage and shortening of the tissues of the anophthalmic orbit resulting in poor retention of the prosthesis (Fig 5-191). This may be secondary to fibrosis from multiple surgeries, implant migration, implant extrusion, infection, chronic inflammation, and conjunctival diseases. Socket contracture may be classified into grades depending on severity

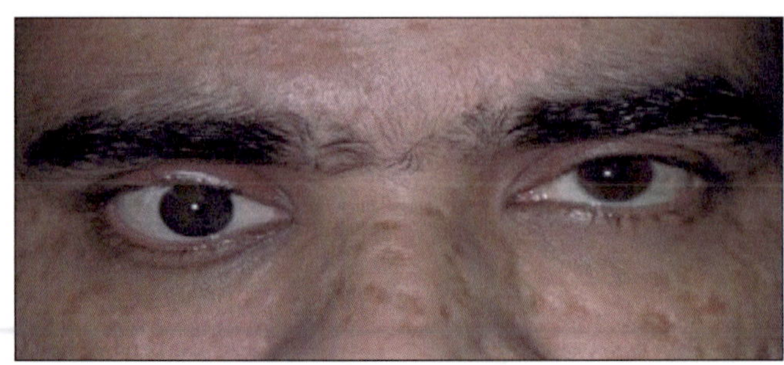

Figure 5-190 Ectropion seen on the right lower eyelid.

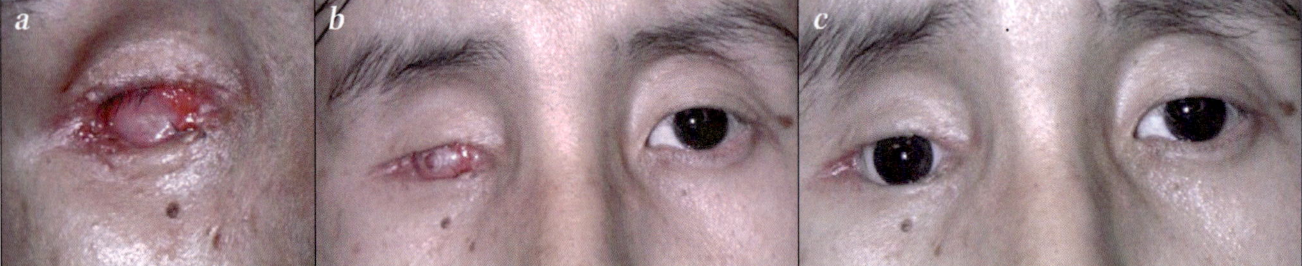

Figure 5-191 *(a)* Right contracted socket reconstructed with a dermis fat graft and deepening of the superior and inferior fornices. *(b)* A customized conformer in place. *(c)* Final outcome with ocular prosthesis.

of contraction, ability to retain the prosthesis, and clinical features (Tawfik et al., 2009). Surgical management of socket contracture is usually required to increase the conjunctival surface area via the addition of mucosal or dermis fat grafts.

Congenital microphthalmia

Congenital anophthalmia is a condition where there is an absence of an eye due to its deficient formation during gestation (Llorente et al., 2011). Microphthalmia is an orbital disorder where the affected eye is abnormally smaller than the natural eye. The exact pathogenesis is not fully known, but possible causes include genetic mutations and chromosomal abnormalities (Dharmasena et al., 2017; Verma and Fitzpatrick, 2007). Environmental factors such as exposure to radiation, chemicals, drugs, toxins, and viruses may also play a role (Dharmasena et al., 2017; Verma and Fitzpatrick, 2007). These factors may adversely affect the differentiation of tissues required for the development of the orbit.

The annual incidence of microphthalmia in 2011 was found to be around 10 per 100,000 infants (Dharmasena et al., 2017). The prevalence between genders is similar. The treatment of microphthalmia varies depending on its severity. Treatment includes the use of different-sized conformers and expanders to stimulate the growth of the socket. Conformers will have to be replaced regularly as the face develops. A definitive prosthesis can be made when the face is fully developed (Fig 5-192).

Stimulation of the continued growth of the orbit is important in microphthalmia patients. This is because the development of the orbit, eyelid, and conjunctival fornices will affect the ability of the patient to wear an ocular prosthesis in the future. Asymmetry of the face due to differential development may also occur, resulting in cosmetic deformity.

Retinoblastoma

Retinoblastoma is an eye tumor that is prevalent in early childhood. The incidence of retinoblastoma ranges from 1 in 15,000 to 1 in 18,000 live births (Pandey, 2014). The malignancy can spread along the nerve to the brain, and removal of the eye is required to prevent its spread. Leukocoria is the most common clinical feature, followed by strabismus, painful blind eye, and loss of vision (Abramson et al., 1998). As significant facial and orbital growth usually occurs during this period of childhood, the enucleation and adjuvant radiation often lead to maldevelopment of the orbit (Fig 5-193) (Oatts et al., 2017).

The loss of an eye has a detrimental impact on the psychosocial well-being and quality of life of patients. Close collaboration between the oculoplastic surgeon and prosthodontist is crucial for the comprehensive planning and execution of the ocular prosthetic rehabilitation. The ideal outcome should consist of a comfortable and properly fitted ocular prosthesis that is centrally positioned with well-supported upper and lower eyelids. It should also look similar to the sighted contralateral globe with good motility. In situations with tissue changes and socket contractures, surgical intervention with or without grafting may be required to improve the prosthetic prognosis. Ongoing developments in digital technology aim to streamline the fabrication workflow of ocular prostheses.

Summary

Although most skin tumors are benign, if they are left untreated for extended periods or if initial treatment is followed by extensive recurrences, large facial defects can be the result. Small facial defects such as loss of an ala are best reconstructed surgically, but

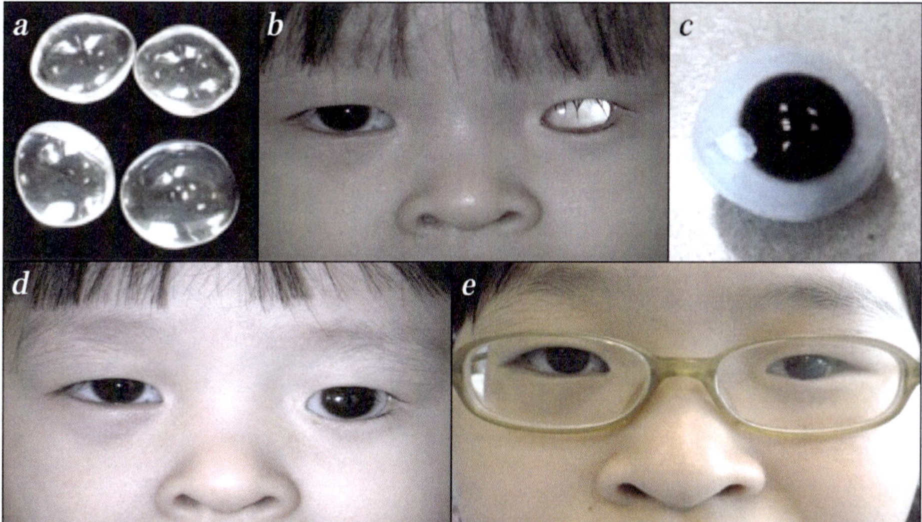

Figure 5-192 *(a)* Expanders of different sizes to stimulate orbital growth. *(b)* Patient at age three with expander in the left eye. *(c)* Aesthetic conformer. *(d)* Patient at age four with aesthetic conformer in place. *(e)* Patient at age five with ocular prosthesis in place.

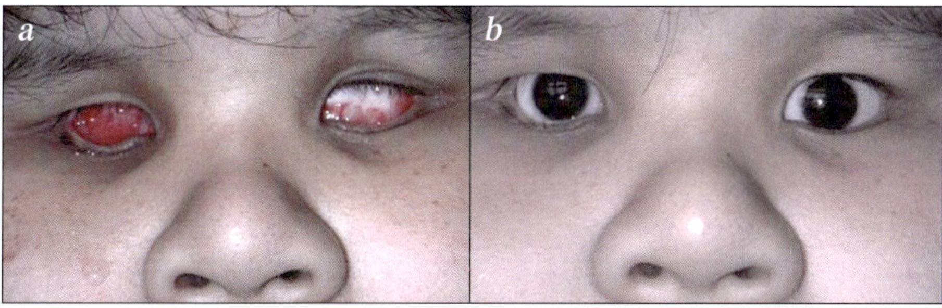

Figure 5-193 Case of a patient with bilateral retinoblastoma, which required enucleation with dermis fat graft to aid in the retention of the ocular prostheses.

large facial defects, such as those arising from auriculectomy, rhinectomy, orbital exenteration, or large midfacial resections, are best rehabilitated with a prosthesis.

Close collaboration between the surgical oncologist and the maxillofacial prosthodontist prior to surgical resection of the tumor is essential because the best results are obtained when there is minimal distortion of adjacent facial structures and when the surgeon prepares the defect to receive a prosthesis following tumor ablation. A successful outcome is enhanced by the placement of skin grafts, properly contoured flaps, and osseointegrated implants.

The silicones remain the material most commonly utilized for facial prostheses. Their physical properties and the workability of the silicone elastomers continue to improve. A successful prosthesis will escape detection by the casual observer and will possess contours, color, and surface texture that are compatible with those of the existing facial features. Lines of juncture between the prosthesis and adjacent skin must be properly positioned and camouflaged.

Osseointegrated implants provide excellent retention for facial prostheses and have dramatically improved patient acceptance. Success rates have been excellent for most sites. Irradiated sites demonstrate lower success rates. CAD/CAM systems are evolving to aid in implant site selection, implant placement, and prosthesis construction.

Techniques have evolved, ensuring excellent outcomes with ocular prostheses. Close collaboration between the maxillofacial prosthodontist/ocularist will optimize outcomes. Digital technologies have been adopted to facilitate designing and streamlining the manufacturing of ocular prostheses. Development on the use of 3D technology using printed resin is ongoing.

References

Ababneh OH, AboTaleb EA, Abu Ameerh MA, et al. Enucleation and evisceration at a tertiary care hospital in a developing country. BMC Ophthalmology 2015;15:120. http://doi.org/10.1186/s12886-015-0108-x.

Abbatucci JS, Boulier N, Laforge T, et al. Radiation therapy of skin carcinomas: Results of a hypofractionated irradiation schedule in 675 cases followed more than 2 years. Radiother Oncol 1989;14:113–119.

Abdelnnabi MM, Moore DJ, Sakumura JS. In vitro comparison study of MDX-4-4210 and polydimethyl siloxane silicone materials. J Prosthet Dent 1984;51:523–526.

Abdullah HA, Abdul-Ameer FM. Evaluation of some mechanical properties of a new silicone elastomer for maxillofacial prostheses after addition of intrinsic pigments. Saudi Dent J 2018;30:330–336.

Abramson DH, Frank CM, Susman M, et al. Presenting signs of retinoblastoma. J Pediatr 1998 Mar;132:505–508.

Adrian T, Lubis RR, Zubaidah TSH. Association between frequency of prosthesis cleaning and the discharge characteristics and the tear film in subjects with anophthalmic socket after evisceration with dermis fat graft. Open Access Maced J Med Sci 2018;6:2012–2016.

Agnese DM, Maupin R, Tillman B, et al. Head and neck melanoma in the sentinel lymph node era. Arch Otolaryngol Head Neck 2007;133:1121–1124.

Akash RN, Guttal SS. Effect of incorporation of nano-oxides on color stability of maxillofacial silicone elastomer subjected to outdoor weathering. J Prosthodont 2015;24:569–575.

Akay C, Cevik P, Karakis D, et al. In vitro cytotoxicity of maxillofacial silicone elastomers: Effect of nano-particles. J Prosthodont 2018;27:584–587.

Alam M, Armstrong A, Baum C, et al. Guidelines of care for the management of cutaneous squamous cell carcinoma. J Am Acad Dermatol 2018;78:560–578.

Alam MS, Sugavaneswaran M, Arumaikkannu G, et al. An innovative method of ocular prosthesis fabrication by bio-CAD and rapid 3-D printing technology: A pilot study. Orbit 2017;36:223–227.

Alexander C. Faces of war. Smithsonian 2007 Feb.

Al-Harbi FA, Ayad NM, Saber MA, et al. Mechanical behavior and color change of facial prosthetic elastomers after outdoor weathering in a hot and humid climate. J Prosthet Dent 2015;113:146–151.

Allen NS, Vasiliou C, Marshall GP, et al. Light stabiliser, antioxidant and pigment interactions in the thermal and photochemical oxidation of polyethylene films. Polymer Degradation and Stability 1989;24:17–31. http://doi.org/10.1016/0141-3910(89)90130-4.

Al-Quarayashi Z, Hassan M, Srivastav S, et al. Risk and survival of patients with head and neck cutaneous melanoma: National perspective. Oncology 2017;93:18–28.

Anderson JD, Johnston DA, Haugh GS, et al. The Toronto outcome measure for craniofacial prosthetics: Reliability and validity of a condition-specific quality-of-life instrument. Int J Oral Maxillofac Implants 2013;28:453–460.

Anderson JD, Szalai JP. The Toronto outcome measure for craniofacial prosthetics: A condition-specific quality-of-life instrument. Int J Oral Maxillofac Implants 2003;18:531–538.

Andres CJ. Survey of materials used in extra-oral maxillofacial prosthetics. In Materials research in maxillofacial prosthetics. Ed. JC Setcos. Trans Acad Dent Mater 1992;5:25–40.

Andres CJ, Haug SP, Brown DT, et al. Effects of environmental factors on maxillofacial elastomers 2: Report of survey. J Prosthet Dent 1992;68:519–522.

Antonucci J, Stansbury J. Polymers and elastomers for extraoral maxillofacial prosthetics (EMFP). In Materials research in maxillofacial prosthetics. Ed. JC Setcos. Trans Acad Dent Mater 1992;5:138–155.

Ariani N, Vissink A, van Oort RP, et al. Microbial biofilms on facial prostheses. Biofouling (Chur, Switzerland) 2012;28:583–591.

Artopoulou II, Chambers MS, Eliades G. Porosity of maxillofacial silicone elastomers and microleakage pattern of the commercially pure Ti-silicone elastomer interface after hydrothermal cycling. J Prosthet Dent 2016a;116:937–942.

Artopoulou II, Chambers MS, Zinelis S, et al. Peel strength and interfacial characterization of maxillofacial silicone elastomers bonded to titanium. Dent Mater 2016b;32(7):e137–e147. http://doi.org/10.1016/j.dental.2016.03.024.

Artopoulou II, Montgomery PC, Wesley PJ, et al. Digital imaging in the fabrication of ocular prostheses. Journal of Prosthetic Dentistry 2006;95:327–330.

Atay A, Piskin B, Akin H, et al. Evaluation of Candida albicans adherence on the surface of various maxillofacial silicone materials. J Mycol Med 2013;23:27–32.

Autian J. Toxicological evaluation of biomaterials: Primary acute toxicity screening program. Artif Organs 1977;1:53–60.

Aziz T, Waters M, Jagger R. Analysis of the properties of silicone rubber maxillofacial prosthetic materials. J Dent 2003a;31:67–74.

Aziz T, Waters M, Jagger R. Development of a new poly(dimethylsiloxane) maxillofacial prosthetic material. J Biomed Mater Res B Appl Biomater 2003b;65:252–261.

Babu AS, Manju V, Gopal VK. Effect of chemical disinfectants and accelerated aging on maxillofacial silicone elastomers: An In vitro Study. Indian J Dent Res 2018;29:67–73.

Bader C, Kolb D, Weaver JC, et al. Data-driven material modeling with functional advection for 3D printing of materially heterogeneous objects. 3D Print Additive Manufact 2016;3(2):71–79.

Baino F, Potestio I. Orbital implants: State-of-the-art review with emphasis on biomaterials and recent advances. Mater Sci Eng C Mater Biol Appl 2016 Dec 1;69:1410–1428.

Balik A, Ozdemir-Karatas M, Peker K, et al. Soft tissue response and survival of extraoral implants: A long-term follow-up. J Oral Implantol 2016;42:41–45.

Bangera BS, Guttal SS. Evaluation of varying concentrations of nano-oxides as ultraviolet protective agents when incorporated in maxillofacial silicones: An in vitro study. J Prosthet Dent 2014;112:1567–1572.

Bankoğlu M, Oral I, Gül EB, et al. Influence of pigments and pigmenting methods on color stability of different silicone maxillofacial elastomers after 1-year dark storage. J Craniofac Surg 2013;24:720–724.

Banks ER, Cooper PH. Adenosquamous carcinoma of the skin: A report of 10 cases. J Cutan Pathol 1991;18:227–234.

Barnhart G. A new material and technic in the art of somato-prosthesis. J Dent Res 1960;39:836–844.

Bates MT, Chow JK, Powers JM, et al. Color stability and mechanical properties of two commonly used silicone elastomers with e-skin and reality coloring systems. Int J Prosthodont 2021;34:204–211.

Bayer A, Goldschmidt A. Silicones: Chemistry and technology. Essen, Germany: Vulkan; 1991. pp. 45–59.

Beatty MW, Mahanna GK, Dick K, et al. Color changes in dry-pigmented maxillofacial elastomer resulting from ultraviolet light exposure. J Prosthet Dent 1995;74:493–498.

Beatty MW, Mahanna GK, Jia W. Ultraviolet radiation-induced color shifts occurring in oil-pigmented maxillofacial elastomers. J Prosthet Dent 1999;82:441–446.

Begum Z, Kola MZ, Joshi P. Analysis of the properties of commercially available silicone elastomers for maxillofacial prostheses. Int J Contemp Dent 2011;2:4.

Bell WT, Chalian VA, Moore BK. Polydimethyl siloxane materials in maxillofacial prosthetics: Evaluation and comparison of physical properties. J Prosthet Dent 1985;54:404–410.

Bellamy K, Limbert G, Waters MG, et al. An elastomeric material for facial prostheses: Synthesis, experimental and numerical testing aspects. Biomater 2003;24:5061–5066.

Bennie KR, Thokoane MG, Owen CP. Metamerism of three different pigments for facial prostheses and a method to improve shade evaluation. Int J Prosthodont 2018;31:607–609.

Berens AM, Newman S, Bhrany AD, et al. Computer-aided design and 3D printing to produce a costal cartilage model for simulation of auricular reconstruction. Otolaryngology—Head and Neck Surgery 2016;155:356–359.

Berg D, Otley CC. Skin cancer in organ transplant recipients: Epidemiology, pathogenesis, and management. J Am Acad Dermatol 2002;47:1–17.

Beumer J, Calcaterra T. Prosthetic restoration of large midfacial defects. Laryngoscope 1976;86:280–285.

Beumer J, Roumanas E, Nishimura R. Facial defects: Alterations at surgery to enhance the prosthetic prognosis. In Proceedings of First International Congress on Maxillofacial Prosthetics. 1995. New York: Sloane Kettering Memorial Hospital; pp. 104–107.

Bibars ARM, Al-Hourani Z, Khader Y, et al. Effect of thixotropic agents as additives on the mechanical properties of maxillofacial silicone elastomers. J Prosthet Dent 2018;119:671–675.

Bishal AK, Wee AG, Barão VAR, et al. Color stability of maxillofacial prosthetic silicone functionalized with oxide nanocoating. J Prosthet Dent 2019;121:538–543.

Bolt RA, Bosch JJ, Coops JC. Influence of window size in small window color measurement, particularly of teeth. Phys Med Biol 1994;39:1133–1142.

Bonatto LDR, Goiato MC, da Silva EVF, et al. Biocompatibility of primers and an adhesive used for implant-retained maxillofacial prostheses: An in vitro analysis. J Prosthet Dent 2017;117:799–805.

Brasier S. Facial prostheses: Maxillofacial laboratory technique and facial prostheses. London: Kimpton; 1954.

Breslow A. Thickness, cross-sectional areas and depth of invasion in the prognosis of cutaneous melanoma. Ann Surg 1970;172:902–908.

Brook M. Platinum in silicone breast implants. Biomaterials 2006;27:3274–3286.

Brunton A, Arikan CA, Urban P. Pushing the limits of 3D color printing: Error diffusion with translucent materials. ACM Transact Graph (TOG) 2015;35(1):4.

Bryant AW, Schaaf NG, Casey DM. The use of a photoprotective agent to increase the color stability of a tinted extraoral prosthetic silicone. J Prosthodont 1994;3:96–102.

Bulbulian AH. An improved technique for prosthetic restoration of facial defects by use of latex compound: Proceedings of staff meeting. Mayo Clin 1939;14:721–727.

Bulbulian AH. Facial prosthetics. Springfield, IL: Thomas; 1973. pp. 364–377.

Cantor R, Curtis T, Rozen R. Prosthetic management of terminal cancer patients. J Prosthet Dent 1968;20:361–366.

Cantor R, Webber RL, Stroud L, et al. Methods for evaluating prosthetic facial materials. J Prosthet Dent 1969;21:324–332.

Cardoso RC, Montgomery PC, Kiat-amnuay S. Extra-oral maxillofacial prosthetic materials: Results of the 2020 International Survey. Int J Prosthodont 2022 Nov 23. http://doi.org/10.11607/ijp.7970. Online ahead of print.

Cevik P, Paravina R, Kenj J, et al. Outdoor and artificial weathering of silicone and CPE maxillofacial prostheses. 2022 IADR abstract.

Cevik P, Yildirim-Bicer AZ. Effect of different types of disinfection solution and aging on the hardness and colour stability of maxillofacial silicone elastomers. Int J Artif Organs 2018;41:108–114.

Chalasani R, Poole-Warren L, Conway RM, et al. Porous orbital implants in enucleation: A systematic review. Survey of Ophthalmology 2007 Mar–Apr;52(2):145–155.

Chalian VA, Drane JB, Metz HH, et al. Extraoral prosthetics. In Maxillofacial prosthetics: Multidisciplinary practice. Ed. VA Chalian, JB Drane, SM Standish. Baltimore: Williams & Wilkins; 1974. pp. 283–329.

Chamaria A, Aras MA, Chitre V, et al. Effect of chemical disinfectants on the color stability of maxillofacial silicones: An in vitro study. J Prosthodont 2019;28:e869–e872. http://doi.org/10.1111/jopr.12768.

Chandra A, Watson J, Rowson JE, et al. Application of rapid manufacturing techniques in support of maxillofacial treatment: Evidence of the requirements of clinical applications. Proc Inst Mech Eng Part B J Eng Manuf 2005;219:469–475.

Chang TL, Garrett N, Roumanas E, et al. Treatment satisfaction with facial prostheses. J Prosthet Dent 2005;94:275–280.

Chang TL, Orellana D, Beumer J. Kratochvil's fundamentals of removal partial dentures. Chicago: Quintessence; 2019.

Chauhan BP, Rathore JS, Chauhan M, et al. Synthesis of polysiloxane stabilized palladium colloids and evidence of their participation in silaesterification reactions. J Am Chem Soc 2003;125:2876–2877.

Chen M, Udagama A, Drane JB. Evaluation of facial prostheses for head and neck cancer patients. J Prosthet Dent 1981;46:538–544.

Cifter ED, Ozdemir-Karatas M, Baca E, et al. Effect of vulcanization temperature and dental stone colour on colour degradation of maxillofacial silicone elastomers. BMC Oral Health 2017;31(17):72.

Ciocca L, De Crescenzio F, Fantini M, et al. CAD/CAM bilateral ear prostheses construction for Treacher Collins syndrome patients using laser scanning and rapid prototyping. Comput Methods Biomech Biomed Eng 2010a;13:379–386.

Ciocca L, Fantini M, De Crescenzio F, et al. New protocol for construction of eyeglasses-supported provisional nasal prosthesis using CAD/CAM techniques. J Rehabil Res Dev 2010b;47:595–604.

Ciocca L, Fantini M, Marchetti C, et al. Immediate facial rehabilitation in cancer patients using CAD-CAM and rapid prototyping technology: A pilot study. Support Care Cancer 2010c;18:723–728.

Ciocca L, Mingucci R, Gassino G, et al. CAD/CAM ear model and virtual construction of the mold. J Prosthet Dent 2007;98:339–343.

Ciocca L, Scotti R. CAD-CAM generated ear cast by means of a laser scanner and rapid prototyping machine. J Prosthet Dent 2004;92:591–595.

Clark WH Jr, From L, Bernardino EA, et al. The histogenesis and biologic behavior of primary human malignant melanomas of the skin. Cancer Res 1969;29:705–727.

Clarke CD. Moulage prosthesis. Am J Orthod Oral Surg 1941;27:214–225.

Colas A, Curtis J. Silicone biomaterials: History and chemistry. In Biomaterials science: An introduction to materials in medicine. 2nd ed. Ed. BD Ratner, AS Hoffman, FJ Schoen, et al. San Diego: Elsevier; 2004. pp. 80–86.

Conroy BF. A brief sortie into the history of cranio-oculofacial prosthetics. Facial Plastic Surgery: FPS 1993;9:89–115.

Cooper J. Undergoing enucleation of the eye: Part 2. Postoperative care. British J Nursing 2010;19:28–34.

Coward TJ, Scott BJJ, Watson RM, et al. Laser scanning of the ear identifying the shape and position in subjects with normal facial symmetry. Int J Oral Maxillofac Surg 2000;29:18–23.

Coward TJ, Seelaus R, Li SY. Computerized color formulation for African-Canadian people requiring facial prostheses: A pilot study. J Prosthodont 2008;17:327–335.

Coward TJ, Watson RM, Scott BJJ. Laser scanning for the identification of repeatable landmarks of the ears and face. Br J Plast Surg 1997;50:308–314.

Craig R, Koran A III, Yu R, et al. Color stability of elastomers for maxillofacial appliances. J Dent Res 1978;57:866–871.

Crump SS. Apparatus and method for creating three-dimensional objects. US Patent No 5,121,329. Washington, DC: US Patent and Trademark Office; 1992.

Cruz RLJ, Ross MT, Powell SK, et al. Advancements in soft-tissue prosthetics part A: The art of imitating life. Front Bioeng Biotechnol 2020a Mar 31;8:121. http://doi.org/10.3389/fbioe.2020.00121. PMID: 32300585; PMCID: PMC7145402.

Cruz RLJ, Ross MT, Powell SK, et al. Advancements in soft-tissue prosthetics part B: The chemistry of imitating life. Front Bioeng Biotechnol 2020b Apr 23;8:147. http://doi.org/10.3389/fbioe.2020.00147. PMID: 32391336; PMCID: PMC7191111.

Curi MM, Oliveira MF, Molina G, et al. Extraoral implants in the rehabilitation of craniofacial defects: Implant and prosthesis survival rates and peri-implant soft tissue evaluation. J Oral Maxillofac Surg 2012;70:1551–1557.

Custer PL, Kennedy RH, Woog JJ, et al. Orbital implants in enucleation surgery: A report by the American Academy of Ophthalmology. Ophthalmology 2003;110:2054–2061.

Custer PL, Trinkaus KM. Porous implant exposure: Incidence, management, and morbidity. Ophthalmic Plast Reconstr Surg 2007;23:1–7.

Dave TV, Kumar S, Vasanthalin J, et al. Development and validation of a grading scale for custom ocular prosthesis. Optom Vis Sci 2016;93:1426–1430.

De Crescenzio F, Fantini M, Ciocca L, et al. Design and manufacturing of ear prosthesis by means of rapid prototyping technology. Proc Inst Mech Eng Part H J Eng Med 2011;225:296–302.

del Pozo JL, Rouse MS, Patel R. Bioelectric effect and bacterial biofilms. A systematic review. Int J Artificial Organs 2008;31:786–795.

de Sousa AA, Mattos BS. Magnetic retention and bar-clip attachment for implant-retained auricular prostheses: A comparative analysis. Int J Prosthodont 2008;21:233–236.

Deng HY, Zwetchkenbaum S, Noone AM. Bond strength of silicone to polyurethane following immersion of silicone in cleaning solutions. J Prosthet Dent 2004;91:582–585.

Dharmasena A, Keenan T, Goldacre R, et al. Trends over time in the incidence of congenital anophthalmia, microphthalmia and orbital malformation in England: Database study. British Journal of Ophthalmology 2017 Jun;101(6):735–739.

Dings JP, Maal TJ, Muradin MS, et al. Extra-oral implants: Insertion per- or post-ablation? Oral Oncol 2011;47:1074–1078.

Dings JP, Verhamme L, Maal JJ, et al. Reliability and accuracy of skin-supported surgical templates for computer-planned craniofacial implant placement, a comparison between surgical templates: With and without bony fixation. J Craniomaxillofac Surg 2019;47:977–983.

Dootz ER, Koran A III, Craig RG. Physical properties of three maxillofacial materials as a function of accelerated aging. J Prosthet Dent 1994;71:379–383.

dos Santos DM, Borgui Paulini M, Silva Faria TG, et al. Analysis of color and hardness of a medical silicone with extrinsic pigmentation after accelerated aging. Eur J Dent 2020;14:634–638.

dos Santos DM, Goiato MC, Moreno A, et al. Influence of pigments and opacifiers on color stability of an artificially aged facial silicone. J of Prosthodont 2011;20:205–208.

dos Santos DM, Goiato MC, Sinhoreti MAC, et al. Color stability of polymers for facial prosthesis. J Craniofac Surg 2010;21:54–58.

dos Santos DM, Goiato MC, Sinhoreti MAC, et al. Influence of natural weathering on colour stability of materials used for facial prosthesis. J Med Engin Technol 2012;36:267–270.

Doubrovski E, Tsai E, Dikovsky D, et al. Voxel-based fabrication through material property mapping: A design method for bitmap printing. Computer-Aided Design 2015;60:3–13.

Douglas RD, Steinhauer TJ, Wee AG. Intraoral determination of the tolerance of dentists for perceptibility and acceptability of shade mismatch. J Prosthet Dent 2007;97:200–208.

Durand ML. Endophthalmitis. Clin Microbiol and Infect 2013 Mar;19:227–234.

Eleni P, Katsavou I, Krokida M, et al. Mechanical behavior of facial prosthetic elastomers after outdoor weathering. Dent Mater 2009a;25:1493–1502.

Eleni PN, Krokida M, Polyzois G, et al. Effects of outdoor weathering on facial prosthetic elastomers. Odontology 2011a;99:68–76.

Eleni PN, Krokida MK, Frangou MJ, et al. Structural damages of maxillofacial biopolymers under solar aging. Mater Sci Mater Med 2007;18:1675–1681.

Eleni PN, Krokida MK, Polyzois GL. The effect of artificial accelerated weathering on the mechanical properties of maxillofacial polymers PDMS and CPE. J Biomed Mater 2009b;4:35001.

Eleni PN, Krokida MK, Polyzois GL. Effects of storage in simulated skin secretions on mechanical behavior and color of polydimethylsiloxanes elastomers. J Cranio Surg 2011b;22:830–836.

Eleni PN, Krokida MK, Polyzois GL, et al. Effect of different disinfecting procedures on the hardness and color stability of two maxillofacial elastomers over time. J Appl Oral Sci 2013a;21:278–283.

Eleni PN, Krokida MK, Polyzois GL, et al. Material properties of a maxillofacial chlorinated polyethylene elastomer stored in simulated skin secretions. J Biomed Mater Res B Appl Biomater 2009b;91:964–974.

Eleni PN, Krokida MK, Polyzois GL, et al. Mechanical behaviour of a polydimethylsiloxane elastomer after outdoor weathering in two different weathering locations. Polymer Degradation Stability 2011c;96:470–476.

Eleni PN, Perivoliotis D, Dragatogiannis DA, et al. Tensile and microindentation properties of maxillofacial elastomers after different disinfecting procedures. J Mech Behav Biomed Mater 2013b;28:147–155.

Eliason C. RPA clasp design for distal-extension removable partial dentures. J Prosthet Dent 1983;49:25–27.

Ellis GL, Corio RL. Spindle cell carcinoma of the oral cavity: A clinicopathologic assessment of fifty-nine cases. Oral Surg Oral Med Oral Pathol 1980;50:523–533.

Ethunandan M, Downie I, Flood T. Implant-retained nasal prosthesis for reconstruction of large rhinectomy defects: The Salisbury experience. Int J Oral Maxillofac Surg 2010;39:343–349.

Euvard S, Kanitakis J, Claudy A. Skin cancers after organ transplantation. N Eng J Med 2003;348:1681–1691.

Falcone MT, Kaylie DM, Labadie RF. Bone anchored hearing aid abutment skin overgrowth reduction with clobetasol. Otolaryngol Head and Neck Surg 2008;139:829–832.

Fantini M, De Crescenzio F, Ciocca L. Design and rapid manufacturing of anatomical prosthesis for facial rehabilitation. Int J Interact Des Manuf 2013;7:51–62.

Farah A, Sherriff M, Coward T. Color stability of nonpigmented and pigmented maxillofacial silicone elastomer exposed to 3 different environments. J Prosthet Dent 2018;120:476–482.

Farah JW, Robinson JC, Hood JA, et al. Force-displacement properties of a modified cross-linked silicone compared with facial tissues. J Oral Rehabil 1988;15:277–283.

Farah JW, Robinson JC, Koran A III, et al. Properties of a modified cross-linked silicone for maxillofacial prostheses. J Oral Rehabil 1987;14:599–605.

Farook TH, Jamayet NB, Abdullah JY, et al. Designing 3D prosthetic templates for maxillofacial defect rehabilitation: A comparative analysis of different virtual workflows. Comput Biol Med 2020 Mar;118:103646. http://doi.org/10.1016/j.compbiomed.2020.103646. Epub 2020 Feb 4. PMID: 32174323.

Feng H, Shuda M, Chang Y, et al. Clonal integration of a polyomavirus in human Merkel cell carcinoma. Science 2008;319:1096–1100.

Feng Z, Dong Y, Zhao Y, et al. Computer-assisted technique for the design and manufacture of realistic facial prostheses. Br J Oral Maxillofac Surg 2010;48:105–109.

Fereshtenejad S, Song J-J. Fundamental study on applicability of powder-based 3D printer for physical modeling in rock mechanics. Rock Mech Rock Eng 2016;49:2065–2074. http://doi.org/10.1007/s00603-015-0904-x.

Fine L. Color and its application in maxillofacial prosthetics. J Prosthet Dent 1978;39:188–192.

Fine L, Robinson JE, Barnhart GW, et al. New method for coloring facial prostheses. J Prosthet Dent 1978;39:643–649.

Firtell DN, Bartlett SO. Maxillofacial prostheses: Reproducible fabrication. J Prosthet Dent 1969;22:247–252.

Firtell DN, Donneau ML, Anderson CR. Lightweight RTV silicone for maxillofacial prostheses. J Prosthet Dent 1976;36:544–549.

Fisher SR. Cutaneous malignant melanoma of the head and neck. Laryngoscope 1989;99:822–836.

Flood T, Downie I. Prosthetic reconstruction following rhinectomy: Evolution of bone-anchored epistheses and adjunctive surgical techniques in nasal reconstruction from one unit. Presented at the Second International Symposium on Bone Conduction—Craniofacial Osseointegration, Gothenburg, Sweden, 11–13 Jun 2009.

Flood TR, Russell K. Reconstruction of nasal defects with implant-retained nasal prostheses. Br J Oral Maxillofac Surg 1998;36:341–345.

Frangou MJ, Polyzois GL, Tarantili PA, et al. Bonding of silicone extraoral elastomers to acrylic resin: The effect of primer composition. Eur J Prosthodont Restor Dent 2003;11:115–118.

Fung YC. Biomechanics: Mechanical properties of living tissues. 2nd ed. New York: Springer-Verlag; 1993.

Gary JJ, Huget EF, Powell LD. Accelerated color change in a maxillofacial elastomer with and without pigmentation. J Prosthet Dent 2001;85:614–620.

Gettleman L. Chlorinated polyethylene and polyphosphazenes. In Materials research in maxillofacial prosthetics. Ed. JC Setcos. Trans Acad Dent Mater 1992;5:156–172.

Gettleman L. Polyphosphazene fluoroelastomer for denture liners and facial prosthetics. Phosphorus Sulfur Silicon 1999;144:205–208.

Gettleman L. Uses of polyphosphazene in dentistry. In Applicative aspects of poly(organophosphazenes). Ed. Mario Gleria and Roger DeJaeger. New York: Nova Science; 2004. pp. 33–47.

Gettleman L, Farris CL, LeBoeuf RJ Jr, et al. Improvement in experimental elastomers for permanent soft denture liners: Physical and biologic properties. In Recent developments in biomedical engineering: Proceedings of the First Southern Biomedical Engineering Conference. Ed. S Saha. New York: Pergamon; 1982. pp. 307–309.

Gettleman L, Gebert P, Ross LM, et al. Extraoral maxillofacial prostheses molded from chlorinated polyethylene. J Dent Res 1958;64:368.

Gettleman L, Goist KC, Vargo JM, et al. Processing and clinical testing of a thermoplastic material for maxillofacial prosthetics. In Oral implantology and biomaterials. Ed. H Kawahara. Amsterdam: Elsevier; 1989a. pp. 7–13.

Gettleman L, Khan Z. Materials research in maxillofacial prosthetics. Ed. L Cochairs, J Setcos. Trans Acad Dental Mater 1992;5:156–172.

Gettleman L, Ross-Bertrand L, Gebert PH, et al. Novel elastomers for denture and maxillofacial prostheses. In Recent developments in biomedical engineering: Proceedings of the Fourth Southern Biomedical Engineering Conference. Ed. B Sauer. New York: Pergamon; 1985. pp. 141–144.

Gettleman L, Vargo JM, Gebert PH, et al. Thermoplastic chlorinated polyethylene for maxillofacial prostheses. In Advances in biomedical polymers: Polymer science and technology series. Vol 35. Ed. CG Gebelein. New York: Plenum; 1987. pp. 31–40.

Gettleman L, Vargo JM, Goist KC, et al. Laboratory and clinical testing of a polyphosphazene resilient denture liner vs. a silicone rubber liner. In Oral implantology and biomaterials. Ed. H Kawahara. Amsterdam: Elsevier; 1989b. pp. 15–20.

Gillman MB. Color matching: Matching skin color in facial prosthesis via the spectrophotometer with special reference to dental restorations demanding color fidelity. Dent Items Interest 1950;72:1250–1255.

Godoy AJ, Lemon JC, Nakamura SH, et al. A shade guide for acrylic resin facial prostheses. J Prosthet Dent 1992;68:120–122.

Goh G, Walradt T, Markarov V, et al. Mutational landscape of MCPyV-positive and MCPyV-negative Merkel cell carcinomas with implications for immunotherapy. Oncotarget 2016;7:3403–3415.

Goiato MC, dos Santos DM, Bannwart LC, et al. Psychosocial impact on anophthalmic patients wearing ocular prosthesis. Int J Oral Maxillofac Surg 2013;42:113–119.

Goiato MC, Pesqueira AA, dos Santos DM, et al. Evaluation of hardness and surface roughness of two maxillofacial silicones following disinfection. Braz Oral Res 2009;23:49–53.

Goiato MC, Pesqueira AA, Moreno A, et al. Effects of pigment, disinfection, and accelerated aging on the hardness and deterioration of a facial silicone elastomer. Polym Degrad Stab 2012;97:1577–1580.

Goiato MC, Zucolotti BCR, Mancuso DN, et al. Care and cleaning of maxillofacial prostheses. J Craniofacial Surg 2010;21:1270–1273.

Goldschmidt MC, Jacob RF, Grant R. Using microwave to sterilize contaminated silicone prostheses. J Dent Res 1993;72:266(abst 1305).

Gonzalez JB. Polyurethane elastomers for facial prostheses. J Prosthet Dent 1978;39:179–187.

Gonzalez JB, Chao EY, An KN. Physical and mechanical behavior of polyurethane elastomer formulations used for facial prostheses. J Prosthet Dent 1978;39:307–318.

Gozalo-Diaz DJ, Lindsey DT, Johnston WM, et al. Measurement of color for craniofacial structures using a 45/0-degree optical configuration. J Prosthet Dent 2007;97:45–53.

Granström G. Osseointegration in irradiated cancer patients: An analysis with respect to implant failures. J Oral Maxillofac Surg 2005;63:579–585.

Green A, Battistutta D. Incidence and determinants of skin cancer in a high-risk Australian population. Int J Cancer 1990;46:356–361.

Groot AL, Remmers JS, Hartong DT. Three-dimensional computer-aided design of a full-color ocular prosthesis with textured iris and sclera manufactured in one single print job. 3D Print Addit Manuf 2021 Dec 1;8(6):343–348. http://doi.org/10.1089/3dp.2021.0048.

Grunewald SJ. Wacker announces new silicone 3D printing technology, in 3D printing materials. 2015 Aug 11. 3DPrint.com.

Guerra ON, Canada K. Open-cast technique for metal molds used in constructing facial prostheses. J Prosthet Dent 1976;36:421–425.

Guerra ON, Kronoveter K. Vinyl chloride concentrations in maxillofacial prosthetics laboratories. J Prosthet Dent 1978;39:200–202.

Guiotti AM, Cunha BG, Paulini MB, et al. Antimicrobial activity of conventional and plant-extract disinfectant solutions on microbial biofilms on a maxillofacial polymer surface. J Prosthet Dent 2016;116:136–143.

Guiotti AM, Goiato MC, dos Santos DM. Evaluation of the Shore A hardness of silicone for facial prosthesis as to the effect of storage period and chemical disinfection. J Cranio Surg 2010;21:323–327.

Guiotti AM, Goiato MC, dos Santos DM, et al. Comparison of conventional and plant-extract disinfectant solutions on the hardness and color stability of a maxillofacial elastomer after artificial aging. J Prosthet Dent 2015;115:501–508.

Güngör MB, Nemli SK, Inal CB, et al. Effect of plasma treatment on the peel bond strength between maxillofacial silicones and resins. Dent Mater J 2020;39:242–250.

Haider YM, Abdullah ZS, Fatalla AA, et al. Corrigendum to "Evaluation of some mechanical properties of a maxillofacial silicon elastomer reinforced with polyester powder." Int J Dent 2020 Sep 28;2020:7187159. http://doi.org/10.1155/2020/7187159. eCollection 2020.

Han AY, Dhanjani S, Pettijohn K, et al. Optimal resection margin for head and neck cutaneous melanoma. Laryngoscope 2019;129:1386–1394.

Han Y, Kiat-amnuay S, Powers JM, et al. Effect of nano-oxide concentration on the mechanical properties of a maxillofacial silicone elastomer. J Prosth Dent 2008;100:465–473.

Han Y, Powers JM, Kiat-amnuay S. Color stability of pigmented maxillofacial silicone MDX4-4210/type a subjected to ten years of dark storage and artificial aging. Trans Amer Academy Maxillofac Prosthet 2010a;58:91–92.

Han Y, Powers JM, Kiat-amnuay S. Effect of opacifiers and UV absorbers on pigmented maxillofacial silicone elastomer, part 1: Color stability after artificial aging. J Prosthet Dent 2013;109:397–401.

Han Y, Zhao Y, Xie C, et al. Color stability of pigmented maxillofacial silicone elastomer: Effects of nano-oxides as opacifiers. J Dent 2010b;38(suppl 2):e100–e105. http://doi.org/10.1016/j.jdent.2010.05.009.

Han Y, Zhao Y-M, Shao L-Q. Evaluation of mechanical properties of ZY-1 maxillofacial prosthetic materials. J US Ch Med Sci 2007;1:30–33.

Harms PW, Vats P, Verhaegen ME, et al. The distinctive mutational spectra of polyomavirus-negative Merkel cell carcinoma. Cancer Res 2015;75:3720–3727.

Hatamleh MM, Polyzois GL, Nuseir A, et al. Mechanical properties and simulated aging of silicone maxillofacial elastomers: Advancements in the past 45 years: Advancements in maxillofacial silicone mechanical properties. J Prosthodont 2016;25:418–426.

Hatamleh MM, Polyzois GL, Silikas N, et al. Effect of extraoral aging conditions on mechanical properties of maxillofacial silicone elastomer. J Prosthodont 2011;20:439–446.

Hatamleh MM, Watts DC. Bonding of maxillofacial silicone elastomers to an acrylic substrate. Dent Mater 2010a;26:387–395.

Hatamleh MM, Watts DC. Mechanical properties and bonding of maxillofacial silicone elastomers. Dent Mater 2010b;26:185–191.

Hatamleh MM, Watts DC. Porosity and color of maxillofacial silicone elastomer. J Prosthodont 2011;20:60–66.

Haug PS, Andres CJ, Muñoz CA, et al. Effects of environmental factors on maxillofacial elastomers: 3. Physical properties. J Prosthet Dent 1992a;68:644–651.

Haug SP, Andres CJ, Moore BK. Color stability of colorant effect on maxillofacial elastomers: 3. Weathering effect on color. J Prosthet Dent 1999a;81:431–438.

Haug SP, Andres CJ, Moore BK. Color stability of colorant effect on maxillofacial elastomers: 1. Colorant effect on physical properties. J Prosthet Dent 1999b;81:418–422.

Haug SP, Andres CJ, Muñoz CA, et al. Effects of environmental factors on maxillofacial elastomers: 4. Optical properties. J Prosthet Dent 1992b;68:820–823.

Haug SP, Moore BK, Andres CJ. Color stability of colorant effect on maxillofacial elastomers: 2. Weathering effect on physical properties. J Prosthet Dent 1999c;81:431–438.

He Y, Xue G, Fu J. Fabrication of low cost soft tissue prostheses with the desktop 3D printer. Sci Rep 2014;4:6973. http://doi.org/10.1038/srep06973.

Henry P. Maxillofacial prosthetic considerations. In Advanced osseointegration surgery. Ed. P Worthington, PI Branemark. Chicago: Quintessence; 1992. pp. 313–326.

Hildrew DM, Guittard JA, Carter JM, et al. Clobetasol's Influence on the management and cost of skin overgrowth associated with the bone-anchored hearing aid. Ochsner J 2015;15:277–283.

Hita-Anton C, Jordano-Luna L, Díez-Villalba R. Eye removal—current indications and technical tips. 2016. http://doi.org/10.5772/61030-Anton.

Hofmann, M. 3D printing gets a boost and opportunities with polymer materials. ACS Macro Lett 2014;3:382–386. http://doi.org/10.1021/mz4006556.

Holzapfel GA. Biomechanics of soft tissue. Biomech Preprint Series 2000 Nov;7:2–3. http://biomechanics.stanford.edu/me338/me338_project02.pdf.

Honavar SG, Rao R. Enucleation and exenteration. In Surgical ophthalmic oncology: A collaborative open access reference. Ed. SS Chaugule, SG Honavar, PT Finger. Cham: Springer International; 2019. pp. 131–139.

Hu X, Gilbert AB, Johnston WM. Interfacial corrections of maxillofacial elastomers for Kubelka–Munk theory using non-contact measurements. Dent Materials 2009a;25:1163–1168.

Hu X, Johnston WM. Concentration additivity of coefficients for maxillofacial elastomer pigmented to skin colors. Dental Materials 2009b;25:1468–1473.

Hu X, Johnston WM. Translucency estimation for thick pigmented maxillofacial elastomer. J Dent 2011 Jul;39(suppl 1):e2–e8. http://doi.org/10.1016/j.jdent.2011.01.002.

Hu X, Johnston W, Seghi R. Measuring the color of maxillofacial prosthetic material. J Dental Res 2010;89:1522–1527.

Hu X, Pan X, Johnston WM. Effects of pigments on dynamic mechanical properties of a maxillofacial prosthetic elastomer. J Prosthet Dent 2014;112:1298–1303.

Huang J, He C, Liu X, et al. Formation and characterization of water-soluble platinum nanoparticles using a unique approach based on the hydrosilylation reaction. Langmuir 2004;20:5145–5148.

Hulterström AK, Ruyter IE. Changes in appearance of silicone elastomers for maxillofacial prostheses as a result of aging. Int J Prosthodont 1999;12:498–504.

Hungerford E, Beatty MW, Marx DB, et al. Coverage error of commercial skin pigments as compared to human facial skin tones. J Dent 2013;41:986–991.

Jacobsson M, Tjellström A, Fine L, et al. A retrospective study of osseointegrated skin-penetrating titanium fixture used for retaining facial prostheses. Int J Oral Maxillofac Implants 1992;7:523–528.

Jacques, LFE. Accelerated and outdoor/natural exposure testing of coatings. Progress Polymer Science 2020;25:1337–1362.

Jindal SK, Sherriff M, Waters MG, et al. Development of a 3D printable maxillofacial silicone: Part I. Optimization of polydimethylsiloxane chains and cross-linker concentration. J Prosthet Dent 2016;116:617–622. http://doi.org/10.1016/j.prosdent.2016.02.020.

Jindal SK, Sherriff M, Waters MG, et al. Development of a 3D printable maxillofacial silicone. Part II. Optimization of moderator and thixotropic agent. J Prosthet Dent 2017;116:617–622. http://doi.org/10.1016/j.prosdent.2017.04.028.

Johnston WM, Hesse NS, Davis BK, et al. Analysis of edge-losses in reflectance measurements of pigmented maxillofacial elastomer. J Dent Res 1996;75:752–760.

Johnston WM, Kao EC. Assessment of appearance match by visual observation and clinical colorimetry. J Dent Res 1989;68:819–822.

Jorba-Garcia A, Gonzalez-Barnadas A, Camps-Font O, et al. Accuracy assessment of dynamic computer-aided implant placement: A systematic review and meta-analysis. Clin Oral Investig 2021 May;25(5):2479–2494.

Jordan DR. Porous versus nonporous orbital implants: A 25-Year retrospective. Ophthalmology 2018;125:1317–1319.

Kagmeni G, Noche CD, Tguefack-Tsague G. Indications for surgical removal of the eye in rural areas in Cameroon. Ophthalmol Eye Dis 2014;9:27–30.

Kale E, Meşe A, Izgi AD. A technique for fabrication of an interim ocular prosthesis. J Prosthodont 2008;17:654–661.

Kaltreider SA. The ideal ocular prosthesis: Analysis of prosthetic volume. Ophthalmic Plast Reconstr Surg 2000;16:388–392.

Kantola R, Lassila L, Vallittu P. Adhesion of maxillofacial silicone elastomer to a fiber-reinforced composite resin framework. Int J Prosthodont 2011;24:582–588.

Kantola RM, Kurunmäki H, Vallittu PK, et al. Use of thermochromic pigment in maxillofacial silicone elastomer. J Prosthet Dent 2013;110:320–325.

Karakoca Nemli S, Bankoğlu Güngör M, Bağkur M, et al. In vitro evaluation of color and translucency reproduction of maxillofacial prostheses using a computerized system. J Adv Prosthodont 2018 Dec;10(6):422–429. http://doi.org/10.4047/jap.2018.10.6.422.

Karakoca S, Aydin C, Yilmaz H, et al. Retrospective study of treatment outcomes with implant-retained extraoral prostheses: Survival rates and prosthetic complications. J Prosthet Dent 2010;103:118–126.

Karakoca S, Aydin C, Yilmaz H, et al. Survival rates and peri-implant soft tissue evaluation of extraoral implants over a mean follow-up period of three years. J Prosthet Dent 2008;100:458–464.

Kashkouli MB, Zolfaghari R, Es'haghi A, et al. Tear film, lacrimal drainage system, and eyelid findings in subjects with anophthalmic socket discharge. Amer J Ophthal 2016;165:33–38.

Kazanjian V, Rowe A, Young H. Prosthesis of the mouth and face: A symposium. J Dent Res 1932;12:651–658.

Keenan TDL, Sargent NJ. Enucleation and evisceration in the Palestinian territories. Middle East Afr Ophthalmol 2011;18:170–172.

Kent K, Zeigel R, Kent K, et al. Controlling the porosity and density of silicone rubber prosthetic materials. J Prosthet Dent 1983;50:230–236.

Khalaf S, Ariffin Z, Husein A, et al. Surface coating of gypsum-based molds for maxillofacial prosthetic silicone elastomeric material: Evaluating different microbial adhesion. J Prosthodont 2017;26:664–669.

Khalaf S, Ariffin Z, Husein A, et al. Surface coating of gypsum-based molds for maxillofacial prosthetic silicone elastomeric material: The surface topography. J Prosthodont 2015;24:419–423.

Khan Z, Gettleman L, Jacobsen C. Conference report: Materials research in maxillofacial prosthetics. J Dent Res 1992;71:1541–1542.

Kheur MG, Kakade D, Trevor CJ, et al. Effect of newly developed pigments and ultraviolet absorbers on the color change of pigmented silicone elastomer. J Indian Prosthodont Soc 2017;17:395–400.

Kheur MG, Sethi T, Coward T, et al. A comparative evaluation of the change in hardness, of two commonly used maxillofacial prosthetic silicone elastomers, as subjected to simulated weathering in tropical climatic conditions. Eur J Prosthodont Restor Dent 2012;20:146–150.

Kiat-amnuay S, Beerbower M, Powers JM, et al. Influence of pigments and opacifiers on color stability of silicone maxillofacial elastomer. J Dent 2009;37(suppl 1):e45–e50. http://doi.org/10.1016/j.jdent.2009.05.004.

Kiat-amnuay S, Gettleman L, Goldsmith LJ. Effect of multi-adhesive layering on retention of extraoral maxillofacial silicone prostheses in vivo. J Prosthet Dent 2004a;92:294–298.

Kiat-amnuay S, Gettleman L, Khan Z, et al. Effect of adhesive retention of maxillofacial prostheses: 2. Time and reapplication effects. J Prosthet Dent 2001;85:438–441.

Kiat-amnuay S, Jacobs RF, Chambers MS, et al. Clinical trial of chlorinated polyethylene for facial prosthetics. Int J Prosthodont 2010;23:263–270.

Kiat-amnuay S, Johnston DA, Powers JM, et al. Color stability of dry earth pigmented maxillofacial silicone A-2186 subjected to microwave energy exposure. J Prosthodont 2005;14:91–76.

Kiat-amnuay S, Leite KSA, Powers JM. Silicone pigments affect color stability of MDX 4-4210/Type A maxillofacial elastomer. Presented at the 82nd General Session and Exhibition of the IADR, Honolulu, 10–13 Mar 2004b.

Kiat-amnuay S, Lemon SC, Powers JM. Effect of opacifiers on color stability of pigmented maxillofacial silicone A-2186 subjected to artificial aging. J Prosthodont 2002;11:109–116.

Kiat-amnuay S, Mekayarajjananonth T, Powers J, et al. Interactions of pigments and opacifiers on color stability of MDX4–4210/Type A maxillofacial elastomers subjected to artificial aging. J Prosthet Dent 2006a;95:249–257.

Kiat-amnuay S, Powers JM. Color stability of silicone A-2000 maxillofacial elastomer. J Dent Res 2006b;85(spec issue B):1551.

Kiat-amnuay S, Waters PJ, Roberts D, et al. Adhesive retention of silicone and chlorinated polyethylene for maxillofacial prostheses. J Prosthet Dent 2008;99:483–488.

Kim JC, Yu B, Lee YK. Influence of surface layer removal of shade guide tabs on the measured color by spectrophotometer. J Dent Res 2008;36:1061–1067.

Kipping F. Organic derivative of silicon. Preparation of alkyl silicon chlorides. Proc Chem Soc 1904;20:15.

Ko JS, Kim SH, Baek SW, et al. Semi-automated fabrication of customized ocular prosthesis with three-dimensional printing and sublimation transfer printing

technology. Sci Rep 2019 Feb 27;9(1):2968. http://doi.org/10.1038/s41598-019-38992-y.
Koran A III, Craig RG. Dynamic mechanical properties of maxillofacial materials. J Dent Res 1975;54:1216–1221.
Koran A III, Powers JM, Lepeak PJ, et al. Stain resistance of maxillofacial materials. J Dent Res 1979a;58:1455–1460.
Koran A III, Powers JM, Raptis CN, et al. Reflection spectrophotometry of facial skin. J Dent Res 1981;60:979–982.
Koran A III, Yu R, Powers JM, et al. Color stability of pigmented elastomer for maxillofacial appliances. J Dent Res 1979b;58:1450–1454.
Kosor BY, Artunç C, Şahan H. Adhesive retention of experimental fiber-reinforced composite, orthodontic acrylic resin, and aliphatic urethane acrylate to silicone elastomer for maxillofacial prostheses. J Prosthet Dent 2015;114:142–148.
Kotha SB, Ramakrishnaiah R, Devang Divakar D, et al. Effect of disinfection and sterilization on the tensile strength, surface roughness, and wettability of elastomers. J Invest Clin Dent 2017;8(4):e12244. http://doi.org/10.1111/jicd.12244.
Kouyoumdjian J, Chalian VA, Moore BK. A comparison of the physical properties of a room temperature vulcanizing silicone/modified and unmodified. J Prosthet Dent 1985;53:388–391.
Koylu MT, Gokce G, Uysal Y, et al. Indications for eye removal surgeries: A 15-year experience at a tertiary military hospital. Saudi Med J 2015;36:1205–1209.
Kratochvil FJ. Influence of occlusal rest position and clasp design on movement of abutment teeth. J Prosthet Dent 1963;13:114–124.
Kuijken I, Bavinck JN. Skin cancer risk associated with immunosuppressive therapy in organ transplant recipients: Epidemiology and proposed mechanism. Bio Drugs 2000;14:319–329.
Kurt M, Nemli S, Güngör M, et al. Visual and instrumental color evaluation of computerized color matching system for color reproduction of maxillofacial prostheses. J Prosthet Dent 2022 Nov;128(5):1121–1127. http://doi.org/10.1016/j.prosdent.2021.01.009.
Kurtoglu C, Ekren O, Powers J, et al. Effect of thixotropic agent on the mechanical properties of three platinum-based silicone maxillofacial elastomers. Int J Anaplastol 2009;3:11–16.
Kurtulmus H, Kumbuloglu O, Özcan M, et al. Candida albicans adherence on silicone elastomers: Effect of polymerisation duration and exposure to simulated saliva and nasal secretion. Dental Mater 2009;26:76–82.
Lai JH, Hodges JS. Effects of processing parameters on physical properties of the silicone maxillofacial prosthetic materials. Dent Mater 1999;15:450–455.
Lai JH, Wang LL, Ko CC, et al. New organosilicon maxillofacial prosthetic materials. Dent Mater 2002;18:281–286.
Lanz J, Bavinck J, Westhuis M, et al. Aggressive squamous cell carcinoma in organ transplant recipients. JAMA Dermatol 2019;155:66–71.
Lanzara R, Thakur A, Viswambaran M, et al. Fabrication of ocular prosthesis with a digital customization technique—a case report. J Family Med Primary Care 2019;8:1239–1242.
LeBlanc KJ, Niemi SR, Bennett AI, et al. Stability of high speed 3D printing in liquid-like solids. ACS Biomaterials Science & Engineering 2016;2:1796–1799.
Lee YC, Zheng J, Kuo J, et al. Binder jetting of custom silicone powder for direct 3D printing of maxillofacial prostheses. 3D Print Addit Manufact 2022 Dec 1;9(6):520–534. http://doi.org/10.1089/3dp.2021.0019. Epub 2022 Dec 13.
Lemon J, Kiat-amnuay S, Gettleman L, et al. Facial prosthetic rehabilitation: Preprosthetic surgical techniques and biomaterials. Curr Opin in Otolaryngol Head and Neck Surg 2005;13:255–262.
Lemon JC, Chambers MS, Jacobsen ML, et al. Color stability of facial prostheses. J Prosthet Dent 1995;74:613–618.
Lewis DH, Castleberry DJ. An assessment of recent advances in external maxillofacial materials. J Prosthet Dent 1980;43:426–432.
Liacouras P, Garnes J, Roman N, et al. Designing and manufacturing an auricular prosthesis using computed tomography, 3-dimensional photographic imaging, and additive manufacturing: A clinical report. J Prosthet Dent 2011;105:78–82.
Lin CW, Liao SL. Long-term complications of different porous orbital implants: A 21-year review. British Journal of Ophthalmology 2017;101(5):681–685.
Liravi F, Toyserkani E. A hybrid additive manufacturing method for the fabrication of silicone bio-structures: 3D printing optimization and surface characterization. Materials & Design 2018;138:46–61.
Liravi F, Vlasea M. Powder bed binder jetting additive manufacturing of silicone structures. Addit Manufact 2018;21:112–124.
Liska JW, Kubon T, Dadjoo S, et al. Color stability of silicone maxillofacial elastomers subjected to artificial aging. J Dent Res 2009;88(spec issue A):1750.
Liu Q, Shao L, Xiang H, et al. Biomechanical characterization of a low density silicone elastomer filled with hollow microspheres for maxillofacial prostheses. J Biomaterials Science Polymer Ed 2013;24:1378–1390.
Llorente-González S, Peralta-Calvo J, Abelairas-Gómez JM. Congenital anophthalmia and microphthalmia: Epidemiology and orbitofacial rehabilitation. Clin Ophthalmol 2011;5:1759–1765.
Lyons KM, Cannon RD, Beumer J, et al. The role of biofilms and material surface characteristics in microbial adhesion to maxillary obturator materials: A literature review. Cleft Palate Craniofac J 2020;57:487–498.
Markt JC, Lemon JC. Extraoral maxillofacial prosthetic rehabilitation at the M. D. Anderson Cancer Center: A survey of patient attitudes and opinions. J Prosthet Dent 2001;85:608–613.
Marunick M, Harrison R, Beumer J. Prosthetic rehabilitation of midfacial defects. J Prosthet Dent 1985;54:553–560.
Maxwell R, Sung W, Solyom D, et al. The effects of [gamma]-radiation on the thermal, mechanical, and segmental dynamics of a silica filled, room temperature vulcanized polysiloxane rubber. Polymer Degradation Stability 2003;80:443–450.
May PD, Farris CL, Gettleman L, et al. New elastomers for soft denture liners. J Dent Res 1981;60:437.
May PD, Guerra LR. Maxillofacial prostheses of chlorinated polyethylene. J Biomed Mater Res 1978;12:421–431.
Mayer MH, Winton GB, Smith AC, et al. Microcystic adnexal carcinoma (sclerosing sweat duct carcinoma). Plast Reconstr Surg 1989;84:970–975.
McBain HB, Ezra DG, Rose GE, et al. The psychosocial impact of living with an ocular prosthesis. Orbit 2014;33:39–44.
McMordie R, King GE. Evaluation of primers used for bonding silicone to denture base material. J Prosthet Dent 1989;61:636–639.
Mehta S, Nandeeshwar DB. A spectrophotometric analysis of extraoral aging conditions on the color stability of maxillofacial silicone. J Indian Prosthodont Soc 2017;17:355–360.
Mendonca JA, Franischone CE, Senna PM, et al. A retrospective evaluation of the survival rates of splinted and non-splinted short dental implants posterior partially edentulous jaws. J Periodontol 2014;85:787–794.
Meran Z, Besinis A, De Peralta T, et al. Antifungal properties and biocompatibility of silver nanoparticle coatings on silicone maxillofacial prostheses in vitro. J Biomed Mater Res B Appl Biomater 2018;106:1038–1051.
Migliori ME. Enucleation versus evisceration. Curr Opin Ophthal 2002;13:298–302.
Mills A, Policarpio-Nicholas ML, Agaimy A, et al. Sclerosing microcystic adenocarcinoma of the head and neck mucosa: A neoplasm closely resembling microcystic adnexal carcinoma. Head Neck Pathol 2016;10:501–508.
Minns RJ, Soden PD, Jackson DS. The role of the fibrous components and ground substance in the mechanical properties of biological tissues: A preliminary investigation. J Biomech 1973;6:153–165.
Misago N, Tanaka T, Kohda H. Trichilemmal carcinoma occurring in a lesion of solar keratosis. J Dermatol 1993;20:358–364.
Mohammed MI, Tatineni J, Cadd B, et al. Advanced auricular prosthesis development by 3D modelling and multi-material printing. KnE Engineering 2017;2:37–43.
Mohite UH, Sandrik JL, Land MF, et al. Environmental factors affecting mechanical properties of facial prosthetic elastomers. Int J Prosthodont 1994;7:479–486.
Mohs FE. Chemosurgery for skin cancer: Fixed tissue and fresh tissue techniques. Arch Dermatol 1976;112:211–215.
Montgomery P, Kiat-amnuay S. Survey of currently used materials for fabrication of extraoral maxillofacial prostheses. J Prosthodont 2010;19:482–490.
Moore DJ, Glaser ZR, Tabacco MJ, et al. Evaluation of polymeric materials for maxillofacial prosthetics. J Prosthet Dent 1977;38:319–326.
Morris-Jones R, Robertson SJ, Ross JS, et al. Dermatitis caused by physical irritants. Br J Dermatol 2002;147:270–275.
Mount J, Singh N, Powers JM, et al. Pigmented maxillofacial silicone elastomer mechanical and color properties after aging. J Dent Res 2018;97(spec issue A):0568.
Mouzakis DE, Papadopoulos TD, Polyzois GL, et al. Dynamic mechanical properties of a maxillofacial silicone elastomer incorporating a ZnO additive: The effect of artificial aging. J Craniofac Surg 2010;21:1867–1871.
Mulcare DC, Coward TJ. Suitability of a mobile phone colorimeter application for use as an objective aid when matching skin color during the fabrication of a maxillofacial prosthesis. J Prosthodont 2019;28:934–943.
Murata H, Hong G, Hamada T, et al. Dynamic mechanical properties of silicone maxillofacial prosthetic materials and the influence of frequency and temperature on their properties. Int J Prosthodont 2003;16:369–374.
Muth JT, Vogt DM, Truby RL, et al. Embedded 3D printing of strain sensors within highly stretchable elastomers. Advanced Materials 2014;26:6307–6312.
Napadensky E. Inkjet 3D printing. The chemistry of inkjet inks. 2010. pp. 255–267. https://doi.org/10.1142/9789812818225_0013.
Nelson BR, Railan D, Cohen S. Mohs' micrographic surgery for nonmelanoma skin cancer. Clin Plast Surg 1997;24:705–718.
Nemli S, Güngör M, Bağkur M. In vitro evaluation of color and translucency reproduction of maxillofacial prostheses using a computerized system. J Adv Prosthodont 2018;10:422–429.
Nemli SK, Aydin C, Yilmaz H, et al. Quality of life of patients with implant-retained maxillofacial prostheses: A prospective and retrospective study. J Prosthet Dent 2013;109:44–52.

Neu TR, Van der Mei HC, Busscher HJ, et al. Biodeterioration of medical-grade silicone rubber used for voice prostheses: A SEM study. Biomaterials 1993;14:459–464.

Nguyen CT, Chambers MS, Powers JM, et al. Effect of opacifiers and UV absorbers on pigmented maxillofacial silicone elastomer, part 2: Mechanical properties after artificial aging. J Prosthet Dent 2013;109:402–410.

Ní Annaidh A, Bruyère K, Destrade M, et al. Characterization of the anisotropic mechanical properties of excised human skin. J Mechan Behav Biomed Mater 2012;5(1):139–148. http://doi.org/10.1016/j.jmbbm.2011.08.016.

Nikawa H, Jin C, Hamada T, et al. Candida albicans growth on thermal cycled materials for maxillofacial prostheses in vitro. J Oral Rehab 2001;28:755–765.

Nishimura R. Implants in irradiated tissues. In Maxillofacial rehabilitation: Prosthodontic and surgical considerations. Ed. J Beumer, T Curtis, M Marunick. St Louis, MO: Ishiyaku EuroAmerica; 1996. pp. 103–106.

Nishimura R, Roumanas E, Lewis S, et al. Craniofacial defects and osseointegrated implants: Nasal defects. J Prosthet Dent 1996;76:597.

Nishimura R, Roumanas E, Lewis S, et al. Craniofacial defects and osseointegrated implants: Orbital defects. J Prosthet Dent 1998;79:304.

Nishimura R, Roumanas E, Moy P, et al. Craniofacial defects and osseointegrated implants: Auricular defects. J Prosth Dent 1995;73:533.

Nobrega AS, Malavazi EM, Melo Neto CLM, et al. Influence of different pigment incorporation methods on color, dimensional stability, and detail reproduction of silicones. Eur J Dent 2019 Jul;13:399–404.

Nuseir A, Hatamleh MM, Alnazzawi A, et al. Direct 3D printing of flexible nasal prosthesis: Optimized digital workflow from scan to fit: 3D printed flexible nose. Journal of Prosthodontics 2019;28(1):10–14. http://doi.org/10.1111/jopr.13001.

Nuutinen J, Kärjä J. Local and distant metastases in patients with surgically treated squamous cell carcinoma of the lip. Clin Otolaryngol Allied Sci 1981;6:415–419.

Oatts JT, Robbins JA, de Alba Campomanes AG. The effect of enucleation on orbital growth in patients with retinoblastoma. Journal of AAPOS 2017;21:309–312.

Ogawa T, Nishimura I. Genes differentially expressed in titanium healing. J Dent Res 2006;85:566–570.

Over LM, Andres CJ, Moore BK, et al. Using a colorimeter to develop an intrinsic silicone shade guide for facial prostheses. J Prosthodont 1998;7:237–249.

Oyasiji T, Tan W, Kane J, et al. Malignant adnexal tumors of the skin: A single institution experience. World J Surg Oncol 2018;16:99.

Pandey AN. Retinoblastoma: An overview. J Saudi Ophthal Soc 2014;28:310–315.

Paravina RD, Majkic G, Del Mar Perez M, et al. Color difference thresholds of maxillofacial skin replications. J Prosthodont 2009;18:618–625.

Parel SM, Tjellström A. The United States and Swedish experience with osseointegration and facial prostheses. Int J Oral Maxillofac Implants 1991;6:75–79.

Paul S, Peter A, Pietrobon N, et al. Visual and spectrophotometric shade analysis of human teeth. J Dent Res 2002;81:578–582.

Pesqueira AA, Goiato MC, dos Santos DM, et al. Effect of disinfection and accelerated aging on color stability of colorless and pigmented facial silicone. J Prosthodont 2011;20:305–309.

Pine K, Sloan B, Jacobs R. History of ocular prosthetics. In Clinical ocular prosthetics. Ed. K Pine, B Sloan, R Jacobs. Clinical Ocular Prosthetics; 2015. pp. 283–312. http://doi.org/10.1007/978-3-319-19057-0_11.

Pine KR, Sloan B, Jacobs RJ. The development of measurement tools for prosthetic eye research. Clin Exp Optom 2013a;96:32–38.

Pine KR, Sloan B, Stewart J, et al. The response of the anophthalmic socket to prosthetic eye wear. Clinical Experimental Optometry 2013b;96:388–393.

Polyzois G, Oilo G, Dahl J. Tensile bond strength of maxillofacial adhesives. J Prosthet Dent 1993;69:374–377.

Polyzois G. Mechanical properties of 2 new addition-vulcanizing silicone prosthetic elastomers. Int J Prosthodont 1999;12:359–362.

Polyzois GL. Evaluation of a new silicone elastomer for maxillofacial prostheses. J Prosthodont 1995;4:38–41.

Polyzois GL, Andreopoulos AG. Some physical properties of an improved facial elastomer: A comparative study. J Prosthet Dent 1993;70:26–32.

Polyzois GL, Eleni PN, Krokida MK. Effect of time passage on some physical properties of silicone maxillofacial elastomers. J Cranio Surg 2011a;22:1617–1621.

Polyzois GL, Eleni PN, Krokida MK. Optical properties of pigmented polydimethylsiloxane prosthetic elastomers: Effect of "outdoor" and "indoor" accelerating aging. J Craniofac Surg 2011b Sep;22:1574–1578.

Polyzois GL, Frangou MJ. Bonding of silicone prosthetic elastomers to three different denture resins. Int J Prosthodont 2002;15:535–538.

Polyzois GL, Frangou MJ, Andreopoulos AG. The effect of bonding agents on the bond strength of facial silicone elastomers to a visible light-activated resin. Int J Prosthodont 1991;4:440–444.

Polyzois GL, Hensten-Pettersen A, Kullmann A. An assessment of the physical properties and biocompatibility of three silicone elastomers. J Prosthet Dent 1994;71:500–504.

Polyzois GL, Pettersen AH. Physicomechanical and cytotoxic properties of room temperature vulcanizing silicone prosthetic elastomers. Acta Odontol Scand 1998;56:245–248.

Polyzois GL, Tarantili PA, Frangou MJ, et al. Physical properties of a silicone prosthetic elastomer stored in simulated skin secretions. J Prosthet Dent 2000;83:572–577.

Preciado DA, Matas A, Adams GL. Squamous cell carcinoma of the head and neck in solid organ transplant recipients. Head Neck 2002;24:319–325.

Qiu J, Gu X, Xiong Y, et al. Nasal prosthesis rehabilitation using CAD-CAM technology after total rhinectomy: A pilot study. Support Care Cancer 2011;19:1055–1059.

Rabek JF. Polymer photodegradation: Mechanisms and experimental methods. Netherlands: Springer; 1994. http://doi.org/10.1007/978-94-011-1274-1.

Ramirez E, Jansat S, Philippot K, et al. Influence of organic ligands on the stabilization of palladium nanoparticles. J Organomet Chem 2004;689:4601–4610.

Ranabhatt R, Singh K, Siddharth R, et al. Color matching in facial prosthetics: A systematic review. J Indian Prosthodont Soc 2017;17:3–7.

Rangert BR, Sullivan RM, Jemt TM. Load factor control for implants in the posterior partially edentulous segment. Int J Oral Maxillofac Implants 1997;12:360–370.

Rasmussen ML. The eye amputated—consequences of eye amputation with emphasis on clinical aspects, phantom eye syndrome and quality of life. Acta Ophthalmol 2010 Dec;88(thesis 2):1–26. http://doi.org/10.1111/j.1755-3768.2010.02039.x.

Reichinger A, Majdak P, Sablatnig R, et al. Evaluation of methods for optical 3D scanning of human Pinnas. In Proceedings of the 2013 International Conference on 3D Vision-3DV. Seattle: IEEE; 2013. pp. 390–397.

Reiffel AJ, Kafka C, Hernandez KA, et al. High-fidelity tissue engineering of patient-specific auricles for reconstruction of pediatric microtia and other auricular deformities. PLoS One 2013;8:e56506. http://doi.org/10.1371/journal.pone.0056506.

Reizner GT, Chuang TY, Elpern DJ, et al. Basal cell carcinoma in Kauai, Hawaii: The highest documented incidence in the United States. J Am Acad Dermatol 1993;29:184–189.

Rennesson JL. A full-range of 3D body scanning solutions. In Proceedings of the Third International Conference on 3D Body Scanning Technology. Lugano; 2012. pp. 16–17.

Ring ME. The history of maxillofacial prosthetics. Plast Reconstr Surg 1991;87:174–184.

Roberts AC. History. In Facial prostheses: The restoration of facial defects by prosthetic means. Ed. AC Roberts. London: Kimpton; 1971. p. 2.

Rodriguez N, Ruelas S, Forien JB, et al. 3D printing of high viscosity reinforced silicone elastomers. Polymers (Basel) 2021 Jul 8;13(14):2239. http://doi.org/10.3390/polym13142239. PMID: 34300996; PMCID: PMC8309234.

Romeu M, Foletti JM, Chossegros C, et al. Malignant cutaneous adnexal neoplasms of the face and scalp: Diagnostic and therapeutic update. J Stomatol Oral Maxillofac Surg 2017;118:95–102.

Ross MT, Cruz R, Brooks-Richards T, et al. Smartphones for frugal three-dimensional scanning of the external ear with application to microtia. J Plast Reconstr Aesthet Surg 2018;71:1362–1380.

Roumanas ED, Freymiller EG, Chang TL. Implant-retained prostheses for facial defects: An up to 14 year follow-up report on the survival rates of implants at UCLA. Int J Prosthet 2002;15:325–332.

Rubenstein JE. Attachments used for implant-supported facial prostheses: A survey of United States, Canada, and Swedish centers. J Prosthet Dent 1995;73:262.

Rubin PA. Enucleation, evisceration, and exenteration. Current Opinion in Ophthalmology 1993;4:39–48.

Ruiters S, De Jong S, Mombaerts I. Measuring quality of care and life in patients with an ocular prosthesis. Graefes Arch Clin Exp Ophthalmol 2021 Jul;259(7):2017–2025. http://doi.org/10.1007/s00417-021-05088-1. Epub 2021 Feb 6.

Ruiters S, Sun Y, de Jong S, et al. Computer-aided design and three-dimensional printing in the manufacturing of an ocular prosthesis. British Journal of Ophthalmology 2016;100:879–881.

Sabol JV, Grant GT, Liacouras P, et al. Digital image capture and rapid prototyping of the maxillofacial defect. J Prosthodont 2011;20:310–314.

Salmi M, Ituarte IF, Chekurov S, et al. Effect of build orientation in 3D printing production for material extrusion, material jetting, binder jetting, sheet object lamination, vat photopolymerisation, and powder bed fusion. International Journal of Collaborative Enterprise 2016;5(3–4):218–231.

Sami D, Young S, Petersen R. Perspective on orbital enucleation implants. Survey of Ophthalmology 2007;52:244–265.

Sanchez RA, Moore DJ, Cruz DL, et al. Comparison of the physical properties of two types of polydimethyl siloxane for fabrication of facial prostheses. J Prosthet Dent 1992;67:679–682.

Santhaveesuk S, Holland JN III, Kiat-amnuay S. Mechanical properties of silicone maxillofacial prostheses subjected to microwave disinfection. IADR Abstract 2022a.

Santhaveesuk S, Kiat-amnuay S, Tribble GD. Microwave disinfection of biofilm contaminated silicone facial prostheses. IADR Abstract 2022b.

Schaaf NG. Color characterizing silicone rubber facial prostheses. J Prosthet Dent 1970;24:198–202.

Schwartz HC, Wollin M, Leake DL, et al. Interface radiation dosimetry in mandibular reconstruction. Arch Otolaryngol 1979;105:293–295.

Seelaus R, Coward TJ, Li S. Coloration of silicone prostheses: Technology versus clinical perception. Is there a difference? Part 2, Clinical evaluation of a pilot study. J Prosthodont 2011;20:67–73.

Sethi T, Kheur M, Coward T, et al. Change in color of a maxillofacial prosthetic silicone elastomer, following investment in molds of different materials. J Indian Prosthodont Society 2015;15:153–157.

Shah RM, Coutinho I, Chitre V, et al. The ocular prosthesis: A novel technique using digital photography. Journal of Indian Prosthodontic Society 2014 Dec;14(suppl 1):248–254.

Singer MT, Mitchell DL, Pelleu GB Jr. Effect of primers on the bond strength of silicone elastomers and polyurethane. J Prosthet Dent 1988;60:602–605.

Sitthi-Amorn P, Ramos JE, Wangy Y, et al. Multifab: A machine vision assisted platform for multi-material 3D printing. ACM Transactions on Graphics (TOG) 2015;34:129.

Smit TJ, Koornneef L, Zonneveld FW, et al. Computed tomography in the assessment of the postenucleation socket syndrome. Ophthalmology 1990;97:1347–1351.

Smith RJ, Prazeres S, Fauquier S, et al. Complications of two scleral flaps evisceration technique: Analysis of 201 procedures. Ophthalmic Plast Reconstr Surg 2011;27:227–231.

Sohaib A, Amano K, Xiao K, et al. Colour quality of facial prostheses in additive manufacturing. Int J Advanced Manufacturing Tech 2018;96:881–894.

Sonnahalli NK, Chowdhary R. Effect of adding silver nanoparticle on physical and mechanical properties of maxillofacial silicone elastomer material-an in-vitro study. J Prosthodont Res 2020;64:431–435.

Spraul CW, Grossniklaus HE. Analysis of 24,444 surgical specimens accessioned over 55 years in an ophthalmic pathology laboratory. International Ophthalmology 1997;21:283–304.

Stathi K, Tarantili PA, Polyzois G. The effect of accelerated ageing on performance properties of addition type silicone biomaterials. Journal of Materials Science Materials in Medicine 2010;21:1403–1411.

Stein J, Lewis LN, Gao Y, et al. In situ determination of the active catalyst in hydrosilylation reactions using highly reactive Pt(0) catalyst precursors. J Am Chem Soc 1999;121:3693–3703.

Stieghorst J, Majaura D, Wevering H, et al. Toward 3D printing of medical implants: Reduced lateral droplet spreading of silicone rubber under intense IR curing. ACS Applied Materials & Interfaces 2016;8:8239–8246.

Subburaj K, Nair C, Rajesh S, et al. Rapid development of auricular prosthesis using CAD and rapid prototyping technologies. Int J Oral Maxillofac Surg 2007;36:938–943. http://doi.org/10.1016/j.ijom.2007. 07.013.

Subramaniam SS, Breik O, Cadd B, et al. Long term outcomes of craniofacial implants for the restoration of facial defects. Int J Oral Maxillofac Surg 2018;47:773–782.

Sugar A, Beumer J III. Reconstructive prosthetic methods for facial defects. Oral Maxillofac Surg Clin North Am 1994;6:755–764.

Sun J, Chen X, Liao H, et al. Template-based framework for nasal prosthesis fabrication. Rapid Prototyp J 2013;19:68–76.

Sun J, Xi J, Chen X, et al. A CAD/CAM system for fabrication of facial prostheses. Rapid Prototyp J 2011;17:253–261.

Sweeney WT, Fischer TE, Castleberry DJ, et al. Evaluation of improved maxillofacial prosthetic materials. J Prosthet Dent 1972;27:297–305.

Taft RM, Cameron SM, Knudson RC, et al. The effect of primers and surface characteristics on the adhesion-in-peel force of silicone elastomers bonded to resin materials. J Prosthet Dent 1996;76:515–518.

Tamareselvy K, Rueggeberg FA. Dynamic mechanical analysis of two crosslinked copolymer systems. Dent Mater 1994;10:290–297.

Tawfik HA, Raslan AO, Talib N. Surgical management of acquired socket contracture. Current Opinion Ophthal 2009;20:406–411.

Taylor R, Liauw CM, Maryan C. The effect of resin/crosslinker ratio on the mechanical properties and fungal deterioration of a maxillofacial silicone elastomer. J Mater Sci Mater Med 2003;14:497–502.

Tjellström A, Granström G. One-stage procedure to establish osseointegration: A zero to five years follow-up report. Int J Oral Maxillofac Implants 1995;109:593–598.

Tjellström A, Linström J, Hallén O, et al. Osseointegrated titanium implants in the temporal bone. Am J Otol 1981;2:304–310.

Toljanic J, Eckert S, Roumanas E, et al. Osseointegrated craniofacial implants in the rehabilitation of orbital defects: An update of a retrospective experience in the United States. J Prosthet Dent 2005;94:177.

Tran NH, Scarbecz M, Gary JJ. In vitro evaluation of color change in maxillofacial elastomer through the use of an ultraviolet light absorber and a hindered amine light stabilizer. J Prosthet Dent 2004;91:483–490.

Tsai F, Xiao C, Koran A, et al. Synthesis of silicone block copolymers for use as maxillofacial materials. In Materials research in maxillofacial prosthetics. Ed. JC Setcos. Trans Acad Dent Mater 1992;5:126–137.

Tso TV, Chao D, Tanner J, et al. Prosthetic reconstruction of a patient with an irradiated total rhinectomy with navigated surgical placement of a single zygomatic implant: A clinical report. J Prosthet Dent 2021;1125:352–356.

Tso TV, Hurwitz M, Margalit DN, et al. Radiation dose enhancement associated with contemporary dental materials. J Prosthet Dent 2019;121:703–707.

Tukmachi MS, Safi IN, Ali MM. Evaluation of mechanical properties and cytotoxicity of maxillofacial silicone material after incorporation of zirconia nanopowder. Materials Today: Proceedings 2021;42:2209–2217.

Turner GE, Fischer TE, Castleberry DJ, et al. Intrinsic color of isophorone polyurethane for maxillofacial prosthetics: 1. Physical properties. J Prosthet Dent 1984a;51:519–522.

Turner GE, Fischer TE, Castleberry DJ, et al. Intrinsic color of isophorone polyurethane for maxillofacial prosthetics: 2. Color stability. J Prosthet Dent 1984b;51:673–675.

Tyers AG, Collin JR. Orbital implants and post enucleation socket syndrome. Transactions of the Ophthalmological Societies of the United Kingdom 1982 Apr;102(Pt 1):90–92.

Udagama A, Drane JB. Use of medical-grade methyl triacetoxy silane crosslinked silicone for facial prostheses. J Prosthet Dent 1982;48:86–88.

Udagama A. Urethane-lined silicone facial prostheses. J Prosthet Dent 1987;58:351–354.

Unkovskiy A, Spintzyk S, Brom J, et al. Direct 3D printing of silicone facial prostheses: A preliminary experience in digital workflow. J Prosthet Dent 2018;120:303–308.

Upham R. Artificial noses and ears. Boston Med Surg J 1901;145:522–523.

Veres EM, Wolfaardt JF, Becker PJ. An evaluation of the surface characteristics of a facial prosthetic elastomer: Part I. Review of the literature on the surface characteristics of dental materials with maxillofacial applications. J Prosthet Dent 1990a;63:193–197.

Veres EM, Wolfaardt JF, Becker PJ. An evaluation of the surface characteristics of a facial prosthetic elastomer: Part II. The surface texture. J Prosthet Dent 1990b;63:325–331.

Veres EM, Wolfaardt JF, Becker PJ. An evaluation of the surface characteristics of a facial prosthetic elastomer: Part III. Wettability and hardness. J Prosthet Dent 1990c;63:466–471.

Verma AS, Fitzpatrick DR. Anophthalmia and microphthalmia. Orphanet J of Rare Diseases 2007 Nov 26;2:47.

Visser A, Raghoebar G, van Oort R, et al. Fate of implant-retained craniofacial prostheses: Life span and aftercare. Int J Oral Maxilofacial Implants 2008;23:89–98.

Viswanathan P, Sagoo MS, Olver JM. UK national survey of enucleation, evisceration and orbital implant trends. British J Ophthalmol 2007;91:616–619.

Viverberg MA, Verhamme L, van de Pol P, et al. Auricular prostheses attached to osseointegrated implants: Multidisciplinary work-up and clinical evaluation. Eur Arch Otorhinolaryngol 2019;276:1017–1027.

Walsh ME, Ostrinskaya A, Sorensen M, et al. 3D-printable materials for microbial liquid culture. 3D Printing and Additive Manufacturing 2016;3(2):113–118.

Walshaw E, Zoltie T, Bartlett P, et al. Manufacture of a high definition ocular prosthesis. British J Oral Maxillofac Surg 2018;56:893–894.

Wang JK. Performance assessment of digital method for skin shade measurement and reproduction [dissertation]. [Houston]: University of Texas School of Dentistry at Houston, ProQuest Master Dissertations; 2016. 10133536.

Wang L, Liu Q, Jing D, et al. Biomechanical properties of nano-TiO(2) addition to a medical silicone elastomer: The effect of artificial ageing. J Dent 2014 Apr;42(4):475–483. http://doi.org/10.1016/j.jdent.2014.01.002.

Wang R, Collard SM, Lemon JC. Adhesion of silicone to polyurethane in maxillofacial prostheses. Int J Prosthodont 1994;7:43–49.

Wang TM, Leu LJ, Wang J, et al. Effects of prosthesis materials and prosthesis splinting on peri-implant bone stress around implants in poor quality bone: A numeric analysis. Int J Oral Maxillofac Implants 2002;17:231–237.

Waters MG, Jagger RG, Polyzois GL. Wettability of silicone rubber maxillofacial prosthetic materials. J Prosthet Dent 1999;81:439–443.

Waters MG, Jagger RG, Polyzois GL, et al. Dynamic mechanical thermal analysis of maxillofacial elastomers. J Prosthet Dent 1997;78:501–505.

Watson J, Hatamleh MM. Complete integration of technology for improved reproduction of auricular prostheses. J Prosthet Dent 2014;111:430–436. http://doi.org/10.1016/j.prosdent.2013.07.018.

Weathering testing guidebook. Mount Prospect, IL: Atlas Electric Devices; 2001.

Wee AG, Beatty MW, Gozalo-Diaz DJ, et al. Proposed shade guide for human facial skin and lip: A pilot study. J Prosthet Dent 2013;110:82–89.

Wee AG, Lindsey DT, Kuo S, et al. Color accuracy of commercial digital cameras for use in dentistry. Dent Mater 2006;22:553–559.

Weifel H, Maier RD, Schiller M. Plastics additives handbook. 6th ed. Munich: Hanser; 2009.

Willett ES, Beatty MW. Outdoor weathering of facial prosthetic elastomers differing in Durometer hardness. J Prosthet Dent 2015;113:228–235.

Wladis EJ, Aakalu VK, Sobel RK, et al. Orbital implants in enucleation surgery: A report by the American Academy of Ophthalmology. Ophthalmology 2018;125:311–317.

Wolfaardt JF, Chandler HD, Smith BA. Mechanical properties of a new facial prosthetic material. J Prosthet Dent 1985;53:228–234.

Wong SQ, Waldek K, Vergara IA, et al. UV-associated mutations underlie the etiology of MCV-negative Merkel cell carcinomas. Cancer Res 2015;75:5228–5234.

Wu G, Bi Y, Zhou B, et al. Computer-aided design and rapid manufacture of an orbital prosthesis. Int J Prosthodont 2009;22:293–295.

Wu G, Zhou B, Bi Y, et al. Selective laser sintering technology for customized fabrication of facial prostheses. J Prosthet Dent 2008;100:56–60.

Xiao K, Zardawi F, van Noort R, et al. Color reproduction for advanced manufacture of soft tissue prostheses. J Dent 2013;41:e15–e23. http://doi.org/10.1016/j.jdent.2013.04.008.

Xiao-na L, Yi-min Z, Shi-bao L, et al. Comparison of mechanical properties of Cosmesil M511 and A-2186 maxillofacial silicone elastomers. J US Ch Med Sci 2007;4:34–37.

Yap Y, Dikshit V, Lionar SP, et al. Investigation of fiber reinforced composite using multi-material 3D printing. Presented at the Annual International Solid Freeform Fabrication Symposium, Austin, TX, 2016.

Yoda N, Gunji Y, Ogawa T, et al. In vivo load measurement for evaluating the splinting effects of implant-supported superstructures: A pilot study. Int J Prosthodont 2013;26:143–146.

Yousuf SJ, Jones LS, Kidwell ED. Enucleation and evisceration: 20 years of experience. Orbit 2012;31:211–215.

Yu R, Koran A III, Craig RG. Physical properties of maxillofacial elastomers under conditions of accelerated aging. J Dent Res 1980a;59:1041–1047.

Yu R, Koran A III, Craig RG. Physical properties of a pigmented silicone maxillofacial material as a function of accelerated aging. J Dent Res 1980b;59:1141–1148.

Yu R, Koran A III, Craig RG, et al. Stain removal from a pigmented silicone maxillofacial elastomer. J Dent Res 1981a;61:993–996.

Yu R, Koran A III, Raptis CN, et al. Cigarette staining and cleaning of a maxillofacial silicone. J Dent Res 1983;627:853–855.

Yu R, Koran A III, Raptis CN, et al. Stain removal from a silicone maxillofacial elastomer. J Dent Res 1981b;60:1754–1758.

Yu R, Koran A. Dimensional stability of elastomers for maxillofacial applications. J Dent Res 1979;58:1908–1909.

Yuan F, LV P, Wang P, et al. Custom fabrication of try-in wax complete denture. Rapid Prototyp J 2016;22:539–543. http://doi.org/10.1108/RPJ-09-2014-0129.

Zardawi FM. Characterisation of implant supported soft tissue prostheses produced with 3D colour printing technology. Sheffield: University of Sheffield; 2013.

Zardawi FM, van Noort R, et al. Mechanical properties of 3D printed facial prostheses compared to handmade silicone polymer prostheses. Eur Sci J 2015b;11:12.

Zardawi FM, Xiao K, van Noort, et al. Investigation of elastomer infiltration into 3D printed facial soft tissue prostheses. Anaplastology 2015;4:1. http://doi.org/10.4172/2161-1173.1000139.

Zeno HA, Sternberger SS, Tuminelli FJ, et al. Combined lower lip prosthesis retained by an intraoral component. J Prosthodont 2013;22:397–401.

Zheng YL, Liu WJ, Li J. Mechanical properties of SEI silicone for maxillofacial prosthesis. J Shanghai Jiaotong Univ Med Sci 2009;29:656–659.

Chapter 6

Rehabilitation of Cleft Lip and Palate and Other Craniofacial Anomalies

Arun B. Sharma, Lawrence E. Brecht, Ting Ling Chang, Satinder Chander, Karen Vargervik, Andrew Weeks

Cleft lip and palate are one of the most common congenital anomalies whose diverse etiologies have made prevention unlikely at this time. Treatment, which is dictated by the severity of the malady, is unique in that it begins at birth and is usually not completed until the end of the patient's second decade. Interdisciplinary management, with interaction among the various specialists of the cleft palate team, is essential to achieving optimum results.

An international review of the interdisciplinary team approach in the management of the patient with cleft lip and palate illustrates the diversity of treatment strategies and techniques (Bardach and Morris, 1990); however, large multicenter trials such as the Eurocleft Study are yielding outcomes data that can help better guide treatments (Semb et al., 2005a, 2005b; Brattstrom et al., 2005; Molsted et al., 2005; Shaw et al., 2005). The treatment philosophy of the Center for Craniofacial Anomalies at the University of California, San Francisco (UCSF), will form the background for this chapter. Other treatment philosophies and their controversies will be discussed with reference to the UCSF model.

The role of the prosthodontist in the management of cleft lip and palate has changed significantly in the past 50 years (Delgado et al., 1992). Definitive prosthodontic treatment is usually one of the final therapies instituted and must attempt to mitigate any anatomical and/or functional deficiencies that may remain after the gamut of other treatments is essentially completed. In the past, large, bulky removable prostheses were often necessary to replace missing teeth, correct horizontal or vertical growth discrepancies, or to provide an obturator extension to restore velopharyngeal function (Figs 6-1 and 6-2). Fortunately, the need for these all-inclusive removable prostheses has diminished significantly in recent years because of more effective surgical and orthodontic treatment and a better understanding of the problems unique to the individuals with clefts.

During the 1960s, treatments became more sophisticated, and prosthodontic intervention with fixed partial dentures was used primarily to replace missing or malformed teeth and stabilize cleft segments following orthodontic therapy (Fig 6-3). These fixed prostheses had to be rigid to hold the cleft segments in position and limit the risk of porcelain fractures. Bulk was often added to the connectors to increase the rigidity of the metal framework. In these young patients with large dental pulps, labial reductions during tooth preparation were often suboptimal because of the risk of pulpal exposure.

Where advances in cleft care have been implemented, the need for these large fixed or fixed-removable prostheses has also diminished. Presently, if the maxillary arch can be united by bone grafting of the alveolar cleft, placement of osseointegrated implants and selective crowns and/or porcelain veneers may be the only prosthetic treatment required.

Younger readers may not realize that some maxillofacial clinics and programs began as cleft palate clinics, especially at university-based hospitals. However, as interdisciplinary treatment for the cleft patient improved, the need for removable prosthodontics especially diminished. The maxillofacial prosthodontist began to treat more and more adult patients with acquired defects, while cleft patients

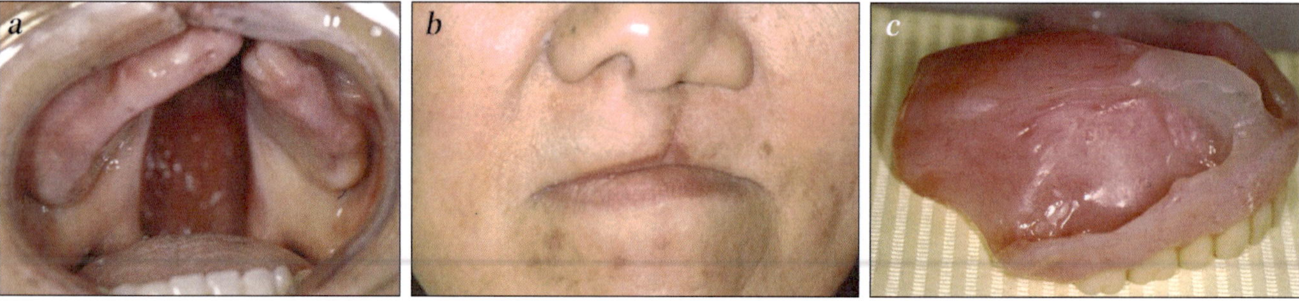

Figure 6-1 Complete dentures. *(a)* Edentulous patient with cleft lip and palate. *(b)* Only the lip was closed surgically, and it was never revised. Note the obvious scar and linear and superior contraction of the lip. *(c)* Maxillary complete denture and obturator. Silicone extensions anteriorly engage undercuts.

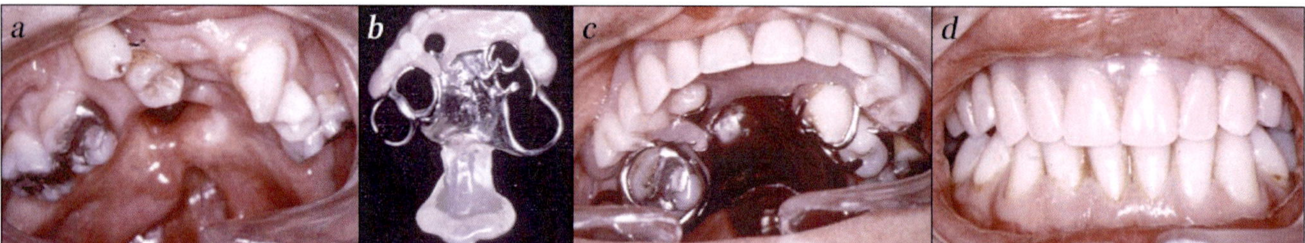

Figure 6-2 Removable partial dentures. *(a)* A patient presented in 1968 with a collapsed maxilla; flat, heavily scarred, and short hard and soft palates; a right premolar that was rotated 180 degrees and anterior and lingual to the canine; and hypernasal speech. Oral hygiene is very good. *(b)* Obturator prosthesis *(c)* The maxillary removable partial denture restores lip support and aesthetics. Prior to prosthetic treatment, the malpositioned premolar was extracted and the soft palate was redivided so that the obturator prosthesis could be positioned in the correct location in the nasopharynx. *(d)* Improved aesthetics.

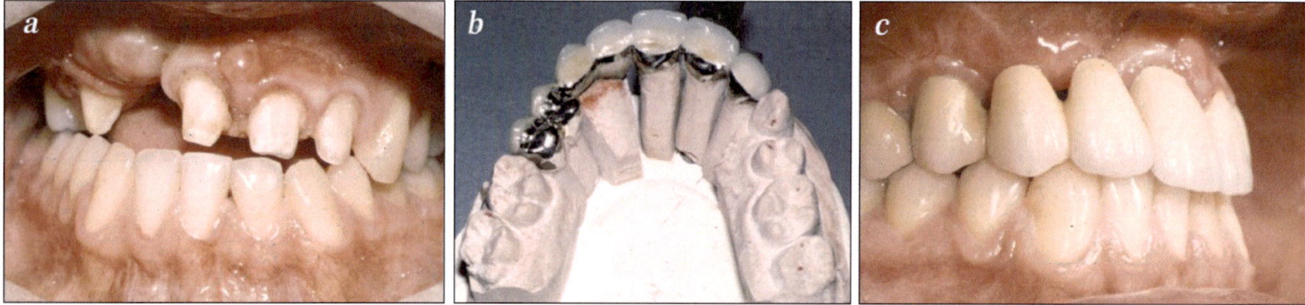

Figure 6-3 Fixed partial dentures. *(a to c)* From the 1950s through the mid-1970s the maxillary fragments were often stabilized with fixed partial dentures. Complete veneer crowns were required to maximize retention. The use of two abutments or more in each cleft segment was recommended.

required less specialized and more routine prosthodontic care. At the same time, the cleft palate team began to examine and to treat more children with other craniofacial anomalies. The purpose of this chapter is to discuss the role prosthodontists still play in the care of patients born with cleft lip and palate and the significant contributions the specialty makes to the care of patients with other congenital deformities.

Palatal Development

Palatogenesis begins in the 5th week and is complete by the 12th week in utero. The palate develops from two primordia: namely, the primary and secondary palates. The primary palate is also called the *medial palatine (nasal) process*. It forms the premaxilla, which includes the incisors and the portion of the hard palate anterior to the incisive foramen. The primary palate develops at the end of the 5th week from the innermost portion of the intermaxillary segment of the maxilla. This segment, formed by merging of the medial nasal prominences, forms a wedge-shaped mass of mesoderm between the internal surfaces of the maxillary prominences of the developing maxilla.

The secondary palate gives rise to the hard (from the incisive foramen posteriorly) and soft palates. It develops from two horizontal mesodermal projections called *lateral palatine (nasal) processes* or *palatine shelves* (Fig 6-4). Initially these processes project inferiorly toward the tongue, but as development occurs, the tongue moves downward, and the palatine shelves become elongated superiorly to the tongue and shift to a more horizontal position (7th week).

The palatine shelves eventually fuse with one another in the midline and with the primary palate and the nasal septum. The fusion begins with the nasal septum anteriorly (9th week) and is completed by the 12th week in the region of the uvula. The posterior portion

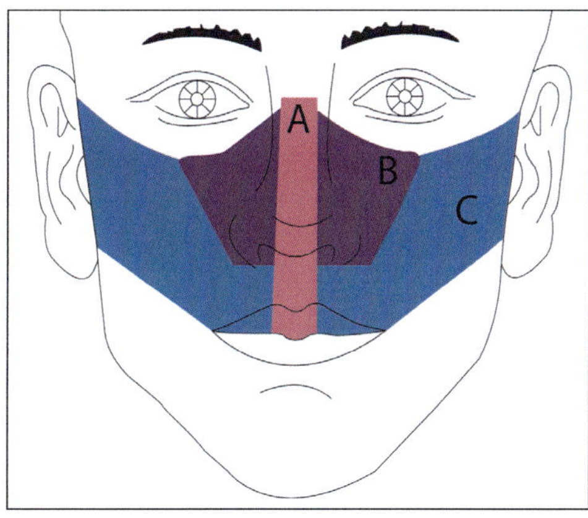

Figure 6-4 Embryologic development of the face. The lack of fusion of embryologic processes leads to formation of clefts. A: medial nasal process; B: lateral nasal process; C: maxillary process.

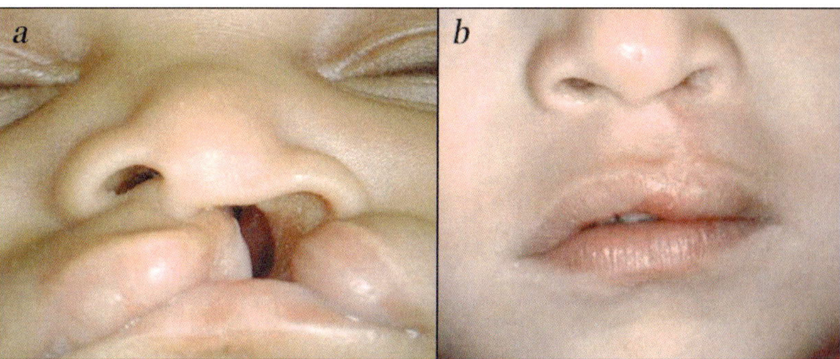

Figure 6-5 Left unilateral cleft lip and palate. *(a)* Prior to lip closure. *(b)* Following lip closure.

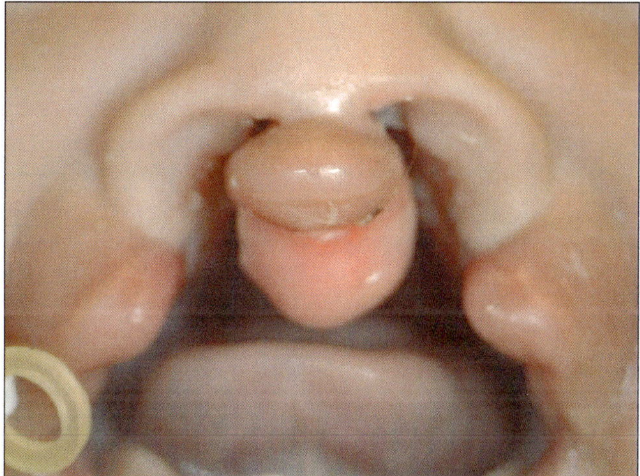

Figure 6-6 Bilateral cleft lip and palate with protruding premaxilla (prolabium).

of the palatine shelves do not become ossified and form the soft palate and uvula. The palatine raphe permanently indicates the line of fusion of the lateral palatine processes. The incisive foramen remains the embryologic border between the primary and secondary palates (Kernahan and Stark, 1958).

Classification of Clefts

Several different classification systems have been proposed over the years. However, we prefer a simple classification, based on embryology, that divides cleft lip and palate patients into three categories: *(1)* cleft lip and alveolus (primary palate), *(2)* cleft of the hard and soft palates (secondary palate), and *(3)* a combination of categories 1 and 2 (primary and secondary palates; Figs 6-5 and 6-6). Clefts can be unilateral or bilateral. Thus, patients can present with a number of combinations (Fig 6-7).

The incisive foramen serves to separate anterior from posterior cleft malformations. Embryologically the anterior and posterior clefts are different. Anterior clefts are caused by defective development of the primary palate due to a mesenchymal deficiency. Posterior clefts result from defective development of the secondary palate due to growth disturbances that interfere with the fusion of the palatine shelves. Anterior clefts include cleft lip with or without a cleft of the alveolus. Posterior clefts involve the soft and/or hard palate up to the incisive foramen.

Cleft patients may also present with other anomalies. Syndromic forms of clefts are those with a medically or surgically relevant abnormality of an organ system outside the anatomical cleft region, including mental retardation. The majority (85%) of patients with clefts have the nonsyndromic form (Jones, 1988). The London Dysmorphology Database lists 215 nonchromosomal syndromes that can include cleft lip, cleft palate, or bifid uvula (Hanson and Murray, 1990).

Incidence and Etiology of Clefting

The incidence of clefting varies in relation to the population studied. Vanderas (1987) has reported the highest rates in American Indians (1 in 278 live births), followed by Japanese, Maoris, Chinese, whites, and African Americans (1 in 3,330 live births). The generally accepted incidence shows that approximately 1 in every 600 infants born in the United States has some form of clefting (Cleft Palate Foundation, 2008). Left-sided clefts (70% of unilateral clefts) are more common than bilateral clefting of the lip and palate, and the right-sided clefts are the least common type (Berkowitz, 1994).

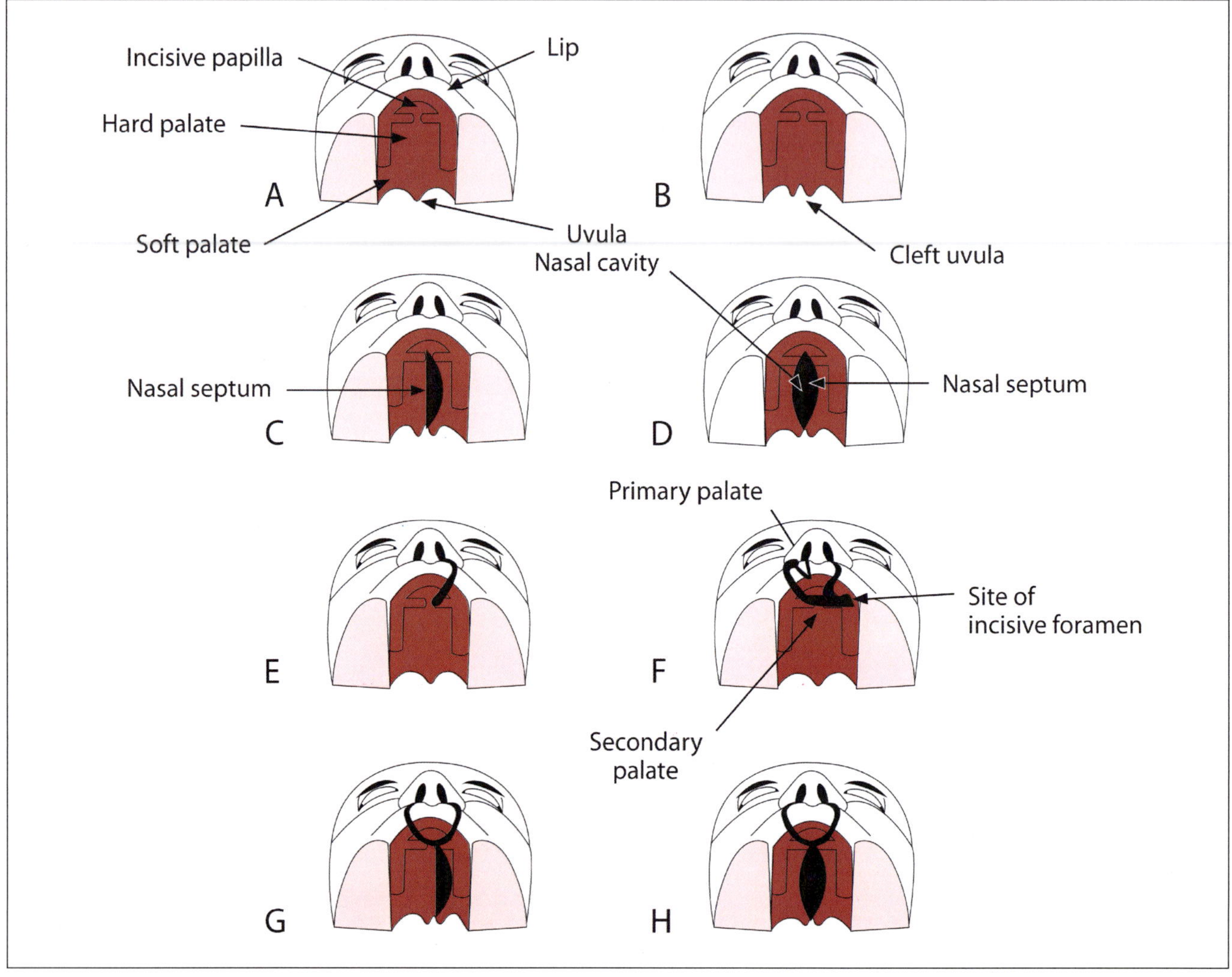

Figure 6-7 Types of cleft lip and palate. *(a)* Normal lip and palate. *(b)* Cleft uvula. *(c)* Unilateral cleft of the posterior or secondary palate. *(d)* Bilateral cleft of the secondary palate. *(e)* Complete unilateral cleft of the lip and alveolar process with a unilateral cleft of the primary palate. *(f)* Complete bilateral cleft of the lip and alveolar process with a bilateral cleft of the primary palate. *(g)* Complete bilateral cleft of the lip and alveolar process with a bilateral cleft of the primary palate and a unilateral cleft of the secondary palate. *(h)* Complete bilateral cleft of the lip and alveolar process with a complete bilateral cleft of the primary and secondary palates.

Cleft lip

Clefts of the upper lip, with or without cleft palate, occur in approximately 1 in 1,000 births; frequency varies among ethnic groups (Thompson and Thompson, 1980). Males are affected twice as frequently as females. The cleft of the primary palate can be unilateral or bilateral and is most commonly found on the left side in patients with unilateral cleft lips.

In a unilateral cleft lip, the maxillary prominence on the affected side fails to unite with the merged medial nasal prominences. If the mesenchymal masses do not proliferate and merge, the overlying lip epithelium is not forced out, and a labial groove will develop and persist. As the epithelium in the labial groove becomes stretched, it ruptures and divides the lip into medial and lateral components.

With a bilateral cleft lip, the mesenchymal masses of the maxillary processes do not merge with the mesenchymal masses of the medial nasal process. The epithelium in both labial grooves stretches and breaks down, resulting in a bilateral cleft. The degree of clefting can vary on the two sides. When the cleft is complete bilaterally and involves the alveolus, the premaxillary segment is free and protrudes anteriorly. The resulting deformity is significant because of the lack of continuity of the orbicularis oris muscle, which is essential for closure of the mouth.

The failure of the medial nasal process to develop and merge results in a rare cleft, the median cleft lip (Fig 6-8). This is a characteristic of Mohr syndrome, transmitted as an autosomal-recessive trait (Goodman and Gorlin, 1970).

Cleft palate

Cleft palate, with or without cleft lip, occurs in about 1 in 2,500 births. Isolated cleft palate is more common in females than in males. The palatine processes fuse about one week later in females than in males, which may explain why isolated clefts of the palate are more common in females (Burdi and Silvey, 1969).

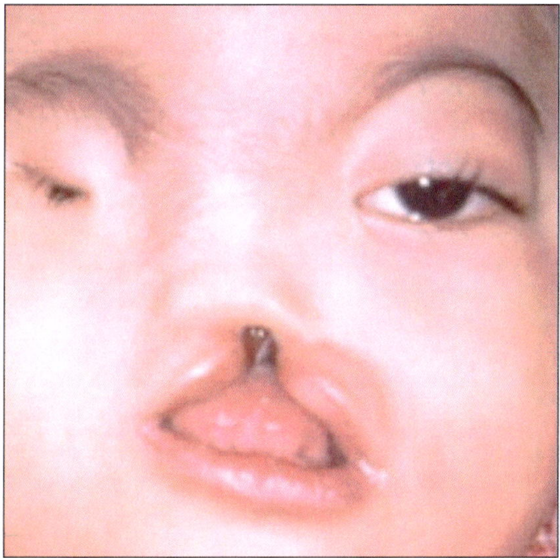

Figure 6-8 Median cleft lip, a rare form of clefting.

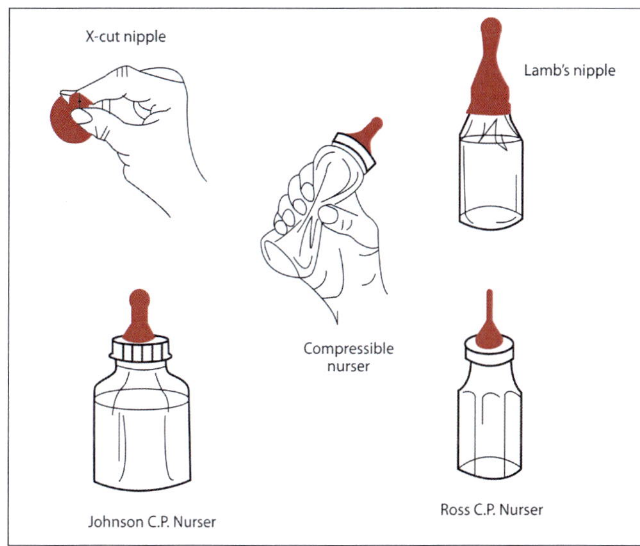

Figure 6-9 Feeding aids.

The embryologic basis of cleft palate is the failure of the mesenchymal masses of the lateral palatine processes to meet and fuse with one another, the nasal septum, and/or with the posterior margin of the primary palate. This could result in a cleft of the primary palate, a cleft of both the primary and the secondary palates, or a cleft of the secondary palate only. Clefts of the secondary palate may involve both the hard and the soft palates or be limited to the soft palate.

Causes

Clefts can be caused by several factors that affect the mother early in the first trimester. These factors include infections and toxicity, poor diet, hormonal imbalances, and genetic factors. Most clefts are caused by multiple genetic and nongenetic factors. The amount of neural crest mesenchyme that migrates to the facial primordia is affected. If this deficiency results in insufficient mesenchyme, clefts of the lip and/or palate occur as part of syndromes that are determined by single mutant genes or as part of chromosomal syndromes such as trisomy 13.

Evaluation of twins indicates that genetic factors play a greater role in cleft lip with or without cleft palate than in clefts of the palate only. Complete clefts involving the lip, alveolus, and palate are usually transmitted through a male sex-linked gene. When the parents of a child with a cleft are not affected, the risk to a subsequent sibling is around 4% (Thompson and Thompson, 1980).

Treatment of Cleft Lip and Palate

Early treatment and evaluation

Early intervention and counseling

When a child is born with a cleft defect, the nurse from a cleft palate team is notified. If the infant is in a hospital with a cleft team, then the team nurse can perform an initial assessment to determine the severity of the cleft and the possibility of other congenital deformities. The nurse then contacts the parents to ascertain their level of understanding of the defect and to clarify the information given to the parents.

At this point, the parents are grief stricken and are usually not prepared to receive detailed information. It is important that the team members assist with the emotional and social adjustment of the family. The nurse should demonstrate an accepting attitude toward the infant and emphasize the positive aspects of the child's appearance. Preoperative and postoperative photographs of patients with similar defects may help considerably in reassuring the parents.

Before leaving the hospital, the parents should be able to feed the infant and to examine and clean the cleft. Appointments should be made for evaluation by the complete team, and follow-up telephone calls should be made by the nurse and/or the social worker to address any problems that may have developed.

Feeding

An infant with a cleft requires special nursing considerations during feeding. Maintenance of nutrition is a priority because adequate nutrition and hydration are essential for growth and development of the infant and for preparation for the first surgery. It is important for the pediatrician to monitor the development of the infant closely.

Depending on the type and severity of the cleft, a variety of feeding devices are available (Fig 6-9). Infants with an isolated cleft lip most often feed normally with a bottle or breast. A broad-based nipple will work well with a regular bottle to provide a seal. The feeding problem is more significant for infants with a cleft palate, with or without a cleft lip. These infants generate a negative pressure when they suck and tire easily, resulting in unfinished feedings. A feeding device that can deliver formula into the mouth is necessary to conserve the infant's energy.

Soft, premature nipples conform better to the palatal defect than do regular hard nipples and can improve sucking. Cross-cut nipples allow for easier flow of formula, thus decreasing the strain on the child. Longer nipples are more successful because they can be positioned posterior to the defect. The squeeze bottle has helped significantly decrease the effort required from the infant, because it allows the parent to squeeze and control the flow of formula into the mouth. This is especially helpful when the sucking reflex is weak. A bulb syringe can also be used to deliver formula without requiring effort from the child.

After a feeding technique has been selected, several modifications may be required to suit the individual situation. Feeding while the infant is in a semiupright position reduces nasal regurgitation. For an infant with a cleft palate, feeding usually requires more time, but the feeding should be unhurried. As the parent and child adjust to the technique, the time required for feeding will usually decrease. If feeding routinely requires more than 45 minutes, the child may be working too hard, and the technique may have to be reevaluated. When feeding is completed, a wet oral swab should be used to clean mucus and formula from the cleft.

If the mother desires to breast-feed her child, she should attempt it. A child with an isolated cleft lip should not have any problem. There may be some leakage of milk when the child is sucking because of the mouth's inability to form a seal on the breast. The mother can improve the seal by placing a finger over the lip defect as the child nurses or by using the areola to fill the lip defect. If there is a unilateral cleft of the alveolus, the nipple should be pointed toward the unaffected side.

When there is a cleft of the palate, breast-feeding is more difficult because of the infant's inability to generate and maintain the necessary vacuum. The mother should position the nipple toward the side of the cleft and support the breast with her fingers to assist the child in grasping the nipple and preventing loss of suction. Chin support for the infant will help stabilize the mandible and press the nipple and areola between the gums. Breast-feeding alone will usually not be adequate, and significant augmentation with formula will be required to ensure adequate nutrition.

Parents should practice feeding their baby while in the hospital and before being sent home. Adequate nutrition is essential for growth and development to prevent delay of the required surgery. The first surgery for the lip is usually performed when the infant is about three months old. At UCSF, the "rule of 10" (10 weeks old, 10 lbs in weight, and a hemoglobin count of 10 g/dL) is used as a rough guideline for surgery.

Genetic evaluation

Genetic evaluation of an infant with a cleft of the lip and/or palate should begin during the first team evaluation. The evaluation includes an accurate prenatal history, including exposure to known teratogens, any family history of known relatives with a cleft, and examination for the presence of lip pits (Fig 6-10), mental retardation, congenital heart disease, limb and ocular abnormalities, bone dysplasia, and other birth defects known to occur with cleft syndromes.

It is important that patients with a cleft be evaluated for the possibility of a syndromic condition. The presence of a cardiac anomaly or chromosome disorders could increase the risk of surgery. A complete physical examination is essential; particular emphasis should be placed on cardiac evaluation and abnormalities associated with the extremities, such as polydactyly, syndactyly, and dwarfing.

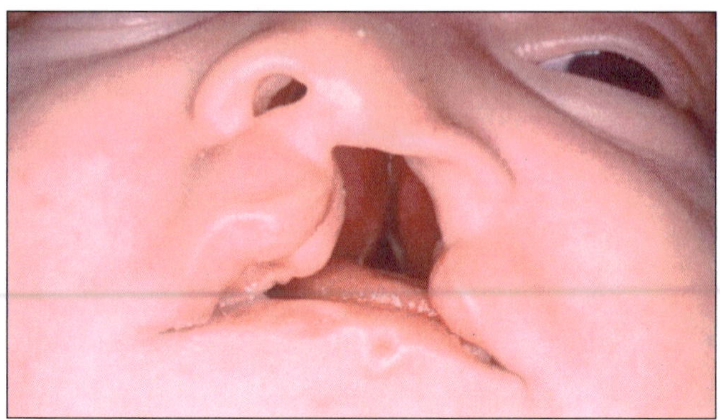

Figure 6-10 Lip pits on the lower lip (Van der Woude syndrome).

An examination of the parents and siblings should also be performed to assess for lip pits, submucous clefts, and so forth, because these conditions may indicate that mendelian disorders are segregating in the family. Trisomy 13, trisomy 18p-, and trisomy 4p- are common chromosomal disorders that include clefting. Chromosomal analysis is essential, especially if other major organ systems are involved. The family should also be informed of the infant's long-term prognosis prior to surgical intervention.

A genetic evaluation is not complete until all medical records are obtained for family members with potential disorders. The patient is examined and referred to specialists in cardiology, ophthalmology, or other services, if required. Once all the information has been evaluated, a diagnosis of a syndromic or nonsyndromic cleft is made. If the diagnosis is syndromic cleft, the parents will require counseling concerning the etiology, incidence, risk to future offspring, and the long-term prognosis.

Distinguishing syndromic from nonsyndromic clefts is important for prognostic reasons and to determine the risk of recurrence in future generations. Clefts can also present with a range of severity. It is important for parents to understand that severely affected children do not necessarily imply a risk of severe defects for future children or that mild defects signify that future children will have a mild disorder. Counseling is very important for the parents, especially about the risk to future generations.

Team evaluation

At the UCSF Center for Craniofacial Anomalies, a patient is initially evaluated by the team. The team members represent the various specialties that will be involved in the care of the patient from birth to adulthood. The team comprises an audiologist, geneticist, genetic counselor, nurse coordinator, oral and maxillofacial surgeon, orthodontist, otolaryngologist, pediatrician, pedodontist, plastic surgeon, prosthodontist, speech pathologist, and social worker. Each patient is initially evaluated by the entire team and, if required, additional referrals are made for completion of the diagnostic workup.

Following the initial evaluation, a treatment plan is outlined and discussed with the family. On recall visits, the team members involved in the current active phase of treatment evaluate the patient. As treatment progresses, modifications are made, as necessary, to the previously outlined treatment sequence (Fig 6-11). Recall visits are scheduled at least once a year until early adulthood.

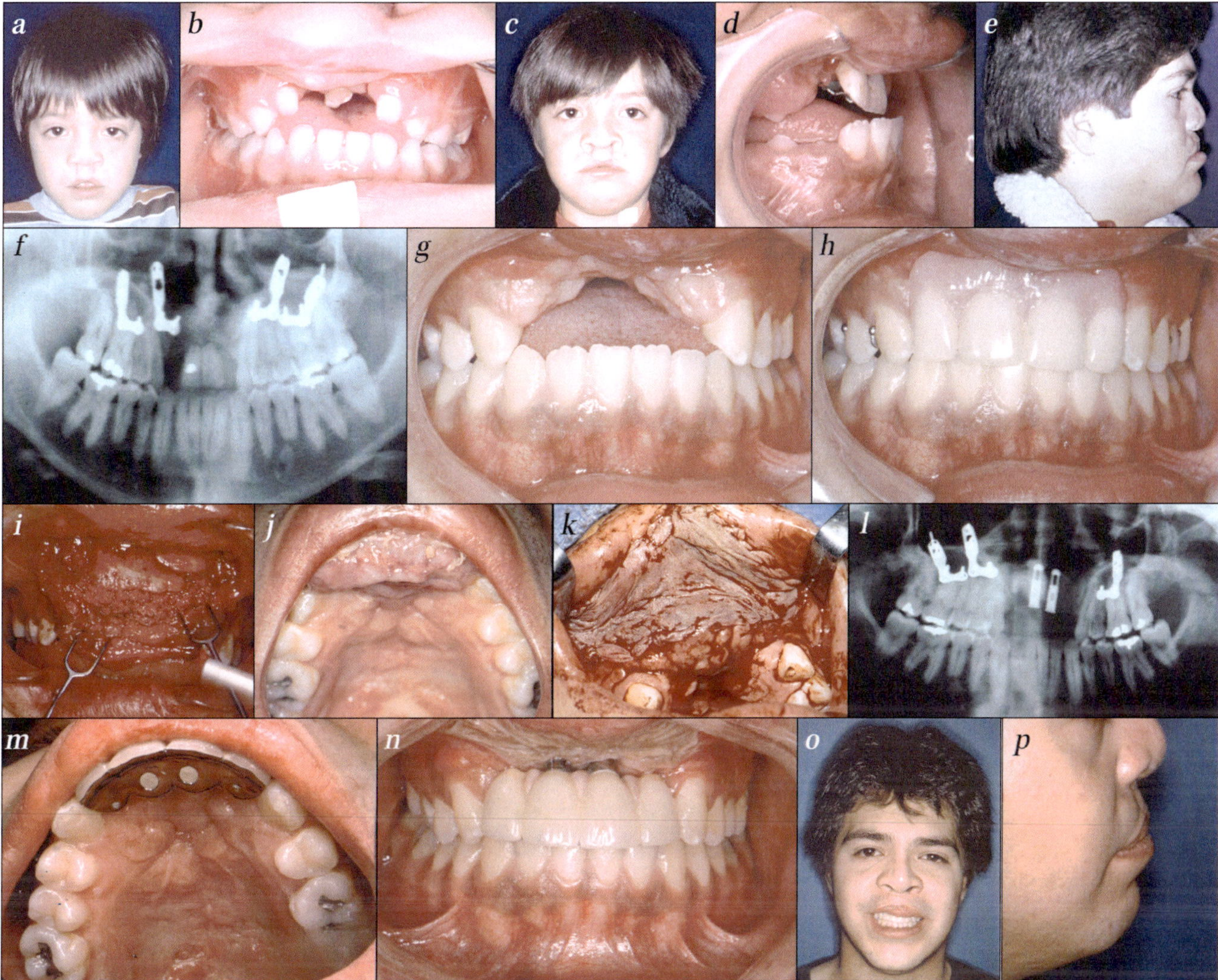

Figure 6-11 Treatment sequence. *(a)* Four-year-old patient with bilateral cleft lip and palate, as presented in 1977 to the Center for Craniofacial Anomalies at UCSF. *(b)* Dentition as presented in 1977. The primary central incisor is malformed and the patient exhibits anterior open bite. *(c)* Patient in 1980. *(d)* Patient in 1983. The maxillomandibular discrepancy is increasing. *(e)* Patient in 1987. He exhibits midfacial retrusion. *(f)* Panoramic radiograph following maxillary advancement and alveolar cleft bone grafting in 1990. The maxillary central incisors show poor root development. *(g)* Occlusion following completion of orthodontic treatment and orthognathic surgery. At this stage, the treatment plan called for bone grafting of the anterior maxilla, skin grafting vestibuloplasty, and implant placement. *(h)* Provisional prosthesis in 1991. *(i)* Autogenous iliac crest marrow bone grafting of the anterior maxilla. *(j)* Reconstructed anterior alveolar ridge three weeks postoperatively. *(k)* Skin grafting. *(l)* Panoramic radiograph showing two implants in the anterior maxilla. *(m and n)* Completed porcelain-fused-to-metal prosthesis incorporating UCLA abutments. *(o and p)* Patient in 1993 after completion of prosthetic treatment. Compare the profile with that in *(e)*. Minor revision surgery may still be required for the lip and nose.

Surgical treatment

Reconstruction of any defect, especially a congenital defect, requires a thorough understanding of the anatomy and embryology of the area. It is also necessary to understand the anatomical and functional relationships of cleft-altered structures to adjacent normal structures.

Lip repair

The reconstruction of a cleft lip requires that the faulty formation of the lip components as well as their defective development be corrected. It is also important to understand the functional relationship between the lip and the adjacent muscles of facial expression and the nose. The upper and lower lips are similar structurally. The major difference is the presence of the philtrum in the upper lip, which originates from the fused medial nasal processes.

The lip can be divided into three zones: *(1)* the external surface covered with skin, *(2)* a transition zone with the vermilion border, and *(3)* the internal aspect of the lip that is covered by mucous membrane. The vermilion zone is covered by thin, nonkeratinized epithelium and appears red because of the abundance of capillaries and increased translucency of the epithelial layers. The central philtrum and its raised adjacent structures, the cristae, join with the medial tubercle to form a curve at the vermilion border. This curve is referred to as the *cupid's bow* of the lip. The lip has many sweat and mucous glands. The vermilion zone does not have any glands, but mucous glands are present in the mucous membrane lining of the inner surface of the lip.

The orbicularis oris muscle, which structurally makes up most of the lip, is firmly attached to both the external skin and the internal mucous membrane. It originates from the second branchial arch, which differentiates during the fifth embryonic week when the facial nerve penetrates this mesenchymal mass. During the second month of normal embryonic development, the orbicularis oris muscle in its primitive form reaches the midline of the lip and joins with its companion muscle on the opposite side.

The muscle consists of external and internal layers and is not covered by fascia. The external layer originates from the periosteum of the maxilla and mandible in the region of the anterior teeth. The muscles of facial expression insert into this external layer (Fig 6-12). The external layer of the orbicularis oris muscle is responsible for opening of the mouth as well as for the facial expressions associated with both the upper and the lower lips. The internal layer passes between both corners of the mouth so that it can perform its primary function of constriction of the lips.

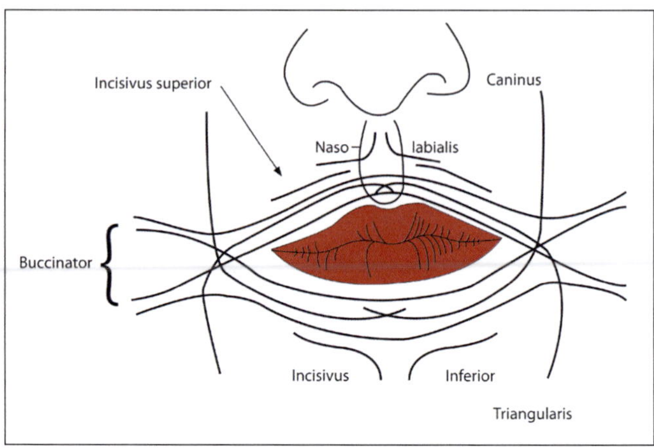

Figure 6-12 Muscle fibers in the lip. The nasolabialis muscle elevates the central part of the lip. The external layer of the orbicularis oris muscle is central to the insertion of these muscles.

The main artery of the upper lip is the superior labial artery, a branch of the facial artery (external maxillary artery). The arteries on both sides meet and anastomose in the midline. The superior labial artery branches off the facial artery just below the corner of the mouth. The facial artery then proceeds superiorly toward the nasolabial crease, where it divides into two branches at the nasal ala. The lateral nasal artery supplies the nasal ala and tip, while the angular artery joins the dorsal nasal artery, a terminal branch of the ophthalmic artery. The superior labial artery in the philtrum produces a small branch that supplies the frontal part of the nasal septum.

The theories of the pathogenesis of a cleft lip deformity include tissue deficiency, malpositioning of the maxillary segments, failure of fusion of the facial processes, and failure of mesodermal penetration of the epithelial layer. Originally it was believed that the cleft lip resulted from a failure of the fusion of the lateral maxillary processes and the frontonasal process. This implied that the deformity was due to a lack of fusion only and that all the tissue components were present. However, it is now accepted that the cleft is a result of failure of mesodermal penetration of the epithelial layer that results in a tissue deficiency in the cleft area. The lack of tissue is an important consideration for the surgeon during repair, because a simple rearrangement of the tissues will not provide a satisfactory result. Studies on the changes in the orbicularis oris muscle in the cleft patient demonstrate that the facial nerve and arteries of the lip follow the course of the muscle bundles (Fara, 1977).

The muscle stumps of the orbicularis oris in the cleft patient do not grow in a lateral to medial direction to meet in the midline. Thus, this mutual insertion with the companion orbicularis muscle is missing. Because the stumps do not meet in the central line of the lip, they seek attachment to firm points in the area. As a result of these atypical insertions, the muscle is not functional and its development is incomplete. In complete bilateral clefts, the prolabium does not have any muscle fibers. To achieve proper lip function following surgery, the surgeon must detach the orbicularis oris from its atypical insertions and bring the muscle bundles together (end to end) or, in patients with complete bilateral clefts, encourage them to grow into the prolabium. This will enhance proper function and foster further growth and development.

It is not the purpose of this chapter to discuss surgical techniques for lip repair (Fig 6-13) but rather to outline the pathogenesis of the cleft lip and the goals for surgery. To enhance proper function of the lip following surgery, it is essential that the surgical repair include isolation of the orbicularis oris muscle bundles, their release from atypical insertions, and their reorientation in a lateral to medial direction. Depending on the tissue deficiency in the area, the bundles could be placed end to end or allowed to grow into the prolabium.

The surgical technique will vary with the severity of the cleft, the greater the tissue deficiency, the more difficult the surgical procedure. In patients with significant tissue deficiencies, multiple procedures may be necessary. The surgical procedure is also complicated by the degree of involvement of the nose.

Adjunctive surgical procedures

A few surgical procedures are commonly performed after lip and palatal closure and continue as the child matures.

Lip adhesion. The lip adhesion operation has been used for many years. According to Randall (1965), lip adhesion converts a wide and difficult to close cleft lip into a much less difficult, incomplete cleft. Johanson and Ohlsson (1961) were the first to perform a lip adhesion procedure. Their protocol suggests a preliminary operation to close the lip and alveolus prior to the primary bone grafting procedure. A second operation is later performed to insert autogenous bone in the alveolar cleft and complete more definitive lip repair. When Randall (1965) followed this protocol, he found during the second procedure that there was frequently little or no space remaining to insert bone in the alveolar cleft, but the lip repair was easier, and the alveolus had been repositioned nicely.

Lip adhesions are most beneficial for patients with a bilateral cleft lip and palate with a protruding premaxilla. The lip adhesion operation helps reposition the protruding premaxilla posteriorly. It provides more underlying bone and reduces tension during lip repair. In bilateral clefts, where the prolabium is small, lip adhesions act as a skin expander, stretching the prolabium and making the definitive lip repair easier to perform.

Lip adhesions are usually combined with the closure of the soft palate. This combined procedure leads to a significant narrowing of the hard palate cleft. Definitive lip repair can then be completed with greater ease, better landmarks, and less tension. A number of

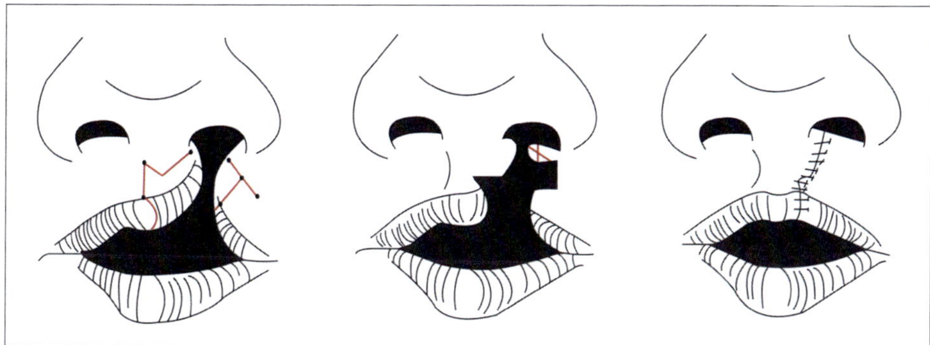

Figure 6-13 Modified Le Mesurier surgical technique for lip closure.

modifications to the lip adhesion procedure have been reported, most notably by Millard (1964) and Walker et al. (1966).

Repair of associated nasal deformities. Some degree of nasal deformity is associated with all clefts of the lip. The nose develops in conjunction with the primary palate, which contributes to not only the premaxilla but also the columella and the anterior nasal septum. Although the exact process of formation of this region is not completely understood, at least two factors are involved in the development of the cleft lip and nose. There is agenesis of tissues in the region of the cleft because of deficiencies of mesoderm and ectoderm; these deficiencies induce a mechanical stress to the developing nose from the progressive separation of the cleft. Mesodermal deficiencies are seen in the lack of bony development at the piriform margin in the floor of the cleft nostril, in the deficiency of septal cartilage, and occasionally in the anterior nasal spine. The nasal ala is always thinner on the cleft side. The ectodermal deficiency is manifested in the underlying dental abnormalities discussed later in this chapter.

The alar cartilage is the focal point of the cleft lip–nasal deformity. Normally, these cartilages are high in the nasal tip and the alar dome is at the level of the junction of the middle and lower thirds of the nasal bridge. On the cleft side, the alar cartilage is spread and rotated downward, while the alar dome is displaced downward, backward, and laterally. This produces a drooping of the nostril rim on the cleft side.

A shortening of the columella occurs as the alar dome is deflected away from the nasal tip. The arch of the nostril is flattened and the ala joins the columella at an oblique angle. The columella is tilted away from the midline toward the noncleft side. The tip of the nose is irregular, broad, and less prominent. In patients with complete clefts the nose is wider than normal.

In patients with bilateral clefts, the nasal tip is flat and broad and the nostril rims may droop and curve downward. The columella appears to be shortened or nonexistent and joined directly to the tip of the nose. The septum is usually in the midline, but the premaxilla can be twisted and/or deviated, especially if the cleft is incomplete on one side.

The goals of cleft lip and nasal repair are to achieve multilayered, anatomical closure of the cleft and to restore lip function by realigning the displaced lip and nasal anatomy while preserving as much tissue as possible. Complete clefts are more difficult to repair. The margins of the cleft lip must be lengthened and aligned without loss of tissue in a transverse dimension, and the nasal dome, ala, and alar base must be aligned atraumatically without causing skin webbing, folds, or vestibular stenosis.

Repair of the cleft lip will improve the nasal appearance. The degree to which surgeons address nasal reconstruction at the time of initial lip repair will vary. Excellent results can be achieved whether the nose is repaired at the time of initial lip repair or delayed to a later date. Even if the nose is repaired at the initial lip repair, most often it will require some revision surgery as growth occurs and the underlying supporting bony skeleton is repositioned surgically or orthodontically.

Revision surgery. The ideal timing for surgery to correct the remaining deformities is not clear. Optimal timing for the surgery is dependent on the nature of the deformity, the amount of scar formation, and the prolonged effects of surgical trauma on facial growth. Surgery for simple problems, such as lip scars and muscle bulging, can be carried out as early as 12 months following the initial repair, although it is preferable to limit the number of revisions and associated burden of care and wait until growth completion.

Structural deformities such as long, tight, or short lips and nasal deformities are related to growth of the facial skeleton. Definitive repair of these structural deformities is best performed once the dental, orthognathic, and maxillary components have been successfully treated. Untreated skeletal and dental asymmetry for both unilateral and bilateral clefts will adversely affect lip repair. Dental and orthognathic bony manipulation can delay lip repair until a satisfactory orthodontic goal is achieved. It is unrealistic to accomplish all these goals with one surgical procedure, and the decision for surgical correction should be made to achieve the most favorable long-term result.

Palatal repair

The principal objectives of cleft palate repair are to enhance normal speech development, to provide anatomical palatal closure, and to minimize maxillary growth inhibition and dentoalveolar deformities (Fig 6-14). The different muscles, their innervation, and their function have been discussed in Chapter 4. The main consideration regarding palatal closure is that surgery on the palatal shelves should not performed too early. As the child grows, the palatal shelves continue to grow and the cleft narrows, especially if lip continuity has been restored. The timing for palatal surgery varies from 12 months to 4 years, depending on the philosophy of the team, the comorbidities, and the width of the cleft. If the cleft is very wide, sufficient tissue may not be available to permit closure with adequate length and function. In this situation, it is better to delay closure.

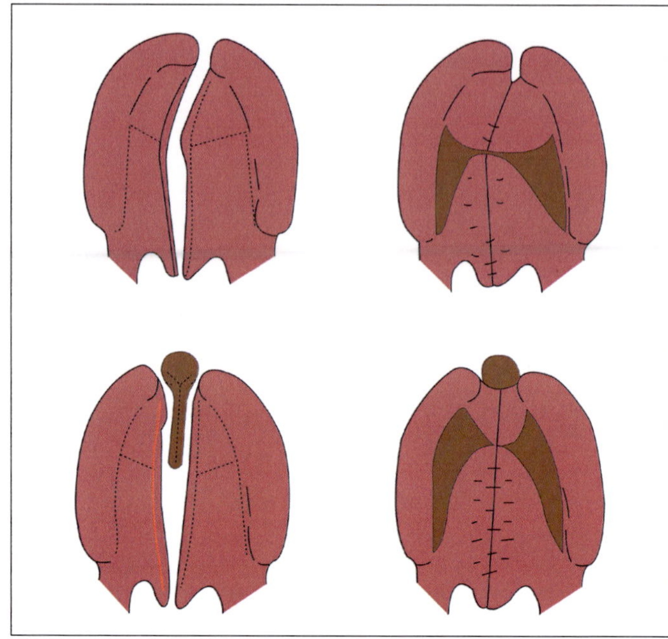

Figure 6-14 Palatal closure and pushback procedure. Flaps are raised in the hard palate area and then rotated posteriorly to increase the length of the reconstructed palate. Denuded areas are allowed to granulate in.

Because of the variability in the extent of the cleft, the availability of tissue, the comorbidities, and the experience of the cleft team, there is no level 1 evidence to support a specific timing or a particular technique of surgical procedure for palatal closure. Proponents of delayed palatal closure (Zurich approach) believe that a delay in palatal surgery will limit the inhibition of maxillary growth and minimize the need for surgery to advance and/or widen the maxilla. Opponents of this approach believe that a delay in closure of the palate will compel the patient to develop compensatory speech and swallowing patterns, which are not easily corrected.

The decision to use a prosthesis during the first few years of life is dictated by the experience of the team and the recommendation of the speech pathologist. At the UCSF Center for Craniofacial Anomalies, prostheses are rarely fabricated for infants. For most patients, the soft palate is closed around 12 months of age.

The only exceptions are for very wide clefts and for patients with Robin sequence (Pierre Robin syndrome). For patients with Robin sequence, the mandible is small and retruded so that the tongue is in a more posterior and superior position. Closure of the soft palate cleft may lead to an inability to breathe through the nose, because the retrusive tongue may close the nasopharynx. The decision as to when to close the cleft must be made individually for these patients. The surgeon must be sure that the mandible has grown sufficiently to allow the tongue to occupy a more normal anterior position.

It is not the purpose of this chapter to discuss surgical techniques, but three of the commonly used procedures will be discussed briefly: the von Langenbeck technique, first described in 1861; the double opposing Z-plasty, or the Furlow palatoplasty; and the two-stage palatoplasty. The von Langenbeck technique consists of the following steps: incision of the edges of the cleft, division of the palatal musculature, detachment of the mucoperiosteal flaps of the palate, and application of sutures.

Most surgeons essentially carry out these same steps today. Opponents of this technique point out that this procedure results in significant scar contracture that tends to pull the soft palate forward, creating palatal insufficiency and preventing velopharyngeal closure. The low rate of fistula occurrence made this procedure widely acceptable. However, dissatisfaction with the functional results has led many surgeons to modify the original procedure by reconstructing an active muscle sling for velopharyngeal closure and for appropriate function of the eustachian tube. To improve function, it is necessary to reconstruct the displaced halves of the levator veli palatini muscles. Today, the levator sling reconstruction is frequently combined with the von Langenbeck procedure.

The double opposing Z-plasty, or Furlow palatoplasty (Furlow, 1986), was first described in 1978 by Dr. Leonard Furlow and has since become one of the most frequently used palatoplasty techniques. It has the advantage of lengthening the palate by virtue of the Z-plasty and has demonstrated relatively good speech outcomes as a result, although it is still contentious as to which palatoplasty technique results in the lowest frequency of fistulas and velopharyngeal insufficiency (Stein et al., 2019).

The two-stage palatoplasty procedure has been used in Zurich since 1969. It is based on interaction and cooperation between maxillary orthopedic treatment and surgery. Orthopedic guidance is initiated at birth and continued until the child is about 16 months old. Its main objectives are to restrict the tongue from the cleft, to normalize feeding, and to allow spontaneous narrowing of the cleft, thus facilitating subsequent soft palate closure and providing more tissue for velar length. The soft palate is closed around 18 months of age and the hard palate when the child is four to five years of age. Individual variations are based on development of the child, particularly in speech.

The Zurich approach was developed as the team found deficiencies in the procedures that were used previously. This group found that the von Langenbeck technique, and its various modifications, resulted in maxillary hypoplasia and poor speech. The group then adopted the two-stage procedure described by Slaughter and Brodie (1946), but this procedure was abandoned because it resulted in poor speech. A one-stage procedure was then used, but many

Nasoalveolar Molding Appliance (NAM)

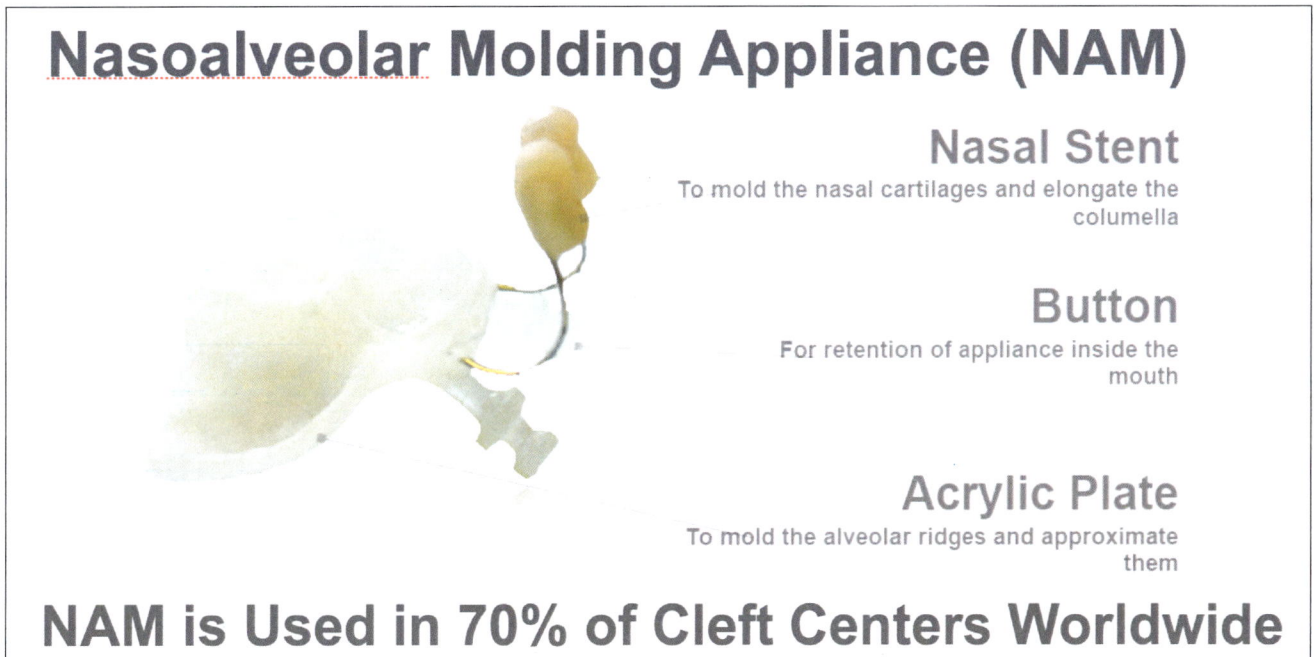

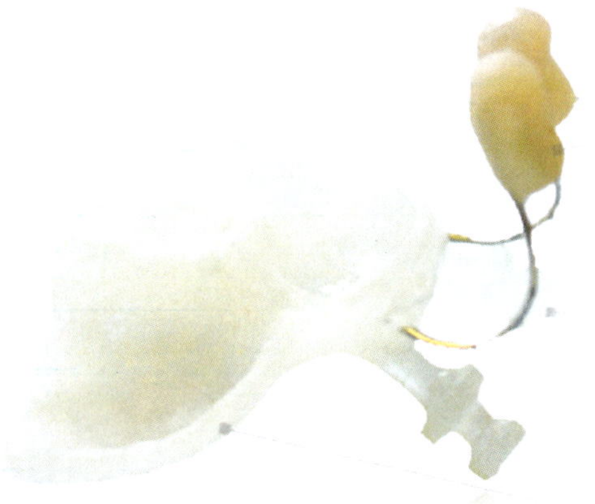
Nasal Stent
To mold the nasal cartilages and elongate the columella
Button
For retention of appliance inside the mouth
Acrylic Plate
To mold the alveolar ridges and approximate them
NAM is Used in 70% of Cleft Centers Worldwide

Figure 6-15 Nasoalveolar molding (NAM) appliance.

residual fistulae and poor development of the maxilla led them to abandon this procedure. It was then that the Zurich two-stage palatoplasty approach was adopted.

Nasoalveolar molding (NAM)

Since its formal introduction into the literature 30 years ago (Grayson et al., 1993), nasoalveolar molding or "NAM" therapy has grown in popularity and is now a technique offered in the majority of cleft centers in the United States (Avinoam et al., 2022) (Fig 6-15). While the technique has evolved over the years and has been modified by various centers providing the treatment modality, the basic goals of NAM therapy remain the same: to nonsurgically reduce the size of the cleft defect and to normalize the anatomy of the oral and nasal structures to facilitate less extensive surgical intervention and hence less scarring and less growth disturbance that may result from scarring.

The precursor techniques to NAM date back nearly 75 years. Since the early 1950s, presurgical infant orthopedics (PSIO) has been used in a variety of ways to reduce the degree of cleft deformity and thereby enhance surgical closure of the lip and palate deformity (McNeil, 1950; Mylin et al., 1968; Latham, 1980). In recent times, this approach has been modified and refined so that the primary focus includes management of the soft tissue deformities of the nasal structures associated with the cleft anomaly (Cutting et al., 1998; Brecht et al., 2000; Grayson and Cutting, 2001). The objective is to better approximate the lip and cleft segments and to mold and expand deficient tissues prior to surgical correction. While some may claim these devices also improve feeding for the infant because they serve to partially obturate the oral defect, the main purpose of these appliances is *not* to improve feeding in the infant with a cleft. There are a variety of innovative nipple-bottle systems that facilitate feeding for the infant with a cleft.

This technique is applicable to both patients with unilateral clefts and those with bilateral clefts. When successfully applied to patients with unilateral clefts, nasoalveolar molding (NAM) results in expanded tissues that reduce tension on wound closures and therefore reduce scarring. Fewer surgical procedures are required, and growth is less negatively affected (Wood et al., 1997; Grayson and Cutting, 2001). In addition, when this technique is successfully employed, the aesthetics and contour of the nasolabial complex are made more ideal. When utilized in patients with a bilateral cleft, NAM lengthens the columella and often eliminates the need for early surgery to further elongate this structure, and the nasal complex displays a growth curve similar to that seen in noncleft patients (Garfinkle et al., 2009). As a result, the nasal tip develops in a more normal fashion and the aesthetics of the entire nasolabial complex is optimized.

Nasoalveolar molding for infants with unilateral cleft lip and palate anomaly

In most situations, the prospective parents have learned that their child will be born with a cleft due to advances in the sensitivity and specificity of current ultrasonography techniques. The cleft team should ideally meet with the parents in the prenatal period and review the advantages and disadvantages of NAM therapy so that when the baby is born, the parents will have already decided whether they will elect to undergo NAM. At this prenatal NAM consultation, it is best if the parents can meet with all the key professionals and support team members who will be caring for their child. This will help in building the bond between the parents and the team and ultimately serve to reduce the "burden of care" often associated

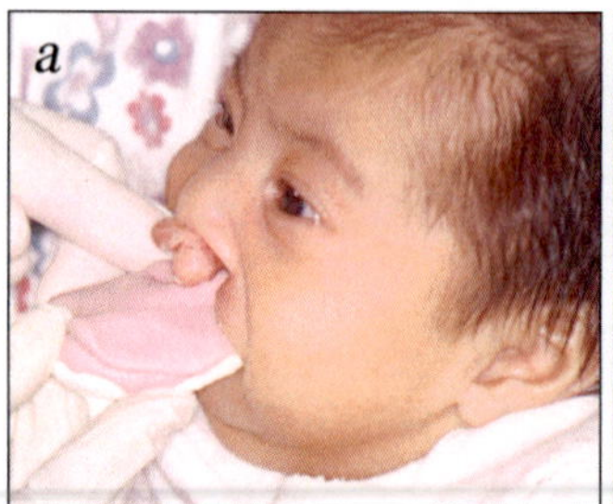
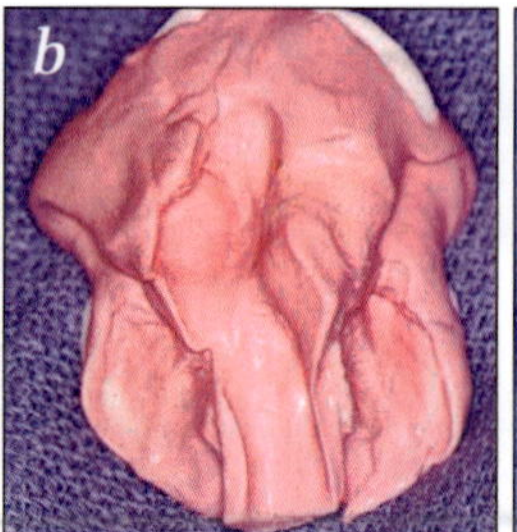
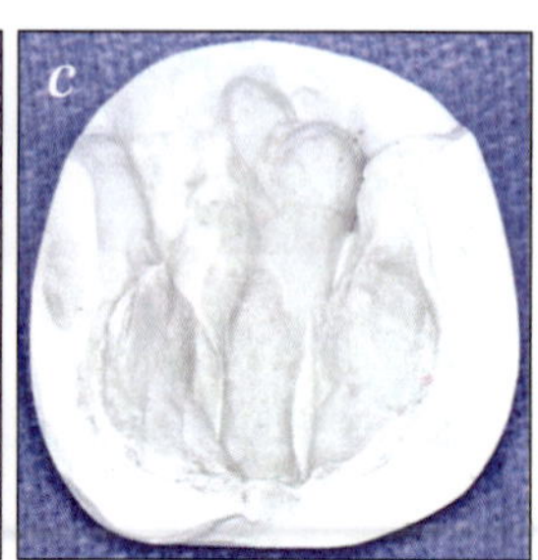

Figure 6-16 *(a)* During impression taking, the infant's head must be in an inverted position and well supported. *(b)* Impression of silicone putty. *(c)* Master cast.

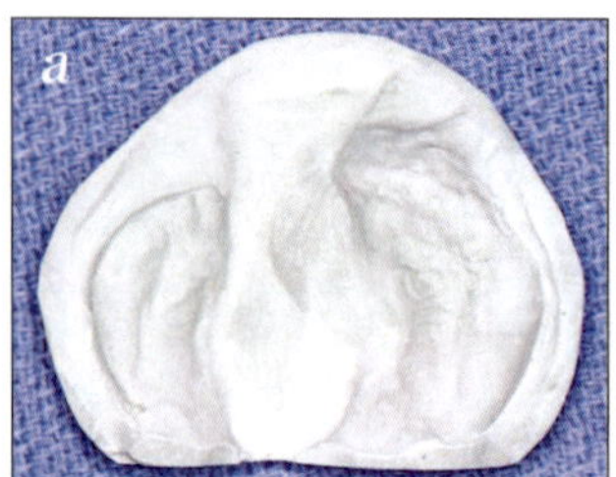
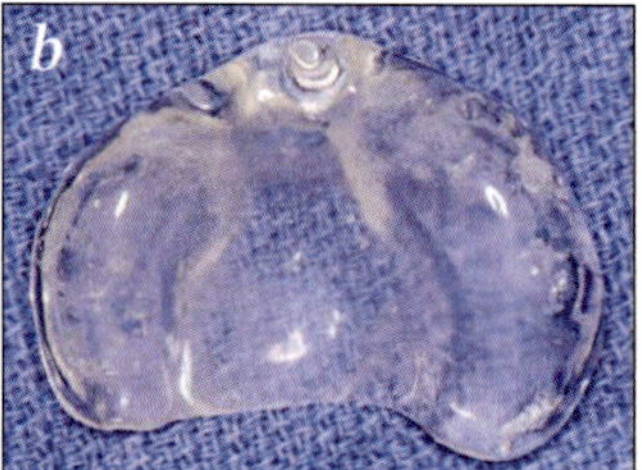
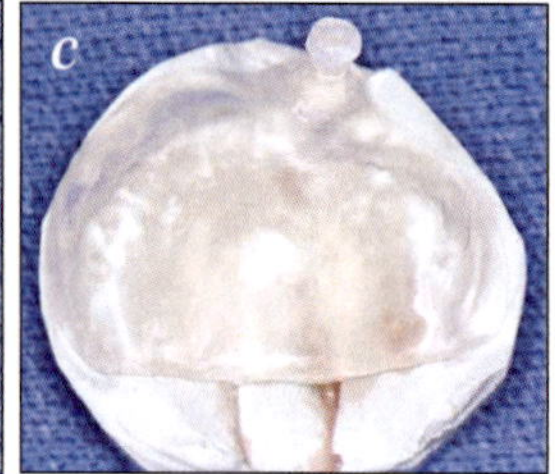

Figure 6-17 *(a)* Cast made from the master cast–wax blockout. *(b)* Oral portion of the NAM device made of clear acrylic resin. *(c)* Completed device on the altered cast. Note the posterior extension. Excessive length in this area will precipitate gagging.

with NAM (Alfonso et al., 2020; Sischo et al., 2015). Subsequently, treatment then commences as soon as possible after birth, ideally within the first week, because as the infant ages, the plasticity of the tissues (particularly the nasal cartilages) diminishes and molding becomes more difficult. A thorough evaluation and oral examination are conducted and, after other team members are consulted, therapy begins. The risks and benefits of NAM must be thoroughly discussed and understood by the parents of the child and appropriate informed consent obtained prior to commencing treatment.

At the initial appointment, the baby is seen by the surgeon and the NAM provider (often on cleft teams, this may be a maxillofacial prosthodontist, craniofacial orthodontist, pediatric dentist, or other dental professional trained in NAM therapy). Photos are obtained of the pretreatment condition, and the size of the cleft defect is noted. The parents are given instruction on the cleft anatomy as it specifically pertains to their child. Often, there is an ulceration present on the oral side of the exposed vomer. It is advisable to note this to the parents *prior to commencing NAM therapy* as the rough dorsal surface of the tongue can rasp away at the delicate nasal mucosa covering the vomer. Often, this ulceration resolves with the introduction of the oral NAM appliance. If natal teeth are found, they are usually removed, as their presence may compromise mucosal healing when the cleft repair is carried out.

In the standard approach to NAM therapy, an impression is obtained using a silicone putty (Fig 6-16) material. The impression putty should be a color that contrasts with the oral mucosa to permit easy identification of any residual impression material that may be lodged in the defect. Irreversible hydrocolloid and flowable elastomeric impression materials should be avoided because these materials can become locked in undercuts in the cleft and may be difficult to remove, or worse, they may flow into the airway.

Care should be taken to maintain the airway. Infants are obligate oral breathers. Ideally, the infant is held facedown or upside down during the impression making to optimize control of the material as it relates to the airway and to provide direct visualization of the oral cavity, cleft defect, and oral airway as the impression is being made and after setting and removal. If the infant does not cry, it may suggest the oral airway is obstructed by the tongue or impression material, and the team must ensure a patent airway.

Impressions are made while the child is awake and in an outpatient setting, preferably a hospital setting in case the airway becomes compromised. The dental professional and the surgeon are usually present at our impression appointments, again in case there is an airway emergency. Multiple impression trays of varying sizes should be available, and suction should be ready if the baby regurgitates. A suitably sized tray is selected, and care is taken to not overload impression putty onto the tray, thereby risking material breaking away from the tray. Care should be taken to maintain the airway while the impression is in the oral cavity, as infants are obligate oral breathers. Ideally, the infant is held face down or upside down while the head is properly supported during the impression making to optimize control of the material as it relates to the airway and to provide direct visualization of the oral cavity, cleft defect, and oral airway as the impression is being made and after setting and removal. If the infant does not cry, it may suggest the oral airway is obstructed by the tongue or impression material, and the team must ensure a patent airway. Positioning of the infant in this manner prevents the tongue from falling back into the oral cavity and will prevent aspiration of regurgitated fluid. This procedure requires two individuals, one to position the baby and the other to support the head and make the impression. Care must be taken to avoid posterior displacement of impression material, because this could partially occlude the oral airway. The border areas of the maxilla and premaxilla must be recorded in the impression (see Fig 6-16b and c).

When silicone putty is used, multiple casts may be obtained. One cast is used to fabricate the NAM device, while the additional cast is stored as a permanent record. The cast is trimmed, and the undercuts in the cleft segments associated with the palate and the alveolar ridges are blocked out with wax to create contours consistent with an intact palate and alveolus. The blocked-out cast may be duplicated, and the oral portion of the device is fabricated from clear acrylic resin (Fig 6-17). Heat-cured methyl methacrylate is preferred. A small button is added anteriorly with cold cure acrylic in the cleft region. The button should be angled at approximately 10 to 15 inferior to the

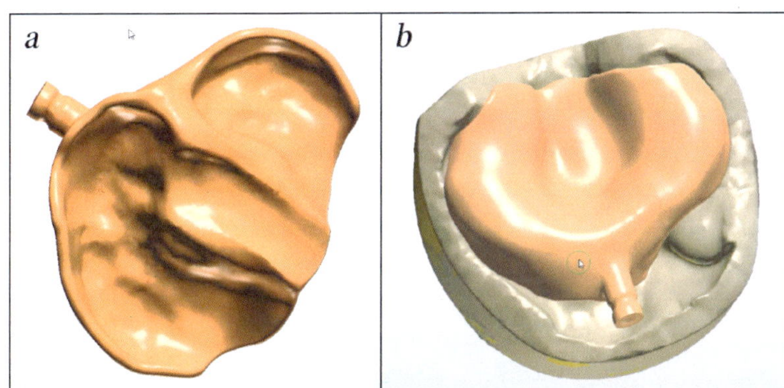

Figure 6-18 *(a and b)* Digitally designed oral molding appliance manufactured by milling.

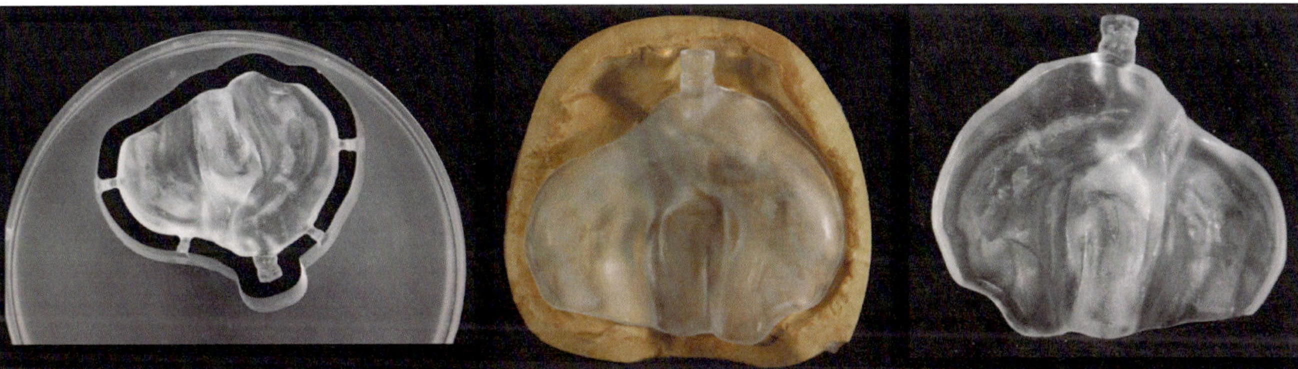

Figure 6-19 Milled PMMA oral molding appliance.

horizontal plane in order to facilitate an upward and posteriorly directed force once the plate is in place. This button will be used to retain the elastic band–tape retention assembly that stabilizes the appliance in place while also applying the necessary traction forces needed to help move the alveolar segments.

There are other methods of generating the oral molding appliance. The goal should be to fabricate the smoothest possible oral appliance without overextension and borders that are approximately 2–3 mm in thickness to allow for adjustments over the course of molding. There are reports in the literature of accurately capturing the oral structures with digital imaging (Shanbhag et al., 2020). These techniques are not currently as accurate and predictable as a well-obtained analog impression of the defect. Digital scanners are currently still relatively bulky in comparison to the size of an infant's oral cavity. Also, digital scanning algorithms poorly capture the movable soft tissue borders of the cleft maxilla, and they cannot read the superior aspects of the cleft defect with the current state of scanning technology. Similarly, while the literature may claim there are "fully digital workflows" to achieving the desired outcomes for NAM therapy, a closer examination of the literature shows a digital workflow only for the oral portion of the therapy, but not for the molding of the soft tissues of the nose, the key to NAM therapy (Gong et al., 2020).

Perhaps the best method of fabricating the oral molding appliance is to obtain a highly accurate intraoral putty impression. Scan the impression using a lab scanner or intraoral scanner, and then design the appliance from the digitized impression (or cast from the poured impression) and mill the appliance from industrially manufactured PMMA (Fig 6-18). The result is a highly predictable and exceedingly smooth appliance that can be reproduced at will (Fig 6-19). Printing of appliances has drawbacks, including a surface that is not as smooth as the milled appliance, and although print resins are approved for oral use, there are concerns that the resins may not have been tested for use for four to six months in newborns.

Irrespective of the method of fabrication, the oral portion of the molding plate is then fitted to the infant to ensure that it is properly adapted and retained. The oral molding plate is delivered as soon as possible after the impression has been obtained. This is usually within a week of the time of the impression to ensure a well-fitting appliance. The appliance should not extend into the cleft because this will prevent proper realignment of the cleft segments during active treatment. The infant should be able to suckle without gagging while the appliance is in position. If the infant does gag, generally it is caused by an excessively thick appliance or one that is overextended posteriorly. Sharp edges or projections should be rounded, and the appliance should be thoroughly polished. A 5 to 7 mm hole should be placed in the midpalatal region to ensure maintenance of the airway if the device is displaced vertically.

Prior to placing the oral molding plate in the infant's mouth for the first time, it is advisable to check the smoothness of the appliance with an ungloved finger to ensure there are no sharp edges or rough spots. Similarly, in order to build trust with the parents, they should be allowed to thoroughly inspect the appliance for them to have an acceptance of the appliance as well. It is also recommended that the parents be instructed by team members on how to properly place and care for the appliance as well as to place the tapes needed to stabilize the appliance and to apply the active traction force. This

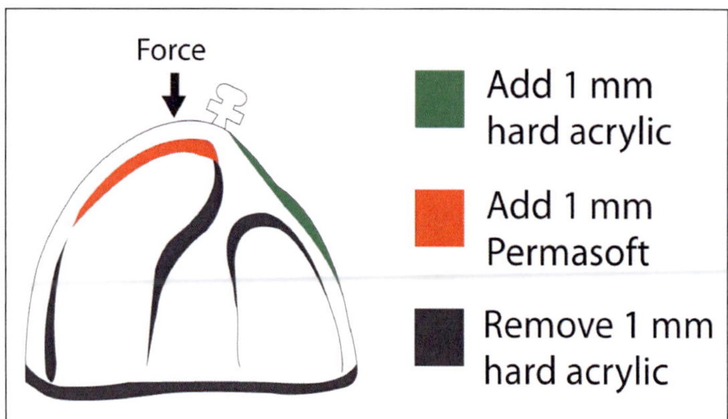

Figure 6-20 Subtractions and additions made to a NAM device (adapted from Brecht et al., 2000, with permission).

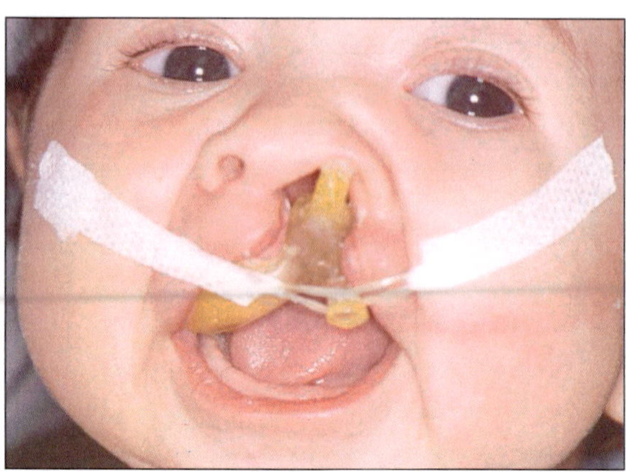

Figure 6-21 Tape and elastics hold the NAM device in position. The anterior button has been modified to retain the elastic band–tape apparatus.

is best accomplished on a life-sized infant doll that may have a cleft made into the lip as well as a small molding device that is easily fabricated for a teaching model.

After the necessary adjustments are made, active *alveolar* molding begins by selective alteration of the tissue surfaces of the device. For a unilateral cleft, acrylic resin is removed from some tissue-bearing surfaces and added to other surfaces (Fig 6-20). The additions and subtractions will permit displacement of the cleft segments into the relieved areas. Provisional or soft denture reline materials are ideal for this task. In most unilateral clefts, the greater alveolar segment is directed medially, and the lesser alveolar segment may be directed laterally. The sequence of additions and subtractions should be customized to each cleft situation as opposed to some formulaic approach, as each cleft will pose a different set of anatomic circumstances (see Fig 6-20). In the end, the goal of the oral phase (the *alveolar molding*) of NAM should be to have the cleft alveolar segments aligned appropriately and the cleft gap reduced to zero.

Additions and subtractions are generally in the order of 1 mm. This process continues at weekly intervals until the cleft segments are in close apposition to one another. Occasionally mucosal ulcerations develop. They usually are the result of an ill-fitting appliance or the addition of too much material in an attempt to move the cleft segments too rapidly. These ulcerations must be resolved and re-epithelialized prior to surgery. Care must be taken to avoid deforming the alveolar segments during molding, especially the buccopalatal dimension. Additions must be equally matched by subtractions. Periodically, the appliance as a whole needs to be widened to allow for posterior transverse palatal growth.

During delivery, the position of the acrylic retentive button used to secure the elastic band–tape apparatus may have to be modified to optimize the force vectors applied to the alveolus through the elastics and the appliance. This button usually is positioned in the middle of the cleft and face downward at a 10–15-degree angle in relation to the occlusal plane (Fig 6-21). It should not impinge on the lip segments as the cleft segments are coapted. If the button is excessively long it will make it difficult for the patient to suckle, can interfere with the approximation of the cleft lip, and will destabilize the apparatus when the elastics are activated.

Appropriate adjustments are made to the button, and the elastic band–tape apparatus is applied. Tape is positioned lateral and superior to the oral commissures and holds the NAM device in position (see Fig 6-21). Ideal retention is achieved if suture strips measuring 0.50 × 1.50 inches are used at the base and connected to long, narrow suture strips (0.25 × 4.00-inch strips). Additional application of wider suture strips may be necessary to facilitate retention. Appropriate taping is necessary for retention; if taping is not done properly, it will compromise the effectiveness of the device. The narrow suture strips are connected to small (red) orthodontic elastics, which in turn are secured to the anterior retention button on the device. The elastics should be activated so that the active dimension of the red elastic loop is equal to 1.5 to 2.0 times the resting diameter of the elastic. *The key to effective reduction of the oral cleft is the consistent application of tapes and elastics with sufficient force to effect movement, but not so tight that they result in tissue ulceration.*

Instructions are provided to the parents, along with an ample supply of taping materials, adhesives, and agents to remove adhesive from the skin of the infant. The device should always be in position. Skin irritation secondary to taping is best addressed by periodic variation in the position of the tape and by the application of hydrocolloid base pads or the use of skin emollient creams. The parents should have access to a team member at all times in order to have the inevitable questions answered as well as to allay any fears and concerns they may have with their newborn!

Adjustments to the device are made weekly but sometimes more frequently if indicated. When the size of the palatal cleft is reduced to 5 mm or less, the nasal portion is added. The purpose of this segment is to mold the nasal cartilage and lengthen and reposition the columella. The appliance is extended superiorly and should project the nasal tip and dome outward and toward the side of the cleft (see Fig 6-21). This movement is achieved with a 0.36-inch round stainless-steel wire with a kidney-shaped acrylic resin component that contacts the nose. The shape of the wire nasal stent may be approximated by taking a piece of rope wax and using it to simulate the curve needed to form a swan-neck shape that connects the undersurface of the molding plate into the nasal aperture to hold the nasal stent. The curve of the wire is the source of the potential energy that is used to apply the force to the nasal structures. Therefore, the curve of the wire stent should not be so short and "tight" as to limit potential force, nor should it be so long and "open" as to

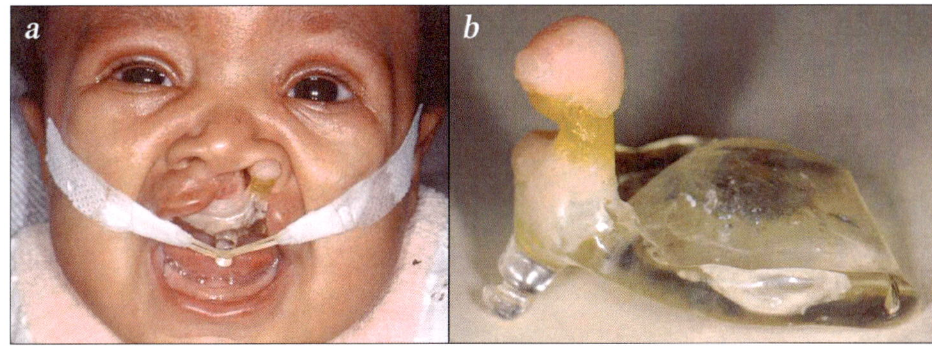

Figure 6-22 *(a)* NAM device for a unilateral cleft. *(b)* NAM is nearly complete. The columella is approaching the midline and the nostril on the cleft side is becoming more symmetric.

pose the possibility of the infant grabbing the wire stent and pulling it out.

With weekly adjustments and additions to the nasal projection of the NAM appliance, the flat nasal dome and medial crus are slowly corrected and the columella is stretched and molded into a more desirable position. When NAM is complete, the columella should approach the midline. For a unilateral cleft deformity, the septum may be corrected by NAM, but the septal defect projects deep caudally. A properly developed nasal projection will also aid in further reducing the width of the intraoral cleft.

When the contours of the nasal extension are developed, attempts should be made to mold the nasal rim and nostril to mimic the contours found in infants without a cleft or to mirror the noncleft nostril (Fig 6-22). When the contours are properly developed, the supporting material will create teardrop-shaped nares similar to those of unaffected infants. It is important that nasal molding be preceded by proper *alveolar molding*. Otherwise, there is danger that the alar rim will be overstretched, resulting in a so-called meganostril, which may only be corrected through reductive surgery.

In some instances, the button retaining the elastic band–tape apparatus may have to be recontoured or repositioned to accommodate the nasal extension. The nasal extension may be developed in acrylic resin or by using 0.036- or 0.050-inch stainless steel orthodontic wire. The wire extension is preferred as a stent material (rather than acrylic) because it is easy to adjust and less prone to breakage.

When a NAM appliance is properly employed and adjusted, for the "average" cleft gap of ~10 mm, the alveolar cleft segments are frequently in contact with one another after four to six weeks. Care must be taken to avoid "locking out" the lesser cleft segment. This occurs when the greater cleft segment is moved too quickly, preventing the lesser segment from moving outwardly. The result is a compromised arch form that may later have to be corrected orthodontically.

On completion of NAM, the alveolar segments should be properly positioned, and the nasal cartilages, columella, and philtrum should be aligned. Proper alignment of these segments may permit a one-stage surgical procedure for primary repair of the lip-nasal defect in combination with a gingivoperiosteoplasty (GPP) to close the alveolar defect (Millard and Latham, 1990; Wood et al., 1997). The NAM device should be worn continuously until the time of the surgical procedure. After surgery, it is returned to the team and maintained as part of the infant's care record. Subsequent palatal repair is usually accomplished when the infant is 10 to 15 months of age, when speech mechanisms normally are beginning to develop. No appliance is used intraorally following the initial lip, nose, or alveolus repair (+/– GPP).

It is often assumed that all infants who undergo NAM are subjected to GGP to repair the alveolar cleft. However, GPP is not indicated for all patients. The cleft segments should be within 2 mm or less of each other for there to be a high probability for the cleft to heal with a bone bridge across the cleft. Also, during the GPP procedure, the developing tooth buds that sit beneath the thin and easily perforated shell of alveolar bone in the young infant should be avoided. As with many other techniques, with NAM and GPP the skill of the surgeon is a most important factor determining the success or failure of the procedure. Even if it has been determined during the NAM process that GPP will not be performed, NAM should be continued because the nasal structures will still benefit from treatment. The nasal benefits of NAM are not dependent on subsequent GPP. Conversely, GPP should not be performed if NAM has not been used to reduce the size of the cleft gap.

Nasoalveolar molding for infants with bilateral cleft lip and palate anomaly

While the application of NAM in the unilateral patient may help turn a large cleft into a small cleft, the real power of the NAM technique is the advantage it provides surgeons in managing the more severe form of clefting—the bilateral cleft. For the patient with a bilateral cleft of the lip, nose, alveolus, and palate, NAM lengthens the columella and often eliminates the need for further early surgery to elongate this structure. As a result, the nasal dome and nasal tip develop in a more normal fashion, and the aesthetics of the entire nasolabial complex is optimized. NAM permits use of a modified surgical technique that allows the surgeon to complete repair of the lip, nose, and alveolus without creating a scar at the lip-columella junction. The result is improved aesthetics of the entire nasolabial complex. In addition, the nose can develop along a trajectory that parallels that of the noncleft infant. During treatment the nasal cartilages are molded, the skin and nasal lining of the columella are expanded, and the premaxilla is repositioned. Expansion of the nasal lining creates additional tissue that facilitates the repair of the nasal deformity. The results are a more symmetric lip and an absence of scars on the nose, columella, or central prolabium after the first surgical correction (Cutting et al., 1998).

Molding of the bilateral clefts consists of three stages. During the first stage, the posterior palatal segments are repositioned, and

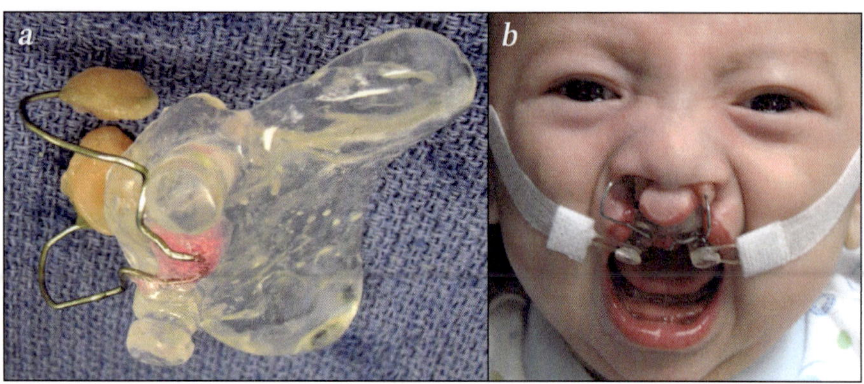

Figure 6-23 *(a)* NAM device for a bilateral cleft. *(b)* Nasal extensions in position.

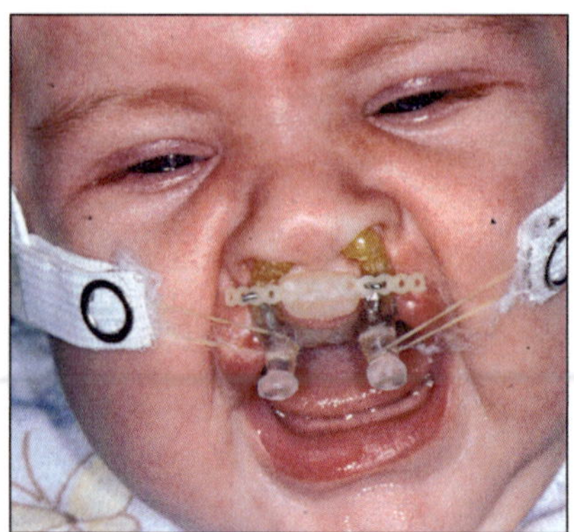

Figure 6-24 NAM device for a bilateral cleft. A columella portion has been added.

the premaxilla is rotated back into a proper midline position. During the second stage, the apices of the flattened alar cartilages are repositioned superiorly toward the nasal tip. The goal of the third stage is to lengthen the columella. Following successful completion of NAM, surgical correction of the lip deformity is carried out in combination with closure of the intraoral alveolar clefts with GPP.

Following a thorough examination and workup by the team, impressions are made, and master casts are retrieved. The NAM device is fabricated as indicated earlier, except retention buttons are placed on both sides. The device is retained with separate elastics and taping (Fig 6-23). In some situations, the elastics may have to be attached to a head cap to provide sufficient traction and/or retention.

The posterior palatal segments are gently displaced laterally to make room for the premaxilla. To produce this movement, material is added to the portion of the device contacting the medial portion (palatal shelves) of these segments and removed from the lateral portions in the areas of the inner buccal flanges. The NAM device is altered in a similar fashion to rotate the upturned and outwardly protruding cleft premaxilla downward into position. In these patients it may be necessary to adjust the appliance twice a week. As the premaxilla rotates down into position, the nasal septum may bend and the NAM device may have to be adjusted if the septum comes in contact with it. As the premaxilla is retracted into a more proper alignment in the keystone position in the arch, it is impossible for the septum not to bend, because it lengthens as the baby's tongue pushes it forward after the cleft is developed in utero. The NAM appliance retracts the premaxilla in a gentler and more predictable fashion than do more active appliances that rely on pins and elastics or screw mechanisms to bring the premaxilla back more rapidly into position. NAM also avoids the damage to the nasal septum often associated with the active techniques.

When the premaxilla attains a reasonable midline position, the nasal molding phase of NAM begins. For bilateral clefts, two nasal extensions are developed (see Fig 6-23). They arise from the undersurface of the oral portion of the device, extend around the prolabium into each nasal aperture, and elevate the nasal cartilage on each side. The tips of these extensions should exert an anterior force under the nasal tip on both sides. They should closely be in contact with the columella on each side to help straighten the columella as it is being lengthened. This also serves to exert a downward and posterior force on the premaxilla that will retract it further and help "dock" it into a more favorable position.

Care must be taken to ensure the tips of the nasal extensions are kept close together. Otherwise, the tip of the nose and the columella will be excessively widened. The object of these extensions is to bring the domes of the nasal cartilages closer together while at the same time expanding the lining of the intranasal tissues (Brecht et al., 2000).

As the position and contours of the nose and nasal cartilages become more normalized, the third phase of treatment, elongation of the columella, commences (Fig 6-24). A horizontal strip of soft acrylic resin, the so-called prolabial band, is secured to the inferior lobes of the two nasal extensions. The band should be configured to displace the base of the columella and direct the expansion forces in way that will preserve the nasolabial angle. The prolabial band "cinches" the columella and provides length rather than width to the columella. The combined forces on these structures, mediated by the NAM device, will lengthen the columella. Care must be taken to ensure an appropriately shaped columella forms, one that is not thick and broad but rather thinner and anatomically correct. Care must also be taken to avoid excessive pressure at the lip-columella junction, or this area will easily ulcerate. If this occurs, the device must be relieved in this area until the ulceration heals, delaying the elongation of the columella and perhaps compromising the result. Similarly, the amount of force applied *intranasally* should be monitored to avoid ulceration of the thin nasal lining and possibly exposing the nasal cartilage. Cartilage being relatively acellular will not heal as rapidly as epithelial lining and hence may result in curtailing of nasal molding and possibly a compromised outcome or delaying of surgery.

This bilateral NAM method, when effectively employed, may lengthen the columella by 4.0 to 7.0 mm (Grayson et al., 1999; Grayson and Cutting, 2001). The patient is now ready for surgical correction (Fig 6-25). The oral and nasal molding phase of care is undertaken for five to six months prior to the surgical repair to optimize tissue molding and elongation. At this age most infants will have developed sufficiently to be able to dislodge the appliance, thereby making molding ineffective or challenging beyond the six-month mark. As was the case for unilateral clefts, the device must be worn continuously prior to surgery. The device is worn by the infant into the operating room, removed by the surgical team, and

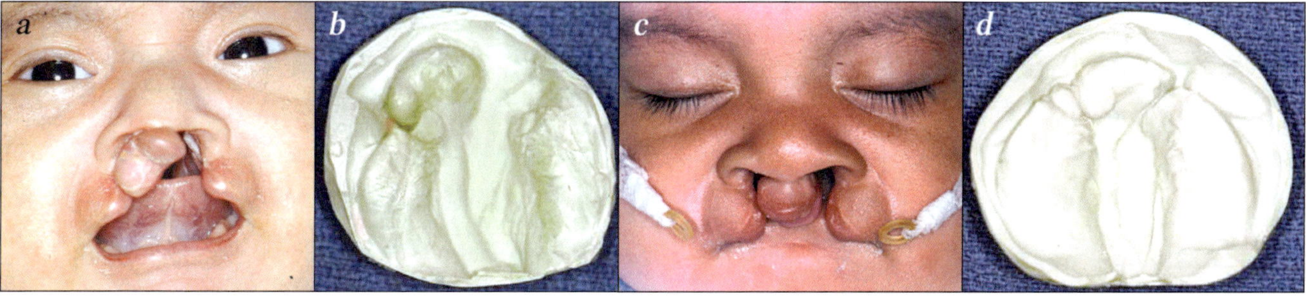

Figure 6-25 Effectiveness of NAM. *(a and b)* Before NAM. *(c and d)* After NAM.

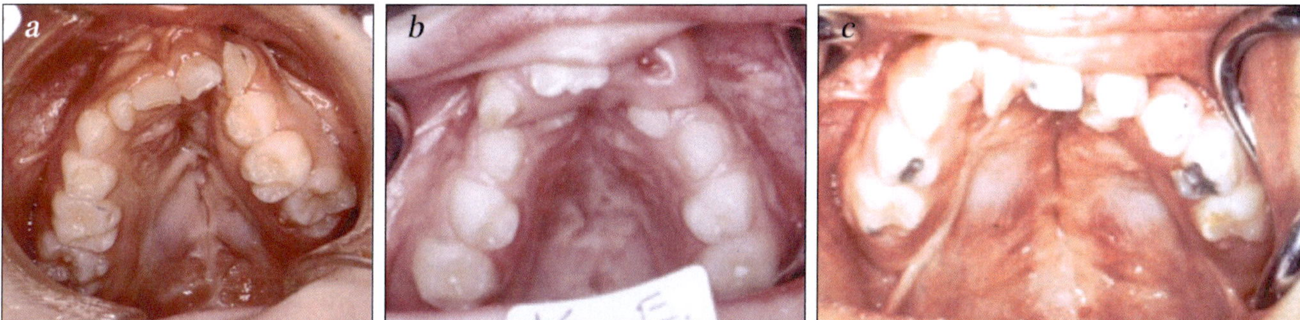

Figure 6-26 Effects of postrepair growth. *(a)* Unilateral cleft. Note the medial displacement of the posterior segment on the cleft side. *(b)* Bilateral cleft. Note the medial displacement of both posterior segments. *(c)* Supernumerary teeth maintain a more normal arch form.

returned to the NAM provider to be incorporated as a part of the patient's treatment record.

During the initial lip closure and surgical correction, the surgeon disrupts the fatty tissue between the widely separated nasal dome cartilages. These nasal cartilages should be sutured together in a more superior position, or the benefits accrued by molding the cartilage in this area will be lost, because it is likely that the alar bases will drift laterally.

An interdisciplinary team approach is advisable to maximize the advantages of NAM. Surgical procedures are altered and should employ a modified GGP as described by Millard and Latham (1990) if the advantages of NAM are to be fully realized. This technique is technically demanding when the cleft segments are in proximity, but when it is performed by skilled and experienced hands, there is a high likelihood that bone will form across the repaired cleft. One center employing this technique reported that 65% of infants born with cleft lip and palate did not require subsequent bone grafting of the cleft (Santiago et al., 1997).

Growth and development

In assessing craniofacial jaw proportions and relationships in a growing child with a cleft condition, the clinician must know that maxillomandibular growth and dentoalveolar development may not follow normal patterns. Knowledge about growth expectations is particularly important for treatment planning. The extent to which growth is inhibited or aberrant depends on many factors, including the degree of intrinsic tissue deficiency and the quality, amount, and location of scar formation because of surgical intervention.

Early, presurgical manipulation of maxillary segments is advocated in some centers to facilitate surgical repair and purportedly also to create an environment for normal tongue position and function. The expectation is that normal function will follow. At the UCSF Center for Craniofacial Anomalies, presurgical orthopedic treatment is generally not initiated in unilateral clefts. It is often necessary, however, to mold a prominent premaxilla back to a position that facilitates lip repair in bilateral clefts (as discussed in the section on NAM).

Following repair of the lip and palate, the anterior alveolar process will be molded by pressure from the lip and by narrowing of the maxillary arch because of scar tissue following palatal repair. The usual findings in a 3-year-old with a repaired unilateral cleft are medial collapse of the cleft segment and crossbite of the canine with or without crossbite of the molars (Fig 6-26a). In patients with repaired bilateral clefts, both lateral segments may be in a medial position (Fig 6-26b).

The cleft margins of the segments usually contact each other by the time the patient is aged four to five years. This contact counteracts further medial movement of the segments unless the teeth on the cleft margin are lost, and the surrounding alveolar bone resorbs. The degree of maxillary width reduction is therefore closely related to the development of the alveolar process; this in turn, is determined to a large extent by the number, position, size, and shape of the teeth in the area (Fig 6-26c). Premature loss or removal of teeth on the cleft margin is therefore undesirable.

Growth during the primary dentition stage

During the primary dentition stage, maxillomandibular relationships, occlusion, and the position of individual teeth usually remain stable, unless there are severe caries and tooth loss. A supernumerary tooth may be present, usually situated on the palatal aspect of the lateral cleft margin. The lateral incisor is often missing.

Studies on skeletal morphology and size in patients with unilateral cleft lip and palate have shown few differences from average values for unaffected children in the late primary and early mixed dentition stages (Mazaheri et al., 1967; Aduss, 1971; Nakamura et al., 1972). As part of a study of orthodontic treatment effects on subjects with unilateral cleft lip and palate at the UCSF Center for Craniofacial Anomalies, pretreatment cephalometric head films of eight girls and eight boys with unilateral cleft lip and palate were studied. The mean ages were eight years one month and seven years two months for the girls and boys, respectively. The mean values for these two groups did not differ significantly from the control values for any of the measurements that were selected to determine unit sizes of the maxilla and mandible and maxillomandibular relationship (Vargervik, 1981).

In children with bilateral cleft lip and palate, the premaxilla is usually protrusive at birth and remains protrusive during the first years of life if surgical intervention in this area is limited to lip closure (Vargervik, 1983).

The transition from the primary to mixed dentition is characterized by an increased discrepancy between maxillary and mandibular sizes and dental arches. The permanent lateral incisor on the side of the cleft is frequently missing, and there is a high incidence of congenital absence of premolars. The central incisor on the cleft side is, on average, 10% narrower than the other central incisor and its shape is often abnormal. The path of eruption of the central incisors is lingual and toward the cleft, and these teeth are usually severely rotated as well. Further medial displacement of the alveolar process on the cleft side and an increased incidence of anterior crossbite usually occur during this stage.

When the maxillary segments are displaced medially, the tongue cannot be accommodated in its normal position in the palate. The position that the tongue acquires becomes decisive for the pattern of further development of the maxilla as well as the mandible. If nasal respiration is adequate, the tongue may be positioned below and in contact with the occlusal surfaces of the maxillary teeth during rest. When this occurs, alveolar height is inhibited even in the absence of restrictive scar tissue. If nasal respiration is impeded, the tongue may assume a low posture to facilitate oral respiration. If the tongue in this low position does not rest under the occlusal surfaces of the maxillary teeth, the alveolar height will increase, resulting in a progressive lowering of the mandible, a more open gonial angle, and a more retruded position of the chin.

Growth during adolescence

The maxilla may become progressively retrusive during later growth. In noncleft children, mandibular length, measured from condyle to pogonion, increases by average yearly increments of 2.5 mm (Vargervik, 1981). The corresponding figure for the maxilla is 1.5 mm. Adjustments for this difference in growth in length of the jaws take place in the alveolar processes, primarily by downward and forward development of the maxillary alveolar process. In a child with cleft lip and palate, this adjustment mechanism is often impeded, and its limitations become an important cause of maxillomandibular disproportions during active growth periods, particularly during adolescent growth.

A tight, scarred lip and scar tissue bands in the palate can impede the forward growth of the entire maxilla as well as the alveolar process. The retrusiveness of the maxilla and maxillary alveolar process generally becomes more pronounced during this stage.

In a study of 16 individuals with unilateral clefts who had received orthodontic treatment and 8 who had only had surgical treatment, Vargervik (1981) reported that the average downward and forward growth and translation of the maxilla were significantly less in the group that did not receive orthodontic treatment than in the treated group. However, the group that did receive orthodontic treatment had significantly less downward and forward growth and translation of the maxilla compared to the noncleft control group.

In a study of patients with bilateral clefts, Vargervik (1983) reported that the premaxillary region stayed more protrusive than normal up to age of 12 years but after that became gradually more retruded as the mandible continued to grow at a normal rate. The premaxilla started out as excessively protrusive but came forward an average of 1.0 mm per year, rather than the normal increment of 1.5 mm per year, from the ages of 6 to 16 years. When treatment is planned for a child with a repaired bilateral cleft, it is therefore important to accept early prominence of the premaxilla and to consider that the forward growth in this area will be less than normal.

Orthodontic treatment

Expansion of the maxilla to correct segment position and crossbite

To achieve lateral movement of the cleft segment, a palatal rather than a labial appliance must be utilized. Several appliance types are available for this purpose, such as a plain lingual wire with auxiliary springs (typically used at UCSF) or a quad helix appliance (also commonly used). This treatment is usually started when the patient is aged about seven years, at the time of eruption of the permanent maxillary incisors and after eruption of the permanent first molars (Fig 6-27).

Because the permanent incisors are almost always malpositioned, they need to be straightened. This is done in conjunction with maxillary expansion. When adequate maxillary width has been achieved and the incisors are aligned, the expansion is retained by a simple lingual archwire and the incisor position is retained by a wire bonded to the lingual surfaces of these teeth.

Monitoring of tooth eruption

Ectopic position of tooth buds and ectopic eruption are not uncommon in the canine and premolar area, and exfoliation of the primary teeth may not proceed normally. It is therefore important to obtain radiographs on a regular basis and extract primary teeth as necessary to facilitate eruption of succedaneous teeth. It is very important to decide if a missing permanent lateral incisor space should be kept open for prosthetic replacement or should be closed by mesial eruption and movement of the canine (Fig 6-28). If the maxilla is judged to be small and/or the canine appears to be too large compared to the other lateral incisor, the lateral space may preferably be kept open for later implant placement. If it is decided that the canine should be moved forward, the alveolar cleft should be bone grafted early, after expansion, but before the canine crown has moved into the bony defect.

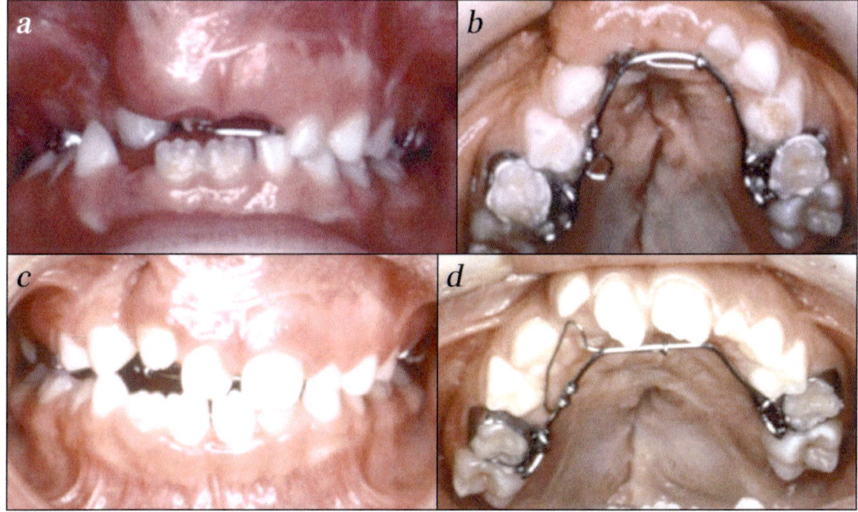

Figure 6-27 Postrepair orthodontic treatment. *(a)* Patient with repaired bilateral cleft, prior to maxillary expansion. *(b)* Palatal view soon after placement of maxillary expansion appliance. *(c and d)* Results one year following expansion of maxilla.

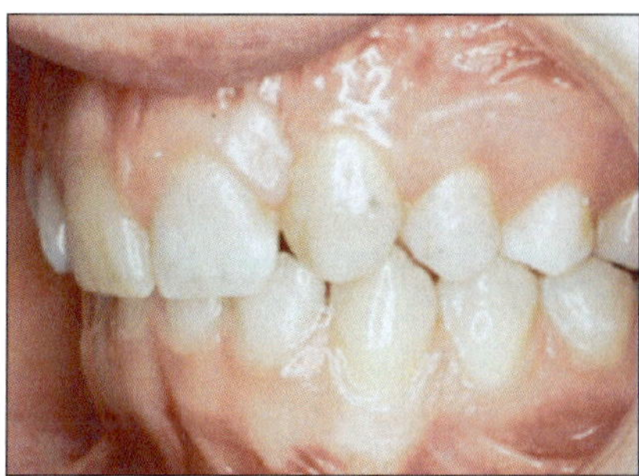

Figure 6-28 Mesial movement of the left canine into the position of the missing lateral incisor.

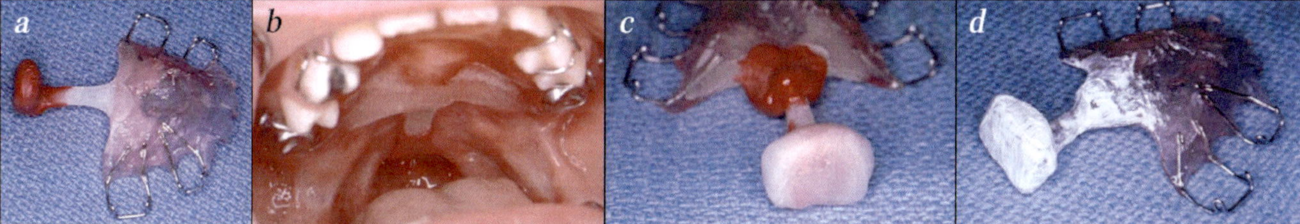

Figure 6-29 Obturator prosthesis. *(a)* Provisional prosthesis with obturator extension during development with modeling compound. Adams retainers have been added. *(b)* Provisional prosthesis in the mouth. *(c)* Fluid wax added and formed functionally after modeling plastic was reduced about 1 mm in all dimensions. *(d)* Finished prosthesis after adjustment with pressure indicator paste. The obturator bulb has been reduced in vertical extension to correspond with area of greatest motion. A trial period with a prosthesis had been recommended before surgical correction with a pharyngeal flap would be considered.

Full orthodontic treatment is begun after eruption of the premolars and canines. Standard orthodontic treatment is performed in the permanent dentition. Long-term retention is necessary because there will be a tendency for loss of maxillary width and shifting of the incisor position.

If occlusal and aesthetic objectives cannot be achieved by orthodontic treatment, orthognathic surgery must be considered. The cause of the jaw size discrepancy is almost always a hypoplastic maxilla. The amount of advancement versus lowering of the maxilla must be determined primarily based on tooth display and other clinical measures of facial balance and aesthetics.

Prosthetic treatment

Although the anatomical and physiologic bases for obturator fabrication and placement are discussed in Chapter 4, a brief discussion of obturators for pediatric cleft palate patients seems appropriate in this chapter. Most velopharyngeal discrepancies for cleft patients are managed surgically, usually with a combination of a pushback and palatal closure procedure initially (9 to 12 months) followed by a superiorly based pharyngeal flap procedure (about three to seven years), if necessary. After surgical treatment has improved the functional aspects of the velopharyngeal mechanism, intensive speech therapy is usually required to refine speech production. The success of these combined therapies has improved the speech of most cleft palate patients to the point where they have acceptable speech.

However, two types of cleft lip and palate patient may require an obturator prosthesis. A very small number of patients, primarily patients with clefts confined to the secondary palate, are best managed prosthodontically without surgery (Fig 6-29). These patients characteristically have an unusually wide posterior maxillomandibular width, a paucity of residual palatal tissues, or poor anesthetic risks. The second group requiring prosthodontic intervention includes those patients who exhibit hypernasality and inadequate speech following pushback and pharyngeal flap surgical procedures.

When velopharyngeal deficiencies and hypernasality are evident, usually because of inadequate length or movement of the soft palate, closure of this sphincteric valve is compromised. Air escapes into the nasopharynx and nasal cavities, and oral pressure is inadequate for proper articulation and oral resonance. To reduce the size of the velopharyngeal orifice, a vertical flap is raised along the midline of the posterior pharyngeal wall, rotated forward, and attached into the nasal surface of the soft palate to reduce the size of the

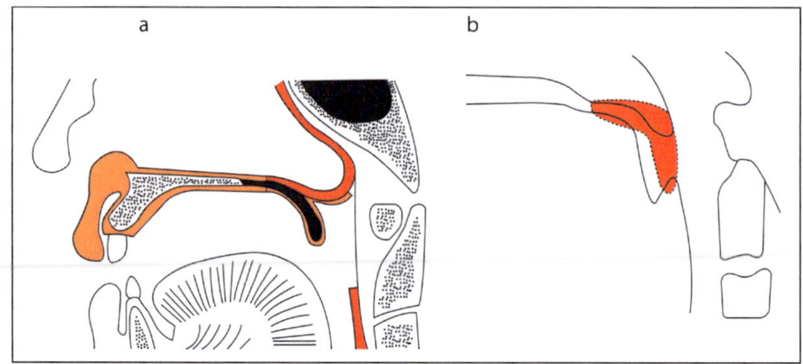

Figure 6-30 High-based pharyngeal flap. *(a)* The soft palate is redivided for access to the posterior pharyngeal wall. Flaps are raised on the nasal surface of the soft palate and from the posterior pharyngeal wall. The pharyngeal flap is rotated into the soft palate and the oral surface is lined with nasal flaps so both surfaces of pharyngeal flap have mucosal covering. *(b)* As organization and contraction occur, the soft palate is pulled toward the area of normal closure.

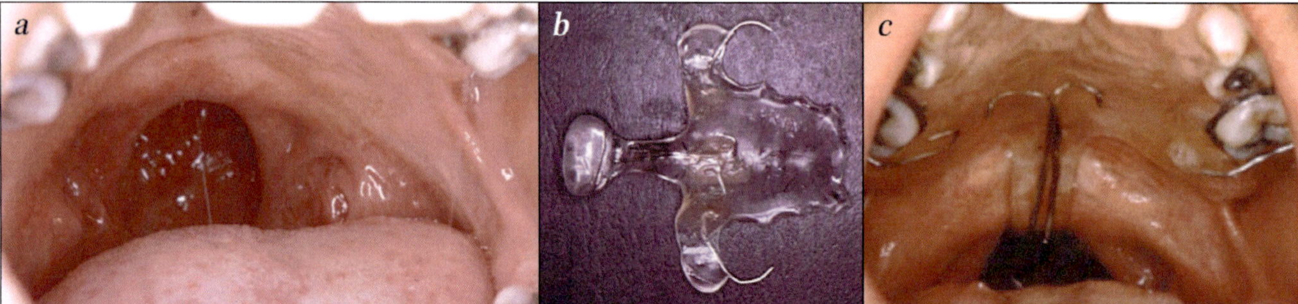

Figure 6-31 Good access to the nasopharyngeal area. *(a)* High-based pharyngeal flap. The right side of the flap has broken down, leading to hypernasality. A trial period with a prosthesis was recommended. Access is now available to the nasopharynx and the area of normal velopharyngeal closure. *(b)* Provisional prosthesis. *(c)* Provisional prosthesis in place.

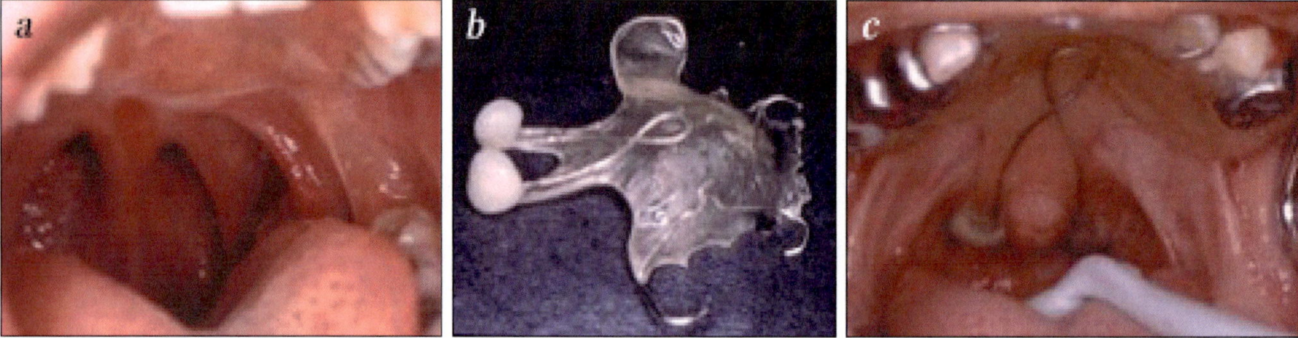

Figure 6-32 Poor access to the nasopharyngeal area. *(a)* Low-based pharyngeal flap with the soft palate tethered inferiorly. The lateral openings are larger than anticipated, resulting in hypernasality. A trial period with provisional prosthesis was recommended. *(b)* Provisional prosthesis. *(c)* Provisional prosthesis in the mouth. Because the soft palate is tethered inferiorly, it was difficult to extend the small obturators superiorly to the area of tissue movement without creating constant contact with inferior immobile pharyngeal tissues, thus creating hyponasality. After this trial period, further pharyngeal surgery was recommended.

orifice. Two small openings are left laterally for nasal breathing. During closure, the lateral pharyngeal walls move medially to contact the flap and to close these lateral openings (Fig 6-30).

There are two types of pharyngeal flap: *(1)* a high-attached and *(2)* a low-attached flap. These are distinguished based on the location of flap attachment to the posterior pharyngeal wall. High-attached pharyngeal flaps are preferred by most surgeons. With healing, these flaps tend to organize and contract and thus pull the soft palate toward the area of flap attachment. Therefore, a high-based flap will tend to elevate and pull the soft palate toward the area of normal closure in the nasopharynx, whereas the low-based flap will tether the soft palate and restrict palatal elevation.

Prostheses for these patients are usually fabricated of acrylic resin with adapted wire retainers. Adams or interproximal ball clasps are effective and require minimal tooth preparation. If retention is or becomes a problem, orthodontic bands with buccal lugs or bonded brackets will provide excellent retention.

One of the problems we have experienced in fabricating obturators for this small group of patients is access to the area of normal closure in the nasopharynx. Access was excellent for the patient depicted in Fig 6-31, because a portion of the flap broke down on the patient's right side, whereas access was restricted for the patient in Fig 6-32. The low-based pharyngeal flap used in this instance required that each of the two small obturators extend superiorly for a considerable distance to reach the area of optimal posterolateral pharyngeal wall movement. For all low-based flaps in this process, it is very difficult to avoid contact with immobile pharyngeal tissues below the level of optimum motion. This constant contact will create hyponasality and restrict nasal breathing.

These prostheses may stimulate additional peripheral motion, so periodic adjustments may be required (Blakeley, 1964).

Bone grafting

The goals for grafting the alveolar cleft are (1) to separate the oral and nasal cavities, (2) to stabilize the maxillary segments with a bony union, (3) to provide normal quality of bone in the alveolus for orthodontic movement and support for the teeth, and (4) to provide adequate three-dimensional bone volume for placement of an osseointegrated implant or implants when this procedure is indicated.

The timing for surgical closure of the alveolar cleft can be divided into three categories: primary, secondary, and delayed. The closure of the oronasal fistula, with or without placement of a bone graft in the alveolar cleft, at the time of lip closure (less than one year of age) would be classified as a primary or "early" closure. Primary alveolar cleft repair with bone grafting has fallen out of favor due to observed detrimental effects on the sagittal growth of the maxilla. Some centers continue to perform gingivoperiosteoplasty, which is a soft tissue repair of the alveolar cleft without bone grafting, at the time of lip repair. This, however, has also been shown to have negative effects on maxillary growth as well (Molsted et al., 2005).

Secondary closure applies to those patients who have a fistula closed by bone grafting the alveolar cleft during the mixed dentition stage. This is typically performed when the maxillary canine root is one-half to two-thirds developed. Secondary bone grafting can also be performed prior to the eruption of the lateral incisor (if present) into the cleft, generally around five to six years of age. However, the large majority of centers graft the alveolar based on the eruption of the canine development (Kaura et al., 2018).

The third group of patients are those who have the alveolar cleft grafted after growth is essentially completed. For these patients the fistula and alveolar cleft are often repaired in combination with a LeFort I osteotomy to correct midfacial retrusion. The surgical technique for alveolar cleft bone grafting is demonstrated in Figs 6-33 and 6-34. When grafting the alveolus on growth completion, one alternative strategy is to perform a sliding segmental LeFort osteotomy to move the cleft maxillary segment anteriorly and close the alveolar cleft simultaneously (Posnick and Thompson, 1992). In moving the posterior maxillary segment anteriorly, canine substitution is usually performed to negate the need for a dental implant (Fig 6-34e).

Newer materials for alveolar cleft repair have emerged, with more centers adopting the use of bone morphogenic protein (BMP-2) in lieu of iliac crest. It has been shown to generate roughly the same amount of bone on post-op CBCT and saves the donor-site morbidity (Hammoudeh et al., 2017). However, the iliac crest continues to be the gold standard for larger defects or more complicated alveolar cleft repairs.

A key consideration in the timing of alveolar cleft repair is its effect on facial growth. Ross (1987) investigated treatment variables affecting facial growth in patients with unilateral cleft lip and palate. Fifteen centers from around the world contributed 1,600 cephalograms of 538 white males with unilateral complete cleft lip and palate. Ross (1987) compared 213 subjects who had various types of alveolar closure and compared them with 226 subjects who underwent no alveolar surgical repair. The results demonstrated that surgical manipulation of the alveolus in patients with unilateral cleft lip and palate prior to completion of growth resulted in a deficiency of vertical growth of the anterior maxilla. If a bone graft or periosteoplasty was used, the vertical growth deficiency of the maxilla increased. There was also a slight anteroposterior maxillary deficiency following bone grafting that was not found in patients who were not bone grafted.

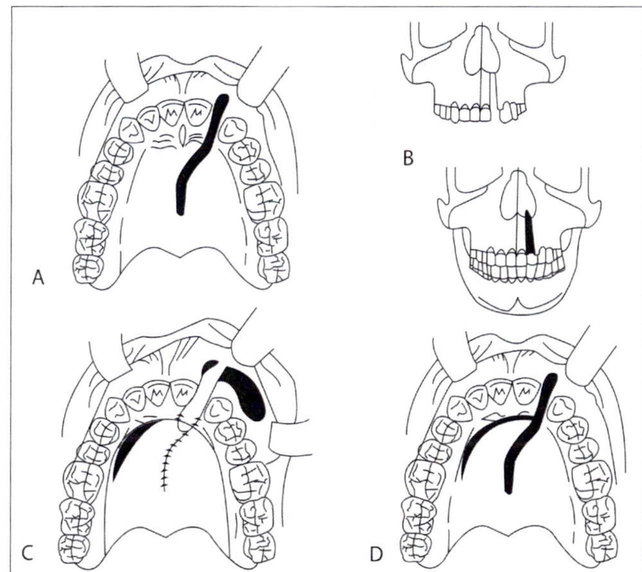

Figure 6-33 Closure of an oronasal fistula. *(a)* The cleft is incised *(dashed line)* at its margin. *(b)* Medial and lateral flaps are elevated for nasal lining *(upper diagram)*. Palatal flaps are mobilized for closure. Iliac cancellous bone and marrow are grafted in the alveolar cleft *(lower diagram)*. *(c)* Alveolar ridge covered with a buccal rotation flap. *(d)* Alveolar ridge covered with a flap of alveolar mucosa and gingiva.

These data are clinically significant regarding the timing and type of operation. The effect of bone grafting an alveolar cleft in infants is different from that of bone grafting performed when patients are in the late mixed dentition. Those patients treated after the age of nine years showed little growth inhibition (Ross, 1987). Friede and Johanson (1982) reported severe maxillary retrognathia and a vertical deficiency that worsened with age in patients who had alveolar cleft bone grafting in infancy. Similar results were reported by Robertson and Jolleys (1983). Rosenstein et al. (1982), in contrast, believed that early alveolar cleft repair and bone grafting does not significantly retard maxillary growth.

The current consensus is to close the oronasal fistula and bone graft the alveolar cleft with iliac cancellous bone and marrow during the late mixed dentition (Kaban, 1990). The maxilla should have achieved its appropriate width, either spontaneously or through orthodontic treatment, by this age. The canine root should be one-half to two-thirds developed. The majority of maxillary canines will spontaneously erupt into the cleft when it is grafted with iliac cancellous bone (Boyne and Sands, 1972; El Deeb et al., 1982; Hall and Psonick, 1983; Turvey et al., 1984). If the canine does not erupt spontaneously, it can be exposed and orthodontically aligned in the arch.

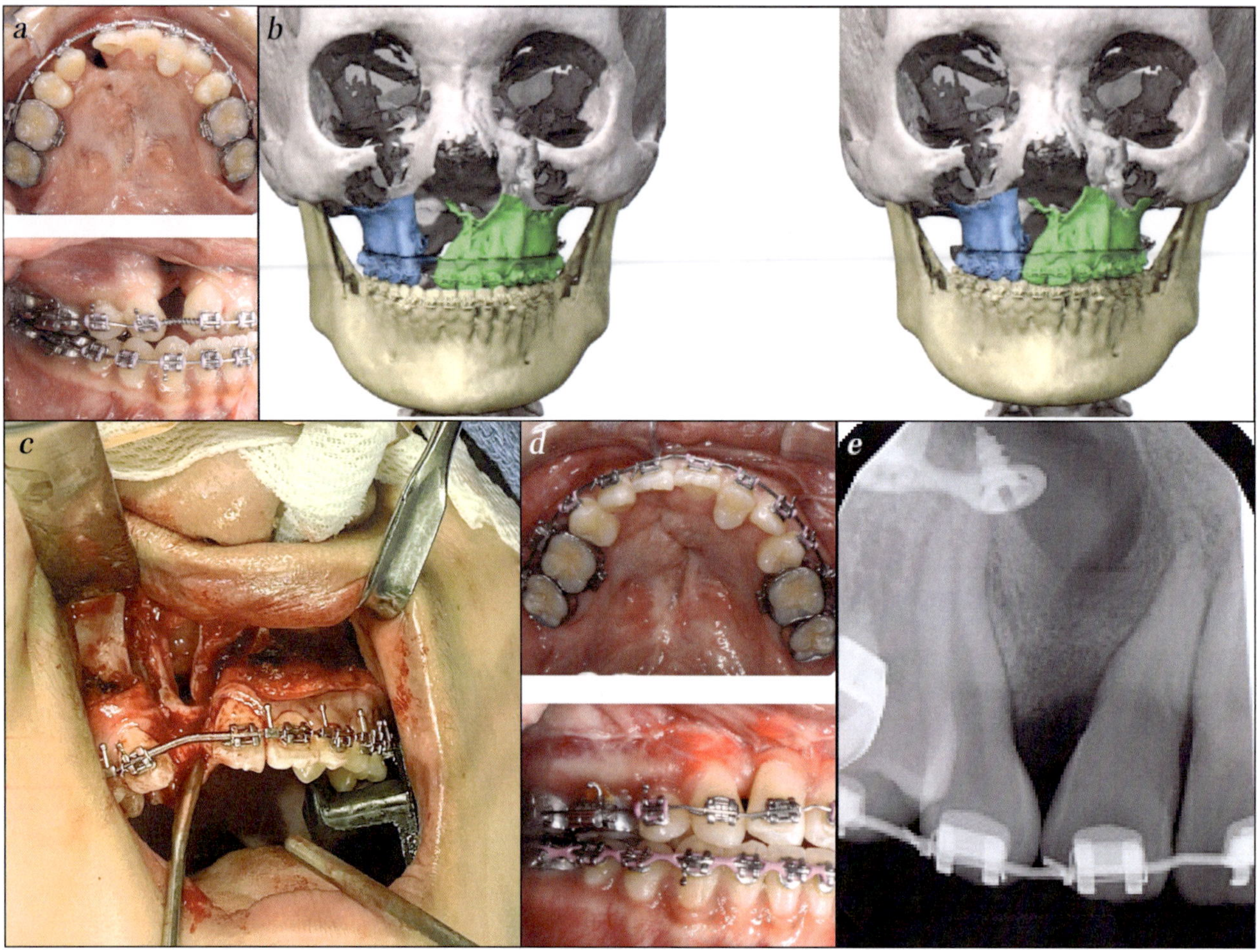

Figure 6-34 *(a)* Preoperative photos of a 17-year-old female planned for LeFort 1 advancement with sliding osteotomy and alveolar cleft repair to close the alveolar cleft defect. *(b)* Virtual surgical plan demonstrating the sliding osteotomy and LeFort advancement. *(c)* Intraoperative photo showing the alveolar cleft defect extending into the nose. *(d)* Postoperative photos showing closure of the alveolar cleft defect and canine substitution. *(e)* Postoperative PA demonstrating bony unity across the alveolar cleft.

Finally, if a midfacial deficiency develops, the maxilla can be moved forward and downward as a single unit with a Le Fort I osteotomy to restore midfacial harmony.

In patients with bilateral cleft lip and palate, the position of the premaxilla and its relationship to the lip and nose must be considered. Vargervik (1983) studied 63 patients with bilateral complete cleft lip and palate who had no premaxillary surgery. The premaxilla was protrusive throughout the primary and mixed dentition periods. By the time the patients reached the age of 12 years, however, the premaxilla became relatively more retrusive as mandibular growth proceeded more normally. At the end of growth, none of these patients had an excessively protrusive premaxilla. Therefore, it is advantageous to maintain the premaxilla in its protrusive position during these formative years to avoid midfacial retrusion as the child approaches maturity.

In 12 subjects who had premaxillary surgery in infancy or early mixed dentition to set back the premaxilla or to stabilize it to the posterior segments, forward growth of the premaxilla was decreased as compared to untreated individuals. All 12 patients developed severe midfacial retrusion (Vargervik, 1983). Surgical procedures that reduce the prominence of the premaxilla should, therefore, be avoided in growing patients, except in extreme cases of premaxillary protrusion where the position of the premaxilla will interfere significantly with the proposed lip and nose surgery.

The use of osseointegrated implants to restore the missing dentition in noncleft patients is well documented (Albrektsson et al., 1988; Jemt et al., 1989; Adell et al., 1990). Patients with cleft lip and palate are frequently missing the lateral incisor on the cleft side. If the treatment plan includes prosthetic replacement of the missing lateral incisor, the surgeon must plan for the placement of an implant by overcorrecting the width and height of the alveolar ridge.

In addition, the timing of implant placement is critical. Perrott et al. (1994) reported that after three months there may be significant resorption that rapidly reduces the width and height of the reconstructed alveolar ridge. Therefore, they recommended placement of endosseous implants in grafted alveolar clefts within three to six months of the grafting procedure.

Restoration of missing dentition

Most cleft lip and palate patients will require more specialized and continuing prosthodontic services than will noncleft patients. There are several reasons for this additional care. If the cleft involves the primary palate, invariably the lateral incisor in the area of the alveolar cleft will be missing or significantly malformed. However, the primary lateral incisor is usually present with relatively normal morphologic development. The maxillary central incisor adjacent to the cleft is often smaller than the companion central incisor (in the case of a unilateral cleft), and the teeth on either side of the cleft characteristically display hypoplastic enamel formation to varying degrees (Fig 6-35). The teeth in the premaxilla usually have shorter and poorly developed roots.

In addition, patients with cleft lip and palate are more likely to have supernumerary teeth or be missing other teeth. A substantially higher incidence of congenitally missing teeth in both the maxillary and the mandibular arches has been reported in children affected by clefting (Olin, 1964). One study found that 24% of patients with cleft lip and palate were congenitally missing premolars, compared with 6.6% in the general population (Valinoti, 1958). Mackey (1958) reported that 49.6% of cleft patients had one or more congenitally missing teeth. Mackey (1958) also found that 21% of patients with cleft lip and palate had one or more supernumerary teeth.

The jaws of clefted individuals tend to be smaller, especially the maxilla. Because of a lack of downward and forward growth of the maxillae and the subsequent underdevelopment of the midface, it is not uncommon for the dental arches to be of insufficient length to accommodate a full complement of succedaneous teeth. The dentition may be crowded and irregularly aligned because of this lack of space. The maxillary canine frequently erupts into the cleft in a diagonal direction and at a level superior to the gingival margin. Occasionally the canine is impacted horizontally in the palate or only the cusp tip will be visible in the alveolar cleft.

Oral hygiene can be compromised because of these alignment and eruptive patterns. Scarring and inflexibility of the upper lip may complicate hygiene in the anterior maxilla. The teeth in the premaxilla may be more prone to caries because of malformation, malalignment, and hypoplastic enamel development. The attached gingiva is often scanty or missing around these maxillary anterior teeth. Therefore, cleft lip and palate patients are likely to require prosthodontic services to replace missing teeth, improve aesthetics, or possibly to provide an obturator prosthesis if palatal surgery is unsuccessful or contraindicated. However, definitive prosthodontic care is customarily one of the final treatment modalities in the progression of treatment from birth to early adulthood.

Early care

Early dental care is usually provided by the pedodontist and orthodontist. The objective of this primary care is to establish a good oral hygiene regimen, to maintain the dentition during these formative years, and to improve alignment and stimulate growth orthodontically during this period. Even malposed, malformed, and supernumerary teeth preserve bone and help maintain arch alignment and occlusal relationships. For example, it is important to maintain the teeth in the premaxillary segment. These teeth can be used as an aid in the early expansion of the maxillae and to correct anterior or posterior crossbite tendencies. If the alignment of the primary teeth can be corrected, they will help guide the permanent teeth into this improved alignment.

Maintenance of alveolar bone during growth and development may enhance future prosthodontic care. For example, adequate alveolar bone may be available in the premaxilla as possible sites for

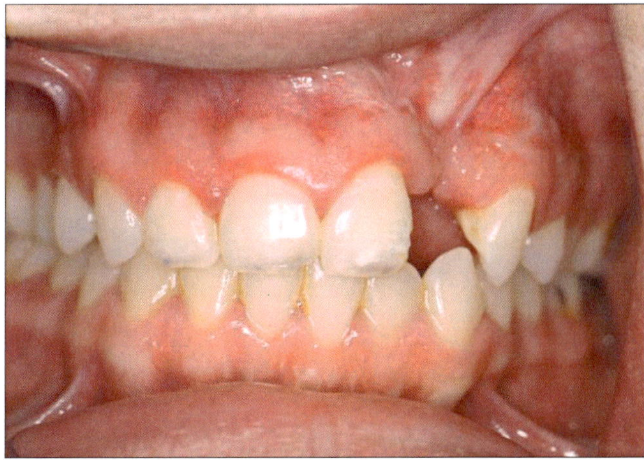

Figure 6-35 Missing left lateral incisor and undersized and hypocalcified left central incisor.

implant placement or to provide stability and support for a removable prosthesis in later years.

Prosthodontic care during the preadolescent years is minimal. Missing teeth, such as missing lateral incisors, are often incorporated into the orthodontic retainer (Fig 6-36). Early prosthodontic treatment may be indicated if the patient has lingering speech problems that are not amenable to surgical intervention (see Chapter 4) or aesthetic problems. However, definitive care is usually indicated after growth and tooth maturation are essentially completed.

Definitive prosthodontic treatment

Definitive prosthodontic care for cleft patients is usually indicated sometime after early adolescence, when the gamut of treatment during the formative years has essentially been completed. If there are missing, malposed, or unesthetic anterior teeth, the motivating factor for referral is customarily aesthetics. It is not uncommon for the replacement tooth or teeth attached to the orthodontic retainer to be less than optimal from the perspective of the maturing patient and his or her family, and the orthodontist often makes the referral. Also, there may be aesthetic concerns about the remaining teeth in the premaxilla, so the patient and parents are looking for direction and guidance.

Mounted diagnostic casts and appropriate radiographs are essential for establishing a diagnosis and for the development of a long-range treatment plan. Prior to the next consultation appointment, the clinician should consult with the patient's other health care providers, such as the plastic surgeon, orthodontist, and the family internist or pediatrician, regarding their thoughts and suggestions for future treatment.

As previously discussed, bone grafting of the alveolar cleft of the primary palate exerts a very significant and positive influence on the treatment plan. A consolidated and mature bone graft unites and stabilizes the cleft segments and simplifies future treatment. If a maxillary alveolar bone graft is contemplated, the prosthodontist should alter and delay the definitive treatment plan accordingly.

If the ultimate treatment plan includes selected porcelain-fused-to-metal or porcelain veneer restorations in addition to the possible placement of osseointegrated implants in the grafted cleft,

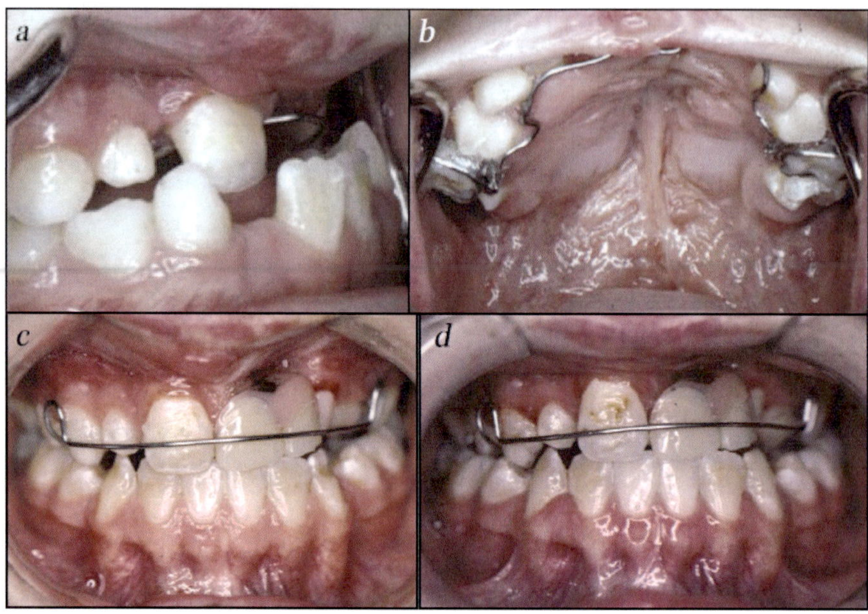

Figure 6-36 Provisional prosthodontic treatment. *(a)* Patient with bilateral cleft lip and palate in 1980. The patient has anterior crossbite and needs maxillary expansion. *(b)* Expander in place in 1980. *(c)* Status in 1986, following orthognathic surgery and completion of orthodontic treatment. *(d)* Patient in the retention phase. Prosthetic left central and lateral incisors are attached to the orthodontic retainer.

then a diagnostic wax-up is required. Indeed, a diagnostic wax-up can be invaluable as orthodontic realignment is nearing completion. A wax-up will permit both the orthodontist and the prosthodontist to visualize the potential aesthetic arrangement and will allow the orthodontist to make final refinements that will enhance future prosthodontic care. Spacing and relative tooth size can vary. If one or both lateral incisors are missing, the space for the lateral incisor may be either wider or narrower mesiodistally than a normal maxillary lateral incisor, while the adjacent central incisor will usually have a smaller than normal mesiodistal width. A diagnostic wax-up will help the prosthodontist proportion the anterior space appropriately, is an excellent educational tool for the patient and parents and can serve as a template for future provisional restorations. With this information, the clinician can provide the family with some idea of the sequence of the proposed treatment and how this treatment might interact with treatment by other health care providers.

Interim prostheses. Often the initial prosthodontic care is the fabrication of a well-fitting interim removable partial denture to replace any missing teeth. This type of partial denture is especially appropriate if a bone graft is scheduled in the future. Ideally, most prosthodontists would prefer to fabricate all anterior fixed units at the same time, including any implant-supported crowns. The ideal time to perform this definitive treatment is when the patient is around 25 years of age, when the alveolar cleft bone grafts are mature and well consolidated. The proposed treatment will be very similar to the treatment for a noncleft patient. At this age, more aesthetic restorations can be fabricated for the natural teeth because these teeth can be prepared so that adequate thickness is available for both porcelain and metal, allowing more ideal crown contours. An interim removable partial denture will fill this void until this definitive treatment is indicated.

Contemporary restorative dentistry offers other alternatives at an earlier age for the cleft patient who has undergone successful alveolar cleft bone grafting. Because implants may serve as anchors for the replacement of missing teeth in the premaxillary segment (or possibly in other areas as well), bonding and/or porcelain veneer restorations are viable options to correct size, space, or aesthetic deficiencies associated with the remaining maxillary anterior teeth. The size of the pulp chamber is not such a limiting factor so restorative treatment may be accomplished at an earlier age. As mentioned previously, the remaining teeth in the premaxillary segment may have short and poorly developed root systems. Therefore, implants, bonding, porcelain veneers, or possibly a resin-bonded fixed partial denture can be a viable alternative.

If the decision is for an interim removable partial denture, the clinician should consult with the orthodontist and the plastic surgeon and inform them of the proposed short- and long-term treatment plans. The orthodontist may have concerns regarding possible relapse of the realigned maxillary cleft segments, especially if a bone graft has not been performed. If grafting has been accomplished, many times the proposed partial denture design will be akin to the design for a noncleft patient. If orthodontic treatment was completed quite recently, the orthodontist is usually concerned about a collapse of the maxillary arch in a lingual direction. If necessary, the partial denture framework must also act as a lingual retainer and the framework should contact most maxillary teeth.

A removable partial denture could even be the treatment of choice if a residual alveolar cleft remains after bone grafting. A long replacement tooth or pontic can be an aesthetic liability. Replacement tooth length can be controlled easier with a removable prosthesis because pink acrylic resin can be added gingivally to maintain the gingival margin at a level consistent with that of adjacent teeth. The upper lip of many cleft patients may display limited mobility superiorly, so the smile line should always be checked during the diagnostic process and prior to treatment.

If there are no arch-retaining requirements, we prefer to fabricate a simple cast chrome removable partial denture framework requiring minimal tooth preparation because of the age of the patient (Fig 6-37). The major connector should be kept well away from nonabutment teeth and gingiva to make the prosthesis as self-cleansing as possible. Adolescents adapt to these prostheses quite well despite

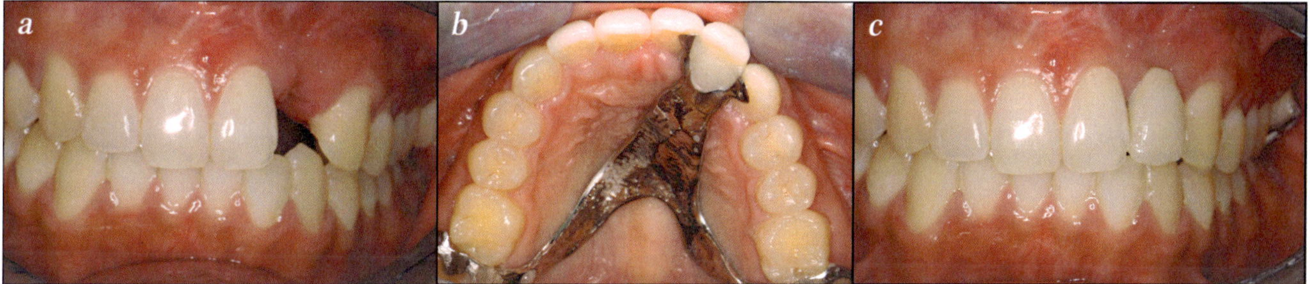

Figure 6-37 *(a)* Teenaged patient after completion of orthodontic treatment. *(b and c)* A removable partial denture restores the missing dentition until an implant can be placed.

their minimal retention. If a lateral incisor or incisors require replacement, the adjacent teeth may exhibit enamel hypoplasia. If bonding or placement of porcelain veneers is not indicated at this time, the acrylic resin replacement tooth or teeth can be stained with resin stains to match the adjacent hypoplastic teeth. This will improve aesthetics and enhance the patient's acceptance of the prosthesis.

Fixed partial dentures. If the patient is functioning quite well with the removable partial denture, further definitive care may not be necessary. However, most cleft patients will prefer some form of fixed replacement. If a bone graft has been performed a single implant-supported tooth replacement may be all that is required. As mentioned previously, if the missing lateral incisor is replaced in this manner, bonding or porcelain veneers are aesthetic options for the adjacent teeth.

If the other adjacent teeth require porcelain-fused-to-metal crowns and if the arch has been stabilized with a bone graft, consideration may be given to fabricating a fixed partial denture with a lateral incisor pontic. A review of the diagnostic wax-up may help the patient understand the options. Extensive fixed partial dentures are not recommended, especially for young patients, because any movement of the cleft segments will tend to rupture the luting bond for the crowns in the more stable segment. In addition, the aggressive tooth preparations required and the large size of the pulps in young children predispose the teeth to a high likelihood of pulpal injury. A more conservative option is bone grafting and the subsequent placement of an implant and crown or a resin-bonded fixed partial denture.

Often the crowns and/or fixed partial dentures will be enhanced with some modest intrinsic staining of the porcelain. However, it can be difficult to match the central incisor abutment of a three-unit fixed partial denture with the adjacent central incisor. Sometimes aesthetics, spacing, and crown contours can be improved by including both central incisors in the fixed partial denture or by placement of a porcelain veneer on the contralateral central incisor. For example, it is not uncommon for the edentulous space for the missing lateral incisor to be wider than the ideal replacement lateral incisor. As noted earlier, the central incisor adjacent to the cleft may be smaller than the other adjacent central incisor, but the overall width of the four units and the relative sizes of the individual teeth (i.e., maxillary canine, lateral incisor, and two central incisors) might be enhanced by including both central incisors so that the matching of shade, size, and contours is improved.

On occasion, it may be difficult to obtain profound local anesthesia of the teeth in the premaxillary segment. The scarring in the labial vestibule makes the anesthetic more painful to administer, and diffusion of the anesthetic may be less effective. Conscious sedation may be an effective adjunct in these situations.

The advent of adhesive dentistry has had a significant impact in the care of the cleft patient who has missing, malformed or discolored dentition. As previously discussed, this group of patients has a higher incidence of size discrepancies, especially in anterior teeth, along with hypoplastic enamel. In the past, a porcelain-fused-to-metal restoration was used to address these aesthetic concerns. Today, however, with significant improvement in composite resins, dentin bonding, and porcelain veneers, the use of porcelain-fused-to-metal restorations is decreasing. Size and color deficiencies can be easily corrected with bonded composite resin restorations or porcelain veneers. Missing teeth may be replaced with a resin-bonded fixed partial denture, provided that the alveolar cleft has been grafted to stabilize the maxillary segments. A resin-bonded fixed partial denture can also be used if an osseointegrated implant is contraindicated.

When adhesive dentistry is the treatment of choice to restore these deficiencies, it is still necessary to have mounted diagnostic casts and a full diagnostic wax-up prior to completion of the orthodontic treatment. This will allow for ideal tooth position with an equitable distribution of spaces between the anterior teeth that will be receiving restorative treatment. The aesthetic results with composite resin and porcelain veneers have been very encouraging. However, the clinician must inform the patient and the parents of the possible discoloration of the composite resin with time as well as the risk of fracture of the porcelain veneers. We believe that the use of adhesive dentistry in this group of patients is less invasive than porcelain-fused-to-metal restorations and more economical.

Very often patients present with hyperplastic gingival tissue and lack of attached gingiva in the premaxillary segment. A periodontal evaluation may also be necessary prior to any definitive restorative treatment. If the observed oral hygiene is marginal or poor, hygiene procedures should be reviewed with the patient and definitive prosthodontic treatment postponed until the patient's motivation and gingival health improve.

Resin-bonded bridges (RBBs)

Historically, conventional fixed or removable prosthodontic replacement of missing teeth was regarded as the standard of care. In modern times, the expectations of patients are centered on longevity, low maintenance, and functional as well as aesthetic restorations. Replacement of missing teeth utilizing more conservative treatment modalities such as resin-bonded bridges (RBBs) has become a reality as they can be an effective means by which teeth can be replaced in patients with dentoalveolar cleft defects.

Resin-bonded bridges have proven to be an effective means by which missing teeth have been replaced for many years (Howe and Denehy, 1977). As with all treatment modalities, careful case selection is imperative to optimize the chance of success. This text is not intended as a comprehensive overview of resin-bonded bridges, but some of the factors that are specific to cleft patients will be addressed. Patients who present with an orofacial cleft that affects the dentoalveolar complex can present with numerous dental issues that can impede their rehabilitation. Below are some of the more common issues that one may encounter when attempting to restore such a dentition.

1. Quality/volume of bone

   This can present somewhat of an unknown entity given the morphological variation of cleft sites. It is not clear how these variations or the use of the plethora of different bone substitute materials may have on the osseointegration of dental implants or soft tissue volume stability over time. As a result, significant bone augmentation may be required to facilitate implant placement. One common example of when an RBB might be indicated is when the patient is unwilling or unable to undergo such surgical treatment. If an RBB is the preferred method of replacement, then consideration should be given to the dimensional stability of any underlying bone graft procedure in the edentulous span. This may influence the choice of bone augmentation substitute materials where dimensional stability beneath a pontic site might be prioritized over the quality of bone such as that required for implant placement.
2. Quality/volume of soft tissue

   Mucogingival issues related to sites of scar tissue in areas of previous surgery/surgeries can resist manipulation and subsequent augmentation. This can especially be the case when there is an attempt to coronally advance scarred and tethered tissues as part of plastic mucogingival surgical procedures or preprosthetic surgery. This can pose an aesthetic as well as a functional issue for some patients. A ridge lap designed pontic of an RBB can be extended in such a way as to optimize the aesthetic outcome. The ability to clean beneath an RBB is not dependent on the presence of keratinized tissue. Where the tissues are heavily scarred one might choose to avoid the use of an ovate pontic unless the site is amenable to surgical preparation prior to making the impression. Some clinicians choose to adjust the cast to compress the soft tissues and develop a more natural emergence profile. As the soft tissues in cleft sites can be variable in their compressibility, it would be prudent for the treating clinician to communicate with the laboratory technician. This is less of an issue for conventional fixed dental prostheses, as the retainers mechanically engage the abutment teeth and hence ensure proper seating. If careful attention is not paid and there is excessive soft tissue resistance to compression of the pontic site, the retainer of an RBB cannot be seated and hence cemented incorrectly.
3. Mobility of the alveolar segments

   Where there is mobility of the alveolar segments, one must be mindful from a prosthodontic perspective when attempting to place splinted restorations that cross a cleft site. The differential movement of multiple abutment teeth can lead to the premature debonding of one of the retainer wings; therefore, cantilever RBBs are the preferred design, as there is evidence that they debond less often than fixed-fixed RBBs (Dejmal et al., 1999). The larger the edentulous span or the presence of a bilateral cleft may result in greater mobility of the alveolar segments. In these cases, one may opt for an alternative to an RBB if the site does not lend itself to a cantilevered solution.
4. Mobility, length, and symmetry of upper lip / lip line

   A cleft-related shallow vestibule (Almeida et al., 2005) as well as an unfavorable lip line can limit ideal prosthetic placement or restoration of replacement teeth. It can also influence the display of teeth. Where there is a significant lack of ridge height the decision may be made to add pink porcelain to the RBB. When more than a single tooth is being replaced and there is a need to prosthetically improve the "pink aesthetics," a fixed-fixed RBB may have to be employed to facilitate a continuous prosthetic gingival margin (two cantilevered RBBs would make it challenging to achieve an uninterrupted pink prosthetic gingival architecture). This is not ideal, as the differential movement of teeth on either side of the span may lead to the debonding of a wing retainer (Dejmal et al., 1999; King et al., 2015). Adding pink porcelain to two cantilever bridges may be the only option if the cosmetic compromise can be accepted.

   If the lip is excessively short or lacks mobility due to a poor outcome following primary surgery, then this issue should be corrected prior to dental rehabilitation. It is not always possible or desirable from a patient's perspective to undergo corrective surgery for this. Lip revision surgery can have a lasting effect that goes beyond aesthetics: the cleanability of the final prosthesis and design from a mechanical point of view, which can have an impact on the maintenance requirements of such a prosthesis.
5. Hypodontia, morphology of teeth adjacent to cleft (Jordan et al., 1966; Schroeder and Green, 1975; Ghaida et al., 2010)

   Adult patients who present with a heavily restored dentition may have reduced enamel available for bonding on the preferred abutment teeth. The surface area available for bonding is a crucial factor for a successful outcome (Dejmal et al., 1999). Malformed teeth either in or adjacent to the cleft site can be unusually small. This will impact the available enamel for bonding and hence can have a deleterious effect on the survival of such a prosthesis. If the desired abutment teeth are bulbous then the resultant height of the metal framework connector may be compromised. On this occasion the proximal area of the tooth can be reduced to produce a guide plane, this should allow for improved connector height and have the subsequent effect of improving the rigidity of the metal framework. The added benefit of proximal reduction is that it can reduce the appearance of black triangles, which may be of particular importance in the anterior region of the mouth (Fig 6-38). Alternatively, the metal wing retainer can be constructed to the dimensions of a diagnostic wax-up. The exposed wing retainer can then be "infilled" labially with a composite resin restorative material. This technique essentially employs the metal wing retainer as a matrix to guide a direct labial resin composite buildup. This technique can also be used to treat a spaced dentition where the metalwork connector would otherwise be exposed. If there is significant crowding present this can affect the path of insertion of the retainer and there are occasions

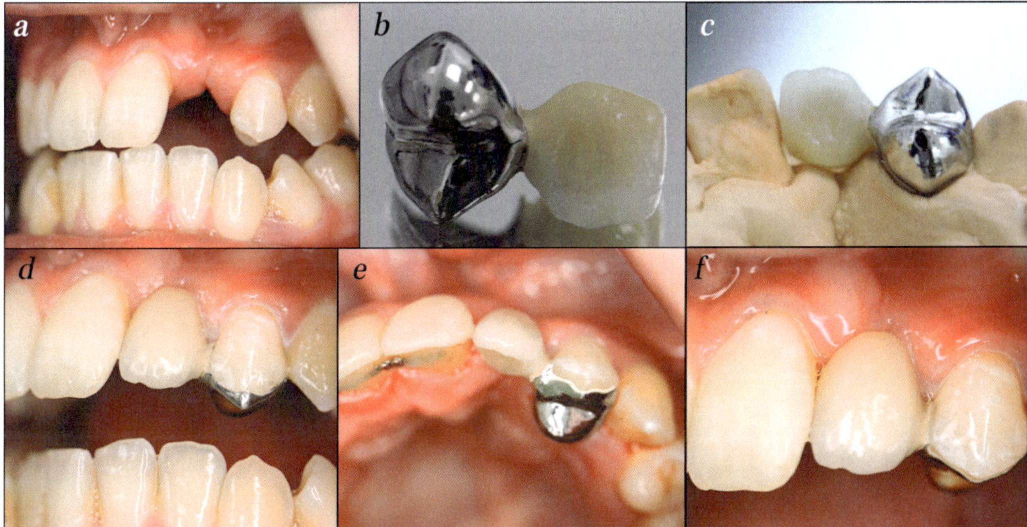

Figure 6-38 *(a)* Missing maxillary left lateral incisor. Note mesial bulbosity of the maxillary premolar. *(b and c)* Palatal view of RBB. *(d)* Full incisal wraparound of wing retainer. *(e)* Adjustment of wing retainer to achieve acceptable aesthetic result. *(f)* Note height of bridge connector to improve rigidity and mesial wraparound of wing retainer due to lack of guide plane and to eliminate black triangle. Orthodontic space reduction and an enameloplasty could have been employed to overcome these issues.

when this can be corrected with minimal preparation within the enamel surfaces to construct a guide plane. If the crowding is severe, orthodontic treatment may be necessary to align the teeth to achieve a common path of insertion.

6. Periodontal/endodontic status of teeth adjacent to cleft

The long-term prognosis of teeth adjacent to clefts can sometimes be challenging given the spectrum of developmental anomalies that can occur. Pathology can go undetected given the potential difficulties in diagnosing disease in or near a cleft site. An apical radiolucency as a result of an alveolar cleft can be misinterpreted as chronic apical periodontitis. A preoperative cone beam computed tomography (CBCT) investigation should be considered in these circumstances. It is important that there is sufficient enamel available for adhesion. This means previously restored teeth, where there is a dearth of enamel available for bonding to, may be a relative contraindication for the provision of an RBB. Where a small restoration is present this may either be replaced with a resin-based composite restoration or, when existing composite restorations are already present, be resurfaced to improve the adhesion. Where an existing restoration is deemed acceptable one should be cognizant of the fact the bond strength of the metal wing retainer to the tooth may be compromised. The accepted school of thought is that the bond strength to enamel is greater than that to dentine, which in turn is greater than that to a composite resin. The bond to glass ionomer and amalgam restorations is weaker still, and therefore, their replacement is usually recommended with a resin composite restoration (Aboush and Jenkins, 1991).

There is a higher prevalence of gingival recession associated with teeth adjacent to the cleft (Almeida et al., 2007, 2010a, 2010b). This can have an impact on the aesthetic outcome of any rehabilitation. In addition to this, the presence of frenula and bands of scar tissue can restrict access to cleaning in the more severe cases (Almeida et al., 2006).

The periodontal status of the abutment teeth should be carefully assessed. It is not uncommon for teeth close to a cleft site to present with either a developmental lack of bone or reduced attachment levels as a result of multiple surgeries. Developmental lack of bone with a stable and intact periodontium can be mistaken for chronic periodontal disease, and in this case, the abutment teeth may present with mobility, which can have an adverse effect on fixed-fixed RBBs. Lack of bone around teeth, especially a deficient labial plate, may complicate orthodontic treatment to optimize spaces for any replacement option.

7. Patient expectations

These often must be managed from the outset of treatment, so patients should be counseled as to what outcomes can be realistically expected. There is evidence to support that maximal enamel coverage of the retainer wing will have a positive effect on the outcome (Dejmal et al., 1999). Some choose to extend the metal retainer over the incisal edge; however, the aesthetic implications of this must be assessed beforehand.

The presence of a metal wing can have a "graying" effect on the abutment tooth. This effect can be mitigated by utilizing a white opaque resin-based cement, extending the wing retainer short of the incisal edge where teeth tend to exhibit the most translucency, and considering the effect of this on the abutment tooth before selecting a shade for the pontic. In some select cases, prescribing a shade map that incorporates gray in the pontic incisal edge can appear harmonious with the affected abutment tooth. A simple test that can easily be performed involves holding a metallic instrument behind the abutment tooth to gauge whether this will be an issue.

8. Occlusal/interarch discrepancy

The resultant occlusal issues may be as follows:

- Class 3 incisal relationship can lead to challenges not only from an occlusal point of view but also from a soft tissue support point of view. A lack of lip support as a result of a flangeless prosthesis can have an undesirable effect on the overall harmony of the facial contour in this region.
- Orthodontic expansion and/or orthognatihic surgery may not correct buccal segment crossbites.
- Buccally tipped posterior teeth can result from orthodontic arch expansion. This in turn can reduce the availability of desirable undercut for clasping as part of a removable prosthesis or a desirable common path of insertion for an RBB.

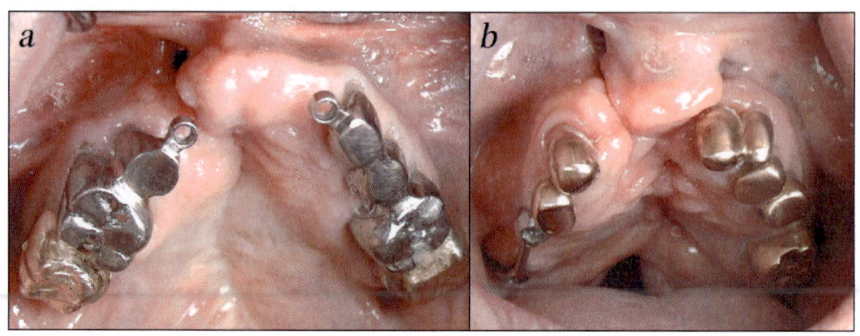

Figure 6-39 *(a and b)* The small openings anteriorly must be occluded with gauze before impressions are made.

Many cleft patients present with an edge-to-edge occlusal scheme, which can lead to premature tooth surface loss or hinder restoration of these teeth if needed. One can choose to take advantage of the retainer wing of an RBB by incorporating sufficient bulk to facilitate canine guidance, while simultaneously, guidance on the pontic should be kept to a minimum if possible. This can prove incredibly useful when one finds the need to alter a patient's occlusal scheme to that which is more desirable. The minimum thickness of a metal retainer should be 0.7 mm in order to impart the desired level of rigidity to the bridge (Ibrahim et al., 1997; Sato et al., 1995). Where a Class 3 incisor relationship with a negative overjet is to be accepted, the loading conditions on the pontic of an RBB can be most favorable. RBBs tend to function very well in these cases.

If excursive or protrusive contacts fall beyond the wing retainer and on one of the two abutment teeth, this can predispose the bridge to debonding. In these cases, it may be necessary to extend the metal wing retainer over the incisal edge to ensure even contact in ICP and protrusive/excursive movements.

Removable partial dentures. Removable partial dentures for patients with repaired cleft lip and palate have similar design and functional requirements as partial dentures for noncleft patients. The exception is for patients with velopharyngeal deficiencies, when the conventional prosthesis must support a palatal lift or obturator prosthesis. As discussed in Chapter 4, the prosthodontist must consider the long lever arm created by this extension. This is especially true for patients requiring a Kennedy Class I or Class II partial denture. Adequate indirect retention is helpful in this situation, but effective indirect retention can be difficult to obtain for Class I patients if only anterior teeth remain and especially for patients with a square arch form.

Two additional precautions should be considered for cleft patients that would not be a consideration for noncleft patients. First, if the primary palate has not been bone grafted, tortuous, fistula-like openings may exist in the alveolar cleft area; these are sometimes difficult to detect as overt openings during examination. A gentle stream of air will aid in the examination process (Fig 6-39). On occasion, slightly larger alveolar and/or palatal openings can be used to enhance retention if acrylic resin or soft silicone materials can be extended into the defect.

These potential openings are of little or no consequence regarding speech, but they should be considered during impression making. When an irreversible hydrocolloid impression is made, the impression material may be forced into these openings. When the impression is removed, the impression material will fracture and remain in the opening. On occasion, the clinician will find the impression material difficult to remove. Usually with patience, this material can be teased out with the aid of cotton pliers.

To avoid this problem, before the impression is made the alveolar cleft area should be blocked out with a gauze strip lubricated with petrolatum. If the gauze protrudes slightly from the cleft, the gauze will be incorporated in the impression material and will be removed with the impression. If the opening is larger than a fistula and is contiguous with the nasal cavity, this aspect of the partial denture should be processed in acrylic resin to provide the potential for adjustments and relining (Fig 6-40).

The second consideration is that repair of a palatal cleft is a soft tissue closure that will display various degrees of scarring and can be quite unyielding. During the fabrication of removable partial dentures, most laboratory technicians will bead the peripheral margins of the tissue surface of the major and minor connectors. The technician should be instructed to follow the ridges of scar tissue rather than cross them, if possible, and to bead the cast only minimally. This situation is analogous to following rather than crossing rugae with the beaded margins of an anterior palatal strap major connector.

Complete dentures. *Treatment concepts.* Complete dentures for patients with clefts of both the primary and the secondary palates are challenging for the clinician to fabricate and for the patient to use effectively. The reasons for this situation are important to recognize:

1. *Reduced size of the cleft maxilla.* In conventional complete denture prosthodontics, edentulous maxillae tend to become both smaller and narrower in all dimensions than the edentulous mandible. As previously explained, dentate cleft maxillae tend to be considerably smaller proportionally than do more normal-sized mandible. This is due to the lack of downward and forward growth of the cleft maxillae. With complete edentulism, this arch disparity becomes even greater (Fig 6-41a).
2. *Excessive interarch space.* Because of the reduced downward and forward growth of the maxillae, cleft patients often have an excessive interocclusal distance. If the patient is edentulous, this disparity is even more significant. This means the denture teeth must be positioned a considerable distance both laterally and inferiorly from the maxillary foundation area, and a Class III tooth relationship is not uncommon.
3. *Lack of a bony palate.* In a noncleft patient, the bony palate and alveolar ridge add to the support and stability of the complete denture, especially in square and ovoid arches. These attributes are eliminated by the lack of a bony palate in cleft palate patients (Fig 6-41b and c).

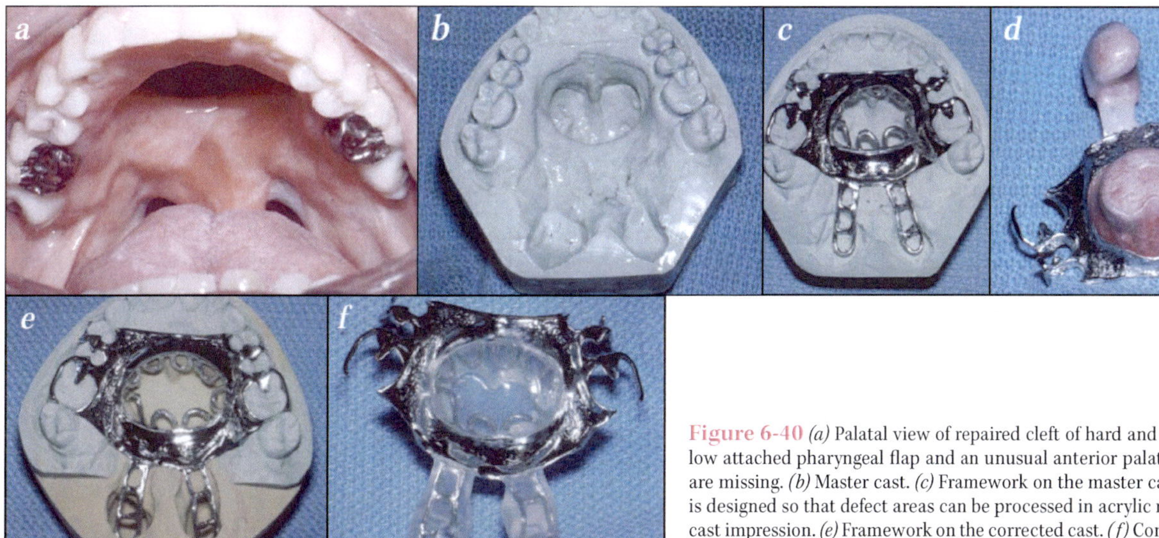

Figure 6-40 *(a)* Palatal view of repaired cleft of hard and soft palates with a low attached pharyngeal flap and an unusual anterior palatal defect. No teeth are missing. *(b)* Master cast. *(c)* Framework on the master cast. The framework is designed so that defect areas can be processed in acrylic resin. *(d)* Corrected cast impression. *(e)* Framework on the corrected cast. *(f)* Completed prosthesis. Clear acrylic resin permits visualization of possible areas of pressure (courtesy of Dr. Eleni Roumanas, Los Angeles, CA).

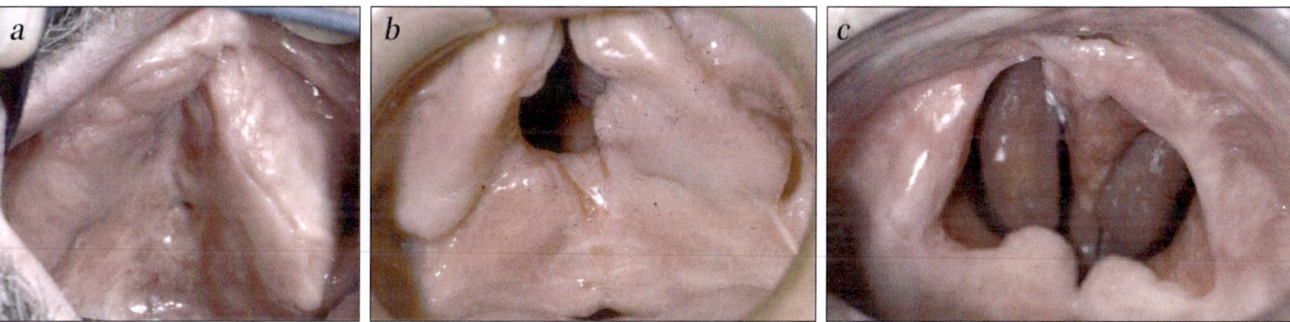

Figure 6-41 Edentulous cleft lip and palate patients. *(a)* Arch collapse and small fistula in posterior palatal seal area. *(b)* Resected premaxilla with large fistula and limited alveolar ridge development. *(c)* Small alveolar ridge with large fistula.

4. *Poor alveolar ridge development and shallow depth of the palate.* Primarily because of the lack of vertical growth, edentulous maxillary alveolar ridges are usually not well developed and the palatal vault may be rather shallow. These conditions will compromise both stability and support of the maxillary complete denture for the edentulous cleft palate patient.
5. *Scarring from lip closure.* Surgical closure of the lip in infancy predisposes the patient to significant and unyielding scar bands in various configurations in the labial vestibule. This scarring in turn reduces the effective depth of the labial vestibule and impairs the stability of the denture.
6. *Scarring in the posterior palatal seal area.* In patients whose palates have been successfully repaired, it may be more difficult to develop an effective posterior palatal seal because of the scarring and varying resiliencies of the residual soft palate (see Fig 6-41a).

Therefore, many of the steps necessary for fabrication of complete dentures for edentulous cleft palate patients are made more difficult for the clinician and ultimately for the patient in adapting to the new prosthesis. Most patients cannot masticate effectively with these dentures. The primary benefits are improved lip contours and aesthetics, improved speech articulation, and the ability to swallow without nasal leakage.

Consultation appointment. Before prosthodontic treatment is commenced, the prosthodontist must discuss the myriad factors related to the treatment to be rendered and the prognosis for the new dentures with the patient. Most patients with a cleft of the lip and palate will realize that they have a problem because they have been living with their condition for all their years. Yet expectations can easily become unrealistic. The prosthodontist should explain these limitations in a realistic manner.

As in conventional prosthodontics, the patient's previous experience with removable prosthesis can be revealing. A favorable history of complete denture use is very encouraging, whereas the opposite scenario is discouraging for both the patient and the clinician. Cleft patients recently rendered edentulous in the maxilla have a very guarded prognosis, especially if the arch is opposed by essentially a complete complement of natural mandibular teeth. A complete history and careful oral examination should be performed. Aspects that would be a negative factor for a noncleft patient take on added significance for cleft patients. An obturator bulb may adversely affect retention, because the additional weight and length of the extension are not centered within the confines of the complete denture.

A word of caution seems in order regarding speech. If the cleft patient is an inexperienced denture wearer, speech may deteriorate modestly with the initial placement of new dentures. Within two to three weeks the patient should begin to adapt to these new contours, and speech should gradually return to pretreatment levels. Rarely will articulation improve with the placement of new dentures.

Impressions. The clinician may use his or her customary denture impression technique for cleft lip and palate patients with only a few exceptions. The need to block out small, bony openings has already been discussed. We prefer a standard technique that includes the fabrication of a custom tray, border molding of the tray with impression compound, and a wash of light-body rubber base impression material. Rubber base material rarely fractures and tends to withdraw completely from small bony defects.

Some clinicians make the corrected impression with impression wax if there are multiple small fistulae, and the tissues are scarred and firm. Occlusal stops are necessary when this technique is used, and some clinicians favor completing the denture before the corrected impression is made.

Two areas require special consideration during border molding. First, care must be taken to avoid overextension in the maxillary labial reflex, especially in relation to the scar bands resulting from lip closure. Low-fusing impression compounds are recommended, and the cleft lip should be manipulated by hand in a downward, forward, and lateral direction several times. Second, the posterior palatal seal should be developed during border molding. The movements of the soft palate should be observed as the patient says *ah*. There may not be a sharp delineation between the immobile and mobile areas of the soft palate.

We prefer not to establish the posterior palatal seal across heavily scarred tissue but to follow the creases or folds of scar tissue in the palate. Therefore, the posterior palatal seal may have an irregular sweep across the palate. However, if the posterior margin terminates in a crease, it will be less obtrusive to the tongue.

To establish the posterior palatal seal, the impression tray is cut back to the desired terminus and the molding process is completed in a customary manner. After the impression is completed, the wash material is cut back to the posterior margin of the impression compound, and the cast is completed in a standard manner. It is helpful to scribe the posterior palatal seal in the cast while the patient is present because the resiliency of the palatal tissues will vary considerably. A posterior bead feathered slightly anteriorly is used instead of the more standard butterfly pattern. Scar tissue has the capacity to rebound if displaced and can have a negative influence on retention.

Vertical dimension of occlusion. Establishing an appropriate vertical dimension of occlusion (VDO) is critical for many edentulous cleft lip and palate patients. Unfortunately, it is difficult to give definitive guidelines for establishing the correct VDO because clinical judgment plays an important role. The clinician is faced with a dilemma in performing this task. The maximum VDO will likely create the best aesthetic arrangement, but the maxillary replacement teeth will be farther from their foundation area, compromising the stability of the denture. We prefer to locate the occlusal platform at the appropriate level for the mandibular teeth and arch and vary the vertical position of the maxillary replacement teeth and arch based on the level of retention, stability, and support available from maxillary structures. For example, if the maxillary structures have limited potential for retention, stability, and support, it is usually beneficial to close the VDO 2 to 4 mm at the incisor point. This may compromise aesthetics; during the insertion of the trial denture, input from the patient should be solicited.

The facebow record is made and the maxillary cast is mounted on the articulator. The final adjustments are made to the wax rims and a centric relation record is made. The flexibility of the upper lip should be considered when the maxillary wax rim is contoured because lip flexibility will vary.

Try-in. If aesthetics is a major concern, the clinician should consider arranging the 12 anterior denture teeth in the operatory while the patient is present. If this tooth arrangement is not satisfactory for either party, consideration should be given to increasing the VDO slightly. If this is done, it is best to make a new centric relation record and remount the mandibular cast. A second try-in appointment should be scheduled to verify both aesthetics and centric relation and to make a protrusive record.

The second try-in appointment is an excellent time to make subtle adjustments in the anterior tooth arrangement related to repair of the cleft lip. The lips tend to frame the anterior arrangement, so if abnormalities in the upper lip are apparent, subtle changes in the tooth arrangement or denture base contours may enhance aesthetic harmony. Because clefts of the lip correspond to the maxillary lateral incisors, most of these adjustments will be related to the replacement lateral incisors or the denture base in this area.

If the denture teeth are set to a relatively even or flat occlusal plane, this arrangement will accentuate slight lip discrepancies. Sometimes scar contracture occurs linearly along the line of the lip scar, so contracture will produce a slight notch in the lip opposite the lateral incisor. If the lateral incisor is raised slightly above the occlusal plane (not an unusual position for the lateral incisor), the irregularity in the lip may be less noticeable.

On occasion, the protruding scar of the upper lip can be made less conspicuous by removing wax from the future denture base. Sometimes moving the lateral incisor slightly lingually will also help. The elevation of the upper lip during smiling, especially for patients with a repaired unilateral cleft lip, should be observed during try-in. Lip elevation may be limited in many cleft patients because of scarring. Adjustments to the future denture base may improve smile harmony. Although these changes are minor, they do improve patient acceptance of the prosthesis, especially if the patient is involved in the decision-making process.

Because of the smaller maxillary edentulous arch, the potential maxillomandibular discrepancies, and the need for rather bulky wax rims, the clinician is often forced to manage two unstable record bases during the recording of VDO and centric relation. Consequently, it is sometimes advisable to scribe the posterior palatal seal and to process the permanent maxillary record base or bases prior to the appointment for maxillomandibular relation records. This will give the clinician the advantage of a more stable record base during this important step. The denture teeth are then processed to these bases (Oh and Roumanas, 2007).

Delivery and adjustment. The complete dentures are processed and delivered in the customary manner. Both laboratory and clinical remounts are used to finalize the occlusion. Thin projections of acrylic resin that extend into the residual cleft are removed and smoothed. Rarely will leakage occur as a result of this maneuver. Disclosing wax is quite effective for relieving the denture base in the labial reflex to accommodate the scar band. Prior to dismissal of the patient, it is advisable to discuss the limitations

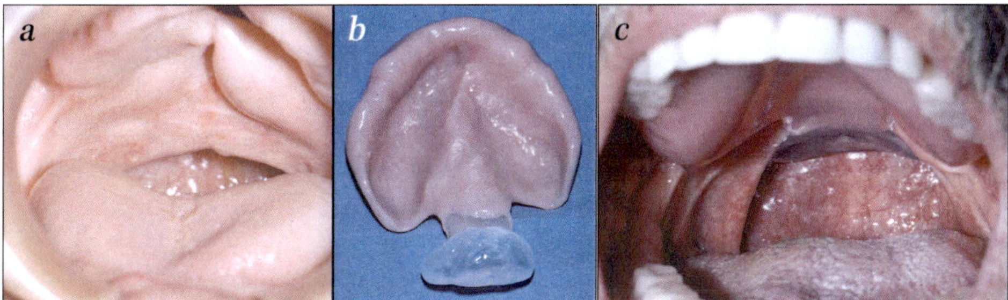

Figure 6-42 *(a)* Edentulous patient with a repaired cleft and an anterior fistula. *(b)* Denture with soft palate obturator added. *(c)* Prosthesis in position. The contour of the soft palate obturator extension is concave to allow for proper tongue elevation during speech and swallowing.

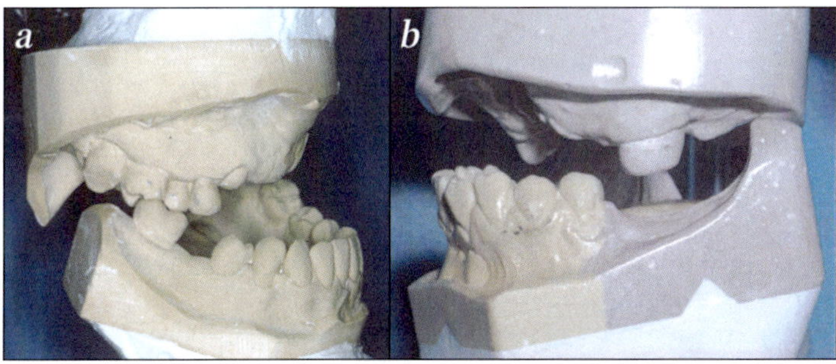

Figure 6-43 *(a and b)* Typical mountings of cleft patients who lacked the benefit of needed orthodontic care, resulting in loss of the premaxilla.

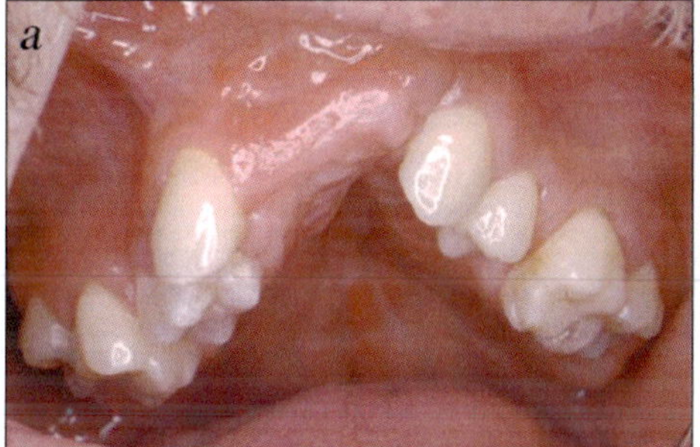

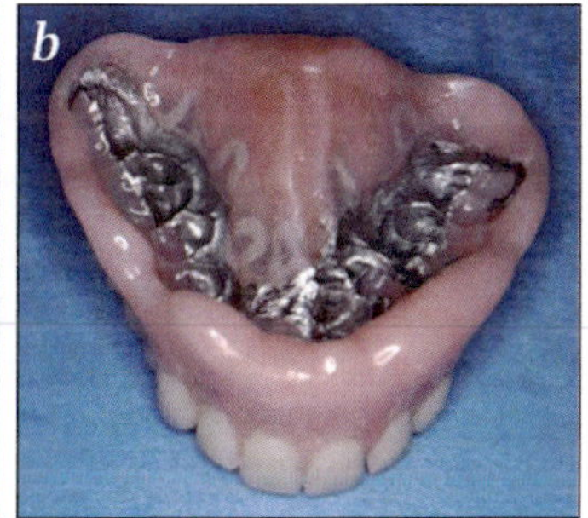

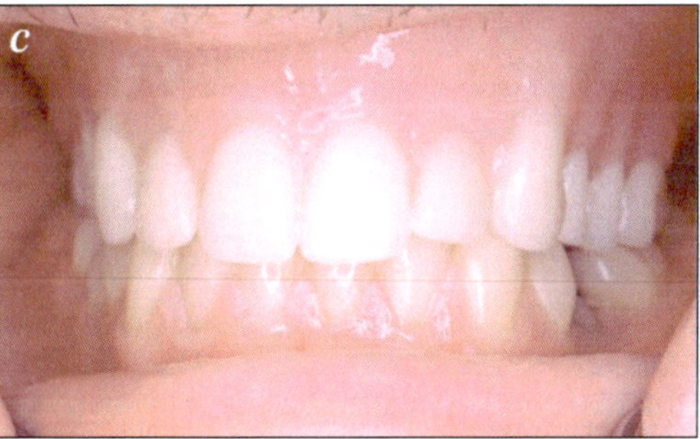

Figure 6-44 *(a)* Bilateral cleft lip and palate with anterior open bite and reduced VDO. Oral hygiene is excellent. *(b)* Overdenture with internal chrome-cobalt framework and retainers. Note the thickness of the labial flange. *(c)* Completed prosthesis.

and expectations for the dentures again. The patient should be scheduled for subsequent recall appointments.

If an obturator is to be attached to the maxillary complete or partial denture, attachment may take place at two different times (Fig 6-42). If the patient has never used an obturator, we prefer to delay its fabrication until the patient has accommodated to the denture (about four to six weeks). If the patient has an existing obturator, the new obturator must be completed prior to delivery of the prosthesis. A wire loop for retention of the obturator segment is attached with wax at the second try-in appointment and checked for position. After the completed dentures are adjusted and the occlusion is refined, the obturator is developed with impression compound and impression wax. The dentures are then delivered at a subsequent appointment.

As discussed in Chapter 4, rarely will speech be markedly improved by the addition of an obturator for adult patients. Nasal resonance and fluid leakage will be reduced, but long-standing articulatory errors will remain.

Single maxillary complete dentures. Single maxillary complete dentures for cleft patients will be a challenge for both the dentist and the patient because of the reduced size of the edentulous maxilla and the difficulty in establishing a reasonable occlusion with the proportionally much larger mandible. Maxillary teeth are often lost at various times and sometimes without replacement. Therefore, the opposing mandibular teeth will often exhibit varying degrees of extrusion and realignment.

The modified Meyer technique (Meyer, 1959) for a single maxillary denture is excellent for establishing a functional occlusion with irregularly positioned mandibular teeth. A bilateral posterior crossbite is not uncommon. Plane of occlusion discrepancies can be addressed with selective crown placement, enameloplasty, or removable partial denture frameworks overlying the dentition in selected areas.

Maxillary overlay dentures. As mentioned previously, although mandibular growth is essentially normal in cleft patients, maxillary growth is restricted in a downward and forward vector when the cleft involves both the primary and the secondary palates. Therefore, some adult patients with cleft lip and palate will exhibit a restricted maxillary arch with an anterior open bite, especially if orthodontic treatment was either not instituted or unsuccessful and/or if the anterior teeth in the premaxilla were lost at a relatively early age (Figs 6-43 and 6-44). Because of these growth deficiencies, some adult patients are candidates for various forms of overlay dentures that may be supported either by the remaining

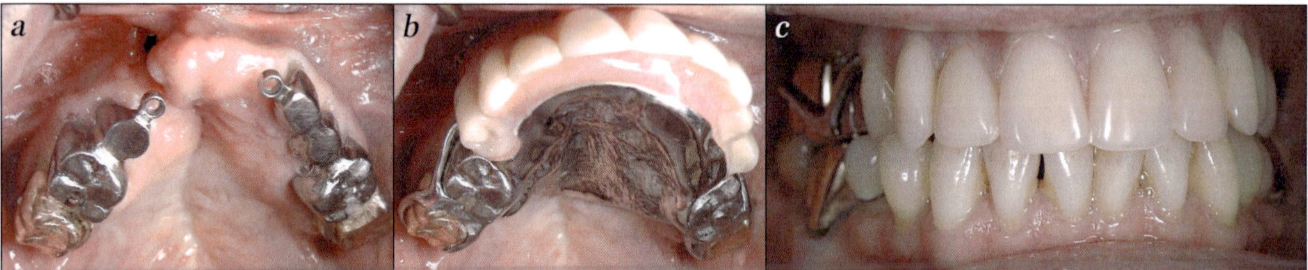

Figure 6-45 Overlay removable partial dentures. *(a)* The patient presents with a collapsed maxilla and a small fistula anteriorly. Velopharyngeal function is normal. Complete veneer crowns are splinted in each segment, and resilient attachments are attached on the mesial side. *(b and c)* An overlay prosthesis restores the premolar occlusion and provides lip support and anterior aesthetics.

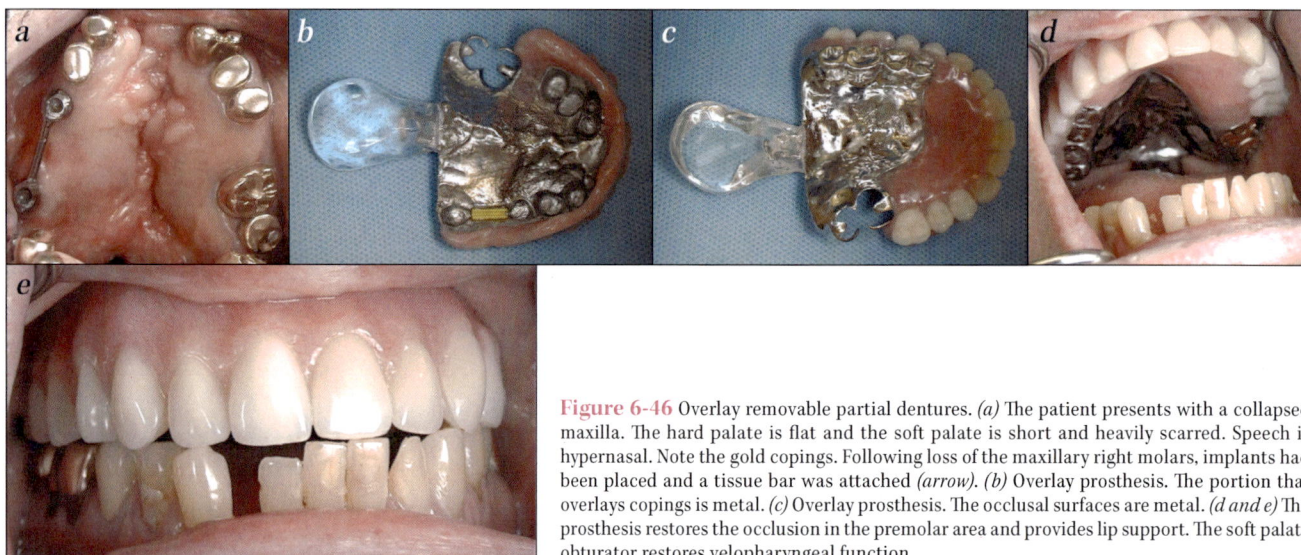

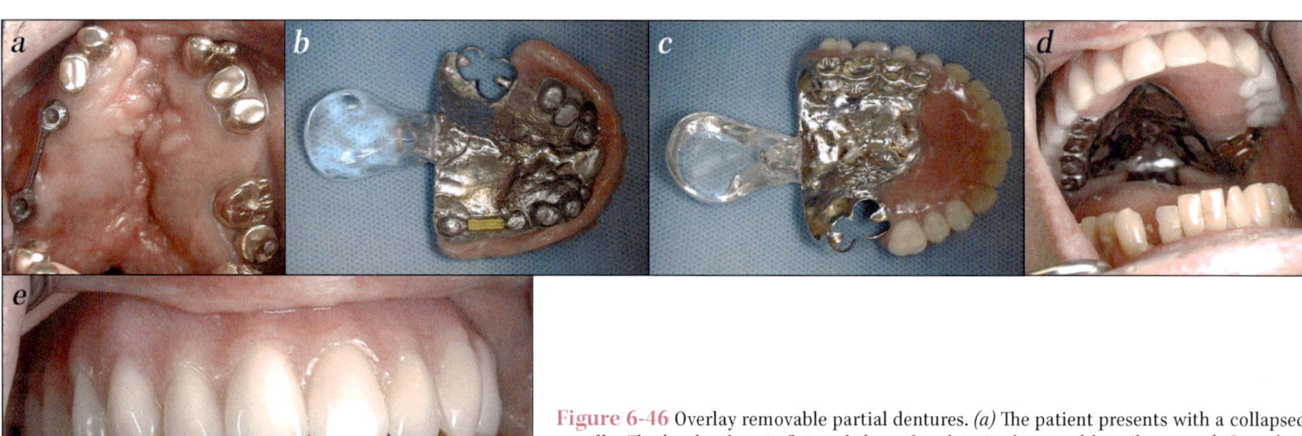

Figure 6-46 Overlay removable partial dentures. *(a)* The patient presents with a collapsed maxilla. The hard palate is flat and the soft palate is short and heavily scarred. Speech is hypernasal. Note the gold copings. Following loss of the maxillary right molars, implants had been placed and a tissue bar was attached *(arrow)*. *(b)* Overlay prosthesis. The portion that overlays copings is metal. *(c)* Overlay prosthesis. The occlusal surfaces are metal. *(d and e)* The prosthesis restores the occlusion in the premolar area and provides lip support. The soft palate obturator restores velopharyngeal function.

teeth (Figs 6-44 and 6-45) or by a combination of remaining teeth and implants (Fig 6-46).

One type of overlay denture, or more appropriately an overlay removable partial denture, is common and reflects this vector of deficient downward and forward growth and development. When few teeth remain in the adult maxillae, they are usually posterior teeth. This is the reverse of the situation in noncleft patients. The occlusion in adults with cleft lip and palate may be limited to posterior molar contact.

If the interocclusal distance seems excessive and if the VDO is overclosed, an improved VDO can be established by placement of crowns on selected molars in occlusal contact (see Fig 6-45a). In addition, solid occlusal stops are created and crown contours can be made ideal for the overlay removable partial denture, which will cover the remaining maxillary teeth and reestablish occlusal contact with the mandibular teeth. If interocclusal space is limited posteriorly, metal occlusal surfaces on the overlay partial denture may be considered (see Fig 6-46c and d). A clinical remount is required.

The portion of the overlay denture in direct contact with the dentition should never be made of acrylic resin. The porous resin harbors multitudes of microorganisms and as a result the overlaid dentition will soon become carious despite good oral hygiene. The risk of caries of the overlaid dentition will be substantially reduced if the portion of the prosthesis that overlays the dentition is fabricated in metal (see Fig 6-46b). Another approach is to place gold copings on the teeth to be overlaid (see Fig 6-46a). Good oral hygiene and patient compliance are essential, and the importance of attending periodic recall visits must be stressed to the patient.

Osseointegrated implants. Osseointegrated implants are of immense value for those with cleft lip and palate, particularly edentulous or partially edentulous patients. In edentulous patients they enhance stability, retention, and support of the prosthesis to enable significant improvement of masticatory performance. In most edentulous patients only posterior sites are available, and the bone volume of the implant sites may be compromised because of the floor of the nose or an enlarged maxillary sinus. However, in these patients, often the cortical layers of bone are more prominent, and the trabecular pattern is relatively dense. Short implant lengths such as 7 to 8 mm, which are generally not used in conventional patients, can be used with reasonable success in cleft patients.

Regardless of the success rates, however, we almost always recommend implants be attempted because of the significant functional benefits derived from a successful outcome. In addition, the so-called microroughened implant surfaces are much more bioreactive than the original machined surfaces and probably will be more successful when sites lack ideal bone volumes (Ogawa et al., 2002; Ogawa and Nishimura, 2003, 2006; Nishimura et al., 2007). Nevertheless, tissue bar designs should be implant assisted rather than

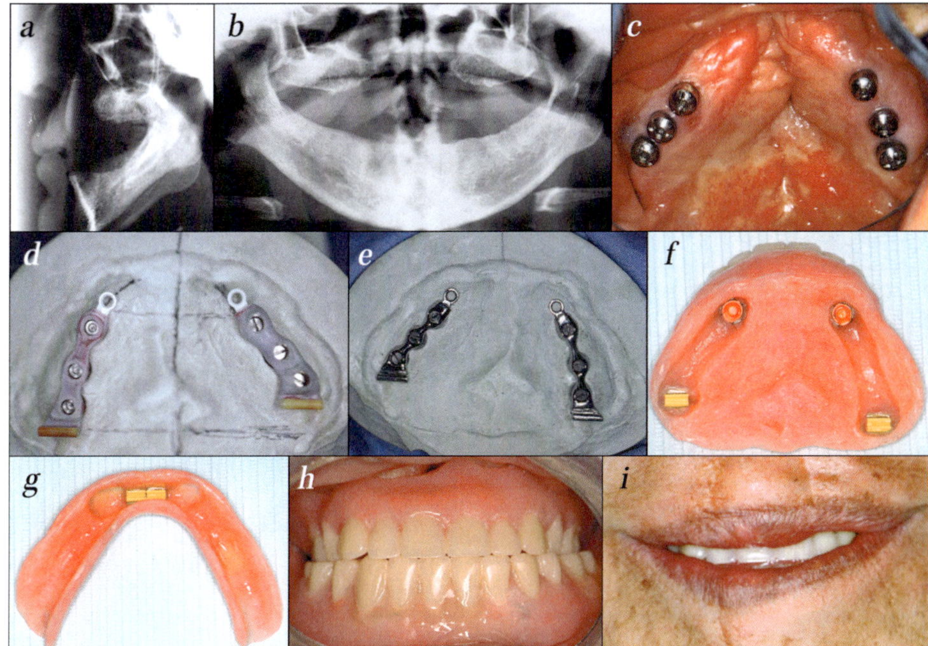

Figure 6-47 *(a)* The premaxillary segment is missing and the cleft has not been reconstructed with a bone graft. There is a profound Class III maxillomandibular relationship. *(b)* Significant bone volume is present in the posterior segments. *(c)* Three implants have been placed in each side. *(d and e)* Implant-assisted tissue bar design. The bar is designed as an anterior extension. When occlusal loads are applied anteriorly, resilient attachments positioned anteriorly permit the prosthesis to rotate around the Hader attachments posteriorly, thereby limiting cantilever forces. *(f and g)* Completed implant-assisted overlay dentures. *(h)* Dentures inserted. *(i)* Final aesthetics. An Abbe flap has been used to provide additional tissue to the upper lip.

implant supported so that the available denture-bearing tissues can be used to maximum advantage to provide appropriate support.

The case of a typical edentulous cleft patient is presented in Fig 6-47. The patient's premaxillary segment had been removed at an early age. Although the cleft has been closed, it had not been bone grafted. Following the loss of the remaining teeth, the patient was fitted with conventional complete dentures. The maxillary denture foundation area was severely compromised, and the maxillary denture was quite unstable and lacked retention. The patient had a profound Class III maxillomandibular relationship (see Fig 6-47a).

Ample bone was available in the residual posterior palatal segments and the mandible (see Fig 6-47b) for placement of osseointegrated implants. Six implants were placed in the two posterior palatal segments (see Fig 6-47c) and two into the mandibular symphysis region. Implant-assisted tissue bar designs were used for both prostheses (see Fig 6-47d–i). The tissue bars in the maxilla were not splinted together. Because the cleft had not been reconstructed with a bone graft, the two residual posterior palatal segments would move independently of one another during function. Splinting the two together with a tissue bar would have exposed the implants to undesirable forces that could compromise their long-term survival.

Implant overload precipitates a resorptive remodeling response of bone anchoring the implants (Hoshaw et al., 1994; Barbier and Schepers, 1997; Miyata et al., 1998; Miyata et al., 2000; Hietz-Mayfield et al., 2004). Because the bone volumes are minimal and the implants are short in most cleft patients, the biomechanics of designs used for the tissue bars must be considered carefully. The two maxillary tissue bars for this patient were designed like an anterior extension removable partial denture (see Fig 6-47d and e). The two Hader bar segments posteriorly functioned like occlusal rests and served as the axis of rotation when occlusal forces were applied anterior to the tissue bars. The resilient attachments anteriorly permitted this rotation but also provided retention.

As is the case for most edentulous cleft patients, the small size of the maxilla relative to the mandible dictated that the posterior teeth be set in crossbite. An Abbe flap was used to supplement the tissues of the upper lip (see Fig 6-47i).

Zygoma implants. If alveolar bone volume is insufficient, another option to consider would be the placement of implants in the zygoma (zygomaticus implants). Zygoma implants, 30 to 50 mm long, have been employed successfully in edentulous patients with large maxillectomy or total palatectomy defects. Schmidt et al. (2004) reported on 28 zygomatic implants placed in 9 patients with large maxillary defects following surgical resection of advanced maxillary or paranasal sinus tumors. Landes et al. (2009) reported on the use of 36 zygomaticus implants in 15 patients, 12 of whom had presented after resection of large tumors of the maxilla and 3 of whom presented with congenital defects.

A 34-year-old recent immigrant presented to the UCSF Center for Craniofacial Anomalies with an unrepaired cleft palate (Fig 6-48a). She was edentulous in both arches. Based on previous success, this patient was treated with zygomaticus implants (Schmidt et al., 2004; Fig 6-48b). After the implants had integrated (Fig 6-48c), an implant-supported tissue bar was fabricated (Fig 6-48d and e). An overlay denture with a soft palate obturator extension was fabricated using traditional methods. The implant-supported tissue bar provided retention, stability, and support for the prosthesis and ensured optimal positioning of the soft palate obturator during speech and swallowing (Fig 6-48f and g).

Implants in grafted alveolar cleft sites. In patients with congenitally missing lateral incisors, implants can be placed after alveolar cleft bone grafting. The timing of implant placement following bone grafting is influenced by the type of bone used for the graft, the developmental stage of the dentition, and the anticipated healing and consolidation of the graft in the alveolar cleft. It is generally accepted that osseous healing of transplants is completed six months after surgery (Jia et al., 2006). The timing between

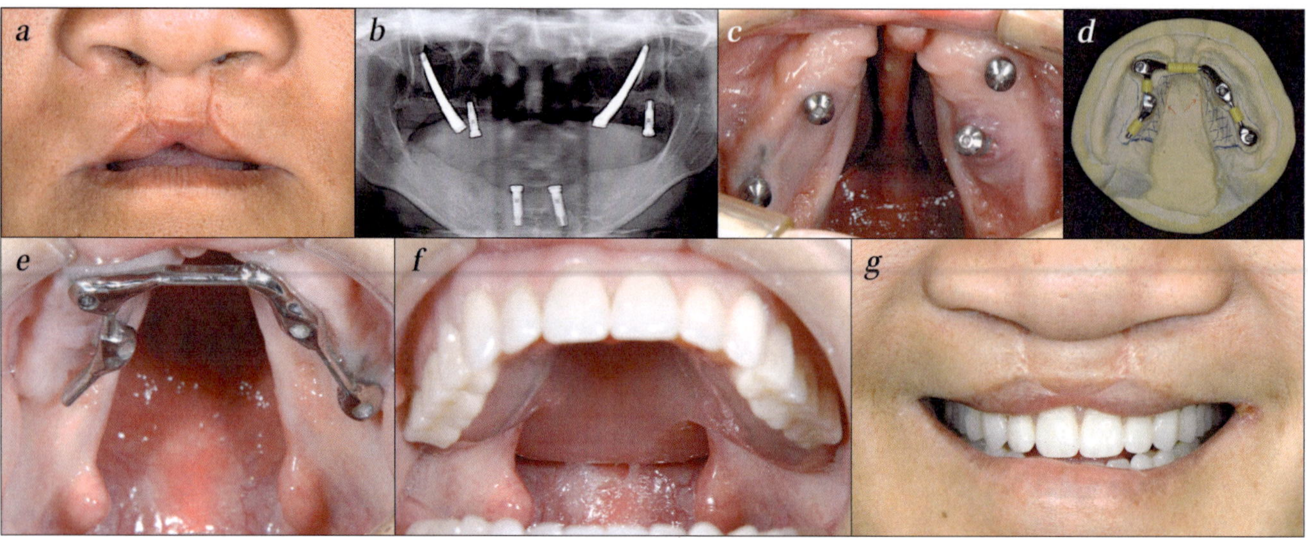

Figure 6-48 *(a)* Edentulous patient with repaired bilateral cleft. *(b and c)* Four implants have been placed in the maxilla: two conventional and two zygomaticus. *(d)* Implant-supported tissue bar on cast. *(e)* Tissue bar placed intraorally. *(f)* Prosthesis with obturator extension in place. *(g)* Final result.

secondary bone grafting and implant placement appears to be an important determinant of implant success or failure (Kearns et al., 1997; Takahashi et al., 1999; Kramer et al., 2005; Matsui et al., 2007).

Alveolar grafting of clefts is often completed sequentially: An initial graft is completed when the patient is between 8 and 11 years of age to help hold the space. The cleft is then often regrafted when the patient is aged 15 to 17 years with autogenous bone from the retromolar area or mental symphysis. The implant is placed four to six months after regrafting. Implants are not usually placed in young patients, because the implant acts as an ankylosed tooth and may become submerged during the rapid growth phase of adolescence (Sharma and Vargervik, 2006).

Patients with alveolar clefts are usually missing the permanent lateral incisor on the side of the cleft. During orthodontic treatment, it is decided whether the lateral space should be restored prosthetically or the space should be closed. If the space is to remain, the prosthetic options include a removable partial denture, a fixed partial denture, a resin-bonded fixed partial denture, or an implant-supported single crown. The UCSF Center for Craniofacial Anomalies has conducted a prospective study (Kearns et al., 1997) to assess the feasibility of using osseointegrated implants to restore alveolar cleft sites reconstructed with bone grafts.

Use of an implant-supported restoration to replace the missing lateral incisor offers many potential advantages over previously available methods: *(1)* abutment tooth preparation is not required, decreasing the possibility of damage to the dental pulp; *(2)* increased loading of the abutment teeth is avoided; and *(3)* the implant in the alveolar cleft may transfer functional forces to the graft, which could decrease resorption of the graft. These potential benefits prompted the study to assess the success rates of osseointegrated implants placed in alveolar clefts following bone grafts.

Twenty-four patients, 15 males and 9 females, were enrolled in the study. Nine patients presented with bilateral clefts and 15 with unilateral clefts. Thirty-three implants have been placed in grafted cleft sites, and 31 of these have been restored with porcelain-fused-to-metal implant crowns. Two implants failed to integrate and were removed at stage-two surgery. Two implants failed in a patient with a bilateral cleft 4 years after implant placement. Another implant failed in a unilateral cleft site after 11 years of service. The remaining 28 implants remain in position and functional.

The follow-up times since implant placement range from 85 to 166 months (median of 130 months). The follow-up times since placement of the restoration range from 74 to 158 months (median of 121 months) for an overall success rate of 93.9 % (Sharma A, unpublished data, 2006).

Most clefts (18 of 33) presented with horizontal or vertical bone deficiencies and required additional bone grafting prior to implant placement. The remaining 15 cleft sites presented with adequate bone for implant placement (Fig 6-49). The most significant challenge was the creation of normal gingival contours. The scarring in the cleft site made this problematic in most patients (Fig 6-50). However, these altered gingival contours were of little clinical significance because the scarring associated with lip closure and grafting of the cleft site prevents most cleft patients from elevating their upper lip sufficiently to expose the gingiva to view (Fig 6-51).

As a result of this study, the UCSF team has recommended the following protocol for restoration of cleft sites:

1. Expand the maxilla orthodontically (7 to 8 years of age).
2. Close the oronasal defect by grafting the alveolar cleft (9 to 12 years of age).
3. Guide the canine into the arch and maintain space for the lateral incisor.
4. If the bone volume in the cleft is inadequate for implant placement, regraft the site.
5. Place an implant to replace the lateral incisor after growth has been completed (15 to 19 years of age).

Overall, the literature substantiates the high clinical success rates of implants placed four to six months after grafting of the alveolar sites. Kearns et al. (1999) reported a success rate of 90% in the two-stage procedure after an average follow-up of 39.1 months. Härtel et al. (1999) reported a success rate of 96% after an average time of 28 months between implantation and follow-up. Matsui et al. (2007)

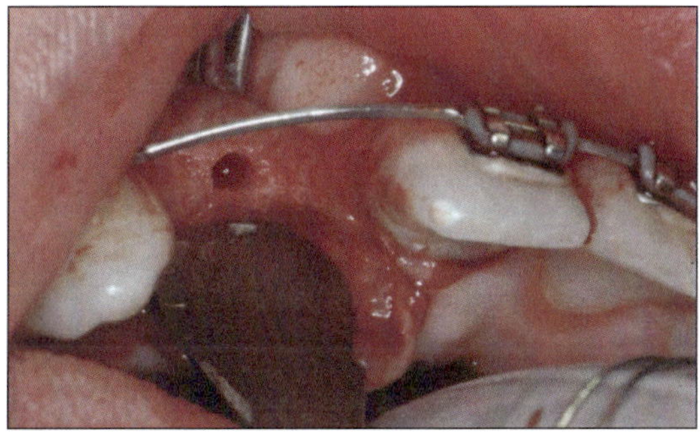

Figure 6-49 Following completion of orthodontic treatment and growth, an implant is placed in a grafted alveolus.

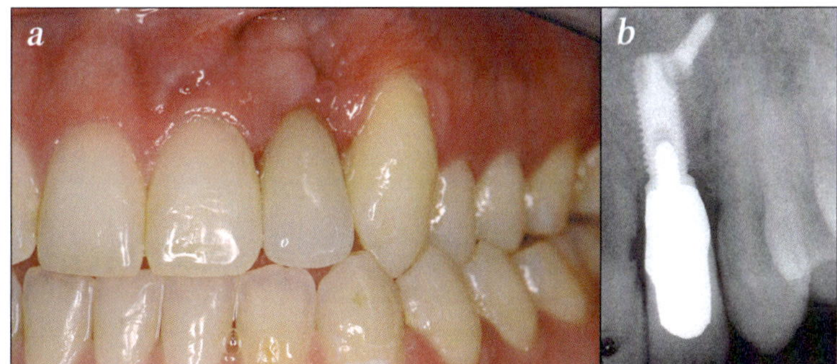

Figure 6-50 *(a and b)* Typical outcome for an implant placed in a grafted cleft site. Note the gingival contours.

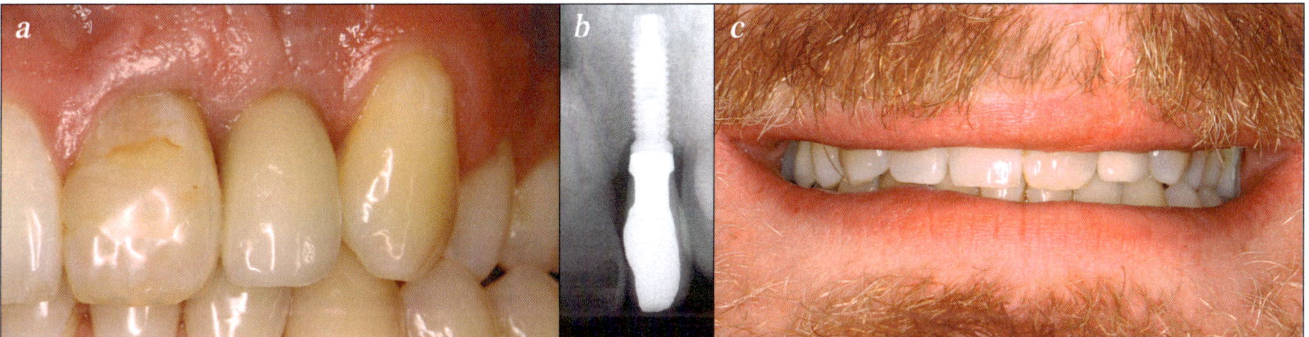

Figure 6-51 *(a and b)* Implant placed in a grafted cleft site. The central incisor is hypocalcified and gingival contours are slightly distorted. *(c)* During a high smile, these areas are not exposed to view.

reported a success rate of 98.6% in a two-stage procedure; their average follow-up time was 60 months. These results suggest that the use of dental implants in combination with an autogenous bone graft is a reliable and clinically effective alternative to the functional and psychologic inconvenience of a prosthetic appliance.

The surface coating of the implant may also play a role in the longevity of implants placed in grafted alveolar sites. In the UCSF study, the three implants that failed after loading were titanium plasma-sprayed press-fit cylindrical implants. Matsui et al. (2007) analyzed the amount of marginal bone loss around three different implant surfaces after one year of follow-up: machined titanium surface, machined surface that has been plasma sprayed, and hydroxyapatite-covered surface. The marginal bone loss was defined as the distance from the implant shoulder to the alveolar crest as measured on a radiograph.

Smooth-surfaced titanium implants had the lowest marginal bone loss among the three fixture surfaces. The average bone loss was 1.60 ± 0.87 mm for smooth-surfaced titanium implants, 2.81 ± 1.91 mm for hydroxyapatite implants, and 3.17 ± 2.30 mm for rough-surfaced titanium implants. The findings of Matsui et al. are consistent with the UCSF findings, in which the three implant failures were press-fit implants.

Treatment of Other Related Anomalies

Two other craniofacial conditions warrant a brief discussion, primarily because of their relationship to cleft palate and because they are representative of the growing interest in craniofacial anomalies. In 1976, fewer than 150 recognized syndromes had been associated with clefting, while today more than 400 have been identified. As a result of this expanded interest, the American Cleft Palate Association has become the American Cleft Palate–Craniofacial Association, and their journal is now the *Cleft Palate–Craniofacial Journal*. In addition, most departments previously named *cleft palate centers* are now known as *craniofacial centers*.

The conditions that will be discussed are *(1)* submucous cleft palate (SMCP) and a variant and related condition, occult submucous cleft palate (OSMCP), and *(2)* Robin sequence (Pierre Robin syndrome). Patients with SMCP and OSMCP have cleft-like symptoms such as hypernasality without overt clefts of the palate, whereas infants with Robin sequence have an interesting triad of anomalies that include a cleft of the hard and soft palates. The primary treatment of choice for both patient groups is surgery, so the indications for prosthetic treatment are limited for either patient group.

Submucous cleft palate and occult submucous cleft palate

SMCP and OSMCP are related both to each other and to cleft lip and palate (Kono et al., 1981) but do not include overt clefting of the palate per se. Patients with SMCP are identified by the triad of a bifid uvula, midline muscular diastasis (zona pellucida), and a notch or other alterations in the contour of the posterior margin of the hard palate (Fig 6-52; Calnan, 1954). The bifid uvula can be detected as

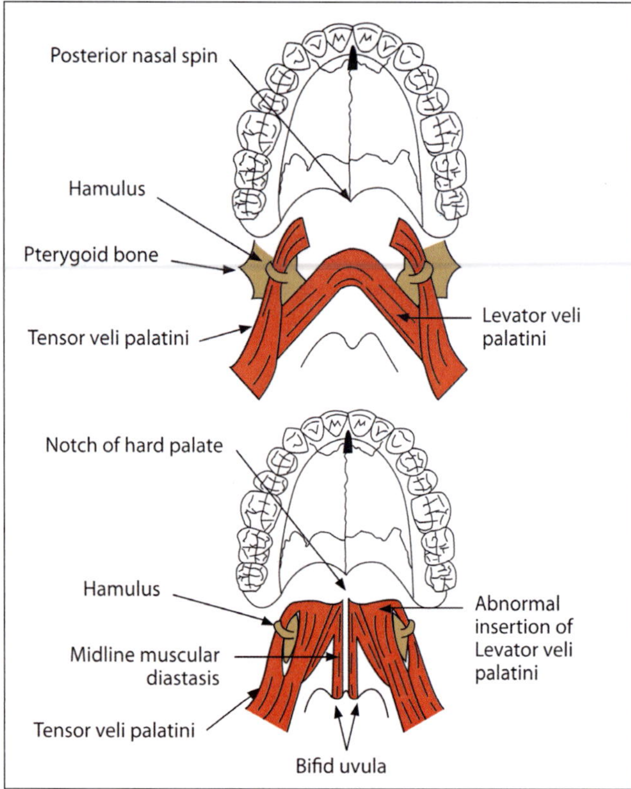

Figure 6-52 SMCP. *(a)* Normal anatomical contours of the soft palate. The levator sling is formed by the anastomosis of levator veli palatini muscles. *(b)* Triad of anatomical abnormalities associated with SMCP: bifid uvula, midline muscular diastasis of the soft palate resulting from abnormal insertion of the levator veil palatini and notching of the hard palate. Several anatomical variations of the levator muscles are possible, such as partial insertion into the hard palate and/or partial anastomosis across the palate.

the SMCP patient says *ah*, and the contour changes of the posterior margin of the hard palate can be detected by palpation.

Patients with OSMCP exhibit only muscular diastasis of the levator veli palatini or hypoplasia of the musculus uvulae, which is responsible for the hypernasality (Kaplan, 1975; Croft et al., 1978; Lewin et al., 1980; Trier, 1983). A careful oral examination will usually reveal the possibility of SMCP, whereas the same examination process may not detect any anatomical limitations of the apparently intact hard and soft palates for patients with OSMCP.

Rarely can muscular diastasis of the levator veli palatini be detected by oral examination, and certainly hypoplasia of the musculus uvulae cannot be detected orally. Multiview videofluoroscopy and/or nasal endoscopy examination are necessary to confirm hypoplasia of the musculus uvulae because these paired muscles occupy the central portion of the nasal surface of the soft palate. On occasion, when the levator veli palatini are aberrantly attached to the posterior margin of the hard palate and do not anastomose and form the levator sling, the clinician may note a pale, bluish cast to the midline of the soft palate that results from the lack of normal musculature beneath the oral mucosa (Fig 6-53). This clinical sign, plus the presence of a bifid uvula and hard palate notch, should lead the clinician to strongly suspect SMCP.

The primary motivating factor for parents to seek consultation and treatment for their child is the development of hypernasal speech, which is caused by velopharyngeal dysfunction as the result of muscular diastasis of the levator veli palatini or hypoplasia of the musculus uvulae. Therefore, it is not uncommon for either of these conditions to go undetected until a child begins speaking.

Normally, the levator veli palatini will insert and anastomose with its counterpart across the medial aponeurosis of the soft palate and posterior to the hard palate border, forming the so-called levator sling. As the normal levators contract, they elevate and retract the central third of the soft palate and, at the same time, move the lateral pharyngeal walls medially to facilitate velopharyngeal closure and create the typical "knee" appearance of the soft palate seen in lateral radiographic projection during closure. With diastasis of the levator veli palatini muscles, at least a portion of each levator muscle inserts instead into the posterior border of the hard palate lateral to the midline. Consequently, the levator sling either does not form or is incompletely formed, and velopharyngeal dysfunction and hypernasal speech result.

The musculus uvulae contribute to velopharyngeal closure, especially with circular closure patterns (see Chapter 4; Croft et al., 1978; Lewin et al., 1980). With hypoplasia of their musculus uvulae and the subsequent lack of development of the velar eminence on the nasal surface of the soft palate, patients with OSMCP also develop hypernasal speech.

Bifid uvula and changes in the bony configuration of the posterior margin of the hard palate have only limited influence on speech problems associated with SMCP. Wharton and Mowrer (1992) examined 709 elementary schoolchildren for bifid uvula. They found that 16 (2.26%) had a bifid uvula. However, only 2 (0.3%) of the children had a full-length uvular cleft and none of the 16 children with bifid uvulae exhibited hypernasality.

The role of the contour changes associated with the posterior border of the hard palate (palatine bones) is undetermined at the present time. As stated previously, the midline notch and/or the absence of the posterior nasal spine can often be palpated. On occasion the posterior margin of the hard palate will exhibit a more U-shaped contour rather than the standard butterfly pattern of the palatine bones. This change in contour would tend to shorten the overall length of the hard palate and thus possibly indirectly shorten the velum because of its more anterior attachment to the shortened hard palate. Kaplan (1975) noted this tendency for a shorter hard palate during surgical treatment for OSMCP.

There is a broad spectrum in the severity of the stigmata associated with both SMCP and OSMCP. The critical assessment is the degree of hypernasality during speech production. If speech is normal or nearly normal, surgical treatment is rarely indicated. Unfortunately, the opposite scenario is also true. If the degree of hypernasality is pervasive, maturity or intensive speech therapy rarely will improve speech or reduce hypernasality.

Some children with SMCP or OSMCP display other symptoms that mimic symptoms in patients with cleft lip and palate, such as middle ear infections and subsequent hearing loss, short hard or soft palate or deep nasopharynx, and a generalized maxillary hypoplasia. Kaplan (1975) suggested that clefts of the secondary palate, SMCP, and OSMCP are "variations of the same embryologic disorder" in a "continuous spectrum of muscle malformation and actual clefting." Trier (1983) suggested that more than 90% of patients with velopharyngeal incompetency without overt cleft of the palate have a microform of cleft palate.

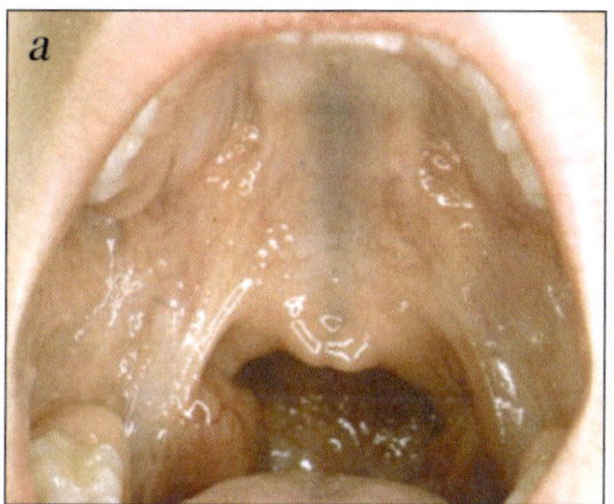

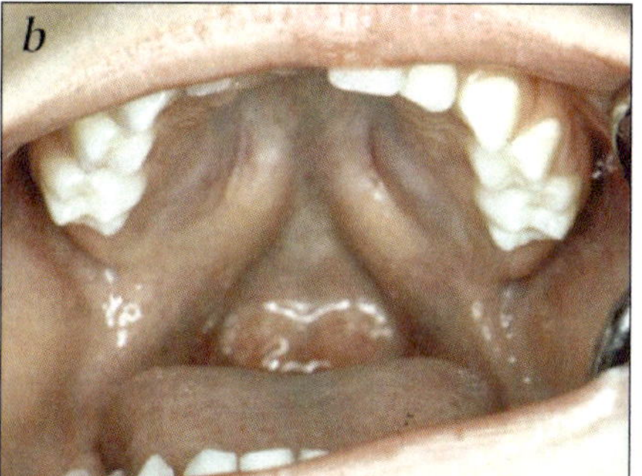

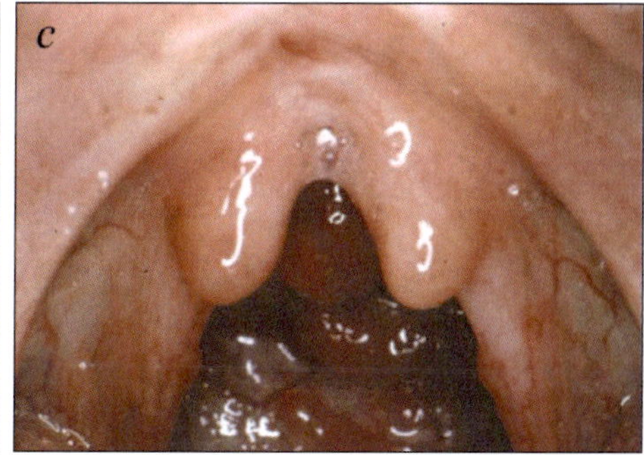

Figure 6-53 SMCP. *(a)* Muscular diastasis of the central soft palate. Note the bluish cast. *(b)* Levator veli palatini during contraction. They insert into the hard palate instead of forming the levator sling. *(c)* Bifid uvula (courtesy of Dr. Karin Vargervik, San Francisco, CA).

A study by Kono et al. (1981) offers some support for these theories. They examined 71 patients with clefts confined to the primary palate (lip and alveolus) for SMCP and OSMCP. These investigators found that 13% of these 71 patients also exhibited the triad of stigmata associated with SMCP. In addition, these 13 patients exhibited other symptoms associated with cleft palate such as hypernasality, middle ear disease, and so forth. The authors suggested that any patient with a cleft confined to the primary palate should always receive a thorough examination for SMCP or OSMCP.

The incidence of SMCP and OSMCP is unknown at the present time because only symptomatic patients with hypernasal speech are referred to craniofacial centers for diagnosis and treatment. Kaplan (1975) examined 240 patients with velopharyngeal incompetence without cleft lip and palate. He found 41 patients with classic overt SMCP and 23 patients with OSMCP among this group of patients. Lewin et al. examined 131 patients without cleft lip and palate, but with velopharyngeal insufficiency, with a nasal endoscope. Of this number, 57 were diagnosed with SMCP, 24 with other neurologic or functional disabilities, and 29 with OSMCP caused by hypoplasia of the musculus uvulae (see Chapter 4 for more details regarding this study).

Symptomatic patients with obvious hypernasality should be treated surgically with a combination of procedures that includes a palatal pushback, a levator muscle reconstruction to reestablish the levator sling, and a superiorly based pharyngeal flap that is inserted into the raw surface of the nasal surface of the soft palate. Kaplan (1975) reported significant speech improvement postoperatively in patients treated with this approach. However, McWilliams (1991) cautioned that surgery is indicated only for patients with demonstrable hypernasality. Among a group of 130 noncleft patients at the Pittsburgh Cleft Palate–Craniofacial Center, 44% of these patients remained asymptomatic into early adulthood and never required surgery. She cautioned that patients with SMCP should not be repaired surgically in infancy unless they exhibit significant feeding problems or unremitting ear disease. Surgery should never be performed on an infant based on the theoretical possibility of the potential effect on speech.

Rarely is prosthodontic treatment indicated for patients with SMCP or OSMCP unless motor or sensory deficits are also associated with the soft palate. Under these circumstances, a palatal lift prosthesis (see Chapter 4) would be indicated, because of the length and position of the anatomically normal appearing palate.

On occasion, persistent hypernasality and either SMCP or OSMCP is diagnosed following a routine tonsillectomy or adenoidectomy in a "normal" patient. The adenoids masked the problem as the intact but compromised soft palate was able to close against the protruding adenoidal pads. Many times, a careful history will reveal feeding problems or persistent middle ear infections and hearing loss during infancy. Therefore, Shprintzen et al. (1985) cautioned that any patient with a bifid uvula or any other marker should be carefully examined for SMCP or OSMCP to avoid the potential for unexpected future problems.

Robin sequence (Pierre Robin syndrome)

The Robin sequence was named after the French stomatologist, Pierre Robin, who first described the triad of anomalies consisting of micrognathia, U-shaped cleft palate, and upper airway obstruction in newborns in 1923 and 1934 (Shprintzen, 1992). Presently the preferred term is *Robin sequence*, because a *sequence* is defined dysmorphologically as multiple anomalies all or some of which are caused by one of the primary anomalies. In contrast, a *syndrome* is caused by a single pathogenesis. In Robin sequence, the mandibular micrognathia secondarily precipitates the development of both the U-shaped cleft palate and the upper airway obstruction, but the mandibular abnormalities may have multiple etiologies (Shprintzen, 1992; Sadewitz, 1992).

The interrelationship between the micrognathic and retrognathic mandible and cleft palate and upper airway obstruction is interesting. It is postulated that the micrognathic mandible forces the embryonic tongue into a superior and more retruded position, which in turn interferes with the midline fusion of the developing palatal shelves (described earlier) during the 7th to 11th weeks of gestation. The retruded mandible is also indirectly responsible for obstruction of the upper airway because the attachment of the tongue to the retrognathic mandible is more posterior than normal. The tongue tends to retrude back into the oral pharynx and blocks the airway through its contact with the posterior and lateral pharyngeal walls. This retropositioning of the tongue is called *glossoptosis*. However, not all newborns with micrognathia will exhibit upper airway obstruction, and the degree of compromise can be quite variable. A thorough pediatric examination is always indicated under these circumstances because there are other causes of infant airway obstruction (Sher, 1992; Singer and Sidoti, 1992). A nasal endoscopic examination is useful to verify the degree of upper airway obstruction.

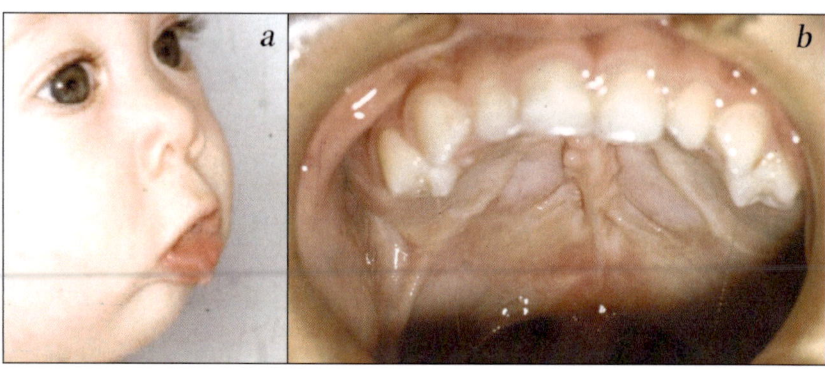

Figure 6-54 *(a)* Patient with Robin sequence at one year of age. Note the retrognathic mandible. *(b)* Palate after closure at age two years six months.

Not only is this triad of anomalies interrelated by cause and effect, but Robin sequence is also related to other primary syndromic conditions. Shprintzen (1992) examined and reviewed the records of 100 children diagnosed with Robin sequence based on the presence of micrognathia, U-shaped cleft palate, and upper airway obstruction. Only 17 of these patients could be diagnosed as nonsyndromic Robin sequence (without other anomalies). Therefore, 83 patients had associated anomalies other than the Robin triad. Stickler syndrome, which occurred in 34 patients of this sample, was by far the most commonly associated syndrome. Stickler syndrome is characterized by myopia, retinal detachment, flat midface, prominent joints with a tendency toward degenerative joint disease, and other abnormalities in addition to the Robin sequence triad.

Airway maintenance is the primary concern in newborns with Robin sequence; these stigmata have the potential to be fatal. Therefore, the infant must be monitored continuously during the first few days and weeks. If the obstructive apnea is not life threatening, less invasive techniques such as prone positioning of the infant and nasopharyngeal and endotracheal tubes are employed initially. The tubes will temporarily maintain the patency of the airway.

If the apnea is or becomes life threatening, a surgical glossopexy procedure is performed to reposition the tongue forward. The tongue tip is surgically attached to the anterior alveolar ridge and lower lip to open the airway. Many times, the attachment of the genioglossus muscle and/or lingual frenum is released at the same time to aid this forward positioning of the tongue (Argamaso, 1992).

This treatment philosophy is based on supporting the infant until mandibular growth and development correct the upper airway obstruction. If the airway and feeding problems are mitigated, many times the tongue is released when the palatal cleft is closed (when the infant is about 9 to 12 months old). LeBlanc and Golding-Kushner (1992) did not find any long-term speech problems in later years after the tongue was released. A tracheotomy, the final treatment option, was necessary in only 9 of 53 patients reviewed by Sher (1992).

Treatment during the first year is complicated by the feeding problems associated with both the cleft palate and the upper airway obstruction. As discussed previously, most infants with a cleft palate will have difficulty nursing because of the palatal opening. Airway obstruction further complicates nursing because the posterior airway obstruction may make the infant a mandatory oral breather. The newborn must pause to breathe, which prolongs feeding time and exhausts the infant. The decision regarding tube placement or surgical intervention is often made on the basis that the infant is not thriving.

A question remains regarding the progression of mandibular growth as the newborn ages. Many times, parents are informed that their child's mandible will "catch up" and have a relatively normal dimension within two years. Shprintzen (1992) cautioned that, if the mandible is intrinsically normal and the micrognathia was caused by positional constriction in utero, the mandible will have the potential to catch up and will be relatively normal at two years. However, in most instances the micrognathia is due to the Robin sequence, so the mandible will remain relatively small as the child continues to grow (Fig 6-54; Shprintzen, 1992; Sadewitz, 1992). If the child is receiving adequate nourishment, some growth does occur, and the patency of the airway improves proportionally.

In contrast, Figueroa and coworkers (1991) found that there was a partial catching up of mandibular growth. These authors conducted a longitudinal cephalometric study during the first 2 years of life of 17 infants with Robin sequence only, 26 matched infants with isolated cleft palate only, and 26 healthy infants without anomalies. They reported that patients with Robin sequence initially had a shorter mandible, narrower airway, and smaller and shorter tongue than did the healthy infants and that the hyoid position of the Robin sequence group was more posterior and inferior to that in the unaffected infants. However, mandibular growth was greater proportionally for infants with Robin sequence than in the other two groups during the first two years of life. Most of the growth occurred early, and the mandibles continued to be smaller than the mandibles of the unaffected group. Thus, there appears to be a partial catching up for patients with Robin sequence.

The incidence of Robin sequence is difficult to determine because the degree of micrognathia and upper airway obstruction may vary, so the criteria for inclusion in any study are important considerations. For example, infants with micrognathia, cleft palate, and borderline upper airway obstruction might not be included in the study unless the infant failed to thrive. Bush and Williams (1983) conducted a carefully controlled study and reported an incidence of 1 in 8,500 live births. Therefore, Robin sequence is not uncommon.

Treatment of Other Craniofacial Anomalies

A prosthodontist in a craniofacial anomalies center is often involved in the treatment of patients with other craniofacial anomalies that have restorative and prosthodontic requirements. Several craniofacial anomalies are associated with congenitally missing dentition (partial or complete anodontia) or malformed teeth. The purpose of this section is not to discuss every condition that potentially could require prosthodontic services but to discuss briefly two conditions that are not related to cleft lip and palate but may require special prosthodontic considerations.

Hemifacial microsomia

Hemifacial microsomia is a variable, progressive, and asymmetric craniofacial deformity. It involves both the skeletal and the soft tissues along with neuromuscular components of the first branchial arches. After cleft lip and palate, it is the most common congenital facial anomaly (1 in 5,600 live births; Kaban et al., 1981; Murray et al., 1984). The mechanism of development in humans is unknown, but Poswillo (1973) has described an animal phenocopy in mice. A hematoma in the area of the first and second branchial arches is produced by hemorrhage of the developing stapedial artery. The size of the hematoma and the resultant tissue destruction explain the morphology and variability of hemifacial microsomia in the experimental model.

Like cleft lip and palate, the patient with hemifacial microsomia requires interdisciplinary treatment that must be integrated by the different specialists in the craniofacial anomalies team. Treatment extends from early childhood to the late teens when growth is completed. An integrated plan that considers all aspects of this complex deformity is essential.

The patient with hemifacial microsomia has a skeletal defect that is classified by the anatomy of the mandibular ramus and the temporomandibular joint (TMJ) along with the soft tissue component. A type I skeletal deformity consists of a small mandible and TMJ. All structures are present, normal in shape and location, but small. A type II skeletal deformity consists of a small and abnormally shaped ramus and hypoplastic TMJ. This group is subdivided into types IIa and IIb. In type IIa, the TMJ hypoplasia is mild and the TMJ does not need to be replaced. In type IIb hemifacial microsomia, the TMJ is hypoplastic and medially, anteriorly, and inferiorly displaced so that a new joint must be constructed. In type III patients, the ramus and TMJ are completely absent. Because condylar growth is an integral component of normal, symmetric mandibular growth, patients with altered or absent condylar growth will exhibit various degrees of facial asymmetry based on the growth potential of the TMJ.

The soft tissue defects include a reduced bulk of subcutaneous tissue, ranging in degree from mild to severe; the degree of soft tissue deficit usually is correlated with the degree of the skeletal defect. Hypoplasia of the muscles of mastication and facial expression is quite common. The patient may have macrostomia and there may be skin tags along a line from the tragus to the commissure of the lip.

The auricular deformity was described by Meurman (1957) as follows:

Grade 1: mild hypoplasia and mild cupping but all structures present
Grade 2: absence of the external auditory canal and variable hypoplasia of the concha
Grade 3: absent auricle, anteriorly and inferiorly displaced lobule

There is usually a conductive hearing loss resulting from hypoplasia of the ear ossicles. More than 25% of patients have cranial nerve abnormalities, usually consisting of facial nerve palsy and/or deviation of the soft palate to the affected side with elevation. Palatal deviation is due to a combination of nerve weakness and muscle hypoplasia. The severity of the seventh nerve palsy correlates with the severity of the ear abnormalities and not the skeletal defect. The most common facial nerve weakness involves the marginal mandibular branch; the second most common weakness involves the branch to the frontalis muscle.

The treatment plan is based on the severity of the skeletal defect; therefore, an accurate classification is essential for optimal treatment. The skeletal type predicts the rate and progression of asymmetry. Treatment of soft tissue deformities begins in infancy. Skin tags are removed and macrostomia can be repaired during the first year. The external ear deformity is not treated until the skeletal correction is completed. This ensures correct positioning of the reconstructed ear. Other soft tissue deficiencies are usually corrected after the skeletal correction. Mild deformities can be corrected with onlay bone grafts, but patients with severe defects require soft tissue augmentation with vascularized tissue transfer.

Prosthodontic treatment is usually limited to the most severe cases (types IIb and III). Following surgery to reconstruct the ramus and condyle, the prosthodontist may be called on to reestablish the mandibular occlusal plane when the permanent dentition is missing on the affected side. The presence of mandibular teeth/occlusal plane is essential to allow the proper positioning of the maxillary dentition. The maxillary teeth will be positioned by a combination of orthognathic surgery and orthodontics.

The patient shown in Fig 6-55 demonstrates the use of osseointegrated implants to support the posterior mandibular dentition. The patient was missing the permanent posterior teeth on the mandibular left side. Following a costochondral graft to reconstruct the TMJ and the ramus as well as the body of the mandible, four osseointegrated implants were placed in the reconstructed mandible. Following stage-two surgery, a provisional implant prosthesis restored the mandibular occlusal plane.

Orthodontic treatment is presently in progress, so the definitive implant-supported restoration will be placed after completion of orthodontic treatment. If the mandibular posterior dentition is not restored, the maxillary dentition may continue to erupt.

Ectodermal dysplasias

The ectodermal dysplasias (EDs) are a group of hereditary diseases that affect the hair, teeth, nails, sweat glands, and other ectodermal derivatives of the body. Medical and dental treatment for these patients can be complicated. Dental treatment is particularly important because it is critical for a normal diet and for the facial appearance, speech, and emotional development of the child (Fig 6-56).

Any part of the body that is formed from ectoderm may be affected in EDs. Hypohidrotic ED was one of the first types of ED to be recognized. It is the most common form of the disorder and is usually transmitted as an X-linked trait; males manifest the disorder more frequently than females (Waggoner, 1987). Individuals with this condition have sparse, lightly pigmented hair, absent or sparse eyebrows and eyelashes, a reduced number of teeth, and a limited ability to sweat. The skin is dry and other body secretions are diminished. The physical appearance varies between individuals and families.

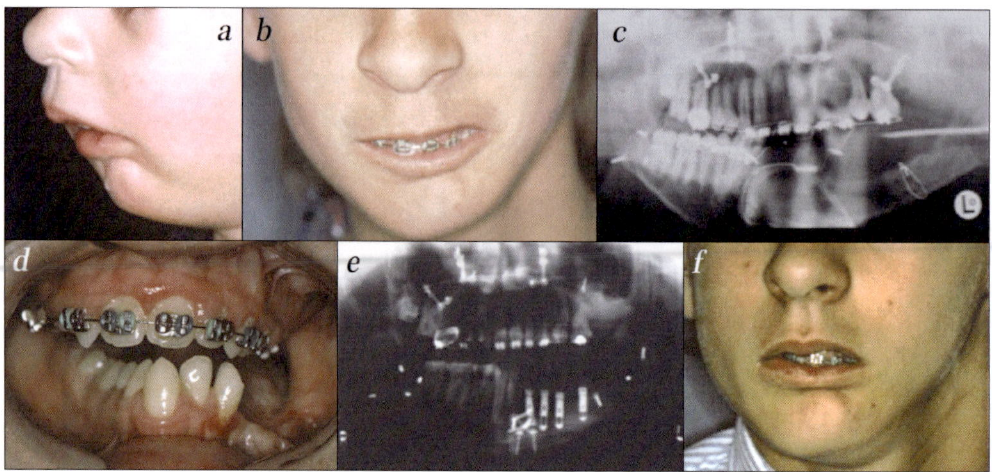

Figure 6-55 *(a)* Patient with left hemifacial microsomia at the time of initial presentation, at the age of two years. *(b)* Patient prior to mandibular reconstruction. He has a short ramus that deviates to the left. *(c)* Panoramic radiograph following mandibular reconstruction with a costochondral rib graft. *(d)* Intraoral view following reconstruction. *(e)* Panoramic radiograph showing four implants in the reconstructed mandible. *(f)* Facial view following surgery.

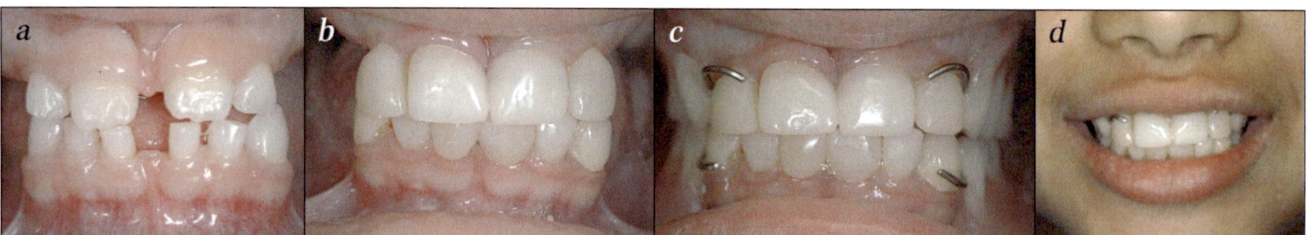

Figure 6-56 Patient with a form of ED. *(a)* Pretreatment appearance. *(b and c)* Transitional dental restorations and treatment partial dentures. *(d)* Excellent anterior aesthetics. Such care eases the transition into definitive care, which in this patient was initiated following completion of growth.

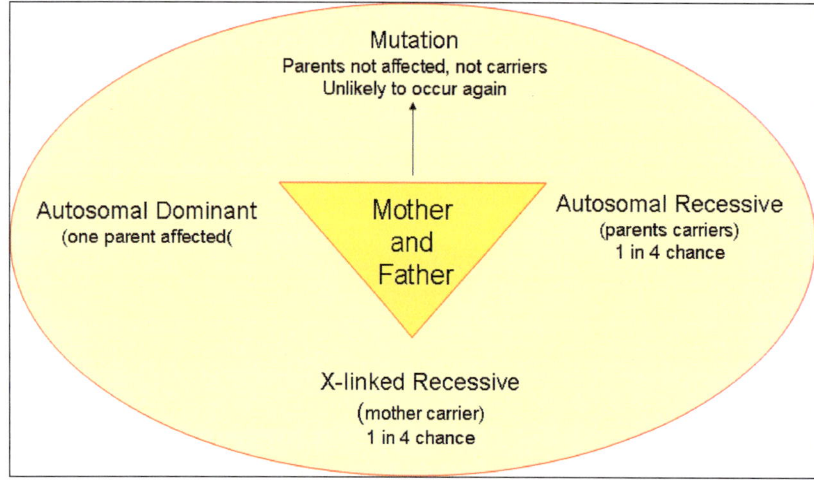

Figure 6-57 Inheritance pattern of ectodermal dysplasias.

Other types of ED have varying degrees of dental malformations. Table 6-1 lists some of the commonly seen malformations and their inheritance patterns. Although some rare forms of ED are associated with mental retardation, the common forms are not. The inheritance patterns of EDs are demonstrated in Fig 6-57.

Depending on the type of ED, the dental problems can vary from unpredictable patterns of tooth eruption and loss, widely spaced teeth, poorly shaped crowns and roots, defective enamel formation, and malformed teeth to partial or complete anodontia. In situations where the teeth are congenitally missing, there is an associated failure of normal development of the corresponding portion of the alveolar process (Sarnat et al., 1953; Sicher and DuBrul, 1970). This leads to underdevelopment of the maxilla compared to the mandible; as a result, most patients present with Class III maxillomandibular relationships. The rudimentary alveolar process is also deficient buccolingually (Figs 6-58 and 6-59).

Once a diagnosis of ED has been made, a dentist should be consulted. An early consultation provides parents with an overview of treatment options and introduces the child to the dentist in a nonthreatening situation. Although early restorative treatment is usually not necessary, regular examinations are important. When indicated, dental treatment for patients with ED can begin as early as two years of age.

Table 6-1 Common Types of ED That Affect Dental Structures

Type	Most obvious features	Inheritance
Book syndrome	White hair, missing teeth, moist palms	AD
Hypertrichosis lanuginosa	Excessive hair, defective tooth enamel	AD
Hypohidrotic ED	Decreased sweating, sparse hair, small teeth, missing teeth	AD, AR, XLR
Incontinentia pigmenti	Absent hair, missing teeth, malformed teeth, marbled pattern of pigmentation	XLD
Marshall ED	Missing teeth, decreased sweating, cataracts, hearing loss	AD
Monilethrix anodontia	Twisted hair, missing teeth	AD
Naegli Franceschetti-Jadassohn syndrome	Defective tooth enamel, thick palms and soles	AD
Otodental dysplasia	Abnormally shaped teeth, hearing loss	AD
Robinson ED	Missing teeth, defective nails, hearing loss	AD
Tooth and nail syndrome	Thin hair, missing teeth, slow nail growth	AD
Tricho-dento-osseous syndrome	Defective enamel, abnormal tooth roots, curly hair	AD
Trichodental syndrome	Thin hair, missing teeth	AD

AD—Autosomal dominant; AR-autosomal recessive; XLD-X-linked dominant; XLR-X-linked recessive.

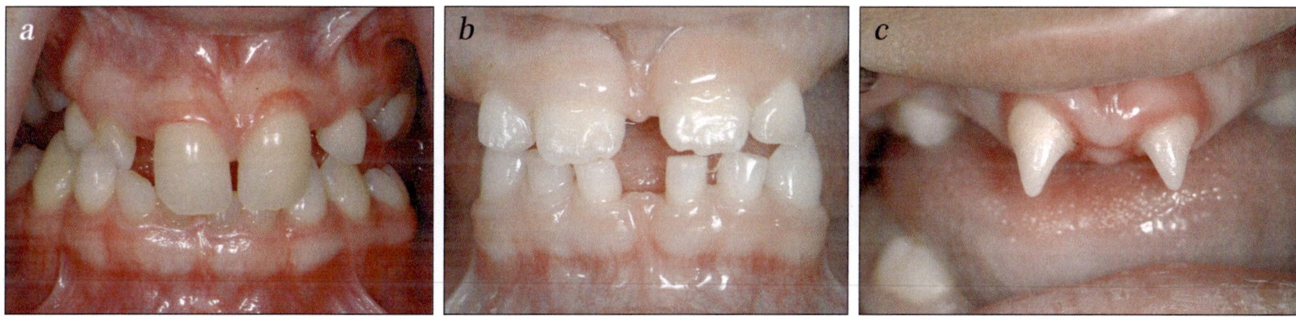

Figure 6-58 *(a to c)* ED is characterized by unpredictable tooth eruption and loss, poorly shaped crowns and roots, defective enamel formation, lack of alveolar development with closed VDO, and in severe cases almost complete anodontia.

Most patients with ED have some permanent teeth, often in the incisor and first molar areas. Often these teeth are small and abnormally shaped. These teeth should not be removed but can be restored with composite resin crowns (see Fig 6-56) or used as overdenture abutments, possibly in combination with implants. Their continued presence also contributes to development of the alveolar process locally, and on extraction of the teeth these sites will be more suitable for implant placement (see Fig 6-59g). The decision to retain the teeth depends on root form, crown morphology, and the position in the arch and the type of prosthetic rehabilitation anticipated.

Many patients also exhibit a closed VDO and deficient lip support. These problems are accentuated when the patient reaches adulthood (see Figs 6-59a and 6-60a). The VDO and support for the lip can be restored with either implant-supported fixed prostheses (see Fig 6-59) or implant-assisted or implant-supported removable overlay prostheses (Fig 6-60).

As children with ED reach school age, they are often ridiculed because of their facial appearance and missing teeth. This may occur as early as kindergarten and can result in significant psychosocial issues for the child. The use of maxillary and mandibular overlay dentures is often an effective treatment for these children at this stage of their development.

If the child is cooperative, the fabrication of overlay dentures is a relatively simple procedure. Because of the conical shape of the primary dentition, there is no need to recontour the clinical crowns to receive overlay dentures. The prostheses are fabricated in the customary fashion, positioning teeth to support the lower third of the face, changing their skeletal prognathic appearance, increasing vertical facial height, and improving the overall appearance (see Fig 6-56). As growth occurs, these prostheses require frequent modifications and/or remakes until more definitive treatment is indicated.

Implants have become invaluable aids in restoring the dentitions of these individuals, but the lack of alveolar process development can limit implant placement. When permanent teeth are present, they can sometimes be manipulated orthodontically to create more bone volume and following extraction of these teeth these sites will be better able to anchor osseointegrated implants. Sinus lift and graft and socket preservation techniques can also be employed to restore or maintain the vertical component of the bone site, and veneer grafts can be used to supplement sites that exhibit horizontal deficiencies.

A sizable group of patients present with nonsyndromic partial anodontia or a form of ED in which significant numbers of permanent teeth are present. When implants are to be used to supplement the available dentition, future alveolar development, the psychologic needs of the patient and family, and the suitability of the residual dentition need to be carefully considered. In such individuals, orthodontic treatment is used to consolidate the residual

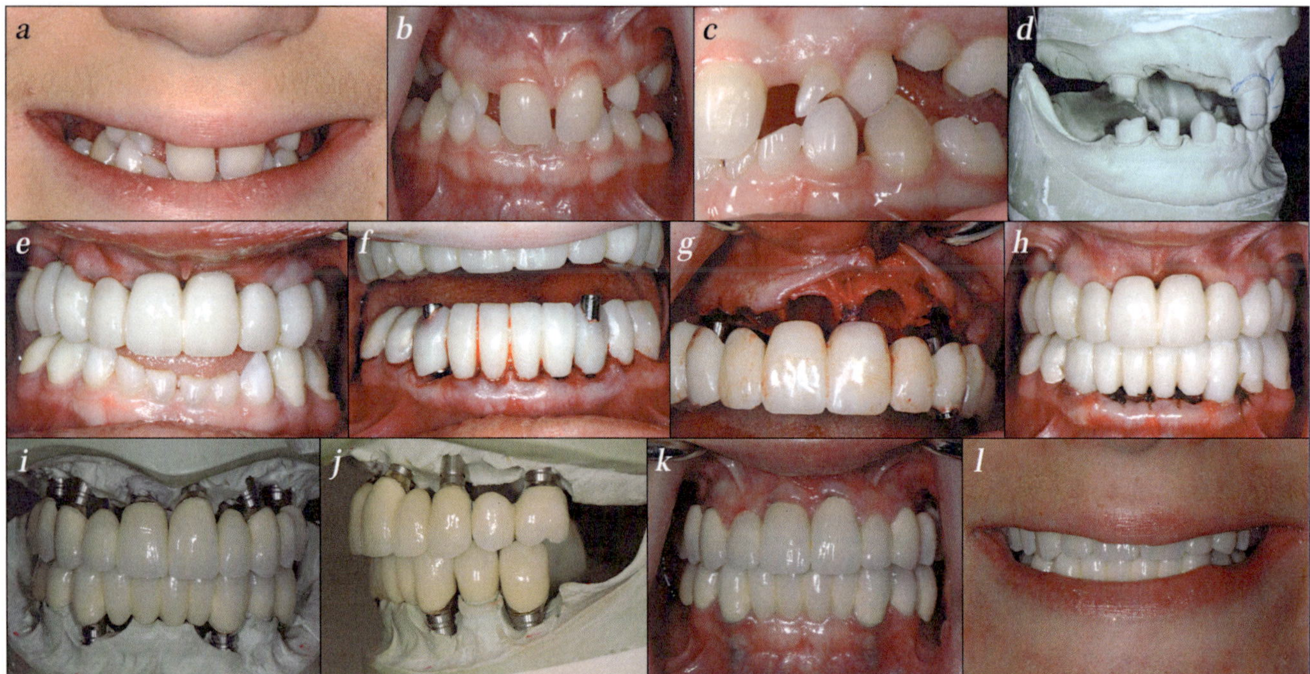

Figure 6-59 Patient presenting with partial anodontia secondary to ED. *(a to c)* In the maxilla, central incisors are well formed but the canines and first molars are misshapen and undersized. In the mandible, the premolars are the only permanent dentition. *(d and e)* Residual dentition is used for provisionalization. Provisional prostheses provide an appropriate aesthetic display and restore the VDO. *(f to h)* Implants are placed in stages. The provisional prostheses are used as a surgical guide for implant placement (six in the maxilla, four in the mandible). *(i and j)* Finished restorations. Custom abutments have been used to correct angulation problems. Implants in each arch are splinted together with rigid frameworks or nonresilient attachments. *(k)* Prostheses inserted. *(l)* Smile line (courtesy of Dr. R. Faulkner, Cincinnati, OH).

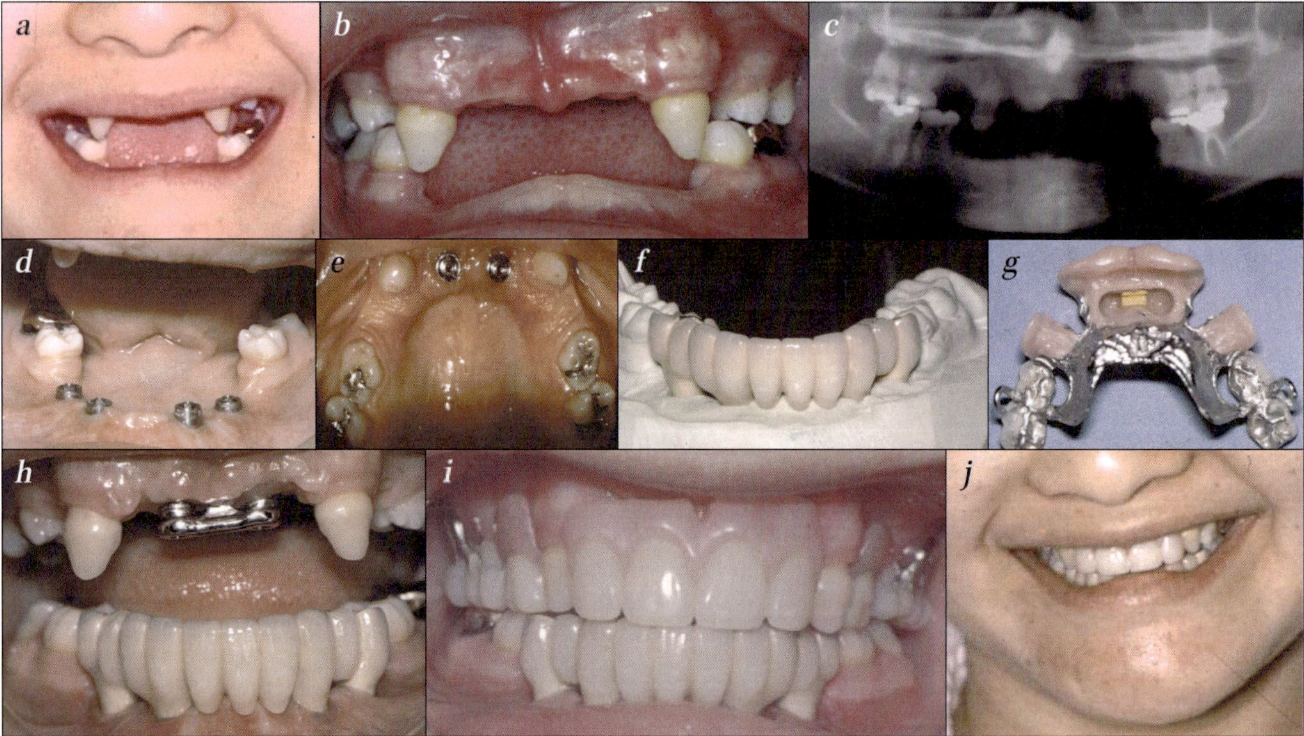

Figure 6-60 Adult with ED. *(a and b)* Clinical views. *(c)* Panoramic radiograph. *(d and e)* Implants placed in the anterior maxilla and mandible. *(f)* Porcelain-fused-to-metal fixed partial denture made with UCLA abutments. *(g)* Completed maxillary overlay prosthesis to restore VDO. *(h)* Tissue bar in the maxilla to retain the overlay removable partial denture. Fixed partial denture placed in the mandible. *(i and j)* Prostheses inserted (courtesy of Dr. Ray Lee, Seattle, WA).

permanent dentition and the edentulous spaces. Removable prostheses are used during this transition stage to restore aesthetics and the posterior occlusion (see Fig 6-56).

In these patients, it is generally preferred to wait until dentoalveolar development is complete before the implants are placed (Sharma and Vargervik, 2006). However, in some individuals it may be prudent to place implants before growth is complete (see the next section of this chapter). The UCSF Craniofacial Biology team is presently conducting a clinical trial assessing the feasibility of using implants in this group of patients, with particular emphasis on those individuals who are essentially edentulous but still possess the potential for growth (ages 7 to 16 years). To date 46 implants have been placed in 7 patients (24 in the mandible and 22 in the maxilla) and all but 2 implants are still in function (2 were lost in the maxilla: 1 before loading and 1 after loading). Follow-up periods from the time of implant placement range from 125 to 170 months (median of 139 months) and follow-up periods from the time of completion of the restoration range from 117 to 162 months (median of 130 months).

In most patients, the mandibular implants were placed anteriorly in the symphyseal region. In these patients, 6 arches were restored with tissue bars and removable overlay dentures and 1 patient was restored with an implant-supported fixed hybrid prosthesis. In most arches, the implants were splinted together but sectioned in the midline to allow normal transverse mandibular growth. In the maxilla, in most patients at least 6 implants were placed. Again, to permit normal transverse maxillary development, the bar did not splint the implants across the midline. Given the lack of maxillary development seen in the most severe forms of ED, all 6 maxillary arches were restored with tissue bars and removable overlay dentures to provide proper lip support and aesthetic display.

Of the 7 patients undergoing implant placement in the mandible, 3 required bone grafts and 7 underwent alveoplasty. In the maxilla (6 patients), 2 patients required sinus lift and graft and 3 others required onlay bone grafts from the iliac crest to increase arch width.

Based on these data, the UCSF team has made the following assumptions: Implants can be successfully placed, restored, and loaded in patients with ED. The most significant problems encountered were poor hygiene compliance and the resulting soft tissue hypertrophy. Although several of the prostheses had to be remade because of growth, growth of the patient does not alter implant position, and the implants as configured did not appear to interfere with the growth of the mandible or maxilla (Hartel et al., 1999).

Implants in Growing Children

For patients with several of the congenital deformities described, it may be advantageous to place implants at an early age. Clinicians can predictably place titanium implants that will, when properly used, presumably last the life of the patient (Lindh et al., 1998). Recent advances in implant surface science have improved implant anchorage, improved success rates, allowed clinicians to place implants into function much earlier than in past years, and implied that clinicians can place implants into sites that are less than ideal (Nishimura et al., 2007; Ogawa et al., 2000; Takeuchi et al., 2005).

Until the study recently conducted by the UCSF team, the following questions regarding the use of implants in growing children remained unanswered: Should implants be placed in growing children? If so, which children? Will the growth of the maxilla, mandible, or alveolar ridges be adversely affected if implants are placed before growth is finished? If implants are considered, under what circumstances and at what age should they be placed? The purpose of this section is to address these questions and to discuss whether there are circumstances under which implant placement might be considered for growing children.

The growth of the maxilla is dependent on sutural apposition and the development and eruption of primary and permanent teeth. However, the growth of the mandible is not dependent on the development of the dentition. Therefore, in patients presenting with hypodontia or anodontia, the size of the mandible will be relatively normal (but lacking normal alveolar ridges where permanent teeth fail to develop), but the maxilla will be considerably undersized. Another key fact is that implants do not change position with growth and do not move vertically with development of the alveolar ridges (Sharma and Vargervik, 2006; Odman et al., 1991).

UCSF team members have published numerous studies reporting their experiences in placing implants in growing children, and they have proposed a useful classification system when implant placement is considered in this patient population:

Group 1: Children who are missing a single tooth but have permanent teeth adjacent to the site (Fig 6-61).

Group 2: Children who are missing multiple teeth anteriorly or posteriorly but have permanent teeth adjacent to the edentulous areas (Fig 6-62).

Group 3: Children who are essentially edentulous. A couple of teeth may be present, but these teeth are poorly developed and in unfavorable positions (Fig 6-63).

Treatment guidelines

Group 1: Single missing tooth

In these patients, skeletal growth is the predominant concern, and the single-tooth defect can be restored satisfactorily with a transitional prosthesis until growth is complete. When an implant is placed in the alveolar ridge before growth is complete, the adjacent teeth will continue to erupt, accompanied by continued vertical development of the alveolar ridges. However, the portion of the alveolar ridge containing the implant will cease to develop, leading to a significant vertical discrepancy between teeth and adjacent implant (Fig 6-64). Eventually these discrepancies would lead to significant prosthodontic complications and difficulties, both aesthetic and biomechanical. Aesthetics would be compromised because of the abnormal position of the gingival margin of the implant crown relative to the adjacent teeth and implant biomechanics would be compromised because of the unfavorable crown-root ratios resulting from premature placement and the resulting growth discrepancies.

Sharma and Vargervik (1970) recommend that implant placement in patients with a single missing tooth be delayed until two annual cephalograms show no change in the position of the adjacent teeth and alveolus. Completion of growth and dentoalveolar development is usually seen as early as 16 years of age in females and as late as 22 years of age in males. In most patients the buccolingual dimension of these single-tooth sites is deficient and must be supplemented with bone grafting (see Fig 6-61). Seldom is soft tissue supplementation required (Fig 6-65).

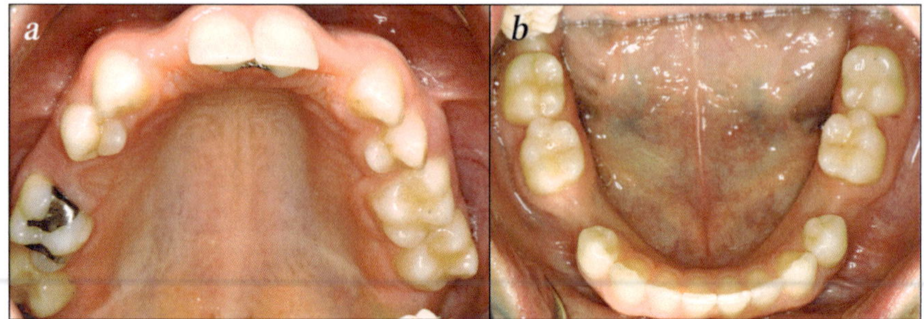

Figure 6-61 *(a and b)* Group I. Children who have single-tooth defects. Permanent dentition is adjacent to all single-tooth defects.

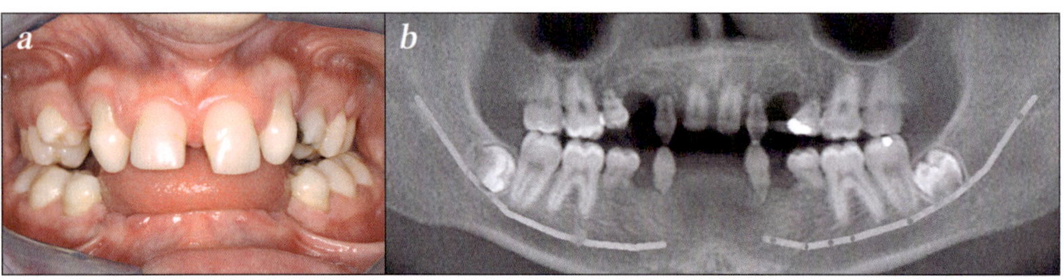

Figure 6-62 *(a and b)* Group II. Children who are missing multiple teeth anteriorly or posteriorly but have permanent teeth adjacent to the edentulous areas.

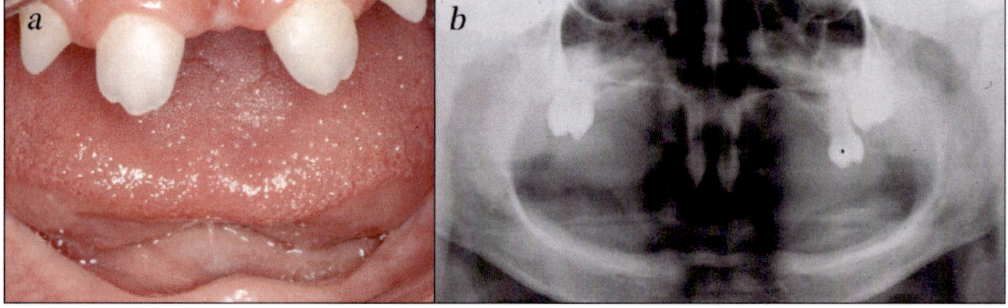

Figure 6-63 *(a to b)* Group III. Children who are essentially edentulous. A couple of teeth may be present, but these teeth are poorly developed and in unfavorable positions.

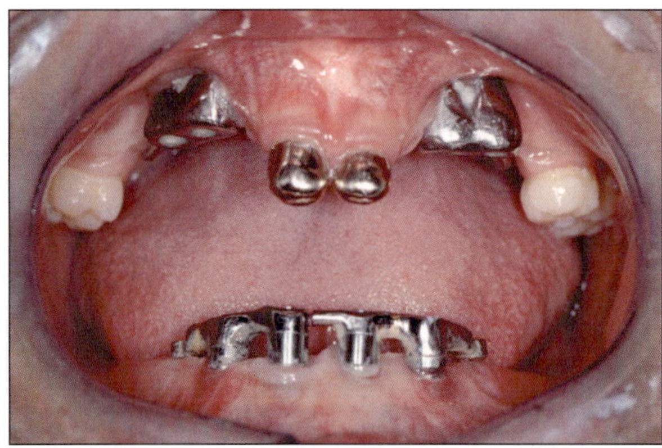

Figure 6-64 Extreme vertical discrepancy between the level of the implants and the level of the natural teeth.

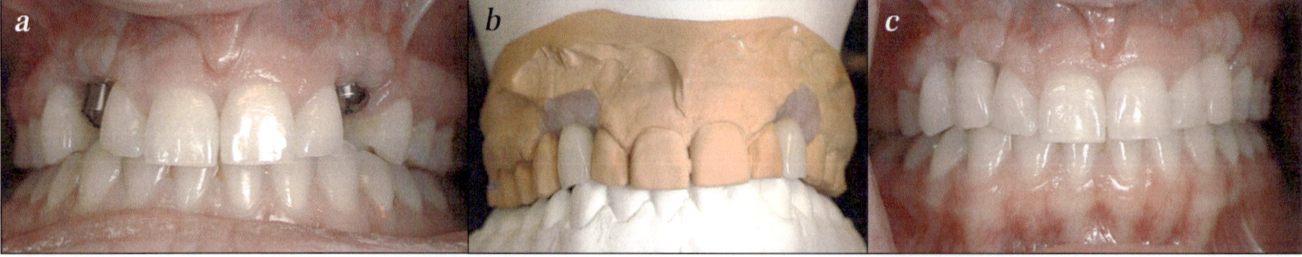

Figure 6-65 *(a to c)* Congenitally missing canines restored with single-tooth implants. Occlusion has been restored with group function.

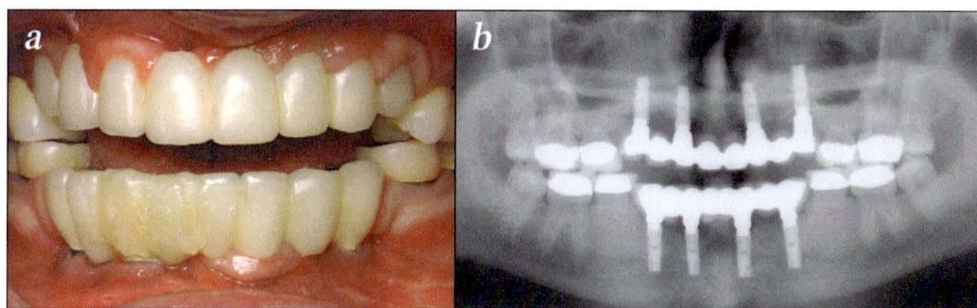

Figure 6-66 *(a and b)* Implants were placed and restored before growth was complete. Anterior open bite developed as the posterior teeth continued to erupt (reprinted from Sharma and Vargervik, 2006, with permission).

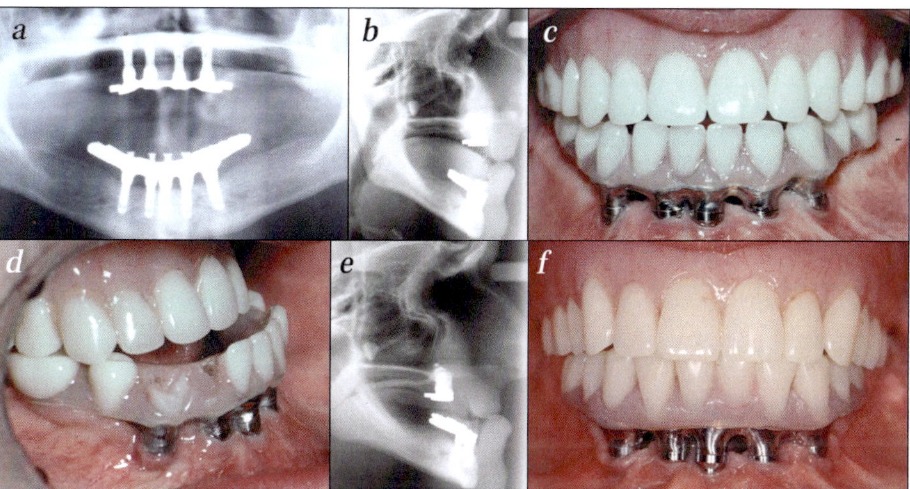

Figure 6-67 *(a to c) Completed prosthesis in place.* Implants were placed when the patient was 11 years old. Note the maxillomandibular relationship. *(d and e)* Patient at 16 years. Note the change in the maxillomandibular relationship. *(f)* Patient at age 19 years. Following orthognathic surgery to move the maxilla downward and forward, an implant retained overlay denture was fabricated for the maxilla and a fixed hybrid prosthesis was fabricated for the mandible (reprinted from Sharma and Vargervik, 2006, with permission).

Group 2: Multiple missing teeth

In this group of patients, we prefer to wait until growth is complete, but implants can be considered prior to completion of growth in selected patients (Fig 6-66). Implants are considered before completion of growth primarily to provide the patient with a more functional, stable, and aesthetic transitional prosthesis. In these situations, the patient and their family must recognize that the restoration will be provisional. When growth is complete, it often is necessary to surgically reposition the implant segments with either distraction osteogenesis or a segmental osteotomy to idealize the aesthetics, function, and serviceability of the definitive prosthesis.

Many of these patients present with various forms of ED. They exhibit unpredictable patterns of tooth eruption and loss, poorly shaped crowns and roots, teeth with defective enamel formation, lack of alveolar development, a closed VDO, and Class III maxillomandibular relationships. A thorough workup is required with study casts mounted on an articulator and a centric relation record. Careful planning is paramount to a successful outcome because these patients present with very complex problems. Treatment is interdisciplinary and requires the collaboration of orthodontists, oral and maxillofacial surgeons, and prosthodontists.

The first tasks are to identify permanent teeth that are suitable for salvage, identify potential implant sites, and consolidate the edentulous spaces by orthodontic means. In some instances, permanent teeth otherwise scheduled for removal are retained to help stabilize, retain, and support provisional removable partial dentures (see Fig 6-56c) or provisional fixed partial dentures (see Fig 6-59d and e) or to further enhance or retain bone of the probable future implant sites.

When growth is complete, either fixed or removable prostheses can be used to restore the dentition definitively. The choice depends on a variety of factors, including the number of permanent teeth available and their distribution, the compliance of the patient, the status of the occlusal plane, the amount of interocclusal space available, and the number, length, and position of the implants.

Group 3: Edentulous

These patients present with virtually no usable teeth, and most are afflicted with severe forms of ectodermal dysplasia. We support the use of implants in this group of patients at an early age if the patient has the potential to be compliant (Fig 6-67a–c).

The use of conventional complete dentures over a long period of time can be destructive to the bone and soft tissues of the denture-bearing regions and may compromise the potential implant sites. Implants provide these patients with an aesthetic and functional prosthesis during their formative years and yield important psychologic and functional benefits. Implants placed in the mandibular symphyseal region will not adversely affect growth of the mandible. Likewise, implants placed in the premaxilla will not affect the downward and forward growth of the maxilla secondary to sutural apposition. However, based on growth studies, implants should not be placed posterior to the mandibular canines (Odman et al., 1991; Thilander et al., 1992).

As the patient continues to grow, significant discrepancies in maxillomandibular relations will develop. Following completion of growth, an orthognathic surgical procedure will be necessary to move the maxilla down and forward into an appropriate position. At this time, the prostheses are remade (Fig 6-67d–f).

Summary

The treatment of cleft lip and palate is a classic example of the success of an interdisciplinary approach to a complex health problem. The principal structural deformities associated with cleft lip and palate are addressed primarily by orthodontic treatment and surgical reconstruction, but disciplines such as speech therapy, otolaryngology, audiology, social services, and others also play important roles. As these treatments have become more predictable and effective, the maxillofacial prosthodontist plays more of a subsidiary role.

Active participation by the maxillofacial prosthodontist begins, at the birth of the patient, with the initiation of NAM. In most situations, the services of a maxillofacial prosthodontist will not be required again until after growth of the patient's mandible and maxilla is completed, and those services will be focused on restoration of the compromised or missing dentition. However, the classic overlay denture, which restores the VDO and lip contours, replaces missing dentition, obturates existing fistulae, and restores velopharyngeal function, is still required for the occasional patient. Missing teeth associated with the cleft sites are restored most often with osseointegrated implants. Implants also are playing an increasing role in the dental rehabilitation of patients with a variety of craniofacial anomalies, including the many variants of ectodermal dysplasia. This practice has focused attention on the growing controversy regarding the use of osseointegrated implants in growing children. We believe that, for most patients, implants should be deferred until growth has been completed. The dentition in these patients can be restored with transitional prostheses. For selected patients, for example, those presenting with essentially an edentulous state, implants should be considered if the patient and family understand the issues and responsibilities involved.

References

Aboush YE, Jenkins CB. The bonding of an adhesive resin cement to single and combined adherends encountered in resin-bonded bridge work: An in vitro study. Br Dent J 1991;171:166–169.

Adell R, Eriksson B, Lekholm U, et al. A long-term follow-up study of osseointegrated implants in the treatment of the totally edentulous jaw. Int J Oral Maxillofac Implants 1990;5:347–359.

Aduss H. Craniofacial growth in complete unilateral cleft lip and palate. Angle Orthod 1971;41:202–213.

Albrektsson T, Dahl E, Enbom L, et al. Osseointegrated oral implants: A Swedish multicenter study of 8139 consecutively inserted Nobelpharma implants. J Periodontol 1988;59:287–296.

Alfonso AR, Ramly EP, Kantar RS, et al. What is the burden of care of nasoalveolar molding? Cleft Palate Craniofac J 2020 Sep;57(9):1078–1092.

Al Jamal GA, Hazza'a AM, Rawashdeh MA. Prevalence of dental anomalies in a population of cleft lip and palate patients. Cleft Palate Craniofac J 2010;47(4):413–420.

Almeida ALPF, Esper LA, Kaizer RO, et al. Surgical treatment of mucogingival alterations in cleft lip and palate patients: A clinical report. Perio 2006;3:31–35.

Almeida ALPF, Esper LA, Pegoraro TA, et al. Gingival recession in individuals with cleft lip and palate: Prevalence and severity. Cleft Palate J 2010a;49:92–95.

Almeida ALPF, Madeira LC, Freitas KC, et al. Cross-sectional evaluation of the presence of gingival recession in individuals with cleft lip and palate. J Periodontol 2007;78:29–36.

Almeida ALPF, Pedro PF, Kogawa EM, et al. Comparative evaluation of two different vestibuloplasty surgical procedures in cleft patients: A pilot study. Cleft Palate Craniofac J 2005;42:439–441.

Almeida ALPF, Sbrana MC, Esper LA, et al. Gingival recession in maxillary canines and central incisors of individuals with clefts. Oral Surg Oral Med Oral Pathol Oral Radiol Endod 2010b;109:37–45.

Argamaso RV. Glossopexy for upper airway obstruction in Robin sequence. Cleft Palate Craniofac J 1992;29:232–238.

Avinoam SP, Kowalski HR, Chaya BF, et al. Current presurgical infant orthopedics practices among American cleft palate association-approved cleft teams in North America. J Craniofac Surg 2022 Nov–Dec;33(8):2522–2528.

Barbier L, Schepers E. Adaptive bone remodeling around oral implants under axial and nonaxial loading conditions in the dog mandible. Int J Oral Maxillofac Implants 1997;12:215–223.

Bardach J, Morris H. Multidisciplinary management of cleft lip and palate. Philadelphia: Saunders; 1990.

Berkowitz S. The cleft palate story. Chicago: Quintessence; 1994.

Blakeley RW. The complementary use of speech prosthesis and pharyngeal flaps in palatal insufficiency. Cleft Palate J 1964;1:194–198.

Boyne PJ, Sands NR. Secondary bone grafting of residual alveolar and palatal clefts. J Oral Surg 1972;30:87–92.

Brattström V, Mølsted K, Prahl-Andersen B, et al. The Eurocleft study: Intercenter study of treatment outcome in patients with complete cleft lip and palate: Part 2. Craniofacial form and nasolabial appearance. Cleft Palate Craniofacial Journal 2005;42(1):69–77.

Brecht LE, Grayson BH, Cutting CB. Nasoalveolar molding in early management of cleft lip and palate. In Clinical maxillofacial prosthetics. Ed. T Taylor. Chicago: Quintessence; 2000. pp. 63–84.

Burdi AR, Silvey RG. Sexual differences in closure of the human palatal shelves. Cleft Palate J 1969;6:1–7.

Bush PG, Williams AJ. Incidence of Robin anomalad (Pierre Robin Syndrome). Br J Plast Surg 1983;36:434–437.

Calnan J. Submucous cleft palate. Br J Plast Surg 1954;6:264–282.

Cleft Palate Foundation. Genetics and you. 2nd ed. Chapel Hill, NC: Cleftline; 2008.

Croft CB, Shprintzen RJ, Daniller AI, et al. The occult submucous cleft palate and musculus uvulae. Cleft Palate J 1978;15:150–154.

Cutting C, Grayson B, Brecht L. Columellar elongation in bilateral cleft lip. Plast Reconstr Surg 1998;102:1761–1762.

Cutting CB, Grayson BH, Brecht LE, et al. Presurgical columellar elongation and primary retrograde nasal reconstruction in one stage bilateral cleft lip and nose repair. Plast Reconstr Surg 1998;101:630–639.

Delgado AA, Schaff NG, Emrich L. Trends in prosthodontic treatment of cleft palate patients at one institution: A twenty-one year review. Cleft Palate Craniofac J 1992;29:425–428.

Djemal S, Setchell D, King P, et al. Long-term survival characteristics of 832 resin-retained bridges and splints provided in a postgraduate teaching hospital between 1978 and 1993. J Oral Rehabil 1999;26:302–320.

El Deeb M, Messer LB, Lehnert MW, et al. Canine eruption into grafted bone in maxillary alveolar cleft. Cleft Palate J 1982;19:9–16.

Fara M. The musculature of cleft lip and palate. In Reconstructive plastic surgery. Vol 4. Ed. JM Converse. Philadelphia: Saunders; 1977.

Figueroa AA, Glupker TJ, Fitz MG, et al. Mandible, tongue, and airway in Pierre Robin sequence: A longitudinal cephalometric study. Cleft Palate Craniofac J 1991;28:425–434.

Friede H, Johanson B. Adolescent facial morphology of early bone grafted cleft lip and palate patients. Scand J Plast Reconstr Surg 1982;16:41–53.

Furlow LT Jr. Cleft palate repair by double opposing Z-plasty. Plast Reconstr Surg 1986 Dec;78(6):724–738.

Garfinkle JS, King TW, Grayson BH, et al. A 12-year anthropometric evaluation of the nose in bilateral cleft lip-cleft palate patients following nasoalveolar molding and cutting bilateral cleft lip and nose reconstruction. Plast Reconstr Surg 2011;127:1659–1667.

Gong X, Dang R, Xu T, et al. Full digital workflow of nasoalveolar molding treatment in infants with cleft lip and palate. J Craniofac Surg 2020 Mar/Apr;31(2):367–371.

Goodman R, Gorlin R. The face in genetic disorders. St Louis, MO: Mosby; 1970.

Grayson BH, Cutting CB. Presurgical nasoalveolar molding in primary correction of the nose, lip, and alveolus of infants born with unilateral and bilateral clefts. Cleft Palate Craniofac J 2001;38:193–198.

Grayson BH, Cutting CB, Wood R. Preoperative columella lengthening in bilateral cleft lip and palate. Plast Reconstr Surg 1993 Dec;92(7):1422–1423.

Grayson BH, Santiago PE, Brecht LE, et al. Presurgical nasoalveolar molding in infants with cleft lip and palate. Cleft Palate Craniofac J 1999;36:486–498.

Hall HD, Posnick JC. Early results of secondary bone grafts in 106 alveolar clefts. J Oral Surg 1983;41:289–294.

Hammoudeh JA, Fahradyan A, Gould DJ, et al. A comparative analysis of recombinant human bone morphogenetic protein-2 with a demineralized bone matrix versus iliac crest bone graft for secondary alveolar bone grafts in patients with cleft lip and palate: Review of 501 cases. Plast Reconstr Surg 2017 Aug;140(2):318e–325e.

Hanson JW, Murray JC. Genetic aspects of cleft lip and palate. In Multidisciplinary management of cleft lip and palate. Ed. J Bardach, H Morris. Philadelphia: Saunders; 1990. pp. 121–124.

Härtel J, Pögl C, Henkel KO, et al. Dental implants in alveolar cleft patients: A retrospective study. J Craniomaxillofac Surg 1999;27:354–357.

Heitz-Mayfield LJ, Schmid B, Weigel C, et al. Does excessive occlusal load affect osseointegration? An experimental study in the dog. Clin Oral Implants Res 2004;15:259–268.

Hoshaw SJ, Brunski JB, Cochran GVB. Mechanical loading of Brånemark implants affects interfacial bone modeling and remodeling. Int J Oral Maxillofac Implants 1994;9:345–360.

Howe DF, Denehy GE. Anterior fixed partial dentures utilizing the acid etch technique and a cast metal framework. J Prosthet Dent 1977;37:28–31.

Ibrahim AA, Byrne D, Hussey DL, et al. Bond strengths of maxillary anterior base metal resin-bonded retainers with different thicknesses. J Prosthet Dent 1997;78:281–285.

Jemt T, Lekholm U, Adell R. Osseointegrated implants in the treatment of partially edentulous patients: A preliminary study of 876 consecutively placed implants. Int J Oral Maxillofac Implants 1989;4:211–217.

Jia YL, Fu MK, Ma L. Long-term outcome of secondary alveolar bone grafting in patients with various types of cleft. Br J Oral Maxillofac Surg 2006;44:308–312.

Johanson B, Ohlsson A. Bone grafting and dental orthopaedics in primary and secondary cases of cleft lip and palate. Acta Chir Scand 1961;122:112–124.

Jones MC. Etiology of facial clefts: Prospective evaluation of 428 patients. Cleft Palate J 1988;25:16–20.

Jordan RE, Kraus BS, Neptune CM. Dental abnormalities associated with cleft lip and/or palate. Cleft Palate J 1966;3:22–55.

Kaban L. Surgical correction of the facial skeleton in childhood. In Pediatric oral and maxillofacial surgery. Ed. LB Kaban. Philadelphia: Saunders; 1990. pp. 425–437.

Kaban LB, Mulliken JB, Murray JE. Three-dimensional approach to analysis and treatment of hemifacial microsomia. Cleft Palate J 1981;18:90–99.

Kaplan EN. The occult submucous cleft palate. Cleft Palate J 1975;12:356–368.

Kaura AS, Srinivasa DR, Kasten SJ. Optimal timing of alveolar cleft bone grafting for maxillary clefts in the cleft palate population. J Craniofac Surg 2018 Sep;29(6):1551–1557.

Kearns G, Perrott DH, Sharma A, et al. Placement of endosseous implants in grafted alveolar clefts. Cleft Palate Craniofac J 1997;34:520–525.

Kearns G, Sharma A, Perrott D, et al. Placement of implants in children and adolescents with hereditary ectodermal dysplasia. Oral Surg Oral Med Oral Path Oral Radiol Endod 1999;88:5–10.

Kernahan DA, Stark RB. A new classification for cleft lip and palate. Plast Reconstr Surg Transplant Bull 1958;22:435–441.

King PA, Foster LV, Yates RJ, et al. Survival characteristics of 771 resin-retained bridges provided at a UK dental teaching hospital. Br Dent J 2015;218:423–428.

Kono D, Young L, Holtmann B. The association of submucous cleft palate and clefting of the primary palate. Cleft Palate J 1981;18:207–209.

Kramer FJ, Baethge C, Swennen G, et al. Dental implants in patients with orofacial clefts: A long-term follow-up study. Int J Oral Maxillofac Surg 2005;34:715–721.

Landes CA, Paffrath C, Koehler C, et al. Zygoma implants for midfacial prosthetic rehabilitation using telescopes: 9-year follow-up. Int J Prosthodont 2009;22:20–32.

Latham RA. Orthopedic advancement of the cleft maxillary segment: A preliminary report. Cleft Palate J 1980;17:227–233.

LeBlanc SM, Golding-Kushner KJ. Effect of glossopexy on speech sound production in Robin sequence. Cleft Palate Craniofac J 1992;29:239–245.

Lewin ML, Croft CB, Shprintzen RJ. Velopharyngeal insufficiency due to hypoplasia of the musculus uvulae and occult submucous cleft palate. Plast Reconstr Surg 1980;65:585–591.

Lindh T, Gunne J, Tillberg A, et al. A meta-analysis of implants in partial edentulism. Clin Oral Implants Res 1998;9:80–90.

Mackey R. Incidence of congenital anomalies in cleft palate patients vs. public health service [undergraduate fellowship study]. Evanston, IL: Northwestern University; 1958.

Matsui Y, Ohno K, Nishimura A, et al. Long-term study of dental implants placed into alveolar cleft sites. Cleft Palate Craniofac J 2007;44:444–447.

Mazaheri M, Nanda S, Sassouni J. Comparison of midfacial development of children with clefts and their siblings. Cleft Palate J 1967;4:334–341.

McNeil C. Orthodontic procedures in the treatment of congenital cleft palate. Dent Rec 1950;70:126–132.

McWilliams BJ. Submucous clefts of the palate: How likely are they to be symptomatic? Cleft Palate Craniofac J 1991;28:247–249.

Meurman Y. Congenital microtia and meatal atresia: Observations and aspects of treatment. AMA Arch Otolaryngol 1957;66:443–463.

Meyer FS. The generated path technique in reconstructive dentistry. J Prosthet Dent 1959;9:354.

Millard DR Jr. Refinements in rotation-advancement cleft lip technique. Plast Reconstr Surg 1964;33:26–38.

Millard DR Jr, Latham RA. Improved primary surgical and dental treatment of clefts. Plast Reconstr Surg 1990;86:856–871.

Miyata T, Kobayashi Y, Araki H, et al. The influence of controlled occlusal overload on peri-implant tissue: A histologic study in monkeys. Int J Oral Maxillofac Implants 1998;13:677–683.

Miyata T, Kobayashi Y, Araki H, et al. The influence of controlled occlusal overload on peri-implant tissue: Part 3. A histologic study in monkeys. Int J Oral Maxillofac Implants 2000;15:425–431.

Mølsted K, Brattström V, Prahl-Andersen B, et al. The Eurocleft study: Intercenter study of treatment outcome in patients with complete cleft lip and palate: Part 3. Dental arch relationships. Cleft Palate-Craniofacial Journal 2005;42(1):78–82.

Murray JE, Kaban LB, Mulliken JB. Analysis and treatment of hemifacial microsomia. Plast Reconstr Surg 1984;74:186–199.

Mylin WK, Hagerty RF, Hess DA. The pin retained prosthesis in cleft palate orthodontics. Cleft Palate J 1968;5:219–227.

Nakamura S, Savara BS, Thomas DR. Facial growth of children with cleft lip and/or palate. Cleft Palate J 1972;9:119–131.

Nishimura I, Huang Y, Ogawa T, et al. Discrete deposition of hydroxyapatite nanoparticles on a titanium implant with predisposing substrate microtopography accelerated osseointegrated. Nanotechnology 2007;18:1–9.

Odman J, Gröndahl K, Lekholm U, et al. The effect osseointegrated implants on dentoalveolar development: A clinical and radiographic study in growing pigs. Eur J Orthod 1991;13:279–286.

Ogawa T, Nishimura I. Different bone integration profiles of turned and acid-etched implants associated with modulated expression of extracellular matrix genes. Int J Oral Maxillofac Implants 2003;18:200–210.

Ogawa T, Nishimura I. Genes differentially expressed in titanium implant healing. J Dent Res 2006;85:566–570.

Ogawa T, Ozawa S, Shih JH, et al. Biomechanical evaluation of osseous implants having different surface topographies in rats. J Dent Res 2000;79:1857–1863.

Ogawa T, Sukotjo C, Nishimura I. Modulated bone matrix-related gene expression is associated with differences in interfacial strength of different implant surface roughness. J Prosthodont 2002;11:241–247.

Oh WS, Roumanas ED. Optimization of maxillary obturator thickness using a double-processing technique. J Prosthodont 2007;17:60–63.

Olin WH. Dental anomalies in cleft lip and palate patients. Angle Orthod 1964;34:119–123.

Perrott DH, Sharma AB, Vargervik K. Endosseous implants for pediatric patients Oral Maxillofac Surg Clin North Am 1994;6:79–88.

Posnick JC, Thompson B. Modification of the maxillary Le Fort I osteotomy in cleft-orthognathic surgery: The unilateral cleft lip and palate deformity. J Oral Maxillofac Surg 1992 Jul;50(7):666–675; discussion 675–676.

Poswillo D. The pathogenesis of 1st and 2nd branchial arch syndrome. Oral Surg Oral Med Oral Pathol 1973;35:302–308.

Randall P. A lip adhesion operation in cleft surgery. Plast Reconstr Surg 1965;35:371–376.

Robertson NR, Jolleys A. An 11-year follow-up of the effects of early bone grafting in infants born with complete clefts of the lip and palate. Br J Plast Surg 1983;36:438–443.

Rosenstein SW, Monroe CW, Kernahan DA, et al. The case of early bone grafting in cleft lip and palate. Plast Reconstr Surg 1982;70:297–309.

Ross RB. Treatment variables affecting facial growth in complete unilateral cleft lip and palate. Cleft Palate J 1987;24:5–77.

Sadewitz VL. Robin sequence: Changes in thinking leading to changes in patient care. Cleft Palate Craniofac J 1992;29:246–253.

Santiago PE, Grayson BH, Cutting CB, et al. Reduced need for alveolar bone grafting by presurgical orthopedics and primary gingivoperiosteoplasty. Cleft Palate Craniofac J 1997;35:77–80.

Sarnat B, Brodie A, Kubacki W. Fourteen-year report of facial growth in a case of complete anodontia with ectodermal dysplasia. AMA Am J Dis Child 1953;86:162–169.

Sato Y, Yuasa Y, Abe Y, et al. Finite element and Weibull analysis to estimate failure risk in resin-bonded retainers. Int J Prosthodont 1995;8:73–78.

Schmidt BL, Pogrel MA, Young CW, et al. Reconstruction of extensive maxillary defects using zygomaticus implants. J Oral Maxillofac Surg 2004;62:82–89.

Schroeder DC, Green LJ. Frequency of dental trait anomalies in cleft, sibling, and noncleft groups. J Dent Res 1975;54:802–807.

Semb G, Brattström V, Mølsted K, et al. The Eurocleft study: Intercenter study of treatment outcome in patients with complete cleft lip and palate: Part 1. Introduction and treatment experience. Cleft Palate Craniofac J 2005a;42(1):64–68.

Semb G, Brattström V, Mølsted K, et al. The Eurocleft study: Intercenter study of treatment outcome in patients with complete cleft lip and palate: Part 4.

Relationship among treatment outcome, patient/parent satisfaction, and the burden of care. Cleft Palate Craniofacial Journal 2005b;42(1):83–92.

Shanbhang G, Pandey S, Mehta N, et al. A virtual noninvasive way of constructing a nasoalveolar molding plate for cleft babies using intraoral scanner, CAD and prosthetic milling. Cleft Palate Craniofac J 2020 Feb;57(2):263–266.

Sharma AB, Vargervik K. Using implants for the growing child. J Calif Dent Assoc 2006;34:719–724.

Shaw WC, Brattström V, Mølsted K, et al. The Eurocleft study: Intercenter study of treatment outcome in patients with complete cleft lip and palate: Part 5. Discussion and conclusions. Cleft Palate Craniofac J 2005;42(1):93–98.

Sher AE. Mechanisms of airway obstruction in Robin sequence: Implications for treatment. Cleft Palate Craniofac J 1992;29:224–231.

Shprintzen RJ, Schwartz RH, Daniller A, et al. Morphologic significance of bifid uvula. Pediatrics 1985;75:553–561.

Shprintzen RJ. The implications of the diagnosis of Robin sequence. Cleft Palate Craniofac J 1992;29:205–209.

Sicher H, DuBrul EL. Oral anatomy. 5th ed. St Louis, MO: Mosby; 1970. p. 108.

Singer L, Sidoti EJ. Pediatric management of Robin sequence. Cleft Palate Craniofac J 1992;29:220–223.

Sischo L, Broder HL, Phillips C. Coping with cleft: A conceptual framework of caregiver responses to nasoalveolar molding. Cleft Palate Craniofac J 2015 Nov;52(67):640–650.

Slaughter WB, Brodie AG. Facial clefts and their surgical management. Plast Reconstr Surg 1946;4:311–332.

Stein MJ, Zhang Z, Fell M, et al. Determining postoperative outcomes after cleft palate repair: A systematic review and meta-analysis. J Plast Reconstr Aesthet Surg 2019 Jan;72(1):85–91. http://doi.org/10.1016/j.bjps.2018.08.019.

Takahashi T, Fukuda M, Yamaguchi T, et al. Placement of endosseous implants into bone grafted alveolar clefts: Assessment of bone bridge after autogenous particulate cancellous bone and marrow graft. Int J Oral Maxillofac Implants 1999;14:86–93.

Takeuchi K, Saruwatari L, Nakamura HK, et al. Enhanced intrinsic biomechanical properties of osteoblastic mineralized tissue on roughened titanium surface. J Biomed Mater Res 2005;72:296–305.

Thilander B, Odman J, Gröndahl K, et al. Aspects of osseointegrated implants inserted in growing jaws: A biometric and radiographic study in young pigs. Eur J Orthod 1992;14:99–109.

Thompson JS, Thompson MW. Genetics in Medicine. 3rd ed. Philadelphia: Saunders; 1980.

Trier WC. Velopharyngeal incompetency in the absence of overt cleft palate: Anatomic and surgical considerations. Cleft Palate J 1983;20:209–217.

Turvey TA, Vig K, Moriarty J, et al. Delayed bone grafting in the cleft maxilla and palate: A retrospective multidisciplinary analysis. Am J Orthod 1984;86:224–256.

Valinoti JR Jr. The congenitally absent premolar problem. Angle Orthod 1958;28:36–46.

Vanderas AP. Incidence of cleft lip, cleft palate and cleft lip and palate among races: A review. Cleft Palate J 1987;24:216–225.

Vargervik K. Growth characteristics of the premaxilla and orthodontic principles in bilateral cleft lip and palate. Cleft Palate J 1983;20:289–302.

Vargervik K. Orthodontic management of unilateral cleft lip and palate. Cleft Palate J 1981;18:256–270.

Waggoner WF. Multidisciplinary treatment of a young child with hypohidrotic ectodermal dysplasia. Spec Care Dent 1987;7:215–217.

Walker JC Jr, Collito MB, Mancusi-Ungaro A, et al. Physiologic considerations in cleft lip closure: The CW technique. Plast Reconstr Surg 1966;37:552–557.

Wharton P, Mowrer DE. Prevalence of cleft uvula among school children in kindergarten through grade five. Cleft Palate Craniofac J 1992;29:10–12.

Wood RJ, Grayson BH, Cutting CB. Gingivoperiosteoplasty and midfacial growth. Cleft Palate Craniofac J 1997;34:17–20.

Moscovitch M. Consecutive cases series of monolithic minimally veneered zirconia restorations on teeth and implants: Up to 68 months. Int J Periodontics Restorative Dent 2015;35:315–323.

Moy PK, Pozzi A, Beumer III J. Fundamentals of implant dentistry: Surgical principles. Chicago: Quintessence; 2016.

Noack EA, Gehrke P. Survival and rates of complication of implant supported lithium disilicate single crowns. J Dent Implantol 2016;32:202–213.

Ogawa T, Nishimura I. Different bone integration profiles of turned and acid-etched implants associated with modulated expression of extracellular matrix genes. Int J Oral Maxillofac Implants 2003;18:200–210.

Pozzi A, Tallarico M, Barlattani A. Monolithic lithium disilicate full-contour crowns bonded on CAD/CAM zirconia complete-arch implant bridges with 3 to 5 years of follow-up. J Oral Implantol 2015;41:450-8.

Takeuchi K, Saruwatari L, Nakamura H, et al. Enhancement of biomechanical properties of mineralized tissue by osteoblasts cultured on titanium with different surface topographies. J Biomed Mater Res 2005;72A:296–305.

Tian H, Wang L, Xie W, et al. Epidemiology and outcome analysis of facial burns: A retrospective multicentre study 2011–2015. Burns 2020;46:718–726.

Tischler M, Patch, Bidra AS. Rehabilitation of edentulous jaws with zirconia complete-arch fixed implant-supported prostheses: An up to 4-year retrospective clinical study. J Prosthet Dent 2018;120:204–209.

Van Ordan AC. Corrosive response of the interface tissues to 316L stainless steel, titanium-based alloys, and cobalt-based alloys. In Dental implant. Eds. McKinney RV, Lemons JE. Littleton, MA: PSG; 1985. pp. 1–24.

Vosselman HH, Glas HH, de Visscher SAHJ, et al. Immediate implant-retained prosthetic obturation after maxillectomy based on zygomatic implant placement by 3D-guided surgery: A cadaver study. Int J Implant Dent 2021 Jun 14;7(1):54. http://doi.org/10.1186/s40729-021-00335-w.

Wiens JP. The use of osseointegrated implants in the treatment of patients with trauma. J Prosthet Dent 1992;67:670–678.

Wiens JP, Hickey A. Maxillofacial trauma. In Maxillofacial rehabilitation: Prosthodontic and surgical considerations. Eds. J Beumer III, TA Curtis, MT Marunick. St Louis, MO: Ishiyaku EuroAmerica Inc; 1996. pp. 479–509.

Wiens R. Psychosocial considerations. In Maxillofacial rehabilitation: Prosthodontic and surgical considerations. Eds. J Beumer III, TA Curtis, MT Marunick. St Louis, MO: Ishiyaku EuroAmerica Inc; 1996. pp. 483–484.

Wu B, Abduo J, Lyons K, et al. Implant biomechanics, screw mechanics, and occlusal concepts for implant patients. In Fundamentals of implant dentistry: Prosthodontic principles. Eds. J Beumer, RF Faulkner, K Shah, B Wu. 2nd ed. Chicago: Quintessence; 2022. pp. 37–59.

Chapter 7

Restoration of Traumatic Defects

John Beumer III, Nadim AbouJoude, Robert M. Taft, Nabil Barakat, Peter K. Moy

Traumatic injuries of the oral facial region pose significant challenges. These injuries vary from localized tooth avulsions and facial fractures to large avulsive wounds with significant loss of hard and soft tissue (Fig 7-1). Reconstruction and rehabilitation of even localized defects can be complex and demanding. For example, patients that present with localized avulsive tooth defects usually exhibit hard and soft tissue deficits that frequently require grafting for optimal results to include possible implant placement. Even more demanding and complex are those patient presentations with misalignment and malunion of facial fractures. These patients usually present with significant occlusal discrepancies and facial deformities that often require an advanced interdisciplinary treatment approach to include orthodontics, surgical support, and prosthodontics. Severe oral facial injuries secondary to gunshot wounds can lead to discontinuity mandibular defects and large avulsive wounds of the maxilla with extensive loss of hard and soft tissue. Closed head injuries often result in central nervous system injury predisposing to compromise of velopharyngeal and tongue function. Burn injuries to the head and neck can also cause significant facial deformity and loss of facial structures such as the ear.

Although surgical disciplines play a major role in the rehabilitation of these patients (implant placement, hard and soft tissue grafting, surgical osteotomies), rehabilitation is primarily prosthodontically driven. Nevertheless, reconstruction and prosthetic restoration of these defects most often require close collaboration between prosthodontists, orthodontists, and reconstructive surgeons with meticulous planning. Significant advances in digital technologies and the use of implants have had a profound impact that has led to improved treatment outcomes. However, in some patients, even the most ideal outcomes fall short, leaving the patient with lingering morbidities, both functional and psychosocial. The purpose of this chapter is to discuss the basic characteristics of frequently encountered traumatic injuries in the oral facial region and the current methods employed in their rehabilitation.

Types of Injuries

Trauma secondary to motor vehicle collisions, gunshot wounds, falls, and athletics

Every year, oral facial trauma from motor vehicle accidents exceeds 1.5 million persons in the United States and several million across the world. Injury severity may vary from simple tooth avulsions to major multiple facial fractures. Frontal vehicular collisions tend to trigger anterior anatomic avulsion defects. However, as discussed below (see section entitled "Condylar fractures"), forces may be directed away from the initial impact area, resulting in fractures at distant sites, such as the condyle and the temporomandibular joint (Wiens, 1992).

Nonfatal facial trauma secondary to firearms is increasing and currently exceeds over 100,000 patients per year in the United States and possibly several million worldwide. These injuries can lead to significant loss of teeth and hard and soft tissue, as well as multiple facial fractures. Gunshot wounds can be penetrating (projectile remains in the body), perforating (projectile exits the body), or avulsive (Kelly, 1977). Perforating injuries are characterized by a small entry and a large nonlinear exit wound with foreign bodies interspersed. The nature of the injuries depends on the type of firearm employed and the ballistics of the projectile (bullet). Some bullets tend to penetrate, while others fragment, expanding at tissue impact and increasing internal damage some distance from its primary pathway. Ultrahigh velocity projectiles increase tissue damage

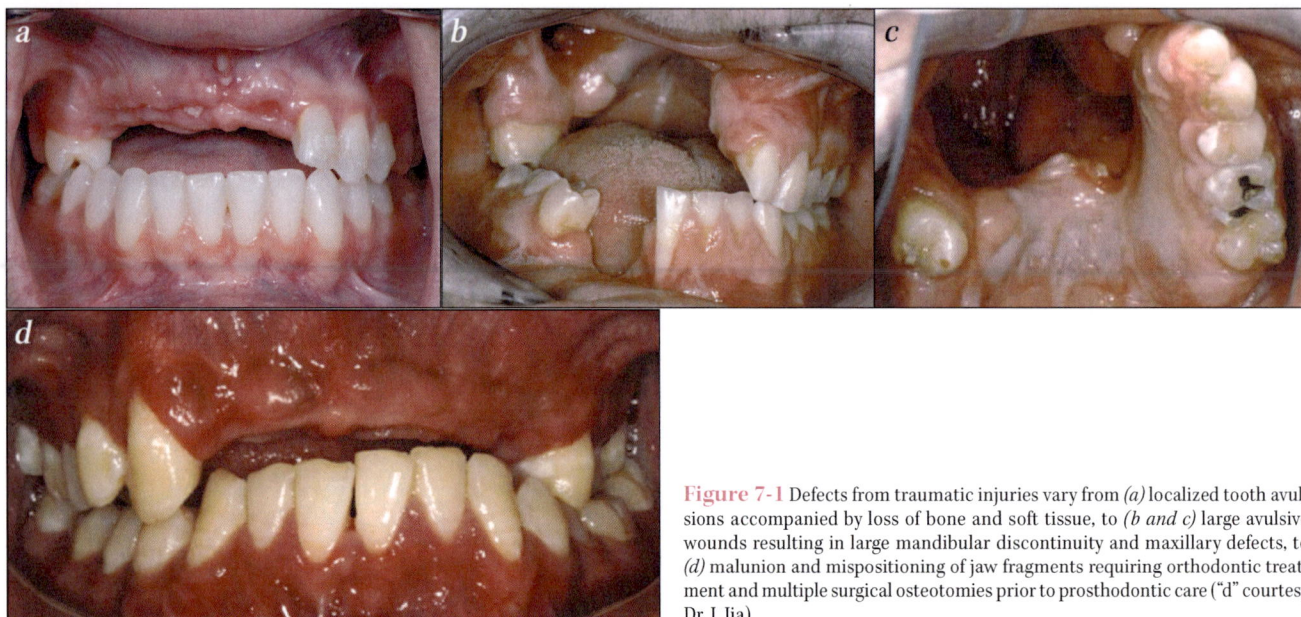

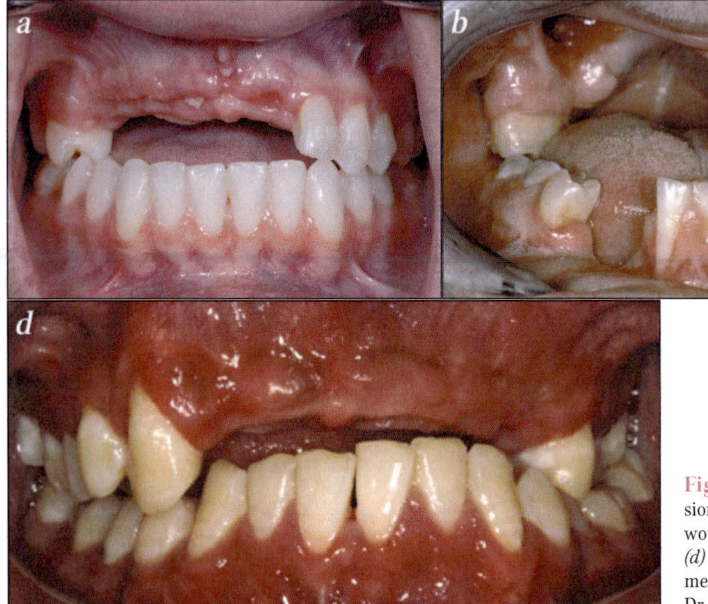

Figure 7-1 Defects from traumatic injuries vary from *(a)* localized tooth avulsions accompanied by loss of bone and soft tissue, to *(b and c)* large avulsive wounds resulting in large mandibular discontinuity and maxillary defects, to *(d)* malunion and mispositioning of jaw fragments requiring orthodontic treatment and multiple surgical osteotomies prior to prosthodontic care ("d" courtesy Dr. J. Jia).

through extensive cavitation of the wound. Shotgun wounds that are self-inflicted produce large avulsive-type wounds (Fig 7-1b and c) (Wiens and Hickey, 1996).

Self-inflicted long gun wounds are unique and generally affect the anterior portion of the maxillofacial region (Fig 7-1b and c). Although challenging to reconstruct and restore, they are typically nonfatal avulsive wounds to the anterior mandible and maxilla. This is based on the gun barrel position under the chin, extended head position, and the distance between the end of the barrel and the trigger mechanism. These patients can present with discontinuity defects of the mandible and large avulsive wounds of the maxilla. Following initial healing, frequently, residual maxillary segments are displaced and often lack bony attachment to the base of the skull. Moreover, the oral mucosa often exhibits significant fibrosis with scarring, and the volume of the oral cavity is reduced (Hickey, 1986).

Contact injuries associated with athletics, falls, and machinery are generally less severe (Fig 7-1a) because contact velocity is low and generally blunt in nature. Most athletic injuries affect the anterior portion of the maxilla or mandible, which often result in tooth loss with adjacent hard and soft tissue and pose significant challenges for the reconstruction team (see below, section entitled "Local avulsive injuries of the dentition and alveolar bone"). Retained teeth adjacent to the defect often exhibit cuspal or root fractures. Some teeth present with undetectable cracks affecting their vitality, and therefore, the remaining dentition must be carefully scrutinized for any signs of injury, especially those teeth that are being considered as abutments for fixed or removable dental prostheses.

Burns

Burn injuries to the head and neck can cause significant deformity and disability that can be divided into two categories: aesthetic and functional. Functional complications include a compromised airway, carbon monoxide poisoning, and corneal/eye burns. Burn injuries can also lead to loss or deformation of facial structures, including the ear and nose. The external ears are particularly vulnerable to thermal burns because of their prominent projecting location on the sides of the face (Fig 7-2). Recent reports indicate that one-half or more of burn injuries affect head and neck structures (Tian et al., 2020; Haddadi et al., 2021). The primary role of the maxillofacial prosthodontist is to restore lost or compromised facial structures, such as the ear and/or the nose, with facial prostheses.

A burn to the oral commissure is a common electrical injury in children (Fig 7-3). They are frequently caused by sucking or biting the end of a live wire or the junction between charged extension and appliance cords. The ionic saliva completes the circuit between the oral mucosa and the electrical components of the cord. Since saliva is an excellent electrical conductor, burns to the oral commissures may be extensive. Localized tissue destruction and subsequent perioral scarring with contracture can result in microstomia, predisposing the patient to a functional and cosmetic deformity of the oral commissure, crossbite, crowding, retrusion, palatal arch contracture, lingually inclined mandibular teeth, and mandibular arch contraction.

Psychosocial perspectives on the care of patients with traumatic injuries to the craniofacial region

Depending on the severity of the injuries and the accompanying cosmetic/functional impact, these patients frequently suffer from anxiety, depression, or posttraumatic stress disorders (PTSD). The prosthodontist must understand that the loss includes not only the alteration of a facial feature but also subsequent deprivation of experiences the individual might have had. Some patients will be subject to rejection by family members, significant others, and business associates. Patient reactions will be like those patients with deformities associated with the treatment for head and neck cancer

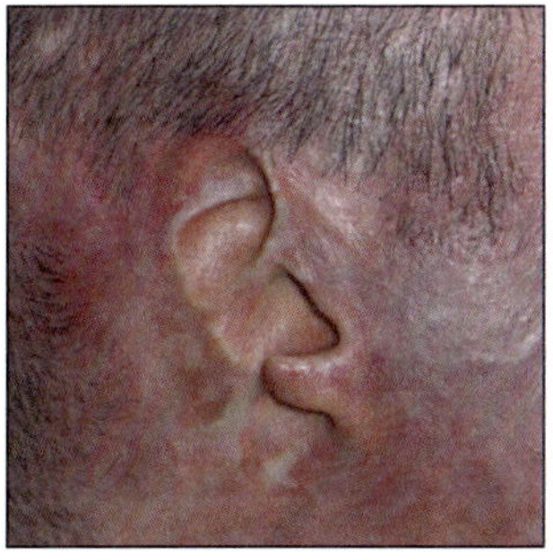

Figure 7-2 An auricular defect secondary to a burn injury.

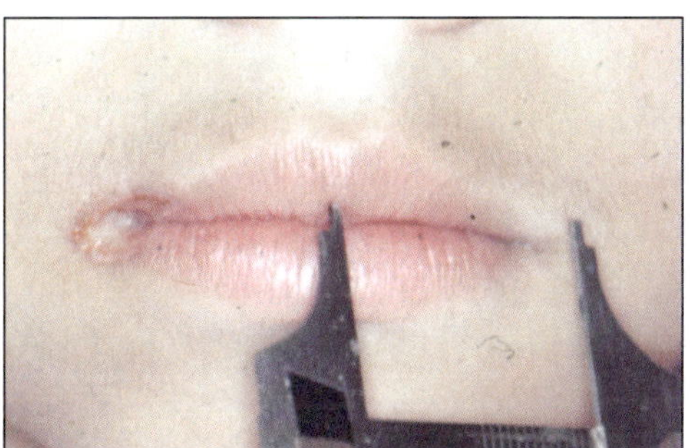

Figure 7-3 Electrical burn of the oral commissure.

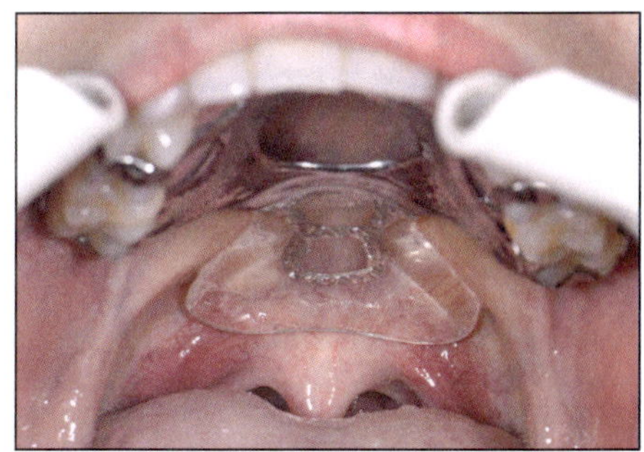

Figure 7-4 Palatal lift prosthesis for a patient with velopharyngeal incompetence secondary to a closed head injury.

and/or war-related injuries. A detailed discussion of the most significant challenges faced by the patient, their social support system, and their caregivers is provided in Chapter 9.

Victims of self-inflicted trauma have complicating psychological factors that need to be processed with a trained psychotherapist. These patients will need to discuss their loss and grief after they work toward ameliorating the factors that led to their destructive or suicidal behavior. Frequently, they will have conflicting thoughts about their nonsuccessful destructive action and acceptance of their new physical self. Previous thoughts and feelings that motivated their behavior may still be present and need to be addressed by a trained psychotherapist (Wiens, 1996).

Maxillofacial Injuries

Closed head injuries

Closed head injuries may result in contusions, intracerebral hematomas, cerebral lacerations, and circulatory deficiencies. These conditions may trigger localized or general brain ischemia that may affect motor control and sensory innervations that sometimes lead to changes in behavioral and cognitive processes. Some patients present with velopharyngeal incompetence and benefit from a palatal lift prosthesis (Fig 7-4). Tongue motor dysfunction often accompanies velopharyngeal incompetence in such patients, and a palatal speech and swallowing aid may be beneficial. The degree of functional impairment varies from patient to patient and depends on the extent of the injuries. Closed head injury patients are typically young, and many have been injured in either motorcycle or automobile accidents. Many patients may be neuromuscularly impaired to the point where they find it difficult to insert and remove a removable prosthesis. The patient's ability to perform routine oral hygiene measures may also be impaired. Under these circumstances, it becomes necessary to train a family member or significant other to aid the patient or otherwise perform these procedures.

Soft tissue trauma

The soft tissues of the head and neck have an abundant blood supply, enabling lacerations to heal quickly. Proper wound management reduces possible complications with minimal scarring and is frequently found acceptable by the patient. Fortunately, it is unusual for portions of the face to be avulsed or sloughed even with severe injuries. Should this occur, local skin flaps are used to reconstruct the area. Large defects may require local regional flaps or possibly a vascularized free flap (Jackson, 1996).

Scalp lacerations are closed in one or two layers depending on the preference of the surgeon. Complications may include the loss of hair in relation to the scars. If there is a loss of a portion of the scalp, a flap can usually be designed to close the defect. Avulsion of large areas of the scalp may require the replacement of the affected part with a vascularized free flap. Lacerations of the ear are common and are carefully repaired. Lacerations of the nose are repaired in layers, while small skin defects can be reconstructed with local flaps. The eyelids are very important functionally and must be carefully repaired in layers. Any defect of the lids must be reconstructed, especially the upper lid, since this lid serves to protect the eye. Local flaps or portions of the lower lid are used in upper-lid reconstruction. An oculoplastic surgeon may be helpful with this very difficult reconstruction. The help of an ophthalmologist is suggested if the eye is damaged in any way (Jackson, 1996).

The lips are an aesthetic area with definite contours and a mucocutaneous junction. Careful closure in layers is indicated with accurate realignment of the skin and vermilion junctions. Small lip defects can be corrected by converting them into a full-thickness, wedge-shaped lip defect and then closing this defect with care. Large lip defects require closure with local flap(s). The tongue has an excellent blood supply, so it should always be repaired even if portions have only a small pedicle or seem ischemic. Watertight closure of the oral mucous membranes during initial treatment is strongly advised even though this practice may lead to some distortion of oral structures (Jackson, 1996).

Local avulsive injuries of the dentition and alveolar bone

Traumatic avulsion of teeth frequently creates extended edentulous areas, which are tooth bound and nonlinear in configuration (Fig 7-5). The associated alveolar bony defects will be more extensive than those that result from routine extractions from dental disease. These anatomical limitations complicate treatment and may limit prosthodontic options.

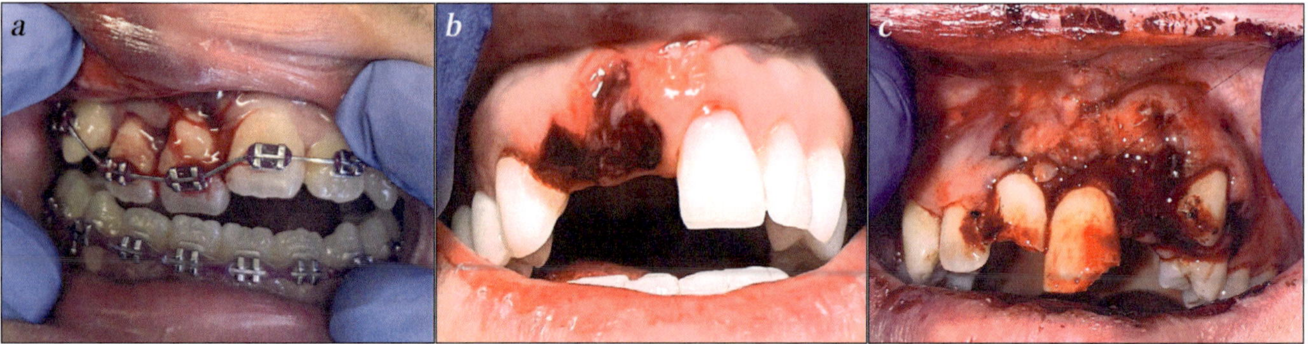

Figure 7-5 Local avulsive injuries vary from *(a)* partial subluxation of teeth, to *(b)* full subluxation of teeth with minimal loss of bone and soft tissue, to *(c)* subluxation of teeth combined with alveolar ridge fractures and significant loss of teeth and adjacent bone (courtesy Dr. E. Sung).

Injuries to the teeth may be categorized into three broad categories: (1) fractures of enamel, dentin, and cementum; (2) irreversible pulpitis; (3) avulsions and/or subluxations resulting in loss of teeth and alveolar bone. Mandibular anterior teeth are more prone to avulsion, while maxillary anterior teeth are more likely to fracture and have pulpal injuries. Periodontal defects are often found with tooth fractures that involve cementum and are immediately adjacent to avulsed regions along displaced jaw fractures. The loss of teeth and alveolar bone often require the use of a removable dental prosthesis, with or without implant support. These prostheses require extensive flanges to replace missing hard and soft tissue while providing adequate facial support. The size and configuration of the edentulous area often preclude the use of conventional fixed prosthodontics.

Jaw fractures

Patients presenting with jaw fractures frequently require an interdisciplinary approach. Often, several teeth are lost and require replacement during the healing period with a provisional prosthesis and after healing with a definitive prosthesis. In addition, the surgeon may be confronted with the management of jaw fractures that are inherently unstable, often resulting in occlusal discrepancies. In such cases, the surgeon requires the support of a maxillofacial prosthodontist to design and fabricate a prosthesis that will aid in the immobilization of the fractured bones to promote rapid and satisfactory healing. Following healing, a definitive prosthesis may be fabricated to address any resultant occlusal discrepancies and restore the missing dentition and adjacent structures.

Anatomic considerations

Traditionally, the facial skeleton has been divided into three components (Fig 7-6). The middle third, frequently referred to as the midface area, comprises a central facial area that includes the nasal complex region. The lateral portion of this middle third area is referred to as the zygoma, malar, or cheek area and should more accurately be called the zygomaticomaxillary complex region. The zygomatic arches lie within this lateral component of the middle third area and often fracture independently. The upper limit of this middle third area is the supraorbital ridge, and the lower (inferior) limit is the occlusal plane. The lower third of the facial skeleton is composed of the mandible and the mandibular teeth.

The midface region is made up of several relatively thin, fragile bones that tend to absorb the fracturing force, resulting in multiple fractures of individual bones. The dissipation of these forces by the fracturing of the facial bones tends to serve as a protection to the orbit and intracranial structures.

Considerable forces are necessary to cause fracture of the jaws. But it must be noted that there are certain inherently weak boney areas of the jaws along which fractures have a greater tendency to occur. This is especially true in the mandible, and fractures occur in the region of the impacted third molar and in the region of the mandibular canine because of its relatively long root structure. The long, slender mandibular condylar neck is another area where fractures frequently occur. In addition, certain pathologic states, such as cysts when they exist in bone, increase the likelihood of a fracture either as a spontaneous event or with a minimum of trauma.

Classification of fractures

Essentially, jaw fractures are of either the closed (simple) or open (compound) variety. Simple fractures occur when the break in the bone is not associated with an open wound. A fracture is referred to as compound when an open wound exists. In the oral and maxillofacial region, a break in the integrity of the skin, mucosal lining of the mouth, nasal passages, or associated paranasal air sinuses constitutes an open wound. It should be appreciated that any fracture of the jaws that occurs in the tooth-bearing area is, by definition, compound intraorally, as there is always some degree of laceration at the gingival crevice.

Fractures in general have been further subdivided to describe the way the ends of the bones have broken. This is usually determined by radiographic studies. A greenstick fracture is one in which the bone is not broken completely through. Because the bones of young children are relatively soft and pliable, it is in this age group that such fractures are generally encountered. Subcondylar fractures in children are generally of this variety. An oblique fracture occurs when the fracture extends diagonally along the bone. This variety of fracture is frequently encountered in the body and ramus of the mandible. A transverse fracture is one in which the fracture exhibits

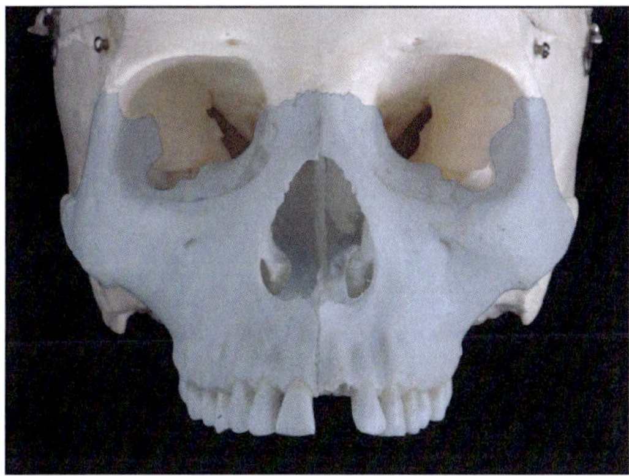

Figure 7-6 Shaded area is shown as the middle (or mid third) of the face. The region lying above this is the upper third, and the lower third is represented by the mandible and mandibular dentition.

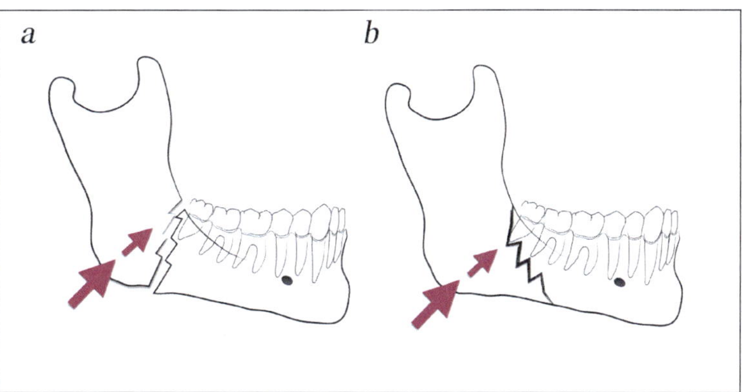

Figure 7-7 *(a)* Unfavorable fracture. Muscular forces are unfavorable. *(b)* Favorable fracture. Muscular forces are favorable.

little or no separation of the broken ends. An impacted fracture is one in which the broken ends of a bone or bony complex are not separate but are actually jammed together. This is a common finding in the mid-maxillofacial region.

General principles of jaw fractures

Fractures can occur singly or in several combinations. A blow to the chin can cause a fracture at the parasymphyseal region (so-called direct fracture), and the fractioning force may be transmitted to the opposite condylar area, causing a subcondylar fracture (so-called indirect fracture). Another commonly seen combination is an injury to the central part of the chin, which often does not fracture itself, in which the force is transmitted to both condylar areas, resulting in bilateral subcondylar fractures (indirect fractures).

Unlike fractures in the midface region, mandibular fractures are frequently influenced by muscular displacing forces. Whether or not the fragments become displaced by the muscular forces depends on the direction of the fracture plane. When it is parallel to the muscular pull, the fracture plane allows displacement of the fragments (unfavorable fracture) (Fig 7-7a). When the fracture plane is in the opposite direction, the muscle pull is advantageous (favorable fracture) (Fig 7-7b). Favorable fractures tend to be self-retaining and facilitate more rapid healing. While displacement of the bony fragments may be the result of the direction of the fracturing force, the degree and severity of the displacement are often greatly influenced by the direction of the muscular pull. Unfavorable fractures usually require the placement of plates or splints to help maintain the position of the fragments.

Fractures of the mandible

The relative prominence of the mandible makes it particularly susceptible to fracture. However, in the absence of an underlying disease process, significant force is required to fracture the mandible. External force—usually in the form of vehicular accidents, sporting injuries, fist fights, falls, industrial accidents, or gunshot injuries—accounts for the fracturing forces in most instances. The mandibular angle, parasymphysis, and condylar neck area are the sites most commonly affected.

Clinical features

The most consistent single clinical finding of a mandibular fracture is a dental malocclusion. Depending on the nature of the fracture, this malocclusion may be obvious, or it may be subtle. If a patient volunteers the information that "the teeth don't meet together properly" after trauma to the jaw, then a fracture must be assumed until proven otherwise. The cardinal clinical features of any fracture (i.e., pain, swelling, deformity, and loss of function) will be seen to varying degrees in any fracture of the mandible. The pain is usually made worse by movements of the fractured segments. Should the fracture be between the lingual and mental foramen, varying degrees of numbness of the lower lip may be present. The site and extent of the swelling are obviously dependent on the location and severity of the fracture. In most fractures of the mandible (other than those in the condylar area), there is evidence of intraoral bruising. A sublingual hematoma is a consistent finding and an important diagnostic sign. Often, there are other areas of hematoma, and if the fracture is in the tooth-bearing area, there is tearing or bruising of the gingivae. The range of deformity varies with the type and severity of the fracture, and the loss of function of the mandible is manifested by inability to chew properly, speech difficulties, dysphagia, inability to control salivation, and occasional respiratory difficulties. Examination of the patient must include gentle palpation of the mandible bimanually, with one finger outside the mouth. Fracture sites and movement of the bones can thus be detected. Most fractures of the mandible can be diagnosed clinically, but radiographs and/or scans must be obtained to confirm the diagnosis.

Location

Region of the symphysis. The anterior region of the mandible that extends from a vertical line just distal to the mandibular canine on each side is called the symphyseal region (Fig 7-8). Fractures in this area are called symphyseal fractures. Fractures that occur exactly through the midline are rare, probably accounting for less than 1% of all mandibular fractures. Fractures in this region are far more likely to occur on either side of the midline and are thus often referred to as parasymphyseal fractures. Such fractures are generally oblique and extend in a posteroinferior direction from the region of the mental fossa to the lower border of the mandible. Because of the

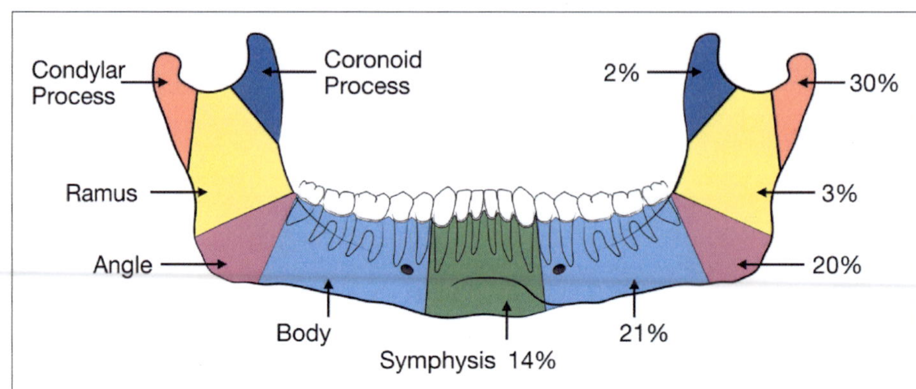

Figure 7-8 Location of mandibular fractures with percentage incidence of occurrence.

nature of the muscle forces acting on such oblique fractures, there is frequently an overlapping or telescoping effect of the fragments.

Region of the body. The body of the mandible has been described as the segment that lies between a vertical line drawn distal to the mandibular canine and a line coinciding with the anterior border of the masseter muscle. This region, which supports the mandibular premolar and molar teeth, is the thickest and strongest portion of the bone, but nonetheless, it is frequently involved in fractures. Fractures in this region, which are by definition compound intraorally, usually exhibit most of the classic signs and symptoms of a mandibular fracture. Paresthesia or anesthesia is a fairly constant finding in these fractures because of injury to the inferior alveolar nerve. Should the proximal segment (i.e., the segment nearest to the temporomandibular joint) be edentulous, and the direction of the fracture is horizontal and unfavorable (as it frequently is), then this fragment is pulled upward and medially by the pterygomasseteric sling of muscles until it impinges on the upper arch or alveolar ridge. If this proximal fragment has teeth, they will occlude with their maxillary counterparts (if present).

Angle fractures. The region of the angle has been defined clinically as the area of the mandible enclosed by the pterygomasseteric sling of muscles. This region accounts for approximately 20–25% of all fractures of the mandible. The possibility of a subcondylar fracture, or fracture of the opposite side of the mandible, should be considered when a fracture of the mandibular angle region occurs. Although the pterygomasseteric muscle complex affords good protection to this area, it is still a common site for fractures because the bone is thinner here than in the body region, and the relatively high incidence of impacted third molars in this region further weakens the bone. The more posterior the angle of the fracture, the more likely it is to be splinted by the muscles and be nondisplaced. More anterior angle fractures frequently produce varying degrees of displacement of the proximal fragment, usually in a superomedial direction.

Ramus fractures. Because of the powerful splinting effect of the pterygomasseteric sling of muscles, fractures in the region are rare and almost never displaced.

Coronoid fractures. The coronoid region is well protected by muscles and by the boney zygomatic arch, and thus, isolated fractures of this region are rare. Fractures of this region generally occur in conjunction with fractures of other parts of the mandible.

Condylar fractures. Fractures in the region of the head of the condyle and the slender condylar neck seldom are the result of direct trauma to the area: they are more likely to be the result of an indirect injury from a direct blow to the parasymphyseal region of the opposite side of the mandible. Fractures of the condyle head are of either the intracapsular or extracapsular variety. Direct trauma to the midline symphyseal area of the mandible can result in bilateral subcondylar fractures, a clinical situation that often poses a difficult management problem. Because of the attachment of the lateral (external) pterygoid muscle (i.e., to the anterior surface of the condylar neck), fractures below this attachment usually result in anteromedial displacement of this proximal (upper) fragment. Clinically, this manifests itself by a deviation to the affected side of the mouth opening and infrequently altered occlusal relationships.

In bilateral subcondylar fractures, there is a shortening of the posterior facial height with an anterior open bite. Intracapsular fractures, which by definition occur above the attachment of the lateral pterygoid muscle, are therefore not subjected to muscular displacing forces. There is often an occlusal disharmony on the affected side as a result of intracapsular bleeding, which forces the condyle downward.

If not managed correctly, subcondylar fractures will lead to a variety of problems. These include an anterior open bite, temporomandibular joint dysfunction, and trismus. The younger the patient the more likely is the possibility of temporomandibular joint ankylosis, especially in an intracapsular fracture.

Fractures of the maxilla and the middle third of the face

General principles—The most common facial fracture, generally the simplest to treat, is the nasal fracture. However, maxillary fractures, often the most demanding facial fractures to treat, also lie within the same middle third area.

Maxillary fractures are often misdiagnosed or underdiagnosed. There are several reasons for this situation. The facial bones are thin and fragile and lie in several planes. Soft tissue swelling often masks the degree of underlying bony deformity. Because of the relative density of the cranial bones that lie behind the midfacial bony skeleton, even a grossly displaced fracture may be difficult to demonstrate radiographically, and therefore, the diagnosis of such fractures is usually determined by clinical evaluation and/or CT scans.

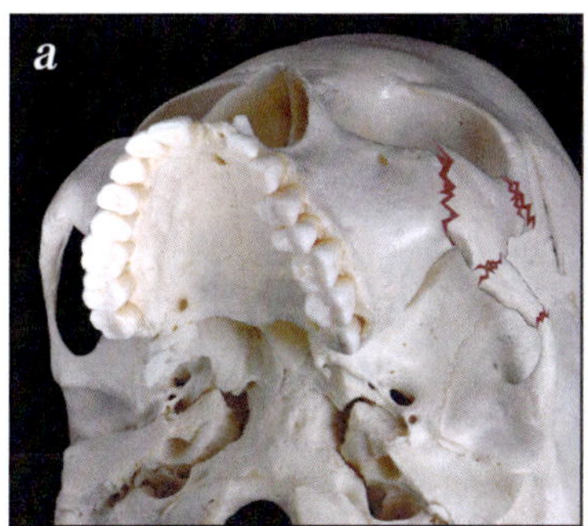

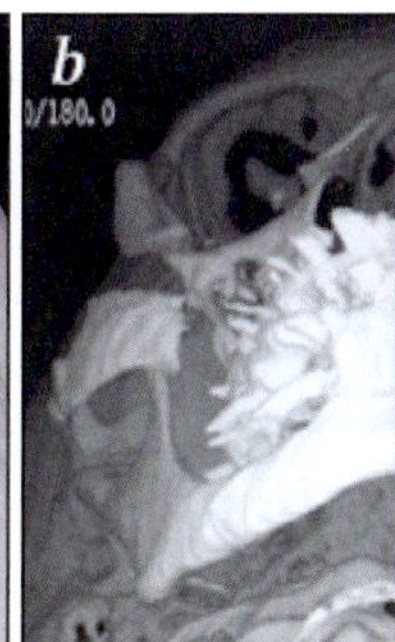

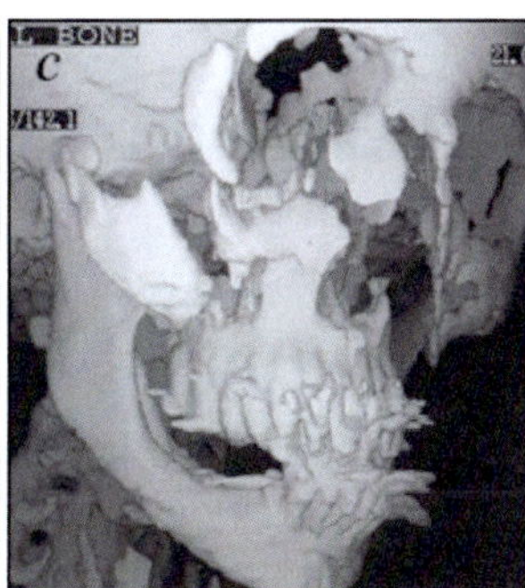

Figure 7-9 *(a, b, and c)* Note the close anatomic relationship between the coronoid process and zygomatic arch. Fractures in these areas result in trismus and restriction of mandibular movement.

Fractures of the zygomaticomaxillary complex

Fractures that are confined to the lateral middle third area are often made more confusing by differences in terminology. The zygoma (malar or cheekbone) and zygomatic arch are composed of three bony entities: the zygomatic process of the temporal bone, the zygoma, and the short zygomatic process of the maxilla. All three form a part of the zygomaticomaxillary complex. Importantly, these bones form part of the bony orbital cavity, and therefore, many of these fractures frequently involve the orbit and its contents.

The orbital blowout fracture is caused by trauma applied to the orbital globe that causes a sudden, sharp rise in the intraorbital pressure. The orbital floor is particularly thin and fragile and is therefore easily fractured by this compressing force. It is of interest to note that fracture and blowout through the equally fragile and thin medial wall of the bony orbit are rare, and this is possibly explained by the fact that this thin wall of bone (lamina papyracea) is composed of honeycombed ethmoidal air sinuses, which may help dissipate the forces.

Clinical features—Of primary importance in evaluating suspected fractures of the zygomaticomaxillary complex is a thorough examination and assessment of the orbit and the orbital contents. In the infant and young child, reliance has often been placed on the physical examination alone. In the older child and adult, correlating the signs with the symptoms makes the diagnosis an easier task. The basic principle of comparing sides is important. The examining doctor should note any periorbital ecchymosis or edema. Should the eyelids be markedly edematous, as they frequently are, difficulty may be experienced in examining the eye adequately. Sterile cotton swabs may prove extremely useful as an aid to examination. Subconjunctival hemorrhage extending to the limbus of the eye is a strong supporting sign of a bony orbital fracture. Edema of the conjunctiva (chemosis) may be seen in many cases. Eye movements should be carefully evaluated and any diplopia noted. Diplopia restricted to the upward gaze usually implies a fracture of the orbital floor with some degree of entrapment of the inferior rectus muscle.

Careful palpation of the orbital rims (comparing both sides) should be carried out, and any "point tenderness" elicited should be noted. Such tenderness in the regions of the frontozygomatic suture and zygomaticomaxillary suture especially is an important diagnostic sign. In addition, any "steps" in the rims should be noted, as these represent a discontinuity in the bony contour. Palpation over the zygomatic arch area for tenderness and any depressions is also important. On occasion, orbital emphysema can be detected as a crackling crepitation sensation by the examining fingers. This sign implies that there is a communication between the nasal passages or paranasal air sinuses and the periorbital soft tissues. The air passes into these soft tissues, usually as the result of blowing the nose sometime after the trauma occurred. This can be an alarming sign but tends to disappear rapidly if simple measures are carried out (Brady et al., 1976).

If the zygomatic arch is depressed and/or the zygomaticomaxillary complex fracture is rotated, there may be an obvious flattening of the normal cheek prominence. However, the inevitable edema that accompanies these fractures often obscures this flattening, and the appearance may be deceptively normal—even though the underlying bony structure may be markedly depressed. Subtle depressions and flattening may be best appreciated if the patient is examined from behind and above. Unilateral epistaxis is often seen in these fractures as a result of bleeding into the maxillary antrum. Because of the close proximity of the infraorbital nerve to the inferior orbital rim, fractures in this region are frequently associated with damage to this nerve and its terminal branches. Clinically, this is manifested by anesthesia (or paresthesia) of the lower eyelid side of the nose and upper lip. Direct trauma to the prominence of the cheek may result in a small area of sensory impairment from the contusion of the zygomaticofacial nerve, a small but consistent branch of the maxillary nerve.

On occasion, these fractures are compound intraorally, with resultant oral bleeding or ecchymosis, and therefore, no examination is complete without a thorough intraoral examination. In addition, the occlusion should be carefully inspected, as a downwardly rotated complex fracture can alter the occlusion in certain circumstances. Trismus and/or restricted lateral excursion of the mandible to the affected side may be seen in depressed arch fractures. This is easily explained when one considers the close anatomic relationship of the zygomatic arch to the coronoid process of the mandible (Fig 7-9).

It is essential to seek consultation from the ophthalmologic service in all cases of fractures involving the bony orbit. Expert preoperative assessment of the eye is essential if serious problems are to be avoided. This obviously is of major importance should any damage to the globe itself be suspected.

Fractures of the central middle third of the facial skeleton

Classic experimental studies by Rene LeFort (1901) broadly subdivided fractures of this region into three main groups (Fig 7-10).

LeFort I (low level)
LeFort II (pyramidal)
LeFort III (high level, craniofacial dysfunction type)

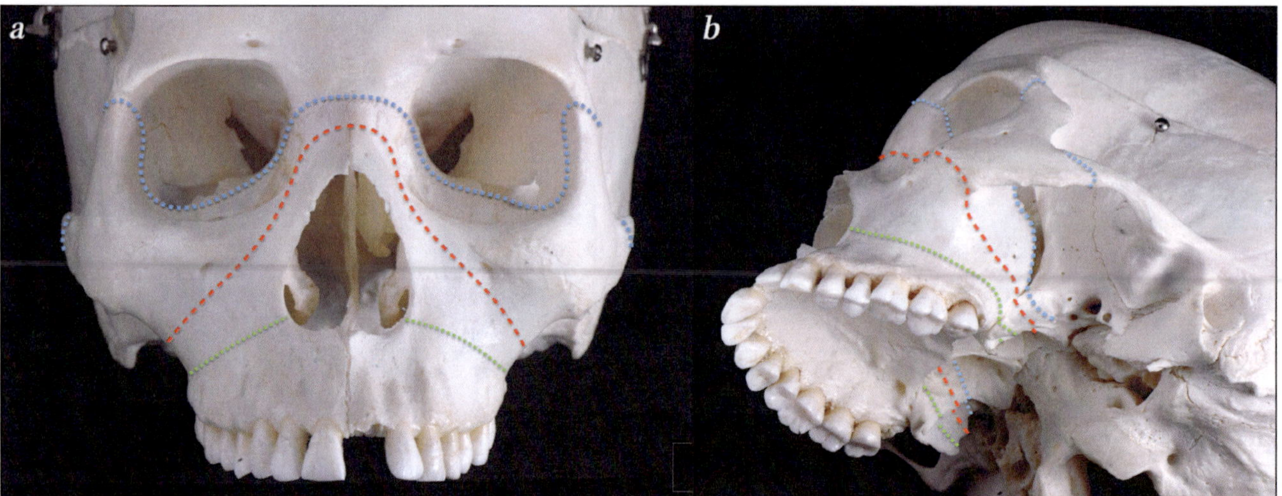

Figure 7-10 *(a and b)* Green line represents the level of LeFort I (low level, Guerin type) fracture; red line represents the level of LeFort II (pyramidal) fracture; blue line represents the level of LeFort III fracture.

Note that LeFort I and II fractures are both subzygomatic, whereas the LeFort III variety is suprazygomatic in nature. Combinations of any of these varieties may occur. Although many different bones compose the facial skeletal framework, from a practical point of view, fractures should be considered in reference to large "blocks" of bone rather than to individual components.

Clinical features—If a LeFort fracture is suspected clinically, important diagnostic signs to look for are mobility of the fractured block of bone and teeth in relation to a fixed point. In a LeFort III fracture (or high-level fracture), such a fixed point is the frontal bone area, whereas in a LeFort I type fracture, the nasal apparatus and zygomatic area are unaffected and therefore stable relative to the mobile fracture. However, such mobility is not always elicited, especially in impacted fractures, and considerable experience is needed to detect subtle movements in some cases. Generalized facial edema is often marked. Bilateral periorbital hematoma and subconjunctival hemorrhage are important signs. Again, massive edema may mask the degree of underlying skeletal disruption. In LeFort III fractures, the tendency is for the entire middle third complex to be pushed posteriorly. As the base of the skull assumes an inclined plane relative to the occlusal plane, such a backward displacement is accompanied by a downward displacement of the posterior portion. This may be represented clinically as an overall flattening of the face, which also becomes elongated and is accompanied by an anterior open bite. Displacement of the middle third facial complex from the cranial base in the region of the cribriform plate of the ethmoid bone may result in the tearing of the olfactory nerve elements, with resultant permanent damage to the sense of smell. Trauma in this area may also be accompanied by a rupture of the meningeal coverings (dura mater and arachnoid) of these first cranial nerves, with the resultant escape of cerebrospinal fluid from the subarachnoid space into the nasal cavity (cerebrospinal fluid rhinorrhea).

Often accompanying such middle third fractures are fractures of the nasal bones and nasoethmoidal complex. Such compression fractures are usually associated with a widening of the nasal bridge area and a resultant traumatic ocular hypertelorism.

Management of facial bone fractures

Early (supportive) management—When fractures of the facial skeleton occur, attention must primarily be directed to basic life-support measures. First, priority must be given to the establishment and maintenance of an adequate airway. Blood, mucous, or vomitus should be removed from the oropharynx, either manually or with the aid of a suction apparatus. The tongue should be prevented from retruding and obstructing the oropharyngeal airway by positioning the head or by utilizing gentle traction with a suture or towel clip placed on the tongue. Placement of an oral airway, a nasoendotracheal airway, or an endotracheal tube may be necessary. Should these measures fail, a tracheostomy may have to be performed. Should any doubt exist about whether to perform a tracheostomy, it is probably best to do one. Once the airway has been established, attention should be directed to arresting any hemorrhage.

Once the airway and hemorrhage have been properly managed, attention should be directed to the patient's general physical condition and any associated injuries, such as trauma to the chest, abdomen, and other bones. Adequate fluid intake is essential. Maintenance of an intravenous line with adequate fluid replacement may prove necessary, as dehydration can easily occur as a result of inadequate oral fluid intake. Once the patient's condition has been stabilized, the nature and extent of the facial injuries are assessed.

As a temporary supportive aid, head bandages may be used. The temporary splinting action can greatly minimize the pain and discomfort. Should it be necessary to sedate the patient, or to administer a short general anesthetic for assessment purposes, this time should be utilized to obtain impressions of the dental arches. Casts made from such impressions often prove invaluable in accurately assessing the occlusion and the condition of the teeth. In addition, these casts can be duplicated and utilized for the construction of various types of splints.

In highly unstable fractures, particularly those that might hamper the airway due to tongue control, it may prove necessary to temporarily wire the jaws together, although this should be avoided unless absolutely necessary. However, a wire passed around the teeth on either side of the fracture, without wiring the jaws together, often proves useful as a temporary measure.

Appropriate analgesics should be administered. Any facial fracture that passes through the tooth socket is, by definition, compounded intraorally—even if the fracture is not displaced and the tooth is firm in the socket. Similarly, fractures that involve the paranasal sinuses should be considered compound, and therefore, all patients with such fractures should receive adequate antibiotic prophylaxis.

The general aim of treatment is to achieve bone healing with the best possible dental occlusion in the shortest possible time. Restoring the bone ends and the proper dental occlusion maintains appearance and symmetry. As soon as the patient's general condition permits, reduction or realignment of the bony fragments should be carried out. This is then followed by a period of immobilization to allow bony healing to take place.

Often, fractured bone fragments can be realigned by manipulation without direct visualization of the fractured bone ends. This closed method of reduction is usually employed when displacement of the fragments is minimal and a good stable result is anticipated. However, it may prove necessary in some instances to surgically expose the fracture site and visualize the bone ends to reduce the fracture. When an open reduction is performed, the reduced fragments are usually secured by intraosseous (transosseous) wires, plates, or metal mesh tray systems. Depending on the individual circumstances, open reduction of a fractured jaw can be performed via either the intraoral or the extraoral route.

As soon as the general condition of the patient permits, reduction and immobilization of the fracture should be carried out. However, it must be emphasized that apart from an acute airway problem or profuse hemorrhage (which is surprisingly rare), fractures of the jaws alone are rarely life-threatening. Therefore, it is generally more prudent to allow time for the patient's condition to be stabilized and utilize this time to obtain satisfactory radiographs, scans, and diagnostic casts.

Temporomandibular joint injuries

Injuries to the temporomandibular joints are common, with traumatic forces directed to the anterior mandible and/or from direct impact on the TMJ. The examination should note the presence of pain, abnormal sounds, and any limitation of rotary and translatory movement, as observed during vertical opening and/or lateral eccentric jaw movements. Evaluation should also include an assessment of the normal range of border movements, with consideration for individual patient variations. Comparisons should be made between restrictions during right and left lateral and protrusive jaw movements, with and without tooth contact. Restrictions to movement may be related to intracapsular injuries, such as adhesions, displaced discs, intracondylar fractures, and so on. Extracapsular injuries may be caused by mandibular-zygoma-maxillary fractures, neuromuscular splinting, or spasms. Deviations will usually occur toward the affected side. The diagnosis is typically supported by restricted lateral jaw movements (lack of translation) that correspond to an ipsilateral deviated protrusive movement. A previous history of temporomandibular joint disorders (TMDs) and their treatment should be carefully noted.

Traumatic injuries may exacerbate a preexisting TMD whose symptomatology may have been subclinical, inconspicuous, and/or longstanding. Initial findings may indicate symptomatology, suggesting subluxation, edema, and sprain of limited duration that may resolve with rest, soft diet, and application of vapocoolant spray with alternating moist heat to the musculature. It is common to find that the posterior teeth cannot achieve maximum intercuspation, as determined by articulating ribbon or shimstock, and the anterior teeth may be in hyperocclusion, as indicated by the patient's awareness and presence of fremitus. The prescription of nonsteroidal anti-inflammatory drugs or muscle relaxants may be indicated.

Unstable disc complexes can result in reciprocal clicking (with anterior displaced disc) with or without reduction and locking. This may indicate a need to provide a stabilizing influence upon the articular disc, with uniform occlusal contact provided by interocclusal splints. Occlusal adjustments may not be indicated during the initial stabilization period, as atypical tooth contacts may resolve with reduction in soft tissue inflammation and spasm, or eliminated with reduction of the bony fractures. Occlusal adjustments may be indicated when attempting to eliminate tooth hyperfunction that may lead to tooth fracture, periodontal injury, and/or migration. After surgical fracture reduction, occlusal adjustments and/or new restorations may be required to reduce excessive tooth contact when the occlusal vertical dimension has been traumatically increased and/or decreased from the residual malposed bony segments. Subcondylar neck fractures are a frequent finding, while intracondylar fractures are less frequent and more difficult to detect radiographically.

Severe trauma may fracture, dislocate, and displace the condylar head from the capsule, causing a severe unresolving mechanical obstruction that prevents mandibular movement. This may necessitate a condylectomy with a resultant discontinuity defect or other additional surgical correction. Aberrant tooth contacts will occur, causing deflection upon closure, and will likely require adjustment. Recontoured or flattened cusps may be necessary to achieve a harmonious or nondeflective occlusion. Reconstructive temporomandibular joint surgery may improve function, but limitations of opening and lateral jaw movements may remain. Consideration may be given to the autogenous grafting of cartilage from the concha of the ear when the disc has been obliterated and a painful bone-to-bone contact exists. The objective is a pain-free joint that permits adequate functional movements at an appropriate occlusal vertical dimension with a repeatable and stable position.

Definitive management of jaw fractures

Mandibular fractures

Many fractures of the mandible can be satisfactorily treated by closed techniques. Provided there are a sufficient number of satisfactory teeth present in both jaws, they may be utilized for the application of arch bars, wire loops, and splints. The maxilla can be used as a stable base for immobilizing the fractured mandible by securing the maxillary and mandibular arch bars together with rubber bands or wires. It is only with the maintenance of proper immobilization in a correct occlusion that will support satisfactory bone healing.

There are several techniques available for the reduction and stabilization of any given mandibular fracture. Most fractures are treated either closed (intermaxillary fixation, splinting, modified diet) or open (plates and screws, interosseous wiring, lag screws). The method chosen depends on a number of variables, including

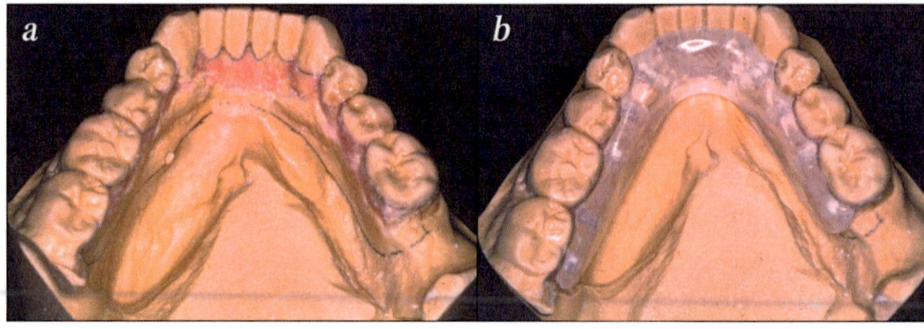

Figure 7-11 *(a)* Cast of a patient with undisplaced parasymphyseal fracture. Note the wax blockout of interproximal areas. *(b)* Completed clear acrylic resin lingual splint on cast.

dental status, fracture characteristics (open, closed, favorable, unfavorable, comminution, bone loss, mechanism of injury, contamination or obvious infection, etc.), fracture location, associated injuries, patient mental status, and patient desires. The most important considerations are the dental status, fracture characteristics, and fracture location.

Impressions

If the patient has an insufficient number of sound teeth available for fixation or is edentulous in either or both arches, it is necessary that impressions be made and duplicated casts be fabricated. In addition to serving as diagnostic study models, the casts allow for the fabrication of various types of fracture splints.

Modifications to standard impression techniques are often required to ensure accurate records are made. The pain, swelling, trismus, and excessive salivation associated with fractures make this task more challenging. However, with careful planning and preparation, good impressions are obtainable. In order not to stress the patient further, local anesthesia using infiltration and block techniques is beneficial. Usually, control of pain reduces trismus, facilitating the impression procedure. Good lighting and suction are essential. The mouth should be gently irrigated and the surfaces of the teeth cleaned. Frequently, stock trays must be modified to meet individual needs. This is usually achieved by trimming the lingual flange of the tray, which greatly facilitates insertion. Care should be taken so that minimum distraction of the fragments occurs. In most cases, irreversible hydrocolloid is the impression material of choice. Should the patient be submitted to a general anesthetic for any other purpose, it is wise to use this opportunity to make impressions.

Lingual splints

Because of adverse muscular forces, parasymphyseal fractures of the mandible tend toward lingual collapse and overlap of the fractured segments with the widening of the posterior sector. Wire loops or arch bars alone that are applied to the teeth on either side of the fracture line frequently cannot control this tendency to collapse. The problem can be overcome by using lingual acrylic resin splints on a corrected sectioned cast of the mandibular dentition (Fig 7-11). The lingual splint is secured to the arch by incorporating it with wires that ligate the buccally placed arch bar to the teeth. The combined effect of the buccal arch bar and the lingual splint is an effective means of immobilization. Parasymphyseal fractures often occur in combination with an indirect fracture of the subcondylar area. Placing the lingual splint supports early removal of the intermaxillary fixation (3–4 weeks postoperatively) so that the chances of fibrous or bony ankylosis can be greatly reduced. Presently, they are primarily used in treating pediatric patients.

Edentulous patients

If an edentulous patient presents with an existing prosthesis, modifications can be made by applying hooks or arch bars secured with autopolymerizing acrylic resin and then secured with circumferential wires. The maxillary denture is retained and stabilized by circumzygomatic and pyriform aperture wires, while circummandibular wires secure the mandibular denture. By occluding the dentures and using interarch wires, the fractured mandible can be immobilized adequately. Even if the dentures were fractured at the time of injury, they should be repaired and then used as fracture splints. If no dentures are available, impressions should be made of the arches, centric records created, the resultant casts mounted on an articulator, and a modified two-piece "Gunning" splint constructed on sectioned and corrected casts. These splints are secured to the jaws in the same manner as the modified dentures. Should the fracture be minimally displaced, especially in older patients, the placement of a lower splint alone, supported by a barrel-type bandage, will suffice. It is less essential to achieve an absolutely perfect reduction in such cases, as subsequently fabricated dentures can compensate for minor bony irregularities. In elderly patients, emphasis must be placed on obtaining bony union in the shortest possible time without compromising the general health of the patient. In the case of the atrophic mandible, the blood supply is generally compromised, requiring closed methods of reduction in most cases. On occasion, open reductions may prove necessary, and the bone ends are secured together with reconstruction plates or metal tray systems.

Condylar fractures

Condylar fractures demand special consideration. There is a general consensus that condylar fractures, when they occur in adults or children, should be treated by closed methods of reduction in the vast majority of cases (Ghasemzadeh et al., 2015; McGoldrick et al., 2019). Indications for an open reduction of such a fracture include a fracture-dislocation that proves impossible to reduce by closed methods alone and bilateral subcondylar fractures associated with midface fractures in which there is a significant loss of posterior face height. It must be emphasized that closed methods of treatment are performed in a majority of cases. Whatever the treatment modality performed, it is important that the patient be

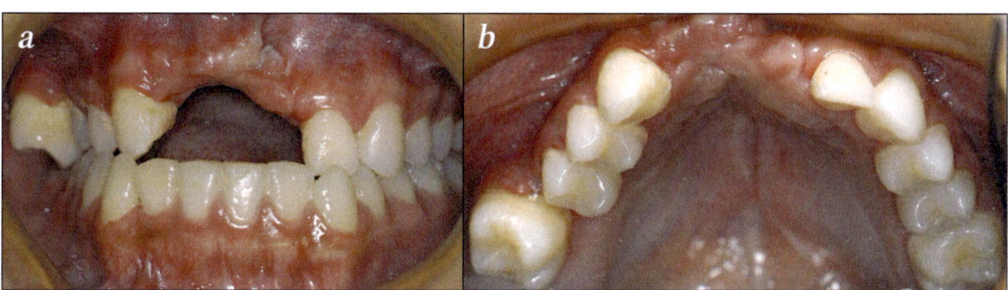

Figure 7-12 *(a and b)* Malunion of maxillary fractures has led to malocclusion and facial disfigurement.

released from intermaxillary fixation approximately three weeks after surgery to prevent trismus, which can often be severe with prolonged fixation. The management of such fractures in the growing child is of particular importance if serious growth deformities are to be avoided. Emphasis should be on early immobilization if a satisfactory occlusion can be consistently registered by the child (Brady and Leak, 1978).

Fractures of the middle third of the facial skeleton

As in fractures of the mandible, the general aim of treatment is to achieve healing with good occlusal and aesthetic outcomes. The complex skeletal union must include the integrity of the orbital apparatus and the nasal airway structures. The correct management of many of these fractures demands the highest diagnostic and surgical skills. Inadequate or incorrectly treated midface fractures can often result in severe facial deformity with aesthetic and functional compromise that often is extremely difficult to treat secondarily.

Unlike fractures of the mandible, there are no strong muscular forces tending to displace the fractures of this region. The downward displacing tendency of the strong masseter muscle is counteracted by the attachment of the equally strong temporalis fascia to the superior aspect of the zygomatic arch. Therefore, unless such a fracture is inherently unstable, once reduced, it generally tends to remain stable. The first step is to restore the occlusion with intermaxillary fixation. When necessary, transosseous wires and miniplates are used to stabilize fractures in this region. LeFort I and II type fractures, once disimpacted and reduced, can be stabilized with circumzygomatic suspension wires and/or titanium miniplates and screws. Following stabilization of all fractures, the intermaxillary wires can be removed and the patient's occlusion checked. Some clinicians prefer to leave the arch bars on for one to two weeks in case training elastics are needed for any occlusal disharmonies that become apparent. The titanium plates and screws are not removed.

Complications of facial fractures

Provided care is taken in the diagnosis and management of facial bone fractures, satisfactory healing with a good functional and aesthetic outcome should be expected in a majority of cases. However, problems in healing can occur. As a result of poor or inadequate treatment or possibly as a result of some intermediate event that occurred during the fixation period, a malunion or nonunion of the fracture may occur. Malunion means that healing has taken place, but the bony union is in poor position (Fig 7-12). The extent of the malunion must be assessed carefully, as the degree of deformity may be acceptable when other considerations are taken into account. This is especially true when the jaws are edentulous, as the primary concern is for the bony union, while the bony irregularities can often be compensated for by adjusting, relining, or remaking the dentures. However, in dentate patients with a significant occlusal discrepancy, it is often necessary to perform the appropriate osteotomies on the jaws to realign the occlusion and to allow the bones to heal in the new, corrected position (see below, section entitled "Rehabilitation of patients with malunion of jaw fractures").

Nonunion (fibrous union) usually occurs from a perpetuation of the delayed healing or delayed union state. Infection affecting the fracture site, especially virulent resisting organisms, is the common culprit. Also, infection is more likely to occur if the overall resistance of the patient is lowered, for example, in diabetes mellitus. Circumstances that permit the establishment and persistence of infection include compound open wounds (especially extraoral), segments of devitalized bone between the fracture, nonvital teeth in the fracture line, interpositional foreign bodies, and improper fixation techniques.

Whereas each case of nonunion must be considered on its own merits, general principles of management include the administration of the appropriate antibiotic in the correct dosage for an adequate period of time, the removal of any necrotic bone and foreign bodies, and the removal of appropriate teeth in the region of the nonunion. After such a thorough debridement of the area, the jaws should be placed in stable intermaxillary fixation. Depending on the individual case, it may prove necessary to bone graft the resultant defect to ensure a firm bony union. If an infection is involved in the nonunion, it is wise to allow this to be fully resolved before bone grafting.

An important complication of fractures in the region of the mandibular condyle is ankylosis (Brady and Leake, 1978). Ankylosis can compromise the development of the mandible on the affected side in the growing child. Additionally, generalized nutritional deficiencies and local deterioration in the health of the teeth and gingiva frequently result. Therefore, careful assessment and correct treatment of such fractures are extremely important.

Treatment during healing and recovery

The period of intermediate management usually extends from two to six months. During this phase, a provisional or treatment prosthesis is usually provided for aesthetic and/or phonetic purposes but also can be used to stabilize the occlusion (Fig 7-13). These prostheses provide the patient with a general sense of well-being and allow them to anticipate future treatment outcomes. They also help

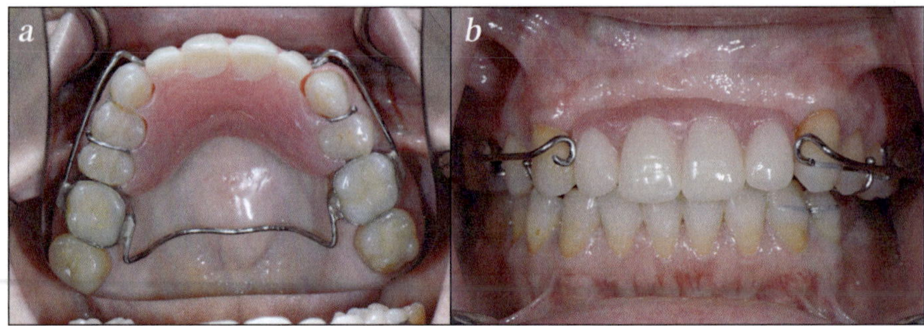

Figure 7-13 *(a and b)* A simple interim RDP can be used as a provisional restoration (reprinted from Beumer et al., 2022, with permission).

define the prosthodontic issues that need to be addressed with the definitive treatment plan, such as tooth position, occlusal scheme, implant position and angulation, and so on.

If the patient presents with a mandibular discontinuity defect, plans are made to restore continuity with appropriate grafts and flaps. Free bone graphs are preferred for most such discontinuity defects, but the soft tissue bed destined to receive the bone graft should be carefully scrutinized. If there has been a significant loss of soft tissue or its vasculature has been compromised, consideration should be given to restoring the defect with a vascularized osteomyocutaneous flap. When free grafts are used, metal lingual splints of cobalt-chrome can be useful adjuncts to supplement fixation during healing (see below, section entitled "Rehabilitation of patients with large avulsive defects of the maxilla and mandible"). They can be designed and cast with the traditional analog method or designed digitally and printed with selective laser melting. Both types of bone grafts (free or vascularized) provide suitable bone volume and density to receive osseointegrated implants.

If the patient presents with malunion of their fractures, plans are made to reposition the residual jaw fragments as necessary with surgical osteotomies in order to restore the occlusion and presurgical facial contours. A cephalometric analysis provides useful information in this endeavor. Presurgical planning can be accomplished with diagnostic casts mounted on a semiadjustable articulator and cast surgery or virtually with CBCT scans and the accompanying software (see below, section entitled "Rehabilitation of patients with malunion of jaw fractures"). Surgical splints are designed as needed and are used to immobilize the jaw segments during consolidation and healing following the surgery.

The maxilla requires careful examination. In patients presenting with multiple fractures or when significant portions of the maxilla have been avulsed, residual fragments are frequently displaced and not attached to the cranial base. Such fragments are repositioned as necessary and reattached to the base of the skull with free bone grafts. In large avulsive defects, consideration should be given to placing implants into the zygoma or the pyriform region when these areas are accessible. These implants can then be used to retain and support an overlay RDP-obturator prosthesis.

It is critical to determine the definitive long-range maxillofacial prosthetic treatment plan during this phase of care and to coordinate this treatment plan with the other treatments being considered. All necessary adjunctive consultations and dental treatment—such as endodontics, periodontics, and orthodontics—should be completed prior to definitive prosthodontic treatment. Customarily, the maxillofacial prosthodontist must coordinate the care of these other specialists, since prosthodontic treatment will be dependent upon the treatment outcomes of these other services. The ability to maintain oral hygiene, keep recall appointments, and develop adequate dexterity for the placement and care of a removable dental prosthesis is another important factor to be considered. The potential influence of other bodily injuries and the level of family support should be assessed. The social worker is essential in this assessment.

Definitive Treatment

Localized defects of the maxilla

Defects secondary to traumatic tooth avulsions differ considerably and vary from loss of just a few teeth and supporting bone of the alveolar ridge to many teeth, creating large tooth-bound and nonlinear edentulous extension defects accompanied by significant loss of soft tissue and supporting bone (Fig 7-14). The alveolar bone defects associated with these injuries are usually clinically significant and, in some instances, quite extensive. These types of injuries occur in both the anterior maxilla and mandible. In some patients, the anterior dentition of both arches is avulsed (Fig 7-15).

These patients may present with significant scarring of the oral mucosa, loss of keratinized attached gingiva, and loss of the facial plate of bone, and in some instances, much of the alveolar ridge, in the affected area. As in Fig 7-16, this finding is especially significant if the use of implants is anticipated. Teeth adjacent to the defect may present with cracks or fractures and be nonvital.

These clinical exam findings will have a significant impact on whether the patient is to be restored with a conventional fixed dental prosthesis using natural tooth abutments, a removable dental prosthesis, or an implant-assisted / implant-supported dental prosthesis. In particular, if an implant-supported fixed dental prosthesis is the objective, the grafting of bone and soft tissues, either prior to implant placement or coincidental with implant placement, will need to be considered.

As implied above, these localized defects can be restored in a variety of ways, including conventional fixed dental prostheses (FDPs), conventional removable dental prostheses (RDPs), implant-supported overlay removable dental prostheses, and implant-supported fixed dental prostheses. The method selected depends on a number of factors, including the size and curvature of the edentulous span, the

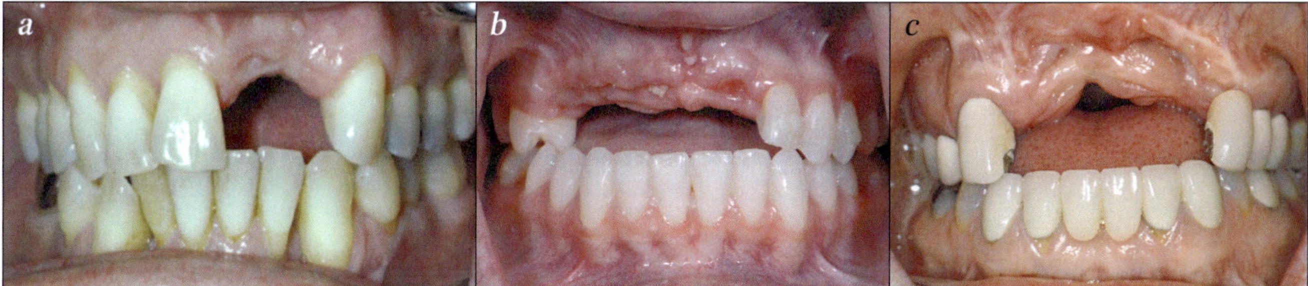

Figure 7-14 *(a)* Complex two-tooth defect secondary to tooth avulsion. There is a significant loss of bone and soft tissue in the edentulous area. *(b and c)* Extensive bone and soft tissue defects have resulted from trauma. Note the soft tissue scarring (reprinted from Beumer et al., 2022, with permission).

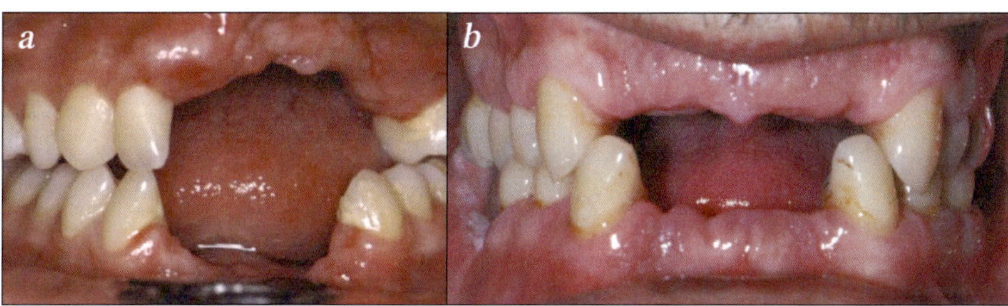

Figure 7-15 *(a and b)* Anterior teeth in both arches have been lost to trauma. One patient *(a)* was restored with implant-supported fixed dental prostheses preceded by bone and soft tissue grafting (see Figure 7-30). The other *(b)* was restored with removable dental prostheses (see Figure 7-20).

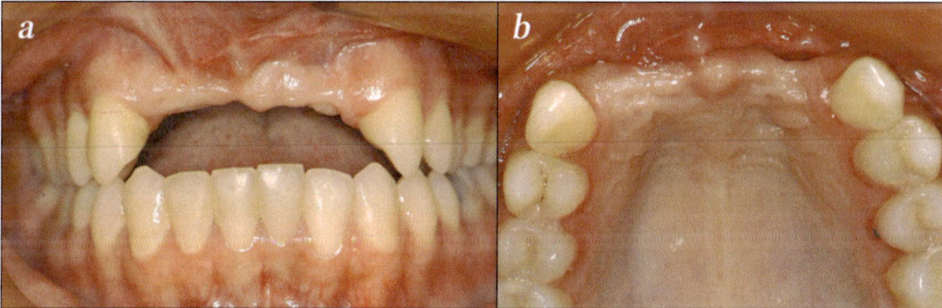

Figure 7-16 *(a)* Traumatic defect with a significant loss of keratinized attached mucosa on the right side. *(b)* Note the loss of the facial plate of bone.

health of potential FDP/RDP abutments, the nature of the hard and soft tissue deficits, the smile line, the predictability of surgical reconstructive procedures, and cost.

These are challenging cases even for the most talented and experienced clinicians. Successful outcomes require careful planning and execution, but it is also important for patients to understand the limits of the proposed method of treatment.

Conventional fixed dental prostheses

This option can be successfully employed when the defects are limited to two to four teeth, are relatively linear, and are accompanied by minimal bone and soft tissue defects. The aesthetic outcome achieved is dependent on the contours of the hard and soft tissue in the edentulous space and the adjacent level of bone associated with the abutment teeth. Patients presenting with large defects and tapered arch forms previously required double abutments to restore from a biomechanical perspective may now be best restored with conventional RDPs, implant-supported overlay RDPs, or implant-supported fixed dental prostheses.

For simple two-to-four tooth defects presenting with reasonable hard and soft tissue contours, a conventional fixed dental prosthesis is cost-effective and predictable. There are several advantages to this approach. Most dentists are familiar with the necessary techniques and are capable of achieving an acceptable outcome. The aesthetic result is quite predictable; however, it is rare to achieve complete bilateral symmetry of tooth form, gingival contours, or perfect restoration of the size/contour of embrasure spaces and the level of interdental papilla, particularly those areas restored by the pontics. The use of pink porcelain will mitigate some of these challenges, providing that the transition between the pink porcelain and the soft tissue is above the smile line (Fig 7-17).

These presentations are challenging, often requiring patients to accept a compromised aesthetic outcome. Tooth forms frequently must be altered, and the interproximal contacts extended to the cervical third to avoid dark spaces in the embrasures are often referred to as black triangles. The use of double abutments is usually necessary when a lateral incisor is adjacent to the edentulous space because its root form and the limited length of the root make this a poor prosthetic abutment. In the areas engaged by the pontics, soft tissue augmentation is often necessary, followed by prolonged use of a provisional restoration to recontour the soft tissues to the desired shape and dimension.

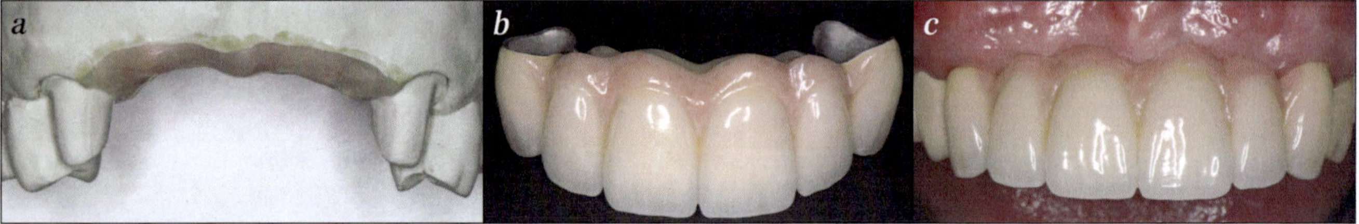

Figure 7-17 *(a)* An anterior defect where all the incisors have been lost. *(b and c)* The gingival tissues have been restored with pink porcelain (courtesy of Dr. C. Goodacre; reprinted from Beumer et al., 2022, with permission).

There are additional issues of concern regarding the conventional approach to these defects that must be taken into account before this method is employed. First, there is a risk of devitalizing the abutments during tooth preparation because the 1.0 to 1.5 mm of tooth reduction on the labial surfaces required for proper thickness of restorative material may inflict irreversible damage to the pulp. Younger individuals with large pulp chambers are particularly susceptible to pulpal injury, but the risk is reduced as the patient ages and the pulp chamber recedes.

If the abutments require endodontic treatment, they become susceptible to fracture. Since these defects are secondary to trauma, the teeth adjacent to the defects often are devitalized and require endodontic treatment, compromising their predictability as abutments. In such defects, many of the remaining teeth exhibit fractures and loss of substantial portions of the abutment clinical crown, making them difficult to prepare with proper retention and resistance forms. Also, occasionally, the abutment teeth are malpositioned, making the required parallel preparation difficult while maintaining appropriate resistance and retention forms without removing excessive amounts of tooth structure and risking injury to the pulpal tissues.

The occlusion scheme should be designed to avoid excessive cantilevering forces on the natural tooth abutments. This is especially important when restoring patients with tapered arch forms. The residual natural dentition should provide tooth support during lateral excursion, either in the form of anterior guidance with residual canines or group function with premolars when canines are absent. In most instances, because of esthetics, prosthetic lateral incisors will be elevated and will not come in contact with the opposing dentition during excursions. However, given that most destruction is caused by parafunctional activity, the prosthetic central incisors should only be in light contact during excursions.

Adequate hygiene may be difficult, given the compromises in hygiene access often necessary to achieve an acceptable aesthetic outcome. Poor access will discourage the noncompliant or marginally compliant patient from attempts at good hygiene, thereby predisposing the abutments to caries and periodontal breakdown, which may limit their life expectancy. Hygiene access is particularly difficult between teeth that have been splinted together. In the past, these patients were required to master the use of dental floss and floss threaders to remove plaque and debris, and few patients were able or willing to make the time and effort necessary to perform this needed daily task. However, a new generation of disposable interproximal brushes has made it much easier to clean these areas, and patient compliance is expected to improve.

Removable dental prostheses

Several factors favor the restoration of such defects with removable dental prostheses. Many patients with traumatically induced defects present with significant loss of the facial plate of bone and keratinized attached mucosa. The size and curvature of the edentulous span, and the availability of suitable tooth abutments, often preclude restoration with a conventional fixed dental prosthesis. Even in more favorable defects—where the size of the span is limited and the edentulous span more linear, and it would seem ideal to restore the defect with a conventional fixed dental prosthesis from a biomechanical perspective—it may not be prudent to do so. For example, the effects of traumatic injuries on abutment teeth often do not become clinically evident for several years. Such teeth may become nonvital and symptomatic and require endodontic therapy several years after an accident, compromising the long-term prognosis of the abutment and the fixed dental prosthesis that they support. The cost of implant dentistry and required preprosthetic surgery may encourage others to seek a less costly option, such as a conventional RDP. Moreover, the RDP provides more favorable aesthetic outcomes because pink acrylic resin can be used to restore the gingival shape to normal form and contour, and a denture flange can be used to provide needed upper lip support, especially in patients who have lost the facial plate of bone.

Rotational path RDPs are ideally suited to restore anterior edentulous extension defects in such patients (King, 1978; Kroll and Finzen, 1988; Chang et al., 2019). They are esthetically pleasing, because with this design, conventional retainers are not needed in the anterior region (Figs 7-18, 7-19, 7-20). The rotational path RDP works in the following manner: it incorporates a curved path of placement, allowing one or more of the rigid components of the framework to engage an undercut area. In a patient with an anterior edentulous extension area, proximal plates of the RDP framework (Fig 7-18) engage undercuts on the mesial guide planes of the anterior abutments.

The anterior abutment teeth adjacent to the edentulous area *must have positive rests* in order to control tooth position and provide support during function. This option restores esthetics, and when canine teeth bound the edentulous spaces, the RDP is essentially tooth supported, effectively restoring the ability to incise the bolus with reasonable occlusal force (Fig 7-20). In these patients, anterior guidance is provided by the natural canines with the prosthetic teeth in passive contact during lateral excursions. If the canine is lacking, the occlusion is designed for group function utilizing the natural premolars.

Implants and overlay RDPs

Since implants were introduced, they have been used in conjunction with RDPs to augment the stability, retention, and support of

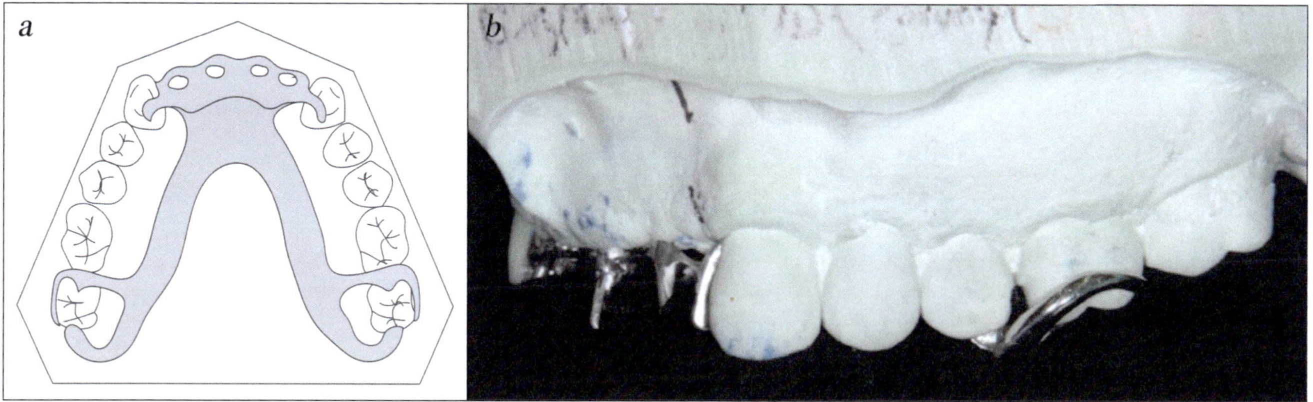

Figure 7-18 *(a)* Rigid proximal plates engage the undercuts on the mesial surfaces of the canines to eliminate the conventional retainers. Positive rests on the canines allow control of the tooth position during function. *(b)* The anterior portion of the rotational path RDP is seated first. Then the RDP rotates around the point where the anterior guide plane contacts the mesial surface of the canine *(a)* and rotates around this point until the molar clasp assembly is completely seated (reprinted from Chang et al., 2019, with permission).

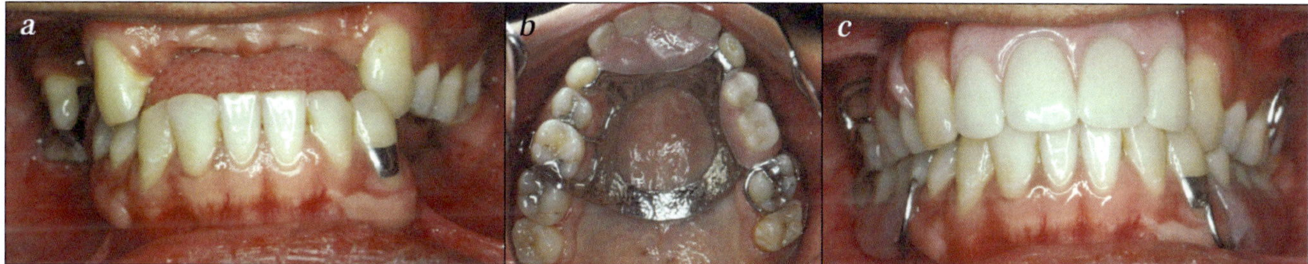

Figure 7-19 *(a)* A large anterior edentulous extension defect secondary to trauma. The anterior dentition was restored with a rotational path RDP. *(b)* Occlusal view of the RDP. Positive cingulum rests were prepared in the two canines. *(c)* Prosthesis in occlusion (courtesy of Dr. E. G. King).

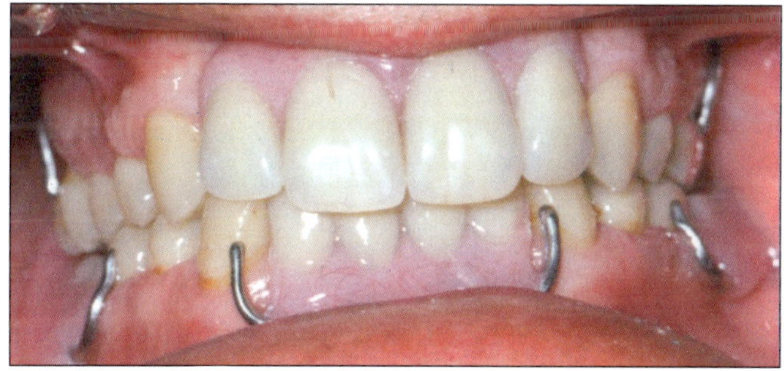

Figure 7-20 The patient presented in Figure 7-15b. The maxillary dentition is restored with a rotational path RDP. The mandibular dentition is restored with a conventional RDP. Cingulum rests were incorporated within all four canines (courtesy of Dr E. G. King).

removable dental prostheses. Large traumatic defects that extend beyond the canine may be best restored with implant-supported overlay RDPs. In such defects, the biomechanics of a conventional fixed dental prosthesis supported by natural tooth abutments may be unfavorable. Moreover, because of the loss of the facial plate and alveolar bone, esthetics and lip support are best restored with a removable dental prosthesis. In such anterior extension defects, two implants provide sufficient support anteriorly so that the patient can incise the bolus. We prefer to use an implant connecting bar in such defects as opposed to individual attachments. Such bars can easily account for divergent implants when present and provide more effective support for the RDP. The RDP engages the natural dentition with positive rests on the abutments adjacent to the anterior edentulous extension area, providing additional support. Stability for the RDP is provided by the minor connectors, associated guide planes, and engagement of the implant connecting bar (Fig 7-21). If individual attachments are preferred, the implants should be placed with the benefit of a surgical template so that the path of insertion of the RDP is compatible with the individual attachments.

In patients presenting with larger traumatic defects, sites for implants may have to be created or augmented with bone grafts. Such grafted bone sites often provide less than ideal implant anchorage. Moreover, the lengths of implants may be suboptimal, and if the implant configuration is linear, lacking A-P spread, the resulting implant configurations will be unfavorable from a biomechanical perspective. Nevertheless, implants can be used effectively in conjunction with overlay RDPs to improve the support in the edentulous extension area.

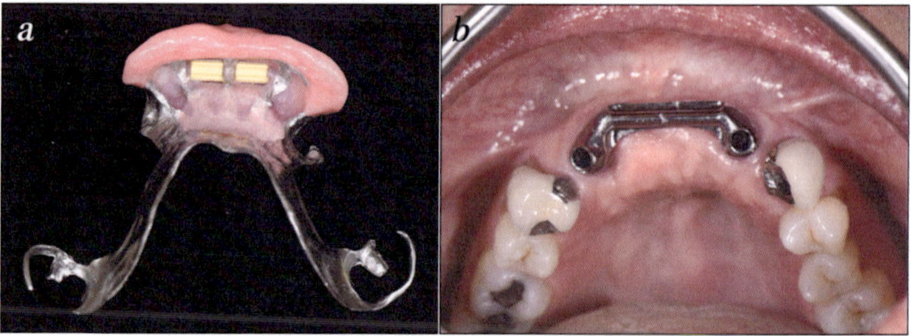

Figure 7-21 *(a and b)* A localized traumatic defect restored with an implant-supported RDP. Note the surveyed crowns bordering the defect with positive rests. The border molded anterior flange provides needed support for the upper lip.

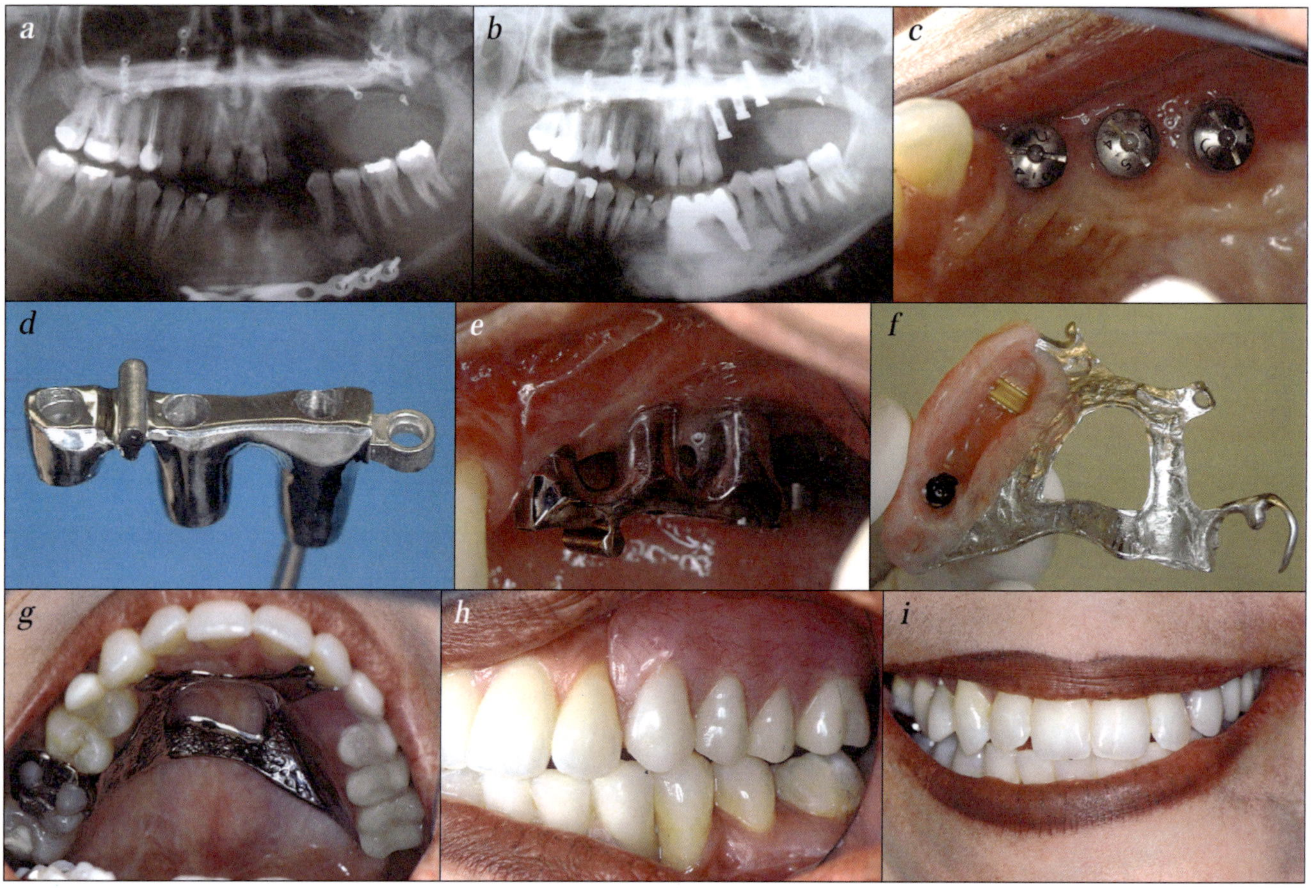

Figure 7-22 *(a)* The patient has suffered multiple facial fractures in an automobile accident and has lost multiple teeth on the left side of the maxilla. *(b and c)* Following a sinus augmentation and additional grafting, three implants have been placed. They are positioned palatally. *(d and e)* Implant connecting bar with a resilient attachment on the distal end. The Hader bar segment is aligned parallel to the axis of rotation. *(f)* Overlay RDP. *(g)* Prosthesis in position. The rests on the anterior teeth are positive. *(h and i)* Prosthesis in position (reprinted from Beumer et al., 2022, with permission).

Such a situation was encountered in the patient shown in Fig 7-22. The patient presented with multiple facial fractures that resulted in the loss of most of the maxillary dentition and much of the alveolar bone posteriorly on the left side. Following the reduction and healing of the fractured mandible and maxilla, a sinus augmentation procedure was performed. An additional grafting procedure was performed to further augment sites for implant placement in the left posterior area of the maxilla. The edentulous region in the mandible was restored with an implant-supported fixed dental prosthesis. However, in the maxilla, only three implants were successfully placed, and the distance between the implant platforms and opposing mandibular dentition was excessive (Fig 7-22b).

Several factors led to the decision to restore the maxilla with an implant-assisted overlay RDP. If an implant-supported fixed dental prosthesis had been fabricated, the biomechanics would have been quite unfavorable, predisposing to implant overload, loss of bone around the implants, and loss of implants. The following factors compromised the biomechanics: unfavorable crown-implant ratios, unfavorable implant positions and angulations, implants anchored primarily in grafted bone, and the linear configuration of the implants, along with the fact that the "corner" of the arch (canine-premolar region) was being restored.

Unfavorable crown-implant ratios. The unfavorable crown-implant ratios were secondary to the loss of teeth and the

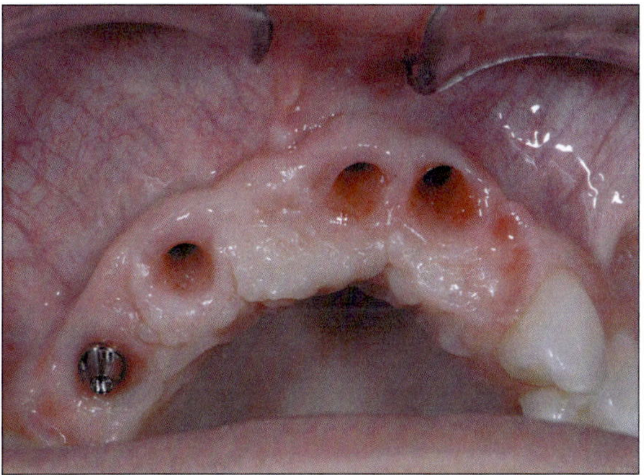

Figure 7-23 Four implants have been placed to restore this large defect secondary to trauma. Note the A-P spread (reprinted from Beumer et al., 2022, with permission).

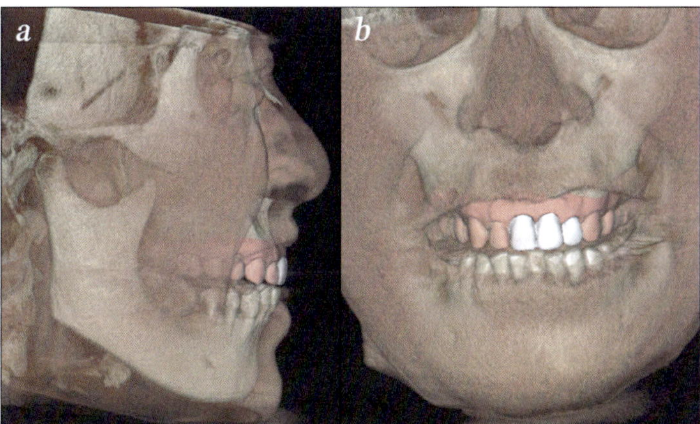

Figure 7-24 *(a and b)* CBCT scans with the associated software permit a three-dimensional representation of the hard and soft tissue anatomy with the proposed prosthetic design superimposed (reprinted from Moy et al., 2016, with permission).

alveolar fractures. Although sinus augmentation was successful, reconstruction of the alveolar ridge with grafting was not possible.

Unfavorable implant positions and angulations. The implants were placed palatally because of anatomical necessity and were angled buccally. This configuration made it virtually impossible to design an implant-supported fixed dental prosthesis that directed occlusal forces along the long axis of the implants.

Anchorage in grafted bone. The implants were anchored in poor-quality (grafted) bone and were insufficient in number to restore the corner of the arch with a fixed dental prosthesis. An overlay RDP was preferred because it provided additional bracing (stability) by engaging abutment teeth on the opposite side of the arch.

Linear configuration and restoration of the corner of the arch. Linear configurations lack the cross-arch stabilization that is achieved with curvilinear implant arrangements. When the other factors are favorable (sufficient numbers of implants of sufficient lengths in favorable bone sites with ideal angulations), a fixed dental prosthesis can be employed predictably. However, in this patient, the authors believed that the implants may not have been able to resist lateral forces without provoking a resorptive remodeling response of the bone anchoring the implants.

The overlay RDP was designed with positive rests on the anterior teeth. The cross-arch stabilization achieved with the dental prosthesis reduced the magnitude of lateral forces delivered to the implants. The implant-assisted implant connecting bar with its resilient attachment allowed the edentulous extension area to enhance the posterior support while minimizing posterior cantilever forces.

Implant-supported fixed dental prostheses

Successful outcomes can be achieved with implant-supported fixed dental prostheses when restoring large traumatic defects in the aesthetic zone. However, adequate bone volume to anchor the implants must be available to place the necessary numbers and with sufficient A-P spread that will withstand the rigors of occlusal function. Moreover, the implants should be circumscribed by keratinized attached mucosa if stable, healthy peri-implant soft tissues are to be sustained over an extended period (Fig 7-23). Given that most trauma patients present with significant hard and soft tissue deficits, it may be necessary to supplement these tissues with grafting. Several surgical techniques have evolved during the last 25 years to address these challenges. Given the aesthetic outcomes that can be achieved with pink porcelain and similar materials, surgical objectives should be driven by the need to create sufficient bone volume to anchor the implants and position them in favorable positions as opposed to restoring peri-implant soft tissue contours.

Bony augmentation of the alveolar ridge in traumatic defects—Several approaches to bone grafting have been proposed in recent years to address the vertical and horizontal deficiencies of bone usually encountered. However, clinicians must realize that when dealing with such tooth loss secondary to trauma, there are significant limitations to each of the techniques, particularly as it relates to soft tissue contours around the prosthetic teeth and in turn the aesthetic outcomes. In most severe tooth loss scenarios, regardless of the surgical outcome, pink porcelain, or a similar material, must be employed to restore gingival architecture. If one accepts this premise, why reconstruct these defects with bone grafts? The answer is to create ample bone volume at the appropriate sites to position and anchor the implants with sufficient A-P spread that will withstand the stress and strain of occlusal function.

The most effective way to assess the bone volume available is with CBCT scans using the associated software (Figs 7-24 and 7-25). This method permits the development of virtual diagnostic wax-ups that can be used to assess the nature of the hard and soft tissue deficits. They also help the clinician determine implant position and alignment and enable the printing of surgical drill guides. Currently, numerous imaging options are employed to identify vital structures, assess the morphology of the potential implant sites, and estimate the bone quantity and bone quality of these sites prior to surgery.

Free bone grafts. If the height of the potential implant sites is sufficient to receive implants, but the width of the site at the ridge crest is deficient, it is possible to widen the alveolus with bone grafts (Fig 7-26). This can be accomplished with a variety of techniques, including veneer grafts, particulate marrow grafts, guided bone tissue regeneration, and osteogenic proteins combined with a tissue scaffold enclosed within a titanium mesh (Moy et al., 2016). These techniques have been shown to predictably provide sufficient

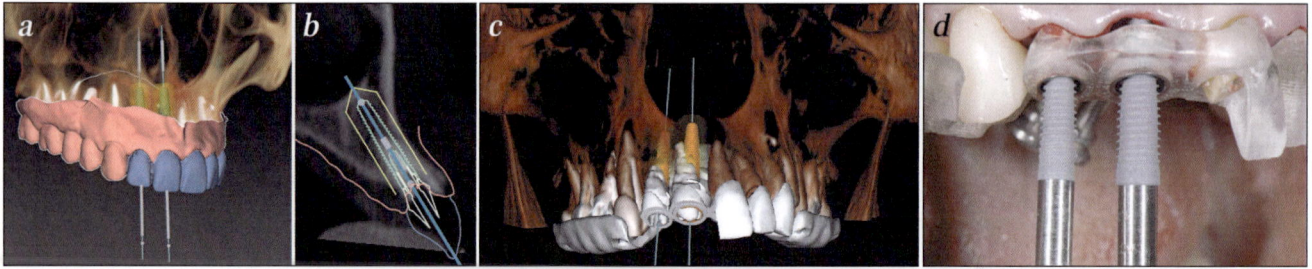

Figure 7-25 *(a)* The contours of the proposed prosthesis can be developed with the software and visualized in three dimensions and in relation to the underlying bone and overlying soft tissues. *(b)* Implant position and angulation also can be determined ensuring that implants are embedded in bone of proper thickness. *(c)* A surgical drill guide can be designed and printed. *(d)* This drill guide is designed to permit fully guided surgical placement (reprinted from Moy et al., 2016, with permission).

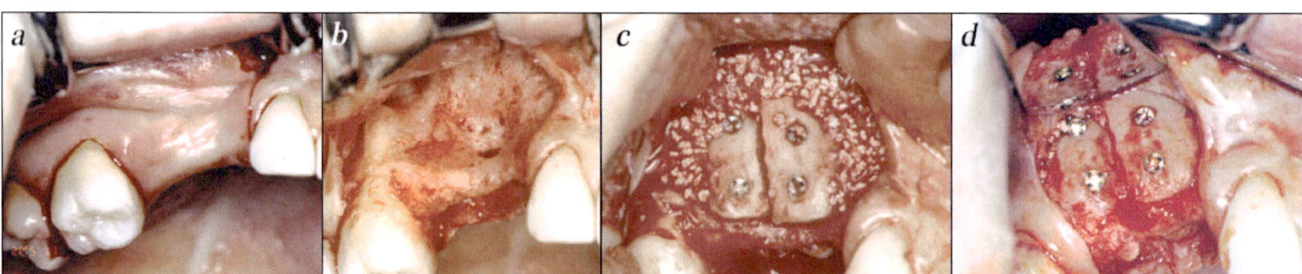

Figure 7-26 *(a and b)* Horizontal defect of the alveolar ridge. *(c)* The site has been reconstructed with marrow and veneer grafts. *(d)* The site six months later (reprinted from Beumer et al., 2022, with permission).

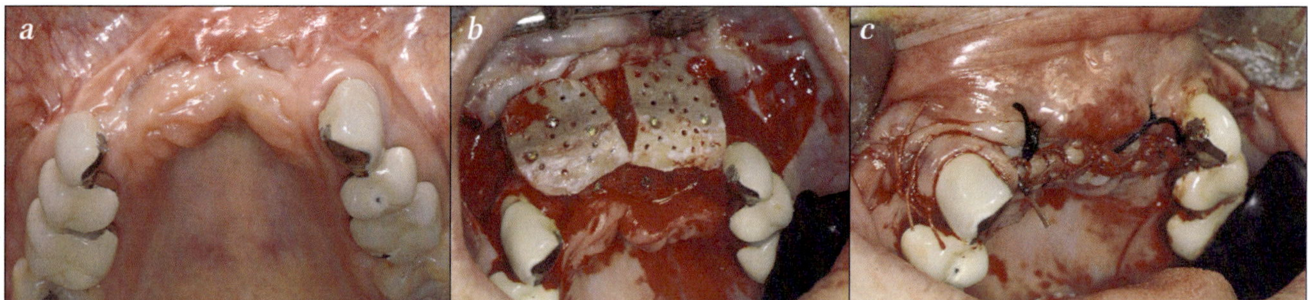

Figure 7-27 Onlay grafts to increase the vertical height of the alveolar ridge of large defects are problematic. *(a)* Presurgical defect. *(b)* Grafts in position. *(c)* Soft tissue closure.

bone volume that permits the placement of implants in appropriate positions and angulation.

However, vertical augmentation of large traumatic defects in anterior alveolar ridges with free autogenous bone grafts (Fig 7-27) is more challenging and less predictable. Several methods have been attempted, including onlay grafts, guided bone regeneration, osteogenic proteins with tissue scaffolds, and interpositional grafts. Following surgery, the resorption rate of these grafts can reach 75%, and this should be taken into account when grafting such defects. Further bone loss may be observed after the implants are placed in function (Aghaloo and Moy, 2007; Moy et al., 2016). The reasons for this are complex and multifactorial and include excessive scarring and poor blood supply, the difficulty in achieving proper fixation of the grafts, and the tension on the wound on soft tissue closure (Moy et al., 2016). Often, the mucogingival junction is repositioned on the crest of the ridge because of the releasing incisions required to effect primary surgical closure. In most instances, substantial soft tissue deficits remain that require grafting. Even when bone grafting is successful, the prosthodontic outcome may be compromised.

Distraction osteogenesis. Distraction osteogenesis can be used in these large traumatic defects in the aesthetic zone of the maxilla to enhance the vertical dimension of the alveolar ridge to create more favorable implant sites (Fig 7-28). However, in almost all cases, following a successful distraction, the horizontal dimension of the alveolar ridge will be deficient and require additional grafting. This procedure is more predictable than conventional onlay grafting techniques. The relapse rate is about 25%, and this should be taken into account during the distraction phase (Aghaloo and Moy, 2007). Clinicians should understand that even with a successful surgical outcome, rarely will ideal soft tissue contours be created around the definitive implant-supported restoration. A typical result, with respect to peri-implant soft tissue contours, is shown in (Fig 7-28), and so when the patient presents with a high smile line,

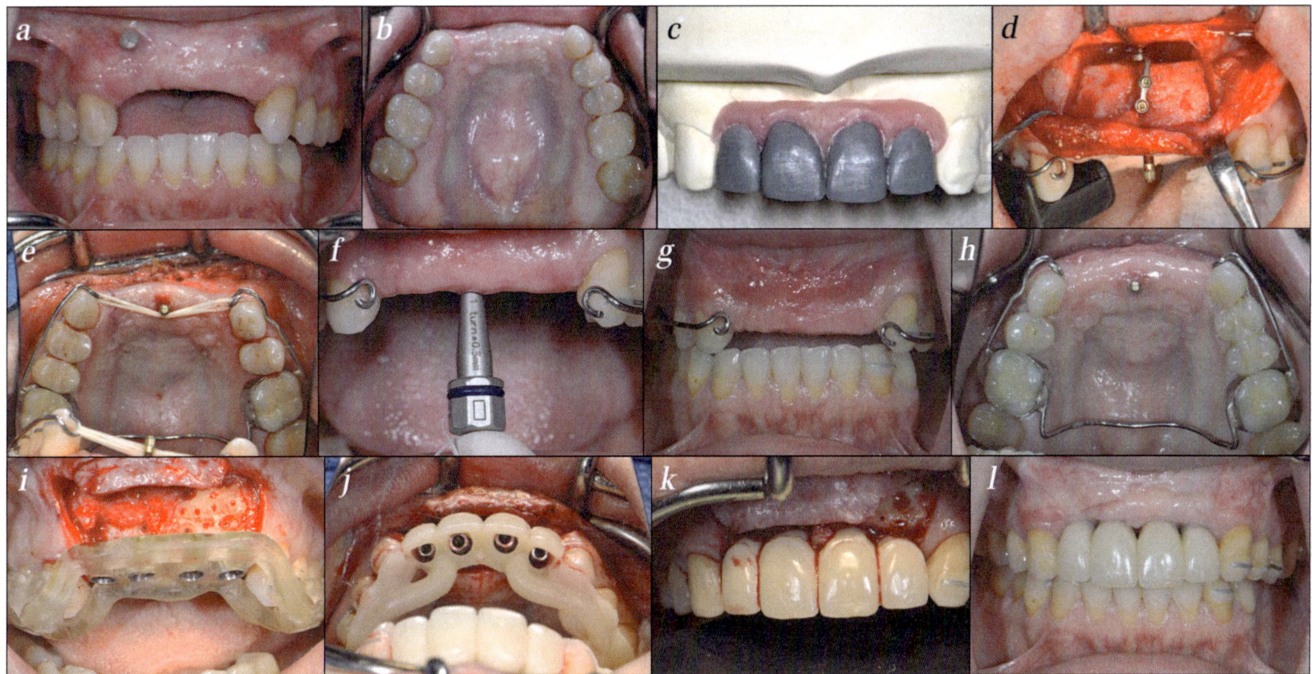

Figure 7-28 Distraction osteogenesis. *(a)* The patient presents with a vertical bone defect. *(b)* The anterior projection of the alveolar ridge is also deficient. A previous bone graft failed to address these deficiencies. *(c)* Diagnostic wax-up. Two-color diagnostic wax-ups make it easier to visualize the bone and soft tissue deficits. *(d)* Osteotomies are made, and the distraction apparatus is connected. *(e)* A modified transpalatal bar has been secured to stabilize the dentition. The elastics, when secured to the distraction screw as shown, provide an anterior vector to the distraction. *(f)* The distraction is about halfway completed by three weeks postsurgery. *(g and h)* The distraction process is completed. *(i)* Several months later, the implants were placed with the aid of a surgical template. *(j)* The temporary abutment cylinders are in position. The provisional restoration is keyed to the temporary abutment cylinders. *(k)* The provisional restoration is in position. *(l)* The provisional is in position after several months of healing. Note the lack of interdental papilla (reprinted from Beumer et al., 2022, with permission).

pink porcelain will usually be necessary to restore the peri-implant gingival architecture, especially the interdental papilla.

Once the surgical osteotomy is completed, the distraction apparatus is attached. The blood supply is maintained by avoiding the reflection of a lingual flap. During the so-called latency phase (seven to ten days), a soft callus is formed. Distraction begins immediately thereafter and takes one to two weeks, depending on the magnitude of regenerated bone needed. The segments are distracted at a rate of 1 mm per day. Following completion of the distraction procedures, three to four months of healing is necessary for the central fibrous and osteoid area to ossify and remodel into dense lamellar bone for implant placement. Instability of the bone fragments or excessively high distraction rates can lead to endochondral ossifications or even the formation of fibrous connective tissue.

Typically, a bone segment can be distracted in both a vertical and horizontal direction with dental implant assistance when appropriately treatment planned. The patient shown in Fig 7-29 is such a presentation. The right side of the palate had been impacted superiorly and medially secondary to vehicular trauma and had not been effectively reduced. The model surgery indicated that the right maxillary segment needed to be distracted both vertically and horizontally. Temporary implants were placed in the segment and allowed to osseointegrate. After the surgical osteotomy was completed, a tooth-borne custom-made distraction apparatus was attached, which distracted the segment laterally. Once the desired outcome laterally had been achieved, a new customized distraction apparatus was fabricated and secured, which distracted the segment vertically. Following the completion of the distraction procedures, and several months later following ossification and remodeling of the distracted bone, definitive implants replaced the temporary implants, and an implant-supported fixed dental prosthesis was eventually fabricated and delivered (Fig 7-29).

Soft tissue grafts and augmentation—The presence of a robust zone of keratinized attached mucosa surrounding the implants is essential for maintaining the long-term stability of the implants and the success of the implant prosthesis. When the peri-implant tissues are mobile and poorly keratinized, hygiene manipulation is compromised, leading to chronic peri-implant mucositis and, if unattended, to peri-implantitis and its associated bone loss. As mentioned above, many patients with trauma-induced defects have lost much of the keratinized attached mucosa on the edentulous alveolar segment. Moreover, frequently, there is considerable scarring of the oral mucosa locally.

The keratinized attached mucosa can be expanded or augmented in a number of ways. If there is a band of keratinized attached tissue available in the extended edentulous area prior to implant placement, during implant placement, or during second-stage surgery when the implants are uncovered, this tissue can be manipulated, via partial thickness flaps, to create appropriate zones of keratinized peri-implant mucosa on the facial side of the implants (Moy et al., 2016).

A suitable zone of keratinized attached mucosa can also be created with the use of free palatal grafts. This procedure can be accomplished prior to or after implant placement (Fig 7-30). After a supraperiosteal dissection, the graft is secured in position. A stent is used to maintain intimate contact of the graft with the underlying

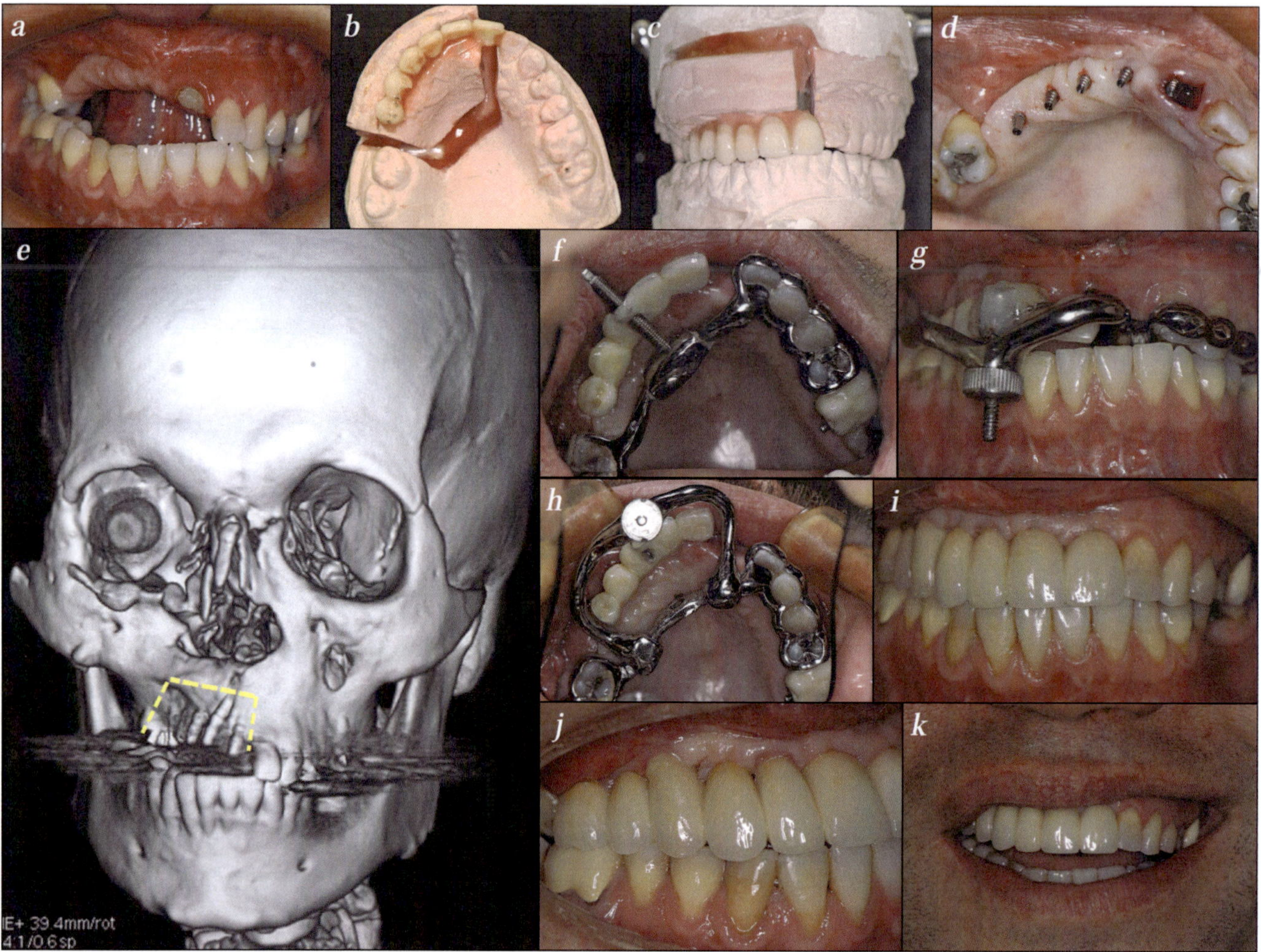

Figure 7-29 *(a)* Patient presents with a malunion of multiple facial fractures of the upper jaw. Note that the right palatal segment has been impacted medially and superiorly. *(b and c)* Model surgery indicates the degree to which this segment must be distracted both vertically and horizontally. *(d)* Temporary implants are in position. *(e)* A 3D representation of the patient prior to distraction and after the temporary implants has been placed. *(f)* The customized distraction apparatus is used to distract the segment laterally. *(g and h)*. The customized distraction apparatus is used to distract the segment vertically. *(i and j)* The definitive implant-supported fixed dental prosthesis is in position. *(k)* Animated smile.

periosteum during initial healing. The stent can be wired to the adjacent dentition or, if implants are present, secured by screws that engage the abutments (Beumer et al., 2022).

Subepithelial connective tissue grafts have been used to increase the thickness and improve the contours of the peri-implant soft tissues around solitary implant crowns and may be useful in specific instances in these large multitooth trauma-inflicted defects. Some clinicians also maintain that these grafts will increase the zone of keratinized tissue encompassing implants (Moy et al., 2016), and there is evidence based on animal studies that this may indeed be the case (Mackenzie and Hill, 1984). They have been primarily employed in the aesthetic zone in patients with thin periodontal phenotypes to enhance an edentulous site either prior to implant placement or simultaneous with tooth extraction and immediate implant placement. The grafted tissue appears stable and does not appear to resorb with time.

Long-term prosthodontic outcomes following augmentation of hard and soft tissue with grafts and/or distraction osteogenesis—As mentioned above, some resorption of bone associated with these augmentation procedures is to be expected and, with it, apical migration of the peri-implant tissues (Aghaloo and Moy, 2007; Moy et al., 2016). However, if prosthetic designs take this into account, by extending the porcelain contact area to the implant platforms, as was done in both these patients, the aesthetic outcomes remain essentially the same (Fig 7-31).

As mentioned above, and it warrants repeating, even when the patient presents with reasonably satisfactory hard and soft tissue contours following conventional bone grafting or distraction, the aesthetic result rarely is ideal when presenting with multiple-tooth, hard and soft tissue loss. In most instances, the lack of interimplant bone and reduced bone levels associated with the adjacent dentition makes it difficult to restore the interdental papilla. As a result, compromises from the ideal tooth forms are often necessary, and the prosthodontist often is forced to lengthen the crowns and elongate the interproximal contact zones to avoid tissue deficits in the interdental papilla region (Figs 7-29 and 7-30) (Faulkner et al., 2022). Another option is to restore the gingival architecture

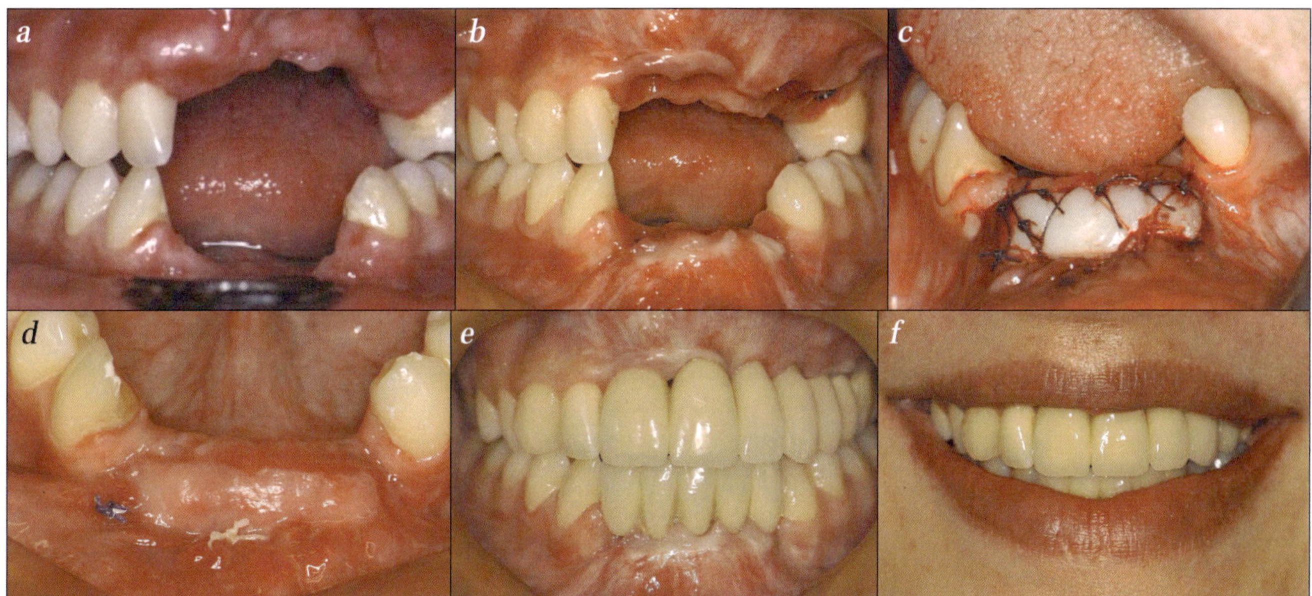

Figure 7-30 *(a)* Avulsive tooth defects affecting both the mandible and maxilla. Note the significant bony deficiency in both arches. *(b)* Much of the alveolar processes have been restored with bone grafts. However, there was very little keratinized attached mucosa available to circumscribe the mandibular implants. Therefore, prior to the placement of the implants, a free palatal graft was used to supplement these tissues. *(c)* The graft is sutured in position. It was held in this position during healing by a surgical stent secured to the adjacent dentition *(d)* The graft after healing. *(e)* The definitive implant-supported fixed dental prostheses. Note that the teeth have been lengthened and the interproximal contacts extended. *(f)* Aesthetic display with an animated smile.

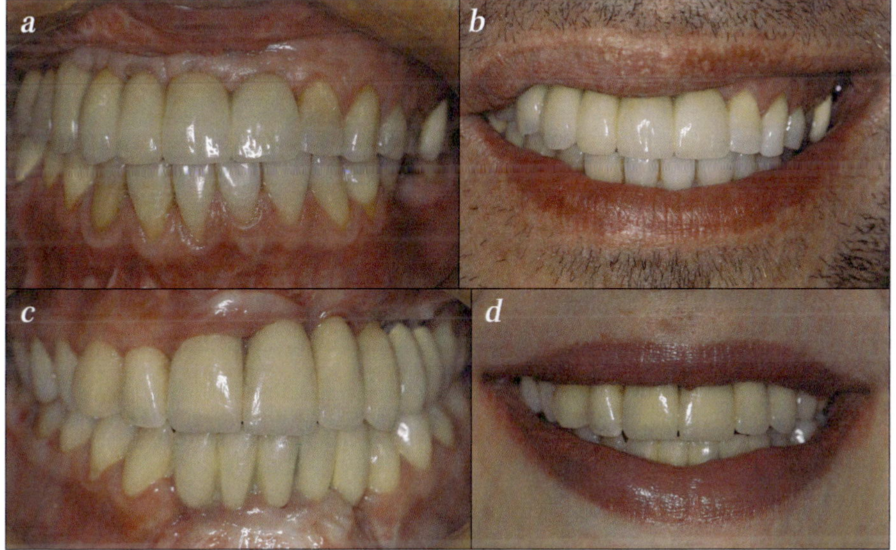

Figure 7-31 *(a and b)* Follow-up of the patient shown in Figure 7-29 (4 years) and *(c and d)* patient shown in Figure 7-30 (12 years). The tissue levels have been relatively stable in both patients. However, there has been some apical migration of the peri-implant tissues in the patient who underwent conventional bone grafting *(c and d)*, but the aesthetic outcome during an animated smile remains essentially the same.

with pink porcelain, and this approach is especially applicable in patients with a high smile line (see below, section entitled "Restoration of gingival tissues with pink porcelain").

Clinical workup and selection of implants

Digital planning tools are rapidly replacing conventional methods and are preferred. As stated in Chapter 3, the precision that can be achieved with these methods represents a sophisticated treatment planning tool and has become more cost-effective. CBCT scans allow visualization of the potential implant site bone contours in three dimensions as well as adjacent structures, including the bony walls of the paranasal sinuses, the floor of the nose, the nasal crest region, and the mental nerve. A separate scan of the radiographic guide allows the digital rendering of the prosthesis and the DICOM data from the scan to be merged, permitting the contours of the proposed prosthesis to be superimposed onto the bony contours of the intended implant sites. When tilted implants are to be placed, these planning programs are invaluable and enable more accurate positioning and angulation of the implants that could otherwise be achieved with free hand surgery.

Implant sites are selected based on an analysis of the three-dimensional bone contours and the probable tooth positions of

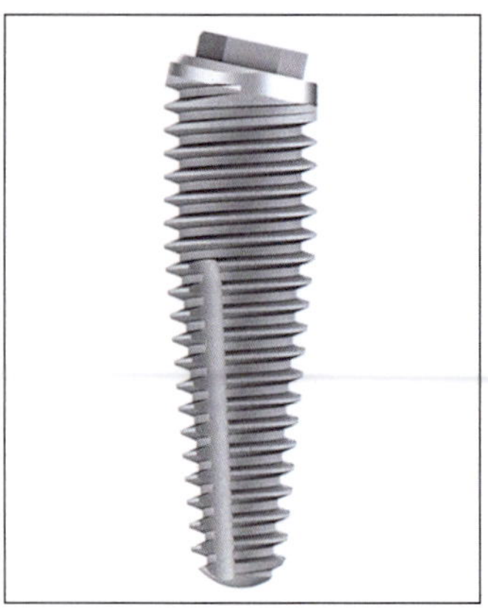

Figure 7-32 Off-axis implant design. They are available in several different angulations and are especially useful when the tilted implant concept is used (courtesy of Southern Implants, Irene, RSA).

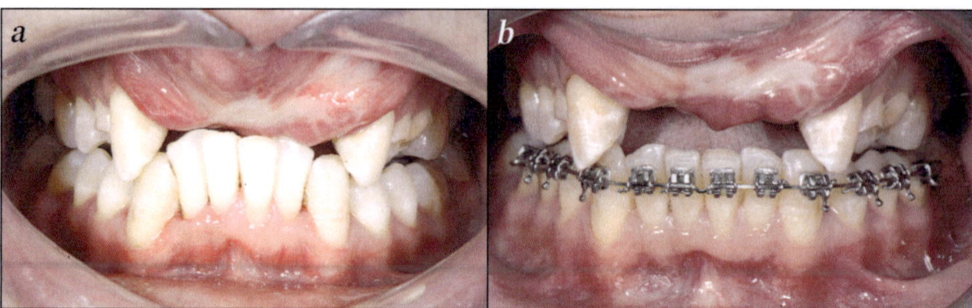

Figure 7-33 *(a)* The anterior teeth have supraerupted. *(b)* The occlusal plane discrepancy was addressed with orthodontic treatment before implants were placed (reprinted from Moy et al., 2016, with permission).

the proposed prosthesis. Positions and angulation of the implants can be determined and a surgical template designed and fabricated that permits either semiguided or fully guided controlled directional drilling, ensuring maximum accuracy of implant placement and alignment. For a detailed description of these procedures, the reader is referred to "Fundamentals of Implant Dentistry: Prosthodontic Considerations," 2nd edition (Beumer J, Faulkner R, Shah K, Wu B. Quintessence; 2022).

Several new implant designs have been introduced that broaden the application and improve the implant success rates, particularly in poor-quality bone, such as ones commonly encountered in grafted sites. Contemporary implants are prepared with microrough surfaces. These microrough surface topographies accelerate the process of osseointegration by upregulating and accelerating the expression of genes of the differentiating mesenchymal stem cells associated with the osseointegration process (Ogawa and Nishimura, 2003) and lead to bone that is harder and stiffer than bone anchoring machined surface implants (Butz et al., 2006; Takeuchi et al., 2005). Tapered, self-tapping implant designs with variable thread patterns are favored, because during insertion of the implant, the trabecular bone of the implant site is compressed around the implant, improving its initial mechanical anchorage. Implants with an off-axis design are particularly well suited for the so-called tilted implant approach when implants are placed along the anterior wall of the maxillary sinus and transit through the residual alveolar ridge and engage the pyriform rim (Fig 7-32). They are available in 12, 24, and 36 degrees of angle correction.

Prosthodontic design issues

Provisional restorations—Provisional restorations are almost always employed when the aesthetic zone is being restored. They can be as simple as an interim RDP (see Fig 7-13) or as sophisticated as a milled polymethyl methacrylate (PMMA) CAD/CAM prosthesis (Fig 7-39f) based on a digital design. These restorations are used to resolve issues associated with the design of the definitive restoration, including inappropriate implant angulation, the need for customized or angle-correcting abutments, hygiene access, the occlusal scheme employed, and so on. Emergence profiles and the contours of the restoration and the enveloping soft tissues can also be fine-tuned. The tooth forms, position of the incisal edges, and phonetics should also be assessed. In addition, the aesthetic concerns of the patient, ease of oral hygiene access, and function are also addressed.

Milled PMMA for provisional or prototype restorations is primarily used when the definitive restoration is destined to be monolithic zirconia. The diagnostic setup or wax-up is scanned or developed digitally and milled from a block of PMMA (see Fig 7-39d–f). This material is denser, stronger, and more color stable than conventional autopolymerizing or heat-curing acrylic resin (Edelhoff et al., 2012) and is preferred when the provisional restoration will be in place for an extended period. If the definitive restoration is to be fabricated from monolithic zirconia, the PMMA prototype is adjusted and contoured to idealize the occlusion and esthetics then scanned, and the data is used to mill the definitive zirconia restoration.

Screw-retained versus cement-retained restorations—When large multiunit prostheses are fabricated for the aesthetic zone, screw retention is advised, particularly when the prosthesis is to be designed with significant ridge laps. Under these circumstances, it is difficult to gain access and remove cement that has become impacted subgingivally during cementation. Even if the restoration is designed without ridge laps, the margins of the implant crowns will be positioned below the gingival margins, and in almost all instances, cement will be impacted subgingivally, making detection and removal difficult (Agar et al., 1997; Linkevicius et al., 2013). Moreover, it is advantageous to design the restoration so that it can be easily retrieved for repair of chips and cracks that may appear after an extended period of use.

Occlusion—It may be necessary to idealize the existing occlusal relationships of the patient in order to create a harmonious and stable occlusion. The plane of occlusion and the position of individual arch quadrants must be carefully assessed. Significant deviations from normal may require orthodontic and/or surgical correction. If significant time has elapsed since the traumatic incident and the loss of teeth, the opposing dentition may supraerupt, disrupting the plane of occlusion requiring correction (Fig 7-33). If teeth are malpositioned in the aesthetic zone, they may need to be restored or repositioned with orthodontic treatment to create pleasing aesthetic and occlusal harmony (Fig 7-34). The amount

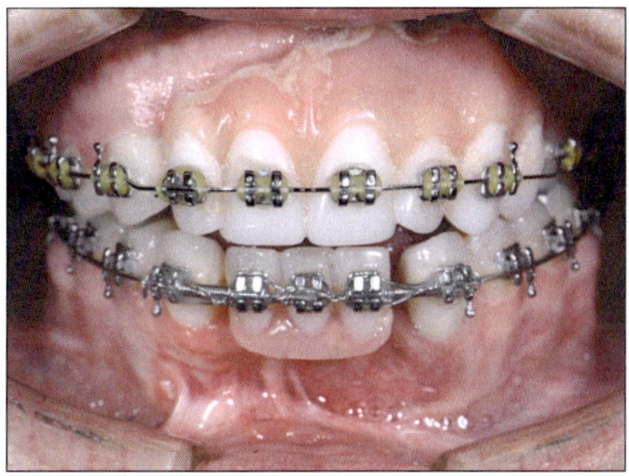

Figure 7-34 The edentulous spaces in both the mandible and maxilla were idealized with orthodontic treatment in conjunction with provisional restorations.

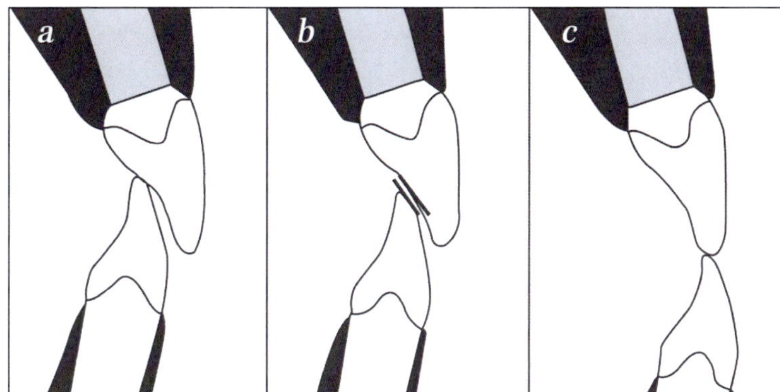

Figure 7-35 Occlusal scheme is suggested when only two implants have been placed to restore an edentulous space in the aesthetic zone in the maxilla. *(a)* Centric contact position of the prosthetic teeth associated with the implant-supported fixed dental prosthesis. *(b)* Along the pathway of anterior guidance, there should not be contact with opposing dentition. *(c)* At the edge-to-edge position contact is reestablished with the opposing natural dentition (reprinted from Beumer et al., 2022, with permission).

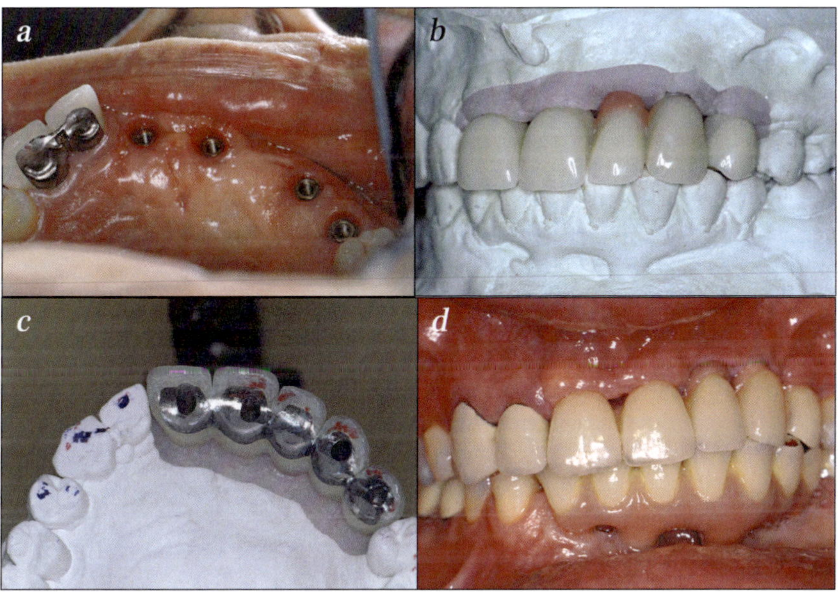

Figure 7-36 A large defect secondary to trauma affected both the mandible and the maxilla. *(a)* A sufficient number of implants have been placed with adequate A-P spread *(b and c)* to permit the implant prosthesis to contact the opposing dentition during left laterotrusion (left working position) without risk of implant overload. *(d)* Note the hygiene access between the implants beneath the mandibular prosthesis (reprinted from Beumer et al., 2022, with permission).

of vertical and horizontal overlap is noted, for this may have an impact on the desired tooth length and chosen occlusal scheme of the future prosthesis, particularly when the "corner" of the arch (canine-premolar region) is restored. Teeth adjacent to the defect are sometimes best removed in order to provide additional implant sites, thus improving the implant configuration (A-P spread) and biomechanics of the proposed implant-supported fixed dental prosthesis (see Fig 7-39a–b) (Wu et al., 2022).

The design of the anterior occlusion is dependent on the number of implants placed, their position in the arch, and their A-P spread. In general, when only two implants have been placed, guidance during excursions is provided by the remaining natural dentition. Such linear configurations are at risk for implant overload, particularly if the patient presents with significant parafunctional activity. For example, when only two implants have been placed, to restore the missing four incisors, a mutually protected occlusal scheme utilizing canine guidance is preferable. Light contact of the incisors associated with the implant-supported fixed dental prosthesis is permitted in centric and at the full extent of protrusion or laterotrusion (Fig 7-35). When three or more implants with suitable A-P spread have been placed, the implants can be employed to provide anterior guidance, sometimes aided by the remaining natural dentition (see Figs 7-36, 7-37, 7-39). The guidance established should be compatible with the condylar guidance of the patient.

Before initiation of treatment, a diagnostic wax-up or setup should be completed to assess whether the residual dentition requires additional restoration and to determine what occlusal adjustments may need to be made to the remaining teeth. A bite plane or occlusal orthotic can be employed prior to treatment to further establish a treatment position that is compatible with the patient's envelope of function.

Restoration of gingival tissues with pink porcelain— Many patients are reluctant to undergo multiple surgical procedures

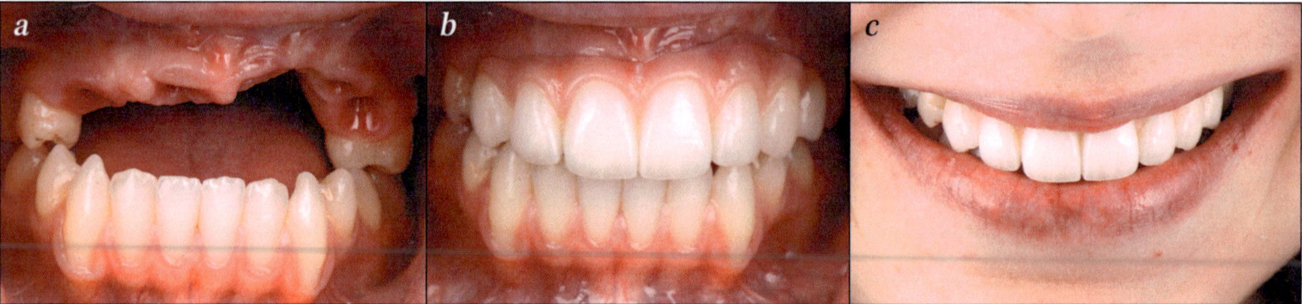

Figure 7-37 *(a)* Large defect in the aesthetic zone. There was sufficient bone available to place implants of sufficient length and number to fabricate an implant-supported fixed dental prosthesis. *(b and c)* Completed metal-ceramic prosthesis. The challenge is to design a prosthesis that provides both pleasing aesthetic contours and adequate access for hygiene (reprinted from Beumer et al., 2022, with permission).

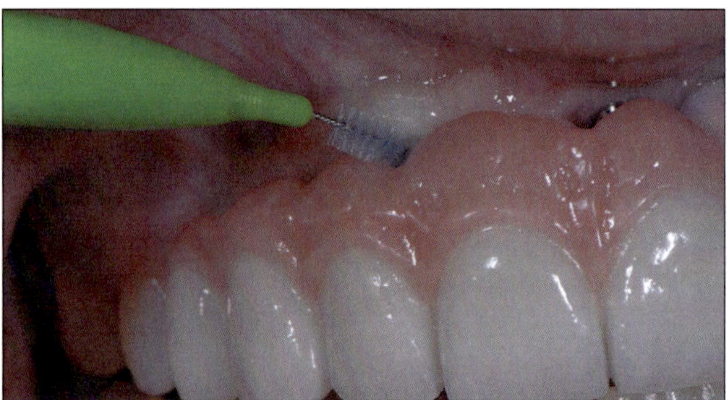

Figure 7-38 The prosthesis should be designed for proxy brush access.

to rebuild the hard and soft tissues for esthetics when there is sufficient bone available to anchor the implants. The authors suggest that when adequate hard and soft tissue architecture is absent, the missing gingival architecture be restored with pink porcelain or an equivalent material. Soft tissue grafting should be limited to improve the quality of the peri-implant tissues. There are several reasons for this. First, bony reconstruction of large hard tissue trauma and soft tissue defects in the aesthetic zone is not especially predictable. Moreover, even if successful, it is unrealistic to be able to design the prosthesis with normal tooth forms with acceptable gingival architecture and interdental papilla. Following completion of the prosthesis, all too frequently, the prosthetic teeth are excessively long, and the interdental papillae between the implants are blunted (see Figs 7-29 and 7-30). Consequently, when the patient displays the gingival tissues during a high smile, it may be aesthetically more advantageous and pleasing to restore these tissues with pink porcelain. These designs are quite aesthetic, as long as the margin (transition zone) between the pink porcelain and the tissues is not exposed during a high, animated smile (Figs 7-37 and 7-39h–k). Note that the challenge with these designs is twofold—that is, to create contours that provide adequate lip support and an aesthetic gingival architecture that also permits appropriate hygiene access. Proximal areas must be designed with proxy brush access, and the intaglio surfaces must be slightly convex to facilitate plaque removal (Fig 7-38).

Selection of materials—Metal ceramic prostheses have been the standard for many years, and esthetically pleasing outcomes can be achieved (see Fig 7-37). However, veneered porcelain restorations fabricated with a layering technique are prone to chipping and fracture when retained by implants (Kinsel and Lin, 2009). Likewise, zirconia restorations that utilize a porcelain layering technique to restore functional surfaces also have the potential for chipping and fracture.

Milled zirconia, in its monolithic state, shows promise as a restorative material for implant-supported fixed dental prostheses in the aesthetic zone (Fig 7-39). The biomechanical properties of this material allow for the design of restorations with minimal or no veneering of feldspathic porcelain. In the monolithic form, this material is very resistant to wear, and little or no chipping and fractures have been reported (Moscovitch, 2015; Abdulmajeed et al., 2016; Bidra et al., 2017). Restorations fabricated from this material can be designed to be screw retained or cement retained. A prototype (provisional restoration) is developed and worn by the patient prior to the fabrication of the definitive zirconia prosthesis. The prototype is designed with computer software, milled from prefabricated blocks of PMMA, delivered, and adjusted as necessary to restore and refine the occlusion and provide appealing aesthetic contours with hygiene access (see Fig 7-39d–f). Once the prototype has been approved by the patient and the clinician, it is retrieved from the patient, placed on the master cast, and scanned. The definitive monolithic zirconia fixed dental prosthesis is milled from the data obtained from the scanned prototype (Fig 7-39g–i). Hence the milled zirconia prosthesis is an exact duplicate of the provisional prototype restoration. A second prototype, milled and adjusted at the same time as the first prototype, is worn by the patient during the fabrication of the definitive prosthesis.

With this technique, only minimal adjustments should be necessary. If required, adjustments should be made with fine diamonds applied with light pressure; a water spray should be used during the

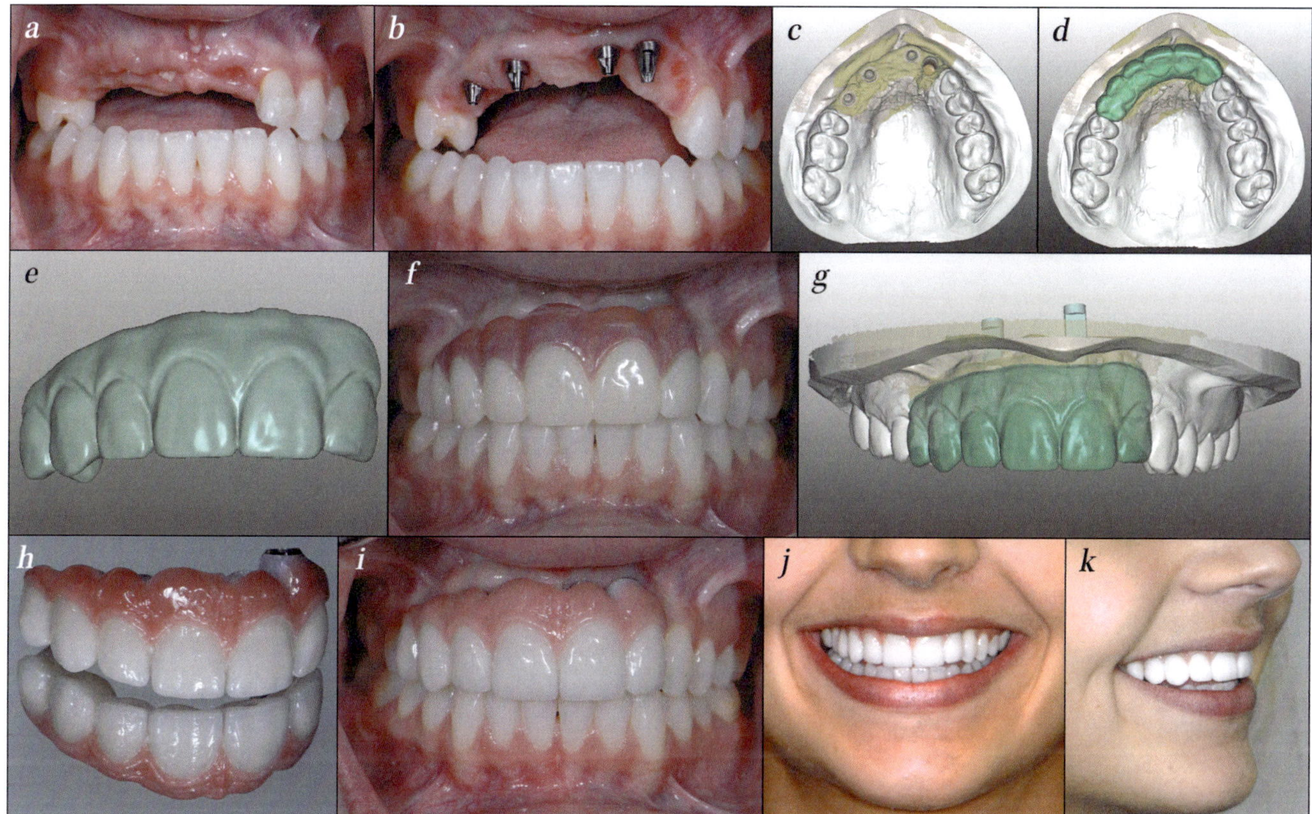

Figure 7-39 *(a)* A large multitooth avulsion defect secondary to trauma. *(b)* Four implants were placed to support an implant-supported fixed dental prosthesis. Note that the left lateral incisor was removed to create an additional implant site. *(c, d, and e)* The provisional restoration is designed using CAD software. *(d)* The provisional (prototype) prosthesis has been milled from a PMMA block. *(f)* The provisional prosthesis. It was worn for several months and adjusted as necessary. During this period, the esthetics and occlusion were refined. *(g)* The scanned provisional. The data developed is used to fabricate the *(h)* definitive prosthesis in monolithic zirconia. *(i)* The definitive prosthesis in position. *(j and k)* View of the prosthesis during a high smile (reprinted from Beumer et al., 2022, with permission).

adjustments to avoid overheating the material. The zirconia is then polished with specially designed zirconia polishing points, again applied with light pressure to avoid overheating of the material. The clinical reports have been favorable (Moscovitch, 2015; Tischler et al., 2018), and in a retrospective analysis (Noack and Gehrke, 2016), chipping was observed in only 1.6% of the cases.

Combinations using zirconia frameworks with lithium disilicate crowns have shown promise and are gaining favor with some clinicians (Pozzi et al., 2015), but long-term follow-up data are not available. When using such materials, screw retention is advised so that the prosthesis can be retrieved for necessary repairs.

Localized defects of the mandible

Localized traumatic defects of the mandible are similar to the defects encountered in the maxilla. The majority of traumatic defects of the mandible involve the avulsive loss of several teeth and associated portions of the alveolar ridge, usually accompanied by some loss of keratinized attached mucosa (Fig 7-40a). Several options are available for the restoration of such defects and include conventional fixed dental prostheses (FDPs), conventional removable dental prostheses (RDPs), implant-supported overlay removable dental prostheses, and implant-supported fixed dental prostheses. The method selected depends on several factors, including the size and curvature of the edentulous span, the health of potential abutment teeth, the nature of the hard and soft tissue deficits, and cost.

When the defects involve significant numbers of teeth, RDPs are a cost-effective option that provide excellent aesthetic and functional outcomes (Fig 7-40). The basic partial removable dental prosthesis design principles should be followed; namely, major connectors should be rigid, rests should be positive and direct occlusal forces along the long axis of the teeth, guiding planes should be designed to facilitate stability and bracing, retention should be within the physiologic limits of the periodontal ligament, and maximum support and stability should be gained from the residual soft tissue denture-bearing surfaces. The authors prefer to use variations of the "I" bar mesial rest (Kratochvil, 1963; Chang et al., 2019) or RPA (Eliason, 1983) concepts of RDP design.

Avulsive tooth defects of the mandible precipitated by trauma pose unique problems if implants are considered. In almost all cases, the quality and quantity of bone are sufficient to place implants of adequate lengths and distribution patterns to support the forces of occlusion. The principal challenge is to develop attached keratinized tissues through which the implants can emerge (Fig 7-41). Often, implants of smaller diameter are employed because of the narrow alveolar ridge and limited space between remaining natural teeth. However, implants at least 3 mm in diameter are required to resist the expected occlusal forces. In many situations, the implants may be angled excessively to the labial, requiring the use of customized

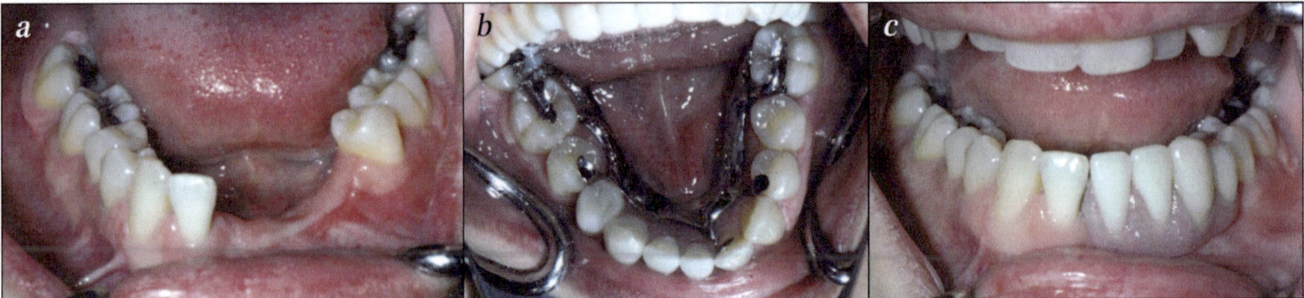

Figure 7-40 *(a)* Large multitooth avulsive defect involving the mandibular dentition. *(b and c)* RDP with a dual path of insertion and lingual retention (courtesy of Dr. E. G. King).

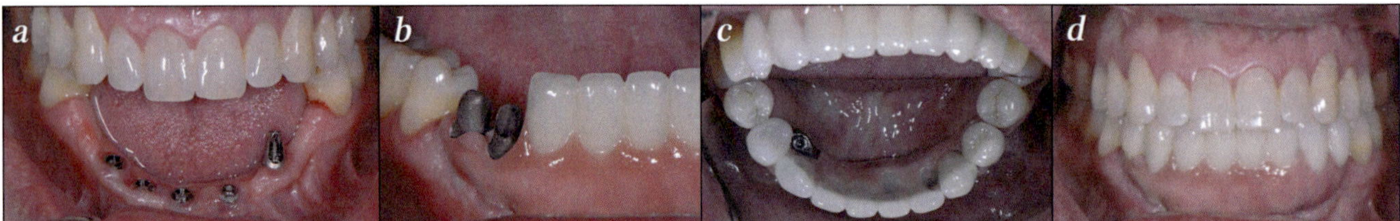

Figure 7-41 *(a)* Despite the large mandibular anterior defect secondary to trauma, the quality of the tissues circumscribing the implants is excellent. *(b)* This prosthesis employed both screw and cement retention. The right first premolar and canine are cemented on custom abutments incorporated within the substructure. *(c and d)* The substructure of the definitive prosthesis is screw retained. The faciolingual contours fit within the restorative space while at the same time providing adequate support for the lower lip and the corners of the mouth (reprinted from Beumer et al., 2022, with permission).

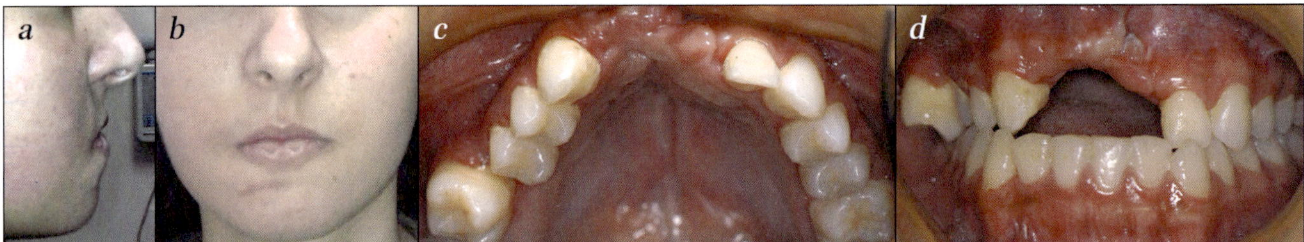

Figure 7-42 Patient presents with malunion of multiple fractures of the upper jaw. *(a and b)* Note the loss of midface support and altered lip contours. *(c and d)* Note the malocclusion secondary to the misalignment of jaw fragments.

milled abutments or substructures (Faulkner et al., 2022). These restorations must be designed with appropriate hygiene access. Screw retention is favored for the reasons mentioned above.

Rehabilitation of patients with malunion of jaw fractures

Interprofessional/disciplinary collaboration from diagnosis and treatment planning through treatment has made possible the correction of many maxillomandibular jaw deformities and malocclusions. These collaborative skills are particularly useful and pertinent when a patient presents with malunion of multiple facial fractures (healing has taken place, but the bony union is in poor position; Fig 7-42). The prosthodontist is well aware of the effect that tooth position and facial contour has on the patient's self-image and is well trained in occlusal analysis. For these reasons, prosthodontists must have significant input when surgical osteotomies are to be performed on the patient presenting with malunion of jaw fractures. An interdisciplinary effort ensures that all hard and soft tissue contours, and occlusal relationships, are thoroughly evaluated to affect the best possible aesthetic, functional, and psychologic outcomes for each patient. The workup can be accomplished with either conventional analog means, digitally, or most likely, a combination of the two methods.

In general, the oral and maxillofacial surgeon is responsible for improving the alveolar and basal bone relationships. The surgeon has further responsibility for evaluating the medical aspects, selecting and performing the appropriate surgical procedures, and supervising the preoperative and postoperative care of the patient. The orthodontist is responsible for locating the site of the anatomic deformity and for the correction of tooth, alveolar bone, and arch-to-arch disharmony. The prosthodontist predetermines the most acceptable occlusal relationships attainable surgically and orthodontically and is relied upon to detail and finalize occlusal relationships to ensure a stable and long-lasting result. The prosthodontist also designs and fabricates the necessary surgical prostheses and provides the necessary restorative care.

One objective of diagnosis is to locate and define the morphology and extent of the malunion deformity. Appropriate radiographs,

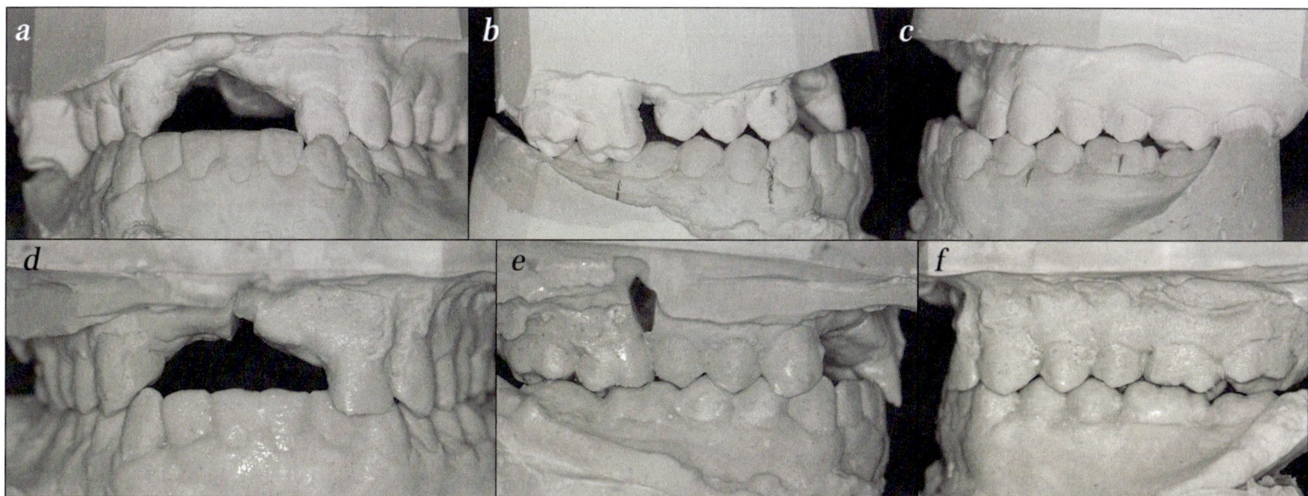

Figure 7-43 *(a, b, and c)* Mounted study casts of the patient with a malunion are shown in Figure 7-42. *(d, e, and f)* Model surgery was performed to correct the malunion. Note the vertical overlap that is to be created with the residual anterior dentition following surgical correction.

CBCT scans, and diagnostic casts mounted on a semiadjustable articulator with a centric relation record are essential for proper evaluation. Cephalometric analysis discloses the location and extent of the skeletal deformity created by malunion. Many cephalometric analyses exist, and the choice of which measurement analysis to select is largely user dependent. This exam reveals the ratio of lower face height to total face height. The occlusal vertical dimension and the soft tissue profile must also be correlated with the skeletal deformity. Predicting changes in facial appearance resulting from therapy is of critical importance. Therefore, a complete diagnostic study must include clinical examination, cephalometric analysis, and evaluation of the mounted diagnostic casts.

Although the clinical exam and cephalometric analysis determine the nature of the deformity, the evaluation of the mounted diagnostic casts discloses the finer points of the functional occlusion and may determine the limits of correction (Fig 7-43). Diagnostic cast evaluation provides information concerning the relationships of teeth in the arch segments that are to be repositioned surgically. The position of the teeth recorded on the diagnostic casts may also determine the need for orthodontic therapy prior to surgical intervention. Orthodontics rarely is used to correct the deformity per se; rather, it attempts to idealize tooth positions and angulations, level the occlusal plane, and improve jaw relationships to facilitate the occlusal position attained at surgery. Also, orthodontic appliances can be used to enhance fixation at the time of surgery. After surgery, minor orthodontic adjustments will improve occlusal relationships in preparation for subsequent prosthodontic therapy. Since many of these patients have lost dentition in association with their injuries and/or subsequent treatment, the orthodontist in coordination with the prosthodontist is often called upon to consolidate dental arch segments and to idealize the edentulous spaces for the placement of implants, in preparation for fabrication of implant-retained dental prostheses.

The prosthodontist examines the mounted diagnostic casts (Fig 7-43) with particular attention to centric relation and centric occlusion. In patients with a malunion of multiple facial fractures, this discrepancy may be quite significant. The presence and extent of anterior guidance or lack thereof should be carefully noted. In partially edentulous patients, the establishment of bilateral posterior tooth-to-tooth stops is essential to preserve the occlusal vertical dimension. Frequently, after surgical osteotomies are completed, potential implant sites need to be grafted and the existing keratinized attached mucosa manipulated or enhanced.

In edentulous patients, the prosthodontist is responsible for properly mounting the diagnostic casts with a centric relation record at the proper occlusal vertical dimension. In cases of surgical correction of segments that have been displaced or supererupted into edentulous spaces, the prosthodontist must predetermine the desired plane of occlusion.

The prosthodontist should take into consideration the possible devitalization of teeth involved and the reorganization of the muscles of mastication and the temporomandibular joint concomitant with healing following surgery to correct jaw malunions. If the surgery avoids encroachment on the root apices of the teeth by at least 4 mm, pulpal vitality is usually not compromised, since the vascular supply to the dental pulp is maintained via capillary diffusion through the surrounding bone and soft tissue attachments (Bell and Levy, 1975). Typical vitality tests, such as electrical stimulation, are often negative up to a year postsurgically and sometimes permanently. Positive signals in some cases may be caused not by the regeneration of pulpal innervation but by the response from the supporting tissues. Accordingly, restoration of these teeth does not usually require endodontic treatment.

One of the major prosthodontic tasks is to restore a stable occlusion coordinated in harmony with the anatomic determinants of occlusion. Following surgery, once the bony union of segments is assured and muscular balance is attained, measurements of mandibular movements may be made and utilized in programming a stable and functional occlusal scheme. It is incumbent on the prosthodontist to allow for reorganization and maturation of the masticatory proprioceptive mechanisms before these records are made and definitive restorations are placed. The use of a maxillary orthopedic appliance (occlusal device) may aid in establishing a treatment position and ensuring joint and muscle balance before commencing with major restorative care.

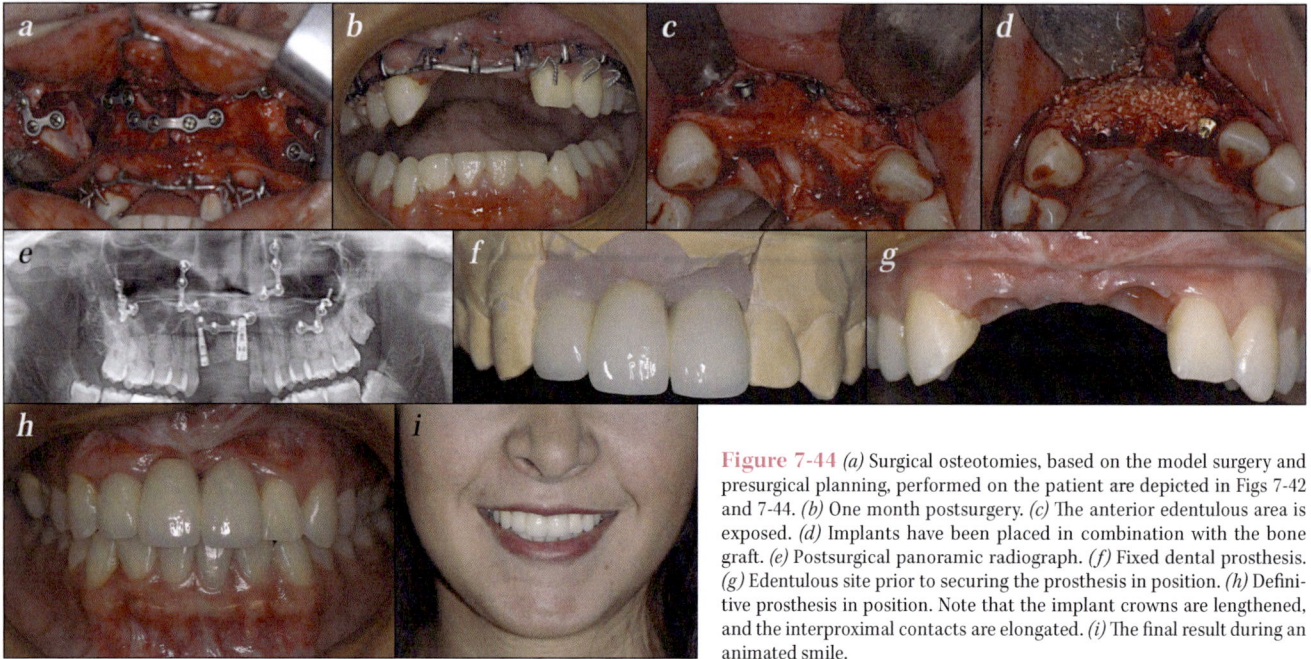

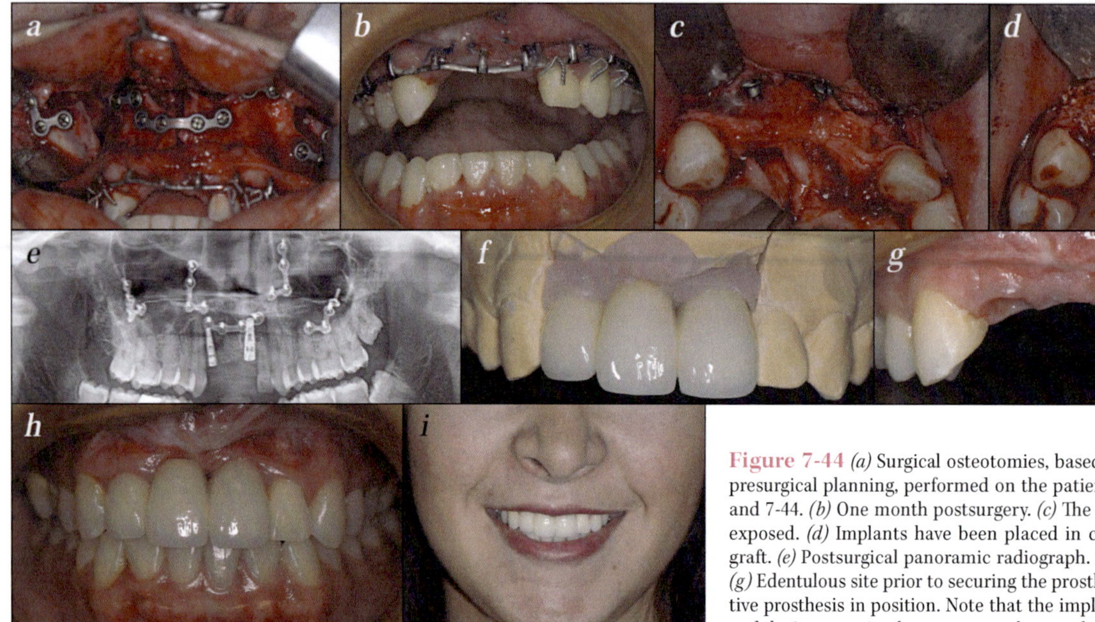

Figure 7-44 *(a)* Surgical osteotomies, based on the model surgery and presurgical planning, performed on the patient are depicted in Figs 7-42 and 7-44. *(b)* One month postsurgery. *(c)* The anterior edentulous area is exposed. *(d)* Implants have been placed in combination with the bone graft. *(e)* Postsurgical panoramic radiograph. *(f)* Fixed dental prosthesis. *(g)* Edentulous site prior to securing the prosthesis in position. *(h)* Definitive prosthesis in position. Note that the implant crowns are lengthened, and the interproximal contacts are elongated. *(i)* The final result during an animated smile.

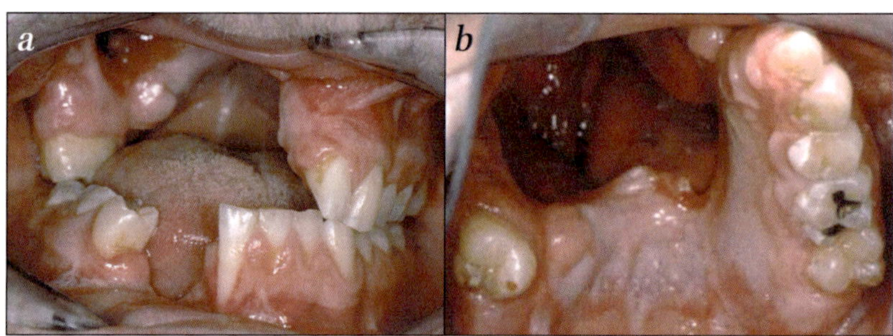

Figure 7-45 *(a and b)* Self-inflicted gunshot wounds resulting in a discontinuity defect of the mandible and a large maxillary defect extending into the paranasal sinuses and nasal cavity.

Likewise, in partially edentulous patients with extensive edentulous segments in the posterior quadrants, critical prosthodontic importance must be placed on establishing tooth-to-tooth stops on each side of the dental arches. These bilateral posterior stops are necessary to maintain and preserve the occlusal vertical dimension. Whereas it is not always possible to achieve these stops with the remaining teeth alone, fixed or removable dental prostheses supported either by implants or existing dentition achieve the same effect.

The patient depicted in Figs 7-42, 7-43, and 7-44 demonstrates the effectiveness of an interdisciplinary approach, and if the guidelines outlined in the previous paragraphs are adhered to carefully, the outcome shown can be expected in most patients. The patient was presented with a malunion of fractures of the upper jaw secondary to trauma. The jaw segments were displaced and had been impacted resulting in a significant midfacial deformity and malocclusion (Fig 7-42). Mounted casts revealed the true nature of the malocclusion (Fig 7-43a–c). Cast surgery was used to determine the proper position of the jaw segments to be osteotomized and repositioned (Fig 7-43d–f). During surgery, fixation of the osteotomized segments is achieved with miniplates and a rigid customized arch bar. Following several months of healing, the edentulous anterior alveolar ridge was exposed, and the implants were positioned in combination with a particulate bone marrow graft. After the implants became osseointegrated, the definitive implant-supported fixed dental prosthesis was fabricated. Note that the implants are circumscribed by a healthy zone of keratinized attached tissue (Fig 7-44g–i), the implant crowns are lengthened, and the interproximal contacts are elongated. The achievement of such an excellent aesthetic outcome is only possible when there is a close professional relationship between all members of the interdisciplinary team.

Rehabilitation of patients with large avulsive defects of the maxilla and mandible

Avulsive wounds of the maxilla that result in large palatal defects often occur in combination with mandibular discontinuity defects (Fig 7-45). Most of these defects are secondary to gunshot wounds and are challenging to restore. Frequently, residual maxillary or mandibular segments in such patients are misaligned, the occlusal plane is irregular, the remaining maxillary segments may be detached from the cranial base, and the maxillomandibular relationship is altered. These issues must be addressed before definitive prosthodontic treatment is considered. Unfavorable maxillomandibular

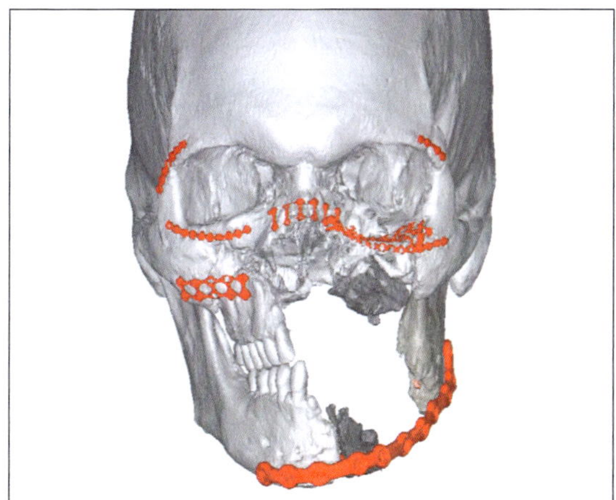

Figure 7-46 This large avulsive defect of the maxilla and mandible is typical of those secondary to a self-inflicted gunshot wound.

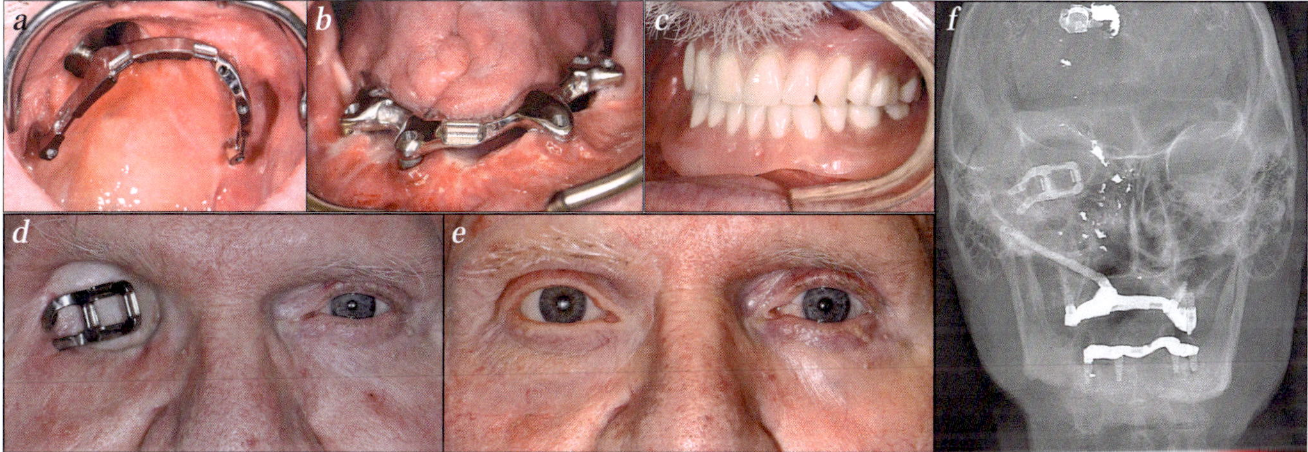

Figure 7-47 Rehabilitation of the patient is shown in Figure 7-48 with multiple defects secondary to a self-inflicted gunshot wound. *(a, b, and c)* The maxilla and mandible were restored with implant-supported overdentures. The OVD was reduced and the occlusal plane lowered because the tongue was slightly immobilized, and also to facilitate lip seal and oral competence. *(d and e)* The orbital defect was restored with an implant-retained orbital prosthesis. *(f)* Radiograph of the dental implants and implant connecting bars.

relationships and displaced alveolar fragments predispose the patient to unfavorable tooth position and alignment, which may compromise future RDP designs and/or implant placement. Study casts, CBCT scans, and 3D models provide useful information at this stage (Figs 7-46 and 7-48).

It is critical to determine the definitive long-range treatment plan during this phase of care and to coordinate this treatment plan with the other appropriate health care disciplines. All necessary adjunctive consultations and dental treatment—such as endodontics, periodontics, and orthodontics—should be completed prior to definitive prosthodontic treatment. Often, the maxillofacial prosthodontist must coordinate the care of these other specialists because prosthodontic treatment will be dependent on the treatment outcomes of these other services. The patient's ability to maintain oral hygiene and willingness to keep recall appointments are important factors to be considered. Psychosocial interventions may be critical at this stage (see Chapter 9).

In the maxilla, the physical configuration of the defect varies considerably and is dependent on the nature of the injury (Figs 7-45 and 7-46). Traumatic defects are generally lined with a combination of pseudostratified columnar epithelium or poorly keratinized squamous epithelium. These types of epithelial lining are more sensitive and do not tolerate the functional contact associated with the prosthesis under function as well as skin-lined or highly keratinized mucosal surfaces do. The soft tissues bordering the traumatic defect are often heavily scarred and cannot be as easily displaced or recontoured by the prosthesis, unlike, for example, the skin-lined cheek of a maxillectomy defect. Thus, facial contours and esthetics are often compromised. The residual maxillary segments in patients with such defects may be displaced and lack a bony attachment to the base of the skull. This scenario compromises support and may subject abutment teeth to unfavorable lateral torquing forces. The arrangement of mandibular dentition, the mandibular arch form, and the occlusal plane of the mandible may be less than ideal, making it difficult to establish proper occlusal relationships in patients with such defects.

Following the usual preprosthetic surgical procedures, such defects can be managed prosthodontically with an RDP-obturator prosthesis, or a complete denture-obturator prosthesis, supplemented by implants if necessary (Fig 7-47). Potential implant sites for oral prostheses include the residual edentulous areas as well as the zygomas and pyriform rim region (Fig 7-48). The challenges encountered

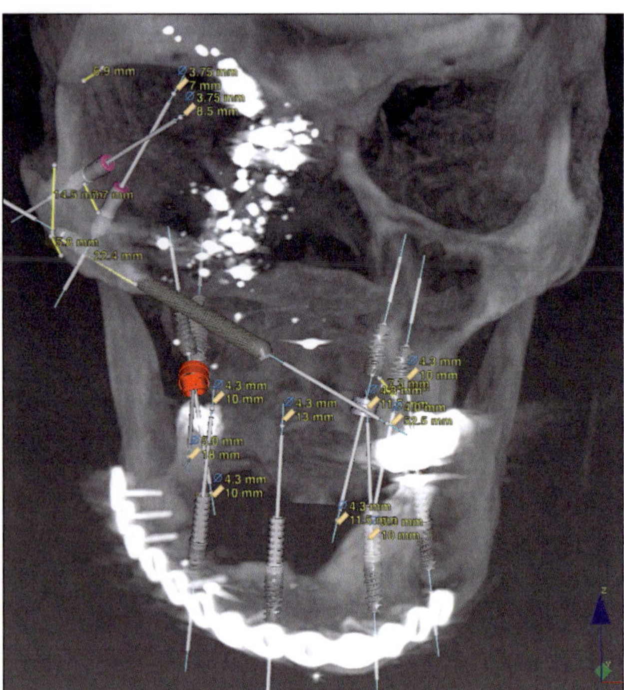

Figure 7-48 Implants were considered for the reconstructed mandible, the malar region, the zygoma, and the residual maxillary alveolar process in this patient with multiple avulsive defects secondary to a self-inflicted gunshot wound.

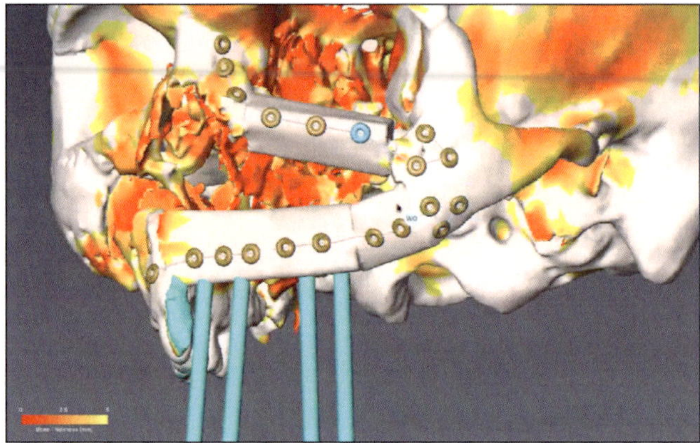

Figure 7-49 This avulsive defect of the maxilla (Fig 7-46) secondary to a self-inflicted gunshot wound is to be reconstructed with a vascularized osteomyocutaneous flap combined with dental implants.

with RDP and implant connecting bar designs for patients with traumatic defects are similar to those already discussed for patients with acquired maxillary defects (see Chapter 3). The basic principles of partial denture design should be followed; namely, major connectors should be rigid, occlusal rests should be positive and direct occlusal forces along the long axis of the teeth, guiding planes should be designed to facilitate stability and bracing, retention should be within the physiologic limits of the periodontal ligament of the abutment teeth, and maximum support and stability should be gained from the residual denture-bearing surfaces, including those accessible in the defect (Kratochvil, 1963; Chang et al., 2019).

If the maxillary defect is of sufficient size, surgical closure and reconstruction with vascularized osteomyocutaneous flaps accompanied by the placement of osseointegrated implants is a viable option (Fig 7-49). The implants should be placed either immediately (see Chapter 3, section entitled "Osteomyocutaneous flaps and conventional implants") or secondarily after the flap has completely healed. Recently, vascularized soft tissue flaps, in combination with the placement of zygomatic implants, have been used in patients with large oncologically triggered defects of the upper jaw (Butterworth and Rogers, 2017; Butterworth et al., 2022). The flap is used to close the palatal defect, and the implants are employed to retain and support either a fixed or removable prosthesis. Customized, digitally designed subperiosteal implants made of titanium have been used in a similar way in combination with vascularized soft tissue flaps (Vosselman et al., 2021; Korn et al., 2021). These methods would seem to be viable options for restoring traumatically induced large avulsive defects of the hard palate.

Large avulsive defects of the mandible secondary to trauma will also challenge the skills of even the most expert of surgical-prosthodontic teams. Sizable segments of the mandible can be lost along with its adjacent and overlying soft tissue. The temporomandibular joint region can be altered, leading to trismus and changes in mandibular movement, and maxillo-mandibular relationships can be altered.

Discontinuity defects should be reconstructed with a bone graft as soon as practical. The goals and principles of bone grafting discussed earlier in reference to patients with tumor resections (see Chapter 2, section entitled "Surgical reconstruction") apply to patients with traumatically induced mandibular discontinuity defects. When free bone grafting such defects, lingual splints made with chrome cobalt alloy can be used to facilitate fixation. The strength and rigidity of the metal permit the fabrication of a hygienic splint, which is advantageous when the splint must remain in place for several months (Fig 7-50). Impressions are made of the maxilla and mandible, and the resulting casts are mounted on a semiadjustable articulator with facebow transfer and centric relation records. Model surgery is performed in order to properly position mandibular segments, and the splint is designed and fabricated. These steps can also be performed digitally and the splint printed with selective laser melting. The splint is secured by wiring it directly to the dentition or by incorporating it with the wires that ligate a buccally placed arch bar to the teeth. The combined effect of the buccal arch bar and the lingual splint is the most efficient means of stabilization. Grafts should be designed so that they possess sufficient volume and density of bone to receive osseointegrated implants.

The presence of foreign bodies is a frequent observation following gunshot trauma and should be taken into consideration when the placement of implants is anticipated. They range from copper/lead bullet fragments to chrome/nickel/iron stainless steel wire used for fixation and at times alloy from dental restorations (Figs 7-48 and 7-51). Bone sites containing metallic foreign bodies should be avoided, if possible, because of the electrolytic interaction between the titanium implant and the foreign body, subsequent corrosion, and unfavorable tissue reaction (Van Ordan, 1985; Geis-Gerstorfer et al., 1989).

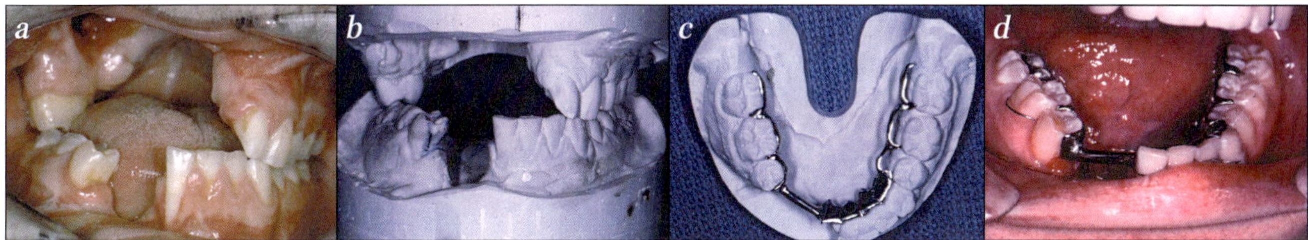

Figure 7-50 *(a)* Patient with a discontinuity defect of the right parasymphyseal region secondary to a self-inflicted gunshot wound. *(b)* Corrected casts mounted on an articulator. *(c)* Lingual splint cast in chrome cobalt alloy. *(d)* Splint wired to the dentition. The splint was left in place for several months to allow time for the bone graft to mature (courtesy of Dr. E. Roumanas).

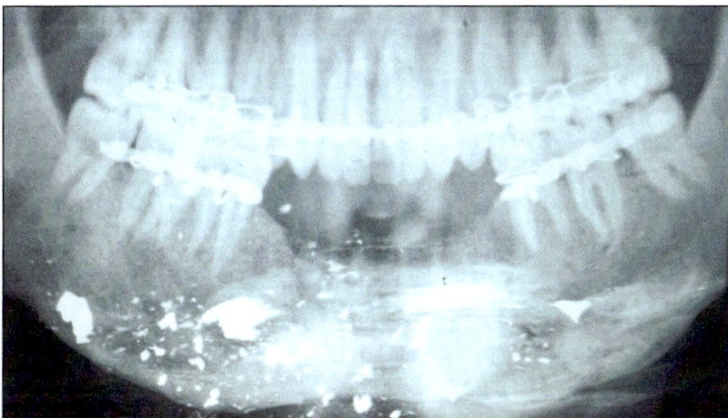

Figure 7-51 Patient suffered a gunshot wound to the anterior mandible. Note multiple metallic fragments. It will be challenging to place implants in this patient and avoid these metallic fragments.

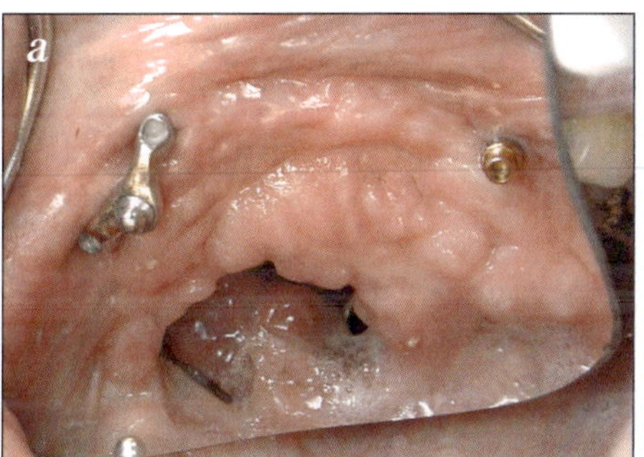

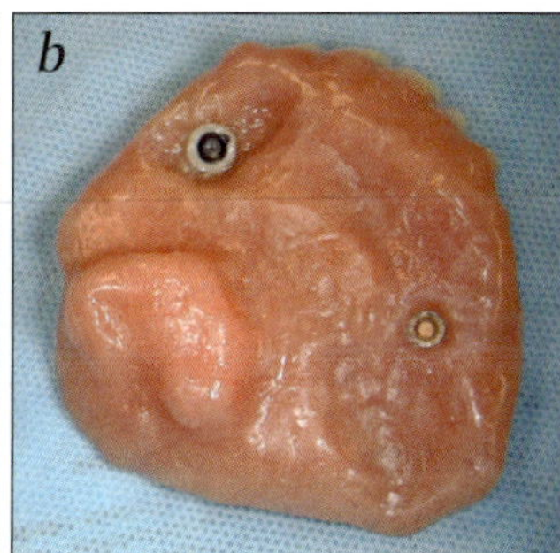

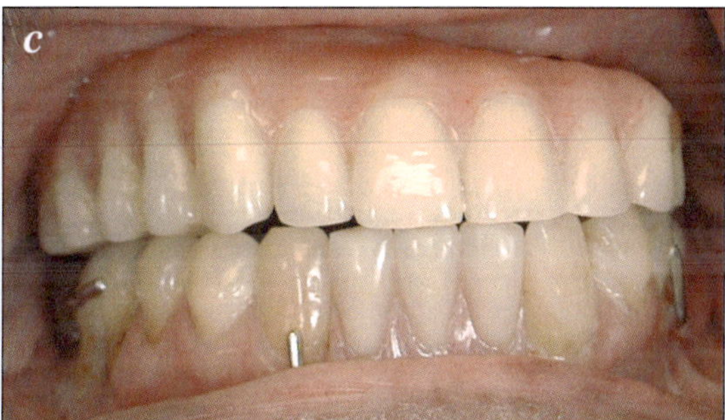

Figure 7-52 Patient suffered from multiple facial fractures, including the maxilla and the mandible. *(a)* Note the loss of alveolar ridges and the communication with the nasal cavity. The maxillary eating surface is essentially flat. Implants have been placed in areas of residual bone and fitted with individual attachments. *(b)* Overlay implant-assisted denture. *(c)* Prosthesis in position. The mandibular dentition was restored with a conventional RDP. A neutrocentric scheme of occlusion was employed.

Edentulous patients

Edentulous patients with a history of jaw fractures present special challenges for the prosthodontist. Discrepancies in edentulous ridge relations are often encountered, and the divergence of denture-bearing surfaces causes denture deflection and instability during function. Scarring and the lack of displaceability of the border tissues may compromise peripheral extensions. On occasion, the alveolar ridge contours are lost or flattened, further compromising the stability of the complete denture. In the edentulous maxilla, oral-antral fistulas or communications with the nasal cavity or paranasal sinuses may be present, making it impossible to obtain/maintain a peripheral seal for a conventional complete denture during function (Fig 7-52a). In the mandibular arch, compromised lingual flange length makes it very difficult for the patient to control their dentures, further impairing retention and stability.

Frequently, the only solution for such patients is the placement of osseointegrated implants (Figs 7-47 and 7-52). The presence of implants provides the retention and stability necessary for effective mastication and also enhances the support provided for the prosthesis. Posterior teeth may need to be arranged in a "reverse articulation" relationship, or an occlusal platform may be needed if mandibular movements are imprecise. Sometimes, the occlusal vertical dimension may need to be decreased to permit lip competency and improve denture base stability.

Burn Injuries

Commissure stents

The prompt application of splint therapy before the initiation of wound contraction will minimize post–burn scarring and the development of microstomia. The commissure stent provides tension,

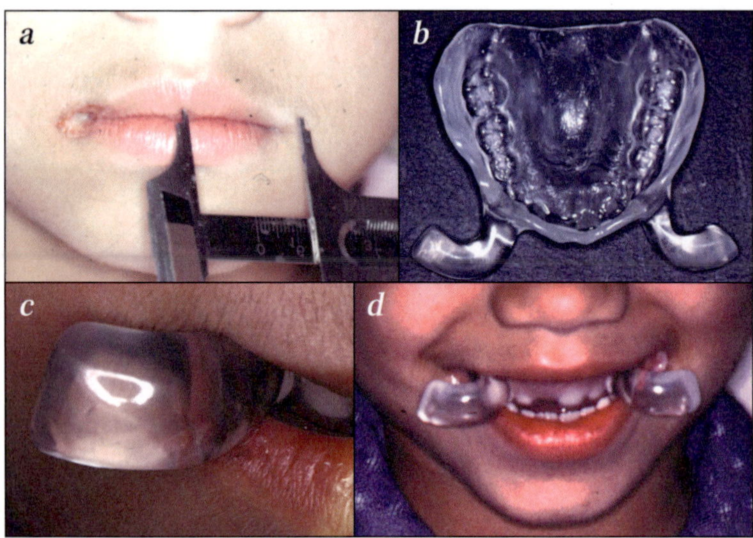

Figure 7-53 *(a)* Patient presents with an electrical burn associated with the right oral commissure. Measurements are made from the midline to the opposite unaffected commissure, and *(b)* the stent is fabricated. The extensions into the commissures must be highly polished. *(c)* The stent is in position, engaging the right commissure. *(d)* The stent must be continued to be worn for 4–6 months after mucosal healing.

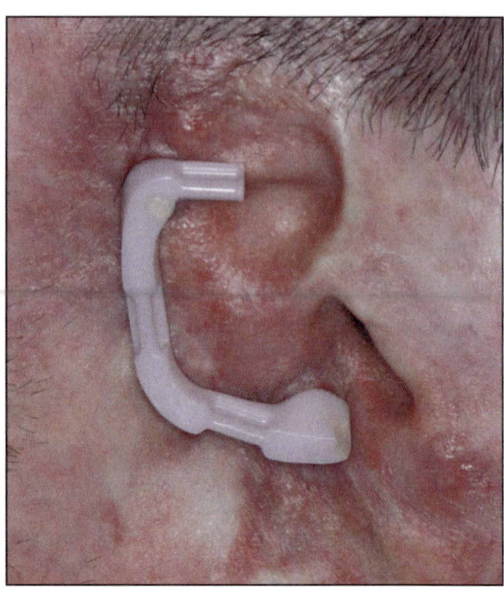

Figure 7-54 The auricle was lost secondary to severe burns. The implant connecting bar was designed digitally and made of monolithic zirconia.

serving as a scaffold during healing, and minimizes scar contracture. Continuous light tension should be employed to avoid decubital ulceration. Patient compliance is critical, and the children will require parental assistance.

Stone casts are obtained from irreversible hydrocolloid impressions and mounted on an articulator using an interocclusal record. A millimeter ruler is used to measure the contour of the mouth from the unaffected side to the midline to determine where the tissue should be placed on the traumatized side. Two layers of baseplate wax are adapted over the maxillary cast covering the palate and the teeth to the level of the sulcus. The occlusal surface of the wax is warmed to index the cusp tips of the mandibular teeth. Wax extensions are adapted to the wax covering the maxillary arch and are molded to curve laterally and posteriorly to retract both corners of the mouth. The internal contours of the extensions should simulate the desired contours of the healed tissue in clear acrylic resin (Fig 7-53). Modifications in contour and extensions can be developed in a soft wax and duplicated in autopolymerizing acrylic resin until the optimal tissue contours are achieved. The prosthesis is worn 24 hours a day for 6–8 months. It is removed for meals and oral hygiene. An additional 4–6 months of nighttime wear is also advised.

Prosthetic restoration of facial defects secondary to burns

Facial defects secondary to burns can be restored with facial prostheses. However, given the damage to the skin, they tolerate skin adhesives poorly, and therefore, most facial prostheses in such patients are retained with implants. However, given the compromised health status of their skin, many patients find it difficult to maintain peri-implant soft tissue health even when they are able to keep the implants free of debris, keratin buildup, and/or sebaceous secretions. Two solutions have emerged, which appear to have successfully addressed the persistent soft tissue irritation in these patients—the use of implant connecting bars fabricated of zirconia (Fig 7-54) and metal-ceramic bars designed such that the ceramic portion of bars interfaces with the peri-implant soft tissues (see Chapter 5, section entitled "Use of metal-ceramic and zirconia bars"). These ceramic surfaces retain debris less readily, which presumably explains why soft tissue health is better maintained.

Summary

Traumatic injuries of the oral facial region pose significant challenges. Facial trauma can be loosely classified into two major groups: a-tissue displacement and b-missing tissue. These injuries vary from localized tooth avulsions, to facial fractures, and to large avulsive wounds with a significant loss of hard and soft tissue. Burn injuries can lead to a loss of facial structures, such as the ear and nose, and so on. Reconstruction and rehabilitation of these patients can be complex and demanding, most often requiring an interdisciplinary effort involving reconstructive surgeons, orthodontists, and prosthodontists. Localized avulsive defects of the dentition and alveolar ridge can be restored with conventional fixed dental prostheses, removable dental prostheses with or without implant support, and implant-supported fixed dental prostheses. Frequently, such defects must be augmented with hard and soft tissue grafting prior to beginning prosthodontic care. Larger, more complex deficits, such as malunion of jaw fractures and avulsive injuries secondary to gunshot wounds, frequently require surgical osteotomies, bone grafting to restore continuity defects, and the placement of implants to retain and/or support fixed or removable dental prostheses. The latter is usually the most challenging. The best outcomes are achieved with well-coordinated interprofessional/interdisciplinary health care teams.

References

Abdulmajeed AA, Lim KG, Narhi To, et al. Complete-arch implant-supported monolithic zirconia fixed dental prostheses: A systematic review. J Prosthet Dent 2016;115:672–677.

Agar J, Cameron SM, Hughbanks JC, et al. Cement removal from restorations luted to titanium abutments with simulated subgingival margins. J Prosthet Dent 1997;78:43–47.

Aghaloo TL, Moy PK. Which hard tissue augmentation techniques are the most successful in furnishing bony support for implant placement? Int J Oral Maxillofacial Implants 2007;22(suppl):49–70.

Bell W, Levy BM. Revascularization and bone healing after total maxillary osteotomy. J Oral Surg 1975;33:253–260.

Beumer J, Faulkner RF, Shah K, et al. Fundamentals of implant dentistry: Prosthodontic principles. 2nd ed. Chicago: Quintessence; 2022.

Bidra AS, Rungruaganunt P, Gauthier M. Clinical outcomes of full arch fixed implant-supported zirconia prostheses: A systematic review. Eur J Oral Implantol 2017;10(Suppl 1):35–45.

Brady FA, Leake DL. Remodeling of the fractured mandibular condyle in a child: Review of the literature and report of a case. J Oral Med 1978;33:57–58.

Brady FA, Roser SN, Hieshima GB. Orbital emphysema. Br J Oral Surg 1976;14:65.

Butterworth CJ, Rogers SN. The zygomatic implant perforated ZIP flap: A new technique for combined surgical reconstruction and rapid fixed dental rehabilitation following low-level maxillary. Int J Implant Dent 2017;3:37. http://doi.org/10.1186/s40729-017-0100-8.

Butterworth CJ, Lowe D, Rogers SN. The zygomatic implant perforated (ZIP) flap reconstructive technique for the management of low-level maxillary malignancy—clinical & patient related outcomes on 35 consecutively treated patients. Head Neck 2022;44:345–358.

Butz F, Aita H, Wang CC, et al. Harder and stiffer osseointegrated bone to roughened titanium. J Dent Res 2006;85:560–565.

Chang TL, Orellana D, Finzen FC. Optimizing esthetics: Attachments and Rotational Path RPD's. In The RPI System per Kratochvil: The principles of removable partial denture design and fabrication. Eds. TL Chang, D Orellana, J Beumer III. Chicago: Quintessence; 2019. pp. 149–160.

Edelhoff D, Beuer F, Schweiger J, et al. CAD/CAM-generated high-density polymer restorations for the pretreatment of complex cases: A case report. Quintessence Int 2012;43:457–467.

Eliason C. RPA clasp design for distal-extension removable partial dentures. J Prosthet Dent 1983;49:25–27.

Faulkner RF, Beumer J, Shah K, et al. Restoration of multiple-tooth defects in the esthetic zone. In Fundamentals of implant dentistry: Prosthodontic principles. 2nd ed. Eds. J Beumer, RF Faulkner, K Shah, B Wu. Chicago: Quintessence; 2022. pp. 444–479.

Geis-Gerstorfer J, Weber H, Sauer KH. In vitro substance loss due to galvanic corrosion in Ti implant/Ni-Cr supraconstruction systems. J Oral Maxillofac Implants 1989;4:119–123.

Ghasemzadeh A, Mundinger GS, Swanson EW, et al. Treatment of pediatric condylar fractures: A 20-year experience. Plast Reconstr Surg 2015;136:1279–1288.

Haddadi S, Parvizi A, Niknama R, et al. Baseline characteristics and outcomes of patients with head and neck burn injuries; a cross-sectional study of 2181 cases. Arch Acad Emerg Med 2021;9(1):e8. Published online 2020 Dec 11. http://doi.org/10.22037/aaem.v9i1.948.

Hickey AJ. Maxillofacial prosthetic rehabilitation following self-inflicted gunshot wounds to the head and neck. J Prosthet Dent 1986;55:78–82.

Jackson I. Soft tissue trauma. In Maxillofacial rehabilitation: Prosthodontic and surgical considerations. Eds. J Beumer, TA Curtis, M Marunick Ishiyaku. St Louis, MO: EuroAmerica; 1996. pp. 486–487.

Kelly JF. Management of war injuries to the jaw and related structures. Washington, DC: US Government Printing Office; 1977.

King GE. Dual path design for removable partial dentures. J Prosthet Dent 1978;39:505–507.

Kinsel RP, Lin D. Retrospective analysis of porcelain failures of metal ceramic crowns and fixed partial dentures supported by 729 implants in 152 patients: Patient-specific and implant-specific predictors of ceramic failure. J Prosthet Dent 2009;101:388–394.

Korn P, Gellrich NC, Jehn P, et al. A new strategy for patient-specific implant bone dental rehabilitation in patient with extended maxillary defects. Front Oncol 2021 Dec 10;11:718872. http://doi.org/10.3389/fonc.2021.718872. eCollection 2021.

Kratochvil FJ. Influence of occlusal rest position and clasp design on movement of abutment teeth. J Prosthet Dent 1963;13:114–124.

Kroll AJ, Finzen F. Rotational path removable partial dentures. Part II. Replacement of anterior teeth. 1988;1:135–142.

LeFort FT. Etude experimentale sur les fractures de Ia machovie superieure. Rev Chir 1901;23:208–227.

Linkevicius T, Vindasiute E, Puisys A, et al. The influence of the cementation margin position on the amount of undetected cement. A prospective clinical study. Clin Oral Implants Res 2013;24:71–76.

Mackenzie IC, Hill MW. Connective tissue influences on patterns of epithelial architecture and keratinization in skin and oral mucosa of the adult mouse. Cell Tissue Res 1984;235:551–559.

McGoldrick DM, Parmar P, Williams R, et al. Treatment of pediatric condylar fractures: A 20-year experience. J Craniofac Surg 2019;30:2045–2047.

Moscovitch M. Consecutive cases series of monolithic minimally veneered zirconia restorations on teeth and implants: Up to 68 months. Int J Periodontics Restorative Dent 2015;35:315–323.

Moy PK, Pozzi A, Beumer III J. Fundamentals of implant dentistry: Surgical principles. Chicago: Quintessence; 2016.

Noack EA, Gehrke P. Survival and rates of complication of implant supported lithium disilicate single crowns. J Dent Implantol 2016;32:202–213.

Ogawa T, Nishimura I. Different bone integration profiles of turned and acid-etched implants associated with modulated expression of extracellular matrix genes. Int J Oral Maxillofac Implants 2003;18:200–210.

Pozzi A, Tallarico M, Barlattani A. Monolithic lithium disilicate full-contour crowns bonded on CAD/CAM zirconia complete-arch implant bridges with 3 to 5 years of follow-up. J Oral Implantol 2015;41:450-8.

Takeuchi K, Saruwatari L, Nakamura H, et al. Enhancement of biomechanical properties of mineralized tissue by osteoblasts cultured on titanium with different surface topographies. J Biomed Mater Res 2005;72A:296–305.

Tian H, Wang L, Xie W, et al. Epidemiology and outcome analysis of facial burns: A retrospective multicentre study 2011–2015. Burns 2020;46:718–726.

Tischler M, Patch, Bidra AS. Rehabilitation of edentulous jaws with zirconia complete-arch fixed implant-supported prostheses: An up to 4-year retrospective clinical study. J Prosthet Dent 2018;120:204–209.

Van Ordan AC. Corrosive response of the interface tissues to 316L stainless steel, titanium-based alloys, and cobalt-based alloys. In Dental implant. Eds. McKinney RV, Lemons JE. Littleton, MA: PSG; 1985. pp. 1–24.

Vosselman HH, Glas HH, de Visscher SAHJ, et al. Immediate implant-retained prosthetic obturation after maxillectomy based on zygomatic implant placement by 3D-guided surgery: A cadaver study. Int J Implant Dent 2021 Jun 14;7(1):54. http://doi.org/10.1186/s40729-021-00335-w.

Wiens JP. The use of osseointegrated implants in the treatment of patients with trauma. J Prosthet Dent 1992;67:670–678.

Wiens JP, Hickey A. Maxillofacial trauma. In Maxillofacial rehabilitation: Prosthodontic and surgical considerations. Eds. J Beumer III, TA Curtis, MT Marunick. St Louis, MO: Ishiyaku EuroAmerica Inc; 1996. pp. 479–509.

Wiens R. Psychosocial considerations. In Maxillofacial rehabilitation: Prosthodontic and surgical considerations. Eds. J Beumer III, TA Curtis, MT Marunick. St Louis, MO: Ishiyaku EuroAmerica Inc; 1996. pp. 483–484.

Wu B, Abduo J, Lyons K, et al. Implant biomechanics, screw mechanics, and occlusal concepts for implant patients. In Fundamentals of implant dentistry: Prosthodontic principles. Eds. J Beumer, RF Faulkner, K Shah, B Wu. 2nd ed. Chicago: Quintessence; 2022. pp. 37–59.

Chapter 8

Tissue Engineering of Maxillofacial Tissues

Min Lee, Minjee Kang, Benjamin M. Wu

Congenital defects, trauma, and tumor resection often produce anatomical defects in the oral and maxillofacial region that may cause severe aesthetic deformity, discomfort, and functional impairment. Radiation damage to specific structures and tissues may render these tissues nonfunctional. These functional and aesthetic deficits can devastate the patient's quality of life and present considerable reconstructive challenges for the surgeon and prosthodontist.

Eradication of tumors often requires irradiation, chemoradiation, and extensive resection for cure. These highly invasive procedures often result in large defects and loss of multiple tissue types, leaving behind tissues that have limited vascularity, significant scarring, and poor healing capacity. Although the use of vascularized free flaps has improved graft survival in these suboptimal healing environments, the need for multiple procedures and hospitalization precludes surgical options for large defects for many patients.

When facial defects are large, maxillofacial prostheses are excellent alternatives that offer the opportunities for routine examination to detect recurrence, while providing retention and superb cosmetic results. However, patient acceptance of large facial prostheses may be impaired because no synthetic material can simulate native tissue motility, color stability, physical-chemical properties, and biologic functionality. Although osseointegrated implants have made a significant impact on the retention, stability, and support provided to oral prostheses, bone of sufficient volume and vitality for implant placement and predictable long-term function may be lacking in this patient population.

In recent years, various approaches based on tissue engineering principles have been explored to regenerate functional tissues that are relevant to maxillofacial rehabilitation. This chapter will begin with a brief review of the tissue engineering triad: *(1)* cells, *(2)* scaffolds, and *(3)* growth factors. Emphasis is placed on components that are particularly relevant for maxillofacial applications. Readers who are interested in other applications are referred to introductory tissue engineering textbooks.

The following section provides the maxillofacial reconstructive team a balanced perspective on the incredible accomplishments to date, and the considerable gaps that remain in the engineering of bone, cartilage, tongue and skeletal muscle, motor neurons, skin, and oral mucosa. Although this section does not cover all tissue types that are commonly lost, the selected examples will provide readers with a general sense of the considerable progress in the hypercompetitive field of tissue engineering.

The third section of this chapter focuses on one of the most significant engineering challenges for the regeneration of large, multilineage tissues that are needed to rehabilitate clinically relevant defects: diffusion-limited nutrient transport. Solution to this fundamental problem requires a much better understanding of stem cell–scaffold interactions and further development in advanced technologies that can manipulate cells, bioactive factors, and carriers in a spatial-specific manner.

The last section presents an overview of computer-aided tissue engineering technologies that are being used to fabricate tissue engineering scaffolds. Some of these technologies are already used for making patient-specific models for presurgical planning, surgical templates, and prosthesis fabrication (see Chapters 2–7). This section will emphasize the ability of these manufacturing technologies to pattern cells and multiple materials along complex three-dimensional (3D) gradients.

Tissue Engineering Overview

The maxillofacial complex contains multiple tissues that are organized in spatially complex cellular arrangements. When injured, healthy natural tissues have the capacity to repair and remodel by orchestrating a highly intricate, time-dependent pattern of cell-cell, cell-matrix, and cell-signal interactions. The temporal-spatial patterning of these cellular interactions involves the efficient use of low-dose growth signals that direct the repair. Even more elaborate patterning and cellular migration are observed in embryogenesis, growth and development, and tumor migration.

Tissue engineering attempts to recapitulate the key temporal-spatial patterning steps by delivering the appropriate signals and microenvironment to promote the desirable cellular activities at specific stages. The field of tissue engineering has evolved dramatically since the early 1960s. Today, it integrates the latest advances in molecular biology, biochemistry, engineering, material science, and medical transplantation (Langer and Vacanti, 1993). Researchers in the basic and medical sciences have identified tissue engineering as an attractive translational target. Clinical problems requiring tissue regeneration are diverse and no single regeneration approach will resolve all injuries.

Recent advances in the field of tissue engineering have included the use of sophisticated biocompatible scaffolds, new postnatal multipotent cell populations, and appropriate cellular stimulation for creation of a permissive microenvironment. In particular, smart synthetic polymer scaffolds allow fast and reproducible construction while still retaining biocompatible characteristics. Additionally, the identification of multipotent mesenchymal precursor cells within numerous tissues has stimulated a new surge of research. Finally, many growth factors have revealed the ability to stimulate tissue regeneration.

The ability to regulate distribution, organization, and function of distinct cell types within 3D matrices that control spatial-temporal growth factor delivery represents an important challenge, and opportunity, in tissue engineering.

Cells in Tissue Engineering

Cells are the engineers that actually do the job of tissue engineering. Many cell-based tissue engineering approaches rely on the delivery of progenitor cells within scaffolds. Although the scaffold microenvironment (e.g., presence of growth factors) may promote cellular differentiation, the implantation of cells that are already committed or differentiated along a particular lineage may significantly shift the microenvironment to favor and/or maintain differentiation by influencing the influx of neighboring cells. Alternatively, the implanted cells may secrete cytokines that may truncate the usual steps of cellular migration, proliferation, and differentiation.

Primary autologous cells

The ideal source for cells is still not well established. At first glance, the use of primary autologous cells would make sense because they can be obtained directly from healthy tissues, and many laboratory-scale experiments have shown that primary cells can be harvested and reimplanted to directly participate in tissue healing without requiring additional growth signals (Psaltis et al., 2008). Therefore, the use of these functional, differentiated cells would relax the constraints on scaffold composition and growth factor delivery.

However, the use of primary cells is not always practical. Beside increasing morbidity associated with the harvesting procedure, the limited number of primary cells imposes the need for ex vivo culture, which exponentially increases the logistics for regulatory approval and the cost for manufacturing. Furthermore, in more advanced cases of organ failure resulting from genetic deficiencies, the harvesting of autologous cells from nonfunctional tissues may be contraindicated. Therefore, primary cells are not always the first choice for cell-based tissue engineering applications that require the use of large numbers of distinct functional cells (e.g., large defects involving multiple tissues).

Embryonic stem cells

Various stem cells are available, ranging in differentiation state from embryonic stem cells (ESCs) to adult stem cells. ESCs are extracted from the inner cell mass of the blastocyst during the early stage of the developing embryo (Fig 8-1). ESCs are the most exciting cell source because of two properties that make them unique among all cell sources for tissue engineering: *(1)* self-renewal and *(2)* true multipotency. ESCs can proliferate continuously under the proper culture conditions for at least hundreds of passages over several years. Under special culture conditions, undifferentiated ESCs can be induced to differentiate along all three embryonic lineages. These two unique attributes give ESCs the potential to be an unlimited cell source that can be differentiated on demand to regenerate any tissue and even organs.

Some fundamental problems must be addressed before this potential is realized. First, although abundant evidence exists to show that ESCs can indeed differentiate into the desirable cell type (Doss et al., 2004), it remains to be shown that the fate of all implanted ESCs can be controlled. Will they all know when to stop dividing and never differentiate into undesirable cell types (e.g., cancer cells)? Indeed, many reports show that cultured ESCs can proliferate and differentiate simultaneously along multiple cell lineages in vitro—a far less complex and infinitely more controllable environment than in vivo (Odorico et al., 2001).

The ability to exert spatial-temporal control of cell fate is a critical issue that is being intensely investigated because it impacts many secondary issues. For example, although ESCs have been shown to alleviate important diseases such as insulin-dependent diabetes, the lack of control makes it difficult to be certain of the immunocompatibility of all implanted cells and their regenerated tissues, although in theory ESCs are able to differentiate properly and develop the same surface antigens as host cells to evade the host immune system.

Exciting developments have been made to address this important concern. For example, somatic cell nuclear transfer can be used

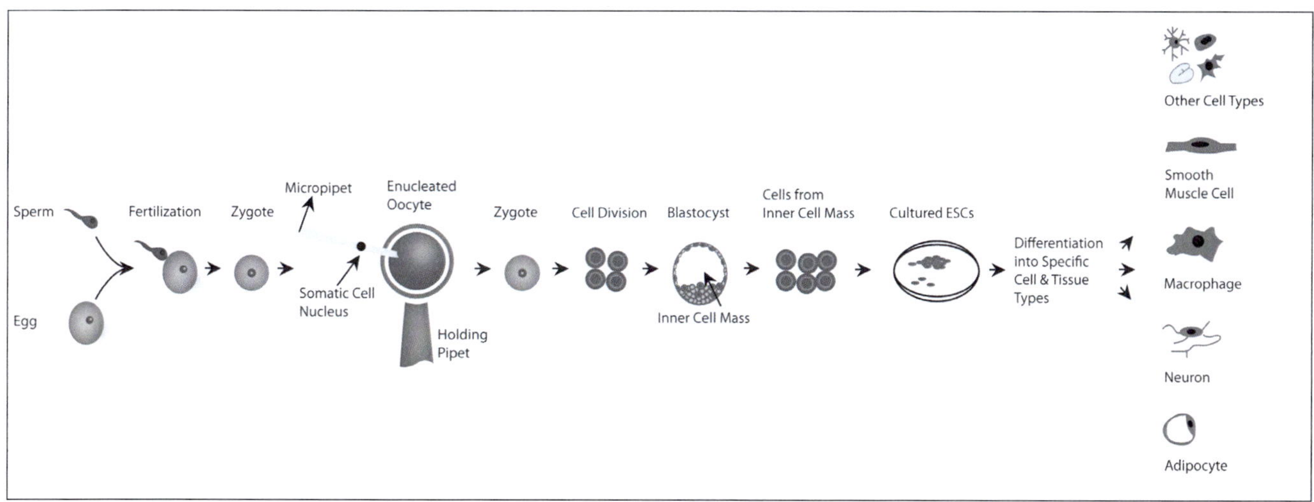

Figure 8-1 Development of the human embryo and somatic cell nuclear transfer (reprinted from the National Academy of Sciences with permission; National Academy of Sciences' Board on Life Sciences. Stem Cells and the Future of Regenerative Medicine. Washington, DC: National Academies, 2002).

to extract the nucleus of a somatic cell from any host tissue and transfer it into an unfertilized egg from which the nucleus has been removed. The resultant cell can self-renew and proliferate indefinitely to produce numerous daughter cells that are multipotent like ESCs (Yamanaka and Blau, 2010). Because they contain exactly the same DNA material as all other host somatic cells, they have a major theoretical advantage of being more histocompatible than ESCs (Yamanaka and Blau, 2010). As exciting as this and other genetic engineering techniques are, having the right DNA is probably not the entire story. The ultimate fate and long-term clinical histocompatibility of these cells in the face of epigenetic regulation and the complex in vivo environment remain to be investigated.

Another limitation of using ESCs is that many of the so-called proper ESC culture conditions involve the use of xenogeneic feeder cells and bovine serum, which may incur the risk of disease transmission. Because it is unknown why ESCs interact with various components of the feeder cells, which release growth factors to support the growth of ESCs, their use in tissue engineering may incur potential complications that may raise concerns from regulatory agencies. If the use of feeder cells cannot be avoided, then care must be taken to ensure that feeder cells are free of animal viruses and prions.

Finally, because the harvesting of ESCs involves the destruction of human embryos, their use in regenerative medicine is somewhat controversial. These ethical concerns have resulted in severe restrictions on federal funding of human ESC research in the United States (National Institutes of Health, U.S. Department of Health and Human Services. National Institutes of Health Guidelines on Human Stem Cell Research. Federal Register 74 [18578], 23 Apr 2009. https://www.govinfo.gov/content/pkg/FR-2009-04-23/pdf/E9-9313.pdf. Accessed 15 Feb 2011). Although former President Barack Obama issued Executive Order 13505, "Removing Barriers to Responsible Scientific Research Involving Human Stem Cells," to expand stem cell research, a Federal District Court ruled that the order violates a federal law that bars federal funding for "research in which a human embryo or embryos are destroyed, discarded or knowingly subjected to risk of injury or death." The fight for innovation will occur outside our American laboratories. As a result, most ESC research has involved the use of mouse ESCs and a few human ESC cell lines. Although great feasibility has been shown with these ESCs (Liu et al., 2011) the genetic and epigenetic controls of cell fate for human ESCs are largely unknown.

The pace of research in this field is expected to pick up significantly as the federal ban becomes more relaxed in the future. Meanwhile, state-funded stem cell programs in California and New York are leading the way to create world-class stem cell research programs (California Institute for Regenerative Medicine. 2010 Report of the External Advisory Panel. https://www.cirm.ca.gov/wp-content/uploads/archive/files/about_cirm/CIRM-EAP_Report.pdf. Accessed 15 Feb 2011; Empire State Stem Cell Board. 2008–2009 Annual Report of the Empire State Stem Cell Board and New York Stem Cell Science Program. https://stemcell.ny.gov/sites/default/files/documents/files/2008-2009_annualreport.pdf. Accessed 15 Feb 2011). The pace must accelerate because the critical control problems are immensely difficult to address. Regardless of whether human ESCs will be used directly for clinical regenerative medicine or whether de-differentiated adult stem cells that exhibit ESC-like behavior will be used, there is no doubt that better understanding of human ESC differentiation will play an important role in advancing the field of tissue engineering.

Hematopoietic adult stem cells

The restriction on federal funding of human ESC research has motivated the search for adult stem cells from numerous tissues. The first successful adult stem cells are the hematopoietic stem cells (HSCs). HSCs are obtained from bone marrow and can self-renew in vivo continuously; under proper culture conditions, they can differentiate into any blood cell without the need for feeder cells. Studies have also suggested that HSCs can differentiate into other cells derived from all three germ layers besides blood cells (Weissman, 2000). Because HSCs are adult stem cells, their use can potentially eliminate the ethical debate surrounding the use of ESCs.

However, only 0.001 percent of marrow cells are HSCs and, although they can self-renew in vivo, the inability to expand HSCs in vitro makes it difficult to obtain enough HSCs for the tissue engineering of large tissues. Although it may appear logical to circumvent the cell number problem by seeding a tissue engineering scaffold with only a limited number of HSCs and expecting them to proliferate in vivo and populate the scaffold, there is no evidence that HSCs can proliferate significantly outside of the marrow environment. On the contrary, there are decades of limited success in stimulating in vitro HSC proliferation outside of the native marrow environment (Ramakrishnan and Torok-Storb, 2010), suggesting that the scaffold microenvironment may have to be highly engineered to produce sequential HSC proliferation and then somehow induce specific differentiation into functional tissues.

As mysterious as HSC proliferation is despite the fact that HSCs have been investigated for decades, the precise conditions to control their cell fate outside of blood cells remain largely unknown. The lack of control over HSC differentiation mirrors the issues discussed earlier for ESCs.

Their small numbers also make it difficult to control the purity using conventional cell-sorting technologies. The impurity of HSCs causes two problems. First, if the impurity contains donor T cells, serious histocompatibility problems can ensue even if the transplanted HSCs are obtained from close blood relatives. The transplanted immune cells within the tissue engineering scaffold may recognize the recipient as foreign and mount an immunologic attack in the recipient. Currently, the incidence of HSC impurity-related graft-versus-host disease after allogeneic bone marrow transplantation ranges from 30% to 80%, depending on the degree of match between the marrow donor and recipient (Wingard et al., 2011). At the present time, recipients of bone marrow transplants take immunosuppressive drugs to reduce the incidence and severity of the immune reaction caused by contaminated cells in the transplant.

These concerns make HSCs from umbilical cord blood more attractive than adult marrow HSCs, because umbilical HSCs are more immature and less immune competent. However, umbilical cord blood is much smaller in volume than marrow and therefore contains even fewer HSCs. The good news is that allogeneic HSCs may not be always necessary for tissue engineering because autologous HSCs may be a viable option. Unlike other indications for bone marrow transplant (e.g., certain types of leukemia and lymphoma), patients with healthy marrow are at far less risk of having defective and cancer cells in their marrow, and therefore the marrow is less likely to deliver these undesirable cells back into the system. Healthy patients with tissue lost due to traumatic injuries or patients who have recovered from surgical resection of local tumors tend to have healthier marrow than those with leukemia and lymphoma. Therefore, autologous cell transplantation is an option for them if their marrow cells are healthy.

The second problem, in addition to the lack of purity of HSCs, is the current inability to reproduce the impurities. The resultant batch-to-batch variations in initial quantity and composition of cells make it difficult to predict the signal required to induce the proper differentiation of HSCs for different tissue engineering applications. Numerous microfluidic cell-sorting techniques with novel biophotonic detection systems are being developed to identify and trap rare cells. Although these techniques cannot compete with the efficiencies of high-throughput multiplex cell-sorting machines, these new engineering tools may prove useful for controlling purity—a necessary prerequisite for improved safety and better understanding of HSC differentiation potential.

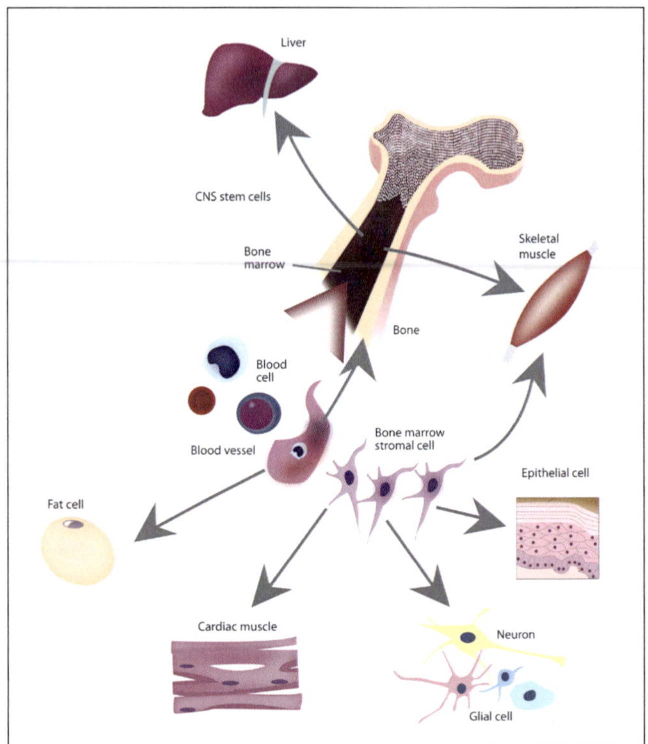

Figure 8-2 Adult stem cell plasticity. CNS—central nervous system (©2001 Terese Winslow, assisted by Lydia Kibiuk and Caitlin Duckwall).

Other adult stem cells

Successful isolation of adult stem cells has been demonstrated from tissues of maxillofacial relevance including teeth, bone, muscles, cartilage, vessels, and skin. Exciting reports have shown that adult stem cells can also be harvested from fat, vessels, heart, liver, kidney, intestine, adrenal glands, neurons, and many others (Ferraro et al., 2010). Their presence in so many tissues suggests that the quantity and potency of adult stem cells within any given adult tissue may contribute to the variation in self-repair ability among different adult tissues (Fig 8-2).

These adult stem cells can differentiate into a variety of cells, but not all of them have been shown convincingly to produce tissue across all three germ layers. Studies have shown that adult stem cells can be coaxed or reprogrammed into a less differentiated, more ESC-like state (O'Brien et al., 2002). Although current understanding is that unmanipulated adult stem cells may not match the multi–germ line potency of ESCs, their limited potency may actually be an advantage for tissue engineering. This limited potency may predispose the adult stem cells harvested from a particular tissue, for example, the salivary gland, to differentiate into only functional cells found in that specific tissue or to secrete the necessary growth factors that promote the desirable tissue development. The primary theoretical benefit is that there may be less chance for them to differentiate into cancer cells.

However, there is no evidence that these localized adult stem cells do not participate in cancer development or differentiate into other cells under various complex in vivo environmental conditions. Furthermore, as with HSCs, their rarity and the inability to purify them makes it difficult to study the fate of these cells. For example, it is not even known how many different types of stem cell are present within a given tissue. It is reasonable that, given their short history and rarity, the mechanistic understanding of these adult stem cells is even more limited than that for HSCs, which have been investigated for decades and already been used clinically.

Despite these limitations, the lack of ethical concern and relative ease of harvesting adult stem cells have resulted in many more translational investigations in tissue engineering. Although few of these studies actually prove that adult stem cells directly become functional cells in regenerated tissues (Chou et al., 2011), their clinical benefit and potential safety may actually bring these cells to be used in clinical trials for regenerative medicine faster than scientific understanding can evolve.

Application of adult stem cells in tissue engineering

The use of adult stem cells for regenerating tissues of maxillofacial relevance is well documented. For instance, bone marrow stromal cells (BMSCs) and adipose-derived adult stromal (ADAS) cells have reproducibly demonstrated the capacity to differentiate down multiple lineages, including the ability to regenerate bone in vivo (Bosch et al., 2000; Krebsbach et al., 2000; Lee et al., 2001b; Lee et al., 2002a; Peng et al., 2002; Wright et al., 2002).

Most cell-based therapies for bone regeneration have focused on the active multipotent precursor cells found in BMSCs (Gundle et al., 1995; Haynesworth et al., 1992; Im et al., 2001; Johnstone et al., 1998; Toquet et al., 1999; Wakitani et al., 1995). Although donating bone marrow may be an unpleasant experience for patients, the richness of the extracted cells aids in many bone tissue engineering strategies, making them a popular choice. In 1999, Pittenger et al. (1999) defined BMSCs as the "gold standard," because under the appropriate conditions they are able to differentiate along three lineages: *(1)* osteoblastic, *(2)* adipocytic, and *(3)* chondrocytic. In vivo, implanted BMSCs have aided in the healing of critical-sized skeletal defects in many animal models, including mice (Cowan et al., 2004; Cowan et al., 2005; Krebsbach et al., 1998), rats (Blum et al., 2003; Lieberman et al., 1999), rabbits (Chang et al., 2004; Dean et al., 2003), swine (Chang et al., 2003), goats (Kruyt et al., 2004), and sheep (Petite et al., 2000; Shang et al., 2001).

Although some research has demonstrated successful bone-defect healing with unstimulated BMSCs, most research has emphasized the need for additional stimulation by growth factors within the microenvironment for timely healing (Lieberman et al., 1999). This is due to the low number of committed osteoprogenitor cells, usually 0.0001% of a bone marrow harvest (Haynesworth et al., 1992; Bruder et al., 1997). Accordingly, growth factor stimulation is required to recruit and expand the number of osteoprogenitor cells in harvested marrow specimens. The reduction of healthy bone marrow cells in aging or diseased adults further diminishes number of osteoprogenitor cells (Egrise et al., 1992; Quarto et al., 1992). Because the success of using bone marrow in vivo is critically dependent on the implantation of sufficient numbers of cells, other cell sources that overcome these limitations may be advantageous.

Adipose tissue has received much attention for its source of multipotent mesenchymal cells. In vitro, ADAS cells can differentiate down osteogenic, chondrogenic, myogenic, adipogenic, and even neuronal pathways (Ashjian et al., 2003; Erickson et al., 2002; Halvorsen et al., 2001a; Halvorsen et al., 2001b; Mizuno et al., 2002; Safford et al., 2002; Tholpady et al., 2003; Wickham et al., 2003; Zuk et al., 2002; Zuk et al., 2001). The greatest advantage of these cells is that they are readily available in large numbers with minimal donor morbidity (i.e., cosmetic liposuction) and attach and proliferate rapidly in culture, making them a very attractive cell source for tissue engineering. Furthermore, use of ADAS cells has the potential to become more popular than use of BMSCs, based on the notion that patients may be more willing to donate adipose tissue than bone marrow.

ADAS cells stimulated by recombinant human bone morphogenetic protein 2 (rhBMP-2) produce more in vitro bone nodules than either osteoblasts or BMSCs cultures under the same conditions (Ashjian et al., 2003; Halvorsen et al., 2001a; Halvorsen et al., 2001b; Tholpady et al., 2003; Zuk et al., 2002; Zuk et al., 2001; De Ugarte et al., 2003; Lee et al., 2003; Ogawa et al., 2004). The in vivo osteogenic capability of ADAS cells placed extraskeletally (Ogawa et al., 2004; Dragoo et al., 2003) or within skeletal defects (Cowan et al., 2004; Cowan et al., 2005) has equaled that of BMSCs and nearly reached that of committed osteoblasts. Local application of ADAS osteoprogenitor cells has successfully aided in the effort to heal skeletal defects.

There is no doubt that the pace of research on all stem cells will accelerate with the relaxation of the federal ban on ESC research. Much more work is needed to focus on human stem cells in clinically relevant in vivo models. In particular, tissue engineers need to know how proliferation and differentiation of stem cells are dictated by their local microenvironment.

Materials in Tissue Engineering

The classic tissue engineering scaffolds are porous sponges that deliver progenitor cells and foster cellular ingrowth after implantation. Subsequently, growth factors are added to provide additional pharmacologic effects. The massive number of scaffold materials indicates the large volume of research conducted in this highly competitive field. The interested reader is referred to general reviews by Geiger et al. (2003) and Rosso et al. (2004) on common materials.

Today, material scientists are developing new biomaterials by engineering chemical moieties that confer molecular specificity to control many biologic processes; these moieties range from adhesion ligands that promote integrin-mediated adhesion, to protease cleavable linkages that release growth factors in response to cellular activity, to unstable bonds that degrade in response to environmental cues including pH, temperature, and electromagnetic energy. It is now common practice to integrate matrix proteins, such as fibronectin or the integrin-binding peptide sequences, to enhance cellular attachment and migration (Nuttelman et al., 2001; Rowley and Mooney, 2002). The development of these molecular-driven biomaterials has been one of the most exciting emerging trends in materials engineering.

Regardless of chemical sophistication, scaffold architecture and surface properties are critical to mass transport and cell-matrix interactions and constitute a key focus of many tissue engineering approaches. The scaffold material not only defines the surface properties of the scaffold in terms of adhesive substrate and physical

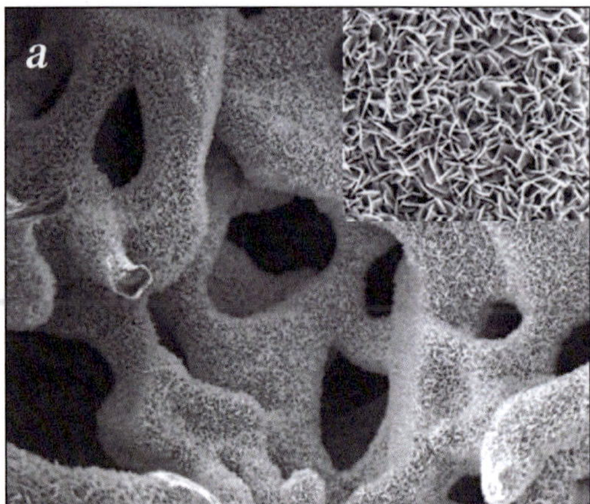

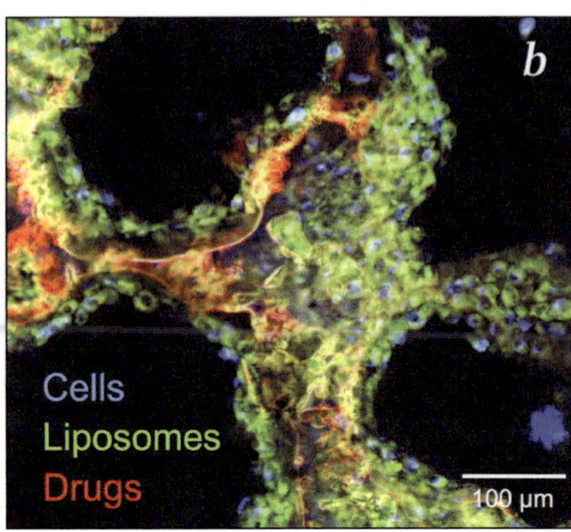

Figure 8-3 Poly(glycolic acid-co-lactic acid; PLGA) scaffolds coated with *(a)* apatite and *(b)* liposomes. The inset in *(a)* shows low magnification image of the scaffold. In *(b)*, the microscopic image shows cells (blue) interacting with liposomes (green) loaded with therapeutic drugs (red) on a scaffold.

support but also provides the surface properties important for cellular signaling (Bottaro et al., 2002). Therefore, it is not surprising that the clinical success of any given biomaterial depends highly on the biologic environment and specific cell types in the surrounding tissues. For each tissue type, there exist materials that are generally considered to be desirable.

An example are the biomaterials for bone regeneration, which are by far the most heavily investigated among all tissue engineering efforts. Orthopedic biomaterials are generally classified as *inert*, *osteoconductive*, or *osteoinductive*. Inert materials may elicit negligible or minor inflammation but do not stimulate or inhibit bone formation. The first evidence of intentional bone tissue engineering using an implantable scaffold occurred in 1969, when Winter and Simpson (1969) implanted a synthetic poly(hydroxyethyl methacrylate) sponge under the skin of young pigs and demonstrated intramembranous ossification.

Osteoconductive scaffolds promote bone cells to attach, migrate, proliferate, and function but do not have the ability to induce nonosteoblasts to differentiate into bone-forming cells. Osteoconductive matrices use biologic materials (e.g., collagen or demineralized bone), and/or nonbiologic materials, including various metals (e.g., titanium), some degradable polymers, and bioglass. Their advantages include controlled construction, minimal immunogenicity, and acceptable biocompatibility.

Osteoinductive scaffolds are able to stimulate undifferentiated cells into osteoblasts. Because very few biomaterials are truly inductive, biomaterials scientists have engineered inductive scaffolds by modifying inert and conductive materials with bioactive coatings or conjugating molecular moieties that directly or indirectly signal growth factor receptors. Creation of microscale or nanoscale features on scaffold surfaces is commonly achieved by adding bioactive coatings. One study has demonstrated that growth factor delivery from collagen-coated polymer scaffold can induce bone regeneration in vivo (Aghaloo et al., 2006). Our group has developed a biomimetic apatite coating process for 3D complex structures and created apatite microenvironments that enhanced the expression of osteoblastic genes (Fig 8-3; Chou et al., 2004; Chou et al., 2005a; Chou et al., 2005b; Fan et al., 2015) Besides enhancing osteoconductivity of scaffolds, the biomimetic apatite coating can produce sustained release of growth factors that can induce bone formation (Lee et al., 2009a).

The bone regenerative performance of scaffolds can be further improved by employing proper delivery systems that protect bioactive cargo (e.g., growth factors, small molecule drugs, and nucleic acids) from fast degradation, burst release, or nonspecific targeting (Xie et al., 2021). Recent approaches to make osteoinductive scaffolds focus on the integration of liposomes or extracellular vesicles into scaffolds (Kang et al., 2021). Bound vesicles serve as an excellent drug delivery vector exerting a controlled and sustained release of bioactive cargo, accelerating bone regeneration at the local defect site. One of the advantages of using liposomes or extracellular vesicles is that their surface can be functionalized to carry specific targeting ligands for cell recruitment or to anchor to a scaffold surface for maintaining a bioactivity of bone-building drugs (Cheng et al., 2020).

Liposomes or extracellular vesicles have been loaded to various types of scaffolds, including β-tricalcium phosphate (β-TCP; Qi et al., 2016; Wu et al., 2019), polycaprolactone (PCL; Yao et al., 2021), polylactic acid (PLA; Gandolfi et al., 2020; Swanson et al., 2020), polyglycolic acid-co-lactic acid (PLGA; Li et al., 2018), and demineralized bone (Xie et al., 2017; Kanwar et al., 2020). To efficiently anchor vesicles to a scaffold surface, biomaterials scientists have introduced molecular moieties or bioactive coatings as an intermediate between vesicles and the scaffold. For example, in a recent study (Lee et al., 2020), bioinspired polymerized dopamine (PDA) coating was applied on the surface of the 3D PLGA scaffold to immobilize vesicles of interest for enhanced cell-scaffold interactions and controlled drug release (Fig 8-3). The vesicles containing purmorphamine drugs were successfully immobilized on the PDA layer by Schiff base formation and Michael-type addition between the PDA and primary amine of the vesicle surface, providing delivery of purmorphamine in a sustained and spatially controlled manner. In a critical-sized mouse calvarial defect model, an average reduction of roughly 50% in the size of the defects was reported after the drug-loaded scaffold was implanted, demonstrating the bone regenerative capability of the liposome-coated scaffold.

Coating scaffolds with extracellular vesicles has received great attention in recent years as a novel cell-free therapy for bone regeneration (Phinney and Pittenger, 2017). Extracellular vesicles carry many constituents of a parent cell, including RNA, lipids, metabolites, and so on. Thus, they are promising as a replacement for ex vivo cultivated cells in bone tissue engineering. Importantly,

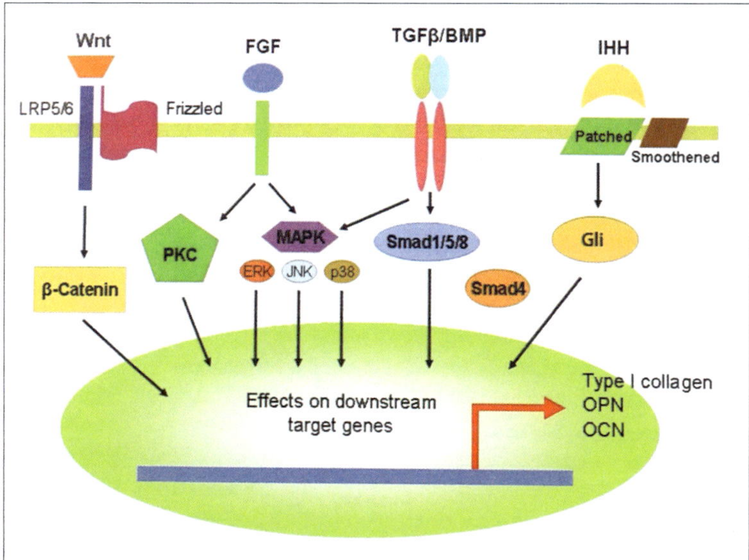

Figure 8-4 Osteoconductive factors and signaling pathways play an important role in regulating osteogenic differentiation. FGF—fibroblast growth factor; TGF-B—transforming growth factor-B; BMP—bone morphogenetic protein; IHH—Indian hedgehog; LRP5/6—low density lipoprotein receptor-related protein 5 and 6; PKC—protein kinase C; MAPK—mitogen-activated protein kinase; ERK—extracellular signal-regulated kinases; JNK—c-Jun N-terminal kinase; OPN—osteopontin; OCN—osteocalcin.

miRNAs encapsulated inside extracellular vesicles have been shown to effectively initiate the signal cascade, exerting an osteoinductive effect on the recipient cells (Zhang et al., 2015). Several studies have demonstrated that extracellular vesicle-loaded scaffolds can stimulate bone regeneration in vivo, ascribed to osteoinductive miRNAs inside extracellular vesicles (Liu et al., 2021a; Fan et al., 2020; Liu et al., 2021b).

Because all materials elicit some level of host inflammatory response, many tissue engineers prefer the use of synthetic degradable polymers that slowly break down into natural metabolites (Chou et al., 2004; Chen et al., 2001; Hollinger and Battistone, 1986; Hollinger et al., 1998). Biodegradable scaffolds have a distinct advantage over nonbiodegradable prosthetic implants, because they allow for bone regeneration, functionality, and eventual elimination of the implant. These biologically compatible and degradable implants allow reproducible and customized therapy that minimizes the duration of foreign body response problems associated with alloplasts (Dupoirieux et al., 1994).

Unfortunately, most degradable materials do not possess the mechanical properties to support weight-bearing tissues, so metal implants or fixation devices are still necessary. The biologic response to these inert materials can be improved by nonmetal coatings (e.g., ceramics) to make them osteoconductive or growth factors (e.g., bone morphogenetic protein 2 [BMP-2]) to make them osteoinductive (Bragdon et al., 2003). Compared to natural extracellular matrix materials, most of the current modifications are rudimentary in terms of biologic interactions and structural organization (Langer and Vacanti, 1993; Geiger et al., 2003; Orban et al., 2002; Parikh, 2002; Ramoshebi et al., 2002; Rose and Oreffo, 2002). Furthermore, long-term adverse effects of foreign materials remain, and over time the materials are susceptible to fatigue, corrosion, stress shielding, and material wear (Slonaker and Goswami, 2004) that can result in bone resorption (Wang et al., 1999). Thus, the ultimate challenge for tissue engineers is to design scaffolding materials that offer the necessary physical, chemical, and biologic properties for the intended implant site.

It is a common misconception that biomaterials must somehow "mimic" all features of native extracellular matrix materials. Some researchers even believe that the ultimate scaffold should recreate the exact in vivo environment. It may be more important, and definitely is more practical, to design scaffolds that exploit the inherent regenerative capability of surrounding tissues by allowing the ingrowth of local progenitor cells to populate and remodel the scaffold. Hence the design rules, and fabrication strategies, of tissue engineering scaffolds can be aimed at producing a microenvironment that induces cells to regenerate the desirable tissues rather than at making materials that resemble the final product. The ability to engineer these scaffolds that promote the development of specific tissues will require better understanding of cell-matrix, cell-cell, and cell-signal interactions in three dimensions.

Growth Factors in Tissue Engineering

Numerous growth factors are employed to control cellular functions and promote natural tissue repair. Growth factors have been tested in attempts to restore salivary gland parenchyma following irradiation and limit the effects of radiation on bone and oral mucous membranes (Lombaert et al., 2008). Tissue engineers have delivered overexpressing cells, gene constructs, proteins, and peptide domains to deliver a plethora of growth factors for tissue regeneration. For instance, BMP, transforming growth factor β (TGF-β), fibroblast growth factor, vascular endothelial growth factor, platelet-derived growth factor, and human growth factor have been studied for bone tissue engineering (Varkey et al., 2004; Fig 8-4).

BMPs are believed to be the most potent among the various osteoinductive factors available (Govender et al., 2002; Kang et al., 2004). The BMP family has at least 15 members (BMP-1 through BMP-15) and belongs to the TGF-β superfamily. They were originally discovered by Urist (1965) in extracts of bovine bone that induced ectopic bone formation subcutaneously in rats. Although first identified because of their ability to induce ectopic bone formation in vivo (Urist, 1965; Hogan, 1996; Wozney and Rosen, 1998; Wozney et al., 1988), BMPs have quickly become known as multifunctional regulators of morphogenesis during embryonic development (Hogan, 1996). In terms of bone formation, BMPs regulate intramembranous as well as endochondral ossification through chemotaxis and mitosis of mesenchymal cells, induction of mesenchymal commitment to osteoblasts or chondrocytes, promotion of further osteoblast or chondrocyte differentiation, and programmed cell death (Reddi, 2001).

BMP-2, BMP-4, BMP-6, BMP-7, and BMP-9 have been deemed the most potent osteogenic BMPs (Hogan, 1996). They stimulate osteogenic differentiation in a variety of cell types including fibroblasts, chondrocytes, osteoprogenitor cells, calvarial cells, periosteal cells, BMSCs, muscle-derived stem cells, and ADAS cells (Lee et al., 2001b; Krebsbach et al., 1998; Dragoo et al., 2003; Hollinger et al., 1998; Lee et al., 2002a; Peng et al., 2002; Boden et al., 1996; Goldstein, 2001; Harland, 1994; Hughes et al., 1995; Mayer et al., 1996; Yamaguchi et al., 1996; Zegzula et al., 1997). Mechanistically, osteogenic BMPs may regulate osteoblast differentiation through increased transcription of Runt-related family 2/core-binding factor 1 (Runx2/Cbfa1)—a molecule deemed essential, but not necessarily sufficient, for osteoblast commitment and differentiation—as well as other modulators in proliferation and differentiation such as Id helix-loop-helix and distal-less homeobox proteins (Enomoto et al., 2000; Gu et al., 2004; Maeda et al., 2004a; Peng et al., 2003; Tou et al., 2003).

BMP-2, in particular, has been extensively studied for its ability to induce many of the events necessary for both intramembranous and endochondral ossification, oftentimes more potently than rhBMP-4 or rhBMP-7 (Urist, 1965). In vitro, BMP-2 (25 to 400 ng/mL) upregulates genes associated with osteogenic differentiation and downregulates genes associated with myogenic differentiation (Peng et al., 2003), as early as the first 24 hours following stimulation (de Jong et al., 2004). Genes upregulated threefold to sixfold include alkaline phosphatase, collagen type I, osteopontin, osteocalcin, *junB*, glial cell–derived neurotrophic factor–inducible transcription factor, latent TGF-β binding protein 2, plasminogen activator inhibitor, and *Runx2/Cbfa1* (Hughes et al., 1995; Peng et al., 2003; Mundy et al., 1995; Rickard et al., 1994; Thies et al., 1992; Wang et al., 1993).

Bone marrow stromal cells display maximal alkaline phosphatase expression when exposed to BMP-2 for at least 14 days, as opposed to only 7 days (Puleo, 1997). BMP-2 also induces bone nodule formation and calcium deposition in BMSC cultures (Hanada et al., 1997). Interestingly, ADAS cells under BMP-2 stimulation produce more bone precursor cells than either osteoblasts or BMSC cultures under the same conditions (De Ugarte et al., 2003), and rhBMP-2 accelerates ADAS cell–mediated bone formation in vivo (Cowan et al., 2005).

However, BMPs are highly pleiotropic molecules exhibiting high functional heterogeneity during growth and development of numerous tissues (Wang et al., 1993; Ducy and Karsenty, 2000). From a clinical perspective, the functional heterogeneity and administration of milligram doses of BMPs may limit their use because of the possibility of unwanted bone formation and other unpredictable side effects and because of cost considerations. Runx2/Cbfa1 is essential for osteoblast formation and function. BMPs are known to upregulate *Runx2/Cbfa1* expression (Komori et al., 1997; Lee et al., 2002; Nakashima and de Crombrugghe, 2003; Yamaguchi et al., 2000), resulting in the induction of osteogenic differentiation of both osseous and nonosseous mesenchymal cells (Ahrens et al., 1993; Katagiri et al., 1994). Therefore, there is a need to identify crucial soluble downstream mediators of Runx2/Cbfa1 for protein-based therapies.

Another protein, Nel-like molecule 1 (Nell-1; Nel [a protein strongly expressed in *n*eural tissue, encoding *e*pidermal growth factor *l*ike domain]), has been investigated for its ability to stimulate osteogenic differentiation and its potential to regenerate bone in vivo (Ting et al., 1999; Zhang et al., 2002). Nell-1 is thought to specifically target cells of the osteogenic lineage, thus reducing the possibility of adverse side effects in other tissues targeted by BMPs. Nell-1 is highly expressed within active bone-forming sites of patients with human craniosynostosis (Ting et al., 1999). Nell-1 is a secretory molecule containing a signal peptide sequence, an NH_2-terminal thrombospondin–like module that may bind heparin and anchor Nell-1 to the extracellular matrix, five von Willebrand factor C domains that may be involved in homotrimeric oligomerization, and six epidermal growth factor–like domains that can bind calcium (Kuroda et al., 1999; Kuroda and Tanizawa, 1999).

Transgenic mice overexpressing *Nell-1* demonstrate calvarial overgrowth and premature suture closure (Zhang et al., 1999). Conversely, a mouse model with mutated *N*-ethyl-*N*-nitrosourea–induced alleles, including *Nell-1*, resulted in cranial and other vertebral skeletal defects (Desai et al., 2006). Furthermore, the *Nell-1* gene is directly regulated by Runx2/Cbfa1, which is essential for osteoblast differentiation, further suggesting its osteogenic specificity (Truong et al., 2007). Taken together, the evidence suggests that Nell-1 has a distinct and specialized role in bone formation.

Moreover, because Nell-1 is a secreted protein that can be delivered extracellularly, controlled delivery systems can be used to maximize biologic efficiency. Indeed, delivery of recombinant Nell-1 protein in preformed polyglycolide-lactide scaffolds has been shown to accelerate osteogenic differentiation in vitro and calvarial bone formation in vivo (Aghaloo et al., 2006). The osteogenic potential of Nell-1 to induce in vivo calvarial regeneration was equivalent to that of BMP-2.

Nell-1 is highly conserved across species. Human and rat Nell-1 share a 93% homology in predicted amino acids. Nell-1 contains several highly conserved motifs, including a secretory signal peptide (black box), NH_2-terminal TSP-1–like module, von Willebrand factor C domains, epidermal growth factor–like domains, and Ca^{2+}-binding–like domains (Kuroda and Tanizawa, 1999).

Growth factor delivery

Ideally, pharmacokinetics analyses facilitate understanding of how factors are released, absorbed, stored, and metabolized in the body. An understanding of these processes allows researchers to better predict signaling effects and improve the outcomes of treatments. BMPs are water-soluble, relatively low–molecular weight molecules that diffuse easily in body fluids. As expected, the concentration of rhBMP-2 greatly affects cellular processes; femtomolar concentrations are optimal for chemotaxis, nanomolar concentrations support mesenchymal cell proliferation, and micromolar concentrations promote bone differentiation (Reddi, 1981; Reddi, 1994). This profile would predict that an effective tissue engineering strategy for bone defects would be to administer lower rhBMP-2 concentrations initially and to increase the concentrations over time.

Despite the availability of rhBMPs (Wozney et al., 1988), their use clinically has been hampered by the lack of detailed pharmacokinetics analyses of various delivery systems. Although BMPs are extremely osteoinductive molecules, their release into the microenvironment must be regulated for optimal bone formation. Thus, the challenge still remains to determine the optimal mix of BMPs, dosage, release dynamics, and matrix carrier that will result in a clinically therapeutic treatment without utilization of superphysiologic doses (Rose and Oreffo, 2002).

In addition to the influence of rhBMP-2, the structural features of biomaterials have also been shown to influence rhBMP-2 pharmacokinetics. Delivery systems evaluated in animal models include hydroxyapatite (HA; Levine et al., 1997), collagen (Yasko et al., 1992), polylactic acid (PLA; Woo et al., 2001), poly(glycolic acid-*co*-lactic acid; PLGA; Woo et al., 2001), and demineralized bone (Schwartz et al., 1998). Binding and interactions between BMPs and carriers play important roles and may contribute to the sustainability of the growth factor. Further understanding of BMP-2–scaffold interactions will aid the progression of research in this field.

Clinically, absorbable collagen sponges (ACSs) have a long-standing safety record as hemostatic agents and wound coverings (Geiger et al., 2003; Chvapil, 1977). Collagen is known to promote cellular invasion and wound healing, exhibit excellent biocompatibility, degrade into nontoxic end products, and exert favorable interaction with cells and factors. ACSs have repeatedly been observed to be an effective carrier for rhBMPs, independent of the site of implantation (Winn et al., 2000). Bovine type I collagen has been used almost exclusively in clinical settings, because it binds BMPs very well.

ACSs have displayed differential binding affinity to BMP-2 and BMP-7. This difference is best illustrated by the US Food and Drug Administration (FDA) requirement that BMP-2 be used in conjunction with a metal cage to prevent load-induced displacement of BMP-2 from the intended space of the ACS (Rengachary, 2002). Generally, cages are not required for BMP-7 delivery, because the binding affinity of ACSs to BMP-7 is significantly stronger and can apparently resist the loss of BMP during similar loads (as will be discussed in the next section).

The release of rhBMP-2 or other growth factors from ACS requires knowledge of protein-collagen interactions, loading, efficacy, and pharmacokinetics. Slower rhBMP-2 release dictates a greater osteoinductive activity (Zhang et al., 2010). Current rhBMP-2 release kinetics from various materials follow a biphasic release profile, in which an early, rapid loss of rhBMP-2 (half-life of 10 minutes to several hours) is followed by a more gradual loss of rhBMP-2 with a half-life of 1 to 10 days (Uludag et al., 1999a; Winn et al., 1999). Thus, the ideal rhBMP-2 concentrations would be released at a rate opposite to what has been demonstrated and be present for prolonged periods of time.

The release rates of rhBMP-2 vary greatly among materials; after 3 hours, ACS retains 59% to 74%, demineralized bone matrix retains 30% to 50%, and HA retains 11% (Uludag et al., 1999a). Experimentally, it is not possible to completely rule out the importance of the initial burst, but the local sustained concentration of rhBMP-2 seems more critical for overall osteoinductive activity in a dose-dependent manner (Hollinger et al., 1998; Kenley et al., 1993). These results suggest that the osteopotency of bone regeneration devices can be improved by using engineered BMPs with superior affinity to scaffold surfaces.

The isoelectric points (pIs) of scaffolds and growth factors are significant determinants of binding and release characteristics (Uludag et al., 1999b). Depending on the manufacturing process, collagen exhibits a pI in the neutral or slightly acidic pH range, whereas rhBMP-2 has a pI of approximately 9. Thus, at a physiologic pH, collagen and rhBMP-2 have opposite charges and yield the greatest binding (0.1 to 0.2 mg of rhBMP-2 per 1.0 mg of collagen; Friess et al., 1999). Thus, electrostatic attractive forces between rhBMP-2 and collagen are believed to be major factors controlling the protein-matrix interactions. On submersion, a collagen scaffold will typically absorb about 90% of a 1.5 mg/mL rhBMP-2 solution at 37°C (Uludag et al., 1999b). Within PLGA microspheres, growth factors can become encapsulated; however, the acidic microclimate is a source of protein instability that can be overcome by using water-soluble basic salts to neutralize the pH of the polymer microclimate (Zhu et al., 2000).

Various techniques can be utilized to enhance rhBMP-2 binding to bone minerals, such as application of heparin conjugates (Gittens et al., 2004). Heparin binds growth factors via electrostatic interactions between its negatively charged sulfate groups and the protein's positively charged amino acid residues. Heparin also increases the stability of the growth factor (that is, biologic half-life). Unlike collagenous carriers, mineral-based carriers appear to bind a fraction of rhBMP-2 (typically 5% to 10% of the implanted dose) irreversibly—that is, without release (Gittens et al., 2004). The biologic consequence of the tightly bound BMP fraction is currently not known.

Additional strategies manipulate scaffold ingredients to finesse the BMP-binding capacity. For example, the addition of glucose to collagen minipellets alters the rate of rhBMP-2 release as desired (Maeda et al., 2004b). Gelatin hydrogels released rhBMP-2 in vivo with a release profile that could be changed by altering the water content of the BMP-2–incorporated hydrogels (Yamamoto et al., 2003).

Other scaffold alterations have attempted to improve and sustain rhBMP-2 release without success. Succinylated collagen sponges have negatively charged residues on their surface to aid in binding to rhBMP-2 and to decrease release rate; unfortunately, these sponges did not alter the rhBMP-2 release profile (Friess et al., 1997). In addition, cross-linking of collagen led to reduced rhBMP-2 incorporation through physical hindrance and a reduction of the collagen's ability to swell on soaking (Uludag et al., 1999b; Friess et al., 1999; Uludag et al., 2001). The rhBMP-2 on cross-linked collagen scaffolds exhibited low initial retention (47.8%) compared to that on non–cross-linked collagen scaffolds (87.1%). Additionally, rhBMP-2 exhibited a biexponential release pattern with $t_{1/2a}$ at 10 minutes followed by $t_{1/2b}$ at 89 and 51 hours for cross-linked and non–cross-linked collagen scaffolds, respectively.

Interestingly, plasmin-cleaved rhBMP-2 resulted in a truncated form and a corresponding pI shift from 9.0 to 6.5 (Uludag et al., 2000). The active site of BMPs, within the cystine knot, was unaffected by the cleavage (Kirsch et al., 2000). This resulted in an increased release rate where 63% of the dose was eliminated in 4.2 days rather than 4.3 days, as it was for uncleaved rhBMP-2.

Because of the importance of controlling protein-material binding interactions, certain materials (e.g., ceramics) with high binding affinity for proteins may not be the optimal carriers. In fact, calcium phosphate composite was found to be a suboptimal carrier (Ruhe et al., 2003). Released rhBMP-2 binds to calcium phosphate cement, delaying release of rhBMP-2 from the composite. Thus, the nanoporosity of the calcium phosphate cement not only did not facilitate the release of rhBMP-2 but also may have further limited it because of the protein adsorption on the ceramic.

Hyaluronic acid scaffolds have been used as delivery vehicles for bioactive rhBMP-2 in bone repair therapies (Hunt et al., 2001; Kim and Valentini, 2002). Hyaluronic acid is a natural polyanionic polysaccharide with structural roles in organizing the cartilage extracellular matrix, cellular motility, and wound healing (Laurent and Fraser, 1992). Hyaluronic acids can be modified to reduce solubility and prolong in vivo half-life. The addition of functional amine groups allows for coupling under physiologic conditions (Prestwich et al., 2008).

Local delivery of rhBMP-2 is achieved through physical or chemical incorporation into the porous hyaluronic acid hydrogels, yielding sustained release (Bulpitt and Aeschlimann, 1999). Interestingly, the presence of collagen was required for the bioactivity of rhBMP-2. Hyaluronic acid hydrogels released low levels of rhBMP-2 in a sustained manner (one-third of initially loaded rhBMP-2 over 28 days) and stimulated pluripotent stem cell differentiation into the osteoblast lineage in vitro and bone formation in vivo (Ruhe et al., 2003).

The need for reliable and clinically relevant delivery vehicles for BMPs has initiated a surge of research investigating the biochemistry of both BMPs and scaffolds. The clinical success of current BMP therapies will undoubtedly motivate further research to elucidate the ideal binding strategy. The success thus far has been sufficient for the transition to clinical trials and promises great success in the near future, when scaffold-BMP interactions are better understood.

FDA-cleared growth factors

Several clinical studies of rhBMP-2 and rhBMP-7 applications have been performed—maxillary sinus floor augmentation (Boyne et al., 1997), alveolar ridge preservation (Howell et al., 1997), fibular defect rehabilitation (Geesink et al., 1999), and spinal fusion (Boden et al., 2002) and superphysiologic doses of rhBMP-2 and rhBMP-7 were needed to induce an effect in each case. Although BMP-2 and BMP-7 seem to be excellent choices for bone tissue engineering stimulation, the transition from an animal model to humans has been only mildly successful. Advances in delivery systems should greatly improve clinical outcomes and eventually allow the development of off-the-shelf devices for clinical application in osseous repair.

Currently, two devices have been cleared by the US FDA for clinical orthopedic applications, one using rhBMP-7 (also called *recombinant human osteogenic protein 1*; Osigraft, withdrawn from the market) and another using rhBMP-2 (Infuse Bone Graft and LT-Cage Lumbar Tapered Fusion Device, Medtronic Sofamor Danek). Osigraft has been approved for the treatment of nonunion tibial fracture of at least 9 months' duration, secondary to trauma, in skeletally mature patients (European Medicines Agency. Osigraft: EPAR–ScientificDiscussion. http://www.eme.europa.eu/docs/en_GB/document_library/EPAR_Scientific_Discussion/human/000293/WC500050378.pdf. Accessed 15 Feb 2011). This device is to be used when previous treatment with autograft has failed or the use of autograft is unfeasible.

Osigraft combines the active ingredient, rhBMP-7, with a bovine type I collagen matrix for in vivo bone formation. Preliminarily studies in rats and nonhuman primates demonstrated that 25% of rhBMP-7 was released within 3 hours Preclinical subcutaneous implantation studies in rats demonstrated that within 24 hours only 20% to 25% of the rhBMP-7 remained in the product and only 6% remained after 6 days; there was no substantial or prolonged tissue or organ uptake Long-term (28-day) toxicology studies in rats injected with rhBMP-7, in doses of 0.035, 0.35, and 3.5 mg/kg/day (0.23 to 23 times that used in humans), demonstrated dose-dependent localized effects, including reduced ovary weight, reduced thymus weight, and increased adrenal weight without changes in the kidney (European Medicines Agency. Osigraft: EPAR–Scientific Discussion. http://www.eme.europa.eu/docs/en_GB/document_library/EPAR_-_Scientific_Discussion/human/000293/WC500050378.pdf. Accessed 15 Feb 2011). The main finding was inflammation, ossification, and necrosis at the injection site but not in other tissues.

The Infuse/LT-Cage device is approved for spinal fusion procedures in skeletally mature patients with degenerative disc disease at one level from L4 to S1 For this device, rhBMP-2 is soaked on an absorbable collagen sponge and placed within a metal device before implantation. Preclinical studies in the rat and the dog demonstrated no related toxicities as well as an absence of remote site bone formation with suprapharmacologic doses. Injected rhBMP-2 cleared rapidly from systemic circulation and none remained after 2 hours. Subcutaneous implantation of Infuse on the ACS resulted in a slow release from the implant; there was a mean residence time of 8 days, and only 0.1% of the implanted dose was found within the blood. Nonhuman primates and humans required doses ranging from 0.4 to 1.5 mg/mL of rhBMP-2, and increasing doses and increasing length of time at the implant site resulted in more bone formation (US Food and Drug Administration. Medical Device Approvals and Clearances: InFUSE Bone Graft/LT-CAGE Lumbar Tapered Fusion Device. http://www.accessdata.fda.gov/cdrh_docs/pdf/P000058b.pdf. Accessed 15 Feb 2011).

Because such high doses of BMP-2 and BMP-7 are necessary for significant bone formation clinically, a variety of concerns have arisen. First, the promotion of uncontrolled bone growth around the implantation site or even cancer would make them unsafe for patients with a history of cancer. This concern is legitimate based on reports linking osteosarcomas with BMP activity (Ravel et al., 1996; Yoshikawa et al., 1994); however, no evidence supports the idea that BMPs play a role as an oncogenic factor. Instead, BMPs play a greater role in recruitment and differentiation than in promoting malignancy. At times, BMP-2 has also been shown to elicit undesirable heterotopic bone formation away from sites of administration (Valentin-Opran et al., 2002).

Second, although the BMPs are extremely conserved, the possibility of a large immune-autoimmune reaction is still questionable. Both Infuse Bone Graft/LT-Cage Lumbar Tapered Fusion Device and Osigraft may initiate a positive antibody response to rhBMP-2 and rhBMP-7, respectively, as well as bovine type I collagen carriers. Some animal models have reported increased blood pressure and even heart attacks. However, this is a rare occurrence and may apply to other growth factors (European Medicines Agency. Osigraft: EPARScientificDiscussion. http://www.eme.europa.eu/docs/en_GB/document_library/EPAR_Scientific_Discussion/human/000293/WC500050378.pdf. Accessed 15 Feb 2011; US Food and Drug Administration. Medical Device Approvals and Clearances: InFUSE Bone Graft/LT-CAGE Lumbar Tapered Fusion Device. http://www.accessdata.fda.gov/cdrh_docs/pdf/P000058b.pdf. Accessed 15 Feb 2011).

Several factors have led to the need for superphysiologic doses of BMPs. Cytokines produced ex vivo typically lack glycosylation and binding proteins, which may result in errors in protein assembly or a loss of functional activity. In addition, delivery of growth factors is insufficient because of the limited knowledge of BMP-scaffold interactions (Centrella et al., 1994; Cook et al., 1994). Viral delivery can generate large quantities of BMPs; however, in vivo complications have hampered the use of viruses (Lee et al., 2001; Peng et al., 2002; Gundle et al., 1995). Moreover, suboptimal BMP protein-peptide binding and immobilization have challenged the ability to deliver substantial quantities; this limitation is magnified because recombinant cytokines are quickly turned over (in approximately 30 minutes; Giannobile et al., 1996) in the harsh environment of a fracture site undergoing repair and may be degraded before cells are stimulated by them (Urist, 1965; Ham, 1930).

Each of these factors further limits the potential success of the clinical therapies available thus far. Future studies will need to elucidate whether BMPs are required throughout the bone regeneration process and the optimal doses necessary for each indication.

Tissue Engineering of Selected Maxillofacial Tissues

Defects in the oral and maxillofacial region often involve the loss of many tissues that perform multiple functions. Tissue engineering represents a paradigm shift away from restoration with synthetic materials toward bioengineering approaches that incorporate stem cells, biomaterials, growth signals, nanotechnology, and bioinformatics (Bayne, 2005, Moioli et al., 2007). The complexity of controlling the regeneration of multiple tissue phenotypes, such as bone, cartilage, tendons, muscles, nerves, salivary glands, and blood vessels, presents special challenges for tissue engineers. This section provides a status update on the incredible accomplishments to date and discusses the considerable gaps that remain in the engineering of bone, cartilage, tongue and skeletal muscle, motor neurons, skin, and oral mucosa. The selected examples do not provide an exhaustive account of all work in each area and do not cover all tissue types that have been regenerated, but they will provide a general sense of the considerable progress in this field.

Bone

Loss of bone structure to bone tumor, trauma, reconstructive surgery, and degenerative disorders remains a significant health problem that impairs patients' quality of life. Current therapeutic options to reconstruct maxillofacial bone consist of synthetic biomaterials and biologic substitutes such as autograft or allograft (Artico et al., 2003; Chen et al., 2002). Fibular transplantation has produced satisfactory long-term outcomes, but the use of bone graft is limited by donor site morbidity, the risk of complication, the resorption of transplanted bone, and the inadequate availability of donor bone for large bone defects. Distraction osteogenesis is another option (Takahashi et al., 2002).

Regeneration via bone grafting is the most frequently used approach for skeletal rehabilitation of bone defects. Autologous bone graft harvested from the iliac crest has been considered the gold standard for bone graft material (see Chapter 2; Canady et al., 1993; Ozaki et al., 1999; Strong et al., 2000). Unfortunately, autografts for craniofacial defects have an unacceptably high failure rate (13% to 30%; Gregory, 1972), and allografts have an even higher failure rate (20% to 35%; Enneking and Mindell, 1991). The availability of donor sites is limited, and harvesting contributes to increased surgical time and hospital stay as well as other complications such as donor site morbidity, pain, infection, pelvic fracture, and wound breakdown. In addition, variations in the osteogenic potential of the graft material make autografts less than ideal (Kline and Wolfe, 1995; Kurz et al., 1989; Laurie et al., 1984; Wolfe, 1996). Prosthetic materials avoid some of these issues, but their effectiveness is limited by unpredictable graft resorption, infection, structural failure, and unsatisfactory aesthetic outcomes (Bostrom and Mikos, 1997; Warren et al., 2003; Mulliken and Glowacki, 1980). Various osteoinductive growth factor–based therapies have been developed in an attempt to provide more effective and safe methods of bone regeneration.

A variety of synthetic bone replacements have been studied to address the shortcomings of existing strategies. Synthetic biomaterials used for reconstruction include titanium (Heissler et al., 1998; Koppel et al., 1999), polymethyl methacrylate (Blum et al., 1997), and HA (Bonucci et al., 1997; Moreira-Gonzalez et al., 2003). These materials are readily available in large amounts and have several advantages over bone graft, such as avoidance of donor site morbidity and shortening of the operation. However, the use of these synthetic biomaterials has been limited because of high infection rates associated with the lack of blood supply (Vasilev et al., 2009).

Among the various osteoinductive factors available, BMPs are believed to be the most potent; they have been studied extensively for the treatment of many bone fractures and bone defects (Govender et al., 2002; Kang et al., 2004). However, BMPs are highly pleiotropic molecules exhibiting high functional heterogeneity during the growth and development of numerous tissues (Komori et al., 1997; Wang et al., 2003). The functional heterogeneity of the BMPs and nonspecificity for osteoblasts may explain in part the clinically documented side effects, including unwanted bone formation, native bone resorption, implant fracture, soft tissue swelling, osseous overgrowth, and other complications in areas away from the implant site (e.g., antibody formation; van den Bergh et al., 2000). Furthermore, the use of collagen sponges as carriers may contribute toward the need for supraphysiologic, milligram-level doses of BMP formulations. Hence, there is a need to develop alternative osteoinductive growth factors and delivery strategies to provide an efficient, safe, and desirable bone-specific effect.

Nell-1 is a novel osteogenic protein believed to specifically target cells committed to the osteogenic lineage. Nell-1 has three Runx2/Cbfa1 binding sites (osteoblast-specific cis-acting element 2) within its promoter. This suggests that Nell-1 acts as a critical downstream mediator of Runx2/Cbfa1 in regulating osteogenic differentiation. Previous in vitro and in vivo data confirm that Nell-1, unlike BMPs, acts specifically on further differentiated osteogenic lineage cells (Truong et al., 2007).

Although very small quantities of Nell-1 are required for osteoinduction, high doses of Nell-1 are necessary in direct therapeutic application. This is due to a short half-life and rapid degradation of the proteins once they are secreted. Technologies that deliver Nell-1 to skeletal defects may accelerate bone regeneration in a timely manner. Collagen is a popular delivery material because it is a major component of the extracellular matrix known to be a reservoir of endogenous growth factors (Lee et al., 2001). The use of collagen to immobilize and release growth factors has been previously employed.

A preliminary study in a rat calvarial defect model demonstrated the potent ability of Nell-1 to regenerate bone (Aghaloo et al., 2006). Subcritical-sized (3 mm) calvarial defects were grafted with collagen-coated PLGA scaffolds enhanced with recombinant rat Nell-1 or rhBMP-2 for a side-by-side comparison of their regenerative abilities. Four weeks after implantation, both Nell-1–enhanced scaffolds (97% healing) and BMP-2–enhanced scaffolds (93% healing) had almost completely healed all defects, whereas control scaffolds (53% healing) had only minimally healed the defects.

Although new bone regenerated by Nell-1 appears woven during early stages, the bone matures and bone marrow pockets are apparent. The pattern of new bone formation indicates a protective healing strategy geared toward coverage of the brain before total volume regeneration (Aghaloo et al., 2006). Most interestingly, Nell-1 induces levels of bone regeneration equivalent to those achieved with BMP-2, one of the most potent known inducers of bone formation (Andriano et al., 2000; Gysin et al., 2002). Nell-1 delivery has been shown to regenerate bone during spinal fusion of the posterolateral lumbar spine in rodents (Lu et al., 2007).

Although gene therapy can provide essential osteoinductive factors, the current status of gene therapy limits actual clinical application. Human application is impractical because of the issues related to virus safety and immunogenicity. Ting group developed a novel growth factor delivery system consisting of polysaccharide-based microparticles and a biomimetic apatite layer on its surface for use as an injectable bone substitute (Lee et al., 2009). Polysaccharides, such as the chitosan and alginate used in the study, are naturally derived polymers. They are cost-effective, biodegradable, and biocompatible. Additionally, they can be easily manipulated into various forms such as beads, microparticles, nanoparticles, and gels under mild conditions (Di Martino et al., 2005; Dodane and Vilivalam, 1998; Rajaonarivony et al., 1993; Tønnesen and Karlsen, 2002).

Nell-1 was incorporated in a moldable putty carrier that can adapt to bony defects to deliver Nell-1 to the local microenvironment (Lee et al., 2009). Moldability was achieved by mixing hyaluronan hydrogel with two types of particles: *(1)* demineralized bone powder for osteoconductivity and *(2)* biomimetic apatite–coated alginate-chitosan microparticles for controlled Nell-1 delivery. Besides enhancing overall osteoconductivity of the carrier, the biomimetic apatite coating also provided a more sustained release (approximately 15% cumulative release over 30 days) and greatly reduced the initial burst release that was observed with noncoated alginate-chitosan microparticles (approximately 40% release after 1 day). The implantation of the microparticles loaded with Nell-1 enhanced spinal fusion rates in rats as detected by manual palpation, radiographs, high-resolution micro–computed tomography, and histology (Lee et al., 2009). This putty formulation for local Nell-1 delivery represents a practical approach to future clinical product development of safe and effective orthobiologic formulations. Progress in this field will benefit from more predictive in vivo models. There are many cases where the damage is too severe or the local environment is suboptimal for adequate self-healing. These nonhealing defects are termed *critical-sized defects* (CSDs); unfortunately, they have been poorly defined. Technically, CSDs are defects that will not heal during the lifetime of the animal, although experimentally a 12-week healing period is acceptable. This definition can be expanded to presume that a defect in which only 50% of the defect area is healed within a 12-week period is a CSD. A review of the literature suggests that models investigating CSD healing observe about 10% healing in control defects during the study period and through at least 12 weeks (Chang et al., 2003; Kruyt et al., 2004; Petite et al., 2000; Shang et al., 2001; Abu-Serriah et al., 2003; Cook et al., 1995; den Boer et al., 2003; Gerhart et al., 1993; Hollinger and Kleinschmidt, 1990; Miki et al., 2000; Schlegel et al., 2004; Warnke et al., 2004). CSDs are age dependent, because infants and juvenile animals can regenerate bone in large skeletal defects deemed critical sized in adults (Aalami et al., 2004).

A recent study demonstrated the feasibility of Nell-1 to improve the clinical safety and efficacy of BMP-2 for bone regeneration (Shen et al., 2016). In a rodent femoral defect model, Nell-1 combined with BMP-2 has been shown to significantly improve bone formation quality by minimizing BMP-2-induced fat-filled cystic bone formation. In vitro studies confirmed that Nell-1 enhances osteogenic differentiation of bone marrow stromal cells induced by BMP-2 at the expense of adipogenesis. The ability of Nell-1 to shift the fate of cells treated with BMP-2 toward osteogenesis was dependent on the canonical Wnt signaling pathway, a major signal transduction pathway regulating mesenchymal stem cell differentiation during bone development and homeostasis. Another study showed that exogenous Nell-1 is able to accelerate BMP-9-induced late-stage osteogenic differentiation while inhibiting BMP-9-upregulated expression of adipogenic regulators/markers in BMSCs (Wang et al., 2017). Interestingly, the overexpression of Nell-1 alone did not lead to any significant osteogenic differentiation in the immortalized mouse embryonic fibroblasts unlike its synergistic osteogenic activity observed in the BMP-9-induced late-stage BMSCs. Such different Nell-1 responsiveness suggests that Nell-1 may be able to potentiate osteogenic activity on the committed or more differentiated pre-osteoblasts but exert a weak influence on cells in higher stemness hierarchy. The combination treatment of Nell-1 with BMP-2/BMP-9 suggests new therapies for improved bone regeneration and the prevention of osteoporotic bone loss through recovering the proper balance between osteogenesis and adipogenesis.

In addition to the local bone regeneration potential of Nell-1, a systemic delivery of Nell-1 for osteoporosis treatment has been investigated in a mouse radial defect model (Tanjaya et al., 2018). Nell-1 was engineered with a Food and Drug Administration–approved polyethylene glycol (PEG) to prolong its short circulation time. PEGylation improved the half-life of Nell-1 threefold without causing considerable toxicity (Kwak et al., 2015). Nell-PEG delivered via systemic administration successfully enhanced bone regeneration and remodeling processes at the fracture site, suggesting its therapeutic potential in the prevention and treatment of fractures.

Cartilage

The temporomandibular joint (TMJ) complex consists of two hyaline cartilage–covered bones that are cushioned by an avascular articular disc and surrounded by a fluid-filled capsule. Arthritis, avascular necrosis, trauma, and bony ankylosis of the TMJ can damage multiple tissues. When autogenous tissue grafts are used to replace only the disc, the clinical success rate is extremely low (8% to 31% over four years; Wolford, 1997). Wear particles from synthetic discs have resulted in extensive foreign body reactions and damage.

The current treatment of choice for advanced TMJ pathosis is total joint replacement with synthetic orthopedic materials. These are susceptible to material wear, component loosening, fatigue failure, and stress shielding.

Tissue engineering of the TMJ complex involves regeneration of multiple tissues, including bone, cartilage, ligaments, muscles, and capsular membrane.

Unfortunately, cartilage has a poor regenerative capacity because of the avascularity and lack of repair cells in this tissue. Spontaneously healed cartilage sometimes undergoes degeneration a few months after repair (Iannone and Lapadula, 2008; Lapadula et al., 1998). Current therapies include chondral shaving, subchondral drilling, microfracturing, mosaicplasty, and prosthetic replacement (Hangody et al., 2001; Martinek and Imhoff, 2003; Spahn et al., 2008). However, these treatments are associated with problems, including an inadequate number of donor organs, donor site morbidity, and limited durability of prosthetics (Jerosch et al., 2000).

Cartilage tissue engineering may offer an alternative treatment approach (Martin et al., 2007; Temenoff et al., 2000). In particular, engineering of osteochondral tissue, simultaneous regeneration of articular cartilage and underlying subchondral bone, can facilitate fixation and integration with the host tissue. A variety of scaffolds for osteochondral tissue regeneration have been developed to meet the complex functional demands of cartilage and bone tissues that have distinctively different structural, chemical, and mechanical properties. One strategy is to engineer two individual cartilage and bone scaffold layers and join the two separately fabricated scaffolds together by suturing, gluing, press fitting, or stabilizing with biodegradable external fixation devices (Brittberg et al., 1997; Kreklau et al., 1999; Schaefer et al., 2002; Shao et al., 2006). However, these methods are limited by the inferior integration between cartilage and bone tissues, which eventually results in separation of the two tissues.

Other studies have reported bilayered scaffolds for engineering cartilage and bone tissue simultaneously on a single integrated construct. These biphasic structures show evidence of integrated cartilage and bone tissues without requiring an additional joining process. Holland et al. (2005) utilized a bilayered scaffold based on the polymer oligo(poly(ethylene glycol) fumarate; OPF). A bilayered scaffold consisted of OPF for the bone layer and OPF/TGF-β loaded gelatin microparticles to promote formation of a cartilage layer. Hyaline cartilage was observed in the chondral region, and the underlying subchondral bone formation completely integrated with the surrounding bone after 14 weeks of implantation.

In another study, Chen et al. (2006) developed a biphasic scaffold from biodegradable synthetic and naturally derived polymers. The upper layer of the scaffold was a collagen sponge to promote cartilage regeneration, while the lower layer of collagen-PLGA was intended to promote bone formation. The PLGA sponge provided mechanical support in the bone layer. The collagen in the PLGA sponge promoted cellular attachment and proliferation and connected the two layers. Although the use of a biphasic scaffold appears to facilitate osteochondral tissue regeneration, an additional design strategy to simulate the biophysical properties of the native cartilage and promote optimized tissue regeneration may be required for successful osteochondral defect regeneration.

Various growth factors and cytokines, such as insulin-like growth factor and members of the TGF-β family, have been employed to induce and maintain expression of type II collagen and aggrecan, or large aggregating proteoglycan, in cartilage (Davies et al., 2008; Joyce et al., 1990; Morales et al., 1991). In particular, BMPs, a subgroup of the TGF-β family, were originally discovered in demineralized bone matrix and were shown to induce ectopic endochondral bone formation in subcutaneous and intramuscular pockets (Hogan, 1996; Celeste et al., 1990). BMPs have also been shown to play important roles in chondrogenesis and to induce chondrocyte differentiation in vitro (Chubinskaya and Kuittner, 2003; Gründer et al., 2004; Yang et al., 2006).

However, BMPs are highly pleiotropic molecules exhibiting high functional heterogeneity during the growth and development of numerous tissues (Ducy and Karsenty, 2000; Moreira-Gonzalez, 2003; Zhao et al., 2003). Specifically, BMPs are reported to signal upstream of Runx2/Cbfa1, a transcription factor essential for differentiation of osteoblasts and hypertrophic chondrocytes (Lee et al., 2002; Yamaguchi et al., 2000; Ahrens et al., 1993), so their effects are not limited to cells in the osteochondral lineage. The nonspecificity of BMPs may limit their therapeutic applications because prolonged exposure can cause unpredictable side effects. In murine models, injection of high doses of BMP-2 into articular cartilage increased cartilage formation but also induced osteophyte formation (van Beuningen et al., 1998; Yeh et al., 2007). Because of the potential for adverse side effects, such as bone formation on the synovial or disk surface, BMPs may not be an optimal growth factor for cartilage repair.

It has also been shown that the introduction of chondrogenic growth factors such as TGF-β induced the intrinsic repair of articular cartilage without the need for cell or tissue transplantation (Pittenger et al., 1999; Blaney et al., 2007). However, there is a high potential for the upgrowth of bone tissue into the cartilage layer, which is undesirable for appropriate cartilage growth. Thus, the interface between the cartilage and bone scaffolding layers must be able to prevent blood vessels and perivascular cells from penetrating the cartilage layer. Blood vessel– and cell-excluding membranes may be helpful to prevent osseous upgrowth into the cartilage layer (Hunziker et al., 2001).

From the perspective of clinical safety, a more specific growth factor that induces cartilage formation with fewer side effects may be advantageous. An *N*-ethyl-*N*-nitrosourea–induced *Nell-1* mutant mouse exhibited vertebral defects with a compressed intervertebral space and altered cervical spine curvature, suggesting a distinct role for Nell-1 in the development of disc fibrocartilage (Desai et al., 2006). Our team has shown that Nell-1 accelerates chondrocyte hypertrophy and endochondral bone formation in the intermaxillary suture of a rat after rapid suture expansion, indicating that Nell-1 can influence chondrogenic differentiation in adult tissues (Cowan et al., 2006).

The stimulatory effects of Nell-1 on chondrocyte differentiation were investigated in 3D alginate hydrogels that contained chitosan-based microparticles (Lee et al., 2010). These microparticles served as local carriers of growth factors within hydrogels to achieve sustained delivery of Nell-1. Tripolyphosphate, a nontoxic multivalent anionic, and chondroitin sulfate, one of the major glycosaminoglycans found in cartilage, were used as a chitosan cross-linker. Over 42 days of culture, chondrocyte proliferation and cluster formation were significantly enhanced by Nell-1 in a dose-dependent manner, demonstrating the ability of Nell-1 to promote chondrocyte proliferation and deposition of cartilage-specific extracellular matrix materials. Future development of injectable formulations of Nell-1 will further enhance the therapeutic potential for the treatment of osteochondral defects.

Further investigation of Nell-1 as the treatment of osteochondral defects has been carried out in *in vivo* cartilage defect models. Siu et al. (2012) utilized a single-site cartilage defect model where circular 3-mm-sized osteochondral defects were created in the femoral condylar cartilage of rabbits. The implants (3D alginate hydrogels containing Nell-1-incorporated chitosan nanoparticles) were press fit into the defects to evaluate the ability of Nell-1 to promote articular cartilage regeneration in vivo. Nell-1-treated osteochondral defects showed remarkable regeneration of cartilage tissues, resembling the high quality of native cartilage as evidenced by histology and immunohistochemistry. The role of Nell-1 in arthritis pathogenesis was demonstrated in a separate study using a loss-of-function *Nell-1*-haploinsufficient (*Nell-1*$^{+/6R}$) mouse model (Li et al., 2020) The absence of Nell-1 caused accelerated and aggravated osteoarthritis (OA) progression with elevated inflammatory markers, implying an anti-inflammatory role of Nell-1. Intra-articular injection of interleukin (IL) 1β promoted more severe inflammation and cartilage degradation in the knee joints of *Nell-1*$^{+/6R}$ mice than in wild-type animals. Notably, exogeneous Nell-1 administration reduced such IL1β-stimulated inflammation and articular cartilage degradation in vivo, suggesting a potential of Nell-1 as a prochondrogenic and anti-inflammatory drug for arthritis-related cartilage damage.

Tongue: Skeletal muscle and motor neurons

Cancer of the oral cavity often necessitates significant resection of tongue tissue, affecting the patient's mastication and speech. The tongue is a complex multifunctional organ and plays an important role in articulation, mastication, and deglutition. The tongue consists of mucosa that contains mucous and serous glands and complex musculature bulk that provides movements. The complexity of tongue anatomy makes it difficult to restore function of the native tongue after partial glossectomy.

Surgical reconstructive approaches are limited by scarring and lack of postoperative morbidity. The currently accepted therapy for glossectomy defects is reconstruction of the tongue with free vascularized flaps, including radial forearm, fibular, lateral thigh, rectus abdominus, and scapular free flaps (see Chapter 2). Although free flap reconstruction represents a significant improvement over previously used methods, functional outcomes vary considerably, depending on the flap chosen and the skill of the surgeon.

Tissue engineering is an alternative therapy that may result in functional neotongue formation. Previous investigators were able to regenerate muscle using isolated myoblasts and collagen as a scaffold material (Kim et al., 2003). Tongue is an ideally suitable bed for transplanted cells because it is a highly vascularized tissue. A collagen hydrogel that contained a suspension of neonatal myoblasts was injected in partial glossectomy defects in rats (Kim et al., 2003). The animals receiving the collagen gel and myoblast injections demonstrated a statistically significant increase in tongue weight and volume after six weeks. Regenerated tissue demonstrated the formation of new muscle tissue and vascularization. In contrast, a group receiving acellular hydrogels showed dense fibrous scarring, lack of neomuscle formation, and dramatic loss of tongue volume and weight. Furthermore, the regenerated muscle tissue was derived from transplanted myoblasts, as identified by fluorescent myoblast labeling, suggesting that myoblast transplantation is a promising strategy for the rehabilitation of glossectomy defects (Luxameechanporn et al., 2006).

A recent study demonstrated that MSCs derived from human gingiva were effective in promoting repair and regeneration of tongue defects by enhancing the function of host skeletal progenitor cells and suppressing fibrosis (Xu et al., 2017). The wounded area of the tongue treated with a small intestinal submucosa (SIS) matrix seeded with gingival MSCs significantly increased the expression of several key myogenic transcriptional factors while suppressing the expression of type I collagen. The findings indicate that MSC/SIS constructs may be a promising myomucosal graft for tongue reconstruction.

The ultimate function of newly formed tongue requires further investigation with clinical trials. Tissue-engineered tongue acquires many of the characteristics and functions of native tongue, such as the generation of directed force and motor nerve supply (van der Bilt et al., 2006). One major issue in tongue tissue engineering is the generation of mature muscular tissue that incorporates motor neurons. A motionless muscle mass can actually incur more energetic cost to the remaining functional muscle mass.

Atrophy can result from lesions of the tongue muscles, the neuromuscular junction, and motor neurons. Immediately after motor nerve transsection, degeneration takes place in the neuron soma, axon, and myelin sheath. Subsequently, the fragments of axon and myelin sheath are eliminated by Schwann cells and macrophages. Schwann cells dedifferentiate, rapidly proliferate, and array along the trunk line of nerve to form a Bungner band. The Bungner band guides axons to grow through the Bungner head and regenerating axons finally form new synapses on denervated muscles. Schwann cells secrete several nerve nutritional factors, including nerve growth factor, ciliary neurotrophic factor, glial cell line–derived neurotrophic factor, brain-derived neurotrophic factor, and neurotrophin, to stimulate axon regeneration. Thus, the introduction of Schwann cells with the appropriate nerve nutritional factors will enhance neotissue functionality.

Zhou et al. (2008) utilized tissue engineering strategies to repair the facial nerve through the application of Schwann cells. Schwann cells transfected with glial cell line–derived neurotrophic factor were injected in tubular PLGA conduits and implanted in the facial skin of rats. Besides minimizing the migration of connective tissue into the conduits, the design also guided axonal regeneration toward the targets without the scar formation that is known to inhibit axonal growth. The regenerated facial nerve exhibited promising electrophysiologic properties.

Collectively, these pioneering studies suggest that tissue engineering approaches can be applied to regenerate integrated neuromotor complexes.

Skin and oral mucosa

Tissue-engineered skin and oral mucosa have been developed to treat and close the surgical wounds of patients disfigured by trauma, tumor ablation, or severe burns. The facial skin is among the most common sites for cutaneous cancer, and postresection defects can be significant. Although skin can self-repair, severely damaged skin (defects greater than 4 cm) will not heal without a graft (MacNeil et al., 2007). The current gold standard for skin graft material is a split-thickness graft containing epidermis and part of the dermis, but skin grafting is limited by availability and donor site morbidity.

Advances in tissue engineering allow skin tissues to be reconstructed by skin cells cultured in vitro. Culturing of keratinocytes has been well established since the late 1970s. Autologous human epidermal cells were cultured into small sheets and grafted on burn wounds (Gallico et al., 1984; Green et al., 1979). However, clinical results have been unsatisfactory when cultured keratinocytes are used in the treatment of full-thickness wounds, where a well-vascularized dermal layer is limited (Compton et al., 1989) In such cases, reconstruction of well-vascularized wound beds that can support epidermal layers is required for successful healing before grafting. Dermal substitutes using collagen have been reported for the treatment of full-thickness burns (Stern et al., 1990). Tissue-engineered skin using autologous keratinocytes and fibroblasts in collagen sheets were successfully combined in dermal substitute–treated wound beds.

Currently available skin replacement products include materials that replace the epidermal layer only, such as an integrated sheet (Epicel, Genzyme Tissue Repair), subconfluent cells on a carrier (Myskin, Altrika), and cells delivered as a spray (CellSpray, Clinical Cell Culture); materials that provide dermal substitutes, such as skin from screened skin (donor skin), bovine collagen sheet (Integra, Integra LifeSciences), and freeze-dried human donor dermis (Alloderm, Lifecell); synthetic materials conditioned with donor fibroblasts (Dermagraft, Advanced Biohealing); and porcine skin for temporary wound dressing (Permacol, Covidien; MacNeil et al., 2007). A number of skin substitutes are being developed for clinical use. Engineered Skin Substitute (EES, previously known as PermaDerm) is a full-thickness skin replacement product prepared from a patient's own skin cells cultured on a collagen substrate to cover large burns. DenovoSkin is another skin substitute for full-thickness skin defects that is currently undergoing clinical trials.

Reconstructed skin tissue can be used for studies of skin biology and pathology, such as pigmentation, skin contraction, melanoma invasion, and various skin diseases, as well as clinical treatment. Tissue-engineered skin also provides in vitro 3D models as alternatives to animals testing for human skin products.

Scar formation after wound healing remains a major challenge in plastic surgery. Previous studies have demonstrated that fetal wounds can heal without scar formation and the overproduction of TGF-β plays an important role in scar formation in adult wounds (Cutroneo, 2007). Understanding the role of TGF-β in wound healing and manipulation of TGF-β in wounds may be keys to scar prevention.

Oral mucosa, like skin, consists of two distinct layers: *(1)* the surface epithelium and *(2)* underlying fibrous connective tissue. However, oral mucosa has physiologic differences from skin, in aspects such as hair growth, adnexal structures, and keratinized pattern. The epithelial layer of the oral mucosa may be keratinized (gingiva and hard palate), nonkeratinized (buccal mucosa, lips, and floor of the mouth), or both (dorsum of the tongue), depending on the region of the mouth. These intraoral regions have distinct functions that require a range of strength and elasticity. Furthermore, engineering of a supportive lamina propria and its supporting vascular components, lymphatic vessels, nerves, and salivary gland ducts will be necessary for generation of full-thickness mucosa that mimics native oral mucosa.

Kinikoglu et al. demonstrated a full-thickness human mucosa equivalent in a porous collagen-glycosaminoglycan-chitosan scaffold (Kinikoglu et al., 2009). Human oral fibroblasts were isolated from the nonkeratinized cheek region of the oral cavity and cultured in a scaffold to create a lamina propria equivalent. Epithelialized full-thickness oral mucosa equivalents were generated by culturing human oral epithelial cells isolated from the same biopsy on top of the created lamina propria equivalent. The epithelium was firmly anchored to the lamina propria, and high amounts of newly synthesized collagen were detected in the subepithelial layer and in the deep lamina propria layer of the reconstructed oral mucosa.

A tissue-engineered oral mucosa was successfully used for the reconstruction of mucosal defects in a pediatric patient with hemifacial microsomia and congenital ankyloglossia (Llames et al., 2014). Mucosal keratinocytes were seeded on a fibrin matrix filled with fibroblasts, and the engineered full-thickness oral mucosa was ready for grafting in three weeks. Autologous cells and plasma are readily available to create the cell-scaffold constructs, indicating the feasibility of using the tissue-engineering approach for oral reconstruction.

Tissue-engineered oral mucosa equivalents can be also used as in vitro models for biocompatibility testing of oral care products, studies of mucosal irritation and disease, and investigation into basic oral biology phenomena.

Engineering of Thick Tissues

Tissue engineering, either with or without stem cell transplantation, offers exciting opportunities for the treatment of lost maxillofacial tissues. However, despite progress in the development of novel progenitor stem cells, growth factors, and carrier materials, limitations in the mass transport of nutrients and waste products remain a major obstacle to the survival, proliferation, and differentiation of the delivered stem cells. The ability of isolated cells to spontaneously reform millimeter-scale cellular networks in vitro has spurred many efforts at constructing functional tissue that eventually may be suitable for human engraftment (Carrier et al., 1999; Eschenhagen et al., 2002; Radisic et al., 2004; Zimmermann et al., 2002a).

The promise of thick tissue engineering has gained momentum in recent years in the scientific community and general public, due in part to dramatic in vitro demonstrations of centimeter-scale synchronously contracting tissue structures assembled from isolated neonatal cells and specialized extracellular matrix components (collagen gels and Matrigel [BD Biosciences], a purified basement membrane extract; Radisic et al., 2004; Zimmermann et al., 2002a). Unfortunately, results in animal models have been disappointing, because of the cell death and potential immunogenicity of the basement membrane extract (Zimmermann et al., 2002b). Although alternative materials and growth factors can be engineered to replace Matrigel, the fundamental problem of cell survival must be addressed before these cell-based approaches can realize therapeutic implementation in humans.

In our experience, the single largest obstacle to engineered thick maxillofacial tissues is the mass transport problem, a multifaceted phenomenon that involves deficient nutrient flux, accumulation of detrimental waste products, and adaptive cellular metabolism. In other words, even if tissue engineers identify the necessary parameters to control stem cell fate, they must still address the mass transport problem caused by a low concentration of critical nutrients and the molecular sequelae of ischemia-like conditions surrounding the progenitor cells. The physical, chemical, and biologic origins of the mass transport–induced hypoxia and acidosis involve complex, time-dependent mechanisms that are modulated by cellular adaptations and multiple modes of cell death.

Consequences of hypoxia

Production of adenosine triphosphate requires molecular oxygen (O_2), the final electron acceptor and energy sink in oxidative phosphorylation, a key step for many major metabolic processes. When oxygen is withdrawn from the culture medium, characteristic biochemical and functional changes quickly ensue in the cells, altering the protein expression pattern through changes in gene expression, messenger RNA stability, rates of translation, and protein degradation (Piacentini and Karliner, 1999).

Shortly after the onset of hypoxia, many mammalian cells are able to adapt transiently and initially by decreasing their oxygen consumption rates to compensate for the reduced oxygen availability. This takes place in an oxygen-dependent manner, resembling a logarithmic or Michaelis-Menten–type curve. In the early stages of hypoxia, many cellular processes are suppressed to decrease the rate of cellular adenosine triphosphate consumption; only critical cellular machinery is preserved in order to modulate nearly constant intracellular phosphocreatine and adenosine triphosphate levels. As hypoxia progresses, phosphocreatine levels begin to decline; this is followed much later by a decline in adenosine triphosphate levels (Casey and Arthur, 2000).

Although hypoxia induces a downregulation of protein synthesis, a number of specific proteins are known to be upregulated. These include cytokines and growth factors, endothelin 1, genes associated with metabolism, nitric oxide synthase, adhesion molecules, antioxidants, heat shock proteins, natriuretic factors, apoptosis genes, adrenergic receptors, and the family of vascular endothelial growth factors.

Among the major nutrients, oxygen seems to be most critical for cell survival. Withdrawal of glucose or fatty acids from the culture medium in normoxic conditions is generally not as toxic as withdrawal of oxygen, evident from the observation that cells cultured under glucose-free or fatty acid–free conditions remain viable and functional for several days (Malhotra and Brosius, 1999). Therefore, many mathematical models focus on the diffusion of molecular oxygen. As discussed in subsequent sections, hypoxia is only one part of the complex cell survival problem.

Consequences of metabolic waste accumulation

Besides delivering nutrients such as oxygen and glucose, transport systems in functional tissues also remove metabolic wastes. A major metabolite is carbon dioxide (CO_2), a major waste product of oxidative metabolism and pH buffer in the extracellular compartment.

In the body, CO_2 is present in three major forms: *(1)* dissolved in plasma, *(2)* bound as bicarbonate (HCO_3^-), or *(3)* bound as carbamate ($NH_2CO_2^-$). Most CO_2 in cellular compartments is present as HCO_3^-, which is related to the pH and amount of dissolved CO_2 by the Henderson-Hasselbalch equation. However, the relative fractions of each of these forms change according to metabolic demand and differ between body compartments, because CO_2 can diffuse faster across membrane barriers, while HCO_3^- is better transported between intracellular and extracellular compartments (Geers and Gros, 2000). Due to the interconversion of dissolved CO_2, water, HCO_3^-, and protons, diffusion of CO_2 is tightly linked to proton diffusion. Although the diffusion coefficient of dissolved CO_2 (17.1×10^{-6} cm^2/s) is twice as great as that of HCO_3^- (8.7×10^{-6} cm^2/s; Remuñán-López, 1997; Shu et al., 2002), HCO_3^- is advantageous in that it will move protons as well as CO_2.

Without buffers, low proton gradients are allowable at physiologic pH levels (10^{-8} to 10^{-7} M; Geers and Gros, 2000). However, physiologic buffers (e.g., phosphate) can create a buffered proton gradient of at least 10^{-3} to 10^{-2} M. Therefore, proton transport can occur by both free diffusion (9.3×10^{-5} cm^2/s at 25 °C; Sandén et al., 2010) and by diffusion of mobile buffers. Although the diffusion coefficients of buffers are usually an order of magnitude less than those of free proton diffusion, the steep gradient of buffered protons allows a much higher flux than is possible with the shallow gradient of free proton (calculated at 10,000 times greater; Geers and Gros, 2000). Therefore, the transport of CO_2 and H^+ essentially occurs by diffusion of HCO_3^- and simultaneous buffer-facilitated H^+ diffusion, and free proton diffusion is negligible.

When these processes are not adequate for CO_2 removal, acidosis can result. Acidosis is a common sequela of ischemia-induced hypoxia and is extremely detrimental to cell viability. Direct measurements of tissue acidity indicate rapid decrease, by 1 to 2 pH units, within 10 minutes of ischemia (Marzouk et al., 2002). The traditional explanation for the pH drop during muscle activity is the formation of lactic acid (pKa = 3.87) during anaerobic glycolysis. Lactic acid, in turn, dissociates almost completely into proton and sodium lactate at most physiologic pH levels. The phenomenon of acidosis induced by accumulation of lactate is termed *lactic acidosis* and is the usual, although not universally accepted, explanation for proton accumulation in the extracellular milieu during hypoxia or ischemia (Robergs et al., 2004).

Regardless of substrate origin, the ensuing acidosis is a potent signal for apoptosis, either alone or in conjunction with hypoxia (Webster et al., 1992; Webster et al., 1999). Within 24 hours of exposure to severe hypoxia (less than 1% oxygen), a pH drop will become evident in standard culture medium with typical pH buffers and the cells will show many of the markers of apoptosis: DNA laddering, positive staining in the terminal deoxynucleotidyl transferase–mediated deoxyuridine triphosphate nick-end–labeling method, and cleavage of the caspase-3 substrate poly(adenosine diphosphate–ribose) polymerase (Malhotra and Brosius, 1999).

Conversely, cultures in 1% oxygen and supplemented with additional buffers to maintain neutral pH did not significantly change in cell numbers after six days, suggesting the dominant role of acidosis over hypoxia. This observation may be related in part to the cell-preserving effects of 2-deoxyglucose (a hexokinase inhibitor) and 4-(2-hydroxyet hyl)-1-piperazineethanesulfonic acid (HEPES) buffer during hypoxia, which prevent the glycolysis-induced pH reduction (Aki et al., 2001). Lactate-induced mild acidosis (pH 6.0) of normoxic culture medium has been shown to stimulate apoptosis in cultured cells, an effect that was not observed in pH-neutralized culture medium containing the same concentration of lactate (Webster et al., 1999).

Collectively, this evidence suggests that successful tissue engineering of large, maxillofacial tissues must simultaneously minimize hypoxia and acidosis, in particular, and possibly deliver antiapoptotic molecules.

Lessons from nature: Organogenesis

In mature tissues, rapid convective transport and slow diffusive transport occur simultaneously. Blood vessels are responsible for the convective transport of nutrients to the capillaries, and then nutrients such as molecular oxygen must diffuse out from the capillary lumen through a thin plasma layer, diffuse down concentration gradient, and diffuse across densely assembled connective tissues, until the nutrients finally reach the cells. In mature tissues, components of the extracellular matrix (e.g., collagen fibers) are spaced tightly together, resulting in small-pore structures with large interstitial hypertension that severely limit convection (Ramanujan et al., 2002).

Therefore, the final transport process occurs primarily via diffusion through the small pores. Because diffusion is slow, the diffusion distance is typically small (generally on the order of 100 μm), and the concentration gradient needs to be high. Indeed, the PO_2 gradient from the capillary to the mitochondria is a major determinant of mitochondrial PO_2 and oxidative phosphorylation (Takahashi and Doi, 1998).

How do developing tissues receive their nutrients prior to the development of connected vessels? During early stages of tissue development, the initial tissues have the necessary architecture to survive by diffusion of nutrients. For example, during organogenesis, the initial myocardium consists of an avascular, thin, spongy structure perfused by an open circulatory system (Poupa, 1994). In the absence of coronary vessels, diffusion alone from the ventricular cavity must nourish the developing myocardium. Although diffusion is a slow process, diffusion can deliver the critical nutrients because of the open spongy structure and short diffusion-length scale in the developing myocardium (Bonarius et al., 1995). These two features must be incorporated into the proposed tissue engineering strategies to maximize cell survival prior to angiogenesis in the injured myocardium.

The subsequent development of coronary circulation is a key step in the evolution of vertebrates. Capillaries originate from vasculogenesis by precursor cells that migrate to the epicardium from the liver-forming region. The fact that these anatomical features do not appear until after the fourth week of development in humans (Obrucník et al., 1972) suggests that diffusion over short-length scale can maintain tissue survival. Over time, the vascular tubes mature, incorporate pericytes, and branch into other vessels by angiogenesis of endothelial cells. The major coronary arteries form by coalescence of microvessels that eventually merge with the aorta, as early as 44 days after conception in humans (Rongish et al., 1994). The coronary arteries continue to grow and increase their branching, while the myocardium develops in size and density.

This successful strategy is repeated in the growth and development of other tissues. Tissue engineering scaffolds must exhibit the open porous structure necessary to facilitate diffusion prior to angiogenesis. While nature starts with small-scale tissues, the challenge for tissue engineers is to control local nutrient transport within much larger scaffolds.

Diffusion in 2D culture and 3D scaffolds

In typical monolayer cell culture, oxygen movement is driven by diffusion-reaction and some convective transport. Adherent cells begin consuming oxygen at the bottom of the culture dish, creating a gradient for oxygen to diffuse from the top of the culture medium downward (Poupa, 1994). Significant convection can be produced by thermal gradients because of cycling of the incubator heater (Baumgardner and Otto, 2003) and the mechanical vibrations from the surrounding environment (Vivian and King, 1964). The oxygen gradient in monolayer cell culture has been found to be 15-fold less than that predicted by diffusion alone, indicating a sizable contribution from convection (Otto et al., 2001). Therefore, although diffusion is the major rate-limiting transport process, diffusion coefficients based on these so-called static cultures tend to overestimate the diffusivity by ignoring convection. Relevant mathematical models of these important processes must utilize more conservative diffusion coefficients.

Whereas most cells can grow well in two-dimensional (2D) cell culture, tissue engineers realized very quickly that seeded cells do not survive within thick 3D carriers in vitro, unless some form of convective transport is provided by bioreactors, flow chambers, and spinner flasks (Freed et al., 1994). In 3D culture, limitations of mass transfer can lead to spatially heterogenous gene expression because of nutrient deprivation and focal concentration of cytokines. This may cause cells on the outer periphery to behave differently from those in the center of the scaffold.

Carrier et al. (1999) modeled oxygen as the limiting substrate within 3D cell-seeded scaffolds and observed cell death at the central core of 3D scaffolds but good cell survival along the outer periphery as long as the cells were within diffusion-length scale from the outer edge. This finding is consistent with repeated observations that cells grew much better at the periphery of tissue constructs, while viable cells were absent in the central region. In addition, thicker scaffolds sustained proportionally fewer cells than thinner scaffolds. These phenomena can all be attributed to limitations in mass transport.

In addition to slow diffusion, cellular consumption of critical nutrients near the bulk fluid-scaffold interface reduces nutrient availability in the inner scaffold core. Galban and Locke (1997, 1999a, 1999b) modeled diffusion-limited cell growth inside engineered tissues using three mathematical arguments. In one model, a moving boundary approach was taken to predict the cell growth as a function of the limiting substrate concentration (Galban and Locke, 1997). A second model combined volume averaging, diffusion-reaction, and three models of growth kinetics (heterogenous kinetics, Moser model, and modified Contois equation). Because the models required changes in their parameters to accurately predict the effects of scaffold thickness on cell growth, it was concluded that other factors besides substrate diffusion may limit cell growth in this type of system (Galban and Locke, 1999a).

They proposed a third model that further considered the effects of competitive product inhibition, spatial variations in cell density, spatial variations in substrate concentration within the scaffold, saturation kinetics of the rate-limiting substrate, and upper limits on cell growth in the scaffold (Galban and Locke, 1999b). This analysis of cell-growth kinetics is certainly applicable to growth of progenitor cells within artificial 3D scaffolding environments, prior to cellular differentiation. However, the models may need to be modified to account for the fact that many terminally differentiated cells do not proliferate significantly.

We developed a mathematical model to predict oxygen levels inside a 3D cell-seeded hydrogel (Brown et al., 2007a). The resultant theoretical predictions were compared to experimental measurements in corresponding experiments with a hypoxia-sensitive stain (pimonidazole). In this model, the hydrogel was cast between two plastic discs, which confined mass transfer to the radial direction only. After 36 hours of culture in the presence of pimonidazole, quantitative image analysis was performed to measure the distance from the culture medium at which hypoxia first occurred under various conditions (Brown et al., 2007a; Ho et al., 2006). Modulation of the design parameters showed that the trends in oxygen profiles predicted by the model were in reasonable agreement with experimental values, although a number of ambiguities related to the specific model parameters led to a general overprediction of oxygen concentrations. Sensitivity analysis showed that diffusion-reaction models offered reasonable predictions of oxygen concentrations in diffusion-limited tissue constructs.

Analysis of pH gradients in engineered tissues

As discussed earlier, an indirect effect of cellular hypoxia is the shunt to the less-efficient glycolytic metabolism, which is accompanied by a reduction in extracellular pH. A four-species, 2D diffusion-reaction mathematical model was developed to predict pH in the aforementioned radial-diffusion model. Experimental validation of the 3D hydrogel demonstrated pH gradients toward the center of the construct, which reached lethal pH values of less than 6.5 at a nominal cell density of 10^6 cells/cm^3. The pH predictions were moderately dependent on O_2 concentration and strongly dependent on cell density, CO_2 concentration, and diffusion length (Brown et al., 2007b). It can be concluded from this study that the diffusion length had the most dominant effect of any experimental parameter modeled. Hypoxia-induced acidosis is an important element in the mass transport problem that must be addressed in the tissue engineering of thick tissues for maxillofacial reconstruction.

Attenuation of hypoxic cell death via pH buffering

The ability of HEPES-buffered culture medium to reduce acidotic cell death in hypoxic monolayer cell cultures and in a diffusion-limited model demonstrates the importance of acidosis and, more importantly, a possible strategy to prevent acidosis-induced cell death. The pH of culture media was measured over time under three different HEPES buffer concentrations (0, 25, and 50 mmol) in normoxic and hypoxic conditions (Brown et al., 2008). Cells that were cultured in severe hypoxia (0% oxygen) exhibited a pH drop to 5.5 after 4 days, but pH drop was eliminated by the addition of 50 mmol of HEPES. Under normoxic conditions, the addition of HEPES did not significantly change the media pH. Under hypoxic conditions, the addition of increasing concentration of HEPES was associated with a decreasing degree of acidosis. This finding supports the notion that acidosis is a main culprit in cell death within engineered tissues. The effects of preventing acidosis on cell viability can be seen by the addition of pH buffers to the 3D hydrogels, which reduced cell death by attenuating acidosis (Brown et al., 2008).

Controlling spatial distribution of cells

Experimental observations suggest that much more uniform cell growth can be expected when cells are not seeded uniformly throughout a 3D volume. In an elegant experiment, cells were seeded within 3D scaffolds in two spatial patterns. Construct A comprised five stacked, alternating layers of cell-seeded (layers 1, 3, and 5) and unseeded (layers 2 and 4) volume. Construct B comprised five cell-seeded layers in which cells were uniformly seeded throughout the volume (Dunn et al., 2006). Each layer was 10 mm in diameter and 1 mm in height (5 mm total).

After 10 days of incubation, cell growth in construct B was limited to the external peripheral border, and there were few cells in the central core. In contrast, the alternating layers in construct A produced more uniform cell growth in the center. Most important, mathematical models predicted that cell growth would be even more uniform if the layer dimension were reduced from 1 mm to the characteristic diffusion-length scale of approximately 140 μm (Dunn et al., 2006), which represents the characteristic distance within which the cells have adequate oxygen to grow. This length scale is similar to that of the normal physiologic environment, where the average intercapillary distance is a few hundred microns.

Thus, direct measurements of hypoxic oxygen levels and pH gradients inside thick tissue scaffolds demonstrate the effects of transport on programmed cell death. Mathematical models and experimental validation of ischemia-imposed metabolite gradients suggest that ischemic cell death is reduced by pH buffering. These mathematical models also show that controlling the microarchitecture of the 3D carrier (Lee et al., 2005) and tailoring the spatial distribution of cells within 3D scaffolds (Dunn et al., 2006) can enhance cell survival.

Advanced Manufacturing Technologies for Tissue Engineering

Malignant neoplasms in the maxillofacial complex often invade underlying structures. As a result, multiple tissues such as muscle, bone, or cartilage are often excised during tumor resection. Patient-specific, highly customizable manufacturing technologies are exceptionally attractive for the fabrication of complex scaffolds to direct 3D tissue ingrowth for the repair of large, complex, multitissue defects. These customizable scaffolds would offer control over macrostructural and microstructural properties that optimize structural and nutrient transport within the scaffolds. Scaffolds designed to promote new bone formation should consider structural properties such as pore size, porosity, pore interconnectivity, mechanical properties, and an environment that provides sufficient nutrient transport. In addition, tissue engineering scaffolds must be an appropriate anatomical shape that matches the patient's exact defect. Control over the macrostructural and microstructural properties of scaffolds is required for the rehabilitation of complex maxillofacial malformations.

A number of different fabrication techniques have been developed to manufacture tissue engineering scaffolds. Conventional fabrication methods include fiber bonding, melt molding, solvent casting, particulate leaching, membrane lamination, phase separation, gas foaming (high-pressure processing), as well as a combination of these techniques.

Although scaffolds produced from conventional techniques address individual issues of structural properties, no single scaffold can meet all required properties. Some conventional fabrication methods, including 3D lamination of precut membranes, melt molding, and sequential solvent casting, can achieve customized production that meets various structural and nutritional issues, but these techniques are labor intensive and time consuming. Virtually all of these conventional techniques can create scaffolds with highly connected microporosity for cell and mass transfer and consequently large surface areas for cell-substrate adhesion. However, none offers simultaneous control over macroscopic shape, oriented channels, and microporosity, and none can work directly with digitized medical imaging data to manufacture patient-specific scaffolds.

The field of computer-aided tissue engineering has evolved over the past decades (Hutmacher et al., 2004; Sun and Lal, 2002). Computer-aided tissue engineering integrates advanced, noninvasive imaging technologies such as computed tomography (CT) and magnetic resonance imaging (MRI), computer-aided design (CAD), and rapid prototyping (RP) and/or solid freeform fabrication (SFF) to construct 3D structures.

SFF technologies fabricate complex objects in a layer-by-layer fashion according to 3D computer models (Leong et al., 2003; Yang et al., 2002). Complicated 3D features such as internal voids, cantilevers, undercuts, and narrow, tortuous paths are simply reduced to a stack of common 2D features such as circles, lines, and points. Exempted from tooling path restrictions, these additive technologies offer much higher levels in shape complexity.

Although these technologies were developed primarily for industrial applications, their flexibility makes them attractive candidates for biomedical engineering. Various SFF techniques were introduced to build objects with controlled macroarchitecture as well as microstructures with biomedical and tissue engineering applications. The freedom in form, combined with the appropriate material deposition technology, offers control over the tissue engineering triad by simultaneously directing the spatial distribution of cells, signals, and scaffolding substrates during fabrication. Furthermore, these technologies allow integration between digitized medical imaging data and CAD models (Colin and Boire, 1997; Winder et al., 1999).

The integration of SFF technologies with patient-specific medical imaging data enables the aseptic manufacturing of tissue engineering grafts that match precisely to a patient's contours. These technologies enable the fabrication of multifunctional scaffolds that meet the structural, mechanical, and nutritional requirements based on optimized models (Hollister et al., 2002). Automated computer-aided fabrication could generate more accurate and consistent scaffolds with minimal workforce and cost requirements. Although most SFF technologies are useful for medical modeling and medical device manufacturing, this section will focus on the biocompatible SFF technologies that have been employed for the fabrication of tissue engineering scaffolds.

Since the initial development of stereolithography (STL) in the 1980s (Dowler, 1989), numerous competing SFF technologies have been developed. In the early 1990s, the introduction of a custom-built 3D printing machine (Cima et al., 1994; Griffith et al., 1997; Wu et al., 1996) allowed the first biomedical devices made directly by SFF. Since then, numerous commercially available SFF technologies, such as fused deposition modeling (FDM; Zein et al., 2002), STL (Fisher et al., 2002), and selective laser sintering (SLS; Leong et al., 2001) have been used in fabricating scaffolds.

In 2004, cell-loaded tissue was presented for the first time using a commercial STL printer (Dhariwala et al., 2004). Since the 2000s, the term *bioprinting* has been widely used to describe 3D printing where living cells, biomaterials, or active biomolecules are being printed to fabricate complex biological constructs, such as multilayered skin, joints, and bone (Dey and Ozbolat, 2020). Bioink can be cross-linked or stabilized during or after the bioprinting process, in which its formulation determines the shape and structure of the biological constructs (Gungor-Ozkerim et al., 2018). Bioink containing photo-cross-linkable biopolymer (e.g., polyethylene glycol diacrylate, gelatin methacryloyl, and methacrylated hyaluronic acid) or ionic cross-linkable biopolymer (e.g., alginate with divalent cations) is commonly used for bioprinting (Hu et al., 2019).

To imitate natural tissue characteristics (e.g., cartilage), it is essential to establish interfaces and gradients of different materials within a single construct. Several approaches have been proposed to generate such biological gradients, especially using polymeric biomaterials. The degree of gelation between deposition of single layers has been controlled using different cross-linking triggers—such as light, ionic, pH, temperature, host-guest interaction, or enzymatic interactions—yielding scaffolds with gradients of mechanical properties across the z-direction (Schwab et al., 2020). However, printing a multimaterial and multigradient scaffold still remains a challenge. Further development of materials that are optimal for bioprinting and next-generation printheads that can separately deposit multiple biofactors and materials on the same platform will provide the potential to create constructs that satisfy the complex biologic requirements of tissue-engineering scaffolds. The following sections will provide more details about these technologies.

Powder 3D printing

Invented at the Massachusetts Institute of Technology, Powder 3D printing (p3DP) fabricates 3D structures using an inkjet that prints liquid binder solution onto a powder bed (Fig 8-5). A wide range of materials has been used in printing because most biomaterials exist in either a solid or liquid state. The process begins with a layer of fine powder material spread evenly across the piston. The x-y positioning system and the printhead are synchronized to print the desired 2D pattern by selective deposition of binder droplets onto the powder layer. The piston, powder bed, and part are lowered, and the next layer of powder is spread. The drop-spread-print cycle is repeated until the entire part is completed. Removal of the unbound powder reveals the fabricated part.

The local composition can be manipulated by specifying the appropriate printhead to deposit the predetermined volume of the appropriate binder. The local microstructure can be controlled by altering the printing parameters during fabrication (Wu and Cima, 1999). The incorporation of microchannels effectively distributes additional seeding surfaces throughout the interior of the device, increasing the effective seeding density and uniformity. Patterned surface chemistry potentially offers spatial control over distribution of multiple cell types.

This technology is limited by the competing needs of printhead reliability and feature resolution, because small nozzles can make finer features but are more prone to clogging. The current limitation

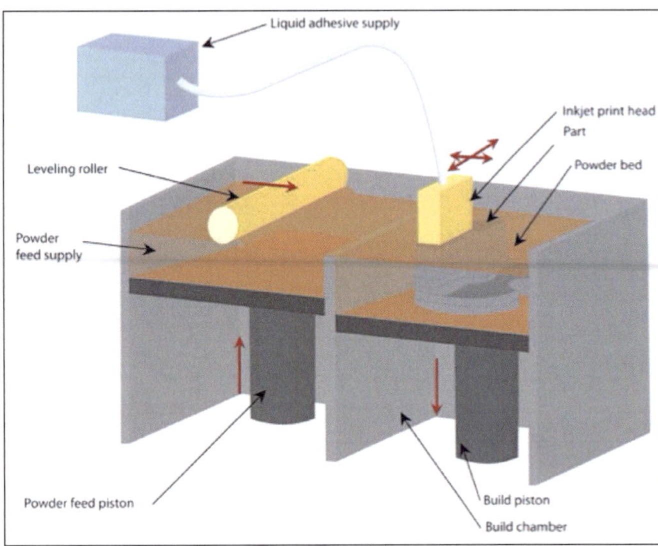

Figure 8-5 3D printing (reprinted from CustomPart.Net with permission; CustomPart.Net http://www.custompartnet.com).

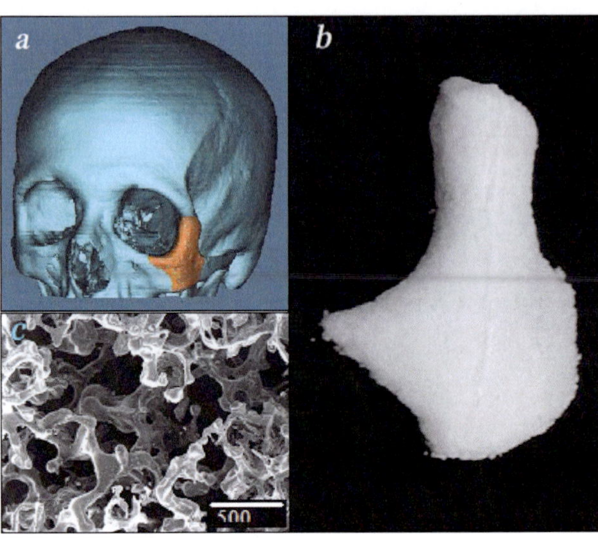

Figure 8-6 *(a)* 3D reconstruction of a zygoma from 2D CT images. *(b)* Zygoma PLGA scaffold. *(c)* Internal pore morphology shows well-interconnected pores with a range of 300 to 500 μm.

is 100 μm for one-dimensional features (lines), and 300 μm for 3D features (walls, etc.).

Fabrication of complex scaffolds such as internal channels or hanging features is easily achievable with this technique, because objects are being supported by surrounding unbound powder. Kim et al. (1998) used p3DP to create highly porous scaffolds in combination with particulate leaching techniques and demonstrated cell ingrowth into the scaffolds. Also, room-temperature processing conditions allow the incorporation of temperature-sensitive materials such as pharmaceutical and biologic agents into scaffolds (Wu et al., 1996). Lam et al. (2002) fabricated starch-based scaffolds by printing distilled water, demonstrating the feasibility of using biologic agents and living cells during fabrication.

Another favorable characteristic of this technology for tissue engineering is multicolor printing, which allows each color ink to be positioned on a precise location. This feature offers the exciting potential to allow simultaneous arrangement of multiple types of cells, deposition of multiple extracellular matrix materials, and exertion of point-to-point control over bioactive agents for biologic tissue manufacturing. In this respect, p3DP may be more flexible for printable material selection than other SFF technologies.

Tissue engineers have used p3DP to fabricate porous ceramic scaffolds with fully interconnected channels directly from HA powder for bone replacement (Seitz et al., 2005). Customized, anatomically shaped HA constructs can be fabricated based on medical information from a patient. This technology also allows construction of a biphasic scaffold to regenerate hybrid tissue systems such as the TMJ. Sherwood et al. (2002) developed osteochondral composite constructs in which the upper region is composed of D,L-PLGA–L-PLA with 90% porosity for cartilage regeneration, and the lower region is composed of a L-PLGA–tricalcium phosphate composite to maximize bone ingrowth.

One drawback of p3DP is a limited available pore size in the final constructs when porogens are incorporated into powders prior to fabrication (Zeltinger et al., 2001). The shape complexity of scaffolds is also limited when the powder material is degradable polymer. This p3DP approach for degradable polymer demands the use of organic solvents as liquid binders. Because organic solvents can dissolve most commercially available drop-on-demand printhead subsystems, the reported studies required the use of custom high-resolution jets depositing through stencils (Zeltinger et al., 2001). However, this approach is inefficient for complicated structures.

This problem was addressed by a practical, indirect p3DP protocol in which molds are printed using commercially available plaster powder and the final materials, biodegradable polymers, are cast in the mold cavity (Lee et al., 2005; Lee et al., 2009). Many different materials can be cast under similar printing parameters, whereas individual processing parameters need to be optimized to maximize the build resolution in a conventional direct p3DP approach.

This technology could be applied to treat patients with zygomatic bone fractures and for other resected structures or tissue enhancement. Lee et al. demonstrated the ability of the indirect p3DP approach to build a zygoma scaffold directly from CT data (Fig 8-6). Medical CT scans were imported into Mimics software (Materialise) to develop a 3D representation. Image data for the zygoma scaffold were virtually repaired using a mirroring tool and exported into STL format for printing on a RP system. Virtual molds, having the negative shape of a reconstructed zygoma model, were created via subtraction of the rendered zygoma structure in CAD software (3D Studio VIZ R3, Autodesk). The objects were sliced into 2D layers, and then each individual sliced layer was built sequentially on a commercially available 3D printing machine (Z402, Zcorp) with plaster powder (ZP100, Zcorp).

To create a porous zygoma polymer scaffold, PLGA solution was mixed with sucrose particles in the range of 300 to 500 μm. The mixture was then cast in plaster molds. Molds and sucrose porogens were removed simultaneously by particulate leaching in deionized water. The internal pore morphology of scaffolds showed well-interconnected pores with the range of 300 to 500 μm (Lee et al., 2005). It has been suggested that a large pore size in a range of 200 to 400 μm is needed to facilitate mineralized bone ingrowth (Boyan et al., 1996), but this range of pore size has not been reported with

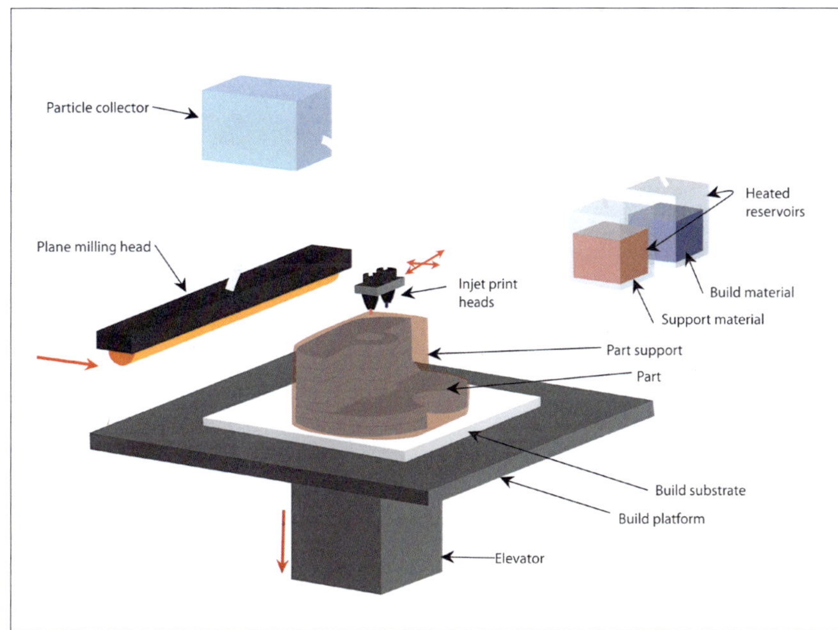

Figure 8-7 Inkjet printing (reprinted from CustomPart.Net with permission; CustomPart.Net).

direct 3D printing, in which the porogen particle size in the powder bed is limited to typical incremental powder layer thickness of about 100 to 150 μm for optimum resolution and integrity of constructs (Wu and Cima, 1999).

Material jetting

Material jetting (MJ) directly prints a build material on a platform (Fig 8-7). This differs from p3DP in two ways: *(1)* The ink is replaced with polymers (or monomers) and *(2)* the powder bed is eliminated. MJ deposits liquid polymer droplets of low viscosity monomer (or polymers) and polymerizes them as soon as they are deposited onto substrates. Polyjet is perhaps the most popular example of material jetting. If the polymer undergoes temperature-dependent phase change, the process is sometimes referred to as *thermal phase change inkjet printing* because a thermoplastic material is heated and ejected, in the form of a liquid drop, from the printhead onto the build platform, where it instantly cools and solidifies.

The advantages of this technique are excellent building resolution and surface finishes. Thus, this process is mostly applicable to investment casting of scaffold materials. However, the use of thermal phase change inkjet printing poses a severe limit on the choice of build materials available for tissue engineering scaffolds and is incompatible with cells and biologics.

The two common thermal phase change systems that are commercially available are ThermoJet Modeler (3D Systems) and ModelMaker (Solidscape). The ThermoJet Modeler utilizes several hundred nozzles for fast building. It uses a hairlike matrix of build material to provide support for overhangs. The ModelMaker system uses single individual heads to print the build material (thermoplastic) and support material (wax). After the object is complete, the wax support material can be melted away. The build speed of this system is much slower than that of the ThermoJet system, but the final resolution of the object is much higher.

Schek et al. (2005) used ModelMaker with indirect SFF techniques to demonstrate the use of biphasic composite scaffolds to engineer osteochondral tissue that can be applied to TMJ repair. HA scaffolds and PLA sponges were fabricated separately from the computer-designed molds created on a ModelMaker. The two phases of the scaffold were then assembled into a biphasic PLA-HA composite scaffold. The researchers differentially seeded the HA phase with fibroblasts that were previously transduced with BMP-7 genes and the PLA sponge with fully differentiated chondrocytes. Following implantation in ectopic sites in mice, the composite scaffolds promoted the simultaneous growth of bone, cartilage, and a mineralized interface.

Stereolithography

STL is regarded as the first RP process (Fig 8-8). The original STL rasters a helium-cadmium laser beam to polymerize photocurable liquid resins to form laminated 2D patterns (Fisher et al., 2002). At the end of each layer, the cured structure is lowered into the liquid resin reservoir. The drop distance represents the thickness of the uncured liquid resin that spreads over the top. The topmost, uncured layer of liquid monomer is ready to be patterned. This laser polymerization process is repeated layer by layer until the entire object is fabricated. Because rastering a laser beam can be slow, the masked lamp technique, in which the entire layer of polymers was patterned, was subsequently introduced to cure photopolymers.

Once the entire layer is built, the excess resin is relatively easy to remove. However, the completed object is weak and needs further curing in an ultraviolet oven (Wang et al., 1996). Typical materials used in STL include acrylics and epoxies; therefore, the use of STL in the tissue engineering scaffold is severely constrained by the scarcity of biocompatible and biodegradable biomaterials that are dimensionally stable during photopolymerization. Furthermore, postcure treatment is necessary because

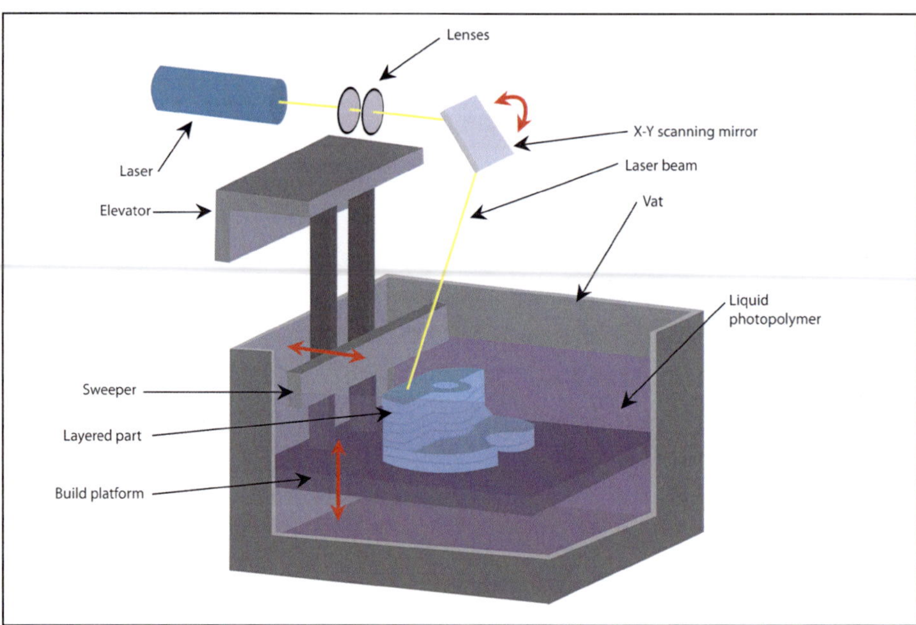

Figure 8-8 Inkjet printing (reprinted from CustomPart.Net with permission; CustomPart.Net. http://www.custompartnet.com).

complete polymerization is usually not achieved during STL. Because polymerization is not instantaneous during STL, temporary support structures must be incorporated into the CAD model to allow production of unsupported features such as cantilevers.

Resins with and without bioceramic dispersions have been processed by STL. Compositional gradients are somewhat impractical, unless the reservoir resin is replaced between layers. Gradients along the horizontal planes are virtually impossible. Biocompatible resins with the proper STL processing properties are also scarce.

Present medical applications of STL include the fabrication of anatomical models for presurgical planning and the indirect fabrication of medical devices by using the STL patterns for molds (see Chapters 2, 3, 5, and 7). Titanium dental implant components have been fabricated by electrical discharge machining of titanium ingot based on an STL model (Schmitt and Chance, 1995).

In the early 2000s, photocurable biopolymer materials with the potential for use in STL tissue engineering processes have been introduced. Photo cross-linkable poly(propylene fumarate) has been used to fabricate complex 3D scaffolds with controlled microstructures for rehabilitation of rabbit cranial defects (Fisher et al., 2002). This resin requires a reactive diluent, such as diethyl fumarate, which introduces significant amounts of a nondegradable component. In addition, photopolymerized resin does not possess the strong mechanical properties that are needed for hard tissue engineering. In another study, photocurable poly(D,L-lactide) resin without the use of reactive diluents has been developed and applied in STL (Melchels et al., 2009). A liquid mixture of polyfunctional acrylic monomers, photoinitiator, and HA has been used to custom-fabricate a composite implant to promote osteogenesis. Polyethylene glycol or natural polysaccharide modified with photo cross-linkable groups such as methacrylates also showed great potential as tissue engineering scaffolds that are fabricated in STL (Arcaute et al., 2010).

This technique also allows fabrication of complex 3D microenvironments with controlled spatial or temporal patterning of biochemical factors. Previous studies have demonstrated precise patterning of various extracellular matrix components in a scaffold, which would allow the growth factors to be sequestered in specific regions (Mapili et al., 2005). Furthermore, polymer microparticles with multiple, defined release kinetics can be spatially incorporated within the scaffolds, indicating creation of temporal patterns of growth factors along with spatial distributions. Such patterned scaffolds might provide a useful adjunct for engineering of complex, hybrid tissue structures from a single stem cell population. Although cell viability is demonstrated on these hydrogels, the ability of these materials to support cellular function remains to be proven.

Selective laser sintering

SLS was developed at the University of Texas in 1989 (Fig 8-9). The SLS technique is based on the sintering of powdered material by a CO_2 laser beam (Leong et al., 2001). SLS directs a laser to pattern each layer by partially fusing thermoplastic particles together. When the laser beam hits the thin layer of powdered polymer materials, the particles are fused to each other at the glass transition temperature to form a solid 2D pattern. At the end of one layer, the piston is lowered, a fresh layer of powder material is rolled evenly across the top surface, and the laser binds the fresh particles to form the appropriate 2D pattern. Subsequent layers are built and fused to the previous layer, and this process is repeated, layer by layer, until the entire object is fabricated. Loose, unbound powder is brushed away on completion of the entire part, and heat treatment is performed to achieve full density.

Unlike STL, SLS does not require temporary support structures because unbound solid particles can serve as supporting struts under cantilevers. It is possible to fabricate scaffolds with irregular shapes, such as channels or hanging features, with this technique. Another advantage of this technique is that it is a solvent-free process.

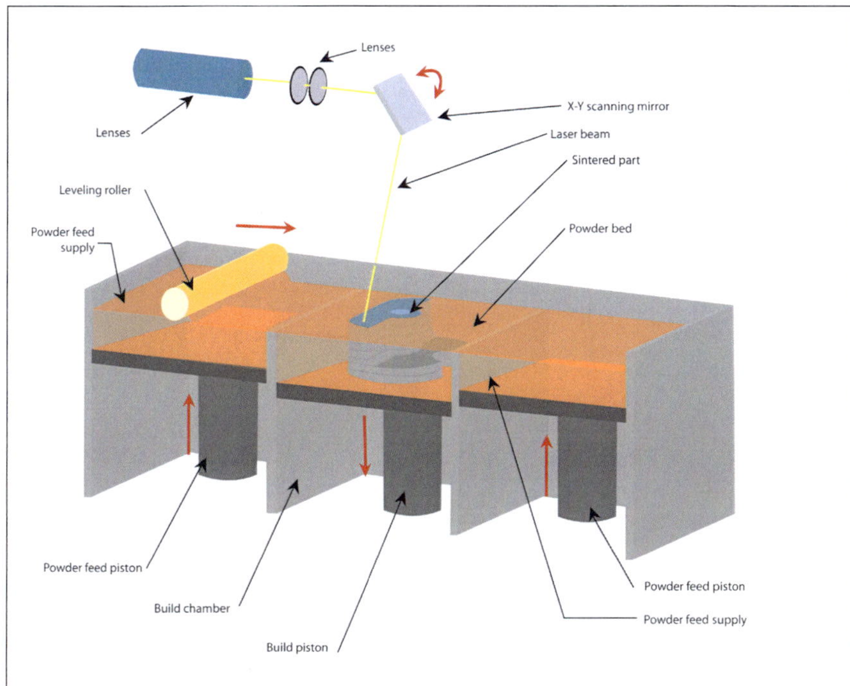

Figure 8-9 Selective laser sintering (reprinted from CustomPart.Net with permission; CustomPart.Net. http://www.custompartnet.com).

Spreading of different powder compositions makes it slightly easier to achieve compositional gradients in SLS than in STL, but compositional gradients along the horizontal planes are virtually impossible in these approaches. The microstructure can be controlled by altering the laser energy, scan speed, and total exposure time. Most of the microstructural control with SLS has relied on postprocessing heat treatments, however. This technique has been used with wax powders to generate wax patterns during the fabrication of facial prostheses (see Chapter 5).

For the use of ceramic powder in SLS techniques, intermediate binding materials are required because of an excessively high glass transition temperature and the melting point of ceramic powder. Tan et al. (2005) fabricated a calcium phosphate bone implant by sintering calcium phosphate powder coated with polymer. Postprocessing such as extra sintering is often required to increase part strengths, but sintering steps cause shrinkage of the parts.

A biocomposite blend comprising polyvinyl alcohol and HA was also sintered in SLS for craniofacial and joint defect applications (Chua et al., 2004). The biocomposite blends were obtained by coating HA with a water-soluble polyvinyl alcohol via a spray-drying technique or physical blending. A previous study also demonstrated the use of SLS to create polycaprolactone scaffolds with porous architecture and sufficient mechanical properties for bone tissue engineering applications (Williams et al., 2005).

This technique also may be used with patients' medical data to create anatomy-specific structures. Use of this technique to fabricate a mandibular condyle scaffold using CT data from a pig condyle (Williams et al., 2005). The integration of computational design and SLS techniques enables fabrication of scaffolds that have anatomically shaped external architectures and porous interior structure.

The use of high processing temperatures limits the incorporation of temperature-sensitive materials in SLS procedures. The conduction and diffusion of laser heat causes unwanted bonding of neighboring powders, and these limit the resolution of final features. Another limitation of SLS is the smaller range of pore sizes in the fabricated structures, because the size of the pores created depends on the particle size of the powder used.

Fused deposition modeling

In FDM, 2D patterns are constructed by selective extrusion of molten thermoplastic materials through two heated extrusion tips (Zein et al., 2002; Fig 8-10). One nozzle deposits the filament modeling material, and the second deposits a temporary material to support cantilevers. In a traditional FDM technique, a thermoplastic polymer feeds into an FDM extrusion head, where it is melted to semiliquid state. The FDM head extrudes the material through a nozzle and deposits it on the build platform. Once a layer is built, molten droplets are deposited and jointed to the previous layer.

With FDM there is no theoretical restriction on compositional gradients, especially when multiple deposition nozzles are available. One variation of FDM uses inkjet printheads to deposit plastic models in a laminated fashion. The use of additional extrusion nozzles for multiple build materials, each depositing different matter, should allow flexible compositional variation in all three dimensions. However, this theoretical possibility has not been developed in practice. Some control of microstructure may be possible during FDM through the manipulation of deposition parameters.

Heat transfer characteristics and rheology are critical to the selection of proper materials for FDM. Thermoplastics such as polyvinyl chloride, nylon, acrylonitrile butadiene styrene, and investment casting wax have been successfully used in FDM. The molten droplet must be hot enough to rapidly induce fusion with previously extruded beads yet solidify fast enough to minimize flow and feature size. The viscosity must be low enough during the molten stage to

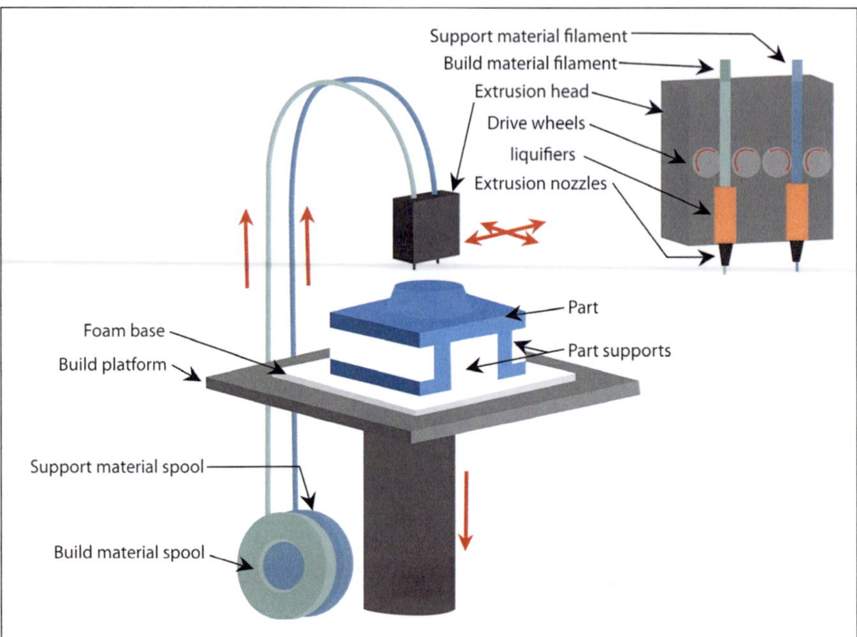

Figure 8-10 Fused deposition modeling (reprinted from CustomPart.Net with permission; CustomPart. Net. http://www.custompartnet.com).

allow reliable extrusion through a fine nozzle to minimize feature size yet high enough during the burnout stage to prevent large-scale collapse in the furnace. Chemical modifiers may be required to facilitate the use of other thermoplastics.

FDM has been employed to construct a carotid lumen model for in vitro flow analysis (Pili et al., 2011). Biocompatibility requirements impose constraints on the type of rheologic modifiers that can be used. Hutmacher et al. (2001) applied FDM to fabricate tissue engineering scaffolds with polycaprolactone, a biodegradable polymer with low glass transition temperature.

Scaffolds with controlled pore size, morphology, and interconnectivity can be obtained if the extrusion head is moved in the horizontal x-y plane. Zein et al. (2002) fabricated polycaprolactone scaffolds with different pore morphologies and different channel sizes by changing the pattern that was deposited. Several composites, such as polycaprolactone-HA or polycaprolactone-tricalcium phosphate, also have been fabricated by FDM to provide favorable mechanical and biochemical properties for bone regeneration (Rai et al., 2004).

FDM is limited by the material range because only thermoplastic materials with low melting transition and low viscosity can be readily extruded through the FDM head. These material limitations have limited the shape complexity of biologic scaffolding materials, which are typically confined to relatively regular structures (Hutmacher et al., 2001). However, the geometric complexity of FDM products is not limited if industrial materials are selected to have optimal thermal and rheologic properties but lack biocompatibility. Even with biocompatible materials, temperature-sensitive biologic agents and living cells cannot be incorporated during the fabrication process because of the high processing temperature.

Use of this technique to fabricate a patient-matched implant for the rehabilitation of large craniofacial defects has been previously reported (Gronet et al., 2003). A CT scan from a patient was sent to FDM, and a 3D craniofacial model was generated from acrylonitrile butadiene styrene plastic resin, which can be easily modified by milling and drilling afterward. The planned extent of bony resection was marked by a surgeon, and then the marked area was removed from the fabricated model. A synthetic molding material was used to fashion an implant prototype based on the estimated defect model. After a casting mold was created around this prototype, the pattern was burned out completely and replaced with titanium or other bone tissue replacement polymers. The fabricated implant was then checked for fit from the craniofacial defect model. The implant was found to be well adapted to the bony margins of the defect.

Recent developments in multibiomaterial 3D printing with FDM and MJ enable the bioengineer to design beyond complex geometry and microarchitecture. Besides introducing novel scaffold functionality by controlling material properties from point-to-point within the same build, simultaneous printing of multiple materials can also greatly simplify the manufacturing process and, in turn, the quality assurance systems and regulatory checkpoints. The next section focuses on printing with cells.

Bioprinting

Direct Writing is a variation of FDM in which molten thermoplastics are replaced with gels and pastes. Usually, these are too viscous to be printed by MJ but can be extruded without heating, making it ideal for depositing cells. When cells are being deposited, the process is commonly termed *Bioprinting*, which can be defined as the process of manipulating cell-laden bioink to create cell-containing constructs with structural organization. In 3D bioprinting, bioink should be biocompatible, printable, and mechanically stable to hold live cells.

Hydrogel precursor formulations are the most common bioink component because they provide a suitable environment to sustain live cells as well as adjustable mechanical and biodegradable properties (Schwab et al., 2020). Bioprinting utilizes conventional

3D printing technologies, most commonly inkjet, microextrusion, laser-assisted, and stereolithography printing (Fig 8-11). Because of the specific biomaterial and biological requirements for bioink, each technique has its own strengths and weaknesses in bioprinting.

In inkjet printing, low viscosity liquid bioinks with the appropriate surface tension profile are required to enable droplet formation (Groot et al., 2021) After printing, the ink in a liquid form should transition into a solid 3D structure in order to provide the essential biological and structural functions as a tissue-engineering scaffold. To meet such requirements, researchers utilized hydrogels that can be cross-linked after deposition via light or controlled ionic, pH, temperature, host-guest interaction, and enzymatic interactions (Murphy and Atala, 2014). Cell suspensions or colloidal solutions are deposited with patterns of single drops in lines of ~50 μm wide (Nakamura et al., 2005).

Xu et al. (2005) demonstrated that inkjet printing technology can precisely place the cells and proteins in 3D alginate structures. This technology provides a controlled spatial distribution of cell or growth factors as well as the scaffold structures. Cui et al. (2012) used a modified HP Deskjet 500 thermal inkjet printer to deposit human articular chondrocytes and poly(ethylene glycol) dimethacrylate (PEGDMA) into a cartilage defect within osteochondral plugs. Simultaneous photopolymerization during layer-by-layer deposition enhanced the viability of printed human chondrocytes by 26% compared with the case of postpolymerization. The printed cartilage implant was successfully integrated into the surrounding tissue and showed a compressive modulus comparable to that of a native human articular cartilage. In another study, a modified HP Deskjet 550C printer was used to fabricate bone constructs, made by layer-by-layer printing of human and rodent amniotic fluid-derived stem cells into an alginate/collagen composite gel (De Coppi et al., 2007). After osteogenic differentiation in vitro for one week, the scaffold/cell constructs were subcutaneously implanted into mice. The printed scaffolds were shown to form bone over a period of several months in vivo.

The inkjet printing technology allows high printing speed, enabling a direct deposition of cells and materials into cartilage or bone defects. However, inkjet-based bioprinting is limited to low cell concentration (fewer than 10 million cells/ml; Xu et al., 2005); high cell concentration can cause nozzle clogging and high shear stress. Further studies are needed to print biologically relevant cell concentrations but without intervening the hydrogel cross-linking mechanisms.

In extrusion-based bioprinting, the bioinks are deposited as small beads of material in two dimensions rather than liquid droplets. The hydrogel precursors, biocompatible copolymers, and cell spheroids can be extruded via a small-sized nozzle through a pneumatic, piston, or thermal extrusion-driven method. Hydrogel precursors with sheer-thinning properties are often employed in extrusion bioprinting to form shape-stable gels upon deposition. The advantages of extrusion bioprinting include high resolution, high cell densities, and the capability of the controlled deposition of a variety of inks.

Bittner et al. (2019) fabricated porous PCL and PCL-hydroxyapatite scaffolds exhibiting vertical gradients in porosity and ceramic content for osteochondral tissue engineering. Kuzucu et al. (2021) employed a static mixer positioned before the printing nozzle to blend native agarose and carboxylated agarose where the number of carboxylic acid groups along the polymer backbone is a function of hydrogel stiffness. The static mixer allowed objects to print with a gradient of stiffness, cell concentration, and immobilized peptides mimicking complex anisotropic osteochondral interface. Sun et al. (2020) successfully built MSC-laden constructs for cartilage repair using a multimaterial extrusion system equipped with a multicartridge module. PCL from syringe A was coprinted with BMSC-laden hydrogel containing PLGA microspheres from syringe B into the microchannels. The PCL fiber spacing was controlled to generate scaffolds with mechanical gradients (from 150 μm to 750 μm). BMP4 and TGFβ3 were encapsulated within PLGA microspheres for a spatiotemporal growth factor release at the defect site. These gradient-structured scaffolds showed enhanced cartilage repair in a rabbit knee cartilage defect model in vivo.

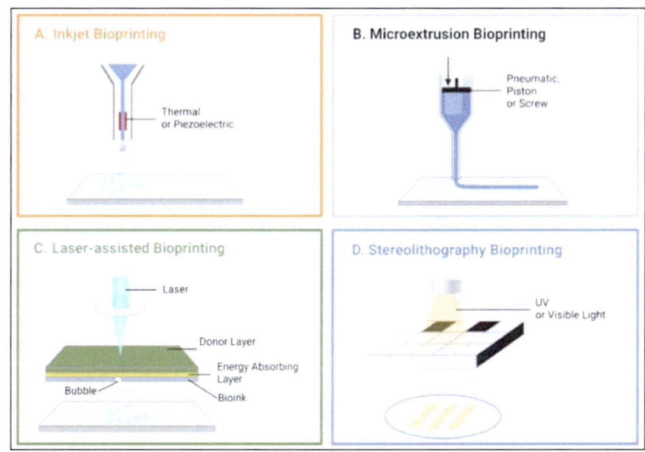

Figure 8-11 Examples of bioprinting techniques (created with BioRender.com permission).

One major challenge in extrusion bioprinting is low cell viability compared with inkjet-based bioprinting. Widening the nozzle diameter can ease shear stress inflicted on cells, but it compromises printing resolution. The optimization of the nozzle, syringe, and stage module could increase the biocompatibility of printed cell-laden scaffolds in extrusion bioprinting.

Laser-assisted bioprinting is a nozzle-free printing mode that can relax the bioinks requirement for viscosity and surface tension. In laser-induced forward transfer (LIFT) technology, a pulsed laser is focused toward a laser-absorbing biomaterial layer, which helps in developing a local pressure to propel biomaterial onto a collector substrate. This technology has been used to deposit nanohydroxyapatite in a mouse calvarial defect model (Keriquel et al., 2010). A 3 mm diameter and 600 μm-deep calvarial hole was filled in situ, demonstrating a proof-of-concept that in vivo bioprinting is possible. The high cost and time-consuming procedures required in laser-assisted bioprinting need to be further addressed for future tissue engineering applications.

Stereolithography bioprinting is a light-based technique where controlled illumination selectively transforms liquid bioinks into solid features via photo-cross-linking in a layer-by-layer manner, offering high spatial resolution. The bioink for stereolithography should possess photocurable moieties, such as PEG or PEGDMA, to generate constructs. In a recent study (Amier et al., 2021), human jawbone model constructs containing primary jawbone-derived osteoblasts and vasculature-like channel structures were fabricated. Over the 28 days of cultivation, both osteoblasts and endothelial cells survived and expressed cell type–specific markers. Constructs showed mineralization with hinted osteocyte differentiation, demonstrating the successful biofabrication of an in vitro model of the human jawbone.

Summary

Once considered an esoteric and anecdotal field, tissue engineering has challenged conventional understanding of cell biology and has attracted engineers, basic scientists, and medical practitioners to solve highly intricate problems that were once thought insurmountable. If successful, tissue-engineered maxillofacial replacements will obviate some of the current shortcomings of synthetic materials and the limited availability of tissue grafts.

Despite the exciting progress summarized in this chapter, further studies are needed to address the remaining challenges. Much work is needed to gain better understanding and controlling of stem cell differentiation, to improve the predictability of host-implant interactions, and to ensure proper delivery of bioactive molecules to promote regeneration around irradiated tissues with poor vasculature and healing capacity. The emergence of stem cells, coupled with the development of new gene editing tools, such as CRISPR, and gene regulation tools, such as noncoding RNA, will undoubtedly accelerate the pace of discovery in these areas.

However, even if these biologic challenges are addressed, the critical problem of nutrient transport must be resolved to allow regeneration of large maxillofacial tissues. Advanced material deposition technologies that can orchestrate the spatial distribution of cells, signals, and scaffolding materials to guide cellular ingrowth, proliferation, and differentiation will go a long way toward addressing some of these challenges. Several 3D manufacturing technologies have already been employed for the fabrication of patient-specific scaffolds based on digitized medical imaging data. Research that elucidates cell-environment interactions will provide critical information that is needed to refine the mathematical models. These models, in turn, can be used to develop the bioinspired design rules for regenerating large complex maxillofacial tissues.

Computer-driven RP technologies offer exciting opportunities for the tissue engineering of highly complex maxillofacial tissues. These technologies have a range of material constraints, postprocessing requirements, cellular compatibilities, and abilities to selectively position multiple materials in 3D patterns. Novel technologies that overcome these limitations can have broad-based impact on tissue engineering as well as other biomedical applications.

Since the last edition of this textbook, SFF techniques have vastly improved in terms of controlling microscopic features, but none can manipulate nanoscale features because of the limited resolution of the deposition technology. Control over the structural properties of scaffolds at the nanoscale may promote cellular attachment and proliferation. Integration of nanofabrication techniques with SFF technologies will provide great capabilities in fabricating 3D constructs for complex tissue regeneration.

These technological accomplishments will expand the treatment options for patients with large defects of the head and neck. While surgical rehabilitation is currently preferable for small, simple defects in patients who prefer to repair defects with their own tissues, the ability to graft larger and more complex tissues will expand the indications for tissue replacements. Although the regenerated tissues may not match the astounding cosmetic results that can be achieved by state-of-the-art maxillofacial prosthesis, tissue grafts may offer functional and biologic benefits that enhance clinical success if patient expectations are also managed properly. The bright future of tissue engineering illuminates the tremendous challenges ahead. It is exciting that the National Institute of Dental and Craniofacial Research has committed tens of millions of dollars to establish two national consortia to create the critical infrastructure to accelerate the clinical translation of innovative regenerative therapies to replace dental, oral, and craniofacial tissues or organs lost to congenital disorders, traumatic injuries, diseases, and medical procedures. These funds have attracted scientists from other fields to focus on oral and craniofacial tissue regeneration with support from industry experts to push highly competitive projects toward human clinical studies and commercialization.

References

Aalami OO, Nacamuli RP, Lenton KA, et al. Applications of a mouse model of calvarial healing: Differences in regenerative abilities of juveniles and adults. Plast Reconstr Surg 2004;114:713–720.

Abu-Serriah M, Ayoub A, Boyd J, Paterson C, Wray D. The role of ultrasound in monitoring reconstruction of mandibular continuity defects using osteogenic protein-1 (rhOP-1). Int J Oral Maxillofac Surg 2003;32:619–627.

Aghaloo T, Cowan CM, Chou YF, et al. Nell-1-induced bone regeneration in calvarial defects. Am J Pathol 2006;169:903–915.

Ahrens M, Ankenbauer T, Schröder D, Hollnagel A, Mayer H, Gross G. Expression of human bone morphogenetic proteins-2 or proteins-4 in murine mesenchymal progenitor C3h10t1/2 cells induces differentiation into distinct mesenchymal cell lineages. DNA Cell Biol 1993;12:871–880.

Aki T, Mizukami Y, Oka Y, et al. Phosphoinositide 3-kinase accelerates necrotic cell death during hypoxia. Biochem J 2001;358:481–487.

Amier AK, Thomas A, Tuzuner S, et al. 3D bioprinting of tissue-specific osteoblasts and endothelial cells to model the human jawbone. Sci Rep 2021;11:4876.

Andriano KP, Chandrashekar B, McEnery, et al. Preliminary in vivo studies on the osteogenic potential of bone morphogenetic proteins delivered from an absorbable puttylike polymer matrix. J Biomed Mater Res 2000;53:36–43.

Arcaute K, Mann B, Wicker R. Stereolithography of spatially controlled multi-material bioactive poly(ethylene glycol) scaffolds. Acta Biomater 2010;6:1047–1054.

Artico M, Ferrante L, Pastore FS, et al. Bone autografting of the calvaria and craniofacial skeleton: Historical background, surgical results in a series of 15 patients, and review of the literature. Surg Neurol 2003;60:71–79.

Ashjian PH, Elbarbary AS, Edmonds B, et al. In vitro differentiation of human processed lipoaspirate cells into early neural progenitors. Plast Reconstr Surg 2003;111:1922–1931.

Baumgardner JE, Otto CM. In vitro intermittent hypoxia: Challenges for creating hypoxia in cell culture. Respir Physiol Neurobiol 2003;136:131–139.

Bayne SC. Dental biomaterials: Where are we and where are we going? J Dent Educ 2005;69:571–585.

Bittner SM, Smith BT, Diaz-Gomez L, et al. Fabrication and mechanical characterization of 3D printed vertical uniform and gradient scaffolds for bone and osteochondral tissue engineering. Acta Biomater 2019;90:37–48.

Blaney Davidson EN, van der Kraan PM, van den Berg WB. TGF-β and osteoarthritis. Osteoarthritis Cartilage 2007;15:597–604.

Blum JS, Barry MA, Mikos AG, et al. In vivo evaluation of gene therapy vectors in ex vivo-derived marrow stromal cells for bone regeneration in a rat critical-size calvarial defect model. Hum Gene Ther 2003;14:1689–1701.

Blum KS, Schneider SJ, Rosenthal AD. Methyl methacrylate cranioplasty in children: Long-term results. Pediatr Neurosurg 1997;26:33–35.

Boden SD, Kang J, Sandhu H, et al. Use of recombinant human bone morphogenetic protein-2 to achieve posterolateral lumbar spine fusion in humans: A prospective, randomized clinical pilot trial: 2002 Volvo Award in clinical studies. Spine 2002;27:2662–2273.

Boden SD, McCuaig K, Hair G, et al. Differential effects and glucocorticoid potentiation of bone morphogenetic protein action during rat osteoblast differentiation in vitro. Endocrinology 1996;137:3401–3407.

Bonarius HPJ, de Gooijer CD, Tramper J, et al. Determination of the respiration quotient in mammalian-cell culture in bicarbonate buffered media. Biotechnol Bioeng 1995;45:524–535.

Bonucci E, Marini E, Valdinucci F, et al. Osteogenic response to hydroxyapatite-fibrin implants in maxillofacial bone defects. Eur J Oral Sci 1997;105:557–561.

Bosch P, Musgrave DS, Lee JY, et al. Osteoprogenitor cells within skeletal muscle. J Orthop Res 2000;18:933–944.

Bostrom R, Mikos A, editors. Tissue Engineering of Bone, vol 1. Boston: Birkhauser; 1997.

Bottaro DP, Liebmann-Vinson A, Heidaran MA. Molecular signaling in bioengineered tissue microenvironments. Ann NY Acad Sci 2002;961:143–153.

Boyne PJ, Marx RE, Nevins M, et al. A feasibility study evaluating rhBMP-2/absorbable collagen sponge for maxillary sinus floor augmentation. Int J Periodontics Restorative Dent 1997;17:11–25.

Bragdon CR, Doherty AM, Rubash HE, et al. The efficacy of BMP-2 to induce bone ingrowth in a total hip replacement model. Clin Orthop 2003;417:50–61.

Brittberg M, Sjögren-Jansson E, Lindahl A, et al. Influence of fibrin sealant (Tisseel) on osteochondral defect repair in the rabbit knee. Biomaterials 1997;18:235–242.

Brown DA, MacLellan WR, Dunn JC, et al. Hypoxic cell death is reduced by pH buffering in a model of engineered heart tissue. Artif Cells Blood Substit Immobil Biotechnol 2008;36:94–113.

Brown DA, MacLellan WR, Laks H, et al. Analysis of oxygen transport in a diffusion-limited model of engineered heart tissue. Biotechnol Bioeng 2007a;97:962–975.

Brown DA, MacLellan WR, Wu BM, et al. Analysis of pH gradients resulting from mass transport limitations in engineered heart tissue. Ann Biomed Eng 2007b;35:1885–1897.

Bruder SP, Jaiswal N, Haynesworth SE. Growth kinetics, self-renewal, and the osteogenic potential of purified human mesenchymal stem cells during extensive subcultivation and following cryopreservation. J Cell Biochem 1997;64:278–294.

Boyan BD, Hummert TW, Dean DD, Schwartz Z. Role of material surfaces in regulating bone and cartilage cell response. Biomaterials 1996;17:137–146.

Bulpitt P, Aeschlimann D. New strategy for chemical modification of hyaluronic acid: Preparation of functionalized derivatives and their use in the formation of novel biocompatible hydrogels. J Biomed Mater Res 1999;47:152–169.

California Institute for Regenerative Medicine. 2010 Report of the external advisory panel. Accessed 15 Feb 2011. https://www.cirm.ca.gov/wp-content/uploads/archive/files/about_cirm/CIRM-EAP_Report.pdf.

Canady JW, Zeitler DP, Thompson SA, et al. Suitability of the iliac crest as a site for harvest of autogenous bone grafts. Cleft Palate Craniofac J 1993;30:579–581.

Carrier RL, Papadaki M, Rupnick M, et al. Cardiac tissue engineering: Cell seeding, cultivation parameters, and tissue construct characterization. Biotechnol Bioeng 1999;64:580–589.

Casey TM, Arthur PG. Hibernation in noncontracting mammalian cardiomyocytes. Circulation 2000;102:3124–3129.

Celeste AJ, Iannazzi JA, Taylor RC, et al. Identification of transforming growth-factor-beta family members present in bone-inductive protein purified from bovine bone. Proc Natl Acad Sci USA 1990;87:9843–9847.

Centrella M, Horowitz MC, Wozney JM, et al. Transforming growth factor-beta gene family members and bone. Endocr Rev 1994;15:27–39.

Chang SC, Chuang HL, Chen YR, et al. Ex vivo gene therapy in autologous bone marrow stromal stem cells for tissue-engineered maxillofacial bone regeneration. Gene Ther 2003;10:2013–2019.

Chang SC, Chuang H, Chen YR, et al. Cranial repair using BMP-2 gene engineered bone marrow stromal cells. J Surg Res 2004;119:85–91.

Chen G, Ushida T, Tateishi T. Poly(DL-lactic-co-glycolic acid) sponge hybridized with collagen microsponges and deposited apatite particulates. J Biomed Mater Res 2001;57:8–14.

Chen GP, Sato T, Tanaka J, et al. Preparation of a biphasic scaffold for osteochondral tissue engineering. Mater Sci Eng C 2006;26:118–123.

Chen TM, Wang HJ. Cranioplasty using allogeneic perforated demineralized bone matrix with autogenous bone paste. Ann Plast Surg 2002;49:272–277.

Cheng R, Liu L, Xiang Y, et al. Advanced liposome loaded scaffolds for therapeutic and tissue engineering applications. Biomaterials 2020 Feb;232:119706. http://doi.org/10.1016/j.biomaterials.2019.119706. Epub 2019 Dec 23.

Chou YF, Chiou WA, Xu YH, et al. The effect of pH on the structural evolution of accelerated biomimetic apatite. Biomaterials 2004;25:5323–5331.

Chou YF, Dunn JC, Wu BM. In vitro response of MC3T3-E1 preosteoblasts within three-dimensional apatite-coated PLGA scaffolds. J Biomed Mater Res B 2005a;75:81–90.

Chou YF, Huang WB, Dunn JC, et al. The effect of biomimetic apatite structure on osteoblast viability, proliferation, and gene expression. Biomaterials 2005b;26:285–295.

Chou YF, Zuk PA, Chang TL, et al. Adipose-derived stem cells and BMP2: Part 1. BMP2-treated adipose-derived stem cells do not improve repair of segmental femoral defects. Connect Tissue Res 2011;52(2):109–118. http://doi.org/10.3109/03008207.2010.484514. Epub 2010 Aug 11.

Chua CK, Leong KF, Tan KH, et al. Development of tissue scaffolds using selective laser sintering of polyvinyl alcohol/hydroxyapatite biocomposite for craniofacial and joint defects. J Mater Sci Mater Med 2004;15:1113–1121.

Chubinskaya S, Kuettner KE. Regulation of osteogenic proteins by chondrocytes. Int J Biochem Cell B 2003;35:1323–1340.

Chvapil M. Collagen sponge: Theory and practice of medical applications. J Biomed Mater Res 1977;11:721–741.

Cima LG, Sachs E, Cima LG, et al. Computer-derived microstructure by 3D printing: Bio- and structural materials. In Proceedings of the solid freeform fabrication symposium. Ed. Marcus HL. Austin: University of Texas; 1994. pp. 41–54.

Colin A, Boire JY. A novel tool for rapid prototyping and development of simple 3D medical image processing applications on PCs. Comput Methods Programs Biomed 1997;53:87–92.

Compton CC, Gill JM, Bradford DA, et al. Skin regenerated from cultured epithelial autografts on full-thickness burn wounds from 6 days to 5 years after grafting. A light, electron microscopic and immunohistochemical study. Lab Invest 1989;60:600–612.

Cook SD, Baffes GC, Wolfe MW, et al. The effect of recombinant human osteogenic protein-1 on healing of large segmental bone defects. J Bone Joint Surg Am 1994;76:827–838.

Cook SD, Wolfe MW, Salkeld SL, et al. Effect of recombinant human osteogenic protein-1 on healing of segmental defects in non-human primates. J Bone Joint Surg Am 1995;77:734–750.

Cowan C, Shi Y, Aalami O, et al. Adipose-derived adult stromal cells heal critical-sized mouse calvarial defects. Nature Biotechnol 2004;22:560–567.

Cowan CM, Aalami O, Shi Y, et al. Bone morphogenetic protein-2 and retinoic acid accelerate in vivo bone formation, osteoclast recruitment, and bone turnover. Tissue Eng 2005;11:645–658.

Cowan CM, Cheng S, Ting K, et al. Nell-1 induced bone formation within the distracted intermaxillary suture. Bone 2006;38:48–58.

Cui X, Breitenkamp K, Finn MG, et al. Direct human cartilage repair using three-dimensional bioprinting technology. Tissue Eng Part A 2012;18(11–12):1304–1312.

CustomPart.Net. Accessed 15 Feb 2011. http://www.custompartnet.com/.

Cutroneo KR. TGF-β-induced fibrosis and SMAD signaling: Oligo decoys as natural therapeutics for inhibition of tissue fibrosis and scarring. Wound Repair Regen 2007;15(suppl 1):S54–S60.

Davies LC, Blain EJ, Gilbert SJ, et al. The potential of IGF-1 and TGF-β 1 for promoting adult articular cartilage repair: An in vitro study. Tissue Eng Part A 2008;14:1251–1261.

Dean D, Topham NS, Meneghetti SC, et al. Poly(propylene fumarate) and poly(DL-lactic-co-glycolic acid) as scaffold materials for solid and foam-coated composite tissue-engineered constructs for cranial reconstruction. Tissue Eng 2003;9:495–504.

De Coppi P, Bartsch G, Siddiqui, et al. Isolation of amniotic stem cell lines with potential for therapy. Nat Biotechnol 2007;5:100–106.

de Jong DS, Vaes BL, Dechering KJ, et al. Identification of novel regulators associated with early-phase osteoblast differentiation. J Bone Miner Res 2004;19:947–958.

den Boer FC, Wippermann BW, Blokhuis TJ, et al. Healing of segmental bone defects with granular porous hydroxyapatite augmented with recombinant human osteogenic protein-1 or autologous bone marrow. J Orthop Res 2003;21:521–528.

Desai J, Shannon ME, Johnson MD, et al. *Nell1*-deficient mice have reduced expression of extracellular matrix proteins causing cranial and vertebral defects. Hum Mol Genet 2006;15:1329–1341.

De Ugarte DA, Morizono K, Elbarbary A, et al. Comparison of multi-lineage cells from human adipose tissue and bone marrow. Cells Tissues Organs 2003;174:101–109.

Dey M, Ozbolat I. 3D bioprinting of cells, tissues and organs. Sci Rep 2020;10:14023.

Dhariwala B, Hunt E, Boland T. Rapid prototyping of tissue-engineering constructs, using photopolymerizable hydrogels and stereolithography. Tissue Eng 2004;10(9–10):1316–1322.

Di Martino A, Sittinger M, Risbud MV. Chitosan: A versatile biopolymer for orthopaedic tissue-engineering. Biomaterials 2005;26:5983–5990.

Dodane V, Vilivalam VD. Pharmaceutical applications of chitosan. Pharm Sci Technol Today 1998;1:246–253.

Doss MX, Koehler CI, Gissel C, et al. Embryonic stem cells: A promising tool for cell replacement therapy. J Cell Mol Med 2004;8:465–473.

Dowler CA. Automatic model building cuts design time, costs. Plastics Eng 1989;45:43–45.

Dragoo JL, Choi JY, Lieberman JR, et al. Bone induction by BMP-2 transduced stem cells derived from human fat. J Orthop Res 2003;21:622–629.

Ducy P, Karsenty G. The family of bone morphogenetic proteins. Kidney Int 2000;57:2207–2214.

Dunn JC, Chan WY, Cristini V, et al. Analysis of cell growth in three-dimensional scaffolds. Tissue Eng 2006;12:705–716.

Dupoirieux L, Costes V, Jammet P, et al. Experimental study on demineralized bone matrix (DBM) and coral as bone graft substitutes in maxillofacial surgery. Int J Oral Maxillofac Surg 1994;23:395–398.

Egrise D, Martin D, Vienne A, et al. The number of fibroblastic colonies formed from bone marrow is decreased and the in vitro proliferation rate of trabecular bone cells increased in aged rats. Bone 1992;13:355–361.

Empire State Stem Cell Board. 2008–2009 Annual report of the empire state stem cell board and New York stem cell science program. Accessed 15 Feb 2011. https://stemcell.ny.gov/sites/default/files/documents/files/2008-2009_annualreport.pdf.

Enneking WF, Mindell ER. Observations on massive retrieved human allografts. J Bone Joint Surg Am 1991;73:1123–1142.

Enomoto H, Enomoto-Iwamoto M, Iwamoto M, et al. Cbfa1 is a positive regulatory factor in chondrocyte maturation. J Biol Chem 2000;275:8695–8702.

Erickson GR, Gimble JM, Franklin DM, et al. Chondrogenic potential of adipose tissue-derived stromal cells in vitro and in vivo. Biochem Biophys Res Commun 2002;290:763–769.

Eschenhagen T, Didié M, Heubach J, et al. Cardiac tissue engineering. Transpl Immunol 2002;9:315–321.

European Medicines Agency. Osigraft: EPAR Scientific Discussion. Accessed 15 Feb 2011. https://www.ema.europa.eu/en/documents/scientific-discussion/osigraft-epar-scientific-discussion_en.pdf.

Fan J, Im CS, Cui ZH, et al. Delivery of phenamil enhances BMP-2-induced osteogenic differentiation of adipose-derived stem cells and bone formation in calvarial defects. 2015 Jul;21(13–14):2053–2065. http://doi.org/10.1089/ten.TEA.2014.0489. Epub 2015 May 20.

Fan J, Lee CS, Kim S, et al. Generation of small RNA-modulated exosome mimetics for bone regeneration. ACS Nano 2020 Sep 22;14(9):11973–11984. http://doi.org/10.1021/acsnano.0c05122. Epub 2020 Sep 11.

Ferraro F, Celso CL, Scadden D. Adult stem cells and their niches. Adv Exp Med Biol 2010;695:155–168.

Fisher JP, Vehof JWM, Dean D, et al. Soft and hard tissue response to photocrosslinked poly(propylene fumarate) scaffolds in a rabbit model. J Biomed Mater Res 2002;59:547–556.

Freed LE, Marquis JC, Langer R, et al. Kinetics of chondrocyte growth in cell-polymer implants. Biotechnol Bioeng 1994;43:597–604.

Friess W, Uludag H, Biron RJ, et al. Recombitant human bone morphogenetic protein-2/collagen sponge combinations—in vitro and phamacokinetic performance. Pharm Res 1997;14:S155.

Friess W, Uludag H, Foskett S, et al. Characterization of absorbable collagen sponges as recombinant human bone morphogenetic protein-2 carriers. Int J Pharm 1999;185:51–60.

Galban CJ, Locke BR. Analysis of cell growth in a polymer scaffold using a moving boundary approach. Biotechnol Bioeng 1997;56:422–432.

Galban CJ, Locke BR. Analysis of cell growth kinetics and substrate diffusion in a polymer scaffold. Biotechnol Bioeng 1999a;65:121–132.

Galban CJ, Locke BR. Effects of spatial variation of cells and nutrient and product concentrations coupled with product inhibition on cell growth in a polymer scaffold. Biotechnol Bioeng 1999b;64:633–643.

Gallico GG III, O'Connor NE, Compton CC, et al. Permanent coverage of large burn wounds with autologous cultured human epithelium. N Engl J Med 1984;311:448–451.

Gandolfi MG, Gardin C, Zamparini F, et al. Mineral-doped poly(L-lactide) acid scaffolds enriched with exosomes improve osteogenic commitment of human adipose-derived mesenchymal stem cells. Nanomaterials (Basel) 2020 Feb 29;10(3):432. http://doi.org/10.3390/nano10030432.

Geers C, Gros G. Carbon dioxide transport and carbonic anhydrase in blood and muscle. Physiol Rev 2000;80:681–715.

Geesink RG, Hoefnagels NH, Bulstra SK. Osteogenic activity of OP-1 bone morphogenetic protein (BMP-7) in a human fibular defect. J Bone Joint Surg Br 1999;81:710–718.

Geiger M, Li RH, Friess W. Collagen sponges for bone regeneration with rhBMP-2. Adv Drug Deliv Rev 2003;55:1613–1629.

Gerhart TN, Kirker-Head CA, Kriz MJ, et al. Healing segmental femoral defects in sheep using recombinant human bone morphogenetic protein. Clin Orthop 1993;293:317–326.

Giannobile WV. Periodontal tissue engineering by growth factors. Bone 1996;19(1 suppl):23S–37S.

Gittens SA, Bagnall K, Matyas JR, et al. Imparting bone mineral affinity to osteogenic proteins through heparin-bisphosphonate conjugates. J Control Release 2004;98:255–268.

Goldstein JA. The use of bioresorbable material in craniofacial surgery. Clin Plast Surg 2001;28:653–659.

Govender S, Csimma C, Genant HK, et al. Recombinant human bone morphogenetic protein-2 for treatment of open tibial fractures—a prospective, controlled, randomized study of four hundred and fifty patients. J Bone Joint Surg Am 2002;84-A:2123–2134.

Green H, Kehinde O, Thomas J. Growth of cultured human epidermal cells into multiple epithelia suitable for grafting. Proc Natl Acad Sci USA 1979;76:5665–5568.

Gregory CF. The current status of bone and joint transplants. Clin Orthop 1972;87:165–166.

Griffith L, Wu BM, Cima MJ, et al. In vitro organogenesis of liver tissue. Ann NY Acad Sci 1997;831:382–397.

Gronet PM, Waskewicz GA, Richardson C. Preformed acrylic cranial implants using fused deposition modeling: A clinical report. J Prosthet Dent 2003;90:429–433.

Groot AL, Remmers JS, Hartong DT. Three-dimensional computer-aided design of a full-color ocular prosthesis with textured iris and sclera manufactured in one single print job. 3D Printing and Additive Manufacturing 2021;10:1089.

Gründer T, Gaissmaier C, Fritz J, et al. Bone morphogenetic protein (BMP)-2 enhances the expression of type II collagen and aggrecan in chondrocytes embedded in alginate beads. Osteoarthritis Cartilage 2004;12:559–567.

Gungor-Ozkerim P, Inci I, Zhang YS, et al. Bioinks for 3D bioprinting: An overview. Biomater Sci 2018;6:915–946.

Gu K, Zhang L, Jin T, et al. Identification of potential modifiers of Runx2/Cbfa1 activity in C2C12 cells in response to bone morphogenetic protein-7. Cells Tissues Organs 2004;176:28–40.

Gundle R, Joyner CJ, Triffitt JT. Human bone tissue formation in diffusion chamber culture in vivo by bone-derived cells and marrow stromal fibroblastic cells. Bone 1995;16:597–601.

Gysin R, Wergedal JE, Sheng MH, et al. Ex vivo gene therapy with stromal cells transduced with a retroviral vector containing the *BMP4* gene completely heals critical size calvarial defect in rats. Gene Ther 2002;9:991–999.

Halvorsen YD, Bond A, Sen A, et al. Thiazolidinediones and glucocorticoids synergistically induce differentiation of human adipose tissue stromal cells: Biochemical, cellular, and molecular analysis. Metabolism 2001a;50:407–413.

Halvorsen YD, Franklin D, Bond AL, et al. Extracellular matrix mineralization and osteoblast gene expression by human adipose tissue-derived stromal cells. Tissue Eng 2001b;7:729–741.

Ham A. A histological study of the early phases of bone repair. J Bone Joint Surg Am 1930;12:827–844.

Hanada K, Dennis JE, Caplan AI. Stimulatory effects of basic fibroblast growth factor and bone morphogenetic protein-2 on osteogenic differentiation of rat bone marrow-derived mesenchymal stem cells. J Bone Miner Res 1997;12:1606–1614.

Hangody L, Kish G, Módis L, et al. Mosaicplasty for the treatment of osteochondritis dissecans of the talus: Two to seven year results in 36 patients. Foot Ankle Int 2001;22:552–558.

Harland RM. The transforming growth factor beta family and induction of the vertebrate mesoderm: Bone morphogenetic proteins are ventral inducers. Proc Natl Acad Sci USA 1994;91:10243–10246.

Haynesworth SE, Goshima J, Goldberg VM, et al. Characterization of cells with osteogenic potential from human marrow. Bone 1992;13:81–88.

Heissler E, Fischer FS, Bolouri S, et al. Custom-made cast titanium implants produced with CAD/CAM for the reconstruction of cranium defects. Int J Oral Maxillofac Surg 1998;27:334–338.

Ho W, Tawil B, Dunn JC, et al. The behavior of human mesenchymal stem cells in 3D fibrin clots: Dependence on fibrinogen concentration and clot structure. Tissue Eng 2006;12:1587–1595.

Hogan BL. Bone morphogenetic proteins: Multifunctional regulators of vertebrate development. Genes Dev 1996;10:1580–1594.

Holland TA, Bodde EWH, Baggett LS, et al. Osteochondral repair in the rabbit model utilizing bilayered, degradable oligo(poly(ethylene glycol) fumarate) hydrogel scaffolds. J Biomed Mater Res A 2005;75:156–167.

Hollinger JO, Battistone GC. Biodegradable bone repair materials. Synthetic polymers and ceramics. Clin Orthop 1986;207:290–305.

Hollinger JO, Kleinschmidt JC. The critical size defect as an experimental model to test bone repair materials. J Craniofac Surg 1990;1:60–68.

Hollinger JO, Uludag H, Winn SR. Sustained release emphasizing recombinant human bone morphogenetic protein-2. Adv Drug Deliv Rev 1998;31:303–318.

Hollister SJ, Maddox RD, Taboas JM. Optimal design and fabrication of scaffolds to mimic tissue properties and satisfy biological constraints. Biomaterials 2002;23:4095–4103.

Howell TH, Fiorellini J, Jones A, et al. A feasibility study evaluating rhBMP-2/absorbable collagen sponge device for local alveolar ridge preservation or augmentation. Int J Periodontics Restorative Dent 1997;17:124–139.

Hu W, Wang Z, Xiao Y, et al. Advances in crosslinking strategies of biomedical hydrogels. Biomater Sci 2019;7:843–855.

Hughes FJ, Collyer J, Stanfield M, et al. The effects of bone morphogenetic protein-2, -4, and -6 on differentiation of rat osteoblast cells in vitro. Endocrinology 1995;136:2671–2677.

Hunt DR, Jovanovic SA, Wikesjö UM, et al. Hyaluronan supports recombinant human bone morphogenetic protein-2 induced bone reconstruction of advanced alveolar ridge defects in dogs. A pilot study. J Periodontol 2001;72:651–658.

Hunziker EB, Driesang IMK, Saager C. Structural barrier principle for growth factor-based articular cartilage repair. Clin Orthop Relat Res 2001;(391 suppl):S182–S189.

Hutmacher DW, Schantz T, Zein I, et al. Mechanical properties and cell cultural response of polycaprolactone scaffolds designed and fabricated via fused deposition modeling. J Biomed Mater Res 2001;55:203–216.

Hutmacher DW, Sittinger M, Risbud MV. Scaffold-based tissue engineering: Rationale for computer-aided design and solid free-form fabrication systems. Trends Biotechnol 2004;22:354–362.

Iannone F, Lapadula G. Phenotype of chondrocytes in osteoarthritis. Biorheology 2008;45:411–413.

Im GI, Kim DY, Shin JH, et al. Repair of cartilage defect in the rabbit with cultured mesenchymal stem cells from bone marrow. J Bone Joint Surg Br 2001;83:289–294.

Jerosch J, Filler T, Peuker E. Is there an option for harvesting autologous osteochondral grafts without damaging weight-bearing areas in the knee joint? Knee Surg Sports Traumatol Arthrosc 2000;8:237–240.

Johnstone B, Hering TM, Caplan AI, et al. In vitro chondrogenesis of bone marrow-derived mesenchymal progenitor cells. Exp Cell Res 1998;238:265–272.

Joyce ME, Roberts AB, Sporn MB, et al. Transforming growth factor-beta and the initiation of chondrogenesis and osteogenesis in the rat femur. J Cell Biol 1990;110:2195–2207.

Kang Q, Sun MH, Cheng H, et al. Characterization of the distinct orthotopic bone-forming activity of 14 BMPs using recombinant adenovirus-mediated gene delivery. Gene Ther 2004;11:1312–1320.

Kang M, Lee CS, Lee M. Bioactive scaffolds integrated with liposomal or extracellular vesicles for bone regeneration. Bioengineering (Basel) 2021 Oct 1;8(10):137. http://doi.org/10.3390/bioengineering8100137.

Kanwar R, Prevost S, Mehta SK. Reply to the "Comment on 'Physicochemical stimuli as tuning parameters to modulate the structure and stability of nanostructured lipid carriers and release kinetics of encapsulated antileprosy drugs'" by J. Kang and A. M. Kang. J Mater Chem B 2020 Nov 18;8(44):10209–10210. http://doi.org/10.1039/d0tb02155e.

Katagiri T, Yamaguchi A, Komaki M, et al. Bone morphogenetic protein-2 converts the differentiation pathway of C2c12 myoblasts into the osteoblast lineage. J Cell Biol 1994;127:1755–1766.

Kenley RA, Yim K, Abrams J, et al. Biotechnology and bone graft substitutes. Pharm Res 1993;10:1393–1401.

Keriquel V, Guillemot F, Arnault I, et al. In vivo bioprinting for computer- and robotic-assisted medical intervention: Preliminary study in mice. Biofabrication 2010;2(1):014101.

Kim HD, Valentini RF. Retention and activity of BMP-2 in hyaluronic acid-based scaffolds in vitro. J Biomed Mater Res 2002;59:573–584.

Kim J, Hadlock T, Cheney M, et al. Muscle tissue engineering for partial glossectomy defects. Arch Facial Plast Surg 2003;5:403–407.

Kim SS, Utsunomiya H, Koski JA, et al. Survival and function of hepatocytes on a novel three-dimensional synthetic biodegradable polymer scaffold with an intrinsic network of channels. Ann Surg 1998;228:8–13.

Kinikoglu B, Auxenfans C, Pierrillas P, et al. Reconstruction of a full-thickness collagen-based human oral mucosal equivalent. Biomaterials 2009;30:6418–6425.

Kirsch T, Sebald W, Dreyer MK. Crystal structure of the BMP-2-BRIA ectodomain complex. Nat Struct Biol 2000;7:492–496.

Kline RM, Wolfe SA. Complications associated with the harvesting of cranial bone-grafts. Plast Reconstr Surg 1995;95:5–13.

Komori T, Yagi H, Nomura S, et al. Targeted disruption of Cbfa1 results in a complete lack of bone formation owing to maturational arrest of osteoblasts. Cell 1997;89:755–764.

Koppel DA, Moos KF, Walker FS. Skull reconstruction with a two-part interlocking custom-made titanium plate. Br J Oral Maxillofac Surg 1999;37:70–72.

Krebsbach PH, Gu K, Franceschi RT, Rutherford RB. Gene therapy-directed osteogenesis: BMP-7-transduced human fibroblasts form bone in vivo. Hum Gene Ther 2000;11:1201–1210.

Krebsbach PH, Mankani MH, Satomura K, Kuznetsov SA, Robey PG. Repair of craniotomy defects using bone marrow stromal cells. Transplantation 1998;66:1272–1278.

Kreklau B, Sittinger M, Mensing MB, et al. Tissue engineering of biphasic joint cartilage transplants. Biomaterials 1999;20:1743–1479.

Kruyt MC, Dhert WJ, Yuan H, et al. Bone tissue engineering in a critical size defect compared to ectopic implantations in the goat. J Orthop Res 2004;22:544–551.

Kuroda S, Oyasu M, Kawakami M, et al. Biochemical characterization and expression analysis of neural thrombospondin-1-like proteins NELL1 and NELL2. Biochem Biophys Res Commun 1999;265:79–86.

Kuroda S, Tanizawa K. Involvement of epidermal growth factor-like domain of NELL proteins in the novel protein-protein interaction with protein kinase C. Biochem Biophys Res Commun 1999;265:752–757.

Kurz LT, Garfin SR, Booth RE. Harvesting autogenous iliac bone grafts. A review of complications and techniques. Spine 1989;14:1324–1331.

Kuzucu M, Vera G, Beaumont M, et al. Extrusion-based 3D bioprinting of gradients of stiffness, cell density, and immobilized peptide using thermogelling hydrogels. ACS Biomater Sci Eng 2021;7(6):2192–2197.

Kwak JH, Zhang Y, Park J, et al. Pharmacokinetics and osteogenic potential of PEGylated NELL-1 in vivo after systemic administration. Biomaterials 2015;57:73–83.

Lam CXF, Mo XM, Teoh SH, Hutmacher DW. Scaffold development using 3D printing with a starch-based polymer. Mater Sci Eng C 2002;20:49–56.

Langer R, Vacanti JP. Tissue engineering. Science 1993;260:920–926.

Lapadula G, Iannone F, Zuccaro C, et al. Chondrocyte phenotyping in human osteoarthritis. Clin Rheumatol 1998;17:99–104.

Laurent TC, Fraser JR. Hyaluronan. FASEB J 1992;6:2397–2404.

Laurie SWS, Kaban LB, Mulliken JB, Murray JE. Donor-site morbidity after harvesting rib and iliac bone. Plast Reconstr Surg 1984;73:933–938.

Lee CH, Singla A, Lee Y. Biomedical applications of collagen. Int J Pharm 2001a;22:1–22.

Lee CS, Kim S, Fan J, et al. Smoothened agonist sterosome immobilized hybrid scaffold for bone regeneration. Sci Adv 2020 Apr 22;6(17):eaaz7822. http://doi.org/10.1126/sciadv.aaz7822. eCollection 2020 Apr.

Lee JA, Parrett BM, Conejero JA, et al. Biological alchemy: Engineering bone and fat from fat-derived stem cells. Ann Plast Surg 2003;50:610–617.

Lee JY, Musgrave D, Pelinkovic D, et al. Effect of bone morphogenetic protein-2-expressing muscle-derived cells on healing of critical-sized bone defects in mice. J Bone Joint Surg Am 2001b;83:1032–1039.

Lee JY, Peng H, Usas A, et al. Enhancement of bone healing based on ex vivo gene therapy using human muscle-derived cells expressing bone morphogenetic protein 2. Hum Gene Ther 2002a;13:1201–1211.

Lee KS, Hong SH, Bae SC. Both the Smad and p38 MAPK pathways play a crucial role in Runx2 expression following induction by transforming growth factor-beta and bone morphogenetic protein. Oncogene 2002b;21:7156–7163.

Lee M, Dunn JCY, Wu BM. Scaffold fabrication by indirect three-dimensional printing. Biomaterials 2005;26:4281–4289.

Lee M, Li WM, Siu RK, et al. Biomimetic apatite-coated alginate/chitosan microparticles as osteogenic protein carriers. Biomaterials 2009a;30:6094–6101.

Lee M, Siu RK, Ting K, et al. Effect of Nell-1 delivery on chondrocyte proliferation and cartilaginous extracellular matrix deposition. Tissue Eng Part A 2010;16:1791–1800.

Lee M, Wu BM, Dunn JC. Effect of scaffold architecture and pore size on smooth muscle cell growth. J Biomed Mater Res A 2009b;87:1010–1016.

Leong KF, Cheah CM, Chua CK. Solid freeform fabrication of three-dimensional scaffolds for engineering replacement tissues and organs. Biomaterials 2003;24:2363–2378.

Leong KF, Phua KKS, Chua CK, et al. Fabrication of porous polymeric matrix drug delivery devices using the selective laser sintering technique. Proc Inst Mech Eng H 2001;215:191–201.

Levine JP, Bradley J, Turk AE, et al. Bone morphogenetic protein promotes vascularization and osteoinduction in preformed hydroxyapatite in the rabbit. Ann Plast Surg 1997;39:158–168.

Li C, Zheng, Ha P, et al. Neural EGFL like 1 as a potential pro-chondrogenic, anti-inflammatory dual-functional disease-modifying osteoarthritis drug. Biomaterials 2020;226:119541.

Li W, Liu Y, Zhang P, et al. Tissue-engineered bone immobilized with human adipose stem cells-derived exosomes promotes bone regeneration. ACS Appl Mater Interfaces 2018 Feb 14;10(6):5240–5254. http://doi.org/10.1021/acsami.7b17620. Epub 2018 Feb 2.

Lieberman JR, Daluiski A, Stevenson S, et al. The effect of regional gene therapy with bone morphogenetic protein-2-producing bone-marrow cells on the repair of segmental femoral defects in rats. J Bone Joint Surg Am 1999;81:905–917.

Liu A, Lin D, Zhao H, et al. Optimized BMSC-derived osteoinductive exosomes immobilized in hierarchical scaffold via lyophilization for bone repair through Bmpr2/Acvr2b competitive receptor-activated Smad pathway. Biomaterials 2021a May;272:120718. http://doi.org/10.1016/j.biomaterials.2021.120718. Epub 2021 Mar 27.

Liu W, Huang J, Chen F, et al. MSC-derived small extracellular vesicles overexpressing miR-20a promoted the osteointegration of porous titanium alloy by enhancing osteogenesis via targeting BAMBI. Stem Cell Res Ther 2021b Jun 16;12(1):348. http://doi.org/10.1186/s13287-021-02303-y.

Liu W, Yin Y, Jiang Y, et al. Genetic and epigenetic X-chromosome variations in a parthenogenetic human embryonic stem cell line. J Assist Reprod Genet 2011 Apr;28(4):303–313. http://doi.org/10.1007/s10815-010-9517-1. Epub 2010 Dec 15.

Llames S, Recuero I, Romance A, et al. Tissue-engineered oral mucosa for mucosal reconstruction in a pediatric patient with hemifacial microsomia and ankyloglossia. Cleft Palate Craniofac J 2014;51(2):246–251.

Lombaert IM, Brunsting JF, Wierenga PK, et al. Cytokine treatment improves parenchymal and vascular damage of salivary glands after irradiation. Clin Cancer Res 2008;14:7741–7750.

Lu SS, Zhang X, Soo C, et al. The osteoinductive properties of *Nell-1* in a rat spinal fusion model. Spine J 2007;7:50–60.

Luxameechanporn T, Hadlock T, Shyu J, et al. Successful myoblast transplantation in rat tongue reconstruction. Head Neck 2006;28:517–524.

MacNeil S. Progress and opportunities for tissue-engineered skin. Nature 2007;445:874–880.

Maeda H, Sano A, Fujioka K. Controlled release of rhBMP-2 from collagen minipellet and the relationship between release profile and ectopic bone formation. Int J Pharm 2004b;275:109–122.

Maeda S, Hayashi M, Komiya S, et al. Endogenous TGF-β signaling suppresses maturation of osteoblastic mesenchymal cells. EMBO J 2004a;23:552–563.

Malhotra R, Brosius FC III. Glucose uptake and glycolysis reduce hypoxia-induced apoptosis in cultured neonatal rat cardiac myocytes. J Biol Chem 1999;274:12567–12575.

Mapili G, Lu Y, Chen S, et al. Laser-layered microfabrication of spatially patterned functionalized tissue-engineering scaffolds. J Biomed Mater Res B Appl Biomater 2005;75:414–424.

Martin I, Miot S, Barbero A, et al. Osteochondral tissue engineering. J Biomech 2007;40:750–765.

Martinek V, Imhoff AB. Treatment of cartilage defects. Deutsch Z Sportmed 2003;54:70–76.

Marzouk SA, Buck RP, Dunlap LA, et al. Measurement of extracellular pH, K(+), and lactate in ischemic heart. Anal Biochem 2002;308:52–60.

Mayer H, Scutt AM, Ankenbauer T. Subtle differences in the mitogenic effects of recombinant human bone morphogenetic proteins -2 to -7 on DNA synthesis on primary bone-forming cells and identification of BMP-2/4 receptor. Calcif Tissue Int 1996;58:249–255.

Melchels FPW, Feijen J, Grijpma DW. A poly(D,L-lactide) resin for the preparation of tissue engineering scaffolds by stereolithography. Biomaterials 2009;30:3801–3809.

Miki T, Masaka K, Imai Y, et al. Experience with freeze-dried PGLA/HA/rhBMP-2 as a bone graft substitute. J Craniomaxillofac Surg 2000;28:294–299.

Mizuno H, Zuk PA, Zhu M, et al. Myogenic differentiation by human processed lipoaspirate cells. Plast Reconstr Surg 2002;109:199–209.

Moioli EK, Clark PA, Xin XJ, et al. Matrices and scaffolds for drug delivery in dental, oral and craniofacial tissue engineering. Adv Drug Deliver Rev 2007;59:308–324.

Morales TI, Joyce ME, Sobel ME, et al. Transforming growth factor-beta in calf articular-cartilage-organ cultures—synthesis and distribution. Arch Biochem Biophys 1991;288:397–405.

Moreira-Gonzalez A, Jackson IT, Miyawaki T, et al. Augmentation of the craniomaxillofacial region using porous hydroxyapatite granules. Plast Reconstr Surg 2003;111:1808–1817.

Mulliken JB, Glowacki J. Induced osteogenesis for repair and construction in the craniofacial region. Plast Reconstr Surg 1980;65:553–560.

Mundy GR, Boyce B, Hughes D, et al. The effects of cytokines and growth factors on osteoblastic cells. Bone 1995;17(2 suppl):71S–75S.

Murphy SV, Atala A. 3D bioprinting of tissues and organs. Nat Biotechnol 2014;32:773–785.

Nakamura M, Kobayashi A, Takagi F, et al. Biocompatible inkjet printing technique for designed seeding of individual living cells. Tissue Eng 2005;11:1658–1666.

Nakashima K, de Crombrugghe B. Transcriptional mechanisms in osteoblast differentiation and bone formation. Trends Genet 2003;19:458–466.

National Academy of Sciences' Board on Life Sciences. Stem Cells and the future of regenerative medicine. Washington, DC: National Academies; 2002.

National Institutes of Health, U.S. Department of Health and Human Services. National Institutes of Health Guidelines on Human Stem Cell Research. Federal Register 74 (18578), 23 Apr 2009. Accessed 15 Feb 2011. https://www.govinfo.gov/content/pkg/FR-2009-04-23/pdf/E9-9313.pdf.

Nuttelman CR, Mortisen DJ, Henry SM, et al. Attachment of fibronectin to poly(vinyl alcohol) hydrogels promotes NIH3T3 cell adhesion, proliferation, and migration. J Biomed Mater Res 2001;57:217–223.

O'Brien K, Muskiewicz K, Gussoni E. Recent advances in and therapeutic potential of muscle-derived stem cells. J Cell Biochem Suppl 2002;38:80–87.

Obrucník M, Malinsky J, Lichnovsky V. The early stages of differentiation of the vascular bed in the ventricular wall of the human embryonic heart as seen in the electron microscope. Folia Morphol (Praha) 1972;20:49–51.

Odorico JS, Kaufman DS, Thomson JA. Multilineage differentiation from human embryonic stem cell lines. Stem Cells 2001;19:193–204.

Ogawa R, Mizuno H, Watanabe A, et al. Osteogenic and chondrogenic differentiation by adipose-derived stem cells harvested from GFP transgenic mice. Biochem Biophys Res Commun 2004;313:871–877.

Orban JM, Marra KG, Hollinger JO. Composition options for tissue-engineered bone. Tissue Eng 2002;8:529–539.

Otto CM, Baumgardner JE. Effect of culture PO2 on macrophage (RAW 264.7) nitric oxide production. Am J Physiol Cell Physiol 2001;280:C280–C287.

Ozaki W, Buchman SR, Goldstein SA, et al. A comparative analysis of the microarchitecture of cortical membranous and cortical endochondral onlay bone grafts in the craniofacial skeleton. Plast Reconstr Surg 1999;104:139–147.

Parikh SN. Bone graft substitutes: Past, present, future. J Postgrad Med 2002;48:142–148.

Peng H, Wright V, Usas A, et al. Synergistic enhancement of bone formation and healing by stem cell-expressed VEGF and bone morphogenetic protein-4. J Clin Invest 2002;110:751–759.

Peng Y, Kang Q, Cheng H, et al. Transcriptional characterization of bone morphogenetic proteins (BMPs)-mediated osteogenic signaling. J Cell Biochem 2003;90:1149–1165.

Petite H, Viateau V, Bensaïd W, et al. Tissue-engineered bone regeneration. Nat Biotechnol 2000;18:959–963.

Phinney DG, Pittenger MF. Concise review: MSC-derived exosomes for cell-free therapy. Stem Cells 2017;35:851–858.

Piacentini L, Karliner JS. Altered gene expression during hypoxia and reoxygenation of the heart. Pharmacol Ther 1999;83:21–37.

Pili R, Murgia F, Pusceddu G, et al. Physical human lumen carotid reconstruction: Life-size models and rapid prototyping. CRS4. Accessed 15 Feb 2011. http://www.crs4.it/Publications/cgi-bin/tr/repository/crs4_826.pdf.

Pittenger MF, Mackay AM, Beck SC, et al. Multilineage potential of adult human mesenchymal stem cells. Science 1999;284:143–147.

Poupa O. Cardiac muscle and its blood supply: Palaeophysiological notes. Cell Mol Biol Res 1994;40:153–165.

Prestwich GD, Kuo JW. Chemically-modified HA for therapy and regenerative medicine. Curr Pharm Biotechnol 2008;9:242–245.

Psaltis PJ, Zannettino AC, Worthley SG, et al. Concise review: Mesenchymal stromal cells: Potential for cardiovascular repair. Stem Cells 2008;26:2201–2210.

Puleo DA. Dependence of mesenchymal cell responses on duration of exposure to bone morphogenetic protein-2 in vitro. J Cell Physiol 1997;173:93–101.

Qi X, Zhang J, Yuan H, et al. Exosomes Secreted by human-induced pluripotent stem cell-derived mesenchymal stem cells repair critical-sized bone defects through enhanced angiogenesis and osteogenesis in osteoporotic rats. Int J Biol Sci 2016 May 25;12(7):836–849. http://doi.org/10.7150/ijbs.14809. eCollection 2016.

Quarto R, Thomas D, Liang CT. Bone progenitor cell deficits and the age-associated decline in bone repair capacity. Calcif Tissue Int 1992;5:123–129.

Radisic M, Park H, Shing H, et al. Functional assembly of engineered myocardium by electrical stimulation of cardiac myocytes cultured on scaffolds. Proc Natl Acad Sci USA 2004;101:18129–18134.

Rai B, Teoh SH, Ho KH, et al. The effect of rhBMP-2 on canine osteoblasts seeded onto 3D bioactive polycaprolactone scaffolds. Biomaterials 2004;25:5499–5506.

Rajaonarivony M, Vauthier C, Couarraze G, et al. Development of a new drug carrier made from alginate. J Pharm Sci 1993;82:912–917.

Ramakrishnan A, Torok-Storb BJ. The role of the marrow microenvironment in hematopoietic stem cell transplantation. Cell Ther Transplant 2010;2:7–12.

Ramanujan S, Pluen A, McKee TD, et al. Diffusion and convection in collagen gels: Implications for transport in the tumor interstitium. Biophys J 2002;83:1650–1660.

Ramoshebi LN, Matsaba TN, Teare J, Renton L, Patton J, Ripamonti U. Tissue engineering: TGF-β superfamily members and delivery systems in bone regeneration. Expert Rev Mol Med 2002;2:4(20):1–11.

Ravel P, Hsu HHT, Schneider MP, et al. Expression of bone morphogenetic proteins by osteoinductive and non-osteoinductive human osteosarcoma cells. J Dent Res 1996;75:1518–1523.

Reddi AH. Bone and cartilage differentiation. Curr Opin Genet Dev 1994;4:737–744.

Reddi AH. Bone morphogenetic proteins: From basic science to clinical applications. J Bone Joint Surg Am 2001;83A suppl 1(pt 1):S1–S6.

Reddi AH. Cell biology and biochemistry of endochondral bone development. Coll Relat Res 1981;1:209–226.

Remuñán-López C, Bodmeier R. Mechanical, water uptake and permeability properties of crosslinked chitosan glutamate and alginate films. J Control Release 1997;44:215–225.

Rengachary SS. Bone morphogenetic proteins: Basic concepts. Neurosurg Focus 2002;13:e2.

Rickard DJ, Sullivan TA, Shenker BJ, et al. Induction of rapid osteoblast differentiation in rat bone marrow stromal cell cultures by dexamethasone and BMP-2. Dev Biol 1994;161:218–228.

Robergs RA, Ghiasvand F, Parker D. Biochemistry of exercise-induced metabolic acidosis. Am J Physiol Regul Integr Comp Physiol 2004;287:R502–R516.

Rongish BJ, Torry RJ, Tucker DC, et al. Neovascularization of embryonic rat hearts cultured in oculo closely mimics in-utero coronary vessel development. J Vasc Res 1994;31:205–215.

Rose FR, Oreffo RO. Bone tissue engineering: Hope vs hype. Biochem Biophys Res Commun 2002;292:1–7.

Rosso F, Giordano A, Barbarisi M, et al. From cell-ECM interactions to tissue engineering. J Cell Physiol 2004;199:174–180.

Rowley JA, Mooney DJ. Alginate type and RGD density control myoblast phenotype. J Biomed Mater Res 2002;60:217–223.

Ruhe PQ, Hedberg EL, Padron NT, et al. rhBMP-2 release from injectable poly(DL-lactic-*co*-glycolic acid)/calcium-phosphate cement composites. J Bone Joint Surg Am 2003;85A(suppl 3):75–81.

Safford KM, Hicok KC, Safford SD, et al. Neurogenic differentiation of murine and human adipose-derived stromal cells. Biochem Biophys Res Commun 2002;294:371–379.

Sandén T, Salomonsson L, Brzezinski P, et al. Surface-coupled proton exchange of a membrane-bound proton acceptor. Proc Natl Acad Sci USA 2010;107:4129–4134.

Schaefer D, Martin I, Jundt G, et al. Tissue-engineered composites for the repair of large osteochondral defects. Arthritis Rheum 2002;46:2524–2534.

Schlegel KA, Donath K, Rupprecht S, et al. De novo bone formation using bovine collagen and platelet-rich plasma. Biomaterials 2004;25:5387–5393.

Schmitt SM, Chance DA. Fabrication of titanium implant-retained restorations with nontraditional machining techniques. Int J Prosthodont 1995;8:332–336.

Schwab A, Levato R, D'Este M, et al. Printability and shape fidelity of bioinks in 3D bioprinting. Chem Rev 2020;120(19):11028–11055.

Schwartz Z, Somers A, Mellonig JT, et al. Addition of human recombinant bone morphogenetic protein-2 to inactive commercial human demineralized freeze-dried bone allograft makes an effective composite bone inductive implant material. J Periodontol 1998;69:1337–1345.

Schek RM, Taboas JM, Hollister SJ, et al. Tissue engineering osteochondral implants for temporomandibular joint repair. Orthod Craniofac Res 2005;8:313–319.

Seitz H, Rieder W, Irsen S, et al. Three-dimensional printing of porous ceramic scaffolds for bone tissue engineering. J Biomed Mater Res B Appl Biomater 2005;74:782–788.

Shang Q, Wang Z, Liu W, et al. Tissue-engineered bone repair of sheep cranial defects with autologous bone marrow stromal cells. J Craniofac Surg 2001;12:586–593.

Shao XX, Hutmacher DW, Ho ST, et al. Evaluation of a hybrid scaffold/cell construct in repair of high-load-bearing osteochondral defects in rabbits. Biomaterials 2006;27:1071–1080.

Shen J, James AW, Zhang X, et al. Novel Wnt regulator NEL-like molecule-1 antagonizes adipogenesis and augments osteogenesis induced by bone morphogenetic protein 2. Am J Pathol 2016;186(2):419–434.

Sherwood JK, Riley SL, Palazzolo R, et al. A three-dimensional osteochondral composite scaffold for articular cartilage repair. Biomaterials 2002;23:4739–4751.

Shu XZ, Zhu KJ. Controlled drug release properties of ionically cross-linked chitosan beads: The influence of anion structure. Int J Pharm 2002;233:217–225.

Siu RK, Zara JN, Hou Y, et al. NELL-1 promotes cartilage regeneration in an in vivo rabbit model. Tissue Eng Part A 2012;18(3–4):252–261.

Slonaker M, Goswami T. Wear mechanisms in ceramic hip implants. J Surg Orthop 2004;13:94–105.

Spahn G, Kahl E, Mückley T, et al. Arthroscopic knee chondroplasty using a bipolar radiofrequency-based device compared to mechanical shaver: Results of a prospective, randomized, controlled study. Knee Surg Sports Traumatol Arthrosc 2008;16:565–573.

Stern R, McPherson M, Longaker MT. Histologic study of artificial skin used in the treatment of full-thickness thermal injury. J Burn Care Rehabil 1990;11:7–13.

Strong EB, Moulthrop T. Calvarial bone graft harvest: A new technique. Otolaryngol Head Neck 2000;123:547–552.

Sun W, Lal P. Recent development on computer aided tissue engineering—a review. Comput Methods Programs Biomed 2002;67:85–103.

Sun Y, You Y, Jiang W, et al. 3D bioprinting dual-factor releasing and gradient-structured constructs ready to implant for anisotropic cartilage regeneration. Sci Adv 2020;6:eaay1422.

Swanson WB, Zhang Z, Xiu K, et al. Scaffolds with controlled release of pro-mineralization exosomes to promote craniofacial bone healing without cell transplantation. Acta Biomater 2020 Dec;118:215–232. http://doi.org/10.1016/j.actbio.2020.09.052. Epub 2020 Oct 13.

Takahashi E, Doi K. Impact of diffusional oxygen transport on oxidative metabolism in the heart. Jpn J Physiol 1998;48:243–252.

Takahashi T, Fukuda M, Aiba T, et al. Distraction osteogenesis for reconstruction after mandibular segmental resection. Oral Surg Oral Med Oral Pathol Oral Radiol Endod 2002;93:21–26.

Tan KH, Chua CK, Leong KF, et al. Selective laser sintering of biocompatible polymers for applications in tissue engineering. Biomed Mater Eng 2005;15:113–124.

Tanjaya J, Lord EL, Wang C, et al. The effects of systemic therapy of PEGylated NEL-like protein 1 (NELL-1) on fracture healing in mice. Am J Pathol 2018;188(3):715–727.

Temenoff JS, Mikos AG. Review: Tissue engineering for regeneration of articular cartilage. Biomaterials 2000;21:431–440.

Thies RS, Bauduy M, Ashton BA, et al. Recombinant human bone morphogenetic protein-2 induces osteoblastic differentiation in W-20-17 stromal cells. Endocrinology 1992;130:1318–1324.

Tholpady SS, Katz AJ, Ogle RC. Mesenchymal stem cells from rat visceral fat exhibit multipotential differentiation in vitro. Anat Rec 2003;272:398–402.

Ting K, Vastardis H, Mulliken JB, et al. Human NELL-1 expressed in unilateral coronal synostosis. J Bone Miner Res 1999;14:80–89.

Tønnesen HH, Karlsen J. Alginate in drug delivery systems. Drug Dev Ind Pharm 2002;28:621–630.

Toquet J, Rohanizadeh R, Guicheux J, et al. Osteogenic potential in vitro of human bone marrow cells cultured on macroporous biphasic calcium phosphate ceramic. J Biomed Mater Res 1999;44:98–108.

Tou L, Quibria N, Alexander JM. Transcriptional regulation of the human Runx2/Cbfa1 gene promoter by bone morphogenetic protein-7. Mol Cell Endocrinol 2003;205:121–129.

Truong T, Zhang XL, Pathmanathan D, et al. Craniosynostosis-associated gene Nell-1 is regulated by Runx2. J Bone Miner Res 2007;22:7–18.

Uludag H, D'Augusta D, Golden J, et al. Implantation of recombinant human bone morphogenetic proteins with biomaterial carriers: A correlation between protein pharmacokinetics and osteoinduction in the rat ectopic model. J Biomed Mater Res 2000;50:227–238.

Uludag H, D'Augusta D, Palmer R, et al. Characterization of rhBMP-2 pharmacokinetics implanted with biomaterial carriers in the rat ectopic model. J Biomed Mater Res 1999a;46:193–202.

Uludag H, Friess W, Williams D, et al. rhBMP-collagen sponges as osteoinductive devices: Effects of in vitro sponge characteristics and protein pI on in vivo rhBMP pharmacokinetics. Ann NY Acad Sci 1999b;875:369–378.

Uludag H, Gao T, Porter TJ, et al. Delivery systems for BMPs: Factors contributing to protein retention at an application site. J Bone Joint Surg Am 2001;83-A suppl 1(pt 2):S128–S135.

Urist MR. Bone: Formation by autoinduction. Science 1965;150:893–899.

US Food and Drug Administration. Medical device approvals and clearances: InFUSE™ bone graft/LT-CAGE™ lumbar tapered fusion device. Accessed 15 Feb 2011. http://www.accessdata.fda.gov/cdrh_docs/pdf/P000058b.pdf.

Valentin-Opran A, Wozney J, Csimma C, et al. Clinical evaluation of recombinant human bone morphogenetic protein-2. Clin Orthop 2002;395:110–120.

van Beuningen HM, Glansbeek HL, van der Kraan PM, et al. Differential effects of local application of BMP-2 or TGF-β 1 on both articular cartilage composition and osteophyte formation. Osteoarthritis Cartilage 1998;6:306–317.

van den Bergh JP, ten Bruggenkate CM, Groeneveld HH, et al. Recombinant human bone morphogenetic protein-7 in maxillary sinus floor elevation surgery in 3 patients compared to autogenous bone grafts—a clinical pilot study. J Clin Periodontol 2000;27:627–636.

van der Bilt A, Engelen L, Pereira LJ, et al. Oral physiology and mastication. Physiol Behav 2006;89:22–27.

Varkey M, Gittens SA, Uludag H. Growth factor delivery for bone tissue repair: An update. Expert Opin Drug Deliv 2004;1:19–36.

Vasilev K, Cook J, Griesser HJ. Antibacterial surfaces for biomedical devices. Expert Rev Med Devices 2009;6:553–567.

Vivian JE, King CJ. Diffusivities of slightly soluble gases in water. AIChE J 1964;10:220–221.

Wakitani S, Saito T, Caplan AI. Myogenic cells derived from rat bone marrow mesenchymal stem cells exposed to 5-azacytidine. Muscle Nerve 1995;18:1417–1426.

Wang EA, Israel DI, Kelly S, et al. Bone morphogenetic protein-2 causes commitment and differentiation in C3H10T1/2 and 3T3 cells. Growth Factors 1993;9:57–71.

Wang J, Liao J, Zhang F, et al. NEL-like molecule-1 (Nell1) is regulated by bone morphogenetic protein 9 (BMP9) and potentiates BMP9-induced osteogenic differentiation at the expense of adipogenesis in mesenchymal stem cells. Cell Physiol Biochem 2017;41:484–500.

Wang JC, Kanim LEA, Yoo S, et al. Effect of regional gene therapy with bone morphogenetic protein-2-producing bone marrow cells on spinal fusion in rats. J Bone Joint Surg Am 2003;85A:905–911.

Wang JC, Yu WD, Sandhu HS, et al. Metal debris from titanium spinal implants. Spine 1999;24:899–903.

Wang WL, Cheah CM, Fuh JY, et al. Influence of process parameters on stereolithography part shrinkage. Mater Design 1996;17:205–213.

Warnke PH, Springer IN, Wiltfang J, et al. Growth and transplantation of a custom vascularised bone graft in a man. Lancet 2004;364:766–770.

Warren SM, Greenwald JA, Nacamuli RP, et al. New strategies for craniofacial repair and replacement: A brief review. J Craniofac Surg 2003;14:363–370.

Webster KA, Bishopric NH. Molecular regulation of cardiac myocyte adaptations to chronic hypoxia. J Mol Cell Cardiol 1992;24:741–751.

Webster KA, Discher DJ, Kaiser S, et al. Hypoxia-activated apoptosis of cardiac myocytes requires reoxygenation or a pH shift and is independent of p53. J Clin Invest 1999;104:239–252.

Weissman IL. Stem cells: Units of development, units of regeneration, and units in evolution. Cell 2000;100:157–168.

Wickham MQ, Erickson GR, Gimble JM, et al. Multipotent stromal cells derived from the infrapatellar fat pad of the knee. Clin Orthop 2003;412:196–212.

Williams JM, Adewunmi A, Schek RM, et al. Bone tissue engineering using polycaprolactone scaffolds fabricated via selective laser sintering. Biomaterials 2005;26:4817–4827.

Winder J, Cooke RS, Gray J, et al. Medical rapid prototyping and 3D CT in the manufacture of custom made cranial titanium plates. J Med Eng Technol 1999;23:26–28.

Wingard JR, Hsu J, Hiemenz JW. Hematopoietic stem cell transplantation: An overview of infection risks and epidemiology. Hematol Oncol Clin North Am 2011;25:101–116.

Winn SR, Hu Y, Sfeir C, et al. Gene therapy approaches for modulating bone regeneration. Adv Drug Deliv Rev 2000;42:121–138.

Winn SR, Uludag H, Hollinger JO. Carrier systems for bone morphogenetic proteins. Clin Orthop Relat Res 1999;(367 suppl):S95–S106.

Winter GD, Simpson BJ. Heterotopic bone formed in a synthetic sponge in the skin of young pigs. Nature 1969;223:88–90.

Wolfe SA. Complications of harvesting cranial bone grafts. Plast Reconstr Surg 1996;98:567.

Wolford LM. Temporomandibular joint devices: Treatment factors and outcomes. Oral Surg Oral Med Oral Pathol Oral Radiol Endod 1997;83:143–149.

Woo BH, Fink BF, Page R, et al. Enhancement of bone growth by sustained delivery of recombinant human bone morphogenetic protein-2 in a polymeric matrix. Pharm Res 2001;18:1747–1753.

Wozney JM, Rosen V. Bone morphogenetic protein and bone morphogenetic protein gene family in bone formation and repair. Clin Orthop 1998;346:26–37.

Wozney JM, Rosen V, Celeste AJ, et al. Novel regulators of bone formation: Molecular clones and activities. Science 1988;242:1528–1534.

Wright V, Peng H, Usas A, et al. BMP4-expressing muscle-derived stem cells differentiate into osteogenic lineage and improve bone healing in immunocompetent mice. Mol Ther 2002;6:169–178.

Wu BM, Borland SW, Giordano RA, et al. Solid free-form fabrication of drug delivery devices. J Control Release 1996;40:77–87.

Wu BM, Cima MJ. Effects of solvent-particle interaction kinetics on microstructure formation during three-dimensional printing. Polym Eng Sci 1999;39:249–260.

Wu J, Chen L, Wang R, et al. Exosomes secreted by stem cells from human exfoliated deciduous teeth promote alveolar bone defect repair through the regulation of angiogenesis and osteogenesis. ACS Biomater Sci Eng 2019 Jul 8;5(7):3561–3571. http://doi.org/10.1021/acsbiomaterials.9b00607. Epub 2019 Jun 7.

Xie C, Ye J, Liang R, et al. Advanced strategies of biomimetic tissue-engineered grafts for bone regeneration. Adv Healthc Mater 2021;10:2100408.

Xie H, Wang, Zhang, et al. Extracellular vesicle-functionalized decalcified bone matrix scaffolds with enhanced pro-angiogenic and pro-bone regeneration activities. Sci Rep 2017 Apr 3;7:45622. http://doi.org/10.1038/srep45622.

Xu Q, Shanti RM, Zhang Q, et al. A gingiva-derived mesenchymal stem cell-laden porcine small intestinal submucosa extracellular matrix construct promotes myomucosal regeneration of the tongue. Eng Part A 2017;23(7–8):301–312.

Xu T, Jin J, Gregory C, et al. Inkjet printing of viable mammalian cells. Biomaterials 2005;26:93–99.

Yamaguchi A, Ishizuya T, Kintou N, et al. Effects of BMP-2, BMP-4, and BMP-6 on osteoblastic differentiation of bone marrow-derived stromal cell lines, ST2 and MC3T3-G2/PA6. Biochem Biophys Res Commun 1996;220:366–371.

Yamaguchi A, Komori T, Suda T. Regulation of osteoblast differentiation mediated by bone morphogenetic proteins, hedgehogs, and Cbfa1. Endocr Rev 2000;21:393–411.

Yamamoto M, Takahashi Y, Tabata Y. Controlled release by biodegradable hydrogels enhances the ectopic bone formation of bone morphogenetic protein. Biomaterials 2003;24:4375–4383.

Yamanaka S, Blau HM. Nuclear reprogramming to a pluripotent state by three approaches. Nature 2010;465:704–712.

Yang SF, Leong KF, Du ZH, et al. The design of scaffolds for use in tissue engineering. Part II. Rapid prototyping techniques. Tissue Eng 2002;8:1–11.

Yang WD, Gomes RR, Brown AJ, et al. Chondrogenic differentiation on perlecan domain I, collagen II, and bone morphogenetic protein-2-based matrices. Tissue Eng 2006;12:2009–2024.

Yao Z, Li Y, Lin T, et al. Progenitor cell-derived exosomes endowed with VEGF plasmids enhance osteogenic induction and vascular remodeling in large segmental bone defects. Theranostics 2021 Jan 1;11(1):397–409.

Yasko AW, Lane JM, Fellinger EJ, et al. The healing of segmental bone defects, induced by recombinant human bone morphogenetic protein (rhBMP-2). A radiographic, histological, and biomechanical study in rats. J Bone Joint Surg Am 1992;74:659–670.

Yeh TT, Wu SS, Lee CH, et al. The short-term therapeutic effect of recombinant human bone morphogenetic protein-2 on collagenase-induced lumbar facet joint osteoarthritis in rats. Osteoarthritis Cartilage 2007;15:1357–1366.

Yoshikawa H, Rettig WJ, Takaoka K, et al. Expression of bone morphogenetic proteins in human osteosarcoma. Immunohistochemical detection with monoclonal antibody. Cancer 1994;73:85–91.

Zegzula HD, Buck DC, Brekke J, et al. Bone formation with use of rhBMP-2 (recombinant human bone morphogenetic protein-2). J Bone Joint Surg Am 1997;79:1778–1790.

Zein I, Hutmacher DW, Tan KC, et al. Fused deposition modeling of novel scaffold architectures for tissue engineering applications. Biomaterials 2002;23:1169–1185.

Zeltinger J, Sherwood JK, Graham D, et al. Effect of pore size and void fraction on cellular adhesion, proliferation, and matrix deposition. Tissue Eng 2001;7:557–572.

Zhang H, Migneco F, Lin CY, et al. Chemically-conjugated bone morphogenetic protein-2 on three-dimensional polycaprolactone scaffolds stimulates osteogenic activity in bone marrow stromal cells. Tissue Eng Part A 2010;16:3441–3448.

Zhang J, Li S, Li L, et al. Exosome and exosomal MicroRNA: Trafficking, sorting, and function. Genom Proteom Bioinform 2015;13:17–24.

Zhang XL, Kuroda S, Carpenter D, et al. Craniosynostosis in transgenic mice overexpressing *Nell-1*. J Clin Invest 2002;110:861–870.

Zhao GQ. Consequences of knocking out BMP signaling in the mouse. Genesis 2003;35:43–56.

Zhou L, Du HD, Tian HB, et al. Experimental study on repair of the facial nerve with Schwann cells transfected with GDNF genes and PLGA conduits. Acta Otolaryngol 2008;128:1266–1272.

Zhu G, Mallery SR, Schwendeman SP. Stabilization of proteins encapsulated in injectable poly(lactide-co-glycolide). Nat Biotechnol 2000;18:52–57.

Zimmermann WH, Didié M, Wasmeier GH, et al. Cardiac grafting of engineered heart tissue in syngenic rats. Circulation 2002b;106(12 suppl 1):I151–I157.

Zimmermann WH, Schneiderbanger K, Schubert P, et al. Tissue engineering of a differentiated cardiac muscle construct. Circ Res 2002a;90:223–230.

Zuk PA, Zhu M, Ashjian P, et al. Human adipose tissue is a source of multipotent stem cells. Mol Biol Cell 2002;13:4279–4295.

Zuk PA, Zhu M, Mizuno H, et al. Multilineage cells from human adipose tissue: Implications for cell-based therapies. Tissue Eng 2001;7:211–228.

Chapter 9

Biopsychosocial Perspectives and Survivorship in the Maxillofacial Prosthodontic Treatment of Head and Neck Cancer

David A. Rapkin, PhD

Introduction

Health care providers' (HCP) conceptualizations of the fundamental nature of head and neck cancer (HNC) and its treatment greatly influence their approach to clinical practice, the success of their efforts, and the experience of patients, their caregivers and families (PCF), and the community. HCP professional gratification and stress levels are similarly affected. A profound and consequential transformation of these foundational views has occurred since the middle of the previous century, culminating in a new consensus that cancer care generally and HNC care specifically should be organized around the concept of "survivorship."

As the consensus regarding the nature of cancer and cancer care evolved from a reductive, biomedical view (BM) to one in which treatment of the patient as a whole person was the goal, essentially all the specialties involved in HNC care have come to recognize the importance of addressing psychosocial (PS) needs of PCF and their communities. Although less widely recognized, the needs and vulnerabilities of HCP themselves have come to be seen as a topic worthy of attention. This shift to a biopsychosocial (BPS) perspective has spurred awareness of and research on PS morbidities and the development of interventions (the interventions being still in their early stages). The BPS perspective offers maxillofacial prosthodontists and other HCP insights, encouragement, and suggestions to increase sensitivity and attunement to the needs of their PCF and themselves, to improve communication and collaboration with PCF and colleagues, to reduce cost while increasing quality of care, and to enhance the success of and satisfaction with their work.

This chapter has two main sections. The first briefly traces the history of the evolution noted above in foundational conceptions of HNC and its treatment. The second section explores the implications of the newer BPS conceptualizations for the work of the entire provider-patient-caregiver-family (PPCF) team. The evolving views affect the understanding and implementation of the organization, functioning, and scope of responsibility of the entire HNC care team. In this context, particular consideration will be given to the intersection of maxillofacial prosthodontic practice and PS morbidities arising from HNC and its treatments (Rapkin and Garrett, 2011).

The Biopsychosocial (BPS) Perspective, Survivorship, and Caring for the Whole Patient: A Brief History of the Emerging Paradigm

During most of the latter half of the twentieth century, fundamental understandings of the nature of HNC and its treatment differed among the disciplines involved in providing care. Early on, HCP who focused on ablative aspects of cancer treatment tended to conceptualize cancer from a narrower perspective, while HCP who focused on rehabilitative aspects tended to conceptualize cancer from a more inclusive point of view. Head and neck surgeons (Healey, 1970), radiation oncologists, and medical oncologists, who were primarily concerned with treatment and management, tended to view their work using a BM perspective. That is, they conceptualized the illness and the scope of their work narrowly in terms of eliminating, reducing, or stabilizing malignant tumors and, where possible, preventing recurrence. Though consideration was given to morbidities of treatment, outcomes such as goals of care and measurement of efficacy were predominantly conceptualized in terms of disease-free interval and overall quantity of life following treatment (conventionally measured in terms of five-year survival rates). HCP who focused on rehabilitation—most prominently maxillofacial prosthodontists, reconstructive surgeons, speech and language pathologists, and clinical social workers—conceptualized their work (sometimes implicitly) using a BPS perspective. That is, their efforts were directed toward ameliorating effects of the disease and its treatment across a broad spectrum of function—including biological and physical health and functioning (e.g., patients' abilities to breathe and to eat), psychological well-being (e.g., appearance and body image, emotional state, and life satisfaction), and social functioning (e.g., viability of patients' relationships, social acceptability, capacity to communicate, and capacity to function in close relationships, socially and at work)—and tended to focus on post-treatment adaptation and quality of life (QOL; Beumer et al., 1996).

Limitations in the narrower BM model were noted early (Rozen et al., 1972; Engel, 1977; Conley, 1981). During the decades from the 1980s through the early 2000s, a perspective emerged that identified inadequacies of a strictly BM approach to cancer and its treatments and which integrated BM and BPS conceptualizations under the rubric of "survivorship" (Hewitt et al., 2005; Hewitt and Ganz, 2006; Rowland et al., 2006; LaMonte, 2016; Ringash, 2015).

A representative definition of survivorship is as follows: "Survivors of cancer and cancer-directed therapies may encounter substantial medical, psychosocial, interpersonal, financial, and functional consequences. This collective experience of the diagnosis, therapies, and resultant consequences has been dubbed *survivorship*" (Miller and Shuman, 2016).

During this latter period, when the value of the BPS perspective and a shift to survivorship-oriented care was being promoted, the cohort of HNC patients surviving for longer durations increased, so the need for care beyond the immediate administration of definitive therapies became increasingly evident and compelling for all HNC providers. Factors promoting this significant change in HNC-related survival appear to include success in the national campaign to reduce tobacco use, increased efficacy of all three major treatment modalities, and recognition that human papillomavirus (HPV) infection can create a "second" pathway to the development of squamous cell carcinomas (SCCA) in the upper aero-digestive tract (UADT)—the "first" or more classically known pathway arising from extensive use of substances, such as alcohol, tobacco, and (especially in Asia) betel. Appropriately treated patients with stage III or IV HPV positive ("P-16" positive) oropharyngeal SCCA generally have significantly better cure rates than do patients with P-16 negative SCCA (Haddad and Limaye, 2021a; Haddad and Shin, 2008).

With the confluence of these two trends—promotion of the BPS perspective and the increasing survival of patients—a focus on survivorship and the associated idea of "patient-centered care" have gradually become accepted as the consensus perspective and basis for understanding and implementing standards of care in oncology generally and in head and neck oncology in particular (Hewitt and Ganz, 2006; Rowland et al., 2006; Ringash, 2015; Chan and Nekhlyudoc, 2021; Tevaarwerk et al., 2021; Goyal et al., 2021; Heineman et al., 2017; St. John, 2017).

Implications of the Survivorship Paradigm

As noted, a comprehensive and inclusive approach to cancer care, embracing awareness of biological, psychological, and social arenas of the impact of cancer and its treatment, is not new to maxillofacial prosthodontists and other HCP focused on oncologic rehabilitation (Strong, 1996). However, the consensus embrace of survivorship as the guiding conceptualization of HNC care does have implications worth noting for the maxillofacial prosthodontist and the entire HNC team. Implications of survivorship and patient-centered care discussed in this chapter include duration or period of survivorship and phases of survivorship; the necessity of multidisciplinary care and composition of the multidisciplinary provider team (MDT); expanded scope of provider responsibility, including surveillance for PS morbidities and vulnerabilities, intervention, and referral; and self-care for the provider.

The arc and phases of survivorship

The period of survivorship has been defined as beginning at the time of cancer diagnosis and lasting through the end of life (Chan and Nekhlyudov, 2021). This scope readily gives rise to the idea of phases of survivorship and associated care-related concerns, such as the following (Morris et al., 2022).

Phase 1: Pretreatment

- Diagnostic workup (typically including history and physical examination, biopsy, and imaging studies)
- Prehabilitation (BPS preparation for treatment, which can include, for example, BPS distress screening and referral for PS treatment of PCF; assessment of BM frailty; dental examinations and pretreatment dental care; fabrication of fluoride stents for dentate patients to be irradiated; preparation for fabricating obturators,

facial prostheses, and other appliances; planning intraoperative placement of implantable devices and extraction of problematic teeth; nutritional evaluation, nutritional treatment, and feeding tube placement; physical therapy; and clarification of patient's priorities and goals of care)
- Case formulation and treatment planning by a multidisciplinary case conference (MDC)

Phase 2: Peri-treatment

- Ablative oncologic treatment (which can include neoadjuvant chemo- or immune therapy, cytoreductive surgery, or radiation therapy; definitive surgery, radiation or chemo-radiation; systemic therapy; and palliative therapies)
- Reconstructive surgery (e.g., creation and placement of tissue flaps and intra-operative placement of dental implants and other prosthetic devices)
- Assessment and management of morbidities arising in the course of treatment or immediately after treatment (e.g., postoperative hospitalization; treatment of nausea, pain, xerostomia, or oral mucositis concurrent with radiation therapy; peri-operative inpatient counseling, individual and/or family psychotherapy)
- Initiation of educational and other rehabilitative interventions (e.g., delivery of temporary obturators, training in tracheostomy self-care, and speech and swallowing therapy)

Phase 3a: Post-treatment, early phase

- Treatment of acute morbidities (including PS interventions for anxiety, depression, sleep disturbance, sexual and intimacy problems; pain; lymphedema; nausea; persistent oral mucositis; financial distress; etc.)
- Initiating care of long-term, treatment-related morbidities
- Subacute medical and physical care (e.g., support for activities of daily living, housing)
- Rehabilitation (e.g., delivery of prosthetic appliances, speech and swallowing therapy)
- Initiating surveillance for long-term and late-arising morbidities (e.g., recurrence, metastases, and second primary tumors and BPS distress screening of PCF for possible problems with health literacy for treatment effects such as dysphagia, trismus, pain, nutritional problems, depression, anxiety, sleep disorders, intimacy and sexual problems, and financial stress)

Phase 3b: Post-treatment, mid-phase

- Functional and cosmetic rehabilitation and/or treatment for defects, deformities, and lasting and late-arising morbidities (e.g., delivery of permanent obturators, dental implants, and facial appliances; treatment for dysphagia; treatment for trismus; treatment for chronic pain; treatment for lymphedema; and treatment for neck and movement disabilities)
- Subacute medical and physical care (e.g., support for activities of daily living, housing)
- Maintenance and replacement of aged or deteriorated appliances and prostheses
- Psychotherapy for intimacy and other relationship issues
- Ongoing surveillance for and treatment and management of lasting and emerging (late arising) morbidities (recurrent, metastatic, and/or second primary tumors and BPS distress screening of PCF for treatment effects, such as xerostomia, dysphagia, trismus, pain, radiation caries, movement disorders, eating and nutritional problems, depression, anxiety, sleep disorders, intimacy and sexual problems, financial stress, employment problems, and other factors diminishing quality of life)

The aim of definitive treatment is that Phase 3b continues for years or decades and constitutes the preponderance of the survivorship arc. In the event of recurrence, metastases, or new disease, the patient cycles through Phases 1 and 3, perhaps multiple times.

Phase 4: End of life care

- Palliative and/or hospice care (especially pain and symptom management)
- Spiritual and psychotherapeutic interventions with PCF (e.g., end-of-life counseling and psychotherapy, along with psychotropically facilitated altered-state experiences)
- Grief and loss counseling for caregivers (e.g., adult children), family (especially spouse and young children), extended family, and community (social friends, work friends)

Although the varied specialists composing the HNC MDT will naturally focus their efforts and attention more on some phases than others, *all HCP should be mindful of the impact of their efforts on the patient's, caregiver's, and family's personal, social, and work relationships, functioning, and QOL within all phases and across the entire arc of survivorship.*

The head and neck cancer (HNC) multidisciplinary provider team (MDT): Composition and functioning

Recognizing the multidimensional morbidities of HNC and its treatments leads to the view that adequate treatment of HNC requires an MDT (Hewitt and Ganz, 2006; Haddad and Limaye, 2021a; Heineman et al., 2017; St. John, 2017; Taberna et al., 2020; Dharmarajan et al., 2020; Nekhlyudov et al., 2018). However, good team functioning is not automatic (Haddad and Limaye, 2021a; Forsythe et al., 2012). In many situations, specialists that make up an HNC care team are habituated to practicing independently (i.e., can be functionally siloed). It is important to recognize that to be effective, the work of team members must be coordinated, necessitating patterns of adequate communication. This requires time and effort on the part of specialists who are likely very busy in their own practices and who may not be trained or used to putting effort into developing and maintaining team consciousness and culture. Appreciating that good teamwork is essential for capitalizing on the advantages of multidisciplinary care—and recognizing that inadequate coordination among provider team members can easily result in substandard care—can motivate team members to make the additional effort required for building and maintaining effective care teams.

Specialties composing the HNC MDT typically include the following (Morris et al., 2022; Taberna et al., 2020; Dharmarajan et al., 2020):

- Audiology
- Dentistry (Maxillofacial Prosthodontics, Oral Oncology, Hospital Dentistry, Oral and Maxillofacial Surgery)
- Medicine and Surgery (Medical Nutrition, Medical Oncology, Otolaryngology—Head and Neck Surgery including ablative and reconstructive surgeons, Pain, Primary Care, Palliative Care, Pathology, Radiation Oncology, Radiology)
- Nutrition
- Psychosocial Oncology (Clinical Social Work, Clinical and Health Psychology, Consultation-Liaison Psychiatry)
- Rehabilitative Specialists (Occupational Therapy, Physical Therapy)
- Translational Research Scientists
- Speech and Language Pathology
- Treatment Navigation (Nurse Coordinators and Practitioners, Physician Assistants, Patient Navigators)

As noted, clear communication is one essential element of good MDT functioning. An important instance of this relates to preoperative education regarding treatment choices, deformities, loss of function, and other daunting treatment and rehabilitative limitations and effects. Under the stress and anxiety induced by the necessity of coping with information regarding their treatment and diagnosis, patients may dissociate or otherwise fail to remember pretreatment briefings by their medical providers, even when briefings are extensive. Alternatively, medical providers, affected by the same stressors as patients, may avoid explicitly or thoroughly informing HNC PCF regarding difficult choices and challenges that lie ahead. It is not unusual for patients to reproach their maxillofacial prosthodontists for a perceived lack of adequate, preparatory information (e.g., "No one told me. If I had known it would be like this, I never would have had that treatment"), from either other members of the MDT (e.g., surgeons, radiation oncologists, medical oncologists) or by the maxillofacial prosthodontists themselves.

In the circumstance of a particular patient's complaint, it may be impossible to determine if the patient actually forgot or was inadequately prepared. It is very helpful, to both reduce the frequency of such events and to manage them when they do occur, if specialists from different disciplines within the MDT can develop mutual trust based on a willingness to give and receive honest communication, inquiry, and potentially, constructive criticism. Though such communications among MDT members can require some courage and may be stressful, if approached with goodwill and mutual respect, they can result in a strengthened team culture and increased team resiliency. Absent such efforts, fissures in mutual confidence and diminished teamwork can easily develop, potentially harming the patient's care and stressing collegial relations.

Patient complaints of inadequate foreknowledge often resolve as they engage in the work of rehabilitation. However, some may be unable to successfully grieve and integrate their losses of function and/or appearance and, consequently, may chronically revert to complaining, develop a critical, passive, or depressed avoidance of their self-care and recovery tasks, and/or become unable to adopt a realistic revision of their expectations from rehabilitation. Such patients can experience significant dissatisfaction with their maxillofacial prosthodontic or preventive dental care and can become sources of considerable stress for their prosthodontists and restorative dentists. In such situations, psychosocial oncologists on the MDT can provide consultation to the prosthodontist and/or to the PCF.

Ideally, coordination among MDT members occurs in the setting of an MDC or tumor board, in either a face-to-face or video conferencing format, where the impact of the team approach on case management decision-making is significant and treatment outcomes are optimized (Dharmarajan et al., 2020; Brunner et al., 2015; Badran et al., 2018). Coordinating the work of the MDT can be easier if the HCP are based in the same institution. When the patient is being treated by HCP practicing within the same health care system but who are geographically dispersed, or when treatment is given by community-based HCP, assembling a sufficiently complete MDT and coordinating team discussions, treatment planning, interventions, and follow-up can be more difficult to accomplish. When the patient is treated at different sites but within the same system, MDCs using a video conferencing format may be feasible and effective (Dharmarajan et al., 2020). In the community setting, a significant amount of time and effort may be needed to create and maintain an MDT. Challenges to the formation and continuity of functioning of a suitable MDT are real, but that reality does not change the fact that treatment and rehabilitation of HNC, which meet the standards of care, require an MDT (Nekhlyudov et al., 2017).

In the case where an HNC MDT has not previously existed and where one needs to be assembled, psychosocial oncologists (mental health professionals—clinical social workers, clinical and health psychologists, and psychiatrists—trained in cancer patient care), especially psychosocial oncologists sub-subspecialized in HNC, can be the most difficult specialty to locate.

The following resources might be helpful: within a health care system, there is usually a clinical social work service and a psychiatry service (which might include health psychologists, consultation-liaison [CL] psychologists, and/or CL psychiatrists). Many health care systems, especially academic ones, now have "Integrative Medicine" or "Wholistic Medicine" centers or departments, which usually contain mental health professionals and sometimes psychosocial oncologists. If the health care system is within a university, there may be a clinical psychology program within the Department of Psychology and a School or Department of Social Work.

In the community setting, some exploration may be needed to locate a psychosocial oncologist or mental health professional to join an MDT. It may be useful to contact local professional societies or associations for social work, psychology, and/or psychiatry. Local psychosocial oncologists may be located through the American Psychosocial Oncology Society (APOS, 615-432-0090, https://apos-society.org/) or the International Psychosocial Oncology Society (IPOS, 416-968-0260, https://ipos-society.org/). In the United States, the American Cancer Society (800-227-2345, https://www.cancer.org/) and the Cancer Support Community (888-793-9355, https://www.cancersupportcommunity.org/) provide free support services to cancer patients and their families and may have volunteer psychosocial oncologists who could be interested in participating in a community-based HNC MDT. Finally, the national (U.S.) and international professional hypnosis societies, whose memberships are restricted to licensed health care professionals, may have members with medical hypnosis or even psychosocial oncology training who might wish to participate. Those are the Society for Clinical and Experimental Hypnosis (508-598-5553, https://mam.memberclicks.net/), the American Society of Clinical Hypnosis (410-940-6585, https://www.asch.net/aws/ASCH/pt/sp/home_page), and the International Society of Hypnosis (info@ishhypnosis.org, https://www.ishhypnosis.org/).

Expanded scope of health care providers' (HCP) responsibility

Approaching cancer care as "care for the whole person" expands the scope of responsibility for all disciplines involved in providing care to include biological/biomedical (BM) and psychological and social/sociological (PS) challenges and morbidities for patients, caregivers (Longacre et al., 2012), families, and significant others and notably *expands the scope of responsibility and concern to include challenges and stressors affecting the community of HCP.* The current section will consider some practical implications of this expansion of scope for maxillofacial prosthodontic practice, including surveillance for BPS morbidities and referrals to psychosocial oncology specialists.

Surveillance for psychosocial (PS) morbidities of head and neck cancer (HNC) and its treatment

Before turning to specific considerations regarding the implementation of surveillance for PS morbidities in HNC care, four general notes regarding BPS and especially PS morbidities, their assessment, and treatment should be made along with a brief enumeration of recognized PS morbidities. First, there is consensus that BPS morbidities associated with HNC and its treatment can be severe for PCF—more so than for most cancers (Rozen et al., 1972; Hewitt et al., 2005; Hewitt and Ganz, 2006; Ringash, 2015; Haddad and Limaye, 2021a; Goyal et al., 2021; Strong, 1996; Morris et al., 2022; Longacre et al., 2012; Argerakis, 1990; Devins et al., 2013; Graboyes, 2020; Jacobson, 2018; Moschopoulou et al., 2018; Osazuwa-Peters et al., 2018; Ross, 1996; Taher, 2016; Chen et al., 2013; Lin et al., 2016; Dunne et al., 2017; Krebber et al., 2016; Fang and Heckman, 2016). *The severity of BPS morbidities can impact everyone involved in HNC care, including HCP, increasing stress and degrading QOL and ability to perform needed activities.*

Second, as researchers have turned their attention to longer durations of survivorship (Phase 3b, post-treatment, mid-phase care; and Phase 4, end-of-life care), evidence has accumulated that many significant BPS morbidities persist (long-term effects) and/or arise (late effects) 5 to 10 years or longer after the time of initial treatment (Phase 2, peri-treatment; Haddad and Limaye, 2021a; Graboyes et al., 2020; Chen et al., 2013; Chen et al., 2014; Duke et al., 2005; El-Deiry et al., 2005; Funk et al., 2012; Payakachat et al., 2013; Wijers, 2002; Westgaard et al., 2021; Bozec et al., 2021). *HCP should remain alert for long-term and late effects, which can severely impact quantity of life and QOL.*

Third, BPS morbidities appear to be frequently overlooked and undertreated (Ringash, 2015; Krebber et al., 2016; Fang and Heckman, 2016; Giuliani et al., 2017; Henry et al., 2014; Werner et al., 2012; Breen et al., 2017). A contributing factor may be the fact that PCF are generalists—they experience all aspects of care—while HCP on their HNC MDT are specialists. This asymmetry can become problematic. PCF can have questions and concerns about diagnosis and care and can encounter challenging BPS morbidities throughout the entirety of the survivorship arc—that is, from diagnosis through end of life (Hewitt et al., 2005; Rowland et al., 2006; Jacobson, 2018; Haddad and Limaye, 2021a; Gomes et al., 2020). They may attempt to make these concerns and challenges known to HCP regardless of whether the issue falls within or outside the scope of expertise of the MDT specialist they are interacting with during any particular appointment. Further, PCF may communicate information about BPS morbidities obliquely, in ways that may be difficult for the provider to understand or address. In the setting of a busy and demanding practice, specialists may find such expressions of concern to be distractions from their main focus of care, may perceive them as otherwise inconvenient or burdensome, or may elicit a sense of helplessness or impotence in the provider. Yet another contributing factor may be the general level of stress, noted above, arising from the severity of BPS morbidities. All members of the HNC MDT should maintain alertness and receptivity to patients' communications about their concerns. *Treating the whole patient implies that HCP have a responsibility to address or refer every patient concern and challenge that is raised or implied, regardless of whether or not the concern falls within their own specialty or may require extra time to clarify.*

Fourth, PS morbidities tend to be mutually synergistic with (i.e., tend to mutually amplify and attenuate) each other and synergistic with BM morbidities (Ringash, 2015; Haddad and Limaye, 2021a; Jacobson, 2018; Dunne et al., 2017). For example, stress, depression, anxiety, body image distress, pain, alcohol and tobacco use, and/or poor self-care tend to exacerbate one another and can cause, can be caused by, and/or worsen with xerostomia; thickened, sticky saliva; eating and swallowing problems and associated loss of lean muscle mass; reduced range of motion; cosmetic deformities; communication problems; the presence of feeding and/or tracheostomy tubes; and cancer recurrence (Haddad and Limaye, 2021a; Jacobson, 2018; Chen et al., 2013; Duke et al., 2005; El-Deiry et al., 2005; Funk et al., 2012; Payakachat et al., 2013). *One implication of this pattern of synergy is that the detection of any of these morbidities should alert the provider to the possible presence of others. Another important implication is that efforts to treat or manage these mutually reinforcing morbidities can be thwarted if they are treated in isolation.* As noted, PCF experience multiple morbidities globally, irrespective of the fact that their HCP skill sets are specialized. Effective treatment and management can require coordination of care with other specialists in the HNC MDT.

Biopsychosocial (BPS) morbidities of head and neck cancer (HNC) and its treatment affecting patients

What are the particular symptoms that may afflict patients? The list is long and impressive. BM morbidities can include (but are not limited to) dental complications and oral health problems; xerostomia and thickened, sticky saliva; radiation caries; dental pain; osteoradionecrosis; trismus; dysphagia; complications of feeding tube placement; complications of tracheostomy tube placement; neuromuscular morbidities, including difficulty speaking, hearing loss, dizziness, near syncope, and peripheral neuropathy; aspiration of food and/or saliva; drooling; loss of appetite; diminished or lost sense of taste or smell; weight loss or gain; difficulty exercising; complications of total laryngectomy; fistula formation; fibrotic changes in irradiated tissues, including neck stiffness and limitation in range of motion; lymphedema; neurocognitive effects, such as "chemo-brain"; fatigue; damage to vital structures, such as the carotid artery and kidney; cosmetic deformity and disfigurement; and recurrent or new primary tumors. PS morbidities can include (but again, are not limited to) depression; anxiety; agoraphobia and social withdrawal; intimacy and sexual dysfunction; body image distress; suicidality; sleep disorders; financial distress, including problems in or loss of employment; substance use and abuse, including alcohol and tobacco; lowered self-esteem and belief in self-efficacy; and chronic pain (Miller et al., 2016; Haddad and Limaye, 2021a; Morris et al.,

2022; Devins et al., 2013; Moschopoulou et al., 2018; Osazuwa-Peters, 2018; Chen et al., 2013; Fang and Heckman, 2016; Chen et al., 2014; Duke et al., 2005; El-Deiry et al., 2005; Funk et al., 2012; Payakachat, 2013; Wijers et al., 2002; Ganzer et al., 2015; Howren et al., 2013; Martino and Ringash, 2008; Rao et al., 2021; Verdonschot et al., 2017). It is important to note that some morbidities, such as drooling or cosmetic deformity, which may not appear to be terribly significant from a BM perspective, can have devastating PS impact.

Jacobson (2018) has given a moving and useful general description of the multidimensional morbidities of an HNC diagnosis and treatment from the patient's perspective:

> It turns out for HNC survivors, that the diseased anatomical apparatus supporting cosmesis and upper aerodigestive tract (UADT) functions is inseparable from the human experience: HNC has invaded the machinery underlying spoken and emotional communication essential to self-expression and socialization; the intricate pleasures of deriving nutrition associated with tasting, eating, and drinking; the effortless capacity for oronasal breathing and sense of smell; the automaticity of coughing, sneezing, and laughing; and the hormonal mechanisms underlying emotional and physical comfort. Furthermore, associated physical disruptions, such as scars, disfigurement, or a stoma for neck-breathing, may be bared to the world, frequently being outside of the areas typically covered by clothing. Moreover, UADT functions have substantial significance: inability to breathe, speak or eat normally may drastically impact quality of life (QOL), affecting nutritional and communication status, relationships, societal roles, and work, profoundly influencing the greater survivorship experience.

Psychosocial (PS) morbidities of head and neck cancer (HNC) and its treatment affecting caregivers and families

Every one of the BPS morbidities listed above can cause secondhand or vicarious distress in caregivers and family members. Some BPS morbidities create firsthand distress, anxiety, and depression in caregivers and family (Haddad and Limaye, 2021a; Longacre et al., 2011; Fang and Heckman, 2016; Ross et al., 2009; Sterba et al., 2016; Richardson et al., 2015; Kassir et al., 2021; Richardson et al., 2016; Hodges and Humphris, 2009; Verdonck-de Leeuw et al., 2007; Drabe et al., 2008; Gondivkar et al., 2021; Wang et al., 2021; Goswami and Gupta, 2020; Dri et al., 2020). An example is financial stress, which may directly affect the entire family, particularly if the patient is a primary source of income (Longacre et al., 2011). Financial stress can be exacerbated if family resources are slim and if the caregiver needs to cut back on their own employment to provide for the patient's needs. Of course, such stress can trigger or worsen anxiety and depression. If the patient's ability to accomplish activities of daily living (ADLs) and contribute to running a household are diminished, those responsibilities can increase requirements for caregivers and family. Fear of future illness (including recurrence), disability, and death can beset the patient and can be a direct and major source of anxiety for the caregiver and other family (Longacre et al., 2011; Lin et al., 2016; Hodges and Humphris, 2009). This anxiety can intensify in anticipation of appointments when bad news might be given by the doctor.

The sheer emotional burden, practical workload, and expenditure of time involved in keeping the family going, managing the patient's care at home, coordinating multiple health care–related appointments, and a resulting steep decrease in access to rewarding and pleasurable experiences can swamp a caregiver's life and create a spiraling degradation in their capacity to support the patient and other family members. Further, the caregiver and family members can feel they are not entitled to or must hide from the patient their own needs and distress, lest they strain the parent-patient's ability to cope or hasten the patient's deterioration or death. The author's clinical impression, formed over years of experience with the HNC population, is that the primary caregiver (often the spouse or adult child of the patient) experiences the most psychological stress of anyone in the patient-caregiver-family-provider system.

For children of HNC patients, witnessing the parent-patient's pain, struggles, disfigurement, impairment, or loss of function; stress and deterioration in the putatively well, caregiving parent and in the spousal relationship; and death of the parent-patient can be traumatizing and can produce lifelong psychological damage, including distrust of HCP. Young children, because of age-appropriate identification with the parent-patient and because of beliefs in their own omniscience, can create deeply held beliefs that they will become ill as their parent did, and/or they can think that they can or should somehow protect their parents, prevent or heal the illness, and prevent death. Consequently, young children in cancer-afflicted families can be vulnerable to deep confusion, anxiety, and intense guilt. As noted, all HCP on the HNC MDT should "keep an eye out," maintaining alertness for these easily overlooked morbidities affecting caregivers and family members.

Psychosocial (PS) morbidities of head and neck cancer (HNC) and its treatment affecting health care providers (HCP)

This section describes evolving conceptualizations of PS morbidities affecting HCP generally, oncology HCP, and HNC HCP specifically. With the gradual acceptance of the BPS model and its emphasis on a wholistic or systemic view of health care and of cancer care, there has been a significant shift in perspective on the role and vulnerabilities of HCP. From the more reductionistic perspective inherent in the BM model, the HCP appears as an external and objective agent, outside of the pathological circumstances and so unaffected by those circumstances. But from a BPS perspective, the HCP role is understood as an intrinsic element functioning within an ecology, which can produce illness, healing, and health. So from a BPS perspective, it is natural to consider ways in which morbidities arising from cancer diagnosis and treatment may affect any participant in the ecology, including HCP.

Definition of burnout (BO)—Burnout (BO) is classified as an "occupational phenomenon" within ICD-11 and is defined as follows: "'Burn-out' is a syndrome conceptualized as resulting from chronic workplace stress that has not been successfully managed. Burn-out refers specifically to phenomena in the occupational context and should not be applied to describe experiences in other areas of life" (WHO, 2022).

It is characterized by three dimensions:

- Feelings of energy depletion or exhaustion
- Increased mental distance from one's job or feelings of negativism or cynicism related to one's job
- Reduced professional efficacy

Seriousness and progression—BO is a serious condition with "negative repercussions for organisations, clinics and companies, resulting in poor service to patients, increased absenteeism, clinical errors, and financial losses, as well as negative consequences for the individual in question that are very similar to the symptoms of depression, potentially even leading to suicide" (Gómez-Polo et al., 2022). BO appears to begin subtly and, often, progress insidiously (Gómez-Polo et al., 2022; Maslach and Jackson, 1981).

Prevalence—Although the precise prevalence varies among HCP specialties and studies may be somewhat affected by response bias, it appears that 40% to 50% of physicians report some degree of BO (Kane, 2020), that the rate may be considerably higher among dentists (Gómez-Polo et al., 2022; Ahola and Hakanen, 2007), and that physicians are at higher risk of BO and report lower job satisfaction than other working adult subpopulations (Shanafelt, 2019). Given the demanding nature of HNC care, there is every reason to presume that the prevalence of BO among HNC HCP falls within this range or is higher.

Risk factors—Risk factors appear to be related to conditions that modulate work-related stress and to factors that limit HCP abilities to discharge or release that stress (Gómez-Polo et al., 2022; Ahola and Hakanen, 2007; Gibson et al., 2021; Johns, 2005; Golub et al., 2007; Golub et al., 2008; Girgis et al., 2008; Swetz et al., 2009; Contag et al., 2010; Eelen et al., 2014; Porto et al., 2014; Singh et al., 2015; Hlubocky et al., 2016; Maslach and Leiter, 2016; Shanafelt and Noseworthy, 2016; Chiu, 2017; Hlubocky et al., 2017; Lamiani et al., 2017; Talbot and Dean, 2019; Winner and Knight, 2019; Laor-Maayany et al., 2020; LeNoble et al., 2020; Alabi et al., 2021; Bui et al., 2021; Kazmi, 2021; HaGani et al., 2022). Factors that may increase or decrease the likelihood of BO appear at all levels of the health care delivery system, from large-scale institutions with multiple facilities to departments, to provider teams, and to individual HCP and their support staff. Specific risk factors tend to be identified similarly across reports and include structural factors, such as a lack of organizational support; excessive work demands and impediments to adequately fulfilling them; compensation levels; dealing with high uncertainty, trauma, and death; student status, younger age, and years in practice (less experienced HCP at higher risk); nonpartnered marital status; and personality factors, such as compulsiveness, neuroticism, excessive conscientiousness, alexithymia, limited psychological hardiness, and type A behavior (Singh et al., 2015; Hlubocky et al., 2016; HaGani et al., 2022). Some studies and reviews report that women are at a higher risk of BO (Hlubocky et al., 2016; HaGani et al., 2022), while others report men to be at higher risk (Singh et al., 2015).

Research and conceptual evolution—Early work on adverse reactions to occupational stressors appears to have begun in the 1970s (Maslach and Jackson, 1981; Figley, 1978), and by the mid-1990s, literature had developed around the recognition that HCP treating trauma survivors were themselves vulnerable to PS distress and injury (Figley, 1995; Stamm, 1995; Maslach et al., 1997; Pearlman and Saakvitne, 1995). This vulnerability was termed "burnout" by some authors (Maslach and Jackson, 1981; Maslach et al., 1997), "compassion fatigue" (Figley, 1995), "secondary traumatic stress" (Figley, 1995; Stamm, 1995), and "vicarious traumatization" (Pearlman and Saakvitne, 1995) by others. Since its beginnings, the research literature related to BO has proliferated extensively and continues to expand (Gómez-Polo et al., 2022; Maslach and Jackson, 1981; Maslach and Leiter, 2016; Lamiani et al., 2017; Talbot and Dean, 2019; Winner and Knight, 2019; HaGani et al., 2022; Figley, 1995; Maslach et al., 1997; Pearlman and Saakvitne, 1995; Figley, 2002a; Figley, 2002b; Maslach and Leiter, 2021; Stamm, 2010; Esplen et al., 2022; Lazar et al., 2022; Prevost et al., 2022; Zhang et al., 2022).

Two major research lineages will be discussed here, one emerging from the work of Figley, Stamm, and Pearlman and colleagues, and one emerging from the work of Maslach and colleagues. Each lineage has produced a distinctive family of questionnaire-based methods of measuring PS morbidity in HCP, and both families of instruments have been extensively used in research studies (Maslach and Leiter, 2021; Lazar et al., 2022), though a given study will typically use an instrument from one or the other lineage. Studies will typically approach BO using (implicitly or explicitly) the theoretical framework associated with the particular instrument they employ.

These two research traditions differ somewhat in their conceptualizations of provider vulnerability and in their approaches to measuring it, and while findings from each lineage differ in detail, overall, there is considerable convergence and agreement on important findings: both lines of BO research strongly agree that the prevalence of BO among HCP is high, that it represents a major problem, and that addressing it requires interventions at multiple levels (i.e., effectively addressing BO requires interventions at the level of the health care organization or system; individual facilities, clinics, and practices; individual HCP; and professional cultures, values, and expectations of HCP; Gómez-Polo et al., 2022; Kane, 2020; Ahola and Hakanen, 2007; Shanafelt et al., 2019; Gibson et al., 2021; Johns, 2005; Golub et al., 2007; Golub et al., 2008; Girgis et al., 2009; Swetz et al., 2009; Contag et al., 2010; Eelen et al., 2014; Porto et al., 2013; Singh et al., 2015; Hlubocky et al., 2016; Maslach and Leiter, 2016; Shanafelt, 2016; Chiu, 2017; Laor-Maayany et al., 2020; LeNoble et al., 2020; Alabi et al., 2021; Bui et al., 2021; Brake et al., 2008; Gillman et al., 2015). The two lineages also make similar recommendations for preventing, mitigating, and fostering resilience to BO (Swetz et al., 2009; Hlubocky et al., 2016; Shanafelt and Noswworthy, 2017; Chiu, 2017; Winner and Knight, 2019; LeNoble et al., 2020; Alabi et al., 2021; Bui et al., 2021; Figley, 2002a; Esplen et al., 2022; Prevost et al., 2022; Gillman et al., 2015; Delaney, 2018; Moore et al., 2018; Vercio et al., 2021; Watts et al., 2021).

An important idea, emphasized by both research lineages, is that BPS toxicity in HCP should be understood not as originating in the individual HCP but rather as *resulting from exposure to morbidities in a particular work setting*. That is, negative effects are seen as fundamentally occupational in nature rather than intrapsychic, arising from interactions between risk factors in the workplace and predisposing susceptibilities in the HCP. Endorsement of this distinction is also evident in the ICD-11 classification of BO as an "occupational phenomenon" and not as a disease. An intended effect of this distinction is to reduce the stigma associated with BO and to support the development and use of multilevel prevention and mitigation strategies.

The research lineage beginning with Figley and Stamm (The ProQOL-20, Burnout [BO], compassion fatigue [CF], secondary traumatic stress [STS], vicarious trauma, and psychological balance). Figley developed the construct "compassion fatigue" (CF; Figley, 1995; Figley, 2002a; Figley, 2002b). In his initial conceptualization, CF was seen as consisting of two factors: BO and a second factor relating to "the costs of caring, empathy, and emotional investment in helping the suffering." The second factor was subsequently characterized as "secondary traumatic stress" (Laor-Maayany et al., 2020; Stamm, 2010).

The development of scales to assess CF was begun by Figley in the late 1980s. He subsequently collaborated with Stamm, who gradually took the lead in the development of a CF measure. By the late 1990s, this project produced what became an extensively researched and employed instrument to assess overall professional quality of life, the ProQOL (Stamm, 2010). The ProQOL defined professional quality of life in terms of two factors, "compassion satisfaction" (CS) and CF. CS was seen as a unitary or integrated factor, while CF was seen as having two subfactors, "burnout" and "secondary traumatic stress" (STS; Stamm, 2010). Implicit in this model is the idea that CS and CF can vary independently (e.g., an HCP could simultaneously experience high CS and high CF). Stamm considered that, while CF, STS, and vicarious trauma appear to differ in nuanced ways (perhaps they emphasize different features of the same underlying phenomenon), psychometric research attempting to differentiate them has largely failed to do so, and the terms can be regarded as essentially interchangeable (Stamm, 2010).

A modernized revision of the ProQOL, the ProQOL-20 (Lazar et al., 2022), has recently been published, which, based on factor analytic and other psychometric considerations, uses two unitary factors, CS and CF (thus assimilating the two subfactors of CF in the earlier version, BO and STS, into the new version's unitary CF factor). The ProQOL-20 combines its two subscales into a more intuitively accessible, single parameter, its "Psychological Balance" ratio, in which a positive value indicates greater satisfaction (CS) on balance and a negative value indicates greater fatigue (CF) and greater related morbidity (Lazar et al., 2022).

The research lineage beginning with Maslach (the MBI and the three-factor model of BO). The Maslach Burnout Inventory (MBI; Maslach et al., 1997; Maslach and Leiter, 2021), originally developed in the early 1980s (Maslach and Jackson, 1981), is an extensively studied and widely used clinical and research tool to assess BO in a number of groups, including dentists (Gómez-Polo et al., 2022; Ahola and Hakanen, 2007; Porto et al., 2014; Brake et al., 2008), oncology HCP (Eelen et al., 2014), and HNC HCP (Gibson et al., 2021; Johns, 2005; Golub et al., 2007; Golub et al., 2008; Contag et al., 2010; Porto et al., 2014; HaGani et al., 2022). The MBI conceptualizes BO using three factors, measured with subscales labeled emotional exhaustion, depersonalization (or cynicism), and personal accomplishment (or professional efficacy; HaGani et al., 2022; Maslach and Leiter, 2021). Of note, the definition of Burnout Syndrome appearing in the ICD-11 classification is based on the three-factor conceptualization of BO developed in MBI research and clinical applications.

Prevention, protective factors, mitigation, and resilience—BO is conceptualized as being multilevel in its causes (i.e., arises from factors at institutional, team, and individual HCP levels; Maslach et al., 1997; Stamm, 2010) and multifactorial in its manifestations (Gómez-Polo et al., 2022; Maslach and Leiter, 2016; Winner and Knight, 2019; Stamm, 2010; Lazar et al., 2022). This naturally suggests that interventions targeting particular manifestations of BO or targeting combinations of BO manifestations could be effective. A further implication is that the more comprehensive interventions can be made (in terms of levels of intervention), the more effective they are likely to be in preventing or mitigating BO and in fostering resilience at all levels.

The fact that relatively few studies have been reported testing such interventions specifically with HNC HCP (Gibson et al., 2021) does not reduce the need for actively coping with BO in HNC HCP. Reported interventions at the institutional, team, and individual HCP levels targeting BO in oncology HCP and HCP more generally tend to identify very similar risk factors; are notably similar in the approaches they explore for BO prevention, mitigation, and resilience; and generally report tested interventions as being well received and beneficial to participants (Hlubocky et al., 2016; Shanafelt and Noseworthy, 2017; Hlubocky et al., 2017; LeNoble et al., 2020; Alabi et al., 2021; Bui et al., 2021; Eslplen et al., 2022; Prevost et al., 2022; Gillman et al., 2015; Vercio et al., 2021; Watts et al., 2021; Beckman et al., 2012; Hlubocky, 2022). So it is reasonable to draw on research and practice across a wide range of levels and HCP groups to identify interventions, which have promise for HNC HCP in particular.

Institutional-level interventions described in the literature tend to focus on changing attitudes and priorities on the part of institutional leaders and on demonstrating the effectiveness of particular educational programs. Institutional leaders, at all levels, are encouraged to acknowledge the reality of BO and to actively promote a culture and institute programs, which directly affect BO (Hlubocky et al., 2016; Shanafelt and Noseworthy, 2017; Hlubocky et al., 2017; Winner and Knight, 2019; LeNoble et al., 2020; Alabi et al., 2021; Vercio et al., 2021; Hlubocky, 2022), such as reducing the burden of documentation and ensuring fair compensation rules (Winner and Knight, 2019). Directly addressing the highest levels of institutional decision-makers, an article in Mayo Clinic Proceedings describes organizational strategies developed at that institution to target BO and to support systemic well-being (Shanafelt and Noseworthy, 2017). Their blueprint includes an acknowledgment by executive leaders of the reality, prevalence, and severity of BO's impact on a hospital system and includes mobilizing leadership at all levels to address BO, providing resources for developing and implementing interventions and then evaluating their effectiveness, supporting the development of community spirit in work settings, incentivizing effective action and behaviors, supporting flexibility in working arrangements and work-life integration, and committing resources to promotion of resilience and care.

The BO literature contains a number of papers describing evaluations of educational and psycho-educational programs designed to legitimate BO prevention and strengthen resiliency skills. These are institutional interventions in the sense that they require institutional recognition and support for development and implementation, are usually conducted in group formats, and target skill development in teams and in individual HCP (Hlubocky et al., 2016; Hlubocky et al., 2017; Lenoble et al., 2020; Alabi et al., 2021; Bui et al., 2021; Esplen et al., 2022; Prevost et al., 2022; Gilman et al., 2015; Vercio et al., 2021; Watts et al., 2021; Beckman et al., 2012). These programs—lasting from several weeks to several months, often meeting weekly or more frequently—include a wide variety of didactic and experiential components, such as support groups (sharing personal experiences), meditation and mindfulness training (developing attentional skills, compassion, and for stress reduction), promotion of self-awareness (especially awareness of emotions) and self-regulation, development of communication skills (empathic listening and authentic self-expression), clinical supervision, use of telemedicine and software applications, stress management (including self-care activities such as exercise, nutrition, and cognitive skill training, such as reframing and proportionalizing), guided imagery, art therapy, team activities, managing grief and loss, and gratitude practice. As noted, these reports present data consistent with the efficacy of their programs.

Team-level interventions generally involve educational and psycho-educational programs, such as those described for institutional interventions but implement training within established working groups (Hlubocky et al., 2017; Winner and Knight, 2019; Lenoble et al., 2020; Alabi et al., 2021; Bui et al., 2021; Esplen et al., 2022; Prevost et al., 2022; Gilman et al., 2015; Vercio et al., 2021; Watts et al., 2021; Beckman et al., 2012; Hlubocky, 2022). Team-oriented interventions aim to reduce intra-group factors that promote BO, such as feelings of isolation and group fragmentation, and enhance resilience by promoting team cohesiveness, coordination, supportiveness, and effectiveness in the provision of care. They do this by mobilizing the potential of small working groups to provide powerful emotional support within and across professional disciplines through informal (casual) interactions and formal structures (such as team meetings focused on creating emotional connection and safety). Reports describe effective implementation of team-level programs using techniques such as mentoring; a buddy system; mindfulness and meditation; active cultivation of compassion and gratitude; cognitive techniques, such as reframing to put experiences in proportion and in perspective; advanced communication skills training; debriefing, trauma sensitivity training, and collective emotional processing of difficult or traumatic experiences; and clinical supervision. The necessity of institutional support for team-level interventions is frequently emphasized (Hlubocky et al., 2017; Winner and Knight, 2019; Lenoble et al., 2020; Alabi et al., 2021; Gillman et al., 2015; Vercio et al., 2021; Hlubocky, 2022).

Individual-level interventions tend to emphasize skill development, provided in institutional and team-oriented training programs, and adoption of attitudes, expectations, and behaviors that are realistic and emotionally encouraging (Swetz et al., 2009; Hlubocky et al., 2016; Shanfelt and Noseworthy, 2017; Hlubocky et al., 2017; Winner and Knight, 2019; Alabi et al., 2021; Bui et al., 2021; Prevost et al., 2022; Gillman et al., 2015; Vercio et al., 2021; Watts et al., 2021; Hlubocky, 2022). Individual HCP are encouraged to take a proactive stance toward their own well-being and toward adverse aspects of their workplace. HCP are encouraged to support themselves by valuing and maintaining work-life balance, including rewarding and refreshing activities outside of work; strong relationships; adequate sleep, exercise, and nutrition; use of humor; and by "taking a transcendental perspective" (Swetz et al., 2009). HCP are encouraged to cope actively with difficult work factors by directly addressing them, cultivating a sense of empowerment through accepting personal responsibility, and applying their personal power and skills to change circumstances and norms, which increase the likelihood of BO. At the same time, HCP are encouraged to assess and transform perfectionistic expectations or self-denying attitudes they may hold (Swetz et al., 2009; Hlubocky et al., 2016; Hlubocky et al., 2017; Winner and Knight, 2019).

Recognizing BO: Personal observations and recommendations—In the author's experience, oncology HCP at all levels of experience and training tend to have a great deal of confidence and pride in their own resilience and capacity to tolerate stress. While this attitude may be well earned, can be beneficial, and provides some protection against morbidities encountered in HCP roles, it also creates a bias toward ignoring indications of stress and BO and can increase vulnerability. This may particularly be so because recognition of vulnerabilities can feel like an acknowledgment of weakness and a degree of failure. Given the high prevalence of BO, such expectations and judgments are potentially hazardous, not only for HCP and for success and longevity in their careers, but for PCF and for families of HCP as well.

Realistic acknowledgment that stress and BO are, in fact, risks of being an HCP generally and an HNC provider specifically is important. Cultivation of a work culture and norms that support this realistic recognition of actual limitations and vulnerabilities, simply as matters of fact, can encourage collegial consultation and support for recognition and engagement with appropriate stress management strategies.

Summary: Burnout—Burnout (BO) is understood as an occupational problem arising from interactions between workplace risk factors and worker characteristics (including worker needs and vulnerabilities). BO poses a significant risk for HCP, PCF, and health care delivery organizations and systems. There is a consensus in the research literature that, as is the case with oncology HCP generally (Girgis et al., 2009; Eelen et al., 2014), burnout is prevalent and is of significant concern for HNC HCP in particular (Gibson et al., 2021). Since its articulation in the 1970s, the construct of BO itself has evolved toward increasing the recognition of its social systemic context and causes (Maslach and Leiter, 2016; Winner and Knight, 2019). Risk factors appear at all levels of health care delivery systems and include excessive demands by the work setting, such as demands relating to patient care and documentation. Additional risk factors include insufficient institutional support for developing positive collegial relations and opportunities to release stress at work, inadequate work-life balance, and unrealistic or perfectionistic self-expectations by HCP. Recognition of indications of BO by individual HCP is often made difficult due to a deeply held adherence to professional values of hard work and provision of service, regardless of personal cost and effort, and a misguided sense that BO symptoms are manifestations of personal weakness or failure (Winner and Wright, 2019).

Interventions designed to prevent or mitigate BO and to promote resilience in organizations, teams, and individual HCP have been reported. A wide variety of approaches have been shown to be effective and well received in oncology and other health care provision settings, which should work well in the setting of HNC. Effective interventions target multiple levels of the health care delivery system, including the institution, the immediate setting of health care delivery, and the self-care decisions of individual HCP. At the individual level, effective interventions address early recognition of BO and emphasize active stress management, taking advantage of the support from colleagues and institutional resources, and commitment to engaging in rewarding social and other activities outside of work.

Guidelines for surveillance of psychosocial (PS) morbidities of head and neck cancer (HNC) and its treatment

Guidelines for HNC surveillance, including PS morbidities, have been published by a number of major organizations (Tevaarwerk et al., 2021; Goyal et al., 2021; Nekhlyudov et al., 2018; ASCO, 2017; Masroor et al., 2019; Cohen et al., 2016). Haddad and Limaye (2021a) provide an especially useful and concise source of recommendations for survivorship care of HNC patients, including PS surveillance and links to society guidelines (Haddad and Limaye, 2021b).

As the patient progresses from Phase 2, the peri-treatment period, through Phase 3a, early posttreatment phase, and into Phase 3b, midphase, in most models of survivorship, the patient's primary care provider (PCP) is increasingly relied upon as the main provider of surveillance for recurrent disease, new primaries, and long-term and late-arising morbidities (Tevaarwerk et al., 2021; Goyal et al., 2021; ASCO, 2017). It is therefore important that communication links be maintained between the PCP and the oncology specialists, including the maxillofacial prosthodontist. Typical recommended surveillance intervals are every one to three months during the first year following Phase 2 (peri-treatment), every two to six months in year two, every four to eight months in years three to five, and once per year beyond five years (ASCO, 2017). In addition to providing early detection of BM needs, it appears that patients experience PS benefits (reassurance) from surveillance visits, especially when visits are in person (McLaren et al., 2021; Alders and Hermens, 2017; Szturz et al., 2020).

In situations where the patient does not have a strong, effective, or dependable relationship with their PCP, or when visits with the PCP are primarily conducted using telemedicine or other non-face-to-face formats, more of the responsibility for surveillance falls to the specialists within the MDT. This possibility underscores the importance of maintaining good communication among all members of the oncology team.

Within the HNC MDT, the maxillofacial prosthodontist and the SLP are particularly well positioned to surveil for PS morbidities. As noted, specialists focused on rehabilitation, such as maxillofacial prosthodontists and speech and language pathologists (SLPs), have historically been oriented to treating the whole patient and, to some degree, treating their PS "ecosystem," and so have been alert for morbidities that can affect patient's QOL. In contrast to other disciplines within the HNC MDT, these two disciplines tend to have continuous contact with PCF throughout the entire arc of survivorship (i.e., from shortly after diagnosis nearly through to end of life). Further, the primary focus of technical attention for these groups extends naturally and easily to include PCF's QOL (e.g., exploring problems of a patient's compliance with their oral hygiene regime can naturally extend to a discussion about their emotional state and patterns of relating to their caregiver, spouse, and/or adult children).

In the author's experience, PCF tend to have positive levels of trust and strong emotional bonding with their maxillofacial prosthodontists and their SLPs. Perhaps this is facilitated by the continuity of relationships with their maxillofacial prosthodontists and with their SLPs, helped by the naturally elevated level of interest these HCP have in their patients' overall experience.

These factors all combine to create an exceptionally good fit between the roles of the maxillofacial prosthodontist and the SLP and the critically important function of ongoing surveillance for BPS morbidities. For these specialists, an expanded scope of responsibility means developing a greater sensitivity to detecting morbidities they would not normally address themselves, particularly PS morbidities, and either addressing them or making appropriate referrals. In a circumstance in which the PCP-patient relationship does not support sufficient surveillance, the maxillofacial prosthodontist may become an even more important source of ongoing psychological support for the PCF and a source of surveillance data for the entire MDT team.

Conducting surveillance for psychosocial (PS) morbidities of head and neck cancer (HNC)

If consistent surveillance is not available from the patient's PCP, how can the maxillofacial prosthodontist and other specialized members of the MDT integrate surveillance for PS toxicities into busy practices and tightly scheduled clinic visits? Consensus intervals for the frequency of follow-up examinations, as HNC PCF move through the arc of survivorship, are described in the previous section on guidelines. (As noted in the guidelines section, Haddad and Limaye [2021a] provide a highly concise, readable, and therefore very useful summary of care guidelines.) In terms of sources of data for screening, three basic modalities for gathering PS data are available for the specialist HNC HCP: history, observation of PCF behavior during their appointment, and brief, standardized psychological instruments.

History—While acknowledging the absence of published, quantitative evidence on which to base guidelines for continuing surveillance of HNC patients (Haddad and Limaye, 2021a; Alders and Hermens, 2017), recommendations can be made for areas to be covered in a history. The following PS and related issues are known to occur in HNC patients during survivorship and so can be reviewed: interval changes in life events; chronic and acute pain; mobility; autonomic dysfunction, especially dizziness and near syncope; neurocognitive effects including "chemo brain" and cognitive impairment; sexual dysfunction and intimacy issues; social withdrawal; financial and employment changes and problems; body and self-image issues; emotional and mood issues, including distress, depression, suicidality, and anxiety; behaviors and behavior patterns relating to health promotion, including healthy weight maintenance, physical activity, nutrition, tobacco cessation, e-cigarette use, vaping, and alcohol consumption (ASCO, 2017; Haddad and Limaye, 2021a). Haddad and Limaye (2021a) recommend encouraging patients regarding healthy lifestyle choices (nutrition, exercise, and sleep) and suggest offering education regarding the importance of abstinence from tobacco and limiting alcohol consumption to reduce the likelihood of recurrence. They also recommend screening caregivers and family members for changes in QOL and levels of energy and exhaustion.

Observation of behavior during the appointment—Direct, respectful, and compassionate observation during the appointment of the PCF—considered as individuals and as a working group or team, coupled with self-observation by the HCP—can provide a rich source of information regarding the PCF's ability to deal with challenges of survivorship and to identify unmet needs. Therefore, HCP should pay attention to—and not discount—what they notice about PCF and how they experience themselves during appointments. Departures from expected or functional deportment or behavior, when thoughtfully and nonjudgmentally contemplated, can provide valuable hints about aspects of BPS status and PCF coping that may require further investigation or clarification and possible intervention or referral.

How to observe? Many HCP are highly perceptive regarding PCF deportment and behaviors, but it may be useful to make explicit some observational goals and techniques. In terms of observational goals, it is vitally important for the HCP to maintain visceral contact with the purpose of their contemplation of a PCF, which is to be of help by identifying PCF strengths and skills, vulnerabilities and dysfunctions, and needs—voiced and unexpressed. Maintaining contact with this overarching purpose ("feeling it in the bones") will protect HCP from many of the stresses that naturally arise when interacting with people who themselves may be in distress and will support HCPs' intuitive nimbleness and empathic attunement with PCF. For example, maintaining such a visceral connection with the goal of observation will support sustaining a compassionate attitude and feeling toward the PCF, even when their behavior is dysfunctional, defensive, or off-putting.

In terms of observational techniques, it can be helpful to recall that contrasts with and departures from expectations tend to be noticed. Being conscious of and purposeful with such observational presuppositions is important in at least two ways. Judgmental, bigoted, prejudiced, and therefore harmful behavior and attitudes on the part of HCP arise from beliefs and expectations, which are often habitual, unconscious, or if conscious, have not been thoughtfully challenged. It is, of course, essential that HCP protect PCF from any tendencies that HCP may have to relate to them in such ways. Beyond avoiding destructive interactions with PCF, thoughtfully choosing the expectations employed to orient observations greatly enhances the effectiveness and utility of those observations.

One useful set of contrasts to track observationally involves what psychologists have called "manner of approach." When people are confronted with a challenge or problem that really matters to them, are in touch with their own sense of agency, and have a realistic appraisal of their ability to successfully deal with the situation, they approach the issue with a combination of readily perceivable qualities: a situationally appropriate balance of caution, courage, and confidence; appropriate degrees of perseverance, determination, and grit; efficiency and practicality; openness to genuinely helpful collaboration; perceptiveness and alertness regarding unhelpful avenues of effort or advice; and proportionality regarding the importance of the current issue relative to their overall values, principles, and goals (i.e., they show good judgment about how important the current issue actually is in the larger scheme of things). Fundamentally, when people are in touch with their sense of agency, they work to solve the problem. When PCF have this manner of approach, the internal experience of HCP can be one of feeling privileged to participate in a meaningful collaboration in which the skill and knowledge they have worked so long and hard to acquire can be brought to bear. The HCP may feel deeply moved and gratified, uplifted, and inspired—even when a cure or a desired level of rehabilitation cannot be achieved.

In contrast, some PCF groups enter their survivorship arc with weak, dysfunctional, or nonexistent connections to their sense of personal agency and empowerment, and some lose an otherwise functional connection with their agency as the result of the BPS distress they encounter in survivorship. When PCF are not in touch with a realistic sense of their own agency—either over- or underestimating it—they will experience this internally and communicate it externally in a number of ways that contrast with expectations of problem-solving attitudes, emotions, and behavior, and so be noticeable to the HCP.

PCF conduct that avoids, slows, or disrupts their own care and the work of HCP constitutes both a challenge and an opportunity for HCP. The challenging aspect for HCP is to find a way to acknowledge and tolerate the distress that arises in themselves while continuing to stay connected—behaviorally, emotionally, and intellectually—with their healing role and tasks and continuing to relate to the PCF in ways that are professional, helpful, and honest (in psychotherapy, this is referred to as "containing" disturbing responses elicited in the therapist). As was suggested at the beginning of this section, the opportunity for HCP is to use these observations to perform some "psychological alchemy," transforming the lead of problematic PCF behavior into the gold of accurately targeted care and strengthened working alliance with the PCF. This can be done by using HCP observations of PCF experience and of their own internal experience to better understand what the PCF's underlying needs or desires are and what obstacle(s) they have encountered that triggered their behavior.

HCP can view the PCF's unhelpful behavior as a communication of sorts, a metaphorical outreach for assistance with a problem they may or may not recognize, that is important to them and which they have been unable to solve. Depending on their personal style, the HCP can attempt to generate a hypothesis about the PCF's unmet need and what to do about it and then present their understanding to the PCF in a way that the PCF can integrate and possibly use to join (or rejoin) the HCP in the work of their cancer care (e.g., "You seem frustrated today. Are you feeling that I'm not hearing what you're saying? Is something else getting in your way?"). Alternatively, the HCP can share their observation and invite the PCF to join them in exploring what the observation might suggest regarding legitimate needs the PCF may have (e.g., "To me, you seem to be having difficulty in expressing yourself today, and I feel concerned about it. Am I perceiving you rightly? Do you understand why?"). It should be noted that figuring out what the problem is that is being obliquely expressed is not always easy or even possible; sometimes requires HCP thought, reflection, and consultation with colleagues after the appointment; sometimes should trigger consultation with or direct intervention by a psychosocial oncologist on the MDT; and sometimes requires the HCP to set limits on inappropriate or disruptive PCF behavior.

The following are more specific domains and behaviors, *interval changes*, that may indicate a disruption in a PCF's working connection with their sense of agency and that may deserve further exploration.

In the domain of appointment-related behavior, notable behaviors are lateness or inconsistency in making or keeping appointments; inability to use appointment time effectively; dress that is unusual or inconsistent with professional settings; impolite, abrasive, disruptive, or otherwise difficult interactions with front office staff, clinic staff, or other HCP; and failure to keep agreements regarding payment.

PCF patterns of physical behavior and movements can arise from distress and/or a lack of sense of agency: they may move and gesture in ways that are slow, ineffective or inefficient, awkward, rushed, repetitive, tense, or stiff (such movement patterns can, of course, have BM causes and simultaneously can express PS distress and imply loss of or a diminished sense of agency).

Any member of the PCF group may speak and interact in ways that indicate inadequate coping and a loss of sense of agency. Speech may be poorly articulated or poorly expressed or organized and, as a result, difficult for the HCP to follow. Poorly organized speech can arise from neurocognitive factors (e.g., so-called chemobrain) and/or from anxiety, suspiciousness, or depression. The PCF may show a reduced ability to focus or to stay on topic, forgetting or losing track of what was said, or using odd or inappropriate expressions.

Distressed mood and affect in the PCF can be expressed directly and can be "radiated" to those around them ("emotional contagion"). Commonly felt distressed affect and emotions are feelings of despair, defeat, fear, tenseness, anxiety, and depression. Less commonly, PCF may experience and communicate guilt, emotional numbness, inappropriate neutrality (so-called *belle indifférence*), emotional withdrawal, or suicidality.

A PCF may express inappropriate aggression or anger, negativity, suspiciousness or distrust, distress, sadness, hopelessness, or helplessness or attempt to be very controlling in their speech or demeanor. They may be perfectionistic or unrealistic in their expectations of cure or rehabilitation. For example, some PCF will express inability or inconsistent ability to be satisfied with aspects of their care. Some PCF will express perfect satisfaction with an appliance when it is first delivered, such as the fit and feeling of an obturator or the appearance of a prosthesis. Then at the next appointment, they may express complete dissatisfaction. After adjustments are made by the maxillofacial prosthodontist, they may once again express perfect satisfaction but, again, at the next appointment, be unsatisfied and repeat this cycle interminably regardless of further adjustments that the maxillofacial prosthodontist may make.

Members of the PCF other than the patient may interact with one another in ways that are overly critical, overly protective or solicitous, detached, bullying, or manipulative. Any member of the PCF group may engage with HCP and support staff in these ways or engage in ways that are overly dependent, passive-aggressive, overtly uncooperative, suspicious or distrustful, demanding and devaluing, combative, hostile, distracted, or inattentive.

PCF who are out of contact with a realistic sense of their own agency can have great difficulty in comprehending the actual extent of what their HCP can do for them and what the limits of care and rehabilitation actually are. Under these conditions, PCF may project onto their HCP unlimited agency and, at one extreme, feel betrayed or dissatisfied when the results of care are less than what they want or, at another extreme, may inappropriately venerate their HCP. A particularly difficult manifestation of the experience of lack of "felt" or experienced agency within the PCF can manifest as PCF who promote conflict among their HCP team by praising an individual HCP in person while disparaging them to another HCP on the MDT.

The internal experience of the HCP is likely to be affected, sometimes subtly and sometimes powerfully, when PCF have lost contact with a realistic sense of their agency. The HCP or support staff may find themselves dreading or wishing to avoid the next appointment, being confused about or being overly critical of the adequacy of the care they are providing, losing access to their own competence and providing substandard care, spending too little or too much time in an appointment with a particular PCF, or disliking or feeling disdainful toward the PCF, individually or collectively. Interacting with the PCF, the HCP may find themselves less articulate than usual, impatient, intolerant of, or overly compliant with PCF requests.

To summarize, this section has discussed direct observation of PCF behavior and self-observation of their own internal experience and outward behavior as one mode of surveillance for PS distress in HNC survivorship. When a person is in contact with their sense of agency, it becomes easier for them to identify, communicate, and work toward their goals and to collaborate with others who can genuinely assist them. Ideas, emotions, actions, and interactional styles within the PCF group, between PCF and HCP, and within the HCP—which are incompatible with HNC treatment and rehabilitation, if changed from baseline—can indicate that one or more members of the PCF group are having difficulty coping with a challenge that they have encountered in survivorship and has lost contact with their own sense of agency. They may need thoughtful, respectful assistance and attention to identify and engage with the area where they need more support. If the problematic behavior or attitude doesn't represent an interval change, this can indicate a more chronic difficulty for the patient in connecting with and acting from their sense of agency. The goal for HCP in either case is to expend a degree of time and effort that is consistent with their personal style of delivering care and the time and energy they have available for the provision of PS support. If the maxillofacial prosthodontist or other HNC HCP is unable to assist the PCF member, given the resources of time and energy that are appropriate to expend, then consultation with one of the MDT's psychosocial oncologists is indicated.

Brief PS screening instruments—In addition to taking a history, making observations of the PCF, and conducting self-observation by the HCP, a third modality for the surveillance of PS needs and morbidities during HNC survivorship is the use of psychological tests. Two parameters of BPS toxicity and well-being, BPS distress (BPSD) and QOL, are of particular interest to the project of surveillance because they are intuitively meaningful; have been well-researched; have validated, practical screening tools, which are reasonably compatible with the constraints of a busy practice (i.e., are quick to administer in either electronic tablet or paper formats, score, and interpret) and so could feasibly be incorporated as part of routine office visits; and can be efficiently documented in the patient's paper or electronic medical record (EMR). Both types of BPS morbidity measures are patient-reported outcome measures (PROMs).

Biopsychosocial distress screening (BPS-DS). A widely accepted definition of BPSD in cancer survivorship is that by the National Comprehensive Cancer Network (NCCN): "Distress is a multifactorial unpleasant experience of a psychological (i.e., cognitive, behavioral, emotional), social, spiritual, and/or physical nature that may interfere with one's ability to cope effectively with cancer, its physical symptoms, and its treatment. This concept exists along a continuum, ranging from normal feelings of vulnerability, sadness, and fears to problems that can become disabling, such as depression, anxiety, panic, social isolation, and existential and spiritual crises" (Riba et al., 2019).

Routine distress screening (DS) for PS morbidities throughout survivorship for cancer patients has been the standard of care since the 2012 Commission on Cancer Program Standards (2012). An example is shown in Fig 9-1. A number of societies and authors have advocated that BPSD be considered the sixth vital sign (Bultz et al., 2005; Holland et al., 2007; Turner, 2015) and that it be routinely and repeatedly assessed just as any other vital sign would. One influential author has emphasized that DS is especially important at "pivotal medical visits" (Pirl et al., 2014), such as appointments when diagnosis and recommended treatment plans are presented to a PCF following an MDC and the completion of each stage of treatment. In the context of survivorship encounters for HNC patients, this would correspond to every visit and particularly to visits occurring at transitions of phases of survivorship.

A model DS program has been proposed consisting of recurring cycles of five steps per cycle: DS using a validated tool, evaluation of the patient's current BPSD level and needs based on the screening instrument, referral to an appropriate member of the MDT or other resource if needed, follow-up to see if the PCF acted on the referral, and documentation of the previous steps in the dental or medical record and revision of the program as is needed to improve it (Lazenby et al., 2015).

A number of validated and widely used tools are available for DS in cancer patients, most considered "ultrashort," having a low response burden for patients and requiring little time or special skills to score or evaluate (Mitchell, 2007). Examples include the NCCN

UCLA Health

HNCP DISTRESS SCREENER FOR PATIENTS

Instructions: First please circle the number (0-10) that best describes how much distress you have been experiencing in the PAST WEEK including today.

Extreme distress 10 9 8 7 6 5 4 3 2 1 0 No distress

Second, please indicate if any of the following has been a problem for you in the PAST WEEK including today. Be sure to check YES or NO for each.

Yes	No	Practical Problems	Yes	No	Physical Problems
☐	☐	Child Care	☐	☐	Appearance
☐	☐	Housing	☐	☐	Breathing
☐	☐	Insurance/Financial	☐	☐	Eating
☐	☐	Transportation	☐	☐	Changes in Swallowing
☐	☐	Work/School	☐	☐	Changes in Speech
☐	☐	Treatment Decisions	☐	☐	Constipation/Diarrhea
		Family Problems	☐	☐	Fatigue
☐	☐	Dealing with Children	☐	☐	Getting Around
☐	☐	Dealing with Partner	☐	☐	Memory/Concentration
☐	☐	Ability to Have Children	☐	☐	Nausea
☐	☐	Family Health Issues	☐	☐	Pain
☐	☐	Isolation/Loneliness	☐	☐	Mouth Sores
☐	☐	Lack of Support	☐	☐	Sexual
			☐	☐	Sleep
☐	☐	Spiritual/Religious Concerns	☐	☐	Substance Abuse

Other: ______________________

Over the LAST TWO WEEKS how often have you been bothered by the following problems? (Use ✓ to indicate your answer)	Not At All	Several Days	More Than Half the Days	Nearly Every Day
1. Feeling nervous, anxious or on edge.	☐ 0	☐ 1	☐ 2	☐ 3
2. Not being able to stop or control worrying.	☐ 0	☐ 1	☐ 2	☐ 3
3. Little interest or pleasure in doing things.	☐ 0	☐ 1	☐ 2	☐ 3
4. Feeling down, depressed, or hopeless.	☐ 0	☐ 1	☐ 2	☐ 3

Patient or Representative Signature:

______________________ Date __________ Time ______

If signed by someone other than the patient, please specify relationship to the Patient: ______________

Interpreter Signature:

______________________ ID # ________

Date __________ Time __________

Figure 9-1 **UCLA HNCP Distress Screener (HNCP-DS) Questionnaire.** The questionnaire is comprised of three brief screening tools: (1) the NCCN Distress Thermometer (DT; left), (2) a modified version of the DT Problem List (PL; upper right), and (3) the Patient Health Questionnaire-4 (PHQ-4; lower right). A DT score of >4 indicated clinically significant distress and triggered same-day evaluation by the Mind-Body Team (Brauer et al., 2022).

Distress Thermometer (NCCN DT), consisting of a single, graphical item and a short problem checklist tailored to survivorship issues frequently encountered by cancer patients (Jacobson et al., 2005). the Hospital Depression and Anxiety Scale (HADS; Mitchell et al., 2010; Hartung et al., 2017; Ryan et al., 2012), and the Patient Health Questionnaire (PHQ), which comes in two- and four-item versions (Ryan et al., 2012; Brauer et al., 2022). Our group at the UCLA Head and Neck Cancer Program (UCLA HNCP) has combined several of these instruments together into a single page, paper (hardcopy), and ultrashort tool and has adapted the problem checklist items specifically for an HNC population (Brauer et al., 2022; a copy of our instrument is appended). We have found it to be well received by patients, easy to administer by our nursing staff, easy to interpret by our MDT, and quite useful for structured interviews with PCF in our HNCP.

Assessment of quality of life (QOL). Health-related quality of life (QOL and HRQOL) measures have been thoroughly developed psychometrically and extensively employed in research going back at least to the 1970s. Major instruments in this category have been adapted and validated for use with specific cancer subpopulations, including HNC. Noteworthy among this group are the Functional Assessment of Cancer Therapy—Head and Neck Cancer Symptom Index (FACT-HN; Pearman et al., 2013), the University of Washington Quality of Life Revised Version 4 (UW-QOL-R4) (Weymuller et al., 2000), the European Organization for Research and Treatment of Cancer Quality of Life Questionnaire Head and Neck Module (EORTC QLQ-HN43; Singer et al., 2013; AAO-HNS, 2021), and the Edmonton-33 (Mendez et al., 2020).

These are powerful instruments and provide excellent quality, high-resolution data for detecting BPS morbidity. They have undergone much more thorough and sophisticated psychometric development than the DS tools mentioned above. Though they are typically smaller and easier to administer and score than their QOL progenitor versions, which were not specialized for specific cancer groups, they are not ultrashort, involving a considerably greater response burden than the DS tools described above. For the most part, these QOL measures have been designed for and used in research applications rather than as clinical, screening tools. If there is a need for a more detailed and precise assessment of survivorship status than the ultrashort instruments can provide, any of these QOL measures could serve well as BPS morbidity screens, assuming sufficient resources are available in terms of staff time and skill level, data entry and storage, and patient tolerance for a greater response burden.

Of note, specialized PROM instruments have been developed for more specific morbidities, such as dysphagia (Chen et al., 2001) and body-image distress (Graboyes et al., 2020a; Macias et al., 2021). Somewhat more information regarding these issues is available in Morris et al. (2022).

Effectively referring to psychosocial oncologists

The composition within and the recruitment of psychosocial oncologists for the MDT were discussed in the earlier section on the HNC MDT. This section gives suggestions to other MDT specialists for making use of subspecialized mental health professionals on the MDT. As with all interdisciplinary collaborations, the development of effective working relationships between nonmental health specialists and psychosocial oncologists requires time and shared experience for the necessary levels of mutual trust and confidence to emerge. This familiarity and trust seem especially important in the realm of PS morbidities. Psychosocial oncologists can make considerable contributions to the BPS welfare of PCF through psychotherapeutic, behavioral, and cognitive-behavioral interventions and help reduce stress levels and time pressures for their MDT colleagues through a combination of relieving them from some potentially burdensome PS support functions (when PCF need more PS support than a nonmental health clinician can or should provide) and by providing consultation to other MDT members. (If an MDT colleague would benefit themselves from therapy, for example, in a situation where they were experiencing symptoms of burnout or for any other reason, the psychosocial oncologists on the MDT would typically make a referral to an outside therapist and not provide that treatment within the MDT.)

Although referrals to psychosocial oncologists are frequently formulated in a more generalized way (e.g., "I think Mr. Jones would really benefit from talking with one of our psychosocial oncologists"), it is always helpful when the MDT colleague who is referring a PCF can provide as much specificity as possible (e.g., "Mr. Jones, who is scheduled for surgery in two weeks, has reported that he is depressed, and his wife is reporting that he has resumed drinking and smoking").

PS resources in the community and beyond

If the MDT cannot recruit a psychosocial oncologist, which, as noted above, may be difficult to do if the MDT is composed of community-based HCP, there are a number of resources that might be of help for a PCF needing PS support and for HCP needing consultation regarding PS morbidities and support (Morris et al., 2022).

Resources for PCF include community-based organizations, which generally provide PS services (frequently in the form of support groups, for which there is usually no charge, and sometimes in the form of referrals to qualified mental health providers, often on a fee-for-service basis) and which also provide helpful information and educational materials. Additionally, there are national organizations that provide authoritative information, often tailored for specific patient groups. Here are some suggestions:

- Direct provision of PS support services
    - If there is an integrative medicine (IM) center associated with a facility where the PCF is receiving care, this would usually be an excellent resource. Contact information for IM centers or departments is often prominently displayed on the facility's website or can be located through an internet (Google) search.
    - The American Cancer Society (ACS)
        - https://www.cancer.org/
        - https://www.cancer.org/cancer/head-neck-cancer.html
    - Cancer Support Community
        - https://www.cancersupportcommunity.org/
- A number of national organizations provide authoritative information and written materials for PCF, including
    - The American Cancer Society (ACS)
        - https://www.cancer.org/
        - https://www.cancer.org/cancer/head-neck-cancer.html
    - The American Head and Neck Society (AHNS)
        - https://www.ahns.info/for-patients/
    - The National Comprehensive Cancer Network (NCCN)
        - Guidelines for patient subgroups
            - Nasopharyngeal cancer
                - https://www.nccn.org/patientresources/patient-resources/guidelines-for-patients/guidelines-for-patients-details?patientGuidelineId=43
            - Oral cancers
                - https://www.nccn.org/patientresources/patient-resources/guidelines-for-patients/guidelines-for-patients-details?patientGuidelineId=31
            - Oropharyngeal cancer
                - https://www.nccn.org/patientresources/patient-resources/guidelines-for-patients/guidelines-for-patients-details?patientGuidelineId=44
    - The National Cancer Institute (NCI)
        - https://www.cancer.gov/types/head-and-neck/head-neck-fact-sheet
    - A recommended book for PCF who have had a laryngectomy is Brook I. The laryngectomee guide. Expanded edition. Raleigh (NC): Lulu Press; 2017.

PS resources for HCP include the following:

- Professional societies
    - American Head and Neck Society (AHNS)
        - https://www.ahns.info/
    - American Psychosocial Oncology Society (APOS)
        - https://apos-society.org
            - APOS road map for psychosocial care
                - Kennedy V, Padgett L. APOS research & practice imperatives for psychosocial care: A roadmap in a new era of value-based cancer care. 2020. https://apos-society.org/wp-content/uploads/2020/08/APOS-Roadmap_FINAL8.19.20.pdf
    - American Society of Clinical Oncology (ASCO)
        - https://asco.org
    - American Society for Radiation Oncology (ASTRO)
        - https://www.astro.org/
    - International Psychosocial Oncology Society (IPOS)
        - https://www.ipos-society.org/
    - Society for Integrative Oncology (SIO)
        - https://integrativeonc.org/
- Information and standards
    - American Academy of Otolaryngology—Head and Neck Surgery (AAO)

    - https://www.entnet.org/
- American Cancer Society (ACS)
    - https://www.cancer.org/
    - https://www.cancer.org/cancer/head-neck-cancer.html
- American Head and Neck Society (AHNS)
    - https://www.ahns.info/
- American Society of Clinical Oncology (ASCO)
    - https://asco.org
- American Society for Radiation Oncology (ASTRO)
    - https://www.astro.org/
- Committee on Cancer (COC), American College of Surgeons (ACOS)
    - Standards and resources
        - https://www.facs.org/quality-programs/cancer/coc/standards/2020
- National Comprehensive Cancer Network (NCCN)
    - https://www.nccn.org/
        - NCCN guidelines for HNC
            - https://jnccn.org/view/journals/jnccn/18/7/article-p873.xml?ArticleBodyColorStyles=inline%20pdf
- "UpToDate" online review articles
    - UpToDate is an excellent online source, which may require an institutional or personal subscription.
        - Home page
            - https://www.wolterskluwer.com/en/solutions/uptodate
        - HNC articles
            - https://www.uptodate.com/contents/search?search=head%20and%20neck%20cancer

Summary

Since the mid-twentieth century, cancer care generally and HNC care in particular have undergone a deep transition in philosophy and approach. Early on, a reductionistic perspective was employed by HCP, especially those focused on treatment and management of disease, including surgeons, radiation oncologists, and medical oncologists. This point of view was derived from a BM model of disease and treatment. Over time, the BM model has been assimilated into an inclusive, systems-oriented perspective, which views cancer as emerging in a complex ecology characterized by interacting biomedical, psychological, and sociological processes, the so-called BPS model of care.

While a BPS perspective had been the basis of approaches to care by HCP focused on rehabilitation—such as maxillofacial prosthodontists, speech and language pathologists, and psychosocial oncologists—it has taken decades for this view to become widely accepted and for implications of the philosophical shift to become clear in practice and in emphasis in the field. By the second decade of the twenty-first century, the implications of this fundamental shift had become widely understood and explicitly articulated in standards of care and care guidelines. An organic consequence of this transition has been the inclusion within the accepted scope of HNC care of the experiences of PCF and HCPs from the time of diagnosis to the end of life for the patient, extending through the period of bereavement for the caregiver, family, and community. The term "survivorship" has been used to identify the collective journey through these experiences.

The purpose of this chapter has been to identify some implications of this shift to a view of HNC care in which survivorship is the central, organizing concept. It is hoped that having a fuller and more vivid sense of the meaning of survivorship will assist maxillofacial prosthodontists and all members of the multidisciplinary team who join with patients, caregivers, and their families in their shared journey through HNC care to engage more efficaciously, creatively, and with less distress and suffering in their profound endeavor.

References

Ahola K, Hakanen J. Job strain, burnout, and depressive symptoms: A prospective study among dentists. Journal of Affective Disorders 2007 Dec 1;104(1):103–110. https://doi.org/10.1016/j.jad.2007.03.004.

Alabi RO, Hietanen P, Elmusrati M, et al. Mitigating burnout in an oncological unit: A scoping review. Review. Frontiers in Public Health 2021 Oct 1;9. http://doi.org/10.3389/fpubh.2021.677915.

Alders ST, Hermens R. Towards personalized surveillance for head and neck cancer patients. Journal of Clinical Oncology 2017;35(31 suppl):116. http://doi.org/10.1200/JCO.2017.35.31_suppl.116.

American Academy of Otolaryngology-Head and Neck Surgery (AAO-HNS). Head and neck surgery outcome tool: UW-QOL-R4. 2021. https://www.entnet.org/resource/head-and-neck-surgery-outcome-tool-uw-qol-r4/.

American College of Surgeons. Cancer program standards 2012: Ensuring patient-centered care. Chicago: American College of Surgeons; 2012.

American Society of Clinical Oncology (ASCO). Head and neck cancer survivorship care guideline: American Society of Clinical Oncology clinical practice guideline endorsement of the American Cancer Society guideline. 2017. https://www.asco.org/sites/new-www.asco.org/files/content-files/practice-and-guidelines/documents/2017-HNC-survivorship-slides.pdf.

Argerakis GP. Psychosocial considerations of the post-treatment of head and neck cancer patients. Dental Clinics of North America 1990;34(2):285–305.

Badran KW, Heineman TE, Kuan EC, et al. Is multidisciplinary team care for head and neck cancer worth it? Laryngoscope 2018;128(6):1257–1258. http://doi.org/10.1002/lary.26919.

Beckman HB, Wendland M, Mooney C, et al. The impact of a program in mindful communication on primary care physicians. Academic Medicine 2012;87(6):815–819. http://doi.org/10.1097/ACM.0b013e318253d3b2.

Beumer J III, Curtis TA, Marunick MT, eds. Maxillofacial rehabilitation: Prosthodontic and surgical considerations. Ishiyaku EuroAmerica; 1996.

Bozec A, Boscagli M, Serris M, et al. Long-term functional and quality of life outcomes in laryngectomized patients after successful voice restoration using tracheoesophageal prostheses. Surgical Oncology 2021 Sep 1;38:101580. https://doi.org/10.1016/j.suronc.2021.101580.

Brake J, Bouman AM, Gorter RC, et al. Using the Maslach Burnout Inventory among dentists: Burnout measurement and trends. Community Dentist Oral Epidemiol 2008 Feb;36(1):69–75. http://doi.org/10.1111/j.1600-0528.2007.00372.x.

Brauer ER, Lazaro S, Williams CL, et al. Implementing a tailored psychosocial distress screening protocol in a head and neck cancer program. Laryngoscope 2022;132:1600–1608. http://doi.org/https://doi.org/10.1002/lary.30000.

Breen LJ, O'Connor M, Calder S, et al. The health professionals' perspectives of support needs of adult head and neck cancer survivors and their families: A Delphi study. Supportive Care in Cancer 2017 Aug 1;25(8):2413–2420. http://doi.org/10.1007/s00520-017-3647-2.

Brunner M, Gore SM, Read RL, et al. Head and neck multidisciplinary team meetings: Effect on patient management. Head & Neck 2015;37(7):1046–1050. http://doi.org/10.1002/hed.23709.

Bui S, Pelosi A, Mazzaschi G, et al. Burnout and oncology: An irreparable paradigm or a manageable condition? Prevention strategies to reduce Burnout in oncology health care professionals. Acta Biomed 2021 Jul 1;92(3):e2021091. http://doi.org/10.23750/abm.v92i3.9738.

Bultz BD, Carlson LE. Emotional distress: The sixth vital sign in cancer care. J Clin Oncol 2005;23(26):6440–6441.

Chan R, Nekhlyudov L. Overview of cancer survivorship care for primary care and oncology providers. UpToDate.com. Accessed 12 Dec 2021. https://www.uptodate.com/contents/overview-of-cancer-survivorship-care-for-primary-care-and-oncology-providers?topicRef=89977&source=see_link.

Chen AM, Daly ME, Farwell D, et al. Quality of life among long-term survivors of head and neck cancer treated by intensity-modulated radiotherapy. JAMA Otolaryngology Head & Neck Surgery 2014;140(2):129–133. http://doi.org/10.1001/jamaoto.2013.5988.

Chen AM, Daly ME, Vazquez E, et al. Depression among long-term survivors of head and neck cancer treated with radiation therapy. JAMA Otolaryngol Head Neck Surg 2013 Sep;139(9):885–889. http://doi.org/10.1001/jamaoto.2013.4072.

Chen AY, Frankowski R, Bishop-Leone J, et al. The development and validation of a dysphagia-specific quality-of-life questionnaire for patients with head and neck cancer: The M.D. Anderson dysphagia inventory. Archives of Otolaryngology Head & Neck Surgery 2001;127(7):870–876. http://doi.org/10-1001/pubs.Arch.

Chiu A. The topsy-turvy world of modern healthcare: Strategies to adapt and flourish. Paper presented at: Paul H Ward MD Society, 29th Annual Scientific Session. Session Keynote Address; 2017; Los Angeles, CA.

Cohen EEW, LaMonte SJ, Erb NL, et al. American Cancer Society head and neck cancer survivorship care guideline. CA: A Cancer Journal for Clinicians 2016;66(3):203–239. https://doi.org/10.3322/caac.21343.

Conley JJ. Ethics in head and neck surgery. Archives of Otolaryngology 1981;107(11):655–657. http://doi.org/10.1001/archotol.1981.00790470003002.

Contag SP, Golub JS, Teknos TN, et al. Professional burnout among microvascular and reconstructive free-flap head and neck surgeons in the United States. Archives of Otolaryngology Head & Neck Surgery 2010;136(10):950–956. http://doi.org/10.1001/archoto.2010.154.

Delaney MC. Caring for the caregivers: Evaluation of the effect of an eight-week pilot mindful self-compassion (MSC) training program on nurses' compassion fatigue and resilience. PLOS ONE 2018;13(11):e0207261. http://doi.org/10.1371/journal.pone.0207261.

Devins GM, Payne AYM, Lebel S, et al. The burden of stress in head and neck cancer. Psycho-Oncology 2013;22(3):668–676. http://doi.org/10.1002/pon.3050.

Dharmarajan H, Anderson JL, Kim S, et al. Transition to a virtual multidisciplinary tumor board during the COVID-19 pandemic: University of Pittsburgh experience. Head & Neck 2020;42(6):1310–1316. https://doi.org/10.1002/hed.26195.

Drabe N, Zwahlen D, Büchi S, et al. Psychiatric morbidity and quality of life in wives of men with long-term head and neck cancer. Psycho-Oncology 2008;17(2):199–204. http://doi.org/https://doi.org/10.1002/pon.1199.

Dri E, Bressan V, Cadorin L, et al. Providing care to a family member affected by head and neck cancer: A phenomenological study. Support Care Cancer 2020 May;28(5):2105–2112. http://doi.org/10.1007/s00520-019-05026-2.

Duke RL, Campbell BH, Indresano AT, et al. Dental Status and quality of life in long-term head and neck cancer survivors. Laryngoscope 2005;115(4):678–683. https://doi.org/10.1097/01.mlg.0000161354.28073.bc.

Dunne S, Mooney O, Coffey L, et al. Psychological variables associated with quality of life following primary treatment for head and neck cancer: A systematic review of the literature from 2004 to 2015. Psychooncology 2017 Feb;26(2):149–160. http://doi.org/10.1002/pon.4109.

Eelen S, Bauwens S, Baillon C, et al. The prevalence of burnout among oncology professionals: Oncologists are at risk of developing burnout. Psycho-Oncology 2014;23(12):1415–1422. https://doi.org/10.1002/pon.3579.

El-Deiry M, Funk GF, Nalwa S, et al. Long-term quality of life for surgical and non-surgical treatment of head and neck cancer. Arch Otolaryngol Head Neck Surg Oct 2005;131(10):879–885. http://doi.org/10.1001/archotol.131.10.879.

Engel GL. The need for a new medical model: A challenge for biomedicine. Science 1977;196(4286):129–136. http://doi.org/10.1126/science.847460.

Esplen MJ, Wong J, Vachon MLS, et al. Continuing educational program supporting health professionals to manage grief and loss. Current Oncology 2022;29(3):1461–1474.

Fang CY, Heckman CJ. Informational and support needs of patients with head and neck cancer: Current status and emerging issues. Cancers of the Head & Neck 2016;1(1). http://doi.org/10.1186/s41199-016-0017-6.

Funk GF, Karnell L, Christensen A. Long-term health-related quality of life in survivors of head and neck cancer. Archives of Otolaryngology Head & Neck Surgery 2012;138(2):123. http://doi.org/10.1001/archoto.2011.234.

Figley CR. Compassion fatigue: Psychotherapists' chronic lack of self care. Journal of Clinical Psychology 2002b;58(11):1433–1441. https://doi.org/10.1002/jclp.10090.

Figley CR. Stress disorders among Vietnam veterans: Theory, research, and treatment. Brunner/Mazel; 1978.

Figley CR, ed. Compassion fatigue: Coping with secondary traumatic stress disorder in those who treat the traumatized. Brunner/Mazel; 1995.

Figley CR, ed. Treating compassion fatigue. 1st ed. Brunner-Routledge; 2002a. Brunne-Routledge psychosocial stress series.

Forsythe LP, Alfano CM, Leach CR, et al. Who provides psychosocial follow-up care for post-treatment cancer survivors? A survey of medical oncologists and primary care physicians. J Clin Oncol 2012 Aug 10;30(23):2897–2905. http://doi.org/10.1200/jco.2011.39.9832.

Ganzer H, Touger-Decker R, Byham-Gray L, et al. The eating experience after treatment for head and neck cancer: A review of the literature. Oral Oncology 2015 July 1;51(7):634–642. https://doi.org/10.1016/j.oraloncology.2015.04.014.

Gibson C, O'Connor M, White R, et al. Burnout or fade away; experiences of health professionals caring for patients with head and neck cancer. European Journal of Oncology Nursing 2021 Feb;50:8. http://doi.org/10.1016/j.ejon.2020.101881.

Gillman L, Adams J, Kovac R, et al. Strategies to promote coping and resilience in oncology and palliative care nurses caring for adult patients with malignancy: A comprehensive systematic review. JBI Evidence Synthesis 2015;13(5):131–204.

Girgis A, Hansen V, Goldstein D. Are Australian oncology health professionals burning out? A view from the trenches. European Journal of Cancer 2009 Feb 1;45(3):393–399. https://doi.org/10.1016/j.ejca.2008.09.029.

Giuliani M, Milne R, McQuestion M, et al. Partner's survivorship care needs: An analysis in head and neck cancer patients. Oral Oncology 2017 Aug 1;71:113–121. https://doi.org/10.1016/j.oraloncology.2017.06.011.

Golub JS, Johns III MM, Weiss PS, et al. Burnout in academic faculty of otolaryngology—head and neck surgery. Laryngoscope 2008;118(11):1951–1956. https://doi.org/10.1097/MLG.0b013e31818226e9.

Golub JS, Weiss PS, Ramesh AK, et al. Burnout in residents of otolaryngology—head and neck surgery: A national inquiry into the health of residency training. Academic Medicine 2007;82(6):596–601. http://doi.org/10.1097/ACM.0b013e3180556825.

Gomes EPAdA, Aranha AMF, Borges ÁH, et al. Head and neck cancer patients' quality of life: Analysis of three instruments. Journal of Dentistry 2020;21:31–41.

Gómez-Polo C, Casado AMM, Montero J. Burnout syndrome in dentists: Work-related factors. Journal of Dentistry 2022 Jun 1;121:104143. https://doi.org/10.1016/j.jdent.2022.104143.

Gondivkar SM, Gadbail AR, Sarode SC, et al. Oral psychosomatic disorders in family caregivers of oral squamous cell carcinoma patients. Asian Pac J Cancer Prev 2021 Feb 1;22(2):477–483. http://doi.org/10.31557/apjcp.2021.22.2.477.

Goswami S, Gupta SS. How cancer of oral cavity affects the family caregivers?—A cross-sectional study in Wardha, India, using the Caregiver Quality of Life Index—cancer questionnaire. South Asian J Cancer 2020 Jan–Mar;9(1):62–65. http://doi.org/10.4103/sajc.sajc_331_18.

Goyal N, Day A, Epstein J, et al. Head and neck cancer survivorship consensus statement from the American Head and Neck Society. Laryngoscope Investigative Otolaryngology 2021 Nov 30:1–23. https://doi.org/10.1002/lio2.702.

Graboyes EM. Late and long-term psychosocial morbidity among head and neck cancer survivors. PowerPoint presented at: 35th Annual F Johnson Putney Lecture in Head & Neck Cancer; Dec 11, 2020; Medical University of South Carolina. https://medicine.musc.edu/-/sm/medicine/departments/otolaryngology/f/cme-2020-putney/graboyes-late-and-longterm-psychosocial-morbidity-among-head-and-neck-cancer-survivors.ashx.

Graboyes EM, Hand BN, Ellis MA, et al. Validation of a novel, multidomain head and neck cancer appearance- and function-distress patient-reported outcome measure. Otolaryngology—Head and Neck Surgery 2020;163(5):979–985. http://doi.org/10.1177/0194599820927364.

Haddad RI, Limaye S. Overview of approach to long-term survivors of head and neck cancer. UpToDate, Inc., Wolters Kluwer. Accessed 18 Oct 2021a. https://www.uptodate.com/contents/overview-of-approach-to-long-term-survivors-of-head-and-neck-cancer.

Haddad RI, Limaye S. Society guideline links: Head and neck cancer. UpToDate, Inc. Accessed 18 Oct 2021b. https://www.uptodate.com/contents/society-guideline-links-head-and-neck-cancer?topicRef=89977&source=see_link.

Haddad RI, Shin DM. Recent advances in head and neck cancer. N Engl J Med 2008 Sep 11;359(11):1143–1154. http://doi.org/10.1056/NEJMra0707975.

HaGani N, Yagil D, Cohen M. Burnout among oncologists and oncology nurses: A systematic review and meta-analysis. Health Psychology 2022 Jan;41(1):53–64. http://doi.org/10.1037/hea0001155.

Hartung TJ, Friedrich M, Johansen C, et al. The Hospital Anxiety and Depression Scale (HADS) and the 9-item Patient Health Questionnaire (PHQ-9) as screening instruments for depression in patients with cancer. Cancer 2017;123(21):4236–4243. https://doi.org/10.1002/cncr.30846.

Healey JE Jr., ed. Ecology of the cancer patient; proceedings of three interdisciplinary conferences on rehabilitation of the patient with cancer. Interdisciplinary Communications Associates; 1970.

Heineman T, St. John MA, Wein RO, et al. It takes a village: The importance of multidisciplinary care. Otolaryngologic Clinics of North America 2017 Aug 1;50(4):679–687. https://doi.org/10.1016/j.otc.2017.03.005.

Henry M, Habib L-A, Morrison M, et al. Head and neck cancer patients want us to support them psychologically in the posttreatment period: Survey results. Palliative and Supportive Care 2014;12(6):481–493. http://doi.org/10.1017/S1478951513000771.

Hewitt M, Ganz PA, eds. From cancer patient to cancer survivor: Lost in transition: An American Society of Clinical Oncology and Institute of Medicine Symposium. National Academies Press; 2006.

Hewitt M, Greenfield S, Stovall E, eds. From cancer patient to cancer survivor: Lost in transition / Committee on Cancer Survivorship: Improving care and quality of life, National Cancer Policy Board, Institute of Medicine and National Research Council. National Academies Press; 2005.

Hlubocky FJ. Attending to oncology team well-being. JCO Oncology Practice 2022;18(8):541–542. http://doi.org/10.1200/op.22.00432.

Hlubocky FJ, Back AL, Shanafelt TD. Addressing burnout in oncology: Why cancer care clinicians are at risk, what individuals can do, and how organizations can respond. American Society of Clinical Oncology Educational Book 2016;(36):271–279. http://doi.org/10.1200/edbk_156120.

Hlubocky FJ, Rose M, Epstein RM. Mastering resilience in oncology: Learn to thrive in the face of burnout. Am Soc Clin Oncol Educ Book 2017;37:771–781. http://doi.org/10.1200/edbk_173874.

Hodges LJ, Humphris GM. Fear of recurrence and psychological distress in head and neck cancer patients and their carers. Psycho-Oncology 2009;18(8):841–848. https://doi.org/10.1002/pon.1346.

Holland JC, Bultz BD. The NCCN guideline for distress management: A case for making distress the sixth vital sign. Journal of the National Comprehensive Cancer Network J Natl Compr Canc Netw 2007 Jan 1;5(1):3–7. http://doi.org/10.6004/jnccn.2007.0003.

Howren MB, Christensen AJ, Karnell LH, et al. Psychological factors associated with head and neck cancer treatment and survivorship: Evidence and opportunities for behavioral medicine. Journal of Consulting and Clinical Psychology 2013;81(2):299–317. http://doi.org/10.1037/a0029940.

Jacobson MC. The experience of head and neck cancer survivorship (including laryngectomy): An integrated biopsychosocial model. Curr Opin Support Palliat Care Mar 2018;12(1):65–73. http://doi.org/10.1097/spc.0000000000000322.

Jacobsen PB, Donovan KA, Trask PC, et al. Screening for psychologic distress in ambulatory cancer patients. Cancer 2005;103(7):1494–1502. https://doi.org/10.1002/cncr.20940.

Johns MM III, Ossoff RH. Burnout in academic chairs of otolaryngology: Head and neck surgery. Laryngoscope 2005 Nov;115(11):2056–2061. http://doi.org/10.1097/01.Mlg.0000181492.36179.8b.

Kane L. Medscape national physician burnout & suicide report 2020: The generational divide. Medscape. https://www.medscape.com/slideshow/2020-lifestyle-burnout-6012460#1.

Kassir ZM, Li J, Harrison C, et al. Disparity of perception of quality of life between head and neck cancer patients and caregivers. BMC Cancer 2021 Oct 20;21(1):1127. http://doi.org/10.1186/s12885-021-08865-7.

Kazmi SM. Burnout is cancer. American Society of Clinical Oncology (ASCO). 25 May 2021. https://connection.asco.org/blogs/burnout-cancer.

Krebber A-MH, Jansen F, Cuijpers P, et al. Screening for psychological distress in follow-up care to identify head and neck cancer patients with untreated distress. Supportive Care in Cancer 2016 Jun 1;24(6):2541–2548. http://doi.org/10.1007/s00520-015-3053-6.

Lamiani G, Borghi L, Argentero P. When healthcare professionals cannot do the right thing: A systematic review of moral distress and its correlates. Journal of Health Psychology 2017;22(1):51–67. http://doi.org/10.1177/1359105315595120.

LaMonte SJ. Addressing survivorship issues in head and neck cancers—it's about time. JAMA Otolaryngology—Head & Neck Surgery. 2016;142(10):1008–1009. http://doi.org/10.1001/jamaoto.2016.1641.

Lazar F, Gaba D, Munch S, et al. The ProQol-20, a restructured version of the professional quality of life scale (ProQOL). Curr Psychol 2022:12. http://doi.org/10.1007/s12144-022-02755-2.

Lazenby M, Ercolano E, Grant M, et al. Supporting commission on cancer-mandated psychosocial distress screening with implementation strategies. Journal of Oncology Practice 2015 Mar 10. http://doi.org/10.1200/jop.2014.002816.

Laor-Maayany R, Goldzweig G, Hasson-Ohayon I, et al. Compassion fatigue among oncologists: The role of grief, sense of failure, and exposure to suffering and death. Supportive Care in Cancer 2020 Apr 1;28(4):2025–2031. http://doi.org/10.1007/s00520-019-05009-3.

LeNoble CA, Pegram R, Shuffler ML, et al. To address burnout in 2022. Oncol Pract 2020 Apr;16(4):e377–e383. http://doi.org/10.1200/jop.19.00631.

Lin C-R, Chen S-C, Chang JT-C, et al. Fear of cancer recurrence and its impacts on quality of life in family caregivers of patients with head and neck cancers. Journal of Nursing Research 2016;24(3):240–248. http://doi.org/10.1097/jnr.0000000000000169.

Longacre ML, Ridge JA, Burtness BA, et al. Psychological functioning of caregivers for head and neck cancer patients. Oral Oncology 2012;48(1):18–25. http://doi.org/10.1016/j.oraloncology.2011.11.012.

Macias D, Hand BN, Maurer S, et al. Factors associated with risk of body image–related distress in patients with head and neck cancer. JAMA Otolaryngology—Head & Neck Surgery 2021. http://doi.org/10.1001/jamaoto.2021.1378.

Martino R, Ringash J. Evaluation of quality of life and organ function in head and neck squamous cell carcinoma. Hematology/Oncology Clinics of North America 2008 Dec 1;22(6):1239–1256. https://doi.org/10.1016/j.hoc.2008.08.011.

Maslach C, Jackson SE. The measurement of experienced burnout. Journal of Organizational Behavior 1981;2(2):99–113. https://doi.org/10.1002/job.4030020205.

Maslach C, Leiter MP. How to measure burnout accurately and ethically. Harvard Business Review 2021 Mar 19.

Maslach C, Leiter MP. Understanding the burnout experience: Recent research and its implications for psychiatry. World Psychiatry 2016;15(2):103–111. https://doi.org/10.1002/wps.20311.

Maslach C, Jackson SE, Leiter MP. Maslach burnout inventory. Scarecrow Education; 1997.

Masroor F, Corpman D, Carpenter DM, et al. Association of NCCN-recommended posttreatment surveillance with outcomes in patients with HPV-associated oropharyngeal squamous cell carcinoma. JAMA Otolaryngol Head Neck Surg 2019 Oct 1;145(10):903–908. http://doi.org/10.1001/jamaoto.2019.1934.

McLaren O, Perkins C, Zhu Y, et al. Patient perspectives on surveillance after head and neck cancer treatment: A systematic review. Clin Otolaryngol 2021 Nov;46(6):1345–1353. http://doi.org/10.1111/coa.13846.

Mendez A, Seikaly H, Eurich D, et al. Development of a patient-centered functional outcomes questionnaire in head and neck cancer. JAMA Otolaryngol Head Neck Surg 2020 May 1;146(5):437–443. http://doi.org/10.1001/jamaoto.2019.4788.

Miller MC, Shuman AG. Survivorship in head and neck cancer: A primer (the American Head and Neck Society's committee on survivorship). JAMA Otolaryngology—Head & Neck Surgery 2016;142(10):1002–1008. http://doi.org/10.1001/jamaoto.2016.1615.

Mitchell AJ. Pooled results from 38 analyses of the accuracy of distress thermometer and other ultra-short methods of detecting cancer-related mood disorders. Journal of Clinical Oncology 2007;25(29):4670–4681. http://doi.org/10.1200/jco.2006.10.0438.

Mitchell AJ, Meader N, Symonds P. Diagnostic validity of the Hospital Anxiety and Depression Scale (HADS) in cancer and palliative settings: A meta-analysis. Journal of Affective Disorders 2010 Nov 1;126(3):335–348. https://doi.org/10.1016/j.jad.2010.01.067.

Moore PM, Rivera S, Bravo-Soto GA, et al. Communication skills training for healthcare professionals working with people who have cancer. Cochrane Database of Systematic Reviews 2018;2018(7). http://doi.org/10.1002/14651858.cd003751.pub4.

Morris JRS, Rapkin DA, Nilsen ML, et al. Surviving and thriving: Survivorship in the 21st century. In Essential Head and Neck Oncology and Surgery. 13th ed. Ed. Judson BL and St. John MA; 2022. Essential Medicine Series.

Moschopoulou E, Hutchison I, Bhui K, et al. Post-traumatic stress in head and neck cancer survivors and their partners. Supportive Care in Cancer 2018;26(9):3003–3011. http://doi.org/10.1007/s00520-018-4146-9.

Nekhlyudov L, Lacchetti C, Siu LL. Head and neck cancer survivorship care guideline: American Society of Clinical oncology clinical practice guideline endorsement summary. Journal of Oncology Practice 2018;14(3):167–171. http://doi.org/10.1200/JOP.2017.029041.

Osazuwa-Peters N, Simpson MC, Zhao L, et al. Suicide risk among cancer survivors: Head and neck versus other cancers. Cancer 2018;124(20):4072–4079. http://doi.org/10.1002/cncr.31675.

Payakachat N, Ounpraseuth S, Suen JY. Late complications and long-term quality of life for survivors (>5 years) with history of head and neck cancer. Head Neck 2013 Jun;35(6):819–25. http://doi.org/10.1002/hed.23035.

Pearlman LA, Saakvitne KW. Trauma and the therapist: Countertransference and vicarious traumatization in psychotherapy with incest survivors. 1st ed. Norton; 1995. p. 451.

Pearman TP, Beaumont JL, Paul D, et al. Evaluation of treatment- and disease-related symptoms in advanced head and neck cancer: Validation of the national comprehensive cancer network-functional assessment of cancer therapy-head and neck cancer symptom index-22 (NFHNSI-22). Journal of Pain and Symptom Management 2013;46(1):113–120. http://doi.org/10.1016/j.jpainsymman.2012.06.004.

Pirl WF, Fann JR, Greer JA, et al. Recommendations for the implementation of distress screening programs in cancer centers: Report from the American Psychosocial Oncology Society (APOS), Association of Oncology Social Work (AOSW), and Oncology Nursing Society (ONS) joint task force. Cancer 2014;120(19):2946–2954. http://doi.org/10.1002/cncr.28750.

Porto GG, Carneiro SC, Vasconcelos BC, et al. Burnout syndrome in oral and maxillofacial surgeons: A critical analysis. Int J Oral Maxillofac Surg 2014 Jul;43(7):894–899. http://doi.org/10.1016/j.ijom.2013.10.025.

Prevost V, Lefevre-Arbogast S, Leconte A, et al. Shared meditation involving cancer patients, health professionals and third persons is relevant and improves well-being: IMPLIC pilot study. BMC Complementary Medicine and Therapies 2022 May 18;22(1):138. http://doi.org/10.1186/s12906-022-03599-w.

Rao D, Behzadi F, Le RT, et al. Radiation induced mucositis: What the radiologist needs to know. Current Problems in Diagnostic Radiology 2021 Nov 1;50(6):899–904. https://doi.org/10.1067/j.cpradiol.2020.10.006.

Rapkin DA, Garrett N. Psychosocial perspectives on the care of head and neck cancer patients. In Maxillofacial rehabilitation: Surgical and prosthodontic management of cancer-related, acquired, and congenital defects of the head and neck. 3rd ed. Eds. Beumer J III, Marunick MT, Esposito SJ. Quintessence; 2011:403–424. Vol. 9.

Riba MB, Donovan KA, Andersen B, et al. Distress management, version 3.2019, NCCN clinical practice guidelines in oncology. J Natl Compr Canc Netw 2019 Oct 1;17(10):1229–1249. http://doi.org/10.6004/jnccn.2019.0048.

Richardson AE, Morton R, Broadbent E. Caregivers' illness perceptions contribute to quality of life in head and neck cancer patients at diagnosis. J Psychosoc Oncol 2015;33(4):414–432. http://doi.org/10.1080/07347332.2015.1046011.

Richardson AE, Morton RP, Broadbent EA. Changes over time in head and neck cancer patients' and caregivers' illness perceptions and relationships with quality of life. Psychol Health 2016 Oct;31(10):1203–1219. http://doi.org/10.1080/08870446.2016.1203686.

Ringash J. Survivorship and quality of life in head and neck cancer. Journal of Clinical Oncology 2015;33(29):3322–3327. http://doi.org/10.1200/jco.2015.61.4115.

Ross BR. The dental clinician and the head and neck cancer patient: Psychodynamic interactions. In Maxillofacial rehabilitation: prosthodontic and surgical considerations. Eds. Beumer J, Curtis TA, Marunick MT. Ishiyaku EuroAmerica; 1996. pp. 15–23:chap 2.

Ross S, Mosher CE, Ronis-Tobin V, et al. Psychosocial adjustment of family caregivers of head and neck cancer survivors. Supportive Care in Cancer 2009 Apr 24;18(2):171. http://doi.org/10.1007/s00520-009-0641-3.

Rowland JH, Hewitt M, Ganz PA. Cancer survivorship: A new challenge in delivering quality cancer care. Journal of Clinical Oncology 2006 Nov 10;24(32):5101–5104.

Rozen RD, Ordway DE, Curtis TA, et al. Psychosocial aspects of maxillofacial rehabilitation. Part 1. The effect of primary cancer treatment. Journal of Prosthetic Dentistry 1972;28(4):423–428.

Ryan DA, Gallagher P, Wright S, et al. Sensitivity and specificity of the Distress Thermometer and a two-item depression screen (Patient Health Questionnaire-2) with a "help" question for psychological distress and psychiatric morbidity in patients with advanced cancer. Psycho-Oncology 2012;21(12):1275–1284. http://doi.org/10.1002/pon.2042.

Shanafelt TD, Noseworthy JH. Executive leadership and physician well-being: Nine organizational strategies to promote engagement and reduce burnout. Mayo Clinic Proceedings 2017 Jan 1;92(1):129–146. https://doi.org/10.1016/j.mayocp.2016.10.004.

Shanafelt TD, West CP, Sinsky C, et al. Changes in burnout and satisfaction with work-life integration in physicians and the general US working population between 2011 and 2017. Mayo Clinic Proceedings 2019;94(9):1681–1694. http://doi.org/10.1016/j.mayocp.2018.10.023.

Singer S, Arraras JI, Chie WC, et al. Performance of the EORTC questionnaire for the assessment of quality of life in head and neck cancer patients EORTC QLQ-H&N35: A methodological review. Qual Life Res 2013 Oct;22(8):1927–1941. http://doi.org/10.1007/s11136-012-0325-1.

Singh P, Aulak DS, Mangat SS, et al. Systematic review: Factors contributing to burnout in dentistry. Occupational Medicine 2015;66(1):27–31. http://doi.org/10.1093/occmed/kqv119.

Stamm BH. The concise ProQOL manual. 2nd ed. ProQOL.org; 2010.

Stamm BH, ed. Secondary traumatic stress: Self-care issues for clinicians, researchers, and educators. In Secondary traumatic stress: Self-care issues for clinicians, researchers, and educators. Ed. Stamm BH. Sidran Press; 1995.

St. John MA. Multidisciplinary approach to head and neck cancer. Otolaryngologic Clinics of North America 2017 Aug 1;50(4):xvii–xviii. https://doi.org/10.1016/j.otc.2017.06.002.

Sterba KR, Zapka J, Cranos C, et al. Quality of life in head and neck cancer patient-caregiver dyads: A systematic review. Cancer Nurs 2016 May–Jun;39(3):238–50. http://doi.org/10.1097/ncc.0000000000000281.

Strong EW. Foreword in Maxillofacial rehabilitation: Prosthodontic and surgical considerations. Eds. Beumer J, Curtis TA, Marunick MT. Ishiyaku EuroAmerica; 1996.

Swetz KM, Harrington SE, Matsuyama RK, et al. Strategies for avoiding burnout in hospice and palliative medicine: Peer advice for physicians on achieving longevity and fulfillment. Journal of Palliative Medicine 2009;12(9):773–777. http://doi.org/10.1089/jpm.2009.0050.

Szturz P, Van Laer C, Simon C, et al. Follow-up of head and neck cancer survivors: Tipping the balance of intensity. Front Oncol 2020;10:688. http://doi.org/10.3389/fonc.2020.00688.

Taberna M, Gil Moncayo F, Jané-Salas E, et al. The Multidisciplinary Team (MDT) approach and quality of care. Front Oncol 2020;10:85–85. http://doi.org/10.3389/fonc.2020.00085.

Taher AN. Head and neck cancer: Closer look at patients quality of life. Journal of Cancer Therapy 2016;7(2):121–128. http://doi.org/10.4236/jct.2016.72014.

Talbot SG, Dean W. Beyond burnout: The real problem facing doctors is moral injury. Medical Economics Journal 2019;96(10).

Tevaarwerk A, Denlinger CS, Sanft T, et al. Survivorship, version 1.2021: Featured updates to the NCCN guidelines. Journal of the National Comprehensive Cancer Network 2021 Jun 1;19(6):676–685. http://doi.org/10.6004/jnccn.2021.0028.

Turner J. The changing landscape of cancer care—the impact of psychosocial clinical practice guidelines. Psycho-Oncology 2015 Apr;24(4):365–370. http://doi.org/10.1002/pon.3803.

Vercio C, Loo LK, Green M, et al. Shifting focus from burnout and wellness toward individual and organizational resilience. Teaching and Learning in Medicine 2021 Oct 20;33(5):568–576. http://doi.org/10.1080/10401334.2021.1879651.

Verdonck-de Leeuw IM, Eerenstein SE, et al. Distress in spouses and patients after treatment for head and neck cancer. Laryngoscope 2007 Feb;117(2):238–41. http://doi.org/10.1097/01.mlg.0000250169.10241.58.

Verdonschot RJCG, Baijens LWJ, Vanbelle S, et al. Affective symptoms in patients with oropharyngeal dysphagia: A systematic review. Journal of Psychosomatic Research 2017 Jul 1;97:102–110. https://doi.org/10.1016/j.jpsychores.2017.04.006.

Wang T, Mazanec SR, Voss JG. Needs of informal caregivers of patients with head and neck cancer: A systematic review. Oncology Nursing Forum 2021;48(1):11–29. http://doi.org/10.1188/21.ONF.11-29.

Watts KJ, O'Connor M, Johnson CE, et al. Mindfulness-based compassion training for health professionals providing end-of-life care: Impact, feasibility, and acceptability. J Palliat Med 2021 Sep;24(9):1364–1374. http://doi.org/10.1089/jpm.2020.0358.

Werner A, Stenner C, Schüz J. Patient versus clinician symptom reporting: How accurate is the detection of distress in the oncologic after-care? Psycho-Oncology 2012;21(8):818–826. http://doi.org/10.1002/pon.1975.

Westgaard KL, Hynne H, Amdal CD, et al. Oral and ocular late effects in head and neck cancer patients treated with radiotherapy. Scientific Reports 2021;11(1):4026–4026. http://doi.org/10.1038/s41598-021-83635-w.

Weymuller EA Jr, Yueh B, Deleyiannis FWB, et al. Quality of life in patients with head and neck cancer: Lessons learned from 549 prospectively evaluated patients. Archives of Otolaryngology—Head & Neck Surgery 2000;126(3):329–335. http://doi.org/10.1001/archotol.126.3.329.

WHO. Burn-out an "occupational phenomenon": International classification of diseases. World Health Organization. Accessed 14 Aug 2022. https://www.who.int/news/item/28-05-2019-burn-out-an-occupational-phenomenon-international-classification-of-diseases.

Wijers OB, Levendag PC, Braaksma MM, et al. Patients with head and neck cancer cured by radiation therapy: A survey of the dry mouth syndrome in long-term survivors. Head Neck 2002 Aug;24(8):737–747. http://doi.org/10.1002/hed.10129.

Winner J, Knight C. Beyond burnout: Addressing system-induced distress. Fam Pract Manag 2019;26(5):4–7.

Zhang Z, Leong Bin, Abdullah MFI, et al. Acceptance and commitment therapy versus mindfulness-based stress reduction for newly diagnosed head and neck cancer patients: A randomized controlled trial assessing efficacy for positive psychology, depression, anxiety, and quality of life. PLOS ONE 2022;17(5):e0267887. http://doi.org/10.1371/journal.pone.0267887.

Chapter 10

Oral Management of Chemotherapy Patients

Evelyn M. Chung, Wanxing Chai-Ho, Eric C. Sung, John Beumer III

Treatment of cancer combines surgery, radiation therapy, and systemic therapy. Chemotherapy has been and remains the mainstay of systemic therapy, but in recent years, novel approaches such as gene therapy, immunotherapy, cellular therapy (chimeric antigen receptor T-cell therapy), biologic agents, and targeted therapy have emerged. Approximately 50% of all cancer patients are also treated with chemotherapeutic agents during some phase of their cancer therapy, and this percentage is likely to increase in future years (DePaola et al., 1986; Rosenberg, 1990; Subramanian et al., 2011; Perez-Herrero and Fernandez-Medarde, 2015; Avula and Grodzinski, 2022).

Surgery and radiation remain the primary modes of treatment for most tumors. Both modalities have adverse effects, but the morbidity is usually limited to the tumor area.

Chemotherapeutic treatments alone are unable to match the success of surgery or radiation but are being used increasingly for palliation, prolongation of life, and in a few cases, a curative intent. It has been a key factor responsible for the increased long-term survival of patients with acute lymphocytic leukemia, Burkitt lymphoma, choriocarcinoma, Hodgkin disease, Wilms tumor, and other cancers. Moreover, during the last decade, targeted chemotherapy has transformed the treatment of many other cancers, including breast, colorectal, lung, lymphoma, leukemia, and multiple myeloma (Carrozzo et al., 2019).

Adjuvant chemotherapeutics has not become the panacea that it was originally thought to be. Although many theories attempt to explain this lack of complete success, most likely an amalgamation of reasons can be cited. Chemotherapy by itself is unable to eradicate the tumor volume completely because of a combination of intrinsic resistance of cancer cells and developed resistance to repeated doses of the same agent. In addition, the maximum tolerated dose may not be sufficient to completely kill all cancer cells. This is especially true in large tumors, in which dormant tumor cells with greater resistance to cytotoxic drugs are more likely to exist.

The effectiveness of chemotherapeutic agents is based on their ability to destroy or to slow the growth of rapidly dividing tumor cells. Unfortunately, these agents are not selective and therefore are unable to distinguish between normally dividing cells and malignant cells. Thus, normal cells are vulnerable and subject to the destructive effects of these drugs. The normal cells most adversely affected by chemotherapeutic agents are those found in bone marrow and those lining the oral cavity and gastrointestinal tract, because of their high proliferation rates. Bone marrow contains a multitude of stem cells that are constantly differentiating and multiplying to replenish circulating hematopoietic cells and to continue the stem cell line. The epithelial basal cell lining of the oral cavity and the gastrointestinal tract have a high cell turnover rate to replace old and damaged lining tissues.

Mechanisms of Action of Chemotherapy

Chemotherapeutic agents can be categorized in many different ways. Development in this field is constantly evolving and the list of therapies is expanding. These drugs can be divided into *cell cycle–specific* and *cell cycle–nonspecific* agents. Cell cycle–specific drugs are most commonly used in treatment of leukemias and

Table 10-1 Indications and Side Effects of Common Chemotherapeutic Agents

Chemotherapeutic agent	Examples	Indications	Side effects
Alkylating agents	Cyclophosphamide Cisplatin Carboplatin Oxaliplatin Mechlorethamine Chlorambucil Ifosfamide	Lymphomas; leukemias; myeloma; advanced solid tumors (Breast, testicular, ovarian, and head and neck cancers)	Nausea and vomiting; leukopenia; thrombocytopenia; possibly sterility and secondary malignancies with prolonged use
Nitrosureas	Carmustine Lomustine Semustine Streptozotocin	Brain tumors	Development of interstitial lung disease; possible bone marrow toxicity
Antimetabolites	Purine analogs Pyrimidine analogs Antifolates Adenosine deaminase inhibitors	Childhood leukemias; breast cancer; lung cancer; osteogenic sarcoma; non-Hodgkin's lymphoma; head and neck cancers	Leukopenia; flulike symptoms; anemia; diarrhea, nausea and vomiting; stomatitis (All antimetabolites)
Plant alkaloids	Vinca alkaloids • Vincristine • Vinblastine Taxanes • Paclitaxol • Docetaxel Podophyllotoxins Camptothecins • Irinotecan • Topotecan • Camptothecin • Etoposide	Ovarian, breast, and small-cell and large-cell lung cancers; Kaposi sarcoma; leukemia; Hodgkin lymphoma; neuroblastoma; rhabdomyosarcoma; Wilm's tumor	Neuropathy; constipation, nausea and vomitis; hair loss; headache; muscle loss; leukopenia; anemia; stomatitis (Vinca alkaloids and camptothecins); xerostomia (Camptothecins)
Hormones	Tamoxifen Toremifene citrate Aromatase inhibitors • Exemestane • Anastrozole	Breast, prostate, and testicular cancers as adjuvant therapy	Hot flashes and sweating; decrease libido; painful joints; mood changes; fatigue
Biologic agents	Antibiotics • Bleomycin • Actinomycin D • Doxorubicin Interferons Interleukins Colony-stimulating factors • rG-CSF Monoclonal antibodies • Rituximab	Lymphomas; head and neck cancers; colon cancer; malignant melanoma; renal cell carcinoma	Increased levels of cytokines (alpha); hypersensitivity reactions (beta); immune imbalance/impaired function (gamma); cross reactivity with normal cells (delta); nonimmunologic side effects (epsilon)

lymphomas. Cell cycle–nonspecific drugs combine with the DNA in a lethal manner, regardless of cell division. Drugs used in chemotherapy can be categorized into five general categories, depending on their mechanism of action: *(1)* alkylating agents and nitrosureas, *(2)* antimetabolites, *(3)* plant alkaloids, *(4)* steroid hormones, and *(5)* biologic agents. Table 10–1 lists common examples of different types of chemotherapeutic agents in each of these categories and their most common uses and side effects.

Alkylating agents and nitrosureas

Alkylating agents are not cell cycle specific but are most effective during DNA synthesis and act by cross-linking strands of DNA. Examples of these alkylating agents are cyclophosphamide, mechlorethamine, busulfan, and cisplatin. These drugs are used to treat Hodgkin disease, lymphomas, chronic leukemias, and carcinomas of the lung, breast, prostate, and ovary. Alkylating agents depress bone marrow function, resulting in anemia, neutropenia, and thrombocytopenia. Patients also develop gastrointestinal disturbances such as nausea and vomiting.

Nitrosureas are in a class similar to alkylating agents and inhibit changes necessary for DNA repair. Examples are carmustine, lomustine, and streptozotocin. Because drugs of this class can cross the blood-brain barrier, they are particularly useful in treating brain tumors. Side effects are similar to those of alkylating agents, but reports of an increased incidence of interstitial fibrosis have raised concern about long-term effects on the pulmonary system in children (Lohani et al., 2004; Huang et al., 2014).

Antimetabolites

The antimetabolites are organic substances that are similar in structure to normal substances in the cell. Once the cell incorporates these substances, it is no longer capable of division. These agents are cell cycle specific. There are four general subcategories of antimetabolites, classified according to the substance they interfere with: *(1)* folic acid antagonist, *(2)* pyrimidine antagonist, *(3)* purine antagonist, and *(4)* adenosine deaminase inhibitor.

Antifolates were one of the first antineoplastic drugs used. Antifolates mimic folic acid so that the cell will attempt to use them, but they inhibit the activity of dihydrofolate reductase, an enzyme that catalyzes the conversion of folic acid to tetrahydrofolic acid, a key precursor in the synthesis of the purines and pyrimidines, which are required for nucleic acid synthesis. The induced folic acid deficiency hinders the division of cells, growth, and production.

Methotrexate is the most widely utilized and well known of the antifolates. Clinically, the major role of methotrexate has been in the treatment of acute lymphoblastic leukemia in children. It has been used in part for the treatment of breast carcinoma, bronchogenic carcinoma, non-Hodgkin lymphoma, osteogenic sarcoma, squamous cell carcinoma of the head and neck, and testicular carcinoma. The most frequent manifestations of methotrexate toxicity include bone marrow depression, extensive oral ulcerations, diarrhea, and skin rash. The incidence and severity of oral mucositis induced by methotrexate are greater than those observed with other stomatotoxic agents and can interrupt therapy (Valer et al., 2021). Other examples of folic acid antagonists include aminopterin, trimetrexate, lometrixol, and leucovorin.

Pyrimidine antagonists function by inhibiting activity of thymidylate synthetase, an enzyme active in the production of a DNA precursor, thymadylic acid, thus preventing production of finished nucleotides. The principal pyrimidine antagonist, 5-fluorouracil (5-FU), is the antimetabolite that enjoys the greatest popularity in the treatment of solid tumors. Its usefulness is enhanced by the fact that uracil is used to a higher degree by tumor cells than by normal cells. 5-FU alters cell function by its effect on DNA and RNA synthesis.

5-FU has been used successfully to eradicate superficial basal cell and squamous cell carcinomas of the skin when applied topically (Peris et al., 2019). It has also been employed in the treatment of colorectal carcinoma, gastric adenocarcinoma, and pancreatic adenocarcinoma. Thrombocytopenia, leukopenia, anemia, oral and gastrointestinal ulcerations, and diarrhea are common side effects. Leukopenia occurs within 7 to 14 days after the initial dose. Arabinosylcytosine, cytarabine, capecitabine, gemcitabine, and decitabine are other types of pyrimidine antagonists.

Purine antagonists inhibit nucleic acid synthesis by interfering with the enzymes responsible for purine metabolism. The prototype for the purine antagonists is 6-mercaptopurine (6-MP), which has been used in the treatment of acute myelogenous leukemia, acute lymphoblastic leukemia, and chronic myelogenous leukemia. The major toxic side effect of 6-MP is bone marrow depression, including thrombocytopenia, leukopenia, and anemia. Oral ulcerations are only seen occasionally. Other purine antagonists include fludarabine, cladribine, and thioguanine.

Adenosine deaminase inhibitors are similar in structure to other antimetabolites, but act by inhibiting adenosine deaminase in lymphocytes, resulting in apoptosis (Toso and Lindley, 1995). They have been recognized as potent immunosuppressive agents and have been used to treat lymphatic leukemias (O'Dwyer et al., 1988). Ongoing research has looked at the efficacy of this agent for treatment of other types of cancer. Examples of adenosine deaminase inhibitors are pentostatin, cladribine, and fludarabine (Barry and Lind, 2000).

Plant alkaloids

Plant alkaloids are chemotherapeutic agents derived from certain specific plants. There are generally four categories of plant alkaloids and they are cell cycle specific: *(1)* vinca alkaloids, *(2)* taxanes, *(3)* podophyllotoxins, and *(4)* camptothecin analogs. The vinca alkaloids are derived from the periwinkle plant (*Catharanthus rosea*) and interfere with the formation of microtubules of the mitotic spindle during metaphase. Vincristine and vinblastine are vinca alkaloids that are used in the treatment of Hodgkin disease, breast carcinoma, non-Hodgkin lymphoma and acute lymphocytic leukemia. Vincristine therapy is associated with severe jaw pain, loss of deep tendon reflexes, ataxia, and muscle wasting and peripheral neuropathy (McCarthy and Skillings, 1992; Van de Velde et al., 2017). The severity of these effects determines the dose limitations of vincristine therapy.

Taxanes are made from the bark of the Pacific yew tree (*Taxus*) and are also antimicrotubule agents. The two most common types of taxanes are paclitaxel and docetaxel. Taxanes are used in the adjuvant treatment of lung, ovarian, breast, and tumors of the head and neck.

The podophyllotoxins are derived from the May apple plant and camptothecin analogs are derived from the Asian happy tree (*Camptotheca acuminate*). Both of these drugs are known as *topoisomerase inhibitors* and prevent DNA replication by preventing the unwinding of the DNA double helix (Binaschi et al., 1995). Commonly used topoisomerase inhibitors are irinotecan, topotecan, camptothecin, and etoposide. Chemotherapeutic agents from this category of plant alkaloids are used to treat malignancies such as Ewing sarcoma, lymphoma, nonlymphocytic leukemias, and lung and testicular cancers.

The principal side effects of plant alkaloids include alopecia, peripheral neuritis, muscle weakness, and mild to moderate bone marrow depression. The oral mucous membranes are rarely affected directly by the plant alkaloids. Gastrointestinal toxicities include nausea, vomiting, abdominal pain, and diarrhea. Leukopenia occurs in 5 to 10 days, but the white blood cell count recovers after 7 to 14 days. Thrombocytopenia is uncommon.

Hormones

Sex hormones (androgens, estrogens, progestins, and testosterone) and adrenocorticosteroids have been used extensively in the treatment of neoplastic disease, especially in tumors derived from normal tissues sensitive to hormonal influences. Mammary and prostate gland tumors tend to retain the properties of the original tissue and may be inhibited or stimulated by changes in the balance of sex hormones. They either suppress hormone production or interfere with the molecular action of the hormone once it is bound to the cell. Hormone therapy is used often in the management of breast cancer. Common hormone therapy drugs used to treat breast cancer are tamoxifen, toremifene citrate, and anastrozole. These selective estrogen receptor modulators work by binding to the estrogen receptor and inhibiting breast cancer growth.

Hormone therapy in the management of prostate cancer, also known as *androgen deprivation therapy*, works by decreasing the body's production of testosterone. Luteinizing hormone–releasing hormone agonists such as leuprolide acetate and goserelin acetate and antiandrogens such as bicalutamide and nilutamide work together to prevent testosterone from reaching cancer cells. Adrenocorticosteroids have also been used in the treatment of acute leukemia, lymphomas, and myelomas. These steroids produce lysis of lymphocytes and compromise delayed hypersensitivity reactions. Principal side effects of hormonal chemotherapeutic agents include fluid retention, masculinization or feminization, and hypertension. Their cytotoxic effect on normal tissues is minimal, and the oral mucous membranes are rarely affected by hormone therapy.

Biologic agents

Biologic therapy is also known as *immunotherapy, biologic response modifier therapy, or biotherapy*. This group of agents is composed of proteins such as cytokines, monoclonal antibodies, and fusion proteins (solubilized receptors). The general approach of biologic therapy has been to use the body's immune system to fight the cancer. These agents work by making cancer cells more recognizable as cancer cells to the immune system and thus more susceptible to destruction by the immune system. They also boost the killing power of the immune system by changing the way cancer cells grow, stopping the process of cancer cell formation, or preventing the dissemination of cancer cells throughout the body.

The mechanism of action, indications for use, and toxicity profiles of antitumor antibiotics differ for each agent. Biologic therapies can be nonspecific immunomodulating agents or biologic response modifiers. Nonspecific immunomodulating agents increase production of cytokines and antibodies to fight the cancer as well as infections during treatment. Biologic response modifiers change the defense system's interaction with cancer cells by increasing the body's ability to fight the disease, directing the immune system's ability to attack cancer cells, and strengthening a weakened immune system. Biologic response modifiers include interferons, interleukins, colony-stimulating factors, monoclonal antibodies, cytokine therapy, and vaccines.

Bleomycin is an antibiotic that is nonspecific in terms of the cells it targets but is cell cycle specific and therefore targets rapidly dividing cells such as tumor cells. It consists of numerous antibiotic peptides that inhibit both mitosis and DNA synthesis. Bleomycin has been used for lymphomas and squamous cell carcinomas of the head and neck, testicular cancer, and cervical cancer. It is often given in combination with radiation therapy. The principal side effects include pulmonary fibrosis, alopecia, hyperpigmentation, desquamation of hands and feet with hardening and tenderness of the fingertips, nausea, vomiting, and stomatitis. The oral ulcerations are quick to develop and can be quite severe.

Both actinomycin D and doxorubicin are also cell cycle–nonspecific antibiotics; they inhibit DNA-dependent RNA synthesis by intercalating between DNA base pairs, similar in action to the plant alkaloids mentioned earlier. They are indicated and useful in the treatment of Ewing sarcoma, osteogenic sarcoma, rhabdomyosarcoma, and Wilms tumor. Doxorubicin has a wider spectrum of indications, including acute leukemia, bladder carcinoma, breast carcinoma, Hodgkin disease, non-Hodgkin lymphoma, soft tissue sarcomas, and thyroid carcinoma. The gastrointestinal side effects of actinomycin D and doxorubicin include anorexia, nausea, vomiting (usually within hours of administration), diarrhea, stomatitis, glossitis, cheilitis, and proctitis. Bone marrow depression results in thrombocytopenia and leukopenia within seven days of therapy. Alopecia, erythema, desquamation, and hyperpigmentation may also be noted after administration. In addition to these adverse effects, doxorubicin turns urine red (not hematuria) and may cause diffuse cardiomyopathy with congestive heart failure. Cardiomyopathy becomes the dose-limiting factor in the use of doxorubicin.

Interferons are cell-signaling proteins produced by the immune systems to fight viruses, parasites and tumor cells. Interferons activate signal transducers to boost production of macrophages and natural killer cells. Interferon therapy has been used for a variety of diseases, depending on the type of immune response desired. Interferon beta 1a and beta 1b are used to treat autoimmune disorders such as multiple sclerosis, while interferon alpha is used in conjunction with other antivirals for hepatitis B and C (Paolicelli et al., 2009; Cooksley, 2004). Interferon therapy is also used in combination with chemoradiation for hematologic malignancies and lymphomas (Borden, 2019). Side effects of interferon therapy consist of flulike symptoms, fatigue, weight loss, depression and irritability, sleep disturbances, sexual dysfunction, suicidal thoughts, bone marrow suppression, and hepatotoxicity. Interferon has not been reported to have oral side effects.

Interleukins, such as interleukin-2, are cytokines expressed by white blood cells. The interleukins help the body's immune system to discriminate between foreign and normal cells by binding to the cell membranes and forming a complex that stimulates the growth, differentiation, and survival of cytotoxic T cells. Aldesleukin is a recombinant form of interleukin-2 that is used to treat malignant melanoma and renal cell carcinoma (Petrella et al., 2007). Side effects of interleukin therapy are dependent on the dose and scheduling of the drug, which is given intravenously or subcutaneously. The most common side effects are nausea, vomiting, hepatotoxicity, neurotoxicity, renal toxicity, and pulmonary damage.

In recent years, immune check point inhibitor therapy, a novel form of immunotherapy, has demonstrated remarkable success in treating various types of cancer—for example, melanoma, non–small cell lung cancer, head and neck cancer, and certain types of gastrointestinal malignancies—and gained popularity in clinical use (Hargadon et al., 2018). Monoclonal antibody blockade of CTLA-4, PD-1, and PD-L1 function by unmasking the "stop signal" on T cells, to allow the immune system to attack the cancer at full speed. These agents are often well tolerated, with minimum effect on a patient's functional status. However, severe side effects could occur and manifest as a profound immune activation, such as endocrine dysfunction, pneumonitis, colitis, severe skin toxicities, and so on.

Colony-stimulating factors are glycoproteins given to patients to stimulate stem cell growth in the bone marrow. The recombinant granulocyte colony-stimulating factor (rG-CSF), also known as filgrastim, is administered in conjunction with other chemotherapeutic agents to allow higher doses of chemotherapy in order to maintain functional levels of white blood cells, platelets, and red blood cells and to prevent febrile neutropenia during myelosuppressive therapy (Nabholtz et al., 2002; Pettengell et al., 2009; Dale et al., 2018; Bongiovanni et al., 2019). Filgrastim is a support medication only and does not directly treat cancer. This drug is given either subcutaneously or as an intravenous infusion. No consistent side effects of the use of filgrastim have been reported, but some patients have reported bone pain, temporary blood abnormalities, and tenderness at the site of injection (Dale et al., 2018; Bongiovanni et al., 2019).

Monoclonal antibodies are widely used in cancer immunotherapy. Researchers have identified specific antigens linked with cancer cells. The monoclonal antibody works by attaching to the surface of the cancer cell, making it more visible for the body's immune system to recognize and attack. In some instances, monoclonal antibodies can be conjugated to radioisotopes or toxins to permit the specific delivery of these agents to the intended cancer cell population. Rituximab works in this manner and is used to treat B-cell lymphomas. Side effects of rituximab include fever, chills, infection, lack of energy, and leukopenia. There have also been significantly severe reactions, which include infusion reactions, tumor lysis syndrome, mucocutaneous reactions, progressive multifocal leukoencephalopathy, and reactivation of hepatitis B and other viral infections. Patients can also suffer from cardiac arrhythmias and renal toxicities.

Monoclonal antibodies such as cetuximab can work to block growth factors secreted by existing tumor cells, preventing the proliferation of cancers such as colon cancer and head and neck cancers. Other types of monoclonal antibodies such as ibritumomab tiuxetan, approved for non-Hodgkin lymphoma, are combined with a radioactive particle so that radiation can be delivered directly to cancer cells. In addition, chemotherapeutic agents are now being attached to some monoclonal antibodies, such as gemtuzumab ozogamicin for the treatment of acute myelogenous leukemia, in order to specifically target cancer cells and lower the chance that normal cells will be harmed.

In general, the side effects for this class of drugs consist of constipation, diarrhea, nausea, vomiting, headache, pain, swelling or redness at the injection site, sleep disturbances, and weakness. Cetuximab is also known for causing dry skin and xerostomia. Gemtuzumab ozogamicin can also cause oral mucosal ulcerations.

The side effects of biologic agents may present similarly to those resulting from other chemotherapeutic agents but tend to vary in form. Recently, clinical researchers have strived to classify side effects and reactions to this drug class. Their aim is to develop a better understanding of these drugs and more effective means of treating side effects. It may also help define risk factors and give direction to future research in this novel area (Kimiz-Gebologlu et al., 2018; Wahid et al., 2018).

Oral Effects of Chemotherapy

The direct effects of the oral manifestations of chemotherapy are secondary to tissue necrosis and desquamation. The indirect effects arise from a decreased number and function of platelets and neutrophils and may be exacerbated by preexisting conditions unrelated to cancer, such as periodontal disease, caries, and defective restorations. Direct oral complications of cancer chemotherapy are usually dose dependent and present as mucositis, xerostomia, and pain with associated neurologic symptoms. Indirect oral complications that may present in the chemotherapy patient are bleeding, infection, and nutritional deficiency.

Oral mucositis

Mucositis is one of the most common side effects associated with chemotherapy and radiation therapy (Lalla and Peterson, 2005; Sonis, 2011; Sroussi et al., 2017; Lalla et al., 2019). The oral mucosa is particularly vulnerable to breakdown because of its high turnover rate and because it is constantly subjected to trauma as a consequence of mastication, oral hygiene procedures, and exposure to chemical and thermal stimuli. In addition, the oral cavity hosts a milieu of microorganisms with the potential to cause infection and delay healing, making it a major site of chemotherapeutic toxicity. The effects are more severe in patients undergoing therapy in preparation for bone marrow transplantation (BMT). Ulcerative oral mucositis affects the patient's ability to maintain appropriate hydration and nutrition and increases the risk of secondary infections and frequently leads to delays or interruptions in cancer treatment (Rosenthal, 2007). All these factors may worsen the overall prognosis as well as increase treatment costs by necessitating multiple and prolonged hospitalizations (Pico et al., 1998; Sonis et al., 2001; Elting et al., 2003).

The occurrence and severity of oral mucositis vary greatly among patients. The patient's age, the type of malignancy, and the concomitant use of radiation can have an effect on the degree of stomatotoxicity. Younger patients are more likely to have ulcerations than are older patients undergoing the same treatment, but younger patients tend to heal more quickly. The reason for both is that younger patients have a more rapid basal cell turnover rate than older patients. Patients with hematologic malignancies tend to have more ulcerations than do patients who are being treated for solid tumors.

Oral mucositis is a complex and multistep process and is the result of damage to tissue mechanisms associated with both the epithelium and the underlying submucosa. It is more than a simple inflammatory process brought on by chemotherapy. Because it is often a great source of pain and has the potential to interfere with the overall care and prognosis of the patient, research has focused on alleviating the symptoms of oral mucositis. Thus, an understanding of how and why it occurs is essential. Sonis (1998, 2004, 2009) suggests that oral mucositis occurs in five stages (Fig 10-1):

1. Initiation
2. Upregulation and message generation
3. Signal amplification
4. Ulceration
5. Healing

Each phase is interdependent, overlapping, and multifactorial in its development and presentation. Initiation occurs when DNA and other cellular components are damaged directly from exposure to radiation and/or chemotherapy, generating reactive oxygen species and free radicals that lead to further damage to DNA. In the upregulation and message generation phase, there is increased synthesis of cytokines such as nuclear factor—kappa B (NF-*κ*B) that increase the rate of cell apoptosis or cell death. Cytokines such as interleukin-1 and tumor necrosis factor-alpha are released from the epithelium, resulting in local tissue damage and increased vascularity.

In the signal amplification phase, there are multiple positive feedback loops that further increase the number and levels of activating signals. The net result is an ongoing cycle of amplification of cell injury and death even after the initial insult of radiation or

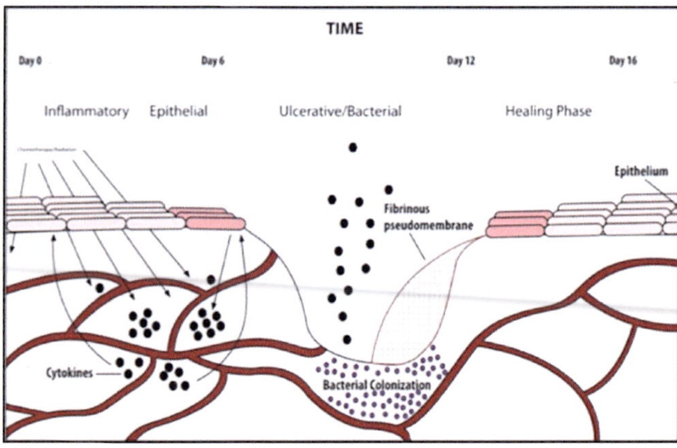

Figure 10-1 Mucositis model according to Sonis (2004).

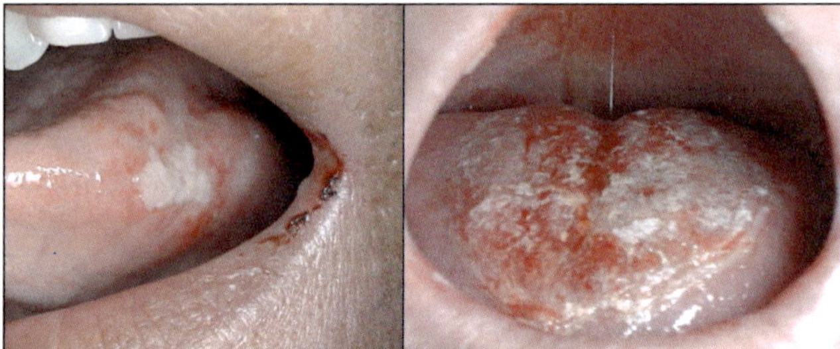

Figure 10-2 Chemotherapy-induced mucositis, seen as generalized ulceration.

Box 10-1

Bland Rinses
- "Magic mouthwash"
- 0.9% Saline
- Sodium bicarbonate solution

Topical anesthetics: Sprays, ointments, gels, and rinses
- Lidocaine or benzocaine
- Diclonine
- Capsaicin

Mucosal protectants
- Gelclair
- Cellulose
- Kaolin
- Sucralfate (Carafate, Axcan Pharma)
- Aluminum hydroxide

Analgesics
- Benzydamine rinse (Not available in the United States)
- Opioids (Nonsteroidal anti-inflammatory drugs contraindicated)

Other
- Allopurinol rinse
- Chlorhexidine rinse
- Pentoxifylline

chemotherapy. Thinning and atrophy of the epithelium and marked degeneration of collagen are observed histologically. Erythematous changes may also appear at this stage. Erythema is most likely due to a combination of increased vascularity and thinning of the overlying epithelium (Kolbinson et al., 1988). The patient is relatively asymptomatic or only mildly symptomatic at this phase, which usually occurs in the first six days of treatment.

In the ulcerative phase, the damage and destruction of basal cells precludes maintenance of continuity of the oral mucosa. This process progresses over a two-week period to erythema, ulceration, and denudation (Fig 10-2). Subsequently, the ulcerated and denuded surfaces collect debris and become vulnerable to secondary infections. Overgrowth of microorganisms around breaks in the mucosa prolongs healing and invites microbial invasions that may lead to severe systemic infections particularly associated with streptococcal species (Elting et al., 1992; Gamis et al., 2000; Facchini et al., 2012). Patients are neutropenic at this stage, and their white blood cell counts will continue to decrease to a nadir in about two weeks following initiation of chemotherapy (Sonis et al., 1990a; Facchini et al., 2012). This is one of the most complex stages of oral mucositis, because there are combined areas of ulcerations, ongoing inflammatory processes, and secondary colonization of bacteria and fungi. Patients will be most symptomatic during this phase and suffer considerably from pain, inflammation, and loss of function. This phase can also add to the overall costs of treatment because of the need to manage pain and an increase in the number of hospitalizations (Pico et al., 1998; Sonis et al., 2001; Elting et al., 2003).

Oral mucositis is most often seen in drug protocols involving alkylating agents and antimetabolites (Greenwald, 1973; Frei, 1974). The antimetabolite, methotrexate, is associated with severe mucositis (Oliff et al., 1979; Driezen et al., 1981). The severity of methotrexate mucositis was originally thought to be related to its excretion in the saliva. However, in a study of salivary concentrations, methotrexate levels did not correlate with the degree of oral mucositis (Oliff et al., 1979). Antitumor antibiotics, such as bleomycin, have a particularly adverse effect on the squamous epithelium and may cause serious mucosal ulceration. The combination of cisplatin and 5-FU, when used with radiation therapy, can also cause severe oral mucositis (Peterson, 2006).

Mucosal healing occurs spontaneously, approximately two to four weeks following the completion of cancer treatments. The healing phase consists of a renewal of epithelial proliferation and differentiation as the white blood cell counts normalize. The control of local bacterial flora also plays a key role in the rapidity of this phase. As the healing progresses, the symptoms begin to abate.

Palliation, prevention and treatment

In past years, the pain and irritation of oral mucositis caused by cancer chemotherapy were managed palliatively, although in recent times, preventive and therapeutic approaches have been studied. Numerous remedies have been advocated for relief of pain. If the mucositis is relatively mild, patients are given a topical anesthetic or a mucosal coating agent with which to rinse or gargle (Box 10-1). Cryotherapy is also used in patients with mild to moderate mucositis (Cascinu et al., 1994; Peterson et al., 2013; Johansson et al., 2019). Moderate to severe pain associated with mucositis is usually treated with a combination of topical and systemic analgesics. The analgesics can be narcotic or nonnarcotic. Agents that bind to oral mucosa (mucosal protective agents), such as sulcrafate, have been largely ineffective (Lalla et al., 2019).

If severe pain and dysfunction are associated with oral mucositis, chemotherapeutic doses may be reduced or discontinued until sufficient tolerance is regained by the patient. If the patient is unable to nutrify or hydrate orally, total parenteral nutrition may be necessary. Severe oral mucositis pain, especially when complicated by a local

Table 10-2 Proposed Oral Mucositis Assessment Scales

Scale	Grade 0	Grade 1	Grade 2	Grade 3	Grade 4
World Health Organization	None	Soreness and erythema	Erythema and ulcers Can eat solid foods	Ulcers: liquid diet only	Ulcers: alimentation not possible
Radiation Therapy Oncology Group	None	Erythema of mucosa	Patchy reaction, ≤1.5 cm, noncontiguous	Confluent reaction, >1.5 cm, contiguous	Necrosis or deep ulceration, with bleeding
National Cancer Institute Common Toxicity Criteria	None	Painless ulcers: erythema or mild soreness in absence of lesions	Painful erythema, edema, or ulcers: can eat and swallow	Painful erythema, edema, or ulcers requiring intravenous hydration	Severe ulceration or requires parenteral/enteral nutritional support or prophylactic intubation
Oral Mucositis Assessment Scale: • Ulceration • Erythema	 • None • None	 • <1 cm^2 • Not severe	 • 1 to 3 cm^2 • Severe	 • >3 cm^2 • NA	 • NA • NA

herpes simplex virus infection, may require a morphine-type narcotic analgesic administered via an intravenous patient-controlled analgesia pump.

Recent research has focused on strategies, based on the model proposed by Sonis, that inhibit the development of tissue injury at the molecular level. Radioprotective agents such as amifostine, which act as reactive oxygen species inhibitors, have been tested. These agents act as free radical and reactive oxygen species scavengers, prevent the upregulation of inflammatory pathways, and theoretically should minimize many of the deleterious effects of irradiation. Intravenous administration of amifostine has been tested the most, but the evidence is conflicting regarding its efficacy (Nicolatou-Galitis et al., 2013).

These drugs are also potent anti-inflammatory agents. As discussed earlier, the inflammatory response plays an important role in the initiation and progression of oral mucositis; drugs that suppress the inflammatory response theoretically should be beneficial. Benzydamine has received the most attention in recent years. It is a nonsteroidal anti-inflammatory drug with analgesic properties and has been shown to inhibit inflammatory cytokine production as well as to be a reactive oxygen species scavenger. It is administered as a mouthwash during radiotherapy, has been tested at a number of centers, and has been shown to reduce the severity of oral mucositis as well as the associated pain and dysphagia (Epstein et al., 2001; Cheng et al., 2006; Kazemian et al., 2009; Roopashri et al., 2011; Rastogi et al., 2017).

Growth factors, such as human keratinocyte growth factor (Palifermin), exercise cytoprotective effects on epithelial cells by reducing the levels of reactive oxygen species and have been shown to reduce the incidence and severity of oral mucositis in patients with hematologic malignancies who are treated with chemotherapy to prepare for stem cell transplantation (Niscola et al., 2009; Raber-Durlacher et al., 2013).

As mentioned previously, a secondary infection probably increases the severity of oral mucositis. As a result, several topical antimicrobial agents have been used in an attempt to reduce severity. However, the results have been disappointing, and MASCC/ISOO (Multinational Association of Supportive Care in Cancer) guidelines recommend against the routine use of antimicrobial lozenges, chlorhexidine mouthrinse, and Eisenmann mouthrinse (McGuire et al., 2013; Saunders et al., 2013).

One of the difficulties faced in designing appropriate clinical outcome studies has been the lack of a standardized method of measuring the severity of oral mucositis. An objective, psychometrically sound examination instrument must be developed to classify and quantify oral mucosal changes accurately and reliably. Several grading systems have been developed to score the severity of oral mucositis (Dyck, 1991; Schubert et al., 1992; Donnelly et al., 1992). While some scales have multiple gradations, and others simply have three or four grades, each is limited in its description, depending on the method of evaluation. Other scales look at the objective findings in the mouth, such as the size and number of lesions in the oral cavity, while others only assess levels of pain and dysfunction, such as the inability to eat, drink, or swallow.

To address this problem, in 1996, oral medicine specialists, oncologists, and oncology nurses from the United States developed a scoring system to evaluate both the anatomical extent and severity of oral mucositis. The resulting scale was the Oral Mucositis Assessment Scale (OMAS), which classifies different areas of the oral cavity for tissue changes, presence and size of ulcerations, and pain and assesses the patient's ability to swallow and masticate.

Schubert et al. (1992) suggested that an ideal mucositis grading system should rate subjective complaints (pain, taste, and dryness), functional performance (speech, chewing, and swallowing), and objective changes (edema, atrophy, pseudomembrane, and ulceration). They developed the Oral Mucositis Rating Scale (OMRS), which considers changes in the oral mucosa during therapy along with subjective complaints and functional performance. Unfortunately, none of these systems have been adopted universally.

The more detailed scoring systems appeal to researchers, while the simpler, less cumbersome scoring systems tend to be favored by clinicians. Table 10-2 compares some of the more commonly used oral mucositis assessment scales.

In summary, as mentioned in Chapter 1, oral mucositis is a complex multifactorial phenomenon, and the palliative, preventive, and therapeutic measures that have been employed to date have proven to be largely ineffective. We are beginning to understand the pathogenesis of oral mucositis, but unfortunately, many of the cellular pathways involved are analogous to those in play in the destruction of tumor cells, which poses a dilemma. Will some of the strategies of mitigation that evolve from our increased level of understanding of these processes increase the risk of protecting tumor cells? Because of this risk, it follows that progress in this field must, by necessity, be slow and deliberate and based on specifically targeting the cellular pathways unique to oral mucositis.

Table 10-3 Effects of Chemotherapy

Cell counts	Normal values	Effects of chemotherapy	Consequences
White Blood Cell Count (WBC)	4,000–10,000 cells/mm³	Decreased WBC	Increased risk of infection: <1,500 cells/mm³
Absolute neutrophil count (ANC): ANC=WBC X (% segs + % bands)*	>2,000	Decreased ANC	Increased risk of infection: • Low risk: ≥1,000 to <2,000 • Moderate risk: >500 to <1,000 • High risk: 0 (Nadir) to 500
Erythrocyte count:	Males: 4.7–6.1 million/mm³ Females: 4.2–5.4 million/mm³	Decreased erythrocyte count:	Increased risk of anemia: <3.5 million/mm³
• Hemoglobin	• Males: 18g/dL • Females: 16g/dL	• Decreased hemoglobin value (<10.8g/dL)	
• Hematocrit	• Males: 42–52% • Females:37–47%	• Decreased hemoglobin value (<31.1g/dL)	
Platelet count	150,000–400,000/mm³	Decreased platelet count	Increased risk of bleeding: • Low risk of prolonged bleeding ≥50,000 • Moderate risk of prolonged bleeding: 20,000 to <50,000/mm³ • Risk of spontaneous bleeding: <20,000/mm³

*Segs are mature neutrophils that appear segmented on a slide; *bands* are immature neutrophils that are less segmented on the slide.

Xerostomia

Dry mouth is a common complaint of patients undergoing chemotherapy. It is not readily apparent until later in the treatment or, more commonly, following treatment. Xerostomia is thought to be caused by the direct effects of chemotherapy on major and minor salivary glands. Lockhart and Sonis (1981) demonstrated histologically that minor salivary glands degenerated in 50% of these patients. A similar degeneration appears to occur in major salivary glands. Chemotherapy-induced xerostomia tends to be much less severe and usually is more transient than radiation-induced xerostomia (see Chapter 1, section entitled "Salivary gland dysfunction").

Saliva is an effective lubricant, and therefore xerostomia can increase the pain and discomfort associated with oral mucositis (Main et al., 1984). In the absence of saliva, the soft tissues of the tongue, floor of the mouth, palate, buccal mucosa, and oropharynx cling to one another, the teeth, and prosthetic appliances. Xerostomia can also exacerbate the oral pain resulting from chemotherapy-induced neuralgia. Neurologic side effects of chemotherapy present as pain and paresthesia in the head and neck region and most commonly occur with the administration of the plant alkaloids.

Intact salivary function is an important component of oral host defenses against infection. Decreased salivary flow renders the patient at an increased risk of secondary infections because of a decrease in the amount of immunoglobulin A secreted, limitations of natural cleansing, and alterations in the oral environment.

Saliva has many beneficial functions in the mouth in addition to acting as a part of the host defense system. It is also responsible for lubrication, mucosal hydration, taste perception, and prevention of dental caries. Acids generated by bacteria are buffered by saliva, and saliva aids in remineralization of tooth structure. Without the buffering and remineralizing capacity of saliva, teeth can quickly become demineralized and susceptible to dental caries.

Although chemotherapy-induced xerostomia is usually reversible and salivary secretion levels can return to near normal levels following cessation of medical therapy, it can be extremely uncomfortable and damaging during treatment.

Because of their increased susceptibility to dental caries, patients should avoid using products with sugar to increase salivary flow. Chewing gum and candies must be sugarless. Saliva stimulants such as pilocarpine may increase salivary flow and are beneficial for some patients. It is recommended that patients adopt diets that are moist and less cariogenic. If salivary flow is extremely compromised, daily fluoride applications of either stannous or neutral sodium fluoride are indicated. The daily use of remineralizing agents is also recommended. (Management of salivary gland dysfunction is discussed in greater detail in Chapter 1.)

Malaise, xerostomia, and the discomfort secondary to oral mucositis may affect the patient's outlook on and tolerance of treatment. Oral mucositis, pharyngitis, and esophagitis are painful, often rendering the patient dysphagic. Some patients are unable or unwilling to communicate verbally, to perform oral hygiene procedures, or to consume food or liquids. As a result, the patient regresses and becomes more vulnerable to the indirect effects of cancer chemotherapy, such as bleeding, infection, and nutritional deficiencies.

Oral hemorrhage

Bleeding in the oral cavity is a direct result of thrombocytopenia and an indirect result of mucositis. The frequency and severity of hemorrhage are directly related to the severity of mucositis and degree of thrombocytopenia. Thrombocytopenia results from inadequate production of megakaryocytes, which decreases the number of platelets, and can be manifested in patients with diseases such as acute leukemia, aplastic anemia, and idiopathic thrombocytopenic purpura or associated with antineoplastic chemotherapy.

A quantitative diagnosis of thrombocytopenia is based on the concentration of circulating platelets. Normal platelet counts can range from 150,000 to 400,000/mm³. Platelet levels of less than 60,000/mm³ put the patient at increased risk of bleeding. At

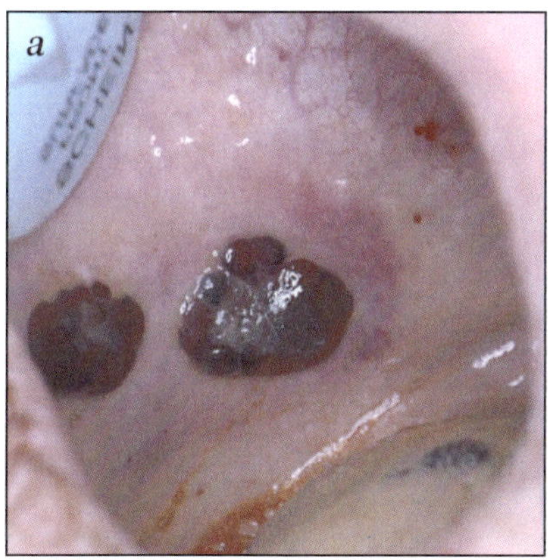

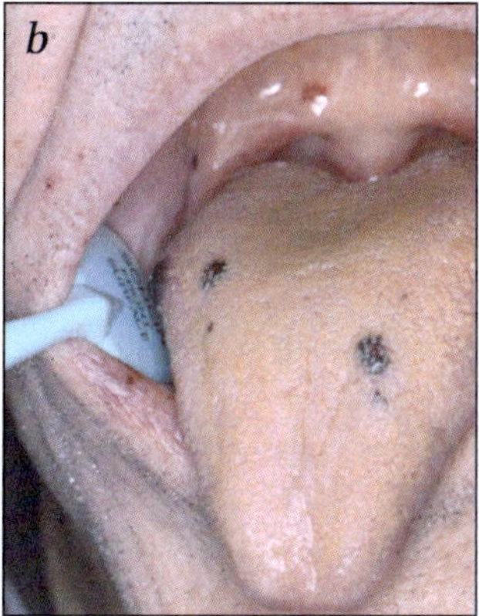

Figure 10-3 Ecchymosis, which results from submucosal bleeding and microvascular incompetence, on the buccal mucosa *(a)* and the tongue *(b)*. Note the petechiae.

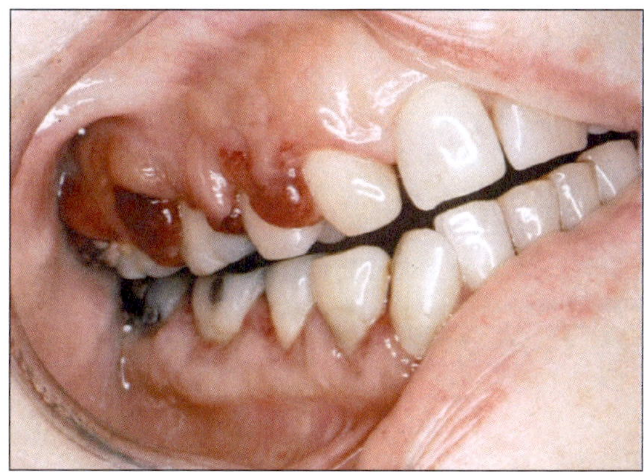

Figure 10-4 Patient who bled continuously through the gingival sulcus while thrombocytopenic. Bleeding persists when the integrity of small vessels is more severely damaged and the platelets are inadequate.

platelet levels of 25,000/mm^3 or less, there is a 75% chance of spontaneous or induced severe, possibly uncontrollable, hemorrhage (Gaydos et al., 1962). The risk drops to 41% at a level of 25,000 to 60,000/mm^3 and to 16% at platelet levels higher than 60,000/mm^3 (Table 10-3) (Bodey et al., 1966). Therefore, accurate monitoring of platelet levels is critical prior to the initiation of any potentially traumatic procedure.

The need to gain control of spontaneous hemorrhage may necessitate platelet transfusion when a patient is thrombocytopenic. The average half-life of host platelets is 8 to 10 days, while that of donor platelets is only 5 days or less after being stored for several days. For this reason, chemotherapy patients with thrombocytopenia often require multiple platelet transfusions to prevent hemorrhage. Platelet transfusions are expensive, however, and can be associated with negative side effects such as febrile nonhemolytic transfusion reactions, infections from the transfusion, and platelet refractoriness (Heal and Blumberg, 2004). Platelet refractoriness occurs when the increase in platelet count is significantly less than expected (≤2,000/µL per unit of platelet concentration given to an average-sized adult) (Schiffer et al., 2001). This results from increased destruction of the transfused platelets by the recipient.

The clinical signs of hemorrhage include petechiae, ecchymosis, and bleeding. Petechiae are characterized by pinpoint red spots on the tissue that are 1 to 3 mm in size. Damage to cells lining small vessels in the submucosa allows erythrocytes to escape into the connective tissues. Ecchymosis is more diffuse and results from submucosal bleeding and microvascular incompetence (Fig 10-3).

Bleeding persists when the integrity of the small vessels is more severely damaged and platelets are inadequate to maintain hemostasis. Intraoral petechiae and/or ecchymosis should be considered an indicator of potential bleeding problems. Hemorrhage most often occurs from areas of traumatic injury or ulceration. The trauma can be physical (toothbrush injury), chemical (strong mouthrinses), thermal (hot food or drink), or microbial (endogenous or exogenous). Ulcerations may be visible breaks in the oral mucosa or microscopic breaks in the sulcular epithelium.

Spontaneous intraoral bleeding is most common from the gingival crevice. The increased vulnerability of this area stems from the fact that the epithelium is only a few cell layers thick in the sulcus. When inflamed, as in gingivitis or periodontal disease, the sulcular epithelium thins and develops numerous microscopic ulcerations. Gingivitis and periodontitis therefore increase the risk for gingival bleeding (Schroeder and Listgarten, 2000).

If the gingival sulcus is identified as the bleeding site, pressure should be applied over the facial and lingual or palatal gingiva with cold gauze. Pressure to the area should be gentle yet firm and consistent. Periodontal dressings do not provide sufficient pressure for the extended periods necessary to stop gingival sulcular bleeding. Topical hemostatic agents can be used in the gingival sulcus to aid in hemostasis. However, it can be difficult to deliver a hemostatic agent to the site of hemorrhage within the gingival sulcus (Fig 10-4). Customized soft silicone stents may be useful as carriers of the hemostatic agent.

Because local management of bleeding can be difficult in the thrombocytopenic patient, any potential cause of bleeding, such as sharp edges on prostheses or abrasive toothbrushing, should be eliminated or modified. Identification of the site of hemorrhage is essential. All blood clots and debris should be gently removed from the mouth. Suction is helpful to remove pooling blood and saliva. Adequate light and proper positioning of the patient are essential in this endeavor.

The size and location of the bleeding area dictate management. Large diffuse areas that are difficult to isolate can be managed with topical hemostatic agents such as topical thrombin or antifibrinolytic rinses. Small, pinpoint areas of bleeding can be controlled with direct application of pressure for a prolonged period (30 minutes or more). Cooling the tissues with intraoral ice packs, placement of gauze, and application of pressure will reduce blood flow to the area and may aid in hemostasis.

If traumatic injury has caused a significant wound or if previous extraction sites are bleeding, management may involve local anesthesia and suturing. However, most bleeding in the thrombocytopenic patient will not benefit from suturing. In fact, suturing and local anesthetic injections may be contraindicated in these patients because the needle punctures can create additional sites of bleeding. Ultimately, correction of thrombocytopenia with platelet transfusion and/or recovery is necessary for control of hemorrhage.

Infection

Infection is the most common and potentially the most serious complication in chemotherapy patients with bone marrow suppression. Leukocytes are reduced, rendering the host unable to resist microbial colonization, invasion, and infection by opportunistic microorganisms. *Leukopenia* is defined as any situation in which the total number of circulating granulocytes or polymorphonuclear leukocytes is less than normal. The normal granulocyte level varies with the individual but generally falls within the range of 5,000 to 6,000/mm^3. The potential for infection is very low at white blood cells levels greater than or equal to 1,500/mm^3 (Bodey et al., 1966). Polymorphonuclear leukocytes (neutrophils) make up 50% to 70% of the circulating white blood cells. These are the most numerous of all blood cell types found in the acute phase of the inflammatory reaction and the most important to prevent infection.

There are many sources of microorganisms for opportunistic infections. The most common are the endogenous oral and skin microbial flora. Microorganisms that are normally kept in check by other microorganisms and the functioning immune system become pathogenic through changes in the microbial balance and a loss of immune function. Many chemotherapeutic agents interfere with the action and numbers of neutrophils, thereby inhibiting phagocytosis (Armstrong, 1973).

Chemotherapy-induced immunosuppression renders the patient susceptible to infection by microorganisms that would normally be controlled. Oral ulcerations induced by chemotherapy are not solely responsible for infections. The immune response must also be compromised. This is evidenced by the fact that normal patients with oral ulcerations (whether traumatically, idiopathically, or virally induced) do not become infected like immunocompromised patients. This profound immunosuppression places the patient at extreme risk of infectious complications. The risk escalates as the degree and duration of myelosuppression increase. The hospital environment can also be a source of potentially lethal exogenous microorganisms that may infect the immunocompromised patient because these microorganisms often have resistance to many antibiotics and can be extremely challenging to manage.

Antineoplastic drugs, such as adrenocorticoids and cytotoxic drugs, lower patients' immunity to infection by inducing leukopenia, inhibiting antibody responses, blocking the mononuclear phase of the inflammatory reaction, and compromising delayed hypersensitivity (Hersh et al., 1965). When delayed hypersensitivity is impaired, there is an increase in host susceptibility to intracellular parasites and a further reduction in host resistance. These drugs also adversely affect macrophage function and diapedesis of granulocytes.

Primary disease processes can also be responsible for lowering host resistance. Patients with acute leukemia who are undergoing chemotherapy are particularly susceptible to frequent and severe infections because of the presence of immature, incompetent myeloblasts.

As previously mentioned, many chemotherapeutic agents directly cause mucositis with ulcerations that become portals of entry for microorganisms into the underlying connective tissues. Ultimately, microorganisms gain access to the systemic vasculature in hosts with compromised cellular and humoral immunity. Continual bacterial seeding (bacteremias) leads to septicemias that are potentially fatal in the immunocompromised patient. Patients can be at risk for developing any combination of bacterial, fungal, and viral infections.

Oral bacterial infections are often associated with periodontal and endodontic disease. Examples include gram-positive organisms such as viridans streptococci and *Streptococcus mutans*. Other pathogens, including *Pseudomonas aeruginosa*, *Staphylococcus aureus*, and *Escherichia coli*, can also cause infections in the oral cavity. It is essential to target antimicrobial therapy to the specific bacterial organism to minimize antibiotic resistance; however, broad-spectrum antibiotics can be administered while the culture results are pending. In addition to taking systemic antibiotics, patients can also be instructed on mechanical reduction of the bacterial population through toothbrushing, flossing, and rinsing with antimicrobial or hydrogen peroxide–based mouthrinses, if tolerated by the patient.

Fungal infections, primarily with *Candida albicans*, are probably the most frequent oral infection. Candidiasis arises when immunosuppression and xerostomia are present and can be exacerbated if the patient is taking antibiotic medications as well. The alteration in the shift of the oral flora and being immunocompromised lead to the clinical disease.

Candida infections may present as pseudomembranous, erythematous (atrophic), or hyperplastic candidiasis. In pseudomembranous candidiasis, white creamy plaques can be rubbed off the mucosal surface. The plaques are foci of fungal organisms. In erythematous candidiasis, there are few obvious fungal organisms, but there is diffuse redness of the oral mucosa. Hyperplastic candidiasis is less common and presents as tenacious white plaques on mucosal surfaces (Fig 10-5). Lesions in severely immunosuppressed patients can be quite extensive, with all forms presenting at the same time. The most common complaint from patients with oral candidiasis is a burning sensation of the oral mucosa.

In cases of profound immunosuppression, the patient is susceptible to infection by more invasive and aggressive fungal organisms, such as *Aspergillus* infections, histoplasmosis, and mucormycosis (Fig 10-6). Systemic fungal infections are very difficult to manage and potentially fatal in the immunosuppressed patient. Although not a common finding, fungal infections in the severely immunosuppressed patient can invade tissues.

Mucormycosis is a locally destructive infection with an often fatal outcome (Kurrasch et al., 1981; Riley et al., 2016). Patients who survive usually suffer facial disfigurement and loss of parts of the maxilla secondary to local tissue loss (see Chapter 3). Treatment consists of the use of local antifungal topical agents in milder forms and systemic treatment for severe cases. Topical medications can include amphotericin B oral suspensions. In severe cases, when the fungal infection is no longer localized to just the oral cavity, systemic fluconazole or intravenous amphotericin B can be prescribed. The infection does not abate until bone marrow recovers to normal levels and xerostomia no longer exists.

Outbreaks of viral infections typically occur in patients with previous exposures. Herpes simplex virus reactivation is common in the BMT patient population (Montgomery et al., 1986; Meyers et al., 1980; Saral, 1990; Liesveld et al., 2002; Blackstock et al., 2005). Meyers et al. (1980) reported an 82% incidence of oral herpes simplex virus infections in seropositive (herpes simplex virus antibody titer) BMT patients. Exogenous viral infections are less common. Herpetic infections are particularly troublesome in patients undergoing intensive chemotherapy. The oral and circumoral lesions can be particularly widespread and quite symptomatic. Resolution of these lesions

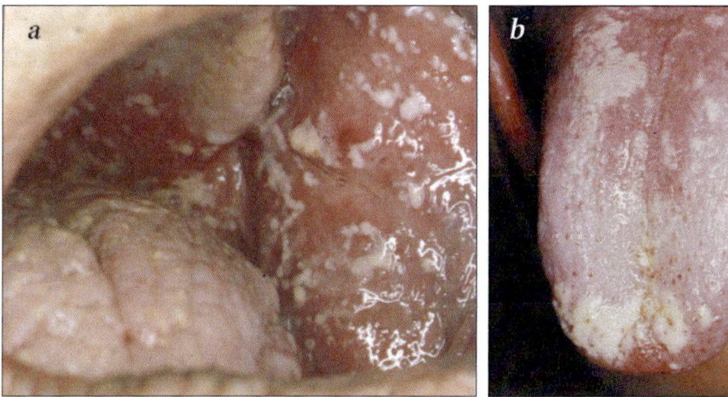

Figure 10-5 *(a and b)* Typical white plaques of candidiasis on the oral mucosa of an immunosuppressed patient during chemotherapy. The white plaques can be rubbed off, exposing an erythematous base (courtesy of Dr. Sol Silverman, Jr.).

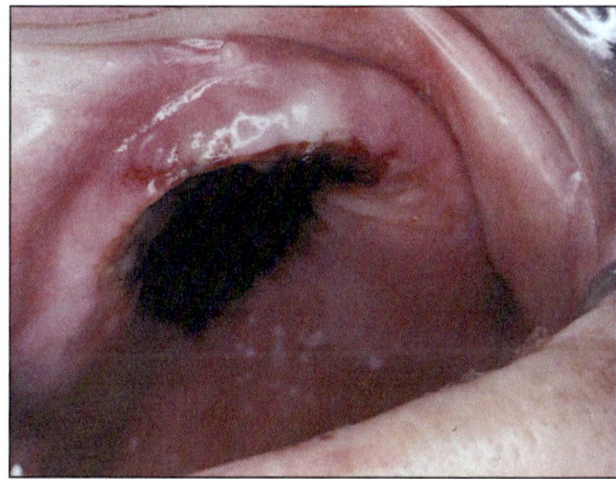

Figure 10-6 Mucormycosis in an immunosuppressed patient.

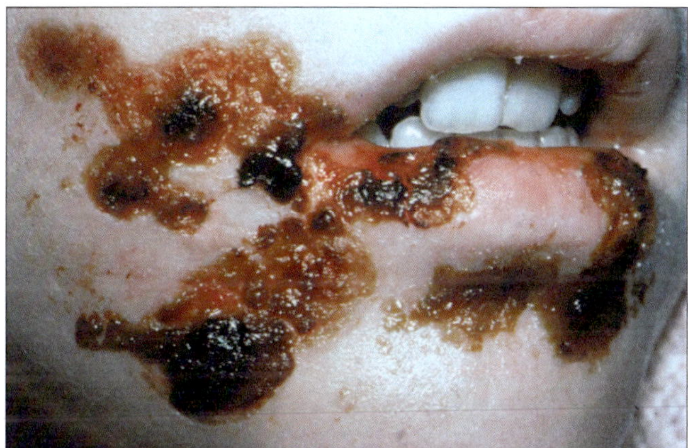

Figure 10-7 Herpes simplex virus. The crusty lesions in this patient are confined primarily to the circumoral region.

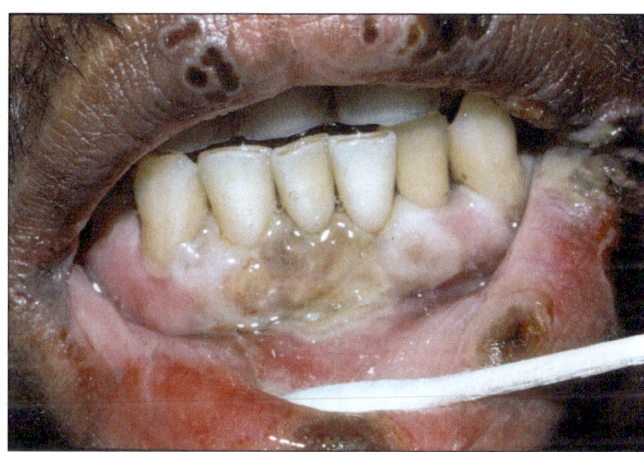

Figure 10-8 Herpes simplex virus. Lesions in this patient undergoing BMT are not confined to keratinized mucosa.

may require five to six weeks, depending on host defense and medical management. The circumoral lesions present as circular, crusty ulcerations, which may form large, painful lesions when they coalesce (Fig 10-7). The oral lesions are likewise quite painful and can be widespread, although most are confined to the keratinized mucosa (Fig 10-8). Other viruses that can present in this patient population are the varicella zoster virus, cytomegalovirus, adenovirus, and coxsackievirus. Treatment consists of use of antiviral agents such as valacyclovir for herpes outbreaks, famciclovir for varicella zoster virus infections, and ganciclovir for treatment of cytomegalovirus.

Although efficacious, some antiretroviral agents are used with reservation in chemotherapy patients because of the toxicity of these agents to vital organs. Acyclovir can be nephrotoxic and neurotoxic, especially in patients exposed to other chemotherapy agents with similar toxicities. This factor is important because treatment time is typically longer in the immunocompromised patient than in the healthy host and may persist until immune function has recovered.

Neurologic changes

Peripheral neuropathy is a debilitating and common occurrence in patients undergoing chemotherapy for malignancies. It is often a dose-limiting factor in cancer treatment. In particular, antineoplastic agents—such as vincristine, cisplatin, oxaliplatin, paclitaxel, and docetaxel—have been known to cause peripheral neuropathy (Staff et al., 2017; Loprinzi et al., 2020; Was et al., 2022). Patients suffer from dysesthesias and pain. Neuropathy can be distal, perioral, and pharyngolaryngeal. Likewise, peripheral motor nerves may also be affected by some drugs, leading to motor impairments (Zajączkowska et al., 2019). Drugs such as oxaliplatin, a third-generation platinum derivate, have short-term effects, but these effects can often be avoided by prolongation of the infusion of the drug (Park et al., 2009). However, drugs such as paclitaxel and cisplatin, which are often used in conjunction with radiation to treat head and neck cancers, can cause severe dysesthesias, weakness, and possible long-term damage. Neuroprotective agents and nerve growth factors are being tested with the hope of minimizing neurotoxic effects (Hu et al., 2019). However, none has gained wide acceptance.

Oral symptoms of peripheral neuropathy include severe, throbbing pain that may mimic dental pain secondary to dental disease such as irreversible pulpitis. Therefore, it is important for the dental clinician to accurately rule out the overt causes of dental, periodontal, or muscular maladies. Chemotherapy patients may also develop a transient mild to moderate dental hypersensitivity within weeks of initiation of chemotherapy, most probably due to the decrease of the sensitivity threshold for nonnoxious and noxious stimuli. The etiology is not well understood, but symptoms can be alleviated with opioid-containing analgesics for pain and application of fluoride, remineralizing agents, or dentinal desensitizers to the exposed dentin. The dentinal hypersensitivity usually resolves shortly after the cessation of chemotherapy treatment.

Chemotherapy-induced neurotoxicity can also cause dysgeusia, resulting from temporary disruption of taste bud regeneration in combination with xerostomia. Other possible alterations in taste can be because of the direct diffusion of chemotherapeutic agents into the oral cavity. There can also be olfactory disturbances (Silverman et al., 2002; Schubert et al., 2003).

Growth and development

Alterations in growth and development have been reported in association with high-dose chemotherapy in young patients (Van Leeuwen et al., 2000). In particular, the permanent dentition may exhibit shortened and conical roots, impaired alveolar development, incomplete enamel formation, and in some instances complete agenesis of teeth The growth centers associated with the development of the mandible and the maxilla may also be affected, resulting in underdevelopment of these structures. The addition of radiotherapy compounds these difficulties (Sonis et al., 1990b; Kaste et al., 2009; Vesterbacka et al., 2012).

Dental Management of the Chemotherapy Patient

Prevention and treatment prior to chemotherapy

Diagnosis and treatment of the oral manifestations of chemotherapy are oriented toward prevention of infection during medical treatment. A complete oral examination, including appropriate radiographs, is essential for any patient scheduled to receive chemotherapy to identify dental pathoses that may interfere with therapy. Without a thorough examination, oral problems can go unrecognized, complicating the clinical course of the disease or even becoming life threatening.

As mentioned above, intensive chemoradiation predisposes to severe neutropenia, which predisposes patients to a high risk of infection, sepsis, and septic shock (Walsh et al., 2020). However, once chemotherapy is completed, neutrophil counts return to normal. It follows that acute oral foci of infection should be eliminated, if possible, before the onset of chemotherapy. A distinction should be made between acute and chronic infectious foci. Chronic periodontitis and asymptomatic endodontic lesions are best deferred until after therapy (Spijkervet et al., 2021). Schuurhuis and colleagues (2016) have shown in a prospective study that such chronic oral foci can be left untreated, as this does not increase infectious complications during chemotherapy.

Dental treatment such as prophylaxis, dental restorations, endodontic therapy, surgical debridement, or extraction may be indicated. If sufficient time is available prior to the start of chemotherapy, such problems should be treated definitively to prevent exacerbation during chemotherapy.

Before any of these dental treatments is rendered, the patient's medical condition and ability to tolerate the proposed procedures must be assessed in consultation with the patient's physician. The primary disease status and secondary medical conditions should be discussed, along with their implications for treatment. The basic quantifiable risk assessment values are white blood cell and platelet counts. They provide a relative assessment for the patient's risk of developing infection and bleeding, respectively. Because polymorphonuclear leukocytes (neutrophils) provide the primary cellular immune defense against invading microorganisms, the absolute neutrophil count should be used to assess the patient's risk of developing infection and bleeding. If the risk is excessively high, the best option may be to perform no dental treatment.

Preventive management of the patient with reduced immune capacity (low white blood cell count) may include premedication with antibiotics or transfusion with granulocytes. In patients with thrombocytopenia, preventive management may include transfusion with platelets and/or admission to the hospital for observation and management of anticipated bleeding.

Carious teeth should be treated by excavation and restoration. If the dental pulp is exposed during excavation, appropriate endodontic care should be provided. Sharp edges on teeth, restorations, and prostheses must be smoothed and eliminated. Rough surfaces and sharp edges can become major sources of injury and irritation to the patient during immunosuppressive chemotherapy because the oral mucosa will be more vulnerable to ulceration and irritation.

Prosthetic appliances should be thoroughly examined for proper fit, function, and smoothness. Inadequacies and defects in prostheses to which a patient has previously adapted may become the source of problems during chemotherapy. Complete and/or partial dentures should be adjusted and relined if indicated. Dentures that do not have proper vertical dimension, occlusal balance, stability, fit, and function should be removed to prevent traumatic ulcerations (DePaola et al., 1983, 1986). Following recovery of the patient between courses of chemotherapy, adjustments, relines, or new dentures can be provided as necessary.

Teeth that present with endodontic problems should be definitively treated whenever possible. Nonvital pulps and/or canals that are avascularized "dead spaces" can provide a nidus for infection. Teeth that are symptomatic and periapically infected should be definitively treated with endodontic therapy or, in more urgent cases, extraction. Some patients who have asymptomatic teeth that show signs of infection—such as abscess formation, fistulas, or purulent drainage—can and should have endodontic treatment completed before chemotherapy. Otherwise, extraction may be a better option. However, there is no data to compare the risk of treatment versus no treatment under such circumstances. For those patients without obvious signs of infection or who cannot complete endodontic therapy prior to chemotherapy, therapy can be completed between treatment courses while the patient's immune system is minimally suppressed. A survey of dental clinicians who often manage leukemic patients revealed that infectious processes that invade bone pose the highest risk if left untreated or unresolved prior to chemotherapy (Wong and Toljanic, 2009). Ultimately, though, if the infection cannot be definitely resolved with endodontic therapy prior to chemotherapy, extraction should be considered.

When the patient undergoes total immunosuppression, such as in BMT/PBSCT, some clinicians prefer extractions of pulpally involved teeth, the premise being that removal of the infected teeth eliminates the potential source of infection, while endodontic therapy may fail to completely eliminate the infection. This risk of endodontic failure is of greater concern in the severely immunosuppressed patient because the resistance to infection is compromised. The decision to extract or treat endodontically remains an empirical choice of the treating dentist and treating physician. Studies are lacking that define the risk of extraction versus the risk of infection following endodontic therapy in the immunosuppressed patient.

Dental extractions should only be performed when retention of the tooth or teeth carries the risk of systemic infection. Extractions should be done at least seven days prior to the start of chemotherapy for proper mucosalization of the wound. Dental extraction immediately prior to the commencement of intensive chemotherapy increases the risk of infection, bleeding, and delayed wound healing and may delay oncologic treatment (Yamagata et al., 2006). Extractions are considered for abscessed teeth, severely periodontally compromised teeth with active periodontal infection, partially erupted third molars, and grossly carious teeth. If time does not permit extractions prior to chemotherapy, treatment can be rendered between cycles of chemotherapy, during periods of minimal bone marrow suppression. The objective is to reduce the potential of infection during periods of profound immunosuppression. Follow-up visits should be scheduled to ensure that surgical sites have healed sufficiently without dehiscence of the mucosal flaps.

There are times that medical treatment needs to be initiated urgently. In such cases, it may not be possible to treat compromised teeth properly. The risks and possible complications of leaving these teeth untreated should be raised with the oncology team.

A thorough oral prophylaxis and oral hygiene instructions should be provided for all patients scheduled to receive cancer chemotherapy. Patients should be instructed to use a soft or extra-soft bristle toothbrush unless bleeding, pain, or infection becomes evident. Patients should be instructed not to use dental floss unless they floss on a regular basis and show excellent manual dexterity. Improper use of dental floss can cause serious injury that may lead to bleeding and/or infection. If toothbrushing precipitates excessive bleeding, pain, or infection, patients should immediately discontinue brushing with a bristle brush. An alternative hygiene aid, such as a cotton swab, a gauze pad, or an oral swab should be substituted to avoid additional injury. The alternative oral hygiene aid should be soft, sterile, and disposable.

Treatment during chemotherapy

During this period, most dental treatment consists of palliative care. Typical symptoms are oral discomfort and pain secondary to mucositis. Xerostomia also becomes apparent during this stage of treatment. The importance of good oral hygiene should be reinforced with the patient, especially because compliance will decrease during this difficult time. Good oral hygiene during chemotherapy helps decrease the severity of mucositis as well as reduce the probability of sepsis due to oral infections (Ferretti et al., 1987).

If an odontogenic or periodontal infection arises, options for treatment should be discussed with the oncologist. If definitive treatment is necessary, it should be done as atraumatically as possible, and the patient, who is in a myelosuppressed state, should be prescribed the appropriate antibiotic regimen for at least a week following treatment. Ideally, it would be best to delay any necessary dental treatment until the patient has completed the chemotherapy cycle and the blood cell counts have returned to more manageable levels to avoid further infection, bleeding problems, and delayed healing.

With so many difficult changes occurring in the mouth, patients experience loss of appetite, dehydration, and subsequent weight loss. Enriched dietary supplements or total parenteral nutrition may be indicated. However, supplemental dietary liquids often contain high levels of sugar, which can lead to increased risk of caries, especially if the patient is xerostomic and has poor oral hygiene.

Treatment following chemotherapy

Immediately following chemotherapy, patients require palliative support because mucositis often is persistent and requires several weeks to resolve. Once sufficient healing has occurred, the patient should return for evaluation. The soft tissues of the oral cavity and the salivary flow of the patient should be evaluated. Any dental caries should be addressed and restored appropriately. It is advisable that patients be scheduled at more frequent dental maintenance intervals immediately following completion of chemotherapy. As the tissues heal and the oral environment normalizes, the interval can be increased.

If the patient has received chemotherapy and has not received radiation to the head and neck, routine dental care can be rendered without the same risks associated with radiation therapy (see Chapter 1). However, invasive or surgical dental procedures may require consultation with the patient's oncologist to ensure that the patient's health is sufficiently recovered to allow the dental procedure.

Dental Considerations for the BMT/PBSCT Patient

BMT/PBSCT is a procedure that effectively uses multiple chemotherapeutic agents, often in combination with total body irradiation. It includes all forms of blood and marrow stem cell transplants. The aim of treatment is to achieve a maximum anticancer effect without the limitations imposed by marrow toxicity. The purpose of BMT is to rescue or replace the recipient's stem cells that were obliterated by the chemotherapy and/or radiation used to eradicate the malignancy. These approaches have been widely used in the treatment of leukemias and lymphomas, but are also used in the treatment of neuroblastomas, multiple myeloma, and various other types of cancer as well as some autoimmune diseases such as pemphigus.

There are three types of transplant: *(1) autologous*, in which patients receive their own stem cells; *(2) syngeneic*, in which patients receive stem cells from their identical twin; and *(3) allogeneic*, in which a patient receives stem cells from a relative or an unrelated donor. Stem cells are intravenously transfused into the bone marrow–suppressed patient, and marrow function is restored following subsequent engraftment.

One of the major improvements in BMT/PBSCT has been in the use of peripheral collection of hematopoietic stem and progenitor

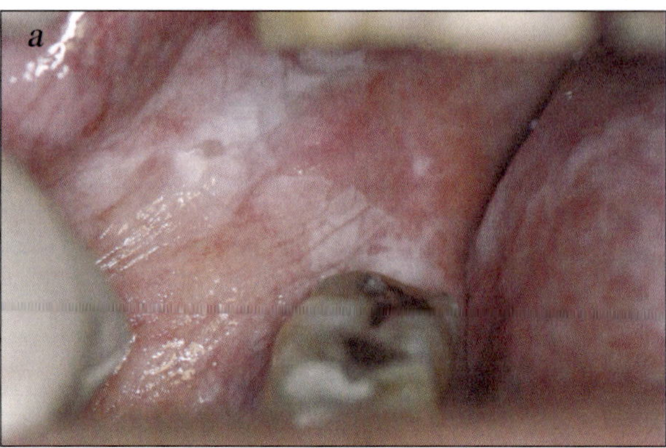

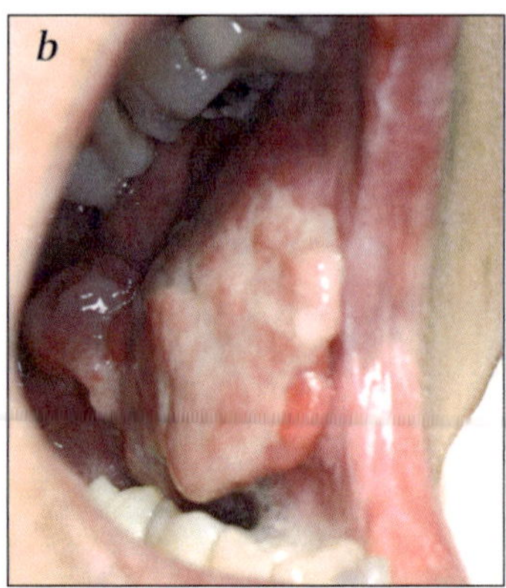

Figure 10-9 Chronic GVHD. *(a)* Chronic lichenoid changes in the buccal mucosa. Similar changes are also seen on the tongue, accompanied by depapillation and a glossy erythema. *(b)* Denuded exophytic mass, occasionally found on the buccal mucosa, tongue, and interdental papilla.

cells (Armitage, 1994; Russel et al., 1996). This approach has been used to decrease the mortality associated with infection, bleeding, and incidence of graft-versus-host disease (GVHD), which only occurs after allogeneic BMT (Tyndall and Gratwohl, 1997).

The complications secondary to BMT/PBSCT are generally more severe than those arising from other forms of chemotherapy. The epithelial lining of the oral cavity and the gastrointestinal tract suffer the greatest effects of combination chemotherapy cytotoxicity. Oral complications include, but are not limited to, mucositis, xerostomia, bleeding, and secondary infections. BMT/PBSCT carries significant risks not shared by chemotherapy alone. The process risks fatal infection during a period of total immunosuppression pending marrow engraftment.

Patients receiving allogeneic BMT/PBSCT have the added risk of GVHD. GVHD occurs when the donor tissue (marrow with donor immunologic memory) rejects the recipient (host antigenic) tissues and mounts an inflammatory response. A graft-versus-host reaction can manifest in any tissue or organ but often occurs intraorally. Acute GVHD occurs within the first 100 days after transplantation and manifests intraorally as mucosal desquamation, erythema, and ulceration. The tongue is often the first and most sensitive intraoral site to be affected.

Chronic GVHD develops 100 days after the transplantation. Approximately 40% of patients who receive an allogeneic BMT eventually develop chronic GVHD (Demarosi et al., 2007). Chronic GVHD appears intraorally in a variety of forms. The most common manifestation is denudation of mucosa with a glossy erythema with associated white areas (Fig 10-9).

There is also a higher incidence of secondary solid tumors in transplanted patients who suffer from chronic GVHD (Demarosi et al., 2005a; Demarosi et al., 2005b). Solid tumors include squamous cell carcinoma of the skin, melanoma, glioblastoma, and sarcoma (Deeg et al., 1984). Studies have reported that patients with a history of allogeneic BMT have a four to seven times greater chance of developing solid tumors than the general population and males may be at greater risk than females (Gluckman et al., 1991; Demarosi et al., 2005a; Demarosi et al., 2005b; Bhatia et al., 1996).

Patients with GVHD often have lichen planus present in the oral cavity, which may be a premalignant lesion. Why lichen planus occurs with greater frequency in patients with GVHD has not been definitively determined, but possible hypotheses include a contribution from total-body irradiation combined with immunosuppressive agents such as cyclosporine or azathioprine. The development of oral squamous cell carcinoma may be dependent on the development of oral lichen planus in patients with GVHD. Therefore, it is important for the dental clinician to perform thorough oral examinations for these patients and offer them adequate therapy, as appropriate (Kruse and Grätz, 2009).

Summary

Chemotherapy remains the mainstay of systemic cancer therapy, but in recent years, novel approaches such as gene therapy, immunotherapy, cellular therapy (chimeric antigen receptor T-cell therapy), biologic agents, and targeted therapy have emerged. The effectiveness of these agents is based on their ability to destroy or slow the growth of rapidly dividing tumor cells. Unfortunately, these drugs are not selective and are unable to distinguish between normally dividing cells and malignant cells. As a result, these patients are subject to significant acute short-term side effects, such as oral mucositis, and chronic long-term side effects, such as peripheral neuropathy and the impairment of growth and development of the craniofacial skeleton, in the case of growing children. Oral mucositis is the most significant acute side effect. It is a complex multifactorial phenomenon, and the palliative, preventive, and therapeutic measures that have been employed to date have proven to be largely ineffective. When evaluating the dentition prior to chemotherapy, a distinction should be made between acute and chronic infectious foci. Whereas acute infections are addressed prior to the initiation of therapy, conditions such as chronic periodontitis and asymptomatic endodontic lesions are best deferred until after therapy.

References

Armitage JO. Bone marrow transplantation. N Engl J Med 1994;330:827–838.

Armstrong D. Infectious complications in cancer patients treated with chemical immunosuppressive agents. Transplant Proc 1973;5:1245–1248.

Avula LR, Grodzinski P. Nanotechnology-aided advancement in the combating of cancer metastasis. Cancer Metastasis Rev 2022 Apr 2;1–22. http://doi.org/10.1007/s10555-022-10025-7.

Barry CP, Lind SE. Adenosine-mediated killing of cultured epithelia cancer cells. Cancer Res 2000;60:1887–1894.

Bhatia S, Ramsay NK, Steinbuch M, et al. Malignant neoplasms following bone marrow transplantation. Blood 1996;8:3633–3639.

Binaschi M, Zunino F, Capranico G. Mechanism of action of DNA topoisonerase inhibitors. Stem Cells 1995;13:369–379.

Blackstock JL, Parikh SH, Talbert JG, et al. Herpes simplex virus in the pediatric bone marrow and stem cell transplantation patient. Transplant Nursing 2005;11:97–98.

Bodey G, Buckley M, Sathe YS, Freireich EJ. Quantitative relationships between circulating leukocytes and infection in patients with acute leukemia. Ann Intern Med 1966;64:328–340.

Bongiovanni A, Recine F, Fausti V, et al. Clinical role of filgrastim in the management of patients at risk of prolonged severe neutropenia: An evidence-based review. Int J Clin Pract 2019 Nov;73(11):e13404. http://doi.org/10.1111/ijcp.13404. Epub 2019 Sep 13.

Borden EC. Interferons α and β in cancer: Therapeutic opportunities from new insights. Rev Drug Discov 2019 Mar;18(3):219–234.

Carrozzo M, Eriksen JG, Bensadoun RJ, et al. Oral mucosal injury caused by targeted cancer therapies. JNCI Monographs 2019 Aug;53. https://doi.org/10.1093/jncimonographs/lgz012.

Cascinu S, Fedeli A, Fedeli SL, et al. Oral cooling (cryotherapy), an effective treatment for the prevention of 5-fluorouracil-induced stomatitis. Eur J Cancer B Oral Oncol 1994;30B4:234–236.

Cheng KKF, Ka Tsui Yuen J. A pilot study of chlorhexidine and benzydamine oral rinses for the prevention and treatment of irradiation mucositis in patients with head and neck cancer. Cancer Nurs 2006;29:423–430.

Cooksley WG. The role of interferon therapy in hepatitis B. Med Gen Med 2004;6:16.

Dale DV, Crawford J, Klippel Z, et al. A systematic literature review of the efficacy, effectiveness, and safety of filgrastim. Support Care Cancer 2018 Jan;26(1):7–20.

Deeg HJ, Sanders J, Martin P, et al. Secondary malignancies after marrow transplantation. Exp Hematol 1984;12:660-666.

Demarosi F, Lodi G, Carrassi A, et al. Clinical and histopathological features of the oral mucosa in allogeneic haematopoietic stem cell transplantation patients. Exp Oncol 2007;29:304–308.

Demarosi F, Lodi G, Carrassi A, et al. Oral malignancies following HSCT: Graft versus host disease and other risk factors. Oral Oncol 2005b;41:865–877.

Demarosi F, Soligo D, Lodi G, et al. Squamous cell carcinoma of the oral cavity associated with graft versus host disease: Report of a case and review of the literature. Oral Surg Oral Med Oral Pathol Oral Radiol Endod 2005a;100:63–69.

DePaola LG, Leupold RJ, Peterson DE, et al. Prosthodontic considerations for patients undergoing cancer chemotherapy. J Am Dent Assoc 1983;107:48–51.

DePaola LG, Peterson DE, Overholser CD Jr, et al. Dental care for patients receiving chemotherapy. J Am Dent Assoc 1986;112:198–203.

Donnelly JP, Muus P, Schattenberg A, et al. A scheme for daily monitoring of oral mucositis in allogeneic BMT recipients. Bone Marrow Transplant 1992;9:409–413.

Driezen S, McCredie KB, Keating MJ. Chemotherapy-induced oral mucositis in adult leukemia. Postgrad Med 1981;69:103–108, 111–112.

Dyck S, Brett K, Davies B, et al. Development of a staging system for chemotheraopy-induced stomatitis. Cancer Nurs 1991;14:6–12.

Elting LS, Bodey GP, Keefe BH. Septicemia and shock syndrome due to viridans streptococci: A case-control study of predisposing factors. Clin Infect Dis 1992;14:1201–1207.

Elting LS, Cooksley C, Chambers MD, et al. The burdens of cancer therapy. Clinical and economic outcomes of chemotherapy-induced mucositis. Cancer 2003;98:1531–1539.

Epstein JB, Silverman S Jr, Paggiarino DA, et al. Benzydamine HCl for prophylaxis of radiation-induced oral mucositis: Results from a multicenter, randomized, double-blind, placebo-controlled clinical trial. Cancer 2001;92:875–885.

Facchini L, Martino R, Ferrari A, et al. Degree of mucositis and duration of neutropenia are the major risk factors for early posttransplant febrile neutropenia and severe bacterial infections after reduced-intensity conditioning. Eur J Haematol 2012;881:46–51.

Ferretti GA, Ash RC, Brown AT, et al. Chlorhexidine for prophylaxis against oral infections and associated complications in patients receiving bone marrow transplants. J Am Dent Assoc 1987;114:461–467.

Frei E III. The clinical use of actinomycin. Cancer Chemother Rep 1974;58:49–54.

Gamis AS, Howells WB, DeSwarte-Wallace J, et al. Alpha hemolytic streptococcal infection during intensive treatment for acute myeloid leukemia: A report from the children's cancer group study CCG-2891. J Clin Oncol 2000;189:1845–1855.

Gaydos LA, Freireich EJ, Mantel N. The quantitative relationship between platelet count and hemorrhage in patients with acute leukemia. N Engl J Med 1962;266:905–909.

Gluckman E, Socie G, Devergie A, et al. Bone marrow transplantation in 107 patients with severe aplastic anemia using cyclophosphamide and thoraco-abdominal irradiation for conditioning: Long-term follow-up. Blood 1991;78:2451–2455.

Greenwald E. Cancer chemotherapy. 2nd ed. New York: Medical Examination; 1973.

Hargadon KM, Johnson CE, Williams CJ. Immune checkpoint blockade therapy for cancer: An overview of FDA-approved immune checkpoint inhibitors. Int Immunopharm 2018;62:29–39.

Heal JM, Blumberg N. Optimizing platelet transfusion therapy. Blood Rev 2004;18:149–165.

Hersh E, Bodey GP, Nies BA, et al. Causes of death in acute leukemia: A ten-year study of 414 patients from 1954–1963. JAMA 1965;193:105–109.

Hu LY, Wu WL, Yan QW, et al. Prevention and treatment for chemotherapy-induced peripheral neuropathy: therapies based on CIPN mechanisms. Curr Neuropharmacol 2019;17(2):184–196.

Huang TT, Chen Y, Dietz AC. Pulmonary outcomes in survivors of childhood central nervous system malignancies: A report from the Childhood Cancer Survivor Study. Pediatr Blood Cancer 2014 Feb;61(2):319–325.

Johansson JE, Bratel J, Hardling M, et al. Cryotherapy as prophylasis against oral mucositis after high-dose melphalan and autologous stem cell transplantation for myeloma: A randomized, open label, phase 3, noninferiority trial. Bone Marrow Transplant 2019. http://doi.org/10.1038/s41409-019-0468-6.

Kaste SC, Goodmand P, Leisenring W, et al. Impact of radiation and chemotherapy on risk of dental abnormalities: A report from the Childhood Cancer Survivor Study. Cancer 2009;115:5817–5827.

Kazemian A, Kamian S, Aghili M, et al. Benzydamine for prophylaxis of radiation-induced oral mucositis in head and neck cancers: A double-blind placebo-controlled randomized clinical trial. Eur J Cancer Care (Engl) 2009;18:174–178.

Kimiz-Gebologlu I, Gulce-Iz S, Biray-Avci C. Monoclonal antibodies in cancer immunotherapy. Mol Biol Rep 2018 Dec;45(6):2935–2940.

Kolbinson DA, Schubert MM, Flournoy N, et al. Early oral changes following bone marrow transplantation. Oral Surg Oral Med Oral Pathol 1988;66:130–138.

Kruse AL, Grätz KW. Oral carcinoma after hematopoietic stem cell transplantation: New classification based on a literature review over 30 years. Head Neck Oncol 2009 Jul 22;1:29. http://doi.org/10.1186/1758-3284-1-29.

Kurrasch M, Beumer J, Kagawa T. Mucormycosis. Oral and prosthodontic implications. J Prosthet Dent 1981;47:422–429.

Lalla RV, Brennan MT, Gordon SM, et al. Oral mucositis due to high-dose chemotherapy and/or head and neck radiation therapy. JNCI Monographs 2019;53:lgz011. http://doi.org/10.1093/jncimonographs/lgz011.

Lalla RV, Peterson DE. Oral mucositis. Dent Clin North Am 2005;491:167–184.

Liesveld JL, Abboud CN, Ifthikhanruddin JJ, et al. Oral valacyclovir versus intravenous acyclovir in preventing herpes simplex virus infections in autologous stem cell transplant recipients. Transplant Cell Ther 2002;8:662–665.

Lockhart PB, Sonis ST. Alterations in the oral mucosa caused by chemotherapeutic agents. A histologic study. J Dermatol Surg Oncol 1981;7:1019–1025.

Lohani S, O'Driscoll BR, Woodcock AA. 25-year study of lung fibrosis following carmustine therapy for brain tumor in childhood. Chest 2004;126:1007.

Loprinzi CL, Lacchetti C, Bleeker J, et al. Prevention and management of chemotherapy-induced peripheral neuropathy in survivors of adult cancers: ASCO guideline update. J Clin Oncol 2020;38:3325–3348.

Main BE, Calman KC, Ferguson MM, et al. The effect of cytotoxic therapy on saliva and oral flora. Oral Surg Oral Med Oral Pathol 1984;58:545–548.

McCarthy GM, Skillings JR. Jaw and other orofacial pain in patients receiving vincristine for the treatment of cancer. Oral Surg Oral Med Oral Pathol 1992;74:299–304.

McGuire DB, Fulton JS, Park J, et al. Systematic review of basic oral care for the management of oral mucositis in cancer patients. Support Care Cancer 2013;2111:3165–77.

Meyers JD, Flournoy N, Thomas ED. Infection with herpes simplex virus and cell-mediated immunity after marrow transplant. J Infect Dis 1980;142:338–346.

Montgomery MT, Redding SW, LeMaistre CF. The incidence of oral herpes simplex virus infection in patients undergoing cancer chemotherapy. Oral Surg Oral Med Oral Pathol 1986;61:238–242.

Nabholtz JM, Cantin J, Chang J. Phase III trial comparing granulocyte colony-stimulating factor to leridistim in the prevention of neutropenic complications in breast cancer patients treated with docetaxel/doxorubinic/cyclophosphamide: Results of the BCIRG 004 trial. Clin Breast Cancer 2002;3:268–275.

Nicolatou-Galitis O, Sarri T, Bowen J, et al. Systematic review of amifostine for the management of oral mucositis in cancer patients. Support Care Cancer 2013;21:357–364.

Niscola P, Scaramucci L, Giovannini M, et al. Palifermin in the management of mucositis in hematological malignancies: Current evidences and future perspectives. Cardiovac Hematol Agents Med Chem 2009;7:305–312.

O'Dwyer PJ, Wagner B, Leyland-Jones B, et al. 2'-Deoxycoformycin (pentostatin) for lymphoid malignancies. Rational development of an active new drug. Ann Intern Med 1988;108:733–743.

Oliff A, Bleyer WA, Poplack DG. Methotrexate-induced oral mucositis and salivary methotrexate concentrations. Cancer Chemother Pharmacol 1979;2:225–226.

Paolicelli D, Direnzo V, Trojano M. Review of interferon blb in the treatment of early and relapsing multiple sclerosis. Biologics 2009;3:369–376.

Park SB, Lin CS, Krishnan AV, et al. Oxaliplatin-induced neurotoxicity: Changes in axonal excitability precede development of neuropathy. Brain 2009;132:2712–2723.

Perez-Herrero E, Fernandez-Medarde A. Advanced targeted therapies in cancer: Drug nanocarriers, the future of chemotherapy. Eur J Pharm Biopharm 2015;93:52–79.

Peris K, Fargnoli MC, Garge C, et al. Diagnosis and treatment of basal cell carcinoma: European consensus-based interdisciplinary guidelines. J Cancer 2019 Sep;118:10–34.

Peterson DE. New strategies for management of oral mucositis in cancer patients. J Support Oncol 2006;4(suppl):9–13.

Peterson DE, Ohrn K, Bowen J, et al. Systematic review of oral cryotherapy for management of oral mucositis caused by cancer therapy. Cancer 2013;211:327–332.

Petrella T, Quirt I, Verma S, et al. Single-agent interleukin-2 in the treatment of metastatic melanoma. Curr Oncol 2007;14:21–26.

Pettengell R, Aapro M, Brusamolino E, et al. Implications of the European Organisation for Research and Treatment of Cancer (EORTC) guidelines on the use of granulocyte colony-stimulating factor (G-CSF) for lymphoma care. Clin Drug Investig 2009;29:491–513.

Pico JL, Avila-Garavito A, Naccache P. Mucositis: Its occurrence, consequences, and treatment in the oncology setting. Oncologist 1998;3:446–451.

Raber-Durlacher JE, von Bultzingslowen I, Logan RM, et al. Systematic review of cytokines and growth factors for management of oral mucositis in cancer patients. Support Care Cancer 2013;211:343–355.

Rastogi M, Khurana R, Revannasiddaiah S, et al. Role of benzydamine hydrochloride in the prevention of oral mucositis in head and neck cancer patients treated with radiotherapy (>50 Gy) with or without chemotherapy. Support Care Cancer 2017;25:1439–1443.

Riley TT, Muzny CA, Swiato E, et al. Breaking the mold: A review of mucormycosis and current pharmacological treatment options. Ann Pharmacother 2016;50:747–757.

Roopashri G, Jayanthi K, Guruprasad R. Efficacy of benzydamine hydrochloride, chlorhexidine, and povidone iodine in the treatment of oral mucositis among patients undergoing radiotherapy in head and neck malignancies: A drug trail. Contemp Clin Dent 2011;2:8–12.

Rosenberg SW. Oral care of chemotherapy patients. Dent Clin North Am 1990;34:239–250.

Rosenthal DI. Consequences of mucositis-induced treatment breaks and dose reductions on head and neck treatment outcomes. J Support Oncol 2007;5(suppl 4):23–31.

Russel N, Gratwohl A, Schmitz N. The place of blood stem cells in allogeneic transplantation. Br J Haematol 1996;93:747–753.

Saral R. Oral complications of cancer therapies. Management of acute viral infections. NCI Monogr 1990;(9):107–110.

Saunders DP, Epstein JB, Elad S, et al. Systematic review of antimicrobials, mucosal coating agents, anesthetics, and analgesics for the management of oral mucositis in cancer patients. Support Care Cancer 2013;2111:3191–3207.

Schiffer C, Anderson KC, Bennett CL, et al. Platelet transfusion for patients with cancer: Clinical practice guidelines of the American Society of Clinical Oncology. J Clin Oncol 2001;19:1519–1538.

Schroeder HE, Listgarten MA. The gingival tissues: The architecture of periodontal protection. Periodontol 2000;13:91–120.

Schubert M, Peterson D, Silverman S. Leukemia and lymphoma. In Oral Cancer. 5th ed. Ed. Silverman S Jr. Hamilton, ON: BC Decker; 2003. pp. 152–173.

Schubert MM, Williams BE, Lloid ME, et al. Clinical assessment scale for the rating of oral mucosal changes associated with bone marrow transplantation. Development of an oral mucositis index. Cancer 1992;69:2469–2477.

Schuurhuis JM, Span LF, Stokman MA, et al. Effect of leaving chronic oral foci untreated on infectious complications during intensive chemotherapy. Brit J Cancer 2016;114:972–978.

Silverman S, Eversole LR, Truelove EL. Essentials of oral medicine. Hamilton, ON: BC Decker; 2002.

Sonis AL, Tarbell N, Valachovic RW. Dentofacial development in long-term survivors of acute lymphoblastic leukemia: A comparison of three treatment modalities. Cancer 1990a;66:2645–2652.

Sonis ST. Mucositis as a biological process: A new hypothesis for the development of chemotherapy-induced stomatotoxicity. Oral Oncol 1998;34:39–43.

Sonis ST. Mucositis: The impact, biology and therapeutic opportunities of oral mucositítis. Oral Oncol 2009;45:1015-1020.

Sonis ST. Oral mucositis. Anticancer Drugs 2011;227:607–612.

Sonis ST, Elting LS, Keefe D, et al. Perspectives on cancer therapy-induced mucosal injury: Pathogenesis, measurement, epidemiology, and consequences for patients. Cancer 2004;100:1995–2025.

Sonis ST, Oster G, Fuchs H, et al. Oral mucositis and the clinical and economic outcomes of hematopoietic stem-cell transplantation. J Clin Oncol 2001;198:2201–2205.

Sonis ST, Tracey C, Shklar G, et al. An animal model for mucositis induced by cancer chemotherapy. Oral Surg Oral Med Oral Pathol 1990b;69:437–443.

Spijkervet FK, Schuurhuis JM, Stokman MA, et al. Should oral foci of infection be removed before the onset of radiotherapy or chemotherapy. Oral Diseases 2021;27:7–13.

Sroussi HY, Epstein JB, Bensadoun RJ, et al. Common oral complications of head and neck cancer radiation therapy: Mucositis, infections, saliva change, fibrosis, sensory dysfunctions, dental caries, periodontal disease, and osteoradionecroisis. Cancer Med 2017;612:2918–2931.

Staff NP, Grisold A, Grisold W, et al. Chemotherapy-induced peripheral neuropathy: A current review. Ann Neurol 2017;81:772–781.

Subramanian J, Vlahiotis A, Frazee S, et al. Real world utilization of targeted-therapy in cancer treatment. J Clin Oncol 2011;29: e16618.

Toso C, Lindley C. Viorelbine: A novel vinca alkaloid. Am J Health Syst Pharm 1995;52:1287–1304.

Tyndall A, Gratwohl A. Bone marrow transplantation in the treatment of autoimmune diseases. Br J Rheumatol 1997;36:1–3.

Valer JB, Curra M, de Farias Gabriel A, et al. Oral mucositis in childhood cancer patients receiving high-dose methotrexate: Prevalence, relationship with other toxicities and methotrexate elimination. Int J Paediatr Dent 2021;31(2):238–246.

Van de Velde M, Kaspers GL, Abbink FC et al. Vincristine-induced peripheral neuropathy in children with cancer: A systematic review. Crit Rev Oncol Hematol 2017 Jun;114:114–130.

Van Leeuwen BL, Kamps WA, Jansen HW, et al. The effect of chemotherapy on the growing skeleton. Cancer Treat Rev 2000;26:363–376.

Vesterbacka M, Ringden M, Remberger M, et al. Disturbances in dental development and craniofacial growth in children treated with hematopoietic stem cell transplantation. Orthodont Craniofac Res 2012;15:21–29.

Wahid B, Ali A, Rafique S, et al. An overview of cancer immunotherapeutic strategies. Immunotherapy 2018 Aug;10(11):999–1010.

Walsh LJ. Clinical assessment and management of the oral environment in the oncology patient. Australian Dent J 2020;55(suppl 1):55–77.

Was H, Borkowska A, Bagues A, et al. Mechanisms of Chemotherapy-Induced Neurotoxicity. Review Front Pharmacol 2022 Mar 28;13:750507. http://doi.org/10.3389/fphar.2022.750507. eCollection 2022.

Wong F, Toljanic JA. A survey of clinicians: Prioritization of dental treatment in leukemia patients prior to chemotherapy. Int J Prosthodont 2009;22:303–306.

Yamagata K, Onizawa K, Yanagawa T, et al. A prospective study to evaluate a new dental management protocol before hemopoietic stem cell transplantation. Bone Marrow Transplantation 2006;38:237–242.

Zajączkowska R, Kocot-Kępska M, Leppert W, et al. Mechanisms of chemotherapy-induced peripheral neuropathy. Int J Mol Sci 2019;20:1451. http://doi.org/10.3390/ijms20061451.

www.ingramcontent.com/pod-product-compliance
Lightning Source LLC
Chambersburg PA
CBRC090248230326
41458CB00109B/6521